A Practical Dictionary of
Chinese Medicine

Second Edition

Nigel Wiseman

Feng Ye

Paradigm Publications   1998   Brookline, Massachusetts

A PRACTICAL DICTIONARY OF
CHINESE MEDICINE

Second Edition, Fourth Printing

Nigel Wiseman
Feng Ye

copyright ©1998 Paradigm Publications
www.paradigm-pubs.com

Library of Congress Cataloging-in-Publication Data:
Wiseman, Nigel. 1954–

    A practical dictionary of chinese medicine/Nigel Wiseman. Feng
Ye

    p. cm.
Text in English and Chinese, with Pinyin
ISBN 0-912111-54-2
1. Medicine, Chinese-Dictionaries. I. - Feng, Ye, 1967-.
II. Title.

    (DNLM: 1. Medicine, Chinese Traditional-dictionaries-Chinese.
W 13 W 814p 1997J
R601.W57   1997
610;.951-DC20

94-18575
CIP

Library of Congress Number 94-18575
International Standard Book Number (ISBN): 0-912111-54-2
Printed in the United States of America
Fourth Printing, 2002

Published by Paradigm Publications, Brookline, MA and Taos, NM

Table of Contents

Foreword by Hen-Hong Chang	ii
Compilers' Preface	iv
A Guide to the Use of This Dictionary	xi
Single Characters with English Equivalents	xiii
A PRACTICAL DICTIONARY OF CHINESE MEDICINE	1

A	1	F	193	K	324	P	423	U	636
B	14	G	234	L	338	Q	475	V	645
C	53	H	251	M	382	R	492	W	658
D	108	I	295	N	405	S	511	X/Y	698
E	166	J	322	O	418	T	602	Z	718

Appendix I: Weights and Measures	719
Appendix II: A Classified List of Medicinals	720
Appendix III: A Classified List of Formulas	729
Appendix IV: A Classified List of Acupuncture Points	746
References	750
Index	753

Designation

Paradigm Publications is a participant in the Council of Oriental Medical Publishers and supports their effort to inform readers of how works in Chinese medicine are prepared.

A Practical Dictionary of Chinese Medicine is an original work compiled from the Chinese sources cited in the bibliography. Please see the Compilers' Preface for details.

Foreword by Hen-Hong Chang

The transmission and development of Chinese medicine has a style of its own; reference works have been few. Since the founding of the Republic of China, the burgeoning of schools has brought change in education methods and in knowledge itself. In the early years of the Republic, Hsieh Kuan of the Shanghai Chinese Medical School compiled *The Comprehensive Chinese Medical Dictionary* (*zhōng yī dà cí diǎn*). His work, as some would have it, was an answer to the challenge of modern sciences, yet from a broader perspective, it was "following Heaven and responding to Man"—a natural response to the changing times. Seventy years later, Wiseman and Feng's English dictionary represents a new milestone in the development of Chinese medicine.

The creation of dictionaries is the work of "rectifying the names." When the names are not right, discourse is foiled. Academic study must have a common language. However, in Chinese medicine, with its vast academic history, it is exceedingly difficult to establish a common language. Nigel Wiseman, by his own account, has poured ten years of sweat into his research on the subject. He journeyed east to obtain the scriptures and fathomed the riddle of words in the magic books. It takes little to imagine his assiduity. The author's powerful command of English is a call to study, and his insistent expression of the hope that Western students will take up the study of Chinese so as to be able to "enter the hall and behold the wonders within" is an admonition that naturally springs from deep inquiry, and is one mark of his sincerity and rigor.

Any academic discipline that moves onto the world stage receives worldwide contributions and challenges that infuse it with life and promote its transformation through development. This is implicit in Kuhn's notion of paradigms in the evolution of science. This English dictionary of Chinese medicine is a brave start in the progression from a common language to a world language. What is more, in its scope and in the standards it sets, it will reflect the sophistication of Chinese medicine after its reception in the West, which with persevering innovative effort will undergo constant development. Scholars should view this book as a bridge and, even more, as a path.

Hen-Hong Chang
China Medical College, Taiwan, Summer 1997

Compilers' Preface

The dictionary has an important and thus far undeveloped role to play in the expansion of Western knowledge of Chinese Medicine. In compiling the present work, we set ourselves the somewhat daunting task of making a dictionary that would be useful to practitioners, students, and teachers of Chinese medicine in the English-speaking world, whether or not they know Chinese or are familiar with the terminology presented.

Over recent decades, a number of English dictionaries of Chinese medicine have appeared, but in general they have not been popular. Chinese-English translator's lists have naturally only attracted the interest of the limited usership for whom they have been intended. Dictionaries containing definitions and other information in English have apparently failed to provide teachers, students, and practitioners not possessing linguistic access to Chinese texts with a useful tool to learn about Chinese medical concepts. Owing to the current lack of standardization of Chinese medical terminology in English, terms are difficult to access, and given the lack of useful information provided, even a successful lookup is poorly rewarded.

Deficiencies of particular bilingual dictionaries of Chinese medicine published to date may account for their lack of popularity, but they do not explain why the dictionary has not been developed to perform the role that it nowadays regularly plays in the interlingual transmission of specialist knowledge in other fields. In the interlingual context, the specialist dictionary, in addition to being able to provide definitions and other information about concepts as regular monolingual specialist dictionaries, also performs the function of establishing relationships between source-language and target-language terms—those intended principally for translators, indeed, serving only this function. The bilingual specialist dictionary has played an important role in the transmission of Western scientific and technical knowledge to non-Western communities. However, it has apparently not been identified as a useful tool for acquiring Chinese medical knowledge.

The lack of importance accorded to the bilingual dictionary in Chinese medicine is one sign that the recipient community is currently not geared to large-scale transmission of knowledge from China. Little attention has been paid to learning Chinese, which would give more students of Chinese medicine access to primary texts, and create more potential translators. Chinese medical texts translated from Chinese are still outnumbered by texts written by Westerners without access to primary texts, who use English terms at their face value without being able to consider whether they represent original concepts. A substantial proportion of the literature translated and compiled from primary sources is the work of Chinese people, whose command of English is forgivably limited and who very often take a "conservative" approach of translating terms with the nearest Western medical equivalents. Greater accuracy in translation and greater conformity in the presentation of Chinese medical information can only be achieved by a thoroughgoing, informed debate. So far, unfortunately, few people have seen value in such a debate, and even fewer have made any contribution to it.

Failure to come to grips with the linguistic problems facing the transmission of Chinese medical knowledge is rooted in various misconceptions of the nature of Chinese medicine and the possibilities for its adoption in the West. Chinese medicine has been identified, in contrast to Western medicine, as a holistic and natural medicine that puts healer-patient interaction firmly in the foreground. With this, Chinese medicine is tacitly assumed to have little of the complex detail and "book knowledge" seen in Western medicine (e.g., the huge complexity of modern anatomical knowledge, of which any doctor in his career only uses a minor portion), and that, unlike Western medicine, it does not need and therefore does not have a large and complex technical vocabulary. These conceptions derive not so much from actual evidence as from expectations of a desirable alternative to Western medicine. In actual fact, the learning of Chinese medicine traditionally involved much book learning, including the memorization of classical texts, and the Chinese terminology that has amassed over two thousand years is colossal (the larger dictionaries of Chinese medicine compiled in this century contain up to 40,000 or more entries).

The freedom that has generally been allowed for the practice of acupuncture and Chinese medicine in the West has allowed the possibility for professionalization, which has—somewhat precociously—encouraged many to assume that training provided by Western schools of acupuncture and Chinese medicine is comprehensive, if not practically complete. Yet, given, among other things, the absence of full translations of classical texts (texts which, despite modernization of Chinese medical education in China, still constitute a major part of modern curricula there), such an assumption is indefensible.

The issues surrounding the accurate transmission of original Chinese medical knowledge have been eclipsed by the argument that a premodern medicine of a distant culture must undergo adaptation before it can be of use to modern Western society. Yet, until the West has a comprehensive understanding of Chinese medicine, which can be gained only through attention to such issues, no debate concerning possible or desirable adaptations can be well informed or democratic.

All of these misconceptions exist only because of the language barrier, which not only prevents Chinese medicine from advancing beyond its initial stage of transmission westward, but also deprives the majority of Western teachers, students and practitioners of the ability to assess how much knowledge has been transmitted and how much remains to be made available.

The key to acquiring Chinese medical knowledge—as indeed any foreign body of knowledge—lies in mastering the language that has traditionally served as the vehicle of transmission from one generation to the next. Without this key, the recipient community is prey to the tendency to form ideas about Chinese medicine not from direct knowledge of it, but from expectations prompted by a 20th-century Western world view. The work of investigating Chinese terminology, developing a rational approach to translation, and presenting terminology in dictionary format form a necessary first step toward developing a language of Chinese medicine in English that is designed to ensure maximum fidelity in the translation of original texts. Ideally, such an effort should go hand in hand with the development of Chinese-language teaching to enable more students to escape the tangle of words and meanings that unavoidably results from an unsystematic approach to translation.

If there is any justification for the view that the westward transmission of Chinese medical knowledge can dispense with any attempt to ensure terminological parity through the creation of bilingual glossaries and foreign-language dictionaries, it must lie in the traditional inattention to the terminology of Chinese medicine in China. Indeed, Chinese medicine traditionally never developed its own specialist lexicography. The reasons for this are to be sought in the nature of the expression of Chinese medical concepts in language and in the nature of Chinese medical knowledge itself.

In the traditional conception, derived from classical Chinese, the single character constitutes the basic element of meaning corresponding to our notion of a "word" (loosely defined as a string of letters demarcated by space). Unlike the modern Western sciences that have created new "words" in profusion, often combining Latin and Greek word-roots, Chinese medicine uses few "words" that are not to be found in general dictionaries, and consequently the notion of a technical term as a word formally distinct from any word used in the ordinary language never arose. Most of the terms of Chinese medicine are ordinary words used in special senses and in combinations unfamiliar to the lay. Unsurprisingly, the first dictionary of Chinese medicine did not appear until the notion developed in general lexicography in China—apparently as a result of Western influence—that combinations of characters constituted "words." The 中国中医大辞典 *Zhōngguó Zhōngyī Dàcídiǎn* (*Comprehensive Dictionary of Chinese Medicine*) compiled under the editorship of Xiè Guān (谢观), which contains single-character and multiple-character terms, appeared six years after the 辞源 *Cí Yuán*, which is generally taken to be the first dictionary to include combinations of characters as entries.

An equally if not more important reason for the traditional absence of dictionaries of Chinese medicine lies in the lack of integration of its knowledge. In the pure and applied sciences of the modern age, knowledge is constantly revised and expanded by the community of researchers as a whole on the basis of an agreed methodology. The unequivocal linguistic expression of knowledge at any given time is ensured by terminological rigor oriented to the (not always achieved) ideal of a single term denoting one and no other concept. Within this framework, a technical dictionary displaying all terms together with precise definitions provides both a key to understanding terms and a standard for their usage. As Paul U. Unschuld has demonstrated, Chinese medicine at no time in its entire history developed an agreed methodology for determining reliable knowledge. It continually gave birth to new ideas, but never laid older ones permanently to rest. Because authority was always considered to lie in particular authors and works, certain concepts—and hence certain terms—continued to appear in literature, ensuring great continuity of thought down to the present. Consequently, in modern texts, many terms are used as they were in much-revered early texts such as the 黄帝内经 *Huáng Dì Nèi Jīng* or the 伤寒论 *Shāng Hán Lùn*. Nevertheless, many terms were used again and again in different senses, and a single idea accrued different linguistic expressions. Terms were, as already said, composed of the lexical material of the ordinary language, and were interpreted against the background of context. No urge ever arose to isolate terms from context and give clear definitions of the concepts they represent (as in a dictionary), let alone to standardize their usage. Yet, somewhat paradoxically, the failure to link terms to clearly define concepts in some respects raised the importance of the term above that of the concept, turning the word into a concept in itself. In the literary tradition that is based on the doctrines of the early medical classics, there is a certain slavery to words, which is evinced by the eternal annotation and re-annotation of ancient texts. It might surprise some Westerners that in some Chinese medical traditions there is actually much more "book knowledge" involved in the process of learning Chinese medicine than there is in learning Western medicine.

The traditional absence of Chinese medical dictionaries cannot be taken to mean that Chinese medicine does not possess a terminology, that is, a set of words and expressions that either do not exist in the ordinary language or are used in senses unfamiliar to the lay. The existence of concepts such as the 三焦 *sān jiāo*, 'triple burner', 痹 *bì*, 'impediment', 马勃 *mǎ bó*, 'puffball', and 一贯煎 *yī guàn jiān*, 'All-the-Way-Through Brew', which are just as obscure to lay Chinese as the English equivalents are to lay English speakers, is certain evidence of this fact. The belief widely held among Westerners that Chinese medicine does not really possess a terminology beyond a handful of specialist terms cannot be substantiated. In the modern age, the word "terminology" is associated with certain notions that have arisen in the modern sciences and technologies, namely that every term should have a clear, concise and unequivocal definition and that each concept should be represented by a single term not used to denote any other concept. Chinese medicine traditionally never perceived the need for this degree of rationalization; writers tended to define only those terms that were not self-explanatory in context, and rarely paid attention to the possibility that they might be using terms differently from other writers. Yet this in no way lessens the technical, that is, non-lay, status of words and word meanings in the language of Chinese medicine. Especially in highly-revered texts, where the concept attached to the word may be unclear, the word takes on importance that it is not accorded in the modern sciences.

Recognition of the technical status of Chinese medical terms explains why Chinese medical lexicography, despite its traditional absence, has undergone considerable development during this century. With the new importance given to Chinese medicine in the People's Republic (PRC), dictionary-making activity has increased. Over recent years, there has been a veritable profusion of Chinese medical dictionaries, the largest one, similar in size to Xiè Guān's, being the 中医大辞典 *Zhōngyī Dàcídiǎn* (*Dictionary of Chinese Medicine*), which finally appeared in 1995 after publication of a trial version (*Zhōngyī Dàcídiǎn, Shìyòngběn*) and a concise version 简明中医辞典 *Jiǎnmíng Zhōngyī Cídiǎn* (*Concise Dictionary of Chinese Medicine*). Numerous other general dictionaries as well as single-character dictionaries and specialist dictionaries of acupuncture, warm disease (温病 *wēn bìng*), manipulation (推拿 *tuī ná*), and so on, have also been published. In addition, there are a number of dictionaries and concordances on particular classical works such as 黄帝内经 *Huángdì Nèijīng* and the 伤寒论

Shānghánlùn, reflecting a continuing preoccupation with words in the absence of clearly defined concepts. Furthermore, given the priority accorded by the PRC Government to the internationalization of Chinese medicine, PRC scholars have also created a number of bilingual dictionaries of Chinese medicine.

Chinese medical dictionaries are not merely an additional tool in the study of traditional Chinese medicine. They are part of the change that Chinese medicine has undergone in the modern era. With the decreasing reliance on classical texts in the teaching of Chinese medicine during recent decades, the dictionary helps to maintain a link by indicating the source and usage of terms in classical literature—a function that could be further developed. In the long-term process of conceptual rationalization that the principles of modern science have unleashed, it may also contribute to a new standardized usage of Chinese medical terms that would reduce the polysemy of the past. However, the stride in this direction falters since it would entail a break with the past insofar as new definitions would fail to reflect the more varied usage of the past.

As has already been noted, bilingual dictionaries perform the important function of pegging target-language terms to source-language terms. During the initial transmission of knowledge from one culture to another, when target-language equivalents have not been standardized or have not been devised for source-language terms, the bilingual dictionary most naturally serves a normative function, making a set of target-language equivalents for source-language terms available to all translators. Insofar as translators adopt these terms, it encourages the standardization of the target-language terms; insofar as translators reject the terms and offer rational alternatives, the target-language terminology is refined. It is for this reason that we began our terminological work 15 years ago with the creation of a bilingual list of terms. The list was first published by Paradigm Publications in 1990 under the title of *A Glossary of Chinese Medical Points and Acupuncture Points*, and a very much revised version with the addition of drug and formula names was published in China by Hunan Science and Technology Press under the title of *An English-Chinese Chinese-English Dictionary of Chinese Medicine*. The computer database from which both publications have been generated continues to be revised and expanded for future editions. Because the absence of a unified English terminology of Chinese medicine is not only due to chance differences in choice of terms but also to completely different approaches to translation, both of the above-mentioned publications have accorded considerable introductory space to the discussion of translation principles and term choices.

Until terminological conventions are established in the target-language (in our case, English), any attempt to devise an English-language dictionary of Chinese medicine intended for users with no knowledge of the source language, that serves the general functions of specialist dictionaries, such as providing definitions and other information, encounters accessing difficulties. When alphabetical order of English terms is chosen, a reader who knows a given concept by one name may fail to access it if it is listed under a name with which she or he is not familiar. The alternative is the thematic order, whereby items are arranged according to subject matter. In theory, the thematic order is seemingly preferable since it presupposes less knowledge on the part of the user. This probably explains why makers of bilingual dictionaries of Chinese medicine have invariably chosen it. In practice, however, the concepts of Chinese medicine do not form a closely integrated conceptual system; the task of devising a logical thematic order is problematic, perhaps impossible, especially when larger numbers of terms are included (to date, most bilingual dictionaries of Chinese medicine have been very small). The thematic order of course can be supplemented by an index of foreign-language (in our case English) equivalents, which would be useful insofar as the English terms are familiar to readers. However, bilingual dictionaries of Chinese medicine published to date lack English term indexes. On the other hand, since Chinese indexes are often included, the intended readership is clearly not foreign readers without linguistic access to primary texts, but rather people with linguistic access to primary texts wishing to translate or create texts for a Western readership.

The disadvantage of the alphabetical order has not been proven by practice. Chinese medicine has a large and complex terminology, but many key concepts such as organs, body parts, and disease-causing entities are not only relatively standardized in translation, but also form the first element in a vast number of terms. For example, entries beginning with 'liver', 'heart', 'spleen', 'wind', 'cold', 'vacuity', 'repletion', and so forth, comprise a significant share of terms.

In devising the present dictionary, we have rejected any attempt to categorize concepts, and have sought to overcome the difficulty of accessing by providing copious references (printed in SMALL CAPITALS). For example, under the entry header 'eye', there are numerous references to terms denoting parts of the eye, eye signs, and eye diseases. Users familiar with Chinese terms or researching concepts in texts that have provided Pinyin transliterations may access definitions through the Pinyin index entries.

Any chosen arrangement of terms has its defects. However, a factor that is probably more important than choice of order in determining utility of the dictionary is the nature and amount of the information contained. Although term definitions are the main item of information in most dictionaries, these are not the only interest of clinicians. In the present dictionary, therefore, we have maximized rewards for consultation by including large amounts of clinical information. For example, disease term entries provide signs and possible treatments, and term entries denoting physiological functions indicate symptoms that arise when the said function fails. We hope that this information will encourage the use of this dictionary, and thereby enable it to perform its function of increasing awareness of terminological issues among users.

We have rejected the completely bilingual format whereby all information in the entry is provided in Chinese as well as English. This format is observed in a number of bilingual dictionaries produced in the PRC, in which definitions and clinical information tend to be written in a modernized idiom of Chinese to minimize translation problems. We take the view that the traditional expression and terminology can be duplicated in English, even if this involves coining new terms. When, as in this work, all terms, or at least all the major and potentially problematic terms that appear in the definitions and clinical information are included as separate entries, the value of including original Chinese text declines.

Given the present state of transmission, an English dictionary as comprehensive as the large monolingual dictionaries would be of limited utility, since it would contain too many terms unfamiliar to readers. We have limited our selection to fewer than 6,000 terms commonly used in modern literature. In selecting terms, emphasis has been placed, for example, on modern pattern identification, and in fact we have included many patterns that have not yet appeared in Chinese monolingual dictionaries. Our selection of terms nonetheless is wide enough to embrace many terms of lower frequency literature, notably a substantial inventory of disease categories much neglected in English literature published to date. It is hoped that copious clinical information and interreferencing between entries will encourage readers to look beyond the bounds of their current focus into the broader realm of Chinese medical concepts. Ideally, readers will find this dictionary to be not only a book of definitions of terms, but an encyclopedic dictionary that invites browsing.

The decision to accommodate a Western focus of interest has led to one novelty not seen in monolingual dictionaries. Most Chinese dictionaries include treatments for pathological states, but these are mostly medicinal therapies, and acupuncture treatments are rarely given, reflecting the much greater importance accorded to drug therapy than to acupuncture in China. Since Westerners have a greater interest in acupuncture, we have included treatments given in modern acupuncture literature. In so doing, we may be courting the danger of giving the false impression that Chinese medicine is a single body of theory with two distinct treatment modalities for each pathological state, but at the present time an English dictionary that failed to take account of this Western focus of interest would probably attract fewer potential users.

The information under entries has been gathered from numerous sources (the texts consulted are listed at end of each entry). This information is not necessarily a translation of a particular text. Definitions have sometimes been conformed to modern terminological conventions when Chinese definitions are unclear or insufficient. This is the most significant area in which we have prioritized comprehension over fidelity to a specific Chinese text. Key concepts given little or no coverage in Chinese dictionaries have been explained from our own research. Detailed information given in source texts (especially textbooks containing large amounts of detailed information) has often been compressed for the sake of brevity. Information has been reorganized to comply with the format adopted in the present text. Medicinal formulas likely to be more familiar to readers have in some cases been substituted for more obscure ones. Generally, however, we have tried to ensure that the information given is expressed in the terminology of Chinese medicine, so that even English text created by the authors could be easily and meaningfully translated into Chinese.

Finally, mention should be made of translation issues. We have discussed these in detail in previous works, but given the normative nature of this dictionary, it is fitting to sketch here the basic approach adopted in the selection of English terms.

Many terms in Chinese medicine are are simple everyday words used in their primary senses, with very close equivalents in everyday English. Examples of such close equivalents can be seen in physiology (眼 *yǎn*, eye; 鼻 *bí*, nose; 心 *xīn*, heart; 涎 *xián*, drool; 尿 *niào*, urine); in pathology (风 *fēng*, wind; 寒 *hán*, cold; 热 *rè*, heat); and in treatment (清 *qīng*, clear; 泻 *xiè*, drain).

Once equivalents for basic words have been chosen, many compounds can be constructed in English much as they are in Chinese. Thus, 'clear heat and drain fire' is a word-for-word literal translation of 清热泻火 *qīng rè xiè huǒ* (only the word 'and' being added in English); 'liver fire flaming upward' is a literal translation of 肝火上炎 *gān huǒ shàng yán*. (For more about the translation of single characters, see Single Characters with English Equivalents on page xiii.)

Some terms are everyday Chinese words used in extended senses, whose English equivalents do not share same literal meaning. For example, 崩 *bēng*, literally 'collapse', 'landslide', is used in medicine to denote heavy non-menstrual discharge of blood via the vagina, which in everyday English is commonly referred to as 'flooding'. In some, but not many, cases, a Chinese term composed of more than one character has a ready-made English expression of different composition. For example, 麻木 *má mù*, whose English equivalent is 'numbness' literally means 'linen and wood' (presumably from the numbing effect of linen clothing and the insensitivity of wood). The Chinese 带下 *dài xià*, translated in this text as 'vaginal discharge', literally means 'below the belt' (and originally referred to all gynecological diseases).

Some Chinese terms that have no ready-made equivalents can be translated etymologically. For example, 疔 *dīng* is a disease (疒), in this case a lesion, that, having a small head on the surface of the body and a long root penetrating the flesh, is likened to a nail or clove (丁). This is rendered in this text as 'clove sore' ('nail' having been rejected because, having two specific meanings in English, fingernails and iron nails, it is ambiguous). By the same procedure, 痿 *wěi*, denoting any condition characterized by atony, wasting, and in severe cases, paralysis of the limbs is rendered as 'wilting' since the character is none other than 萎 *wěi*, wilting or withering [of plants], rewritten with the sickness signifier 疒 *chuáng* instead of the grass signifier 艹 *cǎo*.

We have avoided translations of terms that might encourage readers to attach any modern Western ideas to them. Thus, for example, we render 风火眼 *fēng huǒ yǎn* as 'wind-fire eye' rather than as 'acute conjunctivitis' as many PRC translators have proposed. This literal translation preserves for the Western reader the Chinese medical etiology of the disease and avoids the impression that Chinese medicine has either the anatomical concept of the conjunctiva or the pathological concept of inflammation ('-itis'), as well as obviating the need to establish whether *fēng huǒ yǎn* corresponds in all cases to the Western medical notion of conjunctivitis. Terms used in Western medicine have only been chosen where they per se reflect no uniquely Western medical view. For example, we have chosen 'strangury' to render 淋 *lín*, as the English term, like the Chinese, means 'dripping'.

We have rejected not only term translations that introduce Western medical connotations but also any terms that might invite interference of ideas alien to Chinese medicine. We translate 泻 *xiè*, an acupuncture stimulus used to treat repletion patterns, as 'to drain'. The commonly used 'sedate' implies a notion that is not only alien to Chinese medicine since it rests on the interpretation of qi as some kind of energy, but also confuses the learner's understanding of the concept because its connotations of quiescence and non-movement are precisely opposite those of the Chinese *xiè*.

In a few cases, either for want of a better word or in deference to current usage among English speakers, we have adopted an unsatisfactory translation. For example, we have rendered 穴 *xué* as 'point' rather than by a more literal translation such as 'hole'. We have rendered 证 *zhèng* as 'pattern' or 'sign' depending on the context, rather than by a literal rendering such as 'evidence'.

A common method of dealing with the seemingly untranslatable is to borrow a word from the foreign language. In translation from English to Chinese, this naturally takes the form of representing a Chinese sound in the English alphabet. We have adopted transcriptions only where they are already established in the English language or where no English word or words can cover the meaning of the original term adequately. Thus, we have adopted yin-yang and qi (previously chi, or, according to Wade-Giles Romanization, ch'i), which entered our language centuries ago, but we have otherwise resorted to Pinyin transcriptions sparingly. Although many Chinese medical translators and writers use Pinyin transliterations for 精 *jīng* and 神 *shén*, we believe that 'essence' and 'spirit' reflect the meaning of the Chinese terms more adequately than 'jing' and 'shen', which without clear definitions are meaningless to English speakers.

This maximally word-for-word literal approach to translation has two great advantages that it does not necessarily possess in other realms of translation (e.g., literary). First, it ensures faithful English equivalents that shed light on the Chinese understanding of the concept(s) they represent and that cover the various senses in which the original terms might be used. Second, such an approach provides an English terminology that can be mastered easily by translators by memorizing the equivalents of key Chinese characters. It is well worth noting that the translation of Western medical terminology into Chinese has adopted a similar approach in having standard Chinese translations for Greek and Latin morphemes used in compound terms.

Finally, we would point out some term changes. Ideally, a terminology is devised and then adhered to, without chopping and changing. However, adequate terms are not always found immediately, so that errors have to be corrected and improvements made. Since we began compiling this dictionary we have found superior choices for many terms. Insofar as the concepts in question are as yet largely unfamiliar to English writers or are not represented by any well-established English term, this should cause readers little inconvenience. We have, for example, substituted 'excrescence' for 'outcrop' as our rendering of 胬肉 *nǔ ròu* since it is a more meaningful expression in the pathological context, and 'center burner' for 'middle burner' as our translation of 中焦 *zhōng jiāo* since 'center' is the word that best renders 中 *zhōng* in most contexts. We have replaced 'deep pulse' with 'sunken pulse' because 沉 has the primary meaning of sink and because this pulse is traditionally described as like a stone cast into the water. 'Sunken', rather than 'deep', is the natural opposite of 'floating', so that 'sunken pulse' better expresses the relationship of this pulse to the 'floating pulse'. For 消渴 *xiāo kě*, we have changed 'wasting-thirst' to 'dispersion thirst' since we have not found any traditional explanations of the term that interpret 消 *xiāo* as 消瘦, emaciation or wasting. Traditional commentators argue that *xiāo* refers to the dispersion (or disappearance) of grain and water that causes increased intake of food and fluids.

The boldest term change we have made is the substitution of 'heat (effusion)' for 'fever' in the rendering of （发）热 *(fā) rè*. The primary meaning of 热 *rè* is heat. In Chinese medicine, the term can denote both a manifestation of sickness or a cause of disease. As a manifestation of sickness, it can mean objectively palpable heat or heat that is only felt subjectively. Heat is a manifestation of disease (wind-cold can manifest in palpable heat), and naturally invites us to equate it with our word 'fever'. However, the word 'fever' in its lay usage tends to refer to palpable excessive bodily heat occurring in acute diseases (notably influenza); patients suffering from chronic illness in which there is palpable heat are more commonly described in English as 'hot' rather than 'feverish'. The technical modern medical usage of 'fever' as denoting a higher than normal body temperature has no correspondence in Chinese medicine since it is measured in the interior of the body (oral cavity or anus), taking no account of body surface temperature or the patient's subjective feelings, precisely the factors on which the Chinese medical judgment is based. The exclusion of the word 'fever' from an English-language medical text might contradict the notion of using clear, simple language wherever possible. Nevertheless, the notion of fever is to some extent culturally defined. Chinese describes hot states of the body in terms of 'heat' and sometimes specifically as 'heat effusion' (giving off heat), and Chinese medicine's particular attention to hot states that we might not describe as 'fever' either in lay or modern medical language calls for the more generic concept of *rè* to be reflected in translation as 'heat'. The choice of term is not without clinical significance, since an English-speaking learner or practitioner of Chinese medicine who applies a narrow definition to a common English term (one for which he supplies his own definition when reading) might fail to categorize a patient as suffering from 'fever' where a Chinese person reading (*fā*) *rè* would not.

Acknowledgements

This dictionary has taken nearly ten years to compile. Such a time-consuming project would have been impossible without the continual moral, technical, and, not least, financial support of the publisher, Robert Felt. Special thanks go to Prof. Paul U. Unschuld for sharing his expertise in the historical meanings of terms, and to Lawrence Grinnell and Martha Fielding for proofreading. We would also thank Hong-chien Ha (哈鴻潛), Hen-Hong Chang (張恆鴻), Mason Chen (陳梅生), Chiung-Chung Wang (王炯忠), and Robert Liu Chung-Min (劉重民) for their indispensable support for this project.

N. Wiseman and Feng Y.

A Guide to the Use of This Dictionary

1. Entry Headers

Each English entry term, or entry header, is printed in bold letters flush with the left-hand margin of each column. It is followed by the original Chinese term and Pinyin transliteration.

arched-back rigidity 角弓反张 *jiǎo gōng fǎn zhāng*:

Where the English term is an equivalent for two or more variant Chinese terms, the Chinese variants are also given.

ear acupuncture 耳针 *ěr zhēn*, 耳针疗法 *ěr zhēn liǎo fǎ*:

2. Arrangement of Entries

The entries are arranged in alphabetical order of the letters, regardless of space, hyphen, or punctuation that may occur between letters, and regardless of upper and lower case.

dry lips	qi-moving technique
dry mouth	Qin
dryness	Qing
dryness damage cough	qi occlusion

Homographs and English terms serving as equivalents for distinct Chinese terms are listed separately, preceded by a superscript number.

[1]**moxa** 艾叶 *ài yè*: The prepared leaves of mugwort (*ài yè*) used in the technique of moxibustion, and...

[2]**moxa** 艾灸 *ài jiǔ*: *vb.* moxaing, moxaed. To perform moxabustion; to treat with moxibustion.

[1]**depression** 郁 *yù*: Stagnation; reduced activity.

[2]**depression** 宛宛 *wǎn wǎn*: A concavity or indentation, as in the surface of the body.

[1]**needle** 针 *zhēn*, 鍼 *zhēn*: *n.* Any instrument, usually of metal, used to puncture the skin and flesh in acupuncture...

[2]**needle** 针 *zhēn*, 鍼 *zhēn*, 刺 *cì*: *vb. trans.* To puncture with a needle as in acupuncture. *vb. intrans.* To perform acupuncture. ◇ Chin *zhēn*, to needle; *cì*, to prick, stab.

[1]**scab** 痂 *jiā*: The crust that forms over a wound and protects it until the flesh has grown back. [43:355]

[2]**scab** 疥 *jiè*, 疥疮 *jiè chuāng*: A disease characterized by small papules the size of a pinhead that are associated with insufferable penetrating itching...

3. Information under Main Entries

The entry header may be followed by a synonym or synonyms.

dryness evil invading the lung 燥邪犯肺 *zào xié fàn fèi*: Synonym: *dryness qi damaging the lung*.

Synonyms marked as (*obs*) (obsolete) are terms previously, but no longer used by the compilers.

controlling vessel 任脉 *rèn mài*: Synonym: *conception vessel* (*obs*). Abbreviation: CV.

In some cases, it might be followed by a book title in which the term was first noted.

strangury 淋 *lín*: From *Elementary Questions* (*sù wèn, liù yuán zhèng jì dà lùn*). A disease pattern characterized by...

After any synonyms and source books comes the definition. Multiple definitions are highlighted in bold Arabic numerals, **1.**, **2.**, **3.**, etc.

mammary toxin sore 乳毒 *rǔ dú*: **1.** A boil of the breast unassociated with pregnancy or breast-feeding. **2.** A postpartum MAMMARY WELLING-ABSCESS. [26:377]

Definitions are often followed by clinical information. Large amounts of information are often broken down into sections, e.g., **Pathway**, **Method**, **Application**, etc. Modern medical equivalents of pathological states (which are often only rough) are given under WMC (Western medical correspondences). Therapeutic information is introduced with MED (Medication), ACU (Acupuncture), and occasionally TRT (Treatment).

Where a pattern analysis is given, the pattern name often appears in **bold** type.

abdominal pain 腹痛 *fù tòng*: Pain in the stomach duct, in the umbilical region, in the smaller abdomen, or in the lesser abdomen. Abdominal pain is attributable to external contraction of one of the six excesses... **Cold** pain is pain that is exacerbated by exposure to cold and likes warmth, and... **Heat** pain is pain that...

4. Cross References

References to other entries are set in SMALL CAPITALS. A term written in small capitals can be found as an individual entry.

bladder damp-heat bloody urine 膀胱湿热尿血 *páng guāng shī rè niào xuè*: Synonym: *lower burner damp-heat bloody urine*. BLOODY URINE attributed to bladder damp-heat.

See introduces references to terms that relate to the originating term in different ways.

1. It refers to an entry containing the definition of the originating entry.

   sound of cicadas in the ear 耳作蝉鸣 *ěr zuò chán míng*: See TINNITUS.

2. It refers to more specific or more generic terms.

> **malodor** 臭气 *chòu qì*: Any unpleasant or offensive odor. See ANIMAL ODOR; FISHY SMELL; PUTRID SMELL; FOUL SMELL. [48:284]

3. It refers to an entry that provides more information about the term or related concepts.

See also indicates another term whose relationship with the originating term is more tangential.

Compare provides a reference to terms of similar, but distinct meaning, or to terms of opposite meaning.

> **smaller abdomen** 小腹 *xiǎo fù*: Lower abdomen, i.e., the part of the abdomen below the navel is referred to as the smaller abdomen. Compare LESSER ABDOMEN.
>
> **scant menstruation** 月经过少 *yuè jīng guò shǎo*: Smaller menstrual flow (in some cases reduced to spotting) or shorter menstrual period than normal.... Compare PROFUSE MENSTRUATION.

References are often given in tables.

5. Word Origins and Meanings

Explanations of word origins have been provided for some terms, and are introduced by ◇ . The etymology of Chinese terms (introduced by CHIN) has been given where it illuminates a concept (especially one that is represented by a new coinage in English), or where literal meaning of the English term differs from that of the Chinese (e.g., *xué*, unlike the English point, meaning a hole or cave). English etymologies (Eng) have been given in a few cases to elucidate difficult words (e.g., cholera, glans) or to explain translation choices (e.g., scab, glomus).

6. Abbreviations

Word-classes of English terms have been abbreviated as follows:

n.   noun (or noun phrase)
vb.   verb (or verb phrase)
pp.   past participle
adj.   adjective
prep.   preposition
comb.   combining form
root   word-root
pl.   plural

The word-class of a term is given where it is not clear from the context, and for terms that are used in distinct word-classes (e.g., *clear* as an adjective and as a noun).

NB: signals a note by the compilers. Very often it signals a problem in defining the term in question or interpreting the concept.

Gk.   Greek

F.   French
L.   Latin
Jap.   Japanese
MF.   French
Du.   Dutch
Swed.   Swedish
ⓜ   apply moxibustion

Channel Name Abbreviations

BL	bladder (channel)	LR	liver (ch.)
CV	controlling (vessel)	LU	lung (ch.)
GB	gallbladder (ch.)	PC	pericardium (ch.)
GIV	girdling (ves.)	SI	small intestine (ch.)
GV	governing (ves.)	SP	spleen (ch.)
HT	heart (ch.)	ST	stomach (ch.)
KI	kidney (ch.)	TB	triple burner (ch.)
LI	large intestine (ch.)		

7. The Names of Medicinals, Formulas, and Points

Medicinals are referred to by English names, with Pinyin enclosed in parenthesis. In lists of medicinals, the Chinese terms are also provided. English names, chosen in preference to Latin pharmaceutical names for their brevity and their ease of spelling and pronunciation, are common names (e.g., pear peel, oyster shell, stinkbug, earthworm), simplified Latin names (e.g., angelica, crataegus, veratrum, coptis), or, rarely, literal translations of the Chinese (e.g., dragon bone).

Names of formulas are written in English with a parenthesized Pinyin transliteration.

Acupuncture point names follow a similar format. Channel points are written in alphanumeric code, with Pinyin transliteration and English rendering in parenthesis. Non-channel points are given in their English rendering with Pinyin in parenthesis. The alphanumeric codes are those used in other works by the compilers. They largely coincide with the alphanumeric codes proposed by the World Health Organization, but not in cases where the WHO term goes against the translation principles applied in this text (e.g., TE, triple energizer).

8. Bibliographic References

References to sources translated or consulted are given at the end of each entry in brackets, e.g., [26:98]which means page 98 of [chen] in the bibliography at the end of the book.

The index can be used to locate Chinese (Pinyin) terms, Latin, biomedical and acupoint nomenclature. English entries are not included and may be directly accessed alphabetically in the text.

Single Characters with English Equivalents

Following is a list of commonly used key single characters commonly appearing in Chinese terms. The characters are ordered by their Pinyin pronunciation. The commonly used English equivalent or equivalents are marked in **bold face** type. The word-class of the English term (not necessarily the same as the Chinese) is given in italic (*n.*, *vb.*, *adj.*, etc.). Other forms of the same English word belonging to other word-classes appear in regular type. Example compounds in which the term appears are given in Chinese, Pinyin and English, with the English key term highlighted in *slanted roman* type.

ài 嗳 **belching** *n.* 嗳气 *ài qì*, *belching*.

ān 安 **quiet** *vb.* 安神 *ān shén*, *quiet* the spirit; 心神不安 *xīn shén bù ān*, disquieted heart spirit.

bái 白 **white** *adj.*, *n.* color associated with lung-metal. 面白 *miàn bái*, *white* face.

bài 败 **bad** *adj.* 败血冲心 *bài xuè chōng xīn*, *bad* blood surging into the heart.

bān 斑 **macule** *n.* 斑疹 *bān zhěn*, *maculo*papular eruption.

bào 暴 **sudden** *adj.* 暴盲 *bào máng sudden* blindness. **fulminant** *adj.* 暴脱 *bào tuō*, *fulminant* desertion.

bēi 悲 **sorrow** *n.* one of the seven affects. 悲则气消 *bēi zé qì xiāo*, *sorrow* causes qi to disperse.

bèi 背 **back** *n.* 背痛 *bèi tòng*, *back* pain; 背寒 *bèi hán*, cold *back*.

bèi 焙 **stone-bake** *vb.*

bèi 臂 **forearm** *n.*

bēn 奔 **run** *vb.* 奔豚 *bēn tún*, *running* piglet.

běn 本 **root** *n.* 标本 *biāo běn*, *root* and tip; 肝者，罢极之本 *gān zhě, pí jí zhī běn*, liver is the *root* of resistance to fatigue.

bēng 崩 **flooding** *n.* 崩漏 *bēng lòu*, *flooding* and spotting.

bí 鼻 **nose** *n.* 酒齄鼻 *jiǔ zhā bí*, drinker's *nose*. **nasal** *adj.* 鼻渊 *bí yuān*, deep-source *nasal* congestion.

bì 秘 **constipation** *n.* lit. dense. 便秘 *biàn bì*, *constipation*.

bì 闭 **block** *vb.*, *n.* 热闭 *rè bì*, heat *block*.

bì 辟 **repel** *vb.* 辟秽 *bì huì*, *repel* foulness.

bì 蔽 **cloud** *vb.* lit. cover. 痰浊蒙蔽心包 *tán zhuó méng bì xīn bāo*, phlegm turbidity *clouding* the pericardium.

bì 痹 **impediment** *n.* 风痹 *fēng bì*, wind *impediment*.

biàn 便 **stool** *n.* lit. convenience. 便溏 *biàn táng*, sloppy *stool*. **urine** *n.*urinate *vb.*, urination *n.* 小便 *xiǎo biàn*, *urination*; 小便清长 *xiǎo biàn qīng cháng*, long voidings of clear *urine*.

biàn 变 **transmute** *vb.* **transmutation** *n.*

biāo 标 **tip** *n.* 标本 *biāo běn*, *root* and *tip*.

biǎo 表 **exterior** *adj.*, *n.* 解表 *jiě biǎo*, resolve the *exterior*.

bìng 病 **disease** *n.* 心病 *xīn bìng*, heart *disease*. **illness** *n.* 久病 *jiǔ bìng*, enduring *illness*. **sickness** *n.* **morbid** *adj.* 病癫 *bìng kuí (tuí)*, *morbid* prominence.

bó 薄 **thin** *adj.* 大便溏薄 *dà biàn táng bó*, *thin* stool, 苔薄 *tāi bó*, *thin* tongue fur.

bǔ 补 **supplement** *vb.*, supplementation *n.* 补气 *bǔ qì*, *supplement* qi. 补法 *bǔ fǎ*, *supplementation*.

cáng 藏 **store** *vb.*, storage *n.* 肝藏血 *gān cáng xué*, the liver *stores* the blood.

cāo 糙 **rough** *adj.* 糙苔 *cāo tāi*, *rough* tongue fur.

chǎn 产 **childbirth** *n.*, 生产 *shēng chǎn*, *childbirth*. **delivery** *n.* 早产 *zǎo chǎn*, premature *delivery*. **par-** *tum* *n.* 产后 *chǎn hòu*, post*partum*. **birth** *n.* 产门 *chǎn mén*, *birth* gate.

cháng 长 **long** *adj.* 长脉 *cháng mài*, *long* pulse, 小便清长 *xiǎo biàn qīng cháng*, *long* voidings of clear urine.

cháng 常 **normal** *adj.* 常脉 *cháng mài*, *normal* pulse.

cháng 肠 **intestine** *n.* 大肠 *dà cháng*, large *intestine*.

cháo 潮 **tidal** *adj.* 潮热 *cháo rè*, *tidal* heat [effusion].

chǎo 炒 **stir-fry** *vb.* 微炒 *wēi chǎo*, light *stir-frying*.

chén 臣 **minister** *n.* 君臣佐使 *jūn chén zuǒ shǐ*, sovereign, *minister*, assistant, and courier.

chén 沉 **deep** *adj.* 沉脉 *chén mài*, *deep* pulse. **sink** *vb.* 沉降药 *chén jiàng yào*, down-*sinking* medicinal.

chéng 乘 **overwhelm** *vb.* 木乘土 *mù chéng tǔ*, wood *overwhelming* earth. **exploit** *vb.* 外邪乘虚 *wài xié chéng xū*, external evil *exploiting* vacuity.

chī 眵 **eye discharge** *n.* 多眵 *duō chī*, copious *eye discharge*.

chí 迟 **slow** *adj.*, slowness *n.* 沉脉 *chén mài*, *slow* pulse; 五迟 *wǔ chí*, the five *slownesses*.

chǐ 齿 **tooth** *n.* 齿痛 *chǐ tòng*, *tooth*ache; 齿龂 *chǐ xiè*, grinding of *teeth*.

chì 赤 **red** *adj.* color associated with heart-fire. 目赤 *mù chì*, *red* eyes.

chì 炽 **intense** *adj.* 心火炽盛 *xīn huǒ chì shèng*, *intense* heart fire.

chōng 充 **fullness** *n.* 肾，其充在骨 *shèn, qí chōng zài gǔ*, the kidney, its *fullness* is in the bone.

chōng 冲 **drench** *vb.* 冲服 *chōng fú*, make *drenched*.

chōng 冲 **hub** *n.* 中冲 *zhōng chōng*, Central *Hub* (PC-9). **thoroughfare** *n.* 冲脉 *chōng mài*, *thoroughfare* vessel.

chóng 虫 **worm** *n.* 蛔虫 *huí chóng*, roundworm. **insect** *n.* 百虫入耳 *bǎi chóng rù ěr*, *insects* in the ear. **chong** *n.* 虫类 *chóng lèi*, *chong* products.

chóu 稠 **thick** *adj.* 痰黄黏稠 *tán huáng nián chóu*, *thick* sticky yellow phlegm.

chòu 臭 **malodorous** *adj.* 臭涕 *chòu tì*, *malodorous* snivel. **malodor** *n.* 腥臭 *xīng chòu*, fishy *malodor*.

chú 除 **eliminate** *vb.*, elimination *n.* 除湿 *chú shī*, *eliminate* dampness.

chuán 传 **pass** *vb.*, passage *n.* 传经 *chuán jīng*, channel *passage*. **convey** *vb.*, conveyance *n.* 大肠主传化 *dà cháng zhǔ chuán huà*, the large intestine governs *conveyance* and transformation.

chuǎn 喘 **pant** *vb.*, panting *n.* 喘急 *chuǎn jí*, rapid *panting*.

chuāng 疮 **sore** *n.* 蓐疮 *rù chuāng*, bedsore.

chún 唇 **lip** *n.* 唇风 *chún fēng*, *lip* wind.

cì 痓 **tetany** *n.* 痰火痓 *tán huǒ cì*, phlegm-fire *tetany*.

cì 刺 **needle** *n.*, *vb.*, needling *n.* 九刺 *jiǔ cì*, nine *needling* methods. **insert** *vb.*, insertion *vb.* 直刺 *zhí cì*, perpendicular *insertion*.

cū 粗 **rough** *adj.* 气粗 *qì cū*, rough breathing.

cù 促 **skipping** *adj.* 促脉 *cù mài*, skipping pulse. **hasty** *adj.* 气促 *qì cù*, hasty respiration.

cuàn 窜 **scurry** *vb.* 窜痛 *cuàn tòng*, scurrying pain.

cún 存 **preserve** *vb.*, preservation *n.* 急下存阴 *jí xià cún yīn*, emergency precipitation to *preserve* yin.

cùn 寸 **inch** *n.* 脐下三寸 *qí xià sān cùn*, three *inches* below the umbilicus; 寸口 *cùn kǒu*, inch opening. **cun** *n.*

dá 达 **outthrust** *vb.*, *n.* 木郁达之 *mù yù dá zhī*, depressed wood is treated by *outthrust*.

dà 大 **large** *adj.* 大脉 *dà mài*, large pulse. **great** *adj.* 大汗 *dà hàn*, great sweating. **major** *adj.* 大承气汤 *dà chéng qì tāng*, Major Qi-Coordinating Decoction. **massive** *adj.* 大头瘟 *dà tóu wēn*, massive head scourge. **enlarged** *adj.* 腹大 *fù dà*, enlarged abdomen.

dāi 呆 **feeble-minded** *adj.*, feeble-mindedness *n.* 痴呆 *chī dāi*, feeble-mindedness. **dull** *adj.* 表情呆滞 *biǎo qíng dāi zhì*, dull expression. **torpid** *adj.* 纳呆 *nà dāi*, torpid intake.

dài 代 **intermittent** *adj.* 代脉 *dài mài*, intermittent pulse. **regularly interrupted** *adj.* **changing** *adj.* 脾脉代 *pí mài dài*, the spleen pulse is *changing*.

dài 怠 **fatigue** *n.*, fatigued *adj.* 倦怠乏力 *juàn dài fá lì*, fatigue and lack of strength.

dài 带 **girdle** *n.*, *vb.*, girdling *adj.* 带脉 *dài mài*, girdling vessel. nonliteral: 带下 *dài xià*, vaginal discharge.

dān 丹 **cinnabar** *n.* 赤游风 *chì yóu fēng*, red wandering *cinnabar*, 丹毒 *dān dú*, cinnabar toxin. **elixir** *n.* 紫雪丹 *zǐ xuě dān*, Purple Snow Elixir.

dān 瘅 **pure heat** *n.* 瘅疟 *dān nüè*, pure-heat malaria.

dǎn 疸 **jaundice** *n.* 酒疸 *jiǔ dǎn*, liquor *jaundice*.

dǎn 胆 **gallbladder** *n.* 肝胆湿热 *gān dǎn shī rè*, liver-gallbladder damp-heat. **GB.**

dàn 淡 **pale** *adj.* 面色淡白 *miàn sè dàn bái*, pale white facial complexion. **bland** *adj.*, blandness *n.* 淡渗利水药 *bland* percolating water-disinhibiting medicinals.

dǎo 捣 **pound** *vb.* 捣烂 *dǎo làn*, pound to a pulp.

dǎo 导 **abduct** *vb.*, abduction *n.* 消食导滞 *xiāo shí dǎo zhì*, disperse food and *abduct* stagnation.

dí 涤 **flush** *vb.* 涤痰 *dí tán*, flush phlegm.

dì 地 **earth** *n.* 天地 *tiān dì*, heaven and earth.

diān 颠 **vertex** *n.* 颠顶头痛 *diān dǐng tóu tòng*, vertex headache.

diān 巅 **vertex** *n.* 巅顶头痛 *diān dǐng tóu tòng*, vertex headache.

diān 癫 **withdrawal** *n.* 癫狂 *diān kuáng*, mania and *withdrawal*.

diào 掉 **shaking** *n.* 诸风掉眩，皆属于肝 *zhū fēng diào xuàn, jiē shǔ yú gān*, all wind with *shaking* and dizzy vision is ascribed to the liver.

dīng 疔 **clove sore** *n.* 红丝疔 *hóng sī dīng*, red-thread clove sore.

dǐng 顶 **vertex** *n.* 颠顶头痛 *diān dǐng tóu tòng*, vertex headache.

dìng 锭 **lozenge** *n.*

dòng 动 **stir** *n.* 肝风内动 *gān fēng nèi dòng*, liver wind *stirring* internally.

dòu 痘 **pox** *n.* 痘疮 *dòu chuāng*, pox sores.

dū 督 **governing** *adj.* governing vessel.

dú 毒 **toxin** *n.*, toxic *adj.*, toxicity *n.* 热毒 *rè dú*, heat *toxin*; 微毒 *wēi dú*, slightly *toxic*, slight *toxicity*. **venom** *n.* 蛇毒 *shé dú*, snake venom. **toxin [sore]** *n.*

duàn 煅 **calcine** *vb.*, calcination *n.* 煅牡蛎 *duàn mǔ lì*, calcined oyster shell.

dùn 炖 **double-boil** *vb.*

duō 多 **copious** *adj.* 痰多 *tán duō*, copious phlegm. **profuse** *n.* 多梦 *duō mèng*, profuse dreaming. **increased** *adj.* 多食善肌 *duō shí shàn jī*, increased eating with rapid hungering

duó 夺 **despoliate** *vb.*, despoliation *n.* 夺精 *duó jīng*, despoliation of essence.

ě 恶 **nausea** *n.* 恶心 *ě xīn*, nausea; 泛恶 upflow nausea See also *è* 恶, *wù* 恶.

è 恶 **malign** *adj.*, malignity *n.* 恶血 *è xuè*, malign blood; 恶色 *malign* complexion; 恶阻 *malign* obstruction; 中恶 *zhòng è*, malignity stroke. See also *ě* 恶, *wù* 恶.

ěr 耳 **ear** *n.* 耳痛 *ěr tòng*, ear pain; 耳聤 purulent *ear*.

fā 发 **effuse** *vb.*, effusion *n.* 发表 *fā biǎo*, effuse the exterior; 发背 *fā bèi*, effusion of the back. **erupt** *vb.*, eruption *n.* **emerge** *vb.*, emergence *n.* 晚发 *wǎn fā*, late emergence.

fá 乏 **lack** *vb.*, *n.* 倦怠乏力 *juàn dài fá lì*, fatigue and *lack* of strength.

fǎ 法 **method** *n.* 八法 *bā fǎ*, eight *methods*.

fān 翻 **evert** *vb.* 翻花痔疮 *fàn huā zhì chuāng*, everted-flower hemorrhoids.

fán 烦 **vex** *vb.*, vexation *n.* 烦热 *fán rè*, heat vexation; 五心烦热 *wǔ xīn fán rè*, vexing heat in the five hearts.

fán 燔 **blaze** *vb.*, ablaze *adj.* 气营两燔 *qì yíng liǎng fán*, qi and construction both *ablaze*.

fǎn 反 **reflux** *n.* 反胃 *fǎn wèi*, stomach reflux. **paradoxical** *adj.* 反治 *fǎn zhì*, paradoxical, treatment. nonliteral: 角弓反张 *jiǎo gōng fǎn zhāng*, arched-back rigidity.

fàn 犯 **invade** *vb.*, invasion *n.* 肝气犯胃 *gān qì fàn wèi*, liver qi *invading* the stomach. **assail** *vb.*, assailment *n.*

fàn 泛 **flood** *vb.* 肾虚水泛 *shèn xū shuǐ fàn*, kidney vacuity water *flood*. **upflow** *n.* 泛酸 *fàn suān*, acid upflow. 泛酸 *fàn suān*, acid *upflow*.

fāng 方 **remedy** *n.* **formula** *n.*

féi 肥 **obese** *adj.*, obesity *n.* 肥人多痰 *féi ré duō tán*, obese people tend to have copious phlegm. **fat** *adj.*, fatness *n.* 肥疮 *féi chuāng*, fat sore.

fěi 痱 **disablement** *n.*

fèi 肺 **lung** *n.* 心肺气虚 *xīn fèi qì xū*, heart-lung qi vacuity. **pulmonary** *adj.* 肺痈 *fèi yōng*, pulmonary welling-abscess. **LU.**

fèi 痱 **prickly heat** *n.* 痱子 *fèi zǐ*, prickly heat.

fēn 分 **candareen** *n.* equal to one tenth of a qian. **fen** *n.* equal to one tenth of a body inch or qian.

fén 焚 **deflagrate** *vb.*, deflagration *n.* 心火内焚 *xīn huǒ nèi fén*, heart fire deflagrating internally.

fèn 分 **aspect** *n.* 气分 *qì fèn*, qi aspect.

fèn 粪 **feces** *n.*, fecal *adj.* 吐粪 *tù fèn*, fecal vomiting.

fēng 风 **wind** *n.* 外风 *wài fēng*, external wind.

fēng 蜂 **bee** *n.* 蜂蜜 *fēng mì*, bee's honey. **hornet** *n.* 蜂房 *fēng fáng*, hornet's nest. **wasp** *n.*

fú 伏 **deep-lying** *adj.* 伏饮 *fú yǐn*, deep-lying rheum. **latent** *adj.* 伏瘕 *fú jiǎ*, latent conglomeration. **hidden** *adj.* 伏脉 *fú mài*, hidden pulse. **soaking and standing** *n.* a method of processing medicinal materials.

fú 扶 **support** *vb.* 祛邪扶正 *qū xié fú zhèng*, dispel evil and *support* right.

fú 服 **take** *vb.* 日服三次 *rì fú sān cì*, take three times a day. **dose** *n.* 一服散 *yī fú sǎn*, One *Dose* Powder.

fú 浮 **float** *vb.* 虚阳浮越 *xū yáng fú yuè*, vacuous yang *floating* astray. **superficial** *adj.* 浮络 *fú luò*, superficial network vessel. **puffy** *adj.* 浮肿 *fú zhǒng*, puffy swelling.

fǔ 俯 **prone** *adj.* posture. **bend forward** *adj.*

fǔ 腑 **bowel** *n.* 六腑 *liù fǔ*, the six *bowels*. **storehouse** *n.* as *fǔ* 府. **house** *n.* 府.

fǔ 腐 **putrid** *adj.*, putridity *n.*, putrefy *vb.*, putrefaction *n.* **bean curd** *n.* abbreviation of 豆腐 *dòu fǔ*, bean curd. 苔腐 *tāi fǔ*, bean curd tongue fur.

fù 腹 **abdomen** *n.*, abdominal *adj.* 少腹 *shào fù*, lesser *abdomen*; 腹痛 *fù tòng*, abdominal pain.

gān 干 **dry** *adj.* 口干 *kǒu gān*, dry mouth; 目干涩 *mù gān*, dry eyes.

gān 甘 **sweet** *adj.*, sweetness *n.* 甘草味甘 *gān cǎo wèi gān*, licorice is *sweet* in flavor; 甘入脾 *gān rù pí*, sweetness enters the spleen.

gān 肝 **liver** *n.* 肝肾亏损 *gān shèn kuī sǔn*, liver-kidney depletion. **LR.**

gān 疳 **gan** *n.* 眼疳 *yǎn gān*, eye gan.

gāng 肛 **anus** *n.* 肛漏 *gāng lòu*, anal fistula.

gāng 纲 **principle** *n.* 八纲 *bā gāng*, eight *principles*.

gāo 膏 **paste** *n.* medical preparation. **unctuous** *adj.* 膏淋 *gāo lín*, unctuous stranguary.

gé 膈 **diaphragm** *n.*, diaphragmatic *adj.* **occlusion** *n.* 噎膈 *yē gé*, dysphagia-occulusion.

gēn 根 **root** *n.* 舌根 *shé gēn*, root of the tongue.

gēng 更 **watch** *n.* period of two hours.

gōng 攻 **attack** *vb.*, *n.* 先补后攻 *xiān bǔ hòu gōng*, supplementation followed by *attack*. **offensive treatment** *n.*

gòu 垢 **grime** *n.*, grimy *adj.* 胎垢 *tāi gòu*, fetal grime; 苔垢 *tāi gòu*, grimy tongue fur.

gū 孤 **solitary** *adj.* 孤阳浮越 *gū yáng fú yuè*, solitary yang floating astray.

gǔ 谷 **grain** *n.* 水谷 *shuǐ gǔ*, grain and water.

gǔ 骨 **bone** *n.* 筋骨 *jīn gǔ*, sinew and *bone*.

gǔ 鼓 **drum** *n.* 鼓胀 *gǔ zhàng*, drum distention; 血鼓 *xuè gǔ*, blood *drum*.

gǔ 蛊 **gu** *n.* 蛊毒 *gǔ dú*, gu toxin.

gǔ 臌 **drum distention** *n.* 臌胀 *gǔ zhàng*, drum distention.

gù 固 **secure** *vb.*, security *n.* 益气固表 *yì qì gù biǎo*, boost qi and *secure* the exterior; 肾气不固 *shèn qì bú gù*, insecurity of kidney qi. **stem** *vb.* 涩肠固脱 *sè cháng gù tuō*, astringe the intestines and *stem* desertion.

guān 关 **gate** *n.* 四关 *sì guān*, the four *gates*. **pass** *n.* as in 'mountain pass'. 喉关 *hóu guān*, throat *pass*. **bar** *n.* 寸关尺 *cùn guān chǐ*, inch, bar, and cubit; 风关 *fēng guān*, wind bar.

guǎn 脘 **stomach duct** *n.* see *wǎn* 脘.

guāng 光 **bare** *adj.* 光剥舌 *guāng bō shé*, tongue peeled bare of fur.

guāng 胱 **bladder** *n.* 膀胱 *páng guāng*, bladder.

guī 龟 **tortoise** *n.* 龟头 *guī tóu*, *tortoise's* head (glans penis).

guī 归 **return** *vb.* 引火归原 *yǐn huǒ guī yuán*, return fire to its source.

guǐ 鬼 **ghost** *n.* 十三鬼穴 *shí sān guǐ xué*, the thirteen *ghost* points.

guó 腘 **back of the knee** *n.* popliteal fossa.

hán 涵 **moisten** *vb.* 水不涵木 *shuǐ bù hán mù*, water failing to *moisten* wood.

hàn 汗 **sweat** *n.*, *vb.*, sweating *n.* 黄汗 *huáng hàn*, yellow *sweat*; 自汗 *zì hàn*, spontaneous *sweating*; 盗汗 *dào hàn*, night *sweating*; 汗法 *hàn fǎ*, sweating. **perspire** *vb.*, perspiration *n.*

hào 耗 **wear** *vb.* 心营过耗 *xīn yíng guò hào*, excessive *wearing* of heart construction.

hé 合 **combine** *vb.*, combination *n.* 合病 *hé bìng*, combination disease. **unite** *vb.*, uniting *adj.*, union *n.* 合穴 *hé xué*, uniting point; 合谷 *hé gǔ*, union valley. **connect** *vb.* 肺合皮毛 *fèi hé pí máo*, the lung is *connected* to the skin and [body] hair.

hé 和 **harmonize** *vb.*, harmonization *n.*, harmonious *adj.* 和解少阳 *hé jiě shào yáng*, harmonize [and resolve] the lesser yang; 和法 *hé fǎ*, harmonization; 胃气不和 *wèi qì bù hé*, disharmony of stomach qi.

hé 核 **node** *n.* 乳核 *rǔ hé*, mammary *node*.

hé 涸 **desiccate** *vb.*, desiccated *adj.*, desiccation *n.*

hēi 黑 **black** *adj.*, *n.* color associated with kidney-water.

héng 胻 **lower leg** *n.* **shin** *n.*

hōng 烘 **bake** *vb.* 烘干 *hōng gān*, bake dry; 烘热 *hōng rè*, baking heat [effusion].

hóng 红 **red** *adj.*, *n.* color associated with heart-fire. 舌红 *shé hóng*, red tongue.

hóu 喉 **throat** *n.* 喉风 *hóu fēng*, throat wind. **larynx** *n.*, laryngeal *adj.*

hòu 厚 **thick** *adj.* 舌苔厚 *shé tāi hòu*, thick tongue fur. **rich** *n.* 厚味 *hòu wèi*, rich (in) flavor.

hòu 候 **indicator** *n.* 诸病源候论 *zhū bìng yuán hòu lùn*, The Origin and Indicators of Disease. **indicate** *vb.*

hú 狐 **fox** *n.*, foxy *adj.* 狐臭 *hú chòu*, foxy smell.

hǔ 虎 **tiger** *n.* 白虎汤 *bái hǔ tāng*, White Tiger Decoction.

hù 户 **door** *n.* 阴户 *yīn hù*, the yin doors (the opening of the vagina).

huá 华 **luster** *n.* 面色无华 *miàn sè wú huá*, lusterless complexion. **bloom** *n.* 肝，其华在爪 *gān, qí huá zài zhǎo*, the liver, its *bloom* is in the nails.

huá 滑 **glossy** *adj.* 舌苔滑 *shé tāi huá*, glossy tongue fur. **slippery** *adj.* 滑脉 *huá mài*, slippery pulse. **efflux** *n.* uncontrolled flow from the body. 滑精 *huá jīng*, seminal *efflux*. **lubricate** *vb.* 滑肠 *huá cháng*, lubricate the intestines.

huà 化 **transform** *vb.*, transformation. 舌苔不化 *shé tāi bú huà*, non-transforming tongue fur; 化痰 *huà tán*, transform phlegm.

huǎn 缓 **slack** *adj.*, slacken *vb.* 筋缓 *jīn huǎn*, slack sinews; 舌缓 *shé huǎn*, slack tongue; 喜则气缓 *xǐ yé qì huǎn*, joy causes qi to *slacken*. **moderate** *adj.* 缓脉 *huǎn mài*, moderate pulse. **mild** *adj.* 缓下 *huǎn xià*, mild precipitation; 缓补 *huǎn bǔ*, mild supplementation. **relax** *vb.* 缓急 *huǎn jí*, relax tension.

huáng 黄 **yellow** *adj.*, *n.* color associated with spleen-earth. 面色黄 *miàn sè huáng*, yellow facial complexion. **jaundice** *n.* 阴黄 *yīn huáng*, yin jaundice.

huǎng 㿠 **bright (white)** *adj.* 面色㿠白 *miàn sè huǎng bái*, bright white facial complexion.

huī 灰 **ash** *n.*, ashen *adj.* 灰指甲 *huī zhǐ jiǎ*, ashen nail. **gray** *adj., n.* 灰苔 *huī tāi*, gray tongue fur.

huí 回 **return** *vb.* 回阳救逆 *huí yáng jiù nì*, return yang and stem counterflow.

huí 蛔 **roundworm** *n.* 蛔虫 *huí chóng*, roundworm.

huì 会 **meet** *n.* 会穴 *huì xué*, meeting points.

huì 秽 **foul** *adj.*, foulness *n.* 辟秽 *bì huì*, repel foulness.

hūn 昏 **cloud** *vb.* 神昏 *shén hūn*, clouded spirit; 昏睡 *hūn shuì*, clouding sleep.

hún 魂 **ethereal soul** *n.* 肝藏魂 *gān cáng hún*, the liver stores the *ethereal soul*.

huó 活 **quicken** *vb.* 活血化瘀 *huó xuè huà yū*, quicken the blood and transform stasis.

huǒ 火 **fire** *n.* 痰火 *tán huǒ*, phlegm-fire.

huò 豁 **sweep** *vb.* 豁痰 *huò tán*, sweep phlegm. **gaping** *adj.* 豁豁然空 *huò huò rán kong*, gapingly empty.

jī 肌 **flesh** *n.* 肌表 *jī biǎo*, fleshy exterior.

jī 饥 **hunger** *n., vb.*, hungering *n.* 善食易饥 *shàn shí yì jī*, large appetite with rapid *hungering*.

jī 机 **dynamic** *n.* 气机 *qì jī*, qi *dynamic*. **mechanism** *n.* 病机 *bìng jī*, pathomechanism.

jī 积 **accumulate** *vb.*, accumulation *n.* 积热 *jī rè*, accumulated heat; 癥瘕积聚 *zhēng jiǎ jī jù*, concretions, conglomerations, accumulations and gatherings.

jí 急 **tense** *adj.*, tension *n.* 缓急 *huǎn jí*, relax tension. **acute** *adj.* 急则治标 *jí zé zhì biāo*, in acute conditions, treat the tip. **urgent** *adj.*, urgency *n.* 尿急 *niào jí*, urinary urgency. **rapid** *adj.* 呼吸急促 *hū xī jí cù*, hasty *rapid* breathing.

jí 疾 **disease** *n.* 疾病 *jí bìng*, disease; 疟疾 *nüè jí*, malaria. **racing** *adj.* 疾脉 *jí mài*, racing pulse.

jǐ 脊 **vertebrae** *n.* 夹脊 *jiā jí*, paravertebrals. **spine** *n.*

jì 剂 **preparation** *n.* 丸剂 *wán jì*, pill preparation.

jì 济 **help** *vb.* 水火相济 *shuǐ huǒ xiāng jì*, fire and water *helping* each other.

jiá 颊 **cheek** *n.* 面颊 *miàn jiá*, cheek; 颊车 *jiá chē*, cheek carriage.

jiǎ 瘕 **conglomeration** *n.* 癥瘕积聚 *zhēng jiǎ jī jù*, concretions, *conglomerations*, accumulations, and gatherings.

jiān 肩 **shoulder** *n.* 漏肩风 *lòu jiān fēng*, leaky shoulder wind.

jiān 坚 **hard** *adj.* 软坚 *ruǎn jiān*, soften *hardness*.

jiān 煎 **decoct** *vb.*, decoction *n.* 鳖甲煎丸 *biē-jiǎ jiān wán*, Turtle Shell *Decocted* Pill. **brew** *n.* 济川煎 *jì chuān jiān*, Ferry Brew.

jiǎn 睑 **eyelid** *n.* 睑废 *jiǎn fèi*, drooping *eyelid*.

jiàn 健 **fortify** *vb.* 健脾 *jiàn pí*, fortify the spleen.

jiàng 降 **downbear** *vb.*, downbearing *adj., n.* 和胃降逆 *hé wèi jiàng nì*, harmonize the stomach and *downbear* counterflow.

jiāo 交 **interact** *vb.*, interaction *n.* 心肾相交 *xīn shèn xiāng jiāo*, the heart and kidney *interact*. **intersect** *vb.*, intersection *n.* 交会穴 *jiāo huì xué*, intersection point. **confluence** *n.* 八脉交会穴 *bā mài jiāo huì xué*, confluence points of the eight vessels.

jiāo 焦 **parch** *vb.*, parched *adj.* 唇焦 *chún jiāo*, parched lips. **scorch** *vb.* 肺热叶焦 *fèi rè yè jiāo*, lung heat *scorching* the lobes. **burn** *vb.*, burnt *adj.*, burner *n.* 苔焦黄 *tāi jiāo huáng*, burnt-yellow tongue fur; 三焦 *sān jiāo*, triple burner.

jiāo 胶 **glue** *n.* 阿胶 *ē jiāo*, ass hide glue.

jiǎo 脚 **foot** *n.* 脚湿气 *jiǎo shī qì*, foot damp qi. **leg** *n.* 脚气 *jiǎo qì*, leg qi.

jié 结 **bind** *vb., n.*, bound *pp., adj.* 热结 *rè jié*, heat bind; 大便秘结 *dà biàn mì jié*, dry bound stool; 结脉 *jié mài*, bound pulse.

jié 截 **interrupt** *vb.* 截疟 *jié nüè*, interrupt malaria.

jié 竭 **exhaust** *vb.*, exhaustion *n.* 阴竭阳脱 *yīn jié yáng tuō*, exhaustion of yin and desertion of yang.

jié 洁 **cleanse** *vb.* 洁净腑 *jié jìng fǔ*, cleanse the clear bowel.

jié 疖 **boil** *n.* 暑疖 *shǔ jié*, summerheat boil.

jiě 解 **resolve** *vb.*, resolution *n.* 解表 *jiě biǎo*, resolve the exterior, exterior *resolution*.

jiè 疥 **scab** *n.* 疥癣 *jiè xiǎn*, scab and lichen.

jīn 金 **metal** *n.* 木火刑金 *mù huǒ xíng jīn*, wood fire tormenting *metal*.

jīn 津 **liquid** *n.* 气津两伤 *qì jīn liǎng shāng*, damage to both qi and *liquid*.

jīn 筋 **sinew** *n.* 肝主筋 *gān zhǔ jīn*, the liver governs the *sinews*. **vein** *n.* 腹露青筋 *fù lù qīng jīn*, prominent [green-blue] abdominal veins.

jǐn 紧 **tight** *adj.* 紧脉 *jǐn mài*, tight pulse.

jīng 茎 **penis** *n.* lit. stem. 阴茎 *yīn jīng*, penis; 茎中痛 *jīng zhōng tòng*, pain in the penis.

jīng 睛 **eye** *n.* 眼睛 *yǎn jīng*, eye.

jīng 经 **channel** *n.* 太阳经 *tài yáng jīng*, greater yang *channel*. **menstruation** *n.* 月经 *yuè jīng*, menstruation; 经行腰痛 *jīng xíng yāo tòng*, menstrual lumbar pain. **canon** *n.* 黄帝内经 *huáng dì nèi jīng*, *The Yellow Emperor's Inner Canon*. **river** *n.* 经穴 *jīng xué*, river point.

jīng 精 **essence** *n.* 肾藏精 *shèn cáng jīng*, the kidney stores *essence*. **semen** *n.*, seminal *adj.* 遗精 *yí jīng*, seminal emission.

jīng 惊 **fright** *n.* 肝主惊 *gān zhǔ jīng*, liver governs fright; 易惊 *yì jīng*, susceptibility to *fright*.

jǐng 井 **well** *n.* 井穴 *jǐng xué*, well point.

jìng 痉 **tetany** *n.* 痉病 *jìng bìng*, tetanic disease.

jìng 胫 **lower leg** *n.* **lower leg bone** *n.*

jiǔ 久 **enduring** *adj.* 久病 *jiǔ bìng*, enduring disease.

jiǔ 灸 **moxibustion** (also moxabustion) *n.* 针灸 *zhēn jiǔ*, acupuncture and *moxibustion*.

jiǔ 酒 **wine** *n.* 药酒 *yào jiǔ*, medicinal wine. **liquor** *n.* 酒疸 *jiǔ dǎn*, liquor jaundice.

jiù 救 **rescue** *vb.* 清燥救肺 *qīng zào jiù fèi*, clear dryness and *rescue* the lung. **stem** *vb.* 回阳救逆 *huí yáng jiù nì*, return yang and stem counterflow.

jū 拘 **hypertonicity** *n.* 四肢拘急 *sì zhī jū jí*, hypertonicity of the limbs.

jū 疽 **flat abscess** *n.* 痈疽 *yōng jū*, welling-abscesses and *flat-abscesses*.

jù 拒 **refuse** *vb.* 腹痛拒按 *fù tòng jù àn*, abdominal pain that *refuses* pressure.

jù 沮 **sweating** *n.* 偏沮 *piān jù*, hemilateral sweating.

jù 聚 **gather** *vb.*, gathering *n.* 宗脉所聚 *zōng mài suǒ jù*, gathering place of the ancestral sinews; 积聚 *jī jù*, accumulations and gatherings.

juàn 倦 **fatigue** *n.* 倦怠 *juàn dài*, fatigue. **lassitude** *n.* 神倦 *shén juàn*, lassitude of spirit.

jué 厥 **reversal** *n.* 热厥 *rè jué*, heat reversal. **reverting** *adj.* 足厥阴肝经 *zú jué yīn gān jīng*, foot reverting yin liver channel.

jué 绝 **expire** *vb.*, **expiry** *n.* 绝汗 *jué hàn*, *expiry* sweating; 上厥下竭 *shàng jué xià jié*, upper body reversal and lower body *expiry*.

jūn 君 **sovereign** *n.* 君火 *jūn huǒ*, *sovereign* fire.

jùn 峻 **drastic** *adj.* 峻补 *jùn bǔ*, *drastic* supplementation.

jùn 菌 **mushroom** *n.* 耳菌 *ěr jùn*, ear *mushroom*.

kāi 开 **open** *vb.*, *adj.*, **opening** *n.* 开窍 *kāi qiào*, *open* the orifices; 凉开 *liáng kāi*, cool *opening*.

kàng 亢 **hyperactive** *adj.*, **hyperactivity** *n.* 肝阳上亢 *gān yáng shàng kàng*, ascendant *hyperactivity* of liver yang.

ké 咳 **cough** *vb.*, *n.* sound without matter. 干咳 *gān ké*, dry *cough*. **non-productive cough** *n.*

kě 渴 **thirst** *n.*, **thirsty** *adj.* 口渴 *kǒu kě*, *thirst*.

kè 克 **restrain** *vb.* 木克土 *mù kè tǔ*, wood *restrains* earth.

kè 客 **visit** *vb.*, **visiting** *adj.* 小儿客忤 *xiǎo ér kè wǔ*, child *visiting* hostility; 客色 *kè sè*, *visiting* complexion. **settle** *vb.* of evils in the body. 风温客表 *fēng wēn kè biǎo*, wind-warmth *settling* in the exterior. **guest** *n.* 客主 *kè zhǔ*, Guest-Host (GB-3).

kǒng 恐 **fear** *n.* mind associated with kidney; also one of the seven affects. 肾主恐 *shèn zhǔ kǒng*, the kidney governs *fear*.

kōu 芤 **scallion-stalk** *n.* 芤脉 *kōu mài*, *scallion-stalk* pulse.

kǒu 口 **mouth** *n.* 口干 *kǒu gān*, dry *mouth*; 口眼喎斜 *kǒu yǎn wāi xié*, deviated eyes and *mouth*; 口苦 *kǒu kǔ*, bitter taste in the *mouth*. nonliteral: 口噤 *kǒu jìn*, clenched jaws; 口渴 *kǒu kě*, thirst.

kū 枯 **desiccate** *vb.*, **desiccated** *pp.*, *adj.*, **desiccation** *n.* 牙齿干燥如枯骨 *yá chǐ gān zào rú kū gǔ*, teeth dry as *desiccated* bones; 肾阴枯涸 *shèn yīn kū hé*, *desiccation* of kidney yin.

kuāi 喎 **deviated** *adj.*, **deviation** *n.* 口眼喎斜 *kǒu yǎn kuāi xié*, *deviated* eyes and mouth.

kuài 块 **clot** *n.*, *vb.* 经血夹块 *jīng xuè jiā kuài*, *clotted* menstrual flow. **lump** *n.* 痞块 *pǐ kuài*, *lump* glomus.

kuān 宽 **loosen** *vb.* lit. widen. 宽胸 *kuān xiōng*, *loosen* the chest; 宽中 *kuān zhōng*, *loosen* the center.

kuáng 狂 **mania** *n.*, **manic** *adj.* 癫狂 *diān kuáng*, *mania* and withdrawal.

kuàng 眶 **eye socket** *n.* 目眶 *mù kuàng*, *eye socket*.

kuī 亏 **deplete** *vb.*, **depleted** *pp.*, *adj.*, **depletion** *n.* 肝肾亏损 *gān shèn kuī sǔn*, liver-kidney *depletion*.

kuí 癀 **prominent** *adj.* 癀疝 *kuí shàn*, *prominent* mounting.

kuì 溃 **open** *adj.* 疮疡溃烂 *chuāng yáng kuì làn*, *open* ulcerated sores. **rupture** *n.* 溃后 *kuì hòu*, after *rupture*.

kùn 困 **cumbersome** *adj.*, **encumber** *vb.*, **encumbrance** *n.* 肢体困重 *zhī tǐ kùn zhòng*, heavy *cumbersome* limbs; 脾为湿困 *pí wéi shī kùn*, the spleen *encumbered* by dampness; 脾虚湿困 *pí xū shī kùn*, spleen vacuity damp *encumbrance*.

lài 癞 **lai** *n.* denotes various diseases marked by loss of hair; graph composition (赖) suggests 'repudiation'. 鸡屎癞 *jī shǐ lài*, chicken's-droppings *lai*; 癞大风 *lài dà fēng*, *lai* great wind (leprosy).

làn 烂 **putrefy** *vb.*, **putrefaction** *n.* 烂喉沙 *làn hóu shā*, *putrefying* throat sand. **erode** *vb.*, **erosion** *n.* 糜烂 *mí làn*, *erosion*.

láo 牢 **confined** *adj.* lit. pen; prison; firm and durable. 牢脉 *láo mài*, *confined* pulse.

láo 劳 **taxation** *n.* 虚劳 *xū láo*, vacuity-*taxation*.

láo 痨 **consumption** *n.* 肺痨 *fèi láo*, pulmonary *consumption*; 传尸痨 *chuán shī láo*, corpse-transmitted *consumption*.

lǎo 老 **tough** *n.* 老嫩 *lǎo nèn*, [degree of] *toughness* or tenderness.

léi 雷 **thunder** *n.* 雷头风 *léi tóu fēng*, *thunder* head wind; 龙雷之火 *lóng léi zhī huǒ*, dragon and *thunder* fire; 雷火神针 *léi huǒ shén zhēn*, *thunder* and fire spirit needle.

lèi 泪 **tears** *n.* 泪为肝液 *lèi wéi gān yè*, *tears* are the humor of the liver.

lǐ 里 **interior** *adj.*, *n.* 表里 *biǎo lǐ*, *interior* and exterior.

lǐ 理 **rectify** *vb.*, **rectification** *n.* 理气 *lǐ qì*, *rectify* qi.

lì 疬 **scrofula (large)** *n.* 瘰疬 *luǒ lì*, *scrofula*.

lì 力 **force** *n.*, 有力 *yǒu lì*, **forceful** *adj.* 脉滑数有力 *mài huá shuò yǒu lì*, the pulse is slippery, rapid, and *forceful*.

lì 利 **disinhibit** *vb.*, **uninhibited** *adj.* 利水 *lì shuǐ*, *disinhibit* water; 利咽 *lì yān*, *disinhibit* the throat. 小便自利 *xiǎo biàn zì lì*, *uninhibited* urination.

lì 戾 **perverse** *adj.* 乖戾之气 *guāi lì zhī qì*, *perverse* qi; 戾气 *lì qì*, *perverse* qi.

lì 疠 **pestilence** *n.*, **pestilential** *adj.* 天行疫疠 *tiān xíng yì lì*, heaven-current epidemic *pestilence*. **leprosy** *n.* 疠风 *lì fēng*, *pestilential* wind, leprosy.

liǎn 敛 **constrain** *vb.* 敛阴 *liǎn yīn*, *constrain* yin. **close** *vb.* 敛疮 *liǎn chuāng*, *close* sores.

liáng 凉 **cool** *vb.* 凉血 *liáng xuè*, *cool* the blood.

lín 淋 **strangury** *n.* 血淋 *xuè lín*, blood *strangury*. **dribble** *vb.* 小便淋漓不禁 *xiǎo biàn lín lí bú jìn*, *dribbling* urinary incontinence.

líng 凌 **intimidate** *vb.* 水气凌心 *shuǐ qì líng xīn*, water-qi *intimidating* the heart.

líng 灵 **spirit** *n.* 灵台 *líng tái*, Spirit Tower (GB-10). **magic** *adj.* 灵药 *líng yào*, *magic* medicine; 灵枢 *líng shū*, Magic Pivot.

liú 流 **flow** *vb.*, *n.* 下肢流火 *xià zhī liú huǒ*, lower limb fire *flow*. 流鼻涕 *liú bí tì*, runny nose. 流泪 *liú lèi*, tearing.

liú 留 **lodge** *vb.* 邪留三焦 *xié liú sān jiāo*, evil *lodged* in the triple burner. **retain** *vb.*, **retention** *n.* 留针五分钟 *liú zhēn wǔ fēn zhōng*, *retain* the needles for five minutes.

liú 瘤 **tumor** *n.* 肉瘤 *ròu liú*, flesh *tumor*.

lóng 龙 **dragon** *n.* 龙泉疔 *lóng quán dīng*, *dragon*-spring clove sore.

lóng 聋 **deaf** *adj.*, **deafness** *n.* 耳聋 *ěr lóng*, *deafness*.

lóng 癃 **dribbling block** *n.* 癃闭 *lóng bì*, *dribbling* urinary *block*.

lòu 瘘 **fistula** *n.* 瘘疮 *lòu chuāng*, *fistula*.

lòu 漏 **spotting** *n.* 崩漏 *bēng lòu*, flooding and *spotting*. **fistula** *n.* same as 瘘 *lòu*. 漏疮 *lòu chuāng*, *fistula*.

lù 露 **distillate** *n.*

luǒ 瘰 **scrofula (small)** *n.* 瘰疬 *luǒ lì*, *scrofula*.

luò 咯 **expectorate** *vb.*, **expectoration** *n.* 痰稠不易咯出 *tán chóu bú yì luò chū*, thick phlegm that is difficult to *expectorate*.

luò 络 **network (vessel)** *n.* 经络 *jīng luò*, channels and *network* vessels; 十五络 *shí wǔ luò*, the fifteen *network vessels.* **net** *vb.* 心经络于小肠 *xīn jīng luò yú xiǎo cháng,* the heart channel *nets* the small intestine.

má 麻 **tingling** *adj., n.* **numbness** *n.* 麻木 *má mù,* numbness [and tingling].

mài 脉 **vessel** *n.* 任脉 *rèn mài,* controlling *vessel.* **pulse** *n.* 脉浮数 *mài fú shuò,* the *pulse* is floating and rapid.

mǎn 满 **fullness** *n.* 腹满 *fù mǎn,* abdominal *fullness.*

máng 盲 **blindness** *n.* 雀盲 *què máng,* sparrow *blindness* (night blindness).

mèi 寐 **sleep** *vb., n.* 不寐 *bú mèi,* sleeplessness.

mén 门 **gate** *n.* 产门 *chǎn mén,* birth *gate.*

mèn 闷 **oppression** *n.* 胸闷 *xiōng mèn,* oppression in the chest.

méng 蒙 **cloud** *vb.* 痰浊蒙蔽心包 *tán zhuó méng bì xīn bāo,* phlegm turbidity *clouding* the pericardium.

mí 迷 **confound** *vb.* 痰迷心窍 *tán mí xīn qiào,* phlegm *confounding* the orifices of the heart.

mí 糜 **erode** *vb.,* **erosion** *n.* 糜烂 *mí làn,* erosion; 糜点 *mí diǎn,* erosion speckles.

miàn 面 **face** *n.,* **facial** *adj.* 面痛 *miàn tòng,* facial pain; 面色 *miàn sè,* facial complexion.

míng 明 **bright** *n.,* **brightness** *n.,* **brighten** *vb.* 明堂 *míng táng,* bright hall; 阳明经 *yáng míng jīng,* yang brightness channels; 明目 *míng mù,* brighten the eyes.

míng 鸣 **ringing** *n.* 耳鸣 *ěr míng,* ringing in the ears. **tinnitus** *n.* 耳鸣 *ěr míng,* tinnitus. **rale** *n.* 痰鸣 *tán míng,* phlegm *rale.* **rumbling** *n.* 肠鸣 *cháng míng,* rumbling intestines.

mìng 命 **life** *n.* 命门 *mìng mén,* life gate.

mù 木 **wood** *n.* 肝木 *gān mù,* liver-wood. **numbness** *n.* 麻木 *má mù,* numbness and tingling.

mù 目 **eye** *n.* 肝开窍于目 *gān kāi qiào yú mù,* the liver opens at the eye.

mù 募 **alarm** *n.* lit. muster. 募穴 *mù xué,* alarm point.

nà 纳 **intake** *n.* 胃主受纳 *wèi zhǔ shòu nà,* the stomach governs *intake;* 纳呆 *nà dāi,* torpid *intake.* **absorb** *vb.,* **absorption** *n.* 肾虚不纳气 *shèn xū bú nà qì,* a vacuous kidney failing to *absorb* qi.

nǎi 奶 **breast** *n.,* **mammary** *adj.* 奶吹 *nǎi chuī,* mammary blowing. **breast milk** *n.* 奶少 *nǎi shǎo,* scant breast milk. **milk** *n.*

náng 囊 **sac** *n.* 肾囊 *shèn náng,* kidney sac, i.e., the scrotum. **scrotum** *n.*

nǎo 脑 **brain** *n.* 脑风 *nǎo fēng,* brain wind; 脑为髓之海 *nǎo wéi suǐ zhī hǎi,* the brain is the sea of marrow.

nèi 内 **inner (body)** *n.* 邪气在内 *xié qí zài nèi,* the evil qi is in the *inner body.* **internal** *adj.* 内风 *nèi fēng,* internal wind; 肝风内动 *gān fēng nèi dòng,* liver wind stirring *internally.* **inward** *adj., adv..* 内陷 *nèi xiàn,* inward fall.

nì 䘌 **invisible worm** *n.* 鼻䘌疮 *bí nì chuāng,* invisible worm sore of the nose.

nì 逆 **abnormal** *adj.* 逆传心包 *nì chuán xīn bāo,* abnormal passage to the pericardium. **unfavorable** *n.* 逆证 *nì zhèng,* unfavorable pattern.

nì 腻 **slimy** *adj.,* **sliminess** *n.* 苔腻 *tāi nì,* slimy [tongue] fur.

nián 黏 **sticky** *adj.* 痰黄黏稠 *tán huáng nián chóu,* thick *sticky* yellow phlegm.

nián 粘 **sticky** *adj.* same as 黏 *nián.*

niǎn 捻 **rotate** *vb.,* **rotation** *n.* 捻针 *niǎn zhēn,* rotate the needle. **twirl** *vb.,* **twirling** *n.* 捻针 *niǎn zhēn,* twirl the needle.

niào 尿 **urine** *n.,* **urinate** *vb.,* **urination** *n.* 尿血 *niào xuè,* bloody urine; 夜间多尿 *yè jiān duō niào,* frequent urination at night; 尿痛 *niào tòng,* painful urination.

niào 溺 **urine** *n.* same as 尿 *niào.*

niè 嚼 **bite** *vb.,* **biting** *n.* 嚼舌 *niè shé,* tongue *biting.* **grind** *vb.,* **grinding** *n.* 嚼齿 *niè chǐ,* grinding of the teeth.

níng 宁 **quiet** *vb.* 宁心 *níng xīn,* quiet the heart.

nóng 脓 **pus** *n.* 大便脓血 *dà biàn nóng xuè,* pus and blood in the stool.

nǔ 胬 **outcrop** *n.* 胬肉攀睛 *nǔ ròu pān jīng,* outcrop creeping across the eye.

nù 怒 **anger** *n.* mind associated with liver; also one of the seven affects. 怒伤肝 *nù shāng gān,* anger damages liver.

nǔ 衄 **spontaneous (external) bleeding** *n.* 舌衄 *shé nǔ,* spontaneous bleeding of the tongue.

nuǎn 暖 **warm** *vb.* 暖胃 *nuǎn wèi,* warm the stomach.

nüè 疟 **malaria** *n.* 疟疾 *nüè jí,* malaria.

ǒu 呕 **retching** *n.* 干呕 *gān ǒu,* dry retching.

pái 排 **expel** *vb.* 排脓 *pái nóng,* expel pus.

páng 膀 **bladder** *n.* 膀胱 *páng guāng,* bladder.

pāo 脬 **bladder** *n.* 脬气不固 *pāo qì bú gù,* insecurity of *bladder* qi.

páo 炮 **blast-fry** *vb.* 炮姜 *páo jiāng,* blast-fried ginger.

péi 痦 **miliaria** *n.* 白痦 *bái péi,* miliaria alba.

péi 培 **bank up** *vb.* 培土生金 *péi tǔ shēng jīn,* bank up earth to engender metal.

pí 皮 **skin** *n.* 肺主皮毛 *fèi zhǔ pí máo,* the lung governs the *skin* and [body] hair.

pí 疲 **fatigue** *n.* 神疲乏力 *shén pí fá lì,* fatigued spirit and lack of strength.

pí 脾 **spleen** *n.* 脾土 *pí tǔ,* spleen-earth. **splenic** *adj.* **SP.**

pǐ 痞 **glomus** *n.* 胸脘痞满 *xiōng wǎn pǐ mǎn,* glomus and fullness in the chest and stomach duct.

pì 癖 **aggregation** *n.* 痃癖 *xián pì,* strings and aggregations.

pì 澼 **afflux** *n.* 肠澼 *cháng pì,* intestinal afflux.

piàn 片 **tablet** *n.* 片剂 *piàn jì,* tablet preparation.

pín 频 **frequent** *adj.* 尿频 *niào pí,* frequent urination.

píng 平 **calm** *vb.* 平肝熄风 *píng gān xī fēng,* calm the liver and extinguish wind. **balanced** *adj.* drug nature. 五倍子性平味酸 *wǔ bèi zǐ xìng píng wèi suān,* sumac gallnut is *balanced* in nature and sour in flavor.

pò 迫 **distress** *vb.* 热迫大肠 *rè pò dà cháng,* heat distressing the large intestine.

pò 破 **break** *vb.* 破血 *pò xuè,* break blood.

qì 气 **qi** *n.* 中气 *zhōng qì,* center qi. **flatus** *n.* 失气 *shī qì,* passing of *flatus.* **breath** *n.* 气微 *qì wēi,* faint *breath.* **breathing** *n.* 气急 *qì jí,* rapid breathing. **smell** *n.* 腥臭气 *xīng chòu qì,* fishy smell.

qì 瘛 **tugging** *n.* 瘛疭 *qì zòng,* tugging and slackening.

qián 潜 **subdue** *vb.* 潜阳 *qián yáng,* subdue yang.

qiàn 欠 **yawn** *vb., n.* 呵欠 *hē qiàn,* yawning.

qiáng 强 **strong** *adj.* 胃强脾弱 *wèi qiáng pí ruò,* strong stomach and weak spleen. **strengthen** *vb.* 强阴 *qiáng yīn,* strengthen yin. **rigid** *adj.,* **rigidity** *n.* 强中 *qiáng zhōng,* rigid center; 项强 *xiàng qiáng,* rigidity of the neck. **stiff** *adj.*, stiffness *n.* 舌强 *shé qiáng, stiff* tongue.

qiāo 跷 **springing** *n.* 跷脉 *qiāo mài, springing* vessel.

qiāo 蹻 **springing** *n.* 蹻脉 *qiāo mài, springing* vessel.

qiào 窍 **orifice** *n.* 九窍 *jiǔ qiào,* nine *orifices.*

qiē 切 **cut** *vb.* 切片 *qiē piàn, cut* into slices.

qiè 切 **palpation** *n.* 切诊 *qiè zhěn, palpation.*

qiè 怯 **timid** *adj.*, timidity *n.* 胆虚气怯 *dǎn xū qì qiè,* gallbladder vacuity and qi *timidity.*

qīn 侵 **invade** *n.*, invasion *n.* 白膜侵睛 *bái mó qīn jīng,* white membrane *invading* the eye.

qīng 青 **green-blue** *adj.* color associated with liver-wood. 面色青 *miàn sè qīng, green-blue* facial complexion.

qīng 清 **clear** *adj.*, *vb.*, clearing *n.* 清阳不升 *qīng yáng bù shēng,* non-upbearing of *clear* yang; 清热泻火 *qīng rè xiè huǒ, clear* heat and drain fire; 小便清长 *xiǎo biàn qīng cháng,* long voidings of *clear* urine; 清法 *qīng fǎ, clearing.* **plain** *n.* 清炒 *qīng chǎo, plain* stir-frying.

qīng 轻 **light** *adj.* in weight. 头重脚轻 *tóu zhòng jiǎo qīng,* heavy head and *light* feet.

qíng 情 **affect** *n.* 七情 *qī qíng,* the seven *affects;* 情志 *qíng zhì, affect*-mind.

qiú 鼽 **sniveling** *n.* 鼻鼽 *bí qiú, sniveling* nose.

qū 屈 **bend** *vb.* 屈伸不利 *qū shēn bú lì,* inhibited *bending* and stretching. **curved** *adj.* 屈骨 *qū gǔ,* Curved Bone (CV-2). **crooked** *adj.*

qū 驱 **expel** *vb.* 驱虫 *qū chóng, expel* worms.

qǔ 龋 **decay** *n.* 龋齿 *qǔ chǐ,* tooth *decay.*

qù 去 **remove** *vb.* 去节 *qù jié, remove* the nodes (e.g., of ephedra). **minus** *prep.* 去桂枝 *qù guì zhī, minus* cinnamon twig. **away from** *prep.*

quán 颧 **cheek** *n.* region of the cheek bone. 两颧发红 *liǎng quán fā hóng,* reddening of [both] the *cheeks.*

rǎo 扰 **harass** *vb.* 痰浊上扰 *tán zhuó shàng rǎo,* phlegm turbidity *harassing* the upper body.

rè 热 **hot** *adj.* 附子性热 *fù zǐ xìng rè,* aconite is *hot* in nature; 头热 *tóu rè, hot* head. **heat [effusion]** *n.* 热退 *rè tuì,* the *heat [effusion]* abates.

róng 荣 **luxuriant** *adj.*, luxuriance *n.* 失荣 *shī róng,* loss-of-*luxuriance.* **construction** *n.* same as 营 *yíng.*

róu 柔 **soft** *adj.* 柔痉 *róu jìng, soft* tetany. **emolliate** *vb.* 柔肝 *róu gān, emolliate* the liver.

ròu 肉 **flesh** *n.* 筋肉 *jīn ròu,* sinew and *flesh.*

rú 濡 **moisten** *vb.* 燥者濡之 *zào zhě rú zhī,* dryness is treated by *moistening.* **soggy** *adj.* 濡脉 *rú mài, soggy* pulse.

rǔ 乳 **breast** *n.* 乳房 *rǔ fáng, breast.* **mammary** *adj.* 乳痈 *rǔ yōng, mammary* welling-abscess. **breast milk** *n.* 缺乳 *quē rǔ,* scant *breast milk.* **milk** *n.* **suckle** *vb.* 乳子 *rǔ zǐ, suckle* a child; 乳癣 *rǔ xiǎn, suckling* lichen. **lactation** *n.* 乳难 *rǔ nán,* difficult *lactation.*

rù 入 **enter** *vb.*, entry *n.* 入里 *rù lǐ, enter* the interior; 入经 *rù jīng,* channel *entry.* **inward movement** *n.* **ingest** *vb.*, ingestion *n.* 食入即吐 *shí rù jí tù,* immediate vomiting of *ingested* food.

ruǎn 软 **soft** *adj.* 脉软 *mài ruǎn,* the pulse is *soft.*

rùn 䐃 **twitch** *vb.*, twitching *n.* 筋惕肉䐃 *jīn tì ròu rùn,* jerking sinews and *twitching* flesh; 目䐃 *mù rùn, twitching* of the eyes.

rùn 润 **moist** *adj.*, moisten *vb.* 润苔 *rùn tāi, moist* [tongue] fur; 润肺 *rùn fèi, moisten* the lung.

ruò 弱 **weak** *adj.* 弱脉 *ruò mài, weak* pulse; 胃强脾弱 *wèi qiáng pí ruò,* strong stomach and *weak* spleen.

sǎ 撒 **sprinkle** *vb.* as powder.

sǎ 洒 **sprinkle** *vb.* as liquid.

sāi 塞 **blockage** *n.* **congestion** *n.* 鼻塞 *bí sāi,* nasal *congestion.*

sǎn 散 **powder** *n.* 平胃散 *píng wèi sǎn,* Stomach-Calming *Powder.*

sāo 臊 **animal odor** *n.* 臊味 *sāo wèi, animal odor.*

sè 色 **color** *n.* 五色 *wǔ sè,* the five *colors.* **complexion** *n.* 面色 *miàn sè,* facial *complexion.*

sè 涩 **rough** *adj.* 涩脉 *sè mài, rough* pulse; 小便短涩 *xiǎo biàn duǎn sè,* short *rough* voidings of urine. **inhibited** *adj.* 小便短涩 *xiǎo biàn duǎn sè,* short *inhibited* voidings of urine. **dry** *adj.* 目干涩 *mù gān sè,* dry eyes. **astringe** *vb.*, astringent *adj.* 涩肠 *sè cháng,* astringe the intestine; 涩剂 *sè jì, astringent* formula.

shā 沙 **sand** *n.* 沙炒 *shā chǎo, sand*-fry.

shā 砂 **sand** *n.* 砂淋 *shā lín, sand* stranguory.

shā 杀 **kill** *vb.* 杀虫 *shā chóng, kill* worms.

shā 痧 **sand** *n.* 痧气 *shā qì, sand* qi.

shān 山 **mountain** *n.* 山岚瘴气 *shān lán zhàng qì, mountain* forest miasm; 烧山火 *shāo shān huǒ,* burning *mountain* fire method.

shān 煽 **fan** *vb.* 风火相煽 *fēng huǒ xiāng shān,* wind and fire *fanning* each other.

shàn 善 **susceptible to** *adj.prep.*, susceptibility to *n.-prep.* lit. good at, tend to. 善惊 *shàn jīng, susceptibility to* fright. **frequent** *adj.* 善呕 *shàn ǒu, frequent* retching.

shàng 上 **up** *adv.*, upward *adv.*, upper (body) *n.* 子上冲心 *zǐ shàng chōng xīn,* the fetus surging *up* into the heart; 心火上炎 *xīn huǒ shàng yán,* heart fire flaming *upward;* 上虚下实 *shàng xū xià shí, upper body* vacuity and lower body repletion. **ascend** *vb.*, ascendant *adj.*, ascent *n.* 肝阳上亢 *gān yáng shàng kàng, ascendant* hyperactivity of liver yang; 胃气上逆 *wèi qì shàng nì,* counterflow *ascent* of stomach qi; 胃气上逆 *wèi qì shàng nì,* counterflow *ascent* of stomach qi.

shǎo 少 **scant** *adj.* 精少 *jīng shǎo, scant* semen. **reduced** *adj.* 纳少 *nà shǎo, reduced* food intake.

shào 少 **lesser** *adj.* 少阳 *shào yáng, lesser* yang; 少腹 *shào fù, lesser* abdomen.

shé 舌 **tongue** *n.* 舌质 *shé zhì, tongue* body.

shè 摄 **contain** *vb.*, containment *n.* 气不摄血 *qì bú shè xuè,* qi failing to *contain* the blood.

shēn 身 **body** *n.* 肺主一身之气 *fèi zhǔ yì shēn zhī qì,* the lung governs the qi of the whole *body.* **generalized** *adj.* 身热 *shēn rè, generalized* heat [effusion]; 半身不遂 *bàn shēn bù suì,* hemiplegia.

shén 神 **spirit** *n.* 心藏神 *xīn cáng shén,* heart stores the *spirit;* 神昏 *shén hūn,* clouded *spirit.*

shèn 肾 **kidney** *n.* 肝肾阴虚 *gān shèn yīn xū,* liver-kidney yin vacuity. **KI.**

shèn 渗 **percolate** *vb.*, percolation *n.* 淡渗利水药 *dàn shèn lì shuǐ yào, bland* percolating water-disinhibiting medicinals.

shēng 升 **bear upward** *vb.* 清阳不升 *qīng yáng bù shēng, clear* yang failing to *bear upward.* **upbear** *vb.*, upbearing *n.* 脾主升,胃主降 *pí zhǔ shēng, wèi zhǔ jiàng,* the spleen governs *upbearing;* the stomach governs downbearing. **sheng** *n.* unit of volume.

shēng 生 **engender** *vb.*, engenderment *n.* 火生土 *huǒ sheng tǔ*, fire *engenders* earth. **raw** *adj.* of animal and vegetable products. 生甘草 *shēng gān cǎo*, raw licorice. **crude** *adj.* of minerals and shells. 生石膏 *shēng shí gāo*, crude gypsum.

shēng 声 **voice** *n.* 语声 *yǔ shēng*, voice. **sound** *n.* 痰声漉漉 *tán shēng lù lù*, gurgling *sound* of phlegm; nonliteral: 郑声 *zhèng shēng*, mussitation.

shèng 盛 **exuberant** *adj.*, exuberance *n.* 邪气盛 *xié qì shèng*, exuberant evil qi; 阴盛阳衰 *yīn shèng yáng shuāi*, yin exuberance with yang debilitation.

shèng 胜 **overcome** *vb.* 胜湿 *shēng shī*, overcome dampness.

shī 湿 **damp** *adj.*, *n.*, dampness *n.* 湿气 *shī qì*, damp qi; 湿热下注 *shī rè xià zhù*, damp-heat pouring downward; 芳香化湿 *fāng xiāng huà shī*, transform dampness with aroma.

shí 石 **stone** *n.*, stonelike *adj.* 石淋 *shí lín*, stone strangury; 冬脉石 *dōng mài shí*, the winter pulse is stonelike.

shí 食 **eat** *vb.* 食已即吐 *shí yǐ jí tù*, vomiting immediately after eating. **food** *vb.* 食滞 *shí zhì*, food stagnation; 伤食 *shāng shí*, food damage; 食咳 *shí ké*, food cough. **meal** *vb.* 食后服 *shí hòu fú*, take after meals. **diet** *n.*, dietary *adj.* 食治 *shí zhì*, diet(ary) therapy. nonliteral: 嗜食异物 *shì shí yì wù*, predilection for strange foods.

shí 时 **season** *n.*, seasonal *adj.* 四时 *sì shí*, four seasons; 时气 *shí qì*, seasonal qi. **watch** *n.* two-hour period. **period** *n.*, periodic *adj.* **frequent** *adj.*, frequently *adv.* 时时惊醒 *shí shí jīng xǐng*, frequent awakening from fright. **intermittent** *adj.*, intermittently. 时时发热 *shí shí fā rè*, intermittent heat effusion.

shí 实 **replete** *adj.*, repletion *n.*, replenish *vb.* 实脉 *shí mài*, replete pulse; 实热 *shí rè*, repletion heat; 正虚邪实 *zhèng xū xié shí*, right vacuity and evil *repletion*; 虚虚实实 *xū xū shí shí*, evacuate vacuity and replenish repletion.

shǐ 矢 **feces** *n.*, fecal *adj.* 矢气 *shǐ qì*, fecal qi, flatus.

shǐ 使 **courier** *n.* 君臣佐使 *jūn chén zuǒ shǐ*, sovereign, minister, assistant, and courier.

shōu 收 **withdraw** *vb.*, withdrawal *n.* **disappear** *vb.*, disappearance *n.* 斑出即收 *bān chū jí shōu*, disappearance of patches immediately after eruption.

shū 俞 **acupuncture point** *n.* **transport point** *n.* 背俞穴 *bèi shū xué*, back transport point. **stream** *n.* one of the five transport points. 俞穴 *shū xué*, stream point.

shū 疏 **course** *vb.* 肝主疏泄 *gān zhǔ shū xiè*, the liver governs free *coursing*; 疏肝 *shū gān*, course the liver; 疏风 *shū fēng*, course wind; 疏表 *shū biǎo*, course the exterior.

shū 舒 **soothe** *vb.* 舒肝 *shū gān*, soothe the liver.

shū 枢 **pivot** *n.* 灵枢 *líng shū*, Magic Pivot; 少阳为枢 *shào yáng wéi shū*, the lesser yang is the pivot.

shū 输 **acupuncture point** *n.* 输穴 *shū xué*, acupuncture point. **transport** *n.* 输穴 *shū xué*, transport point.

shū 腧 **acupuncture point** *n.* 腧穴 *shū xuè*, acupuncture point. **transport point** *n.* 腧穴 *shū xuè*, transport point.

shú 熟 **cooked.** of animal and vegetable products. 熟大黄 *shóu dà huáng*, cooked rhubarb.

shǔ 暑 **summerheat** *n.* 暑湿 *shǔ shī*, summerheat-damp.

shǔ 属 **belong to** *vb.prep.* 肾属水 *shèn shǔ shuǐ*, the kidney *belongs to* water. **home (to)** *vb. prep.* of channels to their respective organs. 手阳明属于大肠 *shǒu yáng míng shǔ yú dà cháng*, the hand yang brightness channel *homes* to the large intestine. **be** *vb.* 湿邪属阴 *shī xié shǔ yīn*, damp evil *is* yin.

shù 束 **leash** *n.* 束筋骨 *shù jīn gǔ*, leash sinews and bones.

shuāi 衰 **debilitate** *vb.*, debilitation *n.* 阴盛阳衰 *yīn shèng yáng shuāi*, prevalence of yin with *debilitation* of yang; 命门火衰 *mìng mén huǒ shuāi*, debilitation of the life gate fire; 盛衰 *shèng shuāi*, exuberance and debilitation.

shuāng 霜 **frost** *n.*, *vb.*, frosting *n.* 柿霜 *shì shuāng*, persimmon frost; 制霜 *zhì shuāng*, frosting.

shuǐ 水 **water** *n.* 水谷 *shuǐ gǔ*, grain and *water*; 水湿 *shuǐ shī*, water-damp; 水道 *shuǐ dào*, the waterways; 水煎服 *shuǐ jiān fú*, take decocted with water.

shuì 睡 **sleep** *vb.*, *n.* 睡眠 *shuì mián*, sleep 睡中自醒 *shuì zhōng zì xǐng*, sudden waking from sleep.

shùn 顺 **favorable** *adj.* 顺证 *shùn zhèng*, favorable pattern. **normal** *adj.*, normalize *vb.* 顺传 *shùn chuán*, normal passage; 顺气 *shùn qì*, normalize qi.

shuò 数 **frequent** *adj.* 便意频数 *biàn yì pín shuò*, frequent desire to defecate. **rapid** *adj.* 数脉 *shuò mài*, rapid pulse.

sī 思 **thought** *n.* mind associated with spleen; also one of the seven affects. 思则气结 *sì zé qì jié*, thought causes qi to bind.

sōu 搜 **track (down)** *vb.* 搜风 *sōu fēng*, track down wind.

sù 宿 **abide** *vb.*, abiding *adj.* 宿食 *sù shí*, abiding food.

suān 酸 **sour** *adj.*, sourness *n.* 酸入肝 *suān rù gān*, sourness enters the liver; **acid** *adj.*, acidity *n.* 吞酸 *tūn suān*, swallowing of upflowing acid; 吐酸 *tù suān*, acid vomiting; 泛酸 *fàn suān*, acid upflow. Also used as 痠, see next entry.

suān 痠、酸 **ache** *vb.*, *n.* 腰痠（酸）膝软 *yāo suān xī ruǎn*, aching lumbus and limp knees.

suǐ 髓 **marrow** *n.* 髓海 *suǐ hǎi*, sea of marrow.

sǔn 损 **detriment** *n.* 虚损 *xū sǔn*, vacuity detriment. **reduce** *vb.* 损其有余 *sǔn qí yǒu yú*, reduce the superabundance.

suō 缩 **retracted** *adj.* 囊缩 *náng suō*, retracted scrotum.

tāi 胎 **fetus** *n.*, fetal *n.* 胎死不下 *tāi sǐ bú xià*, retention of dead *fetus*, 胎气 *tāi qì*, fetal qi. **tongue fur** *n.* same as 苔 *tāi*.

tāi 苔 **tongue fur** *n.* 苔白 *tāi bái*, white tongue fur.

tài 太 **greater** *adj.* 太阴 *tài yīn*, greater yin. **supreme** *adj.* 太冲 *tài chōng*, Supreme Surge (LR-3).

tān 瘫 **paralysis** *n.* 瘫痪 *tān huàn*, paralysis.

tán 痰 **phlegm** *n.* 脾虚生痰 *pí xū shēng tán*, spleen vacuity engendering *phlegm*; 痰湿 *tán shī*, phlegm-damp; 湿痰 *shī tán*, damp phlegm.

tàn 炭 **char** *vb.*, charred *pp.*, *adj.* 炒炭 *chǎo tàn*, char-fry; 艾叶炭 *ài yè tàn*, charred mugwort.

tāng 汤 **decoction** *n.* 桂枝汤 *guì zhī tāng*, Cinnamon Twig *Decoction*.

tàng 烫 **scald** *vb.* 烫火伤 *tàng huǒ shāng*, burns and scalds.

téng 疼 **pain** *n.*, painful *adj.* 胃脘疼痛 *wèi wǎn téng tòng*, stomach duct *pain*; 肢节疼痛 *zhī jié téng tòng*, limb joint *pain*.

tí 提 **raise** *vb.* 升提中气 *shēng tí zhōng qì*, upraise center qi. **lift** *vb.* 提插补泻 *tí chā bǔ xiè*, lifting and thrusting supplementation and draining.

tǐ 体 **body** *n.* 体态 *tǐ tài*, bearing of the *body*; 形体消瘦 *xíng tǐ xiāo shòu*, emaciation [of the *body*]. **constitutional body** *n.*

tì 涕 **snivel** *n.* 涕黄 *tì huáng*, yellow *snivel*.

tiān 天 **heaven** *n.*, heavenly *adj.* 天地 *tiān dì*, heaven and earth. **celestial** *adj.* 天府 *tiān fǔ*, celestial storehouse.

tián 甜 **sweet** *adj.* 甜杏仁 *tián xìng rén*, sweet apricot kernel.

tián 填 **replenish** *vb.* 填精 *tián jīng*, replenish essence.

tiáo 调 **regulate** *vb.*, regulation *n.* 调经 *tiáo jīng*, regulate menstruation. **mix** *vb.* 调服 *tiáo fú*, take mixed (with fluid).

tíng 停 **collect** *vb.* 水液内停 *shuǐ yì nèi tíng*, water-humor *collecting* internally; 停饮胁痛 *tíng yǐn xié tòng*, collecting rheum rib-side pain.

tōng 通 **free** *vb.* 通可去滞 *tōng kě qù zhì*, freeing can eliminate stagnation; 通淋 *tōng lín*, free stranguary; 活血通络 *huó xuè tōng luò*, quicken the blood and free the network vessels. **unstop** *vb.* 通因通用 *tōng yīn tōng yòng*, treat the unstopped by stopping; 不通则痛 *bù tōng zé tòng*, when there is stoppage, there is pain.

tǒng 统 **manage** *vb.* 脾不统血 *pí bù tǒng xuè*, spleen failing to manage the blood. **control** *vb.* 脾不统血 *pí bù tǒng xuè*, spleen failing to control the blood.

tòng 痛 **pain** *n.*, painful *adj.* 腹痛 *fù tòng*, abdominal pain; 腰痛 *yāo tòng*, lumbar pain. **sore** *adj.* 咽痛 *yān tòng*, sore throat. **ache** *adj.* 头痛 *tóu tòng*, headache; 牙齿痛 *yá chǐ tòng*, toothache.

tóu 头 **head** *n.* 头痛 *tóu tòng*, headache; 头胀 *tóu zhàng*, distention in the head; 头重 *tóu zhòng* heavy-headedness; 头晕 *tóu yūn*, dizzy head.

tòu 透 **thrust out(ward)** *vb.* **outthrust** *n.* 透表 *tòu biǎo*, outthrust the exterior.

tǔ 土 **earth** *n.* 土生金 *tǔ shēng jīn*, earth engenders metal; 培土生金 *péi tǔ shēng jīn*, bank up earth to engender metal; 脾土 *pí tǔ*, spleen-earth.

tù 吐 **vomit** *vb.*, vomiting *n.* 呕吐 *ǒu tù*, vomiting (and retching). **eject** *vb.*, ejection *n.* 吐法 *tù fǎ*, ejection.

tuí 㿗 **prominence** *n.*, prominent *adj.* 㿗疝 *tuí shàn*, prominent mounting.

tuí 癞 **bulging** *n.* 癞 *tuí shàn*, bulging mounting.

tuǐ 腿 **leg** *n.* 腰酸腿弱 *yāo suān tuǐ ruò*, aching lumbus and weak *legs*.

tūn 吞 **swallow** *vb.* 吞酸 *tūn suān*, swallowing of upflowing acid; 吞咽困难 *tūn yàn kùn nán*, difficulty in swallowing.

tuō 托 **express** *vb.*, expression *n.* 托毒透脓 *tuō dú tòu nóng*, expressing toxin and outthrusting pus.

tuō 脱 **desert** *vb.*, desertion *n.* 气随血脱 *qì suí xuè tuō*, qi deserting with the blood; 气脱 *qì tuō*, qi deserting with the blood. **slough** *vb.* 脱疽 *tuō jū*, sloughing flat-abscess.

tuò 唾 **spittle** *n.*

wāi 歪 **deviated** *adj.*, deviation *n.* of face.

wài 外 **external** *adj.* 外感 *wài gǎn*, external contraction; 外邪 *wài xié*, external evil; 外吹 *wài chuī*, external blowing.

wán 丸 **pill** *n.* 蜜丸 *mì wán*, honey *pill*.

wǎn 脘 **stomach duct** *n.* 胃脘虚痞 *wèi wǎn xū pǐ*, stomach duct vacuity glomus.

wàn 腕 **wrist** *n.*

wáng 亡 **collapse** *vb.*, *n.* 亡阳虚脱 *wáng yáng xū tuō*, yang-collapse vacuity desertion.

wàng 妄 **frenetic** *adj.* 血热妄行 *xuè rè wàng xíng*, frenetic movement of hot blood.

wàng 旺 **effulgent** *adj.*, effulgence *n.* 阴虚火旺 *yīn xū huǒ wàng*, effulgent yin vacuity fire.

wàng 望 **inspect** *vb.*, inspection *n.* 望齿 *wàng chǐ*, inspect the teeth; 望诊 *wàng zhěn*, inspection.

wēi 微 **mild** *adj.* 微风 *wēi fēng*, mild wind. **slight** *adj.* 微微出汗 *wēi wēi chū hàn*, slight sweating. **faint** *n.* 微脉 *wēi mài*, faint pulse. **debilitation** *n.* 衰微 *shuāi wēi*, debilitation.

wéi 维 **link** *vb.* 维脉 *wéi mài*, linking vessel.

wěi 痿 **wilting** *n.* 肺痿 *fèi wěi*, lung wilting. **limp** *n.* 舌痿 *shé wěi*, limp tongue.

wèi 味 **flavor** *n.* 五味 *wǔ wèi*, five flavors. **ingredient** *n.* 六味地黄丸 *liù wèi dì-huáng wán*, Six-Ingredient Rehmannia Pill.

wèi 胃 **stomach** *n.* 胃气上逆 *wèi qì shàng nì*, counterflow ascent of stomach qi. **gastric** *adj.*, gastro- *comb.* 胃肠气滞 *wèi cháng qì zhì*, gastrointestinal qi stagnation. **ST.**

wèi 卫 **defense** *n.*, defensive *adj.* 卫气不固 *wèi qì bú gù*, insecurity of defense qi; 卫气营血 *wèi qì yíng xuè*, defense, qi, construction, and blood.

wēn 瘟 **scourge** *n.* 大头瘟 *dà tóu wēn*, massive head scourge; 疫瘟 *yè wēn*, epidemic scourge.

wén 闻 **smell** *vb.* **hear** *vb.* **listening and smelling** *n.* 闻诊 *wén zhěn*, listening and smelling.

wèn 问 **inquire** *vb.*, inquiry *n.* 问大便 *wèn dà biàn*, inquire about stool; 问诊 *wèn zhěn*, inquiry.

wò 卧 **lie** *vb.* 向里蜷卧 *xiàng lǐ quán wò*, curled-up lying posture. **sleep** *vb.* 胃不和则卧不安 *wèi bù hé zé wò bù ān*, when the stomach is in disharmony, there is unquiet sleep.

wǔ 侮 **rebellion** *n.* 相侮 *xiāng wǔ*, rebellion; 反侮 *fǎn wǔ*, rebellion (five-phase cycle).

wù 物 **agent** *n.* 四物汤 *sì wù tāng*, Four Agents Decoction.

wù 恶 **averse to** *adj.+prep.*, aversion to *n.+prep.* 脾恶湿 *pí wù shī*, the spleen is averse to dampness. 恶风 *wù fēng*, aversion to wind; 恶寒 *wù hán*, aversion to cold. See also *ě* 恶, *è* 恶.

xī 郄 **cleft** *n.* 郄穴 *xī xué*, cleft point.

xī 息 **breathing** *n.* 息粗 *xī cū*, rough breathing. **respiration** *n.* 一息 *yī xī*, one respiration (one inhalation and exhalation).

xī 熄 **extinguish** *n.* 熄风 *xī fēng*, extinguish wind.

xī 膝 **knee** *n.*

xī 瘜 sometimes simplified as （息） **polyp** *n.* 鼻瘜肉 *bí xī ròu*, nasal polyp.

xí 袭 **assail** *vb.*, assailment *n.* 风邪袭表 *fēng xié xí biǎo*, wind evil assailing the exterior.

xǐ 喜 **joy** *n.* mind associated with heart; also one of the seven affects. 心主喜 *xīn zhǔ xǐ*, the heart governs joy. **like** *vb.* 土喜温燥 *tǔ xǐ wēn zào*, earth likes warmth and dryness; 腹痛喜按 *fù tòng xǐ àn*, abdominal pain that *likes* pressure.

xì 细 **fine** *adj.* 脉细而数 *mài xì ér shuò*, the pulse is *fine* and rapid.

xià 下 **down** *adv.*, downward *adv.*. 湿热下注 *shī rè xià zhù*, damp-heat pouring *downward*. **descend** *vb.*, descent *n.* 下行 *xià xíng*, descend. **precipitate** *vb.*, precipitation *n.* to cause to descend (forcefully). 下气 *xià qì*, precipitate qi. **lower** *adj.*, lower body *n.* 下元 不足 *xià yuán bù zú*, insufficiency of the *lower* origin; 上虚下实 *shàng xū xià shí*, upper body vacuity and *lower* body repletion.

xián 痃 **string** *n.* 痃癖 *xián pǐ*, strings and aggregations.

xián 弦 **stringlike** *adj.* 弦脉 *xián mài*, *stringlike* pulse.

xián 咸 **salty** *adj.*, saltiness *n.*, salted *adj.* 咸入肾 *xián rù shèn*, *saltiness* enters the kidney; 咸附子 *xián fù zǐ*, *salted* aconite.

xián 涎 **drool** *n.* 涎为脾液 *xián wéi pí yè*, *drool* is the humor of the spleen. 流涎 *liú xián*, drooling.

xián 痫 **epilepsy** *n.* 痫病 *xián bìng*, epilepsy.

xiǎn 癣 **lichen** *n.* 松皮癣 *sōng pí xiǎn*, pine bark *lichen*; 圆癣 *yuán xiǎn*, coin lichen; 牛皮癣 *niú pí xiǎn*, oxhide *lichen*.

xiàn 陷 **fall** *vb.*, *n.* 中气下陷 *zhōng qì xià xiàn*, center qi *fall*; 邪气内陷 *xié qì nèi xiàn*, inward *fall* of evil qi.

xiāng 香 **fragrant** *adj.*, fragrance *n.* 不知香臭 *bù zhī xiāng chòu*, inability to sense *fragrance* or fetor (loss of smell). **aromatic** *adj.*, aroma *n.* 芳香开窍 *fāng xiāng kāi qiào*, to open the orifices with aroma.

xiàng 相 **minister** *n.*, ministerial *adj.* 相火 *xiàng huǒ*, *ministerial* fire.

xiàng 象 **sign** *n.* 热象 *rè xiàng*, heat *signs*.

xiāo 哮 **wheezing** *n.* 热哮 *rè xiāo*, heat *wheezing*.

xiāo 消 **disperse** *vb.*, dispersion *n.* 消食导滞 *xiāo shí dǎo zhì*, *disperse* and abduct stagnation; 消痞 *xiāo pǐ*, *disperse* glomus; 消瘀 *xiāo yū*, *disperse* stagnation; 消痔 *xiāo zhì*, *disperse* hemorrhoids. **dispersion** *n.* 消渴 *xiāo kě* dispersion-thirst.

xiǎo 小 **small** *adj.*, smaller *adj.* 小脉 *xiǎo mài*, *small* pulse; 小腹 *xiǎo fù* smaller abdomen. **minor** *adj.* 小青龙汤 *xiǎo qīng lóng tāng*, *Minor* Green-Blue Dragon Decoction.

xié 邪 **evil** *n.* 邪气 *xié qì*, *evil* qi.

xié 胁 **rib-side** *n.* 胁痛 *xié tòng*, *rib-side* pain; 胸胁胀 满 *xiōng xié zhàng mǎn*, distention and fullness in the chest and *rib-side*.

xié 斜 **oblique** *adj.* 斜刺 *xié cì*, *oblique* insertion. **deviated** *adj.*, deviation *n.* 口眼歪斜 *kǒu yǎn wāi xié*, *deviated* eyes and mouth.

xiè 泄 **discharge** *vb.*, *n.* 泄热 *xiè rè*, *discharge* heat.

xiè 泻 **drain** *vb.*, drainage *n.* 清热泻火 *qīng rè xiè huǒ*, clear heat and *drain* fire.

xīn 心 **heart** *n.* 心藏神 *xīn cáng shén*, the *heart* stores the spirit. **HT**.

xīn 辛 **acrid** *adj.*, acridity *n.* 辛入肺 *xīn rù fèi*, *acridity* enters the lung.

xìn 囟 **fontanel** *n.* 囟填 *xìn tián*, bulging *fontanels*; 囟 陷 *xìn xiàn*, depressed *fontanels*.

xīng 腥 **fishy-smelling** *adj.* 腥味 *xīng wèi*, *fishy* smell.

xíng 刑 **torment** *vb.* 木火刑金 *mù huǒ xíng jīn*, wood fire *tormenting* metal.

xíng 行 **move** *vb.* 行气 *xíng qì*, *move* qi. **phase** *n.* 五 行 *wǔ xíng*, five *phases*. **current** *n.* 天行 *tiān xíng*, heaven *current*.

xíng 形 **form** *n.* physical **form/body** *n.*

xǐng 醒 **arouse** *vb.* 醒脾 *xǐng pí*, *arouse* the spleen.

xiōng 胸 **chest** *n.* 胸痹 *xiōng bì*, *chest* impediment; 胸 痛 *xiōng tòng*, *chest* pain; 胸满 *xiōng mǎn*, fullness in the *chest*; 胸闷 *xiōng mèn*, oppression in the *chest*.

xiù 嗅 **insufflate** *vb.*, insufflation *n.* 嗅鼻 *xiù bí*, *insufflate* into the nose; nasal *insufflation*.

xū 虚 **vacuous** *adj.*, vacuity *n.* 虚脉 *xū mài*, *vacuous* pulse; 心脾气虚 *xīn pí qì xū*, heart-spleen qi *vacuity*.

xù 蓄 **amass** *vb.*, amassment *n.* 蓄血 *xù xuè*, blood *amassment*.

xuān 宣 **diffuse** *vb.*, diffusion *n.* 宣肺 *xuān fèi*, *diffuse* the lung. **perfuse** *vb.*, perfusion *n.* 宣通阳气 *xuān tōng yáng qì*, *perfuse* yang qi.

xuán 玄 **mysterious** *adj.* common substitute for 元 *yuán*.

xué 穴 **acupuncture point** *n.* 穴道 *xué*, acupuncture point. **point** *n.* 经穴 *jīng xué*, channel *point*. **hole** *n.*

xuè 血 **blood** *n.*, bloody *adj.* 气血 *qì xuè*, qi and *blood*; 尿血 *niào xuè*, *bloody* urine.

xuè 削 **whittle** *vb.*

yā 鸭 **duck** *n.* 大便鸭溏 *dà biàn yā táng*, *duck's* slop stool.

yá 牙 **tooth** *n.* 牙齿 *yá chǐ*, *tooth*.

yān 咽 **pharynx** *n.*, pharyngeal *adj.* 咽干 *yān gān*, dry *pharynx*.

yán 岩 **rock** *n.* 肾岩 *shèn yán*, kidney *rock*.

yǎn 眼 **eye** *n.* 眼睛红肿 *yǎn jīng hóng zhǒng*, red swollen *eyes*.

yàn 咽 **swallow** *vb.* 吞咽困难 *tūn yuàn kùn nán*, difficulty in *swallowing*; 咽酸 *yàn suān*, acid *swallowing*.

yáng 阳 **yang** *n.*, *adj.* 阳气 *yáng qì*, *yang* qi. nonliteral: 阳痿 *yáng wěi*, impotence.

yáng 疡 **sore** *n.* **open sore** *n.*

yǎng 养 **nourish** *vb.*, nourishment *n.* 养阴 *yǎng yīn*, *nourish* yin.

yǎng 痒 **itch** *vb.*, *n.*, itchy *adj.* 阴痒 *yīn yǎng*, pudendal *itch*; 耳痒 *ěr yǎng*, *itchy* ear.

yāo 夭 **perish** *vb.*, perished *pp.*, *adj.* 夭色 *yāo sè*, *perished* complexion.

yāo 腰 **lumbus** *n.*, lumbar *adj.* 腰为肾之府 *yāo wéi shèn zhī fǔ*, the *lumbus* is the house of the kidney; 腰 痛 *yāo tòng*, *lumbar* pain; 腰痛 *yāo tòng*, *lumbar* pain.

yào 药 **medicinal** *n.*, *adj.* 补药 *bǔ yào*, supplementing *medicinal*. **drug** *n.*

yè 液 **humor** *n.* 津液 *jīn yè*, liquid and *humor*; 五液 *wǔ yè*, five *humors*.

yè 腋 **armpit** *n.* 腋下痈 *yì xià yōng*, *armpit* welling-abscess. **axilla** *n.*, axillary *adj.* 腋下痛 *yì xià tòng*, *axillary* pain.

yǐ 乙 **second heavenly stem** *n.*

yì 抑 **repress** *vb.* 抑肝 *yì gān*, *repress* the liver.

yì 疫 **epidemic** *n.*, *adj.* 瘟疫 *wēn yì*, scourge *epidemic*.

yì 益 **boost** *vb.* 益气生津 *yì qì shēng jīn*, *boost* qi and engender liquid.

yì 溢 **spill** *vb.*, spillage *n.* 溢饮 *yì yǐn*, *spillage* rheum.

yì 翳 **screen** *n.* 目翳 *mù yì*, eye *screen*. **shroud** *n.* 益 火之原以消阴翳 *yì huǒ zhī yuán yǐ xiāo yīn yì*, boost the source of fire to disperse the *shroud* of yin.

yīn 因 **cause** *n.* 三因 *sān yīn*, the three causes (of disease).

yīn 音 **note** *n.* 五音 *wǔ yīn*, the five *notes*. **sound** *n.* 声音 *shēng yīn*, sound.

yīn 阴 **yin** *n., adj.* 阴邪 *yīn xié*, yin evil. **genitals** *n.*, genital *adj.* 阴蜃 *yīn ni*, invisible worm sore of the *genitals*. **pudenda** *n.*, pudendal *adj.* 阴痒 *yīn yǎng*, pudendal itch.

yīn 暗 **loss of voice** *n.*

yīn 瘖 **loss of voice** *n.*

yín 淫 **excess** *n.* excessive or untimely environmental qi. 六淫 *liù yín*, the six *excesses*. **spread** *vb.* 浸淫疮 *jìn yín chuāng*, wet spreading sore.

yín 龈 **gum** *n.* 牙龈 *yá yín*, gum.

yǐn 饮 **rheum** *n.* 痰饮 *tán yǐn*, phlegm-rheum. **beverage** *n.* 甘露饮 *gān lù yǐn*, Sweet Dew *Beverage*. **fluid intake** *n.* 渴饮 *kě yǐn*, thirst with *fluid intake*.

yǐn 隐 **dull** *adj.* 隐隐作痛 *yǐn yǐn zuò tòng*, dull pain.

yǐn 瘾 **dormant papules** *n.* 瘾疹 *yǐn zhěn*, dormant papules.

yíng 营 **construction** *n.* 营气 *yíng qì*, construction qi.

yíng 荥 **brook** *n.* one of the five transport points. 荥穴 *yíng xué*, brook point.

yǐng 瘿 **goiter** *n.* 气瘿 *qì yǐng*, qi goiter; 肉瘿 *ròu yǐng*, flesh goiter.

yōng 壅 **congest** *vb.*, congestion *n.* 饮邪壅肺 *yǐn xié yōng fèi*, rheum evil *congesting* the lung; 痰涎壅盛 *tán xián yōng shèng*, phlegm-drool congestion.

yōng 痈 **welling abscess** *n.* 肠痈 *cháng yōng*, intestinal welling-abscess.

yǒng 涌 **eject** *vb.*, ejection *n.*

yōu 忧 **anxiety** *n.* mind or emotion of the lung; also one of the seven affects.

yóu 疣 **wart** *n.*

yóu 游 **wandering** *n.* 赤游风 *chì yóu fēng*, red wandering wind.

yū 瘀 **stasis** *n.*, static *adj.* 血瘀 *xuè yū*, blood *stasis*; 瘀血 *yū xuè*, static blood.

yú 余 **surplus** *n.* 发为血之余 *xiè qí yǒu yú*, the hair is the *surplus* of the blood. **superabundant** *adj.*, superabundance *n.* 泻其有余 *xiè qí yǒu yú*, drain the *superabundance*. **residual** *adj.* 余热 *yú rè*, residual heat.

yù 育 **foster** *vb.* 育阴 *yù yīn*, foster yin.

yù 郁 **depression** *n.* 肝郁 *gān yù*, liver depression.

yù 欲 **desire** *vb., n.* 欲吐 *yù tù*, desire to vomit. **verging on** *vb. prep.* 脉微欲绝 *mài wēi yù jué*, faint pulse verging on expiry.

yuán 元 **origin** *n.*, original *adj.* 下元 *xià yuán*, lower origin; 元气 *yuán qì*, original qi.

yuán 原 **source** *n.* 原气 *yuán qì*, source qi. **principle** *n.* 原则 *yuán zé*, principle.

yuē 约 **retain** *vb.* **constrain** *vb.* **straiten** *vb.* 脾约 *pí yuē*, straitened spleen.

yuě 哕 **vomit** *vb.* **hiccough** *n., vb.* **dry retching** *n.*

yuè 月 **month** *n.*, monthly *adj.* 月经 *yuè jīng*, the monthly courses (periods). **menstruation** *n.*, menstrual *adj.*(from L. *mensis*, month), 月经 *yuè jīng*, menstruation; 痛经 *tòng jīng*, menstrual pain.

yuè 越 **stray** *vb.*, astray *adj.* 孤阳浮越 *gū yáng fú yuè*, solitary yang floating astray.

yūn 晕 **dizzy** *adj.*, dizziness *n.* 头晕目眩 *tóu yūn mù xuàn*, dizzy head and vision.

yùn 孕 **pregnant** *adj.*, pregnancy *n.* 孕妇 *yùn fù*, pregnant women.

yùn 运 **move** *vb.* 运脾 *yùn pí*, move the spleen.

yùn 蕴 **brew** *vb.* 湿热蕴结 *shī rè yùn jié*, damp-heat brewing (and binding).

zàng 脏 **viscus** *n.*, viscera *pl.*, visceral *adj.* plural viscera. 五脏 *wǔ zàng*, the five viscera; 脏气 *zàng qì*, visceral qi.

zào 燥 **dry** *adj.*, dryness *n.* 口干咽燥 *kǒu gān yān zào*, dry throat and mouth; 燥邪 *zào xié*, dryness evil.

zào 躁 **agitation** *n.*, agitated *adj.* 烦躁 *fán zào*, vexation and *agitation*; 脏躁 *zàng zào*, visceral agitation.

zēng 增 **increase** *vb.* 增液行舟 *zēng yè xíng zhōu*, increase humor to move the grounded ship.

zhài 瘵 **consumption** *n.* 痨瘵 *láo zhài*, consumption.

zhān 谵 **delirium** *n.*, delirious *adj.* 谵言 *zhān yán*, delirious speech.

zhàn 战 **shiver** *vb.* 战汗 *zhàn hàn*, shiver sweating.

zhàng 胀 **distention** *n.*, distended *adj.*, distending *adj.* 腹胀 *fù zhàng*, abdominal *distention*.

zhàng 瘴 **miasma** *n.*, miasmic *adj.* 山岚瘴气 *shān lán zhàng qì*, mountain forest miasmic qi.

zhēn 针 **needle** *n., vb.* 毫针 *háo zhēn*, filiform *needle*; 三棱针 *sān léng zhēn*, three-edged needle.

zhěn 疹 **papule** *n.* 斑疹 *bān zhěn*, macules and papules.

zhěn 诊 **examine** *vb.*, examination *n.* 四诊 *sì zhěn*, the four examinations.

zhèn 震 **tremor** *n.* 震颤 *zhèn chàn*, tremor.

zhèn 镇 **settle** *vb.* 镇肝熄风 *zhèn gān xī fēng*, settle the liver and extinguish wind; 镇惊 *zhèn jīng*, settle fright; 重镇药 *zhòng zhèn yào*, heavy *settling* medicinals.

zhēng 癥 **concretion** *n.* 癥瘕 *zhēng jiǎ*, concretions and conglomerations; 酒癥 *jiǔ zhēng*, drinker's concretion.

zhēng 蒸 **steam** *vb.* 骨蒸潮热 *gǔ zhēng cháo rè*, steaming bone tidal heat [effusion]; 酒蒸 *jiǔ zhēng*, steam with liquor; 暑湿郁蒸 *shǔ shī yù zhēng*, depressed steaming summerheat-damp.

zhèng 正 **right** *adj., n.* 正气 *zhèng qì*, right qi. **regular** *adj.* 正经 *zhèng jīng*, regular channel. **straight** *adj.* treatment. 正治 *zhèng zhì* straight treatment. **medial** *adj.* 正头痛 *zhèng tóu tòng*, medial headache.

zhèng 症 **pathocondition** *n.* interchangeable with 证 *zhèng*. 热症 *rè zhèng*, heat pathocondition.

zhèng 证 **sign** *n.* 热证 *rè zhèng*, heat sign. **pattern** *n.* 热证 *rè zhèng*, heat pattern.

zhī 支 **prop** *n.* 支满 *zhī mǎn*, propping fullness.

zhī 肢 **limb** *n.* 四肢 *sì zhī*, the [four] limbs.

zhǐ 止 **suppress** *vb.* 止咳 *zhǐ ké*, suppress cough. **check** *vb.* 止带 *zhǐ dài*, check vaginal discharge. **allay** *vb.* 止渴 *zhǐ kě*, allay thirst. **stanch** *vb.* 止血 *zhǐ xuè*, stanch bleeding.

zhì 志 **mind** *n.* will, power of concentration, memory; one of the five minds. 五志化火 *wǔ zhì huà huǒ*, fire formation due to excesses among the five minds, five-mind fire formation.

zhì 制 **restrain** *vb.* 壮水制阳 *zhuàng shuǐ zhì yáng*, invigorate water to restrain yang. **dam** *vb.* 培土制水 *péi tǔ zhì shuǐ*, bank up earth to dam water.

zhì 治 **treat** *vb.*, treatment *n.* 治法 *zhì fǎ*, method of treatment; 治疗 *zhì liáo*, treat. **control** *vb.* 治风化痰 *zhì fēng huà tán*, control wind and transform phlegm.

zhì 炙 **mix-fry** *vb.* 炙甘草 *zhì gān cǎo*, mix-fried licorice.

zhì 痔 **hemorrhoid** *n.*, usually *pl.*, hemorrhoids. 葡萄痔 *pú táo zhì*, grape *hemorrhoids*. **pile** *n.* 耳痔 *ěr zhì*, ear *pile*.

zhì 滞 **stagnate** *vb.*, stagnation *n.*, stagnant *adj.* 气滞 *qì zhì*, qi *stagnation*.

zhì 瘛 **tugging** *n.* see *qì* 瘛.

zhōng 中 **center** *n.*, central *n.* in the five phases, position associated with earth; in the body, the stomach and spleen. 补中益气 *bǔ zhōng yì qì*, supplement the *center* and boost qi. **middle** *n.*, *adj.* 中焦 *zhōng jiāo*, *middle* burner.

zhǒng 肿 **swelling** *n.* 水肿 *shuǐ zhǒng*, water *swelling*; 咽喉肿痛 *yān hóu zhǒng tòng*, sore *swollen* throat.

zhòng 中 **strike** *vb.*, *n.*, stroke *n.* 直中三阴 *zhí zhòng sān yīn*, direct *strike* on the triple yin. 中风 *zhòng fēng*, wind *stroke*.

zhòng 重 **heavy** *adj.*, heaviness *n.* 重镇安神 *zhòng zhèn ān shén*, to quiet the spirit with *heavy* settlers; 四肢困重 *sì zhī kùn zhòng heavy* cumbersome limbs; 头重 *tóu zhòng heavy*-headedness; 头重如裹 *tóu zhòng rú guǒ*, head *heavy* as if swathed.

zhōu 粥 **gruel** *n.* 龙眼肉粥 *lóng yǎn ròu zhōu*, Longan *Gruel*.

zhú 逐 **expel** *vb.* 逐水 *zhú shuǐ*, *expel* water.

zhǔ 主 **govern** *vb.*, governing *n.*, governor *n.* 心主血脉 *xīn zhǔ xiè mài*, the heart *governs* the blood and vessels; 脾之主运化 *pí zhū zhǔ yùn huà*, the spleen's *governing* of movement and transformation; **host** *n.* 客主 *kè zhǔ*, Guest-*Host* (GB-3). **chief** *n.* 主辅佐引 *zhǔ fǔ zuǒ yǐn*, *chief*, support, assistant, and conductor.

zhù 助 **assist** *vb.* 助阳 *zhù yáng*, *assist* yang. **reinforce** *vb.* 助阳 *zhù yáng*, *reinforce* yang.

zhù 注 **pour** *vb.* 湿热下注 *shī rè xià zhù*, damp-heat *pouring* downward. **influx** *n.* 注夏 *zhù xià*, summer *influx*; 注心痛 *zhù xīn tòng*, *influx* heart pain.

zhù 疰 **infixation** *n.* 夏疰 *xià zhù*, summer *infixation*.

zhuǎ 爪 **nail** *n.* see *zhǎo* 爪.

zhuàng 壮 **vigorous** *adj.*, invigorate *vb.* 壮火 *zhuàng huǒ*, *vigorous* fire; 壮热 *zhuàng rè*, *vigorous* heat [effusion]; 壮阳 *zhuàng yáng*, *invigorate* yang; 壮火 *zhuàng huǒ*, *invigorate* fire. **strengthen** *vb.* 壮筋强骨 *zhuàng jīn qiáng gǔ*, *strengthen* sinew and bone. **cone** *n.* of moxa, sequentially burnt on one spot; 灸三壮 *jiǔ sān zhuàng*, burn three *cones* of moxa.

zhuì 坠 **sag** *vb.*, sagging *adj.* 少腹坠胀 *shào fù zhuì zhàng*, *sagging* distention in the lesser abdomen.

zhuó 灼 **scorch** *vb.* 灼热 *zhuó rè*, *scorching* heat.

zhuó 着 **fixed** *adj.*, fixity *n.* 着痹 *zhuó bì*, *fixed* impediment; 肾着 *shèn zhuó* kidney *fixity*.

zhuó 浊 **turbid** *adj.*, turbidity *n.* 痰浊 *tán zhuó*, phlegm *turbidity*; 白浊 *bái zhuó*, white *turbidity*; 声音重浊 *zhēng yīn zhòng zhuó*, heavy *turbid* voice.

zī 滋 **enrich** *vb.* 滋阴 *zī yīn*, *enrich* yin.

zōng 宗 **ancestor** *n.*, ancestral *adj.* 宗气 *zōng qì*, ancestral qi; 宗筋所聚 *zōng jīn suǒ jù*, gathering place of the ancestral sinews.

zú 足 **foot** *n.* 足少阴肾经 *zú shào yīn shèn jīng*, foot lesser yin kidney channel; 足痛 *zú tòng*, foot pain. **sufficient** *adj.*, sufficiency *n.* 肾气不足 *shèn qì bù zú*, insufficiency of kidney qi.

zǔ 阻 **obstruct** *vb.*, obstruction *n.* 痰阻心窍 *tán zǔ xīn qiào*, phlegm *obstructing* the orifices of the heart; 痰热阻肺 *tán rè zǔ fèi*, phlegm-heat *obstructing* the lung; 恶阻 *è zǔ*, malign *obstruction*.

zuǒ 佐 **assist** *vb.*, assistant *n.* 君臣佐使 *jūn chén zuǒ shǐ*, sovereign, minister, *assistant*, and courier.

A

abating heat 退热 *tuì rè*: CLEARING HEAT or reducing heat effusion (fever).

abdomen 腹 *fù*: *Synonym: belly.* The anterior aspect of the body from the ribs down to the genitals, considered yin in relationship to the back, which is yang. The abdomen is divided into the GREATER ABDOMEN (the part above the UMBILICUS) and the SMALLER ABDOMEN (the part below the umbilicus). A small part of the greater abdomen immediately below the breastbone is variously referred to as the [REGION] BELOW THE HEART or the HEART [REGION]. The central part of the upper abdomen is called the STOMACH DUCT. The LESSER ABDOMEN usually refers to the lateral areas of the lower abdomen, but is sometimes used to mean smaller abdomen. [27: 68] [97: 603]

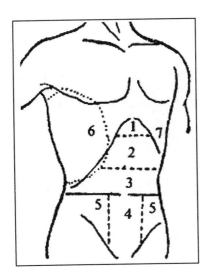

1. [Region] below the heart
2. Stomach duct
1, 2, and 3. Greater abdomen
4. Smaller abdomen
5. Lesser abdomen
6. Rib-side
7. Vacuous li

abdominal distention 腹胀 *fù zhàng*: **1.** Enlargement of the abdomen (objective sign). See DRUM DISTENTION. **2.** A subjective feeling of fullness. See ABDOMINAL FULLNESS (subjective sign). [26: 798] [97: 603] [27: 408] [22: 382]

abdominal fullness 腹满 *fù mǎn*, 腹胀满 *fù zhàng mǎn*: A subjective feeling of fullness in the abdomen without pronounced visible or palpable expansion. Abdominal fullness may be observed in vacuity and repletion patterns. Continued fullness without relief, associated with hard stool or continued fullness relieved by passing of flatus, belching, or defecation indicates repletion. Periodically abating fullness that likes pressure, associated with sloppy stool or with fullness following defecation is a vacuity pattern. *Essential Prescriptions of the Golden Coffer* (*jīn guì yào lüè*) describes the former as "abdominal fullness with little or no relief," and the latter as "abdominal fullness recurring after periods of relief." Abdominal fullness commonly occurs in the cold-damp, spleen-stomach vacuity, damp-heat, food stagnation, and heat bind patterns. **Cold-damp** abdominal fullness is attributable to cold evil directly striking the interior, living in damp places or eating unclean cold foods. The fullness is unrelieved by pressure (repletion), and is accompanied by poor appetite, nausea, vomiting, diarrhea, pain in the stomach duct or abdomen, thirst without desire for fluids, and a slimy tongue fur and stringlike pulse. MED Warm and transform cold-damp using Stomach-Calming Poria (Hoelen) Five Decoction (*wèi líng tāng*) or Magnolia Bark Center-Warming Decoction (*hòu pò wēn zhōng tāng*). ACU Base treatment for abdominal fullness mainly on ST and CV, selecting ST-25 (*tiān shū*, Celestial Pivot), CV-6 (*qì hǎi*, Sea of Qi), PC-6 (*nèi guān*, Inner Pass), and ST-36 (*zú sān lǐ*, Leg Three Li) as the main points. For cold-damp, add SP-9 (*yīn líng quán*, Yin Mound Spring) and LI-4 (*hé gǔ*, Union Valley); needle with drainage and large amounts of moxa. **Spleen-stomach vacuity cold** abdominal fullness arises from usual presence of spleen-stomach yang vacuity, excessive consumption of cold and fatty foods, or excess use of cold or cool medicinals in treatment, imbalance following major illness, and lack of nourishment due to enduring illness. The fullness is intermittent and likes warmth and pressure (and sometimes warm drinks or food), and is accompanied by lassitude of spirit and lack of strength, a pale tongue possibly with dental impressions, a thin white tongue fur, and a slow pulse. MED Use Center-Rectifying Decoction (*lǐ zhōng tāng*) or Magnolia Bark, Fresh Ginger, Pinellia, Licorice, and Ginseng Decoction (*hòu pò shēng jiāng bàn xià gān cǎo rén shēn tāng*). ACU To the main points given above add BL-20 (*pí shū*, Spleen Transport), BL-21 (*wèi shū*, Stomach Transport), CV-4 (*guān yuán*, Pass Head), and LR-13 (*zhāng mén*, Camphorwood Gate); needle with supplementation and add moxa. CROSS MOXA and the Five Pillar Points (*wǔ zhù xué*) can also be used to warm the center and dispel cold. **Brewing damp-heat** abdominal fullness is associated with distention stomach duct glomus, nausea and vomiting, vexation and oppression in the heart, thirst without desire to drink much, periodic sweating, sloppy diarrhea, short voidings of reddish urine, slimy yellow tongue fur, and a soggy rapid pulse. [MED] Transform dampness and clear heat using Wang's Coptis and Magnolia Bark Beverage (*wáng shì lián pò yǐn*). [ACU] To the main points given above, add LI-11 (*qū chí*, Pool at the Bend), LI-4 (*hé gǔ*, Union Valley), SP-9 (*yīn líng quán*, Yin Mound Spring), and ST-44 (*nèi tíng*, Inner Court); needle with drainage. **Food stagnation** abdominal fullness is relieved by the passing of flatus or belching, and is associated with sour belching, swallowing of upflowing acid, diarrhea smelling like rotten eggs, thick slimy tongue fur, and a slippery sunken pulse. [MED] Disperse food and abduct stagnation using Harmony-Preserving Pill (*bǎo hé wán*). [ACU] To the main points given above, add Li Inner Court (*lǐ nèi tíng*), CV-12 (*zhōng wǎn*, Center Stomach Duct), and CV-10 (*xià wǎn*, Lower Stomach Duct); needle with drainage. **Heat bind** abdominal fullness, which occurs in heat (febrile) disease, is fullness without relief sometimes associated with hardness and pain, pain around the umbilicus, constipation, STREAMING SWEAT on the hands and feet, tidal heat [effusion], delirious speech, a sunken replete pulse or forceful slow pulse, and a dry yellow tongue fur. [MED] Drain and precipitate the heat bind with Major Qi-Coordinating Decoction (*dà chéng qì tāng*). [ACU] To the main points given above, add LI-4 (*hé gǔ*, Union Valley), LI-11 (*qū chí*, Pool at the Bend), ST-37 (*shàng jù xū*, Upper Great Hollow), and SP-14 (*fù jié*, Abdominal Bind); needle with drainage. Compare ABDOMINAL DISTENTION; GLOMUS. [92: No. 207] [27: 408] [97: 603] [46: 597, 602, 662, 670]

abdominal pain 腹痛 *fù tòng*: Pain in the stomach duct, in the umbilical region, in the smaller abdomen, or in the lesser abdomen. Abdominal pain is attributable to external contraction of one of the six excesses, dietary irregularities, affect damage, stagnation of qi dynamic, blood stasis obstructing the vessels, or worm accumulations, etc. In pattern identification, it is first of all important to identify cold, heat, vacuity, and repletion, qi stagnation, and blood stasis. **Cold** pain is pain that is exacerbated by exposure to cold and likes warmth, and is accompanied by physical cold and fear of cold, absence of thirst, white tongue fur, and a pulse that is either sunken and slow or sunken and tight. **Heat** pain is pain that is periodic and accompanied by thirst, dry tongue, reddish urine, constipation or diarrhea, a red tongue with yellow fur, and a

rapid surging pulse. **Vacuity** pain is a continual pain that likes pressure. **Repletion** pain is pain accompanied by fullness and comes in violent attacks. **Qi stagnation** pain (often simply called qi pain) is also a pain that comes in bouts, and is characteristically of unfixed location. **Blood stagnation** pain (often simply called *stasis pain*) is a stabbing pain of fixed location. As to location, pain in the greater abdomen (upper abdomen) is a sign of spleen or stomach morbidity; pain in the umbilical region is attributable to large or small intestinal morbidity; pain in the center of the abdomen below the umbilicus itself is attributable to bladder or kidney diseases; pain on both sides of the abdomen below the umbilicus is usually related to the liver. See entries listed below. [26: 798] [97: 603]

Abdominal Pain

QI VACUITY ABDOMINAL PAIN (*qì xū fù tòng*)

BLOOD VACUITY ABDOMINAL PAIN (*xuè xū fù tòng*)

COLD ABDOMINAL PAIN (*hán lěng fù tòng*)

COLD ACCUMULATION ABDOMINAL PAIN (*hán jī fù tòng*)

DAMP-HEAT ABDOMINAL PAIN (*shī rè fù tòng*)

FOOD ACCUMULATION ABDOMINAL PAIN (*shí jī fù tòng*)

PHLEGM-RHEUM ABDOMINAL PAIN (*tán yǐn fù tòng*)

WORM ACCUMULATION ABDOMINAL PAIN (*chóng jī fù tòng*)

QI STAGNATION ABDOMINAL PAIN (*qì zhì fù tòng*)

STATIC BLOOD ABDOMINAL PAIN (*yū xuè fù tòng*)

SMALLER-ABDOMINAL PAIN (*shào fù tòng*)

abdominal pain in pregnancy 妊娠腹痛 *rèn shēn fù tòng*: UTERINE OBSTRUCTION. [26: 341]

abdominal urgency and heaviness in the rectum 里急后重 *lǐ jí hòu zhòng*: Synonym: *tenesmus*. From *The Classic of Difficult Issues* (*nàn jīng, 56*). Urge to defecate with abdominal pain, pressure in the rectum, and difficult defecation. Abdominal urgency and heaviness in the rectum is mostly caused by damp-heat, and is one of the main signs of dysentery. ◇ Chin 里 *lǐ*, interior; 急 *jí*, urgency; 后 *hòu*, posterior, 重 *zhòng*, heaviness. [27: 363] [26: 761]

abduct 导 *dǎo*: To carry away; specifically to carry stagnant food down the digestive tract. See DISPERSING FOOD AND ABDUCTING STAGNATION. ◇ Eng from L. *abducere*, lead away.

abductive dispersion 消导 *xiāo dǎo*: See DISPERSING FOOD AND ABDUCTING STAGNATION.

abhorrence of cold 憎寒 *zēng hán*: External shivering with internal heat vexation arising when a deep-lying internal heat evil blocks yang qi and prevents it from reaching the exterior. Abhorrence of cold occurs, for example, in deep-lying rheum, pestilential qi epidemic toxin hidden in the membrane source, thunder head wind, and gan of the lung. [27: 355]

abiding ailment 宿疾 *sù jí: Synonym: long-standing ailment.* Any disease that persists over many months or years. [97: 539] [27: 378]

abiding food 宿食 *sù shí:* From *Essential Prescriptions of the Golden Coffer* (*jūn guì yào lüè*). Food and drink accumulating in the stomach and intestines. Abiding food arises when, in FOOD DAMAGE, food accumulation remains untransformed for days. It is usually caused by voracious eating or spleen vacuity. It is characterized by abdominal pain and distention, belching of sour fetid qi, nausea, aversion to food, constipation or diarrhea, slimy tongue fur, and in some cases, aversion to cold, heat effusion, and headache. Abiding food can cause phlegm, which in turn can engender heat. Such conditions are known by the compound term *phlegm-food.* MED Treat by fortifying the spleen and stomach and by dispersing food and abducting stagnation. Use Harmony-Preserving Pill (*bǎo hé wán*) or Center-Ordering Decoction (*zhì zhōng tāng*) and variations. For lodged food in the upper stomach duct, characterized by oppression, glomus, and distention in the stomach duct and nausea, mechanical ejection may be used. For heat effusion and aversion to cold, headache, constipation, or diarrhea with ungratifying defecation, use formulas such as Major Bupleurum Decoction (*dà chái hú tāng*) and Unripe Bitter Orange Stagnation-Abducting Pill (*zhǐ shí dǎo zhì wán*). ACU Base treatment mainly on CV and ST. Select CV-12 (*zhōng wǎn,* Center Stomach Duct), CV-10 (*xià wǎn,* Lower Stomach Duct), ST-25 (*tiān shū,* Celestial Pivot), CV-6 (*qì hǎi,* Sea of Qi), and ST-36 (*zú sān lǐ,* Leg Three Li) as the main points. For voracious eating, add Li Inner Court (*lǐ nèi tíng*); and ST-37 (*shàng jù xū,* Upper Great Hollow); needle all points with drainage. For spleen-stomach vacuity, add BL-20 (*pí shū,* Spleen Transport), BL-21 (*wèi shū,* Stomach Transport), CV-4 (*guān yuán,* Pass Head), and SP-4 (*gōng sūn,* Yellow Emperor); needle all points with supplementation, adding moxa. Selection of points according to signs: For constipation, add BL-25 (*dà cháng shū,* Large Intestine Transport). For diarrhea with ungratifying defecation, add PC-6 (*nèi guān,* Inner Pass) and LR-2 (*xíng jiān,* Moving Between). For glomus and oppression, add SP-4 (*gōng sūn,* Yellow Emperor). For putrid belching and swallowing of upflowing acid, add GB-40 (*qiū xū,* Hill Ruins) and GB-34 (*yáng líng quán,* Yang Mound Spring). Compare FOOD DAMAGE, FOOD STAGNATION, and FOOD ACCUMU-

LATION. [26: 563] [97: 538] [25: 283] [46: 662] [13: 328] [113: 223]

abnormal passage to the pericardium 逆传心包 *nì chuán xīn bāo:* In warm diseases, the passage of evils directly to the pericardium without passing through construction. Abnormal passage to the pericardium occurs in febrile disease that is not a regular common cold or flu, e.g., in what Western medicine calls encephalitis B. See HEAT ENTERING THE PERICARDIUM; PERICARDIAC PATTERN. [27: 133] [97: 440]

abnormal qi 异气 *yì qì:* PESTILENTIAL QI. [27: 108]

absence of sweating 无汗 *wú hàn:* The absence of normal sweating. In externally contracted febrile (heat) disease, absence of sweating with aversion to cold is a sign of external wind-cold or cold-damp fettering the exterior, i.e., cold evil blocking the interstices of the flesh (sweat ducts and pores) and thereby preventing normal sweating. This is an exterior repletion pattern that can often be treated with Ephedra Decoction (*má huáng tāng*). Absence of sweating with heat effusion is a sign of blood and fluid depletion or of cold in the exterior and heat in the interior. It stems from a lack of sweat rather than blockage in the sweating function and forms part of a vacuity pattern or a vacuity-repletion complex. See SWEATING. [26: 743] [97: 66]

absence of thirst 口不渴 *kǒu bù kě:* Absence of normal desire for fluids. Absence of thirst or intake of warm fluids in small amounts indicates a cold pattern. In cold patterns, normal sweating is reduced, and diminished fluid loss can be compensated with lesser amounts of fluid. Compare THIRST.

abstraction 恍惚 *huǎng hū:* Inattention to present objects or surroundings, or low powers of mental concentration. It is a sign of HEART DISEASE.

accumulated cold stomach duct pain 积冷胃脘痛 *jī lěng wèi wǎn (guǎn) tòng:* See INTERNAL DAMAGE STOMACH DUCT PAIN.

accumulated heat stomach duct pain 积热胃脘痛 *jī rè wèi wǎn (guǎn) tòng:* See INTERNAL DAMAGE STOMACH DUCT PAIN.

accumulation 积 *jī:* Gathering, amassment; specifically: (1) a type of abdominal lump (see CONCRETIONS, CONGLOMERATIONS, ACCUMULATIONS, AND GATHERINGS); (2) accumulation of food in the digestive tract (see FOOD ACCUMULATION). [97: 480]

aching bones 骨酸 *gǔ suān:* From *The Magic Pivot* (*líng shū, běn shén*). Aching pain in the bones. Aching bones are usually attributable to kidney vacuity and damage to essence, and are accompanied by limp weak lumbus and knees.

Less commonly, this sign occurs in repletion patterns caused by wind-damp and turbid toxin may. Aching bones are observed in WILTING, IMPEDIMENT. and in VACUITY TAXATION. Compare BONE PAIN. See [50: 1089]

aching lumbus 腰酸 *yāo suān*: Continual dull pain and discomfort in the lumbus as distinct from LUMBAR PAIN, which generally denotes more acute pain. Aching lumbus is attributed either to a) kidney vacuity arising from insufficiency of kidney qi in advancing years or from damage to kidney qi by sexual intemperance, or b) TAXATION DETRIMENT, i.e., wear and tear from physical strain or poor posture. Kidney vacuity lumbar pain is a continual pain exacerbated by physical strain and relieved by rest. In severe cases, there is distinct pain and lack of strength associated with cold knees, and heel pain. In some cases, there may also be hair loss, loosening of the teeth, impotence, and seminal emission. The tongue is pale and the pulse is sunken and fine. When from vacuity detriment, the aching is located in a specific spot, is exacerbated by strain but not markedly relieved by rest, is worse on rising in the morning, and abates with light exercise. The two patterns are mutually conducive and hence not clearly distinguishable. MED Kidney vacuity lumbar pain can be treated by warming, supplementing, and nourishing the kidney with formulas such as Young Maid Pill (*qīng é wán*) and Seven-Jewel Beard-Blackening Elixir (*qī bǎo měi rán dān*). Vacuity taxation can be treated with the same formulas. Compare LUMBAR PAIN. ACU Base treatment mainly on BL and GV. Main points: BL-23 (*shèn shū*, Kidney Transport)ⓜ and BL-40 (*wěi zhōng*, Bend Center). For kidney vacuity add KI-3 (*tài xī*, Great Ravine), BL-52 (*zhì shì*, Will Chamber), and GV-4 (*mìng mén*, Life Gate)ⓜ, needling with supplementation. For vacuity detriment, add GV-26 (*shuǐ gōu*, Water Trough) and BL-17 (*gé shū*, Diaphragm Transport), needling with supplementation. [92: No. 165] [113: 229] [4: 146]

aching lumbus and limp knees 腰酸膝软 *yāo suān xī ruǎn*: See LIMP ACHING LUMBUS AND KNEES.

aching lumbus and limp legs 腰酸腿软 *yāo suān tuǐ ruǎn*, 腰酸足软 *yāo suān zú ruǎn*: See LIMP ACHING LUMBUS AND LEGS.

aching pain 酸痛 *suān tòng*: Pain of continuous duration, felt in the sinews and bones. See PAIN.

acid regurgitation 吞酸 *tūn suān*: SWALLOWING OF UPFLOWING ACID.

acid upflow 泛酸 *fàn suān*: The upflow of acid from the stomach into the mouth, that may be ejected or swallowed before it can be ejected. If it is expelled from the body, it is called ACID VOM-

ITING; if it is swallowed, it is called SWALLOWING OF UPFLOWING ACID. [92: No. 85]

acid vomiting 吐酸 *tù suān*: From *Elementary Questions* (*sù wèn, zhì zhēn yào dà lùn*). Expulsion through the mouth of sour fluid that flows up from the stomach. Acid vomiting is similar to SWALLOWING OF UPFLOWING ACID, in which sour water flowing up from the stomach is swallowed before it is ejected, but differs in that the sour water is actually ejected. Acid vomiting is attributed to ABIDING FOOD, phlegm-fire, liver fire invading the stomach, or spleen-stomach vacuity cold. **Lodged food** causes acid vomiting or swallowing of upflowing acid with belching of putrid qi. MED Treat by harmonizing the center, dispersing food, and abducting stagnation with Medicated Leaven and Atractylodes Pill (*qū zhú wán*). ACU Base treatment mainly on the alarm and lower uniting points of the stomach channel, selecting CV-12 (*zhōng wǎn*, Center Stomach Duct), PC-6 (*nèi guān*, Inner Pass), and ST-36 (*zú sān lǐ*, Leg Three Li) as the main points. For lodged food, add CV-10 (*xià wǎn*, Lower Stomach Duct), ST-25 (*tiān shū*, Celestial Pivot), CV-6 (*qì hǎi*, Sea of Qi), GB-34 (*yáng líng quán*, Yang Mound Spring), and GB-40 (*qiū xū*, Hill Ruins); needle with drainage. **Phlegm-fire** causes acid vomiting with heart vexation, and oppressed breath and copious phlegm. MED Transform phlegm and clear fire using Gardenia and Coptis Two Matured Ingredients Decoction (*zhī lián èr chén tāng*). ACU To the main points given above, add ST-40 (*fēng lóng*, Bountiful Bulge), SP-4 (*gōng sūn*, Yellow Emperor), LI-4 (*hé gǔ*, Union Valley), and GB-34 (*yáng líng quán*, Yang Mound Spring); needle with drainage. **Liver fire invading the stomach** causes heart vexation and acid vomiting with stabbing pain in both rib-sides, bitter taste in the mouth, dry throat, and a rapid stringlike pulse. MED Discharge the liver and clear fire using Left-Running Metal Pill (*zuǒ jīn wán*). ACU To the main points given above, add CV-13 (*shàng wǎn*, Upper Stomach Duct); ST-44 (*nèi tíng*, Inner Court), LR-3 (*tài chōng*, Supreme Surge), LR-2 (*xíng jiān*, Moving Between), and GB-34 (*yáng líng quán*, Yang Mound Spring); needle with drainage. **Spleen-stomach vacuity cold** causes acid vomiting with distention and oppression in the chest and stomach duct, belching, white tongue fur, and fine stringlike pulse. MED Warm the spleen and stomach using Saussurea and Amomum Six Gentlemen Decoction (*xiāng shā liù jūn zǐ tāng*). ACU To the main points given above, add BL-20 (*pí shū*, Spleen Transport), BL-21 (*wèi shū*, Stomach Transport), CV-4 (*guān yuán*, Pass Head), LR-13 (*zhāng mén*, Camphorwood Gate), and SP-4 (*gōng sūn*, Yellow Emperor); needle with supplementation and add moxa. CROSS MOXA and the Five Pillar Points (*wǔ zhù xué*) can also be used to warm the center and dispel cold. [26: 259] [97: 186] [46: 596, 597, 658, 662] [113: 223]

acne 粉刺 *fěn cì*: Blackheads (comedones) or red papules ("pimples") on the face that can be squeezed to produce an oily, chalky substance, and that can develop into pustules. Acne is most common in young people. In severe cases, pimples may be large, red, and swollen, and coalesce and spread to the neck, shoulders, and back. Acne is attributed to brewing lung-stomach heat fuming the face, causing heat and stagnation of the blood. It is often found to be related to consumption of rich food. MED Diffuse the lung and clear heat, taking Loquat Leaf Lung-Clearing Beverage (*pí pá qīng fèi yǐn*) orally and applying Reversal Powder (*diān dǎo sǎn*) mixed with cold water topically. ACU Base treatment mainly on back transport points, ST, and LI. Select LI-20 (*yíng xiāng*, Welcome Fragrance), LI-4 (*hé gǔ*, Union Valley), LI-11 (*qū chí*, Pool at the Bend), BL-13 (*fèi shū*, Lung Transport), BL-20 (*pí shū*, Spleen Transport), ST-44 (*nèi tíng*, Inner Court), and ST-36 (*zú sān lǐ*, Leg Three Li), and needle with drainage. For pronounced heat signs, pick BL-40 (*wěi zhōng*, Bend Center) and prick LU-11 (*shào shāng*, Lesser Shang) to bleed. See also DRINKER'S NOSE. ◇ Chin 粉 *fěn*, powder; 刺 *cì*, thorn, prickle. [26: 493] [42: 159]

acquired constitution 后天 *hòu tiān*: LATER HEAVEN.

acrid 辛 *xīn*: See ACRIDITY.

acridity 辛 *xīn*: Synonym: *pungency*. One of the FIVE FLAVORS. Acridity enters the lung; it can dissipate and move. See FIVE FLAVORS; FIVE-FLAVOR ENTRIES. [97: 308]

acridity enters the lung 辛入肺 *xīn rù fèi*: Acrid medicinals act upon the lung. Examples of acrid medicinals that enter the lung are Platycodon (*jié gěng*), ephedra (*má huáng*), borneol (*bīng piàn*), silkworm (*bái jiāng cán*), tribulus (*cì jí lí*), dried ginger (*gān jiāng*), tangerine peel (*chén pí*), peucedanum (*qián hú*), radish seed (*lái fú zǐ*), and gleditsia (*zào jiá*). [27: 62]

acrid opening and bitter discharging 辛开苦泄 *xīn kāi kǔ xiè*: See OPENING WITH ACRIDITY AND DISCHARGING WITH BITTERNESS.

acrid opening and bitter downbearing 辛开苦降 *xīn kāi kǔ jiàng*: See OPENING WITH ACRIDITY AND DOWNBEARING WITH BITTERNESS.

act(ion) according to person 因人制宜 *yīn rén zhì yí*: To determine what is suitable for patients according to their constitution, sex, age, lifestyle, and history. For example, males and females have physiological differences that have to be considered when deciding treatment; children tend to have tender, weak bowels and viscera, whereas elderly people suffer from debilitation of qi and blood so that treatment must be adjusted according to age. [26: 259]

act(ion) according to place 因地制宜 *yīn dì zhì yí*: To determine what is suitable for the patient in accordance with the geographic location. For example, in China, damp-heat patterns are common in the hot, rainy south, whereas dryness patterns are common in the dry north. [26: 259]

action 功效 *gōng xiào*: The manner in which a medicinal acts on the body. For example, poria skin (*fú líng pí*) has the action of disinhibiting water and dispersing swelling, whereas red peony has the action of moving stasis, relieving pain, cooling the blood, and dispersing swelling. Traditionally, acupuncture points were selected according to their ability to eliminate or alleviate particular disease patterns, and since World War II have been ascribed actions in a manner similar to medicinals. Thus, HT-7 (*shén mén*, Spirit Gate), traditionally said to treat heart vexation, mania and withdrawal, forgetfulness, heart palpitations and fearful throbbing, is now also said to quiet the heart and spirit, clear fire and cool construction, and clear heart heat.

act(ion) according to time 因时制宜 *yīn shí zhì yí*: To determine what is suitable for the patient in accordance with the time of the year. The seasons are associated with different types of weather that can all affect the human body. For example, in summer the weather is hot, the interstices loosen and open, so that when treating patients suffering from wind-cold, warm acrid medicinals should not be used to excess if copious sweating and damage to yang qi and the fluids is to be avoided. In the winter, the interstices respond to cold weather by tightening, so that in treating patients with wind-cold, warm acrid medicinals must be used in larger quantities to ensure enough sweating to resolve the evil. [26: 259]

acuanesthesia 针刺麻醉 *zhēn cì má zuì*: A method of acupuncture in which needles are inserted at specific points and manipulation or electrical current is applied to enable surgical operations to be performed painlessly while the patient is conscious. [26: 329] [27: 329]

acumoxatherapy 针灸 *zhēn jiǔ*: Synonym: *acupuncture*.[2] ACUPUNCTURE,[1] MOXIBUSTION, and other related techniques such as magnetic acupuncture.

acupressure 指针 *zhǐ zhēn*: Synonym: *shiatsu*. A method of treatment involving the application of finger pressure at acupuncture points. [27: 330]

acupuncture 针灸 *zhēn jiǔ*: **1.** The practice of puncturing the body with metal needles (steel, gold, or silver) at specific points in order to regulate construction, defense, qi, and the blood.

2. ACUMOXATHERAPY. See MOXIBUSTION. [26: 532] [97: 291] [27: 328]

acupuncture point 穴位 *xué wèi*, 穴道 *xué dào*, 腧 (俞、输) *shū*, 孔穴 *kǒng xué*: Abbreviation: point. A place on the surface of the body where qi and blood of the channels and network vessels gather or pass. Through the channels and network vessels, points are connected to other parts of the body and notably the bowels and viscera, whose state of health they can reflect. Various stimuli such as needling, moxibustion, massage, acupressure, and electroacupuncture can be applied at points to regulate internal functions. A distinction is made between CHANNEL POINT, NONCHANNEL POINT, and OUCH POINT. See also POINT COMBINATION and POINT SELECTION for use of points. ◊ Chin 穴 *xué*, cave, hole; 位 *wèi*, position; 道 *dào*, way, tract; 腧、俞、输 *shū* are all explained as 输, transport; 孔 *kǒng*, hole. The Chinese *xuè* reflects the notion that acupuncture points are usually depressions or crevices between bones, sinews, etc.; this notion is not properly conveyed by the English word "point." [27: 97] [26: 172]

acute fright wind 急惊风 *jí jīng fēng*: Febrile disease in infants and children characterized by clenched jaw and by convulsions of the limbs. The appearance of clenched jaw and convulsions in high fever with vexation and agitation, red face and limbs, and hasty breathing due to phlegm congestion marks the development of an acute fright wind pattern. Clenched jaw is the first fright wind sign to appear. This is often followed by convulsions of the limbs, and in more severe cases by rigidity of the neck or arched-back rigidity (opisthotonos) with clouded spirit. Spasm may come in intermittent bouts. Fright wind is a manifestation of extreme heat engendering wind, occurring when intense internal heat is depressed and blocked by externally contracted wind (see BLOCK PATTERN) and exacerbated by congealing phlegm and stagnant qi. MED Acupuncture or acupressure is the best emergency treatment. Subsequent treatment involves settling the liver and extinguishing wind, clearing the heart and flushing phlegm, using Fright-Disinhibiting Pill (*lì jīng wán*), Green-Blue–Draining Pill (*xiè qīng wán*), or Dragon-Embracing Pill (*bào lóng wán*). ACU For emergency treatment, do not stretch contracted limbs; apply finger pressure at GV-26 (*rén zhōng*, Human Center) at the philtrum and LI-4 (*hé gǔ*, Union Valley) or at Hall of Impression (*yìn táng*) and KI-1 (*yǒng quán*, Gushing Spring). If needles are available, base emergency treatment on GV and LR. Select GV-26 (*shuǐ gōu*, Water Trough), GV-14 (*dà zhuī*, Great Hammer), LI-4 (*hé gǔ*, Union Valley), LR-3 (*tài chōng*, Supreme Surge), and GB-34 (*yáng líng quán*, Yang Mound Spring) as main points; needle with drainage and prick the Ten Dif-

fusing Points (*shí xuān*) to bleed. Further points may be selected according to cause: For external contractions, add LI-11 (*qū chí*, Pool at the Bend). For phlegm-heat, add CV-12 (*zhōng wǎn*, Center Stomach Duct), ST-40 (*fēng lóng*, Bountiful Bulge), and HT-7 (*shén mén*, Spirit Gate). For fright and fear, add Hall of Impression (*yìn táng*), HT-7 (*shén mén*, Spirit Gate), and KI-1 (*yǒng quán*, Gushing Spring). See FRIGHT WIND. Compare CHILD VISITING HOSTILITY. [26: 466] [27: 432] [46: 700] [113: 330]

acute jaundice 急黄 *jí huáng*: **1.** From *The Origin and Indicators of Disease* (*zhū bìng yuán hòu lùn, jí huáng hòu*). Jaundice mostly caused by damp-heat toxin evil scorching construction-blood and characterized by sudden yellowing together with fullness in the heart [region] and panting that threaten the patient's life. The body swiftly turns to the color of tangerines, and, in severe cases, there is clouded spirit and delirious raving, high fever, vexation and thirst, fullness in the chest and abdominal distention, blood ejection and spontaneous external bleeding, bloody stool, and ascites. The pulse is stringlike, slippery, and rapid. The tongue is red or crimson with a dry yellow fur. MED Clear heat and resolve toxin; cool the blood and open the orifices. Use Coptis Toxin-Resolving Decoction (*huáng lián jiě dú tāng*) or Spirit-Like Rhinoceros Horn Elixir (*shén xī dān*). **2.** SCOURGE JAUNDICE. [26: 465]

acute throat wind 急喉风 *jí hóu fēng*: Synonym: *constricting throat wind*. A form of throat wind that develops swiftly, soon making the throat swollen and blocked. It occurs in patients given to excessive consumption of fat meat, fine grain, and strong flavors (i.e., rich food), and liquor and fried foods, or who have brewing lung-stomach heat. Acute throat wind arises when contraction of wind-heat stirs fire and engenders phlegm, the combined evil toxin becoming congested in the throat. At onset, the throat quickly becomes swollen, inhibiting normal swallowing. Subsequently, the whole throat becomes scorching red, hot swollen, and congested with phlegm-drool. There is a constricted sensation, phlegm rale, hasty labored breathing, and hoarse voice. Blockage of the throat hampers the swallowing of liquids, and, in severe cases, can lead to death by asphyxiation. MED Disperse swelling and resolve toxin; clear heat and disinhibit the throat. Use Scourge-Clearing Toxin-Vanquishing Beverage (*qīng wēn bài dú yǐn*). If there is heart vexation and clouded spirit, open the orifices and sweep phlegm with Peaceful Palace Bovine Bezoar Pill (*ān gōng niú huáng wán*). When pus has formed, lance and drain, and insufflate Borneol and Borax Powder (*bīng péng sǎn*). Where asphyxiation is threatened, modern surgery is necessary to maintain respiration. WMC edema of the throat;

retropharyngeal abscess. See THROAT WIND. [26: 465]

add at end 后下 *hòu xià*: Add a medicinal toward the end of the process of decocting the other medicinals in the formula. Some exterior-resolving medicinals such as mint (*bò hé*), agastache/patchouli (*huò xiāng*), and eupatorium (*pèi lán*) loose their qi and flavor when boiled for a long time (i.e., they loose their volatile oils). They are therefore added after the other medicinals have boiled for 15 minutes for the final 5–10 minutes. Uncaria (*gōu téng*) is added just a few seconds before the end. Rhubarb (*dà huáng*) may be first soaked in a small amount of water and likewise added a few seconds before the decoction process is complete. [27: 319] [97: 209]

advanced menstruation 月经先期 *yuè jīng xiān qī*, 经行先期 *jīng xíng xiān qī*: The arrival of the menstrual period eight days or more before the normal time (i.e., within 20 days of the onset of the previous period in women who normally have a standard 28-day cycle). See BLOOD HEAT ADVANCED MENSTRUATION; LIVER DEPRESSION ADVANCED MENSTRUATION; QI VACUITY ADVANCED MENSTRUATION. [26: 813] [27: 440] [97: 111]

affect 情 *qíng*: **1.** Any natural movement of the heart, such as joy, anger, or grief. For example, *The Book of Rites* (礼记 *lǐ jì*, *lǐ yùn*) states, "What are the human affects? [They are] the seven things—joy, anger, grief, fear, love, loathing, and desire—of which a person is capable without learning." **2.** The seven specific emotional and mental activities joy, anger, anxiety, thought, sorrow, fear, and fright, which in excess can cause disease. See INTERNAL DAMAGE BY THE SEVEN AFFECTS. NB: Five of seven bear the same name as the FIVE MINDS. ◇ Chin 情 *qíng*, fact, reason; emotion; affection; affinity; relationship. See also SEVEN RELATIONS.

affect damage 内伤七情 *nèi shāng qī qíng*: INTERNAL DAMAGE BY THE SEVEN AFFECTS.

affect-mind binding depression 情志郁结 *qíng zhì yù jié*: Depression of general mental or emotional activity that results from a dominant mental or emotional activity or response and that causes depression of the activity of qi in the body, ultimately affecting normal functioning of the bowels and viscera and causing disease. In Chinese medicine, mental and emotional activity is viewed in terms of the FIVE MINDS (joy, anger, anxiety, thought, sorrow, fear) or SEVEN AFFECTS (joy, anger, thought, sorrow, fear, fright, anxiety), which, when prolonged or excessive, have a narrowing, dampening, stultifying effect on mental life that can depress normal physiological function. For example, anger, which is frequently associated with frustration, can cause BINDING DE-

PRESSION OF LIVER QI, manifesting as chest and rib-side pain, goiter, gastrointestinal problems, or menstrual irregularities. Excessive thought (cogitation, preoccupation) can damage the spleen and cause digestive tract problems. Affective binding depression often leads to development of fire; see FIVE MINDS FORMING FIRE.

affect-mind internal damage 情志内伤 *qíng zhì nèi shāng*: INTERNAL DAMAGE BY THE SEVEN AFFECTS.

affects causing binding depression 情志郁结 *qíng zhì yù jié*: See AFFECT-MIND BINDING DEPRESSION.

afflux pouch 癖囊 *pǐ náng*: An accumulation of fluid; a sign of PHLEGM LODGED IN THE CHEST AND RIB-SIDE. ◇ Chin 癖 *pǐ*, accumulation, stagnation (cf. INTESTINAL AFFLUX); 囊 *náng*, bag, pouch. See also AGGREGATION. [6: 10] [48: 448]

afterbirth 胞衣 *bāo yī*: The matter discharged from the uterus after childbirth, corresponding in Western medicine to the placenta and fetal membranes discharged with it. ◇ Chin 胞 *bāo*, uterus; 衣 *yī*, tunic, clothing. [50: 1124]

afterpains 产後腹痛 *chǎn hòu fù tòng*: POSTPARTUM ABDOMINAL PAIN.

agent 药 *yào*: MEDICINAL.

aggregation 癖 *pǐ*: An accumulation or amassment, as INTESTINAL AGGREGATION and STRINGS AND AGGREGATIONS. ◇ Chin 癖 *pǐ*, *pī*, unhealthy accumulation, a bad habit, addiction, akin to 澼 *pì*, stagnation or accumulation of fluid. See AFFLUX POUCH. [27: 417] [97: 656] [48: 472]

agitated vexation 躁烦 *zào fán*: A feeling of unease or disquietude accompanied by a cold body and unconscious movement of the limbs, physical fatigue and lassitude of spirit, dry mouth with intake of fluid, and a weak fine pulse; a vacuity cold sign of vacuous yang causing a disturbance. See VEXATION AND AGITATION. [27: 372] [97: 659]

agitation 躁 *zào*: A subjective feeling of vexation outwardly expressed by pronounced abnormal movement. See VEXATION AND AGITATION.

alarm point 募穴 *mù xué*: Synonym: *mustering point* Any of a group of points on the abdomen or chest, each of which is the collecting point of the qi of a bowel or viscus in whose vicinity it lies. The alarm points are listed below. Application: Disease in a given bowel or viscus may be reflected in tenderness, lumps, gatherings, depressions, or other aberrant signs at its alarm point, and can be treated by applying a stimulus at the point. In clinical practice, the alarm points of each bowels is commonly used in the treatment of that bowel, e.g., CV-3 (*zhōng jí*, Central Pole), the alarm point of the bladder, is almost always used in the treatment of urinary diseases; ST-25 (*tiān shū*, Celestial Pivot), the alarm point of the large intestine, is frequently used to treat constipation. The alarm points of the viscera are infrequently employed, the back transport points being the preferred points for treatment of diseases of the viscera. The alarm points are often used in combination with the back transport points. See BACK TRANSPORT POINT. ◇ Chin 募 *mù*, muster, gather. 'Mustering point' is closer to the meaning of the Chinese term than 'alarm point'. [27: 102] [97: 504]

Alarm Points

Lung alarm: LU-1 (*zhōng fǔ*, Central Treasury)
Heart: CV-14 (*jù què*, Great Tower Gate)
Liver: LR-14 (*qī mén*, Cycle Gate)
Spleen: LR-13 (*zhāng mén*, Camphorwood Gate)
Kidney: GB-25 (*jīng mén*, Capital Gate)
Pericardium: CV-17 (*shān zhōng*, Chest Center)
Gallbladder: GB-24 (*rì yuè*, Sun and Moon)
Stomach: CV-12 (*zhōng wǎn*, Center Stomach Duct)
Large intestine: ST-25 (*tiān shū*, Celestial Pivot)
Small intestine: CV-4 (*guān yuán*, Pass Head)
Triple burner: CV-5 (*shí mén*, Stone Gate)
Bladder: CV-3 (*zhōng jí*, Central Pole)

allaying thirst 解渴 *jiě kě*: Eliminating thirst. See THIRST.

alternating fever and chills 寒热往来 *hán rè wǎng lái*, 往来寒热 *wǎng lái hán rè*, 寒热 *hán rè*: ALTERNATING HEAT [EFFUSION] AND [AVERSION TO] COLD.

alternating heat [effusion] and [aversion to] cold 寒热往来 *hán rè wǎng lái*, 往来寒热 *wǎng lái hán rè*, 寒热 *hán rè*: Synonym: *alternating fever and chills* (obs). HEAT EFFUSION without AVERSION TO COLD and aversion to cold without heat effusion occurring in regular or irregular alternating succession, associated with lesser yang (*shào yáng*) midstage patterns, malaria, or damp-heat obstructing the triple burner. **Lesser yang patterns:** Alternating heat effusion and aversion to cold occurring in lesser yang (*shào yáng*) patterns is accompanied by heart vexation, retching, bitter taste in the mouth, dry throat, dizzy vision, [suffering of] chest and rib-side fullness, red tongue margins, thin yellow tongue fur and a stringlike pulse. ACU Base treatment mainly on GV and BL. GV-14 (*dà zhuī*, Great Hammer), and PC-5 (*jiān shǐ*, Intermediary Courier) can be selected as main points to treat alternating heat [effusion] and [aversion to] cold. To these, add LR-14 (*qī mén*, Cycle Gate), GB-41 (*zú lín qì*, Foot Overlooking Tears), TB-5 (*wài guān*, Outer Pass), GB-20 (*fēng chí*, Wind Pool), and TB-6 (*zhī gōu*, Branch Ditch)

to clear lesser yang (*shào yáng*) exterior-interior evil; needle with drainage or with even supplementation and drainage. **Malaria:** In malaria, bouts of aversion to cold followed by high fever that abates with sweating occur once every two or three days. ACU Base treatment mainly on GV and BL. GV-14 (*dà zhuī*, Great Hammer), PC-5 (*jiān shǐ*, Intermediary Courier), GV-13 (*táo dào*, Kiln Path), Malaria Gate (*nüè mén*), and Lofty Bone (*chóng gǔ*) can be selected as main points to treat alternating heat [effusion] and [aversion to] cold. To these, SI-3 (*hòu xī*, Back Ravine) can be added to free yang and eliminate malaria. Needle with drainage. **Damp-heat obstructing the triple burner:** In damp-heat obstructing the triple burner, aversion to cold alternating with heat effusion that is unrelieved by sweating is associated with oppression in the chest and abdominal distention, retching and vomiting, headache, heart vexation, dry mouth, short voidings of reddish urine, red tongue margins, and thick slimy or white mealy tongue fur and a soggy pulse. ACU Base treatment mainly on TB, GV, SP, and ST. GV-14 (*dà zhuī*, Great Hammer) and PC-5 (*jiān shǐ*, Intermediary Courier) can be selected as main points to treat alternating heat [effusion] and [aversion to] cold. To these, add TB-6 (*zhī gōu*, Branch Ditch), SP-9 (*yīn líng quán*, Yin Mound Spring), LI-11 (*qū chí*, Pool at the Bend), LI-4 (*hé gǔ*, Union Valley), ST-36 (*zú sān lǐ*, Leg Three Li), SP-6 (*sān yīn jiāo*, Three Yin Intersection), and ST-44 (*nèi tíng*, Inner Court) to clear and disinhibit triple burner damp-heat. [97: 574] [46: 597, 649] [113: 12, 169] [71: 172]

ambilateral headache 正头痛 *zhèng tóu tòng*: MEDIAL HEADACHE.

amenorrhea 经闭 *jīng bì*: MENSTRUAL BLOCK.

anal desertion 脱肛 *tuō gāng*: PROLAPSE OF THE RECTUM.

anal fistula 肛漏 *gāng lòu*: Synonym: *fistula*. Long pipe-like ulcerations from the perimeter or surrounding area of the anus. They may develop from hemorrhoids, welling- and flat-abscesses (*yōng jū*) of the anus, or splitting of the anus. Fistulas discharge pus-like fluid, are sore and itchy, and heal with difficulty. Distinction is made between vacuity and repletion patterns. Hardness and swelling of the local area, discharge of thick pus, and strong body constitute repletion; softness and depression in the area of the opening, discharge of thin pus, and weakness and emaciation constitute vacuity. MED Fistulas are treated by THREADED LIGATION and other surgical methods, combined with oral medication. For repletion, clear heat and disinhibit dampness. Use variations of Mysterious Two Pill (*èr miào wán*), or Fish Poison Yam Dampness-Percolating Decoction (*bì xiè shèn shī tāng*). For vacuity, support right and promote INTERNAL EXPRESSION. Use variations of Internal Expression Toxin-Dispersing Powder (*tuō lǐ xiāo dú sǎn*) or Six-Ingredient Rehmannia Pill (*liù wèi dì huáng wán*). Compare COMMUNICATING BOWELS. [26: 334] [27: 484] [97: 291]

anal welling-abscess 肛门痈 *gāng mén yōng*: Synonym: *visceral toxin*. A WELLING-ABSCESS (*yōng*) on the inside or outside of the anus; attributable to damp-heat pouring downward. Anal welling-abscesses heal with difficulty, and after bursting easily form fistulas. Distinction is made between repletion and vacuity. Repletion patterns stem from excessive consumption of liquor and rich food and the development of damp turbidity that pours downward to the anus. Repletion patterns are characterized by heat, redness, swelling and pain in the anus and the emergence of a plum-shaped welling-abscess. WMC perianal abscess. Vacuity patterns arise as a result of spleen, lung, and kidney depletion with damp-heat exploiting the vacuity to pour downward to the anus, and are characterized by flat swelling and slight pain. MED Repletion patterns are treated by clearing heat, resolving toxin, and disinhibiting dampness; vacuity patterns are treated by enriching yin and eliminating dampness combined with clearing vacuity heat. See EXTERNAL WELLING-ABSCESS. [26: 334]

ancestral qi 宗气 *zōng qì*: Synonym: *gathering qi* (*obs*). The qi that converges or concentrates in the "sea of qi," which is the chest, pervades the respiratory tract and controls breathing, and penetrates the heart and vessels. Ancestral qi drives the heart and regulates the pulses; its health is reflected in the strength of breathing and in the voice. ◇ Chin 宗 *zōng*, ancestor; clan; root, source; gather, collect, converge; a collection or set; sect, faction, school. *Zōng qì* may be so called because it gathers in the chest, or because it is the fundamental driving force of the heart and lung. Compare the meaning of *zōng* in the term *sinew gathering*. [97: 370]

ancestral sinew 宗筋 *zōng jīn*: **1.** The gathering point of the three yin and three yang channel sinews at the pubic region. **2.** The penis. See SLACKNESS OF THE ANCESTRAL SINEW. ◇ Chin 宗 *zōng*, ancestor; gathering, convergence; *jīn*, sinew. The notion of convergence appears to derive from the idea of lines of lineage converging on an ancestor. Whether in the second meaning the notion of "ancestor" highlights the reproductive significance of the penis is unclear; in the analogously composed terms "ancestral vessel" and "ancestral qi," this notion is absent. [27: 26] [97: 370]

ancestral vessels 宗脉 *zōng mài*: See GATHERING PLACE OF THE ANCESTRAL VESSELS.

andriatric diseases 男科疾病 *nán kē jí bìng*: MEN'S DISEASES.

anger 怒 *nù*: One of the FIVE MINDS, associated with the liver; also one of the SEVEN AFFECTS.

anger causes qi to rise 怒则气上 *nù zé qì shàng*: Liver qi thrives by orderly reaching and is averse to repression. Excessive emotional stimulus can cause excessive upbearing and effusion of liver qi, causing distention and fullness in the rib-side, headache and dizziness, and red sore swollen eyes. Since the liver stores the blood, liver qi ascending counterflow can carry the blood with it, giving rise to CLOUDING REVERSAL or retching of blood. [27: 145] [97: 466]

anger damages the liver 怒伤肝 *nù shāng gān*, 怒气伤肝 *nù qì shāng gan*: Continual anger causes liver qi to rise, carrying blood with it, causing red facial complexion, qi ascent, headache, and dizziness, and in severe cases, blood ejection or CLOUDING REVERSAL. [26: 474]

anguish 懊憹 *ào nóng*: From *On Cold Damage* (*shāng hán lùn*). A feeling of heat and clamoring stomach. Because it is located in the pit of the stomach, it is also called *anguish in the heart*. It arises when, after exterior patterns have been treated by an inappropriate form of sweating or have been wrongly treated by draining precipitation, the external evil enters the interior and lodges in the chest and diaphragm, thus harassing the stomach. In modern clinical practice, it is seen in febrile disease or in acute gastroenteritis. ◇ Chin 懊 *ào* and 憹 *nóng* both mean vexation, annoyance. [27: 372] [27: 372]

animal odor 臊味 *sāo wèi*: The odor of or similar to that of sheep and foxes.

animal soul 魄 *pò*: CORPOREAL SOUL.

ankle-boring phlegm 穿踝痰 *chuān huái tán*: Flowing phlegm of the ankle. See FLOWING PHLEGM.

anterior yin 前阴 *qián yīn*: *lower yin*. The exterior genitals (male or female).

anus 肛门 *gāng mén*: Synonyms: *posterior yin*; *lower extreme*; *corporeal soul gate*. The lower opening of the large intestine through which stool is discharged. Diagnosis: A burning sensation in the anus during defecation is a sign of large intestinal damp-heat. Bleeding from the anus can be attributed either to hemorrhoids or to splitting of the anus by the passage of hard stool in blood heat intestinal dryness patterns. Diseases of the anus include ANAL FISTULA; ANAL WELLING-ABSCESS; HEMORRHOIDS; SPLITTING OF THE ANUS; PROLAPSE OF THE RECTUM. [97: 291]

anxiety 忧 *yōu*: One of the FIVE MINDS; associated with the lung; also one of the SEVEN AFFECTS.

apical pulse 虚里 *xū lǐ*: VACUOUS LI.

appetite 食欲 *shí yù*, 胃口 *wèi kǒu*: The desire to eat. Appetite is considered principally to be a reflection of the state of the stomach and spleen. *The Magic Pivot (líng shū, hǎi lùn piān)* states, "The stomach is the sea of grain and water." The stomach governs intake and decomposition of grain and water (i.e., food); the spleen governs movement and transformation of grain and water and the distribution of their essence (i.e., nutrients). The stomach and spleen together form the "root of the later heaven," i.e., the basis of the acquired constitution. When the spleen and stomach are in harmony, the spleen provides adequate nutrients for the body and the stomach signals the need for food by the sensation of hunger. A good appetite is generally a sign of health, and lack of appetite is a sign of disease. "The presence of stomach qi means life; the absence of stomach qi is death." In disease, a good appetite is a sign of a mild condition, and its return is a sign of recovery. Sudden return of an appetite in critical illness is described as the "LAST RADIANCE OF THE SETTING SUN," and bodes death. See POOR APPETITE. [6: 134]

apply mixed 调敷 *tiáo fū*: To apply topically a powder blended with fluid.

arched-back rigidity 角弓反张 *jiǎo gōng fǎn zhāng*: Synonym: *opisthotonos*; *arched rigidity of the neck*. Rigidity of the neck and back causing them to arch or bow backward. Arched-back rigidity occurs in CHILD FRIGHT WIND, LOCKJAW (tetanus), and other forms of TETANY, which may be attributable to wind, cold, damp or fire stagnating in the channels, or to insufficiency of blood, fluid and qi, allowing vacuity wind to stir internally. WMC opisthotonos (occurring in encephalitis, meningitis and tetanus). ◇ Chin 角 *jiǎo*, horn; 弓 *gōng*, bow; 反 *fǎn*, back; 张 *zhāng*, tensed. Tensed backward like a horn and bow. [27: 374] [97: 294]

arched rigidity of the neck 颈项反张 *jǐng xiǎng fǎn zhāng*: ARCHED-BACK RIGIDITY.

areola 乳晕 *rǔ yūn*: The area around the nipple that is normally darker in color than the breast and lighter in color than the nipple. **Diagnosis**: Darkening of the areolae is one indication of pregnancy. [26: 379]

armpit odor 腋臭 *yì chòu*: See FOXY ODOR.

aromatic 芳香 *fāng xiāng*: Strong smelling. Aromatic turbidity transforming medicinals include agastache/patchouli (*huò xiāng*), eupatorium (*pèi lán*), amomum (*shā rén*), and magnolia bark (*hòu pò*). Aromatic orifice-opening medicinal include acorus (*shí chāng pú*) and liquid storax (*sū hé xiāng*).

arousing the spleen 醒脾 *xǐng pí*: A method of treatment that involves fortifying spleen qi using aromatic medicinals to that is applied when spleen is encumbered by dampness and unable to perform normal transformation, characterized by poor appetite, glomus and fullness after eating, dull abdominal pain, thin stool, pale tongue, and soggy weak pulse. Saussurea and Amomum Six Gentlemen Decoction (*xiāng shā liù jūn zǐ tāng*) is an example of a spleen-arousing formula. [27: 263] [97: 643]

ascendant hyperactivity of liver yang 肝阳上亢 *gān yáng shàng yàng*: Synonyms: *ascendant liver yang*; *effulgent liver yang*. An imbalance of the liver's yin and yang aspects occurring when vacuity of liver-kidney yin lets liver yang get out of control and stir upward excessively. This pathomechanism may be exacerbated when depression, anger, and anxiety impair free coursing, since when free coursing is impaired, depressed qi transforms into fire, fire damages yin-blood, and yin has no power to restrain yang. Ascendant liver yang is identifiable by signs of upper body exuberance and by signs of yin blood insufficiency from which this condition stems. The main signs are dizziness, tinnitus, pressure and pain in the head, and upbearing fire flush with baking heat in the face. Other signs include insomnia and profuse dreaming, heart vexation, agitation and irascibility, heavy head and light feet, limp aching lumbus and knees, dry throat and mouth. In some cases, there is sudden clouding collapse and unconsciousness. The pulse is stringlike and may also be fine. The tongue is red. Predominance of ascendant yang and yin vacuity signs varies from case to case. In some cases, both are equally pronounced. WMC hypertension. **Analysis**: Liver-kidney yin vacuity causes limp aching lumbus and knees. Where there is binding depression of liver qi with depressed qi transforming into fire, vexation, agitation, and irascibility are observed. Counterflow hyperactive yang qi gives rise to a red face, generalized heat [effusion], headache, and dizziness. When hyperactive yang stirs wind, qi and blood ascend counterflow, and phlegm-drool congests, causing sudden clouding collapse and unconsciousness that marks a wind stroke block pattern. **Comparison**: *Liver fire flaming upward:* Ascendant liver yang and liver fire flaming upward are both associated with manifestations of upsurge of fire heat such as red face, red eyes, headache, dizziness, red tongue, and rapid pulse. Ascendant liver yang is at root a vacuity pattern, and is associated with limp aching lumbus and knees, dry eyes, and tinnitus. Furthermore, the tongue fur is scant and the pulse tends to be fine. The condition develops gradually, and is exacerbated by stress. Liver fire flaming upward is a repletion pattern, and develops more rapidly. It is associated with bitter taste in the mouth, dry mouth, constipation, reddish urine, a yellow tongue fur, and forceful rapid pulse. When heat is pronounced, there may be blood ejection or spontaneous external bleeding. [MED] Enrich yin, calm the liver, and subdue yang. Use Gastrodia and Uncaria Beverage (*tiān má gōu téng yǐn*) or Lycium Berry, Chrysanthemum, and Rehmannia Pill (*qǐ jú dì huáng wán*). [ACU] Base treatment mainly on LR, GB, and KI. Needle with drainage at LR-3 (*tài chōng*, Supreme Surge), LR-2 (*xíng jiān*, Moving Between), and GB-43 (*xiá xī*, Pinched Ravine); and with supplementation at BL-18 (*gān shū*, Liver Transport), BL-23 (*shèn shū*, Kidney Transport), KI-3 (*tài xī*, Great Ravine), and SP-6 (*sān yīn jiāo*, Three Yin Intersection). Selection of points according to signs: For irascibility, add PC-6 (*nèi guān*, Inner Pass). For dizziness, add GB-20 (*fēng chí*, Wind Pool). For distention and pain in the head, add Greater Yang (*tài yáng*) and LI-4 (*hé gǔ*, Union Valley). For tinnitus, add TB-17 (*yì fēng*, Wind Screen) and GB-39 (*jué gǔ*, Severed Bone). For insomnia, add HT-7 (*shén mén*, Spirit Gate), PC-6 (*nèi guān*, Inner Pass), and Alert Spirit Quartet (*sì shén cōng*). For heart palpitations, add HT-7 (*shén mén*, Spirit Gate), PC-6 (*nèi guān*, Inner Pass), and BL-15 (*xīn shū*, Heart Transport). For lumbar pain, add GV-3 (*yāo yáng guān*, Lumbar Yang Pass), BL-40 (*wěi zhōng*, Bend Center), and ouch points (*ā shì xué*). For weakness in the legs, add GB-34 (*yáng líng quán*, Yang Mound Spring), ST-36 (*zú sān lǐ*, Leg Three Li), and GB-39 (*jué gǔ*, Severed Bone). [27: 151] [97: 287] [57: 47] [46: 618, 621, 648] [113: 14, 203] [13: 428]

ascendant liver yang 肝阳上亢 *gān yáng shàng kàng*: ASCENDANT HYPERACTIVITY OF LIVER YANG.

ashen nail 灰指甲 *huī zhǐ jiǎ*: *Synonyms: goose-claw wind; oily ashen nail.* A disease of the fingers and toes that starts with itching around the nail and that deprives the nail of nourishment of the blood, causing it gradually to thicken, loose its luster, take on an ashen appearance, and eventually to crumble and become deformed. Ashen nail can be treated by soaking in Vinegar Soaking Formula (*cù pào fāng*) or applying pig's bile or crushed fresh garden balsam flower (*fèng xiān huā*). Compare also GOOSE-FOOT WIND. [26: 345]

a-shi point 阿是穴 *ā shì xué*: OUCH POINT.

assail 袭 *xí*, 侵袭 *qīn xí*: Intrude, as of evils into the exterior of the body. See EXUBERANCE AND DEBILITATION.

assistant 佐 *zuǒ*: See SOVEREIGN, MINISTER, ASSISTANT, AND COURIER.

assisting bone 辅骨 *fǔ gǔ*: The smaller of the two bones of the forearm and lower leg. [WMC] radius and fibula. These bones are so named because they provide support to the main bones (ulna and tibia). [27: 70] [97: 511]

assisting yang 助阳 *zhù yáng*: SUPPLEMENTING YANG. [27: 282] [97: 281]

assisting yang and resolving the exterior 助阳解表 *zhù yáng jiě biǎo*: To treat yang qi vacuity in external contractions with signs such as pronounced aversion to cold with mild heat effusion, absence of sweating, lack of warmth in the extremities, desire to wrap up well to keep warm, fatigued essence-spirit, headache, somnolence, somber white facial complexion, faint low voice, white tongue fur, and a forceless sunken pulse. An example of a yang-assisting exterior-resolving formula is Renewal Powder (*zài zào sǎn*), which contains astragalus (*huáng qí*), codonopsis (*dǎng shēn*), cinnamon twig (*guì zhī*), licorice (*gān cǎo*), cooked aconite (*shú fù zǐ*), asarum (*xì xīn*), notopterygium (*qiāng huó*), ledebouriella (*fáng fēng*), ligusticum (*chuān xiōng*), fresh ginger (*shēng jiāng*), peony (*sháo yào*), and jujube (*dà zǎo*). [27: 250] [97: 281]

associated point 背俞 *bèi shū*: BACK TRANSPORT POINT.

astringent formula 涩剂 *sè jì*: One of the TEN FORMULA TYPES. Astringent [medicinals] can eliminate desertion, i.e., they can treat efflux desertion and insecurity patterns. Formulas in which such medicinals predominate are called astringent formulas. For example, Oyster Shell Powder (*mǔ lì sǎn*), which contains oyster shell (*mǔ lì*), ephedra root (*má huáng gēn*), and astragalus (*huáng qí*), treats spontaneous sweating after disease due to insecurity of defense qi, whereas Golden Lock Essence-Securing Pill (*jīn suǒ gù jīng wán*) containing complanate astragalus seed (*shā yuàn zǐ*), euryale (*qiàn shí*), dragon bone (*lóng gǔ*), and oyster shell (*mǔ lì*) treats kidney vacuity with seminal emission. [27: 306] [97: 485]

astringent [medicinals] can eliminate desertion 涩可去脱 *sè kě qù tuō*: Astringent medicinals such as dragon bone (*lóng gǔ*) and oyster shell (*mǔ lì*) can treat efflux desertion and insecurity patterns. See ASTRINGENT FORMULA. [27: 174]

astringing essence 涩精 *sè jīng*: SECURING ESSENCE.

astringing essence and checking seminal emission and enuresis 涩精止遗 *sè jīng zhǐ yí*: A method of treatment addressing SEMINAL EMISSION or SEMINAL EFFLUX attributed to kidney vacuity with insecurity of the ESSENCE GATE or enuresis or frequent urination due to kidney vacuity with bladder retention failure. For kidney vacuity seminal emission, kidney-supplementing essence-astringing medicinals such as complanate astragalus seed (*shā yuàn zǐ*), dragon bone (*lóng gǔ*), oyster shell (*mǔ lì*), lotus stamen (*lián xū*), mantis egg-case (*sāng piāo xiāo*), euryale (*qiàn shí*), cornus (*shān zhū yú*), and Cherokee rose fruit (*jīn yīng zǐ*) are used. For enuresis or frequent urination, a similar range of medicinals are used: mantis egg-case (*sāng piāo xiāo*), rubus (*fù pén zǐ*), and alpinia (*yì zhì rén*). Representative formulas include Golden Lock Essence-Securing Pill (*jīn suǒ gù jīng wán*), designed for seminal emission, but also used for enuresis, Mantis Egg-Case Powder (*sāng piāo xiāo sǎn*) originally designed for enuresis, but also used for seminal emission, and Stream-Reducing Pill (*suō quán wán*), mainly used for enuresis, frequent urination, and child bedwetting. [16: 355]

astringing the intestines 涩肠 *sè cháng*: See *astringing the intestines and stemming desertion.*

astringing the intestines and checking diarrhea 涩肠止泻 *sè cháng zhǐ xiè*: ASTRINGING THE INTESTINES AND STEMMING DESERTION. [27: 286] [97: 485]

astringing the intestines and stemming desertion 涩肠固脱 *sè cháng gù tuō*: Synonym: *astringing the intestines and checking diarrhea.* The method of treating enduring diarrhea and fecal incontinence, or persistent pus and blood in the stool with dark red blood, conditions that culminate in efflux desertion and prolapse of the rectum, abdominal pain that likes warmth and pressure, and a weak slow pulse. Intestine-astringing medicinals include ones that are warm and supplement the spleen and kidney such as codonopsis (*dǎng shēn*), ovate atractylodes (*bái zhú*), aconite (*fù zǐ*), cinnamon twig (*guì zhī*), and dried ginger (*gān jiāng*). To these should be added securing astringent medicinals to astringe the bowels and stem desertion, such as psoralea (*bǔ gǔ zhī*), nutmeg (*ròu dòu kòu*), schisandra (*wǔ wèi zǐ*), poppy husk (*yīng sù ké*), halloysite (*chì shí zhī*), limonite (*yǔ yú liáng*), dioscorea (*shān yào*), euryale (*qiàn shí*), and lotus seed (*lián ròu*). A representative formula is True Man Viscus-Nourishing Decoction (*zhēn rén yǎng zàng tāng*). [50: 1316] [6: 267] [16: 349]

atony 痿 *wěi*: WILTING.

¹**attack** 攻 *gōng*: Synonym: *offensive treatment.* **1.** To treat repletion, especially with drastic draining precipitants. **2.** (Of evils) to affect forcefully, e.g., fire toxin attacking the inner body.

²**attack** 发作 *fā zuò*: EPISODE.

attack followed by supplementation 先攻后补 *xiān gōng hòu bǔ*: The principle of destroying evil (attack) before any vacuity is supplemented. The principle of attack followed by supplementation is applied when an extremely strong evil urgently needs to be dispelled, and right qi, though markedly weakened, can still withstand attack, especially where the weakness of right qi is attributable to the evil. This principle may apply in the treatment of gastrointestinal heat bind, and

other externally contracted heat (febrile) diseases characterized by constipation and painful fullness in the abdomen. Such conditions may be treated with Major Qi-Coordinating Decoction (*dà chéng qì tāng*) even though yin may have been damaged; indeed, failure to precipitate the heat bind would cause further damage to yin. [27: 257] [6: 244]

attacking phlegm 攻痰 *gōng tán*: A method of treatment used to address stagnant, binding phlegm such as occurs in epilepsy, mania, and withdrawal, or in child fright wind characterized by gurgling phlegm congesting the throat, and convulsions of the limbs. The main medicinals used are chlorite/mica (*méng shí*) and tingli (*tíng lì zǐ*) A commonly used formula is Chlorite/Mica Phlegm-Rolling Pill (*méng shí gǔn tán wán*).

audio-olfactory examination 闻诊 *wén zhěn*: LISTENING AND SMELLING.

auricle 耳廓 *ěr kuò*: The trumpet-shaped flap of the ear used to catch sounds. [26: 250]

autumn dryness 秋燥 *qiū zào*: A disease attributable to contraction of dryness qi in autumn, and usually manifesting as mild conditions that undergo relatively few SHIFTS. Distinction is made between cool dryness and warm dryness. Cool dryness is characterized by heat effusion, headache, aversion to cold, absence of sweating, dry lips and throat, ungratifying coughing of phlegm, and dry thin white tongue fur. Warm dryness is marked by heat effusion, mild aversion to cold, headache, dry skin, cough with sticky phlegm, dry nose and throat, thirst, and yellow urine. Wu Gen-Chu states, "In the depth of autumn when cold weather begins and the west wind kills and depurates, wind-dryness is what is mostly contracted; this is cool dryness.... If there are long spells of clear, rainless weather and exposure to the autumn sun, warm dryness is mostly what is contracted; this is dryness-heat." This suggests that the distinction is made on the basis of weather conditions. The warm disease school places greater emphasis on warm dryness. MED Cool dryness is treated by acrid opening and warm moistening, and by coursing the evil and diffusing the lung. Apricot Kernel and Perilla Powder (*xìng sū sǎn*) or Scallion and Fermented Soybean Decoction (*cōng chǐ tāng*) may be used. Warm dryness is treated by acrid cooling and sweet moistening with formulas such as Mulberry Leaf and Apricot Kernel Decoction (*sāng xìng tāng*). ACU For cool dryness, base treatment mainly on LU, LI, KI, and BL. Select BL-13 (*fèi shū*, Lung Transport), BL-12 (*fēng mén*, Wind Gate), LU-5 (*chǐ zé*, Cubit Marsh), LU-7 (*liè quē*, Broken Sequence), LI-4 (*hé gǔ*, Union Valley), and KI-6 (*zhào hǎi*, Shining Sea); needle with drainage. For pronounced external cold, use moxa. For warm dryness, base treatment mainly on LU and KI. Drain BL-13 (*fèi shū*, Lung Transport), CV-17 (*shān zhōng*, Chest Center), LU-5 (*chǐ zé*, Cubit Marsh), LI-11 (*qū chí*, Pool at the Bend), and CV-22 (*tiān tú*, Celestial Chimney); and supplement KI-6 (*zhào hǎi*, Shining Sea). See also DRYNESS EVIL INVADING THE LUNG. [26: 443] [27: 352]

aversion 相恶 *xiāng wù*: See SEVEN RELATIONS.

aversions of the five viscera 五脏所恶 *wǔ zàng suǒ wù*: *Synonym: five aversions*. The notion contained in *Elementary Questions* (*sù wèn*) that the five viscera are each averse to a particular evil. See HEART IS AVERSE TO HEAT; LUNG IS AVERSE TO COLD; LIVER IS AVERSE TO WIND; SPLEEN IS AVERSE TO DAMPNESS; KIDNEY IS AVERSE TO DRYNESS. See these individual entries. [27: 61] [97: 56]

aversion to cold 恶寒 *wù hán*: *Synonyms: fear of cold*. A pronounced sensation of cold. With heat effusion, it is a sign of wind-cold; without heat effusion, it is associated with cold arising from within due to yang qi vacuity. External cold striking the bowels and viscera directly can also manifest in aversion to cold without heat effusion, in which case it is accompanied by cold signs in the affected area such as cold stomach duct pain and clear-food diarrhea. Compare ABHORRENCE OF COLD; SHIVERING. ◇ Chin 恶 *wù*, averse (aversion) to (otherwise read as *ě*; see NAUSEA); 寒 *hán*, cold. NB: The English 'chill' has connotations of sudden onset and hence does not adequately cover the sensation of cold associated with yang qi vacuity. 'Aversion to cold', a literal translation of the Chinese, is the preferred term. [27: 355] [97: 462] [26: 685]

aversion to cold in the back 背恶寒 *bèi wù hán*: COLD BACK.

aversion to food 厌食 *yàn shí*, 恶食 *wù shí*: **1.** Absence of appetite and sickness at the thought or sight of food. Aversion to food is most commonly observed when voracious eating and drinking impairs decomposition, causing food to stagnate in the stomach. Hence, it is said, "Food damage is invariably characterized by aversion to food." If aversion to food occurs with vomiting, ab-

sence of menstruation, and a rapid slippery pulse in sexually active women, it is a sign of pregnancy vomiting which arises when an upsurge of thoroughfare vessel qi causes disharmony of stomach qi. Aversion to food differs from poor appetite, which is a reduced feeling of hunger. See POOR APPETITE. **2.** MALIGN OBSTRUCTION. [26: 685] [29: 198] [24: 148]

aversion to heat 恶热 *wù rè*: Abnormal intolerance of heat. Aversion to heat is observed in externally contracted heat (febrile) disease and in internal damage. (1) In externally contracted heat (febrile) disease, aversion to heat is associated with yang brightness (*yáng míng*) disease. (2) In internal damage disease, aversion to heat is associated with yin vacuity and with repletion fire in the stomach. [27: 356] [97: 462] [26: 685]

aversion to light 恶光羞明 *wù guāng xiū míng*: *Synonyms: photophobia; aversion to lights and fire*. Abnormal insensitivity to or intolerance of light—and sometimes also of warmth (aversion to lights and fire)—causing a desire to close the eyes. Aversion to light, in addition to being experienced after prolonged deprivation of light and during resuscitation after drowning, is observed in some eye diseases. In wind-cold fettering the exterior, aversion is associated with red sore eyes, copious thick discharge, distention in the brow, and nasal congestion and runny nose. In qi vacuity with wind-heat, it is associated with soreness of the eyes, and tension in the canthi, tearing on exposure to wind, and flowery vision. In dual vacuity of qi and yin, it is associated with flowery vision, tendency to close the eyes, slight redness of the whites of the eyes, dizziness and tinnitus, dry throat, sloppy stool, and fear of cold in the lower limbs. In this context, it is specifically observed, for example, in GAN OF THE LIVER. [27: No. 455]

aversion to lights and fire 恶见灯火 *wù jiàn dēng huǒ*: See AVERSION TO LIGHT.

aversion to wind 恶风 *wù fēng*: *Synonym: fear of wind*. Sensation of cold on exposure to a wind or draft; mild aversion to cold. Aversion to wind is usually a sign of external evils assailing the FLESHY EXTERIOR. Compare AVERSION TO COLD. [97: 461] [26: 685]

B

baby moth 乳蛾 *rǔ é*, 蛾子 *é zǐ*: *Synonyms: nipple moth*; *throat moth*. Redness, swelling, and soreness of either or both of the throat nodes (tonsils) with a yellowish white discharge visible on their surface. Baby moth is attributable to a) congesting lung-stomach heat with fire toxin steaming upward; b) qi stagnation and congealing blood together with old phlegm and liver fire binding to form malign blood; or c) liver kidney yin-liquid depletion with vacuity fire flaming upward. Accompanying signs include constipation, a thick slimy tongue fur, difficulty in swallowing fluids, and alternating heat [effusion] and [aversion to] cold. WMC tonsillitis. MED Congesting lung-stomach heat is treated by coursing wind and diffusing the lung, and by dispersing swelling and resolving toxin; formulas such as Throat-Clearing Diaphragm-Disinhibiting Decoction (*qīng yān lì gé tāng*) can be used. Liver fire patterns are treated by clearing heat and expelling phlegm with formulas such as Pathfinder Poria (Hoelen) Pill (*zhǐ mí fú líng wán*). Effulgent yin vacuity fire patterns are treated by enriching yin and downbearing fire with formulas such as Anemarrhena, Phellodendron, and Rehmannia Pill (*zhī bǎi dì huáng wán*). Nipple moth assuming a nipple-like shape without severe pain and brought on by contraction of cold is called STONE MOTH, a condition that is difficult to treat. ACU For lung-stomach heat, base treatment mainly on LU, LI, and ST. Select LI-4 (*hé gǔ*, Union Valley), LI-11 (*qū chí*, Pool at the Bend), LU-5 (*chǐ zé*, Cubit Marsh), ST-44 (*nèi tíng*, Inner Court), ST-43 (*xiàn gǔ*, Sunken Valley), and CV-22 (*tiān tú*, Celestial Chimney); needle with drainage, and prick TB-1 (*guān chōng*, Passage Hub), LU-11 (*shào shāng*, Lesser Shang), and LI-1 (*shāng yáng*, Shang Yang) to bleed. For phlegm turbidity and liver fire, base treatment mainly on LR, GB, and ST. Select LI-4 (*hé gǔ*, Union Valley), LR-3 (*tài chōng*, Supreme Surge), LR-2 (*xíng jiān*, Moving Between), GB-34 (*yáng líng quán*, Yang Mound Spring), SP-6 (*sān yīn jiāo*, Three Yin Intersection), ST-36 (*zú sān lǐ*, Leg Three Li), and ST-40 (*fēng lóng*, Bountiful Bulge); needle with drainage. For effulgent yin vacuity fire, base treatment mainly on KI and LU. Select KI-3 (*tài xī*, Great Ravine), KI-6 (*zhào hǎi*, Shining Sea), and LU-10 (*yú jì*, Fish Border); needle with even supplementation and drainage, and prick LU-11 (*shào shāng*, Lesser Shang) to bleed. ◇ Chin 乳 *rǔ*, breast, milk, suckle, suckling; 蛾 *é*, moth. The name is usually understood as a double metaphor (a swelling both like a nipple and like a moth) although, as has been pointed out [98], "suckling moth" (i.e., baby moth) is an equally plausible interpretation, which is supported by the alternate name *é zǐ*. [26: 379] [27: 497] [97: 358] [46: 723] [113: 505]

back 背 *bèi*: The rear aspect of the trunk from the shoulder to the buttocks, especially the part excluding the lumbus. The back is considered yang in relationship to the chest and abdomen, which are yin. [27: 69] [97: 401]

back associated point 背俞 *bèi shū*: BACK TRANSPORT POINT.

back pain 背痛 *bèi tòng*: Pain in the upper part of the back, as distinct from lumbar (low back) pain. The two main patterns are wind-cold and qi stagnation and blood stasis. **Wind-cold** back pain is pain and stiffness in the back stretching into the nape, with inhibited movement of the shoulder blade, or heaviness and stiffness in the back with aversion to cold. MED Dispel wind and dissipate cold using Notopterygium Dampness-Overcoming Decoction (*qiāng huó shèng shī tāng*). Channel conductors such as ledebouriella (*fáng fēng*) and notopterygium (*qiāng huó*) can be used according to the precise location of discomfort. ACU Base treatment mainly on GV, BL, and GB. Select GB-20 (*fēng chí*, Wind Pool), GV-16 (*fēng fǔ*, Wind Mansion), TB-5 (*wài guān*, Outer Pass), LI-4 (*hé gǔ*, Union Valley), GV-26 (*rén zhōng*, Human Center), GV-12 (*shēn zhù*, Body Pillar), GV-4 (*mìng mén*, Life Gate), GV-3 (*yāo yáng guān*, Lumbar Yang Pass), BL-60 (*kūn lún*, Kunlun Mountains), and BL-40 (*wěi zhōng*, Bend Center); needle with drainage and add moxa. **Qi stagnation and blood stasis** back pain is most common in the elderly and in patients left weak after enduring disease, and is marked by aching back pain with numbness in the elbow after waking from sleep, where discomfort is relieved by physical activity. MED Treat by boosting qi and nourishing the blood, assisted by quickening the blood. Use Impediment-Alleviating Decoction (*juān bì tāng*) combined with Minor Network-Quickening Elixir (*xiǎo huó luò dān*). The channel conductors given above may be used. ACU Base treatment mainly on GV, BL, CV, SP, and LR. Select CV-6 (*qì hǎi*, Sea of Qi), LR-3 (*tài chōng*, Supreme Surge), LI-4 (*hé gǔ*, Union Valley), BL-17 (*gé shū*, Diaphragm

Transport), SP-10 (*xuè hǎi*, Sea of Blood), SP-6 (*sān yīn jiāo*, Three Yin Intersection), GV-26 (*rén zhōng*, Human Center), BL-43 (*gāo huāng shū*, Gao-Huang Transport), GV-12 (*shēn zhù*, Body Pillar), GV-3 (*yāo yáng guān*, Lumbar Yang Pass), and BL-40 (*wěi zhōng*, Bend Center); needle with even supplementation and drainage or with supplementation, and add moxa. [92: No. 161] [46: 629, 633] [113: 228] [4: 144]

back transport point 背俞 *bèi shū*: Any of a group of points on the bladder channel, 1.5 body-inches either side of the spinal column, each associated with, and named after, an organ whose qi is said to pass through their locations. The back transport points of the bowels and viscera are given in the list below. **Application:** Back transport points are used to diagnose and treat the bowels and viscera with which they are associated. When the qi of a particular bowels or viscus is inhibited, qi collects at the transport point, and tenderness or other abnormalities can be detected by palpation. Thus, the transport points are primarily used to treat diseases of the five viscera and the tissues and sense organs to which they are related. This usage accords with *The Classic of Difficult Issues* (*nàn jīng*), which states that "yin disease moves to the yang," i.e., disease in the yin aspect of the body, the viscera, manifests in the yang aspect of the body, the back. Back transport points are also appropriate for the treatment of acute diseases. They are drained to treat repletion of the bowel or viscus with which they are associated, and supplemented to treat vacuity. **Combinations:** The transport points may be combined with alarm points of the respective bowels and viscera. See COMBINING TRANSPORT AND ALARM POINTS. [27: 102]

Back Transport Points

Lung: BL-13 (*fèi shū*, Lung Transport)
Heart: BL-15 (*xīn shū*, Heart Transport)
Liver: BL-18 (*gān shū*, Liver Transport)
Spleen: BL-20 (*pí shū*, Spleen Transport)
Kidney: BL-23 (*shèn shū*, Kidney Transport)
Gallbladder: BL-19 (*dǎn shū*, Gallbladder Transport)
Stomach: BL-21 (*wèi shū*, Stomach Transport)
Bladder: BL-28 (*páng guāng shū*, Bladder Transport)
Triple burner: BL-22 (*sān jiāo shū*, Triple Burner Transport)
Large intestine: BL-25 (*dà cháng shū*, Large Intestine Transport)
Small intestine: BL-27 (*xiǎo cháng shū*, Small Intestine Transport)

bad breath 口臭 *kǒu chòu*: Fetid breath. When poor oral hygiene or tooth decay, which are com-

mon causes, have been ruled out, bad breath is attributable to stomach heat steaming upward, phlegm heat congesting the lung, or gastrointestinal food accumulation. **Stomach heat** steaming upward causes bad breath with thirst as well as intake of cold drinks, red lips, mouth sores, erosion of the mouth or red sore swollen gums, reddish urine, constipation, yellow tongue fur, and a forceful rapid pulse. MED Clear the stomach and discharge heat with Stomach-Clearing Decoction (*qīng wèi tāng*) or Gastrodia and Astragalus Decoction (*shēng má huáng qí tāng*). If there is bowel repletion with constipation, use Diaphragm-Cooling Powder (*liáng gé sǎn*). ACU Base treatment mainly on ST, LI, and PC. Select ST-44 (*nèi tíng*, Inner Court), ST-36 (*zú sān lǐ*, Leg Three Li), LI-4 (*hé gǔ*, Union Valley), and PC-7 (*dà líng*, Great Mound). Needle with drainage. **Phlegm-heat congesting the lung** causes fishy-smelling breath with pain or fullness in the chest, cough with ejection of turbid phlegm, coughing up of blood, dry throat, bitter taste in the mouth and dry tongue with no desire to drink, a slimy yellow tongue fur, and a slippery rapid pulse. MED Treat by dispersing accumulations and abducting stagnation with Harmony-Preserving Pill (*bǎo hé wán*) or Unripe Bitter Orange Stagnation-Abducting Pill (*zhǐ shí dǎo zhì wán*). ACU Base treatment mainly on LU, ST, LI and PC. Select BL-13 (*fèi shū*, Lung Transport), LU-5 (*chǐ zé*, Cubit Marsh), ST-40 (*fēng lóng*, Bountiful Bulge), LI-4 (*hé gǔ*, Union Valley), LI-11 (*qū chí*, Pool at the Bend), ST-44 (*nèi tíng*, Inner Court), and PC-7 (*dà líng*, Great Mound). Needle with drainage. **Gastrointestinal food accumulation** causes sour bad breath with distention and fullness in the stomach duct and abdomen, frequent belching, no thought of food and drink, constipation or uninhibited stool, foul-smelling flatus, thick slimy or putrid slimy tongue fur, and a slippery rapid pulse. MED Use White-Draining Powder (*xiè bái sǎn*) or Thousand Gold Pieces Phragmites Decoction (*qiān jīn wěi jīng tāng*). ACU Base treatment mainly on CV, ST, and PC. Select Li Inner Court (*lǐ nèi tíng*), CV-21 (*xuán jī*, Jade Swivel), CV-10 (*xià wǎn*, Lower Stomach Duct), ST-25 (*tiān shū*, Celestial Pivot), CV-6 (*qì hǎi*, Sea of Qi), ST-36 (*zú sān lǐ*, Leg Three Li), ST-37 (*shàng jù xū*, Upper Great Hollow), ST-44 (*nèi tíng*, Inner Court), and PC-7 (*dà líng*, Great Mound). Needle with drainage. [26: 61] [92: No. 86] [4: 98] [46: 597, 653, 662, 725] [113: 51, 223, 508]

bad odor 臭气 *chòu qì*: See MALODOR.

bag-over-the-head sensation 头重如裹 *tóu zhòng rú guǒ*: HEAD HEAVY AS IF SWATHED.

baking heat [effusion] 烘热 *hōng rè*: Pronounced, persistent heat effusion associated with damage to yin, and usually attended by vexation, insomnia, and oppression. See HEAT EFFUSION.

bald scalp sore 禿疮 *tū chuāng*: BALD WHITE SCALP SORE.

bald white scalp sore 白禿疮 *bái tū chuāng*, 白禿 *bái tū*: Synonyms: *white perverse crop*; *lai scalp sore*. A disease of the scalp mostly seen in children and characterized by white crusts that spread and coalesce, and that are associated with unbearable itching and hair loss on the affected area. The hair usually grows back once the sores heal. Bald white scalp sores are attributed to wind evil invading the interstices of the scalp or to the use of unclean hair-dressing implements. ⎡MED⎤ Treat with Chinaberry Root Bark Paste (*kǔ liàn gāo*) or Bald Sores Oil (*tū chuāng yóu*). ⎡ACU⎤ Needle with drainage bilaterally at LI-11 (*qū chí*, Pool at the Bend), with supplementation bilaterally at KI-2 (*rán gǔ*, Blazing Valley), and with even supplemenation and drainage at BL-18 (*gān shū*, Liver Transport), BL-23 (*shèn shū*, Kidney Transport), and ST-36 (*zú sān lǐ*, Leg Three Li). [26: 220] [27: 473] [97: 155] [15: 384]

banking up earth 培土 *péi tǔ*: Supplementing spleen-earth to restore normal movement and transformation. The method of banking up earth is used to treat spleen vacuity with reduced food intake and diarrhea. [27: 263]

banking up earth and repressing wood 培土抑木 *pí tǔ yì mù*: FORTIFYING THE SPLEEN AND COURSING THE LIVER. [27: 263]

banking up earth to dam water 培土制水 *péi tǔ zhì shuǐ*: A method of treatment used to address water swelling by fortifying the spleen and boosting qi. Here, earth refers to the spleen, but water refers not to the kidney but to water-damp. [6: 34]

banking up earth to engender metal 培土生金 *péi tǔ shēng jīn*: A method of treatment that involves fortifying the spleen to treat diseases of the lung. Banking up earth and engendering metal is used, for example, in the treatment of phlegm that arises when water-damp gathers and concentrates as a result of impaired splenic movement and transformation. See SUPPLEMENTING THE SPLEEN TO BOOST THE LUNG. [6: 33] [27: 263] [97: 512]

bar 关 *guān*: **1.** The pulse position between the inch and cubit. See WRIST PULSE. **2.** Any one of the segments in the INFANT'S FINGER EXAMINATION.

base joint 本节 *běn jié*: The joint at which a digit springs from the hand or foot. [27: 74] [97: 137]

basket-steam 笼蒸 *lóng zhēng*: To steam in steaming baskets.

bean curd tongue fur 腐苔 *fǔ tāi*: Synonym: *tofu tongue fur*. A lumpy, easily removable fur like crumbs of bean curd (tofu). A bean curd tongue fur indicates the development of sweltering damp-heat in patterns of damage to yin by stomach vacuity. This generally occurs in enduring or severe illnesses and indicates complex patterns that are difficult to treat. ◇ Chin 腐 *fǔ*, rot, rotten, here an abbreviation for 豆腐 (*dòu fǔ*), bean curd (lit. bean rot, so called because it is soft like things that have turned rotten); *tāi*, moss. [27: 182] [97: 631] [27: 124]

¹**bearing** 态 *tài*, 姿态 *zī tài*, 动态 *dòng tài*: Posture and movement. Examining a patient's bearing is an important part of diagnosis. Flailing of the limbs, agitation and talkativeness, or manic agitation and desire to throw off clothing and bedclothes usually indicates a yang disease, i.e., a disease due to heat or repletion. A patient who sleeps curled up, is uncommunicative, who suffers from a general feeling of heaviness and difficulty in movement, and who keeps his body well wrapped, is ordinarily suffering from a yin disease, i.e., a disease of cold or vacuity. GROPING IN THE AIR AND PULLING AT INVISIBLE STRINGS and PICKING AT BEDCLOTHES indicate that the illness has reached its most advanced stage and that the condition is severe. Deviated eyes and mouth, convulsions of the limbs, shaking of the head, and twitching of the lips or cheeks are conditions mostly attributable to LIVER WIND STIRRING INTERNALLY. Pronounced forceful spasm is usually seen in repletion heat patterns, whereas milder forms usually indicate vacuity wind. RIGIDITY OF THE NECK, ARCHED-BACK RIGIDITY (opisthotonos), and CLENCHED JAW (trismus) indicate TETANY (*jìng*). HYPERTONICITY OF THE LIMBS inhibiting normal bending and stretching, and rigidity, distention, and deformation of the joints usually indicate IMPEDIMENT (*bì*). Weakness and limpness of the limbs that deprives the patient of the ability to grasp things and move about freely indicates WILTING (*wěi*). If the patient suffers from rapid breathing while lying, and is thus forced to sit up, an exuberant evil is present and right qi is vacuous. Dizziness experienced when sitting up, confining the patient to a lying posture, usually indicates either a vacuity pattern or PHLEGM TURBIDITY HARASSING THE UPPER BODY. [6: 116]

²**bearing** 升降 *shēng jiàng*: Upward and downward bearing of qi, e.g., upbearing of clear yang and downbearing of the turbid. See, for example, SPLEEN GOVERNS UPBEARING OF THE CLEAR and STOMACH GOVERNS DOWNBEARING OF THE TURBID.

³**bearing** 升降浮沉 *shēng jiàng fú chén*: The direction of medicinal action, including upbearing, downbearing, floating, and sinking. Upbearing means ascending to the upper body; downbear-

ing means descending to the lower body. Floating means effusing and dissipating; sinking means draining and disinhibiting. Upbearing and floating medicinals (upfloaters) move upward and outward, and have actions such as upbearing yang, effusing the exterior, and dispersing cold. Downbearing and sinking medicinals (downsinkers) move downward and inward, have actions such as subduing yang, downbearing counterflow, astriction, clearing heat, percolating dampness, and draining. Most yang medicinals, which are warm or hot in nature and sweet and acrid in flavor, such as ephedra (*má huáng*), cinnamon twig (*guì zhī*), and astragalus (*huáng qí*), are upfloaters. Most yin medicinals, which are cold in nature and bitter or sour in nature, such as rhubarb (*dà huáng*), mirabilite (*máng xiāo*), and phellodendron (*huáng bǎi*), are downsinkers. Generally, flowers and leaves and other light medicinals such as asarum (*xì xīn*), mint (*bò hé*), and cimicifuga (*shēng má*), are upfloaters—inula flower (*xuán fù huā*) being an exception, whereas seeds, fruits, and heavy items, such as white perilla seed (*bái sū zǐ*), unripe bitter orange (*zhǐ shí*), and glauberite (*hán shuǐ shí*), are downsinkers—vitex (*màn jīng zǐ*) being an exception. Bearing can be imparted to other medicinals. Stir-frying with wine causes medicinals to bear upward; stir-frying with bran causes medicinals to downbear; stir-frying with ginger causes medicinals to dissipate; and stir-frying with vinegar causes medicinals to astringe. ◇ Chin 升 *shēng*, rise or cause to rise; 浮 *fú*, float (to the surface of the body); 沉 *chén*, sink, heavy; 降 *jiàng*, fall or cause to fall. [27: 315]

⁴**bearing** 所载 *suǒ zài*: The environment conducive to supporting the fetus in the uterus.

bedsore 蓐（褥）疮 *rù chuāng*: Synonym: *yin sores*. A sore on the back, sacrum, heels etc., that develops in comatose, paralyzed, or weak patients confined to bed. Bedsores start as red patches which gradually develop into ulcerations that are difficult to heal. They are attributable to major depletion of qi and blood in enduring illness with confinement to bed that causes friction and prevents the normal movement of qi and blood, thus depriving the skin of nourishment. MED Oral: Commonly used medicinals include astragalus (*huáng qí*), ovate atractylodes (*bái zhú*), codonopsis (*dǎng shēn*), poria (*fú líng*), tangkuei (*dāng guī*), red peony (*chì sháo yào*), white peony (*bái sháo yào*), salvia (*dān shēn*), lonicera (*jīn yín huā*), dandelion (*pú gōng yīng*), and raw licorice (*shēng gān cǎo*). Topical: Prior to ulceration, apply an alcohol compress, and then sprinkle with talcum (*huá shí*). After ulceration has started, apply Red Oil Paste (*hóng yóu gāo*) sprinkled with Nine-to-One Elixir (*jiǔ yī dān*). In the healing stage, use Flesh-

Engendering Jade and Red Paste (*shēng jī yù hóng gāo*). [96: 443]

bedwetting 尿床 *niào chuáng*: See ENURESIS.

begrudging milk 妒乳 *dù rǔ*: A condition attributable to the accumulation of breast milk arising after delivery when either there is no child to feed or the mother produces more milk than the child can take and characterized by hard painful distended breasts that cannot bear even the slightest touch. Small sores may grow on the nipples that may be sore or itchy and that, when scratched, exude yellow water that causes them to spread. MED Clear heat and resolve toxin. Use Forsythia Powder (*lián qiào sǎn*) from *The Golden Mirror of Medicine* (*yī zōng jīn jiàn*). If ruptured, apply Deerhorn Powder (*lù jiǎo sǎn*) which consists of deerhorn (*lù jiǎo*) and licorice (*gān cǎo*) ground to a powder and mixed with egg yolk (*jī zǐ huáng*). See MAMMARY WELLING-ABSCESS. ◇ Chin 妒 (same as 妬) *dù*, jealous; begrudge; 乳 *rǔ*, milk, breast. Possibly so called because the breast is, as it were, reluctant to release milk. [26: 396] [19: 3581]

begrudging semen sore 妒精疮 *dù jīng chuāng*: GAN SORE. ◇ Chin 妒 (same as 妬) *dù*, jealous; begrudge; 精 *jīng*, essence, semen; 疮 *chuāng*, sore. Possibly so called because of a popular belief that it is caused by withholding semen in order to preserve the body's essence.

belching 嗳气 *ài qì*, 噫气 *yī qì*: Synonym: *belching*. Expulsion of gas (qi) from the stomach that occurs after eating to satiation or eating too quickly, and in stomach diseases. It is one manifestation of STOMACH QI ASCENDING COUNTERFLOW. ACU Base treatment mainly on ST and CV. Select CV-6 (*qì hǎi*, Sea of Qi), PC-6 (*nèi guān*, Inner Pass), ST-36 (*zú sān lǐ*, Leg Three Li), CV-12 (*zhōng wǎn*, Center Stomach Duct), and BL-21 (*wèi shū*, Stomach Transport); needle with even supplementation and drainage, add moxa if appropriate. [26: 916] [27: 410] [97: 600, 644] [113: 82] [46: 602]

belching of putrid qi 嗳腐 *ài fǔ*: PUTRID BELCHING.

bell healer 铃医 *líng yī*: itinerant healer. [27: 516] [97: 474]

belly 肚 *dù*, 肚子 *dù zi*: ABDOMEN.

bencao 本草 *běn cǎo*: HERBAL FOUNDATION.

bend-center toxin [sore] 委中毒 *wěi zhōng dú*: Synonym: *bend-center welling-abscess*. A WELLING-ABSCESS (*yōng*) located at BL-40 (*wěi zhōng*, Bend Center), i.e., on the back of the knee (popliteal fossa). A bend-center toxin is attributed to accumulated heat in the gallbladder channel binding in the bladder channel or to stagnation of qi and blood in the kidney channel. Sometimes it develops from other sores at the site. The back of the knee becomes as hard as stone, is slightly red and swollen or scorching hot and red with generalized heat [effusion] and aversion to cold. It makes bending and stretching difficult and causes flexing. When the pain and swelling grows more severe day by day and the heat effusion and aversion to cold do not abated, this is a sign that pus has formed. [MED] Quicken the blood and transform stasis. Use Blood-Quickening Stasis-Dissipating Decoction (*huó xuè sàn yū tāng*). [26: 382] [27: 462]

bend-center welling-abscess 委中痈 *wěi zhōng yōng*: bend-center toxin (*sore*). [27: 462]

bent needle 弯针 *wān zhēn*: A needle that, owing to poor needle manipulation skill or physical movement by the patient, becomes bent after insertion in the human body. **Management:** Gently move the patient into the original posture in which the needle was inserted. Then gradually work the needle out. Do not under any circumstances use forceful or brisk movement, otherwise the needle may break. [27: 339] [27: 339] [97: 443]

beverage 饮 *yǐn*: A decoction that is left to cool before being taken, e.g., Elsholtzia Beverage (*xiāng rú yǐn*). Compare DRINK. [27: 441] [97: 295]

bi 痹 *bì*: IMPEDIMENT.

bian toxin [sore] 便毒 *biàn dú*: **1.** BUBO SORE. **2.** A BUBO SORE on right side of the body, as distinct from a FISH MOUTH, which is one on the left. ◇ The meaning of 便 *biàn* in this term is unclear. [27: 487] [26: 466] [97: 422] [19: 1014]

biaoju 瘭疽 *biāo jū*: TIP-ABSCESS.

bind 结 *jié*: **1.** To become tight, hard, or stiff. **2.** To cohere or make cohere. **3.** To constipate. *Bind* denotes a concentration of evils in a specific location, that causes hardness. When phlegm and qi bind, phlegm nodes form. When heat binds in the intestines, the stool becomes dry, solid, and difficult to evacuate. For example, large intestinal heat can cause heat bind, which is characterized by hard bound stool (i.e., constipation). When damp-heat gathers and binds in the lower burner, urinary stones form. In the term "binding depression of qi dynamic," it refers to frustrated movement of qi that can cause accumulation of phlegm or static blood. See STOPPAGE. ◇ Chin 结 *jié*, to knot, freeze, congeal, form, bear fruit.

binding depression of liver qi 肝气郁结 *gān qì yù jié*: *Synonyms: liver depression (depressed liver); liver qi depression (depressed liver qi).* Stagnation in the liver and liver channel resulting from impairment of the liver's function of free coursing. It arises when affect-mind frustration leads to depression and anger that damage the liver and impair free coursing. Other factors include invasion of external damp-heat and insufficiency of yin-blood depriving the liver of nourish-

ment. The chief signs are affect-mind depression, vexation, agitation, and irascibility. There is also distention and pain in the rib-side, oppression in the chest, and sighing. Other signs include distention and pain in the breasts before menstruation, distention and pain in the lesser abdomen, menstrual irregularities, plum-pit qi, goiter, accumulations and gatherings under the rib-side, jaundice, and epilepsy. The tongue body may be normal. The tongue fur is thin and white. The pulse is stringlike. **Analysis:** The liver channel skirts around the genitals, passes through the lesser abdomen, spreads over the rib-side and breasts, and passes up the neck. Binding depression of liver qi manifests in signs along this part of the liver channel pathway. Qi stagnation in the chest and rib-side region causes distending pain in the rib-side and frequent sighing. Liver qi depression may also ascend counterflow, carrying phlegm upward and causing plum-pit qi (the sensation of a lump in the throat that can neither be swallowed nor ejected). It can cause phlegm to bind at the neck, causing goiter (thyroid enlargement), characterized by soft swellings on both sides of the laryngeal prominence that move up and down when the patient swallows. Enduring depression of liver qi can cause blood stasis that develops into accumulations and gatherings under the rib-side. Blood stasis can cause water to collect, further giving rise to drum distention. When liver qi is depressed, it can affect other bowels and viscera. Liver qi invading the stomach manifests as nausea, vomiting, swallowing of upflowing acid, and acute abdominal pain and distention, or as painful distention and diarrhea. This can develop into liver-spleen disharmony with diarrhea. When caused by damp-heat, it can disrupt bile secretion, manifesting in jaundice and vomiting of bitter fluid or yellow bile (see *damp-heat brewing the liver and gallbladder*). It may also affect the thoroughfare (*chōng*) and controlling (*rèn*) vessels, leading to menstrual pain, menstrual block, premenstrual swelling of the breast, breast lumps, and menstrual irregularities. Whatever form liver qi depression takes, it can always manifest in or be caused by emotional disturbances such as anger, frustration, rashness and impatience. Severe depression of liver qi may lead to fire formation and the emergence of a liver fire flaming upward pattern or to damage to liver yin-blood, which manifests as a vacuity pattern. When patients with binding depression of liver qi also suffer from spleen vacuity with phlegm turbidity arising from within, liver qi can carry the phlegm turbidity upward to cloud the clear orifices, causing epileptic fits. Extreme depression may cause a counterflow upsurge of liver qi, one form of QI REVERSAL. **Comparison:** *Liver fire flaming upward:* Binding depression of liver qi and liver fire flaming upward are both associated with inhibition of liver channel qi causing rib-side pain and distention of the breasts. However, liver fire flaming upward is associated with heat signs not observed in simple binding depression of liver qi. Binding depression of liver qi is often associated with diarrhea from a strong liver that restrains the spleen and poor appetite. Liver fire flaming upward is associated with heat signs such as scorching pain in the rib-side, as well as headache, dizziness, tinnitus, deafness, red face and red ears. When liver fire scorches the blood network vessels, there may be blood ejection or spontaneous external bleeding. MED Binding depression of liver qi is treated by coursing the liver and rectifying qi. Medicinals commonly used to treat binding depression of liver qi include bupleurum (*chái hú*), curcuma (*yù jīn*), unripe tangerine peel (*qīng pí*), bitter orange (*zhǐ ké*), cyperus (*xiāng fù zǐ*), toosendan (*chuān liàn zǐ*), corydalis (*yán hú suǒ*), perilla stem (*zǐ sū gěng*), akebia (*bā yuè zhá*), liquidambar fruit (*lù lù tōng*), lindera (*wū yào*), and tangerine pip (*jú hé*). Bupleurum Liver-Coursing Powder (*chái hú shū gān sǎn*) or Depression-Overcoming Pill (*yuè jú wán*) may be used as a basic formula and varied according to need. Counterflow Cold Powder (*sì nì sǎn*) plus cyperus (*xiāng fù zǐ*), curcuma (*yù jīn*), and unripe tangerine peel (*qīng pí*) is a further option. When depressed qi transforms into fire, Moutan and Gardenia Free Wanderer Powder (*dān zhī xiāo yáo sǎn*) combined with Left-Running Metal Pill (*zuǒ jīn wán*) can be used, adding gentian (*lóng dǎn*) and rhubarb (*dà huáng*) for constipation. Liver qi invading the stomach can be treated with Left-Running Metal Pill (*zuǒ jīn wán*). Liver-spleen disharmony can be treated with Free Wanderer Powder (*xiāo yáo sǎn*) or Pain and Diarrhea Formula (*tòng xiè yào fāng*). Plum-pit qi is treated by downbearing qi and transforming phlegm with formulas such as Four-Seven Decoction (*sì qī tāng*) or Pinellia and Magnolia Bark Decoction (*bàn xià hòu pò tāng*). Goiter is treated by rectifying qi and dispersing goiter with Sargassum Jade Flask Decoction (*hǎi zǎo yù hú tāng*). Menstrual problems arising when binding depression of liver qi affects the thoroughfare (*chōng*) and controlling (*rèn*) vessels can be treated with variations of Free Wanderer Powder (*xiāo yáo sǎn*). Epilepsy can be treated with Fit-Settling Pill (*dìng xián wán*). Accumulations and gatherings can be treated with Bupleurum Liver-Coursing Powder (*chái hú shū gān sǎn*) combined with Toosendan Powder (*jīn líng zǐ sǎn*) or Saussurea Qi-Normalizing Decoction (*mù xiāng shùn qì tāng*). Drum distention can be treated with Bupleurum Liver-Coursing Powder (*chái hú shū gān sǎn*) combined with Stomach-Calming Powder (*píng wèi sǎn*), or Free Wanderer Powder (*xiāo yáo*

sǎn) combined with Harmony-Preserving Pill (*bǎo hé wán*). Most liver-coursing qi-rectifying medicinals are dry and aromatic, and therefore readily damage yin-blood. This effect can be reduced by the inclusion of liver-emolliating medicinals such as white peony (*bái sháo yào*), tangkuei (*dāng guī*), dried/fresh rehmannia (*shēng dì huáng*), and lycium berry (*gǒu qǐ zǐ*). ACU Base treatment mainly on LR, PC, SP and back transport points. Select BL-18 (*gān shū*, Liver Transport), PC-6 (*nèi guān*, Inner Pass), LR-3 (*tài chōng*, Supreme Surge), SP-6 (*sān yīn jiāo*, Three Yin Intersection), LR-13 (*zhāng mén*, Camphorwood Gate), ST-36 (*zú sān lǐ*, Leg Three Li), LR-2 (*xíng jiān*, Moving Between), TB-6 (*zhī gōu*, Branch Ditch), and GB-34 (*yáng líng quán*, Yang Mound Spring); needle with even supplementation and drainage and add moxa. Selection of points according to the signs: For mental depression, add HT-7 (*shén mén*, Spirit Gate) and GV-26 (*rén zhōng*, Human Center). For oppression in the chest, add CV-17 (*shān zhōng*, Chest Center). For rib-side pain and distention, add LR-14 (*qī mén*, Cycle Gate), GB-40 (*qiū xū*, Hill Ruins), and TB-5 (*wài guān*, Outer Pass). For pain and distention of the breasts, add CV-17 (*shān zhōng*, Chest Center) and LR-14 (*qī mén*, Cycle Gate). For pain and distention in the lesser abdomen, add LR-5 (*lǐ gōu*, Woodworm Canal), and LR-6 (*zhōng dū*, Central Metropolis). GB-32 (*zhōng dú*, Central River). For plum-pit qi, add CV-17 (*shān zhōng*, Chest Center), PC-5 (*jiān shǐ*, Intermediary Courier), and CV-22 (*tiān tú*, Celestial Chimney). [6: 185] [116: 98] [57: 56] [27: 152] [113: 14, 210, 267] [46: 594, 646] [37: 445]

binding depression of phlegm and qi 痰气郁结 *tán qì yù jié*: PHLEGM AND QI BINDING TOGETHER.

binding in yang 结阳 *jié yáng*: From *Elementary Questions* (*sù wèn, yīn yáng bié lùn*). A pathomechanism of swelling of the limbs. The four limbs are the root of yang, and when yang qi of the limbs congeals and binds, water collects. [27: 131] [27: 131] [97: 444]

binding in yin 结阴 *jié yīn*: From *Elementary Questions* (*sù wèn, yīn yáng bié lùn*). Evil qi binding in the yin channels. The liver belongs to reverting yin (*jué yīn*) and stores the blood; the spleen belongs to greater yin (*tài yīn*) and manages the blood. When evil qi binds in the yin channels, and is not moved by yang qi, in time the yin network vessels are damaged and the blood spills internally causing bloody stool. [27: 131] [26: 754]

birth 分娩 *fēn miǎn*, 分解 *fēn jiě*, 分诞 *fēn dàn*, 免身 *miǎn shēn*, 产 *chǎn*: CHILDBIRTH. [26: 171]

birth gate 产门 *chǎn mén*: **1.** YIN DOOR. **2.** The cervix of the uterus. The *Wings to the Classified Canon* (*lèi jīng fù yìqiú zhèng lù, sān jiāo bāo luò* *mìng mén*) states, "At the bottom of the uterus is a door, which in women can be felt with the hand. This is what is commonly called *chǎn mén*." [50: 608] [36: 102]

bitter 苦 *kǔ*: See BITTERNESS.

bitterness 苦 *kǔ*: The flavor of burnt things; the flavor associated with fire. Bitterness enters the heart; it can drain and dry. See FIVE FLAVORS and FIVE FLAVOR ENTRIES. [19: 12131]

bitterness enters the heart 苦入心 *kǔ rù xīn*: Bitter medicinals act on the heart. Examples of bitter medicinals that enter the heart are coptis (*huáng lián*), scutellaria (*huáng qín*), gardenia (*shān zhī zǐ*), forsythia (*lián qiào*), moutan (*mǔ dān pí*), polygala (*yuǎn zhì*), dried rehmannia (*gān dì huáng*), salvia (*dān shēn*), madder (*qiàn cǎo gēn*), and peach kernel (*táo rén*).

bitter taste in the mouth 口苦 *kǒu kǔ*: Experience of a bitter flavor not attributable to foodstuffs. Bitter taste is the most commonly reported deviation from "harmony of mouth." It is explained in terms of bile in the mouth. *The Magic Pivot* (*líng shū, sì shí qì piàn*) states, "When bile is discharged, there is a bitter taste in the mouth." It is a sign of liver or gallbladder disease and most commonly reflects steaming of gallbladder qi when there is heat in the liver and gallbladder. *Elementary Questions* (*sù wèn, qí bìng lùn*) states, "When there is illness marked by a bitter taste in the mouth... the disease is called 'gallbladder pure heat'... the person [affected] is one who plots and schemes indecisively, so that the gallbladder becomes vacuous and qi spills upward to make the mouth bitter." **Lesser yang disease** causes bitter taste in the mouth with dry throat, headache, dizzy vision, alternating heat [effusion] and [aversion to] cold, bitter fullness in the chest and rib-side, heart vexation and frequent vomiting, reduced intake of food, yellow urine, thin white or yellow tongue fur, and a forceful floating stringlike pulse. *On Cold Damage* (*shāng hán lùn*) states, "Lesser yang (*shào yáng*) disease: bitter taste in the mouth, and dizzy vision." MED Harmonize the lesser yang with variations of Minor Bupleurum Decoction (*xiǎo chái hú tāng*). ACU Base treatment mainly on TB, PC, GB, and LR. Select TB-4 (*yáng chí*, Yang Pool), PC-6 (*nèi guān*, Inner Pass), GB-40 (*qiū xū*, Hill Ruins), LR-5 (*lǐ gōu*, Woodworm Canal), and GB-38 (*yáng fǔ*, Yang Assistance); needle with even supplemenation and drainage or with drainage. **Depressed liver-gallbladder heat** can cause bitter taste in the mouth with heart vexation, dry mouth with desire to drink, sighing and irascibility, dizzy head and headache, red eyes and dizzy vision, distention and pain in the rib-sides, yellow urine, stool tending to be dry, red margins of

the tongue, thin yellow or slimy yellow tongue fur, and a rapid stringlike pulse. MED Clear and resolve depressed liver-gallbladder heat using Gentian Liver-Draining Decoction (*lóng dǎn xiè gān tāng*). If there is phlegm-heat harassing the inner body, use Coptis Gallbladder-Warming Decoction (*huáng lián wēn dǎn tāng*). ACU Base treatment mainly on LR and GB. Select BL-18 (*gān shū*, Liver Transport), LR-2 (*xíng jiān*, Moving Between), GB-43 (*xiá xī*, Pinched Ravine), GB-34 (*yáng líng quán*, Yang Mound Spring), GB-40 (*qiū xū*, Hill Ruins), ST-36 (*zú sān lǐ*, Leg Three Li), PC-6 (*nèi guān*, Inner Pass), and GB-38 (*yáng fǔ*, Yang Assistance); needle with drainage. [92: No. 81] [26: 61] [46: 646] [113: 14] [4: 98] [75: 206]

bitter vomiting 呕苦 *ǒu kǔ*: *Synonyms: vomiting of bitter water; vomiting of bile.* Vomiting of bitter-tasting fluid. Bitter vomiting is usually a sign of disease in the liver channel. MED Treat with Bupleurum Gallbladder-Clearing Decoction (*chái hú qīng dǎn tāng*), which is comprised of bupleurum (*chái hú*), scutellaria (*huáng qín*), pinellia (*bàn xià*), tangerine peel (*chén pí*), licorice (*gān cǎo*), or bamboo shavings (*zhú rú*). Alternatively use Left-Running Metal Pill (*zuǒ jīn wán*). ACU Base treatment on PC, ST, and CV, and on alarm and lower uniting points of GB. Select CV-12 (*zhōng wǎn*, Center Stomach Duct), PC-6 (*nèi guān*, Inner Pass), ST-36 (*zú sān lǐ*, Leg Three Li), LR-3 (*tài chōng*, Supreme Surge), GB-24 (*rì yuè*, Sun and Moon), and GB-34 (*yáng líng quán*, Yang Mound Spring); needle with drainage. [26: 846] [46: 659]

BL 膀胱经 *páng guāng jīng*, 足太阳膀胱经 *zú tài yáng páng guāng jīng*: Abbreviation for the bladder or the foot greater yang (*tài yáng*) bladder channel.

black 黑 *hēi*: Color associated with water and the kidney in the five phases.

black face 面黑 *miàn hēi*: BLACK FACIAL COMPLEXION.

black facial complexion 面色黑 *miàn sè hēi*: *Synonym: black face.* A sign of severe or intractable disease, associated with kidney vacuity and blood stasis. A complexion that is soot-black (black with a tinge of yellow), dark gray, or purple-black may occur in enduring diseases, patterns characterized by kidney essence depletion or in static blood accumulation patterns. [6: 117] [92: No. 101]

blackhead 黑头粉刺 *hēi tóu fěn cì*: See ACNE.

black jaundice 黑疸 *hēi dǎn*: From *Essential Prescriptions of the Golden Coffer* (*jīn guì yào lüè, huáng dǎn mài zhèng bìng zhì*). JAUNDICE characterized by a blackish facial complexion. Black jaundice arises in persistent jaundice as a result of liver-kidney debilitation and stasis turbidity causing internal obstruction. The body is yellow and lusterless, while the eyes and face are blackish. There is anguish in the heart, dry skin that is insensitive to scratching, black stool, bladder tension (smaller-abdominal distention and fullness), heat in the underside of the feet, and a weak floating pulse. In severe cases, the abdomen is distended as if containing water, the face is puffy, and pain in the spine prevents the patient from standing erect. MED Treat by supporting right and supplementing the liver and kidney, supported by attacking evil and transforming stasis. Niter and Alum Powder (*xiāo shí fán shí sǎn*) can be combined with liver-kidney–enriching medicinals. [26: 728] [49: 448]

black mole 黑痣 *hēi zhì*: A black or dark brown spot, from the size of a millet seed to the size of a soybean, either flat or raised, often growing string-like hairs. Black moles are found on the face and other parts of the body, and are attributed to turbid qi in the kidney channel binding in the skin. Normally, they require no treatment, but when they gradually grow larger as a result of friction, they can be treated with Water Crystal Paste (*shuǐ jīng gāo*). Swift appearance or sudden increase in size may indicate what is termed malignancy in Western medicine. Compare BLOOD MOLE. [26: 728]

black stool 大便黑色 *dà biàn hēi sè*: Stool that is extremely dark in color; a sign of static blood. [26: 127]

black teeth 齿黑 *yá hēi*: Sudden blackening of the teeth is sign of impending death. If the gums of black, this is expiration of the heart and liver. Black teeth with lumbar pain and reversal cold of the feet is observed in steaming bones. [29: 83]

black tongue fur 黑苔 *hēi tāi*: A tongue fur presenting a blackish or grayish coloration. Black fur may occur in cold, heat, repletion, and vacuity patterns, but most commonly indicates exuberant evil. A rough dry black fur somewhat parched in appearance, on a red or deep red tongue body indicates damp-heat transforming into dryness or damage to yin by intense heat. A thick slimy black fur usually indicates a phlegm-damp complication. A glossy black fur signifies either stomach or kidney vacuity. A slimy yellow fur with a grayish black coloring generally indicates exuberant damp-heat. A mixed gray and white fur or a gray fur that is thin, slimy, and glossy generally means cold-damp. [6: 124]

black vaginal discharge 黑带 *hēi dài*: See LIVER CHANNEL DAMP-HEAT VAGINAL DISCHARGE.

bladder 膀胱 *páng guāng*: One of the SIX BOWELS; the organ in the smaller abdomen that stores and discharges urine. The bladder stands in exterior-interior relationship with the kidney. *Elementary*

Questions (*sù wèn, líng lán mì diǎn lùn*) states, "The bladder holds the office of river island (or Regional Rectifier), stores fluid, and by qi transformation lets it out." The qi transformtion in this context is seen as kidney qi transformation. See KIDNEY GOVERNS WATER. [26: 849] [27: 166] [97: 455] [36: 120]

bladder channel 膀胱经 *páng guāng jīng*: FOOT GREATER YANG BLADDER CHANNEL.

bladder cough 膀胱咳 *páng guāng ké*: From *Elementary Questions* (*sù wèn*). Cough with urinary incontinence. See COUGH. [26: 849]

bladder damp-heat 膀胱湿热 *páng guāng shī rè*: Synonym: *damp-heat brewing in the bladder*; *downpour of damp-heat into the bladder*. A disease pattern that arises when damp-heat causes INHIBITED BLADDER QI TRANSFORMATION and that manifests in frequent urination, urinary urgency, inhibited urination, painful urination, red or yellow murky urine, or bloody urine. Other signs of bladder damp-heat include heat effusion, lumbar pain, and sand or stones in the urine. The tongue is red with slimy yellow fur. The pulse is rapid and slippery. WMC observed in acute urinary tract infections or urinary calculus. MED Clear heat and disinhibit dampness; disinhibit water and free strangury. Commonly used medicinals include mutong (*mù tōng*), plantago (*chē qián*), knotgrass (*biǎn xù*), talcum (*huá shí*), dianthus (*qū mài*), gardenia (*shān zhī zǐ*), moneywort (*jīn qián cǎo*), cephalanoplos (*xiǎo jì*), typha pollen (*pú huáng*), polyporus (*zhū líng*), alisma (*zé xiè*), and fish poison yam (*bì xiè*). A general formula is Eight Corrections Powder (*bā zhèng sǎn*). Pyrrosia Powder (*shí wéi sǎn*) and its variations can be used to treat sand and stone strangury. ACU Base treatment mainly on BL and CV. Select CV-3 (*zhōng jí*, Central Pole), BL-28 (*páng guāng shū*, Bladder Transport), SP-9 (*yīn líng quán*, Yin Mound Spring), and SP-6 (*sān yīn jiāo*, Three Yin Intersection); needle with drainage. For short voidings of reddish urine, add GV-27 (*duì duān*, Extremity of the Mouth). For pain on urination, add LR-5 (*lǐ gōu*, Woodworm Canal), and LR-2 (*xíng jiān*, Moving Between). For bloody urine, add SP-10 (*xuè hǎi*, Sea of Blood) and BL-60 (*kūn lún*, Kunlun Mountains). See STRANGURY. [6: 210] [26: 850] [27: 139] [97: 582] [46: 675] [113: 118] [37: 375]

bladder damp-heat bloody urine 膀胱湿热尿血 *páng guāng shī rè niào xuè*: Synonym: *lower burner damp-heat bloody urine*. BLOODY URINE attributed to bladder damp-heat. Bladder damp-heat bloody urine is marked by dry pharynx and mouth, tense fullness in the lesser abdomen, rough voidings of reddish urine, dribbling urinary blockage, slimy yellow tongue fur, and a rapid pulse.

MED Clear heat and disinhibit dampness. Cephalanoplos Drink (*xiǎo jì yǐn zi*). ACU Base treatment mainly on BL, CV, and SP. Select BL-28 (*páng guāng shū*, Bladder Transport), CV-3 (*zhōng jí*, Central Pole), SP-9 (*yīn líng quán*, Yin Mound Spring), SP-6 (*sān yīn jiāo*, Three Yin Intersection), SP-10 (*xuè hǎi*, Sea of Blood), and BL-60 (*kūn lún*, Kunlun Mountains). Needle with drainage. [37: 377] [46: 675] [113: 118]

bladder disease 膀胱病 *páng guāng bìng*: Any morbid state of the bladder. Bladder disease manifests in changes in urine and urination. It may take the form of vacuity or repletion. Vacuity patterns are attributable to insufficiency of kidney qi affecting bladder qi transformation (voiding of urine) and take the form of frequent urination, dribbling incontinence, or enuresis. Repletion patterns are usually attributable to damp-heat and are characterized by short voidings of reddish urine, murky urine, frequent urination with difficulty in voiding, heat pain during urination, stones, pus, or bloody urine, and urinary block with painful distention of the lesser abdomen. Vacuity patterns are treated by supplementing the kidney and securing the bladder; damp-heat patterns are treated by clearing heat and disinhibiting dampness. [26: 849]

bladder distention 膀胱胀 *páng guāng zhàng*: Fullness of the lower abdomen with inhibited urination, usually attributed to bladder cold. MED Treat with formulas such as Complementarity Decoction (*jì jì tāng*). Bladder distention may also be observed in drum distention patterns, for which bladder channel conductors such as talcum (*huá shí*) and notopterygium (*qiāng huó*) are added to the formula treating the principal pattern. [26: 850]

bladder governs fluid storage 膀胱主藏津液 *páng guāng zhǔ cáng jīn yè*: The bladder is the collecting point of water passing through the triple burner, from where it is discharged by kidney qi transformation. [27: 57] [97: 625]

bladder heat bind 热结膀胱 *rè jié páng guāng*: HEAT BINDING IN THE BLADDER.

bladder holds the office of the river island; it stores fluids 膀胱者，州都之官，津液藏焉 *páng guāng zhě, zhōu dū zhī guān, jīn yè cáng yān*: From *Elementary Questions* (*sù wèn, líng lán mì diǎn lùn*). The bladder stores urine. The "office of the river island" is one interpretation of 州都之官 (*zhōu dū zhī guān*), by which 州都 is taken to mean 洲渚 (*zhōu dǔ*). Other interpretations claim 渚 to be a confluence of waters. P.U. Unschuld suggests that 州都 should be interpreted literally to mean Regional Rectifier, an official title in ancient China. [36: 120]

bladder impediment 膀胱痹 *páng guāng bì*, 胞痹 *bāo bì*, 脬痹 *pāo bì*: From *Elementary Questions* (*sù wèn, bì lùn*). A condition characterized by smaller-abdominal distention with pain exacerbated by pressure and difficult urination, and attended by runny nose with clear snivel (nasal mucus). Bladder impediment arises when wind-cold-damp settles in the bladder, causes bladder vacuity cold, and disrupts normal qi transformation. A pattern of similar smaller-abdominal signs may be the result of damp-heat brewing in the bladder. MED Wind-cold-damp patterns are treated by warming and freeing with formulas such as Kidney Fixity Decoction (*shèn zhuó tāng*); damp-heat patterns are treated by clearing and disinhibiting with formulas like Eight Corrections Powder (*bā zhèng sǎn*) and variations. See IMPEDIMENT. [26: 452] [27: 407] [97: 414]

bladder qi block 膀胱气闭 *páng guāng qì bì*: Impairment of bladder qi transformation (the action of the bladder) mostly related to inhibited qi transformation of the kidney, lung, or triple burner, resulting in inhibited urination, difficult urination, or urinary block with smaller-abdominal distention. Bladder qi block is a functional disorder of the bladder preventing normal flow of urine, and differs from blockage caused by stones, which is of a mechanical nature. MED For inhibited qi transformation of the bladder due to kidney vacuity, use variations of Life Saver Kidney Qi Pill (*jì shēng shèn qì wán*). For inhibited qi transformation of the bladder due to lung qi congestion, use the method of "raising the pot and removing the lid" (causing the patient to sneeze or vomit) to open lung qi; if after a long time heat develops, Lung-Clearing Beverage (*qīng fèi yǐn*) with urine-disinhibiting medicinals can be used. ACU Base treatment mainly on KI and BL. Select BL-23 (*shèn shū*, Kidney Transport), BL-22 (*sān jiāo shū*, Triple Burner Transport), KI-10 (*yīn gǔ*, Yin Valley), BL-39 (*wěi yáng*, Bend Yang), and SP-6 (*sān yīn jiāo*, Three Yin Intersection), needle with supplementation and add moxa. For pronounced smaller-abdominal fullness and distention, add CV-6 (*qì hǎi*, Sea of Qi). Selection of points according to pattern: For kidney vacuity and inhibited qi transformation, add CV-4 (*guān yuán*, Pass Head) and GV-4 (*mìng mén*, Life Gate). For lung-metal dryness-heat and impaired downbearing of qi, needle with drainage at LU-5 (*chǐ zé*, Cubit Marsh), LI-11 (*qū chí*, Pool at the Bend), and LU-7 (*liè quē*, Broken Sequence). See BLOCK. [26: 850] [27: 165] [97: 624] [46: 672] [113: 12, 17] [37: 383]

bladder qi transformation failure 膀胱气化失司 *páng guāng qì huà shī sī*: Impairment of bladder function. *Qi transformation* in its widest sense denotes all transformations of qi, blood, fluids, and essence in the body. *Bladder qi transformation* denotes the function of ensuring the regular uninhibited discharge of urine. Breakdown of bladder qi transformation can result in any of the following: FREQUENT URINATION; PROFUSE URINATION AT NIGHT; ENURESIS; URINARY INCONTINENCE; DRIBBLE AFTER VOIDING; URINARY URGENCY; INHIBITED URINATION; and PAINFUL URINATION. *Inhibited bladder qi transformation* is a term often used specifically to denote the pathomechanism that explains frequent urination, dribble after voiding, urinary urgency, inhibited urination, and painful urination, as well as signs such as turbid urine or the passage of sand or stones that frequently accompany them. 320]zfzz

bladder vacuity cold 膀胱虚寒 *páng guāng xū hán*: Loss of the retentive power of the bladder due either to insufficiency of qi transformation or to contraction of external cold evil. The main signs of bladder vacuity cold are frequent voidings of clear urine, enuresis, dribble after voiding, or incontinence. Other signs include white turbidity after urination, ungratifying dribbling urination, inability to achieve a full stream, and smaller-abdominal cold pain. Lumbar pain and other kidney yang vacuity signs are usually present. The tongue is pale with a thin moist white fur. The pulse is sunken and fine. [MED] Stream-Reducing Pill (*suō quán wán*) or Dyke-Strengthening Pill (*gǒng tí wán*). [ACU] Base treatment mainly on BL and CV. Select CV-3 (*zhōng jí*, Central Pole), BL-28 (*páng guāng shū*, Bladder Transport), CV-4 (*guān yuán*, Pass Head), SP-6 (*sān yīn jiāo*, Three Yin Intersection), and BL-23 (*shèn shū*, Kidney Transport); needle with supplementation and add moxa. For pronounced vacuity cold, add CV-6 (*qì hǎi*, Sea of Qi) and CV-4 (*guān yuán*, Pass Head), and apply a large amount of moxa. For concurrent kidney yang vacuity, add GV-4 (*mìng mén*, Life Gate), and KI-3 (*tài xī*, Great Ravine). [27: 165] [97: 625] [46: 588] [113: 12, 114]

bland 淡 *dàn*: See BLANDNESS.

blandness 淡 *dàn*: Mild flavor, or the absence of a predominating flavor. The flavor associated with damp-percolating and water-disinhibiting medicinals. See FIVE FLAVORS; FIVE FLAVOR ENTRIES. [19: 8230]

bland taste in the mouth 口淡 *kǒu dàn*: Lack of taste in the mouth. Patients suffering from bland taste in the mouth differ from normal individuals with HARMONY OF MOUTH in that food lacks flavor and eating leaves no pleasant taste in the mouth. It is attributed to spleen-stomach vacuity or to dampness obstructing the center burner. It may also be observed in patients suffering from aversion to cold and heat effusion due to external contraction of wind-cold. **Spleen-stomach vacuity** causes bland taste in the mouth with

no desire for food and drink, lassitude of spirit, shortness of breath, lack of strength, stomach duct glomus and abdominal distention, sloppy stool, a pale tongue with thin fur, and a weak moderate pulse. [MED] Boost qi, fortify the spleen, and harmonize the stomach. Use Saussurea and Amomum Six Gentlemen Decoction (*xiāng shā liù jūn zǐ tāng*) plus scorch-fried rice sprout (*gǔ yá*) or barley sprout (*mài yá*). **Dampness obstructing the center burner** causes inability to taste food, bland taste in the mouth associated with stickiness and sliminess, torpid intake, glomus and oppression in the chest and stomach duct, nausea and vomiting, sloppy stool, white slimy or yellow slimy tongue fur and a soggy pulse. [MED] Repel turbidity with aroma; transform dampness and awaken the stomach. Use Agastache/Patchouli, Magnolia Bark, Pinellia, and Poria (Hoelen) Decoction (*huò pò xià líng tāng*) and Three Kernels Decoction (*sān rén tāng*). [92: No. 87] [97: 31]

blast-frying 炮 *páo*: Stir-frying (medicinal materials) vigorously in an iron wok over a fierce fire 'until they give off smoke and their surface becomes scorched, swollen, and cracked. Dried ginger (*gān jiāng*), aconite (*fù zǐ*), and tianxiong aconite (*tiān xióng*) may be processed in this way to reduce their harshness. Compare CHAR-FRYING. ◊ Chin 炮 *páo*, burn, blast. [97: 524]

blaze 燔 *fán*: To burn furiously. Describes heat in the exuberant heat stage of warm diseases. See HEAT.

blazing bone 然骨 *rán gǔ*: A bone on the inside of the foot. [WMC] navicular bone. [27: 72] [97: 569]

blazing of both qi and blood 气血两燔 *qì xuè liǎng fán*: QI AND BLOOD BOTH ABLAZE.

blazing of both qi and construction 气营两燔 *qì yíng liǎng fán*: QI AND CONSTRUCTION BOTH ABLAZE

bleed 出血 *chū xuè*, 血 *xuè*: To put or bring forth blood.

bleeding 出血 *chū xuè*, 血 *xuè*: The escape of blood from vessels. See BLOOD SPILLAGE.

bleeding gums 牙龈出血 *yá yín chū xuè*, 齿衄 *chǐ nǜ*: SPONTANEOUS BLEEDING OF THE GUMS.

bleeding hemorrhoids 血痔 *xuè zhì*: HEMORRHOIDS with pronounced bleeding. [26: 280]

blister 水疱（泡）*shuǐ pào*: 1. *Synonym: vesicle*. An elevation in the skin containing fluid; attributable to friction, heat, or to certain heat (febrile) diseases. Blistering occurs in SCARRING MOXIBUSTION; MEDICINAL-INDUCED BLISTER MOXIBUSTION. GIRDLING FIRE CINNABAR; HEAVEN-BORNE BLISTERS; TONGUE BLISTER; LACQUER SORE; PALM HEART TOXIN SORE; PLASTER WIND; WIND RED SORE; 2. CHICKEN POX.

block 闭 *bì*: Blockage. The term block occurs in the terminology of signs and pathomechanisms: (1) blockage of normal discharge from the body, as in MENSTRUAL BLOCK (amenorrhea), FECAL BLOCK (constipation), and DRIBBLING URINARY BLOCK (retention of urine). (2) blockage or disturbance of the pathways of qi as in QI BLOCK. See also STOPPAGE. [6: Ch. 6] [26: 606] [27: 217] [97: 227]

blockage 不通 *bù tōng*: See STOPPAGE.

block and repulsion 关格 *guān gé*: **1.** URINARY STOPPAGE (block) and continuous vomiting (repulsion) caused by insufficiency of the spleen and kidney with depressed lodged damp turbidity transforming into heat and thrusting upward. MED Treatment involves the use of Golden Coffer Kidney Qi Pill (*jīn guì shèn qì wán*) to provide warming supplementation and boost kidney qi and to warm yang and transform water, and Left-Running Metal Pill (*zuǒ jīn wán*) to harmonize the stomach and downbear turbidity. Where enduring depression has given way to heat transformation, abdominal distention and diarrhea, vexation and agitation, dry lips, a taste of urine in the mouth, and a thick turbid tongue fur are observed, and the treatment is to free yang and downbear turbidity with Rhubarb and Aconite Decoction (*dà huáng fù zǐ tāng*) combined with Coptis Gallbladder-Warming Decoction (*huáng lián wēn dǎn tāng*). If there is a pronounced yang brightness (*yáng míng*) bowel pattern, formulas such as Major Qi-Coordinating Decoction (*dà chéng qì tāng*) and Yellow Dragon Decoction (*huáng lóng tāng*) may be used. **2.** Vomiting with the gradual appearance of fecal and urinary stoppage, accompanied by a sense of blockage in the throat. This is a severe form of dysphagia-occlusion (*yē gé*). **3.** Exuberance of both yin and yang. When yin qi is overexuberant and yang qi is not nourished, this is called block. When yang qi is overexuberant and yin qi is not nourished, this is called repulsion. When yin and yang are both overexuberant and fail to nourish each other, this is called block and repulsion. **4.** Extremely exuberant wrist and man's prognosis pulses, which are a sign of impending separation of yin and yang. ◇ Chin 观 *guān*, shut, close; a narrow pass; 格 *gé*, fight, resist. [26: 975] [27: 412] [97: 222]

block pattern 闭证 *bì zhèng*: See BLOCK. [27: 217]

blood 血 *xuè* (*xiě*): The red fluid of the body that according to traditional explanations is derived from the essential qi derived from food by the stomach and spleen, which becomes red blood after being transformed by construction qi and the lung. Blood flows to all parts of the body, and is governed by the heart. By the action of the heart and lung, it flows through the vessels, carrying nourishment to the whole of the body. All the bowels and viscera and all parts of the body rely on the blood for nourishment. The heart and liver are said to have their own blood, the terms *heart blood* and *liver blood* meaning blood in relation to the functions of those two viscera. See HEART QI AND HEART BLOOD; LIVER BLOOD. [27: 75] [97: 187]

blood accumulation 血积 *xuè jī*: An accumulation of static blood due to qi counterflow and blood depression or due to injury from knocks and falls. Blood accumulation is accompanied by a withered-yellow facial complexion with CRAB CLAW MARKINGS, a lump in the abdomen of rib-side that does not move and frequently causes pain, and constipation or black stool. MED Quicken the blood and transform stasis with formulas like Dead-On Pill (*dǐ dàng wán*), Peach Kernel and Carthamus Four Agents Decoction (*táo hóng sì wù tāng*), Peach Kernel Qi-Coordinating Decoction (*táo hé chéng qì tāng*), or Rhubarb and Wingless Cockroach Pill (*dà huáng zhè chóng wán*). ACU Main points are blood-quickening stasis-dispelling points such as BL-17 (*gé shū*, Diaphragm Transport), SP-10 (*xuè hǎi*, Sea of Blood), LI-4 (*hé gǔ*, Union Valley), LR-3 (*tài chōng*, Supreme Surge), SP-6 (*sān yīn jiāo*, Three Yin Intersection), and Glomus Root (*pǐ gēn*); needle with even supplementation and drainage or bleed with a three-edged needle. For qi counterflow and blood depression, add CV-6 (*qì hǎi*, Sea of Qi), PC-6 (*nèi guān*, Inner Pass), and BL-18 (*gān shū*, Liver Transport). [26: 286]

blood amassment 蓄血 *xù xuè*: **1.** A greater yang (*tài yáng*) COLD DAMAGE pattern in which evil heat enters the interior to contend with the blood, causing stasis heat amassing and binding internally and manifesting in the form of smaller-abdominal pain and distention, heat effusion and aversion to cold, clear-mindedness in the daytime that gives way to delirious raving, mania, confused speech, and vociferation and violent behavior at night. MED Blood amassment is treated by offensive precipitation of static blood using Dead-On Pill (*dǐ dàng wán*), Peach Kernel Qi-Coordinating Decoction (*táo hé chéng qì tāng*), Infradiaphragmatic Stasis-Expelling Decoction (*gé xià zhú yū tāng*), plus rhubarb (*dà huáng*), or Rhinoceros Horn and Rehmannia Decoction (*xī jiǎo dì huáng tāng*). **2.** Any substantial or insubstantial blood stasis accumulation due to internal causes or to external injury. [26: 841] [27: 119] [97: 596]

blood amassment yellowing 蓄血发黄 *xù xuè fā huáng*: Synonym: *static blood yellowing*. From *Cold Damage Life-for-All Collection* (*shāng hán quán shēng jí*). JAUNDICE due to stasis heat amassing internally. *On Cold Damage* (*shāng hán* *lùn, biàn tài yáng bìng mài zhèng bìng zhì*) states "Greater yang (*tài yáng*) disease with yellow body, bound sunken pulse, lesser-abdominal hardness and inhibited urination indicates a lack of blood; if there is uninhibited urination and the patient acts like a maniac, this is definitely a blood pattern." MED Treat by offensive expulsion of stasis heat. Peach Kernel Qi-Coordinating Decoction (*táo hé chéng qì tāng*) or Dead-On Decoction (*dǐ dàng tāng*). [26: 842]

blood arrow 血箭 *xuè jiàn*: **1.** SPONTANEOUS EXTERNAL BLEEDING of the flesh, attributable to exuberant fire in the heart channel that causes frenetic movement of the blood. Blood arrow is characterized by red macules and bleeding from the pores, in severe cases with blood spurting out like an arrow. MED Enrich yin, downbear fire, and cool the blood using Blood-Cooling Rehmannia Decoction (*liáng xuè dì huáng tāng*). If bleeding is profuse, use Tangkuei Blood-Supplementing Decoction (*dāng guī bǔ xuè tāng*). Peach Blossom Powder (*táo huā sǎn*) may be applied topically. **2.** INTESTINAL AGGREGATION. [26: 286] [27: 189] [61: 346]

blood aspect 血分 *xuè fèn*: DEFENSE, QI, CONSTRUCTION, AND BLOOD.

blood-aspect heat toxin 血分热毒 *xuè fèn rè dú*: **1.** Heat evil in the blood-aspect, characterized by high fever, clouded spirit, macules and papules, and in some cases blood ejection, spontaneous external bleeding, or bloody stool, and a deep crimson or purple-crimson tongue. WMC severe measles; scarlet fever; exanthematous typhus. MED Cool and dissipate the blood. Use Rhinoceros Horn and Rehmannia Decoction (*xī jiǎo dì huáng tāng*). ACU Base treatment mainly on HT and PC. Select PC-3 (*qū zé*, Marsh at the Bend), PC-9 (*zhōng chōng*, Central Hub), HT-9 (*shào chōng*, Lesser Surge), LI-11 (*qū chí*, Pool at the Bend), BL-40 (*wěi zhōng*, Bend Center), SP-10 (*xuè hǎi*, Sea of Blood), and SP-6 (*sān yīn jiāo*, Three Yin Intersection); needle with drainage or prick to bleed. For high fever, add the Ten Diffusing Points (*shí xuān*) and GV-14 (*dà zhuī*, Great Hammer). For clouded spirit, add HT-7 (*shén mén*, Spirit Gate), Alert Spirit Quartet (*sì shén cōng*), and PC-7 (*dà líng*, Great Mound). **2.** Generally denotes what Western medicine describes as recurrent or multiple acute pyogenic infections. [26: 277] [27: 137] [97: 191] [83: 110] [50: 587] [46: 595, 732] [113: 19]

blood-aspect pattern 血分证 *xuè fèn zhèng*: Any warm disease pattern arising when an evil enters the blood aspect. Signs include a deep crimson tongue coloring and signs of frenetic movement of the blood such as bleeding and purple maculopapular eruptions. The tongue may, in addition

to being crimson, be bare and smooth like a mirror, indicating damage to yin and fluid desertion. Such a condition may include signs of vacuity stirring internal wind such as convulsions of the limbs or TETANIC REVERSAL. These latter signs are nevertheless differentiated from the tetanic reversal and convulsions associated with extreme heat engendering wind. The accent in blood-aspect patterns may be on repletion signs such as frenetic blood movement; or it may be on vacuity of right with a lodged evil, where signs such as desiccated tongue and teeth, dry pharynx and mouth, heart vexation, and a rapid fine pulse indicate that although the heat has abated, the evil is still present and yin humor is severely damaged. TRT See COOLING THE BLOOD. [27: 225] [97: 182] [84: 37]

blood chamber 血室 *xuè shì*: **1.** The uterus. **2.** The thoroughfare (*chōng*) vessel. **3.** The LIVER. [26: 278]

blood chest bind 血结胸 *xuè jié xiōng*: A yang-natured cold damage pattern arising when blood ejection is incomplete and blood amasses in the upper burner. It is characterized by distention, fullness, hardness and pain in the chest and abdomen, generalized heat [effusion] with only a desire to wet the mouth rather than swallow fluid, forgetfulness, black stool, and inhibited urination. MED Use formulas such as Rhinoceros Horn and Rehmannia Decoction (*xī jiǎo dì huáng tāng*) or Dead-On Decoction (*dǐ dàng tāng*). ACU Base treatment on CV, PC, SP, and LR. Select CV-17 (*shān zhōng*, Chest Center), PC-6 (*nèi guān*, Inner Pass), SP-10 (*xuè hǎi*, Sea of Blood), SP-6 (*sān yīn jiāo*, Three Yin Intersection), LR-3 (*tài chōng*, Supreme Surge), PC-5 (*jiān shǐ*, Intermediary Courier), and HT-7 (*shén mén*, Spirit Gate); needle with drainage. [26: 283] [27: 376]

blood cold 血寒 *xuè hán*: Congealing cold and qi stagnation inhibiting movement of blood causing stasis. Blood cold is observed in MOUNTING QI (*shàn qì*), CONCRETIONS, CONGLOMERATIONS, ACCUMULATIONS, AND GATHERINGS, DELAYED MENSTRUATION, and SCANT MENSTRUATION, FROSTBITE, and SLOUGHING FLAT-ABSCESS (*jū*). Blood cold mostly arises through blood congealing in the liver vessel. *Elementary Questions* (*sù wèn*) states, "The reverting yin (*jué yīn*) vessel connects with the yin organs (genitals) and ties to the liver; when cold qi settles in [this] vessel, the blood congeals and the pulse because urgent; hence there is pain from the rib-side to the lesser abdomen." [29: 363] [57: 20]

blood cold delayed menstruation 血寒经行后期 *xuè hán jīng xíng hòu qī*: DELAYED MENSTRUATION due to blood cold, most commonly observed in postpartum patients who contract external cold that seizes a vacuity and storms the uterus, where it causes stagnation of the blood. Arrival of periods is delayed and flow is dark, clotted, and scant. The condition is associated with gripping abdominal pain relieved by warmth, green-blue or white facial complexion, physical cold, and aversion to cold. If flow is scant and pale and accompanied by dull abdominal pain relieved by warmth and pressure, a bright white facial complexion, dizziness and shortness of breath, the pattern is one of thoroughfare (*chōng*) and controlling (*rèn*) vessel vacuity cold making the blood powerless to move. MED Repletion cold is treated by warming the channels and moving stagnation using Channel-Warming (Menses-Warming) Decoction (*wēn jīng tāng*); vacuity cold is treated by warming the channels and nourishing the blood with Major Construction Brew (*dà yíng jiān*). ACU Base treatment on the CV and the three yin channels of the foot. Main points: CV-6 (*qì hǎi*, Sea of Qi), KI-13 (*qì xué*, Qi Point), SP-6 (*sān yīn jiāo*, Three Yin Intersection), needle with supplementation and add moxa. To warm the channels and move stagnation, add ST-29 (*guī lái*, Return), ST-25 (*tiān shū*, Celestial Pivot), and LR-3 (*tài chōng*, Supreme Surge); to warm the channels and nourish the blood, add BL-20 (*pí shū*, Spleen Transport), BL-17 (*gé shū*, Diaphragm Transport), GV-4 (*mìng mén*, Life Gate), and KI-3 (*tài xī*, Great Ravine), See DELAYED MENSTRUATION. [26: 282] [46: 683]

blood cold scant menstruation 血寒月经过少 *xuè hán yuè jīng guò shǎo*: SCANT MENSTRUATION due to yang vacuity engendering internal yin cold, insufficient production of blood due to reduced qi transformation and shortage of blood in the thoroughfare (*chōng*) and controlling (*rèn*) vessels. A scant thin pale or dark pale or dark flow is accompanied by physical cold and aversion to cold, cold pain in the smaller abdomen relieved by warmth. MED Warm the channels and nourish the blood with formulas such as Major Construction Brew (*dà yíng jiān*) with the addition of blast-fried ginger (*páo jiāng*) and, if necessary, aconite (*fù zǐ*). ACU The CV, back transport points, SP, and ST provide the main basis for treatment. Select CV-6 (*qì hǎi*, Sea of Qi), SP-6 (*sān yīn jiāo*, Three Yin Intersection), BL-20 (*pí shū*, Spleen Transport), BL-17 (*gé shū*, Diaphragm Transport), ST-36 (*zú sān lǐ*, Leg Three Li), CV-4 (*guān yuán*, Pass Head), GV-4 (*mìng mén*, Life Gate), and KI-3 (*tài xī*, Great Ravine), and needle with supplementation and use large amounts of moxa. [26: 282]

blood collapse 亡血 *wáng xuè*: Acute, critical vacuity of the blood. See COLLAPSE.

blood concretion 血癥 *xuè zhēng*: An abdominal lump attributable to accumulation of static blood congesting the channels. Concretions may occur in the rib-side or below the abdomen. They feel hard to the touch, do not move when pushed, and are associated with local stasis pain. Patients suffering from them also reveal signs such as gradual emaciation, fatigue and lack of strength, reduced food intake, and in women menstrual irregularities or menstrual block. MED Quicken the blood and dissipate stasis. If visceral qi is weak, support right and dispel the evil. Formulas that may be used include Turtle Shell Decocted Pill (*biē jiǎ jiān wán*), Concretion-Transforming Return-to-Life Elixir (*huà zhēng huí shēng dān*), Infradiaphragmatic Stasis-Expelling Decoction (*gé xià zhú yū tāng*), and Lesser Abdomen Stasis-Expelling Decoction (*shào fù zhú yū tāng*). ACU Base treatment on back transport points, SP, and LR. Main points are blood-quickening stasis-dispelling points such as BL-17 (*gé shū*, Diaphragm Transport), SP-10 (*xuè hǎi*, Sea of Blood), LI-4 (*hé gǔ*, Union Valley), LR-3 (*tài chōng*, Supreme Surge), SP-6 (*sān yīn jiāo*, Three Yin Intersection), and Glomus Root (*pǐ gēn*). Selection of points according to affected area: Chest and abdomen: add CV-17 (*shān zhōng*, Chest Center) and ST-36 (*zú sān lǐ*, Leg Three Li). Rib-side: add SP-21 (*dà bāo*, Great Embracement) and GB-34 (*yáng líng quán*, Yang Mound Spring). Below the umbilicus: add CV-3 (*zhōng jí*, Central Pole), SP-8 (*dì jī*, Earth's Crux), and ST-29 (*guī lái*, Return); needle with even supplementation and drainage or pricking and cupping. For vacuity of visceral qi, add CV-4 (*guān yuán*, Pass Head), BL-20 (*pí shū*, Spleen Transport), and ST-36 (*zú sān lǐ*, Leg Three Li), and needle with supplementation and add moxa. [26: 287] [27: 417] [97: 189] [113: 19] [46: 688]

blood depletion menstrual block 血亏经闭 *xuè kuī jīng bì*: MENSTRUAL BLOCK (absence of menstruation) due to blood depletion arising when loss of blood, early marriage, excessive number of births, or excessive breast feeding causes damage to essence-blood. Blood depletion menstrual block appears gradually, and menstrual flow gradually becomes increasingly scant until it finally ceases. It is accompanied by no thought of food and drink, dry skin, and emaciation. MED Supplement the blood and boost qi using formulas such as Ginseng Construction-Nourishing Decoction (*rén shēn yǎng róng tāng*) or Perfect Major Supplementation Decoction (*shí quán dà bǔ tāng*). ACU Base treatment on CV and back transport points, selecting CV-4 (*guān yuán*, Pass Head), BL-18 (*gān shū*, Liver Transport), BL-23 (*shèn shū*, Kidney Transport), BL-17 (*gé shū*, Diaphragm Transport), BL-20 (*pí shū*, Spleen Transport), ST-36 (*zú sān lǐ*, Leg Three Li), SP-6 (*sān yīn jiāo*, Three Yin Intersection), and the Four Flowers (*sì huā*). Needle with supplementation and add moxa. [26: 286] [46: 686]

blood depression 血郁 *xuè yù*: A condition that results from sudden violent flights of anger, sprains, or irregular eating and that is characterized by stabbing pain in the chest and ribside accompanied by lack of strength in the limbs, dribbling urination, bloody stool or a pulse sunken, scallion-stalk, rough, bound, or skipping and scallion-stalk. MED Harmonize the blood and resolve depression with Blood Depression Decoction (*xuè yù tāng*), Four Agents Depression-Transforming Decoction (*sì wù huà yù tāng*) or Toosendan Powder (*jīn líng zǐ sǎn*) with the judicious addition of peach kernel (*táo rén*), tangkuei tails (*dāng guī wěi*), curcuma (*yù jīn*), and dalbergia (*jiàng zhēn xiāng*). [26: 287]

blood desertion 血脱 *xuè tuō*, 脱血 *tuō xuè*: Depletion of true yin and emptiness of the sea of blood resulting from insufficiency of the congenital constitution, anxiety, taxation fatigue, sexual taxation, damage by food and liquor, or massive or chronic loss of blood. Blood desertion is characterized by somber white facial complexion that is sheenless and perished, as well as dizziness and flowery vision, heart palpitations or fearful throbbing, shortness of breath and faint breathing, cold limbs, CLOUDING REVERSAL and loss of consciousness. The tongue is pale; the pulse is empty and vacuous, or scallion-stalk, or faint and fine, verging on expiration. Loss of blood deprives the skin and flesh of nourishment, hence the somber white perished complexion and pale tongue. When it deprives the clear orifices of nourishment, there is dizziness and flowery vision. When it deprives the heart-spirit of nourishment, there are heart palpitations or fearful throbbing. The blood is the mother of qi, and qi is the commander of the blood. Massive loss of blood deprives qi of its support, causing qi to desert with the blood and giving rise to signs such as cold limbs and, in severe cases, CLOUDING REVERSAL and loss of consciousness. With the sudden reduction in the volume of blood that results from excessive loss of blood, construction-blood is insufficient and fails to fill the vessels; hence the pulse is empty and vacuous, or faint and verging on desertion. If yang qi loses its support and dissipates outward, there is a scallion-stalk pulse. MED Boost yin and supplement the blood using Construction-Supplementing Decoction (*bǔ róng tāng*) or Ginseng Construction-Nourishing Decoction (*rén shēn yǎng róng tāng*). For acute hemorrhage, supplement qi, nourish the blood, and stem desertion, using Pure Ginseng Decoction (*dú shēn tāng*) or Ginseng and Aconite Decoction (*shēn fù tāng*). ACU Base treatment mainly on back transport points, CV, and SP; select points such as CV-6 (*qì hǎi*, Sea of Qi),

ST-36 (*zú sān lǐ*, Leg Three Li), SP-6 (*sān yīn jiāo*, Three Yin Intersection), BL-17 (*gé shū*, Diaphragm Transport), BL-20 (*pí shū*, Spleen Transport), and BL-21 (*wèi shū*, Stomach Transport); needle with supplementation and add moxa. Point selection according to signs: For dizzy head and flowery vision, add GV-20 (*bǎi huì*, Hundred Convergences), BL-1 (*jīng míng*, Bright Eyes), and BL-2 (*zǎn zhú*, Bamboo Gathering). See also QI DESERTING WITH THE BLOOD. For acute massive hemorrhage, see YIN COLLAPSE. [26: 282] [116: 172] [27: 423] [97: 188]

blood desertion with qi desertion 血脱气脱 *xuè tuō qì tuō*: QI DESERTING WITH THE BLOOD. [26: 282]

blood desiccation 血枯 *xuè kū*: **1.** Blood vacuity manifesting in emaciation, scant semen, and menstrual block. **2.** Insufficiency of the blood due to massive bleeding. [27: 144] [97: 192]

blood desiccation menstrual block 血枯经闭 *xuè kū jīng bì*: MENSTRUAL BLOCK (absence of menses) due to desiccation of the blood. Distinction is made between vacuity and repletion patterns. **Vacuity** patterns arise from loss of blood, early marriage, excessive number of births, or excessive breast-feeding cause damage to the blood that leads to emptiness of the thoroughfare (*chōng*) and controlling (*rèn*) vessels. Signs include reduced food intake, lusterless bright white facial complexion, gradual emaciation, reddening of the cheeks, and sometimes postmeridian heat effusion and steaming bone. MED When due to excessive blood loss, treat by supplementing the blood, using Ginseng Construction-Nourishing Decoction (*rén shēn yǎng róng tāng*). When due to damage to essence through early marriage, treat by enriching yin and supplementing the blood, using Six-Ingredient Rehmannia Decoction (*liù wèi dì huáng tāng*). When due to excessive breast feeding, treat by dual supplementation of qi and the blood, with Perfect Major Supplementation Decoction (*shí quán dà bǔ tāng*). ACU Base treatment mainly on back transport points, CV, and SP. Select BL-23 (*shèn shū*, Kidney Transport), BL-17 (*gé shū*, Diaphragm Transport), BL-20 (*pí shū*, Spleen Transport), CV-7 (*yīn jiāo*, Yin Intersection), CV-6 (*qì hǎi*, Sea of Qi), SP-10 (*xuè hǎi*, Sea of Blood), SP-6 (*sān yīn jiāo*, Three Yin Intersection), and ST-36 (*zú sān lǐ*, Leg Three Li); needle with supplementation and add moxa. **Repletion** patterns are usually attributed to heat evil entering the stomach, scorching the blood, and thereby causing liquid depletion and dryness of the thoroughfare (*chōng*) vessel. They are characterized by a red facial complexion and generalized heat [effusion], dry mouth and desire for cool drinks, dry stool, and yellow urine. MED Drain stomach heat and regulate the blood vessels using Jade Candle Powder (*yù zhú săn*). ACU Base treatment mainly on ST, SP, and LI. Select ST-36 (*zú sān lĭ*, Leg Three Li), LI-4 (*hé gŭ*, Union Valley), ST-44 (*nèi tíng*, Inner Court), SP-10 (*xuè hăi*, Sea of Blood), SP-6 (*sān yīn jiāo*, Three Yin Intersection), and KI-2 (*rán gŭ*, Blazing Valley); needle with drainage. [26: 278] [46: 686]

blood disease pattern 血病证候 *xuè bìng zhèng hòu*: Any abnormal condition of the blood. See the entries listed below. [116: 170] [57: 15]

Blood Disease Patterns

> BLOOD VACUITY (*xuè xū*)
>
> BLOOD DESERTION (*xuè tuō*)
>
> BLOOD STASIS (*xuè yū*)
>
> BLOOD HEAT (*xuè rè*)
>
> BLOOD DRYNESS (*xuè zào*)
>
> BLOOD COLD (*xuè cold*)

---

blood drum 血鼓 *xuè gŭ*: *Synonyms: blood drum distention*; *blood gu*. DRUM DISTENTION (pronounced abdominal distention), arising when blood stasis and qi stagnation hamper the movement of water-damp. Blood drum is characterized by enlargement of the abdomen with green-blue prominent vessels (caput medusae), and red-thread marks (spider nevi), black stool, short voidings of reddish urine, and a scallion-stalk pulse. In some cases there is spontaneous external bleeding or blood ejection. MED Quicken the blood and move stasis; fortify the spleen and disinhibit dampness. Use formulas such as Dead-On Pill (*dĭ dàng wán*) and Spleen-Firming Beverage (*shí pí yĭn*). WMC ascites due to schistosomiasis (blood fluke infestation) or other causes. ACU Two sets of points may be used: (1) CV-12 (*zhōng wăn*, Center Stomach Duct), ST-25 (*tiān shū*, Celestial Pivot), ST-36 (*zú sān lĭ*, Leg Three Li), BL-17 (*gé shū*, Diaphragm Transport), KI-9 (*zhú bīn*, Guest House), and KI-16 (*huāng shū*, Huang Transport). (2) SP-15 (*dà hèng*, Great Horizontal), CV-6 (*qì hăi*, Sea of Qi), SP-6 (*sān yīn jiāo*, Three Yin Intersection), BL-17 (*gé shū*, Diaphragm Transport), KI-9 (*zhú bīn*, Guest House), and KI-16 (*huāng shū*, Huang Transport). The sets may be alternated, needling with drainage. Pole CV-12 (*zhōng wăn*, Center Stomach Duct), CV-4 (*guān yuán*, Pass Head), and bilateral SP-15 (*dà hèng*, Great Horizontal) for 30–60 minutes each time after needling. [26: 284] [42: 194] [27: 413]

blood drum distention 血臌 *xuè gŭ*: BLOOD DRUM.

blood dryness 血燥 *xuè zào*: Blood vacuity manifesting in signs of dryness. Blood dryness may occur when essence-blood is depleted in old age or when nutritional disturbances or static blood binding internally reduce the nutritive power of the blood. Blood dryness is characterized by emaciation, rough dry skin (ENCRUSTED SKIN), brittle nails, dry lusterless hair, hard stool, and dry tongue. Itchy and scaling skin, occurring either alone or with the above signs, is known as blood dryness (or blood vacuity) engendering wind. MED Nourish the blood and moisten dryness with dried/fresh rehmannia (*shēng dì huáng*), cooked rehmannia (*shú dì huáng*), flowery knotweed (*hé shŏu wū*), tangkuei (*dāng guī*), salvia (*dān shēn*), white peony (*bái sháo yào*), lycium berry (*gŏu qĭ zĭ*), biota seed (*băi zĭ rén*), black sesame (*hēi zhī má*), etc. Blood-nourishing dryness-moistening formulas include Dryness-Enriching Construction-Nourishing Decoction (*zī zào yăng yíng tāng*). ACU Base treatment mainly on ST, SP, LR and KI. Select ST-36 (*zú sān lĭ*, Leg Three Li), LR-3 (*tài chōng*, Supreme Surge), SP-6 (*sān yīn jiāo*, Three Yin Intersection), KI-3 (*tài xī*, Great Ravine), KI-6 (*zhào hăi*, Shining Sea), BL-20 (*pí shū*, Spleen Transport), and BL-17 (*gé shū*, Diaphragm Transport); needle with supplementation. For blood dryness engendering wind, add SP-10 (*xuè hăi*, Sea of Blood), GB-31 (*fēng shì*, Wind Market), and LR-8 (*qū quán*, Spring at the Bend), needling these points with drainage. [6: 213] [46: 594] [113: 20, 436]

blood dryness engendering wind 血燥生风 *xuè zào shēng fēng*: BLOOD VACUITY ENGENDERING WIND. [6: 213]

blood dysentery 血痢 *xuè lì*: *Synonym: red dysentery*. Dysentery characterized by bright bloody stool or passing of pure blood, associated with tenesmus and an exuberant pulse. WMC amebic dysentery; ulcerative colitis; chronic schistosomiasis (blood fluke infestation); bacillary dysentery. MED Clear the intestines and resolve toxin with formulas such as Pulsatilla Decoction (*bái tóu wēng tāng*). For persistent passage of blood, use Coptis and Ass Hide Glue Decoction (*huáng lián ē jiāo tāng*) with the judicious addition of blood-cooling blood-quickening medicinals like lonicera (*jīn yín huā*), dried/fresh rehmannia (*shēng dì huáng*), tangkuei (*dāng guī*), and sanguisorba (*dì yú*). Persistence of the condition can cause center qi vacuity cold, which is characterized by passage of grayish blood, withered-yellow facial complexion, and a soggy pulse, and is treated by warming the spleen and containing the blood with Yellow Earth Decoction (*huáng tŭ tāng*). ACU To clear the intestines and resolve toxin, base treatment mainly on ST and LI; select BL-17 (*gé shū*, Diaphragm Transport), LI-4 (*hé gŭ*, Union Valley), ST-25 (*tiān shū*, Celestial Pivot), ST-37 (*shàng jù xū*, Upper Great Hollow), ST-36 (*zú sān lĭ*, Leg Three Li) SP-4 (*gōng sūn*, Yellow Emperor), GV-1 (*cháng qiáng,* Long Strong), LI-11 (*qū chí,* Pool at the Bend), and GV-14 (*dà zhuī,* Great Hammer); needle with drainage. For persistent passing of blood, needle with even supplementation and drainage and, if appropriate, use moxa at GV-20 (*bǎi huì,* Hundred Convergences), SP-1 (*yǐn bái,* Hidden White), SP-6 (*sān yīn jiāo,* Three Yin Intersection), and LR-3 (*tài chōng,* Supreme Surge). For enduring disease causing center qi vacuity cold, base treatment on CV, ST, LI and back transport points. Select CV-12 (*zhōng wǎn,* Center Stomach Duct), CV-4 (*guān yuán,* Pass Head), ST-36 (*zú sān lǐ,* Leg Three Li), LI-4 (*hé gǔ,* Union Valley), ST-25 (*tiān shū,* Celestial Pivot), ST-37 (*shàng jù xū,* Upper Great Hollow), BL-20 (*pí shū,* Spleen Transport), and BL-21 (*wèi shū,* Stomach Transport); needle with supplementation and use moxa. See DYSENTERY. [26: 282] [46: 666, 667]

blood ejection 吐血 *tù xuè:* Ejection of blood through the mouth; vomiting or expectoration of blood (i.e., respiratory tract or digestive tract bleeding); sometimes defined as being associated with neither the sound of retching or of coughing. Blood ejection is attributed liquor damage, food damage, or taxation fatigue causing exuberant heat in the bowels and viscera, effulgent yin vacuity fire, or qi vacuity and spleen cold. The main patterns are accumulated heat in the stomach, intense liver fire, effulgent yin vacuity fire, spleen-stomach vacuity cold, and qi vacuity verging on desertion. **Accumulated heat in the stomach** causes blood ejection marked by fresh or dark purple blood, distending pain in the stomach duct and abdomen, constipation, yellow tongue fur, and a slippery rapid pulse. MED Clear the stomach and drain fire. Use variations of Firewood-Removing Beverage (*xǐ xīn yǐn*) or Heart-Draining Decoction (*xiè xīn tāng*). ACU Base treatment mainly on ST, LI, and PC. Select CV-13 (*shàng wǎn,* Upper Stomach Duct), ST-44 (*nèi tíng,* Inner Court), LI-11 (*qū chí,* Pool at the Bend), PC-6 (*nèi guān,* Inner Pass), SP-10 (*xuè hǎi,* Sea of Blood), ST-37 (*shàng jù xū,* Upper Great Hollow), and PC-4 (*xī mén,* Cleft Gate). Needle with drainage. **Intense liver fire** blood ejection is characterized by bright red blood with purple stasis, bitter taste in the mouth, rib-side pain, heart vexation, irascibility, red tongue, and rapid stringlike pulse. MED Drain the liver and harmonize the stomach with variations of Moutan and Gardenia Free Wanderer Powder (*dān zhī xiāo yáo sǎn*). ACU Base treatment mainly on ST, LR, and CV. Select ST-34 (*liáng qiū,* Beam Hill), LR-3 (*tài chōng,* Supreme Surge), LR-2 (*xíng jiān,* Moving Between), LR-14 (*qī mén,* Cycle Gate), CV-12 (*zhōng wǎn,* Center Stomach Duct), PC-6 (*nèi guān,* Inner Pass), BL-18 (*gān shū,* Liver Transport), and BL-17 (*gé shū,* Diaphragm Transport). Needle with drainage.

Effulgent yin vacuity fire blood ejection is associated with heat effusion, night sweating, tinnitus, insomnia, and a rapid fine pulse. MED Enrich yin and downbear fire; cool the blood and stanch bleeding. Use formulas such as Blood-Cooling Rehmannia Decoction (*liáng xuè dì huáng tāng*). ACU Base treatment on back transport points, KI, and HT. Needle with supplementation at BL-23 (*shèn shū,* Kidney Transport), KI-3 (*tài xī,* Great Ravine), and SP-6 (*sān yīn jiāo,* Three Yin Intersection) and with drainage at KI-6 (*zhào hǎi,* Shining Sea), KI-2 (*rán gǔ,* Blazing Valley), BL-17 (*gé shū,* Diaphragm Transport), ST-36 (*zú sān lǐ,* Leg Three Li), ST-44 (*nèi tíng,* Inner Court), and HT-7 (*shén mén,* Spirit Gate). If fire signs are pronounced, prick HT-8 (*shào fǔ,* Lesser Mansion) to bleed. **Spleen-stomach vacuity cold** blood ejection is characterized by ejection of dark, dull, purple blood, fear of cold, cold limbs, and a faint pulse. MED Warm the center and stanch bleeding. Use Aconite Center-Rectifying Decoction (*fù zǐ lǐ zhōng tāng*). ACU Base treatment mainly on CV, ST, BL, and SP. Select CV-12 (*zhōng wǎn,* Center Stomach Duct), ST-36 (*zú sān lǐ,* Leg Three Li), BL-20 (*pí shū,* Spleen Transport), BL-17 (*gé shū,* Diaphragm Transport), SP-1 (*yǐn bái,* Hidden White), and ST-25 (*tiān shū,* Celestial Pivot). Needle with supplementation and moxa. **Qi vacuity verging on desertion** blood ejection is characterized by exhaustion of essence-spirit, and faint weak soft vacuous pulse. MED Boost qi and contain the blood with formulas such as Pure Ginseng Decoction (*dú shēn tāng*). ACU See BLOOD DESERTION. ◇ Chin 吐 *tù,* spit, vomit, belch, eject; 血 *xuè,* blood. [26: 258] [46: 738] [37: 308] [14: 166]

blood failing to nourish the sinews 血不养筋 *xuè bù yǎng jīn:* Insufficiency of liver blood manifesting in HYPERTONICITY of the sinews, numbness or wilting (*wěi*) of limbs, or brittle nails. The liver stores the blood and governs the sinews, and the nails are the surplus of the sinews. Hence, insufficiency of liver blood depriving the sinews of nourishment manifests in abnormalities of the sinews and nails. [26: 277]

blood failing to stay in the channels 血不归经 *xuè bù guī jīng,* 血不循经 *xuè bù xún jīng:* Escape of blood from the vessels. Examples of blood failing to stay in the channels include flooding and spotting, blood ejection, spontaneous external bleeding, bloody stool, bloody urine, and stasis macules, which may be due to qi vacuity, qi counterflow, blood stasis, fire or heat. [26: 277]

blood falling with qi 血随气陷 *xuè suí qì xiàn:* Bleeding due to qi vacuity fall. For example, spleen-stomach vacuity can cause qi vacuity fall and deprive qi of the ability to contain the blood, so that blood becomes depressed in the lower body and seeps out. It is accompanied by devitalized essence-spirit, fatigued limbs, somber white facial complexion, pale tongue with scant fur, and a rapid vacuous or forceless fine sunken pulse. [WMC] In modern clinical practice, blood falling with qi is seen in dysfunctional uterine bleeding and some forms of bloody stool. [26: 286]

blood flying to the eye 目飞血 *mù fēi xuè*: The development of red vessels in the whites of the eye. Blood flying into the eye occurs in a number of eye diseases such as PEPPERCORN SORE, MILLET SORES, and FIRE GAN. ◇ Chin 目 *mù*, eye; 飞 *fēi*, to fly; 血 *xuè*, blood. [26: 200]

blood goiter 血瘿 *xuè yǐng*: A GOITER on the neck characterized by purple red coloration of the skin and red intersecting veins. It arises when blood heat stemming from fulminant exuberance of liver fire contends with an externally contracted evil. [WMC] angioma of the neck. [MED] Enrich yin and suppress fire; nourish the blood and transform stasis. Use Scutellaria, Coptis, Anemarrhena, and Fritillaria Pill (*qín lián èr mǔ wán*) or combine sargassum (*hǎi zǎo*), clamshell (*hǎi gé ké*), kelp (*kūn bù*), alisma (*zé xiè*), pig's thyroid gland (*zhū yè*), scutellaria (*huáng qín*), coptis (*huáng lián*), and fritillaria (*bèi mǔ*) with Four Agents Decoction (*sì wù tāng*). [ACU] Base treatment on TB, GB, LI, ST, SP, and LR. Needle with even supplementation and drainage at TB-13 (*nào huì*, Upper Arm Convergence), LI-4 (*hé gǔ*, Union Valley), ST-36 (*zú sān lǐ*, Leg Three Li), KI-6 (*zhào hǎi*, Shining Sea), SP-6 (*sān yīn jiāo*, Three Yin Intersection), CV-22 (*tiān tú*, Celestial Chimney), SI-17 (*tiān róng*, Celestial Countenance), LI-17 (*tiān dǐng*, Celestial Tripod), BL-17 (*gé shū*, Diaphragm Transport), and SP-10 (*xuè hǎi*, Sea of Blood), and with drainage at LR-3 (*tài chōng*, Supreme Surge), LR-2 (*xíng jiān*, Moving Between), and GB-34 (*yáng líng quán*, Yang Mound Spring). [26: 287] [27: 413]

blood gu 血蛊 *xuè gǔ*: BLOOD DRUM. [26: 287]

blood heat 血热 *xuè rè*: A condition characterized by heat and blood signs, mostly occurring in externally contracted heat (febrile) diseases, though not uncommon in miscellaneous diseases. When blood heat scorches the vessels causing extravasation of the blood, there is retching of blood, expectoration of blood, bloody stool or urine, nosebleed, or menstrual irregularities (see following entries). This pathomechanism is called FRENETIC BLOOD HEAT (or frenetic movement of hot blood). Bleeding is often profuse and the blood is either bright red or purple-black in color. Blood heat can also cause red papules and macules. General signs of blood heat such as heart vexation, thirst, red or sunken red tongue, and rapid pulse all indicate heat. Coma may occur in severe cases. [WMC] anaphylactoid and thrombocytopenic purpura; aplas-

tic anemia; leukemia. [MED] Cool the blood, clear heat, and resolve toxin using medicinals such as dried/fresh rehmannia (*shēng dì huáng*), fresh imperata (*xiān máo gēn*), puccoon (*zǐ cǎo*), moutan (*mǔ dān pí*), red peony (*chì sháo yào*), typha pollen (*pú huáng*), sanguisorba (*dì yú*), and cephalanoplos (*xiǎo jì*). Among commonly used formulas, Rhinoceros Horn and Rehmannia Decoction (*xī jiǎo dì huáng tāng*) treats blood heat with generalized signs such as clouded spirit, delirious mania, red or crimson tongue, and maculopapular eruptions, whereas Cephalanoplos Drink (*xiǎo jì yǐn zi*) is a general blood-cooling blood-stanching formula. [ACU] The following points are considered to clear heat and cool the blood: KI-2 (*rán gǔ*, Blazing Valley), LR-2 (*xíng jiān*, Moving Between), SP-6 (*sān yīn jiāo*, Three Yin Intersection), SP-10 (*xuè hǎi*, Sea of Blood), PC-7 (*dà líng*, Great Mound), HT-7 (*shén mén*, Spirit Gate), PC-3 (*qū zé*, Marsh at the Bend), and BL-17 (*gé shū*, Diaphragm Transport). Needle with drainage or with even supplementation and drainage. For exuberant heat, prick and bleed with a three-edged needle. When blood heat scorches the vessels causing extravasation of the blood, points such as PC-7 (*dà líng*, Great Mound), PC-4 (*xī mén*, Cleft Gate), LU-6 (*kǒng zuì*, Collection Hole), LU-9 (*tài yuān*, Great Abyss), KI-3 (*tài xī*, Great Ravine), LR-3 (*tài chōng*, Supreme Surge), SP-6 (*sān yīn jiāo*, Three Yin Intersection), SP-1 (*yǐn bái*, Hidden White), and ST-44 (*nèi tíng*, Inner Court) can be drained to clear heat and stanch bleeding. [46: 595] [6: 167]

blood heat advanced menstruation 血热经行先期 *xuè rè jīng xíng xiān qī*: ADVANCED MENSTRUATION (i.e., premature arrival of periods) due to blood heat. Blood heat advanced menstruation occurs in women who usually have internal heat or like hot spicy food; it may result from contracting heat evil; it may stem from excessive anger causing qi depression that transforms into fire; it can also be the result of yin vacuity internal heat. In all cases, the heat harasses the thoroughfare (*chōng*) and controlling (*rèn*) vessels and causes frenetic movement of the blood. **Blood heat** advanced menstruation is characterized by early periods with copious thick sticky purple red flow, heart vexation, thirst with desire for cool drinks, constipation, and yellow urination. [MED] Clear heat and cool the blood using Scutellaria and Coptis Four Agents Decoction (*qín lián sì wù tāng*). [ACU] Treatment is based on the CV and the three yin channels of the foot. Main points: CV-4 (*guān yuán*, Pass Head) and SP-10 (*xuè hǎi*, Sea of Blood). For blood heat, add LR-3 (*tài chōng*, Supreme Surge), and LI-11 (*qū chí*, Pool at the Bend), needling with drainage. **Qi depression transforming into fire** causes advanced menstruation with purple clotted flow, distending pain in the chest and rib-side, vexation and irascibility. MED Calm the liver and clear heat, using formulas like Moutan and Gardenia Free Wanderer Powder (*dān zhī xiāo yáo sǎn*). ACU Add to the main points given above PC-6 (*nèi guān*, Inner Pass), LR-3 (*tài chōng*, Supreme Surge), GB-34 (*yáng líng quán*, Yang Mound Spring), PC-8 (*láo gōng*, Palace of Toil), and SP-8 (*dì jī*, Earth's Crux), needling with drainage. **Yin vacuity blood heat** advanced menstruation is marked by a scant dribbling red thick sticky flow, reddening of the cheeks, and heat in the soles and palms. MED Nourish yin and clear heat using Rehmannia and Lycium Root Bark Decoction (*liǎng dì tāng*) or Lycium Root Bark Beverage (*dì gǔ pí yǐn*). ACU Add to the main points given above SP-6 (*sān yīn jiāo*, Three Yin Intersection), and KI-2 (*rán gǔ*, Blazing Valley), needling with even supplemenation and drainage. See ADVANCED MENSTRUATION. [26: 285] [46: 682]

blood heat flooding and spotting 血热崩漏 *xuè rè bēng lòu*: FLOODING AND SPOTTING (abnormal discharge of blood via the vagina) due to blood heat. Blood heat flooding and spotting forms a repletion pattern when due to constitutional internal heat, excessive consumption of hot spicy food, or contraction of heat evil. It may stem from excessive anger causing qi depression that transforms into fire. It can also be the result of yin vacuity internal heat. In all cases, the heat harasses the thoroughfare (*chōng*) and controlling (*rèn*) vessels and causes frenetic movement of the blood. **Repletion pattern blood heat** flooding and spotting is characterized by sudden bleeding from the vagina that is copious or dribbling. The flow is deep red or purple in color and thick and sticky in consistency. General signs include a red facial complexion, thirst, vexation and agitation, and irascibility. MED Clear heat, cool the blood, and stanch bleeding with Heat-Clearing Channel-Securing (Menses-Securing) Decoction (*qīng rè gù jīng tāng*). **Qi depression transforming into fire** giving rise to blood heat flooding and spotting is marked by chest and rib-side distention and pain, heart vexation and irascibility. MED Calm the liver and clear heat, using formulas like Moutan and Gardenia Free Wanderer Powder (*dān zhī xiāo yáo sǎn*). **Yin vacuity blood heat** is characterized by a scant dribbling flow that is red, thick and sticky, as well as by reddening of the cheeks and heat in the soles and palms. MED Nourish yin and clear heat, using Rehmannia and Lycium Root Bark Decoction (*liǎng dì tāng*). ACU Base treatment on the CV and SP. Main points: CV-6 (*qì hǎi*, Sea of Qi), SP-6 (*sān yīn jiāo*, Three Yin Intersection), and SP-1 (*yǐn bái*, Hidden White). For repletion pattern blood heat, add SP-10 (*xuè hǎi*, Sea of Blood), and KI-5 (*shuǐ quán*, Water Spring), needling with

drainage. For qi depression transforming into fire, add LR-3 (*tài chōng*, Supreme Surge), TB-6 (*zhī gōu*, Branch Ditch), and LR-1 (*dà dūn*, Large Pile). LR-2 (*xíng jiān*, Moving Between), needling with drainage. For yin vacuity blood heat, add KI-6 (*zhào hǎi*, Shining Sea), KI-2 (*rán gǔ*, Blazing Valley), KI-3 (*tài xī*, Great Ravine), and HT-7 (*shén mén*, Spirit Gate), needling with even supplementation and drainage. [26: 285] [27: 406] [27: 189] [46: 688]

blood heat habitual miscarriage 血热滑胎 *xuè rè huá tāi*: HABITUAL MISCARRIAGE due to blood heat lying latent in the thoroughfare (*chōng*) and controlling (*rèn*) vessels, causing frenetic movement of the blood that damages the fetal origin. The patient experiences smaller-abdominal pain, heart vexation, thirst, and desire for cool drinks. Bleeding from the vagina portends stirring fetus and impending miscarriage. MED Clear heat and quiet the fetus with Yin-Safeguarding Brew (*bǎo yīn jiān*). See HABITUAL MISCARRIAGE. [26: 285]

blood heat profuse menstruation 血热月经过多 *xuè rè yuè jīng guò duō*: PROFUSE MENSTRUATION due to blood heat damaging the thoroughfare (*chōng*) and controlling (*rèn*) vessels and causing frenetic movement of the blood. Distinction is made between vacuity heat and repletion heat. **Repletion heat** is characterized by profuse menstrual flow that is deep red or purple in color, thick in consistency, and sometimes bears a foul smell, in addition to which a red facial complexion, dry mouth, thirst, and periodic vexation and agitation are observed. MED Clear heat and cool the blood with Channel-Clearing Decoction (*qīng jīng tāng*) plus ass hide glue (*ē jiāo*). ACU Base treatment on the CV, SP, LR, ST, and LI, selecting CV-4 (*guān yuán*, Pass Head), SP-10 (*xuè hǎi*, Sea of Blood), LR-3 (*tài chōng*, Supreme Surge), LI-11 (*qū chí*, Pool at the Bend), LI-2 (*èr jiān*, Second Space), ST-44 (*nèi tíng*, Inner Court), and LR-2 (*xíng jiān*, Moving Between), and needling with drainage. **Vacuity heat** is marked by postmeridian heat in the soles and palms. MED Enrich yin, clear heat, and cool the blood with Rehmannia and Lycium Root Bark Decoction (*liǎng dì tāng*) or Lycium Root Bark Beverage (*dì gǔ pí yǐn*). ACU Base treatment on CV and three yin channels of the foot. Select CV-4 (*guān yuán*, Pass Head), SP-10 (*xuè hǎi*, Sea of Blood), KI-6 (*zhào hǎi*, Shining Sea), KI-2 (*rán gǔ*, Blazing Valley), SP-6 (*sān yīn jiāo*, Three Yin Intersection), and HT-7 (*shén mén*, Spirit Gate); needle with even supplementation and drainage. [26: 285] [46: 682] [37: 438]

blood impediment 血痹 *xuè bì*: **1.** From *Elementary Questions* (*sù wèn, jiǔ zhēn*). An IMPEDIMENT (*bì*) pattern that results from evil entering the blood aspect in patients suffering from qi-blood vacuity, often traceable to sleeping in drafts or sweating from exertion. Blood impediment is characterized by numbness, pain in the limbs, and a faint rough pulse that is fine and tight at the cubit. MED Boost qi and harmonize construction; free yang and move impediment (*bì*). Use formulas such as Tangkuei Decoction (*dāng guī tāng*) or Astragalus and Cinnamon Twig Five Agents Decoction (*huáng qí guì zhī wǔ wù tāng*). ACU Use the same basic formulas as given for WIND IMPEDIMENT, and add points such as ST-36 (*zú sān lǐ*, Leg Three Li), BL-17 (*gé shū*, Diaphragm Transport), BL-20 (*pí shū*, Spleen Transport), and LR-3 (*tài chōng*, Supreme Surge) to boost qi and nourish the blood. **2.** Wind impediment migrating from place to place with no fixed location. [26: 284]

blood in the stool 便血 *biàn xuè*: BLOODY STOOL.

blood in the urine 尿血 *niào xuè*: BLOODY URINE.

blood is the mother of qi 血为气之母 *xuè wéi qì zhī mǔ*: The nourishing action of blood is necessary for the activity of qi. The capacity of qi to enable all parts of the body to carry out their various activities is attributable to the adequate supply of nutrition from the blood. Blood is to qi as a mother is to a child. This is one aspect of the yin-yang relationship between qi and blood. See QI IS THE COMMANDER OF THE BLOOD. [27: 80] [97: 181]

bloodletting 放血 *fàng xuè*: *Synonym: network vessel pricking.* An acupuncture method whereby the skin is punctured with a stabbing or picking action, usually with a THREE-EDGED NEEDLE (or nowadays, especially in the West, with disposable lancets) and a few drops of blood are squeezed out in order to drain heat, quicken the blood, move qi, and reduce swelling. It is performed at the site of a point or at the small veins in the area surrounding a point (such as BL-40). First, pressure is applied to restrict the blood flow of the area, to increase the visibility of the veins and to cause the blood to flow out more easily when the vein is pricked. The point is then swiftly and decisively pricked to a superficial depth of about 0.1 body-inches and a few drops of blood are allowed to escape. Lastly, the point is pressed with sterile cotton until the bleeding ceases. Before bloodletting, explain the procedure to the patient thoroughly to allay any fears. This method is inappropriate for weak, pregnant, or postpartum patients, or those suffering from bleeding, anemia or low blood pressure. Bloodletting is often indicated in this text by the term "PRICK TO BLEED" or "PICK TO BLEED." See also DIFFUSE PRICKING; THREE-EDGED NEEDLE. [80: 502]

blood loss 失血 *shī xuè*: Reduction in blood due any form of BLEEDING, notably SPONTANEOUS EXTERNAL BLEEDING, BLOOD EJECTION, RETCHING OF BLOOD, EXPECTORATION OF BLOOD, COUGHING OF BLOOD, SPITTING OF BLOOD, SPONTANEOUS EXTERNAL BLEEDING, BLOODY STOOL, BLOODY URINE, or BLEEDING FROM WOUNDS (see INCISED WOUND). Blood loss is attributed fire heat, vacuity cold, blood stasis, or external injury. [26: 209]

blood loss dizziness 失血眩晕 *shī xuè xuàn yūn*: DIZZINESS due to loss of blood through blood ejection, nosebleed, flooding and spotting, or external injury, and accompanied by somber white facial complexion, heart palpitations, spontaneous sweating, pale tongue, and, in severe cases, REVERSAL DESERTION (i.e., shock). MED Supplement the blood and boost qi with Ginseng Construction-Nourishing Decoction (*rén shēn yǎng róng tāng*) or Spleen-Returning Decoction (*guī pí tāng*). ACU Base treatment mainly on GV, CV, ST, and SP. Select GV-20 (*bǎi huì*, Hundred Convergences), ST-8 (*tóu wéi*, Head Corner), CV-12 (*zhōng wǎn*, Center Stomach Duct), ST-36 (*zú sān lǐ*, Leg Three Li), BL-20 (*pí shū*, Spleen Transport), and SP-1 (*yǐn bái*, Hidden White); needle with supplementation and add moxa. For reversal desertion, add GV-26 (*rén zhōng*, Human Center), GV-25 (*sù liáo*, White Bone-Hole), PC-6 (*nèi guān*, Inner Pass), CV-4 (*guān yuán*, Pass Head), and KI-1 (*yǒng quán*, Gushing Spring). See DIZZINESS. [26: 209]

blood management failure 脾不统血 *pí bù tǒng xuè*: SPLEEN FAILING TO MANAGE THE BLOOD.

blood mole 血痣 *xuè zhì*: A clearly delineated smooth shiny purple-red patch or swelling on the skin, usually of the face, neck or trunk, that bleeds fresh blood when forcefully ruptured. It is congenital, or attributable to binding depression of fire and anger in the liver channel. WMC vascular nevus. MED Topical: Apply Borneol and Freshwater Snail Powder (*bīng sī sǎn*). When the mole has disappeared, apply Pearl Powder (*zhēn zhū sǎn*). Oral: If there is pronounced bleeding, take Blood-Cooling Rehmannia Decoction (*liáng xuè dì huáng tāng*). [26: 282] [27: 485] [97: 188] [61: 346]

blood mounting 血疝 *xuè shàn*: **1.** Painful binding of static blood in the smaller abdomen manifesting as hard fullness that is palpably circumscribed, and, in severe cases, associated with black stool, inhibited urination, and menstrual irregularities. MED Use Cinnamon Twig and Poria (Hoelen) Pill (*guì zhī fú líng wán*) or Lesser Abdomen Stasis-Expelling Decoction (*shào fù zhú yū tāng*). ACU Base treatment mainly on LR and SP. Select LR-2 (*xíng jiān*, Moving Between), SP-10 (*xuè hǎi*, Sea of Blood), SP-6 (*sān yīn jiāo*, Three Yin

Intersection), CV-3 (*zhōng jí,* Central Pole), and GB-41 (*zú lín qì,* Foot Overlooking Tears); needle with drainage. **2.** Blood swelling of the scrotum following external injury. [26: 2772] [27: 430] [97: 187] [37: 455]

blood network vessel 血络 *xuè luò*: See NETWORK VESSEL.

blood pattern 血证 *xuè zhèng*: Any manifestation of disease in the blood. The main blood patterns are BLOOD VACUITY, BLOOD STASIS, and BLOOD HEAT. See also BLOOD DRYNESS; BLOOD DESICCATION; BLOOD COLD. [6: 164]

blood pouring into the pupil spirit 血灌瞳神 *xuè guàn tóng shén*: A condition characterized by a blood spot in the pupil that obstructs vision. Blood pouring into the pupil spirit may be the result of exuberant liver-gallbladder heat or yin vacuity fire flaming upward and causing FRENETIC MOVEMENT OF HOT BLOOD. It may also be the result of external injury or surgery. MED Clear heat and cool the blood with Rhinoceros Horn and Rehmannia Decoction (*xī jiǎo dì huáng tāng*) and variations, by enriching yin and downbearing fire with Anemarrhena, Phellodendron, and Rehmannia Pill (*zhī bǎi dì huáng wán*), or by clearing heat, cooling the blood, and dissipating stasis with Rhubarb and Tangkuei Powder (*dà huáng dāng guī sǎn*). WMC hyphema. See PUPIL SPIRIT. [26: 287] [27: 507] [97: 193]

blood reversal 血厥 *xuè jué*: **1.** CLOUDING REVERSAL (clouding of consciousness and cold limbs) due to blood loss (blood desertion) or to sudden violent anger causing qi to move counterflow and blood to become depressed in the upper body. **Blood desertion** blood reversal is observed in severe flooding and spotting or blood ejection, and is characterized by sudden dizziness, bright white facial complexion, reversal cold of the limbs, and a faint pulse on the verge of expiration. MED Boost qi and stem desertion with formulas such as Pure Ginseng Decoction (*dú shēn tāng*). ACU Base treatment on CV, GV, SP, and back transport points. Select CV-6 (*qì hǎi,* Sea of Qi), GV-26 (*shuǐ gōu,* Water Trough), GV-25 (*sù liáo,* White Bone-Hole), PC-6 (*nèi guān,* Inner Pass), GV-20 (*bǎi huì,* Hundred Convergences), CV-4 (*guān yuán,* Pass Head), and KI-1 (*yǒng quán,* Gushing Spring) to stem vacuity desertion, combined with ST-36 (*zú sān lǐ,* Leg Three Li), SP-6 (*sān yīn jiāo,* Three Yin Intersection), BL-17 (*gé shū,* Diaphragm Transport), BL-20 (*pí shū,* Spleen Transport), and BL-21 (*wèi shū,* Stomach Transport) to supplement qi and contain the blood. Needle with supplementation and use large amounts of moxa. **Qi counterflow and blood depression** blood reversal is characterized by sudden collapse with clenched jaw, unconsciousness,

and green-blue or purple lips. MED Downbear counterflow and free stasis, using formulas such as Liver-Transforming Brew (*huà gān jiān*) or Stasis-Freeing Brew (*tōng yū jiān*). ACU Base treatment mainly on PC, LR, SP, GV and Twelve Well Points (*shí èr jǐng xué*); select PC-6 (*nèi guān,* Inner Pass), LR-3 (*tài chōng,* Supreme Surge), SP-6 (*sān yīn jiāo,* Three Yin Intersection), BL-18 (*gān shū,* Liver Transport), BL-17 (*gé shū,* Diaphragm Transport), ST-36 (*zú sān lǐ,* Leg Three Li), SP-10 (*xuè hǎi,* Sea of Blood), and CV-17 (*shān zhōng,* Chest Center) to downbear qi and free stasis, combined with GV-26 (*shuǐ gōu,* Water Trough), Twelve Well Points (*shí èr jǐng xué*), PC-8 (*láo gōng,* Palace of Toil) and LI-4 (*hé gǔ,* Union Valley). Needle with drainage or prick to bleed. See REVERSAL. **2.** The sudden appearance of a death-like condition in an otherwise healthy person. The patient does not move, cannot open his eyes, does not recognize people, and cannot open his mouth to speak. In some cases, he may show slight recognition of people, and may perceive sounds dimly. MED Use Baiwei Decoction (*bái wēi tāng*). ACU Base treatment mainly on back transport points and GV. Select BL-15 (*xīn shū,* Heart Transport), BL-17 (*gé shū,* Diaphragm Transport), BL-20 (*pí shū,* Spleen Transport), CV-6 (*qì hǎi,* Sea of Qi), and GV-20 (*bǎi huì,* Hundred Convergences); needle with supplementation and use moxa. See REVERSAL. [26: 283] [37: 402] [27: 400] [97: 188]

blood spillage 血溢 *xuè yì*: The escape of blood from the vessels; bleeding; hemorrhage. Blood leaving its channels and flowing out of the body. Although the causes of blood spillage are numerous, they are all embraced by two pathomechanisms: damage to the nextwork vessels due to external injury and QI FAILING TO CONTAIN THE BLOOD. SPONTANEOUS EXTERNAL BLEEDING is blood spillage not attributable to external injury. Severe blood spillage gives rise to BLOOD COLLAPSE. [50: 584]

blood stagnation abdominal pain 血滞腹痛 *xuè zhì fù tòng*: STATIC BLOOD ABDOMINAL PAIN. [26: 284]

blood stagnation menstrual block 血滞经闭 *xuè zhì jīng bì*: MENSTRUAL BLOCK (absence of menses) attributable to qi depression and blood stagnation obstructing the thoroughfare (*chōng*) and controlling (*rèn*) vessels and preventing blood from reaching the uterus. Blood stagnation menstrual block often stems from constrained emotions. Attending signs include purple somber facial complexion, smaller-abdominal pain exacerbated by pressure, with pain sometimes reaching to the rib-sides. MED Resolve depression and move qi; quicken the blood and free the channels. Use

Stasis-Freeing Brew (*tōng yū jiān*) or Amber Powder (*hǔ pò sǎn*). ACU Base treatment on CV, SP, and LR; select CV-3 (*zhōng jí*, Central Pole), SP-8 (*dì jī*, Earth's Crux), SP-10 (*xuè hǎi*, Sea of Blood), LI-4 (*hé gǔ*, Union Valley), LR-3 (*tài chōng*, Supreme Surge), and SP-6 (*sān yīn jiāo*, Three Yin Intersection); needle with drainage and add moxa. Point selection according to signs: For smaller-abdominal pain and distention, add CV-6 (*qì hǎi*, Sea of Qi) and KI-14 (*sì mǎn*, Fourfold Fullness). For pain in both rib-sides, add LR-14 (*qī mén*, Cycle Gate) and TB-6 (*zhī gōu*, Branch Ditch). [46: 687]

blood stasis 血瘀 *xuè yū*: Impairment or cessation of the normal free flow of blood. Blood stasis may arise when knocks and falls, bleeding, qi stagnation, qi vacuity, blood cold, or blood heat impair free flow, causing local blood stasis. It manifests in a variety of ways including pain, abdominal masses, bleeding (especially from the vagina), and abdominal distention. The observable signs of blood stasis may be discussed under five headings: **Pain:** Static blood obstructs the channels impeding the flow of blood. Since "when there is stoppage, there is pain," pain is the outstanding feature of blood stasis. The pain associated with blood stasis differs from the acute and scurrying pain characterizing qi stagnation since it is of fixed location and confined to the locality of the obstruction, and is stabbing in nature. **Masses and swellings:** When static blood accumulates, it forms masses and swellings. When resulting from knocks and falls, it gives rise to local green-blue or purple swellings (bruises). When occurring internally, it may cause hard swellings that can develop into concretions and accumulations. **Bleeding:** Since static blood obstructs the vessels, blood may extravasate when unable to pursue its normal course. Periodic bleeding is a common sign of blood stasis, particularly in menstrual irregularities and postpartum diseases, and is generally characterized by dark purple clotted blood. **General signs:** The complexion tends to be soot-black. The tongue is dark and purple, with stasis speckles. The pulse is fine and rough. The skin may be rough, dry, and lusterless (encrusted skin) with red speckles and purple macules (both due to subcutaneous bleeding), red thread marks (spider nevi), and prominent green-blue veins on the abdomen (caput medusae). Such signs are observed in enduring sickness. **Miscellaneous:** When blood stasis overwhelms the heart, raving, delirious speech and mania are observed. Static blood obstructing the vessels may also affect the free flow of fluids, causing internal water accumulations, e.g., blood drum. The etiology of such conditions is described in *Essential Prescriptions of the Golden Coffer* (*jīn guì yào*

lüè) by the phrase, "inhibited blood flow may give rise to water." WMC cardiovascular diseases, hepatosplenomegaly, menstrual disorders, heterotopic pregnancy, and postpartum disorders often present as blood stasis patterns. MED Quicken the blood and transform stasis. Commonly used medicinals include peach kernel (*táo rén*), carthamus (*hóng huā*), tangkuei (*dāng guī*), salvia (*dān shēn*), red peony (*chì sháo yào*), leonurus (*yì mǔ cǎo*), and lycopus (*zé lán*). In severe enduring conditions, blood-breaking hardness-dispersing medicinals such as sparganium (*sān léng*), zedoary (*é zhú*), pangolin scales (*chuān shān jiǎ*), and wingless cockroach (*zhè chóng*) may be used. Where a draining precipitant action is also required as in heat stasis patterns such as cold damage blood amassment patterns, rhubarb (*dà huáng*), and mirabilite (*máng xiāo*) may be added. Where blood stasis causes bleeding, medicinals that have both a blood-stanching and blood-quickening action such as notoginseng (*sān qī*), typha pollen (*pú huáng*), cephalanoplos (*xiǎo jì*), and madder (*qiàn cǎo gēn*) are used. Stasis-dispelling blood-quickening formulas include Peach Kernel and Carthamus Four Agents Decoction (*táo hóng sì wù tāng*), House of Blood Stasis-Expelling Decoction (*xuè fǔ zhú yū tāng*), Peach Kernel Qi-Coordinating Decoction (*táo rén chéng qì tāng*), and Rhubarb and Wingless Cockroach Pill (*dà huáng zhè chóng wán*). ACU Treatment varies according to cause and affected area. Points used to dispel stasis include: CV-17 (*shān zhōng*, Chest Center), BL-17 (*gé shū*, Diaphragm Transport), SP-10 (*xuè hǎi*, Sea of Blood), LI-4 (*hé gǔ*, Union Valley), LR-3 (*tài chōng*, Supreme Surge), LR-2 (*xíng jiān*, Moving Between), SP-6 (*sān yīn jiāo*, Three Yin Intersection), BL-60 (*kūn lún*, Kunlun Mountains), SP-8 (*dì jī*, Earth's Crux), PC-3 (*qū zé*, Marsh at the Bend), BL-40 (*wěi zhōng*, Bend Center), and Glomus Root (*pǐ gēn*). Needle with even supplementation and drainage or bleed with a three-edged needle. See STATIC BLOOD; DISPELLING STASIS AND QUICKENING THE BLOOD. ◇ Chin 血 *xuè*, blood; 瘀 *yū*, related to 淤 *yū*, sediment, silt up. [6: 166] [27: 387] cite[594]zyzj [113: 19] [14: 161]

blood stasis delayed menstruation 血瘀经行后期 *xuè yū jīng xíng hòu qī*: DELAYED MENSTRUATION (late periods) due to blood stasis arising when qi stagnation or congealing cold obstruct the thoroughfare (*chōng*) and controlling (*rèn*) vessels and prevent the timely arrival of blood to the uterus. **Qi stagnation** gives rise to blood stasis delayed menstruation associated with scant inhibited flow, smaller-abdominal distention and pain exacerbated by pressure and relieved by passing of clots. MED Move qi, quicken the blood, and transform stasis using Overdue Beverage (*guò qī* *yĭn*). **Congealing cold** causes blood stasis delayed menstruation attended by lesser-abdominal cold pain exacerbated by pressure. MED Warm the channels, quicken the blood, and transform stasis using Lesser Abdomen Stasis-Expelling Decoction (*shào fù zhú yū tāng*). ACU Base treatment on the CV and the three yin channels of the foot. Main points: CV-6 (*qì hăi*, Sea of Qi), KI-13 (*qì xué*, Qi Point), SP-6 (*sān yīn jiāo*, Three Yin Intersection), CV-3 (*zhōng jí*, Central Pole), and SP-8 (*dì jī*, Earth's Crux). Needle with even supplementation and drainage. Selection of points according to pattern: For qi stagnation, needle with drainage at LR-3 (*tài chōng*, Supreme Surge) and LR-5 (*lĭ gōu*, Woodworm Canal). For congealing cold, needle with drainage and moxa at ST-29 (*guī lái*, Return) and ST-25 (*tiān shū*, Celestial Pivot), and moxa CV-4 (*guān yuán*, Pass Head) for smaller-abdominal cold pain. [26: 284] [46: 683]

blood stasis flooding and spotting 血瘀崩漏 *xuè yū bēng lòu*: FLOODING AND SPOTTING (abnormal discharge of blood via the vagina) due to static blood, which arises when internal damage by the seven affects or externally contracted evils cause static blood to collect before menstrual or postpartum blood has been fully discharged, so that static blood fails to be discharged and new blood fails to stay in the channels. Blood stasis flooding and spotting is characterized by either a sometimes scant, sometimes copious flow or by a dribbling inhibited flow that is dark in color, and thick and clotted in consistency. It is accompanied by abdominal pain exacerbated by pressure and relieved by the passing of clots. MED Quicken the blood and move stasis using Hand-of-Buddha Powder (*fó shŏu săn*), Sudden Smile Powder (*shī xiào săn*), or Leonurus (Motherwort) Paste (*yì mŭ căo gāo*). ACU Base treatment mainly on CV and SP. Select CV-6 (*qì hăi*, Sea of Qi), SP-6 (*sān yīn jiāo*, Three Yin Intersection), SP-1 (*yĭn bái*, Hidden White), SP-8 (*dì jī*, Earth's Crux), ST-30 (*qì chōng*, Qi Thoroughfare), and SP-12 (*chōng mén*, Surging Gate); needle with drainage. [26: 283] [46: 688]

blood stasis infertility 血瘀不孕 *xuè yū bù yùn*: INFERTILITY is due to blockage of the thoroughfare (*chōng*) and controlling (*rèn*) vessels and the blood vessels of the uterus by static blood that arises when affect-mind internal damage causes inhibited movement of qi and blood, or when contraction of cold evil causes blood to congeal and prevents receptivity to male essence (semen). It is attended by delayed menstruation, inhibited menstrual flow, clotted flow, and abdominal pain exacerbated by pressure. **Qi stagnation and blood stasis** gives rise to infertility that, in addition to the above signs, is characterized by distention and fullness in the chest and rib-side, agitation,

vexation, and irascibility, distending pain in the breasts. MED Quicken the blood, move stasis, and regulate menstruation. Use House of Blood Stasis-Expelling Decoction (*xuè fŭ zhú yū tāng*). **Cold evil settling in the uterus** gives rise to lack of warmth in the extremities and small-abdominal cold pain in addition to the general signs. MED Warm the channels and dissipate cold. Use Lesser Abdomen Stasis-Expelling Decoction (*shào fù zhú yū tāng*). ACU Base treatment mainly on CV, ST, SP, KI, and LR. Main points: CV-6 (*qì hăi*, Sea of Qi), ST-30 (*qì chōng*, Qi Thoroughfare), SP-6 (*sān yīn jiāo*, Three Yin Intersection), KI-14 (*sì măn*, Fourfold Fullness), LR-3 (*tài chōng*, Supreme Surge), BL-17 (*gé shū*, Diaphragm Transport), and SP-10 (*xuè hăi*, Sea of Blood), and needle with even supplementation and drainage. Selection of points according to pattern: For qi stagnation and blood stasis, add PC-6 (*nèi guān*, Inner Pass), BL-18 (*gān shū*, Liver Transport), and HT-7 (*shén mén*, Spirit Gate). For cold evil settling in the uterus, add LI-4 (*hé gŭ*, Union Valley), CV-4 (*guān yuán*, Pass Head)ⓜ, and GV-4 (*mìng mén*, Life Gate)ⓜ. See INFERTILITY. [50: 589] [26: 283] [46: 595] [46: 685] [37: 416]

blood stasis lumbar pain 血瘀腰痛 *xuè yū yāo tòng*: STATIC BLOOD LUMBAR PAIN.

blood stasis menstrual pain 血瘀痛经 *xuè yū tòng jīng*: MENSTRUAL PAIN attributed to blood stasis obstructing the thoroughfare (*chōng*) and controlling (*rèn*) vessels and the uterine vessels and is characterized by stabbing pain in the smaller abdomen prior to or during menstruation, scant clotted menstrual flow, and relief from discomfort after passing clots. MED Move stasis and quicken the blood using Infradiaphragmatic Stasis-Expelling Decoction (*gé xià zhú yū tāng*), Amber Powder (*hŭ pò săn*), or Leonurus (Motherwort) Paste (*yì mŭ căo gāo*). ACU Base treatment on the CV, SP, and LR. Select CV-3 (*zhōng jí*, Central Pole), BL-32 (*cì liáo*, Second Bone-Hole), SP-8 (*dì jī*, Earth's Crux), SP-10 (*xuè hăi*, Sea of Blood), ST-29 (*guī lái*, Return), CV-6 (*qì hăi*, Sea of Qi), LR-3 (*tài chōng*, Supreme Surge), and SP-6 (*sān yīn jiāo*, Three Yin Intersection); needle with drainage. If there are purple clots in the menstrual flow, add LR-2 (*xíng jiān*, Moving Between). [26: 283] [113: 280] [46: 685] [59: 71]

blood stasis scant menstruation 血瘀月经过少 *xuè yū yuè jīng guò shăo*: SCANT MENSTRUATION due to blood stasis, usually caused by congealing cold and stagnant qi causing internal blood stasis inhibiting the movement of blood in the thoroughfare (*chōng*) and controlling (*rèn*) vessels. **Congealing cold** causes scant menstruation with dark clotted flow, cold, pain, and sometimes distention in the smaller abdomen relieved by warmth and the passing of clots and exacerbated by pressure. MED Warm the channels, quicken the blood, and move stasis using with Lesser Abdomen Stasis-Expelling Decoction (*shào fù zhú yū tāng*) or Overdue Beverage (*guò qī yǐn*). ACU Base treatment on the CV and the three yin channels of the foot. Main points: CV-6 (*qì hǎi*, Sea of Qi), KI-13 (*qì xué*, Qi Point), SP-6 (*sān yīn jiāo*, Three Yin Intersection), BL-17 (*gé shū*, Diaphragm Transport), CV-3 (*zhōng jí*, Central Pole), and SP-8 (*dì jī*, Earth's Crux). Needle with even supplementation and drainage. In addition, to address the congealing cold, needle with drainage and large amounts of moxa at ST-29 (*guī lái*, Return) and ST-25 (*tiān shū*, Celestial Pivot). **Qi stagnation** causes scant menstruation associated with purple clotted flow, abdominal distention and sometimes pain relieved by the passing of flatus. MED Move qi and quicken the blood with formulas like Infradiaphragmatic Stasis-Expelling Decoction (*gé xià zhú yū tāng*) or Sevenfold Processed Cyperus Pill (*qī zhì xiāng fù wán*). ACU Use the same basic points that are given above, and to address the qi stagnation, needle with drainage at LR-3 (*tài chōng*, Supreme Surge) and LR-5 (*lǐ gōu*, Woodworm Canal). For cold pain in the smaller abdomen, moxa CV-4 (*guān yuán*, Pass Head). [26: 283] [59: 70–1] [46: 682–3] [113: 276, 280]

blood stasis wilting 血瘀痿 *xuè yū wěi*: WILTING (*wěi*) (severe weakness of the sinews that hampers normal movement) due to blood stasis resulting from injuries from knocks and falls or arising after childbirth when static blood flows into the lumbus and knees before the LOCHIA has been fully eliminated. Blood stasis wilting is characterized by wilting, limpness, and pain of the limbs preventing normal movement and a rough pulse. MED Quicken blood and move stasis using Peach Kernel and Carthamus Four Agents Decoction (*táo hóng sì wù tāng*) and variations. ACU Use the basic treatments given under WILTING with points that dispel stasis such as BL-17 (*gé shū*, Diaphragm Transport), SP-10 (*xuè hǎi*, Sea of Blood), LR-3 (*tài chōng*, Supreme Surge), SP-6 (*sān yīn jiāo*, Three Yin Intersection), and BL-40 (*wěi zhōng*, Bend Center); needle with even supplementation and drainage or prick to bleed with a three-edged needle. If blood stasis is due to incomplete elimination of the LOCHIA, see PERSISTENT FLOW OF LOCHIA. [26: 284]

blood strangury 血淋 *xuè lín*: STRANGURY (dribbling urination) with blood in the urine. Distinction is made between blood vacuity, blood cold, blood heat, and blood stasis. **Blood vacuity** causes strangury with nonacute pain on urination, pale red urine, and a rapid vacuous pulse. MED Enrich yin and nourish the blood using Six-

Ingredient Rehmannia Decoction (*liù wèi dì huáng tāng*) plus biota leaf (*cè bǎi yè*), plantago seed (*chē qián zǐ*), and white peony (*bái sháo yào*), or swallowing Origin-Boosting Powder (*yì yuán sǎn*) with Eight-Gem Decoction (*bā zhēn tāng*). **Blood cold** causes strangury with dark-colored bloody urine, dry-white facial complexion, and a slow sunken pulse. MED Warm the kidney using either Golden Coffer Kidney Qi Pill (*jīn guì shèn qì wán*) plus achyranthes (*niú xī*), a decoction of zanthoxylum root (*huā jiāo gēn*) taken cold. **Blood heat** causes strangury marked by scorching heat and stabbing pain with bright red bloody urine, and forceful pulse. MED Cool the blood and clear heat using formulas such as Cephalanoplos Drink (*xiǎo jì yǐn zi*), Red-Abducting Powder (*dǎo chì sǎn*), or Anemarrhena, Phellodendron, and Rehmannia Decoction (*zhī bǎi dì huáng tāng*). **Blood stasis** causes strangury marked by pain in the penis like the cutting of a knife, dark clots in the urine, hard fullness of the smaller abdomen, and a sunken stringlike or rapid pulse. MED Quicken the blood and dispel stasis using a paste made of achyranthes (*niú xī*), or formulas such as Peach Kernel and Carthamus Four Agents Decoction (*táo hóng sì wù tāng*) or Peach Kernel Qi-Coordinating Decoction (*táo hé chéng qì tāng*). ACU Base treatment mainly on the three yin channels of the foot and alarm and back transport points of BL (CV-3 and BL-28). Main points: BL-28 (*páng guāng shū*, Bladder Transport), CV-3 (*zhōng jí*, Central Pole), SP-9 (*yīn líng quán*, Yin Mound Spring), LR-2 (*xíng jiān*, Moving Between), and KI-3 (*tài xī*, Great Ravine). Selection of points according to pattern: For blood vacuity, add KI-2 (*rán gǔ*, Blazing Valley), SP-6 (*sān yīn jiāo*, Three Yin Intersection), BL-20 (*pí shū*, Spleen Transport), and ST-36 (*zú sān lǐ*, Leg Three Li), needling with supplementation. For blood cold, add BL-23 (*shèn shū*, Kidney Transport), GV-4 (*mìng mén*, Life Gate), CV-4 (*guān yuán*, Pass Head), and ST-36 (*zú sān lǐ*, Leg Three Li), needling with drainage and adding moxa. For blood heat, add SP-10 (*xuè hǎi*, Sea of Blood), SP-6 (*sān yīn jiāo*, Three Yin Intersection), and BL-27 (*xiǎo cháng shū*, Small Intestine Transport), needling with drainage. For blood stasis, add BL-17 (*gé shū*, Diaphragm Transport), SP-10 (*xuè hǎi*, Sea of Blood), SP-6 (*sān yīn jiāo*, Three Yin Intersection), and LR-3 (*tài chōng*, Supreme Surge), needling with drainage or with even supplementation and drainage. [26: 279] [27: 426] [97: 188]

blood swelling 血肿 *xuè zhǒng*: WATER SWELLING due to BLOOD STASIS inhibiting the transformation of WATER-DAMP. Blood swelling is characterized by swelling, red filiform marks under the skin, and long voidings of clear urine. In women, there may be sudden water swelling after a sudden interruption in the menstrual flow with abdominal pain exacerbated by pressure. MED Use Peach Kernel and Carthamus Four Agents Decoction (*táo hóng sì wù tāng*) or Substitute Dead-On Pill (*dài dǐ dàng wán*) and variations. ACU Base treatment mainly on the CV, back transport points, and the three yin channels of the foot, selecting BL-17 (*gé shū*, Diaphragm Transport), SP-10 (*xuè hǎi*, Sea of Blood), LR-3 (*tài chōng*, Supreme Surge), CV-9 (*shuǐ fēn*, Water Divide), CV-6 (*qì hǎi*, Sea of Qi), BL-22 (*sān jiāo shū*, Triple Burner Transport), ST-36 (*zú sān lǐ*, Leg Three Li), BL-20 (*pí shū*, Spleen Transport), and SP-9 (*yīn líng quán*, Yin Mound Spring). Needle with even supplementation and drainage. [26: 284]

blood thirst 血渴 *xuè kě*: THIRST due to BLOOD VACUITY and diminished liquid stemming from loss of blood. MED Treat by major supplementation of the blood with formulas such as Four Agents Decoction (*sì wù tāng*) or Tangkuei Blood-Supplementing Decoction (*dāng guī bǔ xuè tāng*) and variations. ACU Base treatment mainly on the back transport points, ST, SP, and LR. Select Gold Liquid and Jade Humor (*jīn jīn yù yè*), Sea Source (*hǎi quán*), TB-2 (*yè mén*, Humor Gate), BL-17 (*gé shū*, Diaphragm Transport), BL-20 (*pí shū*, Spleen Transport), BL-21 (*wèi shū*, Stomach Transport), LR-3 (*tài chōng*, Supreme Surge), ST-36 (*zú sān lǐ*, Leg Three Li), and SP-6 (*sān yīn jiāo*, Three Yin Intersection); needle with supplementation. [26: 282]

blood tumor 血瘤 *xuè liú*: A TUMOR (a growth on the outside of the body) attributed to blood bind and qi stagnation that block the channels and network vessels and are exacerbated by contraction of external evil. The tumor is purple or red in color, has hard and soft spots, and is surrounded by dimly visible red threads. If accidentally ruptured by grazing, it bleeds persistently. It may grow on the lips, neck, or limbs. WMC angioma. MED Cool and nourish the blood; enrich yin and repress fire. Use Scutellaria, Coptis, Anemarrhena, and Fritillaria Pill (*qín lián èr mǔ wán*). See TUMOR. [26: 285] [27: 480] [97: 189]

blood vacuity 血虚 *xuè xū*: The manifestation of insufficiency of the blood. Blood vacuity may develop from excessive loss of blood before replenishment is complete. It may also be caused by insufficiency of blood formation stemming from splenic movement and transformation failure. A further cause is failure to eliminate static blood and engender new blood. Blood vacuity is characterized by a pale white or withered-yellow facial complexion, dizzy head, flowery vision, relatively pale tongue, and a fine pulse. Other commonly observed signs include heart palpitations or fearful

throbbing, insomnia, and numbness of the extremities. Blood vacuity signs can reflect the insufficient supply of blood to nourish specific organs and channels. Thus, general signs must be correlated with organ-specific data to determine the focus of the vacuity. Since the blood is governed by the heart, stored by the liver, and produced and managed by the spleen, blood vacuity is intimately related to diseases of these viscera. Heart blood vacuity is characterized by signs of insufficiency of heart blood and disquieted heart spirit. Heart-spleen blood vacuity is characterized by signs of insufficiency of heart blood and the spleen failing to manage the blood. Liver blood vacuity is characterized by signs of insufficient supply of nourishment to the eyes and sinews or by diseases of the thoroughfare (*chōng*) and controlling (*rèn*) vessels. Since blood is yin in nature, blood vacuity and yin vacuity have much in common, both presenting such signs as dizzy head, flowery vision, heart palpitations, and a fine pulse. Blood vacuity, however, is not generally associated with heat signs, and may even be accompanied by cold signs when occurring with qi vacuity. It is readily distinguished from yin vacuity (vacuity of fluids in general), which is characterized by signs of heat and dryness such as upbearing fire flush, a rapid fine stringlike pulse, and a distinctly red tongue, all of which indicate internal heat or hyperactivity of yang. MED Supplement the blood. Blood-supplementing medicinals include tangkuei (*dāng guī*), cooked rehmannia (*shú dì huáng*), white peony (*bái sháo yào*), flowery knotweed (*hé shǒu wū*), ass hide glue (*ē jiāo*), and eclipta (*mò hàn lián*). Spirit-quieting blood-nourishing medicinals used to treat heart blood vacuity include salvia (*dān shēn*), spiny jujube (*suān zǎo rén*), and longan flesh (*lóng yǎn ròu*). These medicinals may be combined with spleen-fortifying medicinals to treat heart-spleen blood vacuity. Liver-nourishing medicinals use to treat liver blood vacuity include lycium berry (*gǒu qǐ zǐ*), mulberry (*sāng shèn*), and millettia (*jī xuè téng*). Blood-supplementing formulas include Four Agents Decoction (*sì wù tāng*) for insufficiency of liver blood and menstrual irregularities, Celestial Emperor Heart-Supplementing Elixir (*tiān wáng bǔ xīn dān*) for insufficiency of yin-blood and disquieted spirit, and Spleen-Returning Decoction (*guī pí tāng*) for heart-spleen blood vacuity. ACU General blood-supplementing points are LR-3 (*tài chōng*, Supreme Surge), LR-13 (*zhāng mén*, Camphorwood Gate), ST-36 (*zú sān lǐ*, Leg Three Li), SP-6 (*sān yīn jiāo*, Three Yin Intersection), BL-17 (*gé shū*, Diaphragm Transport), BL-20 (*pí shū*, Spleen Transport), and BL-21 (*wèi shū*, Stomach Transport). Needle with supplementation and moxa. [6: 168] [27: 143] [97: 188]

blood vacuity abdominal pain 血虚腹痛 *xuè xū fù tòng*: ABDOMINAL PAIN due to BLOOD VACUITY that results from excessive loss of blood or when excessive thought and anxiety cause wear on yin blood. Blood vacuity abdominal pain is a mild pain of unfixed location, and is exacerbated by hunger and taxation. It is accompanied by a withered-yellow facial complexion, fatigue and lack of strength, and a rough fine or rapid fine pulse. MED Supplement the blood and relieve the center using formulas such as Four Agents Decoction (*sì wù tāng*) plus saussurea (*mù xiāng*) and tangerine peel (*chén pí*), or Tangkuei Center-Fortifying Decoction (*dāng guī jiàn zhōng tāng*) and variations. ACU Base treatment mainly on the back transport points and CV, selecting BL-20 (*pí shū*, Spleen Transport), BL-21 (*wèi shū*, Stomach Transport), BL-17 (*gé shū*, Diaphragm Transport), ST-36 (*zú sān lǐ*, Leg Three Li), CV-12 (*zhōng wǎn*, Center Stomach Duct), CV-4 (*guān yuán*, Pass Head), and SP-6 (*sān yīn jiāo*, Three Yin Intersection). Needle with supplementation. See ABDOMINAL PAIN. [26: 281]

blood vacuity deafness 血虚耳聋 *xuè xū ěr lóng*: DEAFNESS due to liver-kidney essence-blood depletion depriving the ear orifices of nourishment. Blood vacuity deafness is of gradual onset, and is accompanied by limp aching lumbus and knees, tinnitus, night sweating, reddening of the cheeks, and dizziness. MED Enrich yin, supplement the blood, and open the orifices using Lycium Berry, Chrysanthemum, and Rehmannia Pill (*qǐ jú dì huáng wán*) and variations. ACU See DEAFNESS. [26: 280] [46: 734]

blood vacuity delayed menstruation 血虚经行后期 *xuè xū jīng xíng hòu qī*: DELAYED MENSTRUATION (late periods) due to blood vacuity and insufficiency of the thoroughfare (*chōng*) and controlling (*rèn*) vessels preventing the timely filling of the uterus. Blood vacuity delayed menstruation is associated with thin pale menstrual flow, withered-yellow facial complexion, emaciation, and continual abdominal pain relieved by pressure. MED Supplement the blood, nourish construction, and boost qi with formulas such as Ginseng Construction-Nourishing Decoction (*rén shēn yǎng róng tāng*). ACU Base treatment mainly on CV, back transport points, and the three yin channels of the foot. Select CV-6 (*qì hǎi*, Sea of Qi), KI-13 (*qì xué*, Qi Point), SP-6 (*sān yīn jiāo*, Three Yin Intersection), BL-20 (*pí shū*, Spleen Transport), BL-17 (*gé shū*, Diaphragm Transport), and ST-36 (*zú sān lǐ*, Leg Three Li); needle with supplementation and add moxa. See DELAYED MENSTRUATION. [26: 280] [46: 683]

blood vacuity dizziness 血虚眩晕 *xuè xū xuàn yūn*: DIZZINESS attributable to yin-blood depletion, which may stem from blood loss, from damage to construction-blood in heat (febrile) disease, from intense vacuity fire, or from heart-spleen qi vacuity. Blood vacuity dizziness is accompanied by vexing heat in the five hearts, insomnia, emaciation, a red tongue, and a fine pulse, which indicate yin vacuity. Signs such as bright white facial complexion, lassitude of spirit and lack of strength, heart palpitations, and reduced food intake indicate dual vacuity of the heart and spleen. MED Enrich yin and nourish the blood or boosting qi and engendering blood. Use Tangkuei Blood-Supplementing Decoction (*dāng guī bǔ xuè tāng*), Anemarrhena and Phellodendron Four Agents Decoction (*zhī bǎi sì wù tāng*), or Spleen-Returning Decoction (*guī pí tāng*). ACU Base treatment on SP, ST, and back transport points. Select GV-20 (*bǎi huì*, Hundred Convergences), CV-6 (*qì hǎi*, Sea of Qi), ST-36 (*zú sān lǐ*, Leg Three Li), SP-6 (*sān yīn jiāo*, Three Yin Intersection), BL-15 (*xīn shū*, Heart Transport), BL-20 (*pí shū*, Spleen Transport), and BL-21 (*wèi shū*, Stomach Transport); needle with supplementation and add moxa. See DIZZINESS. [26: 280]

blood vacuity engendering wind 血虚生风 *xuè xū shēng fēng*: See LIVER WIND STIRRING INTERNALLY.

blood vacuity habitual miscarriage 血虚滑胎 *xuè xū huá tāi*: HABITUAL MISCARRIAGE due to blood vacuity. Signs include lassitude of spirit and lack of strength, pale yellow facial complexion, water swelling, aching lumbus, and abdominal pain. Blood vacuity habitual miscarriage occurs when blood vacuity is exacerbated by pregnancy. Miscarriage is heralded by bleeding. MED Supplement the blood and boost qi with Fetal Origin Beverage (*tāi yuán yǐn*), adding ass hide glue (*ē jiāo*) and charred mugwort (*ài yè tàn*) if there is bleeding. See HABITUAL MISCARRIAGE. [26: 281]

blood vacuity headache 血虚头痛 *xuè xū tóu tòng*: HEADACHE attributable to blood vacuity failing to nourish the upper body. Blood vacuity headache is characterized by pulling pain from the eyebrows to the corners of the head or dull pain in the head, dizzy head and flowery vision, bright white facial complexion and heart palpitations. MED Supplement the blood using formulas such as Four Agents Decoction (*sì wù tāng*). ACU Base treatment mainly on GV, back transport points, SP and ST. Select GV-20 (*bǎi huì*, Hundred Convergences), BL-15 (*xīn shū*, Heart Transport), BL-20 (*pí shū*, Spleen Transport), ST-36 (*zú sān lǐ*, Leg Three Li), SP-6 (*sān yīn jiāo*, Three Yin Intersection), and CV-6 (*qì hǎi*, Sea of Qi). Needle with supplementation and add moxa according to need. For selection of points according to affected area, see HEADACHE. [26: 280] [46: 621] [37: 363]

blood vacuity heart palpitations 血虚心悸 *xuè xū xīn jì*: HEART PALPITATIONS due to blood vacuity depriving the heart of nourishment. It is associated with lusterless facial complexion, somber white nails, lack of strength in the limbs, dizziness, insomnia, pale tongue, and weak fine pulse. ⟦MED⟧ Nourish the blood and boost yin. Use Cinnabar Spirit-Quieting Pill (*zhū shā ān shén wán*) or Spleen-Returning Decoction (*guī pí tāng*). ⟦ACU⟧ Base treatment mainly on back transport points, CV, HT, PC, and ST. Select BL-15 (*xīn shū*, Heart Transport), CV-14 (*jù què*, Great Tower Gate), BL-17 (*gé shū*, Diaphragm Transport), BL-20 (*pí shū*, Spleen Transport), HT-7 (*shén mén*, Spirit Gate), PC-6 (*nèi guān*, Inner Pass), ST-36 (*zú sān lǐ*, Leg Three Li), SP-6 (*sān yīn jiāo*, Three Yin Intersection), and HT-5 (*tōng lǐ*, Connecting Li); needle with even supplementation and drainage. See HEART PALPITATIONS. [50: 588] [26: 280]

blood vacuity heat effusion 血虚发热 *xuè xū fā rè*, 血虚热 *xuè xū rè*: HEAT EFFUSION due to BLOOD VACUITY. Blood vacuity heat effusion is attributed most commonly to blood ejection, bloody stool, or postpartum flooding and spotting, but sometimes to internal damage to the spleen and stomach from dietary irregularities or taxation fatigue. Signs include heat in the flesh, a red facial complexion, thirst, and sometimes vexation and agitation, and unquiet sleep. The pulse is large and vacuous and is forceless under pressure. ⟦MED⟧ Enrich yin and nourish the blood or nourish the blood and boost qi. Use formulas such as Four Agents Decoction (*sì wù tāng*), Tangkuei Blood-Supplementing Decoction (*dāng guī bǔ xuè tāng*), or Sagacious Cure Decoction (*shèng yù tāng*). ⟦ACU⟧ Base treatment mainly on the back transport points, SP, ST, and LI, selecting ST-36 (*zú sān lǐ*, Leg Three Li), SP-6 (*sān yīn jiāo*, Three Yin Intersection), BL-17 (*gé shū*, Diaphragm Transport), BL-20 (*pí shū*, Spleen Transport), BL-21 (*wèi shū*, Stomach Transport), LI-4 (*hé gǔ*, Union Valley), and LI-11 (*qū chí*, Pool at the Bend). Needle with supplementation or even supplemenation and drainage. [26: 280]

blood vacuity impediment 血虚痹 *xuè xū bì*: BLOOD VACUITY depriving the limbs of nourishment, sometimes with contraction of wind-damp evil. Blood vacuity impediment is characterized by numbness of the skin, or inability to lift the limbs, and a scallion-stalk pulse. ⟦MED⟧ Apply the method of nourishing the blood, combined as necessary with boosting qi and dispelling wind. Use formulas such as Tangkuei Center-Fortifying Decoction (*dāng guī jiàn zhōng tāng*). ⟦ACU⟧ Use the ba-

sic treatments for impediment (*bì*) combined with qi-supplementing blood-nourishing points such as LR-3 (*tài chōng*, Supreme Surge), ST-36 (*zú sān lǐ*, Leg Three Li), SP-6 (*sān yīn jiāo*, Three Yin Intersection), BL-17 (*gé shū*, Diaphragm Transport), BL-20 (*pí shū*, Spleen Transport), and BL-21 (*wèi shū*, Stomach Transport). Needle with supplementation and add moxa. See IMPEDIMENT. [26: 281]

blood vacuity infertility 血虚不孕 *xuè xū bù yùn*: Female INFERTILITY due to emptiness of the thoroughfare (*chōng*) and controlling (*rèn*) vessels, preventing the nourishment of essence needed for conception. Blood vacuity infertility stems from spleen-stomach vacuity, from enduring illness, from loss of blood, or from damage to yin, and is accompanied by emaciation, withered-yellow facial complexion, fatigue and lack of strength. ⟦MED⟧ Supplement the blood, nourish yin, and enrich the kidney using Essence-Nourishing Jade-Planting Decoction (*yǎng jīng zhòng yù tāng*), comprising cooked rehmannia (*shú dì huáng*), tangkuei (*dāng guī*), white peony (*bái sháo yào*), and cornus (*shān zhū yú*). ⟦ACU⟧ Base treatment on back transport points, SP, and ST. Select BL-20 (*pí shū*, Spleen Transport), BL-23 (*shèn shū*, Kidney Transport), CV-4 (*guān yuán*, Pass Head), SP-10 (*xuè hǎi*, Sea of Blood), ST-36 (*zú sān lǐ*, Leg Three Li), SP-6 (*sān yīn jiāo*, Three Yin Intersection), ST-13 (*qì hù*, Qi Door), and Infant's Palace (*zǐ gōng*); needle with supplementation and add moxa. [26: 280] [37: 415] [59: 101]

blood vacuity lumbar pain 血虚腰痛 *xuè xū yāo tòng*: LUMBAR PAIN due to loss of blood or general blood vacuity depriving the sinews of nourishment. ⟦MED⟧ Nourish the blood using variations of Four Agents Decoction (*sì wù tāng*). ⟦ACU⟧ Base treatment mainly on the back transport points, BL, SP and ST. Needle with even supplemenation and drainage at BL-23 (*shèn shū*, Kidney Transport), GV-3 (*yāo yáng guān*, Lumbar Yang Pass), BL-40 (*wěi zhōng*, Bend Center), and ouch points (*ā shì xué*), and with supplementation and moxa at BL-17 (*gé shū*, Diaphragm Transport). BL-20 (*pí shū*, Spleen Transport) LR-3 (*tài chōng*, Supreme Surge), ST-36 (*zú sān lǐ*, Leg Three Li), and SP-6 (*sān yīn jiāo*, Three Yin Intersection). See LUMBAR PAIN. [26: 280]

blood vacuity night sweating 血虚盗汗 *xuè xū dào hàn*: NIGHT SWEATING due to insufficiency of yin-blood. See YIN VACUITY NIGHT SWEATING. [26: 280]

blood vacuity scant menstruation 血虚月经过少 *xuè xū yuè jīng guò shǎo*: SCANT MENSTRUATION resulting from constitutional vacuity, damage to yin through enduring sickness or blood loss, or insufficiency of the source of engendering transformation from damage to the spleen and stomach.

Blood vacuity scant menstruation is marked by a scant thin pale flow, and is accompanied by empty pain in the smaller abdomen, headache, dizziness, heart palpitations, and withered-yellow facial complexion. ⃞MED Supplement the blood, boost qi, and fortify the spleen using formulas such as Ginseng Construction-Nourishing Decoction (*rén shēn yǎng róng tāng*). ⃞ACU Base treatment mainly on SP, ST, and back transport points, selecting ST-36 (*zú sān lǐ*, Leg Three Li), SP-6 (*sān yīn jiāo*, Three Yin Intersection), CV-6 (*qì hǎi*, Sea of Qi), BL-17 (*gé shū*, Diaphragm Transport), BL-20 (*pí shū*, Spleen Transport), BL-21 (*wèi shū*, Stomach Transport), and LR-3 (*tài chōng*, Supreme Surge). Needle with supplementation and add moxa. [26: 280]

blood vacuity spontaneous sweating 血虚自汗 *xuè xū zì hàn*: SPONTANEOUS SWEATING stemming from blood vacuity. Spontaneous sweating is essentially associated with qi vacuity, but since blood vacuity invariably causes some degree of qi vacuity, it is also observed in blood vacuity patterns, especially when due to major blood loss where it is a sign of qi deserting with the blood. ⃞MED Enrich yin and supplement the blood using Four Agents Decoction (*sì wù tāng*) plus astragalus (*huáng qí*). If blood vacuity is accompanied by heat, Tangkuei Six Yellows Decoction (*dāng guī liù huáng tāng*) can be used. Spontaneous sweating due to major blood loss requires emergency qi supplementation with Pure Ginseng Decoction (*dú shēn tāng*) followed up with blood-supplementing formulas. See SPONTANEOUS SWEATING. ⃞ACU For general blood vacuity, base treatment mainly on back transport points, SP, ST, LI, HT, and SI. Select LI-4 (*hé gǔ*, Union Valley), HT-6 (*yīn xī*, Yin Cleft), SI-3 (*hòu xī*, Back Ravine), ST-36 (*zú sān lǐ*, Leg Three Li), SP-6 (*sān yīn jiāo*, Three Yin Intersection), BL-17 (*gé shū*, Diaphragm Transport), and BL-20 (*pí shū*, Spleen Transport); needle with supplementation and moxa to enrich yin and supplement the blood. Add LI-11 (*qū chí*, Pool at the Bend) for blood vacuity with heat. For major blood loss, base treatment mainly on back transport points, CV, and SP. Select CV-6 (*qì hǎi*, Sea of Qi), ST-36 (*zú sān lǐ*, Leg Three Li), SP-6 (*sān yīn jiāo*, Three Yin Intersection), BL-17 (*gé shū*, Diaphragm Transport), BL-20 (*pí shū*, Spleen Transport), and BL-21 (*wèi shū*, Stomach Transport); needle with supplementation and large amounts of moxa; needle LI-4 (*hé gǔ*, Union Valley), HT-6 (*yīn xī*, Yin Cleft), and SI-3 (*hòu xī*, Back Ravine) to check sweating. [26: 280] [46: 602] [14: 174]

blood vacuity wilting 血虚痿 *xuè xū wěi*: WILTING (*wěi*) (weakness, limpness, withering) attributable to blood vacuity from postpartum or other major blood loss depriving the sinews of nourishment, characterized by wilting and lack of strength in the extremities hampering movement, and associated with a withered-yellow facial complexion and a weak fine pulse. ⃞MED Nourish the blood using Four Agents Decoction (*sì wù tāng*) combined with Mysterious Two Pill (*èr miào wán*) and Yin-Supplementing Pill (*bǔ yīn wán*), or Blood-Supplementing Sinew-Enhancing Pill (*bǔ xuè róng jīn wán*). ⃞ACU Use the general treatments given under WILTING, and add CV-6 (*qì hǎi*, Sea of Qi), LR-3 (*tài chōng*, Supreme Surge), and BL-17 (*gé shū*, Diaphragm Transport); needle with supplementation and add moxa. [26: 281]

blood wheel 血轮 *xuè lún*: The canthi; related to the heart. [27: 65, 500] [97: 187]

bloody stool 便血 *biàn xuè*: Synonym: *precipitation of blood; blood in the stool*. Loss of blood through the anus, with varying amounts of stool. ⃞WMC Bloody stool is attributable either to the spleen failing to manage the blood or to damp-heat pouring down into the large intestine and damaging the network vessels. Bright red blood indicates heat, whereas dark red blood indicates qi vacuity or damp toxin. **Fire evil and heat toxin** causing the frenetic movement of the blood gives rise to fresh thick blood. ⃞MED Cool the blood and drain fire with formulas such as Coptis Pill (*huáng lián wán*). ⃞ACU Base treatment mainly on BL, ST, and LI. Select ST-25 (*tiān shū*, Celestial Pivot), BL-25 (*dà cháng shū*, Large Intestine Transport), ST-37 (*shàng jù xū*, Upper Great Hollow), GV-1 (*cháng qiáng*, Long Strong), BL-57 (*chéng shān*, Mountain Support), BL-32 (*cì liáo*, Second Bone-Hole), SP-6 (*sān yīn jiāo*, Three Yin Intersection), LR-3 (*tài chōng*, Supreme Surge), and PC-8 (*láo gōng*, Palace of Toil); needle with drainage. See HEAT TOXIN PRECIPITATION OF BLOOD. **Damp toxin** brewing and binding in the large intestine causes passage of dull-colored blood that may be blackish purple like the juice of (cooked) rice-bean (*chì xiǎo dòu*). ⃞MED Transform damp toxin with formulas such as Sophora Flower Powder (*huái huā sǎn*). ⃞ACU Base treatment mainly on ST and SP. Select ST-25 (*tiān shū*, Celestial Pivot), BL-25 (*dà cháng shū*, Large Intestine Transport), ST-37 (*shàng jù xū*, Upper Great Hollow), BL-20 (*pí shū*, Spleen Transport), SP-10 (*xuè hǎi*, Sea of Blood), SP-6 (*sān yīn jiāo*, Three Yin Intersection), SP-9 (*yīn líng quán*, Yin Mound Spring), and LR-2 (*xíng jiān*, Moving Between); needle with drainage and add moxa. **Wind evil binding in the yin aspect:** See BINDING IN YIN. **Spleen-stomach yang vacuity** bloody stool is marked by pale blood. ⃞MED Warm and supplement the spleen and stomach with Perfect Major Supplementation Decoction (*shí quán dà bǔ tāng*). ⃞ACU Base treatment on back transport points, CV, SP, and ST. Select BL-20 (*pí shū*, Spleen Transport), BL-21 (*wèi shū*, Stomach

Transport), CV-4 (*guān yuán*, Pass Head), SP-3 (*tài bái*, Supreme White), ST-36 (*zú sān lǐ*, Leg Three Li), BL-35 (*huì yáng*, Meeting of Yang), and SP-6 (*sān yīn jiāo*, Three Yin Intersection); needle with supplementation and add moxa. **Spleen vacuity** bloody stool is due to damage by thought and preoccupation and qi vacuity fall is marked by reduced eating, fatigue, withered-yellow facial complexion, pale tongue, and fine pulse. When the heart is deprived of nourishment, there are heart palpitations and insomnia. [MED] Supplement qi and contain the blood with Spleen-Returning Decoction (*guī pí tāng*). [ACU] Base treatment mainly on CV, ST, SP, and GV. Select CV-12 (*zhōng wǎn*, Center Stomach Duct), ST-36 (*zú sān lǐ*, Leg Three Li), BL-20 (*pí shū*, Spleen Transport), SP-1 (*yǐn bái*, Hidden White), CV-4 (*guān yuán*, Pass Head), CV-6 (*qì hǎi*, Sea of Qi), and GV-20 (*bǎi huì*, Hundred Convergences); needle with supplementation and add moxa. Apart from the above pattern types, a different method of differentiation is to determine whether blood is passed before or after stool. Blood followed by stool is called DISTAL BLEEDING, whereas stool followed by blood is called PROXIMAL BLEEDING. Distal bleeding is a sign of vacuity or visceral toxin, whereas proximal bleeding is a sign of INTESTINAL WIND. Finally, bloody stool associated with diarrhea, abdominal pain, and tenesmus indicates DYSENTERY. [26: 466] [27: 421]

bloody urine 尿血 *niào xuè*, 溺血 *niào xuè*, 溲血 *sōu xuè*: *Synonym: blood in the urine*. The presence of liquid blood or blood clots in the urine, without any pronounced discomfort. [WMC] hematuria. Bloody urine is distinguished from BLOOD STRANGURY by the absence of pain on urination. It is also distinct from REDDISH URINE, which is urine darker in color than normal. Bloody urine is usually attributed to insufficiency of kidney yin with effulgent heart-liver fire spreading to the small intestine or to dual depletion of the spleen and kidney preventing the blood from being contained. **Effulgent yin vacuity fire** patterns are marked by red urine or passing of pure blood attended by limp aching lumbus and legs, tinnitus and flowery vision, vexation and dry mouth, red tongue, and a fine rapid pulse. [MED] Enrich yin and clear fire; cool the blood and stanch bleeding. Use with formulas such as Ass Hide Glue Powder (*ē jiāo sǎn*), Red-Abducting Powder (*dǎo chì sǎn*), Anemarrhena, Phellodendron, and Rehmannia Pill (*zhī bǎi dì huáng wán*) combined with Cephalanoplos Drink (*xiǎo jì yǐn zi*). [ACU] Base treatment on back transport points, HT, and the three yin channels of the foot; select BL-23 (*shèn shū*, Kidney Transport), CV-4 (*guān yuán*, Pass Head), KI-3 (*tài xī*, Great Ravine), SP-6 (*sān yīn jiāo*, Three Yin Intersection), KI-10 (*yīn gǔ*, Yin Valley), KI-3

(*tài xī*, Great Ravine), LR-1 (*dà dūn*, Large Pile), HT-7 (*shén mén*, Spirit Gate); needle with even supplemenation and drainage. **Dual depletion of the spleen and kidney** gives rise to pale red urine, withered-yellow facial complexion, reduced food intake, aching lumbus and cold limbs, pale tongue, and a soft vacuous pulse. [MED] Fortify the spleen and supplement the kidney; boost qi and contain the blood. Use Center-Supplementing Qi-Boosting Decoction (*bǔ zhōng yì qì tāng*) or Matchless Dioscorea Pill (*wú bǐ shān yào wán*). [ACU] Base treatment on the back transport points, BL-23 (*shèn shū*, Kidney Transport), BL-20 (*pí shū*, Spleen Transport), BL-17 (*gé shū*, Diaphragm Transport), BL-27 (*xiǎo cháng shū*, Small Intestine Transport), CV-4 (*guān yuán*, Pass Head), KI-3 (*tài xī*, Great Ravine), ST-36 (*zú sān lǐ*, Leg Three Li), SP-6 (*sān yīn jiāo*, Three Yin Intersection), and SP-10 (*xuè hǎi*, Sea of Blood); needle with supplementation. [26: 314] [27: 422]

blown blossom lichen 吹花癣 *chuī huā xiǎn*: *Synonym: peach-blossom lichen*. Reddening of the skin of the face with small papules that form into clearly circumscribed plaques covered with thin scales, slightly itchy and dry. [WMC] pityriasis of the face. [MED] Apply a tincture of golden larch (root) bark (*tǔ jīng pí*). [26: 474] [27: 474] [97: 277]

blue whites of the eye 白睛青蓝 *hēi jīng qīng lán*: Whites of the eyes bearing a bluish coloration; observed in the later stages of FIRE GAN, when pain and redness abate to leave purple-blue or blue-gray patches. See FIRE GAN. [26: 227]

bobble wind 绣球风 *xiù qiú fēng*: SCROTAL WIND. [26: 693] [27: 475] [97: 503] ◇ Chin 绣 *xiù*, embroider(ed); 球 *qiú*, ball; 风 *fēng*, wind.

body 形体 *xíng tǐ*: The physical body and constitution. [27: 83] ◇ Chin 形 *xíng*, shape or form; the body as outwardly manifest; 体 *tǐ*, the body as an unified, organic whole or as a constitutional entity; part of the body; corpus or system.

body-inch 同身寸 *tóng shēn cùn*, 寸 *cùn*: *Synonym: cun*. From *A Thousand Gold Pieces Prescriptions* (*qiān jīn yào fāng*). A proportional unit of measurement used to determine the location of acupuncture points on the body, calculated from the length of specific body parts according to the FINGER STANDARD and BONE STANDARD. ◇ Chin 同 *tóng*, same; 身 *shēn*, body; 寸 *cùn*, inch. [26: 259] [27: 104] [97: 186]

body odor 体臭 *tǐ chòu*: See FOXY ODOR.

body palpation 触诊 *chù zhěn*: Palpation of the body surface, palpation of the chest and abdomen, and palpation of the acupuncture points. **Body surface:** The chief aim of palpating the body surface is to ascertain the presence of heat and cold, so as to judge the relative strength of the right and evil. Exuberant evil qi is generally characterized by generalized heat in the body surface, especially at the forehead, whereas debilitation of yang qi is reflected in a cold body surface. Palpation of the fleshy exterior does not simply aim to judge the temperature; the degree of heat can help identify exterior and interior, vacuity and repletion. If the patient has heat effusion, pronounced heat felt on initial palpation that abates with extended palpation indicates heat in the exterior; if the heat becomes more pronounced with extended palpation, it is steaming out from the inner body, i.e., the heat is in the interior. If the body surface feels soft and the patient feels comforted by palpation, the pattern is one of vacuity; if an area is hard and painful, and the pain is exacerbated by palpation, the pattern is one of repletion. If pain is felt by light pressure, there is disease in the surface of the body (e.g., a superficial injury from a knock or fall); if the pain is only felt when heavy pressure is applied, the disease is at a deeper location. By touching the fleshy exterior lightly, the practitioner can determine the degree of moisture and whether or not there is sweating. In an externally contracted heat (febrile) disease of recent onset, the dryness or moistness tells whether sweating has commenced or not. A dry body surface indicates the absence of sweating, whereas a moist surface indicates that the patient is sweating. In enduring conditions, dry skin lacking natural moisture indicates insufficiency of the fluids; severely dry rough hardened skin in patients that are usually emaciated is called ENCRUSTED SKIN, and indicates damage to yin or dry blood in the inner body. In external medicine, sores that are felt to be swollen, hard and numb constitute a cold pattern. Sores that are swollen and scorching hot to the touch indicate heat. Sores with flat bases and diffuse swelling are attributable to vacuity, whereas those with a well-confined base and high swelling are due to repletion. If the affected area is hard, but not markedly hot, or only feels swollen but not painful under heavy pressure, pus has not formed. If, by contrast, there is marked heat, and application of pressure reveals hard outer surface enclosing a soft center, the sore contains pus. **Extremities:** The main aim of palpating the extremities is to determine the presence of heat or cold. At the onset of disease, cold extremities indicate yang vacuity and exuberant cold, whereas hot extremities indicate exuberant yang and intense heat. Heat and cold in the extremities can also differentiate externally contracted febrile disease from internal damage. If the dorsal aspects of the hands and feet are hotter than the palms and soles, the disease is an external contraction; if the palms and soles are hotter, the heat effusion is due to internal damage. The relative degree of heat of the palms and forehead tells whether the heat is in the exterior or interior. If heat in the forehead is more pronounced than heat in the palms, the pattern is one of exterior heat; if the reverse is true, the pattern is one of interior heat. In infants and children, cold fingertips indicate FRIGHT REVERSAL. If the middle finger alone is hot, this is an indication of externally contracted wind-cold; if the middle finger alone is cold, measles or pox is about to erupt. Warmth and cold in the extremities are useful in determining the severity of yang vacuity. If in yang vacuity patterns, there is still warmth in the extremities, yang qi has not collapsed. By contrast, REVERSAL COLD OF THE EXTREMITIES is an unfavorable sign indicating a poor prognosis. **Chest and abdomen:** Palpation of the chest and abdomen can help to determine interior and exterior patterns, and vacuity and repletion of the bowels and viscera. A light touch can establish the degree of moisture of the skin, so as to determine the presence of heat and cold. By applying medium pressure along the muscle grain or the lines of the channels and by asking the patient when he or she feels discomfort, it is possible to determine the presence of evil qi. By heavy pressing and pushing, it is possible to feel hardness and softness and so identify vacuity or repletion in the bowels and viscera and the degree of accumulation of evils. The main points of palpation of the chest and abdomen are as follows: (1) Vacuous Li (虚里 *xū lǐ*, the apical pulse): Vacuous li is located at a point between the fourth and fifth rib below the nipple, and reflects the pulsation of the heart. Formerly, it was accorded great importance as a convergence point of all channels and the GREAT NETWORK VESSEL OF THE STOMACH. Examination of the apical pulse can help to determine the severity of disease. If it strikes the fingers when palpated, is stirring but not tight, is moderate and not urgent, ancestral qi is accumulated in the chest and there is no disease. If the pulsation is faint or cannot be felt at all, ancestral qi is vacuous. A pulsation felt to beat against the clothing indicates ancestral qi discharging through the outer body. In some cases, such as in states of fright, fear or anger, intoxication or after hard running, marked pulsation is only temporary, and quickly returns to normal. If the pulsation is on the verge of expiration, but there are no fatal signs, the pattern is usually one of phlegm-rheum or food accumulation. Expiration of the apical pulse together with all other pulses is a fatal sign. (2) Chest and rib-side: The chest contains the lung and heart, whereas the rib-side on the right-hand side of the body protects the liver. If the anterior chest is elevated, a sign known as *raised chest*, and the patient responds to local palpation with panting, the condition is PULMONARY DISTENTION. If palpation of the chest and rib-side produces a feeling of distention and pain, the cause may be phlegm-heat qi bind or water-rheum. The liver is covered by the ribs and normally cannot be felt. If it is swollen and either hard or soft to the touch, the cause is qi stagnation and blood stasis. It is known from Western medicine that if the liver is felt to have an uneven surface, there may be cancer. If the patient complains of distending pain in the right rib-side, and the local body surface feels hot, but cannot be pressed without causing pain, the cause is a LIVER WELLING-ABSCESS (*gān yōng*). A mass felt under the ribs may be felt in chronic malaria and is referred to as MOTHER-OF-MALARIA. (3) Region below the heart: The area below the breast bone is the point at which the stomach can be felt. If the patient complains of a subjective feeling of fullness or blockage in this area, referred to as GLOMUS, palpation can provide additional information. If the area feels soft and is not tender, the pattern is one of vacuity; if hard, resistant to pressure, and tender, the pattern is one of repletion. Commonly observed repletion patterns include CHEST BIND, which includes minor and major patterns. Tenderness below the heart constitutes minor chest bind pattern, whereas hardness, fullness, and pain stretching into the chest and abdomen constitutes a major chest bind pattern. When there is fullness below the heart and palpation reveals a tangible mass that moves and produces a gurgling sound when pushed, there is water-rheum in the stomach. (4) Abdomen: Abdominal palpation is conducted to detect cold and heat, hardness, distention, lumps, and tenderness. A cold abdomen that likes warmth and pressure is a vacuity cold pattern, whereas scorching heat relieved by cold objects is a repletion heat pattern. Abdominal pain is ascribed to vacuity if it likes pressure and to repletion if it refuses pressure. An area of scorching heat that cannot be pressed without causing severe pain indicates an INTERNAL WELLING-ABSCESS. Abdominal distention feels solid, is tender, and produces a dull heavy turbid sound when tapped is ascribed to repletion. Distention that does not feel solid, is not tender, and produces a hollow sound when tapped is QI DISTENTION. A highly enlarged abdomen with a projecting umbilicus is a severe condition called DRUM DISTENTION. Distinction is made between water drum and qi drum. In water drum, the abdomen feels like a bag of water, pressure leaves an indentation, and a gentle patting by one hand on one side of the abdomen produces a wave that can be felt by the other hand resting on the opposite side. In qi drum, tapping produces a hollow drumlike sound, pressure leaves no indentation, and patting produces no wave. The large abdomen of obese people differs from this drum distention by being soft to the touch and having a normal umbilicus. Abdominal lumps can also be felt by palpation. Accumulations and gatherings are lumps that may or many not be painful. Accumulations have a clearly defined shape, do not move, and are associated with pain of fixed location; they are ascribed to disease in the blood aspect. Gatherings are amorphous, move, and are associated with pain of unfixed location, and a clearly defined shape; they are ascribed to disease in the qi aspect. In the lower abdomen, traditionally referred to as the smaller abdomen, a stringlike formation of lumps is a sign of old stool in the intestine. A palpable lump in the smaller abdomen with pain that refuses pressure is an INTESTINAL WELLING-ABSCESS (*cháng yōng*), i.e., appendicitis. Palpation can reveal three signs that indicate the presence of worms: a) an abdominal lump that is tough as sinew, and is felt to move after long palpation; b) the wriggling sensation felt under the fingers with careful palpation; c) an uneven abdominal wall with a constantly changing topography (constant rising, sinking, gathering and dispersing). **Acupuncture points:** The back transport points can be used in diagnosis. If there is disease in one of the bowels or viscera, pressure can produce a pain or even a pleasant sensation at its corresponding back transport point. Transport point palpation finds its earliest mention in *The Magic Pivot* (*líng shū*): "If pressing a spot relieves internal pain, the spot is a transport point." Any channel point, particular the source points, may become a tender spot when its associated bowel or viscus is diseased. *The Magic Pivot* (*líng shū*) states, "When there is disease in the viscera, it is reflected in the sources [i.e., source points] of which there are twelve. The sources each have an exit point. By knowing sources and observing their responses, it is possible to understand disease in the viscera." Thus, disease of the liver is reflected at LR-3 (*tài chōng,* Supreme Surge); lung disease at LU-9 (*tài yuān,* Great Abyss); heart disease at HT-7 (*shén mén,* Spirit Gate) and PC-7 (*dà líng,* Great Mound); spleen disease at SP-3 (*tài bái,* Supreme White); and kidney disease at KI-3 (*tài xī,* Great Ravine). The modern MERIDIOMETER is used for assessment of the channels, of qi and blood, and in electroacutherapy. Modern research shows that channel and nonchannel points have different cutaneous electrical resistance values, which are affected when there is disease in the organs or channels. These changes in resistance are understood to reflect changes in the flow of qi and blood at acupoints. The meridiometer can thus provide information about the flow of qi and blood at various acupoints, the location of disease, and the presence of vacuity and repletion. The use of the meridiometer in diagnosis is, however, still at an experimental stage. [29: 266] [6: 145] [27: 187]

boil 疖 *jié*: A small, round, superficial swelling that is hot and painful, suppurates within a few days, and easily bursts. It is attributable to heat toxin or to summerheat-heat and usually occurs in the summer and autumn. [WMC] furuncle (boil). [MED] Clear heat and resolve toxin as for EX-TERNAL WELLING-ABSCESS. [ACU] Base treatment mainly on local and affected channel points. One of a number of methods may be applied individually or combined: (1) Encirclement needling: For boils in the initial stage of swelling prior to suppuration, select 2–4 ouch points (*ā shì xué*) around the sites and insert needles at a slight oblique angle pointing toward the root of the boil. If the boil is over 4 cm in diameter, an appropriate number of needles can be inserted in the center. If it is hard and painful, it should be needled in the center. Points can be needled with supplementation or drainage depending on whether the condition is one of vacuity or repletion; generally, draining is called for. Moxa can also be used at points around the boil. If the boil has already become painful, moxa until the pain abates; if not, moxa until slight pain is felt. (2) Selection of distant points on the affected channel: Select one or two affected-channel points. For example, if the boil is on the hand yang brightness (*yáng míng*) channel, select points such as LI-4 (*hé gǔ*, Union Valley), and LI-11 (*qū chí*, Pool at the Bend), needling with drainage. (3) Heat-clearing toxin-resolving formula: Prick BL-40 (*wěi zhōng*, Bend Center) and LU-5 (*chǐ zé*, Cubit Marsh) to bleed, and needle with drainage at LI-11 (*qū chí*, Pool at the Bend), and LI-4 (*hé gǔ*, Union Valley). Prick GV-14 (*dà zhuī*, Great Hammer) to bleed and fire-cup. (4) Selection of points according to location of the boil: For head and face, needle LI-4 (*hé gǔ*, Union Valley) and LI-11 (*qū chí*, Pool at the Bend). For chest and abdomen, needle ST-36 (*zú sān lǐ*, Leg Three Li) and SP-6 (*sān yīn jiāo*, Three Yin Intersection). For neck, needle GV-14 (*dà zhuī*, Great Hammer) and GV-10 (*líng tái*, Spirit Tower). For lumbus and back, needle BL-40 (*wěi zhōng*, Bend Center), needling with drainage. Compare WELLING-ABSCESS. See SORE. [26: 950] [27: 456] [97: 312] [42: 231] [15: 363]

boiling 煮 *zhǔ*: Cooking (foods or medicines) in boiling water or other liquid. Boiling, as a method of processing individual medicinals, has the aim of eliminating toxicity and irritants, preventing side-effects, increasing effectiveness, or facilitating storage. For example, boiling genkwa (*yuán huā*) in vinegar can reduce its toxicity; boiling impure mirabilite (*pò xiāo*) with radish can remove impurities, making it into refined mirabilite (*xuán míng fěn*). Boiling is also the method of making a formula into a *decoction*. See PROCESSING OF MEDIC-INALS. [27: 326] [74: 10] [11: 20]

boiling reversal 煎厥 *jiān jué*: An ancient disease name denoting internal heat that scorches yin fluids, giving rise to CLOUDING REVERSAL. It arises in patients suffering from depletion of yin essence and hyperactivity of yang qi, when they contract summerheat-heat qi. Signs include tinnitus, deafness, blindness, and, in severe cases, sudden CLOUDING REVERSAL. [WMC] cerebrovascular spasm, cerebral hemorrhage, subarachnoid hemorrhage. See REVERSAL PATTERN and WIND STROKE. [27: 400]

boil swelling 疖肿 *jié zhǒng*: A swelling of a boil. See BOIL.

bolt bone 楗骨 *jiàn gǔ*: SEAT BOARD BONE. [27: 70]

bone 骨 *gǔ*: The hardest substance of the body that holds the body up and defines the body's shape. Since bone stores marrow, it is an EX-TRAORDINARY ORGAN. See KIDNEY GOVERNS THE BONES AND ENGENDERS MARROW.

bone-clinging flat-abscess 附骨疽 *fù gǔ jū*: *Synonym*: *bone flat-abscess*. A headless FLAT-ABSCESS (*wú tóu jū*) located on a bony and sinewy part of the body, usually caused by congealing stagnation of qi and blood that develops from wind-cold and damp in the sinew and bone. Bone flat-abscess is characterized at onset by alternating heat [effusion] and [aversion to] cold, and subsequently by sinew and bone pain with difficulty in bending and stretching, but without any localized heat or redness. When depressed heat transforms into fire, the flesh becomes putrid and suppuration begins. The flat-abscess takes the form of a broad swelling without a head, and without any change in skin color. After rupturing, there is a persistent dribbling discharge of pus from the opening, which does not heal easily. Any pieces of dead bone must be removed before healing is possible. [WMC] pyogenic osteomyelitis. Compare HEADLESS FLAT-ABSCESS; FLAT-ABSCESS; SORE. [26: 370] [97: 321] [61: 208]

bone-clinging tumor 贴骨疽 *tiē gǔ jū*: See BONE TUMOR.

bone damage 骨伤 *gǔ shāng*: Any damage to a bone or bones, notably including fracture.

bone-eating flat-abscess 咬骨疽 *yǎo gǔ jū*: BONE FLAT-ABSCESS.

bone erosion 骨蚀 *gǔ shí*: A disease characterized by bone pain, atrophy of the muscles, shrinking of the affected limb, and limping gait. Bone erosion arises when evils entering the body in the presence of vacuity or damage to the sinew and bone causes stagnation of qi and blood and obstruction of the channels. [MED] Treat with oral formulas such as Harmonious Yang Decoction (*yáng hé tāng*) or Golden Coffer Kidney Qi Pill (*jīn guì shèn qì wán*) and topical application of Harmonious Yang Decongealing Plaster (*yáng hé jiě níng gāo*). WMC epiphysitis; osteochondritis. [26: 531]

bone flat-abscess 骨疽 *gǔ jū*: BONE-CLINGING FLAT-ABSCESS.

bone fracture 骨折 *gǔ zhé*: Any break in a bone. Bone fractures result from knocks and falls or pulling of sinews and flesh. They occur more easily in old age, vacuity detriment, and disease affecting the bone. They are characterized by local blood stasis, painful swelling, displacement or deformity, the sound of bones grating against each other, and abnormal movement. TRT Bone-righting manipulation is used to put the affected bone or parts thereof back into place. The fracture is then set with splints and bandages. Medication aims to quicken the blood and transform stasis and to disperse swelling and relieve swelling. Oral: Bone-Righting Purple Gold Elixir (*zhèng gǔ zǐ jīn dān*) and Origin-Restorative Blood-Quickening Decoction (*fù yuán huó xuè tāng*). Topical: Erythrina Decoction (*hǎi tóng pí tāng*) can be used as an external wash. [97: 400] [26: 528] [27: 487] [97: 400]

bone-hole 髎 *liáo*: A hole through or crevice in a bone. This term is used in acupuncture point names located at such sites, including BL-31 through BL-34 (*bā liáo*, Eight Bone-Holes), LI-19 (*hé liáo*, Grain Bone-Hole), and ST-3 (*jù liáo*, Great Bone-Hole). [26: 529] [97: 497]

bone impediment 骨痹 *gǔ bì*: IMPEDIMENT (*bì*) patterns characterized by pronounced joint signs such as pain and swelling. The bones feel heavy and difficult to lift and there is aching pain in the bone and marrow. It is attributed to wind-cold-damp that seizes vacuity and invades the bones. Distinction is made between repletion and vacuity patterns. Repletion patterns are treated with Five Impediments Decoction (*wǔ bì tāng*) with extra tiger bone (*hǔ gǔ*) and the addition of duhuo (*dú huó*), quilled cinnamon (*guān guì*), achyranthes (*niú xī*), astragalus (*huáng qí*), and fish poison yam (*bì xiè*). Vacuity patterns are treated with Minor Life-Prolonging Decoction (*xiǎo xù mìng tāng*). ACU Select BL-11 (*dà zhù*, Great Shuttle) as the main point. For repletion patterns, select points according to pattern (wind, cold, dampness, or complications). See WIND IMPEDIMENT; COLD IMPEDIMENT; DAMP IMPEDIMENT. For vacuity patterns, apply the basic treatments for impediment patterns, and needle with supplementation and moxa at points such as BL-23 (*shèn shū*, Kidney Transport), CV-4 (*guān yuán*, Pass Head), GV-4 (*mìng mén*, Life Gate), KI-3 (*tài xī*, Great Ravine), and SP-6 (*sān yīn jiāo*, Three Yin Intersection). See IMPEDIMENT for selection of points according to location. [26: 529] [27: 404] [97: 400]

bone juncture 岐骨 *qí gǔ*: Seventh costosternal articulation. [27: 73] [97: 281]

bone pain 骨痛 *gǔ tòng*: Pain felt to come from the bone. It is observed in IMPEDIMENT (*bì*) patterns, bone fractures, and vacuity taxation. *Incisive Light on the Source of Miscellaneous Disease* (*zá bìng yuán liú xī zhú*) states, "Pain in the human body may be caused by wind spreading and dampness stagnating, or by blood pricking and phlegm attacking. When shallow, it is no deeper than the skin and [body] hair; when deep, it penetrates as far as the channels and network vessels. If it enters the interior and stretches into the bone, causing aching and pain, although it differs depending on whether the cause is cold or heat... It is treated with Tiger Bone Powder (*hǔ gǔ sǎn*) or Mysterious Three Powder (*sān miào sǎn*). If prolonged standing has damaged the bone, or if there is bone damage, causing pain or gradually giving rise to wilting, this urgently requires treatment at onset, using psoralea (*bǔ gǔ zhī*), beef marrow (*niú gǔ suǐ*), velvet deerhorn (*lù róng*), and drynaria (*gǔ suì bǔ*)." Compare ACHING BONES. [50: 1089] [26: 529]

bone righting 正骨 *zhèng gǔ*: Treatment of bone fractures and dislocations by manipulating bones into their correct positions and fixing them with splints and bandages, and providing medication to aid healing. [26: 182] [27: 487] [27: 141]

bones stuck in the throat 骨鲠 *gǔ gěng*: The condition in which fish or splintered animal bones become lodged in the flesh of the throat. Fish bones and splintered chicken bones may get stuck in the throat if accidentally swallowed. They can give rise to a feeling of blockage, difficulty in swallowing, and bleeding. Nowadays, bones stuck in the throat that fail to dislodge themselves are usually removed by pincers. Traditionally, they were often freed with the aid of decoctions. Clematis (*wēi líng xiān*) is particularly noted for this action. It can be combined with tsaoko (*cǎo guǒ*), amomum (*shā rén*), and white sugar (*bái shā táng*), and decocted in half water half vinegar and sipped slowly. [26: 531] [97: 141]

bone standard 骨度 *gǔ dù*: *The Magic Pivot* (*líng shū, gǔ dù*). A proportional standard for measuring parts of the body based on the size of bones. See Table on following page. [26: 530] [27: 32]

1. The Bone Standard			
Body part	From to	Body inches	Area applied
Head	Anterior hairline to posterior hairline	12	Forehead and nape
and	Anterior hairline to point between eyebrows (Hall of Impression)	3	
Neck	Posterior hairline to T7	3	
	From one mastoid process (completion bone) to other	9	Horizontally between points on head
	From one frontal angle (ST-8) to other	9	
Chest	Xiphoid process to navel	8	Upper abdomen
and	Navel to pubic bone (transverse bone)	5	Lower abdomen
Abdomen	Armpit to 11th rib	12	Lateral thoracic region
	Nipple to nipple	8	Chest & abdomen
	Clavicle to clavicle	8	Chest and abdomen in women
Upper	Anterior crease of armpit to elbow crease	9	Upper arm
Limbs	Elbow crease to wrist crease	12	Forearm
Lower	Upper horizontal of public bone to medial epicondyle of femur	18	Inside of thigh
Limbs	Ball of femur to lower extremity of kneecap	19	Outside of thigh
	Lower gluteal crease (BL-36) to center of popliteal crease	15	Back of thigh
	Below external epicondyle of tibia (SP-9) to inner ankle bone	13	Medial aspect of lower leg
	Lower extremity of the kneecap to the outer ankle bone	16	Lateral aspect of lower leg

bone trough wind 骨槽风 *gǔ cáo fēng*: A sore in front of the ear that eventually affects the "bone trough," i.e., the tooth bed. It is heralded by dull pain under the skin stretching into the sinew and bone; it starts as a small node that grows to the size of a walnut. If it bursts, it does not heal easily, and discharges pus that is foul-smelling and sometimes clear and thin. If it persists, rotten bone is discharged, and the gums swell and become purple-black in color, and bleed. In severe cases, the movement of the jaw is inhibited, the tooth bed putrefies, and teeth fall out. It is attributable to wind-fire toxin in the hand lesser yang (*shào yáng*) or foot yang brightness (*yáng míng*) stomach channel, which can be exacerbated by spleen yang vacuity that prevents expulsion of the toxin. MED Dispel wind, dissipate fire, and resolve toxin with Yang-Upbearing Fire-Dissipating Decoction (*shēng yáng sàn huǒ tāng*). Persistent cases can be treated with Aconite Center-Rectifying Decoction (*fù zǐ lǐ zhōng tāng*) or Harmonious Yang Decoction (*yáng hé tāng*) to expressing the toxin. [26: 531] [61: 320]

bone tumor 骨瘤 *gǔ liú*: A TUMOR (growth on the outside of the body) that grows on bone. A disease called "bone flat-abscess" possibly fitting the description of bone tumor was mentioned in *The Inner Canon* (*nèi jīng*). The term *gǔ liú* first appeared in the in *A Unified Treatise on Diseases, Patterns, and Remedies According to the Three Causes* (*sān yīn jí yī bìng zhèng fāng lùn*) in the Song Dynasty, but without any description. *Pivot of External Medicine* (*wài kē shū yào*) states, "If there is taxation damage to kidney water preventing it from giving luxuriance to the bone, there is swelling which rises from the bone and which is hard to the touch. This is called a bone tumor." *Life-for-All Compendium of External Medicine, Patterns and Treatment* (*wài kē zhèng zhì quán shēng jí*) of the Qing dynasty states, "There is also a bone-clinging tumor that grows on the bone and is extremely painful." This latter description may be that of what Western medicine calls an advanced malignant bone tumor. Bone tumor is attributed to insufficiency of kidney qi and cold-damp carrying phlegm into the bone, causing qi and blood to congeal. In mild (in Western medicine, benign) cases, it develops slowly and is not marked by pronounced signs. In severe cases, onset is characterized by a dull pain that gradually worsens until it becomes unbearable, especially at night; the tumor grows swiftly, and is attached to the bone, immovable, and hard as stone, while the skin becomes purple brown in color with dilated vessels. Accompanying signs include low fever, emaciation, lassitude of spirit, and poor appetite. MED Supplement kidney qi, disperse swelling, and break hardness. Use Kidney Qi Pill (*shèn qì wán*) as oral medication and apply Harmonious Yang Decongealing Plaster (*yáng hé jiě níng gāo*) topically. [26: 531] [27: 480] [96: 201]

bone wilting 骨痿 *gǔ wěi*: *Synonym: kidney wilting.* Desiccation of the bone and vacuity of the marrow characterized by limp aching lumbar spine preventing normal movement, weak wilting lower limbs preventing the patient from getting out of bed, desiccated teeth, and a somber black facial complexion; attributed to damage to the kidney by heat evil. MED Enrich yin and clear heat; supplement the kidney and boost essence. Use formulas such as Hidden Tiger Pill (*hŭ qián wán*) or Metal Strength Pill (*jīn gāng wán*). [ACU] Base treatment mainly on KI and GB. Select BL-23 (*shèn shū*, Kidney Transport), KI-3 (*tài xī*, Great Ravine), KI-6 (*zhào hăi*, Shining Sea), KI-1 (*yŏng quán*, Gushing Spring), GB-30 (*huán tiào*, Jumping Round), GB-31 (*fēng shì*, Wind Market), GB-34 (*yáng líng quán*, Yang Mound Spring), and GB-39 (*xuán zhōng*, Suspended Bell). Needle with supplementation. See WILTING. [26: 531] [27: 403] [97: 400] [113: 242] [46: 638]

boost 益 *yì*: See SUPPLEMENT. ◇ Chin 益 *yì*, increase, more.

boosting (and supplementing) lung qi 补益 肺气 *bŭ yì fèi qì*: A method of treating lung qi vacuity characterized by feeble speech, cough and panting and shortness of breath, using medicinals such as codonopsis (*dăng shēn*), astragalus (*huáng qí*), licorice (*gān căo*), and schisandra (*wŭ wèi zĭ*). A representative lung-qi–boosting formula is Lung-Supplementing Decoction (*bŭ fèi tāng*). [6: 176]

boosting fire and dispersing yin 益火消阴 *yì huŏ xiāo yīn*: BOOSTING THE SOURCE OF FIRE TO DISPERSE THE SHROUD OF YIN. [27: 238]

boosting fire and engendering earth 益火生土 *yì huŏ shēng tŭ*: Warming and supplementing kidney yang to treat spleen-kidney yang vacuity with signs such as clear-food diarrhea, enduring diarrhea, or early morning diarrhea. In this context, "fire" refers to kidney yang, not to the heart. [6: 32]

boosting qi and engendering liquid 益气生津 *yì qì shēng jīn*: A method of treating qi vacuity and liquid depletion arising from excessive sweating, and characterized by fatigue, shortness of breath, dry mouth and thirst, and a vacuous pulse. An example of a qi-boosting liquid-engendering formula is Pulse-Engendering Powder (*shēng mài săn*), which contains ginseng (*rén shēn*), ophiopogon (*mài mén dōng*), and schisandra (*wŭ wèi zĭ*). [ACU] Base treatment mainly on CV, ST, SP, back transport points, and KI. Select CV-6 (*qì hăi*, Sea of Qi), ST-36 (*zú sān lĭ*, Leg Three Li), BL-20 (*pí shū*, Spleen Transport), BL-21 (*wèi shū*, Stomach Transport), LU-9 (*tài yuān*, Great Abyss), SP-6 (*sān yīn jiāo*, Three Yin Intersection), KI-3 (*tài xī*, Great Ravine), and KI-6 (*zhào hăi*, Shining Sea); needle with supplementation and moxa. For excessive sweating, add LI-4 (*hé gŭ*, Union Valley), and KI-7 (*fù liū*, Recover Flow), [27: 283] [97: 486] [46: 594] [113: 20]

boosting qi and harmonizing the stomach 益气和胃 *yì qì hé wèi*: A method of treatment used to address qi vacuity stomach problems characterized by glomus and oppression in the chest and stomach duct, no thought of food and drink, and, in severe cases, vomiting of food after inges-

tion. [MED] A commonly used qi-boosting stomach-harmonizing formula is Saussurea and Amomum Six Gentlemen Decoction (*xiāng shā liù jūn zĭ tāng*). [ACU] Base treatment mainly on ST, CV, and back transport points. Select BL-20 (*pí shū*, Spleen Transport), BL-21 (*wèi shū*, Stomach Transport), CV-6 (*qì hăi*, Sea of Qi), ST-36 (*zú sān lĭ*, Leg Three Li), ST-25 (*tiān shū*, Celestial Pivot), and PC-6 (*nèi guān*, Inner Pass), needle with supplementation and large amounts of moxa. [6: 179] [46: 586, 594, 602]

boosting qi and resolving the exterior 益气 解表 *yì qì jiě biăo*: Synonym: *supplementing qi and resolving the exterior*. A method of treatment used to address continual common colds and copious sweat from qi vacuity that increases vulnerability to external evils and reduces the body's ability to expel an evil once it has entered. In such cases, qi-boosting medicinals may be combined with exterior-resolving medicinals. An example of such a formula is Ginseng and Perilla Beverage (*shēn sū yĭn*), which contains codonopsis (*dăng shēn*), white perilla leaf (*bái sū yè*), pueraria (*gé gēn*), peucedanum (*qián hú*), ginger pinellia (*jiāng bàn xià*), tangerine peel (*chén pí*), platycodon (*jié gĕng*), poria (*fú líng*), saussurea (*mù xiāng*), bitter orange (*zhĭ ké*), and licorice (*gān căo*). [ACU] Use points given under EXTERIOR RESOLUTION in combination with qi-boosting points such as ST-36 (*zú sān lĭ*, Leg Three Li), CV-6 (*qì hăi*, Sea of Qi), CV-4 (*guān yuán*, Pass Head), BL-20 (*pí shū*, Spleen Transport), BL-21 (*wèi shū*, Stomach Transport), and LU-9 (*tài yuān*, Great Abyss). Needle with supplementation, and for pronounced qi vacuity, add moxa. [27: 250] [50: 1297]

boosting the source of fire to disperse the shroud of yin 益火之原以消阴翳 *yì huŏ zhī yuán yĭ xiāo yīn yì*: A method of treatment involving supplementation of kidney yang to treat cold patterns. This term is actually a comment by Wang Bing of the Tang dynasty on the line in *Elementary Questions* (*sù wèn*) that reads "Wherever heat [is applied], but cold [remains], treat the yang." The implication of this comment is that wherever the use of warm or hot medicinals to treat cold patterns produces no effect or makes the cold worse, the cold pattern is one of yang vacuity with exuberant yang, i.e., the condition is essentially one of yang vacuity that is treated by supplementing kidney yang (the true fire of the life gate). According to this principle, insufficiency of kidney yang with aching lumbus and weak legs, cold sensation in the lower half of the body, impotence, and seminal cold is treated with Eight-Ingredient Rehmannia Pill (*bā wèi dì huáng wán*), which contains cooked rehmannia (*shú dì huáng*), cornus (*shān zhū yú*), dioscorea (*shān yào*), poria (*fú líng*), moutan (*mŭ dān pí*), alisma (*zé xiè*), prepared cooked aconite (*shú fù zǐ*), and cinnamon bark (*ròu guì*). Boosting the source of fire to disperse the shroud of yin is now often referred to as *boosting fire to disperse yin* or *supporting yang to abate yin.* [27: 238]

boosting the spleen 益脾 *yì pí*: FORTIFYING THE SPLEEN.

boosting the stomach 益胃 *yì wèi*: Supplementing stomach vacuity, which means a) to warm the stomach and fortify the center to treat stomach qi vacuity cold or b) to enrich stomach yin in the treatment of insufficiency of stomach yin. [27: 279] [97: 486]

boosting yin 益阴 *yì yīn*: SUPPLEMENTING YIN.

borborygmus 肠鸣 *cháng míng*: *pl.* borborygmi. RUMBLING INTESTINES.

borderland 蕃 *fān*: Region anterior to the ear and inferolateral to the cheek bone. [27: 64] [48: 437]

border of the red and white flesh 赤白肉际 *chì bái ròu jì*: The division between the darker suntanned flesh and paler flesh of the backs of the arms and legs. The "red" (sun-tanned) flesh forms the yang side, whereas the "white" (paler) flesh is the yin side. The dividing line between the two represents one of the landmarks in acupuncture point location. [26: 302] [27: 74] [97: 247]

bound 结 *jié*: See BIND.

bound or intermittent (pulse) 结代（脉）*jié dài (mài)*: Any pulse that is moderate and interrupted. *The Magic Pivot (líng shū, suì lù lùn)* states, "These two evils become conglomerated, and channel qi becomes bound or intermittent. See BOUND PULSE; INTERMITTENT PULSE. [50: 1196]

bound pulse 结脉 *jié mài*: *Synonym: slow irregularly interrupted pulse.* A pulse that is moderate or slow and pauses at irregular intervals. *The Pulse Canon (mài jīng)* states that it "indicates exuberant yin and bound qi, congested qi and stagnant phlegm, or concretions, conglomerations, accumulations, and gatherings." See PULSE CONDITION. [50: 1196] [6: 142]

bowel 腑 *fǔ*: Any of the organs of the exterior (stomach, small and large intestines, gallbladder, bladder, and triple burner). See BOWELS AND VISCERA. ◇ Chin 腑 *fǔ*, derived from 府 *fǔ*, mansion, by addition of the flesh signifier.

bowel and visceral fright pattern 脏腑惊证 *zàng fǔ jīng zhèng*: Patterns of fright convulsions of the extremities associated with the bowels and viscera. *Children's Diseases: Remedies and Sources (xiǎo ér bìng yuán fāng lùn)* states, "In liver fright, the eyes are red and the stool is green-blue; In gallbladder fright, the face is green-blue and white below; in heart fright, the face is red; in small intestinal fright, there is night crying through to dawn; in spleen fright, there is heat in the five hearts and dry retching; in stomach fright, there is abdominal distention and inability to eat; in lung fright, there is panting and swallowing of water (吃水 *chī shuǐ*); in large intestinal fright, there is phlegm rale in the throat; in kidney fright, there is grinding of the teeth in sleep; in triple burner [fright], there is fright crying during sleep. [50: 1276]

bowel and visceral pattern identification 脏腑辨证 *zàng fǔ biàn zhèng*: The correlation of information derived from the four examinations with doctrine of visceral manifestation to determine what bowels or viscera are affected by disease, and identify morbid changes in their qi-blood and yin-yang aspects. The first step of bowel and visceral pattern identification involves identifying the affected organ on the basis of its physiopathological characteristics. **Heart:** The heart governs the blood vessels and stores the spirit. Therefore, heart palpitations, interrupted (结代 *jié dài*) pulses, and derangement of the heart spirit all point to disease of the heart. **Lung:** The lung is connected with the surface skin and governs qi, and lung qi diffuses, depurates, and bears downward; hence signs such as cough, panting, and insecurity of the defensive exterior are seen to be lung disorders. **Spleen:** The spleen governs movement and transformation of the food, the stomach governs ingestion, and the intestines govern the conveyance and transformation of waste; hence vomiting, abdominal distention and fullness, and diarrhea are associated with diseases of the spleen, stomach and intestines. **Liver:** The liver governs free coursing and stores blood, and liver yang is prone to upbearing and stirring; hence rib-side pain, blood loss, dizziness, and spasms indicate liver disease. **Kidney:** The kidney governs water, stores essence, governs the bones and engenders marrow; hence water swelling, urinary block, enuresis, seminal emission, limp aching lumbus and knees, and sluggish movement are associated with kidney disease. **Yin-yang and qi-blood:** Once the affected bowel or viscus has been identified, the relative states of yin, yang, qi, and blood can be determined with the information derived from eight-principle and qi-blood pattern identification. Each bowel and viscus is associated with characteristic pathologies of yin, yang, qi, and blood. The heart and the liver are associated with disease of all four aspects, whereas the lung is mainly susceptible to pathologies of yin and qi; the spleen is primarily affected by disorders of qi and yang, whereas kidney diseases include yin-yang and essential qi pathologies. Determining the affected aspect of an organ is of vital importance in treatment. Thus, identifying heart palpitations as a sign of heart disease provides an inadequate basis for prescribing treatment, since it may be attributable to vacuity of heart yin, heart blood, heart yang, or heart qi.

The bowels and viscera are each closely related not only to one another but also to the other organs and tissues of the body. Therefore, understanding the development of diseases, making a correct diagnosis, and determining appropriate treatment are all dependent on a holistic approach. For example, once insomnia has been identified as the result of heart blood or heart yin vacuity, it is important to determine whether the spleen or kidney is also affected, since the dual disorders, heart-spleen blood vacuity and noninteraction of the heart and kidney, are treated in different ways. See under the HEART, LUNG, SPLEEN, LIVER, KIDNEY, etc., for more detail. [6: 169]

bowel and visceral qi 脏腑之气 *zàng fǔ zhī qì*: The qi of the bowels and viscera. Each organ has its own qi, which is the basis of its physiological activity and manifests as a major aspect of its physiological function. The heartbeat is the manifestation of heart qi, and bowel movements are a manifestation of large intestine qi. [6: 38]

bowel and visceral stroke 中脏腑 *zhòng zàng fǔ*: WIND STROKE taking the form of bowel stroke or visceral stroke. See WIND STROKE. [26: 142]

bowel of center clearness 中清之腑 *zhōng qīng zhī fǔ*: The gallbladder; so named because the gall is considered a clear or pure fluid, rather than waste. [27: 21]

bowel of center essence 中精之腑 *zhōng jīng zhī fǔ*: The gallbladder. See BOWEL OF CENTER CLEARNESS. [27: 21]

bowels and viscera 脏腑 *zàng fǔ*: Organs of the chest and abdomen. The five viscera are the heart, lung, spleen, liver, and kidney. The pericardium is considered a sixth viscus in channel theory. The six bowels (paired by functional relationship with the viscera respectively) are the stomach, small intestine, large intestine, gallbladder, bladder, and triple burner. The function of the viscera is to produce and store essence, that of the bowels is to decompose food and convey waste. Thus, *Elementary Questions* (*sù wèn*) states, "The so-called five viscera store essential qi and do not discharge waste. Thus they are full, but cannot be filled. The six bowels process and convey matter, and do not store. Thus, they are filled, but are not full." ◇ Chin 脏 *zàng* and 腑 *fǔ*, deriving from 藏 *zàng*, *cáng* and 府 *fǔ* without the flesh signifier, originally denoted grain collection centers, the former generally denoting a storehouse, and the latter a locus of administration. [6: 78]

bowel stroke 中腑 *zhòng fǔ*: WIND STROKE not quite as severe as visceral stroke and marked by sudden clouding collapse that after regaining of consciousness leaves the patient with hemiplegia, deviated eyes and mouth, difficult speech, and pos-

sibly urinary and fecal stoppage. [26: 140] [27: 397] [97: 80]

brain 脑 *nǎo*: Synonym: *head marrow*. Extraordinary organ located in the skull. According to traditional doctrine of visceral manifestation, "the brain is the sea of marrow; all marrow belongs to the brain, flowing up to the brain and down to the coccyx." The brain is most closely related to the kidney, which engenders the marrow. Modern observation shows that diminished cerebral function can manifest in signs of insufficiency of kidney essence. *The Magic Pivot* (*líng shū*), "If the sea of marrow is insufficient, the brain turns and the ears ring, there is aching in the neck, dizziness, poor vision, and lethargy." Later, Li Shi-Zhen (1518–1593), Jin Zheng-Xi, and others explicitly stated, "The brain is the seat of the original spirit," and believed that the senses and control of physical movement were related to the brain. However, the main functions of the brain as perceived by Western medicine are ascribed in the doctrine of visceral manifestation to the heart, liver, kidney, and other viscera. The HEART STORES THE SPIRIT refers basically to the brain's function of mental activity and thought. Such conditions as heat entering the pericardium and phlegm confounding the orifices of the heart correspond to what Western medicine describes as disorders of the central nervous system. Imbalance of heart yin and heart yang, and heart qi and heart blood, are explained in Western medicine as disturbance of the brain function. The LIVER GOVERNS FREE COURSING and the LIVER GOVERNS THE SINEWS corresponds to what in Western medicine are brain functions. Disease patterns such as liver qi depression and ascendant liver yang may also be partly explained in Western medicine as being associated with the nervous system. [27: 24] [97: 476] [6: 97]

brain-gripping sand 控脑痧 *kòng nǎo shā*: **1.** A disease marked by runny nose with yellow watery discharge associated with dryness in the nose, impaired sense of smell, and occasional nosebleeds, and attributed to damp-heat. MED Treat with Dryness-Clearing Lung-Rescuing Decoction (*qīng zào jiù fèi tāng*) minus gypsum (*shí gāo*). WMC atrophic rhinitis. Compare WITHERED NOSE. **2.** Severe DEEP-SOURCE NASAL CONGESTION. ◇ Chin 控 *kòng*, grasp, control, accuse; 脑 *nǎo*, brain; 痧 *shā*, "sand sickness," see SAND *shā*. [26: 602]

brain is the house of the original spirit 脑为元神之府 *nǎo wéi yuán shén zhī fǔ*: From *The Comprehensive Herbal Foundation* (*běn cǎo gāng mù*). The brain is the seat of mental function. [36: 127]

brain is the sea of marrow 脑为髓之海 *nǎo wéi suǐ zhī hǎi*: From *The Magic Pivot* (*líng shū, hǎi lùn*). The ancient Chinese considered the brain and the marrow to be the same in substance. Since the kidney engenders marrow, the brain, as the sea of marrow, is closely related to the kidney. See KIDNEY ENGENDERS BONE AND MARROW. [36: 127]

brain leak 脑漏 *nǎo lòu*: A severe form of DEEP-SOURCE NASAL CONGESTION. [61: 327] ◇ Chin 脑 *nǎo*, brain; 漏 *lòu*, leak, ooze.

brain-squeezing wind 夹脑风 *jiá nǎo fēng*: See HEAD WIND. ◇ Chin 夹 *jiá*, pinch, clasp, squeeze; 脑 *nǎo*, brain; 风 *fēng*, wind.

brain wind 脑风 *nǎo fēng*: A disease similar to HEAD WIND, attributed to wind evil entering the brain, and characterized by aversion to cold on the nape and neck and extreme cold of GV-17 (*nǎo hù*, Brain's Door) area with unbearable pain. ⎡MED⎤ Warm and dissipate using formulas such as Tangkuei Counterflow Cold Decoction (*dāng guī sì nì tāng*). ⎡ACU⎤ Base treatment mainly on points of the three yang channel, GV and LU. Select GB-20 (*fēng chí*, Wind Pool), GV-20 (*bǎi huì*, Hundred Convergences), GV-22 (*xìn huì*, Fontanel Meeting), Greater Yang (*tài yáng*), GV-23 (*shàng xīng*, Upper Star), LI-4 (*hé gǔ*, Union Valley), LU-7 (*liè quē*, Broken Sequence), and SI-3 (*hòu xī*, Back Ravine). Needle with drainage, and use large amounts of moxa. See HEADACHE; HEAD WIND. [26: 800] [27: 393] [97: 469]

branch 支 *zhī*: See HEAVENLY STEMS AND EARTHLY BRANCHES.

bran-frying 麸炒 *fū chǎo*: Stir-frying medicinal materials in a wok with bran until a thick yellow-black smoke is given off. This process increases a medicinal's capacity to fortify the spleen and stomach and causes oils that would otherwise cause side effects and unpleasant smells to be absorbed by the bran. The same method is used to process ovate atractylodes (*bái zhú*) and bitter orange (*zhǐ ké*). [27: 274] [97: 463]

breakdown of heart-kidney interaction 心肾不交 *xīn shèn bù jiāo*: NONINTERACTION OF THE HEART AND KIDNEY.

breaking blood 破血 *pò xuè*: Dispelling static blood with drastic stasis-dispelling medicinals such as rhubarb (*dà huáng*), peach kernel (*táo rén*), pangolin scales (*chuān shān jiǎ*), and wingless cockroach (*zhè chóng*). See DISPERSE. [27: 274]

breaking qi 破气 *pò qì*: Rectifying qi with drastic medicinals such as unripe tangerine peel (*qīng pí*) and unripe bitter orange (*zhǐ shí*), which dissipate binds and abduct stagnation. [27: 271]

breaking stasis and dispersing concretions 破瘀消癥 *pò yū xiāo zhēng*: See DISPELLING STASIS AND QUICKENING THE BLOOD. [27: 274]

breast 乳房 *rǔ fáng*: Either of two fleshy protruberances of the female chest each headed by a nipple and whose function is produce milk for breast-

feeding. The breasts lie on the foot yang brightness (*yáng míng*) channel. The nipples belong to the liver. See also AREOLA; NIPPLE. [26: 377]

breast blowing 吹奶 *chuī nǎi*, 吹乳 *chuī rǔ*: MAMMARY WELLING-ABSCESS.

breastbone 髆骭 *hé gàn*: **1.** The vertical bone of the center of the chest that joins the ribs. ⎡WMC⎤ sternum. See also HEART-COVERING BONE; TURTLE-DOVE'S TAIL. **2.** Any bone of the chest. [27: 68]

breast milk stoppage 乳汁不行 *rǔ zhī bù xíng*, 乳汁不通 *rǔ zhī bù tōng*, 乳汁不下 *rǔ zhī bù xià*: SCANT BREAST MILK.

breast node 乳核 *rǔ hé*: MAMMARY NODE. [26: 377]

breath gate 吸门 *xī mén*: One of the SEVEN GATES. The organ that covers the opening of the wind-pipe in the throat when swallowing; hence the name. ⎡WMC⎤ epiglottis. [26: 324]

breathing 呼吸 *hū xī*: Synonym: respiration. The taking of air into and putting of air out of the lung. Normal breathing depends on the diffusion and depurative downbearing of lung qi. The principal disturbances of normal breathing include PANTING, SHORTAGE OF QI, HASTY BREATHING, QI ASCENT, SHORTNESS OF BREATH, and ROUGH BREATHING. See also LUNG DISEASE. [26: 375]

¹**brew** 煎 *jiān*: **1.** *n.* DECOCTION; a term occurring in names of decoctions, e.g., Ferry Brew (*jì chuān jiān*). **2.** *vb.* DECOCT. [27: 311]

²**brew** 蕴 *yùn*: To gather, ferment (usually in a concealed or inconspicuous way); describes certain forms of internal (and especially lung) heat. See HEAT.

brightening the eyes 明目 *míng mù*: Enhancing visual acuity.

bright hall 明堂 *míng táng*: **1.** The nose. **2.** Any of the marks on an acupuncture model that indicate an acupuncture point. [27: 66] [26: 376]

bright white facial complexion 面色㿠白 *miàn sè huǎng bái*: See WHITE FACIAL COMPLEXION. ◇ Chin 㿠 *huǎng*, bright, white and bright. This character is not included in most standard non-medical dictionaries; it is believed to have originally been a miswriting of 晃 *huàng* and is sometimes pronounced in the same way. [6: 116] [48: 331]

brittle foot 脆脚 *cuì jiǎo*: A form of swelling in pregnancy. The swelling of the foot is marked by pitting and thin shiny appearance of the skin, and is not associated with other discomforts. It arises in women ordinarily suffering from devitalized spleen yang when the growing fetus hampers the spread of spleen-yang, which causes water-damp to pour downward. ⎡MED⎤ Fortify the spleen and percolate dampness. Use Life-for-All Ovate Atractylodes Powder (*quán shēng bái zhú sǎn*).

Compare WRINKLY FOOT; SWELLING AND DISTENTION IN PREGNANCY. [26: 550] [24: 154]

broad and bright 广明 *guǎng míng*: The anterosuperior region of the body. [27: 73]

broken metal failing to sound 金破不鸣 *jīn pò bù míng*: **1.** Damage to lung qi causing a hoarse voice. The lung governs the voice; in the doctrine of the five phases, it belongs to metal, a substance frequently utilized, as in bells and gongs, for its sonorous qualities. When lung qi is damaged, the voice looses its normal sonorous quality just as a broken bell fails to ring. The lung governs the movement of qi, whereas the kidney governs qi absorption. The voice is therefore dependent not only on the lung but also the kidney. **2.** Enduring loss of voice. [26: 391] [27: 162] [97: 347]

bruise 青紫 *qīng zǐ*: Local purple or green-blue coloring of the skin due to external injury. ◇ Chin 青 *qīng*, green-blue; 紫 *zǐ*, purple. [97: 325]

bruxism 啮齿 *niè chǐ*: GRINDING OF THE TEETH.

bubo sore 横痃 *héng xián*: Swelling in the groin. At onset, it is the size of an almond; it can grow to the size of a goose's egg, becoming hard, painful, and either red and scorching hot or mildly reddened and warm. It ruptures to exude pus. [WMC] corresponds to various kinds of lymphadenectasis (dilation or distention of a lymph node). See RED BAYBERRY SORE. Compare FISH MOUTH; BIAN TOXIN [SORE]. [27: 162] [97: 347]

bulging 癞 *tuí* (*tui*): Synonym: *prominence* A general name for diseases of the anterior yin, including, in males, swelling of the testicles and sagging of one testicle etc, and in females, vaginal protrusion, etc. [48: 471]

bulging fontanel 囟填 *xìn tián*, 囟门高凸 *xìn mén gāo tú*: From *The Origin and Indicators of Disease* (*zhū bìng yuán hòu lùn*). A condition characterized by bulging at the anterior fontanel (traditionally called the "fontanel gate," see FONTANEL). Distinction is made between heat and cold patterns. A hard bulging fontanel associated with absence of heat effusion and lack of warmth in the limbs is attributable to congealing cold and stagnant qi. A soft bulging fontanel associated with red facial complexion and limbs and with purple finger veins is due to upsurge of fire qi. [WMC] hydrocephalus. [MED] For congealing cold and stagnant qi, dissipate cold using Ginseng and Perilla Beverage (*shēn sū yǐn*). For upsurge of fire qi, clear heat using Green-Blue–Draining Pill (*xiè qīng wán*). [26: 288] [27: 437] [97: 213]

bulging mounting 癞疝 *tuí shàn*: From *Elementary Questions* (*sù wèn, yīn yáng bié lùn*). **1.** Swelling of the scrotum. Described by Yang Zi-He as follows: "Bulging mounting takes the form of a scrotum swollen and pendulous like a dipper, without pain or itching; it arises from being in low

places with damp qi." [MED] Use Tangerine Pip Pill (*jú hé wán*). [ACU] Base treatment mainly on LR, CV, and SP. Select LR-5 (*lǐ gōu*, Woodworm Canal), GB-34 (*yáng líng quán*, Yang Mound Spring), CV-4 (*guān yuán*, Pass Head), SP-6 (*sān yīn jiāo*, Three Yin Intersection), and LR-12 (*jí mài*, Urgent Pulse); needle with drainage and add moxa. **2.** From *Elementary questions* (*sù wèn, mài jiě piān*). A pattern of abdominal swelling in women. **3.** Protrusion of the vagina. ◇ Chin 癞 *tuí*, swollen, bulging, sagging. [26: 989][37: 455]

bundle bone 束骨 *shù gǔ*: The fifth metatarsophalangeal articulation (lateral aspect). [27: 72] [97: 268]

¹**burn** 烧 *shāo*: *vb.* To undergo or subject to the destructive or transformative action of fire or heat. In medicinal processing, medicinal materials may be burned (calcined or charred) to enhance certain of their properties.

²**burn** 烧伤 *shāo shāng*: *n.* Injury to the body by burning action of fire, or hot fluids or objects, those specifically being caused by hot liquids being called *scalds*. Mild burns are characterized by local redness, blistering or erosion of the skin. Severe burns cause damage to deeper tissue, and when the fire toxin attacks the inner body there are general signs such as thirst, heat effusion, clouding of the spirit, constipation, and inhibited urination. [MED] Treat mild cases by topical application of medicinals such as powdered sanguisorba (*dì yú*) and rhubarb (*dà huáng*) in equal proportions with a pinch of borneol (*bīng piàn*), blended with sesame oil (*má yóu*). For severe burns, oral administration of heat-clearing toxin-resolving and construction-cooling wind-extinguishing formulas such as Coptis Toxin-Resolving Decoction (*huáng lián jiě dú tāng*), Rhinoceros Horn and Rehmannia Decoction (*xī jiǎo dì huáng tāng*), or Antelope Horn and Uncaria Decoction (*líng jiǎo gōu téng tāng*) is necessary. In recent years, a number of new Chinese medical techniques have been developed to treat burns and reduce scarring. [26: 904] [27: 497]

burning mountain fire method 烧山火 *shāo shān huǒ*: A complex needle manipulation technique that combines a number of simple supplementing techniques such as lifting and thrusting and open and closed needle extraction to treat vacuity cold diseases such as the three yin stages of cold damage disease, impotence, incontinence, vaginal protrusion, and swelling and sagging of one testicle. Method: (1) Determine the depth to which the needle will be inserted. Divide this depth into three equal segments. Proceeding from the surface of the skin, these depths are labeled the level of heaven, the level of human, and the level of earth, respectively. (2) Ask the patient to inhale deeply.

Steps 2, 3, and 4 are performed during exhalation. Upon exhalation, thrust the needle quickly and lift slowly nine times to the level of heaven. (3) Thrust the needle quickly and lift slowly nine times in the level of human. (4) Thrust the needle quickly and lift slowly nine times in the level of earth. (5) Ask the patient to exhale, and slowly withdraw the needle. If the procedure is to be repeated, withdraw the needle to the level of heaven and repeat steps 2, 3, and 4; if not, withdraw the needle fully from the skin. (6) Press the site gently with a cotton swab after the needle has been withdrawn. [27: 314] [27: 497]

burning preserving nature 烧存性 *shāo cún xìng*: See CHAR-FRYING. [27: 325] [97: 497]

burns and scalds 水火烫伤 *shuǐ huǒ tàng shāng*: See ²BURN.

burnt-yellow tongue fur 舌苔焦黄 *shé tāi jiāo huáng*: A dark yellow or brown tongue fur that is dry and bears the look of having been burnt; a sign of repletion heat bind. [6: 124]

C

cadaverous odor 尸臭 *shī chòu*: From *On Warm Epidemics Expanded* (*guǎng wēn yì lùn*). An odor attributed to exuberant toxic heat in the inner body. WMC Possibly equivalent to hepatic odor. [6: 128]

calcination 煅 *duàn*: A medicinal processing method whereby medicinal materials are heated until red hot by charcoal, coal, or the like, in order to make them crisp, soft, and easily crushed, and to facilitate the extraction of their active constituents in decoction. Materials such as dragon bone (*lóng gǔ*), oyster shell (*mǔ lì*), gypsum (*shí gāo*), and chlorite/mica (*méng shí*) that come in large lumps that do not crumble under heat are calcined by being placed directly in the fire. Materials such as hematite (*dài zhě shí*), and pyrite (*zì rán tóng*) that easily crumble are calcined in crucibles called DULU. Some materials such as borax (*péng shā*), smithsonite (*lú gān shí*), and alum (*bái fán*) may be simply heated in a wok. Soft materials such as juncus (*dēng xīn cǎo*) and old trachycarpus (*chén zōng pí*) are calcined in a mud-sealed wok to char. Especially hard materials such as hematite (*dài zhě shí*), white quartz (*bái shí yīng*), pyrite (*zì rán tóng*), tortoise plastron (*guī bǎn*), and loadstone (*cí shí*) are dipped in vinegar after heating to make them softer; actinolite (*yáng qǐ shí*) can be dipped in wine. See CALCINING AND QUENCHING. [27: 323]

calcining and quenching 淬 *cuì*: To heat (medicinal materials) to a high temperature and then dip them in water or vinegar. See CALCINATION. [27: 533] [82: 15]

calf 腓肠 *féi cháng*, 腨 *chuài*, 腓腨 *féi nào*, 腓肠 *féi cháng*: The fleshy rear part of the lower leg. [27: 72]

callus 胼胝 *pián zhī*: A thickening and hardening of the skin on protuberant parts of the feet that arises when long-term pressure and friction from footwear causes local blockage of qi and blood depriving the skin of nourishment. It is unclearly circumscribed and may range in color from white or yellow to brown. MED Treat by pairing away dead skin with a knife and applying Water Crystal Paste (*shuǐ jīng gāo*). ACU Treatment is based on ouch points (*ā shì xué*). Compare CORN. [26: 548] [27: 485] [97: 473] [50: 1279]

calm 平 *píng*: To reduce certain disturbances (ascendant hyperactivity of liver yang, panting).

calm breathing 平息 *píng xī*: Regular breathing at normal speed. To ensure maximum accuracy when taking a patient's pulse, practitioners should make sure that their own respiration is natural and even. This ensures accurate timing of the pace of the pulse, and facilitates the mental composure required to detect even the slightest changes. [27: 190] [97: 144]

calm dawn 平旦 *píng dàn*: The third of the twelve watches (two hour periods); B3 watch; 3–5 a.m. According to *Elementary Questions* (*sù wèn, mài yào jīng wéi lùn*), calm dawn is the best time to take the pulse. [6: 137]

calming and extinguishing internal wind 平熄内风 *píng xī nèi fēng*: EXTINGUISHING WIND.

calming panting 平喘 *píng chuǎn*: Synonym: *stabilizing panting*. Elimination or reduction of panting. See DISPERSING PHLEGM AND CALMING PANTING; DIFFUSING THE LUNG AND TRANSFORMING PHLEGM.

calming the liver and extinguishing wind 平肝熄风 *píng gān xī fēng*: Synonyms: *settling the liver and extinguishing wind*; *subduing yang and extinguishing wind*. A method of treatment used to address ascendant liver yang stirring internal wind with pulling pain in the head, dizziness, deviated eyes and mouth, numbness or tremor of the limbs, stiffening of the tongue, deviated trembling tongue, unclear speech, red tongue with thin fur, a stringlike pulse, and, in severe cases, clouding collapse, hypertonicity or convulsions of the limbs. MED Medicinals used include uncaria (*gōu téng*), gastrodia (*tiān má*), tribulus (*cì jí lí*), chrysanthemum (*jú huā*), earthworm (*dì lóng*), mother-of-pearl (*zhēn zhū mǔ*), oyster shell (*mǔ lì*), and abalone shell (*shí jué míng*). Formulas include Liver-Settling Wind-Extinguishing Decoction (*zhèn gān xī fēng tāng*), Antelope Horn and Uncaria Decoction (*líng jiǎo gōu téng tāng*), and Sweeping Down Decoction (*jiàn líng tāng*). ACU Base treatment mainly on GV, GB, and LR. Needle with drainage at GV-20 (*bǎi huì*, Hundred Convergences), GB-20 (*fēng chí*, Wind Pool), PC-6 (*nèi guān*, Inner Pass), and LR-3 (*tài chōng*, Supreme Surge), and with supplementation at BL-18 (*gān shū*, Liver Transport), BL-17 (*gé shū*, Diaphragm Transport), SP-6 (*sān yīn jiāo*, Three Yin Intersection), and KI-1 (*yǒng quán*, Gushing Spring). See also EXTINGUISHING WIND. [26: 178] [27: 267] [97: 144] [46: 596] [37: 338]

Liver-Calming Wind-Extinguishing Medicinals

羚羊角 (*líng yáng jiǎo*) antelope horn (Antelopis Cornu)

山羊角 (*shān yáng jiǎo*) goral horn (Naemorhedi Goral Cornu)

石决明 (*shí jué míng*) abalone shell (Haliotidis Concha)

牡蛎 (*mǔ lì*) oyster shell (Ostreae Concha)

生牡蛎 (*shēng mǔ lì*) crude oyster shell (Ostreae Concha Cruda)

珍珠 (*zhēn zhū*) pearl (Margarita)

珍珠母 (*zhēn zhū mǔ*) mother-of-pearl (Concha Margaritifera)

玳瑁 (*dài mào*) hawksbill shell (Eretmochelydis Carapax)

紫贝 (*zǐ bèi*) purple cowrie (Mauritiae, Erosariae seu Cypraeae Testa)

代赭石 (*dài zhě shí*) hematite (Haematitum)

钩藤 (*gōu téng*) uncaria (Uncariae Ramulus cum Unco)

天麻 (*tiān má*) gastrodia (Gastrodiae Rhizoma)

刺蒺藜 (*cì jí lí*) tribulus (Tribuli Fructus)

黑大豆 (*hēi dà dòu*) black soybean (Glycines Semen Atrum)

全蝎 (*quán xiē*) scorpion (Buthus)

蜈蚣 (*wú gōng*) centipede (Scolopendra)

白僵蚕 (*bái jiāng cán*) silkworm (Bombyx Batryticatus)

地龙 (*dì lóng*) earthworm (Lumbricus)

铁落 (*tiě luò*) iron flakes (Ferri Frusta)

---

calming the liver and relieving pain 平肝止痛 *píng gān zhǐ tòng*: A method of treatment used to address headache due to ascendant liver yang.

calming the liver and subduing yang 平肝潜阳 *píng gān qián yáng*: SUBDUING YANG.

candareen 分 *fēn*: FEN.

canthus 眦 *zì*: *pl.* canthi. The point at which the upper and lower lids meet at either extremity of the eye; the corner or angle of the eye. The inner canthus is the point where the lids meet beside the nose; the outer canthus is the point where they meet on the lateral aspect of the face. The canthi are also known as the BLOOD WHEEL. Diseases affecting the canthi include EXCRESCENCE CREEPING OVER THE EYE and WEEPING CANTHUS. ◇ Eng 眦 *canthus*, from Gk. *kanthos*, cant, angle. [26: 636]

carphology 循衣摸床 *xún yī mō chuáng*: PICKING AT BEDCLOTHES. ◇ Eng from Gk. karphos, *stalks; legein,* to pluck—picking of dry stalks from mud walls.

catgut embedding 埋线疗法 *mái xiàn liáo fǎ*: A method of treatment whereby acupuncture points are stimulated by catgut embedded in the skin. It is used in modern clinical practice to treat WHEEZING AND PANTING, STOMACH PAIN, DIARRHEA, ENURESIS, DEVIATED EYES AND MOUTH, EPILEPSY, and WILTING (*wěi*). [46: 537]

catty 斤 *jīn*: JIN.

celestial court 天庭 *tiān tíng*: Center of the forehead. [27: 63] [97: 500]

center 中 *zhōng*: The spleen and stomach; the center burner.

center burner 中焦 *zhōng jiāo*: *Synonym: middle burner.* The middle section of the triple burner, comprising the spleen and stomach. See TRIPLE BURNER. [26: 140]

center burner damp-heat 中焦湿热 *zhōng jiāo shī rè*: SPLEEN-STOMACH DAMP-HEAT.

center burner damp obstruction 湿阻中焦 *shī zǔ zhōng jiāo*: DAMP OBSTRUCTION.

center burner governs transformation 中焦主化 *zhōng jiāo zhǔ huà*: The center burner comprises the stomach and spleen, which move and transform the essence of grain and water. More at SPLEEN GOVERNS MOVEMENT AND TRANSFORMATION and TRIPLE BURNER. [27: 58] [97: 81]

center burner is like foam 中焦如沤 *zhōng jiāo rú ōu*: The center burner is like a fermentation turning the ingested foods into a form from which their essence can be extracted. More at TRIPLE BURNER. [27: 58] [97: 81]

center cold 中寒 *zhōng hán*: Center burner vacuity cold arising from insufficiency of yang qi and impaired splenic movement and transformation, and marked by abdominal pain that likes pressure, cold limbs and fear of cold, bland taste in the mouth, upflow nausea, reduced eating, and sloppy stool. [26: 139] [27: 112]

center dispersion 中消 *zhōng xiāo*: *Synonyms: spleen dispersion; stomach dispersion; heart dispersion.* A dispersion-thirst pattern characterized by thirst, increased eating and rapid hungering, emaciation, frequent urination, and hard stool, and attributed to spleen-stomach dryness-heat. MED Treat by clearing heat and draining fire complemented by enriching yin and moistening dryness. Use White Tiger Decoction (*bái hǔ tāng*), Firewood-Raking Beverage (*chōu xīn yǐn*), or Stomach-Regulating Qi-Coordinating Decoction (*tiáo wèi chéng qì tāng*). ACU Base treatment mainly on CV, ST, and SP. Select CV-12 (*zhōng wǎn*, Center Stomach Duct), ST-25 (*tiān shū*, Celestial Pivot), SP-2 (*dà dū*, Great Metropolis), ST-43 (*xiàn gǔ*, Sunken Valley), SP-6 (*sān yīn jiāo*, Three Yin Intersection), and KI-3 (*tài xī*, Great Ravine); needle with drainage. See DISPERSION-THIRST.[1] [26: 138] [27: 424] [97: 79] [22: 42] [37: 392]

center fullness is treated by draining the inner body 中满者泻之于内 *zhōng mǎn zhě xiè zhī yú nèi*: From *Elementary Questions* (*sù wèn, yīn yáng yìng xiàng lùn*). To disinhibit qi dynamic to relieve distention and fullness caused by internal stagnation of qi. For distention and fullness in the chest and abdomen due to stagnation of qi and phlegm-damp in the middle stomach duct, for example, the method of HARMONIZING THE STOMACH AND RECTIFYING QI can be used. For distention and pain in the stomach duct and abdomen, ABDUCTIVE DISPERSION can be used. [27: 243]

center qi 中气 *zhōng qì*: **1.** The qi of the spleen and stomach (center burner) and other bowels and viscera insofar as they are involved in the digestion and the upbearing of the clear and downbearing of the turbid. **2.** Spleen qi. Spleen qi governs upbearing, and impairment of the function can take the form of spleen vacuity fall manifesting as prolapse of the anus or uterus. See CENTER QI FALL. [26: 138] [27: 80] [97: 78]

center qi fall 中气下陷 *zhōng qì xià xiàn*: *Synonym: qi vacuity fall; spleen qi fall; qi fall.* Insufficiency of spleen yang qi in which its uplift is diminished and that manifests in sinking effects such as prolapse of the anus, enduring diarrhea, prolapse of the uterus, or, in infants, depressed fontanel. The spleen occupies the center, its qi governs upbearing; damage to the spleen by diet or taxation fatigue or enduring illness can cause spleen qi to fall. MED Supplement the center and boost qi; upbear yang and raise the fall. Use formulas such as Center-Supplementing Qi-Boosting Decoction (*bǔ zhōng yì qì tāng*). ACU Base treatment mainly on CV, GV, back transport points and ST, selecting GV-20 (*bǎi huì*, Hundred Convergences), CV-6 (*qì hǎi*, Sea of Qi), CV-12 (*zhōng wǎn*, Center Stomach Duct), ST-36 (*zú sān lǐ*, Leg Three Li), BL-20 (*pí shū*, Spleen Transport), and BL-21 (*wèi shū*, Stomach Transport). Needle with supplementation and add moxa. [26: 138] [46: 575] [27: 156] [97: 81]

ceruminal congestion 耵耳 *dīng ěr*: Accumulation of earwax in the ear. [27: 494] [97: 355]

change of teeth 齿更 *chǐ gēng*, 换齿 *huàn chǐ*: The replacement of the milk teeth (deciduous) teeth by the permanent teeth at the age of six to seven. Change of teeth is considered a manifestation of kidney qi. *Elementary Questions* (*sù wèn, shàng gǔ tiān zhēn lùn*) states, "When a male is eight years old and his kidney qi is replete, the hair grows and the teeth change." [26: 886] [27: 84] [97: 377]

channel 经 *jīng*, 经脉 *jīng mài*: Any of the main pathways of qi and blood. Distinction is made between regular channels, usually referred to as the twelve channels, and extraordinary vessels. See TWELVE CHANNELS; EXTRAORDINARY VESSELS; CHANNELS AND NETWORK VESSELS.

channel [and network] qi 经络之气 *jīng luò zhī qì*: Qi that flows through the channels and network vessels. Its movement is seen in the channels' function of transmission and conveyance. The sensation produced by needling an acupuncture point, known as "obtaining qi," demonstrates the presence of channel qi.

channel and network stroke 中经络 *zhòng jīng luò*: WIND STROKE taking the form of a CHANNEL STROKE or NETWORK STROKE, and marked by signs such as deviated eyes and mouth, numbness of the skin, hemiplegia, and impeded speech, but not by spirit-mind changes that characterize bowel and visceral stroke. [26: 141]

channel conductor 引经药 *yǐn jīng yào*: A medicinal that conducts the action of other medicinals to specific channels of the body. Channel conduction is one aspect of the actions of conductors. The main conductors for each of the channels are presented below. See SOVEREIGN, MINISTER, ASSISTANT, AND COURIER. [26: 133] [27: 94] [97: 376]

Channel Conductors

Greater yang (*tài yáng*)
羌活 (*qiāng huó*) notopterygium (Notopterygii Rhizoma)
防风 (*fáng fēng*) ledebouriella (Ledebouriellae Radix)
藁本 (*gǎo běn*) Chinese lovage (Ligustici Sinensis Rhizoma et Radix)

Yang brightness (*yáng míng*)
升麻 (*shēng má*) cimicifuga (Cimicifugae Rhizoma)
葛根 (*gé gēn*) pueraria (Puerariae Radix)
白芷 (*bái zhǐ*) angelica (Angelicae Dahuricae Radix)

Lesser yang (*shào yáng*)
柴胡 (*chái hú*) bupleurum (Bupleuri Radix)
蔓荆子 (*màn jīng zǐ*) vitex (Viticis Fructus)

Greater yin (*tài yīn*)
苍术 (*cāng zhú*) atractylodes (Atractylodis Rhizoma)

Lesser yin (*shào yīn*)
独活 (*dú huó*) duhuo (Angelicae Duhuo Radix)

Reverting yin (*jué yīn*)
细辛 (*xì xīn*) asarum (Asiasari Herba cum Radice)
川芎 (*chuān xiōng*) ligusticum (Ligustici Rhizoma)
青皮 (*qīng pí*) unripe tangerine peel (Citri Exocarpium Immaturum)

channel divergence 经别 *jīng bié*: Any of the TWELVE CHANNEL DIVERGENCES.

channel entry 归经 *guī jīng*, 入经 *rù jīng*: Action (of a medicinal) on a particular channel and the organ to which the channel homes. For example, platycodon (*jié gěng*) and tussilago (*kuǎn dōng huā*), treat cough and panting and are said to enter the lung channel; gastrodia (*tiān má*), scorpion (*quán xiē*), and antelope horn (*líng yáng jiǎo*) treat convulsions and are said to enter the liver channel. Some medicinals enter two channels or more, indicating that they have a broad scope of action. For example, apricot kernel (*xìng rén*) enters the lung and the large intestine, and treats both cough and constipation. Alisma (*zé xiè*) enters the kidney, bladder, and triple burner channels, and treats water-damp problems. [26: 969] [27: 316]

channel-freeing manipulation 循摄法 *xún shè fǎ*: A technique used acupuncture to help obtain qi, involving the application of light pressure along the course of the channel above and below the point being needled; this hastens the movement of qi and blood in the channel. [46: 465]

channel needling 经刺 *jīng cì*: From *The Magic Pivot* (*líng shū, guān zhēn piān*). **1.** The needling of a channel affected by disease. **2.** One of the NINE NEEDLING METHODS. To needle a blocked area on a channel that passes through the affected area. [27: 334] [27: 344] [97: 377]

channel passage 传经 *chuán jīng*: The movement of evils from one channel to another in doctrine of cold damage. [27: 92] [97: 376]

channel point 经穴 *jīng xué*: **1.** *Synonym:* FOURTEEN-CHANNEL POINT. Any point on the fourteen channels. **2.** *Synonym: river point.* See TRANSPORT POINTS. [26: 812]

channel qi 经气 *jīng qì*: *Synonym: vessel qi.* The qi that flows through the channels. Channel qi is composed of earlier and later heaven essential qi (congenital and acquired elements) and moves through the entire body. Channel qi has both activating and nourishing functions, and reflects the functions of the whole body. *Elementary Questions* (*sù wèn, lí hé zhēn xié lùn*) states, "True qi is channel qi." [26: 816]

channel rubbing 循 *xún*: A technique by which the acupuncturist rubs the course of a channel at an acupuncture point prior to needle insertion in order to diffuse qi and blood in the area. [27: 333]

channels and network vessels 经络 *jīng luò*: The pathways of blood and qi pervading the whole the body, connecting the bowels and viscera, the limbs and joints. The channels are the main pathways of qi and blood, whereas the network vessels are smaller branches ensuring supply of qi and blood to all localities. Disturbances in the channels are reflected in abnormalities along their course. Acupuncture, acupressure, and cupping are largely based on the theory of the channels and network

vessels. See TWELVE CHANNELS; FOURTEEN CHANNELS. [27: 84] [97: 377]

channel sinew 经筋 *jīng jīn*: Any of the TWELVE CHANNEL SINEWS.

channel stroke 中经 *zhòng jīng*: WIND STROKE in which evil is in the channels; characterized by hemiplegia, deviated eyes and mouth, and difficult speech. It is distinguished from organ stroke by the absence of spirit-mind signs like clouding collapse, and differs from network stroke by including hemiplegia and difficult speech. [26: 141] [27: 397] [97: 79]

channel theory 经络学说 *jīng luò xué shuō*: All theories concerning the channels, their pathways, functions, and diseases. ◇ Chin Lit. channel and network [vessel] theory. [26: 817]

chaotic menstruation 经乱 *jīng luàn*: MENSTRUATION AT IRREGULAR INTERVALS.

chaotic red-thread vessels 赤丝乱脉 *chì sī luàn mài*: TANGLED RED-THREAD VESSELS.

chaotic vessels in the white of the eye 白睛乱脉 *bái jīng luàn mài*: TANGLED RED-THREAD VESSELS.

characteristic 性能 *xìng néng*: The qi, flavor, and bearing of a medicinal. See FOUR QI; FIVE FLAVORS; BEARING. [27: 316]

char-frying 炒炭 *chǎo tàn*: A medicinal processing method similar to scorch-frying, but using an even higher flame. The aim of char-frying is to make the materials charred and black on the outside, brown on the inside, and brittle. Although a large proportion of the material is charred, the original properties are still present. This is what is known as "nature-preservative burning." To ensure that the nature is partially preserved in this way, it is important that the material should not be completely carbonized. Because of the high temperature used in char-frying, materials easily catch fire. In this event, water should be sprinkled over the material until no sparks are seen. Some materials, such as typha pollen (*pú huáng*) require particularly vigorous stirring to clear the smoke they produce. Char-frying moderates the properties of a medicinal, and increases its ability to promote contraction and check bleeding. Some modern experiments show that blood-stanching properties may in some cases be destroyed through the process. [27: 324] [82: 46]

checking diarrhea 止泻 *zhǐ xiè*: A method of treatment used to address diarrhea. Checking diarrhea takes a variety of forms depending on the pattern in which it occurs. Specific methods include: CLEARING HEAT AND DISINHIBITING DAMPNESS; DISPERSING FOOD AND ABDUCTING STAGNATION; WARMING THE STOMACH AND FORTIFYING THE CENTER; WARMING AND SUPPLEMENTING THE LIFE GATE; FORTIFYING THE SPLEEN

AND HARMONIZING THE STOMACH. See also DIARRHEA.

checking tetany 止痉 *zhǐ jìng*: RESOLVING TETANY.

checking vaginal discharge 止带 *zhǐ dài*: A method of treatment used to address vaginal discharge. Checking vaginal discharge usually denotes securing and astringing to treat vaginal discharge due to vacuity and characterized by persistent clear thin white vaginal discharge without foul smell, often accompanied by gradually developing physical weakness. It involves the use of qi-supplementing and kidney-supplementing medicinals combined with securing astringents such as calcined cuttlefish bone (*duàn wū zéi gǔ*), calcined oyster shell (*duàn mǔ lì*), euryale (*qiàn shí*), ginkgo (*bái guǒ*), and yellow wax (*huáng là*). A representative vaginal-discharge–checking formula is Discharge-Checking Tablet (*zhǐ dài piàn*). ACU Base treatment mainly on CV, SP, GIV, and KI. Main points: GB-26 (*dài mài*, Girdling Vessel), BL-30 (*bái huán shū*, White Ring Transport), CV-6 (*qì hǎi*, Sea of Qi), and SP-6 (*sān yīn jiāo*, Three Yin Intersection); needle with supplementation and add moxa. For continuous vaginal discharge, add SP-12 (*chōng mén*, Surging Gate) and ST-30 (*qì chōng*, Qi Thoroughfare). For copious discharge, add KI-12 (*dà hè*, Great Manifestation) and KI-13 (*qì xué*, Qi Point). See VAGINAL DISCHARGE. [6: 268]

checking vomiting 止呕 *zhǐ ǒu*: Suppression of vomiting. Vomiting occurs in a wide variety of stomach diseases and is treated in different ways accordingly. See VOMITING (AND RETCHING). [27: 64] [97: 661]

cheek bone 颧骨 *quán gǔ*: The prominent bone beneath the eye. WMC zygomatic bone. [27: 64] [26: 1009]

cheek carriage 颊车 *jiá chē*: **1.** The joint of the lower jaw. **2.** A point name, ST-6. ◇ Chin 颊 *jiá*, cheek (the area in front of the ear); 车 *chē*, vehicle; carriage, a mobile support. The use of "carriage" in this term derives from the notions a) that the lower jaw bone is the bone that bears all the teeth and b) that the joint of the jaw carries or supports the jaw. [25: 292] [81: 564] [76: 33] [79: 913]

cheek carriage bone 颊车骨 *jiá chē gǔ*: Synonyms: *tooth carriage*; *tooth bed*. The lower jaw. WMC The mandible. ◇ Chin 颊 *jiá*, cheek (the area in front of the ear); 车 *chē*, vehicle; carriage, support; *gǔ*, bone. [25: 292]

Chen 陈 *chén*: Name of a dynasty (A.D. 557–589).

chest 胸 *xiōng*, 胸部 *xiōng bù*: The upper part of the trunk, enclosed by the ribs and breastbone. *adj.* thoracic. See CHEST AND RIB-SIDE.

chest and rib-side 胸胁 *xiōng xié*: The anterior chest and the sides of the body from the armpit to the lowest rib. Signs associated with this part of the body are CHEST PAIN, glomus in the chest, [suffering of] chest and rib-side fullness, (CHEST AND RIB-SIDE FULLNESS, PROPPING FULLNESS IN THE CHEST AND RIB-SIDE), FULLNESS IN THE CHEST, and OPPRESSION IN THE CHEST.

chest and rib-side fullness 胸胁苦满 *xiōng xié kǔ mǎn*, 胸胁满 *xiōng xié mǎn*: *Synonym: suffering of chest and rib-side suffering fullness.* From *On Cold Damage* (*shāng hán lùn, biàn shào yáng bìng mài zhèng bìng zhì*). Fullness and oppression in the chest and rib-side associated with disturbance of qi dynamic in the foot lesser yang (*shào yáng*) gallbladder channel and with gallbladder fire. MED Use Minor Bupleurum Decoction (*xiǎo chái hú tāng*) or Bupleurum Liver-Coursing Powder (*chái hú shū gān sǎn*). ACU Base treatment mainly on GB and PC. Select PC-6 (*nèi guān*, Inner Pass), LR-3 (*tài chōng*, Supreme Surge), LR-14 (*qī mén*, Cycle Gate), GB-34 (*yáng líng quán*, Yang Mound Spring), ST-36 (*zú sān lǐ*, Leg Three Li), and SP-6 (*sān yīn jiāo*, Three Yin Intersection); needle with drainage. ◇ Chin 苦 *kǔ*, bitter, causing suffering; to suffer. [26: 459] [51: 374]

chest and rib-side pain 胸胁痛 *xiōng xié tòng*: See CHEST PAIN; RIB-SIDE PAIN. [26: 549] [26: 516]

chest and rib-side suffering fullness 胸胁苦满 *xiōng xié kǔ mǎn*: CHEST AND RIB-SIDE FULLNESS.

chest bind 结胸 *jié xiōng*: A pattern arising when evil qi binds in the chest, causing pain below the heart with hard fullness that can be felt under pressure. It occurs when offensive precipitation is administered too early in greater yang (*tài yáng*) disease and causes exterior heat to fall into the inner body to bind with water-rheum. It may also occur (without inappropriate precipitation) when greater yang disease passes to yang brightness (*yáng míng*) and yang brightness repletion heat combines with preexisting water-rheum. See entries listed below. [26: 754] [27: 376]

Chest Bind

MAJOR CHEST BIND (*dà jié xiōng*)

MINOR CHEST BIND (*xiǎo jié xiōng*)

COLD REPLETION CHEST BIND (*hán jié xiōng*)

WATER CHEST BIND (*shuǐ jié xiōng*)

BLOOD CHEST BIND (*xuè jié xiōng*)

chest bones 胸骨 *xiōng gǔ*: The breast bone and ribs. [26: 549]

chest center 膻中 *shān zhōng*: **1.** The center of the chest between the nipples. *The Magic Pivot* (*líng shū, hǎi lùn*) states, "The chest center is the sea of qi." **2.** The pericardium. *Elementary Questions* (*sù wèn, líng lán mì diǎn lùn*) states, "The chest center holds the office of minister and courier; from it joy and pleasure emanate." [26: 943]

chest impediment 胸痹 *xiōng bì*: *Synonym: thoracic impediment.* From *The Magic Pivot* (*líng shū, běn zàng*) **1.** In *Emergency Standby Remedies* (*zhǒu hòu bèi jí fāng*) and *Essential Prescriptions of the Golden Coffer* (*jīn guì yào lüè*), chest impediment is described as a disease pattern characterized by fullness and oppression in the anterior chest, in severe cases with pain stretching to the back, and panting that prevents the patient from lying down. It is caused by yin evils like phlegm turbidity and static blood that congeal and bind, preventing diffusion of chest yang. Depending on severity, chest impediment may take the form of FULLNESS IN THE CHEST or CHEST PAIN. WMC Observed in what Western medicine classes as heart disease, pulmonary emphysema, and pleurisy. MED Warm yang and boost qi; course qi and sweep phlegm. In enduring cases, blockage of the network vessels by static blood can be addressed by freeing the network vessels. Formulas such as Trichosanthes, Chinese Chive, and White Liquor Decoction (*guā lóu xiè bái bái jiǔ tāng*), Trichosanthes, Chinese Chive, and Pinellia Decoction (*guā lóu xiè bái bàn xià tāng*) or Aconite Main Tuber and Halloysite Pill (*wū tóu chì shí zhī wán*). ACU Base treatment mainly on HT, PC, and CV. Main points: BL-15 (*xīn shū*, Heart Transport), BL-14 (*jué yīn shū*, Reverting Yin Transport), CV-14 (*jù què*, Great Tower Gate), CV-17 (*shān zhōng*, Chest Center), PC-6 (*nèi guān*, Inner Pass), and HT-5 (*tōng lǐ*, Connecting Li). Selection of points according to pattern: For phlegm turbidity congestion, add ST-40 (*fēng lóng*, Bountiful Bulge), ST-36 (*zú sān lǐ*, Leg Three Li), and SP-6 (*sān yīn jiāo*, Three Yin Intersection), needling with drainage. For qi stagnation and blood stasis, add BL-18 (*gān shū*, Liver Transport) BL-17 (*gé shū*, Diaphragm Transport), LR-3 (*tài chōng*, Supreme Surge), ST-36 (*zú sān lǐ*, Leg Three Li), and SP-6 (*sān yīn jiāo*, Three Yin Intersection), needling with even supplementation and drainage and adding moxa. For yin evil obstruction with pronounced cold signs, add CV-6 (*qì hǎi*, Sea of Qi), and CV-4 (*guān yuán*, Pass Head), needling with supplementation and large amounts of moxa. **2.** In *Pathoconditions, Causes, Pulses, and Treatments* (*zhèng yīn mài zhì*), stomach impediment (*wèi bì*); characterized by fullness and oppression in the anterior chest, pain on swallowing, and in some cases occasional vomiting. Compare HEART IMPEDIMENT. [50: 1272] [26: 549] [80: 208] [113: 265]

chest pain 胸痛 *xiōng tòng*: From *Elementary Questions* (*sù wèn*). Any pain in any part of the chest. Chest pain is attributable to a variety of diseases including HEART IMPEDIMENT, HEART PAIN, TRUE HEART PAIN, REVERSAL HEART PAIN, PHLEGM-RHEUM, PULMONARY WELLING-ABSCESS,

and PULMONARY CONSUMPTION. The chest corresponds to the upper burner and contains the heart and lung, and chest pain is the manifestation of heart or lung disease, especially heart disease; hence chest pain includes heart pain and in some contexts the two terms are synonymous. The stomach duct is contiguous to the chest, and in the past "heart pain" was often used to denote pain in the pit of the stomach. As a result, the terms "chest pain," "heart pain," and "stomach duct pain" have been confused. Chest pain proper (not including stomach duct pain) is attributed to heart qi vacuity, congealing cold and stagnant qi, heart blood stasis obstruction, dual vacuity of qi and yin, phlegm turbidity obstruction, or pulmonary welling-abscess. For scorching pain in the chest and rib-side, see LIVER FIRE INVADING THE LUNG. WMC pneumonia; pleurisy; intercostal neuralgia; coronary heart disease. **Heart qi vacuity:** Chest pain due to heart qi vacuity is an intermittent dull pain of varying severity, with oppression in the chest, heart palpitations, shortness of breath, spontaneous sweating, and fatigue, all exacerbated following physical exertion, as well as bright white facial complexion, pale tongue, and a pulse that is fine or forceless, vacuous, and large. MED Supplement heart qi. Use variations of Origin-Preserving Decoction (*bǎo yuán tāng*). If there is concurrent blood vacuity, add tangkuei (*dāng guī*) and ass hide glue (*ē jiāo*); if there is blood stasis add ligusticum (*chuān xiōng*) and red peony (*chì sháo yào*). ACU Base treatment mainly on CV and PC. Main points: CV-17 (*shān zhōng*, Chest Center), PC-4 (*xī mén*, Cleft Gate), and PC-6 (*nèi guān*, Inner Pass). For heart qi vacuity, add BL-15 (*xīn shū*, Heart Transport), CV-14 (*jù què*, Great Tower Gate), HT-7 (*shén mén*, Spirit Gate), CV-4 (*guān yuán*, Pass Head), CV-6 (*qì hǎi*, Sea of Qi), BL-20 (*pí shū*, Spleen Transport), and ST-36 (*zú sān lǐ*, Leg Three Li); needle with supplementation and add moxa. **Congealing cold and stagnant qi:** Congealing cold and stagnant qi is due to heart yang vacuity. It is therefore similar to heart qi vacuity, but is marked by pronounced cold signs. It causes chest pain of varying severity, with distention and oppression. In severe cases, the pain stretches into the back, left shoulder, and arm. Other signs include somber white complexion, spontaneous sweating, fear of cold, cold limbs (or REVERSE-FLOW), a moist pale tongue that may be enlarged and have dental impressions, and a deep slow or bound intermittent pulse. MED Warm and free heart yang. Use Trichosanthes, Chinese Chive, and White Liquor Decoction (*guā lóu xiè bái bái jiǔ tāng*). In severe cases, with yang vacuity on the verge of desertion, pain like the cutting of a knife, dripping cold sweat, REVERSE-FLOW of the limbs, and a faint pulse on the verge of expiration, use Ginseng and Aconite Decoction (*shēn fù tāng*) or Ginseng, Aconite, Dragon Bone, and Oyster Shell Decoction (*shēn fù lóng mǔ tāng*) to return yang and stem counterflow. ACU To the main points given above, add BL-15 (*xīn shū*, Heart Transport), BL-14 (*jué yīn shū*, Reverting Yin Transport), CV-14 (*jù què*, Great Tower Gate), CV-6 (*qì hǎi*, Sea of Qi), CV-4 (*guān yuán*, Pass Head), LI-4 (*hé gǔ*, Union Valley), and LR-3 (*tài chōng*, Supreme Surge); needle with drainage and large amounts of moxa. **Heart blood stasis obstruction:** Heart blood stasis obstruction is a pattern of right vacuity and evil repletion, developing as a result of heart qi or heart yang vacuity. It causes acute, usually stabbing chest pain of fixed location. In severe cases, it comes in sudden attacks, like the cutting of a knife, accompanied by a cold sweat, heart palpitations or fearful throbbing, and fear. After attacks, the patient is fatigued and listless. The tongue is green-blue or purple, dark and dull, sometimes with stasis macules. The pulse is sunken and fine, or rough, or bound and intermittent. MED Quicken the blood and transform stasis. Use House of Blood Stasis-Expelling Decoction (*xuè fǔ zhú yū tāng*) combined with Sudden Smile Powder (*shī xiào sǎn*). ACU To the main points given above, add BL-15 (*xīn shū*, Heart Transport), CV-14 (*jù què*, Great Tower Gate), BL-17 (*gé shū*, Diaphragm Transport), SP-10 (*xuè hǎi*, Sea of Blood), LR-3 (*tài chōng*, Supreme Surge), and SP-6 (*sān yīn jiāo*, Three Yin Intersection); needle with drainage. **Dual vacuity of qi and yin:** Chest pain from dual vacuity of qi and yin is a continuous pain of varying severity associated with palpation, profuse dreaming and insomnia, spontaneous sweating, shortness of breath, and panting that are markedly exacerbated by physical exertion. There is a subjective feeling of heat effusion, a dry red tongue with scant fur and little liquid, yellow or reddish urine, and a forceless fine or rapid or bound or intermittent pulse. MED Boost qi and nourish yin. Use Pulse-Engendering Powder (*shēng mài sǎn*) or Honey-Fried Licorice Decoction (*zhì gān cǎo tāng*). ACU To the main points given above, add BL-15 (*xīn shū*, Heart Transport), CV-14 (*jù què*, Great Tower Gate), BL-20 (*pí shū*, Spleen Transport), BL-23 (*shèn shū*, Kidney Transport), CV-6 (*qì hǎi*, Sea of Qi), ST-36 (*zú sān lǐ*, Leg Three Li), SP-6 (*sān yīn jiāo*, Three Yin Intersection), KI-6 (*zhào hǎi*, Shining Sea), and KI-3 (*tài xī*, Great Ravine); needle with supplementation. **Phlegm turbidity obstruction:** Chest pain due to phlegm turbidity obstruction is associated with cough and copious phlegm (clear thin phlegm-drool or thick and sticky), and shortness of breath or panting. In severe cases, the pain stretches through to the back and prevents the patient from lying flat. The tongue fur is white and moist or glossy, and the pulse is slippery. MED Transform phlegm and free yang. Use Trichosanthes, Chinese Chive, and Pinellia Decoction (*guā lóu xiè bái bàn xià tāng*) or Unripe Bitter Orange, Chinese Chive, and Cinnamon Twig Decoction (*zhǐ shí xiè bái guì zhī tāng*). For phlegm-stasis obstruction use Trichosanthes, Chinese Chive, and Pinellia Decoction (*guā lóu xiè bái bàn xià tāng*) plus peach kernel (*táo rén*), carthamus (*hóng huā*), typha pollen (*pú huáng*), and ark shell (*wǔ léng zǐ*), to transform stasis. ACU To the main points given above, add ST-40 (*fēng lóng*, Bountiful Bulge), CV-12 (*zhōng wǎn*, Center Stomach Duct), and ST-36 (*zú sān lǐ*, Leg Three Li), to transform phlegm, and BL-17 (*gé shū*, Diaphragm Transport), SP-10 (*xuè hǎi*, Sea of Blood), LR-3 (*tài chōng*, Supreme Surge), and SP-6 (*sān yīn jiāo*, Three Yin Intersection), to transform stasis. Needle with drainage and add moxa. **Pulmonary welling-abscess:** The main characteristics are a dull pain and coughing up of yellow phlegm that may contain pus and blood and that is fishy smelling. There is a dry mouth and thirst with no desire to drink. There may also be vexation and fullness, sweating, and sudden bouts of aversion to cold and heat effusion. The tongue is red and the pulse is slippery or slippery and rapid. MED Clear heat and push out pus. Use Thousand Gold Pieces Phragmites Decoction (*qiān jīn wěi jīng tāng*). [26: 549] [92: No. 177] [46: 594, 597, 602] [113: 20] [37: 333–36] [14: 148]

chest yang 胸阳 *xiōng yáng*: Synonym: *thoracic yang*. The yang qi of the chest.

ch'i 气 *qì*: QI.

chicken breast 鸡胸 *jī xiōng*: Synonym: *pigeon chest*. A deformity in infants in which the chest protrudes at the center, giving it the appearance of a chicken's breast; hence the name. This condition is attributed to congenital insufficiency and/or poor nourishment after birth and manifests as spleen-kidney depletion and softness of the bones. WMC pectus carinatum (pectus gallinatum). [27: 436]

chicken pox 水痘 *shuǐ dòu*: A contagious disease of children first recorded in *On Pox Formulas* (*dòu zhěn fāng lùn*) (A.D. 1518) by Cai Wei-Fan. It is characterized by heat effusion, and bursts of macular and papular eruptions, and is attributed to seasonal wind-toxin and brewing internal damp-heat harassing the defense aspect. MED Course wind, clear heat, and resolve toxin using Lonicera and Forsythia Powder (*yín qiào sǎn*) as the main formula. Where pox papules burst and erode, Indigo Powder (*qīng dài sǎn*) can be applied topically. ◇ Chin 水 *shuǐ*, water; 痘 *dòu*, pox. [26: 152]

chicken's-claw wind 鸡爪风 *jī zhuǎ (zhǎo) fēng*: ASHEN NAIL.

chief 主 *zhǔ*: See SOVEREIGN, MINISTER, ASSISTANT, AND COURIER.

chief, support, assistant, and conductor 主辅佐引 *zhǔ fǔ zuǒ yǐn*: See SOVEREIGN, MINISTER, ASSISTANT, AND COURIER.

child bedwetting 尿来 *niào lái*: See ENURESIS.

childbed wind 蓐风 *rù fēng*: Synonym: *wind tetany*. Arched-back rigidity and clenched jaw from wind stroke after childbirth. MED Use Hua Tuo's Wind-Healing Powder (*huá tuó yù fēng sǎn*). See POSTPARTUM WIND STROKE; LOCKJAW. ◇ Chin 蓐 *rù*, straw mat or mattress; 风 *fēng*, wind. [26: 842]

childbirth 分娩 *fēn miǎn*, 分解 *fēn jiě*, 分诞 *fēn dàn*, 免身 *miǎn shēn*, 产 *chǎn*: Synonym: *birth*; *delivery*. The separation of the child from the mother's body, after 28th week of pregnancy. [97: 112]

child dysentery 小儿痢疾 *xiǎo ér lì jí*: DYSENTERY in infants and children, usually resulting from contraction of damp-heat and damage by raw, cold, or unclean food in summer. Child dysentery is characterized by heat effusion, abdominal pain and, in the initial stage, diarrhea with watery stool, which gives way to the standard signs of dysentery, i.e., stool containing pus and blood with tenesmus and frequent defecation. Distinction is made between cold and heat pattern. [26: 71]

child enuresis 小儿遗尿 *niào lái*: Synonym: *child bedwetting*. See ENURESIS.

child eye gan 小儿疳眼 *xiǎo ér gān yǎn*: Synonyms: *eye gan*; *gan toxin eye*; *gan disease ascending to the eye*. Dryness, aversion to light, screens on the dark of the eyes (iris and cornea), possibly causing CRAB'S-EYE, or, in severe cases, withering of the eyeball and blindness. It is attributed to spleen-stomach depletion with essence-blood depletion depriving the eye of nourishment and liver heat attacking the upper body. WMC keratomalacia. MED Treat by fortifying the spleen and clearing heat, by killing worms and dispersing gan, and by nourishing the liver and brightening the eyes, or other methods depending on the condition of the patient. Use variations of Chubby Child Pill (*féi ér wán*) from *The Golden Mirror of Medicine* (*yī zōng jīn jiàn*). ACU The above medicinal treatment can also be combined with spine pinching and needling of the Four Seams (*sì fèng*), and burning moxa at ST-36 (*zú sān lǐ*, Leg Three Li), BL-18 (*gān shū*, Liver Transport), and BL-23 (*shèn shū*, Kidney Transport). See GAN. [26: 69]

child fright reversal 小儿惊厥 *xiǎo ér jīng jué*: FRIGHT REVERSAL.

child fright wind 小儿惊风 *xiǎo ér jīng fēng*: FRIGHT WIND.

children's diseases 小儿杂病 *xiǎo ér zá bìng*: Synonym: *infants' and children's diseases*. Diseases to which infants and children are prone. In general, small children are susceptible to external contractions and disease of the lungs and spleen. See LUNG IS OFTEN IN INSUFFICIENCY. A comprehensive list of children's diseases is given under DISEASE.

child visiting hostility 小儿客忤 *xiǎo ér kè wǔ*: Synonyms: *visiting hostility*; *strike-on-person*. Crying, fright, disquietude, or even changes in complexion in infants brought on by seeing a stranger or strange sight, or being exposed to unfamiliar surroundings or circumstances. The condition often involves contention between wind and phlegm and affects the spleen and stomach's functions of intake, movement, and transformation, giving rise to vomiting, diarrhea, abdominal pain, and convulsions similar to those of epilepsy. MED Use Soul-Quieting Decoction (*ān hún tāng*), which contains spiny jujube kernel (*suān zǎo rén*), root poria (*fú shén*), polygala (*yuǎn zhì*), tangkuei (*dāng guī*), bile arisaema (*dǎn xīng*), and juncus (*dēng xīn cǎo*), with variations according to need. For cases of exuberant phlegm, see ACUTE FRIGHT WIND. ◇ Chin 客 *kè*, visit, intrude, lodge; 忤 *wǔ*, hostility, unruliness. [26: 64]

child wilting pattern 小儿痿证 *xiǎo ér wěi zhèng*: Any limpness of the limbs and inability to grasp objects in children. Chinese medicine traditionally had no disease name corresponding to 'infantile paralysis' in modern medicine. 'Child wilting pattern' is a modern Chinese medical term that corresponds in Western medicine to infantile paralysis as the sequela of poliomyelitis or resulting from other causes such as infantile myodystrophy. Child wilting patterns are attributed to dual depletion of qi and humor and LUNG HEAT SCORCHING THE LOBES after heat (febrile) disease, depriving the skin and sinews of nourishment, or to warm heat sweltering the yang brightness *yáng míng*, with slackness of the ancestral sinews. They may also be attributed to insufficiency of the earlier heaven constitution with depletion of the liver and kidney. MED See WILTING. ACU Base treatment mainly on yang brightness (*yáng míng*) channel points. Main points: LI-4 (*hé gǔ*, Union Valley), LI-11 (*qū chí*, Pool at the Bend), ST-36 (*zú sān lǐ*, Leg Three Li), and SP-6 (*sān yīn jiāo*, Three Yin Intersection). For lung heat scorching the lobes, add LU-7 (*liè quē*, Broken Sequence), GB-20 (*fēng chí*, Wind Pool), and KI-6 (*zhào hǎi*, Shining Sea). needling with drainage. For insufficiency of earlier heaven constitution with depletion of the liver and kidney, add BL-18 (*gān shū*, Liver

Transport), BL-23 (*shèn shū*, Kidney Transport), GB-39 (*xuán zhōng*, Suspended Bell), GB-34 (*yáng líng quán*, Yang Mound Spring), and KI-3 (*tài xī*, Great Ravine), needling with supplementation. Selection of points according to affected area: For difficulty raising the shoulder, add GB-21 (*jiān jǐng*, Shoulder Well), LI-15 (*jiān yú*, Shoulder Bone), TB-14 (*jiān liáo*, Shoulder Bone-Hole), LI-16 (*jù gǔ*, Great Bone), and SI-11 (*tiān zōng*, Celestial Gathering). For limp wrists, add TB-5 (*wài guān*, Outer Pass), SI-5 (*yáng gǔ*, Yang Valley), and Central Spring (*zhōng quán*). For paralysis of the lower limbs, add GV-4 (*mìng mén*, Life Gate), GB-33 (*xī yáng guān*, Knee Yang Joint), ST-31 (*bì guān*, Thigh Joint), BL-37 (*yīn mén*, Gate of Abundance), GB-30 (*huán tiào*, Jumping Round), GB-34 (*yáng líng quán*, Yang Mound Spring), and GB-39 (*xuán zhōng*, Suspended Bell). For paralysis of the abdominal muscles, add CV-12 (*zhōng wǎn*, Center Stomach Duct) and ST-25 (*tiān shū*, Celestial Pivot). [50: 137] [39: 233] [46: 638] [40: 90]

Chinese medicinal 中药 *zhōng yào*: Any medicinal used in the orthodox literary tradition. See MEDICINAL.

Chinese medicinals and herbs 中草药 *zhōng cǎo yào*: Any medicinals of traditional orthodox medicinal therapy and herbs locally used in folk medicine in China. See MEDICINAL. [27: 314]

cholera 霍乱 *huò luàn*: Synonym: *sudden turmoil*. A disease characterized by simultaneous vomiting and diarrhea, usually followed by severe cramps. Dry cholera is characterized by an ungratified urge to vomit and defecate at the same time. Cholera in Chinese medicine includes what modern Western medicine calls cholera and as well as acute gastroenteritis presenting with the same signs. WMC See COLD CHOLERA; HEAT CHOLERA; DRY CHOLERA; DAMP CHOLERA; CHOLERA CRAMPS. ◇ Chin 霍 *huò*, sudden, fulminant; 乱 *luàn*, chaos, turmoil; possibly from Gk. *kholera*. Eng L. from Gk. *kholera* (*kholē*, bile, anger). [26: 905] [27: 365] [97: 641]

cholera cramps 霍乱转筋 *huò luàn zhuǎn jīn*: Synonym: *leg-hoisting sand*. Cramps occurring when vomiting and diarrhea in cholera (sudden turmoil) causes fulminant loss of fluids and damage to qi and yin, thereby depriving the sinews of nourishment. Contraction of the legs in severe cases may be accompanied by hypertonicity of the abdomen, retracted scrotum and curled tongue. MED Determine whether the condition is heat cholera or cold cholera. Use formulas such as Chaenomeles Decoction (*mù guā tāng*) or Center-Rectifying Decoction (*lǐ zhōng tāng*), or administer one (rice) bowl of fresh lablab leaf (*biǎn dòu yè*) juice obtained by crushing and squeez-ing. Crushed garlic can be applied at the heart of the soles of the feet. ACU Apply treatments for heat or cold cholera, and needle with drainage at GB-34 (*yáng líng quán*, Yang Mound Spring), BL-57 (*chéng shān*, Mountain Support), GB-38 (*yáng fǔ*, Yang Assistance), SP-3 (*tài bái*, Supreme White), SP-2 (*dà dū*, Great Metropolis), LR-4 (*zhōng fēng*, Mound Center), and BL-60 (*kūn lún*, Kunlun Mountains); for severe cases, add moxa. [26: 905] [27: 365] [97: 641]

chong product 虫类 *chóng lèi*: Any medicinal product derived from reptiles, arthropods, or shellfish. ◇ Chin 虫 *chóng*, worm, insect, reptile, animal.

chronic fright wind 慢惊风 *màn jīn fēng*: A disease of infants and children characterized by intermittent mild convulsions associated with pale yellow facial complexion of mixed blue-green and white facial complexion and in most cases the absence of heat effusion. Most chronic fright wind patients exhibit signs such as CLOUDING SLEEP, either with the eyes fully closed or with the eyeballs exposed, as well as fatigue and laziness to speak. Stool may be slightly green-blue in color or there may be CLEAR-FOOD DIARRHEA. The pulse is sunken and moderate or sunken, slow, and forceless. Chronic fright wind is attributed to insufficiency of qi and blood and exuberance of the liver with vacuity of the spleen, and often occurs in the advanced stages of severe chronic disease when right qi is greatly weakened. MED Treatment should focus on supporting right and rectifying the liver and spleen, supported by clearing the heart and flushing phlegm. Formulas that can be used include Center-Rectifying Decoction (*lǐ zhōng tāng*), Clever Powder (*xīng xīng sǎn*), Spleen-Arousing Pill (*xǐng pí wán*), and Cinnabar Spirit-Quieting Pill (*zhū shā ān shén wán*). ACU Base treatment mainly on CV, ST, and LR, needling with supplementation and moxa at CV-12 (*zhōng wǎn*, Center Stomach Duct), LR-13 (*zhāng mén*, Camphorwood Gate), CV-6 (*qì hǎi*, Sea of Qi), ST-25 (*tiān shū*, Celestial Pivot), and ST-36 (*zú sān lǐ*, Leg Three Li), and needling with even supplementation and drainage without moxa at GB-20 (*fēng chí*, Wind Pool), LR-3 (*tài chōng*, Supreme Surge), and LR-2 (*xíng jiān*, Moving Between). Selection of points according to signs: For no thought of food and drink, add BL-20 (*pí shū*, Spleen Transport) and Four Seams (*sì fèng*), applying moxa at the former. For clear-food diarrhea, add BL-25 (*dà cháng shū*, Large Intestine Transport) and Five Pillar Points (*wǔ zhù xué*), applying moxa at all the points. For rigidity of the nape and neck, add GV-14 (*dà zhuī*, Great Hammer) and GV-12 (*shēn zhù*, Body Pillar). For convulsions, add LI-11 (*qū chí*, Pool at the Bend), SI-3 (*hòu xī*, Back Ravine), GB-34 (*yáng líng quán*, Yang Mound Spring), and BL-57 (*chéng shān*, Mountain Support). [27: 432] [113: 332] [46: 596] [79: 171]

chronic spleen wind 慢脾风 *màn pí fēng*: A disease pattern in young children arising when excessive vomiting or diarrhea weakens right qi, causing closed eyes and shaking head, dark green-blue face and lips, sweating brow, clouded spirit, somnolence, reversal cold of the limbs, and wriggling of the extremities. It is a form of chronic fright wind characterized by spleen yin vacuity and spleen yang debilitation. MED Warm the center and supplement the spleen; secure the root and restore yang. Administer Ginseng and Aconite Decoction (*shēn fù tāng*) in frequent small doses, and later use Aconite Center-Rectifying Decoction (*fù zǐ lǐ zhōng tāng*) with additional medicinals. ACU Base treatment mainly on CV, ST, and LR. Select BL-20 (*pí shū*, Spleen Transport), CV-12 (*zhōng wǎn*, Center Stomach Duct), LR-13 (*zhāng mén*, Camphorwood Gate), CV-6 (*qì hǎi*, Sea of Qi), ST-25 (*tiān shū*, Celestial Pivot), ST-36 (*zú sān lǐ*, Leg Three Li), and LR-3 (*tài chōng*, Supreme Surge); needle with supplementation and a large amount of moxa. [26: 831] [113: 334]

cinnabar eye 眼丹 *yǎn dān*: A condition in which the eyelid becomes red, swollen, hot, and painful, and which in the later stages may suppurate and rupture and cause pronounced generalized signs. Cinnabar eye can develop from sties or damage to skin, and is traced to brewing accumulation of spleen-stomach heat toxin and externally contracted wind evil, combining to transform into fire, which binds in the eyelid, obstructs the network vessels, and scorches the fluids. At onset, the upper eyelid suddenly becomes red, swollen, and painful. Gradually, the whole of the area of the eyelids is affected by diffuse swelling that prevents full opening of the eye. The skin is red or purplish red in color, and is tender. Other signs include heat effusion and aversion to cold, headache, and general discomfort. As pus gathers, the skin gradually becomes thinner and turns a yellow white in color, and rippling can be felt under the touch. After rupture, it heals. If pus is excessively abundant and is not discharged easily, the condition may spread. WMC palpebral cellulitis. **Wind-toxin fettering the outer body:** Signs include diffuse swelling soft to the touch, diffuse redness, pain, and itching. These signs are accompanied by aversion to wind, headache, dizziness, general discomfort, pale tongue with yellow fur, and tight floating pulse. MED Course wind and resolve toxin with variations of Schizonepeta and Ledebouriella Toxin-Vanquishing Powder (*jīng fáng bài dú sǎn*). ACU Base treatment mainly on LI. Select GB-20 (*fēng chí*, Wind Pool), LI-4 (*hé gǔ*, Union Valley), LI-11 (*qū chí*, Pool at the Bend), TB-5 (*wài guān*, Outer Pass), GV-14 (*dà zhuī*, Great Ham-

mer), and BL-2 (*zǎn zhú*, Bamboo Gathering); needle with drainage and prick Greater Yang (*tài yáng*), LU-11 (*shào shāng*, Lesser Shang), GV-23 (*shàng xīng*, Upper Star), SP-10 (*xuè hǎi*, Sea of Blood), and BL-40 (*wěi zhōng*, Bend Center) to bleed. **Heat toxin congesting internally:** Signs include hard diffuse swelling that is red in color as though smeared with cinnabar and with fire-like scorching pain. General signs include thirst and constipation, a red tongue with yellow fur, and large surging pulse. MED Clear heat and resolve toxin with Immortal Formula Life-Giving Beverage (*xiān fāng huó mìng yǐn*). ACU Base treatment mainly on LI, ST, and PC. Select LI-4 (*hé gǔ*, Union Valley), LI-11 (*qū chí*, Pool at the Bend), PC-6 (*nèi guān*, Inner Pass), ST-36 (*zú sān lǐ*, Leg Three Li), SP-6 (*sān yīn jiāo*, Three Yin Intersection), needle with drainage and prick BL-40 (*wěi zhōng*, Bend Center), SP-10 (*xuè hǎi*, Sea of Blood), and Greater Yang (*tài yáng*) to bleed. [27: 501] [97: 517] [46: 595, 720] [113: 353] [4: 125] [125: 125]

cinnabar field 丹田 *dān tián*: **1.** An area three body-inches (*cùn*) below the umbilicus, believed by Daoists to be the chamber of essence (semen) in males and the uterus in females. **2.** Any of three mustering positions in qi-gong, including the lower cinnabar field (*xià dān tián*) located below the umbilicus, the middle cinnabar field (*zhōng dān tián*) located in the pit of the stomach (scrobiculus cordis), and the upper cinnabar field (*shàng dān tián*) located in the center of the brow. [27: 34] [27: 112]

cinnabar sand 丹痧 *dān shā*: EPIDEMIC THROAT SAND.

cinnabar toxin 丹毒 *dān dú*: *Synonym: fire cinnabar*. A condition characterized by sudden localized reddening of the skin, giving it the appearance of having been smeared with cinnabar. Cinnabar toxin usually affects the face and lower legs, is most common among children and the elderly, and usually occurs in spring and summer. Cinnabar toxin is known by different names according to form and location. When it affects the head, it is called *head fire cinnabar* (*bào tóu huǒ dān*). When it assumes a wandering pattern, it is called *wandering cinnabar* (*chì yóu dān*), as is observed in newborns. Cinnabar toxin of the lower legs is called *fire flow* (*liú huǒ*) or *fire cinnabar leg* (*huǒ dān jiǎo*). Cinnabar toxin arises when damaged skin and insecurity of defense qi allow evil toxin to enter the body and gives rise to heat in the blood aspect, which becomes trapped in the skin. If the toxin is accompanied by wind, the face is affected; if accompanied by dampness, the lower legs are affected. Thus the facial type tends to be wind-heat, whereas the lower leg type is damp-heat. The disease develops swiftly. The onset of heat effusion and aversion to cold is followed by the rapid outbreak of red patches on the skin. These patches are clearly defined, and slightly raised at the edges; they feel painful and are scorching hot to the touch. They quickly spread in all directions, turn from a bright to a darker red, and may scale. In some cases, there are also vesicles that leak yellow fluid on bursting and cause pain and itching. Other signs include vexing thirst, generalized heat [effusion], constipation, reddish urine, and other general heat signs. Development of a vigorous heat [effusion] with vomiting, clouded spirit, delirious speech, or even TETANIC REVERSAL are signs of the toxin attacking the body's interior. WMC Mostly corresponds to erysipelas. MED Clear heat and resolve toxin; cool the blood and transform stasis. Oral: For head fire cinnabar, use Universal Aid Toxin-Dispersing Beverage (pǔ jì xiāo dú yǐn). For fire flow, use Gentian Liver-Draining Decoction (lóng dǎn xiè gān tāng) supplemented with additional medicinals. For wandering cinnabar in newborns, treat by cooling the blood, clearing construction, and resolving toxin. Rhinoceros Horn and Rehmannia Decoction (xī jiǎo dì huáng tāng) combined with Coptis Toxin-Resolving Decoction (huáng lián jiě dú tāng). Topical: Four Colors Powder (sì sè sǎn). ACU Base treatment mainly on LI and SP. Main points: Apply diffuse pricking at ouch points (ā shì xué) and prick SP-10 (xuè hǎi, Sea of Blood), and BL-40 (wěi zhōng, Bend Center) to bleed with three-edged needle. Needle with drainage at LI-11 (qū chí, Pool at the Bend), LI-4 (hé gǔ, Union Valley), SP-9 (yīn líng quán, Yin Mound Spring), and SP-6 (sān yīn jiāo, Three Yin Intersection). Selection of points according to causes: For wind-heat transforming into fire, add GB-20 (fēng chí, Wind Pool), TB-5 (wài guān, Outer Pass), GV-14 (dà zhuī, Great Hammer), LU-11 (shào shāng, Lesser Shang), and LI-1 (shāng yáng, Shang Yang). For damp-heat, add SP-6 (sān yīn jiāo, Three Yin Intersection) and SP-5 (shāng qiū, Shang Hill). For evil toxin attacking the inner body, add PC-6 (nèi guān, Inner Pass), prick Twelve Well Points (shí èr jǐng xué) to bleed. Selection of points according to signs: For headache, add GB-20 (fēng chí, Wind Pool) Greater Yang (tài yáng). For vigorous heat [effusion] with vexation and agitation, add GV-14 (dà zhuī, Great Hammer). For clouded spirit and delirious speech, add GV-26 (rén zhōng, Human Center), PC-7 (dà líng, Great Mound) and KI-1 (yǒng quán, Gushing Spring). For nausea and vomiting, add PC-6 (nèi guān, Inner Pass) and ST-36 (zú sān lǐ, Leg Three Li). ◇ Chin 丹 dān, cinnabar, elixir; 毒 dú, toxin. [26: 166] [50: 298] [46: 707] [96: 110] [27: 461] [97: 1131] [61: 360]

civil flame 文火 *wén huǒ*: A low flame. When decocting formulas, the water is first brought to the boil, and then the flame is reduced so that the medicinals are decocted slowly. Richly flavored supplementing medicinals in particular require long boiling over a civil flame. Compare MARTIAL FLAME. [26: 89]

clamoring stomach 嘈杂 *cáo zá*: A sensation of emptiness and burning in the stomach duct or heart [region] described as being like hunger but not hunger, and like pain but not pain, and accompanied by belching, nausea, swallowing of up flowing acid, and fullness. WMC Associated with conditions classed in Western medicine as chronic gastritis and ulcers. Distinction is sometimes made between fire clamor, phlegm clamor, water soaking the heart clamor, chest and diaphragm qi depression clamor, and roundworm clamor. **Fire clamor** is characterized by hunger immediately after eating and insatiety despite eating. MED Treat by downbearing fire with formulas such as Left-Running Metal Pill (zuǒ jīn wán). ACU Base treatment mainly on ST and LI. Select ST-44 (nèi tíng, Inner Court), ST-36 (zú sān lǐ, Leg Three Li), and LI-4 (hé gǔ, Union Valley); needle with drainage. **Phlegm clamor** is characterized by oppressed breath and copious phlegm, a sensation like hunger but not hunger, and no desire for food and drink. MED Harmonize the stomach and transform phlegm with Medicated Leaven and Atractylodes Pill (qū zhú wán). For phlegm-fire, use Triple Supplementation Pill (sān bǔ wán) plus pinellia (bàn xià) and atractylodes (cāng zhú). ACU Base treatment mainly on ST, PC, CV, and back transport points. Select ST-36 (zú sān lǐ, Leg Three Li), PC-6 (nèi guān, Inner Pass), ST-25 (tiān shū, Celestial Pivot), CV-12 (zhōng wǎn, Center Stomach Duct), BL-20 (pí shū, Spleen Transport), BL-17 (gé shū, Diaphragm Transport), and ST-40 (fēng lóng, Bountiful Bulge); needle with even supplementation and drainage. For phlegm-fire, add ST-44 (nèi tíng, Inner Court) and LI-4 (hé gǔ, Union Valley), needling with drainage. **Clamor from sour water soaking the heart** is usually attributed to spleen-stomach vacuity cold with nontransformation of food. MED Warm the center and harmonize the stomach. Use Stomach-Warming Beverage (wēn wèi yǐn) or Six Gentlemen Decoction (liù jūn zǐ tāng). If the yin aspect has been damaged, use Yin-Rectifying Brew (lǐ yīn jiān) or Six Gentlemen Metal and Water Brew (jīn shuǐ liù jūn jiān). ACU Base treatment mainly on PC, ST, and SP. Main points: PC-6 (nèi guān, Inner Pass), ST-36 (zú sān lǐ, Leg Three Li), and BL-20 (pí shū, Spleen Transport). For spleen-stomach vacuity cold, add CV-12 (zhōng wǎn, Center Stomach Duct) and SP-4 (gōng sūn, Yellow Emperor); needle with supplementation and add moxa. For damage to the yin aspect, add SP-6 (*sān yīn jiāo*, Three Yin Intersection) and SP-3 (*tài bái*, Supreme White). **Chest and diaphragm qi depression clamor** is accompanied by glomus and oppression in the chest and diaphragm and rough sunken pulse. MED Rectify qi and loosen the chest. Use Qi Depression Decoction (*qì yù tāng*). ACU Base treatment mainly on CV and PC. Selecting CV-6 (*qì hǎi*, Sea of Qi), CV-17 (*shān zhōng*, Chest Center), PC-6 (*nèi guān*, Inner Pass), LI-4 (*hé gǔ*, Union Valley), LR-3 (*tài chōng*, Supreme Surge), and TB-6 (*zhī gōu*, Branch Ditch); needle with drainage. **Roundworm clamor** is characterized by vomiting and bouts of acute pain, and, in severe cases, vomiting of roundworm. MED Expel roundworm using formulas such as Mume Pill (*wū méi wán*) or Worm-Transforming Pill (*huà chóng wán*). ACU Base treatment mainly on SP and ST. Select SP-15 (*dà hèng*, Great Horizontal), LI-4 (*hé gǔ*, Union Valley), ST-36 (*zú sān lǐ*, Leg Three Li), and Hundred Worm Nest (*bǎi chóng wō*); needle with drainage. ◇ Chin 嘈 *cáo*, noise; 杂 *zá*, sundry, hodgepodge, impurity. [26: 845] [27: 411] [97: 621]

clavicle 巨骨 *jù gǔ*: The shoulder bone. [27: 67] [97: 77]

clean bowel 净腑 *jìng fǔ*: The bladder.

clean tongue fur 净苔 *jìng tāi*: An extremely fine fur with a grainy appearance. It is a normal healthy fur. [6: 123]

clear 清 *qīng*: **1.** *adj.* Pure and insubstantial (e.g., clear yang qi) in opposition to turbid. **2.** *adj.* Not properly decomposed. See CLEAR-FOOD DIARRHEA. **3.** *n.* That which is clear (usually "the clear"). See CLEAR YANG. **4.** *vb. trans.* To eliminate heat or fire, e.g., clear the heart (eliminate heart heat), clear the lung (eliminate lung heat), and clear qi (eliminate heat from the qi aspect), and specifically to clear heat as opposed to draining fire. See CLEARING. **5.** *vb. trans.* To excrete (same as 圊 *qīng*). [48: 305] ◇ Chin 清 *qīng*, clear, clean, pure, fresh, cool.

clear-eye blindness 青盲 *qīng máng*: Gradual blindness that in severe cases can be total. It is attributable to insufficiency of the liver and kidney and depletion of essence blood, combined with spleen-stomach vacuity preventing essential qi from reaching up to the eyes. WMC optic atrophy. MED Enrich the liver and kidney; replenish essence and supplement the marrow; open the orifices and brighten the eyes. Formulas include Lycium Berry, Chrysanthemum, and Rehmannia Pill (*qǐ jú dì huáng wán*) or variations of Long Vistas Pill Variant Formula (*zhù jǐng wán jiā jiǎn fāng*) with the addition of fresh pig's spine marrow (*zhū jǐ suǐ*). ACU Base treatment mainly on BL, ST, and back transport points, selecting BL-1 (*jīng*

míng, Bright Eyes), ST-1 (*chéng qì*, Tear Container), BL-18 (*gān shū*, Liver Transport), BL-23 (*shèn shū*, Kidney Transport), GB-37 (*guāng míng*, Bright Light), and GB-1 (*tóng zǐ liáo*, Pupil Bone-Hole). For liver-kidney depletion, add GV-4 (*mìng mén*, Life Gate)ⓜ. For spleen-stomach vacuity, add ST-36 (*zú sān lǐ*, Leg Three Li), BL-20 (*pí shū*, Spleen Transport), and BL-17 (*gé shū*, Diaphragm Transport). Use a weak stimulus for points around the eyes. Other points should be needled with supplementation. ◇ Chin 青 *qīng*, green-blue; 盲 *máng*, blind. Note that in the Chinese term, the character *qīng*, green-blue, also has the meaning of black or any dark color. It appears to be used here to suggest blindness without any white or other pale-colored eye screen; hence it is rendered more clearly in English as "clear-eye." [37: 465] [27: 505] [97: 234]

clear-food diarrhea 下利清谷 *xià lì qīng gǔ*: Diarrhea characterized by watery, light brown stool containing partially digested food and having no malodor. Clear-food diarrhea is accompanied by aversion to cold and cold limbs, and is a sign of kidney and spleen yang vacuity. MED Warm the center and dissipate cold using Vessel-Freeing Counterflow Cold Decoction (*tōng mài sì nì tāng*). ACU Base treatment mainly on back transport points, CV, GV and ST. Select BL-23 (*shèn shū*, Kidney Transport), CV-4 (*guān yuán*, Pass Head), GV-4 (*mìng mén*, Life Gate), BL-20 (*pí shū*, Spleen Transport), CV-12 (*zhōng wǎn*, Center Stomach Duct), LR-13 (*zhāng mén*, Camphorwood Gate), ST-25 (*tiān shū*, Celestial Pivot), and ST-36 (*zú sān lǐ*, Leg Three Li); needle with supplementation and add moxa. Compare COLD DIARRHEA; SWILL DIARRHEA. [26: 36] [27: 365] [97: 26] [46: 666] [37: 323,324]

clearing 清法 *qīng*: One of the EIGHT METHODS. See CLEARING HEAT. [27: 252] [97: 529]

clearing and depurating lung qi 清肃肺气 *qīng sù fèi qì*: Synonyms: *clearing metal; clearing metal and downbearing fire.* A method of treatment used to address lung heat with LUNG QI ASCENDING COUNTERFLOW. Lung qi normally descends, but when the lung is distressed by fire, there are heat signs such as expectoration of yellow phlegm, dry mouth, heat effusion without aversion to cold, red tongue, and a rapid floating pulse. Fire also disrupts the normal downward movement of qi, causing counterflow ascent of qi and cough. MED The method of clearing and depurating the lung makes use of medicinals that clear lung heat and downbear lung qi such as mulberry root bark (*sāng bái pí*), houttuynia (*yú xīng cǎo*), phragmites (*lú gēn*), isatis root (*bǎn lán gēn*), lonicera (*jīn yín huā*), white perilla seed (*bái sū zǐ*), peucedanum (*qián hú*), and loquat leaf (*pí* *pá yè*). [ACU] Base treatment mainly on LU, LI, and ST. Select BL-13 (*fèi shū*, Lung Transport), LU-10 (*yú jì*, Fish Border), LU-7 (*liè quē*, Broken Sequence), LI-11 (*qū chí*, Pool at the Bend), LI-4 (*hé gǔ*, Union Valley), ST-40 (*fēng lóng*, Bountiful Bulge), and GV-14 (*dà zhuī*, Great Hammer); needle with drainage. [27: 272] [97: 530]

clearing and disinhibiting 清利 *qīng lì*: CLEARING HEAT AND DISINHIBITING DAMPNESS. [26: 925]

clearing blood heat 清血热 *qīng xuè rè*: COOLING THE BLOOD.

clearing both qi and construction 气营两清 *qì yíng liǎng qīng*: A method of treatment used to address febrile disease in which heat evil has entered the qi aspect and the construction aspect, causing high fever, heart vexation, unquiet sleep, thirst, sweating, crimson tongue with dry yellow tongue fur, and a rapid surging pulse. [MED] Medicinals that clear qi and construction include gypsum (*shí gāo*), anemarrhena (*zhī mǔ*), tender bamboo leaf (lophatherum) (*zhú yè xīn*), forsythia (*lián qiào*), scutellaria (*huáng qín*), dendrobium (*shí hú*), dried/fresh rehmannia (*shēng dì huáng*), and scrophularia (*xuán shēn*). A representative formula is Scourge-Clearing Toxin-Vanquishing Beverage (*qīng wēn bài dú yǐn*). [ACU] Base treatment mainly on HT, PC, and LI. Needle with drainage at GV-14 (*dà zhuī*, Great Hammer), LI-11 (*qū chí*, Pool at the Bend), LI-4 (*hé gǔ*, Union Valley), PC-3 (*qū zé*, Marsh at the Bend), PC-9 (*zhōng chōng*, Central Hub), HT-9 (*shào chōng*, Lesser Surge), and prick them to bleed with a three-edged needle if necessary. Pricking the Twelve Well Points (*shí èr jǐng xué*) to bleed can also clear construction-aspect heat. [26: 546] [27: 1334] [97: 97]

clearing bowel and visceral heat 清脏腑热 *qīng zàng fǔ rè*: Dispelling heat or fire from any of the bowels and viscera. See the entries listed below. [60: 330]

Clearing Bowel and Visceral Heat

DRAINING THE HEART (*xiè xīn*)

CLEARING THE HEART AND OPENING THE ORIFICES (*qīng xīn kāi qiào*)

DRAINING THE LUNG (*xiè fèi*)

CLEARING AND DEPURATING LUNG QI (*qīng sù fèi qì*)

CLEARING THE LUNG AND MOISTENING DRYNESS (*qīng fèi rùn zào*)

CLEARING DRYNESS AND RESCUING THE LUNG (*qīng zào jiù fèi*)

CLEARING THE LUNG AND SUPPRESSING COUGH (*qīng fèi zhǐ ké*)

DRAINING THE LIVER (*xiè gān*)

CLEARING THE INTESTINES AND MOISTENING DRYNESS (*qīng cháng rùn zào*)

CLEARING THE STOMACH AND DOWNBEARING COUNTERFLOW (*qīng wèi jiàng nì*)

clearing construction 清营 *qīng yíng*: *Synonym: clearing construction and discharging heat.* A method of treatment used to address heat in the construction aspect characterized by high fever, vexation and agitation, unquiet sleep, dry crimson tongue, a rapid fine pulse, and unpronounced thirst. [MED] Clear construction, clear the heart, and resolve toxin. The main formula is Construction-Clearing Decoction (*qīng yíng tāng*) Where there are pericardium signs such as clouded spirit, this formula can be combined with one that opens the orifices, such as Peaceful Palace Bovine Bezoar Pill (*ān gōng niú huáng wán*), Spirit-Like Rhinoceros Horn Elixir (*shén xī dān*), or Purple Snow Elixir (*zǐ xuě dān*). When the pattern comprises stirring wind, Construction-Clearing Decoction can be combined with the liver-clearing and wind-extinguishing method by the admixture of medicinals such as antelope horn (*líng yáng jiǎo*) and uncaria (*gōu téng*). If the evil entering the construction aspect is damp-heat, the basic methods must be combined with that of drying dampness and clearing heat with cold bitter medicinals such as scutellaria (*huáng qín*) and coptis (*huáng lián*). Initial-stage construction-aspect heat patterns, where qi-aspect signs are still present, can be treated by combining the method of clearing construction and engendering liquid with that of promoting diffusion and outthrust with dissipating acridity to outthrust heat to the qi aspect. The basic formula used for such cases is Black Paste (Formula) (*hēi gāo (fāng)*). Broadly speaking, construction-aspect patterns are treated with cold bitter medicinals combined with cold sweet medicinals to drain heat and resolve toxin as well as to nourish yin and engender liquid. Construction-Clearing Decoction (*qīng yíng tāng*) has both these effects. Cold, sweet medicinals engender liquids. They enrich yin and increase humor. But if used alone, they not only fail to produce this effect, but may prevent elimination of the evil. Similarly, cold bitter medicinals used alone can cause dryness to form and damage yin, thus affecting their fire-draining and toxin-resolving effect. [ACU] Base treatment mainly on HT, PC, and LI, Needle with drainage at PC-8 (*láo gōng*, Palace of Toil), HT-8 (*shào fǔ*, Lesser Mansion), PC-3 (*qū zé*, Marsh at the Bend), PC-9 (*zhōng chōng*, Central Hub), HT-9 (*shào chōng*, Lesser Surge), and LI-11 (*qū chí*, Pool at the Bend), and prick them to bleed with a three-edged needle if necessary. Pricking the Twelve Well Points (*shí èr jǐng xué*) to bleed can also clear construction-aspect heat. [27: 254] [97: 529]

clearing construction and cooling the blood 清营凉血 *qīng yíng liáng xuè*: A method of treatment used to address evil heat in the construction-blood aspect using cool-cold medicinals. Clearing construction and cooling the blood treats heat entering construction-blood in warm disease, notably including intense construction heat, heat damaging construction-yin, exuberant heat stirring the blood, and qi and blood (construction) both ablaze. See CLEARING CONSTRUCTION, COOLING THE BLOOD, COOLING AND DISSIPATING THE BLOOD, CLEARING BOTH QI AND CONSTRUCTION, and OUTTHRUSTING MACULES. [83: 110]

clearing construction and discharging heat 清营泄热 *qīng yíng xiè rè*: CLEARING CONSTRUCTION.

clearing damp-heat 清湿热 *qīng shī rè*: A method of treatment used to address damp-heat conditions such as liver channel damp-heat, damp-heat jaundice, and persistent damp-heat in externally contracted heat (febrile) diseases. Medicinals that clear damp-heat include: (1) Cold bitter heat-clearing dampness-drying medicinals such as coptis (*huáng lián*), phellodendron (*huáng bǎi*), scutellaria (*huáng qín*), and gentian (*lóng dǎn*). (2) Warm bitter dampness-drying medicinals such as atractylodes (*cāng zhú*), magnolia bark (*hòu pò*), and pinellia (*bàn xià*). (3) Aromatic dampness-transforming medicinals such as agastache/patchouli (*huò xiāng*), eupatorium (*pèi lán*), and Katsumada's galangal seed (*cǎo dòu kòu*). (4) Water-disinhibiting medicinals such as talcum (*huá shí*), rice-paper plant pith (*tōng cǎo*), poria (*fú líng*), and bamboo leaf (lophatherum) (*dàn zhú yè*). If sign of dampness are more pronounced, warm bitter dampness-drying or aromatic dampness-transforming medicinals are used. An appropriate formula for this is Three Kernels Decoction (*sān rén tāng*). If the heat signs are more pronounced, cold bitter heat-clearing and dampness-drying medicinals are combined in formulas like Sweet Dew Toxin-Dispersing Elixir (*gān lù xiāo dú dān*). Where damp-heat is severe or leads to fire formation, it is treated with cold bitter medicinals that not only clear heat and transform dampness, but also drain fire and resolve toxin. One commonly used method of clearing damp-heat is "acrid opening and bitter discharging," i.e., opening with acridity and discharging with bitterness, using pinellia (*bàn xià*) with scutellaria (*huáng qín*), and magnolia bark (*hòu pò*) with coptis (*huáng lián*), etc., in formulas such as Coptis and Magnolia Bark Beverage (*lián pò yǐn*). Damp-heat skin diseases are frequently treated with flavescent sophora (*kǔ shēn*), and white perilla bark (*bái sū pí*). Gentian Liver-Draining Decoction (*lóng dǎn xiè gān tāng*) treats damp-heat in the liver channel. Capillaris Decoction (*yīn chén hāo tāng*) treats damp-heat jaundice. ACU Base treatment mainly on ST, LI, and SP. Main points: ST-36 (*zú sān lǐ*, Leg Three Li), LI-4 (*hé gǔ*, Union Valley), SP-9 (*yīn líng quán*, Yin Mound Spring), and SP-6 (*sān yīn jiāo*, Three Yin Intersection); needle with drainage. Selection of points according to pattern: If dampness is predominant, add CV-12 (*zhōng wǎn*, Center Stomach Duct) and BL-20 (*pí shū*, Spleen Transport). If heat is predominant, add GV-14 (*dà zhuī*, Great Hammer). For liver channel damp-heat, add LR-2 (*xíng jiān*, Moving Between), GB-43 (*xiá xī*, Pinched Ravine), and GB-34 (*yáng líng quán*, Yang Mound Spring). For damp-heat jaundice, add BL-19 (*dǎn shū*, Gallbladder Transport), GB-34 (*yáng líng quán*, Yang Mound Spring), LR-3 (*tài chōng*, Supreme Surge), and ST-44 (*nèi tíng*, Inner Court). For externally contracted febrile disease, add GB-20 (*fēng chí*, Wind Pool), TB-5 (*wài guān*, Outer Pass), GV-14 (*dà zhuī*, Great Hammer), and LI-11 (*qū chí*, Pool at the Bend), and prick LU-11 (*shào shāng*, Lesser Shang) to bleed. [6: 249]

clearing dryness 清燥 *qīng zào*: MOISTENING DRYNESS. [27: 269]

clearing dryness and rescuing the lung 清燥救肺 *qīng zào jiù fèi*: A method of treatment used to address dryness-heat damaging the lung and causing lung wilting. Clearing dryness and rescuing the lung involves clearing lung-stomach heat with cool sweet and slightly acrid medicinals, boosting stomach qi, and enriching kidney water to protect lung-metal. It avoids the use of both cold bitter and warm-hot medicinals. A representative formula is Dryness-Clearing Lung-Rescuing Decoction (*qīng zào jiù fèi tāng*). [50: 1443]

clearing heart fire 清心火 *qīng xīn huǒ*: CLEARING THE HEART.

Clearing Heat

CLEARING QI-ASPECT HEAT (*qīng qì fèn rè*)

CLEARING CONSTRUCTION AND COOLING THE BLOOD (*qīng yíng liáng xuè*)

CLEARING BOTH QI AND CONSTRUCTION (*qì yíng shuāng qīng*)

CLEARING HEAT AND RESOLVING SUMMERHEAT (*qīng rè jiě shǔ*)

CLEARING HEAT AND RESOLVING TOXIN (*qīng rè jiě dú*)

CLEARING BOWEL AND VISCERAL HEAT (*qīng zàng fǔ rè*)

CLEARING VACUITY HEAT (*qīng xū rè*)

---

clearing heat 清热 *qīng rè*: Synonym: *clearing*. A method of treatment used to address heat using cool and cold medicinals, in accordance with the principle referred to in *Elementary Questions* (*sù wèn*) that "heat is treated with cold." Clearing heat is used in the treatment of interior heat patterns such as qi-aspect heat, blood-aspect heat, damp-heat, and yang sore patterns. *Clearing heat* is a generic term that corresponds to *clearing* among the eight methods. It includes clearing heat (in a more specific sense), draining fire, and resolving toxin. The distinction between *clearing heat* and *draining fire* rests on the distinction between specific senses of the terms *heat* and *fire*. Here, fire denotes a form of repletion heat arising from the transformation of other evils and from the transformation of yang qi (see FIRE). *Resolving toxin* is the removal of any toxin, and *clearing heat and resolving toxin* refers to the method of treating severe redness, swelling and pain, and suppuration. *Clearing heat and draining fire* is poorly distinguished from *clearing heat and resolving toxin*, and in modern literature either term is used to cover the two. When the word *clear* is followed by a word denoting a part of the body, the implication is that heat is removed from that part of the body. Thus, *clear construction* means to clear construction heat. *Clearing blood heat* is conventionally referred to as cooling the blood. In modern clinical practice, the main methods of clearing heat are listed above. See also CLEARING DAMP-HEAT and CLEARING HEAT AND RESOLVING THE EXTERIOR. [27: 352]

Heat-Clearing Medicinals

Heat-Clearing Fire-Draining Medicinals

石膏 (*shí gāo*) gypsum (Gypsum)

生石膏 (*shēng shí gāo*) crude gypsum (Gypsum Crudum)

知母 (*zhī mǔ*) anemarrhena (Anemarrhenae Rhizoma)

芦根 (*lú gēn*) phragmites (Phragmititis Rhizoma)

鲜芦根 (*xiān lú gēn*) fresh phragmites (Phragmititis Rhizoma Recens)

天花粉 (*tiān huā fěn*) trichosanthes root (Trichosanthis Radix)

山栀子 (*shān zhī zǐ*) gardenia (Gardeniae Fructus)

夏枯草 (*xià kū cǎo*) prunella (Prunellae Spica)

淡竹叶 (*dàn zhú yè*) bamboo leaf (lophatherum) (Lophatheri Folium)

竹叶 (*zhú yè*) bamboo leaf (Bambusae Folium)

寒水石 (*hán shuǐ shí*) glauberite (Gypsum seu Calcitum)

鸭跖草 (*yā zhí cǎo*) dayflower (Commelinae Herba)

密蒙花 (*mì méng huā*) buddleia (Buddleiae Flos)

青葙子 (*qīng xiāng zǐ*) celosia (Celosiae Argenteae Semen)

西瓜 (*xī guā*) watermelon (Citrulli Fructus)

西瓜皮 (*xī guā pí*) watermelon rind (Citrulli Exocarpium)

西瓜霜 (*xī guā shuāng*) watermelon frost (Mirabiliti et Citrulli Praeparatio)

Heat-Clearing Dampness-Drying Medicinals

黄芩 (*huáng qín*) scutellaria (Scutellariae Radix)

黄连 (*huáng lián*) coptis (Coptidis Rhizoma)

黄柏 (*huáng bǎi*) phellodendron (Phellodendri Cortex)

龙胆 (*lóng dǎn*) gentian (Gentianae Radix)

苦参 (*kǔ shēn*) flavescent sophora (Sophorae Flavescentis Radix)

马尾连 (*mǎ wěi lián*) meadow rue (Thalictri Rhizoma et Radix)

十大功劳叶 (*shí dà gōng láo yè*) mahonia (Mahoniae Folium)

Heat-Clearing Blood-Cooling Medicinals

犀角 (*xī jiǎo*) rhinoceros horn (Rhinocerotis Cornu)

水牛角 (*shuǐ niú jiǎo*) water buffalo horn (Bubali Cornu)

干地黄 (*gān dì huáng*) dried rehmannia (Rehmanniae Radix Exsiccata)

鲜地黄 (*xiān dì huáng*) fresh rehmannia (Rehmanniae Radix Recens)

玄参 (*xuán shēn*) scrophularia (Scrophulariae Radix)

牡丹皮 (*mǔ dān pí*) moutan (Moutan Radicis Cortex)

赤芍药 (*chì sháo yào*) red peony (Paeoniae Radix Rubra)

牡丹皮 (*mǔ dān pí*) moutan (Moutan Radicis Cortex)

赤芍药 (*chì sháo yào*) red peony (Paeoniae Radix Rubra)

紫草 (*zǐ cǎo*) puccoon (Lithospermi, Macrotomiae, seu Onosmatis Radix)

Heat-Clearing Toxin-Resolving Medicinals

金银花 (*jīn yín huā*) lonicera (Lonicerae Flos)

忍冬藤 (*rěn dōng téng*) lonicera stem and leaf (Lonicerae Caulis et Folium)

连翘 (*lián qiào*) forsythia (Forsythiae Fructus)

蒲公英 (*pú gōng yīng*) dandelion (Taraxaci Herba cum Radice)

紫花地丁 (*zǐ huā dì dīng*) Yedo violet (Violae Yedoensis Herba cum Radice)

地丁 (*dì dīng*) violet (Violae Herba cum Radice)

大青叶 (*dà qīng yè*) isatis leaf (Isatidis Folium)

板蓝根 (*bǎn lán gēn*) isatis root (Isatidis Radix)

青黛 (*qīng dài*) indigo (Indigo Pulverata Levis)

穿心莲 (*chuān xīn lián*) andrographis (Andrographidis Herba)

牛黄 (*niú huáng*) bovine bezoar (Bovis Bezoar)

蚤休 (*zǎo xiū*) paris (Paridis Rhizoma)

半边莲 (*bàn biān lián*) Chinese lobelia (Lobeliae Chinensis Herba cum Radice)

拳参 (*quán shēn*) bistort (Polygoni Bistortae Rhizoma)quán shēn

石指甲 (*shí zhǐ jiǎ*) hanging stonecrop (Sedi Sarmentosi Herba)

土茯苓 (*tǔ fú líng*) smooth greenbrier root (Smilacis Glabrae Rhizoma)

鱼腥草 (*yú xīng cǎo*) houttuynia (Houttuyniae Herba cum Radice)

射干 (*shè gān*) belamcanda (Belamcandae Rhizoma)

山豆根 (*shān dòu gēn*) bushy sophora (Sophorae Subprostratae Radix)

马勃 (*mǎ bó*) puffball (Lasiosphaera seu Calvatia)

马齿苋 (*mǎ chǐ xiàn*) purslane (Portulacae Herba)

白头翁 (*bái tóu wēng*) pulsatilla (Pulsatillae Radix)

秦皮 (*qín pí*) ash (Fraxini Cortex)

鸦胆子 (*yā dǎn zǐ*) brucea (Bruceae Fructus)

大血藤 (*dà xuè téng*) sargentodoxa (Sargentodoxae Caulis)

败酱草 (*bài jiàng cǎo*) baijiang (Baijiang Herba cum Radice)

墓头回 (*mù tóu huí*) heterophyllous patrinia (Patriniae Heterophyllae Radix)

白花蛇舌草 (*hedyotis*) bái huā shé shé cǎo (Hedyotis Herba)

熊胆 (*xióng dǎn*) bear's gall (Ursi Fel)

白蔹 (*bái liǎn*) ampelopsis (Ampelopsis Radix)

白鲜皮 (*bái xiān pí*) dictamnus (Dictamni Radicis Cortex)

漏芦 (*lòu lú*) rhaponticum/echinops (Rhapontici seu Echinopis Radix)

山慈姑 (*shān cí gū*) shancigu (Shancigu Bulbus)

冬青叶 (*dōng qīng yè*) Chinese ilex leaf (Ilicis Chinensis Folium)

天荞麦根 (*tiān qiáo mài gēn*) wild buckwheat root (Fagopyri Cymosi Radix et Rhizoma)

地锦草 (*dì jǐn cǎo*) humifuse euphorbia (Euphorbiae Humifusae Herba)

白毛夏枯草 (*bái máo xià kū cǎo*) bending bugle (Ajugae Decumbentis Herba)

鬼针草 (*guǐ zhēn cǎo*) Spanish needles (Bidentis Bipinnatae Herba)

绿豆皮 (*lǜ dòu pí*) mung bean seed-coat (Phaseoli Aurei Testa)

千里光 (*qiān lǐ guāng*) climbing groundsel (Senecionis Scandentis Herba)

葎草 (*lǜ cǎo*) Japanese hop (Humuli Scandentis Herba)

虎耳草 (*hǔ ěr cǎo*) saxifrage (Saxifragae Herba)

地耳草 (*dì ěr cǎo*) lesser hypericum (Hyperici Japonici Herba)

青叶胆 (*qīng yè dǎn*) pretty swertia (Swertiae Pulchellae Herba)

鸡骨草 (*jī gǔ cǎo*) prayer-beads (Abri Cantoniensis Herba cum Radice)

九节茶 (*jiǔ jié chá*) sarcandra (Sarcandrae Ramulus et Folium)

半枝莲 (*bàn zhī lián*) bearded scutellaria (Scutellariae Barbatae Herba)

天葵子 (*tiān kuí zǐ*) semiaquilegia tuber (Semiaquilegiae Tuber)

龙葵 (*lóng kuí*) black nightshade (Solani Nigri Herba)

白毛藤 (*bái máo téng*) climbing nightshade (Solani Lyrati Herba)

蛇莓 (*shé mé*) snake strawberry (Duchesneae Herba)

凤尾草 (*fèng wěi cǎo*) phoenix-tail fern (Pteridis Multifidi Herba)

白马骨 (*bái mǎ gǔ*) serissa (Serissae Herba)

委陵菜 (*wěi líng cài*) Chinese silverweed (Potentillae Chinensis Radix seu Herba cum Radice)

金莲花 (*jīn lián huā*) globeflower (Trollii Flos)

挂金灯 (*guà jīn dēng*) lantern plant calyx (Physalis Alkekengi Calyx)

蒟蒻 (*jǔ ruò*) devil's tongue (Amorphophalli Tuber)

酸浆 (*suān jiāng*) lantern plant (Physalis Alkekengi Herba)

金果榄 (*jīn guǒ lǎn*) tinospora tuber (Tinosporae Tuber)

橄榄 (*gǎn lǎn*) Chinese olive (Canarii Albi Fructus)

万年青根 (*wàn nián qīng gēn*) rohdea root (Rohdeae Rhizoma et Radix)

藏青果 (*zàng qīng guǒ*) unripe chebule (Chebulae Fructus Immaturus)

Vacuity-Heat–Clearing Medicinals

青蒿 (*qīng hāo*) sweet wormwood (Artemisiae Apiaceae seu Annuae Herba)

白薇 (*bái wēi*) baiwei (Cynanchi Baiwei Radix)

地骨皮 (*dì gǔ pí*) lycium root bark (Lycii Radicis Cortex)

银柴胡 (*yín chái hú*) lanceolate stellaria (Stellariae Lanceolatae Radix)

胡黄连 (*hú huáng lián*) picrorhiza (Picrorhizae Rhizoma)

---

clearing heat and disinhibiting dampness 清热利湿 *qīng rè lì shī*: A method of treatment used to address lower burner damp-heat characterized by urgency and distention of the smaller abdomen, murky reddish urine, pain on urination, dribbling urination, and yellow slimy tongue fur. ⟦MED⟧ Heat-clearing dampness-disinhibiting formulas include Eight Corrections Powder (*bā zhèng sǎn*) and Pyrrosia Powder (*shí wéi sǎn*). ⟦ACU⟧ Base treatment mainly on CV and SP. Needle with drainage at BL-28 (*páng guāng shū*, Bladder Transport), CV-3 (*zhōng jí*, Central Pole), SP-9 (*yīn líng quán*, Yin Mound Spring), and SP-6 (*sān yīn jiāo*, Three Yin Intersection). **Comparison:** Clearing and heat and disinhibiting dampness is a specific form of clearing damp-heat used to treat lower burner damp-heat. See CLEARING DAMP-HEAT. [26: 570] [46: 597, 675]

clearing heat and dispelling dampness 清热祛湿 *qīng rè qū shī*: Any method of treatment used to treat damp-heat. Clearing heat and dispelling dampness is applied to DAMP WARMTH, JAUNDICE, CHOLERA, HEAT STRANGURY, and WILTING or IMPEDIMENT due to damp-heat external contractions, exuberant internal damp-heat, or damp-heat pouring downward. Commonly used heat-clearing dampness-dispelling medicinals include capillaris (*yīn chén hāo*), coix (*yì yǐ rén*), talcum (*huá shí*), and gardenia (*shān zhī zǐ*). Formulas include Three Kernels Decoction (*sān rén tāng*) Capillaris Decoction (*yīn chén hāo tāng*) and Sweet Dew Toxin-Dispersing Elixir (*gān lù xiāo dú dān*). See also CLEARING HEAT AND TRANSFORMING DAMPNESS and CLEARING HEAT AND DISINHIBITING DAMPNESS. [121: 497] [16: 488]

clearing heat and draining fire 清热泻火 *qīng rè xiè huǒ*: See CLEARING.

clearing heat and extinguishing wind 清热熄风 *qīng rè xī fēng*: DRAINING FIRE AND EXTINGUISHING WIND.

clearing heat and freeing strangury 清热通淋 *qīng rè tōng lín*: A method of treatment used to address painful, burning sensations in the urethra, urinary urgency and frequency, and reddish urine. MED Heat-clearing strangury-freeing medicinals include mutong (*mù tōng*), plantago seed (*chē qián zǐ*) or plantago (*chē qián*), knotgrass (*biǎn xù*), pyrrosia (*shí wéi*), dianthus (*qū mài*), and talcum (*huá shí*). These may be combined with heat-clearing medicinals such as andrographis (*chuān xīn lián*), dandelion (*pú gōng yīng*), dayflower (*yā zhí cǎo*), houttuynia (*yú xīng cǎo*), phoenix-tail fern (*fèng wěi cǎo*), lonicera (*jīn yín huā*), and phellodendron (*huáng bǎi*). A representative heat-clearing strangury-freeing formula is Eight Corrections Powder (*bā zhèng sǎn*). ACU Base treatment mainly on the three yin channels of the foot and alarm and back transport points of BL (CV-3 and BL-28). Select BL-28 (*páng guāng shū*, Bladder Transport), CV-3 (*zhōng jí*, Central Pole), SP-9 (*yīn líng quán*, Yin Mound Spring), LR-2 (*xíng jiān*, Moving Between), KI-3 (*tài xī*, Great Ravine), LR-8 (*qū quán*, Spring at the Bend), SP-6 (*sān yīn jiāo*, Three Yin Intersection), LI-4 (*hé gǔ*, Union Valley), and TB-5 (*wài guān*, Outer Pass); needle with drainage. [46: 674] [27: 267]

clearing heat and opening the orifices 清热开窍 *qīng rè kāi qiào*: Synonyms: *cool opening*; *clearing the heart and opening the orifices.* A

method of treatment used to address externally contracted febrile disease patterns, such as heat entering the pericardium, characterized by high fever with clouded spirit and delirious speech, vexation and agitation, parched lips and dry teeth, TETANIC REVERSAL, and convulsions, including child FRIGHT WIND. MED A representative heart-clearing orifice-opening formula is Peaceful Palace Bovine Bezoar Pill (*ān gōng niú huáng wán*), which can be combined with Construction-Clearing Decoction (*qīng yíng tāng*). Others include Purple Snow Elixir (*zǐ xuě dān*), Spirit-Like Rhinoceros Horn Elixir (*shén xī dān*), and Supreme Jewel Elixir (*zhì bǎo dān*). These may be combined with blood-cooling medicinals, heat-clearing medicinals, and toxin-resolving medicinals where necessary. Furthermore, wind stroke can be treated with Supreme Jewel Elixir combined with liver-calming wind-extinguishing medicinals. ACU Base treatment mainly on GV, PC, and Twelve Well Points (*shí èr jǐng xué*). Select GV-26 (*shuǐ gōu*, Water Trough), Twelve Well Points, PC-8 (*láo gōng*, Palace of Toil), GV-14 (*dà zhuī*, Great Hammer), and LI-11 (*qū chí*, Pool at the Bend); needle with drainage or prick to bleed. For convulsions, add GV-20 (*bǎi huì*, Hundred Convergences), GV-16 (*fēng fǔ*, Wind Mansion), and LR-3 (*tài chōng*, Supreme Surge). See OPENING THE ORIFICES. [26: 571] [27: 275] [97: 530] [46: 576]

clearing heat and resolving summerheat 清热解暑 *qīng rè jiě shǔ*: A method of treatment used to address externally contracted SUMMERHEAT-HEAT characterized by headache, generalized heat [effusion], sweating, vexation and thirst, short voiding of reddish urine, thin yellow tongue fur, and a rapid floating pulse. MED Use heat-clearing summerheat-resolving medicinals such as fresh mint (*bò hé*), lablab flower (*biǎn dòu huā*), sweet wormwood (*qīng hāo*), elsholtzia (*xiāng rú*), lonicera (*jīn yín huā*), forsythia (*lián qiào*), phragmites (*lú gēn*), and coptis (*huáng lián*). Representative formulas include Network-Clearing Beverage (*qīng luò yǐn*) and Wang's Summerheat-Clearing Qi-Boosting Decoction (*wáng shì qīng shǔ yì qì tāng*). ACU Needle with drainage at PC-6 (*nèi guān*, Inner Pass), LI-4 (*hé gǔ*, Union Valley), and ST-36 (*zú sān lǐ*, Leg Three Li). For headache, add GV-20 (*bǎi huì*, Hundred Convergences) and GB-20 (*fēng chí*, Wind Pool). For vexation and thirst, add HT-5 (*tōng lǐ*, Connecting Li) and KI-6 (*zhào hǎi*, Shining Sea). [27: 254] [97: 531]

clearing heat and resolving the exterior 清热解表 *qīng rè jiě biǎo*: 1. A method of treatment that uses cool acrid exterior-resolving medicinals to treat wind-warmth exterior patterns. A representative formula is Lonicera and Forsythia Powder (*yín qiào sǎn*). ACU Base treatment mainly on LI, LU, and TB. Needle with drainage at LI-11 (*qū chí*,

Pool at the Bend), TB-5 (*wài guān*, Outer Pass), LI-4 (*hé gǔ*, Union Valley), LU-7 (*liè quē*, Broken Sequence), and GV-14 (*dà zhuī*, Great Hammer). **2.** One form of RESOLVING BOTH EXTERIOR AND INTERIOR, used to address mild exterior heat with more pronounced interior heat characterized by high fever, vexation and thirst, mild aversion to wind or cold, little or no sweating, constipation, yellow urine, dry white or yellow tongue fur, and a slippery rapid pulse. MED A representative heat-clearing exterior-resolving formula is Three Yellows and Gypsum Decoction (*sān huáng shí gāo tāng*), in which gypsum (*shí gāo*), coptis (*huáng lián*), scutellaria (*huáng qín*), and phellodendron (*huáng bǎi*) clear interior heat, and ephedra (*má huáng*) and fermented soybean (*dàn dòu chǐ*) resolve the exterior evil. [50: 1143] [26: 571]

clearing heat and resolving toxin 清热解毒 *qīng rè jiě dú*: A method of treatment used to address any repletion pattern attributed to heat toxin, such as intense HEAT TOXIN in EXTERNALLY CONTRACTED HEAT (FEBRILE) DISEASE, SORE (yang patterns), CINNABAR TOXIN, MACULOPAPULAR ERUPTION, PULMONARY WELLING-ABSCESS (*fèi yōng*), DYSENTERY with blood and pus in the stool, and HEAT STRANGURY with painful urination and reddish urine. Such patterns are characterized by SCORCHING HEAT, heat effusion, swelling and distention, pain, suppuration, and putrefaction. Medicinals used include isatis leaf (*dà qīng yè*), isatis root (*bǎn lán gēn*), dandelion (*pú gōng yīng*), scutellaria (*huáng qín*), coptis (*huáng lián*), phellodendron (*huáng bǎi*), moutan (*mǔ dān pí*), red peony (*chì sháo yào*), lonicera (*jīn yín huā*), forsythia (*lián qiào*), fresh ginger (*shēng jiāng*), and gardenia (*shān zhī zǐ*). A commonly used heat-clearing toxin-resolving formula is Coptis Toxin-Resolving Decoction (*huáng lián jiě dú tāng*). ACU Select BL-40 (*wěi zhōng*, Bend Center), PC-3 (*qū zé*, Marsh at the Bend), Ten Diffusing Points (*shí xuān*), as the main points and, for sores etc., prick ouch points (*ā shì xué*) to bleed. [27: 254] [97: 531]

clearing heat and stanching bleeding 清热止血 *qīng rè zhǐ xuè*: A method of treatment used to address frenetic movement of hot blood, as observed in stomach heat blood ejection with bright colored blood, dry mouth and throat, crimson red tongue, yellow tongue fur, and a surging rapid pulse. MED Use medicinals such as madder (*qiàn cǎo gēn*), ass hide glue (*ē jiāo*), scutellaria (*huáng qín*), biota leaf (*cè bǎi yè*), dried/fresh rehmannia (*shēng dì huáng*), and cephalanoplos (*xiǎo jì*). ACU Select points such as PC-7 (*dà líng*, Great Mound), PC-4 (*xī mén*, Cleft Gate), LU-6 (*kǒng zuì*, Collection Hole), LU-9 (*tài yuān*, Great Abyss), KI-3 (*tài xī*, Great Ravine), LR-3 (*tài chōng*, Supreme Surge), SP-6 (*sān yīn jiāo*,

Three Yin Intersection), and ST-44 (*nèi tíng*, Inner Court), and needle with drainage. [46: 595] [27: 275] [97: 530]

clearing heat and transforming dampness 清热化湿 *qīng rè huà shī*: A method of treatment used to address dampness and heat binding in the upper or middle burner characterized by oppression in the chest, abdominal distention, poor appetite, bitter taste in the mouth, sometimes sore throat, yellow or reddish urine, slimy yellow tongue fur, and soggy rapid pulse. MED Use formulas such as Sweet Dew Toxin-Dispersing Elixir (*gān lù xiāo dú dān*) and Capillaris Decoction (*yīn chén hāo tāng*). ACU Needle with drainage at PC-6 (*nèi guān*, Inner Pass), CV-12 (*zhōng wǎn*, Center Stomach Duct), ST-25 (*tiān shū*, Celestial Pivot), ST-36 (*zú sān lǐ*, Leg Three Li), LI-4 (*hé gǔ*, Union Valley), LI-11 (*qū chí*, Pool at the Bend), SP-9 (*yīn líng quán*, Yin Mound Spring), ST-37 (*shàng jù xū*, Upper Great Hollow), and ST-44 (*nèi tíng*, Inner Court). [27: 260] [97: 531]

clearing heat and transforming phlegm 清热化痰 *qīng rè huà tán*: *Synonym: clearing and transforming heat phlegm.* A method of treatment used to address heat phlegm, which arises when heat congests the lung and manifests as inhibited cough, expectoration of thick yellow phlegm, red facial complexion, heat vexation, red tongue with yellow fur, etc. MED Heat-clearing phlegm-transforming medicinals include tingli (*tíng lì zǐ*), scutellaria (*huáng qín*), mulberry root bark (*sāng bái pí*), trichosanthes rind (*guā lóu pí*), Zhejiang fritillaria (*zhè bèi mǔ*), and phragmites (*lú gēn*). Formulas include Qi-Clearing Phlegm-Transforming Pill (*qīng qì huà tán wán*) and Gallbladder-Warming Decoction (*wēn dǎn tāng*). ACU Base treatment mainly on back transport points, LU, LI, and ST. Needle with drainage at BL-13 (*fèi shū*, Lung Transport), LU-5 (*chǐ zé*, Cubit Marsh), LI-11 (*qū chí*, Pool at the Bend) LI-4 (*hé gǔ*, Union Valley), LU-10 (*yú jì*, Fish Border), LU-9 (*tài yuān*, Great Abyss), SP-3 (*tài bái*, Supreme White), and ST-40 (*fēng lóng*, Bountiful Bulge). [26: 570]

clearing heat, draining fire, and resolving toxin 清热泻火解毒 *qīng rè xiè huǒ jiě dú*: See CLEARING.

clearing heat, transforming phlegm, and opening the orifices 清热化痰开窍 *qīng rè huà tán kāi qiào*: A method of treatment used to address phlegm heat congestion in children, causing heat effusion and clouded spirit, rough breathing, fright reversal, and convulsions of the limbs (an acute fright wind repletion pattern). MED Heat-clearing phlegm-transforming and orifice-opening formulas include Dragon-Embracing Pill (*bào lóng wán*). ACU Use the points given under CLEAR-

ING HEAT AND TRANSFORMING PHLEGM. In addition, drain GV-26 (*shuǐ gōu*, Water Trough), PC-6 (*nèi guān*, Inner Pass), PC-5 (*jiān shǐ*, Intermediary Courier), and GV-14 (*dà zhuī*, Great Hammer), and prick the twelve well points or the ten diffusing points to bleed. For convulsions of the limbs, drain GV-20 (*bǎi huì*, Hundred Convergences), LI-11 (*qū chí*, Pool at the Bend), GV-16 (*fēng fǔ*, Wind Mansion), and LR-3 (*tài chōng*, Supreme Surge). [27: 276] [46: 597, 729]

clearing liver fire 清肝火 *qīng gān huǒ*: DRAINING THE LIVER.

clearing metal 清金 *qīng jīn*: CLEARING AND DEPURATING LUNG QI.

clearing metal and downbearing fire 清金降火 *qīng jīn jiàng huǒ*: CLEARING AND DEPURATING LUNG QI.

clearing organ heat 清脏腑热 *qīng zàng fǔ rè*: CLEARING BOWEL AND VISCERAL HEAT.

clearing qi 清气 *qīng qì*: CLEARING QI-ASPECT HEAT.

clearing qi-aspect heat 清气分热 *qīng qì fèn rè*: Synonym: *clearing qi heat; clearing qi*. A method of treatment used to address QI-ASPECT HEAT patterns with vigorous (surfaced) heat effusion, thirst, dry tongue, and surging pulse. Commonly used medicinals include gypsum (*shí gāo*), anemarrhena (*zhī mǔ*), and gardenia (*shān zhī zǐ*). White Tiger Decoction (*bái hǔ tāng*) and Gardenia and Fermented Soybean Decoction (*zhī zǐ chǐ tāng*) are representative qi-heat-clearing formulas. ACU Base treatment mainly on LI and ST. Select LI-4 (*hé gǔ*, Union Valley), LI-11 (*qū chí*, Pool at the Bend), ST-44 (*nèi tíng*, Inner Court), and PC-6 (*nèi guān*, Inner Pass), needle with drainage. [75: 30–31] [6: 249] [27: 134] [97: 97]

clearing qi heat 清气热 *qīng qì rè*: CLEARING QI-ASPECT HEAT.

clearing qi with coldness and bitterness 苦寒清气 *kǔ hán qīng qì*: A method of treatment used to address qi-aspect heat with cold bitter medicinals in the treatment of warm disease of spring with heat effusion, no (or slight) aversion to cold, joint pain, thirst, scant sweating, yellow urine, red tongue with yellow tongue fur, and a rapid pulse. MED Scutellaria Decoction (*huáng qín tāng*) is an example of a cold bitter qi-clearing formula. [26: 432] [27: 252] [27: 327]

clearing summerheat and boosting qi 清暑益气 *qīng shǔ yì qì*: A method of treatment used to address summerheat in the treatment of contraction of summerheat with damage to liquid characterized by heat effusion, heart vexation, dry mouth, and inhibited urination, principally by boosting qi to engender liquid and secondarily by clearing summerheat. MED Use Summerheat-Clearing Qi-Boosting Decoction (*qīng shǔ yì qì tāng*). ACU Base treatment mainly on PC, LI, ST, KI, and CV. Needle LI-4 (*hé gǔ*, Union Valley), PC-6 (*nèi guān*, Inner Pass), ST-36 (*zú sān lǐ*, Leg Three Li), HT-5 (*tōng lǐ*, Connecting Li), and KI-6 (*zhào hǎi*, Shining Sea), with drainage, and CV-6 (*qì hǎi*, Sea of Qi), and CV-4 (*guān yuán*, Pass Head) with supplementation or with even supplemenation and drainage; if necessary, add moxa. [113: 48] [97: 531] [27: 569] [26: 569]

clearing summerheat and disinhibiting dampness 清暑利湿 *qīng shǔ lì shī*: A method of treatment used to address summerheat-damp characterized by heat effusion, vexation, thirst, inhibited urination. MED A commonly used summerheat-clearing dampness-disinhibiting formula is Six-to-One Powder (*liù yī sǎn*). ACU Base treatment mainly on PC, LI, ST, KI, and CV. Select LI-4 (*hé gǔ*, Union Valley), PC-6 (*nèi guān*, Inner Pass), ST-36 (*zú sān lǐ*, Leg Three Li), HT-5 (*tōng lǐ*, Connecting Li), KI-6 (*zhào hǎi*, Shining Sea), CV-3 (*zhōng jí*, Central Pole), SP-6 (*sān yīn jiāo*, Three Yin Intersection), and SP-9 (*yīn líng quán*, Yin Mound Spring), and needle with drainage. [97: 531] [27: 261] [113: 48] [46: 672]

clearing the heart 清心 *qīng xīn*: Synonym: *clearing the palace*. A method of treatment used to address heat entering the pericardium characterized by high fever, clouded spirit, vexation and agitation, delirious speech, crimson tongue, and a rapid fine pulse. MED A representative heart-clearing formula is Palace-Clearing Decoction (*qīng gōng tāng*). [27: 254] [97: 529]

clearing the heart and boosting the kidney 清心益肾 *qīng xīn yì shèn*: A method of treatment that involves clearing heart fire and supplement kidney water and that is used to address noninteraction of the heart and kidney characterized by dizziness, heart palpitations, fearful throbbing, sleeplessness, limp aching lumbus and legs, and dream emissions in males, and dreaming of intercourse in women. See *promote interaction of the heart and kidney*.

clearing the heart and draining fire 清心泻火 *qīng xīn xiè huǒ*: CLEARING THE HEART.

clearing the heart and flushing heat 清心涤热 *qīng xīn dí rè*: CLEARING THE HEART.

clearing the heart and opening the orifices 清心开窍 *qīng xīn kāi qiào*: See CLEARING HEAT AND OPENING THE ORIFICES.

clearing the intestines and moistening dryness 清肠润燥 *qīng cháng rùn zào*: A method of treatment used to address large intestine heat marked by constipation, bad breath, lip sores, red facial complexion, short voidings of reddish urine, dry yellow tongue fur, and a replete slippery pulse. MED A representative intestine-clearing dryness-moistening formula is Hemp Seed Pill (*má rén* *wán*), which contains hemp seed (*huǒ má rén*), peony (*sháo yào*), unripe bitter orange (*zhǐ shí*), rhubarb (*dà huáng*), magnolia bark (*hòu pò*), and apricot kernel (*xìng rén*). ACU Base treatment mainly on ST and on back transport, alarm, and lower uniting points of LI. Select BL-25 (*dà cháng shū*, Large Intestine Transport), ST-25 (*tiān shū*, Celestial Pivot), ST-37 (*shàng jù xū*, Upper Great Hollow), LI-4 (*hé gǔ*, Union Valley), LI-11 (*qū chí*, Pool at the Bend), ST-44 (*nèi tíng*, Inner Court), SP-14 (*fù jié*, Abdominal Bind), and KI-6 (*zhào hǎi*, Shining Sea); needle with drainage. [26: 569] [27: 269] [97: 530]

clearing the liver and draining fire 清肝泻火 *qīng gān xiè huǒ*: DRAINING THE LIVER.

clearing the lung and moistening dryness 清肺润燥 *qīng fèi rùn zào*: A method of treatment used to address damage to the lung by warm dryness or heat. MED Use formulas such as Dryness-Clearing Lung-Rescuing Decoction (*qīng zào jiù fèi tāng*) or Adenophora/Glehnia and Ophiopogon Decoction (*shā shēn mài dōng tāng*). ACU Base treatment mainly on back transport points, LU, and KI. Select BL-13 (*fèi shū*, Lung Transport), BL-43 (*gāo huāng shū*, Gao-Huang Transport), LU-5 (*chǐ zé*, Cubit Marsh), and KI-6 (*zhào hǎi*, Shining Sea); needle with even supplementation and drainage. [46: 653]

clearing the lung and suppressing cough 清肺止咳 *qīng fèi zhǐ ké*: A method of treatment used to address cough due to lung heat. MED Use formulas like White-Draining Powder (*xiè bái sǎn*).

clearing the palace 清宫 *qīng gōng*: CLEARING THE HEART. See PALACE.

clearing the stomach and downbearing counterflow 清胃降逆 *qīng wèi jiàng nì*: A method of treatment used to address hiccough due to stomach heat. MED Use New Tangerine Peel and Bamboo Shavings Decoction (*xīn zhì jú pí zhú rú tāng*). ACU Base treatment mainly on ST, PC, and LR. Select BL-17 (*gé shū*, Diaphragm Transport), CV-17 (*shān zhōng*, Chest Center), PC-6 (*nèi guān*, Inner Pass), ST-44 (*nèi tíng*, Inner Court), ST-36 (*zú sān lǐ*, Leg Three Li), LI-4 (*hé gǔ*, Union Valley), and LR-3 (*tài chōng*, Supreme Surge); needle with drainage. [26: 567]

clearing vacuity heat 清虚热 *qīng xū rè*: A method of treatment used to address advanced-stage externally contracted heat (febrile) diseases or chronic diseases such as pulmonary consumption presenting with signs such as steaming bone or tidal heat [effusion], night sweating, persistent low fever, reddening of the cheeks, emaciation, and red or crimson tongue with little fur, which indicate that yin humor is damaged and evil heat is lodged in the yin aspect. MED Commonly used vacuity-heat–clearing medicinals include turtle shell (*biē*

jiǎ), sweet wormwood (*qīng hāo*), lycium root bark (*dì gǔ pí*), lanceolate stellaria (*yín chái hú*), large gentian (*qín jiāo*), and baiwei (*bái wēi*). Representative formulas include Sweet Wormwood and Turtle Shell Decoction (*qīng hāo biē jiǎ tāng*) and Bone-Clearing Powder (*qīng gǔ sǎn*). ACU Base treatment mainly on KI. Select KI-6 (*zhào hǎi*, Shining Sea), KI-3 (*tài xī*, Great Ravine), KI-2 (*rán gǔ*, Blazing Valley), and LR-2 (*xíng jiān*, Moving Between). Needle with even supplementation and drainage. For advanced-stage febrile disease, add LI-11 (*qū chí*, Pool at the Bend), LI-4 (*hé gǔ*, Union Valley), and TB-5 (*wài guān*, Outer Pass), needling with drainage. For pulmonary consumption, add BL-13 (*fèi shū*, Lung Transport), BL-43 (*gāo huāng shū*, Gao-Huang Transport), and LU-9 (*tài yuān*, Great Abyss), needling with supplementation. Selection of points according to signs: For tidal heat [effusion], add LU-5 (*chǐ zé*, Cubit Marsh) and LU-10 (*yú jì*, Fish Border). For night sweating, add HT-6 (*yīn xī*, Yin Cleft). Compare ENRICHING YIN AND CLEARING HEAT. [6: 250] [46: 657, 596, 732]

clear orifice 清窍 *qīng qiào*: Any of the UPPER ORIFICES (eyes, ears, nostrils, and mouth), usually referred to collectively. The clear orifices are sometimes called the *seven orifices*. They are described as clear in contradistinction to the lower orifices, usually referred to as the *two yin*, i.e., the anal and genital orifices, through which turbid waste is discharged from the body.

clear qi 清气 *qīng qì*: The clear, light part of the essence of grain and water. *The Magic Pivot* (*líng shū, dòng shū*) states, "The stomach is the sea of the five viscera and six bowels; its clear qi pours upward into the lung." Compare CLEAR YANG. [50: 1435] [27: 80] [26: 568]

clear qi failing to bear upward 清气不升 *qīng qì bù shēng*: CLEAR YANG FAILING TO BEAR UPWARD.

clear uninhibited stool and urine 便溺清利 *biàn niào qīng lì*, 二便清利 *èr biàn qīng lì*: Clean stool composed of improperly digested food with clear urine; a sign of cold.

clear yang 清阳 *qīng yáng*: Yang qi as a clean, light, insubstantial qi that moves upward and outward. It stands in complementary opposition to turbid yin, which is the unclean, heavy, substantial qi (solid waste products). See TURBID YIN. Compare *clear qi*. [27: 81]

clear yang failing to bear upward 清阳不升 *qīng yáng bù shēng*: Synonym: *clear qi failing to bear upward*. The inability of yang qi to warm and nourish the head, flesh, limbs, etc. The main signs are dizzy head and vision, shortness of breath and laziness to speak, fatigue and lack of strength, abdominal distention and diarrhea.

Other signs my be reduced hearing acuity, somnolence, and poor appetite. The tongue is pale with white fur, and the pulse is weak or vacuous. MED Boost qi and upbear yang. Use Center-Supplementing Qi-Boosting Decoction (*bǔ zhōng yì qì tāng*) or Yang-Upbearing Stomach-Boosting Decoction (*shēng yáng yì wèi tāng*). ACU Base treatment mainly on GV and CV. Select GV-20 (*bǎi huì*, Hundred Convergences), CV-6 (*qì hǎi*, Sea of Qi), CV-4 (*guān yuán*, Pass Head), CV-12 (*zhōng wǎn*, Center Stomach Duct), BL-20 (*pí shū*, Spleen Transport), BL-21 (*wèi shū*, Stomach Transport), and ST-36 (*zú sān lǐ*, Leg Three Li), needle with supplementation and large amounts of moxa. Selection of points according to signs: For dizziness, add ST-8 (*tóu wéi*, Head Corner) and LI-4 (*hé gǔ*, Union Valley). For poor food intake and sloppy stool, add ST-25 (*tiān shū*, Celestial Pivot) or moxa Five Pillar Points (*wǔ zhù xué*). For abdominal distention, add PC-6 (*nèi guān*, Inner Pass) and ST-25 (*tiān shū*, Celestial Pivot). [57: 30] [46: 585, 594, 619, 666]

cleft point 郄穴 *xì xué*: Any of a group of points located one on each of the twelve channels and four of the *eight extraordinary vessels* (the yin springing, yang springing, yin linking, and yang linking vessels) at the site of a small cleft or indentation at which qi and blood accumulate. **Application:** The cleft can reflect repletion or vacuity in the channel on which they are located. Sharp or intense pain on pressure, or redness and swelling indicate repletion, whereas dull or mild pain or a depression at the point indicates vacuity. Cleft points are commonly employed in the treatment of either stubborn or acute ailments involving the organs and channels. The effectiveness of cleft points in relieving pain is evidenced by their frequent use in acupuncture anesthesia. **Combinations:** The cleft points are often used in combination with the meeting points. For example, the cleft point of the lung, LU-6 (*kǒng zuì*, Collection Hole), is combined with the meeting point of the blood, BL-17 (*gé shū*, Diaphragm Transport), to treat coughing of blood, whereas the cleft point of the stomach, ST-34 (*liáng qiū*, Beam Hill), is combined with the meeting point of the bowels, CV-12 (*zhōng wǎn*, Center Stomach Duct), to treat acute stomach pain. ◇ Chin 郄 (same as 郤 or 隙) *xì*, cleft or fissure. [27: 103]

clenched jaw 口噤 *kǒu jìn*, 牙关紧闭 *yá guān jǐn bì*: Inability to open the mouth. A sign of TETANIC DISEASE, WIND STROKE, and FRIGHT WIND. When accompanied by foaming at the mouth, clenched jaw is generally a sign of epilepsy. When associated with a phlegm rale in the throat and deviation of the eyes or mouth, it indicates wind stroke. WMC trismus. **Externally contracted wind-cold:** Clenched jaw due to wind-cold results when externally contracted wind, cold, or dampness evils enter the three yang channels causing hypertonicity of the sinews. It appears in patients suffering from heat effusion, aversion to cold, headache, stiff nape and back, either absence of sweating or sweating, white tongue fur, and a tight floating pulse. MED Diffuse external evil with Pueraria Decoction (*gé gēn tāng*). ACU Base treatment for all clenched jaw patterns mainly on ST and LI. Main points: ST-6 (*jiá chē*, Cheek Carriage), ST-4 (*dì cāng*, Earth Granary), ST-7 (*xià guān*, Below the Joint), and LI-4 (*hé gǔ*, Union Valley). For externally contracted wind-cold, add GB-20 (*fēng chí*, Wind Pool) TB-5 (*wài guān*, Outer Pass), LU-7 (*liè quē*, Broken Sequence), and TB-17 (*yì fēng*, Wind Screen); needle with drainage and add moxa. **Exuberant internal heat:** Clenched jaw due to internal heat results when wind-cold enters the exterior and transforms into heat or when warm heat enters the interior causing congestion in the qi aspect or stirring liver wind. It is associated with stiff neck, arched-back rigidity, hypertonicity of the limbs, vigorous heat [effusion], yellow face and eyes, parched lips, constipation and rough urination, red tongue with yellow fur and a stringlike rapid or forceful rapid sunken pulse. MED Clear and drain internal heat. Exuberant yang brightness (*yáng míng*) heat is treated with White Tiger Decoction (*bái hǔ tāng*) or Major Qi-Coordinating Decoction (*dà chéng qì tāng*). If heat toxin scorches qi and blood or congests the throat, use variations of Scourge-Clearing Toxin-Vanquishing Beverage (*qīng wēn bài dú yǐn*), which clears heat and resolves toxin as well as clearing the blood and draining fire. Exuberant liver channel heat stirring wind with convulsions and arched-back rigidity can be treated by clearing heat, draining fire, and extinguishing wind, using variations of Gentian Liver-Draining Decoction (*lóng dǎn xiè gān tāng*) or Antelope Horn and Uncaria Decoction (*líng jiǎo gōu téng tāng*). Clouded spirit and coma can be treated by clearing the heart and opening the orifices using Peaceful Palace Bovine Bezoar Pill (*ān gōng niú huáng wán*). ACU For exuberant yang brightness (*yáng míng*) heat is treated with adding to above main points LI-11 (*qū chí*, Pool at the Bend), ST-44 (*nèi tíng*, Inner Court), ST-25 (*tiān shū*, Celestial Pivot), and ST-37 (*shàng jù xū*, Upper Great Hollow); needle with drainage. If heat toxin scorches qi and blood or congests the throat, adding LI-11 (*qū chí*, Pool at the Bend), TB-5 (*wài guān*, Outer Pass), BL-40 (*wěi zhōng*, Bend Center), and ST-43 (*xiàn gǔ*, Sunken Valley); needle with drainage. and pricking LU-11 (*shào shāng*, Lesser Shang), PC-9 (*zhōng chōng*, Central Hub), and HT-9 (*shào chōng*, Lesser Surge) to bleed. For exuberant liver channel heat stirring wind with convulsions and arched-back rigidity, add LR-2 (*xíng jiān*, Moving Between), LR-3 (*tài chōng*, Supreme Surge), LI-11 (*qū chí*, Pool at the Bend), GV-20 (*bǎi huì*, Hundred Convergences), GV-14 (*dà zhuī*, Great Hammer), and GV-16 (*fēng fǔ*, Wind Mansion); needle with drainage. and pricking Ten Diffusing Points (*shí xuān*) to bleed. For clouded spirit and coma, add PC-8 (*láo gōng*, Palace of Toil), PC-6 (*nèi guān*, Inner Pass), HT-8 (*shào fǔ*, Lesser Mansion), and GV-26 (*shuǐ gōu*, Water Trough); needle with drainage and prick Twelve Well Points (*shí èr jǐng xué*) to bleed. **Yin depletion and blood vacuity:** Clenched jaw due to yin depletion and blood vacuity mostly occurs in the advanced stages of warm disease when heat evil has damaged yin-liquid, or after sweating or precipitation has damaged yin and the evil has abated. It is accompanied by dizzy head and flowery vision, convulsions of the limbs or hypertonicity of the limbs, emaciation, red tongue without fur, and a rapid fine sunken pulse. There may be heat effusion. Enrich yin, nourish the blood, and extinguish wind with Major Wind-Stabilizing Pill (*dà dìng fēng zhū*). ACU To the main points given above add ST-36 (*zú sān lǐ*, Leg Three Li), SP-6 (*sān yīn jiāo*, Three Yin Intersection), KI-1 (*yǒng quán*, Gushing Spring), LR-3 (*tài chōng*, Supreme Surge), GV-20 (*bǎi huì*, Hundred Convergences), GV-8 (*jīn suō*, Sinew Contraction), and GB-20 (*fēng chí*, Wind Pool); needle with supplementation. **Direct strike by cold evil:** Clenched jaw preventing speech due to direct strike by cold evil is accompanied by shivering limbs, hypertonicity, reversal cold of the extremities, abdominal pain and diarrhea, blue-green or purple facial complexion, dark tongue with white fur, and a sunken stringlike and rough pulse. MED Warm the center and dispel cold. Use variations of Counterflow Cold Decoction (*sì nì tāng*) or Great Rectifying Powder (*dà shùn sǎn*). ACU To the main points given above add ST-36 (*zú sān lǐ*, Leg Three Li), CV-6 (*qì hǎi*, Sea of Qi), CV-4 (*guān yuán*, Pass Head), and CV-8 (*shén què*, Spirit Gate Tower)ⓜ; needle with drainage and large amounts of moxa. **Qi depression and phlegm congestion:** Clenched jaw due to qi depression and phlegm congestion is observed in miscellaneous disease when phlegm and qi become depressed and bound, block the clear orifices, and, as happens in some cases, carry wind through the channels and network vessels. It may occur with CLOUDING REVERSAL and convulsions of the limbs, or with physical collapse, phlegm congestion in the throat, hasty panting, thin white or slimy white tongue fur and a sunken stringlike or slippery stringlike pulse. MED Rectify qi, open the orifices, and sweep phlegm. Use Saussurea Qi-Regulating Powder (*mù xiāng tiáo qì sǎn*). For unclear spirit-mind, first use Liquid Storax Pill (*sū hé xiāng wán*) to open the orifices. ACU To the main points given

above add SI-3 (*hòu xī*, Back Ravine), ST-36 (*zú sān lǐ*, Leg Three Li), ST-40 (*fēng lóng*, Bountiful Bulge), PC-6 (*nèi guān*, Inner Pass), and LR-3 (*tài chōng*, Supreme Surge); needle with drainage, and add GV-26 (*shuǐ gōu*, Water Trough) and PC-5 (*jiān shǐ*, Intermediary Courier) for clouded spirit. **External wind toxin damage:** Clenched jaw can arise when wind toxin enters through an open wound or sore. In such cases, it is associated with stiff neck, hypertonicity of the limbs, and even arched-back rigidity, as well as with alternating heat [effusion] and [aversion to] cold, a white slimy tongue fur, and a stringlike pulse. MED Settle tetany and dispel wind. Make use of chong products such as scorpion (*quán xiē*), centipede (*wú gōng*), silkworm (*bái jiāng cán*), and earthworm (*dì lóng*). Use formulas such as True Jade Powder (*yù zhēn sǎn*) or Five-Tigers-Chasing-the-Wind Powder (*wǔ hǔ zhuī fēng sǎn*). ACU To the main points add GV-20 (*bǎi huì*, Hundred Convergences), GB-20 (*fēng chí*, Wind Pool), GV-14 (*dà zhuī*, Great Hammer), GV-12 (*shēn zhù*, Body Pillar), GV-26 (*shuǐ gōu*, Water Trough), GV-1 (*cháng qiáng*, Long Strong), and SI-3 (*hòu xī*, Back Ravine); needle with drainage, and add GV-26 (*shuǐ gōu*, Water Trough) and KI-1 (*yǒng quán*, Gushing Spring), and prick Twelve Well Points (*shí èr jǐng xué*) to bleed for clouded spirit or arched-back rigidity. ◇ Chin 口 *kǒu*, mouth; 噤 *jìn*, closed of the mouth (related to 禁 bar, ban). 牙 *yá*, tooth; 关 *guān*, gate, pass; 紧 *jǐn*, tightly; 闭 *bì*, closed. [50: 104] [26: 62] [27: 398] [97: 31] [46: 595, 596, 615, 732, 733] [113: 29] [4: 142] [42: 143, 213]

clot 血块 *xuè kuài*: A lump of coagulated blood, such as may be observed in the menstrual flow in blood stasis patterns.

clotted menstrual flow 经来成块 *jīng lái chéng kuài*: Menstrual flow containing dark purple lumps of coagulated blood. It is a sign of blood stasis, or of cold or heat causing blood stasis. See BLOOD STASIS SCANT MENSTRUATION; BLOOD STASIS MENSTRUAL PAIN; BLOOD STASIS INFERTILITY; BLOOD STASIS DELAYED MENSTRUATION; CONGEALING COLD-DAMP MENSTRUAL PAIN; BLOOD COLD DELAYED MENSTRUATION; BLOOD HEAT ADVANCED MENSTRUATION; MENSTRUATION AT IRREGULAR INTERVALS; DISPELLING STASIS AND STANCHING BLEEDING.

[1]**cloud** 蒙 *méng*: To cover, cloud, obscure; describes the effect of phlegm turbidity, such as in the term PHLEGM CLOUDING THE PERICARDIUM, a pattern characterized by oppression in the chest, confusion, and, in severe cases, coma. See EXUBERANCE AND DEBILITATION.

[2]**cloud** 昏 *hūn*: Describes severe lack of clarity (of vision or consciousness).

clouded spirit 神昏 *shén hūn*: Stupor or complete loss of consciousness. Occurs in many diseases and may be of sudden or gradual onset. In bowel heat patterns, for example, it develops gradually, and, in severe cases, is associated with DELIRIOUS SPEECH and PICKING AT BEDCLOTHES. See COMA. [27: 371] [97: 424] [50: 1182]

clouded spirit-mind 神志昏糊 *shén zhì hūn hú*: Stupor. See CLOUDED SPIRIT.

clouded vision 目昏 *mù hūn*: Blurred, unclear vision; attributable to the following possible causes: dual depletion of qi and blood in enduring sickness; liver-kidney insufficiency and wearing of essence-blood; depletion of heart construction and vacuity of spirit qi; spleen-stomach vacuity and disturbance of movement and transformation; constrained emotions and disturbance of liver free coursing; qi stagnation and blood stasis; wind, fire, phlegm, or dampness harassing the clear orifices of the upper body; external injury. [26: 200] [27: 150]

clouding reversal 昏厥 *hūn jué*: Sudden loss of consciousness and collapse, sometimes accompanied by reversal cold of the limbs. Clouding reversal is usually of short duration as in various REVERSAL PATTERNS; the patient returns to consciousness without hemiplegia or deviation of the eyes and mouth as occurs in wind stroke. In rare cases, it continues, as in DEATHLIKE REVERSAL. Causes include qi vacuity, blood vacuity, phlegm turbidity harassing the upper body, ascendant liver yang, summerheat stroke, and tetanic diseases such as child fright wind and epilepsy. ◇ Chin 昏 *hūn*, clouded, hazy; 厥 *jué*, invert, turn around. [27: 399] [92: No. 55]

clouding sleep 昏睡 *hūn shuì*: Synonym: *hypersomnia*. A pronounced somnolence that occurs in heat entering the pericardium, whose other signs include generalized heat [effusion] that is most pronounced at night, a crimson tongue, rapid pulse, and sometimes maculopapular eruptions. ◇ Chin 昏 *hūn*, clouded, hazy; 睡 *shuì*, sleep. [97: 363]

clove sore 疔疮 *dīng chuāng*: A small, hard sore with a deep root like a clove or nail, appearing most commonly on the face and ends of the fingers. A clove sore arises when fire toxin enters the body through a wound, and then heat brews and binds in the skin and flesh. It may also arise when anger, anxiety, and preoccupation or excessive indulgence in rich food or alcohol lead to accumulated heat in the organs, which effuses outward to the skin. Sometimes, a clove sore may have a single red threadlike line stretching from the sore toward the trunk. This is known as a RED-THREAD CLOVE SORE. Severe forms are known as toxin clove sores, whose toxin can spread to penetrate the blood aspect and attack the organs, causing clouded spirit. This is called a RUNNING YELLOW. MED Clear

heat and resolve toxin. Use Five-Ingredient Toxin-Dispersing Beverage (*wǔ wèi xiāo dú yǐn*) or Coptis Toxin-Resolving Decoction (*huáng lián jiě dú tāng*) for oral medication, and apply Thoroughly Pounded Paste (*qiān chuí gāo*). Clove sores of the limbs can be lanced to allow pus to drain. However, clove sores that are lanced and squeezed too early can cause running. ACU Base treatment mainly on GV and LI. Select GV-12 (*shēn zhù*, Body Pillar), GV-10 (*líng tái*, Spirit Tower), LI-4 (*hé gǔ*, Union Valley), and BL-40 (*wěi zhōng*, Bend Center); needle with drainage or pricking to bleed with a three-edged needle. Selection of points according to affected area: When lying on the large intestine channel pathway on the face, add LI-1 (*shāng yáng*, Shang Yang) and LI-11 (*qū chí*, Pool at the Bend). When lying on the gallbladder channel pathway on the face, add GB-34 (*yáng líng quán*, Yang Mound Spring), GB-41 (*zú lín qì*, Foot Overlooking Tears), and GB-44 (*zú qiào yīn*, Foot Orifice Yin). Affecting the end of the index finger, add LI-11 (*qū chí*, Pool at the Bend) and LI-20 (*yíng xiāng*, Welcome Fragrance). Affecting the end of the little toe and second toe, add GB-34 (*yáng líng quán*, Yang Mound Spring), and GB-2 (*tīng huì*, Auditory Convergence). When growing on the lower limbs, add KI-9 (*zhú bīn*, Guest House) and SP-10 (*xuè hǎi*, Sea of Blood). Selection of points according to signs: For high fever, add LI-11 (*qū chí*, Pool at the Bend) and GV-14 (*dà zhuī*, Great Hammer). For clove toxin attacking the inner body and clouding the spirit, add GV-26 (*shuǐ gōu*, Water Trough), SI-8 (*xiǎo hǎi*, Small Sea), and HT-7 (*shén mén*, Spirit Gate), and prick Ten Diffusing Points (*shí xuān*) to bleed. ◇ Chin The character 疔 *dīng* is composed of the character 丁 *dīng* meaning a nail or clove with the illness signifier 疒. [27: 467] [97: 311] [26: 297] [61: 95] [96: 89]

clove sore running yellow 疔疮走黄 *dīng chuāng zǒu huáng*: Synonym: *running yellow*. A CLOVE SORE from which the toxin spreads and falls inward (see INWARD FALL) to penetrate the blood aspect. The clove sore is characterized by broad swelling, and is accompanied by high fever, SHIVER SWEATING, headache, vexation and agitation, distention and oppression in the chest and abdomen, lack of strength in the limbs, a red or crimson tongue, a rough yellow tongue fur, and a surging rapid or slippery stringlike pulse. There may also be nausea, vomiting, stiffening of the tongue with dry mouth, constipation or diarrhea, and, in severe cases, clouded spirit, delirious speech, and TETANIC REVERSAL, stasis speckles or macules. In some cases, the whole body turns yellow (which explains the origin of the Chinese term), and the spread of pus toxin can cause pulmonary welling-abscess (*fèi yōng*) or bone flat-abscess (*gǔ jū*). Running yellow occurs when intense heat toxin is spread by inappropriate squeezing, premature lancing, or accidental rupture of the clove sore. WMC septicemia. MED Clear heat, resolve toxin, and cool the blood with formulas such as Rhinoceros Horn and Rehmannia Decoction (*xī jiǎo dì huáng tāng*), Coptis Toxin-Resolving Decoction (*huáng lián jiě dú tāng*), and Five-Ingredient Toxin-Dispersing Beverage (*wǔ wèi xiāo dú yǐn*). For topical treatment, see CLOVE SORE. ACU Use the point given under CLOVE SORE, and prick Twelve Well Points (*shí èr jǐng xué*), GV-14 (*dà zhuī*, Great Hammer), and LI-11 (*qū chí*, Pool at the Bend) to bleed with a three-edged needle. Clove sore running yellow is a critical condition that should be treated vigorously treated with all possible methods (acupuncture and medicinals), or with Chinese-Western integrated methods. ◇ Chin 走 *zǒu*, go, travel; 黄 *huáng*, yellow, possibly confused with 横 *hèng*, reckless, tyrannical [98].

coacting treatment 从治 *cóng zhì*: PARADOXICAL TREATMENT.

cocoon lip 茧唇 *jiǎn chún*: A disease of the mouth that starts with a bean-like hard lump on the lip (usually the lower lip), which gradually grows larger and whose skin becomes white and fissured, giving it the appearance of a cocoon, an everted flower, ganoderma or other fungus. It can rupture to exude bloody fluid, leaving an ulceration with an uneven surface that forms scabs. In the final stages, there is dry mouth and throat, and emaciation. Patterns include intense internal spleen fire, spleen-stomach repletion heat, and intense yin vacuity fire. WMC cancer of the lip. **Intense internal spleen fire:** The swelling is elevated and hard, and may be ulcerated and painful. It is accompanied by thirst, yellow urine, red tongue with yellow fur, and a rapid fine pulse. MED Clear fire and resolve toxin; nourish yin and engender liquid. Use variations of Cool Clearing Sweet Dew Beverage (*qīng liáng gān lù yǐn*). **Spleen-stomach repletion heat:** The swelling is scorching and painful, and the lips are dry and cracked. There is thirst, constipation, yellow urine, and a dry yellow fur, and forceful slippery rapid pulse. MED Free the bowels and discharge heat; resolve toxin and transform phlegm. Use Diaphragm-Cooling Powder (*liáng gé sǎn*) plus silkworm (*bái jiāng cán*) and bearded scutellaria (*bàn zhī lián*). **Intense yin vacuity fire:** The lesion is painful and burns like fire. It is deep dull purple in color and periodically exudes blood water. Other signs include reddening of the checks, heat in the hearts of the palms and soles, a red tongue without fur, and a rapid fine pulse. MED Nourish yin and downbear fire with Anemarrhena, Phellodendron, and Rehmannia Pill (*zhī bǎi dì huáng wán*). [96: 217] [26: 976] [27: 486] [97: 384] [61: 338]

coin lichen 金钱癣 *jīn qián xiǎn*, 圆癣 *yuán xiǎn*: A condition characterized by clearly circumscribed red macules that often heal from the center (Chinese coins traditionally had holes in them), sometimes with papules, vesicles, or pustules at the periphery which crust and scale. It may be observed on the face, neck, trunk, or limbs. WMC tinea corporis. MED Treat by topical application of 3 g of borax blended with 100 ml of vinegar. ACU Base treatment mainly on SP, ST, and LI. Needle with even supplementation and drainage at ST-36 (*zú sān lǐ*, Leg Three Li), SP-6 (*sān yīn jiāo*, Three Yin Intersection), SP-9 (*yīn líng quán*, Yin Mound Spring), and KI-2 (*rán gǔ*, Blazing Valley), and with drainage at LI-4 (*hé gǔ*, Union Valley), and LI-11 (*qū chí*, Pool at the Bend). Apply moxa at ouch points (*ā shì xué*). [26: 792] [15: 385] [37: 450] [42: 157]

coin screen 圆翳 *yuán yì*: *Synonym: silvery internal obstruction.* An internal obstruction of the eye. A round white opacity blocking the pupil. It is usually attributed to insufficiency of the liver and kidney with yin vacuity damp-heat or liver channel wind-heat attacking the upper body. It may affect either or both eyes. WMC cataract. MED Enrich the liver and kidney or nourish yin, clear heat, and eliminate dampness. [26: 792]

¹**cold** 寒 *hán*: **1.** The opposite of heat. **2.** One of the SIX QI; cold weather, normally occurring in winter. **3.** One of the SIX EXCESSES, i.e., cold weather as a cause of disease. **4.** Cold in the body causing disease and classified as "cold" among the eight principles. The nature of cold as an evil and its clinical manifestations are similar to those of cold in the natural environment, e.g., low temperature, deceleration of activity, and congealing. Diseases caused by cold evil result from severe or sudden exposure to cold, e.g., catching cold, excessive consumption of cold fluids, or exposure to frost. They bear the following features: **4a.** Generalized or local signs of cold, such as aversion to cold, desire for warmth, pronounced lack of warmth in the extremities, and cold and pain in the lower abdomen. **4b.** Cold, thin, clear excreta; for example, a runny nose with clear mucus, clear phlegm, watery vomitus, long voidings of clear urine, or clear watery diarrhea. *Elementary Questions* (*sù wèn, zhì zhēn yào dà lùn*) states, "All disease with water humors that are clear, pure, and cold are ascribed to cold." (See NINETEEN PATHOMECHANISMS.) **4c.** Tendency to develop qi stagnation and blood stasis, characterized by severe pain. It has been said, "When cold prevails, there is pain." **4d.** Contracture and hypertonicity of the sinews, indicating invasion of the channels by the evil; hence it is said, "Cold is associated with contracture and tautness." Cold may arise in the body not only as a result of invasion by cold evil, but also

as a result of debilitation of yang qi. This is called vacuity cold, and is characterized by curled-up lying posture, long voidings of clear urine, clear-food diarrhea, counterflow cold of the limbs, and a slow pulse. See also COLD PATTERN. **5.** One of the FOUR QI (heat, cold, warmth, coolness). **6.** *adj.* **6a.** Of or pertaining to the quality cold. **6b.** Of a nature tending to reduce heat, e.g., cold medicinal. See FOUR QI. See also COMMON COLD. [26: 656] [27: 570]

²**cold** 冷 *lěng*: Pronounced, overt, or palpable cold. See COLD. [19: 4028]

cold abdominal pain 寒冷腹痛 *hán lěng fù tòng*: COLD QI ABDOMINAL PAIN.

cold accumulation abdominal pain 寒积腹痛 *hán jī fù tòng*: ABDOMINAL PAIN that arises when spleen-stomach yang vacuity, damage from eating raw and cold foods, and contraction of cold evil cause an accumulation of congealing stagnant cold. It is characterized by continual pain that likes heat and refuses warmth. Bouts of pain are accompanied by diarrhea. The pulse is usually sunken and slow or sunken and tight. MED Warm and move spleen yang; dissipate cold and move qi. Use formulas such as Center-Ordering Decoction (*zhì zhōng tāng*) or Tsaoko Pill (*dòu kòu wán*). Compare the milder COLD QI ABDOMINAL PAIN. ACU Base treatment mainly on CV, ST, SP, and LI. Select CV-12 (*zhōng wǎn*, Center Stomach Duct), CV-8 (*shén què*, Spirit Gate Tower), ST-25 (*tiān shū*, Celestial Pivot), BL-25 (*dà cháng shū*, Large Intestine Transport), ST-36 (*zú sān lǐ*, Leg Three Li), SP-15 (*dà hèng*, Great Horizontal), SP-4 (*gōng sūn*, Yellow Emperor), and LI-4 (*hé gǔ*, Union Valley); needle with drainage and add moxa. Moxibustion on ginger can be performed at CV-8 (*shén què*, Spirit Gate Tower). [26: 661] [46: 662] [37: 316]

cold aching lumbus and knees 腰膝酸冷 *yāo xī suān lěng*: Aching pain and palpable cold in the lumbus and knees attributable to kidney yang vacuity. See LUMBAR PAIN.

cold aggregation 寒癖 *hán pì*: A lump in the ribside that feels like a taut cord, associated with pain on exposure to cold, and a large stringlike pulse. Cold aggregation is attributable to cold evil contending with water-rheum. MED Use Sal Ammoniac Decocted Pill (*náo shā jiān wán*). See STRINGS AND AGGREGATIONS. [26: 662]

cold and heat 寒热 *hán rè*: **1.** Cold and heat in the eight-principle sense. Cold and heat represent the yin and yang of bodily functions. Cold results from contraction of cold evil or insufficiency of yang qi; heat results from contraction of heat evil or yin vacuity. **2.** Heat effusion and aversion to cold. **3.** Alternating heat effusion and aversion to cold. [27: 212] [97: 571] [6: 153]

cold back 背寒 *bèi hán*: Palpable cold or a feeling of cold in the back. Cold back may be observed in a) external contraction of wind-cold with heat effusion, generalized pain, and a tight floating pulse, b) in yang vacuity with yin exuberance, attended by bland taste in the mouth, somber complexion, counterflow cold of the extremities, long voidings of clear urine, sloppy stool, pale tongue with glossy moist tongue fur, and slow sunken pulse, and c) phlegm-rheum with cough or panting, copious thin white phlegm, dizziness, no desire for fluid or desire for warm drinks in small quantities, abdominal distention, reduced food intake, general fatigue and lack of strength, swelling of the limbs, white glossy tongue fur, and slippery sunken pulse. Compare HOT BACK. [92: No. 162]

cold bind 寒结 *hán jié*: COLD CONSTIPATION. [26: 659]

cold causes contracture and tension 寒则收引 *hán zé shōu yǐn*: See COLD CAUSES QI TO CONTRACT. [26: 658] [27: 141] [97: 573]

cold causes qi to contract 寒则气收 *hán zé qì shōu*: Synonym: *cold causes contracture and tension*. From *Elementary Questions* (*sù wèn, jǔ tòng lùn*). When cold qi damages the skin and flesh, the pores close, yang qi contracts, and sweat ceases to flow; when it damages the sinews, the sinews become contracted and tense (hypertonic) and painful. [26: 658]

cold chest bind 寒结胸 *hán jié xiōng*: COLD REPLETION CHEST BIND. [26: 659]

cold cholera 寒霍乱 *hán huò luàn*: Cholera due to consumption of raw or cold foods or contraction of cold-damp in patients with yang qi. Cold cholera is characterized by simultaneous vomiting and diarrhea, with vomitus and stool that is normally without foul smell and that is like clear water or like water in which rice has been washed. Other signs include mild abdominal pain, aversion to cold, cold limbs, green-blue or purple lips and nails, and sunken tight or sunken hidden pulse. WMC acute enteritis, cholera, and paracholera. MED Warm the center, dissipate cold, and transform dampness. Use Agastache/Patchouli Qi-Righting Powder (*huò xiāng zhèng qì sǎn*) for mild cases and Center-Rectifying Decoction (*lǐ zhōng tāng*) or Counterflow Cold Decoction (*sì nì tāng*) for severe cases. ACU Base treatment mainly on CV, LI, ST, and SP. Select CV-12 (*zhōng wǎn*, Center Stomach Duct), ST-25 (*tiān shū*, Celestial Pivot), ST-37 (*shàng jù xū*, Upper Great Hollow), PC-6 (*nèi guān*, Inner Pass), and ST-36 (*zú sān lǐ*, Leg Three Li); needle with supplementation and large amounts of moxa. Moxibustion on ginger can be performed at CV-8 (*shén què*, Spirit Gate Tower). For yang vacuity constitution, add CV-6 (*qì hǎi*, Sea of Qi) and CV-4 (*guān yuán*, Pass

Head). For internal damage by raw cold foods, add BL-20 (*pí shū*, Spleen Transport) and LR-13 (*zhāng mén*, Camphorwood Gate). For external cold-damp contraction, needle with drainage and moxa at BL-12 (*fēng mén*, Wind Gate), LU-7 (*liè quē*, Broken Sequence), and SP-9 (*yīn líng quán*, Yin Mound Spring). See CHOLERA. [26: 661]

cold congealing in the liver vessel 寒凝肝脉 *hán níng gān mài*: See COLD STAGNATING IN THE LIVER VESSEL.

cold constipation 冷秘 *lěng bì*: Synonym: *yin bind*; *cold bind*. Constipation arising when spleen-kidney yang vacuity causes yin cold to congeal and bind, reducing warmth and movement of food. Cold constipation is associated with pale lips, harmony of mouth, lack of warmth in the limbs, cold sensation in the lumbus and abdomen, or cold pain in the abdomen, desire for heat and aversion to cold, long voidings of clear urine, an enlarged tongue with white fur, and a forceless fine pulse. MED Supplement the kidney and warm yang. Use Pinellia and Sulfur Pill (*bàn liú wán*) plus cistanche (*ròu cōng róng*) and achyranthes (*niú xī*). ACU Base treatment on the alarm, back transport, and lower uniting points of LI, and on CV, SP, and KI. Select BL-25 (*dà cháng shū*, Large Intestine Transport), ST-25 (*tiān shū*, Celestial Pivot), ST-37 (*shàng jù xū*, Upper Great Hollow), CV-6 (*qì hǎi*, Sea of Qi), KI-6 (*zhào hǎi*, Shining Sea), KI-18 (*shí guān*, Stone Pass), BL-23 (*shèn shū*, Kidney Transport), and CV-4 (*guān yuán*, Pass Head); needle with supplementation and add moxa. Apply moxa on salt or ginger at CV-8 (*shén què*, Spirit Gate Tower). [26: 297] [46: 671] [37: 325]

cold cough 寒嗽 *hán sòu*: Cough due to damage to the lung by externally contracted cold or damage to the spleen by eating raw and cold foodstuffs. Cold cough is associated with white foamy phlegm, white face, tight pulse, and fine stringlike pulse. In the winter, contraction of cold may also cause aversion to cold and heat effusion, absence of sweating, and nasal congestion. MED Warm the lung and resolve the exterior using formulas like Minor Green-Blue Dragon Decoction (*xiǎo qīng lóng tāng*). ACU Base treatment mainly on LU, LI, and ST. Select BL-13 (*fèi shū*, Lung Transport), LU-7 (*liè quē*, Broken Sequence), LI-4 (*hé gǔ*, Union Valley), BL-12 (*fēng mén*, Wind Gate), BL-11 (*dà zhù*, Great Shuttle), ST-25 (*tiān shū*, Celestial Pivot), and ST-40 (*fēng lóng*, Bountiful Bulge). Needle with drainage and add moxa. See COUGH. [26: 660] [37: 275] [27: 348] [97: 198]

cold damage 伤寒 *shāng hán*: **1.** Externally contracted heat (febrile) diseases. *Elementary Questions* (*sù wèn, rè lùn*) states, "Heat (febrile) diseases are all of the cold damage kind." It also states, "When a person is damaged by cold, the disease is febrile (one of heat)." **2.** A specific form of externally contracted heat (febrile) disease, *The Classic of Difficult Issues* (*nàn jīng*) states, "Cold damage has five [forms]: cold damage, wind stroke, damp warmth, heat disease, and warm disease." This specific form of febrile disease is elaborated on in *On Cold Damage* (*shāng hán lùn*), i.e., a greater yang (*tài yáng*) pattern of externally contracted heat (febrile) disease with absence of sweating, stiff neck, and a tight floating pulse. **3.** A disease caused by catching cold in the winter. ◇ Chin 伤 *shāng*, damage; 寒 *hán*, cold. [26: 808]

cold damage blood amassment pattern 伤寒蓄血证 *shāng hán xù xuè zhèng*: A greater yang (*tài yáng*) bowel pattern arising when stasis heat binds in the lower burner causing lesser-abdominal tension or lower abdominal hardness and fullness, mania-like or manic states, forgetfulness, sloppy stool that is black and slimy like lacquer. The bladder is the greater yang bowel, and when greater yang evil heat passes through the channels into the bowel, it causes stasis heat to bind in the lower burner. Because the evil is in the blood aspect rather than in the qi aspect, urination is uninhibited. MED For mild cases, use Peach Kernel Qi-Coordinating Decoction (*táo hé chéng qì tāng*) to discharge heat and move stasis; for severe cases, use Dead-On Decoction (*dǐ dàng tāng*) or Dead-On Pill (*dǐ dàng wán*). Comparison: Cold damage blood amassment, water amassment, and yang brightness (*yáng míng*) bowel repletion patterns are similar, and care must be taken to differentiate. Lower abdominal fullness that is not painful when pressed and inhibited urination indicate water amassment; pain around the umbilicus that refuses pressure, short rough urination, and fecal stoppage constitutes a yang brightness bowel repletion pattern; lesser-abdominal hardness and black stool like lacquer, mania-like or manic states, and uninhibited urination constitutes a blood amassment pattern. See COLD DAMAGE; GREATER YANG DISEASE. [26: 808]

cold damage exterior pattern 伤寒表证 *shāng hán biǎo zhèng*: Any disease pattern resulting from the presence of cold damage disease evil in the exterior, referred to in the doctrine of cold damage greater yang (*tài yáng*) exterior pattern. See COLD DAMAGE; GREATER YANG DISEASE. [26: 806]

cold damage interior pattern 伤寒里证 *shāng hán lǐ zhèng*: Any cold damage disease pattern resulting when external evils pass from the exterior to the interior. Evils in the yang channels are in the interior when in the yang brightness (*yáng míng*). For example, YANG BRIGHTNESS DISEASE with a slow pulse, heavy body, shortness of breath, abdominal fullness and panting, and tidal heat [effusion] can be treated by attacking the interior with one of the Qi-Coordinating Decoctions (*chéng qì tāng*); yang brightness with sweating from the head only (absence of generalized sweating), inhibited urination, and thirst with intake of fluid is a sign of STASIS HEAT in the interior that is invariably accompanied by yellowing, and is treated with Capillaris Decoction (*yīn chén hāo tāng*). If the evils pass from the yang to the yin channels, or make a direct strike on the lesser yin (*shào yīn*), the resulting patterns are of interior vacuity cold. For example, LESSER YIN DISEASE with sunken rapid fine pulse indicates disease of the interior for which the method of sweating is contraindicated; lesser yin disease with clear-food diarrhea, interior cold and external heat, REVERSE-FLOW OF THE EXTREMITIES, and faint pulse verging on expiration should be treated with Vessel-Freeing Counterflow Cold Decoction (*tōng mài sì nì tāng*). Yang brightness disease and TRIPLE-YIN DISEASE are both interior patterns that are quite different in terms of cold, heat, vacuity, and repletion, so care must be taken in pattern identification and treatment. See COLD DAMAGE. [26: 807]

cold damages the physical body 寒伤形 *hán shāng xíng*: Cold evil can cause injury to the body. Cold is a yin evil, and by nature causes congealing, stagnation, and contracture. External contraction of cold prevents the normal diffusion of yang qi, causing headache, aversion to cold, absence of sweating, generalized pain, and a tight floating pulse. When cold evil lodges in the sinews, it causes tension in the network vessels, which restricts the movement of qi and blood, thereby causing spasm, pain, and numbness. [26: 660] [27: 140]

cold damage water amassment pattern 伤寒蓄水证 *shāng hán xù shuǐ zhèng*: A greater yang (*tài yáng*) bowel pattern arising when greater yang disease fails to resolve, and evil heat passes through the channel into the bowel (the bladder) and binds with water, hampering qi transformation. Signs include floating pulse, heat effusion, thirst, inhibited urination, lesser-abdominal fullness, and in some cases the immediate vomiting of water ingested. [MED] Free yang and promote qi transformation; disinhibit water and resolve the exterior. Use Poria (Hoelen) Five Powder (*wǔ líng sǎn*). See GREATER YANG DISEASE. [26: 807]

cold-damp 寒湿 *hán shī*: **1.** Cold and dampness combining to create stagnation of yang qi and inhibit the flow of blood, causing cold in the flesh and inhibited bending and stretching. **2.** A disease pattern in which dampness encumbers the stomach and spleen and damages spleen yang or in which water-rheum collects as a result of spleen-kidney yang vacuity. It is characterized by cold limbs, abdominal distention, diarrhea, and in some cases water swelling. [26: 661]

cold-damp dizziness 寒湿眩晕 *hán shī xuàn yūn*: See SUMMERHEAT-DAMP DIZZINESS. [26: 661]

cold-damp encumbering the spleen 寒湿困脾 *hán shī kùn pí*: Synonym: *cold-damp obstructing the center*. Impairment of splenic movement arising when excessive consumption of cold food and drinks or of gourds and fruits, or spleen-yang vacuity allows dampness to invade. Signs include distention and fullness in the stomach duct and abdomen, heavy-headedness, fatigue, torpid intake, upflow nausea and desire to vomit, bland taste in the mouth without thirst, sloppy stool, inhibited urination, a gray-white glossy tongue fur, and a slow or moderate, or soggy pulse. In women, there may be a thin white fishy-smelling vaginal discharge. [MED] Treat by warming the center and dispelling cold combined with the method of moving the spleen. Use variations of Center-Rectifying Decoction (*lǐ zhōng tāng*) combined with Stomach-Calming Poria (Hoelen) Five Decoction (*wèi líng tāng*). Compare SPLEEN VACUITY WITH DAMP ENCUMBRANCE. [ACU] Base treatment mainly on CV, GV, SP, and ST. Select BL-20 (*pí shū*, Spleen Transport), CV-12 (*zhōng wǎn*, Center Stomach Duct), ST-36 (*zú sān lǐ*, Leg Three Li), LR-13 (*zhāng mén*, Camphorwood Gate), SP-9 (*yīn líng quán*, Yin Mound Spring), CV-4 (*guān yuán*, Pass Head), and SP-6 (*sān yīn jiāo*, Three Yin Intersection); needle with supplementation and large amounts of moxa. [25: 314] [57: 70] [50: 1580] [46: 597, 666]

cold-damp enduring impediment 寒湿久痹 *hán shī jiǔ bì*: A chronic IMPEDIMENT (*bì*) pattern arising when cold-damp invades the body. Cold evil causes qi and blood to congeal, whereas dampness causes stagnation and fixity. The two evils combined cause persistent morbid states of pain in the flesh and skin, stiffness in the joints, pain of fixed location. [26: 661]

cold-damp headache 寒湿头痛 *hán shī tóu tòng*: HEADACHE due to cold-damp clouding clear yang in the upper body, congealing the blood, and causing hypertonicity of the network vessels. It tends to occur in wet or dull (yin-type) weather and is associated with oppression in the chest, heavy cumbersome limbs, a white slimy tongue fur, and a moderate pulse. [MED] Dissipate cold and dispel dampness using formulas such as Notopterygium Dampness-Overcoming Decoction (*qiāng huó shèng shī tāng*) or Ligusticum and Asarum Decoction (*xiōng xīn tāng*). [ACU] Base treatment mainly on SP, ST, and LI. Select ST-8 (*tóu wéi*, Head Corner), Greater Yang (*tài yáng*), ST-36 (*zú sān lǐ*, Leg Three Li), LI-4 (*hé gǔ*, Union Valley), and SP-9 (*yīn líng quán*, Yin Mound Spring); needle with drainage and use large amounts of moxa. For

selection of points according to affected area, see
HEADACHE. [26: 662] [50: 1580] [46: 595]

cold-damp leg qi 寒湿脚气 *hán shī jiǎo qì*: LEG
QI (beriberi) that arises when external cold invades
to hamper the movement of channel qi and to cause
disharmony of the blood vessels, and that is characterized by weakness of the legs and knees, no
strength to move, persistent numbness, and water swelling. In some cases there is hypertonicity and pain, and sometimes aversion to cold and
cold limbs. MED Treat by warming the channels
and eliminating dampness, supported by quickening the blood, freeing the vessels, and soothing the
sinews. Appropriate formulas include Chaenomeles and Achyranthes Pill (*mù guā niú xī wán*) and
Fenugreek Pill (*hú lú bā wán*). ACU Base treatment mainly on SP, ST, and GB. Select ST-36 (*zú
sān lǐ*, Leg Three Li), SP-6 (*sān yīn jiāo*, Three
Yin Intersection), SP-9 (*yīn líng quán*, Yin Mound
Spring), SP-5 (*shāng qiū*, Shang Hill), GB-34 (*yáng
líng quán*, Yang Mound Spring), GB-39 (*xuán
zhōng*, Suspended Bell), ST-41 (*jiě xī*, Ravine Divide), and Eight Winds (*bā fēng*). Needle with
drainage and use large amounts of moxa. [26: 661]
[27: 574]

cold-damp lumbar pain 寒湿腰痛 *hán shī yāo
tòng*: LUMBAR PAIN attributable to cold-damp obstructing the channels and network vessels, inhibiting the movement of qi and blood. Cold-damp
lumbar pain likes heat and refuses cold, and is
associated with normal eating and drinking, normal stool, and a tight sunken pulse. MED Dispel cold-damp and warm the channels and network
vessels. Use formulas such as Ovate Atractylodes
and Aconite Decoction (*zhú fù tāng*) or Five Accumulations Powder (*wǔ jī sǎn*). Lumbar Rub Elixir
(*mó yāo dān*) can be applied topically. ACU Base
treatment mainly on GV, BL, and SP. Select BL-23
(*shèn shū*, Kidney Transport), GV-3 (*yāo yáng
guān*, Lumbar Yang Pass), BL-40 (*wěi zhōng*, Bend
Center), BL-60 (*kūn lún*, Kunlun Mountains), ouch
points (*ā shì xué*), GV-4 (*mìng mén*, Life Gate),
and SP-9 (*yīn líng quán*, Yin Mound Spring). Needle with drainage and use large amounts of moxa.
[26: 662] [46: 633] [37: 389]

cold-damp obstructing the center 寒湿中阻
hán shī zhōng zǔ: COLD-DAMP ENCUMBERING THE
SPLEEN.

cold diarrhea 寒泄 *hán xiè*, 寒泻 *hán xiè*: DIAR-
RHEA with clear watery stool, or stool like duck's
slop (droppings), or sometimes with nontransformation of food (undigested food is seen in the
stool). *Elementary Questions* (*sù wèn*) "Any disease with watery humors that are clear, pure, and
cold is ascribed to cold." Hence, watery stool is understood to be a cold sign. There is abdominal pain
relieved by both pressure and heat, lack of warmth

in the extremities, and a drop in body temperature.
The tongue fur is white, and the pulse is either
stringlike and tight or sunken and slow. Cold di-
arrhea is often accompanied by signs of dampness.
MED Use formulas like Aconite Center-Rectifying
Decoction (*fù zǐ lǐ zhōng tāng*). ACU Base treatment mainly on CV and ST. Select CV-12 (*zhōng
wǎn*, Center Stomach Duct), LR-13 (*zhāng mén*,
Camphorwood Gate), ST-25 (*tiān shū*, Celestial
Pivot), ST-36 (*zú sān lǐ*, Leg Three Li), CV-4 (*guān
yuán*, Pass Head), CV-3 (*zhōng jí*, Central Pole),
ST-21 (*liáng mén*, Beam Gate), and CV-6 (*qì hǎi*,
Sea of Qi). Needle with supplementation and use
large amounts of moxa. Use cross moxa (*shí zì jiǔ*).
[26: 657-8] [6: 201] [27: 363] [97: 571]

cold distention 寒胀 *hán zhàng*: ABDOMINAL
DISTENTION due to spleen-stomach vacuity cold
or cold-damp obstruction accompanied by no desire for food and drink, vomiting, heart vexation,
reversal cold of the limbs, and a weak sunken
pulse. MED Warm the center and dispel cold using
formulas such as Center Fullness Separating and
Dispersing Decoction (*zhōng mǎn fēn xiāo tāng*).
ACU Base treatment mainly on ST, CV, PC, back
transport points and SP. Main points: ST-25 (*tiān
shū*, Celestial Pivot), CV-6 (*qì hǎi*, Sea of Qi),
PC-6 (*nèi guān*, Inner Pass), and ST-36 (*zú sān lǐ*,
Leg Three Li). For sleen-stomach vacuity cold, add
CV-12 (*zhōng wǎn*, Center Stomach Duct), BL-20
(*pí shū*, Spleen Transport), and BL-21 (*wèi shū*,
Stomach Transport), and needle with supplementation and large amounts of moxa. For cold-damp
obstruction, add SP-9 (*yīn líng quán*, Yin Mound
Spring), and needle with drainage and add moxa.
[26: 659] [46: 666, 602, 596]

cold dysentery 寒痢 *hán lì*: DYSENTERY attributed to damage to spleen yang by congealing
stagnation of cold qi after excessive consumption
of raw, cold, or unclean foods in hot weather. The
stool is largely pure white (i.e., a high content
of pus-like substance) or white with a little red
(blood), and either thin in consistency with a fishy
smell or gluey. The pulse is slow and the tongue
fur is white. MED Use Center-Rectifying Decoction (*lǐ zhōng tāng*) plus chebule (*hē zǐ*), nutmeg
(*ròu dòu kòu*), saussurea (*mù xiāng*), and amomum (*shā rén*). If the stool has the appearance
of duck's droppings, and the sagging sensation in
the abdomen is not pronounced, it can be treated
with Priceless Qi-Righting Powder (*bù huàn jīn
zhèng qì sǎn*) plus mume (*wū méi*), and tangerine peel (*chén pí*). If the stool is clear (i.e., clean)
and the limbs are cold, Center-Rectifying Decoction (*lǐ zhōng tāng*) or Ginger and Aconite Decoction (*jiāng fù tāng*) may be used. ACU Base treatment on ST, LI, and CV, select LI-4 (*hé gǔ*, Union
Valley), ST-25 (*tiān shū*, Celestial Pivot), ST-37
(*shàng jù xū*, Upper Great Hollow), CV-12 (*zhōng*

wǎn, Center Stomach Duct), and CV-6 (*qì hǎi*, Sea of Qi) and needle with drainage with moxa. Selection of points according to sign: For stool bearing the appearance of duck's droppings, add ST-36 (*zú sān lǐ*, Leg Three Li) and SP-4 (*gōng sūn*, Yellow Emperor). For cold limbs and clear stool, add BL-20 (*pí shū*, Spleen Transport) and BL-23 (*shèn shū*, Kidney Transport), applying moxa in large amounts. For persistent conditions needle with supplementation with moxa at ST-36 (*zú sān lǐ*, Leg Three Li), CV-4 (*guān yuán*, Pass Head), and BL-20 (*pí shū*, Spleen Transport). [26: 658] [27: 361] [97: 572]

cold enveloping fire 寒包火 *hán bāo huǒ*: Synonym: *cold enveloping heat*. A pattern of external cold due to contraction of wind-cold with accumulated internal heat. The external cold is understood to "envelope" the depressed internal heat. Cold enveloping fire presents as a wind-cold exterior pattern with cough, panting, loss of voice, red sore swollen eyes, or sore swollen gums. [26: 657]

cold enveloping heat 寒包热 *hán bāo rè*: COLD ENVELOPING FIRE.

cold epilepsy 寒痫 *hán xián*: EPILEPSY attributed to externally contracted wind-cold binding in the chest and diaphragm in children suffering from damage to the spleen and stomach. Cold epilepsy is characterized by sudden collapse and loss of consciousness, and foaming of phlegm and drool at the mouth. MED Warm the center and transform phlegm using Phlegm-Abducting Decoction (*dǎo tán tāng*). ACU Apply the treatments for fits given under EPILEPSY, and apply moxibustion at KI-1 (*yǒng quán*, Gushing Spring), CV-17 (*shān zhōng*, Chest Center), PC-6 (*nèi guān*, Inner Pass), and SP-6 (*sān yīn jiāo*, Three Yin Intersection). [26: 662]

cold evil 寒邪 *hán xié*: COLD as a disease-causing entity.

cold evil dizziness 寒邪眩晕 *hán xié xuàn yūn*: See WIND-COLD DIZZINESS.

cold evil invading the stomach 寒邪犯胃 *hán xié fàn wèi*: See STOMACH REPLETION COLD. [116: 95]

cold extremities 手足寒 *shǒu zú hán*: , 手足清冷 *shǒu zú qīng lěng*: See COLD LIMBS.

cold formula 寒剂 *hán jì*: One of the TWELVE FORMULA TYPES; a formula comprising cold-nature medicinals. Cold [medicinals] can eliminate heat; hence cold formulas are used to treat heat patterns. An example of a cold formula is Coptis Toxin-Resolving Decoction (*huáng lián jiě dú tāng*), which contains coptis (*huáng lián*), scutellaria (*huáng qín*), phellodendron (*huáng bǎi*), and gardenia (*shān zhī zǐ*), and treats exterior-interior heat. [27: 307] [97: 571]

cold gan 冷疳 *lěng gān*: See COLD-HEAT GAN. [26: 297]

cold heart pain 冷心痛 *lěng xīn tòng*, 寒心痛 *hán xīn tòng*: Synonyms: *cold reversal heart pain*; *cold heart pain*. Fulminant HEART PAIN characterized by pain in the heart stretching to the back and pain in the back stretching into the heart, or continual unabating pain. It may be accompanied by REVERSE-FLOW OF THE EXTREMITIES, generalized cold sweating, clear uninhibited stool and urine or uninhibited stool without thirst, faint breath and lack of strength, and a forceless fine sunken pulse. MED Supplement the kidney, support yang, and dissipate cold using formulas such as Ginger and Aconite Decoction (*jiāng fù tāng*) plus cinnamon bark (*ròu guì*). If there is also vomiting, Evodia Decoction (*wú zhū yú tāng*) may be used. ACU Base treatment mainly on back transport points, CV and GV. Select BL-15 (*xīn shū*, Heart Transport), CV-14 (*jù què*, Great Tower Gate), CV-17 (*shān zhōng*, Chest Center), PC-6 (*nèi guān*, Inner Pass), BL-23 (*shèn shū*, Kidney Transport), GV-4 (*mìng mén*, Life Gate), and CV-4 (*guān yuán*, Pass Head); needle with even supplementation and drainage and add moxa. [26: 297, 657]

cold-heat complex 寒热错杂 *hán rè cuò zá*: Any disease characterized by signs of both heat and cold. A common example of a cold-heat complex is upper body heat and lower body cold characterized by signs such as a sensation of heat and feverishness in the chest, pain in the stomach duct, clamoring stomach, and vomiting of sour and bitter matter, occurring at the same time as abdominal pain that likes warmth and pressure, rumbling intestines, and diarrhea with nontransformation of food (as seen from undigested food in the stool). See UPPER BODY HEAT AND LOWER BODY COLD; UPPER BODY COLD AND LOWER BODY HEAT; EXTERIOR HEAT AND INTERIOR COLD; EXTERIOR COLD AND INTERIOR HEAT. [26: 661] [27: 14]

cold-heat gan 冷热疳 *lěng rè gān*: COLD GAN (also called LEAN COLD GAN) and HEAT GAN (also called FAT HEAT GAN.) New gan disease (i.e., recent onset) tends to manifest in external and heat signs, whereas old gan disease tends to manifest in internal and cold signs. Hence, new gan tends to be heat gan, whereas old gan tends to be cold gan. *The Level-Line of Pediatrics* (*yòu kē zhǔn shéng*) states, "Heat gan is mostly external; there is erosion under the nose, head sores and damp itch, vexing heat in the five hearts, rejection of clothing, rough breathing, thirst with intake of cold water, vexation and agitation, tendency to lie on the ground, hot belly and cold feet, and tidal heat [effusion]. These signs all indicate heat gan. Cold gan is mostly internal. Signs include diarrhea of abnormal color with whitish green-blue foam, limp weak limbs, swollen eyes, and soot-black facial complexion. Another pattern is agitation and thirst with a tendency to lie on the ground like the heat pattern, but with inability to eat and continuous efflux diarrhea. This is also cold gan. The heat pattern is one of heat in vacuity; the cold pattern is one of cold in vacuity. In treating the heat pattern, one should not wildly apply cool medicinals for the exterior; in treating the cold pattern, one should not suddenly apply drastic supplementing medicinals." For heat gan, *The Level-Line of Pediatrics* (*yòu kē zhǔn shéng*) prescribes a formula for Coptis Pill (*huáng lián wán*), which comprises coptis (*huáng lián*), trichosanthes root (*tiān huā fěn*), mume (*wū méi*), apricot kernel (*xìng rén*), and lotus fruit (*shí lián zǐ*) blended with ox's gallbladder (*niú dǎn*) and formed into pills. See GAN. [26: 298]

cold hiccough 寒呃 *hán è*: HICCOUGH due to cold evil invading the stomach or due to stomach (or spleen-stomach) vacuity cold. Cold hiccough is a continuous hiccough that is severe in the evening and mild in the morning, cold extremities, and a forceless slow pulse. MED Warm the center and dissipate cold with formulas such as Center-Rectifying Decoction (*lǐ zhōng tāng*) plus clove (*dīng xiāng*). Alternatively, use Clove Powder (*dīng xiāng sǎn*). For cold evil, add agastache/ patchouli (*huò xiāng*) and perilla leaf (*zǐ sū yè*). If the pattern is one of spleen-kidney vacuity cold, the method of warming and supplementing the spleen and kidney with variations of Yin-Rectifying Brew (*lǐ yīn jiān*) can be used. ACU Base treatment mainly on CV, PC, ST, and LR. Select BL-17 (*gé shū*, Diaphragm Transport), CV-17 (*shān zhōng*, Chest Center), PC-6 (*nèi guān*, Inner Pass), CV-6 (*qì hǎi*, Sea of Qi), CV-12 (*zhōng wǎn*, Center Stomach Duct), ST-36 (*zú sān lǐ*, Leg Three Li), and LR-3 (*tài chōng*, Supreme Surge). For cold evil invading the stomach, add TB-5 (*wài guān*, Outer Pass) and LI-4 (*hé gǔ*, Union Valley); needle with drainage and add moxa. For stomach vacuity cold, needle with supplementation and add moxa. [26: 657] [37: 308] [113: 76]

cold impediment 寒痹 *hán bì*: **1.** *Synonym: painful impediment.* An IMPEDIMENT (*bì*) pattern attributed to wind-cold-damp, with a prevalence of cold, invading the joints and channels and characterized by acute pain in the joints exacerbated by exposure to cold and relieved by warmth. There may also be hypertonicity of the extremities. WMC rheumatic arthritis, rheumatoid arthritis, and gout. MED Treat by warming the channels and dissipating cold, assisted by coursing wind and dispelling dampness. Use formulas such as Poria (Hoelen) Decoction (*fú líng tāng*) and Five Accumulations Powder (*wǔ jī sǎn*). ACU Main points: Select BL-23 (*shèn shū*, Kidney Transport), GV-4

(*mìng mén*, Life Gate), and CV-4 (*guān yuán*, Pass Head); apply deep insertion, needle retention, and moxa or warm needle. Apply moxibustion on salt or ginger at CV-8 (*shén què*, Spirit Gate Tower). For selection of points according to affected area, see IMPEDIMENT. **2.** SKIN IMPEDIMENT. [26: 660] [27: 403] [97: 572]

cold is treated with heat 寒者热之 *hán zhě rè zhī*: From *Elementary Questions* (*sù wèn, zhì zhēn yào dà lùn*). Use warm- or hot-natured medicines to treat cold patterns. For example, exterior cold is treated by by RESOLVING THE EXTERIOR WITH WARMTH AND ACRIDITY, while interior cold is treated by methods such as WARMING THE CENTER AND DISSIPATING COLD or RETURNING YANG AND STEMMING COUNTERFLOW. [27: 239]

cold limbs 肢冷 *zhī lěng*: *Synonym: cold extremities.* Any condition of palpable cold in the limbs. Mild cases are referred to as *lack of warmth in the limbs* and severe cases as REVERSAL COLD OF THE EXTREMITIES. See also PHYSICAL COLD. [92: No. 145]

cold malaria 寒疟 *hán nüè*: MALARIA resulting from the contraction of wind-cold when there is deep-lying internal cold. Cold malaria occurs in episodes daily or every other day, which are characterized by heat effusion and aversion to cold, where the aversion to cold is more pronounced than the heat effusion. Heat effusion and aversion to cold are accompanied by headache, little or no sweating, and a forceful tight stringlike pulse. MED Treat by warming resolution using formulas such as Bupleurum, Cinnamon Twig, and Dried Ginger (*chái hú guì jiāng tāng*) and variations. ACU Base treatment mainly on GV, SI, PC, and BL. Select GV-14 (*dà zhuī*, Great Hammer), GV-13 (*táo dào*, Kiln Path), SI-3 (*hòu xī*, Back Ravine), PC-5 (*jiān shǐ*, Intermediary Courier), BL-28 (*páng guāng shū*, Bladder Transport), and BL-67 (*zhì yīn*, Reaching Yin), and needle with drainage and add moxa. For principles and methods of treatment, see MALARIA. [26: 660] [27: 359] [97: 570] [113: 170]

cold [medicinals] can eliminate heat 寒可去 热 *hán kě qù rè*: Cold medicinals such as coptis (*huáng lián*) and scutellaria (*huáng qín*) can treat heat patterns. See COLD FORMULA.

cold mounting 寒疝 *hán shàn*: **1.** Accumulation of cold evil in the abdomen arising from repeated wind-cold contractions that in turn stem either from vacuity cold in the spleen and stomach or from postpartum blood vacuity. Cold mounting is characterized by cold in the umbilical region, cold sweating, and counterflow cold in the limbs. The pulse is sunken and tight. In severe cases there is generalized cold in the body and numbness in the limbs. In blood vacuity patients, the abdominal pain stretches up the rib-side and is accompanied by cramp in the lower abdomen. [MED] Warm the interior and dissipate cold; move qi and disinhibit dampness. Use Tiantai Lindera Powder (*tiān tái wū yào sǎn*). [ACU] Base treatment mainly on CV, ST, SP, and LI. Select CV-12 (*zhōng wǎn*, Center Stomach Duct), CV-8 (*shén què*, Spirit Gate Tower), ST-25 (*tiān shū*, Celestial Pivot), BL-25 (*dà cháng shū*, Large Intestine Transport), ST-36 (*zú sān lǐ*, Leg Three Li), SP-15 (*dà héng*, Great Horizontal), SP-4 (*gōng sūn*, Yellow Emperor), and LI-4 (*hé gǔ*, Union Valley); needle with drainage and add moxa. Moxibustion on ginger can be performed at CV-8 (*shén què*, Spirit Gate Tower). See MOUNTING. **2.** A condition of cold pain in the scrotum attributable to cold evil invading the reverting yin (*jué yīn*) liver channel. The scrotum becomes swollen, hard as stone, cold, and painful. Attending signs may include impotence, desire for warmth and aversion to cold, physical cold and cold limbs. The pulse is sunken, stringlike, and tight. [MED] Warm the liver and dissipate cold using Evodia Decoction (*wú zhū yú tāng*) plus aconite (*fù zǐ*), fenugreek (*hú lú bā*), lindera (*wū yào*), and fennel (*huí xiāng*). [ACU] Base treatment mainly on CV, LR, and SP. Select CV-6 (*qì hǎi*, Sea of Qi), CV-4 (*guān yuán*, Pass Head), SP-6 (*sān yīn jiāo*, Three Yin Intersection), and LR-1 (*dà dūn*, Large Pile), and needle with drainage and add moxa. See MOUNTING; compare YIN MOUNTING. [26: 658] [6: 201] [27: 429] [97: 570]

cold moxibustion 冷灸 *lěng jiǔ*: MEDICINAL-INDUCED BLISTER MOXIBUSTION.

cold night crying 寒夜啼 *hán yè tí*: NIGHT CRYING IN INFANTS attributed to vacuity cold in the organs. Cold night crying is characterized by crying associated with abdominal pain, lying with back bent, green-blue white facial complexion, lack of warmth in the limbs. [MED] Warm the center and dispel cold using Ginseng and Aconite Decoction (*shēn fù tāng*). [ACU] Base treatment mainly on CV, GV, PC, ST, and empirical points. Use large amounts of moxa at PC-6 (*nèi guān*, Inner Pass), CV-12 (*zhōng wǎn*, Center Stomach Duct), and ST-36 (*zú sān lǐ*, Leg Three Li), and pole GV-20 (*bǎi huì*, Hundred Convergences), and needle with even supplementation and drainage at Quiet Sleep (*ān mián*), Hall of Impression (*yìn táng*), and SI-3 (*hòu xī*, Back Ravine). [26: 658] [26: 659]

cold occlusion 寒膈 *hán gé*: From *Emergency Standby Remedies* (*zhǒu hòu bèi jí fāng*). Dysphagia-occlusion (*yē gé*) characterized by distention and fullness in the stomach duct and abdomen, nontransformation of food, hiccough, bitter cold in the abdomen, rumbling intestines, pain around the umbilicus, and emaciation. See DYSPHAGIA-OCCLUSION. [92: No. 260]

cold pain 冷痛 *lěng tòng*: Pain associated with a feeling of cold; attributed to cold evil. See PAIN. [29: 190]

cold pain in the heart [region] and abdomen 心腹冷痛 *xīn fù lěng tòng*: Acute pain in the pit of the stomach and below, associated with a sensation of cold.

cold panting 寒喘 *hán chuǎn*: **1.** PANTING attributable to yang vacuity and exuberant cold, associated with counterflow cold of the limbs, and a fine sunken pulse. [MED] Warm the lung and dissipate cold; assisting yang to absorb qi. Use Nine-Ingredient Center-Rectifying Decoction (*jiǔ wèi lǐ zhōng tāng*) plus aconite (*fù zǐ*). [ACU] Base treatment mainly on back transport points, CV and LU. Select BL-13 (*fèi shū*, Lung Transport), Panting Stabilizer (*dìng chuǎn*), BL-43 (*gāo huāng shū*, Gao-Huang Transport), LU-9 (*tài yuān*, Great Abyss), ST-36 (*zú sān lǐ*, Leg Three Li), BL-20 (*pí shū*, Spleen Transport), BL-23 (*shèn shū*, Kidney Transport), CV-6 (*qì hǎi*, Sea of Qi), GV-4 (*mìng mén*, Life Gate), and CV-4 (*guān yuán*, Pass Head); needle with supplementation, using large amounts of moxa. **2.** PANTING due to wind-cold fettering the exterior, and usually associated with exterior cold signs. [MED] Use Supplemented Rough and Ready Three Decoction (*jiā wèi sān ào tāng*). Alternatively, use variations of Ephedra Decoction (*má huáng tāng*) combined with Florid Canopy Powder (*huá gài sǎn*). [ACU] See WIND-COLD RAPID PANTING; PANTING. [26: 659]

cold pattern 寒证 *hán zhèng*: Any disease pattern characterized by cold signs such as aversion to cold, a somber white or green-blue facial complexion, slow or tight pulse, no thirst or desire for warm fluid, long voidings of clear urine. The complexion and the pulse are explained in terms of the principle that "cold causes contracture and tension" and tightens the blood vessels. Long voidings of clear urine and moist white tongue fur exemplify the general observation that "all disease with watery humors that are clear, pure, and cold is ascribed to cold." Cold patterns may be the result of the influence of yin evils or insufficiency of yang qi, this distinction being apparent in signs. (1) Prevalence of yin due to an exuberant yin evil accounts for pronounced cold signs such as abdominal pain, fulminant (i.e., sudden and violent) vomiting or diarrhea, green-blue facial complexion, and a tight pulse. (2) Yang vacuity accounts for signs more commonly encountered in clinical practice, such as liking for quiet, curled-up lying posture, long voidings of clear urine, clear-food diarrhea, counterflow cold of the limbs, and a slow pulse. Since cold evil may damage yang, and yang vacuity may engender cold, these two forms of cold are interrelated. Cold limbs and somber white facial complexion, which are commonly observed cold signs, are attributed to the debilitation of yang qi and the presence of an exuberant cold evil. MED Since "cold is treated with heat," warming is the chief method of treating cold patterns. Patterns mainly involving invasion by an external evil are treated by dissipating cold evil with warm medicinals. Those patterns primarily characterized by debilitation of yang qi are treated by warming yang and boosting qi. Commonly used medicinals that dissipate cold evil include aconite (*fù zǐ*), cinnamon bark (*ròu guì*), fresh ginger (*shēng jiāng*), dried ginger (*gān jiāng*), evodia (*wú zhū yú*), and lesser galangal (*gāo liáng jiāng*). In addition, aconite (*fù zǐ*) and cinnamon bark (*ròu guì*) possess a yang-warming effect. Ginseng (*rén shēn*), or its more economical substitute codonopsis (*dǎng shēn*), licorice (*gān cǎo*), ovate atractylodes (*bái zhú*), and other qi-supplementing medicinals can be added to boost qi. Cold-dissipating formulas include Lesser Galangal and Cyperus Pill (*liáng fù wán*), which is commonly used where there is pain. Ginseng and Aconite Decoction (*shēn fù tāng*), Counterflow Cold Decoction Plus Ginseng (*sì nì jiā rén shēn tāng*), and Center-Rectifying Pill (*lǐ zhōng wán*) are commonly used to warm yang and boost qi. ACU The use of moxibustion is important in treating cold patterns and conditions characterized by yang debilitation. Commonly used points include the following: CV-6 (*qì hǎi*, Sea of Qi)ⓜ, CV-4 (*guān yuán*, Pass Head)ⓜ, ST-36 (*zú sān lǐ*, Leg Three Li)ⓜ, SP-6 (*sān yīn jiāo*, Three Yin Intersection)ⓜ, BL-20 (*pí shū*, Spleen Transport)ⓜ, and GV-4 (*mìng mén*, Life Gate)ⓜ. [6: 153] [27: 212] [97: 571]

cold phlegm 寒痰 *hán tán*: PHLEGM with cold signs. Three patterns are observed: contraction of cold, vacuity phlegm, and phlegm-damp in the kidney channel. **Contraction of external wind-cold** causing cough, panting, and expectoration in patients usually suffering from phlegm disease is characterized by clear white phlegm, a white moist tongue fur, and a stagnant stringlike pulse. In some cases, there may be physical cold and cold limbs. MED Warm the lung and transform phlegm. Use Cough-Stopping Powder (*zhǐ sòu sǎn*) plus pinellia (*bàn xià*) and poria (*fú líng*). Alternatively, use Poria (Hoelen), Licorice, Schisandra, Ginger, and Asarum Decoction (*líng gān wǔ wèi jiāng xīn tāng*). ACU Base treatment mainly on LU and ST. Select CV-12 (*zhōng wǎn*, Center Stomach Duct), ST-36 (*zú sān lǐ*, Leg Three Li), ST-40 (*fēng lóng*, Bountiful Bulge), BL-13 (*fèi shū*, Lung Transport), LU-7 (*liè quē*, Broken Sequence), LI-4 (*hé gǔ*, Union Valley), BL-12 (*fēng mén*, Wind Gate), and BL-11 (*dà zhù*, Great Shuttle)ⓜ; needle with drainage and add moxa. **Vacuity phlegm,** i.e., yang vacuity with contention be-

tween cold and dampness, is a cold phlegm pattern characterized by limp aching legs and knees, stiff lumbus and back, cold impediment (*hán bì*) in the joints, and bone pain. This condition is sometimes also referred to as *vacuity phlegm*. MED Warm and free the channels and vessels to dissipate cold-damp. Use Impediment-Alleviating Decoction (*juān bì tāng*) plus poria (*fú líng*), pinellia (*bàn xià*), bile arisaema (*dǎn xīng*), and dried bamboo sap (*zhú lì*). For pronounced cold, add cinnamon bark (*ròu guì*) and aconite (*fù zǐ*); For pronounced dampness, add fangji (*fáng jǐ*) and coix (*yì yǐ rén*). ACU Base treatment mainly on GV, CV, ST, and SP. Main points: BL-23 (*shèn shū*, Kidney Transport), GV-4 (*mìng mén*, Life Gate), CV-4 (*guān yuán*, Pass Head), ST-36 (*zú sān lǐ*, Leg Three Li), SP-9 (*yīn líng quán*, Yin Mound Spring), and SP-5 (*shāng qiū*, Shang Hill); needle with drainage and large amounts of moxa. Apply moxibustion on salt or ginger at CV-8 (*shén què*, Spirit Gate Tower). For selection of points according to affected area, see IMPEDIMENT. **Phlegm-damp in the kidney channel** is characterized by a sunken pulse, black face, urinary urgency with pain on voiding, cold lower extremities, and feelings of fear. The phlegm is copious and thin, with black speckles. MED Fortify the spleen, warm the kidney, and transform phlegm. ACU Base treatment mainly on back transport points, CV, KI, and ST. Select BL-20 (*pí shū*, Spleen Transport), BL-21 (*wèi shū*, Stomach Transport), CV-12 (*zhōng wǎn*, Center Stomach Duct), ST-36 (*zú sān lǐ*, Leg Three Li), ST-40 (*fēng lóng*, Bountiful Bulge), BL-23 (*shèn shū*, Kidney Transport), CV-4 (*guān yuán*, Pass Head), and KI-3 (*tài xī*, Great Ravine); needle with supplementation and add moxa. Selection of points according to signs: For urinary urgency and painful urination, add CV-3 (*zhōng jí*, Central Pole), SP-6 (*sān yīn jiāo*, Three Yin Intersection), and LR-2 (*xíng jiān*, Moving Between). [26: 660] [27: 380] [97: 572] [46: 597, 628]

cold phlegm obstructing the lung 寒痰阻肺 *hán tán zǔ fèi*: See COLD PHLEGM. [57: 79]

cold precipitation 寒下 *hán xià*: A method of treating interior heat repletion patterns with signs such as constipation, abdominal fullness, tidal heat [effusion], dry mouth and thirst, parched yellow tongue fur, forceful slippery rapid pulse; also treats food and water accumulations. MED Cold precipitation makes use of cold bitter medicinals such as rhubarb (*dà huáng*), mirabilite (*máng xiāo*), and senna (*fān xiè yè*). Cold precipitating formulas include Major Qi-Coordinating Decoction (*dà chéng qì tāng*), Minor Qi-Coordinating Decoction (*xiǎo chéng qì tāng*), and Stomach-Regulating Qi-Coordinating Decoction (*tiáo wèi chéng qì tāng*). See PRECIPITATION. [26: 656] [27: 256] [97: 570]

cold qi abdominal pain 寒气腹痛 *hán qì fù tòng*:
Synonym: cold abdominal pain. ABDOMINAL PAIN
due to spleen-stomach vacuity cold or to external
cold evil contraction, and characterized by continual pain exacerbated by exposure to cold, relieved slightly by warmth, and accompanied by a
slow sunken pulse. [MED] Warm the center and
dissipate cold; rectify qi and relieve pain. Use
Magnolia Bark Center-Warming Decoction (*hòu pò
wēn zhōng tāng*) or Center-Rectifying Decoction (*lǐ
zhōng tāng*). Compare the more severe COLD AC-
CUMULATION ABDOMINAL PAIN. [ACU] Base treatment mainly on CV, SP, and ST. Select CV-12
(*zhōng wǎn*, Center Stomach Duct), ST-36 (*zú sān
lǐ,* Leg Three Li), SP-15 (*dà hèng*, Great Horizontal), SP-4 (*gōng sūn*, Yellow Emperor), and LI-4
(*hé gǔ*, Union Valley); needle with drainage and
add moxa. [26: 657] [46: 662] [37: 317]

cold repletion 寒实 *hán shí*: Patterns in which
the cold evil stagnates and binds internally, characterized by harmony of the mouth (no particular
taste in the mouth), cold limbs, long voidings of
clear urine, abdominal pain that refuses pressure,
constipation, a white tongue fur, and a stringlike
sunken pulse. ◇ Chin 寒 *hán*, cold; 实 *shí*, repletion. The reason for the difference in order of components from that of 实热 *shí rè* is not clear. [26:
660] [27: 116] [97: 572]

cold repletion chest bind 寒实结胸 *hán shí jié
xiōng*: A CHEST BIND pattern marked by painful
hardness and distention in the stomach duct without generalized heat [effusion] and without thirst,
associated with a sunken tight or slow sunken
pulse. [MED] Dispel cold and open binds with
Three Agents White Powder (*sān wù bái sǎn*). For
patients with a vacuity constitution in whom the
signs are not pronounced, Unripe Bitter Orange
Center-Rectifying Pill (*zhǐ shí lǐ zhōng wán*) can
be used. [ACU] Select PC-6 (*nèi guān*, Inner Pass),
CV-12 (*zhōng wǎn*, Center Stomach Duct), ST-36
(*zú sān lǐ*, Leg Three Li), and SP-4 (*gōng sūn*,
Yellow Emperor); needle with drainage and moxa.
[26: 660] [27: 376] [97: 574]

cold reversal 寒厥 *hán jué*: A REVERSAL PAT-
TERN attributable to yang vacuity and yin exuberance, characterized by reversal cold of the extremities, aversion to cold and lying in curled-up
posture, clear-food diarrhea, and absence of thirst.
In some cases, there is cold body and curled posture, abdominal pain, red face, green-blue nails,
and, in severe cases, CLOUDING REVERSAL. The
tongue body is pale with moist fur, and the pulse is
usually faint and fine. [MED] Warm yang and boost
qi. For patients showing signs of blood vacuity and
congealing cold, also nourish the blood and harmonize construction. Use Counterflow Cold Decoction (*sì nì tāng*), Vessel-Freeing Counterflow Cold

Decoction (*tōng mài sì nì tāng*), Aconite Center-
Rectifying Decoction (*fù zǐ lǐ zhōng tāng*), and
Tangkuei Counterflow Cold Decoction (*dāng guī
sì nì tāng*). [ACU] Base treatment mainly on back
transport points, GV, CV, and ST. Select BL-23
(*shèn shū*, Kidney Transport), GV-4 (*mìng mén*,
Life Gate), CV-4 (*guān yuán*, Pass Head), ST-36
(*zú sān lǐ*, Leg Three Li), CV-6 (*qì hǎi*, Sea of Qi),
and needle with supplementation and add moxa.
Apply moxibustion on ginger or salt at CV-8 (*shén
què*, Spirit Gate Tower). [26: 659] [37: 401] [27:
401] [97: 571]

cold reversal heart pain 寒厥心痛 *hán jué xīn
tòng*: See COLD HEART PAIN. [26: 659]

cold rheum 寒饮 *hán yǐn*: See next entry.

cold rheum lying latent in the lung 寒饮伏
肺 *hán yǐn fú fèi*: One form of PROPPING RHEUM,
characterized by cough counterflow, panting, and
fullness preventing the patient from lying flat, attributable to rheum evil ascending to invade the
lung and preventing normal downbearing of lung
qi. It is a persistent condition, episodes of which
are brought on or exacerbated by exposure to cold
and which are characterized by heat effusion and
aversion to cold, back pain, lumbar pain, and copious foamy white phlegm. The tongue is white
and glossy, and the pulse is stringlike and tight.
There may also be swelling of the face and instep.
[MED] Warm the lung and transform rheum with
formulas such as Minor Green-Blue Dragon Decoction (*xiǎo qīng lóng tāng*). See RHEUM. [80: 151]

cold stagnating in the liver vessel 寒滞肝脉
hán zhì gān mài: Cold evil (usually externally contracted) congealing in the liver channel causing
liver channel qi and blood to stagnate. The chief
signs are lesser-abdominal pain that may stretch
into the testicles, and that may be associated with
RETRACTED SCROTUM. Secondary signs include
bright white facial complexion, physical cold and
cold limbs, green-blue or purple lips, long voidings
of clear urine, and sloppy stool. The tongue is pale
with a glossy white fur. The pulse is sunken and
stringlike, and possibly slow. **Analysis:** The liver
channel spreads over the rib-side, passes through
the lesser abdomen, and connects with the external genitals. When cold evil stagnates in the liver
vessel, there are signs of hypertonicity along the
course of the channel. *Elementary Questions (sù
wèn)* states, "The reverting yin (*jué yīn*) vessel
connects with the yin organs (genitals) and ties to
the liver; when cold qi settles in [this] vessel, the
blood congeals and the pulse because urgent; hence
pain from the rib-side to the lesser abdomen." This
describes the pathomechanism of cold congealing
in the liver vessel. [MED] Warm the liver and dissipate cold. Use Liver-Warming Brew (*nuǎn gān
jiān*). [ACU] Base treatment mainly on CV and LR.

Select CV-4 (*guān yuán*, Pass Head), CV-6 (*qì hǎi*, Sea of Qi), SP-6 (*sān yīn jiāo*, Three Yin Intersection), and LR-1 (*dà dūn*, Large Pile); needle with drainage; moxa can also be used, in large amounts if cold signs are pronounced. For physical cold and cold limbs, add ST-36 (*zú sān lǐ*, Leg Three Li) and CV-8 (*shén què*, Spirit Gate Tower)ⓜ. Compare LIVER COLD. See MOUNTING. [27: 153] [97: 574] [25: 314] [116: 107] [57: 63] [50: 1580] [37: 454] [46: 592, 680]

cold strangury 冷淋 *lěng lín*: **1.** A STRANGURY pattern described in *Sages' Aid Records* (*shèng jì zǒng lù*) as, "It manifests first with cold shivering, then as urinary strangury." It is attributed to kidney vacuity and with cold qi settling in the lower burner. MED Treat by warming the kidney, plus freeing and disinhibiting. Use Cistanche Pill (*ròu cōng róng wán*) or Raw Aconite Powder (*shēng fù sǎn*). ACU Base treatment mainly on the three yin channels of the foot and alarm and back transport points of BL (CV-3 and BL-28). Select BL-28 (*páng guāng shū*, Bladder Transport), CV-3 (*zhōng jí,* Central Pole), SP-9 (*yīn líng quán,* Yin Mound Spring), KI-3 (*tài xī,* Great Ravine), BL-23 (*shèn shū,* Kidney Transport), GV-4 (*mìng mén,* Life Gate), CV-4 (*guān yuán,* Pass Head), and KI-7 (*fù liū,* Recover Flow); needle with supplementation and add moxa. **2.** From *Central Treasury Canon* (*zhōng zàng jīng, lùn lín lì xiǎo biàn bù lì*). A disease pattern marked by frequent urination with urine like rice water. **3.** Blood strangury ascribed to vacuity cold of the lower origin marked by dribbling urination with urine dark with static blood. MED This pattern is exacerbated by the use of cold and cool medicinals. Use Golden Coffer Kidney Qi Pill (*jīn guì shèn qì wán*). ACU Base treatment mainly on the three yin channels of the foot and alarm and back transport points of BL (CV-3 and BL-28). Select BL-28 (*páng guāng shū,* Bladder Transport), CV-3 (*zhōng jí,* Central Pole), SP-9 (*yīn líng quán,* Yin Mound Spring), LR-2 (*xíng jiān,* Moving Between), BL-20 (*pí shū,* Spleen Transport), BL-23 (*shèn shū,* Kidney Transport), GV-4 (*mìng mén,* Life Gate), CV-4 (*guān yuán,* Pass Head), and ST-36 (*zú sān lǐ,* Leg Three Li); needle with drainage and add moxa. [26: 298]

cold stroke 寒中 *hán zhòng*: **1.** A form of WIND-LIKE STROKE that arises when cold evil invades the channels, and that is characterized by rigid body, clenched jaw preventing speech, shaking of the limbs, sudden dizziness, and absence of sweating. MED Warm the interior and dissipate cold using Ginger and Aconite Decoction (*jiāng fù tāng*) or Aconite Center-Rectifying Decoction (*fù zǐ lǐ zhōng tāng*). In severe cases, Liquid Storax Pill (*sū hé xiāng wán*) may be given first to open the block. ACU Base treatment mainly on GV and CV. Apply moxa at GV-20 (*bǎi huì,* Hundred Con-

vergences), CV-8 (*shén què,* Spirit Gate Tower), CV-4 (*guān yuán,* Pass Head), CV-12 (*zhōng wǎn,* Center Stomach Duct), CV-6 (*qì hǎi,* Sea of Qi), and ST-25 (*tiān shū,* Celestial Pivot), until the limbs become warm, the pulse rises, and the patient's spirit-mind becomes clear. **2.** Evil in the spleen and stomach with interior cold signs. It is usually due to spleen-stomach vacuity cold with evils transforming with cold, or develops from taxation fatigue and internal damage. Signs include abdominal pain, diarrhea, and rumbling intestines. MED Warm the center and dissipate cold with Aquilaria Stomach-Warming Pill (*chén xiāng wēn wèi wán*). ACU Base treatment mainly on CV, SP, ST, and LI. Select CV-12 (*zhōng wǎn,* Center Stomach Duct), ST-36 (*zú sān lǐ,* Leg Three Li), PC-6 (*nèi guān,* Inner Pass), SP-4 (*gōng sūn,* Yellow Emperor), and LI-4 (*hé gǔ,* Union Valley); needle with drainage and large amounts of moxa. [26: 657] [50: 1574] [27: 570] [46: 660, 662]

cold sweating 冷汗 *lěng hàn*: **1.** SWEATING due to a) yang vacuity (treated by warming and supplementing), b) heat gathering internally (treated by cooling the blood and clearing heat), or c) phlegm (treated by normalizing qi and transforming phlegm). **2.** YIN SWEATING.

cold tearing 冷泪 *lěng lèi*: TEARING (lacrimation) attributable to dual vacuity of the liver and kidney and depletion of essence blood attracting contraction of external wind. It may also be attributable to MILLET SORES or to nose problems such as nasal congestion. Tearing occurs periodically, is exacerbated or brought on by exposure to wind (see also TEARING ON EXPOSURE TO WIND), and is not associated with any heat or pain. The tear water is clear. MED Liver-kidney vacuity is treated by supplementing the liver and kidney. Use Lycium Berry, Chrysanthemum, and Rehmannia Pill (*qǐ jú dì huáng wán*). [26: 298]

cold tetany 寒痉 *hán jìng*: A disease described by Wu Ju-Tong (1758–1836, Qing) as tetany occurring in children suffering from wind-cold cough. MED Use Apricot Kernel and Perilla Powder (*xìng sū sǎn*). ACU Base treatment mainly on LU, LI, and GV. Select BL-13 (*fèi shū,* Lung Transport), LU-7 (*liè quē,* Broken Sequence), LI-4 (*hé gǔ,* Union Valley), BL-11 (*dà zhù,* Great Shuttle), GV-16 (*fēng fǔ,* Wind Mansion), GV-20 (*bǎi huì,* Hundred Convergences), GV-26 (*shuǐ gōu,* Water Trough), and GV-8 (*jīn suō,* Sinew Contraction). Needle with drainage and add moxa. See TETANY. [26: 658] [42: 188]

cold vomiting 寒呕 *hán ǒu,* 寒吐 *hán tù*: VOMITING attributed to stomach vacuity cold or stomach repletion cold (including excessive consumption of cold, raw foods or external evil invading the stomach). It is characterized by vomiting long after eating, or vomiting on exposure to cold, and is associated with green-blue facial complexion, cold extremities, and a sunken fine slow, sometimes stringlike pulse. [MED] Warm the stomach and dissipate cold with Evodia Decoction (*wú zhū yú tāng*), Center-Rectifying Decoction (*lǐ zhōng tāng*), or Counterflow Cold Decoction (*sì nì tāng*). [ACU] For vacuity cold, base treatment on alarm and lower uniting points of ST, and on PC, CV, SP, and back transport points. Select CV-12 (*zhōng wǎn*, Center Stomach Duct), ST-36 (*zú sān lǐ*, Leg Three Li), PC-6 (*nèi guān*, Inner Pass), BL-21 (*wèi shū*, Stomach Transport), CV-13 (*shàng wǎn*, Upper Stomach Duct), SP-4 (*gōng sūn*, Yellow Emperor), and CV-4 (*guān yuán*, Pass Head)ⓜ; needle with supplementation and add moxa. For repletion cold, base treatment mainly on ST points. Select CV-12 (*zhōng wǎn*, Center Stomach Duct), ST-36 (*zú sān lǐ*, Leg Three Li), ST-44 (*nèi tíng*, Inner Court), ST-21 (*liáng mén*, Beam Gate), and PC-6 (*nèi guān*, Inner Pass). Needle with drainage and large amounts of moxa. For external cold invading the stomach, add GB-20 (*fēng chí*, Wind Pool), TB-5 (*wài guān*, Outer Pass), LI-4 (*hé gǔ*, Union Valley), and LU-7 (*liè quē*, Broken Sequence); needle with drainage and large amounts of moxa. [26: 657, 660] [46: 659] [37: 306] [113: 71]

cold wheezing 冷哮 *lěng xiāo*: WHEEZING due to cold phlegm and water-rheum that arises when externally contracted wind-cold entering the lung collects internally with rheum to obstruct the airways. Cold wheezing is characterized by hasty breathing with a wheezing rale in the throat, coughing of clear thin stick phlegm, stifling oppression in the chest, dull gray facial complexion, a white glossy tongue fur, and a tight floating pulse. [MED] Warm the lung and dissipate cold; sweep phlegm and disinhibit the orifices. Use Belamcanda and Ephedra Decoction (*shè gān má huáng tāng*) or Three-Seed Decoction (*sān zǐ tāng*). [ACU] Base treatment mainly on back transport points, CV, and LU to warm and regulate lung qi. Select BL-13 (*fèi shū*, Lung Transport), BL-12 (*fēng mén*, Wind Gate), CV-17 (*shān zhōng*, Chest Center), BL-43 (*gāo huāng shū*, Gao-Huang Transport), Panting Stabilizer (*dìng chuǎn*), LU-7 (*liè quē*, Broken Sequence), CV-22 (*tiān tú*, Celestial Chimney), CV-12 (*zhōng wǎn*, Center Stomach Duct), and ST-40 (*fēng lóng*, Bountiful Bulge); needle with even supplementation and drainage, followed by large amounts of moxa. For stifling oppression in the chest, add PC-6 (*nèi guān*, Inner Pass) and BL-17 (*gé shū*, Diaphragm Transport). Formerly, the term cold wheezing also included wheezing due to COLD ENVELOPING HEAT, which is now categorized as a form of HEAT WHEEZING. [26: 297] [37: 281] [46: 653]

collapse 亡 *wáng*: Acute, critical forms of vacuity. High fever, great sweating, fulminant vomiting, fulminant diarrhea, and heavy bleeding may all lead to severe depletion of yang qi and yin blood. In such cases, both yang qi and yin humor are damaged. Since yin and yang are interdependent, when yin collapses yang has no support and scatters, and when yang collapses, yin humor is no longer produced and is gradually depleted. Thus, yin collapse may swiftly cause yang collapse, and yang collapse invariably causes damage to yin. See YANG COLLAPSE; YIN COLLAPSE; FLUID COLLAPSE; BLOOD COLLAPSE; EXUBERANCE AND DEBILITATION. ◊ Chin 亡 *wáng*, die, perish, be ruined.

collect 停 *tíng*: Accumulation, as of water, in specific locations; e.g., water collecting around the stomach. See STOPPAGE. ◊ Chin 停 *tíng*, stop, stagnate, remain.

collecting rheum dizziness 停饮眩晕 *tíng yǐn xuàn yūn*: DIZZINESS attributed to the nonmovement of center yang and internal gathering of water-rheum and characterized by fearful throbbing, heart palpitations, or palpitations below the umbilicus, and vomiting of foamy drool. [MED] Treat by freeing yang and transforming rheum with Poria (Hoelen), Cinnamon Twig, Ovate Atractylodes, and Licorice Decoction (*líng guì zhú gān tāng*), Minor Pinellia Decoction Plus Poria (Hoelen) (*xiǎo bàn xià jiā fú líng tāng*), or Alisma Decoction (*zé xiè tāng*). See PHLEGM-RHEUM DIZZINESS; DIZZINESS. [26: 650]

collecting rheum heart palpitations 停饮心悸 *tíng yǐn xī jì*: HEART PALPITATIONS attributable to water-rheum collecting internally. Apart from heart palpitations, other signs include glomus and fullness in the chest and stomach duct, dizziness, nausea, short voidings of scant urine, white tongue fur, and a stringlike pulse. [MED] Free yang and transform rheum. Use Poria (Hoelen), Cinnamon Twig, Ovate Atractylodes, and Licorice Decoction (*líng guì zhú gān tāng*) combined with Major Pinellia Decoction (*dà bàn xià tāng*). [ACU] Base treatment mainly on back transport points, CV, HT, PC, and ST. Select BL-15 (*xīn shū*, Heart Transport), HT-7 (*shén mén*, Spirit Gate), PC-6 (*nèi guān*, Inner Pass), BL-21 (*wèi shū*, Stomach Transport), BL-22 (*sān jiāo shū*, Triple Burner Transport), CV-17 (*shān zhōng*, Chest Center), CV-6 (*qì hǎi*, Sea of Qi), CV-12 (*zhōng wǎn*, Center Stomach Duct), and ST-36 (*zú sān lǐ*, Leg Three Li); needle with even supplementation and drainage. See HEART PALPITATIONS. [26: 650]

collecting rheum rib-side pain 停饮胁痛 *tíng yǐn xié tòng*: Synonym: *phlegm-rheum rib-side pain*. RIB-SIDE PAIN attributed to water-rheum or phlegm-turbidity flowing into the liver channel and obstructing qi dynamic. The pain is a moving or flowing pain in severe cases associated with gurgling sounds. Other signs include cough, rapid breathing, and a stringlike sunken pulse. MED Flush phlegm and free the network vessels using formulas such as Phlegm-Abducting Decoction (*dǎo tán tāng*) or Drool-Controlling Elixir (*kòng xián dān*) and variations. ACU Base treatment mainly on GB/TB and ST/LI. Select ST-40 (*fēng lóng*, Bountiful Bulge), ST-36 (*zú sān lǐ*, Leg Three Li), LI-4 (*hé gǔ*, Union Valley), LU-5 (*chǐ zé*, Cubit Marsh), SP-9 (*yīn líng quán*, Yin Mound Spring), LR-14 (*qī mén*, Cycle Gate), GB-24 (*rì yuè*, Sun and Moon), TB-6 (*zhī gōu*, Branch Ditch), and GB-34 (*yáng líng quán*, Yang Mound Spring). Needle with even supplementation and drainage. Compare PHLEGM-RHEUM RIB-SIDE PAIN. [26: 650]

coma 昏迷（不醒）*hūn mí* (*bù xǐng*): Clouding of the spirit with complete or partial loss of consciousness; usually caused by evil obstructing the clear orifices and clouding the spirit light. Coma may be observed in cold damage, warm disease, wind stroke, inversion patterns, and epilepsy. Whether due to external contraction or to internal damage, it is always a critical sign. MED Treatment should be determined according to cause, but the first step is to open the orifices and arouse the spirit using formulas such as Liquid Storax Pill (*sū hé xiāng wán*), Supreme Jewel Elixir (*zhì bǎo dān*), Purple Snow Elixir (*zǐ xuě dān*), Peaceful Palace Bovine Bezoar Pill (*ān gōng niú huáng wán*), and Bovine Bezoar Heart-Clearing Pill (*niú huáng qīng xīn wán*). ACU To open the orifices and arouse the spirit, needle GV-26 (*rén zhōng*, Human Center), KI-1 (*yǒng quán*, Gushing Spring), HT-7 (*shén mén*, Spirit Gate), and PC-8 (*láo gōng*, Palace of Toil), and prick Ten Diffusing Points (*shí xuān*) to bleed. See OPENING THE ORIFICES. [50: 963] [46: 602]

combination 相兼 *xiāng jiān*: A two- or threefold concurrence of interior, exterior, cold, heat, vacuity and repletion, excluding cold with heat or vacuity with repletion, which, involving contradictions in the nature of the disease, are known as complexes rather than combinations. Most disease patterns are combinations. For example, initial-stage externally contracted heat (febrile) diseases manifest as exterior patterns, which must be further differentiated as exterior cold or exterior heat. Enduring diseases presenting as vacuity patterns must be further differentiated into vacuity cold and vacuity heat. Clearly the principles follow a strict order of importance. Exterior cold and exterior heat patterns are primarily exterior patterns, and secondarily cold or heat patterns. Vacuity cold and vacuity heat patterns are primarily vacuity patterns and secondarily cold or heat patterns. In interior-

exterior combinations, principle precedence varies from case to case. Compare COMPLEX. [6: 148]

combination disease 合病 *hé bìng*: Cold damage disease affecting two or three channels. Compare DRAGOVER DISEASE. [26: 290]

combined treatment of lung and kidney 肺肾同治 *fèi shèn tóng zhì*: Simultaneous treatment of lung yin vacuity and kidney yin vacuity to treat cough with counterflow qi ascent, coughing of blood, loss of voice, steaming bone tidal heat [effusion], dry mouth, night sweating, seminal emission, aching lumbus and limp legs, emaciation, red tongue with scant fur, and rapid fine pulse. Medicinals used include adenophora/glehnia (*shā shēn*), asparagus (*tiān mén dōng*), ophiopogon (*mài mén dōng*), Solomon's seal (*yù zhú*), dried/fresh rehmannia (*shēng dì huáng*), cooked rehmannia (*shú dì huáng*), ligustrum (*nǔ zhēn zǐ*), lycium berry (*gǒu qǐ zǐ*), and eclipta (*mò hàn lián*). ACU Base treatment mainly LU and KI. Select BL-13 (*fèi shū*, Lung Transport), BL-23 (*shèn shū*, Kidney Transport), BL-43 (*gāo huāng shū*, Gao-Huang Transport), LU-5 (*chǐ zé*, Cubit Marsh), KI-6 (*zhào hǎi*, Shining Sea), and KI-3 (*tài xī*, Great Ravine); needle with supplementation. [26: 449] [27: 221] [97: 208]

combining front and back points 俞募配穴法 *shū mù pèi xué fǎ*: COMBINING TRANSPORT AND ALARM POINTS. [46: 600]

combining guest and host points 主客配穴法 *zhǔ kè pèi xué fǎ*: See COMBINING SOURCE AND NETWORK POINTS.

combining left and right points 左右配穴法 *zuǒ yòu pèi xué fǎ*: Combining the corresponding points on either side of the body. For example, bilateral ST-36 (*zú sān lǐ*, Leg Three Li) points can be needled for stomach pain; bilateral Greater Yang (*tài yáng*) or LU-7 (*liè quē*, Broken Sequence) points can be needled for headache; and bilateral SP-6 (*sān yīn jiāo*, Three Yin Intersection) points can be needled for some women's problems. See POINT COMBINATION. [79: 268]

combining local and distant points 远近配穴法 *yuǎn jìn pèi xué fǎ*: Combined needling of points close to the affected area with others at a distance from it. For example, stomach pain can be treated with local points such as CV-12 (*zhōng wǎn*, Center Stomach Duct) and BL-21 (*wèi shū*, Stomach Transport) combined with distant points such as PC-6 (*nèi guān*, Inner Pass) and ST-36 (*zú sān lǐ*, Leg Three Li). More examples of combinations are presented in the list below. See POINT COMBINATION. [26: 835] [46: 610]

Combining Local (L) and Distant (D) Points

Forehead
  L. Hall of Impression (*yìn táng*)
    GB-14 (*yáng bái*, Yang White)
  D. LI-4 (*hé gǔ*, Union Valley)
    ST-44 (*nèi tíng*, Inner Court)

Temples
  L. Greater Yang (*tài yáng*)
    GB-8 (*shuài gǔ*, Valley Lead)
  D. GB-32 (*zhōng dú*, Central River)
    GB-41 (*zú lín qì*, Foot Overlooking Tears)

Back of head
  L. GB-20 (*fēng chí*, Wind Pool)
    BL-10 (*tiān zhù*, Celestial Pillar)
  D. SI-3 (*hòu xī*, Back Ravine)
    BL-65 (*shù gǔ*, Bundle Bone)

Vertex
  L. GV-20 (*bǎi huì*, Hundred Convergences)
  D. LR-3 (*tài chōng*, Supreme Surge)

Eye
  L. BL-1 (*jīng míng*, Bright Eyes)
    ST-1 (*chéng qì*, Tear Container)
    GB-20 (*fēng chí*, Wind Pool)
  D. LI-4 (*hé gǔ*, Union Valley)

Nose
  L. Hall of Impression (*yìn táng*)
    LI-20 (*yíng xiāng*, Welcome Fragrance)
  D. LI-4 (*hé gǔ*, Union Valley)

Mouth and Teeth
  L. ST-6 (*jiá chē*, Cheek Carriage)
    ST-7 (*xià guān*, Below the Joint)
    ST-4 (*dì cāng*, Earth Granary)
  D. LI-4 (*hé gǔ*, Union Valley)

Ear
  L. TB-17 (*yì fēng*, Wind Screen)
    SI-19 (*tīng gōng*, Auditory Palace)
    GB-2 (*tīng huì*, Auditory Convergence)
  D. GB-32 (*zhōng dú*, Central River)
    TB-5 (*wài guān*, Outer Pass)

Tongue
  L. CV-23 (*lián quán*, Ridge Spring)
  D. PC-8 (*láo gōng*, Palace of Toil)

Throat
  L. SI-17 (*tiān róng*, Celestial Countenance)
  D. LI-4 (*hé gǔ*, Union Valley)

Lung
  L. BL-13 (*fèi shū*, Lung Transport)
    CV-17 (*dàn zhōng*, Chest Center)
    SI-17 (*tiān róng*, Celestial Countenance)
  D. LU-7 (*liè quē*, Broken Sequence)
    LU-5 (*chǐ zé*, Cubit Marsh)

Heart
  L. BL-15 (*xīn shū*, Heart Transport)
    BL-14 (*jué yīn shū*, Reverting Yin Transport)
    CV-17 (*dàn zhōng*, Chest Center)
  D. PC-6 (*nèi guān*, Inner Pass)
    HT-7 (*shén mén*, Spirit Gate)

PC-5 (*jiān shǐ*, Intermediary Courier)
PC-4 (*xī mén*, Cleft Gate)

Stomach
  L. BL-21 (*wèi shū*, Stomach Transport)
    CV-12 (*zhōng wǎn*, Center Stomach Duct)
  D. PC-6 (*nèi guān*, Inner Pass)
    ST-36 (*zú sān lǐ*, Leg Three Li)

Liver
  L. BL-18 (*gān shū*, Liver Transport)
  D. LR-3 (*tài chōng*, Supreme Surge)

Gallbladder
  L. BL-19 (*dǎn shū*, Gallbladder Transport)
  D. GB-34 (*yáng líng quán*, Yang Mound Spring)

Intestines
  L. BL-25 (*dà cháng shū*, Large Intestine Transport)
    BL-27 (*xiǎo cháng shū*, Small Intestine Transport)
    ST-25 (*tiān shū*, Celestial Pivot)
    CV-4 (*guān yuán*, Pass Head)
  D. ST-37 (*shàng jù xū*, Upper Great Hollow)
    ST-36 (*zú sān lǐ*, Leg Three Li)
    ST-39 (*xià jù xū*, Lower Great Hollow)

Kidney
  BL-23 (*shèn shū*, Kidney Transport)
  BL-52 (*zhì shì*, Will Chamber)
  KI-3 (*tài xī*, Great Ravine)

Bladder
  L. BL-32 (*cì liáo*, Second Bone-Hole)
    CV-3 (*zhōng jí*, Central Pole)
  D. SP-6 (*sān yīn jiāo*, Three Yin Intersection)

Anus
  L. GV-1 (*cháng qiáng*, Long Strong)
    BL-54 (*zhì biān*, Sequential Limit)
  D. BL-57 (*chéng shān*, Mountain Support)

Upper limbs
  L. TB-14 (*jiān liáo*, Shoulder Bone-Hole)
    LI-11 (*qū chí*, Pool at the Bend)
    LI-4 (*hé gǔ*, Union Valley)
  D. Paravertebrals (*jiā jí*)i C_1–T_1

Lower limbs
  L. GB-30 (*huán tiào*, Jumping Round)
    BL-40 (*wěi zhōng*, Bend Center)
    GB-34 (*yáng líng quán*, Yang Mound Spring)
    GB-39 (*xuán zhōng*, Suspended Bell)
  D. Paravertebrals (*jiā jí*)i C_1–T_1

---

combining same-name channel points 同名
经配穴法 *tóng míng jīng pèi xué fǎ*: Combined
needling of points on the hand and foot channels with the same yin-yang name (e.g., the foot
lesser yang gallbladder channel and the hand lesser
yang triple burner channel).   Combining same-
name channel points is based on the rationale that
the channels of the same name are linked to each

other (the hand and foot yang brightness channels at the side of the nose, the hand and foot lesser yang channels at outer canthus, hand and foot greater yang channels at the inner canthus, the hand and foot greater yin channels in the chest, the hand and foot reverting yin channels in the chest, and the hand and foot lesser yin channel in the heart [region]). Examples of same-channel point combinations include: LI-4 (*hé gǔ*, Union Valley) and ST-41 (*jiě xī*, Ravine Divide) or the yang brightness for frontal headache; TB-5 (*wài guān*, Outer Pass) and GB-41 (*zú lín qì*, Foot Overlooking Tears) of the lesser yang for hemilateral headache; SI-3 (*hòu xī*, Back Ravine) and BL-62 (*shēn mài*, Extending Vessel) for posterior headache; LU-11 (*shào shāng*, Lesser Shang) and SP-1 (*yǐn bái*, Hidden White) of the lesser yin for mania and withdrawal; PC-6 (*nèi guān*, Inner Pass) and LR-3 (*tài chōng*, Supreme Surge) of the reverting yin for epilepsy; and HT-7 (*shén mén*, Spirit Gate) and KI-6 (*zhào hǎi*, Shining Sea) of the lesser yin for insomnia. See POINT COMBINATION. [46: 600]

combining source and network points 原络配穴法 *yuán luò pèi xué fǎ*: Synonym: *combining guest and host points* Simultaneous needling of source points and network points. When both bowel and viscus an exterior-interior pair are diseased, the source of the channel of the one is combined with the network point of the channel associated with the other. The general rule is that the source point of the more severely or more chronically involved organ is coupled with the network point of the less involved organ. For example, severe panting with mild constipation can be treated by needling the source point of the lung, LU-9 (*tài yuān*, Great Abyss), and the network point of the large intestine, LI-6 (*piān lì*, Veering Passageway). The less involved channel is termed the guest, and the more involved channel is termed the host, so this method of treatment is sometimes called guest-host treatment. See the list below and POINT COMBINATION. [46: 600]

Combining Source (S) and Network (N) Points

Lung
　S. LU-9 (*tài yuān*, Great Abyss)
　N. LI-16 (*jù gǔ*, Great Bone)
　　Sore throat, shortness of breath, copious phlegm, sweating, heat in the hearts of the palms and soles, breast pain, lung channel shoulder pain.

Spleen
　S. SP-3 (*tài bái*, Supreme White)
　N. ST-40 (*fēng lóng*, Bountiful Bulge)
　　Stiff tongue, abdominal pain, heavy body, constipation, jaundice, spleen channel leg pain, malaria.

Stomach
　S. ST-42 (*chōng yáng*, Surging Yang)
　N. SP-4 (*gōng sūn*, Yellow Emperor)
　　Nosebleed, facial numbness, stomach channel leg pain, malaria, abdominal distention, general weakness.

Heart
　S. HT-7 (*shén mén*, Spirit Gate)
　N. SI-7 (*zhī zhèng*, Branch to the Correct)
　　Heart pain, palpitation, dry mouth, yellow eyes, heart channel arm pain.

Small Intestine
　S. SI-4 (*wàn gǔ*, Wrist Bone)
　N. HT-5 (*tōng lǐ*, Connecting Li)
　　Pain and swelling under the chin, should pain, neck pain, deafness, small intestine channel arm pain.

Kidney
　S. KI-3 (*tài xī*, Great Ravine)
　N. BL-58 (*fēi yáng*, Taking Flight)
　　Lassitude of spirit, poor appetite, poor visual acuity, aching lumbus and limp legs, gray facial complexion.

Bladder
　S. BL-64 (*jīng gǔ*, Capital Bone)
　N. PC-6 (*nèi guān*, Inner Pass)
　　Eye pain, neck pain, back pain, lumbar and leg pain, epilepsy, nosebleed, prolapse of the rectum, malaria.

Triple Burner
　S. TB-4 (*yáng chí*, Yang Pool)
　N. PC-6 (*nèi guān*, Inner Pass)
　　Deafness, sore throat, conjunctivitis, should and back pain, constipation, urinary block, enuresis.

Pericardium
　S. PC-7 (*dà líng*, Great Mound)
　N. TB-5 (*wài guān*, Outer Pass)
　　Pain or hypertonicity of the forearm or hand, chest pain, palpitation, nausea, vexation, heat in the hearts of the palms, incessant laughing.

Liver
　S. LR-3 (*tài chōng*, Supreme Surge)
　N. GB-37 (*guāng míng*, Bright Light)
　　Painful swelling of the testicles, mounting qi (*shàn qì*) pain, fullness in the chest, vomiting, abdominal pain, diarrhea, enuresis, and urinary block.

Gallbladder
　S. GB-40 (*qiū xū*, Hill Ruins)
　N. LR-5 (*lǐ gōu*, Woodworm Canal)
　　Pain in the chest and rib-side, headache, eye pain, malaria, goiter, swollen lymph nodes.

combining transport and alarm points 俞募配穴法 *shū mù pèi xué fǎ*: Synonym: *combining front and back points*. Simultaneous needling of transport points on the back and alarm points on the chest and abdomen for specific therapeutic purposes. For example, BL-13 (*fèi shū*, Lung Transport), the transport point of the lung, is combined LU-1 (*zhōng fǔ*, Central Treasury), with the alarm point of the lung, to treat respiratory problems such as cough, panting, fullness in the chest. See the list below and POINT COMBINATION. [46: 600]

Combining Transport (T) and Alarm (A) Points

Lung
  T. BL-13 (*fèi shū*, Lung Transport)
  A. LU-1 (*zhōng fǔ*, Central Treasury)
Pericardium
  T. BL-14 (*jué yīn shū*, Reverting Yin Transport)
  A. CV-17 (*dàn zhōng*, Chest Center)
Heart
  T. BL-15 (*xīn shū*, Heart Transport)
  A. CV-14 (*jù què*, Great Tower Gate)
Spleen
  T. BL-20 (*pí shū*, Spleen Transport)
  A. LR-13 (*zhāng mén*, Camphorwood Gate)
Liver
  T. BL-18 (*gān shū*, Liver Transport)
  A. LR-14 (*qī mén*, Cycle Gate)
Kidney
  T. BL-23 (*shèn shū*, Kidney Transport)
  A. GB-25 (*jīng mén*, Capital Gate)
Large Intestine
  T. BL-25 (*dà cháng shū*, Large Intestine Transport)
  A. ST-25 (*tiān shū*, Celestial Pivot)
Triple Burner
  T. BL-22 (*sān jiāo shū*, Triple Burner Transport)
  A. CV-5 (*shí mén*, Stone Gate)
Small Intestine
  T. BL-27 (*xiǎo cháng shū*, Small Intestine Transport)
  A. CV-4 (*guān yuán*, Pass Head)
Stomach
  T. BL-21 (*wèi shū*, Stomach Transport)
  A. LU-1 (*zhōng fǔ*, Central Treasury)
Gallbladder
  T. BL-19 (*dǎn shū*, Gallbladder Transport)
  A. GB-24 (*rì yuè*, Sun and Moon)
Bladder
  T. BL-28 (*páng guāng shū*, Bladder Transport)
  A. CV-3 (*zhōng jí*, Central Pole)

combining transport points 五输配穴法 *wǔ shū pèi xué fǎ*: See TRANSPORT POINT. [46: 600]

combining upper and lower body points 上下配穴法 *shàng xià pèi xué fǎ*: Simultaneous needling of points above and below the waist. For example, stomach pain can be treated by combining PC-6 (*nèi guān*, Inner Pass) on the upper body and ST-36 (*zú sān lǐ*, Leg Three Li) on the lower body. Sore throat or toothache can be treated with LI-4 (*hé gǔ*, Union Valley) on the upper body and ST-44 (*nèi tíng*, Inner Court) on the lower body. Insomnia can be treated by combining HT-7 (*shén mén*, Spirit Gate) on the upper body and SP-6 (*sān yīn jiāo*, Three Yin Intersection) on the lower body. Constipation can be treated by combining TB-6 (*zhī gōu*, Branch Ditch) on the upper body and KI-6 (*zhào hǎi*, Shining Sea) on the lower body. See POINT COMBINATION. [46: 600]

coming and going heart pain 去来心痛 *qù lái xīn tòng*: From *A Thousand Gold Pieces Prescriptions* (*qiān jīn yào fāng*). Heart pain that comes and goes abruptly, sometimes up to ten times a day; attributed to insufficiency of yang qi and damp phlegm stagnating internally. [MED] Supplement qi and warm yang; eliminate dampness and disperse phlegm. Use Coming and Going Decoction (*qù lái tāng*). See HEART PAIN. [26: 183]

common cold 感冒 *gǎn mào*: **1.** A disease that is attributed to contraction of wind-cold or other untimely seasonal qi, and that forms an exterior pattern characterized by nasal congestion, runny nose, headache and distention in the head, fear of wind, pain in the joints, aversion to cold and heat effusion, and in some cases cough and sore throat. NB: The term common cold is potentially confusing in the context of Chinese medicine where distinction is made between cold and heat patterns. [MED] Treat variously according to the nature the offending evil, severity of the condition, constitution of the patient, and climate. For wind-heat, course exterior and discharge heat with Lonicera and Forsythia Powder (*yín qiào sǎn*) or Mulberry Leaf and Chrysanthemum Beverage (*sāng jú yǐn*). For wind-cold, course the exterior and dissipate cold with Schizonepeta and Ledebouriella Toxin-Vanquishing Powder (*jīng fáng bài dú sǎn*). [ACU] For wind-cold, base treatment mainly on LU, LI, and BL. Select LU-7 (*liè quē*, Broken Sequence), LI-4 (*hé gǔ*, Union Valley), BL-12 (*fēng mén*, Wind Gate), and GB-20 (*fēng chí*, Wind Pool). Needle with drainage and, if necessary, moxa. For wind-heat, base treatment mainly on LU, LI and TB. Select LU-10 (*yú jì*, Fish Border), GV-14 (*dà zhuī*, Great Hammer), LU-5 (*chǐ zé*, Cubit Marsh), LI-11 (*qū chí*, Pool at the Bend), ST-44 (*nèi tíng*, Inner Court), GB-20 (*fēng *chí*, Wind Pool), and TB-5 (*wài guān*, Outer Pass). Needle with drainage or prick with a three-edged needle to bleed. For high fever, prick Ten Diffusing Points (*shí xuān*) to bleed. Selection of points according to signs: For runny nose and nasal congestion, add LI-20 (*yíng xiāng*, Welcome Fragrance), GV-23 (*shàng xīng*, Upper Star), and Hall of Impression (*yìn táng*). For headache with distention in the head, add GV-20 (*bǎi huì*, Hundred Convergences), Greater Yang (*tài yáng*), and SI-3 (*hòu xī*, Back Ravine). See also HEADACHE for selection of points according to affected area. For cough, add BL-13 (*fèi shū*, Lung Transport) and LU-9 (*tài yuān*, Great Abyss). For sore throat, add CV-22 (*tiān tú*, Celestial Chimney) and prick LU-11 (*shào shāng*, Lesser Shang) to bleed. **2.** WIND DAMAGE. [26: 778] [97: 595] [46: 650] [46: 724]

common cold headache 感冒头痛 *gǎn mào tóu tòng*: HEADACHE due to contraction of wind evil. Common cold headache is associated with nasal congestion that makes the voice sound heavy, spontaneous sweating, aversion to wind, and a moderate floating pulse. Wind evil in common-cold is usually combined with cold, heat, or dampness. See WIND-COLD HEADACHE; WIND-HEAT HEADACHE; and WIND-DAMP HEADACHE. [26: 778]

communicating bowels 交肠 *jiāo cháng*: A fistula between the rectum and bladder or between the rectum and the vagina. Compare ANAL FISTULA. [27: 413] [97: 221]

completion bone 完骨 *wán gǔ*: *Synonym: longevity platform bone.* The protuberant bone behind the ear. ⃞WMC The mastoid process of the temporal bone. [26: 834] [27: 63] [97: 311]

complex 夹杂 *jiá zá*, 夹错 *jiá cuò*: The simultaneous appearance of signs of the paired principles cold and heat, or vacuity and repletion. The simultaneous appearance of interior and exterior signs, which is referred to as a combination rather than a complex, is an exception. See COLD-HEAT COMPLEX; VACUITY-REPLETION COMPLEX. Compare COMBINATION. [6: 148]

complexion 色泽 *sè zé*: The color and sheen of the skin, especially that of the face, as reflecting health or disease. See FACIAL COMPLEXION. ⋄ Chin 色 *sè*, color; 泽 *zé*, sheen, luster. [6: 116]

conception vessel 任脉 *rèn mài*: CONTROLLING VESSEL.

concretion 癥 *zhēng*: See CONCRETIONS, CONGLOMERATIONS, ACCUMULATIONS, AND GATHERINGS.

concretions and gatherings 癥瘕积聚 *zhēng jiǎ jī jù*: See CONCRETIONS, CONGLOMERATIONS, ACCUMULATIONS, AND GATHERINGS.

concretions, conglomerations, accumulations, and gatherings 癥瘕积聚 *zhēng jiǎ jī jù*: Four kinds of abdominal masses associated with pain and distention. Concretions and accumulations are masses of definite form and fixed location, associated with pain of fixed location. They stem from disease in the viscera and blood aspect. Conglomerations and gatherings are masses of indefinite form, which gather and dissipate at irregular intervals and are attended by pain of unfixed location. They are attributed to disease in the bowels and qi aspect. Accumulations and gatherings chiefly occur in the center burner. Concretions and conglomerations chiefly occur in the lower burner, and in many cases are the result of gynecological diseases. In general, concretions and gatherings arise when emotional depression or dietary intemperance causes damage to the liver and spleen. The resultant organ disharmony leads to obstruction and stagnation of qi, which in turn causes static blood to collect gradually. Most often the root cause is insufficiency of right qi. See Table 2. Concretions, conglomerations, accumulations, and gatherings also include other specific masses such as STRINGS AND AGGREGATIONS. ⋄ Chin 癥 *zhēng* is composed of the the illness signifier 疒 with the phonetic 徵 (sign, proof); *jiǎ*, 瘕 is composed of the illness signifier with the phonetic 假 (false, fake); 积 *jī*, accumulate; 聚 *jù*, gather. [37: 394] [27: 416] [80: 401]

2. Concretions, Conglomerations Accumulations and Gatherings		
	Definite shape	Indefinite shape
Lower burner	Concretion	Conglomeration
Middle burner	Accumulation	Gathering

conductor 引 *yǐn*, 引药 *yǐn yào*, 引子 *yǐn zi*: See SOVEREIGN, MINISTER, ASSISTANT, AND COURIER. [26: 133]

confined pulse 牢脉 *láo mài*: FIRM PULSE.

confluence of the yang [channels] 诸阳之会 *zhū yáng zhī huì*: The place through which all the yang channels pass, i.e., the head. [27: 35] [97: 493]

confluence points of the eight vessels 八脉交会穴 *bā mài jiāo huì xué*: *Synonym: master points of the eight vessels.* Any of eight regular channel points located on the four limbs, each linked, via its home channel, with one of the eight extraordinary vessels. The points are listed below:

The Confluence Points of the Eight Vessels

Yin linking (*yīn wéi*) vessel: PC-6 (*nèi guān*, Inner Pass)

Thoroughfare (*chōng*) vessel: SP-4 (*gōng sūn*, Yellow Emperor)

Yang linking (*yáng wéi*) vessel: TB-5 (*wài guān*, Outer Pass)

Girdling (*dài*) vessel: GB-41 (*zú lín qì*, Foot Overlooking Tears)

Controlling (*rèn*) vessel: LU-7 (*liè quē*, Broken Sequence)

Yin springing (*yīn qiāo*) vessel: KI-6 (*zhào hǎi*, Shining Sea)

Governing (*dū*) vessel: SI-3 (*hòu xī*, Back Ravine)

Yang springing (*yáng qiāo*) vessel: BL-62 (*shēn mài*, Extending Vessel)

Only in one case, that of BL-62, is the confluence point a point of actual intersection with the extraordinary vessel. The confluence points can be employed singly to treat diseases associated with the relevant extraordinary vessels. For example, SI-3 can treat diseases associated with the governing (*dū*) vessel vessel such as stiffness of the spine or arched-back rigidity. They may also be used in pairs of diseases of specific areas of the body. PC-6 (YIL) and SP-4 (PV) are combined to treat problems of the heart, stomach, and chest; TB-5 (YAL) and GB-41 (GIV) are used treat problems of the outer canthus, area behind the ear, shoulder, and neck (front); LU-7 (CV) and KI-6 (YIS) address diseases of the diaphragm, throat, and lung; and SI-3 (GV) and BL-62 (YAS) treat problems of the inner canthus, neck (front and back), ear, and shoulders. [26: 24]

confound 迷 *mí*: To render stuporous; to cloud severely; occurs in the term *phlegm confounding the orifices of the heart*, which denotes a condition characterized, among other signs, by stupor or coma. See EXUBERANCE AND DEBILITATION.

confounding phlegm 痰迷 *tán mí*: Phlegm congesting the orifices causing noisy breathing and stupor. ☐MED☐ Sweep phlegm and open the orifices using Phlegm-Flushing Decoction (*dí tán tāng*). ☐ACU☐ Needle CV-22 (*tiān tú*, Celestial Chimney) and PC-6 (*nèi guān*, Inner Pass). [26: 765] [97: 608]

confused spirit-mind 神志昏乱 *shén zhì hūn luàn*: A confused, stuporous state of mind.

congealed-fat screen 凝脂翳 *níng zhī yì*: An external obstruction of the eye that has the appearance of congealed lard and that in severe cases can cause loss of sight. Congealed-fat screen develops swiftly and is attended by acute eye pain and pain in the brow, redness of the eyes, hot tears, and copious discharge. It is attributable to externally contracted wind-heat toxin invading and contending contending with intense internal liver-gallbladder fire and binding in the eye. ☐MED☐ Use Gentian Liver-Draining Decoction (*lóng dǎn xiè gān tāng*) plus dandelion (*pú gōng yīng*), antelope horn (*líng yáng jiǎo*), rhubarb (*dà huáng*), and moutan (*mǔ dān pí*). ☐WMC☐ observed in suppurative keratitis. ☐ACU☐ Select BL-2 (*zǎn zhú*, Bamboo

Gathering), BL-1 (*jīng míng*, Bright Eyes), GB-1 (*tóng zǐ liáo*, Pupil Bone-Hole), GB-20 (*fēng chí*, Wind Pool), GB-41 (*zú lín qì*, Foot Overlooking Tears), Thumb Bone Hollow (*dà gǔ kōng*), Little Finger Bone Hollow (*xiǎo gǔ kōng*), LR-2 (*xíng jiān*, Moving Between), GB-43 (*xiá xī*, Pinched Ravine), and GB-34 (*yáng líng quán*, Yang Mound Spring). Needle with drainage. [26: 902] [37: 468] [27: 503] [97: 650]

congealing 凝 *níng*: Viscid, or becoming or making viscid; describes the viscid nature of evils such as dampness and their inhibitive effect on normal flow of blood and qi. When applied to the blood, this term denotes thickening but not necessarily coagulation.

congealing cold and stagnant qi 寒气凝滞 *hán qì níng zhì*: Cold giving rise to qi stagnation. Cold tends to congeal and obstruct qi transformation. It is a yin evil that causes congealing and stagnation, contracture and tautness, and easily damages yang qi. *Elementary Questions* (*sù wèn, jǔ tòng lùn*) states, "When cold qi enters the channels, there is a slowing down, congealing, and nonmovement. When it settles outside the vessels, then blood is scant; when it settles inside the vessels, qi is blocked and there is sudden pain." Thus when cold causes illness, there is pain, abdominal distention, swelling of the lower leg, hypertonicity, paralysis, and reversal cold. [25: 315]

congealing cold-damp menstrual block 寒湿凝滞经闭 *hán shī níng zhì jīng bì*: MENSTRUAL BLOCK due to cold-damp contending and binding with the blood and blocking the thoroughfare (*chōng*) and controlling (*rèn*) vessels. Congealing cold-damp menstrual block is characterized by smaller-abdominal cold pain, physical cold and cold limbs, and copious white vaginal discharge. Where cold is prevalent, it is associated with thin watery vaginal discharge and a slow pulse. Where dampness is prevalent, it is usually associated with abdominal distention and sloppy stool, in some cases with swelling of the lower limbs. ☐MED☐ Cold patterns are treated by warming the channels and dissipating cold with Channel-Warming (Menses-Warming) Decoction (*wēn jīng tāng*), whereas dampness patterns are treated by drying dampness and transforming turbidity with Zhu Dan-Xi's Damp Phlegm Formula (*zhū dān xī zhì shī tán fāng*), which contains atractylodes (*cāng zhú*), ovate atractylodes (*bái zhú*), pinellia (*bàn xià*), poria (*fú líng*), talcum (*huá shí*), cyperus (*xiāng fù zǐ*), ligusticum (*chuān xiōng*), and tangkuei (*dāng guī*). ☐ACU☐ Base treatment mainly on CV, SP, and ST. Select CV-3 (*zhōng jí*, Central Pole), GB-26 (*dài mài*, Girdling Vessel), LI-4 (*hé gǔ*, Union Valley), SP-10 (*xuè hǎi*, Sea of Blood), SP-6 (*sān yīn jiāo*, Three Yin Intersection), ST-36 (*zú sān lǐ,* Leg Three Li), SP-9 (*yīn líng quán,* Yin Mound Spring), and LR-3 (*tài chōng,* Supreme Surge). Needle with drainage and large amounts of moxa. Where cold is prominent, add CV-4 (*guān yuán,* Pass Head), and CV-6 (*qì hǎi,* Sea of Qi). Where dampness is prominent, add CV-12 (*zhōng wǎn,* Center Stomach Duct), ST-25 (*tiān shū,* Celestial Pivot), and BL-20 (*pí shū,* Spleen Transport). [26: 662] [46: 596, 686] [59: 43–4] [113: 288]

congealing cold-damp menstrual pain 寒湿凝滞痛经 *hán shī níng zhì tòng jīng:* MENSTRUAL PAIN attributable to cold-damp damaging the thoroughfare (*chōng*) and controlling (*rèn*) vessels and the uterus, congealing the blood and blocking its downward movement to the uterus. Congealing cold-damp menstrual pain is characterized by cold or gripping pain in the lower abdomen that likes warmth, and dark clotted inhibited flow. [MED] Use formulas such as Lesser Abdomen Stasis-Expelling Decoction (*shào fù zhú yū tāng*) or a decoction of leonurus (*yì mǔ cǎo*), dried ginger (*gān jiāng*), and pepper (*hú jiāo*). Vacuity cold with thin pale flow and dull abdominal pain that likes warmth is treated by warming the channels and supplementing vacuity with formulas such as Minor Construction Brew (*xiǎo yíng jiān*) and Tangkuei Center-Fortifying Decoction (*dāng guī jiàn zhōng tāng*). [ACU] Base treatment mainly on CV and SP. Select CV-3 (*zhōng jí,* Central Pole), SP-8 (*dì jī,* Earth's Crux), and ST-28 (*shuǐ dào,* Waterway); needle with drainage and add moxa. Selection of points according to signs: For abdominal distention stretching into the lumbus, add GV-4 (*mìng mén,* Life Gate), and BL-23 (*shèn shū,* Kidney Transport). For acute pain, add BL-32 (*cì liáo,* Second Bone-Hole) and ST-29 (*guī lái,* Return). For vaginal discharge, add GB-26 (*dài mài,* Girdling Vessel), BL-30 (*bái huán shū,* White Ring Transport), CV-6 (*qì hǎi,* Sea of Qi), and SP-6 (*sān yīn jiāo,* Three Yin Intersection). [26: 662] [46: 684]

congealing yin cold 阴寒凝结 *yīn hán níng jié:* A cold pattern arising from debilitation of yang qi and stagnation of cold evil. Signs include somber white facial complexion, aversion to cold and desire for warmth, lack of warmth in the limbs, abdominal pain and bound stool, menstrual irregularities, and local hypertonicity and pain. Enduring cold impediment (*hán bì*) and yin flat-abscess (*yīn jū*) also fall within the scope of congealing yin cold. [26: 621]

congenital constitution 先天 *xiān tiān:* EARLIER HEAVEN.

congest 壅 *yǒng:* To clog (the lung, the throat, the channels, etc.). See STOPPAGE.

conglomeration 瘕 *jiǎ:* A type of abdominal lump. See CONCRETIONS, CONGLOMERATIONS, ACCUMULATIONS, AND GATHERINGS.

conglomeration-mounting 瘕疝 *shàn jiǎ:* MOUNTING-CONGLOMERATION.

connect 络 *luò:* NET.

consolidating yin 坚阴 *jiān yīn:* A method of treatment used to secure kidney essence and calm the ministerial fire. The method of consolidating yin is used in the treatment of frenetic stirring of the ministerial fire and insecurity of kidney qi characterized by seminal emission while dreaming. This condition can be treated with Marrow-Sealing Elixir (*fēng suǐ dān*), a formula whose chief ingredient is phellodendron (*huáng bǎi*), which both calms the ministerial fire and secures kidney essence. Compare SUPPLEMENTING YIN; STRENGTHENING YIN. [27: 266]

constipation 便秘 *biàn bì: Synonyms: fecal block; fecal stoppage.* Stagnation in the intestines lengthening the interval between bowel movements to three or four days or more. Constipation occurs in the following patterns. **Repletion:** Constipation with abdominal distention that refuses pressure, red facial complexion, generalized heat [effusion] that heightens in the afternoon (late afternoon tidal heat [effusion]), copious sweating, reddish urine, rough breathing, thick slimy yellow tongue fur, and a sunken replete pulse is a sign of gastrointestinal heat bind (repletion heat), sometimes referred to as a *yang bind.* Constipation accompanied by frequent belching, glomus and oppression in the chest, rib-side distention, swelling of the breasts, slimy white tongue fur and sunken or stringlike pulse is a sign of liver qi depression affecting the spleen, and is sometimes called *qi constipation.* **Vacuity:** Constipation with long voidings of clear urine and signs of spleen-kidney yang vacuity, sometimes called *yin bind.* Dry bound stool with emaciation, lusterless facial complexion, dizziness, red tongue with little fluid, and a forceless fine pulse is a sign of yin-blood depletion and may occur in the recovery period of externally contracted heat (febrile) diseases, after childbirth, or in old age. Constipation with straining to evacuate that causes sweating and shortness of breath is a sign of lung-kidney vacuity. Compare DIFFICULT DEFECATION. [26: 466] [97: 422]

Constipation

VACUITY CONSTIPATION (*xū bì*)

REPLETION CONSTIPATION (*shí bì*)

COLD CONSTIPATION (*lěng bì*)

HEAT CONSTIPATION (*rè bì*)

WIND CONSTIPATION (*fēng bì*)

PHLEGM CONSTIPATION (*tán bì*)

QI CONSTIPATION (*qì bì*)

INTESTINAL DRYNESS CONSTIPATION (*cháng zào biàn bì*)

---

constitutional body 体 *tǐ*: The human body in its constitutional aspect, as opposed to the physical body, which denotes the purely physical manifestation of human life.

constrain 敛 *liǎn*: Astringe, especially of the lung, as in the terms *constrain the lung and suppress cough* and *constrain sweat*.

constrained liver qi 肝气不舒 *gān qì bù shū*: Deficiency of the liver's free coursing action, usually caused by affect-mind binding depression, and characterized distention and pain in the rib-side, constrained sensation in the chest, sighing, mental depression, and no desire for food and drink. There may be bitter taste in the mouth and retching. The pulse is stringlike. Constrained liver qi is treated by coursing the liver and resolving depression. Compare BINDING DEPRESSION OF LIVER QI and DISHARMONY OF LIVER QI. [25: 164]

constrained spleen qi 脾气不舒 *pí qì bù shū*: Nonmovement of spleen qi caused by impaired liver free coursing, dampness encumbering spleen yang, or congestion of food. Constrained spleen qi is characterized by distention and oppression in the stomach duct and abdomen, nontransformation of food, aversion to food, and hiccough. [26: 748] [97: 562]

constraining sweat 敛汗 *liǎn hàn*: A method of treatment used to address spontaneous or night sweating using securing astringents combined with other medicinals according to need. MED Spontaneous sweating is usually attributable to qi vacuity, and is therefore primarily treated by boosting qi and securing the exterior with medicinals such as astragalus (*huáng qí*). Night sweating is usually a consequence of yin vacuity, and is therefore treated by enriching yin and constraining the lung, using white peony (*bái sháo yào*), mung bean seed-coat (*lǜ dòu pí*), and light wheat (*fú xiǎo mài*). Treatment of both spontaneous and night sweating may include medicinals such as schisandra (*wǔ wèi zǐ*), glutinous rice root (*nuò dào gēn xū*), calcined dragon bone (*duàn lóng gǔ*), and calcined oyster shell (*duàn mǔ lì*). A representative formula is Oyster Shell Powder (*mǔ lì sǎn*). Securing astriction is only one method of checking spontaneous and night sweating. Cinnamon Twig Decoction (*guì zhī tāng*), by harmonizing construction and defense, can also check sweating. Jade Wind-Barrier Powder (*yù píng fēng sǎn*) can check sweating by boosting qi and securing the exterior. Night sweating may also be treated by the yin-nourishing and fire-draining effect of Tangkuei Six Yellows Decoction (*dāng guī liù huáng tāng*). ACU LI-4 (*hé gǔ*, Union Valley), KI-7 (*fù liū*, Recover Flow), SI-3

(*hòu xī*, Back Ravine), and HT-6 (*yīn xī*, Yin Cleft) can all be used to constrain sweating. The first two are used in particular for spontaneous sweating, and the last two for night sweating. [6: 267] [46: 602] [113: 18]

constraining sweat and securing the exterior 敛汗固表 *liǎn hàn gù biǎo*: A method of treatment used to address exterior vacuity with copious sweating. Exterior vacuity may take the form of qi vacuity or yin vacuity. **Qi vacuity** patterns are characterized by spontaneous sweating, heart palpitations, susceptibility to fright, shortness of breath, heart vexation, fatigue, and large forceless pulse. MED Representative sweat-constraining exterior-securing formulas for qi vacuity include Oyster Shell Powder (*mǔ lì sǎn*) and Jade Wind-Barrier Powder (*yù píng fēng sǎn*). **Yin vacuity** patterns are characterized by night sweating, postmeridian tidal heat [effusion], dry lips and mouth, red tongue, and a rapid fine pulse. MED Use formulas such as Tangkuei Six Yellows Decoction (*dāng guī liù huáng tāng*) and Six-Ingredient Rehmannia Decoction (*liù wèi dì huáng tāng*) plus oyster shell (*mǔ lì*), light wheat (*fú xiǎo mài*), and glutinous rice root (*nuò dào gēn xū*). ACU For qi vacuity, base treatment mainly on BL, ST, and LI. Select BL-13 (*fèi shū*, Lung Transport), BL-43 (*gāo huāng shū*, Gao-Huang Transport), ST-36 (*zú sān lǐ*, Leg Three Li), LI-4 (*hé gǔ*, Union Valley), and KI-7 (*fù liū*, Recover Flow); needle with supplementation and moxa, if necessary. For yin vacuity, base treatment mainly on KI, SI, and HT. Select KI-6 (*zhào hǎi*, Shining Sea), KI-3 (*tài xī*, Great Ravine), LU-5 (*chǐ zé*, Cubit Marsh), SI-3 (*hòu xī*, Back Ravine), and HT-6 (*yīn xī*, Yin Cleft), needle with supplementation. See CONSTRAINING SWEAT. [26: 943] [27: 285] [97: 528] [46: 651, 602] [113: 18]

constraining the lung 敛肺 *liǎn fèi*: See CONSTRAINING THE LUNG AND SUPPRESSING COUGH.

constraining the lung and suppressing cough 敛肺止咳 *liǎn fèi zhǐ ké*: A method of treatment used to address enduring cough and lung vacuity characterized by scant phlegm, hasty breathing, spontaneous sweating, dry mouth and tongue, and vacuous rapid pulse. MED Lung-constraining cough-suppressing medicinals such as schisandra (*wǔ wèi zǐ*), chebule (*hē zǐ*), and poppy husk (*yīng sù ké*) can be combined with general cough-suppressing medicinals such as stemona (*bǎi bù*), aster (*zǐ wǎn*), aristolochia fruit (*mǎ dōu líng*), loquat leaf (*pí pá yè*), and tussilago (*kuǎn dōng huā*). A commonly used lung-constraining cough-suppressing formula is Schisandra Decoction (*wǔ wèi zǐ tāng*), which consists of tangkuei (*dāng guī*), schisandra (*wǔ wèi zǐ*), ophiopogon (*mài mén dōng*), apricot kernel (*xìng rén*), red tangerine peel (*jú hóng*), fresh ginger (*shēng jiāng*), and jujube (*dà zǎo*). Another representative formula is Nine Immortals Powder (*jiǔ xiān sǎn*). ACU Base treatment mainly on LU, LI, and back transport points. Main points: LU-7 (*liè quē*, Broken Sequence), LU-9 (*tài yuān*, Great Abyss), LU-5 (*chǐ zé*, Cubit Marsh), and BL-13 (*fèi shū*, Lung Transport). For exterior vacuity, add LI-4 (*hé gǔ*, Union Valley) and ST-36 (*zú sān lǐ*, Leg Three Li). For yin vacuity, add BL-23 (*shèn shū*, Kidney Transport), KI-3 (*tài xī*, Great Ravine), and KI-6 (*zhào hǎi*, Shining Sea), needling with supplementation. [26: 943] [27: 286] [6: 267]

constraining yin 敛阴 *liǎn yīn*: A method of treatment used to prevent loss of yin qi from the body, as in night sweating or after abatement of heat effusion in heat (febrile) disease. Yin-constraining medicinals include cornus (*shān zhū yú*) and schisandra (*wǔ wèi zǐ*). [27: 266]

constricting throat wind 紧喉风 *jǐn hóu fēng*: ACUTE THROAT WIND.

construction 营 *yíng*: An abbreviation for construction qi, which is an essential qi formed from the essence of food and which flows in the vessels. Construction is considered to be an aspect of the blood. ◊ Chin 营 *yíng*, military camp, operate, develop. The English *construction* conveys the original sense of the *yíng* in the medical context, reflecting the analogy to national administration, in which construction or maintenance of infrastructures (the various parts of the body) is paired with defense. Also the character 荣 (*róng*), splendor, glory, luxuriance is also used to denote construction. See LOSS-OF-LUXURIANCE. [26: 930] [27: 76] [97: 508]

construction aspect 营分 *yíng fèn*: DEFENSE, QI, CONSTRUCTION, AND BLOOD.

construction-aspect pattern 营分证 *yíng fèn zhèng*: Warm disease one stage more advanced than a qi-aspect pattern, characterized by red or crimson tongue, a rapid pulse, generalized heat EF-FUSION, heart vexation, and unquiet sleep. The essential characteristic of construction-aspect patterns is a red or crimson tongue, which indicates that evil heat has entered the construction aspect. Identification of construction-aspect patterns poses two requirements. (1) It is important to determine whether the evil entering the construction aspect is warm heat, wind-heat, or damp-heat. Warm heat and wind-heat evils entering the construction aspect are characterized by a red or crimson tongue with either no fur or a very thin fur. Damp-heat evil entering construction is characterized by a red or crimson tongue with a thick slimy or turbid tongue fur (indicating that the dampness evil has not transformed dryness), or a parched, black tongue fur (indicating that dryness formation has occurred). (2) It is essential to deter-mine the degree to which the construction aspect has been penetrated. Initial-stage construction-aspect patterns invariably include qi-aspect signs, such as red to sunken red tongue with a yellow, or mixed yellow-and-white tongue fur. Deep penetration of construction aspect is characterized by a dry sunken red tongue, as well as such signs as clouded spirit-mind (see PERICARDIAC PATTERN) and stirring wind and tetanic reversal. TRT See CLEARING CONSTRUCTION. [6: 235] [26: 930] [84: 37]

construction-defense disharmony 营卫不和 *yíng wèi bù hé*: Exterior patterns characterized by spontaneous sweating and occurring in one of two forms: (1) strong defense and weak construction, where yang qi is depressed in the FLESHY EXTE-RIOR and forces sweat out of the pores, giving rise to sweating whenever, but only when, heat effu-sion occurs; and (2) weak defense and strong con-struction, characterized by spontaneous sweating without heat effusion, where sweat flows forth un-constrained by defense qi. [27: 131] [97: 509]

construction, defense, qi, and blood 营卫气血 *yíng wèi qì xuè*: Four basic aspects of human phys-iology. These four aspects were adopted by the warm disease school as the basis of pattern identi-fication in febrile disease. Compare DEFENSE, QI, CONSTRUCTION, AND BLOOD. [27: 363] [97: 509]

construction qi 营气 *yíng qì*: The qi that forms the blood and flows with it in the vessels, helping to nourish the entire body, is known as construc-tion qi (*yíng qì*). As *The Magic Pivot* (*líng shū*) points out: "Construction qi secretes fluids, dis-charges them into the vessels, and turns them into blood to nourish the limbs and supply the bowels and viscera." More at CONSTRUCTION. [6: 38] [27: 79] [97: 508]

consumption 痨瘵 *láo zhài*: **1.** *Synonym: pul-monary consumption*; *corpse transmission*; *flying corpse*; *corpse influx*; *demonic influx*. A con-tagious disease characterized by cough with ex-pectoration of blood, tidal heat [effusion], night sweating, emaciation. The cough is persistent and chronic, producing blood-flecked phlegm or in se-vere cases mouthfuls of blood. The tidal heat [effu-sion] comes in the afternoon and evening, and abat-ing in B1 watch (11 p.m. to 1 a.m.). Emaciation develops with reduced food intake and fatigue and lack of strength. The pulse is fine and rapid. Con-sumption begins with yin depletion, which causes vacuity fire, and finally, when damage to yin af-fects yang, dual depletion of yin and yang. As early as the Western Jin Dynasty (A.D. 265–316), consumption was recognized to be contagious, and by the Song Dynasty (960–1279), it was posited to be caused by "consumption worms." Predisposing factors include constitutional insufficiency (especially in children), excesses of drink and sex, taxation fatigue from thought and anxiety, as well as poverty poverty and poor living conditions. This disease and the specific forms in which it manifests have been variously labeled over the history of Chinese medicine: The terms *corpse transmission*, *flying corpse*, *corpse influx*, and *demonic influx* emphasize the contagious and deathly nature of the disease (see INFLUX); *worm infixation* indicates knowledge or intuition that the disease was caused by "worms" (see INFIXATION); *taxation influx* emphasizes the weakening of the lung and wasting of the body. Since the late Qing Dynasty in China, consumption has been called popularly called 肺痨 (pulmonary consumption), identified with pulmonary tuberculosis of Western medicine. In traditional literature, consumption is not always clearly differentiated from LUNG WILTING, STEAMING BONE, and TAXATION COUGH, although these three conditions are not only observed in the contagious disease consumption; they may be the result of other causes. MED Enrich yin and downbear fire; clear the lung and kill worms, using formulas such as Spirit-Moistening Powder (*rùn shén sǎn*), Stemona Metal-Clearing Decoction (*bǎi bù qīng jīn tāng*), and Turtle Shell and Rehmannia Decoction (*biē jiǎ dì huáng tāng*). ACU Base treatment mainly on LU and back transport points. Select LU-9 (*tài yuān*, Great Abyss), BL-13 (*fèi shū*, Lung Transport), BL-43 (*gāo huāng shū*, Gao-Huang Transport), ST-36 (*zú sān lǐ*, Leg Three Li), SP-6 (*sān yīn jiāo*, Three Yin Intersection), and KI-3 (*tài xī*, Great Ravine); needle with supplementation. Selection of points according to pattern: For depletion of lung yin, add LU-5 (*chǐ zé*, Cubit Marsh) and KI-6 (*zhào hǎi*, Shining Sea). For effulgent yin vacuity fire, add KI-2 (*rán gǔ*, Blazing Valley) and LR-2 (*xíng jiān*, Moving Between). For dual vacuity of qi and yin, add BL-20 (*pí shū*, Spleen Transport), BL-21 (*wèi shū*, Stomach Transport), and CV-6 (*qì hǎi*, Sea of Qi). Selection of points according to signs: For tidal heat [effusion], add LU-5 (*chǐ zé*, Cubit Marsh) and LU-10 (*yú jì*, Fish Border). For expectoration of blood, add LU-6 (*kǒng zuì*, Collection Hole). For night sweating, add HT-6 (*yīn xī*, Yin Cleft). For seminal emission, add BL-52 (*zhì shì*, Will Chamber). For menstrual block, add SP-10 (*xuè hǎi*, Sea of Blood). **2.** Severe vacuity taxation. [26: 680] [46: 657] [27: 386]

contain 摄 *shè*: To hold in; in physiology, specofically denotes qi's action of keeping the blood flowing within the vessels, and in therapy, the promotion of this and similar functions.

containing the blood 摄血 *shè xuè*: STANCHING BLEEDING.

contend 相搏 *xiāng bó*: Struggle, especially of two evils simultaneously present in the body, such as contention of wind and dampness. See EXUBERANCE AND DEBILITATION.

contracted tongue 舌短 *shé duǎn*: Contraction of the tongue preventing it from being extended. A contracted tongue is a critical sign in most cases. The cause is either damage to yin by extreme heat or fulminant (sudden and violent) yang qi desertion. A congenitally short frenulum may also prevent extension. [27: 179] [97: 196]

¹**contraction** 收 *shōu*: Drawing together, shrinking, withdrawing.

²**contraction** 感 *gǎn*: The act of contracting or state of having contracted (an external evil), e.g., wind-cold contraction, a disease caused by external wind-cold.

contracture and tautness 收引 *shōu yǐn*: Enduring contraction or hypertonicity of the sinews, generally associated with kidney yang vacuity.

contraindications of medicinals in pregnancy 妊娠药忌 *rèn shēn yào jì*: Inappropriateness or inadvisability of taking or prescribing certain medicinals during pregnancy since they may cause miscarriage or harm both the mother and child.

Contraindications of medicinals in Pregnancy

Vegetable

Toxic herbs

附子 (*fù zǐ*) aconite (Aconiti Tuber Laterale)

川乌头 (*chuān wū tóu*) aconite main tuber (Aconiti Tuber)

天雄 (*tiān xióng*) tianxiong aconite (Aconiti Tuber Laterale Tianxiong)

侧子 (*cè zǐ*) small aconite (Aconiti Tuber Laterale Parvum)

钩吻 (*gōu wěn*) yellow jessamine (Gelsemii Herba)

天南星 (*tiān nán xīng*) arisaema (Arisaematis Rhizoma)

姜半夏 (*jiāng bàn xià*) ginger pinellia (Pinelliae Tuber cum Zingibere Praeparatum)

大戟 (*dà jǐ*) euphorbia/knoxia (Euphorbiae seu Knoxiae Radix)

芫花 (*yuán huā*) genkwa (Daphnes Genkwa Flos)

常山 (*cháng shān*) dichroa (Dichroae Radix)

马钱子 (*mǎ qián zǐ*) nux vomica (Nux-Vomicae Semen)

Blood-breaking medicinals

川牛膝 (*chuān niú xī*) cyathula (Cyathulae Radix)

胡桃仁 (*hú táo rén*) walnut (Juglandis Semen)

牡丹皮 (*mǔ dān pí*) moutan (Moutan Radicis Cortex)

茜草根 (*qiàn cǎo gēn*) madder (Rubiae Radix)

干漆 (*gān qī*) lacquer (Lacca Exsiccata)

瞿麦 (*qū mài*) dianthus (Dianthi Herba)

三棱 (*sān léng*) sparganium (Sparganii Rhizoma)

鬼羽箭 (*guǐ yǔ jiàn*) buchnera (Buchnerae Herba)

通草 (*tōng cǎo*) rice-paper plant pith (Tetrapanacis Medulla)

红花 (*hóng huā*) carthamus (Carthami Flos)

藏红花 (*zàng hóng huā*) saffron (Croci Stigma)

莪术 (*é zhú*) zedoary (Zedoariae Rhizoma)

苏木 (*sū mù*) sappan (Sappan Lignum)

Ejecting precipitating and slippery medicinals

藜芦 (*lí lú*) veratrum (Veratri Radix et Rhizoma)

巴豆 (*bā dòu*) croton (Crotonis Semen)

牵牛子 (*qiān niú zǐ*) morning glory (Pharbitidis Semen)

冬葵子 (*dōng kuí zǐ*) mallow seed (Malvae Verticillatae Semen)

薏苡仁 (*yì yǐ rén*) coix (Coicis Semen)

枳实 (*zhǐ shí*) unripe bitter orange (Aurantii Fructus Immaturus)

Warm or hot acrid medicinals

厚朴 (*hòu pò*) magnolia bark (Magnoliae Cortex)

肉桂 (*ròu guì*) cinnamon bark (Cinnamomi Cortex)

干姜 (*gān jiāng*) dried ginger (Zingiberis Rhizoma Exsiccatum)

Animal

Blood-quickening stasis-transforming medicinals

水蛭 (*shuǐ zhì*) leech (Hirudo seu Whitmania)

斑蝥 (*bān máo*) mylabris (Mylabris)

地胆 (*dì dǎn*) oil beetle (Meloë)

蜘蛛 (*zhī zhū*) spider (Aranea)

蝼蛄 (*lóu gū*) mole cricket (Gryllotalpa)

蜈蚣 (*wú gōng*) centipede (Scolopendra)

蛇蜕 (*shé tuì*) snake slough (Serpentis Exuviae)

虻虫 (*méng chóng*) tabanus (Tabanus)

Others

刺猬皮 (*cì wèi pí*) hedgehog's pelt (Erinacei Pellis)

牛黄 (*niú huáng*) bovine bezoar (Bovis Bezoar)

麝香 (*shè xiāng*) musk (Moschus)

龟版 (*guī bǎn*) tortoise plastron (Testudinis Plastrum)

鳖甲 (*biē jiǎ*) turtle shell (Amydae Carapax)

Minerals

代赭石 (*dài zhě shí*) hematite (Haematitum)

水银 (*shuǐ yín*) mercury (Hydrargyrum)

铅粉 (*qiān fěn*) processed galenite (Galenitum Praeparatum)

硇砂 (*náo shā*) sal ammoniac (Sal Ammoniacum)

砒石 (*pī shí*) arsenic (Arsenicum)

芒硝 (*máng xiāo*) mirabilite (Mirabilitum)

石硫黄 (*shí liú huáng*) sulfur (Sulphur)

雄黄 (*xióng huáng*) realgar (Realgar)

轻粉 (*qīng fěn*) calomel (Calomelas)

Some of these medicinals such as arsenic (*pī shí*), croton (*bā dòu*), and mylabris (*bān máo*) are ab-

solutely contraindicated in pregnancy. Others are permitted when suitably processed, e.g., pinellia (*bàn xià*) prepared with ginger juice, which is often used for malign obstruction in the early stages of pregnancy. [26: 342]

controlling malaria 治疟 *zhì nüè*:

controlling vessel 任脉 *rèn mài*: Synonym: conception vessel (*obs*). Abbreviation: CV. One of the EIGHT EXTRAORDINARY VESSELS; the vessel whose principal course ascends from the pelvis along the midline of the body, and splits to skirt around the mouth and nose, and which is the sea of the yin channels, regulates menstruation, and matures the fetus. **Pathway:** The controlling vessel originates in the pelvic cavity, connects with the internal genitourinary organs, and emerges in the perineum at CV-1 (*huì yīn*, Meeting of Yin). It ascends through the pubic hair region and then runs up the midline of the abdomen, chest, and neck to the depression below the lower lip (sauce receptacle). Here it splits into two branches that contour the mouth and ascend to the infraorbital region. A second course arises in the pelvic cavity, enters the spine and ascends up the back. **Functions:** The controlling vessel is the sea of the yin channels. The three yin channels of the foot all join the controlling (*rèn*) vessel, allowing their bilateral courses to communicate. In this way, the controlling (*rèn*) vessel has a regulating effect on the yin channels, for which reason it is said that it regulates all the yin channels of the body. The controlling vessel regulates menstruation and nurtures the fetus. Thus it is said, "The controlling vessel governs the fetus." **Signs:** Menstrual irregularities, menstrual block, white vaginal discharge, miscarriage, infertility, mounting qi (*shàn qì*), enuresis, and abdominal masses. See UTERUS. ◇ Chin 任 *rèn*, be in charge, control. Often translated on as 'conception' on the grounds that 任 was also used in the sense 'pregnancy', (now written as 妊 in this sense). [6: 66] [27: 89] [97: 206]

controlling wind and transforming phlegm 治风化痰 *zhì fēng huà tán*: **1.** Synonym: *extinguishing wind and transforming phlegm*. To eliminate internal wind-phlegm. Phlegm may arise when damp turbidity fails to transform and congeals or when intense internal fire heat condenses humor. It may rise with wind and penetrate the channels and network vessels, causing, in mild cases, numbness or dizziness and headache with spinning head and black vision and, in severe cases, paralysis. It is for this condition that the method of controlling wind and transforming phlegm is used. MED A representative formula is Pinellia, Ovate Atractylodes, and Gastrodia Decoction (*bàn xià bái zhú tiān má tāng*). ACU Base treatment mainly on ST, and LR. Select CV-12 (*zhōng wǎn*, Center Stomach Duct), LI-4 (*hé gǔ*, Union Valley), ST-40 (*fēng lóng*, Bountiful Bulge), GB-20 (*fēng chí*, Wind Pool), and LR-3 (*tài chōng*, Supreme Surge); needle with even supplementation and drainage. For dizziness and headache, add ST-8 (*tóu wéi*, Head Corner), and ST-41 (*jiě xī*, Ravine Divide). **2.** A method of treatment used to eliminate externally contracted wind evil causing expectoration of phlegm. The method of controlling wind and transforming phlegm addresses copious phlegm from wind evil fettering the exterior disinhibiting lung qi and causing qi congestion that cause phlegm. MED A representative formula is Cough-Stopping Powder (*zhǐ sòu sǎn*). ACU Base treatment mainly on LU and ST. Select BL-13 (*fèi shū*, Lung Transport), LU-7 (*liè quē*, Broken Sequence), LI-4 (*hé gǔ*, Union Valley), ST-36 (*zú sān lǐ*, Leg Three Li), and ST-40 (*fēng lóng*, Bountiful Bulge); needle with drainage and moxa. **3.** A method of treating round or oval lumps at the surface of the body that are soft to the touch and neither red nor painful. [50: 989] [27: 271] [97: 265] [46: 596, 597, 619, 652]

conversion 转化 *zhuǎn huà*: In the doctrine of yin and yang, change from yin or yang to its complement. In eight-principle pattern identification, displacement of signs of one principle by those of its opposite. Any pattern may, under given circumstances, convert into its opposite principle. Conversion is often observed in externally contracted heat (febrile) diseases. Such diseases are characterized in the initial stages by signs such as headache, body pain, aversion to cold, and heat effusion. If in such cases the evil enters the interior, either as a result of its own strength, vacuity of right qi, or as a result of inappropriate treatment, the original exterior pattern converts into an interior pattern. Patterns of all the other principles may similarly convert in specific circumstances. The aim of treatment is therefore to foster favorable and prevent unfavorable conversion. [6: 25, 148]

convulsions 抽搐 *chōu chù*, 搐搦 *chù nuò*: TUGGING AND SLACKENING.

cool 凉 *liáng*: **1.** *adj.* **1a.** Not hot, e.g., *cool body*, i.e., absence of generalized heat [effusion]. **1b.** Of a nature mildly tending to reduce heat, e.g., COOL MEDICINAL. See FOUR QI. **2.** *vb.* To make cold or cool, e.g., cool the blood. See DRAIN.

cool acrid exterior resolution 辛凉解表 *xīn liáng jiě biǎo*: See RESOLVING THE EXTERIOR WITH COOLNESS AND ACRIDITY.

cool dryness 凉燥 *liáng zào*: A disease pattern attributable to contraction of dryness evil in the colder weather of autumn, taking the form of dry nose and throat, dry cough with little phlegm, and dry skin with cold signs. Compare WARM DRYNESS. See AUTUMN DRYNESS.

cooling and dissipating the blood 凉血散血 *liáng xuè sàn xuè*: A method of treatment used to clear and resolve blood-aspect heat evil using blood-cooling and blood-quickening products. Cooling and dissipating the blood is used to treat evil heat penetrating deep into the blood aspect and stirring the blood, causing signs such as scorching heat effusion, agitation, in severe cases with manic derangement and delirious raving, dense maculopapular eruption, blood ejection and bloody stool, a deep crimsom or purple crimsom tongue. MED Rhinoceros Horn and Rehmannia Decoction (*xī jiǎo dì huáng tāng*). [83: 110]

cooling dryness 凉燥 *liáng zào*: MOISTENING DRYNESS in the treatment of warm dryness. [27: 269] [27: 352] [97: 495]

cooling the blood 凉血 *liáng xuè*: Synonym: *clearing blood heat*. A method of treatment used to address heat penetrating construction-blood in heat diseases with general signs such as high fever, clouded spirit, and crimson tongue, and specific signs of frenetic movement of hot blood (blood ejection, spontaneous external bleeding, bloody stool, or bloody urine). MED A commonly used blood-cooling formula is Rhinoceros Horn and Rehmannia Decoction (*xī jiǎo dì huáng tāng*). ACU Base treatment mainly on HT and PC. Select PC-3 (*qū zé*, Marsh at the Bend), PC-9 (*zhōng chōng*, Central Hub), HT-9 (*shào chōng*, Lesser Surge), LI-11 (*qū chí*, Pool at the Bend), and BL-40 (*wěi zhōng*, Bend Center); needle with drainage and, if appropriate, prick to bleed. The following points are all blood-cooling points that can be combined with the above: KI-2 (*rán gǔ*, Blazing Valley), LR-2 (*xíng jiān*, Moving Between), SP-6 (*sān yīn jiāo*, Three Yin Intersection), SP-10 (*xuè hǎi*, Sea of Blood), PC-7 (*dà líng*, Great Mound), HT-7 (*shén mén*, Spirit Gate), and BL-17 (*gé shū*, Diaphragm Transport). [26: 564] [27: 255] [97: 495]

coolness 凉 *liáng*: **1.** Mild cold. **2.** One of the FOUR QI. A quality mildly tending to produce cold.

cool opening 凉开 *liáng kāi*: CLEARING HEAT AND OPENING THE ORIFICES.

copious sweat 汗多 *hàn duō*: Large amounts of sweat. See SWEATING.

copious urine 尿多 *niào duō*: Discharge of urine in greater quantities than normal. WMC polyuria. See URINE. Compare PROFUSE URINATION. [29: 204]

cormorant cough 鸬鹚咳 *lù cí ké*: WHOOPING COUGH.

corn 肉刺 *ròu cì*, 鸡眼 *jī yǎn*: A local thickening and hardening of the skin of the foot such as at the distal edge of the sole or between the toes and especially at the base joint of the great toe. A corn is called a "flesh spike" (肉刺 *ròu cì*) or "chicken's eye" (鸡眼 *jī yǎn*) in Chinese; it has a deep root and a hard hollow head, is painful when pressed, and affects walking. It is produced by friction and pressure from footwear, occurring especially in cases where the affected part is abnormally protuberant. [MED] Treat by paring away the dead skin down to red flesh and applying Elephant Skin Paste (*xiàng pí gāo*). [ACU] One method is to apply the fire needle in the center of the corn and four surrounding points, pointing into the root. In mild cases, a week of such treatments performed daily is sufficient; in severe cases, two weeks may be necessary. Alternatively, direct moxibustion can be applied. Five to seven cones can be burned at a time, or 3–5 cones if the feet have been soaked and the surplus dead skin pared away with a knife. Compare CALLUS. ◇ Chin 肉 *ròu*, flesh; 刺 *cì*, prick. 鸡 *jī*, chicken; 眼 *yǎn*, eye; from the appearance. [26: 261] [27: 486] [113: 448] [50: 857]

corporeal soul 魄 *pò*: Synonym: *animal soul*. A nonphysical aspect of the human being. *Pò* is the corporeal soul stored by the lung, as distinct from *hún*, the ethereal soul, stored by the liver. *The Magic Pivot* (*líng shū*) states, "that which enters and exists with essence is called the corporeal soul." *The Classified Canon* (*lèi jīng*) states, "The function of the corporeal soul is to enable the body to move and perform its function; pain and itching are felt by it." These descriptions suggest that the corporeal soul is the animating and sensitizing principle that gives humans the ability of movement and physical sensation. The ability of the newborn to cry and take milk is understood as a manifestation of the corporeal soul. The corporeal soul is believed to be closely related to essence, which in the traditional view, is the foundation of human life. Compare LUNG STORES THE CORPOREAL SOUL; KIDNEY HOLDS THE OFFICE OF LABOR, WHENCE AGILITY EMANATES; ETHEREAL SOUL. [26: 894]

corporeal soul gate 魄门 *pò mén*: The anus. One of the SEVEN GATES. ◇ Chin In older texts 魄 *pò* was interchangeable with the homophone 粕 *pò* meaning "waste," which is conveyed through the large intestine for discharge at the anus; hence the name. [27: 30] [97: 626]

corporeal soul sweating 魄汗 *pò hàn*: From *Elementary Questions* (*sù wèn, shēng qì tōng tiān lùn*). Sweat emanating from the lung. According to traditional understanding, the lung stores the corporeal soul, and governs the skin and hair; hence the name. [26: 892]

corpse influx 尸注 *shī zhù*: CONSUMPTION.

corpse transmission 传尸 *chuán shī*: CONSUMPTION.

cough 咳嗽 *ké sòu*: Sudden expulsion of air from the lung with an explosive noise, usually in a series of efforts. The Chinese term is composed of two characters, 咳 (*ké*) and 嗽 (*sòu*). In *The Inner Canon* (*nèi jīng*), these two characters have the same meaning, and this usage prevailed until the Song Dynasty (A.D. 960–1279), when Liu Wan-Su [He-Jian] (c. A.D. 1120–1200) introduced a distinction: "*Ké* [sonorous cough] means a cough that produces sound but no matter, and arises when lung qi is damaged and loses its clarity; *sòu* [productive cough] is a cough that produces matter without sound, and is attributed to spleen dampness stirring to form phlegm; *ké sòu* [sonorous and productive cough], is one with phlegm and sound, and arises when damage to lung qi stirs dampness in the spleen, so that the *ké* becomes *sòu*." From that time on, some followed *The Inner Canon* (*nèi jīng*) in treating the characters as synonymous, whereas others adopted the distinction made by Liu Wan-Su. In modern literature, the distinct forms are often referred to as *gān ké*, dry cough, and *tán ké*, phlegm cough, and both are referred to together by the combined form *ké sòu*. Cough can be caused by external evils invading the lung or by internal damage to organs affecting the lung; hence the notion that "Cough does not stop at the lung; but never leaves the lung." In other words the pathomechanisms of cough are not limited to the lung but always involve it. Cough may be attributable to an exuberant evil (external evils or phlegm-damp) or to vacuity. External contraction cough may be caused by wind-cold, wind-heat, or dryness. The cough itself can in some cases indicate the cause. For example, a cough that is pronounced in the daytime is usually attributed to heat or dryness; one that gets worse at night is more likely to be attributable to spleen-kidney debilitation or to exuberant phlegm-damp. However, correlation with other signs is necessary for accurate diagnosis. The main patterns can be diagnosed as follows. **Wind-cold** fettering the lung causes a heavy turbid sounding cough with expectoration of thin white phlegm and accompanied by runny nose with clear snivel, heat effusion and aversion to cold, body pains, absence of sweating and a floating pulse. **Wind-heat** invading the lung gives raise to an ungratifying coughing sound, expectoration of thick yellow phlegm, dry mouth and sore throat, aversion to cold and heat effusion. **Dryness evil** damaging the lung is characterized by no phlegm and a clear crisp voice, or phlegm that is difficult to expectorate, a dry mouth and throat, dry skin, hoarse voice, and pain in the chest when coughing. **Phlegm-damp** obstructing the lung is characterized by a cough that ceases after expectoration, and thick sticky phlegm that is easy to bring up, and is accompanied by distention and oppression in the stomach duct and abdomen, nausea and torpid intake, sloppy stool, slimy tongue fur, and slippery pulse. It arises when a vacuous spleen failing to move water-damp allows the gradual collection of phlegm that obstructs the lung. **Liver fire** invading the lung causes cough and counterflow qi, phlegm like rotted threads that is difficult to expectorate, pain in the rib-side when coughing, dry pharynx and mouth, rashness, impatience, irascibility, oppression in the chest, sighing, generalized heat [effusion] and red face, and a rapid stringlike pulse. **Lung-spleen qi vacuity** cough is characterized by copious thin white phlegm, low voice, shortness of breath, reduced eating, sloppy stool, bright white facial complexion, spontaneous sweating and fear of wind, and a forceless vacuous pulse. **Kidney yang vacuity** cough is usually associated with hasty panting and labored breathing, clear thin foamy phlegm, vacuity swelling of the face, soft enlarged tongue, and, in severe cases, enuresis accompanying coughing. **Lung-kidney yin vacuity** is an enduring cough with scant sticky phlegm in some cases flecked with blood, accompanied by emaciation, tidal heat [effusion], vexation and agitation, reddening of the cheeks, night sweating, dry mouth and pharynx, hoarse voice, red tongue with scant fur, and rapid fine pulse. Cough is often classified and labeled according to cause or nature or time, and less commonly nowadays according to bowel or visceral involvement. See entries listed below. [26: 434–5] [27: 378] [97: 402]

Cough

Classification by cause
WIND DAMAGE COUGH (*shāng fēng ké sòu*)
WIND-COLD COUGH (*fēng hán ké sòu*)
WIND-HEAT COUGH (*fēng rè ké sòu*)
DRYNESS DAMAGE COUGH (*shāng zào ké sòu*)
DRYNESS-HEAT COUGH (*zào rè ké sòu*)
PHLEGM-RHEUM COUGH (*tán yǐn ké sòu*)
COLD COUGH (*hán sòu*)
HEAT COUGH (*rè sòu*)
SUMMERHEAT COUGH (*shǔ ké*)
FIRE COUGH (*huǒ ké*)
FOOD COUGH (*shí ké*)
STATIC BLOOD COUGH (*yū xuè ké*)
QI COUGH (*qì sòu*)

Classification by bowels or viscera
LUNG COUGH (*fèi ké*)
HEART COUGH (*xīn ké*)
LIVER COUGH (*gān ké*)
SPLEEN COUGH (*pí ké*)
KIDNEY COUGH (*shèn ké*)
LARGE INTESTINAL COUGH (*dà cháng ké*)
SMALL INTESTINAL COUGH (*xiǎo cháng ké*)
STOMACH COUGH (*wèi ké*)
BLADDER COUGH (*páng guāng ké*)
TRIPLE BURNER COUGH (*sān jiāo ké*)
GALLBLADDER COUGH (*dǎn ké*)

Classification by Time
ENDURING COUGH (*jiǔ ké*)
SEASONAL COUGH (*shí sòu*)
FIFTH-WATCH COUGH (*wǔ gēng sòu*)
NIGHT COUGH (*yè sòu*)
LONG-BOUT COUGH (*dùn ké*)

Miscellaneous
DRY COUGH (*gān ké*)
TAXATION COUGH (*láo ké*)
COUNTERFLOW QI ASCENT COUGH (*ké nì shàng qì*)

---

cough and panting 咳喘 *ké chuǎn*: See COUNTERFLOW QI ASCENT COUGH.

coughing of blood 咳血 *ké xuè*, 咳嗽血 *ké sòu xuè*, 嗽血 *sòu xuè*: The coughing up of pure blood or blood-flecked phlegm; usually attributable to externally contracted wind evil that fails to resolve, transforms into heat and dryness, and damages the network vessels of the lung, or to liver fire invading the lung. **External contraction** patterns are characterized by itchy throat, cough, blood-flecked phlegm, dry mouth and nose, and in some cases generalized heat [effusion] and aching bones. MED Dispel wind and clear the lung, calm the network vessels and stanch bleeding. Use formulas such as Mulberry Leaf and Apricot Kernel Decoction (*sāng xìng tāng*). **Liver fire** invading the lung causes coughing bouts producing pure bright red blood or blood-flecked phlegm, stabbing pain in the chest and rib-side, vexation and irascibility, dry stool, red tongue with yellow fur, and a rapid stringlike pulse. MED Drain the liver and clear the lung; harmonize the network vessels and stanch bleeding. Use White-Draining Powder (*xiè bái sǎn*) combined with Indigo and Clamshell Powder (*dài gé sǎn*). Coughing of blood is also observed in diseases such as CONSUMPTION, LUNG TAXATION, LUNG WILTING, and PULMONARY WELLING-ABSCESS. [26: 434] [27: 421] [97: 402]

cough of pregnancy 子嗽 *zǐ sòu*: Cough during pregnancy. Cough of pregnancy is attributable to impaired depurative downbearing and inhibited qi dynamic arising when blood gathers to nourish the fetus and allows yin vacuity fire stir, or when phlegm-rheum ascends counterflow, or when wind-cold is contracted. **Yin vacuity and stirring fire** causes cough with tidal heat [effusion] and red cheeks, shortness of breath and lack of strength. MED Enrich yin and clear heat. Use Ophiopogon and Rehmannia Pill (*mài wèi dì huáng wán*). **Phlegm-rheum ascending counterflow** causes cough with copious phlegm, oppression in the chest, and heart vexation. MED Rectify qi and transform phlegm. Use variations of Two Matured Ingredients Decoction (*èr chén tāng*). **Contraction of external wind-cold** causes cough with nasal congestion, runny nose, heat effusion and aversion to cold. MED Resolve the exterior and diffuse the lung. Use Apricot Kernel and Perilla Powder (*xìng sū sǎn*). [26: 57]

counteracting treatment 逆治 *nì zhì*: STRAIGHT TREATMENT.

counterflow 逆 *nì*: Flow counter to the normal direction. See QI COUNTERFLOW; REVERSAL and following entries. ◊ Chin 逆 *nì*, contrary, counter, upstream.

counterflow cold of the extremities 手足逆冷 *shǒu zú nì lěng*: REVERSAL COLD OF THE EXTREMITIES.

counterflow cold of the limbs 四肢逆冷 *sì zhī nì lěng*: REVERSAL COLD OF THE EXTREMITIES.

counterflow fullness below the heart 心下逆满 *xīn xià nì mǎn*: Fullness below the heart with a sensation of counterflow qi ascent. [27: 377]

counterflow liver qi 肝气逆 *gān qì nì*: LIVER QI ASCENDING COUNTERFLOW.

counterflow lung qi 肺气逆 *fèi qì nì*: LUNG QI ASCENDING COUNTERFLOW.

counterflow menstruation 逆经 *nì jīng*: Synonym: *inverted menstruation*. Passing of blood through the mouth or nose during or around menstruation; includes MENSTRUAL SPONTANEOUS EXTERNAL BLEEDING and MENSTRUAL BLOOD EJECTION. **Repletion:** Counterflow menstruation occurring before or during menstruation is usually attributable to congestion of internal heat forcing blood to rise and forming a repletion heat pattern. WMC vicarious menstruation. MED Drain heat and cool the blood with Three Yellows Four Agents Decoction (*sān huáng sì wù tāng*). **Vacuity:** Counterflow menstruation occurring after menstruation is attributable to yin vacuity causing internal harassment. MED Nourish the blood and clear heat with Rhinoceros Horn and Rehmannia Decoction (*xī jiǎo dì huáng tāng*). Compare DEVIATED MENSTRUATION. [26: 495] [27: 442]

counterflow qi ascent 气上逆 *qì shàng nì*: A sensation of qi rising in the stomach or chest.

counterflow qi ascent cough 咳逆上气 *ké nì shàng qì*: Synonym: *cough and panting*. Cough and counterflow qi giving rise to panting. Counterflow qi ascent cough stemming from contraction of one or more of the six excesses or from phlegm-rheum collecting internally forms a repletion pattern. Occurring in enduring illness or as a result of major damage to original qi, it takes the form of a vacuity pattern. In all cases, it is associated with disease of the lung, spleen, and kidney, since it can result from congestion or vacuity of lung qi, from impaired splenic movement and transformation, and from the kidney failing to absorb qi. Persistent counterflow qi ascent cough can gradu-

ally give rise to debilitation of heart qi. [26: 434] [27: 384]

counterflow stomach qi 胃气逆 *wèi qì nì*: STOMACH QI ASCENDING COUNTERFLOW.

courier 使 *shǐ*: See SOVEREIGN, MINISTER, ASSISTANT, AND COURIER.

course 疏 *shū*: To enhance flow (of qi, especially depressed liver qi); to free (the liver, digestive tract of qi stagnation and depression); to eliminate (evils such as wind in the exterior); to free (the exterior or channels from evils such as wind). Compare SOOTHE. ◊ Chin 疏 *shū*, free the course of (a river), smooth the flow; sparse; scatter, dissipate. The character 疏 contains a pictorial representation of water, and is used in the combination 疏浚 *shū jùn*, to dredge, which is a common rendering for the *shū* in the medical context. The character 疏 is akin to 梳 *shū*, to comb (i.e., to make the hair "flow" smoothly.) The English word "course" is chosen as the equivalent in the medical context in the sense of freeing the course of qi or freeing the course of wind (out of the body). The homophone 舒 *shū*, to soothe, is sometimes used as a substitute for 疏 in the term 疏肝, as in the formula name Liver-Soothing Pill (*shū gān wán*).

coursing and dissipating external wind 疏散外风 *shū sàn wài fēng*: Any of a number of methods of treatment using mainly acrid dissipating wind-coursing medicinals to treat external wind invading the channels, the flesh, the sinew and bone, and joints. It includes: coursing wind and relieving pain to treat headache or dizziness due to wind invading the head; coursing wind and relieving itching, and clearing heat and eliminating dampness to treat itching, wind papules, or eczema due to wind-heat or wind-damp becoming depressed in the skin and spreading through the blood vessels; dispelling wind and transforming phlegm to treat deviated eyes and mouth due to wind evil with phlegm obstructing the channels network vessels of the face and head; dispelling wind and checking tetany to treat lockjaw arising when "wind evil toxic qi" invades through a wound; dispelling wind and eliminating dampness, quickening the blood and freeing the network vessels to treat numbness of the extremities with inhibited bending and stretching due wind, phlegm-damp, and static blood obstructing the network vessels. The main medicinals used as notopterygium (*qiāng huó*), duhuo (*dú huó*), ledebouriella (*fáng fēng*), angelica (*bái zhǐ*), schizonepeta (*jīng jiè*), and ligusticum (*chuān xiōng*). See COURSING WIND. [16: 432] [60: 351]

coursing and dissipating wind-heat 疏散风热 *shū sàn fēng rè*: See COURSING AND DISSIPATING EXTERNAL WIND. [60: 351]

coursing depression and rectifying qi 疏郁理气 *shū yù lǐ qì*: Synonyms: *resolving depres-*

sion; loosening the chest; loosening the center. A method of treatment used to address qi stagnation due to emotional depression characterized by glomus and oppression in the chest and diaphragm, and pain and distention in the both rib-side and lesser abdomen. Medicinals that course depression and rectify qi include cyperus (*xiāng fù zǐ*), Buddha's hand (*fó shǒu gān*), lindera (*wū yào*), and amomum (*shā rén*). ACU Base treatment mainly on PC, LR, and ST. Select PC-6 (*nèi guān*, Inner Pass), LR-3 (*tài chōng*, Supreme Surge), SP-6 (*sān yīn jiāo*, Three Yin Intersection), BL-18 (*gān shū*, Liver Transport), and ST-36 (*zú sān lǐ*, Leg Three Li); needle with even supplementation and drainage. [26: 711] [27: 270] [46: 646]

coursing the exterior 疏表 *shū biǎo*: A method of treatment used to free the exterior of evil without necessarily making the patient sweat. MED Medicinals used to course the exterior are mild exterior-resolving medicinals such as warm acrid perilla leaf (*zǐ sū yè*) and ledebouriella (*fáng fēng*), and cool acrid mint (*bò hé*), mulberry leaf (*sāng yè*), and pueraria (*gé gēn*). ACU See RESOLVING THE EXTERIOR. [27: 248] [97: 591]

coursing the exterior and transforming dampness 疏表化湿 *shū biǎo huà shī*: A method of treatment used to address dampness in the upper burner and defense aspects, characterized by distention in the head and heavy-headedness, heavy aching body, slimy sensation in the mouth without thirst, slimy white tongue fur, and a soggy floating pulse. MED Use Notopterygium Dampness-Overcoming Decoction (*qiāng huó shèng shī tāng*). ACU Base treatment mainly on LI, LU, SP, and ST. Select GB-20 (*fēng chí*, Wind Pool), LI-4 (*hé gǔ*, Union Valley), LU-7 (*liè quē*, Broken Sequence), LU-5 (*chǐ zé*, Cubit Marsh), SP-9 (*yīn líng quán*, Yin Mound Spring), LI-10 (*shǒu sān lǐ*, Arm Three Li), and ST-36 (*zú sān lǐ*, Leg Three Li); needle with drainage and moxa, if necessary. [27: 260] [46: 597, 650]

coursing the liver 疏肝 *shū gān*: COURSING THE LIVER AND RECTIFYING QI.

coursing the liver and rectifying qi 疏肝理气 *shū gān lǐ qì*: Synonym: *coursing the liver; soothing the liver; discharging the liver.* To restore the normal free coursing of liver qi in the treatment of depression of liver qi, which is characterized by rib-side pain and distention, oppression in the chest, mental depression, pain and distention in the stomach duct, nausea and vomiting, poor appetite, menstrual irregularities, bitter taste in the mouth, stringlike pulse, and thin tongue fur. MED Medicinals that course liver and rectify qi include bupleurum (*chái hú*), tangkuei (*dāng guī*), white peony (*bái sháo yào*), cyperus (*xiāng fù zǐ*), toosendan (*chuān liàn zǐ*), corydalis (*yán hú suǒ*),

and magnolia bark (*hòu pò*). Formulas include Bupleurum Liver-Coursing Powder (*chái hú shū gān sǎn*), Free Wanderer Powder (*xiāo yáo sǎn*), and Counterflow Cold Powder (*sì nì sǎn*). ACU See BINDING DEPRESSION OF LIVER QI. [26: 711] [27: 264] [97: 591]

coursing the liver and resolving depression 疏肝解郁 *shū gān jiě yù*: See COURSING THE LIVER AND RECTIFYING QI.

coursing wind 疏风 *shū fēng*: A method of treatment used to dissipate wind evil with wind-eliminating exterior-resolving medicinals. Wind is a major cause of externally contracted exterior patterns because other evils easily combine with it to enter the body. Hence, treatment of exterior patterns frequently requires wind-coursing action. MED Wind-coursing medicinals used for wind-cold include ledebouriella (*fáng fēng*), cinnamon twig (*guì zhī*), and Chinese lovage (*gǎo běn*); ones used for wind-heat include mint (*bò hé*) and arctium (*niú bàng zǐ*); ones used for wind-damp include notopterygium (*qiāng huó*) and angelica (*bái zhǐ*). Wind-coursing medicinals generally have a mild sweat-effusing effect, and hence differ from powerful sweat-effusing exterior-resolving medicinals such as ephedra (*má huáng*). ACU Base treatment mainly on GB, TB, LU, and LI. Main points: GV-20 (*bǎi huì*, Hundred Convergences), GB-20 (*fēng chí*, Wind Pool), and TB-5 (*wài guān*, Outer Pass). Point selection according to signs: For wind-cold, add LI-4 (*hé gǔ*, Union Valley) and LU-7 (*liè quē*, Broken Sequence); needle with drainage and add moxa. For wind-heat, add GV-14 (*dà zhuī*, Great Hammer), LI-4 (*hé gǔ*, Union Valley), LU-11 (*shào shāng*, Lesser Shang), and LI-1 (*shāng yáng*, Shang Yang); needle with drainage or prick to bleed with a three-edged needle. For wind-damp, add LI-11 (*qū chí*, Pool at the Bend), ST-36 (*zú sān lǐ*, Leg Three Li), and SP-9 (*yīn líng quán*, Yin Mound Spring), needling with drainage. [46: 595] [26: 711] [27: 284] [97: 591]

coursing wind and discharging heat 疏风泄热 *shū fēng xiè rè*: A method of treatment used to address exterior wind-heat with interior heat in colds and flu with sore throat, dry mouth, red tongue, and thin yellow fur. MED Representative wind-coursing heat-discharging formulas include Mulberry Leaf and Chrysanthemum Beverage (*sāng jú yǐn*) and Lonicera and Forsythia Powder (*yín qiào sǎn*). ACU Base treatment mainly on GB, GV, TB, LU, and LI. Select GB-20 (*fēng chí*, Wind Pool), GV-20 (*bǎi huì*, Hundred Convergences), TB-5 (*wài guān*, Outer Pass), GV-14 (*dà zhuī*, Great Hammer), LI-4 (*hé gǔ*, Union Valley), LU-11 (*shào shāng*, Lesser Shang), and LI-1 (*shāng yáng*, Shang Yang); needle with drainage. See COOL ACRID EXTERIOR RESOLUTION. [26: 711]

court 庭 *tíng*: Center of the forehead. [26: 63]

covered moistening 闷润 *mèn rùn*: To allow materials that have been washed or steeped to stand in a receptacle covered with hemp sacking or a bag of moist straw and frequently sprinkle them with water so that they gradually become thoroughly moistened. See WATER PROCESSING. [74: 4] [11: 16]

covering bone 盖骨 *gài gǔ*: LOWER TRANSVERSE BONE.

crab claw markings 蟹爪 *xiè zhuǎ (zhǎo)*: Unnatural lines in the skin like those observed on crab claws; a sign of blood stasis. [95: 90]

crab's-eye 蟹睛 *xiè jīng*, 蟹目 *xiè mù*: A condition characterized by an erosive screen on the DARK OF THE EYE (iris and cornea) from which a bead-like formation resembling the eye of a crab emerges. It is caused by accumulated heat in the liver surging up into the eyes or by external injury. The bead-like formation is surrounded by a white screen and is associated with acute eye pain, aversion to light, and tearing. It leaves a scar on healing, and if the "spirit jelly" (vitreous humor) of the eye escapes, blindness usually ensues. WMC iridoptosis. MED Clear the liver and drain fire. Use variations of Gentian Liver-Draining Decoction (*lóng dǎn xiè gān tāng*). When the redness and pain has abated, treat by nourishing yin and clearing fire with Kidney-Settling Abalone Shell Pill (*zhèn shèn jué míng wán*) and Anemarrhena, Phellodendron, and Rehmannia Pill (*zhī bǎi dì huáng wán*). [27: 504] [97: 658]

cracked dry lips 唇燥裂 *chún zào liè*: See CRACKED LIPS.

cracked lips 唇裂 *chún liè*: Synonym: *cracked parched lips*. Dryness and cracking of the lips with bleeding in severe cases. It is observed in exuberant spleen-stomach heat (yang brightness repletion heat) and effulgent yin vacuity fire. **Exuberant spleen-stomach heat:** In this pattern, cracked lips are accompanied by great thirst and intake of fluid, increased food intake and rapid hungering in cases with bad breath, constipation, large surging, slippery rapid, or sunken replete pulse, and a red tongue with yellow fur. MED Exuberant spleen-stomach heat can be treated by clearing and draining spleen-stomach repletion heat with Cool Clearing Beverage (*qīng liáng yǐn*). **Effulgent yin vacuity fire:** In this pattern, cracked lips are accompanied by reddening of the cheeks, tidal heat [effusion], night sweating, vacuity vexation and insomnia, yellow urine, constipation, red tongue with little fur, and a rapid fine pulse. MED Treat by "invigorating the governor of water to restrain the brilliance of yang" using Six-Ingredient Rehmannia Pill (*liù wèi dì huáng wán*) plus ophiopogon (*mài mén dōng*), tangkuei (*dāng guī*), schisandra

(*wǔ wèi zǐ*), chrysanthemum (*jú huā*), and lycium berry (*gǒu qǐ zǐ*), further adding anemarrhena (*zhī mǔ*) and phellodendron (*huáng bǎi*) if fire signs are pronounced. [26: 512] [92: No. 92] [27: 184] [97: 458]

cracked nipple 乳头破碎 *rǔ tóu pò suì*: NIPPLE WIND.

cramp 转筋 *zhuǎn jīn*: Painful contraction and contortion of the sinews due to insufficiency of qi and blood, fatigue, dampness, or cold. It usually affects the sinews of the calf, and, in severe cases, can affect those of the abdomen, as is commonly the case after vomiting and diarrhea in cholera. See CHOLERA CRAMPS. [27: 374] [97: 330]

crane's-knee phlegm 鹤膝痰 *hè xī tán*: Flowing phlegm of the knee. See FLOWING PHLEGM.

crane's-knee wind 鹤膝风 *hè xī fēng*: Synonym: *knee's eye wind*; *wandering knee wind*. A disease marked by a painful suppurative swelling of the knee associated with emaciation of the lower leg. Crane's-knee wind is attributed to depletion of kidney yin and to depletion of the three yang channels allowing the invasion of cold-damp, which causes congealing stagnation; in most cases it develops from JOINT-RUNNING WIND (*lì jié fēng*). Crane's-knee wind starts with physical cold and heat effusion, slight swelling of knee, difficulty walking, and local pain. As is progresses, the knee becomes red, swollen, and hot or white with diffuse swelling. The thigh and calf become thin, and the swelling at the knee bursts to produce fluid pus or a thick yellow humor. Crane's-knee wind heals with difficulty. MED In the initial stage, use Five Accumulations Powder (*wǔ jī sǎn*) and apply white mustard (*bái jiè zǐ*) topically and apply a scallion hot pack. Alternative topical treatments include moxibustion or application of Yang-Returning Jade Dragon Paste (*huí yáng yù lóng gāo*). In enduring conditions characterized by painful white swelling, treatment should take the form of supporting right and dispelling the evil by warming yang and dispersing dampness with Major Ledebouriella Decoction (*dà fáng fēng tāng*) or Duhuo and Mistletoe Decoction (*dú huó jì shēng tāng*), with judicious addition of frankincense (*rǔ xiāng*) for severe pain. After rupture, 15 g each of cotton rose leaf (*mù fú róng yè*) and chrysanthemum leaf (*jú huā yè*) can be applied crushed and mixed with boiled wheat and steamed bean curd dregs (*dòu fǔ zhā*). ACU Base treatment mainly on GB and local points. Select GB-34 (*yáng líng quán*, Yang Mound Spring), GB-30 (*huán tiào*, Jumping Round), GB-31 (*fēng shì*, Wind Market), ST-34 (*liáng qiū*, Beam Hill), Eye of the Knee (*xī yǎn*) GB-33 (*xī yáng guān*, Knee Yang Joint), and SP-9 (*yīn líng quán*, Yin Mound Spring); needle with drainage and add moxa. Selection of points according to stage: In the initial stage, add to the main points GB-20 (*fēng chí*, Wind Pool), GV-16 (*fēng fǔ*, Wind Mansion), LI-4 (*hé gǔ*, Union Valley), and LI-11 (*qū chí*, Pool at the Bend); needle with drainage and add moxa. In enduring illness, add to the main points BL-23 (*shèn shū*, Kidney Transport), GV-4 (*mìng mén*, Life Gate), CV-4 (*guān yuán*, Pass Head), and ST-36 (*zú sān lǐ*, Leg Three Li); needle with even supplementation and drainage or with supplementation, and add large amounts of moxa. ◇ Chin 鹤 *hè*, crane; 膝 *xī*, knee; 风 *fēng*, wind; so called because the leg is thin while the knee is enlarged as in the crane. [26: 990] [27: 407] [97: 638] [46: 629, 630] [113: 234]

crevice 罅陷 *xià xiàn*: A parting or opening in flesh, sinew, and bone that can be felt by palpation. [48: 470]

crick in the neck 落枕 *luò zhěn*: Stiffness of the neck that results from taxation fatigue (overwork etc.) twisting, sleeping in the wrong posture or from exposure to a draft (wind-cold). MED For twisting, use Sinew-Soothing Decoction (*shū jīn tāng*). For wind-cold, use Pueraria Decoction (*gé gēn tāng*). For kidney vacuity in run-down patients, use Six-Ingredient Rehmannia Pill (*liù wèi dì huáng wán*). ACU Base treatment mainly on GV, hand and foot greater yang (*tài yáng*) SI/BL, and hand and foot lesser yang (*shào yáng*) TB/GB. Select GV-14 (*dà zhuī*, Great Hammer), ouch points (*ā shì xué*), SI-3 (*hòu xī*, Back Ravine), Crick in the Neck Point (*luò zhěn xué*) (0.5 body-inches above the posterior hairline, 1.3 body-inches lateral to the midline), and GB-39 (*xuán zhōng*, Suspended Bell). Needle with drainage followed by moxa or cupping. Selection of points according to cause: For wind-cold, add TB-5 (*wài guān*, Outer Pass), GB-20 (*fēng chí*, Wind Pool), and LI-4 (*hé gǔ*, Union Valley). For kidney vacuity taxation detriment, add BL-23 (*shèn shū*, Kidney Transport) and KI-3 (*tài xī*, Great Ravine). Selection of points according to affected area: When affecting the greater yang (*tài yáng*) channel, add BL-10 (*tiān zhù*, Celestial Pillar), BL-11 (*dà zhù*, Great Shuttle), SI-14 (*jiān wài shū*, Outer Shoulder Transport), BL-60 (*kūn lún*, Kunlun Mountains), and LU-7 (*liè quē*, Broken Sequence). When affecting the lesser yang (*shào yáng*) channel, add GB-20 (*fēng chí*, Wind Pool), TB-17 (*yì fēng*, Wind Screen), and TB-5 (*wài guān*, Outer Pass). [27: 544] [37: 440] [113: 427]

crimson 绛 *jiàng*: A deep shade of red indicating severe heat. Usually describes the tongue body. See CRIMSON TONGUE. [6: 122] [27: 178] [97: 195]

crimson tongue 舌绛 *shé jiàng*: A crimson tongue is deep red tongue. Like the red tongue, it is associated with heat, but the added depth of color indicates a warm evil that has penetrated to the construction or blood aspect. [26: 122]

critical measles pattern 麻疹险证 *má zhěn xiǎn zhèng*: The manifestation of a measles marked by exuberant evil and debilitation of right. See UNFAVORABLE MEASLES PATTERN; MEASLES TOXIN FALLING INTO THE LUNG. [26: 588]

crippling wilt 痿躄 *wěi bì*: See WILTING.

crossed menstruation 错经 *cuò jīng*: MENSTRUAL BLOODY STOOL.

cross moxa 十字灸 *shí zì jiǔ*: Applying moxa pole moxibustion at five points that form a cross: CV-8 (*shén què*, Spirit Gate Tower), which is the umbilicus, CV-6 (*qì hǎi*, Sea of Qi) just above it, bilateral ST-25 (*tiān shū*, Celestial Pivot) beside it, and CV-9 (*shuǐ fēn*, Water Divide) below it. Cross moxa is used to treat enduring spleen vacuity diarrhea and cold-damp diarrhea with abdominal pain. Compare FIVE PILLAR POINTS. [113: 88]

cross needling 缪刺 *miù cì*: A needling method involving the needling of one side of the body to treat disease affecting the other side. It differs from the GREAT NEEDLING in that it involves shallow needling of the network vessels, and in practice mainly involves shallow needling of the well points or pricking of network vessels showing visible blood stasis to bleed. It may also include needling of points at the contralateral point in the position corresponding to that of the affected area. The cross needling method is used in the treatment of disease of the network vessels. Compare GREAT NEEDLING and SELECTION OF CONTRALATERAL POINTS. [26: 947]

crude 生 *shēng*: *Synonym:* raw. Uncooked or unprocessed.

crushing 捣 *dǎo*: *Synonym:* pounding. To damage or destroy the structure of medicinal materials such as with a pestle and mortar. Some small fruits and seeds are crushed just before with a pestle and mortar. Gardenia (*shān zhī zǐ*), amomum (*shā rén*), and Katsumada's galangal seed (*cǎo dòu kòu*), are crushed in small quantities before decoction to ensure that the active constituents are extracted. Medicinals should not be stored for long periods after crushing since they may lose their oil content and other constituents, thus becoming less effective. [27: 322]

crust 痂 *jiā*, 结痂 *jié jiā*: **1.** *n.* A scab. **2.** *vb.* To form a scab. [48: 255]

cubit 尺 *chǐ*: **1.** A unit of measure equal to ten inches. **2.** Of the three positions of the wrist pulse, the one closest to the elbow. See WRIST PULSE. ◇ Chin 尺 *chǐ*, the distance from the elbow to the wrist; Eng *cubit* from L. *cubitum*, the elbow; a unit of measure equal to the distance from the elbow to the tip of the fingers. [48: 35]

cubit pulse 尺脉 *chǐ mài*: A position of the wrist pulse, one inch behind the bar on the line running from the bar to the transverse crease at LU-5 (*chǐ zé*, Cubit Marsh). See WRIST PULSE. [27: 198]

cubit skin 尺肤 *chǐ fū*: The area from LU-5 (*chǐ zé*, Cubit Marsh) to the wrist pulse. Formerly, examination of the cubit skin was a part of diagnosis, and attention was paid to whether the cubit skin was moist or dry and hot or cold. See BODY PALPATION. [27: 203] [26: 133]

cumbersome 困 *kùn*: Heaviness and fatigue felt in the limbs, particularly when the spleen fails to transform water-damp. See SPLEEN VACUITY WITH DAMP ENCUMBRANCE. [48: 121]

cun 寸 *cùn*: INCH.

cupping 拔罐法 *bá guàn fǎ*: Synonym: *horning*; *fire cupping*. Synonym: A method of treatment involving the application of suction to skin to draw out blood and sometimes pus. Cupping is also called *fire cupping* because the suction is produced when, for example, a lighted alcohol swab placed inside the cup burns the oxygen to create a vacuum after the cup has been placed on the skin. The method of treatment now called cupping was mentioned in *Emergency Standby Remedies* (*zhǒu hòu bèi jí fāng*) by Ge Hong (c. 281–361) as *horning*. Fire cups used to be made of animal horn, bamboo, or earthenware, but globe-shaped glass ones are now preferred because they enable the practitioner to see the flame and so prevent it from burning the patient. The recent development of cups with suction pumps (suction cups) makes cupping safer and more convenient than before. **Application**: Cupping is used to treat wind-damp impediment (*bì*) pain, colds, phlegm-rheum, cough and panting; stomach pain, abdominal pain, back and lumbar pain, leg qi pain; initial-stage welling-abscess (*yōng*) and flat-abscess (*jū*). Individual forms of cupping include STATIONARY CUPPING, PUSH-CUPPING, FLASH-CUPPING, and PRICKING AND CUPPING. **Contraindications**: Cupping should not be applied where there is generalized heat [effusion] with headache, clouded vision and heavy head, convulsions, arched-back rigidity, or clenched jaw. It should not be used on parts of the body affected by skin disease or areas where the flesh is thin or bones show through, or on major blood vessels. It should not be applied to the abdomen in pregnancy or to areas affected by water swelling. [37: 235] [27: 345] [97: 333]

cutaneous 皮 *pí*, 皮肤 *pí fū*: Of or relating to the SKIN.

cutaneous needle 皮肤针 *pí fū zhēn*: An instrument traditionally made by binding five or seven sewing needles to a bamboo stick (traditionally called PLUM-BLOSSOM NEEDLE and SEVEN-STAR NEEDLE, now made by mounting needles on a metal or plastic hammer), and used to tap the skin to move qi and quicken the blood in the affected area or on the pathway of an affected channel. The cutaneous needle is especially suitable for treating children and others where pain or fear of needle insertion may be a necessary consideration. The tapping can be light (no bleeding) or heavy (slight bleeding) depending on the patient's condition and the disease being treated. Nowadays in China, heavy tapping is employed to move stagnant blood in a local area. Cupping can be used to treat a number of internal medical diseases including digestive disorders, headache, menstrual pain and some skin diseases. Legal factors limit the applicability of this method in the West since cutaneous needles are difficult to sterilize. **Method**: The needle should be held about two inches above the skin and manipulated by a loose movement of the wrist. The needle must strike the skin perpendicularly and without excessive force to prevent bleeding. In general, tapping is performed from the top downward and from the medial toward the lateral aspect. Cutaneous tapping is contraindicated on ulcerations or external injuries. The two most common types of cutaneous needle now used are the plum blossom and the seven-star needle. [27: 530]

cutaneous region 皮部 *pí bù*: Any of the TWELVE CUTANEOUS REGIONS.

cutting 切 *qiē*: Dividing (medicinal materials) with a knife into two or more pieces. Cutting is a commonly used basic method of medicinal processing. It facilitates drying and storage, increases weighing accuracy, and makes it easier for active constituents to be extracted during preparation processes such as decoction. Cutting is often facilitated by soaking or steeping. Kitchen knives, herb knives, guillotines, and nowadays, cutting machines, are used to cut materials into lumps, slices of various sizes, usually known as *decocting pieces*. Herb cutters save labor time, but cut less cleanly than an experienced hand cutter using a sharp knife. Cutting includes cross-cutting (横切 *héng qiē*), oblique cutting (斜切 *xié qiē*), and lengthwise cutting (纵切 *zòng qiē*). The length or thickness and shape to which materials are cut depends on the material. Roots, rhizomes, stems, vines, and woody materials that are hard in substance are cut into thin slices, i.e., about 0.15 cm, whereas softer, less dense materials are cut into thick slices (about 0.3 cm) slices or in lengths of 1–1.5 cm. Materials that are long and thin, such as imperata (*bái máo gēn*) can be cut into lengths of 1–1.5 cm. Skins and barks, such as phellodendron (*huáng bǎi*), that are hard and thick can be cut into shreds of 0.6 cm. Thinner, less dense barks, such as eucommia (*dù zhòng*) are cut into broad strips of 1–1.5 cm. Brittle, fragile materials like lycium root bark (*dì gǔ pí*) need not be cut. Leaves that are thick and flexible, such as pyrrosia (*shí wéi*) are cut into strips of 1–1.5 cm. Thick ones that are brittle after drying, such as mulberry leaf (*sāng yè*) and perilla leaf (*zǐ sū yè*) are either not cut or are simply rubbed between the hands. Whole plants with thin stems are cut into lengths of 1.5 cm; ones with thicker stems are cut into shorter lengths. Flowers and small fruits and seeds are generally not cut. Large fruits or ones that do not dry easily, such as crataegus (*shān zhā*) are cut into three or four slices. Some pericarps such as trichosanthes rind (*guā lóu pí*) are roughly shredded. [27: 322]

CV 任脉 *rèn mài*: CONTROLLING VESSEL.

D

dai yang 戴阳 *dài yáng*: UPCAST YANG.

damage 伤 *shāng*: Injury of any kind, e.g., damage to liquid.

damage by the five taxations 五劳所伤 *wǔ láo suǒ shāng*: Diseases of qi, blood, sinews, and bones caused by imbalance of work and rest. *The Inner Canon* (*nèi jīng*) states, "Prolonged vision damages the blood; prolonged lying damages qi; prolonged sitting damages the flesh; prolonged standing damages the bones; and prolonged walking damages the sinews. These are the five forms of taxation damage." See TAXATION. [27: 118] [97: 55]

damage to both qi and yin 气阴两伤 *qì yīn liǎng shāng*: DUAL VACUITY OF QI AND YIN. [26: 540]

damage to fluids 津液损伤 *jīn yè sǔn shāng*: Reduction of liquid and humor by the action of heat or fire occurring in internal damage miscellaneous disease when yin humor is depleted as a result of enduring illness, excessive loss of blood, excessive urination, or overuse of water-disinhibiting (diuretic) medicinals. It includes DAMAGE TO LIQUID and the more severe form, DAMAGE TO YIN. [6: 46]

damage to liquid 伤津 *shāng jīn*: A disease pattern resulting from major depletion of fluids following high fever, excessive sweating in externally contracted heat (febrile) disease or from severe vomiting and diarrhea. Signs include thirst with desire to drink, dry throat, lips, tongue, nose, and skin, and a dry red tongue. MED Clear heat and moisten dryness; engender liquid and increase humor. Commonly used medicinals include adenophora/glehnia (*shā shēn*), ophiopogon (*mài mén dōng*), Solomon's seal (*yù zhú*), scrophularia (*xuán shēn*), dried/fresh rehmannia (*shēng dì huáng*), trichosanthes root (*tiān huā fěn*), pseudostellaria (*tài zǐ shēn*), and black sesame (*hēi zhī má*). Formulas include Humor-Increasing Decoction (*zēng yè tāng*), Adenophora/Glehnia and Ophiopogon Decoction (*shā shēn mài dōng tāng*), and Bamboo Leaf and Gypsum Decoction (*zhú yè shí gāo tāng*). [6: 46] [27: 207] [97: 198]

damage to the fetus by toxic medicinals in pregnancy 妊娠毒药伤胎 *rèn shēn dú yào shāng tāi*: Lumbar pain, sagging in the abdomen, and signs of stirring fetus after consumption of toxic medicinals in pregnancy. MED Resolve toxin and quiet the fetus. Make a strong decoction of licorice (*gān cǎo*), black soybean (*hēi dà dòu*), and bamboo leaf (lophatherum) (*dàn zhú yè*) and take in frequent small doses. See also STIRRING FETUS. [26: 340]

damage to the liver by anger 怒伤肝 *nù shāng gān*, 怒气伤肝 *nù qì shāng gan*: See ANGER DAMAGES THE LIVER.

damage to the lung by the dryness qi 燥气伤肺 *zào qì shāng fèi*: DRYNESS QI DAMAGING THE LUNG.

damage to the network vessels of the lung 肺络损伤 *fèi luò sǔn shāng*: A condition manifest in expectoration of blood; caused by severe or enduring cough.

damage to the thoroughfare and controlling vessels 冲任损伤 *chōng rèn sǔn shāng*: *Synonym: emptiness of the thoroughfare and controlling vessels*. Any of various patterns such as menstrual irregularities, lesser-abdominal pain, lumbar pain, flooding and spotting, habitual miscarriage, or infertility attributable to excessive sexual activity, excessive childbirth, or various evils. The thoroughfare (*chōng*) vessel is the sea of blood, whereas the controlling (*rèn*) vessel governs the fetus; both are intimately related to the liver, kidney, qi and blood. [27: 146] [97: 223]

damage to yang 伤阳 *shāng yáng*: Damage to yang qi; it may be a) due to use of cold bitter medicinals, or sweating, or diarrhea during the course of disease; b) due to direct strike by cold evil or prevalence of internal cold yin qi, described in *Elementary Questions* (*sù wèn, yīn yáng yìng xiàng dà lùn*) as "When yin prevails, yang ails"; c) due to sudden joy that causes the heart spirit to float astray and qi to be easily worn and dissipated, causing heart palpitations, fearful throbbing, abstraction, and insomnia. [26: 809] [27: 207] [97: 198] [25: 117]

damage to yin 伤阴 *shāng yīn*: Loss of body fluids. **1.** Scorching of yin fluid by hyperactive yang. **2.** *Synonym: humor desertion*. Loss of fluids more severe than damage to liquid, generally occurring in the later stages of externally contracted heat (febrile) diseases when the patient's general condition is poor and characterized by a desiccated, peeling, or mirror tongue that is dull crimson in color. The throat and mouth, lips, nose, and skin are dry although the thirst is not pronounced. There are also signs such as dry bound stool and short voidings of scant urine. In severe cases, there may be clouded spirit and TETANIC REVERSAL. [26: 805] [27: 207] [97: 198] [25: 117]

damming method 按截法 *àn jié fǎ*: See QI-MOVING TECHNIQUE.

damp 湿 *shī*: See DAMPNESS.

damp cholera 湿霍乱 *shī huò luàn*: **1.** CHOLERA. The principal feature of cholera is simultaneous vomiting and diarrhea. However, desire to vomit without vomiting and desire to defecate without diarrhea constitutes DRY CHOLERA; hence the term damp cholera serves the purpose of differentiation. See CHOLERA. **2.** Synonym: *summerheat cholera*. Summerheat cholera. ⟨WMC⟩ cholera; paracholera; bacillary food poisoning. See COLD CHOLERA; HEAT CHOLERA; CHOLERA CRAMPS. [26: 928] [27: 365] [97: 581]

damp cough 湿咳 *shī ké*, 湿嗽 *shī sòu*: COUGH due to contraction of dampness evil giving rise to damp phlegm that congests the lung. Damp cough is characterized by cough with copious phlegm, joint pain, heavy limbs, swelling of the face and limbs, and inhibited urination. ⟨MED⟩ Transform dampness and dispel phlegm using formulas such as Priceless Qi-Righting Powder (*bù huàn jīn zhèng qì sǎn*) ⟨ACU⟩ Base treatment mainly on LU, SP, and ST. Select BL-13 (*fèi shū*, Lung Transport), LU-9 (*tài yuān*, Great Abyss), SP-3 (*tài bái*, Supreme White), LU-5 (*chǐ zé*, Cubit Marsh), CV-22 (*tiān tú*, Celestial Chimney), ST-40 (*fēng lóng*, Bountiful Bulge), ST-36 (*zú sān lǐ*, Leg Three Li), SP-9 (*yīn líng quán*, Yin Mound Spring), and LI-4 (*hé gǔ*, Union Valley). Needle with drainage and add moxa. [26: 924] [46: 653]

damp depression 湿郁 *shī yù*: One of the SIX DEPRESSIONS. Stagnation of dampness usually arising when dampness causes qi to stagnate. Damp depression is characterized by generalized pain and heaviness, heavy clouded head, fatigue and lassitude, somnolence, thin slimy tongue fur, and a pulse that is sunken, rough, and moderate. Episodes are brought on by yin-type (dull wet) weather. If damp depression is accompanied by heat and prevents the heat from thrusting through to the outer body, the pattern is called DAMPNESS TRAPPING HIDDEN HEAT; if it affects movement and transformation of the spleen, it is called DAMPNESS ENCUMBERING SPLEEN YANG. ⟨MED⟩ Eliminate dampness and resolve depression. Use Damp Depression Decoction (*shī yù tāng*), Dampness-Eliminating Decoction (*chú shī tāng*), or Stomach-Calming Powder (*píng wèi sǎn*). See SIX DEPRESSIONS. ⟨ACU⟩ Base treatment mainly on SP and ST. Select SP-9 (*yīn líng quán*, Yin Mound Spring), ST-36 (*zú sān lǐ*, Leg Three Li), LI-4 (*hé gǔ*, Union Valley), PC-6 (*nèi guān*, Inner Pass), CV-6 (*qì hǎi*, Sea of Qi), and LR-3 (*tài chōng*, Supreme Surge); needle with even supplementation and drainage

and moxa, if appropriate. For dampness trapping hidden heat, drain LI-11 (*qū chí*, Pool at the Bend), ST-44 (*nèi tíng*, Inner Court), and SP-6 (*sān yīn jiāo*, Three Yin Intersection). For dampness encumbering spleen yang, add CV-12 (*zhōng wǎn*, Center Stomach Duct), LR-13 (*zhāng mén*, Camphorwood Gate), and BL-20 (*pí shū*, Spleen Transport). [26: 928] [46: 597, 646]

damp diarrhea 湿泻 *shī xiè*: Synonyms: *soggy diarrhea*; *throughflux diarrhea*. DIARRHEA attributable to dampness qi damaging the spleen. The stool is either watery or sloppy and evacuated several times a day. The tongue fur is slimy and the pulse soggy. ⟨MED⟩ Transform dampness and harmonize the center using formulas like Dampness-Eliminating Decoction (*chú shī tāng*) or Stomach-Calming Poria (Hoelen) Five Decoction (*wèi líng tāng*). If there is heat, Fifth and Sixth Heavenly Stem Pill (*wù jǐ wán*) can be used. ⟨ACU⟩ Base treatment mainly on CV, ST, SP, and back transport points. Select CV-12 (*zhōng wǎn*, Center Stomach Duct), LR-13 (*zhāng mén*, Camphorwood Gate), BL-20 (*pí shū*, Spleen Transport), ST-25 (*tiān shū*, Celestial Pivot), CV-4 (*guān yuán*, Pass Head), SP-9 (*yīn líng quán*, Yin Mound Spring), ST-36 (*zú sān lǐ*, Leg Three Li), and CV-9 (*shuǐ fēn*, Water Divide). Needle with supplementation, adding moxa at these points or cross moxa (*shí zì jiǔ*). [26: 928] [27: 363] [97: 597]

damp-heat 湿热 *shī rè*: A combination of dampness and heat. Damp-heat may be of external or internal origin, or a combination of both. It can cause a variety of different diseases, and is characterized by signs of both dampness and heat. Pain and fullness in the abdomen and poor appetite reflect dampness, whereas heat effusion, hard stool, and short voidings of scant yellow or reddish urine reflect heat. The tongue fur is yellow, thick, and slimy, the yellowness reflecting heat and the thickness and sliminess reflecting dampness. The pulse is rapid, and either soggy or slippery, the rapidness indicating heat and the soggy or slippery quality indicating dampness. Thirst indicates heat, but the lack of desire to actually swallow fluids reflects the clogging effect of dampness. Generally speaking, damp-heat of external origin gives rise to signs such as heat effusion, heart vexation, thirst, spontaneous sweating, painful swollen limb joints, and fullness in the chest. Damp-heat that arises internally by dampness forming with heat tends to affect the middle and lower burner, as well as the skin. This broad range of diseases caused by damp-heat evil may be classified according to the organ or aspect of the organism affected. Damp-heat patterns include: DAMP-HEAT LODGED IN THE QI ASPECT, characterized by low fluctuating heat effusion with fatigued limbs and oppression in the chest; SPLEEN-STOMACH DAMP-HEAT, characterized by nausea, vomiting, and diarrhea. DAMP-HEAT BREWING IN THE LIVER AND GALL-BLADDER, characterized by rib-side pain and distention; DAMP-HEAT POURING DOWN INTO THE BLADDER, characterized by frequent urination, urinary urgency, painful urination, and yellow to reddish urine; DAMP-HEAT POURING DOWN INTO THE LARGE INTESTINE, characterized by diarrhea with ungratifying defecation or by frequent defecation with tenesmus and stool containing pus and blood (dysentery). The latter two categories are forms of DAMP-HEAT POURING DOWNWARD (lower burner damp-heat), which can also manifest in the form of genital itch, vaginal discharge, painful swelling of the joints of the lower limbs, foot damp qi (Hongkong foot), and cinnabar toxin (erysipelas) of the lower leg. MED Damp-heat is treated by the combined method of clearing heat and transforming dampness, emphasis being variously placed on either of its two components depending on whether dampness or heat is prominent. ACU Points are selected according to whether the cause is external or internal. For external causes, use LI-11 (*qū chí*, Pool at the Bend), LI-4 (*hé gǔ*, Union Valley), ST-36 (*zú sān lǐ*, Leg Three Li), GB-34 (*yáng líng quán*, Yang Mound Spring) as the main points, and drain. For internal causes, use SP-9 (*yīn líng quán*, Yin Mound Spring), SP-6 (*sān yīn jiāo*, Three Yin Intersection), LI-11 (*qū chí*, Pool at the Bend), and ST-44 (*nèi tíng*, Inner Court) as the main points, and drain. Although moxa is often used in the treatment of dampness, it should not be used for damp-heat. Treatment varies according to the organ or aspect of the organism affected. [26: 926] [27: 115] [97: 580] [46: 597]

damp-heat abdominal pain 湿热腹痛 *shī rè fù tòng*: ABDOMINAL PAIN due to damp-heat brewing in the spleen and stomach. It is intermittent pain that refuses pressure, and is sometimes associated with retching and vomiting, or heat effusion and aversion to cold, or yellowing of the body and eyes, and with oppression in the chest. Other accompanying signs include bitter taste or slimy sensation in the mouth, constipation or diarrhea, a slimy yellow tongue fur, and a soggy rapid or surging rapid pulse. WMC This pattern is seen in cholecystitis, cholelithiasis (gallstones), intestinal tuberculosis, and chronic bacillary dysentery. MED Clear heat and drain fire; move qi and transform dampness. Use formulas like Fire-Dissipating Decoction (*sàn huǒ tāng*) or Major Bupleurum Decoction (*dà chái hú tāng*). ACU Base treatment mainly on LI, ST, and SP. Select LI-4 (*hé gǔ*, Union Valley), ST-25 (*tiān shū*, Celestial Pivot), CV-12 (*zhōng wǎn*, Center Stomach Duct), ST-36 (*zú sān lǐ*, Leg Three Li), LI-11 (*qū chí*, Pool at the Bend), SP-9 (*yīn líng quán*, Yin Mound Spring), and needle with drainage. See also DAMP-HEAT DYSENTERY. [26: 928]

damp-heat brewing internally 湿热内蕴 *shī rè nèi yùn*: Damp-heat brewing in the spleen and stomach and in the liver and gallbladder. Dampness is a heavy, turbid, and stagnant evil that hampers qi dynamic. Heat, when combining with dampness, is difficult to resolve, and has a damaging effect on yang qi. It is characterized by abiding, high postmeridian fever, generalized heaviness, fatigue and lack of strength, heavy clouded spirit, glomus and fullness in the chest and stomach duct, no thought of food and drink, sticky slimy stool with ungratifying defecation, inhibited urination with yellow or reddish urine. In some cases, there may be jaundice. [26: 927] [27: 132] [97: 582]

damp-heat brewing in the bladder 湿热蕴结膀胱 *shī rè yùn jié páng guāng*: BLADDER DAMP-HEAT.

damp-heat brewing in the liver and gallbladder 湿热蕴结肝胆 *shī rè yùn jié gān dǎn*: LIVER-GALLBLADDER DAMP-HEAT.

damp-heat brewing in the spleen 湿热蕴脾 *shī rè yùn pí*: SPLEEN-STOMACH DAMP-HEAT.

damp-heat diarrhea 湿热泻 *shī rè xiè*: Diarrhea due to damp-heat brewing and binding in the stomach and intestines. Damp-heat diarrhea is thick yellow diarrhea with abdominal pain and heat, red face, and thirst. It mostly occurs in the summer. MED Use Poria (Hoelen) Five Powder (*wǔ líng sǎn*) plus gypsum (*shí gāo*), licorice (*gān cǎo*), and mutong (*mù tōng*). [50: 1559]

damp-heat dizziness 湿热眩晕 *shī rè xuàn yūn*: See SUMMERHEAT-DAMP DIZZINESS. [26: 927]

damp-heat dysentery 湿热痢 *shī rè lì*: DYSENTERY attributed to damp-heat. Damp-heat dysentery arises when damp-heat accumulates in the intestines, causing stagnation of qi and blood and impairing the intestine's function of conveyance. It is associated with the classic signs of dysentery, i.e., red and white stool due to the presence of blood and pus, tenesmus, and abdominal pain; it is characterized by thick sticky, foul-smelling stool that causes a burning sensation in the anus when passed, short voidings of reddish urine, a slimy yellow tongue fur, and slippery rapid pulse. In some cases, heat effusion is present. MED Clear heat and dry dampness; regulate qi and move the blood. Use formulas like Peony Decoction (*sháo yào tāng*), Pulsatilla Decoction (*bái tóu wēng tāng*), or Saussurea and Coptis Pill (*xiāng lián wán*). If there is pronounced generalized heat [effusion], Pueraria, Scutellaria, and Coptis Decoction (*gé gēn qín lián tāng*) can be used. If qi and food stagnation signs such as abdominal pain and tenesmus are pronounced, use Unripe Bitter Orange Stagnation-Abducting Pill (*zhǐ shí dǎo zhì wán*). In addition, humifuse euphorbia (*dì jǐn cǎo*), purslane (*mǎ chǐ xiàn*), andrographis (*chuān xīn lián*), and garlic (*dà suàn*) are also effective. ACU Base treatment on ST and LI. Select LI-4 (*hé gǔ*, Union Valley), ST-25 (*tiān shū*, Celestial Pivot), ST-37 (*shàng jù xū*, Upper Great Hollow), LI-11 (*qū chí*, Pool at the Bend), and ST-44 (*nèi tíng*, Inner Court), needling with drainage. For pronounced generalized heat [effusion], add GV-14 (*dà zhuī*, Great Hammer) and prick the Ten Diffusing Points (*shí xuān*). For pronounced qi stagnation or food stagnation, add CV-12 (*zhōng wǎn*, Center Stomach Duct), CV-6 (*qì hǎi*, Sea of Qi), ST-36 (*zú sān lǐ*, Leg Three Li), PC-6 (*nèi guān*, Inner Pass), and ST-21 (*liáng mén*, Beam Gate). [26: 927] [27: 361] [97: 581]

damp-heat headache 湿热头痛 *shī rè tóu tòng*: HEADACHE due to damp-heat steaming upward and clouding the upper orifices. It is associated with heavy-headedness, heavy body, vexation, pain in the joints, swelling of the limbs and face, slimy yellow tongue fur, and a rapid soggy pulse. MED Clear heat and transform dampness. Use Clear Sky Paste (*qīng kōng gāo*) or Three Kernels Decoction (*sān rén tāng*) and their variations. ACU Base treatment mainly on ST and LI. Select Greater Yang (*tài yáng*), LI-4 (*hé gǔ*, Union Valley), LU-7 (*liè quē*, Broken Sequence), LI-11 (*qū chí*, Pool at the Bend), ST-36 (*zú sān lǐ*, Leg Three Li), and SP-9 (*yīn líng quán*, Yin Mound Spring), and needle with drainage. For selection of points according to affected area, and additional information, see HEADACHE. [26: 928] [46: 597]

damp-heat jaundice 湿热黄疸 *shī rè huáng dǎn*: JAUNDICE due to damp-heat; a form of yang jaundice. Damp-heat is the major cause of jaundice and is identified by signs such as generalized heat [effusion], vexation and thirst, and a forceful surging slippery pulse. Other signs include agitation, swift digestion with rapid hungering, painful rough voidings of red urine, and constipation. WMC Mostly corresponds to acute icteric hepatitis. MED Clear heat and disinhibit dampness; open depression. Use Rhubarb and Niter Decoction (*dà huáng xiāo shí tāng*) or Capillaris Decoction (*yīn chén hāo tāng*). Compare YANG JAUNDICE. More at JAUNDICE. [26: 927] [97: 583]

damp-heat lodged in the qi aspect 湿热留恋气分 *shī rè liú liàn qì fèn*: *Synonym: damp-heat lodged in the triple burner.* An externally contracted heat (febrile) disease pattern characterized by persistent low or remittent heat effusion, fatigued limbs, and oppression in the chest. Thirst without appreciable intake of fluid is accompanied by a bland, bitter taste or slimy sensation in the mouth. Voidings are short with reddish urine. The tongue fur is yellow and slimy. Summerheat-damp and damp obstruction may also be characterized by such signs. More at QI-ASPECT PATTERN. [6: 209]

damp-heat lodged in the triple burner 湿热留恋三焦 *shī rè liú liàn sān jiāo*: DAMP-HEAT LODGED IN THE QI ASPECT.

damp-heat lumbar pain 湿热腰痛 *shī rè yāo tòng*: LUMBAR PAIN due to damp-heat obstructing the channels and network vessels. Damp-heat lumbar pain is characterized by lumbar and hip pain with local sensation of heat, associated with a rapid stringlike pulse and reddish urine. MED Clear heat and disinhibit dampness. Use formulas like Supplemented Mysterious Two Powder (*jiā wèi èr miào sǎn*). ACU Base treatment on SP, BL, and KI. Select SP-9 (*yīn líng quán*, Yin Mound Spring), BL-40 (*wěi zhōng*, Bend Center), BL-37 (*yīn mén*, Gate of Abundance), and KI-3 (*tài xī*, Great Ravine). Needle with drainage or prick to bleed. [26: 928] [46: 633] [37: 390]

damp-heat mounting 湿热疝 *shī rè shàn*: MOUNTING (*shàn*) attributed to damp-heat; characterized by heat, swelling, distention, and pain of the scrotum with constipation, yellow urine, slimy yellow tongue fur, and a rapid stringlike pulse. In some cases there may be heat effusion and aversion to cold. MED Clear heat and transform dampness; disperse swelling and dissipate binds. Use Gentian Liver-Draining Decoction (*lóng dǎn xiè gān tāng*) combined with Tangerine Pip Pill (*jú hé wán*). ACU Base treatment mainly on the CV and the three yin channels of the foot. Select CV-3 (*zhōng jí*, Central Pole), ST-30 (*qì chōng*, Qi Thoroughfare), CV-4 (*guān yuán*, Pass Head), LR-3 (*tài chōng*, Supreme Surge), SP-9 (*yīn líng quán*, Yin Mound Spring), SP-6 (*sān yīn jiāo*, Three Yin Intersection), and LR-1 (*dà dūn*, Large Pile), needling with drainage. Selection of points according to signs: For painful swelling of the scrotum, add LR-8 (*qū quán*, Spring at the Bend), KI-6 (*zhào hǎi*, Shining Sea), and LR-5 (*lǐ gōu*, Woodworm Canal). For heat effusion and aversion to cold, add LI-4 (*hé gǔ*, Union Valley), LI-11 (*qū chí*, Pool at the Bend), and TB-5 (*wài guān*, Outer Pass). [46: 680] [113: 191]

damp-heat obstructing the spleen and stomach 湿热阻滞脾胃 *shī rè zǔ zhì pí wèi*: SPLEEN-STOMACH DAMP-HEAT.

damp-heat pouring down into the bladder 湿热下注膀胱 *shī rè xià zhù páng guāng*: BLADDER DAMP-HEAT.

damp-heat pouring down into the large intestine 湿热下注大肠 *shī rè xià zhù dà cháng*: *Synonym:* LARGE INTESTINAL DAMP-HEAT.

damp-heat pouring downward 湿热下注 *shī rè xià zhù*: LOWER BURNER DAMP-HEAT. [26: 927]

damp-heat rib-side pain 湿热胁痛 *shī rè xié tòng*: RIB-SIDE PAIN due to damp-heat causing stagnation of qi in the liver and gallbladder vessels. Damp-heat rib-side pain is a continuous pain associated with distention or that comes in acute episodes, and and that may stretch into the region below the heart and the back of the chest. It is associated with nausea, vomiting, oppression in the chest, torpid intake, short voidings of reddish urine, and in some cases heat and cold and yellowing of the eye and skin. MED Course the liver and gallbladder; clear heat and transform dampness. Use formulas like Gentian Liver-Draining Decoction (*lóng dǎn xiè gān tāng*) or Capillaris Decoction (*yīn chén hāo tāng*). ACU Base treatment mainly on hand and foot lesser yang (*shào yáng*) TB/GB, LR and SP. Select LR-14 (*qī mén*, Cycle Gate), GB-24 (*rì yuè*, Sun and Moon), TB-6 (*zhī gōu*, Branch Ditch), GB-34 (*yáng líng quán*, Yang Mound Spring), SP-9 (*yīn líng quán*, Yin Mound Spring), and needle with drainage. [26: 927] [46: 636]

damp-heat seminal emission 湿热遗精 *shī rè yí jīng*: SEMINAL EMISSION arising when excessive consumption of liquor and rich food causes spleen-stomach damp-heat, which pours downward to harass the "essence chamber." MED Drain heat, abduct dampness, and fortify the spleen. Use Essence-Containing Pill (*mì jīng wán*). ACU Base treatment mainly on CV and SP to clear heat and disinhibit dampness and to quiet the palace of essence. Select CV-3 (*zhōng jí*, Central Pole), SP-9 (*yīn líng quán*, Yin Mound Spring), SP-6 (*sān yīn jiāo*, Three Yin Intersection), and ST-36 (*zú sān lǐ*, Leg Three Li); needle with drainage. See SEMINAL EMISSION. [26: 928] [46: 678]

damp-heat wilting 湿热痿 *shī rè wěi*: WILTING (*wěi*) attributed to damp-heat damaging the sinews. Damp-heat wilting is characterized by wilting (*wěi*), slight swelling, and numbness of the lower limbs, attended by generalized heaviness, oppression in the chest, inhibited voidings of reddish urine, a slimy yellow tongue fur, and soggy rapid pulse. MED Clear heat and dry dampness; fortify the spleen and percolate dampness. Use formulas like Supplemented Mysterious Two Powder (*jiā wèi èr miào sǎn*). ACU Use the basic points given under WILTING (*wěi*), and add SP-9 (*yīn líng quán*, Yin Mound Spring), SP-5 (*shāng qiū*, Shang Hill), and ST-44 (*nèi tíng*, Inner Court), needling with drainage. [26: 927]

damp impediment 湿痹 *shī bì*: *Synonym: fixed impediment* (*bì*). **1.** An IMPEDIMENT (*bì*) pattern arising when wind, cold, and predominantly dampness invades the channels and joints. Damp impediment is characterized by heaviness of the limbs, stubborn numbness of the skin, pain in the joints of fixed location triggered by yin-type (dull wet) weather. MED Treatment is based primarily

on dispelling dampness, and secondarily on dissipating wind and expelling cold, and supplementing the spleen and moving qi, using formulas such as Dampness-Eliminating Impediment-Alleviating Decoction (*chú shī juān bì tāng*). ACU Main points: ST-36 (*zú sān lǐ*, Leg Three Li), SP-9 (*yīn líng quán*, Yin Mound Spring), and SP-5 (*shāng qiū*, Shang Hill). Needle with drainage and add moxa, or use warm needle technique. Cutaneous needling and cupping may also be used. See IMPEDIMENT for selection of points according to affected area. **2.** LEG QI with pain and numbness in the legs. See DAMP LEG QI. [26: 926] [27: 404] [97: 580]

damp leg qi 湿脚气 *shī jiǎo qì*: LEG QI characterized by severe swelling from the foot to the knee, attended by numbness, heaviness, and limpness of the lower limbs, inhibited urination, slimy white tongue fur, and a soggy moderate pulse. Damp leg qi is attributed to water-damp congesting the channels. WMC beriberi (attributed to vitamin B₁ deficiency). MED Diffuse congestion and expel dampness. Use Cockcrow Powder (*jī míng sǎn*) and variations. Where damp-heat is prevalent with signs such as thirst, reddish urine, slimy yellow tongue fur, and soggy rapid pulse, treat by clearing and disinhibiting with formulas such as Fangji Beverage (*fáng jǐ yǐn*). ACU Base treatment mainly on SP, ST, and GB. Select ST-36 (*zú sān lǐ*, Leg Three Li), SP-6 (*sān yīn jiāo*, Three Yin Intersection), SP-9 (*yīn líng quán*, Yin Mound Spring), SP-5 (*shāng qiū*, Shang Hill), GB-34 (*yáng líng quán*, Yang Mound Spring), GB-39 (*xuán zhōng*, Suspended Bell), ST-41 (*jiě xī*, Ravine Divide), and Eight Winds (*bā fēng*). Needle with drainage. Selection of points according to signs: For pronounced damp-heat, add GB-41 (*zú lín qì*, Foot Overlooking Tears), LI-4 (*hé gǔ*, Union Valley), and LI-11 (*qū chí*, Pool at the Bend), and prick LI-1 (*shāng yáng*, Shang Yang) to bleed. For heat effusion and aversion to cold, add LI-4 (*hé gǔ*, Union Valley), GV-14 (*dà zhuī*, Great Hammer), and TB-5 (*wài guān*, Outer Pass). [46: 668] [26: 925] [97: 581]

damp lichen 湿癣 *shī xiǎn*: LICHEN (*xiǎn*) (skin conditions characterized by slight elevation of the skin, watery discharge, scaling, and itching) arising as a result of wind-damp-heat invading the skin. Damp lichen is characterized by redness, ulceration, itching, a feeling of worms creeping in the skin. Scratching causes exudation of watery discharge and gradual spread of the sore. WMC acute eczema, dermatitis. MED Eliminate dampness and kill worms. Use Dampness-Eliminating Stomach-Calming Poria (Hoelen) Five Decoction (*chú shī wèi líng tāng*) as oral medication and Cnidium Seed Powder (*shé chuáng zǐ sǎn*) mixed with sesame oil. ACU Select ouch points (*ā* *shì xué*), GV-14 (*dà zhuī*, Great Hammer), BL-12 (*fēng mén*, Wind Gate), BL-40 (*wěi zhōng*, Bend Center), LI-11 (*qū chí*, Pool at the Bend), LI-4 (*hé gǔ*, Union Valley), SP-9 (*yīn líng quán*, Yin Mound Spring), SP-10 (*xuè hǎi*, Sea of Blood), and HT-7 (*shén mén*, Spirit Gate). Needle with drainage. For pronounced itching, add Itch Reliever (*zhǐ yǎng*). [26: 928] [97: 581] [113: 434, 445]

damp lumbar pain 湿腰痛 *shī yāo tòng*: See DAMPNESS DAMAGE LUMBAR PAIN. [26: 926]

damp malaria 湿疟 *shī nüè*: **1.** SUMMERHEAT MALARIA. **2.** MALARIA attributed to water-damp collecting internally after exposure to rain or dew. Damp malaria is characterized by aversion to cold with unpronounced heat effusion, generalized pain, heavy limbs, oppression in the stomach duct, nausea and retching, swollen face, scant urine, white slimy tongue fur, and soggy rapid pulse. ⌐MED⌐ Resolve the exterior and eliminate dampness. Use formulas such as Bupleurum Stomach-Calming Brew (*chái píng jiān*), Stomach-Calming Poria (Hoelen) Five Decoction (*wèi líng tāng*), or Atractylodes White Tiger Decoction (*cāng zhú bái hǔ tāng*) plus tsaoko (*cǎo guǒ*). ⌐ACU⌐ Base treatment mainly on GV, PC, SI, SP, and ST. Select GV-14 (*dà zhuī*, Great Hammer), PC-5 (*jiān shǐ*, Intermediary Courier), SI-3 (*hòu xī*, Back Ravine), SP-9 (*yīn líng quán*, Yin Mound Spring), ST-36 (*zú sān lǐ*, Leg Three Li), and CV-12 (*zhōng wǎn*, Center Stomach Duct). Needle with even supplementation and drainage and, if appropriate, moxa. See MALARIA for principles and methods of treatment. [26: 926] [27: 359] [97: 579]

dampness 湿 *shī*: **1.** One of the SIX QI, i.e., dampness as an environmental phenomenon. **2.** One of the SIX EXCESSES, i.e., the environmental qi as a cause of disease. **3.** Dampness as an evil in the body. Dampness in the body is qualitatively analogous and causally related to dampness in the natural environment. It is associated with damp weather or damp climates and with stagnant water in places where ground drainage is poor. To some extent, it is seasonal in nature, tending to occur when the weather is wet or damp. Sitting and lying in wet places, living in damp conditions, working in a damp or wet environment, or wearing sweat-soaked clothing can also cause dampness diseases. *Thorough Knowledge of Medicine* (*yī guàn*) states, "There is dampness in heaven (i.e., in the atmosphere), which comes from rain, dew, and mist. Being in heaven, it gets its nature from qi, so it strikes construction and defense. There is dampness from earth, which comes from mud and water. Being in the earth, it nature comes from [that which possesses] form, hence it damages the flesh, the sinews, the bones, the blood, and ves-

sels. There is the dampness of sweat, which comes from sweat-soaked clothing that is not immediately changed. There is dampness that forms in greater yin (*tài yīn*) spleen-earth, which is not from outside the body. When yang is exuberant, fire is prevails, and transforms into damp-heat; when yin is exuberant, water prevails, and transforms into cold-damp. The signs are heat effusion, aversion to cold, generalized heaviness, sweating, sinew and bone pain, rough urination, sloppy diarrhea, lumbar pain that prevents turning, swelling of instep with flesh [that feels] like mud, not springing back when pressed." Dampness has a number of characteristics: (1) It is clammy, viscous, and lingering. Dampness diseases are persistent and difficult to cure. (2) Dampness tends to stagnate. When dampness evil invades the exterior, the patient may complain of physical fatigue, heavy, cumbersome limbs, and heavy-headedness. If it invades the channels and the joints, the patient may complain of aching joints and inhibited bending and stretching. Dampness can also trap and dampen the effect of heat by causing an UNSURFACED HEAT, one that can be felt only by prolonged palpation. (3) The spleen is particularly vulnerable to dampness evil; signs of dampness encumbering the spleen include poor appetite, glomus and oppression in the chest and stomach duct, upflow nausea, abdominal distention, sloppy stool, short voidings of scant urine, thick and slimy tongue fur, and a soggy moderate pulse. The lack of desire for fluids—though especially in the case of damp-heat there may be thirst—is a sign of the "clogging" or "encumbering" effect of dampness. (4) There may be generalized or local stagnation or accumulation of water-damp, such as water swelling, leg qi, vaginal discharge, or exudating sores such as eczema. Dampness in the body is often referred to as damp turbidity to highlight it as the antithesis of clear yang qi. (5) Over time, dampness can gather to form phlegm. NB: *Damp* may serve as an adjective as in "damp phlegm" or as a noun (equivalent to dampness), e.g., "damp-heat." *Damp* is actually preferable to *dampness* since it denotes moisture in the air, on a surface, diffused through a solid, which over long period can cause mold and cause disease. *Dampness*, by contrast, strictly means the quality of being damp. However, in this text, the form dampness has been used in most cases to avoid the confusion that may arise in terms such as *dampness-drying formula*, which is not to be understood as a "damp, drying formula." See DAMPNESS FORMING WITH HEAT and DAMPNESS FORMING WITH COLD. [27: 113] [97: 579]

dampness damage lumbar pain 伤湿腰痛 *shāng shī yāo tòng*: Synonym: *damp lumbar pain*. LUMBAR PAIN arising from living in a cold-damp place or from exposure to rain or dew. Dampness damage lumbar pain is characterized by cold, painful, heavy lumbus that feels as though one were sitting in water. The pain is exacerbated by yin-type (dull wet) weather and by sitting for long periods. The pulse is moderate, and there may also be generalized swelling. MED Use Priceless Qi-Righting Powder (*bù huàn jīn zhèng qì sǎn*). ACU Base treatment mainly on BL, GV, SP, and ST. Select BL-23 (*shèn shū*, Kidney Transport), BL-40 (*wěi zhōng*, Bend Center), GV-3 (*yāo yáng guān*, Lumbar Yang Pass), ouch points (*ā shì xué*), BL-60 (*kūn lún*, Kunlun Mountains), ST-36 (*zú sān lǐ*, Leg Three Li), and SP-9 (*yīn líng quán*, Yin Mound Spring). Needle with drainage and large amounts of moxa. See LUMBAR PAIN. [26: 810] [37: 390] [46: 596, 163]

dampness damage spontaneous sweating 伤湿 自汗 *shāng shī zì hàn*: SPONTANEOUS SWEATING attributed to obstruction by dampness evil. This pattern is characterized by relatively small amount of sweat, aversion to wind, heavy turbid voice, fatigued heavy body, and joint pain that grows worse in yin-type (dull wet) weather. MED Fortify the spleen and boost qi so that the dampness naturally disappears. Formulas include Fangji and Astragalus Decoction (*fáng jǐ huáng qí tāng*) or Notopterygium Dampness-Overcoming Decoction (*qiāng huó shèng shī tāng*). See SPONTANEOUS SWEATING. ACU Base treatment mainly on SP, ST, and LI. Select ST-36 (*zú sān lǐ*, Leg Three Li), SP-9 (*yīn líng quán*, Yin Mound Spring), CV-12 (*zhōng wǎn*, Center Stomach Duct), LR-13 (*zhāng mén*, Camphorwood Gate), LI-4 (*hé gǔ*, Union Valley), KI-7 (*fù liū*, Recover Flow), and SI-3 (*hòu xī*, Back Ravine); needle with even supplementation and drainage and moxa, if appropriate. [113: 18] [26: 810] [46: 597, 602] [14: 174]

dampness encumbering spleen-earth 湿困 脾土 *shī kùn pí tǔ*: DAMPNESS ENCUMBERING SPLEEN YANG.

dampness encumbering spleen yang 湿困脾 阳 *shī kùn pí yáng*: Synonym: *dampness encumbering spleen-earth*. WATER-DAMP affecting the movement and transformation of SPLEEN YANG. MED Dry or disinhibit dampness. **Comparison:** dampness encumbering spleen yang is similar to *spleen vacuity with damp encumbrance*, which is essentially a vacuity pattern with water-damp as a result. Treatment of spleen vacuity focuses on fortifying the spleen assisted by drying dampness. [26: 924]

dampness evil 湿邪 *shī xié*: DAMPNESS as a disease-causing entity.

dampness forming with cold 湿从寒化 *shī cóng hán huà*: The development of COLD-DAMP in patients suffering from impaired fluid transformation due to DEVITALIZED SPLEEN YANG, giving rise to

abdominal fullness and diarrhea, and sometimes to phlegm-rheum and water swelling. This corresponds to the pathomechanism described in *Elementary Questions* (*sù wèn, zhì zhēn yào dà lùn*) as "All dampness with swelling and fullness is ascribed to the spleen." MED Treat by warming and transforming with formulas such as Spleen-Firming Beverage (*shí pí yǐn*). See DAMPNESS. [6: 211] [29: 318]

dampness forming with heat 湿从热化 *shī cóng rè huà*: The development of damp-heat in patients suffering from intense stomach heat due to excessive consumption of sweet or fatty foods. External dampness or damp-heat may or may not be involved. See DAMPNESS. [6: 211] [29: 318]

dampness obstructing the center burner 湿 阻中焦 *shī zǔ zhōng jiāo*: Dampness evil causing stagnation and obstruction in the spleen and stomach and impairing normal movement and transformation. Dampness obstructing the center burner is characterized by heavy-headedness, fatigue, oppression in the stomach duct, abdominal distention, torpid intake, sticky mouth, thirst with desire for warm drinks, short voidings of reddish urine, thick or slimy white tongue fur, and a moderate pulse. MED Use Stomach-Calming Powder (*píng wèi sǎn*) or Stomach-Calming Poria (Hoelen) Five Decoction (*wèi líng tāng*). ACU Base treatment mainly on SP and ST. Select ST-36 (*zú sān lǐ*, Leg Three Li), SP-9 (*yīn líng quán*, Yin Mound Spring), LI-4 (*hé gǔ*, Union Valley), CV-12 (*zhōng wǎn*, Center Stomach Duct), LR-13 (*zhāng mén*, Camphorwood Gate), ST-25 (*tiān shū*, Celestial Pivot), PC-6 (*nèi guān*, Inner Pass), and CV-6 (*qì hǎi*, Sea of Qi); needle with even supplementation and drainage and moxa. [26: 924] [27: 155] [97: 581] [46: 597, 602]

dampness obstructing the qi aspect 湿阻气分 *shī zǔ qì fèn*: Synonym: *qi-aspect damp obstruction*. Dampness invading the QI ASPECT, causing an unsurfaced heat (i.e., heat effusion felt only after prolonged palpation), head heavy as if swathed (bag-over-the-head sensation), heavy aching body, vexing pain in the joints, oppression in the chest, torpid intake, painful glomus in the abdomen and stomach duct, vomiting and diarrhea, slimy glossy tongue fur, and soggy moderate pulse. [26: 924]

dampness stroke 湿中 *shī zhòng*: See PHLEGM STROKE. [26: 923]

dampness trapping hidden heat 湿遏热伏 *shī è rè fú*: Synonym: *depressed dampness and deep-lying heat*. A condition in which the dampness prevents heat from effusing. Dampness trapping hidden heat is characterized by unsurfaced heat arising in the afternoon to bring about sweating that fails to abate heat effusion. Other signs include lassitude of spirit, heavy-headedness, oppression in the chest and abdominal distention, aversion to food, yellow or reddish urine, white or yellow slimy tongue fur, and a rapid soggy pulse. [26: 926] [27: 139] [97: 583] [6: 207]

damp obstruction 湿阻 *shī zǔ*: Synonym: *center burner damp obstruction.* A frequently observed disease in which the spleen and stomach are obstructed by DAMPNESS EVIL. It mainly occurs in summer and is characterized by impaired spleen-stomach movement and transformation. Signs include oppression in the chest, no thought of food and drink, and a bland or sweet taste or slimy sensation in the mouth. The tongue fur is thick and slimy, and the pulse is soggy. Voidings are short with scant urine; the limbs are cumbersome and fatigued; sometimes a low heat effusion is observed. Damp obstruction includes what in China is known as *summer infixation (zhù xià)*, which is the regular recurrence each summer of signs such as of loss of appetite, fatigue and weakness, and low fever, with gradual recovery in the autumn. The above signs together with sloppy stool or diarrhea are also signs of dampness encumbering the spleen and stomach. A higher body temperature with more pronounced heat signs indicates summerheat-damp, which is a form of damp-heat. [27: 90]

damp phlegm 湿痰 *shī tán*: A condition characterized by copious thin white (or yellow) PHLEGM that is easily expectorated and often associated with other signs of DAMPNESS such as heavy body, cumbersome limbs, fatigue, tendency to lie down, abdominal distention sometimes with pain, diarrhea, and slippery moderate pulse. Damp phlegm is attributed to splenic transformation failure, causing dampness that gathers to form phlegm. Distinction is made between spleen vacuity and spleen repletion by the prevalence of vacuity or dampness signs. WMC chronic inflammatory diseases of the respiratory tract such as chronic bronchitis. MED Treat vacuity patterns with Six Gentlemen Decoction (*liù jūn zǐ tāng*) varied according to pattern, and repletion patterns with Two Matured Ingredients Decoction (*èr chén tāng*) or Phlegm-Rolling Pill (*gǔn tán wán*). ACU Base treatment mainly on SP, ST, and LI. Main points: CV-12 (*zhōng wǎn*, Center Stomach Duct), ST-36 (*zú sān lǐ*, Leg Three Li), LI-4 (*hé gǔ*, Union Valley), and ST-40 (*fēng lóng*, Bountiful Bulge). For vacuity patterns, add SP-9 (*yīn líng quán*, Yin Mound Spring), ST-25 (*tiān shū*, Celestial Pivot), CV-6 (*qì hǎi*, Sea of Qi), and BL-20 (*pí shū*, Spleen Transport); needle with even supplementation and drainage and moxa. For repletion patterns, add LU-5 (*chǐ zé*, Cubit Marsh), CV-17 (*shān zhōng*, Chest Center), and CV-22 (*tiān tú*, Celestial Chimney); needle with drainage. NB: Damp phlegm may manifest in parts of the body other than the

chest. See next entries. Compare PHLEGM-DAMP. [26: 925] [6: 217] [27: 120] [46: 597]

damp phlegm dizziness 湿痰眩晕 *shī tán xuàn yūn*: DIZZINESS due to DAMP PHLEGM congestion. Damp phlegm dizziness is characterized by heavy head and clouded vision, oppression in the chest, nausea, vomiting and retching, slimy white tongue fur, and a soggy pulse. It usually occurs in people who are overweight. MED Dry dampness and transform phlegm. Use Pinellia, Ovate Atractylodes, and Gastrodia Decoction (*bàn xià bái zhú tiān má tāng*) combined with Two Matured Ingredients Decoction (*èr chén tāng*). If there are qi vacuity signs, Six Gentlemen Decoction (*liù jūn zǐ tāng*) may also be given. ACU See PHLEGM-RHEUM DIZZINESS. [26: 926] [27: 120] [97: 580]

damp phlegm leg qi 湿痰脚气 *shī tán jiǎo qì*: LEG QI (beriberi) attributed to exuberant dampness pouring downward and engendering phlegm. In addition to the principal signs of leg qi (e.g., lack of strength in the legs), damp phlegm leg qi is characterized by efflux diarrhea. MED Treat with medicinals such as atractylodes (*cāng zhú*), ledebouriella (*fáng fēng*), areca (*bīng láng*), cyperus (*xiāng fù zǐ*), ligusticum (*chuān xiōng*), scutellaria (*huáng qín*), talcum (*huá shí*), and licorice (*gān cǎo*). ACU Base treatment mainly on SP, ST, and GB. Select ST-36 (*zú sān lǐ*, Leg Three Li), SP-6 (*sān yīn jiāo*, Three Yin Intersection), SP-9 (*yīn líng quán*, Yin Mound Spring), SP-5 (*shāng qiū*, Shang Hill), CV-12 (*zhōng wǎn*, Center Stomach Duct), ST-25 (*tiān shū*, Celestial Pivot), ST-40 (*fēng lóng*, Bountiful Bulge), GB-34 (*yáng líng quán*, Yang Mound Spring), GB-39 (*xuán zhōng*, Suspended Bell), ST-41 (*jiě xī*, Ravine Divide), and Eight Winds (*bā fēng*). Needle with drainage. See LEG QI. [26: 926]

damp phlegm lumbar pain 湿痰腰痛 *shī tán yāo tòng*: Lumbar pain attributable to damp phlegm pouring into the kidney channel, and characterized by cold heavy painful lumbus stretching into the back and rib-side and exacerbated by yin-type (dull wet) weather, and associated with diarrhea and a slippery pulse. MED Use Tortoise Plastron and Ailanthus Bark Pill (*guī shū wán*) or Two Matured Ingredients Decoction (*èr chén tāng*). ACU Base treatment mainly on BL, CV, and ST. Select BL-23 (*shèn shū*, Kidney Transport), BL-40 (*wěi zhōng*, Bend Center), GV-3 (*yāo yáng guān*, Lumbar Yang Pass), ouch points (*ā shì xué*), ST-36 (*zú sān lǐ*, Leg Three Li), CV-12 (*zhōng wǎn*, Center Stomach Duct), and ST-40 (*fēng lóng*, Bountiful Bulge). Needle with drainage and add moxa. [26: 926] [37: 390]

damp phlegm streaming sore 湿痰流注 *shī tán liú zhù*: A deep-seated sore arising in patients suffering from spleen qi vacuity when damp phlegm causing internal obstruction combines with additionally contracted evil toxins to seep into construction and defense. It begins with pain in the flesh, diffuse swelling without a head and without any change in skin color, and attended by cold and heat and generalized joint pain. When pus forms, pain and swelling become more acute, and there is vigorous heat [effusion] with sweating. The sore bursts to exude thin white pus, and heals once the discharge ceases. MED In the initial stage, Saussurea Qi Flow Beverage (*mù xiāng liú qì yǐn*) complemented with spleen-fortifying phlegm-transforming formulas can be used as oral medication, whereas Harmonious Flow Paste (*chōng hé gāo*) can be applied topically. After the sore has burst, use Internal Expression Pus-Expelling Decoction (*tuō lǐ tòu nóng tāng*). If the sore does not close and continues to exude thin pus, formulas like Ginseng Construction-Nourishing Decoction (*rén shēn yǎng róng tāng*) may be given to supplement qi and blood. ACU Moxibustion may be used to help disperse the sore in the initial phase. See STREAMING SORE. [26: 925]

damp phlegm wilting 湿痰痿 *shī tán wěi*: A WILTING (*wěi*) pattern usually affecting overweight people, attributed to damp phlegm lodged in the channel, and characterized by wilting and weakness of the limbs, numbness of the lumbus and knee, and pulse that is sunken and slippery. MED Use Two Matured Ingredients Decoction (*èr chén tāng*) with judicious addition of atractylodes (*cāng zhú*), ovate atractylodes (*bái zhú*), scutellaria (*huáng qín*), phellodendron (*huáng bǎi*), dried bamboo sap (*zhú lì*), and ginger juice (*jiāng zhī*). ACU Use the general points given under WILTING, and add ST-25 (*tiān shū*, Celestial Pivot), CV-6 (*qì hǎi*, Sea of Qi), SP-9 (*yīn líng quán*, Yin Mound Spring), and ST-40 (*fēng lóng*, Bountiful Bulge), needling with drainage. [26: 926]

damp scab 湿疥 *shī jiè*: See SCAB (*jiè*). [26: 924]

damp sores 湿疮 *shī chuāng*: Any of a variety of skin diseases characterized by itching, ulceration, exudation, crusting, and recurrence. It specifically includes: SCROTAL WIND; FOUR BENDS WIND; UMBILICAL DAMP; NIPPLE WIND; INVISIBLE WORM SORE OF THE NOSE. Acute forms are ascribed mainly to damp-heat, very often with external wind. Wind is a yang evil, light and buoyant; it easily invades the interstices of the head, face, and upper body. It is swift and changeable; it often changes location and spreads quickly. Dampness is a yin evil, it is sticky and stagnating, and is spreading and pervasive. It is heavy and turbid, and tends to be found in low places. When it invades the body, it can cause water vesicles, ulceration, and exudation. Wind and dampness easily harbor brewing heat, and the three evils

together cause dampness, scorching heat, itching and soreness of the skin. Chronic damp sores tend to be caused by blood vacuity and wind dryness with damp-heat brewing and accumulating. They are recurrent and persistent, associated with severe itching that prevents the patient from sleeping, and poor stomach intake. Yin blood depletion engenders wind and dryness, depriving the skin of nourishment, and causing dryness, thickening of the skin, and scaling. Persistent damp sores affecting the chest, abdomen, or genitals are associated with liver channel damp-heat. Damp sores affecting the lower body with prominent green-blue veins (varicose veins) are associated with liquor heat brewing internally. Damp sores with nutritional disturbance are ascribed to spleen vacuity with brewing damp-heat. MED For damp-heat, clear heat and disinhibit dampness. Use formulas such as variations of Fish Poison Yam Dampness-Percolating Decoction (*bì xiè shèn shī tāng*) combined with Mysterious Two Pill (*èr miào wán*). For blood heat, cool the blood, clear heat, and disinhibit dampness with medicinals such as fresh rehmannia (*xiān dì huáng*), red peony (*chì sháo yào*), moutan (*mǔ dān pí*), coptis (*huáng lián*), fresh gardenia (*shēng shān zhī*), gardenia (*shān zhī zǐ*), dictamnus (*bái xiān pí*), kochia (*dì fū zǐ*), siegesbeckia (*xī xiān*), flavescent sophora (*kǔ shēn*), erythrina (*hǎi tóng pí*), and raw licorice (*shēng gān cǎo*). For damp obstruction, fortify the stomach and eliminate dampness with formulas such as variations of Dampness-Eliminating Stomach-Calming Poria (Hoelen) Five Decoction (*chú shī wèi líng tāng*). For blood dryness, nourish the blood and dispel wind, and clear heat and transform dampness. Use dried/fresh rehmannia (*shēng dì huáng*), tangkuei (*dāng guī*), white peony (*bái sháo yào*), dictamnus (*bái xiān pí*), kochia (*dì fū zǐ*), fish poison yam (*bì xiè*), poria skin (*fú líng pí*), cnidium seed (*shé chuáng zǐ*), and raw licorice (*shēng gān cǎo*). Selection of medicinals according to location: For the head and face, add ligusticum (*chuān xiōng*), notopterygium (*qiāng huó*), and angelica (*bái zhǐ*). For the breasts and umbilicus, add capillaris (*yīn chén hāo*), Madaio dock root (*tǔ dà huáng*), and plantago seed (*chē qián zǐ*). For the limbs, add mulberry twig (*sāng zhī*), cyathula (*chuān niú xī*), and lonicera stem and leaf (*rěn dōng téng*). For damp sores on the lower leg with prominent green-blue veins and dark-colored skin, quicken the blood and dispel stasis by adding lycopus (*zé lán*), zedoary (*é zhú*), and cyathula (*chuān niú xī*). [96: 277]

damp swelling 湿肿 *shī zhǒng*: WATER SWELLING due to dampness. Damp swelling may arise from sitting for a long time on damp ground, or from being soaked in water. Damp swelling is characterized by swelling of the limbs that engulfs the fingers when pressure is applied, associated with heaviness from the lumbus downward and with distended legs, and is attended by short scant voidings of urine and in some cases by rapid breathing and sloppy stool. [MED] Fortify the spleen, warm yang, and disinhibit water. Use formulas such as Poria (Hoelen) Five Powder (*wǔ líng sǎn*) or Golden Coffer Kidney Qi Pill (*jīn guì shèn qì wán*). [ACU] Base treatment mainly on CV, back transport points, SP, and ST. Select CV-9 (*shuǐ fēn*, Water Divide), CV-6 (*qì hǎi*, Sea of Qi), BL-22 (*sān jiāo shū*, Triple Burner Transport), ST-36 (*zú sān lǐ*, Leg Three Li), BL-20 (*pí shū*, Spleen Transport), CV-12 (*zhōng wǎn*, Center Stomach Duct), BL-23 (*shèn shū*, Kidney Transport), KI-3 (*tài xī*, Great Ravine), BL-39 (*wěi yáng*, Bend Yang), and SP-9 (*yīn líng quán*, Yin Mound Spring); needle with supplementation and add moxa. See YIN WATER; WATER SWELLING. [26: 926] [61: 376]

damp tetany 湿痉 *shī jìng*: A disease commonly affecting children, that is characterized by clouded spirit, TETANIC REVERSAL, unsurfaced heat, oppression in the chest, and a thick white tongue fur, and that is attributed to dampness evil spreading through the triple burner and clouding the clear orifices. [MED] Use Sweet Dew Toxin-Dispersing Elixir (*gān lù xiāo dú dān*). [ACU] Base treatment mainly on ST, SP, GV, PC, TB, and LI. Select ST-36 (*zú sān lǐ*, Leg Three Li), SP-9 (*yīn líng quán*, Yin Mound Spring), BL-20 (*pí shū*, Spleen Transport), GV-26 (*shuǐ gōu*, Water Trough), GV-8 (*jīn suō*, Sinew Contraction), PC-6 (*nèi guān*, Inner Pass), TB-5 (*wài guān*, Outer Pass), LI-4 (*hé gǔ*, Union Valley), and LI-11 (*qū chí*, Pool at the Bend). Needle with drainage. [26: 925]

damp toxin 湿毒 *shī dú*: Toxin arising when damp qi accumulates. Damp toxin accumulating in the intestines causes damp toxin bloody stool. Damp toxin in the skin can cause a damp-heat streaming sore, a pattern of ulceration of the lower leg. Damp toxin patterns are characterized by copious discharge from the focus of the disease, are chronic in nature, and difficult to cure. [26: 924]

damp toxin precipitation of blood 湿毒下血 *shī dú xià xuè*: Bloody stool due to damp toxin brewing in the large intestine. The signs are dull purple or blackish bloody stool, absence of abdominal pain, distention and oppression in the chest and diaphragm, reduced food intake, yellow facial complexion, and inhibited urination. [MED] Use formulas such as Sophora Flower Powder (*huái huā sǎn*). [ACU] Base treatment mainly on ST and SP. Select ST-25 (*tiān shū*, Celestial Pivot), BL-25 (*dà cháng shū*, Large Intestine Transport), ST-37 (*shàng jù xū*, Upper Great Hollow), BL-20 (*pí shū*, Spleen Transport), SP-10 (*xuè hǎi*, Sea of Blood), SP-6

(*sān yīn jiāo*, Three Yin Intersection), SP-9 (*yīn líng quán*, Yin Mound Spring), and LR-2 (*xíng jiān*, Moving Between); needle with drainage and add moxa. [26: 924] [27: 113]

damp toxin sore 湿毒疮 *shī dú chuāng*: Synonym: *downpour sore*. A sore on the lower leg or ankle attributed to wind, dampness, and heat lodged in the skin. Acute forms, attributed to prevalence of damp-heat, begin with flushing of the skin and papules, and with vesicles that itch to exude a yellow discharge. Chronic forms, which are complicated by blood vacuity, are characterized by drying, thickening, and scaling of the skin. [WMC] eczema. [MED] Treat the acute form by clearing heat and disinhibiting dampness. For oral medication use Fish Poison Yam Dampness-Percolating Decoction (*bì xiè shèn shī tāng*) combined with Mysterious Two Pill (*èr miào wán*). For topical treatment, apply a decoction of phellodendron cold; when the skin has absorbed as much as it can, apply Indigo Powder (*qīng dài sǎn*). Treat the chronic form by nourishing the blood and eliminating wind, using Tangkuei Drink (*dāng guī yǐn zi*) combined with Mysterious Three Powder (*sān miào sǎn*) and applying Indigo Powder (*qīng dài sǎn*) mixed as a paste. [ACU] Base treatment mainly on GV, LI, ST, and SP. Main points: GV-14 (*dà zhuī*, Great Hammer), LI-11 (*qū chí*, Pool at the Bend), SP-9 (*yīn líng quán*, Yin Mound Spring), and SP-6 (*sān yīn jiāo*, Three Yin Intersection). For acute cases, needle with drainage to clear heat and disinhibit dampness. For chronic cases, add SP-10 (*xuè hǎi*, Sea of Blood), ST-36 (*zú sān lǐ*, Leg Three Li), and HT-7 (*shén mén*, Spirit Gate), and needle with supplementation to nourish the blood and dispel wind; also apply the pricking and cupping method. Selection of points according to signs: For pronounced itching, add HT-8 (*shào fǔ*, Lesser Mansion) and Itch Reliever (*zhǐ yǎng*). For pronounced dampness, add LI-4 (*hé gǔ*, Union Valley) and moxa. [26: 924] [27: 113] [97: 582]

damp toxin streaming sore 湿毒流注 *shī dú liú zhù*: A sore of the lower leg taking the form of a flat unelevated ulceration, with diffuse purple or blackish swelling that stretches to the heal. The sore exudes pus, which encourages its spread. It takes a long time to heal and is resistant to treatment. [26: 924]

damp toxin vaginal discharge 湿毒带下 *shī dú dài xià*: Malodorous vaginal discharge like rice water (water in which rice has been washed), yellow-green like pus, or multicolored, and attended by pudendal itch and soreness. It occurs during menstrual periods or after childbirth, and is attributed to exploiting vacuity of the uterine vessels and damaging the uterine vessels and the qi and blood of the thoroughfare (*chōng*) and controlling (*rèn*) vessels. MED Use Discharge-Checking Formula (*zhǐ dài fāng*), to which lonicera (*jīn yín huā*), forsythia (*lián qiào*), and houttuynia (*yú xīng cǎo*) may also be added. In modern clinical practice, this kind of vaginal discharge is sometimes associated with cancer. ACU Base treatment mainly on CV, GIV, and SP. Select GB-26 (*dài mài*, Girdling Vessel), BL-30 (*bái huán shū*, White Ring Transport), CV-6 (*qì hǎi*, Sea of Qi), SP-6 (*sān yīn jiāo*, Three Yin Intersection), CV-3 (*zhōng jí*, Central Pole), SP-9 (*yīn líng quán*, Yin Mound Spring), and BL-34 (*xià liáo*, Lower Bone-Hole). Needle with drainage. [26: 924]

damp turbidity 湿浊 *shī zhuó*: Dampness, especially where it is heavy or viscid in nature and obstructs clear light yang qi. See DAMPNESS. [26: 928]

damp ulceration 湿烂 *shī làn*: An ulceration that exudes fluid and is attributable to dampness.

damp warmth 湿温 *shī wēn*: A febrile disease occurring in the summer or autumn that is attributed to damp-heat and characterized by persistent heat effusion, heavy-headedness, generalized pain, glomus and oppression in the chest and stomach duct, white or yellow slimy tongue fur, and a soggy pulse. MED If dampness is prevalent, focus treatment on transforming dampness with formulas like Agastache/Patchouli, Magnolia Bark, Pinellia, and Poria (Hoelen) Decoction (*huò pò xià líng tāng*) or Three Kernels Decoction (*sān rén tāng*). If heat is prevalent, focus on clearing heat with formulas such as Coptis and Magnolia Bark Beverage (*lián pò yǐn*) or Sweet Dew Toxin-Dispersing Elixir (*gān lù xiāo dú dān*). If the condition advances, the evil can enter construction and the blood, causing TETANIC REVERSAL or bloody stool. WMC typhoid fever (ileotyphus), paratyphoid, leptospirosis. ACU Base treatment mainly on LI, ST, SP, and CV. Select LI-11 (*qū chí*, Pool at the Bend), LI-4 (*hé gǔ*, Union Valley), ST-36 (*zú sān lǐ*, Leg Three Li), SP-6 (*sān yīn jiāo*, Three Yin Intersection), SP-9 (*yīn líng quán*, Yin Mound Spring), CV-17 (*shān zhōng*, Chest Center), PC-6 (*nèi guān*, Inner Pass), and CV-12 (*zhōng wǎn*, Center Stomach Duct). For predominance of heat, add GV-14 (*dà zhuī*, Great Hammer). For heat entering the construction-blood, add GV-26 (*shuǐ gōu*, Water Trough) and PC-8 (*láo gōng*, Palace of Toil) and prick Twelve Well Points (*shí èr jǐng xué*) to bleed. See WARM DISEASE. [26: 925] [46: 597]

dark-colored urine 尿赤 *niào chì*: REDDISH URINE.

dark gate 幽门 *yōu mén*: One of the SEVEN GATES. The lower mouth of the stomach. WMC pylorus. [27: 30]

dark of the eye 黑睛 *hēi jīng*, 青睛 *qīng jīng*, 黑珠 *hēi zhū*, 乌珠 *wū zhū*: The anterior central part of the eye that is colorless and transparent. The dark of the eye is so called because the dark-colored iris and pupil can be seen through it. The dark of the eye corresponds to the liver; it is equivalent to the wind wheel among the five wheels. If the dark of the eye looses its transparency, vision can be affected. WMC cornea. [26: 729] [27: 65] [125: 336]

darting shrimp pulse 虾游脉 *xiā yóu mài*: See SEVEN STRANGE PULSES. [27: 199] [27: 199] [97: 409]

dead blood rib-side pain 死血胁痛 *sǐ xuè xié tòng*: Rib-side pain caused by locally lodged static blood. Dead blood rib-side pain is usually attributable to liver-spleen qi stagnation or enduring illness entering the network vessels causing stasis obstruction. Sometimes it is attributed to blood stasis due to knocks or falls. Dead blood rib-side pain is characterized by stabbing pain of fixed location in the ribs that refuses pressure and that gets worse at night. There may also be a glomus lump, constipation and hard black stool. The pulse is usually sunken and rough. MED Dispel stasis and free the network vessels. Use Origin-Restorative Blood-Quickening Decoction (*fù yuán huó xuè tāng*) or Stasis-Precipitating Decoction (*xià yū xuè tāng*). For evil repletion and right vacuity, add blood-supplementing or qi-boosting medicinals. ACU Base treatment mainly on LR, TB, and SP. Select SP-21 (*dà bāo*, Great Embracement), TB-6 (*zhī gōu*, Branch Ditch), LR-3 (*tài chōng*, Supreme Surge), GB-40 (*qiū xū*, Hill Ruins), BL-17 (*gé shū*, Diaphragm Transport), SP-6 (*sān yīn jiāo*, Three Yin Intersection), and GB-34 (*yáng líng quán*, Yang Mound Spring). Needle with drainage or bleed with a three-edged needle. For pronounced pain, add ouch points (*ā shì xué*). For repletion of evil and vacuity of right, add BL-20 (*pí shū*, Spleen Transport), CV-17 (*shān zhōng*, Chest Center), and ST-36 (*zú sān lǐ*, Leg Three Li). [26: 253] [46: 636] [113: 211]

deafness 耳聋 *ěr lóng*, 耳聩 *ěr kuì*: Loss of hearing. Deafness can be congenital; otherwise it is the result of external contractions or internal damage. Sudden deafness usually forms a repletion pattern, whereas deafness of gradual onset is usually due to vacuity. **Repletion** patterns are attributable to wind-heat, wind-cold, or liver fire, and attended by headache, nasal congestion, bitter taste in the mouth, a feeling that the ears are stuffed with cotton, and tinnitus. MED Wind-heat is treated by by coursing wind and clearing heat, using Lonicera and Forsythia Powder (*yín qiào sǎn*); wind-cold is treated by coursing wind and dissipating cold, using formulas such as Nine-Ingredient Notopterygium Decoction (*jiŭ wèi qiāng huó tāng*); and liver is treated by clearing the liver and draining fire, using formulas such as Gentian Liver-Draining Decoction (*lóng dăn xiè gān tāng*). ACU Base treatment mainly on TB, GB, and ST. Main points: TB-17 (*yì fēng*, Wind Screen), TB-3 (*zhōng zhŭ*, Central Islet), GB-2 (*tīng huì*, Auditory Convergence), GB-43 (*xiá xī*, Pinched Ravine), and ST-40 (*fēng lóng*, Bountiful Bulge). Selection of points according to pattern: For wind-heat, add GB-20 (*fēng chí*, Wind Pool), TB-5 (*wài guān*, Outer Pass), SI-19 (*tīng gōng*, Auditory Palace), GV-14 (*dà zhuī*, Great Hammer), LU-5 (*chĭ zé*, Cubit Marsh), and LI-4 (*hé gŭ*, Union Valley). For wind-cold, add GB-20 (*fēng chí*, Wind Pool), BL-12 (*fēng mén*, Wind Gate), SI-19 (*tīng gōng*, Auditory Palace), LU-7 (*liè quē*, Broken Sequence), LI-4 (*hé gŭ*, Union Valley), and apply moxa. For liver-fire, add LR-3 (*tài chōng*, Supreme Surge), LR-2 (*xíng jiān*, Moving Between), and KI-6 (*zhào hăi*, Shining Sea). Needle with drainage. **Vacuity** patterns include qi vacuity and blood vacuity patterns, and are characterized by dizziness, limp aching lumbus and knees, lack of strength, and tinnitus. MED Treat by supplementing the center and boosting qi or by enriching the kidney and nourishing the blood. Use formulas such as Center-Supplementing Qi-Boosting Decoction (*bŭ zhōng yì qì tāng*), Deafness Left-Benefiting Loadstone Pill (*ĕr lóng zuŏ cí wán*), and Lycium Berry, Chrysanthemum, and Rehmannia Pill (*qĭ jú dì huáng wán*). ACU Base treatment mainly on KI, TB, GB, CV, and back transport points. Main points: BL-23 (*shèn shū*, Kidney Transport), CV-4 (*guān yuán*, Pass Head), KI-3 (*tài xī*, Great Ravine), TB-17 (*yì fēng*, Wind Screen), GB-2 (*tīng huì*, Auditory Convergence), TB-3 (*zhōng zhŭ*, Central Islet), and TB-21 (*ĕr mén*, Ear Gate). For blood vacuity, add BL-18 (*gān shū*, Liver Transport), BL-20 (*pí shū*, Spleen Transport), ST-36 (*zú sān lĭ*, Leg Three Li), LR-3 (*tài chōng*, Supreme Surge), and SP-6 (*sān yīn jiāo*, Three Yin Intersection). For qi vacuity, add CV-6 (*qì hăi*, Sea of Qi), ST-36 (*zú sān lĭ*, Leg Three Li), GV-20 (*băi huì*, Hundred Convergences), and CV-12 (*zhōng wăn*, Center Stomach Duct). Needle with supplementation. If there are vacuity cold signs, add moxa. [26: 251] [27: 439] [97: 174] [46: 722]

death in utero 胎死腹中 *tāi sĭ fù zhōng*: Death of the fetus in the uterus, attributable to a) knocks and falls, b) deep-lying heat toxin in the thoroughfare (*chōng*) and controlling (*rèn*) vessels in febrile disease, c) qi-blood vacuity in the thoroughfare (*chōng*) and controlling (*rèn*) vessels vessels due to constitutional vacuity in the mother, d) strangling by the umbilical cord, and e) abortifacient medicines. See RETENTION OF DEAD FETUS. [27: 450] [97: 410]

deathlike reversal 尸厥 *shī jué*: CLOUDING REVERSAL and reversal cold in the limbs giving the patient a deathlike appearance. Though unconscious, the patient has a pulse. ACU Moxa GV-20 (*băi huì*, Hundred Convergences). ◇ Chin 尸 *shī*, a corpse; 厥 *jué*, reversal. [27: 410] [59: 16]

debilitation 衰 *shuāi*: A weakness, usually severe, especially of yang. See EXUBERANCE AND DEBILITATION.

debilitation of kidney yang 肾阳衰微 *shèn yáng shuāi wēi*: Severe kidney yang vacuity. [27: 164] [97: 164]

debilitation of the life gate fire 命门火衰 *mìng mén huŏ shuāi*: Synonym: *insufficiency of the life fire*. Severe kidney yang vacuity. See KIDNEY YANG VACUITY. [27: 164]

debility is treated by supplementing 衰者补之 *shuāi zhĕ bŭ zhī*: Synonym: *vacuity is treated by supplementing*. The principle that weakness, i.e., vacuity, is treated with supplementing medicinals. Different vacuity patterns, such as qi vacuity, blood vacuity, yin vacuity, and yang vacuity, are treated by different forms of supplementation (SUPPLEMENTING QI, SUPPLEMENTING BLOOD, SUPPLEMENTING YIN, SUPPLEMENTING YANG, etc.) [97: 515] [26: 486] [27: 239]

decoct 煎 *jiān*: Synonym: *brew*. To boil (medicinal materials) in water in order to extract their active properties. See DECOCTION. [27: 311]

decocting pieces 饮片 *yĭn piàn*: Medicinal materials cut to size and if necessary processed as by stir-frying in preparation for decoction. ◇ Chin 饮 *yĭn*, drink; 片 *piàn*, piece, slice. [27: 327]

decoction 汤剂 *tāng jì*, 煎剂 *jiān jì*: A medicinal preparation made by boiling the ingredients of a formula in water, and then straining off the dregs. Because it was recognized that decoctions prepared in iron pots could have reduced effects, traditional literature stipulates the use of earthenware pots. Pyrex or enamel may now be used. The decoction is the most common medicinal preparation. Decoctions are quickly absorbed by the body, and so are particularly suitable for acute diseases of recent onset. In contrast to ready-prepared pills and powders, decoctions enable the formula to be tailored to the patient's individual needs. Materials can usually be boiled twice. The first time, add enough water to cover the materials. The pot is brought to the boil and the contents are given an occasional stir over the 20–30 minute boiling period. The decoction is then strained off. Any materials that swell on absorbing water will have done so during the first boiling, so that for the second boiling only enough water is added to cover the materials and a duration of twenty minutes only is required. The two boilings may be mixed together before the patient takes them, in order to ensure even doses. The water quantities, boiling times, and size of flame given above represent a general guide only. Ideally they are varied according to the medicinals used to ensure maximum benefit. Exterior-effusing and qi-rectifying medicinals are used for their qi rather than their flavor, and are cooked over a fierce fire for a relatively short period to prevent loss of active constituents. Supplementing medicinals are used for their flavor, and are therefore boiled for a longer period (about ten minutes longer) over a low flame to ensure complete extraction of active constituents. Compare BEVERAGE; BREW; DRINK. [27: 311] [97: 226]

deep-lying 伏 *fú*: (Of evils or masses) being present in the inner body, latent, or barely perceptible. ◇ Chin 伏 *fú*, crouch, lie low, latent. [48: 79]

deep-lying beam 伏梁 *fú liáng*: Mass below the heart or in the umbilical region, mostly caused by binding stagnation of qi and blood. Old books describe three patterns by the same name: (1) One of the FIVE ACCUMULATIONS; the accumulation of the heart, characterized by a large lump below the heart, causing vexation and insomnia (*The Classic of Difficult Issues* (*nàn jīng*)). (2) Hard distention in the lower abdomen with a lump outside the intestines that does not move when pushed and contains pus and static blood. It is attended by pain in the umbilical region, and generalized swelling (*Elementary Questions* (*sù wèn, fù zhōng lùn*)). (3) From *The Magic Pivot* (*líng shū, xié qì zàng fù bìng xíng piān*). Mass below the heart, with periodic spitting of blood. ◇ Chin 伏 *fú*, crouch, lie low, latent; 梁 *liáng*, roof beam. [27: 415] [97: 205]

deep-lying heat in the thoroughfare and controlling vessels 热伏冲任 *rè fú chōng rèn*: A disease pattern arising when evil heat affects the thoroughfare (*chōng*) and controlling (*rèn*) vessels, causing wear on yin-essence and depletion of kidney yin, and in some cases frenetic movement of the blood. Clinical signs include low fever, lumbar pain, and uterine bleeding, and lower abdominal pain. The heat in this pattern is described as "deep-lying" because overt signs of the heat are not as pronounced as the damage to yin caused by it. [26: 872] [27: 135] [97: 454]

deep-lying rheum 伏饮 *fú yǐn*: From *Essential Prescriptions of the Golden Coffer* (*jīn guì yào lüè, tán yǐn ké sòu bìng mài zhèng bìng zhì*). Phlegm-rheum lying latent in the body or residual lodged rheum. Deep-lying rheum is characterized by frequent episodes of panting and fullness, and coughing and spitting. The episodes are often brought on by contraction of external cold evil, in which case there is abhorrence of cold, heat effusion, back and lumbar pain, spontaneous tearing, and twitching and jerking of the body. [WMC] chronic bronchitis, pulmonary emphysema, pulmogenic heart disease. [MED] Transform yin and expel evil; support right and secure the root. Use Minor Green-Blue Dragon Decoction (*xiǎo qīng lóng tāng*) or Woody Fangji Decoction (*mù fáng jǐ tāng*). [26: 275] [50: 559] [27: 282] [97: 205]

deep pulse 沉脉 *chén mài*: SUNKEN PULSE.

deep-source nasal congestion 鼻渊 *bí yuān*: Persistent nasal congestion with turbid snivel (nasal mucus) attributable to wind-cold, wind-heat, or gallbladder heat. [WMC] paranasal sinusitis, chronic rhinitis. **Wind-cold** patterns are typified by nasal congestion with loss of smell, with a frequent sensation of acrid sour-sore in the nose. [MED] Rectify the lung and open the orifices. Use Magnolia Flower Powder (*xīn yí sǎn*). [ACU] As for all deep-source nasal congestion patterns, base treatment mainly on GV, LU, and LI. Main points: LU-7 (*liè quē*, Broken Sequence), LI-4 (*hé gǔ*, Union Valley), LI-20 (*yíng xiāng*, Welcome Fragrance), Hall of Impression (*yìn táng*), GV-23 (*shàng xīng*, Upper Star), and GB-20 (*fēng chí*, Wind Pool), needling with drainage. For loss of smell, add BL-7 (*tōng tiān*, Celestial Connection) and BL-10 (*tiān zhù*, Celestial Pillar). For wind-cold, add moxa. **Wind-heat** patterns are marked by pronounced runny nose with fishy-smelling yellow snivel (nasal mucus). [MED] Clear and diffuse the orifices of the lung; cool the blood and resolve toxin. Use Xanthium Powder (*cāng ěr zǐ sǎn*) plus moutan (*mǔ dān pí*) and dandelion (*pú gōng yīng*). [ACU] to the basic points add GV-14 (*dà zhuī*, Great Hammer) and LI-11 (*qū chí*, Pool at the Bend). **Gallbladder heat** spreading to the brain usually causes a more severe form of deep-source nasal congestion called BRAIN LEAK, characterized by sourness in the nose and persistent nasal discharge like marrow or pus that has a foul or fishy smell and accompanied by dizziness, headache, and forgetfulness. [MED] Clear the gallbladder and diffuse the orifices of the lung. Use formulas like Deep-Source Decoction (*qǔ yuān tāng*), which contains magnolia flower[1] (*xīn yí*), tangkuei (*dāng guī*), charred gardenia (*hēi shān zhī zǐ*), fritillaria (*bèi mǔ*), bupleurum (*chái hú*), and scrophularia (*xuán shēn*). [ACU] Add to the basic points GB-34 (*yáng líng quán*, Yang Mound Spring), LR-2 (*xíng jiān*, Moving Between), GB-39 (*xuán zhōng*, Suspended Bell), and GB-19 (*nǎo kōng*, Brain Hollow). **Qi vacuity** signs are often concurrent in deep-source nasal congestion. [MED] Supplement the center and boost qi. Use Center-Supplementing Qi-Boosting Decoction (*bǔ zhōng yì qì tāng*) plus magnolia flower[1] (*xīn yí*) and xanthium (*cāng ěr zǐ*). [ACU] Needle with supplementation at ST-36 (*zú sān lǐ*, Leg Three Li). Deep-source nasal congestion characterized by persistent bloody discharge with foul or fishy smell accompanied by dizzy head and vision and general emaciation is called BRAIN-GRIPPING SAND (shā), which nowadays prompts investigation into the possible presence of cancer. [MED] Diffuse the lung and free the network vessels using Luffa Stem Powder (tiān luó sǎn), which is luffa stem (sī guā) ground, and swallowed with yellow wine. Both brain leak and brain-gripping sand (shā) can also be treated with Old Hermit Agastache/Patchouli Pill (qí shòu huò xiāng wán), comprising agastache/patchouli (huò xiāng) combined with pig or ox bile, which can be taken with a decoction of xanthium (cāng ěr zǐ). [26: 855] [27: 494] [97: 623]

deep turbid voice 语声重浊 yǔ shēng zhòng zhuó: A voice or cough sound that is deep and muffled or otherwise unclear. A deep turbid voice is observed in external contraction of wind-cold or internal phlegm-damp obstruction inhibiting the airways. [26: 825] [27: 186] [97: 444]

defense 卫 wèi: An abbreviation for DEFENSE QI. [48: 12]

defense aspect 卫分 wèi fèn: See DEFENSE, QI, CONSTRUCTION, AND BLOOD.

defense-aspect pattern 卫分证 wèi fèn zhèng: Warm disease principally characterized by heat effusion, slight aversion to cold, presence or absence of sweating, and dry mouth. The tongue is distinctly red, and the pulse is floating and rapid. In some cases there may also be headache, cough, and sore, red pharynx, and in others, distention in the head, clouded head, oppression in the chest, and upflow nausea. Defense-aspect patterns include signs common to the initial stage of all external heat diseases. Of these signs, heat effusion with slight aversion to wind and cold is the main indicator of defense-aspect disease. Like greater yang (tài yáng) disease of the doctrine of cold damage, defense-aspect disease is seen as an exterior pattern in terms of the eight principles. However, whereas greater yang disease may generally be classified as caused by cold, defense-aspect disease is classified as caused by heat. Warm evil enters the body through the nose and mouth, invariably invading the lung first. The lung is connected with the [surface] skin and [body] hair, and governs the exterior and defense. Thus, when it is invaded by an external evil, the defensive exterior is "thwarted," and this causes heat effusion and slight aversion to cold. This is the fundamental law applied to defense-aspect disease. Warm evil is hot in nature, so that defense-aspect patterns include heat signs, and as such differ from greater yang exterior patterns, which tend to be marked by cold signs. Once a defense-aspect pattern has been identified, it is usually necessary to determine whether warm evil is accompanied by wind or dampness.

Wind warmth patterns are generally characterized by signs of lung heat such as cough, sore pharynx, and distinctly red tongue. Damp warmth patterns are characterized by signs of damp turbidity obstructing the center, such as general sensations of heaviness, oppression in the chest, upflow nausea, dry throat with no desire for fluid, and a distinctly slimy tongue. Defense-aspect patterns are chiefly treated by the method of resolving the exterior with cool and acrid medicinals that discharge warm evil from the defense aspect. [6: 239] [27: 224] [97: 40]

defense qi 卫气 wèi qì: A qi described as being "fierce, bold, and uninhibited," unable to be contained by the vessels and therefore flowing outside them. In the chest and abdomen it warms the organs, whereas in the exterior it flows through the skin and flesh, regulates the opening and closing of the interstices (i.e., the sweat glands ducts), and keeps the skin lustrous and healthy, thereby protecting the FLESHY EXTERIOR and preventing the invasion of external evils. *The Magic Pivot* (líng shū, běn zàng piān) states, "defense qi warms the flesh and flushes the skin; it keeps the interstices replenished and controls their opening and closing." If defense qi is in harmony, the skin is supple and the interstices are kept tight and sound. [27: 47] [97: 395]

defense, qi, construction, and blood 卫气营血 wèi qì yíng xuè: The four levels of evil penetration in doctrine of warm diseases. See FOUR-ASPECT PATTERN IDENTIFICATION.

defensive exterior 卫表 wèi biǎo: The exterior of the body and defense qi, which defends it against external evils.

deficit 偏衰 piān shuāi: In doctrine of yin and yang, relative weakening (of either yin or yang). Deficit of yin is often referred to as vacuity, whereas that of yang is often termed debilitation.

deflagrate 焚 fén: To burn fiercely; describes heat in the exuberant heat stage of warm diseases. See HEAT.

delayed menstruation 经行后期 jīng xíng hòu qī, 月经后期 yuè jīng hòu qī: Late menstrual periods. The arrival of the menstrual period eight days or more after the normal time (i.e., roughly 36 days after the onset of the previous period in women who normally have a standard 28-day cycle). See entries listed below. [26: 814] [92: No. 250]

Delayed Menstruation

BLOOD VACUITY DELAYED MENSTRUATION (xuè xū jīng xíng hòu qī)

BLOOD COLD DELAYED MENSTRUATION (xuè hán jīng xíng hòu qī)

KIDNEY VACUITY DELAYED MENSTRUATION (shèn xū jīng xíng hòu qī)

QI STAGNATION DELAYED MENSTRUATION (*qì zhì jīng xíng hòu qī*)

BLOOD STASIS DELAYED MENSTRUATION (*xuè yū jīng xíng hòu qī*)

---

delirious speech 谵语 *zhān yǔ*, 谵言 *zhān yán*: Nonsensical talk in patients with unclear spirit-mind occurring in yang brightness repletion heat or when warm evil enters construction blood. Delirious speech is mostly observed in repletion patterns, and is treated by draining heat and clear the heart. See YANG BRIGHTNESS BOWEL PATTERN; COLD DAMAGE BLOOD AMASSMENT PATTERN; HEAT ENTERING THE PERICARDIUM. [26: 982]

delivery 分娩 *fēn miǎn*, 分解 *fēn jiě*, 分诞 *fēn dàn*, 免身 *miǎn shēn*, 产 *chǎn*: CHILDBIRTH. [26: 171]

delivery stagnation 滞产 *zhì chǎn*: DIFFICULT DELIVERY.

dementia 呆病 *dāi bìng*: Synonym: *feeble-mindedness*. A disease characterized by not talking the whole day, not eating, not drinking, sudden laughing or crying, rejection of fine food and acceptance of ordure, and a preference to dress in plant and tree leaves rather than in fine clothes. Some individuals spend the whole day alone, muttering unintelligibly; some sew up all the openings in their clothes; some hide other people's possessions; some do not eat when given food, and may go without food for days without complaining of hunger. Feeble-mindedness results when the orifices of the heart are clouded by phlegm-damp arising internally, when binding depression of liver qi restrains the spleen and stomach, or when an irregular lifestyle causes damage to the spleen and stomach. MED Use formulas such as Dementia-Shifting Elixir (*zhuǎn dāi dān*). [26: 317]

demonic influx 鬼注 *guǐ zhù*: CONSUMPTION.

demon-licked head 鬼舐头 *guǐ shì tóu*: GLOSSY SCALP WIND.

dental impressions on the margins of the tongue 舌边齿痕 *shé biān chǐ hén*: Dental impressions are observed on an enlarged pale tongue. They are a sign of qi vacuity. [26: 120]

depleted water and effulgent fire 水亏火旺 *shuǐ kuī huǒ wàng*: 1. DEPLETED WATER AND FLAMING FIRE[1]. 2. Kidney yin depletion with hyperactivity of the life gate fire, characterized by loosening of and pain in the teeth, excessive libido, and seminal emission. [26: 155]

depleted water and flaming fire 水亏火炎 *shuǐ kuī huǒ yán*: 1. Insufficiency of kidney-water causing effulgent heart fire, characterized by heart vexation, dizziness, insomnia or unquiet sleep, red-tipped tongue, and a rapid fine pulse. 2. A yin-yang imbalance of the kidney characterized by yin

vacuity and yang hyperactivity. See HYPERACTIVE KIDNEY FIRE. [26: 155]

depletion 亏 *kuī*: Severe loss, especially of fluids or kidney yin. See EXUBERANCE AND DEBILITATION.

depletion of the lower origin 下元亏损 *xià yuán kuī sǔn*: See KIDNEY YIN VACUITY. [27: 164]

depressed 郁 *yù*: Stagnant; frustrated. See DEPRESSION.

depressed dampness and hidden (deep-lying) heat 湿郁热伏 *shī yù rè fú*: DAMPNESS TRAPPING HIDDEN HEAT. [26: 929]

depressed fire 郁火 *yù huǒ*: 1. Any pattern arising when yang qi becomes depressed and exuberant heat arises. Signs include headache, red eyes, mouth sores, abdominal pain, constipation, reddish urine, red tongue with yellow fur, and a rapid replete pulse. 2. Any pattern arising when affect-mind depression causes disharmony in the bowels and viscera, allowing internal heat to arise. Signs include headache, rib-side pain, insomnia, irascibility, tongue with red tip or margins, and a rapid stringlike pulse. [27: 115]

depressed fontanel 囟陷 *xìn xiàn*: Synonym: *depressed fontanel gate*. From *The Origin and Indicators of Disease* (*zhū bìng yuán hòu lùn*). A condition in infants in which the anterior fontanel (traditionally called the "fontanel gate," see FONTANEL) forms an indentation. A depressed fontanel is attributed to qi-blood vacuity and vacuous visceral qi failing to rise to nourish the head, stemming from congenital insufficiency, prolonged diarrhea, or chronic fright wind. A slightly depressed fontanel in otherwise healthy infants is not a sign of morbidity. MED Bank up the origin and supplement the kidney. Use True-Securing Decoction (*gù zhēn tāng*). For center qi fall, use Center-Supplementing Qi-Boosting Decoction (*bǔ zhōng yì qì tāng*). [27: 437] [97: 313]

depressed fontanel gate 囟门下陷 *xìn mén xià xiàn*: DEPRESSED FONTANEL.

depressed heat seminal emission 郁热遗精 *yù rè yí jīng*: SEMINAL EMISSION arising when liver-kidney heat depression causes unhindered discharge of essence through the "essence gate." Depressed heat seminal emission is associated with heat in the spine at night, abstraction and heat in the diaphragm, and in some cases a surging pulse and generalized heat [effusion]. MED Clear heat and discharge depression. Use Pig's Stomach Pill (*zhū dǔ wán*) or Kidney-Enriching Pill (*zī shèn wán*) plus dried/fresh rehmannia (*shēng dì huáng*), root poria (*fú shén*), spiny jujube (*suān zǎo rén*), and acorus (*shí chāng pú*). ACU Base treatment mainly on KI, LR, HT, and SP. Needle with drainage at KI-2 (*rán gǔ*, Blazing Valley), KI-6 (*zhào hǎi*, Shining Sea), LR-3 (*tài chōng*,

Supreme Surge), LR-2 (*xíng jiān*, Moving Between), HT-7 (*shén mén*, Spirit Gate), PC-6 (*nèi guān*, Inner Pass), and HT-8 (*shào fǔ*, Lesser Mansion) and with supplementation at KI-3 (*tài xī*, Great Ravine), and SP-6 (*sān yīn jiāo*, Three Yin Intersection). See SEMINAL EMISSION. [26: 1010]

depressed liver 肝郁 *gān yù*: BINDING DEPRESSION OF LIVER QI. [26: 333]

depressed liver qi 肝气郁 *gān qì yù*: BINDING DEPRESSION OF LIVER QI.

depressed wood transforming into fire 木郁化火 *mù yù huà huǒ*: Depressed liver qi causing fire signs such as red face, red eyes, headache, dizziness, vomiting and retching, coughing of blood, and, in severe cases, mania. "Wood" in this context means the liver according to the five-phase understanding that the liver belongs to wood. However, "fire" means fire as an evil, not the viscus that belongs to fire, which is the heart. [26: 114] [27: 12]

depressed wood transforming into wind 木郁化风 *mù yù huà fēng*: Depressed liver qi causing wind signs such as dizziness, numbness of the tongue, tremor, and tetanic reversal, etc. [27: 114]

¹**depression** 郁 *yù*: Stagnation; reduced activity. In physiology, depression refers either to depressed qi dynamic (frustrated physiological activity) or to flow stoppage due to due to congestion. The term also describes inhibition of normal emotional activity, expressing itself in the form of oppression, frustration, and irascibility. In practice, depression is usually qi stagnation due to affect damage, and is therefore more restricted in meaning than qi stagnation, which may be due to other causes. See also SIX DEPRESSIONS; DEPRESSION PATTERN; STOPPAGE. [48: 158]

²**depression** 宛宛 *wǎn wǎn*: A concavity or indentation, as in the surface of the body. [48: 139]

depression pattern 郁证 *yù zhèng*: **1.** Any pattern of qi stagnation (frustration of normal physiological activity). *Elementary Questions* (*sù wèn, liù yuán zhèng jì dà lùn*) speaks of wood depression, fire depression, earth depression, metal depression, and water depression. These were later called the FIVE DEPRESSIONS. *Dan Xi's Experiential Methods* (*dān xī xīn fǎ*) describes qi depression, blood depression, damp depression, heat depression, phlegm depression, and food depression, which together are known as the SIX DEPRESSIONS. *Jing-Yue's Complete Compendium* (*jǐng yuè quán shū*) speaks of depression caused by affect-mind depression: anger depression, thought depression, anxiety depression, sorrow, fright depression, and fear depression. *Mysterious Pearl of Red Water* (*chì shuǐ xuán zhū*) puts forward the notion the qi of the five viscera could become depressed, and speaks of heart depression, liver depression,

earth depression, lung depression, kidney depression, and gallbladder depression. See DEPRESSION. **2.** Specifically, any pattern arising when constrained affect-mind causes binding depression of qi dynamic, and characterized by mental depression, oppression in the chest, and rib-side pain. When liver qi runs cross counterflow and restrains the spleen, signs include abdominal distention, belching, no thought of food and drink, and a fine string-like pulse. When depressed qi transforms into fire, and liver fire ascends counterflow, signs include headache, dizziness, oppression in the chest and rib-side distention, bitter taste in the mouth, dry mouth, red tongue with yellow fur, and a pulse that is usually rapid and stringlike. When phlegm and qi become depressed and bound, there is a feeling of blockage in the throat that can neither be expectorated nor swallowed. MED Liver qi running cross counterflow is treated by coursing the liver and rectifying qi with Counterflow Cold Powder (*sì nì sǎn*). Depressed qi transforming into fire is treated by clearing and draining liver fire with Supplemented Free Wanderer Powder (*jiā wèi xiāo yáo sǎn*). Binding depression of phlegm and qi is treated by disinhibiting qi and transforming phlegm with formulas such as Pinellia and Magnolia Bark Decoction (*bàn xià hòu pò tāng*) or Gallbladder-Warming Decoction (*wēn dǎn tāng*). ACU Base treatment on PC, LR, and SP. Main points: PC-6 (*nèi guān*, Inner Pass), LR-3 (*tài chōng*, Supreme Surge), and SP-6 (*sān yīn jiāo*, Three Yin Intersection). Selection of points according to pattern: For binding depression of liver qi, add BL-18 (*gān shū*, Liver Transport), BL-17 (*gé shū*, Diaphragm Transport), LR-14 (*qī mén*, Cycle Gate), and ST-36 (*zú sān lǐ*, Leg Three Li), needling with even supplementation and drainage. For depressed qi transforming into fire, add GB-34 (*yáng líng quán*, Yang Mound Spring), LR-2 (*xíng jiān*, Moving Between), PC-8 (*láo gōng*, Palace of Toil), and KI-1 (*yǒng quán*, Gushing Spring), needling with drainage. For binding depression of phlegm and qi, add CV-17 (*shān zhōng*, Chest Center), ST-40 (*fēng lóng*, Bountiful Bulge), and CV-22 (*tiān tú*, Celestial Chimney), needling with drainage. WMC These pattern are observed in neurosis, hypertension, chronic gastritis, and ulcers of the digestive tract. [26: 1010]

depurative downbearing 肃降 *sù jiàng*: A function of the lung comprising two aspects: regulating the waterways (i.e., ensuring the passage of fluids down to the kidney) and sending qi absorbed from the air down to the kidney. See LUNG GOVERNS DEPURATIVE DOWNBEARING; KIDNEY GOVERNS QI ABSORPTION. ◇ Chin 肃 *sù*, purge, clean; 降 *jiàng* fall, drop.

deranged speech 言语错乱 *yán yǔ cuò luàn*, 语言错乱 *yǔ yán cuò luàn*: Incoherent unintelligible speech; observed in phlegm turbidity confounding the orifices of the heart, phlegm-fire harassing the heart, mania patterns, and severe cases of leg qi.

deserting qi 脱气 *tuō qì*: Debilitation of yang qi in vacuity taxation disease. *Essential Prescriptions of the Golden Coffer* (*jīn guì yào lüè, xuè bì xū láo bìng mài zhèng bìng zhì*) states, "A pulse that is sunken, small, and slow is called *deserting qi*... counterflow cold of the extremities, abdominal fullness with sloppy stool, and indigestion." MED Warm and supplement the spleen and kidney with Aconite Center-Rectifying Decoction (*fù zǐ lǐ zhōng tāng*). Compare QI DESERTION. [26: 646]

desertion 脱 *tuō*: Any critical loss. *The Magic Pivot* (*líng shū, jué qì*) states, "When essence deserts, there is deafness; when qi desertions, the eyes are not clear; when liquid deserts, the interstices open and there is a great discharge of sweat; when humor deserts, the bending and stretching of the joints is inhibited, the complexion is perished, the brain and marrow wastes away, the lower legs ache, and the ears continually ring; when the blood deserts, the complexion is white, perished, and lusterless, and the pulse is empty and vacuous." These are descriptions of chronic conditions. In modern texts, however, desertion mostly refers to critical acute conditions. See DESERTION PATTERN. ◇ Chin 脱 *tuō*, shed, cast off, escape. [26: 647] [29: 588] [27: 217] [97: 521]

desertion of the flesh 肉脱 *ròu tuō*: Shedding of the flesh, i.e., emaciation. It occurs in depletion of essence-blood and debilitation of center qi, as is observed in vacuity taxation, wilting (*wěi*) patterns, or severe disease. [26: 262]

desertion pattern 脱证 *tuō zhèng*: Any disease pattern arising through critical damage to yin, yang, qi, or blood. Signs include pearly sweat reversal cold of the limbs, open eyes and closed mouth, limp hands and enuresis, and a faint fine pulse verging on expiration. Sudden damage to essential qi as in wind stroke, great sweating, great diarrhea, major blood loss, and great seminal discharge threatening the separation of yin and yang is called *fulminant desertion*. Gradual collapse of essential qi that results when original qi is weakened through enduring illness is called *vacuity desertion*. Such patterns are called "desertion" patterns because they are perceived as arising when essential qi leaves the body. *The Magic Pivot* (*líng shū, tōng dà*) states, "Desertion of yin and yang is a sudden death[-like state] with inability to recognize people." Distinction is made between yin desertion and yang desertion, which are more usually referred to as YIN COLLAPSE and YANG COLLAPSE. The concept of desertion is important in wind stroke pattern identification, in which deser-

tion patterns stand in opposition to block patterns. WMC Fulminant desertion corresponds roughly to shock, whereas vacuity desertion corresponds roughly to heart, lung, liver, or kidney failure. See EXUBERANCE AND DEBILITATION; WIND STROKE; COLLAPSE. [26: 647] [27: 217] [97: 522]

desertion sweating 脱汗 *tuō hàn*: EXPIRATION SWEATING.

desiccated 枯 *kū*: Dried out, dehydrated. See BLOOD DESICCATION; EXUBERANCE AND DEBILITATION.

desiccated teeth 牙齿干枯 *yá chǐ gān kū*, 牙齿枯槁 *yá chǐ kū gǎo*, 齿槁 *chǐ gǎo*: Synonym: *teeth dry as desiccated bones*. Teeth that appear to have lost a fluid content, like old bones that have been exposed to the sun for a long time. Desiccated teeth are a sign of kidney yin depletion. The kidney engenders bone and marrow, and the teeth are the surplus of the bone. [26: 887]

desiccation 枯 *kū*, 干枯 *gān kū*: See DESICCATED.

desiccation of kidney yin 肾阴枯涸 *shèn yin kū hé*: Severe insufficiency of kidney yin manifesting in teeth dry as desiccated bones. [29: 83]

desire only to sleep 但欲寐 *dàn yù mèi*: Somnolence in lesser yin (*shào yīn*) disease. See also WATER TOXIN. [27: 375] [97: 296]

despoliate 夺 *duó*: **1.** (Of blood, fluid, or essence) to be sudden and severely depleted. See EXUBERANCE AND DEBILITATION. **2.** Eliminate (evils) forcefully. ◇ Chin 夺 *duó* lit. to snatch or rest.

determining treatment by patterns identified 辨证论治 *biàn zhèng lùn zhì*: Basing treatment on disease patterns (as opposed to diseases). See DISEASE; PATTERN. [26: 899] [124: 360]

detriment 损 *sǔn*: Loss or damage (to blood, fluids, bowels and viscera, etc.); specifically severe chronic damage. See VACUITY TAXATION.

detriment to yang affects yin 阳损及阴 *yáng sǔn jí yīn*: Any major loss to yang ultimately causes loss to yin. Given the interdependence of yin and yang, major loss to either one ultimately affects the other (see also DETRIMENT TO YIN AFFECTS YANG). When a deficit of yang reaches a peak, the production of yin humor is affected, and a deficit of yin also develops. For example, when kidney yang is weak, inability to transform fluids causes water swelling and, in time, can cause dual depletion of both yin and yang. [26: 624]

detriment to yin affects yang 阴损及阳 *yīn sǔn jí yáng*: Any major loss to yin ultimately causes loss to yang. Given the interdependence of yin and yang, major loss to either one ultimately affects the other (see also DETRIMENT TO YANG AFFECTS YIN). Since yin-humor and yang qi are interdependent in the body, yin vacuity, when reaching a certain peak, can cause yang vacuity in keeping with the principle that "without yin, yang cannot arise." Thus liver-kidney yin vacuity can easily cause ascendant hyperactivity of liver yang or liver wind. [27: 5] [97: 235]

deviated eyes and mouth 口眼喎斜 *kǒu yǎn wāi (kuāi) xié*: Tension in the sinews of one side of the face and relaxation in those of the other side manifesting in skewing of the mouth and inability to close the eyes. Deviated eyes and mouth are attributed to wind or wind-phlegm obstructing the channels. Deviated mouth and surrounding area without deviated eyes, accompanied by hemiplegia (paralysis of one side of the body) and sometimes inability to speak is observed in wind stroke. ⃞WMC facial paralysis (Bell's palsy). ⃞MED Use Pull Aright Powder (*qiān zhèng sǎn*). ⃞ACU Base treatment mainly on LI and ST, supported by TB, GB, and BL. Select GB-20 (*fēng chí*, Wind Pool), TB-17 (*yì fēng*, Wind Screen), ST-4 (*dì cāng*, Earth Granary), ST-6 (*jiá chē*, Cheek Carriage), Pull Aright (*qiān zhèng*), LI-4 (*hé gǔ*, Union Valley), GB-14 (*yáng bái*, Yang White), BL-2 (*zǎn zhú*, Bamboo Gathering), and ST-2 (*sì bái*, Four Whites). In the initial stage, use transverse needling and point joining; for advanced stages, use shallow needling with supplementation. [26: 61] [92: No. 78]

deviated menstruation 差经 *chā jīng*: MENSTRUAL BLOODY STOOL. [26: 492]

deviated mouth 口喎 *kǒu wāi (kuāi)*, 口僻 *kǒu pì*: See DEVIATED EYES AND MOUTH. [81: 102]

deviated tongue 舌歪 *shé wāi (kuāi)*: A tongue that inclines to one side. It occurs in wind stroke due to internal liver wind or phlegm obstructing the network vessels. ⃞ACU Prick Gold Liquid and Jade Humor (*jīn jīn yù yè*), with a three-edged needle to bleed, and drain CV-23 (*lián quán*, Ridge Spring) and GV-16 (*fēng fǔ*, Wind Mansion). [26: 266] [14: 57] [46: 616] [4: 142]

devitalization 不振 *bù zhèn*: Loss of vigor or force. See EXUBERANCE AND DEBILITATION. ◇ Chin 不 *bù*, not; 振 *zhèn*, shake, stir, rouse.

devitalized center yang 中阳不振 *zhōng yáng bù zhèn*: SPLEEN-STOMACH YANG VACUITY.

devitalized heart yang 心阳不振 *xīn yáng bù zhèn*: HEART YANG VACUITY.

devitalized spleen yang 脾阳不振 *pí yáng bù zhèn*: SPLEEN YANG VACUITY.

dew 露 *lù*: DISTILLATE.

diagnosis 诊断 *zhěn duàn*: Identification of disease states. Chinese medical diagnosis is a process of gathering information through the four examinations (inspection, smelling and listening, inquiry, and palpation) and classifying the information according to the various methods of pattern identification (eight-principle pattern identification; qi-

blood pattern identification; bowel and visceral pattern identification; evil pattern identification; six-channel pattern identification; four-aspect pattern identification). NB: The Chinese term *zhěn duàn* is the equivalent of "diagnosis" in Western medicine, and is now commonly used in Chinese medical texts.

diaphoresis 汗法 *hàn fǎ*: SWEATING.[2]

diaphragm 膈 *gé*: The partition between the chest and abdomen. *The Mirror-of-Man Canon* (人镜经 *rén jìng jīng*) states, "The diaphragm membrane is below the heart; it is attached to the spine, the ribside, and abdomen all the way round like a screen that does not leak. It screens out turbid qi and prevents it from fuming the clear paths." *The Classic of Difficult Issues* (*nàn jīng*) states, "...the heart and lung alone are above the diaphragm." All the channels with the exception of the foot greater yang (*tài yáng*) bladder channel pass through the diaphragm. For example, *The Magic Pivot* (*líng shū*) says: "The heart hand lesser yin (*shào yīn*) vessel starts in the center of the heart... goes down [through] the diaphragm and connects with the small intestine. ◇ Chin 膈 *gé*, from 鬲 *gé*, partition. [26: 850] [27: 625]

diaphragmatic dispersion 膈消 *gé xiāo*: UPPER DISPERSION. [27: 423] [97: 625]

diaphragm phlegm 膈痰 *gé tán*: A phlegm pattern of qi counterflow and phlegm congestion arising when phlegm gathers and binds in the chest and diaphragm preventing normal upbearing and downbearing of qi. Signs include glomus and fullness in the abdomen and heart [region], shortness of breath that prevents the patient from lying flat, dizzy head and dim vision, and frequent desire to vomit. ⃞MED Downbear qi and flush phlegm. See PHLEGM. [26: 850]

diarrhea 泄泻 *xiè xiè*: Any deviation from established bowel rhythm characterized by increased frequency of the stool; the semi-liquid or liquid stool characteristic of this condition. Diarrhea occurs in vacuity, repletion, cold, and heat patterns. Fulminant (sudden and violent) diarrhea usually indicates repletion. Enduring diarrhea generally indicates vacuity, or a vacuity-repletion complex. Diarrhea characterized by ungratifying defecation and foul-smelling stool, and associated with abdominal pain indicates damp-heat in the large intestine. Diarrhea characterized by frequent defecation with blood and pus in the stool, abdominal pain, tenesmus, and a burning sensation in the rectum constitutes dysentery, which is another form of large intestinal damp-heat. Abdominal pain followed and relieved by diarrhea is most often attributable to food accumulation. Bouts of diarrhea with abdominal pain that is unrelieved by defecation are brought on by emotional stimuli in patients suffering from liver-spleen disharmony. Diarrhea occurring shortly after eating indicates spleen-stomach qi vacuity. Diarrhea each day before dawn is known as early morning diarrhea (fifth watch diarrhea) and is attributable to spleen-kidney yang vacuity. Diarrhea with loss of voluntary control over bowel movements, sometimes accompanied by prolapse of the rectum, is known as intestinal vacuity efflux desertion, and is attributed to vacuity cold or to center qi fall. Fulminant diarrhea and vomiting is a sign of cholera, which includes what Western medicine calls cholera and some forms of gastroenteritis. Specific types of diarrhea are named in three ways: according to pathomechanism, according to the associated morbid bowel or viscus, and according to signs.

Diarrhea

Classification according to causes
COLD DIARRHEA (*hán xiè*)
HEAT DIARRHEA (*rè xiè*)
SUMMERHEAT DIARRHEA (*shǔ xiè*)
FOOD DAMAGE DIARRHEA (*shāng shí xiè*)
VACUITY DIARRHEA (*xū xiè*)

Classification by morbid bowel or viscus
SPLEEN DIARRHEA (*pí xiè*)
STOMACH DIARRHEA (*wèi xiè*)
SMALL INTESTINE DIARRHEA (*xiǎo cháng xiè*)
LARGE INTESTINE DIARRHEA (*dà cháng xiè*)
KIDNEY DIARRHEA (*shèn xiè*)

Classification according to causes
SLOPPY DIARRHEA (*táng xiè*)
ENDURING DIARRHEA (*jiǔ xiè*)
EARLY MORNING DIARRHEA (*chén xiè*)
EFFLUX DIARRHEA (*huá xiè*)
OUTPOUR DIARRHEA (*zhù xiè*)
SWILL DIARRHEA (*sūn xiè*)
CLEAR-FOOD DIARRHEA (*xià lì qīng gǔ*)

These categories are not mutually exclusive. Food damage diarrhea, for example, is the result of damage to the digestive system by ingested food, as opposed to preexisting dysfunction. It may therefore include certain forms of stomach, large intestine, and small intestine diarrhea, but excludes large intestine diarrhea due to lung qi vacuity. Association between causes and form of diarrhea is variable. For example, kidney diarrhea is always a form of fifth-watch diarrhea, whereas sloppy diarrhea may be part of either heat or cold patterns. ◇ Chin 泄 *xiè* pour, flow, discharge; explained in this context to mean remittent sloppy stool; 泻 *xiè*, flow, drain; explained in this as meaning defecation like the pouring down of water. The two characters therefore cover the various forms of diarrhea. [27: 363] [97: 366]

diarrhea and dysentery 下利 *xià lì*: See DIARRHEA; DYSENTERY. [27: 25]

dietary contraindications 忌口 *jì kǒu*: The inadvisability of eating certain foods in certain diseases or in combination with certain medicines or other foods. *The Magic Pivot* (*líng shū, wǔ wèi*) includes statements such as "acridity is contraindicated in liver disease, saltiness is contraindicated in heart disease, sourness is contraindicated in spleen disease..." Practical experience shows that salt should be avoided in water swelling, whereas oily foods should be avoided in jaundice and diarrhea. Dietary contraindications also include prohibitions about food combinations, e.g., cold and raw foods should not be taken after consumption of fatty foods, tangerines should not be eaten when suffering from the common cold. Some traditional contraindications should not be applied indiscriminately, e.g., complete avoidance of cold or oily foods, meat, and fish in measles can prevent recovery. Finally, certain foods are contraindicated while taking certain medicinals. For example, when taking turtle shell, amaranth (a leaf vegetable not readily available in the West) is contraindicated, and while taking schizonepeta, fish and crab are contraindicated. Generally, traditional dietary contraindications still await statistical proof. [27: 321] [97: 324]

dietary irregularities 饮食失调 *yǐn shí shī tiáo*: A NEUTRAL CAUSE [OF DISEASE]; any excess in the consumption of food, including: ingestion of raw, cold, or unclean foodstuffs; voracious eating; predilection for sweet fatty foods; habitual consumption of liquor or hot, spicy foods. Dietary irregularities may not only affect the spleen and stomach, causing digestive disturbances, food accumulation, stomach pain, diarrhea, etc., but in cases of excessive liquor consumption and overindulgence in sweet and fatty foods, they may create heat, phlegm, and dampness. In addition, improper diet may combine with the six excesses to cause disease, e.g., ingestion of raw or cold foodstuffs in summer. [6: 107]

difficult defecation 大便困难 *dà biàn kùn nán*, 便难 *biàn nán*, 大便艰难 *dà biàn jiān nán*, 大便排出困难 *dà biàn pái chū kùn nán*, 排便困难 *pái biàn kùn nán*: Difficulty in evacuating the bowels with evacuation at long intervals. Difficult defecation differs from constipation on three points. (1) In constipation, evacuation is once every other day, or may occur only after several days, whereas in difficult defecation, stool is passed, usually about once a day. (2) In constipation, the stool is always dry and hard, whereas in difficult defecation, the stool is is not necessarily hard, although it may be dry and bound like jujubes or chestnuts. (3) Constipation is usually associated with abdominal discomfort, whereas difficult defecation usually is not. Difficult defecation occurs in the following patterns: large intestinal heat bind, brewing damp-heat, spleen-lung qi vacuity, liver-spleen qi stagnation, spleen-kidney yang vacuity, and yin vacuity and blood depletion. **Large intestinal heat bind** causes difficult defecation with hard stool or pelleted stool. Accompanying signs include abdominal fullness and distention or distention and pain that refuses pressure, red face and ears, heart vexation, agitation, thirst, and yellow urine. The tongue is dry with slimy fur or rough and yellow. The pulse is sunken, replete, and forceful. MED Drain heat and free the stool. Use Stomach-Regulating Qi-Coordinating Decoction (*tiáo wèi chéng qì tāng*). ACU Base treatment mainly on LI and ST. Select LI-4 (*hé gǔ*, Union Valley), LI-11 (*qū chí*, Pool at the Bend), ST-44 (*nèi tíng*, Inner Court), BL-25 (*dà cháng shū*, Large Intestine Transport), ST-25 (*tiān shū*, Celestial Pivot), SP-14 (*fù jié*, Abdominal Bind), ST-37 (*shàng jù xū*, Upper Great Hollow), and KI-6 (*zhào hǎi*, Shining Sea); needle with drainage. **Brewing damp-heat** causes difficult defecation with sticky grimy turbid stool, or hard stool followed by sloppy stool, or alternating diarrhea and constipation. Other signs include sagging distention in the lesser abdomen, glomus in the stomach duct and oppression in the chest, heavy body, bitter taste in the mouth, absence of thirst, and short voidings of reddish urine. The tongue fur is yellow and slimy. The pulse is rapid and slippery. MED Minor Qi-Coordinating Decoction (*xiǎo chéng qì tāng*) plus anemarrhena (*zhī mǔ*) and phellodendron (*huáng bǎi*). ACU Base treatment mainly on LI, ST, and SP. Select LI-4 (*hé gǔ*, Union Valley), LI-11 (*qū chí*, Pool at the Bend), ST-36 (*zú sān lǐ*, Leg Three Li), SP-9 (*yīn líng quán*, Yin Mound Spring), BL-25 (*dà cháng shū*, Large Intestine Transport), and ST-25 (*tiān shū*, Celestial Pivot); needle with drainage. **Spleen-lung qi vacuity** causes difficult ungratifying defecation associated with straining. Other signs include sweating, shortness of breath, hasty panting, exhaustion of essence-spirit, fatigued limbs, shortage of qi and laziness to speak, low timid voice, empty sagging in the smaller abdomen, in some cases with prolapse of the rectum. The tongue is enlarged and soft with dental impressions at the margins. The pulse is vacuous and forceless. MED Supplement the spleen and lung. Use Center-Supplementing Qi-Boosting Decoction (*bǔ zhōng yì qì tāng*) plus apricot kernel (*xìng rén*) and trichosanthes seed frost (*guā lóu rén shuāng*). ACU Base treatment mainly on back transport points, CV, and TB. Select CV-17 (*shān zhōng*, Chest Center), BL-20 (*pí shū*, Spleen Transport), BL-21 (*wèi shū*, Stomach Transport), BL-25 (*dà cháng shū*, Large Intestine Transport), CV-6

(*qì hǎi*, Sea of Qi), CV-4 (*guān yuán*, Pass Head), ST-36 (*zú sān lǐ*, Leg Three Li), and TB-6 (*zhī gōu*, Branch Ditch); needle with supplementation and moxa. **Liver-spleen qi stagnation** causes difficult defecation with distress and heaviness in the rectum, ungratified desire to defecate, and flatus that relieves abdominal discomfort. Other signs include distention and pain in the rib-side, mental depression, and belching. In women, there is premenstrual distention of the breasts. The pulse is stringlike or sunken and stringlike. MED Normalize qi and abduct stagnation; downbear qi and free the stool. Use Six Milled Ingredients Decoction (*liù mò tāng*). ACU Base treatment mainly on CV and LR. Select CV-12 (*zhōng wǎn*, Center Stomach Duct), GB-34 (*yáng líng quán*, Yang Mound Spring), LR-3 (*tài chōng*, Supreme Surge), ST-25 (*tiān shū*, Celestial Pivot), CV-6 (*qì hǎi*, Sea of Qi), and LR-2 (*xíng jiān*, Moving Between); needle with drainage. **Spleen-kidney yang vacuity** causes difficult defecation with dry or normal stool. It is especially common among the elderly. Accompanying signs include physical cold and fear of cold, exhaustion of essence-spirit, and limp aching lumbus and knees. Urinary signs include long voidings of clear urine, profuse urination at night, and dribble after voiding. The tongue is pale and enlarged with dental impressions at the margins. The tongue fur is white and moist. The pulse is slow or sunken. MED Warm yang and supplement the kidney. Use Ferry Brew (*jì chuān jiān*). ACU Base treatment mainly on CV, SP, KI and back transport points. Select CV-6 (*qì hǎi*, Sea of Qi), ST-25 (*tiān shū*, Celestial Pivot), KI-6 (*zhào hǎi*, Shining Sea), SP-6 (*sān yīn jiāo*, Three Yin Intersection), BL-20 (*pí shū*, Spleen Transport), BL-23 (*shèn shū*, Kidney Transport), and CV-4 (*guān yuán*, Pass Head); needle with supplementation and moxa; also, moxa CV-8 (*shén què*, Spirit Gate Tower). **Yin vacuity and blood depletion** causes difficult defecation with dizzy head and flowery vision, heart palpitations, insomnia, dry mouth and throat, and somber white facial complexion. In some cases, there is postmeridian tidal heat [effusion] with reddening of the cheeks. The tongue is red with little fur and the pulse is fine and rapid. MED When blood vacuity is prominent, nourish the blood and moisten the intestines to free the stool. Use Blood-Boosting Intestine-Moistening Pill (*yì xuè rùn cháng wán*) plus flowery knotweed (*hé shǒu wū*) and black sesame (*hēi zhī má*). If yin vacuity is prominent, nourish yin and engender liquid. Use Blood-Boosting Intestine-Moistening Pill (*yì xuè rùn cháng wán*) combined with Humor-Increasing Decoction (*zēng yè tāng*). ACU Base treatment mainly on back transport points, SP, ST, and KI. Select BL-17 (*gé shū*, Diaphragm Transport), BL-20 (*pí shū*, Spleen

Transport), BL-21 (*wèi shū*, Stomach Transport), BL-25 (*dà cháng shū*, Large Intestine Transport), ST-36 (*zú sān lǐ*, Leg Three Li), CV-4 (*guān yuán*, Pass Head), SP-6 (*sān yīn jiāo*, Three Yin Intersection), KI-3 (*tài xī*, Great Ravine), and KI-6 (*zhào hǎi*, Shining Sea); needle with supplementation. [92: No. 218] [46: 594, 670] [113: 102] [37: 325]

difficult delivery 难产 *nán chǎn*: Synonym: *delivery stagnation*. Difficulty in giving birth; failure to give birth despite labor pains and aching lumbus and sagging sensation in the smaller abdomen, and despite the breaking of the bag of waters. Distinction is made between qi-blood vacuity on the one hand and qi stagnation and blood stasis on the other. **Qi-blood vacuity** patterns may be attributable to a normally weak constitution and insufficiency of right qi; damage to qi by straining too early in delivery; or lack of fluid and exhaustion of blood due to early breaking of the bag of waters. Signs include somber white facial complexion, fatigue, limp limbs, heart palpitations, shortness of breath, pale tongue with thin fur, large vacuous or sunken fine weak pulse. MED Qi-blood vacuity patterns are treated with Cai Song-Ding's Difficult Delivery Formula (*cài sōng dīng nán chǎn fāng*) or Agreeable Birth-Hastening Powder (*cuī shēng rú yì sǎn*). **Qi stagnation and blood stasis** may arise from nervousness and fear of childbirth or idleness during pregnancy, either of which can prevent the normal movement of qi and hamper the flow of blood; it may also result from contraction of cold evil, which causes the blood to congeal and inhibits qi dynamic. Signs include a dark purplish facial complexion, nervousness, distention and oppression in the chest and stomach duct, nausea and vomiting, dark red tongue, normal or thin slimy tongue fur, large stringlike pulse with irregular beats. MED Qi stagnation and blood stasis patterns are treated with Birth-Hastening Beverage (*cuī shēng yǐn*). ACU Base treatment mainly on SP and LI. Main points: LI-4 (*hé gǔ*, Union Valley), SP-6 (*sān yīn jiāo*, Three Yin Intersection), BL-67 (*zhì yīn*, Reaching Yin), and Solitary Yin (*dú yīn*). These are combined with other points according to vacuity and repletion. For qi-blood vacuity, add ST-36 (*zú sān lǐ*, Leg Three Li) and KI-7 (*fù liū*, Recover Flow), needling with supplementation. For qi stagnation and blood stasis repletion patterns, add LR-3 (*tài chōng*, Supreme Surge) and GB-21 (*jiān jǐng*, Shoulder Well), needling with drainage. WMC Western medicine explains difficult delivery as being due to narrowness of the birth canal, malposition of the fetus, oversized fetus, or premature rupture of the amniotic sac (bag of waters). See also MALPOSITION OF FETUS. [26: 973] [46: 692] [67: 257] [27: 449] [97: 500]

diffuse 宣 *xuān*: (Of qi) to spread; to promote the spread (of qi), e.g., *diffusing the lung*, promoting the normal diffusion or spread of lung qi, so that it reaches to the exterior upper parts of the body. ◇ Chin 宣 *xuān*, proclaim, spread abroad.

diffuse pricking 散刺 *sǎn cì*: Light pricking with a three-edged needle over a broad area. See BLOODLETTING.

diffuse swelling 漫肿 *màn zhǒng*: Swelling that is not clearly circumscribed. Diffuse swelling is a feature of a flat-abscess (*jū*) that distinguishes from a welling-abscess (*yōng*).

diffusing formula 宣剂 *xuān jì*: One of the TEN FORMULA TYPES. Diffusing [medicinals] can eliminate congestion. Thus, Two Matured Ingredients Decoction (*èr chén tāng*) by the diffusing action of fresh ginger (*shēng jiāng*) and tangerine peel (*chén pí*) can treat distention and oppression in the chest, vomiting and retching, and nausea. Melon Stalk Powder (*guā dì sǎn*), which ejects phlegm-rheum from the stomach, is another example of a diffusing formula. [27: 305] [97: 433]

diffusing lung qi 宣通肺气 *xuān tōng fèi qì*: DIFFUSING THE LUNG.

diffusing lung qi with lightness 轻宣肺气 *qīng xuān fèi qì*: A method of treatment used to restore diffusion of lung qi using light medicinals and to clear heat and resolve the exterior. The method of diffusing the lung with lightness is used to treat contraction of warm dryness in autumn with slight generalized heat [effusion], dry mouth and thirst, and cough without phlegm. A representative formula is Mulberry Leaf and Apricot Kernel Decoction (*sāng xìng tāng*). [25: 219]

diffusing [medicinals] can eliminate congestion 宣可去壅 *xuān kě qù yōng*: Diffusing and dissipating medicinals such as dried ginger (*gān jiāng*) and tangerine peel (*chén pí*) can eliminate congestion and depression. See DIFFUSING FORMULA.

diffusing the lung 宣肺 *xuān fèi*: Synonyms: *diffusing the white*; *diffusing lung qi*. A method of treatment used to address inhibited lung qi with cough, panting, and copious phlegm using medicinals such as ephedra (*má huáng*), apricot kernel (*xìng rén*), platycodon (*jié gěng*), cicada molting (*chán tuì*), and perilla (*zǐ sū*). ACU Base treatment mainly on LU and LI. Select LU-7 (*liè quē*, Broken Sequence), BL-13 (*fèi shū*, Lung Transport), and LI-4 (*hé gǔ*, Union Valley). Needle with drainage and moxa if appropriate. [27: 272] [97: 433]

diffusing the lung and calming panting 宣肺平喘 *xuān fèi píng chuǎn*: See DIFFUSING THE LUNG AND TRANSFORMING PHLEGM.

diffusing the lung and dispelling phlegm 宣肺祛痰 *xuān fèi qū tán*: See DIFFUSING THE LUNG AND TRANSFORMING PHLEGM.

diffusing the lung and transforming phlegm
宣肺化痰 *xuān fèi huà tán*: Synonyms: *diffusing the lung and dispelling phlegm*; *dissipating cold and transforming phlegm*. A method of treatment used to restore lung qi diffusion and eliminate phlegm from the lung. The method of diffusing the lung and transforming phlegm is used to treat externally contracted wind-cold causing nondiffusion of lung qi with nasal congestion, itchy throat, cough with copious phlegm, and thin white tongue fur. MED Lung-diffusing phlegm-transforming medicinals include ephedra (*má huáng*), platycodon (*jié gěng*), apricot kernel (*xìng rén*), cicada molting (*chán tuì*), magnolia flower[1] (*xīn yí*), tangerine peel (*chén pí*), and licorice (*gān cǎo*). Formulas include Cough-Stopping Powder (*zhǐ sòu sǎn*) and Apricot Kernel and Perilla Powder (*xìng sū sǎn*). ACU Base treatment mainly on LU, LI, and ST. Select LU-7 (*liè quē*, Broken Sequence), BL-13 (*fèi shū*, Lung Transport), LI-4 (*hé gǔ*, Union Valley), and ST-40 (*fēng lóng*, Bountiful Bulge). Needle with drainage. [26: 397] [27: 271] [97: 433]

diffusing the white 宣白 *xuān bái*: DIFFUSING THE LUNG.

diphtheria 白喉 *bái hóu*: A disease characterized by whitening of the throat. It occurs mostly in the autumn or winter after a long period of dryness, and is attributed to seasonal epidemic scourge toxin exploiting vacuity of the lung and stomach. It starts with a sore throat that makes swallowing painful, and with the appearance of white speckles on one or both throat nodes (i.e., the tonsils), which spread quickly to create a white membrane that covers the uvula and stretches into the regions inside and outside the THROAT PASS (isthmus faucium). The membrane does not easily slough off, cannot be forcefully removed without causing bleeding, and if removed always grows back. Other signs include headache, generalized pain, slight heat effusion or alternating heat [effusion] and [aversion to] cold, lack of spirit, oppression in the chest, vexation and agitation, bad breath, and nasal congestion. If the white membrane spreads into the region inside the throat pass and down to the epiglottis and beyond, signs such as labored breathing, flaring nostrils, green-blue lips, heart palpitations or fearful throbbing, and a bound or intermittent pulse may be observed. Distinction is made between yang heat and yin vacuity patterns. Yang heat patterns are attributed to wind-heat or heat toxin, and are characterized by a red sore swollen throat, heat effusion, constipation, and reddish urine; yin vacuity patterns are attributed to dryness-heat damaging the lung and stomach, and are characterized by white putrid throat, low fever, heat in the hearts of the palms and soles, fatigue, shortness of breath, and a fine rapid pulse. MED Yang heat patterns are treated by draining heat and resolving toxin using Spirit Immortal Life-Giving Decoction (*shén xiān huó mìng tāng*). Yin vacuity patterns are treated by nourishing yin and clearing heat with formulas such as Yin-Nourishing Lung-Clearing Decoction (*yǎng yīn qīng fèi tāng*). Diphtheria should not be treated by upraising, sweating, precipitation, or surgery. ACU For yang heat, base treatment mainly on LU, LI, TB, and ST. Select as the main points TB-17 (*yì fēng*, Wind Screen), LU-5 (*chǐ zé*, Cubit Marsh), LI-4 (*hé gǔ*, Union Valley), LI-17 (*tiān dǐng*, Celestial Tripod), LI-18 (*fú tú*, Protuberance Assistant), and ST-36 (*zú sān lǐ*, Leg Three Li), needling with drainage. Prick LU-11 (*shào shāng*, Lesser Shang) and LI-1 (*shāng yáng*, Shang Yang) to bleed. For yin vacuity, use the main points listed above, needling with supplementation or with even supplemenation and drainage at BL-13 (*fèi shū*, Lung Transport), SP-6 (*sān yīn jiāo*, Three Yin Intersection), LU-5 (*chǐ zé*, Cubit Marsh), ST-44 (*nèi tíng*, Inner Court), and KI-6 (*zhào hǎi*, Shining Sea). Selection of points according to signs: For headache, add Greater Yang (*tài yáng*) and GB-20 (*fēng chí*, Wind Pool). For heat effusion and aversion to cold, add GV-14 (*dà zhuī*, Great Hammer) and LI-11 (*qū chí*, Pool at the Bend). For panting, add PC-6 (*nèi guān*, Inner Pass) and CV-22 (*tiān tú*, Celestial Chimney). For heart palpitations or fearful throbbing, add HT-7 (*shén mén*, Spirit Gate), PC-6 (*nèi guān*, Inner Pass), PC-4 (*xī mén*, Cleft Gate), and BL-15 (*xīn shū*, Heart Transport). ◇ Chin 白 *bái*, white; 喉 *hóu*, throat, larynx. Eng *diphtheria*, from Gk. diphthera, a piece of leather, from the toughness of the false membrane that characterizes the disease. [26: 226] [27: 498, 368] [17: 240] [97: 155] [42: 106] [29: 569]

directional supplementation and drainage 迎随补泻 *yíng suí bǔ xiè*: An acupuncture technique whereby the needle is angled with or against the flow of qi in a channel to produce a supplementing or a draining needle stimulus. A needle pointing in the direction of the channel flow produces supplementation, whereas one pointing counter to the direction of the flow produces drainage. See NEEDLE MANIPULATION (TECHNIQUE). ◇ Chin 迎 *yíng*, against, head on, advance to meet (an oncoming or arriving person or thing); 随 *suí*, following, with. [46: 470] [26: 389]

direct moxibustion 直接灸 *zhí jiē jiǔ*: The burning of hand-rolled moxa cones directly on the skin at selected points. This method includes SCARRING MOXIBUSTION and NONSCARRING MOXIBUSTION. [26: 367] [46: 491]

direct strike 直中 *zhí zhòng*: See DIRECT STRIKE ON THE TRIPLE YIN.

direct strike on the triple yin 直中三阴 *zhí zhòng sān yīn*: Direct invasion of the yin channels by disease evils that requires emergency treatment. Normally, disease evils in the early stages give rise to triple-yang patterns, which may then develop into triple-yin patterns. However, if the disease evil is strong and right qi is weak, the disease evil can directly strike the triple yin. In clinical practice, direct strike on the lesser yin (*shào yīn*) is the most commonly seen, and is due to kidney yang debilitation and extreme exuberance of yin-cold. MED Return yang with Counterflow Cold Decoction (*sì nì tāng*). [26: 366] [97: 330] [27: 222]

direct strike on the yin channels 直中阴经 *zhí zhòng yīn jīng*: Disease evil directly invading the yin channels without passing through the triple yang; characterized by absence of heat effusion, by aversion to cold, and by other yin-channel signs. See DIRECT STRIKE ON THE TRIPLE YIN. [26: 366] [97: 330]

disablement 痱 *féi*: Synonym: *wind disablement*. WILTING and loss of the use of the limbs without pain and with loss of mental faculties. *The Magic Pivot (líng shū, rè bìng)* states, "When disablement is the disease, and there is no generalized pain, the limbs cannot contract, cognitive faculties are not seriously confused, and speech is faint, the condition can be treated." This passage would indicate that disablement is a sequela of wind stroke. See HEMILATERAL WITHERING; STROKE. [26: 769]

¹**discharge** 泄 *xiè*, 洩 *xiè*: Release or leakage; spontaneous or induced outward or downward movement. Same as drain. See also DIARRHEA.

²**discharge** 带 *dài*: Abbreviation for vaginal discharge.

discharge defense and outthrust heat 泄卫透热 *xiè wèi tòu rè*: To treat warm disease in which evil heat has reached the qi-aspect, causing generalized heat [effusion], absence of aversion to cold, vexation and thirst, and yellow tongue fur, but in which the exterior is blocked so that there is no sweating (a sign of a defense aspect block). MED Use cool acrid outthrusting medicinals to bring on a mild sweat ("draining defense"), and make the qi-aspect evil thrust outward through the exterior ("outthrusting heat"). This method uses medicinals such as duckweed (*fú píng*), mint (*bò hé*), fermented soybean (*dàn dòu chǐ*), cicada molting (*chán tuì*), chrysanthemum (*jú huā*), lonicera (*jīn yín huā*), forsythia (*lián qiào*), and imperata (*bái máo gēn*). [27: 251] [27: 251] [97: 366]

discharge of stool with flatus 大便随矢气而出 *dà biàn suí shǐ qì ér chū*: Involuntary discharge of stool while passing flatus. Discharge of stool with flatus is observed in qi dysentery (dysentery manifesting as qi vacuity). [26: 542]

discharge the liver 泄肝 *xiè gān*: COURSING THE LIVER.

discharging formula 泄剂 *xiè jì*: One of the TEN FORMULA TYPES. Discharging [medicinals] can eliminate blocks. Formulas containing discharging and draining medicinals treat interior repletion patterns. For example, Tingli and Jujube Lung-Draining Decoction (*tíng lì dà zǎo xiè fèi tāng*) is used to treat lung repletion patterns of cough, rapid breathing, and copious phlegm, whereas Six Milled Ingredients Decoction (*liù mò tāng*) is used to treat constipation due to qi depression accompanied by belching, chest and rib-side distention and fullness (and abdominal pain in severe cases), a slimy yellow tongue fur, and a stringlike pulse. [27: 305] [97: 366]

discharging [medicinals] can eliminate blocks 泄可去闭 *xiè kě qù bì*: Discharging medicinals, i.e., draining medicinals, such as rhubarb (*dà huáng*) and tingli (*tíng lì zǐ*) treat interior repletion patterns. See DISCHARGING FORMULA. [27: 267]

disease 病 *bìng*, 疾 *jí*, 疾病 *jí bìng*: Any sick condition of the body of part of it; either an instance of such a condition (also called *illness*) or a any specific kind of morbidity, as identified by specific signs or specific causes or pathomechanisms common to all individuals affected by it. Wind stroke, for example, is a disease defined by the sudden loss of use of the limbs (hemiplegia), inability to speak, and inability to recognize people. The notion of a disease entity is distinct from that of PATTERN. A specific disease entity may be characterized by different patterns that reflect different pathomechanisms or variations in the disease that are determined by the patient's individual state of health. Measles, for example, may take the form of a *favorable* or *unfavorable* pattern. The principle diseases are listed below.

Internal Diseases

BABY MOTH (*rǔ é*)
CHICKEN POX (*shuǐ dòu*)
CHOLERA (*huò luàn*)
   COLD CHOLERA (*hán huò luàn*)
   CHOLERA CRAMPS (*huò luàn zhuǎn jīn*)
   DAMP CHOLERA (*shī huò luàn*)
   DRY CHOLERA (*gān huò luàn*)
   HEAT CHOLERA (*rè huò luàn*)
CONCRETIONS, CONGLOMERATION, ACCUMULATIONS, AND GATHERINGS (*zhēng jiǎ jī jù*)
   FIVE ACCUMULATIONS (*wǔ jī*)
   STRINGS AND AGGREGATIONS (*xián pǐ*)
CONSUMPTION (*láo zhài*)
DRUM DISTENTION (*gǔ zhàng*)
DIPHTHERIA (*bái hóu*)
DYSENTERY (*lì jí*)

ENDURING DYSENTERY (*jiǔ lì*)

EPIDEMIC DYSENTERY (*yì lì*)

FOOD-DENYING DYSENTERY (*jìn kǒu lì*)

INTERMITTENT DYSENTERY (*xiū xí lì*)

VACUITY DYSENTERY (*xū lì*)

DYSPHAGIA-OCCLUSION (*yē gé*)

EPIDEMIC THROAT SAND (*yì hóu shā*)

EPILEPSY (*xián*)

FOOD DAMAGE (*shāng shí*)

FOOD ACCUMULATION (*shí jī*)

GAN (*gān*)

IMPEDIMENT (*bì*)

WIND IMPEDIMENT (*fēng bì*)

COLD IMPEDIMENT (*hán bì*)

DAMP IMPEDIMENT (*shī bì*)

HEAT IMPEDIMENT (*rè bì*)

JOINT-RUNNING WIND (*lì jié fēng*)

CRANE'S-KNEE WIND (*hè xī fēng*)

JAUNDICE (*huáng dàn*)

ACUTE JAUNDICE (*jí huáng*)

BLOOD AMASSMENT JAUNDICE (*xuè xū huáng dǎn*)

BLACK JAUNDICE (*hēi dǎn*)

DAMP-HEAT JAUNDICE (*shī rè huáng dǎn*)

FIVE JAUNDICES (*wǔ dǎn*)

GALLBLADDER JAUNDICE (*dǎng huáng*)

GRAIN JAUNDICE (*gǔ dǎn*)

LIQUOR JAUNDICE (*jiǔ dǎn*)

SCOURGE JAUNDICE (*wēn huáng*)

VACUITY JAUNDICE (*xū huáng*)

YANG JAUNDICE (*yáng huáng*)

YELLOW SWEAT (*huáng hàn*)

YIN JAUNDICE (*yīn huáng*)

LEG QI (*jiǎo qì*)

DAMP LEG QI (*shī jiǎo qì*)

DRY LEG QI (*gān jiǎo qì*)

COLD-DAMP LEG QI (*hán shī jiǎo qì*)

PHLEGM-DAMP LEG QI (*tán shī jiǎo qì*)

MALARIA (*nüè jí*)

DAMP MALARIA (*shī nüè*)

COLD MALARIA (*hán nüè*)

ENDURING MALARIA (*jiǔ nüè*)

EPIDEMIC MALARIA (*yì nüè*)

FOOD MALARIA (*shí nüè*)

FEMALE MALARIA (*pìn nüè*)

MIASMIC MALARIA (*zhāng nüè*)

PURE-HEAT MALARIA (*dǎn nüè*)

PHLEGM MALARIA (*tán nüè*)

TRIPLE-YIN MALARIA (*sān yīn nüè*)

TAXATION MALARIA (*láo nüè*)

SUMMERHEAT MALARIA (*shǔ nüè*)

WARM MALARIA (*wēn nüè*)

WIND MALARIA (*fēng nüè*)

MANIA AND WITHDRAWAL (*diān kuáng*)

MOUNTING (*shàn*)

BULGING MOUNTING (*tuí shàn*)

BLOOD MOUNTING (*xuè shàn*)

COLD MOUNTING (*hán shàn*)

FOXY MOUNTING (*hú shàn*)

PROMINENT MOUNTING (*tuí (tuí) shàn*)

QI MOUNTING (*qì shàn*)

SINEW MOUNTING (*jīn shàn*)

WATER MOUNTING (*shuǐ shàn*)

MUMPS (*zhà sāi*)

STONE MOTH (*shí é*)

STOMACH REFLUX (*fǎn wèi*)

SMALLPOX (*tiān huā*)

DISPERSION-THIRST (*xiāo kě*)

CENTER DISPERSION (*zhōng xiāo*)

LOWER DISPERSION (*xià xiāo*)

UPPER DISPERSION (*shàng xiāo*)

WHEEZING AND PANTING (*xiào chuǎn*)

WILTING (*wěi*)

BLOOD STASIS WILTING (*xuè yū wěi*)

BLOOD VACUITY WILTING (*xuè xū wěi*)

BONE WILTING (*gǔ wěi*)

DAMP-HEAT WILTING (*shī rè wěi*)

DAMP PHLEGM WILTING (*shī tán wěi*)

DRYNESS-HEAT WILTING (*zào rè wěi*)

FLESH WILTING (*ròu wěi*)

QI VACUITY WILTING (*qì xū wěi*)

SINEW WILTING (*jīn wěi*)

SKIN AND HAIR WILTING (*pí máo wěi*)

VESSEL WILTING (*mài wěi*)

YIN VACUITY WILTING (*yīn xū wěi*)

WIND DAMAGE (*shàng fēng*)

WIND STROKE (*zhòng fēng*)

WORM ACCUMULATION (*chóng jī*)

YELLOW SWELLING (*huáng zhǒng*)

Men's diseases

IMPOTENCE (*yáng wěi*)

PREMATURE EJACULATION (*zǎo xiè*)

SEMINAL EMISSION (*yí jīng*)

FOXY MOUNTING (*hú shàn*)

KIDNEY ROCK (*shèn yán*)

PERSISTENT ERECTION (*yīn zòng*)

RETRACTED GENITALS (*yīn suō*)

SCROTAL ITCH (*yīn náng sāo yǎng*)

SCROTAL WIND (*shèn náng fēng*)

SCROTAL WELLING-ABSCESS (*shèn náng yōng*)

SEMINAL COLD (*jīng lěng*)

SEXUAL TAXATION (*fáng láo*)

RIGID CENTER (*qiáng zhōng*)

SLOUGHING SCROTUM (*tuō náng*)

TESTICULAR WELLING-ABSCESS (*zǐ yōng*)

WHITE TURBIDITY (*bái zhuó*)

Women's diseases

Menstruation and Vaginal discharge

MENSTRUAL IRREGULARITIES (*yuè jīng bù tiáo*)

DELAYED MENSTRUATION (*jīng xíng hòu qí*)

ADVANCED MENSTRUATION (*jīng xíng xiān qí*)

CHAOTIC MENSTRUATION (*jīng luàn*)

MENSTRUAL PAIN (*tòng jīng*)

SCANT MENSTRUATION (*yuè jīng guò shǎo*)

PROFUSE MENSTRUATION (*yuè jīng guò duō*)

See entries beginning with *menstrual*.

FLOODING AND SPOTTING (*bēng lòu*)

VAGINAL DISCHARGE (*dài xià*)

WHITE FLOOD (*bái bēng*)

WHITE LEAK (*bái lòu*)

WHITE OOZE (*bái yín*)

Diseases of pregnancy

BRITTLE FOOT (*cuì jiǎo*)

DIFFICULT DELIVERY (*nán chǎn*)

FAILURE OF THE INTERLOCKING BONES TO OPEN (*jiāo gǔ bù kāi*)

FETAL SPOTTING (*tāi lòu*)

FETAL WATER (*tāi shuǐ*)

HABITUAL MISCARRIAGE (*huá tāi*)

MALIGN OBSTRUCTION (*è zǔ*) (morning sickness)

MALPOSITION OF FETUS (*tāi wèi bù zhèng*)

SHIFTED BLADDER (*zhuǎn bāo*)

WRINKLY FOOT (*zhòu jiǎo*)

Postpartum diseases

BREAST MILK STOPPAGE (*rǔ zhī bù xià*)

INFANT'S-PILLOW PAIN (*ér zhěn tòng*)

NONCLOSURE OF THE BIRTH GATE (*chǎn mén bù bì*)

PAINFUL SWELLING OF THE YIN DOOR (*yīn hù zhǒng tòng*)

RETENTION OF THE AFTERBIRTH (*bāo yī bù xià*)

RETENTION OF THE LOCHIA (*è lù bù xíng*)

Miscellaneous women's diseases

INFERTILITY (*bù yùn*)

INTERCOURSE BLEEDING (*jiāo jiē chū xuè*)

PUDENDAL ITCH (*yīn yǎng*)

VAGINAL FLATUS (*yīn chuī*)

VAGINAL PROTRUSION (*yīn tíng*)

VISCERAL AGITATION (*zàng zào*)

YIN SORE (*yīn chuāng*)

See "External diseases" list, and other entries beginning with *mammary*.

Children's diseases

BULGING FONTANEL (*xìn tián*)

CHILD DYSENTERY (*xiǎo ér lì jí*)

CHILD EYE GAN (*xiǎo ér gān yán*)

CHILD VISITING HOSTILITY (*xiǎo ér kè wǔ*)

DEPRESSED FONTANEL (*xìn xiàn*)

FETAL EPILEPSY (*tāi xián*)

FETAL FEEBLENESS (*tāi ruò*)

FETAL FRIGHT (*tāi jīng*)

FETAL HEAT (*tāi rè*)

FETAL JAUNDICE (*tāi huáng*)

FETAL REDNESS (*tāi chì*)

FETAL MOUNTING (*tāi shàn*)

FETAL OBESITY (*tāi féi*)

FETAL TOXIN (*tāi dú*)

FETAL WIND (*tāi fēng*)

FIVE SLOWNESSES (*wǔ chí*)

FIVE LIMPNESSES (*wǔ ruǎn*)

FRIGHT WIND (*jīng fēng*)

GAN (*gān*)

GOOSE-MOUTH SORE (*é kǒu chuāng*)

MILK ACCUMULATION (*rǔ jī*)

MEASLES (*má zhěn*)

MUMPS (*zhà sāi*)

NIGHT CRYING (*yè tí*)

PIGEON BREAST (*jī xiōng*)

TORTOISE BACK (*guī bèi*)

UMBILICAL WIND (*qí fēng*)

UNUNITED SKULL (*jiě lú*)

WHITE-FACE SAND (*bái miàn shā*)

WHOOPING COUGH (*bǎi rì ké*)

External diseases

BOIL (*jié*)

CLOVE SORE (*dīng chuāng*)

RED THREAD CLOVE SORE (*hóng sī dīng*)

CLOVE SORE RUNNING YELLOW (*dīng chuāng zǒu huáng*)

CINNABAR TOXIN (*dān dú*)

HEAD FIRE CINNABAR (*bào tóu huǒ dān*)

WANDERING CINNABAR (*chì yóu dān*)

FIRE FLOW (*liú huǒ*)

DAMP TOXIN SORE (*shī dú chuāng*)

FLOWING PHLEGM (*liú tán*)

CRANE'S-KNEE PHLEGM (*hē xī tán*)

ANKLE-BORING PHLEGM (*chuān huái tán*)

FIRE-GIRDLE CINNABAR (*chán yāo huǒ dān*)

INWARD FALL (*nèi xiàn*)

POCK PIMPLES (*cuò féi*)

SEAT SORE (*zuò bǎn chuāng*)

SLOUGHING FLAT-ABSCESS (*tuō jū*)

ROCK (*yán*)

TONGUE MUSHROOM (*shé jùn*)

COCOON LIP (*jiǎn chún*)

LOSS-OF-LUXURIANCE (*shī róng*)

MAMMARY ROCK (*rǔ yán*)

KIDNEY ROCK (*shèn yán*)

RUNNING YELLOW (*zǒu huáng*)

SCROFULA (*luǒ lì*)

TUMOR (*liú*)

QI TUMOR (*qì liú*)

BLOOD TUMOR (*xuè liú*)

FLESH TUMOR (*ròu liú*)

SINEW TUMOR (*jīn liú*)

BONE TUMOR (*gǔ liú*)

FATTY TUMOR (*zhī liú*)

WELLING- AND FLAT-ABSCESSES (*yōng jū*)

WELLING-ABSCESS (*yōng*)

FLAT-ABSCESS (*jū*)

EFFUSION (*fā*)

THROAT-LOCKING WELLING-ABSCESS (*yōng*)

HEADED FLAT-ABSCESS (*yǒu tóu jū*)

JOWL EFFUSION (*fā yí*)

STREAMING SORE (*liú zhù*)

DAMP TOXIN STREAMING SORE (*shī dú liú zhù*)

HEADLESS FLAT-ABSCESS (*wú tóu jū*)

JUMPING ROUND FLAT-ABSCESS (*huán tiào jū*)

BONE FLAT-ABSCESS (*fù gǔ jū*)

Skin diseases

ACNE (*fěn cì*)

DORMANT PAPULES (*yǐn zhěn*)

DRINKER'S NOSE (*jiǔ zhā*)

FOOT DAMP QI (*shī jiǎo qì*)

GLOSSY SCALP WIND (*yóu fēng*)

HEAT SORE (*rè chuāng*)

LICHEN (*xiǎn*)

  OXHIDE LICHEN (*niú pí xiǎn*)

  PINE-BARK LICHEN (*sōng pí xiǎn*)

  COIN LICHEN (*yuán xiǎn*)

  MAMMARY LICHEN (*rǔ xiǎn*)

  BLOWN BLOSSOM LICHEN (*chuī huā xiǎn*)

  WIND LICHEN (*fēng xiǎn*)

  CHAMBER POT LICHEN (*mǎ tǒng xiǎn*)

  PLASTER WIND (*gāo yào fēng*)

  BALD WHITE SCALP SORE (*bái tū chuāng*)

  FAT SORE (*féi chuāng*)

  GOOSE-FOOT WIND (*é zhǎng fēng*)

  PALM HEART WIND (*zhǎng xīn fēng*)

  ASHEN NAIL (*huī zhǐ jiǎ*)

  LACQUER SORE (*qī chuāng*)

LIP WIND (*chún fēng*)

MOLE (*zhì*)

PESTILENTIAL WIND (*lì fēng*)

PRICKLY HEAT (*fèi zǐ*)

PURPLE AND WHITE PATCH WIND (*zǐ bái diàn fēng*)

RED FLAMING SORE (*chì yán chuāng*)

SCAB (*jiè*)

WART (*yóu*)

WATER-SOAKING SORE (*shuǐ zì chuāng*)

WIIITE CRUST (*bái bǐ*)

WHITE SCALING WIND (*bái xiè fēng*)

WIND ITCH (*fēng yǎng*)

WIND-HEAT SORE (*fēng rè chuāng*)

YELLOW-WATER (*huáng shuǐ chuāng*)

Genital diseases

LOWER BODY GAN (*xià gān*)

RED BAYBERRY SORES (*yáng méi chuāng*)

Women's external diseases

NIPPLE WIND (*rǔ tóu fēng*)

MAMMARY WELLING-ABSCESS (*rǔ yōng*)

EFFUSION OF THE BREAST (*rǔ fā*)

MAMMARY AGGREGATION (*rǔ pì*)

MAMMARY FISTULA (*rǔ lòu*)

SPONTANEOUS BLEEDING OF THE NIPPLES (*rǔ nǜ*)

Men's external diseases

SCROTAL WELLING-ABSCESS (*yīn náng yōng*)

SCROTAL WIND (*náng fēng*)

SLOUGHING SCROTUM (*tuō náng*)

TESTICULAR WELLING-ABSCESS (*zǐ yōng*)

WATER MOUNTING (*shuǐ shàn*)

Anus

COMMUNICATING BOWELS (*jiāo cháng*)

FISTULA (*lòu chuāng*)

HEMORRHOIDS (*zhì chuāng*)

PROLAPSE OF THE RECTUM (*tuō gāng*)

Miscellaneous

BED SORES (*rù chuāng*)

BUBO (*héng xián*)

BURNS AND SCALDS (*huǒ tàng shāng*)

DAMP SORE (*shī chuāng*)

FRECKLES (*què bān*)

FROSTBITE (*dòng chuāng*)

GAN (*gān*)

INNOMINATE SWOLLEN TOXIN SORE (*wú míng zhǒng dú*)

INTESTINAL WELLING-ABSCESS (*cháng yōng*)

LAI (*lài*)

MOUTH SORES (*kǒu chuāng*)

PHLEGM NODE (*tán hé*)

TIP-ABSCESS (*biāo jū*)

TOXIN SORE (*dú chuāng*)

TOXIN SWELLING (*zhǒng dú*)

SHANK SORES (*lián chuāng*)

SNAKE BITES (*dú shé yǎo shāng*)

WATER-SOAKING SORE (*shuǐ zì chuang*)

WET-SPREADING SORE (*jìn yín chuāng*)

Diseases of the Nose

BRAIN-GRIPPING SAND (*jiā nǎo shā*)

BRAIN LEAK (*nǎo lòu*)

DEEP-SOURCE NASAL CONGESTION (*bí yuā*)

DRINKER'S NOSE (*jiǔ zhā*)

NASAL CONGESTION (*bí sāi*)

NASAL POLYP (*bí xī ròu*)

NOSEBLEED (*bí nǜ*)

SNIVELING NOSE (*bí qiú*)

WITHERED NOSE (*bí gǎo*)

Diseases of the eye

Diseases of the eyelid

DROOPING OF THE UPPER EYELID (*shàng bāo xià chuí*)

CINNABAR TOXIN OF THE EYELID (*yǎn bāo dān dú*)

INGROWN EYELASH (*ingrown eyelash*)

MILLET SORE OF THE EYE (*mù shēng sù chuāng*)

PEPPERCORN SORE OF THE EYE (*mù shēng jiāo chuāng*)

PHLEGM NODE OF THE EYE (*yǎn shēng tán hé*)

STY (*zhēn yǎn*)

TWITCHING OF THE EYELIDS (*yǎn pí tiào*)

ULCERATION OF THE EYELID RIM (*yǎn xián chì lán*)

WEEPING CANTHUS (*lòu jīng*)

Diseases of the eyeball

BLOOD FLYING INTO THE EYE (*mù fèi xuè*)

BLOOD SPILLAGE IN THE WHITE OF THE EYE (*bái jīng yì xuè*)

CHAOTIC RED-THREAD VESSELS (*chì sī luàn mài*)

COIN SCREEN (*yuán yì*)

CONGEALED-FAT SCREEN (*níng zhī yì*)

CRAB'S EYE (*xiè jīng*)

FALLING CURTAIN SCREEN (*chuí lián yì*)

GAN SCREEN (*gān yì*)

GREEN WIND INTERNAL OBSTRUCTION (*lù9 fēng nèi zhàng*)

HANGING RED MEMBRANE (*chì mò xià chuí*)

HEAVEN-CURRENT RED EYE (*tiān xíng chì yǎn*)

EXCRESCENCE CREEPING OVER THE EYE (*nǔ ròu pān jīng*)

RED AREOLA SURROUNDING THE DARK OF THE EYE (*bào lún hóng*)

RED VESSELS SPREADING ACROSS THE EYE (*chì mài chuán jīng*)

RESIDUAL SCREEN (*sù yì*)

STARRY EYE SCREEN (*mù shēng xīng yì*)

TANGLED RED-THREAD VESSELS (*chì sī qiú mài*)

UPSURGING YELLOW HUMOR (*huáng yè shàng chōng*)

WHITE DRY EYE (*bái sè zhèng*)

WHITE MEMBRANE INVADING THE EYE (*bái mó qīn jīng*)

YELLOW WIND INTERNAL OBSTRUCTION (*huáng fēng nèi zhàng*)

Abnormalities of vision

BLINKING (*mù zhá*)

BLOOD POURING INTO THE PUPIL SPIRIT (*xuè guàn tóng shén*)

CLOUDED VISION (*mù hūn*)

FARSIGHTEDNESS (*yuǎn shì*)

FEELING OF DISTENTION IN THE EYES (*mù zì zhàng*)

NEARSIGHTEDNESS (*jìn shì*)

SEEING DIMLY AFAR (*yuǎn shì huāng huāng*)

SPIRITLESS EYES (*mù shì wú shén*)

SQUINT (*mù piān shì*)

SPARROW'S VISION (*què mù*)

Diseases of the Ear

CERUMINAL CONGESTION (*dīng ěr*)

EAR MUSHROOM (*ěr jùn*)

EAR PAIN (*ěr tòng*)

DEAFNESS (*ěr lóng*)

FULMINANT DEAFNESS (*bào lóng*)

HEARING IMPAIRMENT (*zhòng tīng*)

ITCHY EAR (*ěr yǎng*)

TINNITUS (*ěr míng*)

PURULENT EAR (*tíng ěr*)

Diseases of the Head

Internal medicine

BULGING FONTANEL (*xìn tián*)

DEPRESSED FONTANEL (*xìn xiàn*)

DISTENTION IN THE HEAD (*tóu zhàng*)

DIZZINESS (*xuàn yūn*)

HEAT EFFUSION OF THE HEAD (hot head)

HEADACHE (*tóu tòng*)

HEAD WIND (*tóu fēng*)

HEMILATERAL HEADACHE (*piān tóu tòng*)

HEMILATERAL HEAD WIND (*piān tóu fēng*)

SHAKING OF THE HEAD (*tóu yáo*)

THUNDER HEAD WIND (*léi tóu fēng*)

SWEATING HEAD (*tóu hàn*)

UNUNITED SKULL (*jiě lú*)

External medicine

BALD WHITE SCALP SORE (*bái tū chuāng*)

WHITE SCALING WIND (*bái xiè fēng*)

Disease of the Mouth

BONE TROUGH WIND (*gǔ cáo fēng*)

GAPING GUMS (*yā xuān*)

GAN OF THE TEETH AND GUMS (*yá gān*)

GALLOPING GAN OF THE TEETH AND GUMS (*zǒu mǎ yá gān*)

MOUTH SORES (*kǒu chuāng*)

SPONTANEOUS BLEEDING OF THE GUMS (*chì nǜ*)

Injuries

BONE FRACTURE (*gǔ zhé*)

CRICK IN THE NECK (*luò zhěn*)

DISLOCATION (*tuō jiù*)

ELBOW TAXATION (*zhǒu láo*)
(tennis elbow)

INCISED WOUNDS (*jīn chuāng*)

LEAKY SHOULDER WIND (*lòu jiān fēng*)
(frozen shoulder)

SPRAIN (*niǔ shāng*)

WRENCHED LUMBUS PAIN (*shǎn cuò yāo tòng*)

disease correspondences of the five colors 五色主病 *wǔ sè zhǔ bìng*: The diagnostic significance of the five colors (green-blue, red, yellow, white, and black). The five colors have two sets or correspondences: (1) In the doctrine of the five phases, green-blue, red, yellow, white and black facial complexions indicate disease of the liver, heart, spleen, lung, and kidney respectively. (2) The five colors are also have correspondences to the nature of disease. Green-blue is associated with wind, fright, cold and pain; red is associated with heat; yellow is associated with dampness; white is associated with blood vacuity and cold; black is associated with pain, blood stasis, and taxation damage. These correspondence are rough guidelines, not immutable rules. [26: 116] [27: 173] [97: 53]

disease evil 病邪 *bìng xié*: EVIL.

disease-evil pattern identification 病邪辨证 *bìng xié biàn zhèng*: The process of identifying evils present in the body from examination data. Evils are recognized by certain characteristic signs. Heat, for example, is identified by the presence of high fever, palpable heat, red facial complexion, red tongue and rapid pulse. Disease-evil pattern identification is not in itself a basis for treatment. External evils are identified through EXTERNALLY CONTRACTED HEAT (FEBRILE) DISEASE PATTERN IDENTIFICATION, while the internal evils require further scrutiny through BOWEL AND VISCERAL PATTERN IDENTIFICATION. Furthermore, whatever evil is present, treatment can only be prescribed once the relative strength of the evil to right qi has been assessed. [6: 195]

disease of the mother affects the child 母病及子 *mǔ bìng jí zǐ*: The five-phase law that disease can spread from one bowel or viscus to the other according to the engendering sequence. For example, liver-wood is the mother of heart-fire, and ascendant liver yang causing exuberant heart fire is a disease of the mother affecting the child. Spleen-earth is the mother of lung-metal, and spleen-stomach vacuity giving rise to insufficiency of lung qi is another example. See also VACUITY EVIL. [26: 207] [27: 11] [97: 171]

disease pattern 病证 *bìng zhèng*: See PATTERN.

disharmony 不和 *bù hé*: A functional disturbance of any bowel or viscus, qi, blood, etc., e.g., DISHARMONY OF STOMACH QI; or a functional imbalance between bowels and viscera, or qi and blood, etc., e.g., CONSTRUCTION-DEFENSE DISHARMONY, LIVER-SPLEEN DISHARMONY.

disharmony of liver qi 肝气不和 *gān qì bù hé*: Deficiency or excessiveness of the liver's free coursing action. Signs include rashness, impatience, and irascibility, distending pain in the chest and ribside, in severe cases with pain reaching into the lesser abdomen. In women, there may be distention and pain of the breasts, and menstrual irregularities. When the spleen and stomach are affected, there may be digestive tract signs. Compare CONSTRAINED LIVER QI. [25: 164] [97: 286] [50: 787]

disharmony of qi and blood 气血失调 *qì xuè shī tiáo*: Any failure in the mutually complementary relationship of qi and blood. Qi is the commander of the blood, whereas blood is the mother of qi. Disease of qi affects the blood, whereas blood disease affects qi. Qi stagnation can cause blood

stasis. Qi counterflow can cause blood counterflow manifesting in blood ejection, expectoration of blood, or spontaneous external bleeding. Qi vacuity can cause blood management failure characterized by bloody stool, bloody urine, menstrual irregularities, uterine blood, or subcutaneous bleeding. In clinical practice, enduring pain, REVERSEFLOW, menstrual irregularities and chronic hemorrhage are usually associated with disharmony of qi and blood. [26: 537] [27: 142]

disharmony of stomach qi 胃气不和 *wèi qì bù hé*: Synonyms: *disharmony of the stomach*; *stomach disharmony*. Mild upset of the stomach characterized by aversion to food, upflow nausea, sleeplessness, and abnormal stool. Severe nausea and vomiting is a pronounced form of disharmony of stomach qi called STOMACH QI ASCENDING COUNTERFLOW. [26: 438] [27: 132]

disharmony of the stomach 胃不和 *wèi bù hé*: DISHARMONY OF STOMACH QI.

disinhibit 利 *lì*: To promote fluency, movement, or activity, i.e., to treat inhibited flow of qi, blood or fluids, or inhibited physical movement. ◇ Chin The Chinese ideogram was originally a pictorial representation. The left-hand portion, 禾 *hé* represents a grain stock heavy with seed, and right side is a variant form of 刀 *dāo*, a knife. A sharp knife cutting down ripe grain stock, speedily bringing the benefit of the harvest. In its modern usage, the character retains the meaning of sharpness, favorability, profit, and benefit. In Chinese medicine, the meaning is to promote favorable movement, which we render as disinhibit. **Eng** from L. *dis*, not *inhibire*, inhibit.

disinhibiting dampness 利湿 *lì shī*: A method of treatment used to cause dampness evil to pass out in the urine by the use of dampness-percolating water-disinhibiting medicinals. See the entries listed below. [26: 327] [27: 261]

Disinhibiting Dampness

DISINHIBITING WATER AND PERCOLATING DAMPNESS (*lì shuǐ shèn shī*)

DISINHIBITING DAMPNESS BY BLAND PERCOLATION (*dàn shèn lì shī*)

FORTIFYING THE SPLEEN AND DISINHIBIT WATER (*jiàn pí lì shuǐ*)

WARMING YANG AND DISINHIBITING DAMPNESS (*wēn yáng lì shī*)

ENRICHING YIN AND DISINHIBITING DAMPNESS (*zī yīn lì shī*)

CLEARING SUMMERHEAT AND DISINHIBITING DAMPNESS (*qīng shǔ lì shī*)

CLEARING HEAT AND DISINHIBITING DAMPNESS (*qīng rè lì shī*)

WARMING THE KIDNEY AND DISINHIBITING WATER (*wēn yáng lì shuǐ*)

disinhibiting dampness by bland percolation
淡渗利湿 *dàn shèn lì shī*: A method of treatment that makes use of sweet and bland dampness-percolating medicines to facilitate the eliminating of damp evil through the urine. Disinhibiting dampness by bland percolation is used to treat patterns characterized by clear thin diarrhea, inhibited urination, white tongue fur, and a soggy pulse. Bland percolating dampness-disinhibiting medicinals include poria (*fú líng*), polyporus (*zhū líng*), alisma (*zé xiè*), and coix (*yì yǐ rén*). [50: 1453] [26: 565] [27: 261]

disinhibiting qi 利气 *lì qì*: MOVING QI.

disinhibiting water 利水 *lì shuǐ*: See DISINHIBITING WATER AND PERCOLATING DAMPNESS. [6: 265]

disinhibiting water and percolating dampness 利水渗湿 *lì shuǐ shèn shī*: To eliminate dampness by freeing urination in the treatment of of strangury-turbidity, water swelling, and diarrhea due to water-damp congesting in the lower burner. Disinhibiting water and percolating dampness makes use of sweet and bland water-disinhibiting medicinals such as poria (*fú líng*), alisma (*zé xiè*), and polyporus (*zhū líng*). Representative formulas include Poria (Hoelen) Five Powder (*wǔ líng sǎn*) and Five-Peel Powder (*wǔ pí sǎn*). [121: 510] [16: 503]

Water-Disinhibiting Dampness-Percolating Medicinals

茯苓 (*fú líng*) poria (Poria)
茯苓皮 (*fú líng pí*) poria skin (Poriae Cortex)
猪苓 (*zhū líng*) polyporus (Polyporus)
泽泻 (*zé xiè*) alisma (Alismatis Rhizoma)
薏苡仁 (*yì yǐ rén*) coix (Coicis Semen)
薏苡根 (*yì yǐ gēn*) coix root (Coicis Radix)
车前 (*chē qián*) plantago (Plantaginis Herba)
车前子 (*chē qián zǐ*) plantago seed (Plantaginis Semen)
滑石 (*huá shí*) talcum (Talcum)
木通 (*mù tōng*) mutong (Mutong Caulis)
通草 (*tōng cǎo*) rice-paper plant pith (Tetrapanacis Medulla)
灯心草 (*dēng xīn cǎo*) juncus (Junci Medulla)
小金钱草 (*xiǎo jīn qián cǎo*) dichondra (Dichondrae Herba)
金钱草 (*jīn qián cǎo*) moneywort (Jinqiancao Herba)
海金沙 (*hǎi jīn shā*) lygodium spore (Lygodii Spora)
石韦 (*shí wéi*) pyrrosia (Pyrrosiae Folium)
地肤子 (*dì fū zǐ*) kochia (Kochiae Fructus)
萹蓄 (*biǎn xù*) knotgrass (Polygoni Avicularis Herba)

瞿麦 (*qú mài*) dianthus (Dianthi Herba)
萆薢 (*bì xiè*) fish poison yam (Dioscoreae Hypoglaucae Rhizoma)
茵陈蒿 (*yīn chén hāo*) capillaris (Artemisiae Capillaris Herba)
壶芦 (*hú lú*) bottle gourd (Lagenariae Depressae Fructus)
冬瓜子 (*dōng guā zǐ*) wax gourd seed (Benincasae Semen)
冬瓜皮 (*dōng guā pí*) wax gourd rind (Benincasae Exocarpium)
赤小豆 (*chì xiǎo dòu*) rice bean (Phaseoli Calcarati Semen)
泽漆 (*zé qī*) sun spurge (Euphorbiae Helioscopiae Herba)
玉米须 (*yù mǐ xū*) corn silk (Mays Stylus)
冬葵子 (*dōng kuí zǐ*) mallow seed (Malvae Verticillatae Semen)
蝼蛄 (*lóu gū*) mole cricket (Gryllotalpa)
地耳草 (*dì ěr cǎo*) lesser hypericum (Hyperici Japonici Herba)
虎杖 (*hǔ zhàng*) bushy knotweed (Polygoni Cuspidati Rhizoma)

dislocation 脱臼 *tuō jiù*, 脱骱 *tuō jiè*: The displacement of bones of a joint; usually attributed to falls, twisting, pressure or other forms of violence, and, less commonly, the result of wind-cold-damp invasion or liver-kidney debilitation. [27: 488] [27: 488] [97: 521]

dispel 祛 *qū*: Eliminate (evils). See DRAIN.

dispelling cold and transforming phlegm 祛寒化痰 *qū hán huà tán*: A method of treatment used to address cold phlegm arising from spleen-stomach yang vacuity and internal collection of cold rheum characterized by ejection of thin clear phlegm, aversion to cold, lack of warmth in the extremities, and a slimy tongue fur. [MED] Cold-dispelling phlegm-transforming medicinals include cinnamon twig (*guì zhī*), poria (*fú líng*), dried ginger (*gān jiāng*), pinellia (*bàn xià*), and red tangerine peel (*jú hóng*). Formulas include Center-Rectifying Phlegm-Transforming Pill (*lǐ zhōng huà tán wán*) and Cold Wheezing Pill (*lěng xiāo wán*). [ACU] Base treatment mainly on CV, ST, and LI. Select CV-12 (*zhōng wǎn*, Center Stomach Duct), ST-36 (*zú sān lǐ*, Leg Three Li), ST-40 (*fēng lóng*, Bountiful Bulge), CV-6 (*qì hǎi*, Sea of Qi), LI-4 (*hé gǔ*, Union Valley), and ST-25 (*tiān shū*, Celestial Pivot), needling with even supplementation and drainage and large amounts of moxa. **Comparison**: The emphasis of this method is on addressing cold phlegm arising from spleen-stomach yang vacuity; *warming the lung and transforming rheum* is a similar method but its emphasis on addressing cold rheum lying latent in the lung. *Dissipating cold and transforming phlegm* would appear to be synonymous with dispelling cold and transforming phlegm, but is in fact a distinct method used to eliminate external cold with phlegm (see DIFFUSING THE LUNG AND TRANSFORMING PHLEGM). [27: 271] [97: 425]

dispelling dampness 祛湿 *qū shī*: *Synonym: transforming dampness.* Any method of treatment used to eliminate dampness. It includes: TRANSFORMING DAMPNESS (eliminating upper burner dampness), DRYING DAMPNESS (eliminating center burner dampness), and DISINHIBITING DAMPNESS (eliminating lower burner dampness). Dispelling dampness is often combined with treatment to fortify the spleen since the spleen governs movement and transformation of water-damp. NB: The term *transform dampness* is used in the general sense equivalent to *dispel dampness* and in the specific sense of removing dampness from the upper burner. [27: 260] [97: 425]

dispelling evil 祛邪 *qū xié*: Ay method of treatment used to eliminate, e.g., CLEARING HEAT; TRANSFORMING PHLEGM.

dispelling evil and supporting right 祛邪扶正 *qū xié fú zhèng*: To treat evil repletion and minor vacuity of the right mainly by dispelling evil and secondarily by supporting right. Compare SUPPORTING RIGHT AND DISPELLING EVIL. [50: 1180]

dispelling phlegm 祛痰 *qū tán*: *Synonym: transforming phlegm.* Any method of treatment used to eliminate phlegm. The term TRANSFORMING PHLEGM is the most common. The terms *dispersing phlegm, flushing phlegm, expelling phlegm, sweeping phlegm,* and *attacking phlegm* describe more forceful actions. The term *transforming phlegm,* like *dispelling phlegm,* is generic, but is also used in the specific sense of the dispelling phlegm in the upper burner. See TRANSFORMING PHLEGM. The main forms of dispelling phlegm are listed below. [50: 1180] [26: 405] [27: 271] [97: 425] [25: 240]

Dispelling Phlegm

DRYING DAMPNESS AND TRANSFORMING PHLEGM (*zào shī huà tán*)

DIFFUSING THE LUNG AND TRANSFORMING PHLEGM (*xuān fèi huà tán*)

CLEARING HEAT AND TRANSFORMING PHLEGM (*qīng rè huà tán*)

WARMING TRANSFORMING COLD RHEUM (PHLEGM) (*wēn fèi huà yǐn (tán)*)

MOISTENING THE LUNG AND TRANSFORMING PHLEGM (*rùn fèi huà tán*)

CONTROLLING WIND AND TRANSFORMING PHLEGM (*zhì fēng huà tán*)

NORMALIZING QI AND TRANSFORMING PHLEGM (*shùn qì huà tán*)

---

dispelling stasis and dispersing swelling 祛瘀消肿 *qū yū xiāo zhǒng*: A method of treatment used to address blood stasis arising from external injury. The method of dispelling stasis and dispersing swelling can be used for painful swollen bruises due to knocks and falls, or for internal injury with qi and blood stagnation and pain. ▢MED A representative stasis-dispelling swelling-dispersing formula is Seven Pinches Powder (*qī lí sǎn*). ▢ACU Select local points and points at the ends of the channels and needle with drainage, or prick to bleed with a three-edged needle. Selection of points according to location: Shoulder: LI-15 (*jiān yú*, Shoulder Bone) and TB-14 (*jiān liáo*, Shoulder Bone-Hole), and SI-9 (*jiān zhēn*, True Shoulder). Elbow: LI-11 (*qū chí*, Pool at the Bend), SI-8 (*xiǎo hǎi*, Small Sea), and TB-10 (*tiān jǐng*, Celestial Well). Wrist: TB-4 (*yáng chí*, Yang Pool), LI-5 (*yáng xī*, Yang Ravine), and SI-5 (*yáng gǔ*, Yang Valley). Lumbus: BL-23 (*shèn shū*, Kidney Transport), GV-3 (*yāo yáng guān*, Lumbar Yang Pass), and BL-40 (*wěi zhōng*, Bend Center). Thigh and buttock: GB-30 (*huán tiào*, Jumping Round), BL-54 (*zhì biān*, Sequential Limit), and BL-36 (*chéng fú*, Support). Knee: Eye of the Knee (*xī yǎn*) ST-34 (*liáng qiū*, Beam Hill), and GB-33 (*xī yáng guān*, Knee Yang Joint). Ankle: ST-41 (*jiě xī*, Ravine Divide), BL-60 (*kūn lún*, Kunlun Mountains), and GB-40 (*qiū xū*, Hill Ruins). See DISPELLING STASIS AND QUICKENING THE BLOOD; SPRAIN. [27: 274]

dispelling stasis and quickening the blood 祛瘀活血 *qū yū huó xuè*: *Synonyms: quickening the blood and transforming stasis; quickening the blood and dispelling stasis; transforming stasis and moving the blood; eliminating stasis and engendering the new; quickening the blood and engendering the new.* A method of treatment used to restore normal movement of the blood by eliminating blood stasis. On the basis of the power of action, distinction can be made between quickening the blood, transforming stasis, and breaking blood. Quickening the blood is the mildest action, and is performed with medicinals such as salvia (*dān shēn*), red peony (*chì sháo yào*), ligusticum (*chuān xiōng*), moutan (*mǔ dān pí*), and millettia (*jī xuè téng*). Transforming stasis is a stronger action performed with medicinals such as peach kernel (*táo rén*), carthamus (*hóng huā*), and myrrh (*mò yào*). Among stasis-transforming medicinals, lycopus (*zé lán*), leonurus (*yì mǔ cǎo*), typha pollen (*pú huáng*), and flying squirrel's droppings (*wǔ líng zhī*) are especially effective for women's problems; corydalis (*yán hú suǒ*), frankincense (*rǔ xiāng*), myrrh (*mò yào*), and notoginseng (*sān qī*) are effective in relieving pain; and pangolin scales (*chuān shān jiǎ*), typha pollen (*pú huáng*), flying squirrel's droppings (*wǔ líng zhī*), anomalous artemisia (*liú jì nú*), and erythrina (*hǎi tóng pí*) are effective for dispersing swelling in the treatment of knocks and falls. Breaking blood is the most drastic of all stasis dispelling medicinals used to treat enduring menstrual block and abdominal masses, and is performed with medicinals such as leech (*shuǐ zhì*), tabanus (*méng chóng*), wingless cockroach (*zhè chóng*), sparganium (*sān léng*), zedoary (*é zhú*), and dung beetle (*qiāng láng*). Agents in this latter category are contraindicated in bleeding and pregnancy. Blood-quickening stasis-transforming medicinals belonging to the category of *chong* products (worms, insects, reptiles) are often used for ENDURING PAIN ENTERING THE NETWORK VESSELS. Among formulas, Origin-Restorative Blood-Quickening Decoction (*fù yuán huó xuè tāng*) is effective for knocks and falls, whereas Peach Kernel and Carthamus Four Agents Decoction (*táo hóng sì wù tāng*) is used to quicken the blood and regulate menstruation. Sudden Smile Powder (*shī xiào sǎn*) quickens the blood and relieves pain. Seven Pinches Powder (*qī lí sǎn*) dispels stasis and disperses swelling in the treatment of external injuries. Turtle Shell Decocted Pill (*biē jiǎ jiān wán*) is effective in dispersing masses. Generalized Pain Stasis-Expelling Decoction (*shēn tòng zhú yū tāng*) and Fixed Impediment Empirical Formula (*zhuó bì yàn fāng*) treat impediment (*bì*) patterns characterized by "enduring pain entering the network vessels." Specific forms of dispelling stasis and quickening the blood include DISPELLING STASIS AND DISPERSING SWELLING; WARMING AND TRANSFORMING STATIC BLOOD; DISPERSING CONCRETIONS, CONGLOMERATIONS, ACCUMULATIONS, AND GATHERINGS; and DISPELLING STASIS AND STANCHING BLEEDING. ACU Select points such as BL-17 (*gé shū*, Diaphragm Transport), SP-10 (*xuè hǎi*, Sea of Blood), LI-4 (*hé gǔ*, Union Valley), LR-3 (*tài chōng*, Supreme Surge), SP-6 (*sān yīn jiāo*, Three Yin Intersection), and Glomus Root (*pǐ gēn*) as main points. Selection of points according to affected area: On the upper limbs, add LI-4 (*hé gǔ*, Union Valley) joined with SI-3 (*hòu xī*, Back Ravine), TB-5 (*wài guān*, Outer Pass) joined to PC-6 (*nèi guān*, Inner Pass), and LI-11 (*qū chí*, Pool at the Bend) joined to HT-3 (*shào hǎi*, Lesser Sea). On the lower limbs, add GB-34 (*yáng líng quán*, Yang Mound Spring) joined to SP-9 (*yīn líng quán*, Yin Mound Spring), GB-39 (*xuán zhōng*, Suspended Bell) joined to SP-6 (*sān yīn jiāo*, Three Yin Intersection). Needle with even supplementation and drainage or with drainage, or bleed with a three-edged needle. [50: 1180] [6: 261] [113: 19] [46: 594]

Stasis-Dispelling Blood-Quickening Medicinals

川芎 (*chuān xiōng*) ligusticum (Ligustici Rhizoma)

乳香 (*rǔ xiāng*) frankincense (Olibanum)

没药 (*mò yào*) myrrh (Myrrha)

生没药 (*shēng mò yào*) raw myrrh (Myrrha Cruda)

延胡索 (*yán hú suǒ*) corydalis (Corydalis Tuber)

郁金 (*yù jīn*) curcuma (Curcumae Tuber)

姜黄 (*jiāng huáng*) turmeric (Curcumae Longae Rhizoma)

莪术 (*é zhú*) zedoary (Zedoariae Rhizoma)

三棱 (*sān léng*) sparganium (Sparganii Rhizoma)

丹参 (*dān shēn*) salvia (Salviae Miltiorrhizae Radix)

虎杖 (*hǔ zhàng*) bushy knotweed (Polygoni Cuspidati Rhizoma)

益母草 (*yì mǔ cǎo*) leonurus (Leonuri Herba)

茺蔚子 (*chōng wèi zǐ*) leonurus fruit (Leonuri Fructus)

鸡血藤 (*jī xuè téng*) millettia (Millettiae Radix et Caulis)

桃仁 (*táo rén*) peach kernel (Persicae Semen)

红花 (*hóng huā*) carthamus (Carthami Flos)

藏红花 (*zàng hóng huā*) saffron (Croci Stigma)

五灵脂 (*wǔ líng zhī*) flying squirrel's droppings (Trogopteri seu Pteromydis Excrementum)

牛膝 (*niú xī*) achyranthes (Achyranthis Bidentatae Radix)

土牛膝 (*tǔ niú xī*) native achyranthes (Achyranthis Radix)

穿山甲 (*chuān shān jiǎ*) pangolin scales (Manitis Squama)

䗪虫 (*zhè chóng*) wingless cockroach (Eupolyphaga seu Opisthoplatia)

水蛭 (*shuǐ zhì*) leech (Hirudo seu Whitmania)

虻虫 (*méng chóng*) tabanus (Tabanus)

降真香 (*jiàng zhēn xiāng*) dalbergia (Dalbergiae Lignum)

泽兰 (*zé lán*) lycopus (Lycopi Herba)

月季花 (*yuè jì huā*) China tea rose (Rosae Chinensis Flos et Fructus)

凌霄花 (*líng xiāo huā*) campsis flower (Campsitis Flos)

自然铜 (*zì rán tóng*) pyrite (Pyritum)

王不留行 (*wáng bù liú xíng*) vaccaria (Vaccariae Semen)

刘寄奴 (*liú jì nú*) anomalous artemisia (Artemisiae Anomalae Herba)

苏木 (*sū mù*) sappan (Sappan Lignum)

干漆 (*gān qī*) lacquer (Lacca Exsiccata)

毛冬青 (*máo dōng qīng*) hairy holly root (Ilicis Pubescentis Radix)hairy holly root

马鞭草 (*mǎ biān cǎo*) verbena (Verbenae Herba (cum Radice))

积雪草 (*jī xuě cǎo*) centella (Centellae Herb (cum Radice))

石见穿 (*shí jiàn chuān*) Chinese sage (Salviae Chinensis Herba)

夜明砂 (*yè míng shā*) bat's droppings (Vespertilionis Excrementum)

鬼箭羽 (*guǐ jiàn yǔ*) spindle tree wings (Euonymi Lignum Suberalatum)

蜣螂 (*qiāng láng*) dung beetle (Catharsius)

---

dispelling stasis and stanching bleeding 祛瘀止血 *qū yū zhǐ xuè*: A method of treatment used to eliminate blood stasis and to check bleeding in the treatment of patterns such as a) blood stasis flooding and spotting with copious purple-black clotted flow, lower abdominal pain that refuses pressure and is relieved by passing of clots, dark a gray tongue fur, and a rough pulse, or b) dribbling discharge of the LOCHIA due to blood stasis marked by abdominal pain that refuses pressure, purple-black facial complexion, and purple tongue margins. For uterine bleeding, use medicinals such as tangkuei (*dāng guī*), ligusticum (*chuān xiōng*), ovate atractylodes (*bái zhú*), typha pollen (*pú huáng*), charred crataegus (*shān zhā tàn*), peach kernel (*táo rén*), and notoginseng (*sān qī*). For dribbling discharge of the LOCHIA, use tangkuei (*dāng guī*), red peony (*chì sháo yào*), peach kernel (*táo rén*), and blast-fried ginger (*páo jiāng*). ACU Select points such as BL-17 (*gé shū*, Diaphragm Transport), SP-10 (*xuè hǎi*, Sea of Blood), CV-17 (*shān zhōng*, Chest Center) and CV-6 (*qì hǎi*, Sea of Qi). Needle with even supplementation and drainage. [27: 275] [97: 425]

dispelling wind 祛风 *qū fēng*: Any method of treatment used to eliminate wind, especially external wind. See DISPELLING WIND AND ELIMINATING DAMPNESS; EXTINGUISHING WIND; DISPELLING WIND AND RESOLVING TETANY; COURSING WIND AND DISCHARGING HEAT; DISPELLING WIND AND NOURISHING THE BLOOD; TRACKING WIND AND EXPELLING COLD. [27: 268] [97: 425]

dispelling wind and eliminating dampness 祛风除湿 *qū fēng chú shī*: Synonym: *dispelling wind and overcoming dampness*. A method of treatment used to address wind-damp lodged in the channels and network vessels, the flesh, and the joints that causes wandering pain, using medicinals such as duhuo (*dú huó*), notopterygium (*qiāng huó*), ledebouriella (*fáng fēng*), large gentian (*qín jiāo*), clematis (*wēi líng xiān*), mulberry twig (*sāng zhī*), and acanthopanax (*wǔ jiā pí*). ACU Base treatment mainly on GB, TB, LI, ST, and SP. Select GB-20 (*fēng chí*, Wind Pool), GB-31 (*fēng shì*, Wind Market), TB-5 (*wài guān*, Outer Pass), LI-4 (*hé gǔ*, Union Valley) LI-11 (*qū chí*, Pool at the Bend), ST-36 (*zú sān lǐ*, Leg Three Li), LI-10 (*shǒu sān lǐ*, Arm Three Li), GB-34 (*yáng líng quán*, Yang Mound Spring), and SP-9 (*yīn líng quán*, Yin Mound Spring), needling with drainage. [27: 268] [97: 425] [14: 83] [50: 1180] [46: 597]

Wind-Damp–Dispelling Medicinals

独活 (*dú huó*) duhuo (Angelicae Duhuo Radix)

威灵仙 (*wēi líng xiān*) clematis (Clematidis Radix)

防己 (*fáng jǐ*) fangji (Fangji Radix), includes the following 4 items

木防己 (*mù fáng jǐ*) woody fangji (Cocculi Radix)

粉防己 (*fěn fáng jǐ*) mealy fangji (Stephaniae Tetrandrae Radix)

汉中防己 (*hàn zhōng fáng jǐ*) northern fangji (Aristolochiae Heterophyllae Radix)

广防己 (*guǎng fáng jǐ*) southern fangji (Aristolochiae Fangchi Radix)

秦艽 (*qín jiāo*) large gentian (Gentianae Macrophyllae Radix)

豨莶 (*xī xiān*) siegesbeckia (Siegesbeckiae Herba)

臭梧桐 (*chòu wú tóng*) clerodendron (Clerodendri Folium)

木瓜 (*mù guā*) chaenomeles (Chaenomelis Fructus)

络石藤 (*luò shí téng*) star jasmine stem (Trachelospermi Caulis)

徐长卿 (*xú cháng qīng*) paniculate cynanchum (Cynanchi Paniculati Herba cum Radice)

桑枝 (*sāng zhī*) mulberry twig (Mori Ramulus)

桑寄生 (*sāng jì shēng*) mistletoe (Loranthi seu Visci Ramus)

五加皮 (*wǔ jiā pí*) acanthopanax (Acanthopanacis Radicis Cortex)

狗骨 (*gǒu gǔ*) dog's bone (Canis Os)

虎骨 (*hǔ gǔ*) tiger bone (Tigris Os)

豹骨 (*bào gǔ*) leopard's bone (Leopardi Os)

白花蛇 (*bái huā shé*) krait/agkistrodon (Bungarus seu Agkistrodon)

蕲蛇 (*qí shé*) agkistrodon (Agkistrodon)

海桐皮 (*hǎi tóng pí*) erythrina (Erythrinae Cortex)

乌蛇 (*wū shé*) black-striped snake (Zaocys)

蛇蜕 (*shé tuì*) snake slough (Serpentis Exuviae)

原蚕沙 (*yuán cán shā*) silkworm droppings (Bombycis Excrementum)

海风藤 (*hǎi fēng téng*) kadsura pepper stem (Piperis Kadsurae Caulis)

寻骨风 (*xún gǔ fēng*) mollissima (Aristolochiae Mollissimae Rhizoma seu Herba)

千年健 (*qiān nián jiàn*) homalomena (Homalomenae Rhizoma)

松节 (*sōng jié*) knotty pine wood (Pini Lignum Nodi)

青风藤 (*qīng fēng téng*) Orient vine (Sinomenii seu Sabiae Caulis et Rhizoma)

穿山龙 (*chuān shān lóng*) Japanese dioscorea (Dioscoreae Nipponicae Rhizoma)

雷公藤 (*léi gōng téng*) thunder god vine (Tripterygii Wilfordi Radix, Folium et Flos)

夏天无 (*xià tiān wú*) Jilong corydalis (Corydalis Decumbentis Tuber et Herba)

伸筋草 (*shēn jīn cǎo*) ground pine (Lycopodii Clavati Herba cum Radice)

伸筋藤 (*shēn jīn téng*) Chinese tinospora (Tinosporae Sinensis Caulis)

老鹳草 (*lǎo guàn cǎo*) cranesbill (Geranii Herba)

鹿衔草 (*lù xián cǎo*) pyrola (Pyrolae Herba)

dispelling wind and nourishing the blood 祛风养血 *qū fēng yǎng xuè*: A method of treatment used to address persistent wind-damp with disharmony of the blood and vessels and liver-kidney depletion characterized by cold pain of the lumbus and knee using formulas like Duhuo and Mistletoe Decoction (*dú huó jì shēng tāng*). This formula contains not only wind-damp-dispelling medicinals and liver-kidney-supplementing medicinals, but also tangkuei (*dāng guī*), white peony (*bái sháo yào*), ligusticum (*chuān xiōng*), and cooked rehmannia (*shú dì huáng*), which harmonize construction and nourish the blood, and free the vessels, thereby enabling the wind to disperse. Dispelling wind and nourishing the blood is a method of treatment that accords with the principle that "to treat wind, first treat the blood; when the blood moves, wind naturally disappears." ACU Base treatment mainly on back transport points, LR, GB, SP, and ST. Needle with supplementation at BL-17 (*gé shū*, Diaphragm Transport), LR-3 (*tài chōng*, Supreme Surge), SP-6 (*sān yīn jiāo*, Three Yin Intersection), BL-23 (*shèn shū*, Kidney Transport), and BL-18 (*gān shū*, Liver Transport), and with drainage at GB-20 (*fēng chí*, Wind Pool), TB-5 (*wài guān*, Outer Pass), LI-11 (*qū chí*, Pool at the Bend), ST-36 (*zú sān lǐ*, Leg Three Li), and SP-9 (*yīn líng quán*, Yin Mound Spring). [27: 268] [97: 425]

dispelling wind and overcoming dampness 祛风胜湿 *qū fēng shèng shī*: DISPELLING WIND AND ELIMINATING DAMPNESS. [16: 527]

dispelling wind and resolving tetany 祛风解痉 *qū fēng jiě jìng*: A method of treatment used to address tetany using wind-dispelling medicinals. Wind-dispelling tetany-resolving formulas include True Jade Powder (*yù zhēn sǎn*) or Five-Tigers-Chasing-the-Wind Powder (*wǔ hǔ zhuī fēng sǎn*) used to treat lockjaw, and Pull Aright Powder (*qiān zhèng sǎn*) used to treat facial paralysis, and Uncaria Beverage (*gōu téng yǐn*) used to treat exuberant heat engendering wind causing tetany (acute child fright wind). See RESOLVING TETANY.

dispelling wind and transforming phlegm 祛风化痰 *qū fēng huà tán*: A method of treatment used to address deviated mouth and eyes, stiff tongue and impeded speech as in wind stroke, and child fright wind, using wind-dispelling and phlegm-forming medicinals such as aconite/typhonium (*bái fù zǐ*), silkworm (*bái jiāng cán*), bamboo sugar (*tiān zhú huáng*), and bile arisaema (*dǎn xīng*), which are often combined with wind-extinguishing medicinals such as scorpion (*quán xiē*), and centipede (*wú gōng*), and, if necessary, with heat-clearing orifice-opening medicinals. A representative formula is Pull Aright Powder (*qiān zhèng sǎn*). ACU For wind stroke with wind-phlegm obstructing the network vessels, base treatment mainly on LI and ST, supported by TB, GB, and BL. Select GB-20 (*fēng chí*, Wind Pool), LI-4 (*hé gǔ*, Union Valley), ST-36 (*zú sān lǐ*, Leg Three Li), ST-40 (*fēng lóng*, Bountiful Bulge), TB-17 (*yì fēng*, Wind Screen), ST-4 (*dì cāng*, Earth Granary), ST-6 (*jiá chē*, Cheek Carriage), GB-14 (*yáng bái*, Yang White), BL-2 (*zǎn zhú*, Bamboo Gathering), ST-2 (*sì bái*, Four Whites), CV-23 (*lián quán*, Ridge Spring), and HT-5 (*tōng lǐ*, Connecting Li). In the initial stage, use transverse needling and point joining; for advanced stages, use shallow needling with supplementation. For child fright wind, see ACUTE FRIGHT WIND; CHRONIC FRIGHT WIND. [94: 107] [113: 22] [46: 597, 615] [37: 339]

disperse 消 *xiāo*: To break up, dispel. See DISPERSION; DRAIN.

dispersing concretions, conglomerations, accumulations, and gatherings 消癥瘕积聚 *xiāo zhēng jiǎ jī jù*: The method of treating concretions, conglomerations, accumulations, and gatherings, i.e., any masses in the abdomen. This method makes use of channel-freeing stasis-dispelling medicinals such as peach kernel (*táo rén*), carthamus (*hóng huā*), moutan (*mǔ dān pí*), red peony (*chì sháo yào*), and cinnamon twig (*guì zhī*). Representative formulas include Cinnamon Twig and Poria (Hoelen) Pill (*guì zhī fú líng wán*) and Turtle Shell Decocted Pill (*biē jiǎ jiān wán*). [104: 240]

dispersing food 消食 *xiāo shí*: See DISPERSING FOOD AND ABDUCTING STAGNATION.

dispersing food and abducting stagnation 消食导滞 *xiāo shí dǎo zhì*: *Synonym: dispersing food and transforming stagnation*. A method of treatment used to disperse stagnant food and enable it to be carried through the digestive tract. Dispersing food and abducting stagnation, often called *abductive dispersion*, is employed in the treatment of food stagnation causing oppression in the stomach duct and abdominal distention, poor appetite, putrid belching, swallowing of upflowing acid, and nausea and upflow, abdominal pain, constipation, or diarrhea with ungratifying defecation. Commonly used abductive dispersion medicinals include crataegus (*shān zhā*), medicated leaven (*shén qū*), barley sprout (*mài yá*), gizzard lining (*jī nèi jīn*), and rice sprout (*gǔ yá*). Radish seed (*lái fú zǐ*), unripe bitter orange (*zhǐ shí*), and areca (*bīng láng*) may be added to break qi, precipitate phlegm, and free the stool. A formula used for this purpose is Harmony-Preserving Pill (*bǎo hé wán*), which includes crataegus (*shān zhā*), medicated leaven (*shén qū*), pinellia (*bàn xià*), poria (*fú líng*), tangerine peel (*chén pí*), forsythia (*lián qiào*), and radish seed (*lái fú zǐ*). Unripe Bitter Orange Stagnation-Abducting Pill (*zhǐ shí dǎo zhì wán*) has an additional precipitant action. When the food stagnation is due to spleen-stomach vacuity, abductive dispersing medicinals can be combined with supplementing medicinals, which enhance digestive system function, thereby reducing susceptibility to food accumulation in the long term. An example of such a formula is Spleen-Fortifying Pill (*jiàn pí wán*), which contains ovate atractylodes (*bái zhú*), white poria (*bái fú líng*), codonopsis (*dǎng shēn*), licorice (*gān cǎo*), saussurea (*mù xiāng*), forsythia (*lián qiào*), coptis (*huáng lián*), medicated leaven (*shén qū*), tangerine peel (*chén pí*), barley sprout (*mài yá*), amomum (*shā rén*), crataegus (*shān zhā*), nutmeg (*ròu dòu kòu*), and dioscorea (*shān yào*). ACU Base treatment on ST, SP, and CV. Select ST-25 (*tiān shū*, Celestial Pivot), ST-36 (*zú sān lǐ*, Leg Three Li), CV-10 (*xià wǎn*, Lower Stomach Duct), CV-6 (*qì hǎi*, Sea of Qi), SP-4 (*gōng sūn*, Yellow Emperor), Li Inner Court (*lǐ nèi tíng*), and CV-21 (*xuán jī*, Jade Swivel); needle with drainage. [113: 18] [27: 280] [97: 483] [46: 662]

Food-Dispersing Medicinals

山楂 (*shān zhā*) crataegus (Crataegi Fructus)

神麯 (*shén qū*) medicated leaven (Massa Medicata Fermentata)

建神麯 (*jiàn shén qū*) Fujian leaven (Massa Medicata Fermentata Fujianensis)

麦芽 (*mài yá*) barley sprout (Hordei Fructus Germinatus)

谷芽 (*gǔ yá*) rice sprout (Oryzae Fructus Germinatus)

莱菔子 (*lái fú zǐ*) radish seed (Raphani Semen)

鸡内金 (*jī nèi jīn*) gizzard lining (Galli Gigerii Endothelium)

---

dispersing food and transforming phlegm 消食化痰 *xiāo shí huà tán*: A method of treatment used to eliminate phlegm and food stagnation. The method of dispersing food and transforming phlegm is used to treat replete qi and exuberant phlegm causing cough and qi counterflow, oppression in the chest and copious phlegm, indigestion, distention and oppression in the stomach duct and abdomen, a slimy tongue, and a slippery pulse, as is often observed in elderly patients. MED Two commonly used food-dispersing phlegm-transforming formulas Qi-Normalizing Food-Dispersing Phlegm-Transforming Pill (*shùn qì xiāo shí huà tán wán*) and Three-Seed Filial Devotion Decoction (*sān zǐ yǎng qīn tāng*). ACU Base treatment mainly on ST and CV. Select ST-25 (*tiān shū*, Celestial Pivot), ST-36 (*zú sān lǐ*, Leg Three Li), Li Inner Court (*lǐ nèi tíng*), CV-21 (*xuán jī*, Jade Swivel), CV-12 (*zhōng wǎn*, Center Stomach Duct), ST-40 (*fēng lóng*, Bountiful Bulge), PC-6 (*nèi guān*, Inner Pass), LI-4 (*hé gǔ*, Union Valley), and CV-17 (*shān zhōng*, Chest Center), needle with drainage. [113: 18] [6: 481] [27: 280] [97: 482] [46: 597, 662]

dispersing food and transforming stagnation 消食化滞 *xiāo shí huà zhì*: DISPERSING FOOD AND ABDUCTING STAGNATION.

dispersing gan 消疳 *xiāo gān*: A method of treatment used to eliminate GAN ACCUMULATION.

dispersing glomus and transforming accumulations 消痞化积 *xiāo pǐ huà jī*: A method of treatment used to eliminate glomus and accumulations (abdominal masses) by moving qi and transforming stasis, dispersing stagnation, and softening hardness. Dispersing glomus and transforming accumulations may be used, for example, to treat a hard lump of fixed location under the rib-side (hepatosplenomegaly) or GAN ACCUMULATION. [27: 280] [97: 483]

dispersing goiter, scrofula, and phlegm nodes 消瘿瘰痰核 *xiāo yǐng luǒ tán hé*: Any method used to treat goiter, scrofula, and phlegm nodes. Dispersing goiter, scrofula, and phlegm nodes makes use of phlegm-transforming hardness-softening, bind-dispersing medicinals such as sargassum (*hǎi zǎo*), kelp (*kūn bù*), and prunella (*xià kū cǎo*). Representative formulas include Scrofula Internal Dispersion Pill (*nèi xiāo luǒ lì wán*) and Sargassum Jade Flask Decoction (*hǎi zǎo yù hú tāng*). [104: 237]

dispersing phlegm 消痰 *xiāo tán*: A method of treatment used to attack stagnant turbid phlegm. The method of dispersing phlegm can damage original qi, and should be used with care. See DISPERSING PHLEGM AND CALMING PANTING; DISPERSING PHLEGM AND SOFTENING HARDNESS. [50: 1304] [26: 481] [27: 271] [97: 482] [25: 266]

dispersing phlegm and calming panting 消痰平喘 *xiāo tán píng chuǎn*: A method of treatment used to address copious phlegm with qi counterflow, oppression in the chest, reduced food intake, sticky slimy tongue fur, and a slippery pulse due to phlegm-rheum deep-lying in the lung. An example of a phlegm-dispersing panting-calming formula is Three-Seed Filial Devotion Decoction (*sān zǐ yǎng qīn tāng*). ACU Base treatment mainly on LU and ST. Select BL-13 (*fèi shū*, Lung Transport), LU-1 (*zhōng fǔ*, Central Treasury), Panting Stabilizer (*dìng chuǎn*), LU-7 (*liè quē*, Broken Sequence), LU-5 (*chǐ zé*, Cubit Marsh), CV-17 (*shān zhōng*, Chest Center), ST-40 (*fēng lóng*, Bountiful Bulge), and CV-12 (*zhōng wǎn*, Center Stomach Duct); needle with drainage. [26: 481] [46: 654] [113: 63] [37: 278]

dispersing phlegm and softening hardness 消痰软坚 *xiāo tán ruǎn jiān*: A method of treatment used to address binding turbid phlegm or scrofula. An example of a phlegm-dispersing hardness-softening formula is Scrofula-Dispersing Pill (*xiāo luǒ wán*). ACU Apply moxa cones at Hundred Taxations (*bǎi láo*) and moxa pole at Tip of the Elbow (*zhǒu jiān*). Ouch points (*ā shì xué*) can be needled and moxaed. For scrofula on the nape, add TB-17 (*yì fēng*, Wind Screen), GB-41 (*zú lín qì*, Foot Overlooking Tears), and TB-10 (*tiān jǐng*, Celestial Well)ⓜ, needling with supplementation. For scrofula on the neck, add LI-14 (*bì nào*, Upper Arm), ST-5 (*dà yíng*, Great Reception), and LI-10 (*shǒu sān lǐ*, Arm Three Li)ⓜ, needling with supplementation. For scrofula below the armpits, add GB-21 (*jiān jǐng*, Shoulder Well), HT-3 (*shào hǎi*, Lesser Sea), and GB-38 (*yáng fǔ*, Yang Assistance). [26: 481] [113: 383] [27: 271] [97: 483]

²**dispersion** 消法 *xiāo fǎ*: One of the EIGHT METHODS. The gradual breaking up of accumulations of substances in the body, using medicinals that abduct and disperse, soften hardness, and transform accumulations. *Elementary Questions* (*sù wèn*) states, "Hardness is whittled away," and "Binds are dispersed." In practice, dispersion possesses a broad field of application. It can be used for concretions and conglomerations, glomus lumps, food accumulations, water amassment, calculi (stones), scrofula, and phlegm nodes. See DISPERSING FOOD; DISPERSING PHLEGM AND SOFTENING HARDNESS; DISPERSING GLOMUS AND TRANSFORMING ACCUMULATIONS. [26: 480] [27: 272] [97: 483]

²**dispersion** 消 *xiāo*: Abbreviation for DISPERSION-THIRST.

dispersion-thirst 消渴 *xiāo kě*: DISPERSION-THIRST.

dispersion-thirst 消渴 *xiāo kě*: Synonym: *wasting-thirst* (*obs*). **1.** Any disease characterized by thirst, increased fluid intake, and copious urine, and categorized as upper burner, center burner, and lower burner dispersion, depending on the pathomechanism. WMC diabetes mellitus,

diabetes insipidus, and hypoadrenocorticism. For treatment see UPPER DISPERSION; CENTER DISPERSION; LOWER DISPERSION. NB: Dispersion-thirst is often equated with diabetes mellitus, although in actual fact, its scope is larger. *Essential Secrets from Outside the Metropolis* (*wài tái mì yào*) (Tang Dynasty, A.D. 752) describes dispersion-thirst as follows, "Dispersion-thirst... is caused by kidney vacuity, and, in episodes, is characterized by extremely sweet urine." It also says, "When the lumbus and kidney are both affected by vacuity cold, upward steaming is impaired, and grain qi all descends to form urine in such a way as its sweet flavor does not change." This nosology, with its particular mention of sweet urine (= glycosuria), fits the description of diabetes mellitus spoken of in Western medicine. [26: 481] [50: 1304] [27: 423] [80: 564] [97: 482]

disquieted heart spirit 心神不安 *xīn shén bù ān*: Spirit disturbed as a result of the heart's failure to store it. The spirit is stored by the heart, and is often referred to as the heart spirit. Disquieted heart spirit arises in heart disease when the heart fails to store the spirit, and manifests as heart palpitations, fearful throbbing, susceptibility to fright, heart vexation, and insomnia. See DISQUIETING OF HEART QI.

disquieting of heart qi 心气不宁 *xīn qì bù níng*: A term loosely denoting disquieted heart spirit, heart palpitations or fearful throbbing, susceptibility to fright, heart vexation, and insomnia. Disquieting of heart qi is attributed to taxation of the spirit, insufficiency of heart blood, damage to heart qi by fear and fright, and is usually accompanied by fatigue, tender-soft tongue, a vacuous or interrupted (skipping, bound, or intermittent) pulse. It may also occur in patterns of phlegm-damp, blood stasis, or water qi intimidating the heart. Compare HEART VACUITY AND GALLBLADDER TIMIDITY. [26: 92] [27: 147]

dissipate 散 *sàn*: **1.** To spread (of qi). **2.** To break up (evil) and eliminate. See DRAIN.

dissipated pulse 散脉 *sàn mài*: Synonym: *scattered pulse*. A large floating pulse without root. A dissipated pulse is large at the superficial level, but ceases to be felt as soon as the slightest pressure is applied. It indicates the dissipation of qi and blood and the impending expiration of the essential qi of the bowels and viscera. [27: 195] [97: 495]

dissipating cold and transforming phlegm 散寒化痰 *sàn hán huà tán*: DIFFUSING THE LUNG AND TRANSFORMING PHLEGM.

distal bleeding 远血 *yuǎn xuè*: Internal bleeding from a point far from the anus, i.e., in the stomach or small intestine, characterized by the passage of stool followed by blood and by dark blackish stool. Distal bleeding is attributable to

a) spleen-stomach vacuity cold, b) liver depression transforming into fire causing frenetic movement of the blood, c) accumulated heat toxin, or d) spleen vacuity and lung dryness stemming from effulgent yin vacuity fire. MED Spleen-stomach vacuity cold is treated by warming the center and fortifying the spleen, using Yellow Earth Decoction (*huáng tǔ tāng*). Liver depression transforming into fire is treated by clearing the liver and resolving depression with variations of Moutan and Gardenia Free Wanderer Powder (*dān zhī xiāo yáo sǎn*). Accumulated heat toxin, often referred to as VISCERAL TOXIN, is treated by clearing heat and resolving toxin with formulas such as Pig's Intestines and Coptis Pill (*zàng lián wán*). Spleen vacuity and lung dryness is treated by nourishing yin and clearing the stomach, using Ginseng Lung-Clearing Decoction (*rén shēn qīng fèi tāng*). For severe bloody stool and reversal cold of extremities, and a faint weak vacuous floating pulse, the method of treatment is to greatly supplement qi and blood and fortify the spleen and boost the kidney, using formulas such as Ginseng Construction-Nourishing Decoction (*rén shēn yǎng róng tāng*) or Redness-Severing Pill (*duàn hóng wán*). See VISCERAL TOXIN[2]; BLOODY STOOL. Compare PROXIMAL BLEEDING. [26: 835] [27: 422] [97: 261]

distant needling 远道刺 *yuǎn dào cì*: From *The Magic Pivot* (*líng shū, guān zhēn piān*) One of the NINE NEEDLING METHODS. Treating disease of the upper body by needling points on yang channels of the lower body. [27: 334] [97: 261]

distending pain 胀痛 *zhàng tòng*: Pain associated with subjective fullness or objective distention; attributable to qi stagnation. See PAIN. [29: 190]

distention 胀 *zhàng*: **1.** *Synonym: distention disease.* Enlargement of the abdomen. See ABDOMINAL DISTENTION; DRUM DISTENTION. **2.** A subjective feeling of inflation, bloating, or pressure, e.g., RIB-SIDE PAIN AND DISTENTION, ABDOMINAL DISTENTION, and DISTENTION IN THE HEAD. [26: 745] [27: 256]

distention and fullness in the heart [region] and abdomen in pregnancy 妊娠心腹胀满 *rèn shēn xīn fù zhàng mǎn*: Fullness and distention in the upper abdomen during pregnancy. It is observed in women ordinarily suffering from vacuity cold, who contract cold or suffer internal damage by dietary irregularities during pregnancy. The resulting congestion of stomach qi allows turbid evil to cause internal obstruction and disturb upbearing and downbearing. **Cold contraction** is associated with pronounced distention after eating, which likes pressure and heat. MED Warm the center and dissipate cold. Use Saussurea and Amomum Six Gentlemen Decoction (*xiāng shā liù jūn zǐ tāng*). **Food damage** is attended by pain and

distention after eating, putrid belching, and swallowing of upflowing acid. MED Disperse food and transform stagnation. Use Harmony-Preserving Pill (*bǎo hé wán*). [26: 340]

distention disease 胀病 *zhàng bìng*: See DISTENTION.

distention in the head 头胀 *tóu zhàng*: A feeling of pressure and discomfort in the head. Distention in the head is usually caused by external contraction of dampness evil, or nonelimination of summerheat-warmth evil. It is variously treated by resolving the exterior, clearing heat, repelling foulness, and transforming dampness. [26: 910] [97: 165]

distention qi 气胀 *zhàng qì*: Flatulence in the abdomen.

distillate 露剂 *lù jì*, 露 *lù*: *Synonym: medicinal dew; dew.* The condensed vapor obtained when medicinals are boiled in water. Lonicera (*jīn yín huā*), agastache/patchouli (*huò xiāng*), and mint (*bò hé*) can all be made into distillates. Distillates are bland in flavor, and are taken as a beverage in the summer. They rapidly lose their effectiveness and so are best used as soon as possible. [27: 660]

distillation 蒸露 *zhēng lù*: The process of making a DISTILLATE. See PROCESSING OF MEDICINALS.

distress 迫 *pò*: To cause acute disturbance. For example, in the term "heat distressing the large intestine," where damp-heat damages the stomach and large intestine, affecting conveyance of waste, *distress* describes how heat creates abdominal pain, severe diarrhea with yellow malodorous stool, and a burning sensation in the anus.

distress below the heart 心下急 *xīn xià jí*: A feeling of distress associated with slight pain and fullness in the stomach duct. Distress below the heart is caused by evil heat binding in the stomach and occurs after severe vomiting. It may also be associated with heart vexation and constipation. WMC observed in acute gastritis and intestinal flu. [27: 377] [97: 118]

diverging network vessel 别络 *bié luò*: The larger network vessels that branch off from the main channels. The twelve channels, the governing (*dū*) vessel and controlling (*rèn*) vessel each have one diverging network vessel. In addition, there is the great network vessel of the spleen, making a total of fifteen. These are called the *fifteen diverging network vessels* or the *fifteen network vessels*. *The Classic of Difficult Issues* (*nàn jīng, 23*) states, "The fifteen diverging network vessels all return to their origins, as in a ring without end, pouring from one to next; they face the inch opening [wrist pulse] and man's prognosis (*rén yíng*), where the hundred illnesses can be determined and [a person's] death or survival can be judged." See NETWORK VESSEL. [97: 280] [26: 318]

divided flesh 分肉 *fēn ròu*: **1.** Flesh, especially as divisible into red and white parts. Formerly, the outer layer of flesh (subcutaneous fat) was called "white flesh" and the internal layer (muscle) was called "red flesh," and therefore the flesh was divided into red and white parts. **2.** A distinct separation between two masses of flesh (muscles). [50: 295] [26: 171]

divide needling 分刺 *fēn cì*: One of the nine needling methods; needling into a crevice, or parting, in the flesh (i.e., a between two muscles). *The Magic Pivot* (*líng shū, guān zhēn*) states, "Divide needling is needling between divided flesh." [26: 171] [50: 295] [27: 334]

dizziness 眩晕 *xuàn yūn*: Visual distortion with a whirling sensation in the head that, in severe cases, can upset the sense of balance. In some literature, flowery vision causing dizziness is known as "dizzy vision," whereas dizziness giving rise to flowery vision is called "dizzy head." Dizziness can be caused by the six excesses or by internal damage to qi, blood, bowels and viscera, the most common being wind-fire, phlegm-damp, and vacuity of right. See entries listed below. [26: 528] [27: 390] [97: 466]

Dizziness

External contractions

WIND DIZZINESS (*fēng xuàn*)
WIND-HEAT DIZZINESS (*fēng rè xuàn yūn*)
WIND-COLD DIZZINESS (*fēng hán xuàn yūn*)
DRYNESS-FIRE DIZZINESS (*zào huǒ xuàn yūn*)
SUMMERHEAT-DAMP DIZZINESS (*shǔ zhī xuàn yūn*)
SUMMERHEAT STROKE DIZZINESS (*zhòng shǔ xuàn yūn*)

Internal damage

QI VACUITY DIZZINESS (*qì xū xuàn yūn*)
YANG VACUITY DIZZINESS (*yáng xū xuàn yūn*)
BLOOD VACUITY DIZZINESS (*xuè xū xuàn yūn*)
BLOOD LOSS DIZZINESS (*shī xuè xuàn yūn*)
KIDNEY VACUITY DIZZINESS (*shèn xū xuàn yūn*)
QI DEPRESSION DIZZINESS (*qì yù xuàn yūn*)
LIVER YANG DIZZINESS (*gān yáng xuàn yūn*)
LIVER FIRE DIZZINESS (*gān huǒ xuàn yūn*)
DAMP PHLEGM DIZZINESS (*shī tán xuàn yūn*)
PHLEGM-FIRE DIZZINESS (*tán huǒ xuàn yūn*)
COLLECTING RHEUM DIZZINESS (*tíng yǐn xuàn yūn*)
WIND-PHLEGM DIZZINESS (*fēng tán xuàn yūn*)
DIZZINESS IN PREGNANCY (*rèn shēn xuàn yūn*)

---

dizziness in pregnancy 妊娠眩晕 *rèn shēn xuàn yūn*: DIZZINESS during pregnancy. It is observed in insufficiency of the liver and kidney when the gathering of blood to nourish the fetus in pregnancy exacerbates the yin vacuity and causes yang to become hyperactive and harass the clear orifices. Dizziness is accompanied by headache, tinnitus, flowery vision, and vexation and agitation. ⬚MED Nourish yin and clear heat; calm the liver and subdue yang. Use formulas such as All-the-Way-Through Brew (*yī guàn jiān*) and Lycium Berry, Chrysanthemum, and Rehmannia Pill (*qǐ jú dì huáng wán*). [26: 341]

dizzy head 头晕 *tóu yūn*, 晕 *yūn*: See DIZZINESS.

dizzy vision 目眩 *mù xuàn*, 眩 *xuàn*: : See DIZZINESS. [27: 391]

doctrine of periods and qi 运气学说 *yùn qì xué shuō*: The doctrine of five periods and six qi by which incidence of sickness is related to climate. The five periods are the five phases, i.e., wood, fire, earth, metal and water. The six qi are wind, heat, dampness, fire, dryness, and cold. The periods are calculated in terms of the ten heavenly stems, whereas the qi are calculated in terms of the twelve earthly branches. The doctrine aims, by means of the complementary opposition of yin and yang and the engendering and restraining relationship between the five phases, to calculate meteorological features and changes for each year and their effects on the human body. [26: 771]

donkey's-mouth wind 驴嘴风 *lǘ zuǐ fēng*: LIP WIND. [27: 499] [97: 324]

do not harm stomach qi 无犯胃气 *wú fàn wèi qì*: Do not damage stomach qi with the indiscriminate use of attacking and cold bitter agents. Stomach qi is the root of man. For this reason, it is said that "If grain is taken, the body thrives." If stomach qi is sufficient, original qi can be restored; if stomach qi is damaged, recovery is difficult. [27: 244]

do not use cold against cold 寒无犯寒 *hán wú fàn hán*: From *Elementary Questions* (*sù wèn, liù yuán zhèng jì lùn*). In the absence of heat signs in cold winter weather, cold medicinals should not be given indiscriminately since this could damage yang qi, giving rise to a transmuation pattern. However, if there is an interior pattern of binding heat, cold and cool offensive precipitants can be used, but in cold winter whether, they should be carefully chosen and their dosages should be kept to a minimum. [27: 243]

do not use heat against heat 热无犯热 *rè wú fàn rè*: From *Elementary Questions* (*sù wèn, liù yuán zhèng jì lùn*). In the absence of cold signs in hot weather, hot medicinals should not be given indiscriminately since this could damage liquid and promote the formation of dryness giving rise to a transmutation pattern. However, if there is an exterior cold pattern, warm acrid exterior-effusing medicinals may be used, but in hot summer weather, they should be carefully chosen and their dosages should be kept to a minimum. [27: 243]

door gate 户门 *hù mén*: One of the SEVEN GATES. The teeth. [27: 128]

dormant papules 瘾疹 *yǐn zhěn*: *Synonyms: wind dormant papules; papular wind lumps.* Wheals that come and go, so named by their ability to remain latent between eruptions. Being itchy and of unfixed location, they bear the attributes of wind; hence an alternate name *papular wind lumps.* Dormant papules can arise when wind evil invades owing to looseness of the INTERSTICES, or when toxin from insect bites gets trapped in the FLESHY EXTERIOR and flows into the channels. Another cause is accumulated heat in the stomach and intestines that can neither discharge through the bowels nor thrust out through the exterior and so becomes depressed in the skin. In some cases, they are brought on by eating fish or shrimp. Dormant papules usually start abruptly with itchy skin, which, when scratched produces, raised wheals of different sizes. They are most commonly observed on the inner face of the arm and usually disappear without trace. Hot red papules accompanied by a red tongue and floating rapid pulse are wind-heat. White wheals associated with aversion to cold, thin white tongue fur, and a tight floating pulse are wind-cold. Persistent recurrent eruptions indicate qi-blood depletion. WMC urticaria. MED Wind-heat is treated with Wind-Dispersing Powder (*xiāo fēng sǎn*); wind-cold with Schizonepeta and Ledebouriella Toxin-Vanquishing Powder (*jīng fáng bài dú sǎn*), and persistent conditions with Tangkuei Drink (*dāng guī yǐn zi*). ACU Select hand and foot yang brightness (*yáng míng*) and greater yin (*tài yīn*) as the main channels. Main points: LI-4 (*hé gǔ*, Union Valley), SP-10 (*xuè hǎi*, Sea of Blood), SP-6 (*sān yīn jiāo*, Three Yin Intersection), BL-17 (*gé shū*, Diaphragm Transport), BL-40 (*wěi zhōng*, Bend Center), and GB-31 (*fēng shì*, Wind Market). For wind-heat, add LU-5 (*chǐ zé*, Cubit Marsh), GV-14 (*dà zhuī*, Great Hammer), and TB-5 (*wài guān*, Outer Pass), needling with drainage. For wind-cold, add LU-7 (*liè quē*, Broken Sequence) and GB-20 (*fēng chí*, Wind Pool); needling with drainage and adding moxa. For qi-blood depletion, add BL-20 (*pí shū*, Spleen Transport) and ST-36 (*zú sān lǐ*, Leg Three Li), needling with supplementation. Cutaneous needle tapping may also be applied. Selection of points according to signs: If dampness is prominent, add SP-9 (*yīn líng quán*, Yin Mound Spring). If itching is pronounced, add Itch Reliever (*zhǐ yǎng xué*). For food allergy, add ST-36 (*zú sān lǐ*, Leg Three Li) and CV-21 (*xuán jī*, Jade Swivel). [26: 937]

dorsal styloid pulse 反关脉 *fǎn guān mài*: PULSE ON THE BACK OF THE WRIST.

double-boiling 炖 *dùn*, 隔水炖 *gé shuǐ dùn*: To boil in a container placed in boiling water rather than directly over a fire; to cook or heat in a double boiler. See PROCESSING OF MEDICINALS. [27: 326] [97: 649] [11: 20]

double contraction 两感 *liǎng gǎn*: A disease in the interior and exterior (yin and yang channels). MED Treat by methods such as returning yang, warming and freeing, and fortifying movement, using formulas such as Aconite Center-Rectifying Decoction (*fù zǐ lǐ zhōng tāng*) or Cinnamon Twig Decoction Plus Aconite (*guì zhī jiā fù zǐ tāng*). [26: 361] [27: 335] [97: 262]

double vision 视一为二 *shì yī wéi èr*: Seeing one object as two; observed, for example, in drunkenness and WIND-INDUCED DEVIATION. ◇ Chin 视 *shì*, see; 一 *yī*, one; 为 *wéi*, be, as; 二 *èr*, two.

downbear 降 *jiàng*: To descend, or cause to descend.

downbearing counterflow and checking vomiting 降逆止呕 *jiàng nì zhǐ ǒu*: A method of treatment used to downbear counterflow and precipitate qi to treat stomach vacuity cold causing persistent hiccough, discomfort in the chest, and a slow pulse. MED Use Clove and Persimmon Decoction (*dīng xiāng shì dì tāng*). ACU Base treatment on the alarm and lower uniting points of ST. Select CV-12 (*zhōng wǎn*, Center Stomach Duct), PC-6 (*nèi guān*, Inner Pass), and ST-36 (*zú sān lǐ*, Leg Three Li); needle with supplementation and moxa to treat stomach vacuity cold. [60: 348] [26: 429]

downbearing counterflow and precipitating qi 降逆下气 *jiàng nì xià qì*: Synonym: *normalizing qi.* A method of treatment used to address lung or stomach qi ascending counterflow. Downbearing counterflow and precipitating qi falls within the scope of rectifying qi, and is used to treat LUNG QI ASCENDING COUNTERFLOW and STOMACH QI ASCENDING COUNTERFLOW. See DOWNBEARING QI AND CALMING PANTING; DOWNBEARING COUNTERFLOW AND CHECKING VOMITING; [26: 429] [27: 270] [60: 348] [46: 654, 658]

downbearing formula 降剂 *jiàng jì*: One of the TWELVE FORMULA TYPES. Downbearing [medicinals] can eliminate upbearing, i.e., they can treat counterflow ascent. An example of a downbearing formula is Perilla Seed Qi-Downbearing Decoction (*sū zǐ jiàng qì tāng*), which contains the downbearing agent perilla seed (*zǐ sū zǐ*) and treats panting. [97: 382]

downbearing [medicinals] can eliminate upbearing 降可去升 *jiàng kě qù shēng*: Downbearing medicinals such as white perilla seed (*bái sū zǐ*) and inula flower (*xuán fù huā*) can treat counterflow ascent. See DOWNBEARING FORMULA. [97: 382]

downbearing qi 降气 *jiàng qì*: Synonym: *precipitating qi*. A method of treatment used to address counterflow qi ascent manifesting as panting, cough, or hiccough, using medicinals such as perilla seed (*zǐ sū zǐ*), inula flower (*xuán fù huā*), pinellia (*bàn xià*), clove (*dīng xiāng*), and hematite (*dài zhě shí*). Downbearing qi is one method of rectifying qi. See PRINCIPLE OF TREATMENT. [26: 429] [97: 382] [50: 1002]

downbearing qi and calming panting 降逆平喘 *jiàng nì píng chuǎn*: A method of treatment used to downbear counterflow and precipitate qi in the treatment of wheezing and panting or rapid panting breathing, and copious phlegm. MED For repletion patterns, use Panting-Stabilizing Decoction (*dìng chuǎn tāng*), and for repletion patterns, use Six Gentlemen Decoction (*liù jūn zǐ tāng*). ACU For repletion patterns, base treatment mainly on LU and LI. Select Panting Stabilizer (*dìng chuǎn*), LU-7 (*liè quē*, Broken Sequence), LU-5 (*chǐ zé*, Cubit Marsh), LI-4 (*hé gǔ*, Union Valley), and CV-17 (*shān zhōng*, Chest Center); needle with drainage. For vacuity patterns, base treatment mainly on LU and back transport points. Select BL-13 (*fèi shū*, Lung Transport), Panting Stabilizer (*dìng chuǎn*), BL-43 (*gāo huāng shū*, Gao-Huang Transport), LU-9 (*tài yuān*, Great Abyss), and ST-36 (*zú sān lǐ*, Leg Three Li); needle with supplementation and add moxa. [60: 348] [26: 429]

downpour 下注 *xià zhù*: Downward movement (of damp-heat). See DAMP-HEAT POURING DOWNWARD.

downpour diarrhea 注下 *zhù xià*: Diarrhea characterized by stool flowing out like water. [27: 365] [97: 367]

downpour of damp-heat 湿热下注 *shī rè xià zhù*: LOWER BURNER DAMP-HEAT.

downpour of damp-heat into the bladder 湿热下注膀胱 *shī rè xià zhù páng guāng*: BLADDER DAMP-HEAT.

downpour of damp-heat into the large intestine 湿热下注大肠 *shī rè xià zhù dà cháng*: LARGE INTESTINAL DAMP-HEAT.

downpour sore 下注疮 *xià zhù chuāng*: DAMP TOXIN SORE.

downsinker 沉降药 *chén jiàng yào*: A medicinal that downbears or sinks. See ³BEARING.

downward fall 下陷 *xià xiàn*: Downward movement, as of insufficient center qi; frequently abbreviated to *fall*, as in the term *qi fall*. [27: 133] [97: 26]

dragon and thunder fire 龙雷之火 *lóng léi zhī huǒ*: **1.** Excessively effulgent ministerial fire. **2.** Life gate fire (dragon) and lesser yang ministerial fire (thunder) fire. [3: 49] [50: 394]

dragon-spring clove sore 龙泉疔 *lóng quán dīng*: HUMAN-CENTER CLOVE SORE. [27: 468] [97: 137]

dragover disease 并病 *bìng bìng*: In cold damage, the appearance of signs in a channel before those of a previously affected channel have resolved. Compare COMBINATION DISEASE. [26: 386] [27: 220] [97: 361]

drain 泻 *xiè*: **1.** To eliminate evils in the body manifesting in repletion patterns. Words of similar meaning include: **dispel** (祛 *qū*), destroy or drive out (evils from the body); **eliminate** (除 *chú*), destroy or remove (evils, especially phlegm or dampness); **expel** (驱 *qū*), remove (parasites from the body); **resolve** (解 *jiě*), eliminate (evils, especially those affecting the exterior), or free (parts of the body from evils); **clear** (清 *qīng*), eliminate (heat); **cool** (凉 *liáng*), remove heat (from the blood aspect); **dissipate** (散 *sàn*), eliminate (cold) or whittle away (stasis nodes and binds); **disperse** (消 *xiāo*), disintegrate or cause to disappear (glomus, phlegm and food accumulations, and swellings); **break** (破 *pò*), dissipate (static blood) gently but powerfully; **dry** (燥 *zào*), eliminate (dampness by using dry, bitter medicinals); **disinhibit** (利 *lì*), promote the free movement (of fluids, qi, or blood), or the elimination (of dampness, water qi), or free (parts of the body from impeded movement); **expel** (排 *pái*), promote elimination from the body (phlegm, pus, static blood, stones, water, wind, worms); **precipitate** (下 *xià*), to cause to pass downward, especially through the intestines and out of the anus; **attack** (攻 *gōng*), eliminate evils forcefully; in particular, to precipitate. **2.** Specifically, to eliminate fire and lower burner damp-heat. **3.** To cause the stool to flow (note that the character *xiè* appears in the term *xiè xiè* diarrhea). See also DISCHARGE.

drainage 泻法 *xiè fǎ*: In acupuncture, a strong stimulus applied to eliminate repletion. See DRAIN.

draining fire 泻火 *xiè huǒ*: See CLEARING.

draining fire and extinguishing wind 泻火熄风 *xiè huǒ xī fēng*: Synonym: *clearing heat and extinguishing wind*. A method of treatment used to address extreme heat engendering wind (repletion heat), i.e., convulsions, upturned eyes, rigid neck, or, in severe cases, arched-back rigidity and clouded spirit in high fever. MED Fire-draining wind-extinguishing medicinals uncaria (*gōu téng*), earthworm (*dì lóng*), scorpion (*quán xiē*), centipede (*wú gōng*), crude abalone shell (*shēng shí jué míng*), crude oyster shell (*shēng mǔ lì*), coptis (*huáng lián*), and isatis leaf (*dà qīng yè*). ACU Base treatment mainly on GV, GB, and LR. Select GV-20 (*bǎi huì*, Hundred Convergences), GB-20 (*fēng chí*, Wind Pool), LR-3 (*tài chōng*, Supreme Surge), GV-14 (*dà zhuī*, Great Hammer), LI-11 (*qū chí*, Pool at the Bend), PC-8 (*láo gōng*,

Palace of Toil), HT-8 (*shào fŭ*, Lesser Mansion), and Twelve Well Points (*shí èr jĭng xué*); needle with drainage or pricking to bleed. See EXTIN-GUISHING WIND. [27: 267]

draining fire and resolving toxin 泻火解毒 *xiè huŏ jiĕ dú*: See CLEARING. [60: 329]

draining precipitation 泻下 *xiè xià*: See PRE-CIPITATION.

draining the heart 泻心 *xiè xīn*: A method of treatment used to eliminate fire from the heart [region], i.e., from the stomach or the heart itself. This method applies to both a) exuberant stomach fire with sore swollen gums, bad breath, clamoring stomach, constipation, red tongue with yellow fur, and a rapid pulse; and b) exuberant heart fire with frenetic movement of the blood (blood ejection, spontaneous external bleeding), constipation, reddish urine, red eye, mouth sores, yellow tongue fur, and rapid pulse. Both these patterns can be treated with Three Yellows Heart-Draining Decoction (*sān huáng xiè xīn tāng*). ACU Base treatment mainly on HT and PC. PC-8 (*láo gōng*, Palace of Toil), HT-8 (*shào fŭ*, Lesser Mansion), PC-9 (*zhōng chōng*, Central Hub), HT-9 (*shào chōng*, Lesser Surge), or GV-26 (*shuĭ gōu*, Water Trough) can be drained or bled with a three-edged needle to drain heart fire. [27: 255] [97: 365] [46: 596]

draining the liver 泻肝 *xiè gān*: *Synonym: clearing the liver and draining fire.* A method of treatment used to clear and drain liver fire with cold bitter medicinals. Draining the liver is the method used to treat liver fire flaming upward characterized by headache, dizziness, tinnitus, deafness, red face and eyes, dry mouth with bitter taste, rib-side pain, vomiting and retching of bitter fluid or, in severe cases, blood ejection, rashness, impatience, and irascibility, constipation, yellow tongue fur, and rapid stringlike pulse. MED A representative liver-draining formula is Gentian Liver-Draining Decoction (*lóng dăn xiè gān tāng*). ACU Base treatment on the LR and GB. LR-2 (*xíng jiān*, Moving Between), GB-43 (*xiá xī*, Pinched Ravine), or GB-34 (*yáng líng quán*, Yang Mound Spring) can be selected and needle with drainage to drain liver fire.

draining the lung 泻肺 *xiè fèi*: *Synonym: draining the white.* A method of treatment used to eliminate heat from the lung, in the treatment of of conditions such as deep-lying lung heat with cough, panting, persistent heat effusion, steaming hot skin that grows more severe at dusk, red tongue with yellow fur, and thin rapid pulse. MED A commonly used lung-draining formula is White-Draining Powder (*xiè bái săn*) with additions. Since the lung is associated through the five phases with the color white, draining the lung is

sometimes referred to as "draining the white," as is seen in this formula name. ACU Base treatment mainly on LU and LI. LU-10 (*yú jì*, Fish Border), LU-5 (*chĭ zé*, Cubit Marsh), LI-11 (*qū chí*, Pool at the Bend), LU-11 (*shào shāng*, Lesser Shang), or LI-1 (*shāng yáng*, Shang Yang) can be selected and needle with drainage or prick to bleed to drain lung fire. [27: 272] [97: 365] [46: 650, 652]

draining the white 泻白 *xiè bái*: DRAINING THE LUNG. For example, in the name White-Draining Powder (*xiè bái săn*), "white-draining" means "lung-draining."

drastic 峻 *jùn*: Highly powerful, as of medicinal action and methods of treatment; applied most commonly to draining and supplementing.

drawing-pin intradermal needle 图钉型皮内针 *tú dīng xíng pí nèi zhēn*: THUMB-TACK INTRADERMAL NEEDLE.

dream emission 梦遗 *mèng yí*: Spontaneous discharge of semen associated with dreaming. Dream emission arises when sexually stimulating sights and thoughts cause frenetic stirring of the ministerial fire or when excessive mental activity causes exuberant heart fire. As a general rule, the principle of "when there is dreaming, treat the heart; when there is no dreaming, treat the kidney" applies, although dream emission may be attributed to heart-spleen vacuity or heart-kidney vacuity. Damp-heat is a further possible factor. MED Treat by clearing the heart and quieting the spirit, using formulas such as Heart-Clearing Lotus Seed Beverage (*qīng xīn lián zĭ yĭn*), Mysterious Fragrance Powder (*miào xiāng săn*), or Mind-Stabilizing Pill (*dìng zhì wán*). For persistent conditions in which disease of the heart affects the kidney and causes noninteraction of the heart and kidney, combine the method of nourishing yin and clearing the heart with that of boosting the kidney and securing essence, using formulas such as Anemarrhena and Phellodendron Eight-Ingredient Pill (*zhī bái bā wèi wán*), Great Creation Pill (*dà zào wán*), or Golden Lock Essence-Securing Pill (*jīn suŏ gù jīng wán*). ACU To clear the heart and quiet the spirit, base treatment mainly on HT and the three yin channels of the foot. Select BL-15 (*xīn shū*, Heart Transport), HT-7 (*shén mén*, Spirit Gate), GB-44 (*zú qiào yīn*, Foot Orifice Yin), and SP-6 (*sān yīn jiāo*, Three Yin Intersection); needle with drainage. For exuberant heart fire, add PC-8 (*láo gōng*, Palace of Toil) and HT-8 (*shào fŭ*, Lesser Mansion). For heart disease affecting the kidney, base treatment mainly on back transporting points and the three yin channels of the foot. Drain BL-15 (*xīn shū*, Heart Transport), HT-7 (*shén mén*, Spirit Gate), PC-7 (*dà líng*, Great Mound), and LR-3 (*tài chōng*, Supreme Surge); supplement BL-23 (*shèn shū*, Kidney Transport), BL-52 (*zhì* *shì*, Will Chamber), and SP-6 (*sān yīn jiāo*, Three Yin Intersection). Drain the heart and supplement the kidney by needling. Selection of points according to signs: For pronounced yin vacuity, add KI-6 (*zhào hǎi*, Shining Sea), needling with supplementation. For profuse dreaming, add GB-44 (*zú qiào yīn*, Foot Orifice Yin) and ST-45 (*lì duì*, Severe Mouth). See SEMINAL EMISSION; DAMP-HEAT SEMINAL EMISSION. [26: 843] [46: 678] [37: 384] [56: 48]

dreaming of intercourse 梦交 *mèng jiāo*: Dreaming of performing coitus, which in males may involve ejaculation known as DREAM EMISSION. This term is not commonly used in modern literature. See also SEMINAL EMISSION. [44: 1167]

dreaming of intercourse with ghosts 夜梦鬼交 *yè mèng guǐ jiāo*: Dreaming of performing coitus with unnatural or supernatural beings. This term is no longer commonly used in modern literature. Compare DREAMING OF INTERCOURSE; DREAM EMISSION; SEMINAL EMISSION. [44: 1195]

dream talking 梦中呓语 *mèng zhōng yì yǔ*: Talking while apparently dreaming. A sign of unquiet sleep. See HEART HEAT SUSCEPTIBILITY TO FRIGHT.

drench 冲 *chōng*: To saturate or dissolve medicinals in liquid. Formulas often indicate that dry mineral medicinals such as mirabilite (*máng xiāo*) and cinnabar (*zhū shā*) or sticky medicinals such as malt sugar (*yí táng*), which means that they can be mixed with the decoction of the other medicinals in the formula or other fluid to facilitate swallowing.

dribble after voiding 尿后馀沥 *niào hòu yú lì*: Synonym: *post-voiding dribble*. A dribbling discharge of urine after urination. Dribble after voiding falls into three basic patterns: kidney vacuity, insufficiency of center qi, and bladder damp-heat. **Kidney vacuity** dribble after voiding is associated with frequent long voidings of clear urine, lassitude of spirit and general fatigue, limp aching back and lumbus, lack of warmth in the extremities, pale tongue with white tongue fur, and a fine sunken pulse, especially at the cubit position. This is observed most commonly in old age. [MED] Warm the kidney and promote astriction. Use variations of Golden Coffer Kidney Qi Pill (*jīn guì shèn qì wán*) combined with Mantis Egg-Case Powder (*sāng piāo xiāo sǎn*). **Insufficiency of center qi** is characterized intermittent post-voiding dribble often brought on by taxation, and characterized by bright white facial complexion, reduced food intake, sloppy stool, sagging distention in the lesser abdomen, pale tongue with white fur, and a moderate soggy or weak fine pulse. [MED] Supplement the center and boost qi. Use Center-Supplementing Qi-Boosting Decoction (*bǔ zhōng yì qì tāng*). **Bladder damp-heat** is char-

acterized by frequent urination, yellow, sometimes murky urine, burning sensation in the urethra, red tongue with slimy yellow tongue fur, and a soggy rapid pulse. [MED] Clear heat and disinhibit dampness using formulas such as Eight Corrections Powder (*bā zhèng sǎn*). See URINE. [92: No. 226]

dribbling urinary block 癃闭 *lóng bì*, 闭癃 *bì lóng*: Synonyms: *urinary block*; *urinary stoppage*. Dribbling urination or, in severe cases, almost complete blockage of urine flow. Distinction is made between a number of vacuity and repletion patterns. Vacuity patterns include insufficiency of center qi and insufficiency of kidney qi. The repletion patterns include lower burner damp-heat, lung qi congestion, binding depression of liver qi, and urinary tract stasis blockage. [WMC] Ischuria due to spasm of the vesical sphincter, urinary calculus, urethrostenosis, tumor of the urethra, urethral injury, hyperplasia of the prostate in old age, myelitis, or toxemia. **Insufficiency of center qi** is characterized by difficult voiding, fatigue, shortness of breath, reduced food intake, distention and oppression in the stomach duct and abdomen, sagging distention in the smaller abdomen, sloppy stool, pale tongue with thin fur, and a sunken weak pulse. [MED] Supplement the center and boost qi; free urination. Use variations of Center-Supplementing Qi-Boosting Decoction (*bǔ zhōng yì qì tāng*). **Insufficiency of kidney qi** is characterized by forceless voiding, frequent urge to urinate, aching lumbus and knees, lack of warmth in the extremities, pale tongue with dental impressions, thin white tongue fur, and a fine sunken pulse that is weak at the cubit position. [MED] Warm kidney yang and boost qi; supplement the kidney and disinhibit urine. Use variations of Life Saver Kidney Qi Pill (*jì shēng shèn qì wán*). **Lower burner damp-heat** is characterized by urinary block with painful urination, frequent urination, and urinary urgency, bitter taste in the mouth, thirst without desire to drink, inhibited stool, red tongue with slimy yellow fur, and a sunken rapid or soggy rapid pulse. [MED] Clear and disinhibit damp-heat; free urination. Use formulas such as Eight Corrections Powder (*bā zhèng sǎn*). **Lung qi congestion** is marked by oppression in the chest, cough and inhibited rapid breathing, constipation, red tongue or pale tongue, with white or thin yellow tongue fur, and sunken weak pulse. [MED] Treat by "taking the lid off," i.e., by inducing sneezing or by mechanical emesis to open lung qi. For enduring conditions in which heat has developed, Lung-Clearing Drink (*qīng fèi yǐn zi*) can be used with the judicious addition of urine-freeing medicinals. **Binding depression of liver qi** is characterized by dribbling urinary block or ungratifying urination, affect-mind binding depression, tendency to vexation and irascibility, constrained feeling in the rib-sides, unquiet sleep, profuse dreaming, bitter taste in the mouth and swallowing of upflowing acid, red tongue with thin yellow fur, and a stringlike pulse. MED Treat by Aquilaria Powder (*chén xiāng sǎn*), combined with Bupleurum Liver-Coursing Powder (*chái hú shū gān sǎn*) if necessary. **Urinary tract stasis blockage** is characterized by intermittent inability to void urine, lesser-abdominal distention, dark purple tongue with stasis speckles, white or slightly yellow tongue fur, and a rough pulse. MED Move stasis and dissipate binds; disinhibit the waterways. Use Substitute Dead-On Pill (*dài dǐ dàng wán*). ACU For repletion patterns, base treatment mainly on the alarm and back transporting points of BL and SP. Select CV-3 (*zhōng jí*, Central Pole), BL-28 (*páng guāng shū*, Bladder Transport), SP-6 (*sān yīn jiāo*, Three Yin Intersection), SP-9 (*yīn líng quán*, Yin Mound Spring), and LU-5 (*chǐ zé*, Cubit Marsh); needle with drainage. For vacuity patterns, base treatment mainly on KI, SP, and back transporting points. Select BL-23 (*shèn shū*, Kidney Transport), BL-20 (*pí shū*, Spleen Transport), BL-22 (*sān jiāo shū*, Triple Burner Transport), CV-4 (*guān yuán*, Pass Head), KI-10 (*yīn gǔ*, Yin Valley), and SP-6 (*sān yīn jiāo*, Three Yin Intersection); needle with supplementation and add moxa. Compare INHIBITED URINATION; SHIFTED BLADDER; BLOCK AND REPULSION; URINE. ◇ Chin 癃 is composed of 疒, the illness signifier, with 隆 *lóng*, high, prominent, thriving, or intense. The character composition may originally have reflected the fullness in the abdomen associated with urinary stoppage. However, in *The Inner Canon* (*nèi jīng*), 癃 was used interchangeably with 淋 *lín*, dribble. In the Han Dynasty, the given name 隆 of the Emperor Han Shang Di 汉殇帝, invoked the taboo against profane use the emperor's name, and thereafter 癃 was replaced with 淋, until the Ming dynasty when the two characters came to be used in distinct senses. Still to this day, 癃 is commonly explained as "dribbling" or "trickling" and as denoting a mild form of urine retention, whereas 闭 *bì* is explained as denoting severe or complete blockage. [92: No. 224] [26: 929] [27: 426] [97: 648] [80: 533]

dribbling urinary incontinence 小便淋沥不禁 *xiǎo biàn lín lì bù jìn*: See DRIBBLING URINATION. [27: 427]

dribbling urination 小便淋沥 *xiǎo biàn lín lì*: Frequent short rough voidings of urine with a continuous dribble. Distinction is made between vacuity and repletion. Vacuity patterns are mostly attributable to insecurity of kidney qi or dual vacuity of the spleen and kidney. Repletion patterns are mostly due to lower burner damp-heat or urinary calculi. See URINE. [27: 427]

dried-meat nose 鼻藁腊 *bí gǎo là*: WITHERED NOSE. [26: 856]

drink 饮子 *yǐn zi*: A BEVERAGE (a decoction left to cool) that can be taken at any time. [27: 311] [97: 295]

drinker's aggregation 酒癖 *jiǔ pǐ*: Synonym: *drinker's concretion*. A hard lump that arises through drinking of liquor. Through excessiving drinking, water collects in the chest and diaphragm and the rib-side forming into an aggregation. *The Origin and Indicators of Disease* (*zhū bìng yuán hòu lùn*) states: "Drinker's aggregations results from heavy drinking after which [the person] is thirsty and drinks large amounts of fluid. When the liquor and fluid fail to disperse and collect below the rib-side, and bind and aggregation, that is periodically painful..." MED Use formulas such as Major Seven Qi Decoction (*dà qī qì tāng*). WMC alcoholic cirrhosis. [50: 1301] [27: 121] [25: 264]

drinker's concretion 酒癥 *jiǔ zhēng*: DRINKER'S AGGREGATION. [50: 1301]

drinker's nose 酒齇 *jiǔ zhā*: Synonym: *red nose*; *lung wind*; *lung wind acne*. Reddening and thickening of the skin of the bulb of the nose in those fond of drinking. Drinker's nose is understood as local blood stasis occurring when spleen damp-heat fumes up into the lung. The bulb of the nose becomes enlarged and the surface becomes uneven and warty in appearance. Severe conditions, known as lung-wind or lung-wind acne, are characterized by the appearance of red swollen papules that burst to exude a chalky substance and white fluid and that eventually give way to scaling. WMC brandy nose; (acne) rosacea. MED Clear heat, cool the blood, and dissipate stasis using formulas such as Blood-Cooling Four Agents Decoction (*liáng xuè sì wù tāng*). Reversal Powder (*diān dǎo sǎn*) can be applied topically. ACU Base treatment mainly on SP, LI and ST. Select SP-6 (*sān yīn jiāo*, Three Yin Intersection), SP-10 (*xuè hǎi*, Sea of Blood), BL-17 (*gé shū*, Diaphragm Transport), LI-4 (*hé gǔ*, Union Valley), LI-11 (*qū chí*, Pool at the Bend), ST-44 (*nèi tíng*, Inner Court); needle with drainage, and prick LI-20 (*yíng xiāng*, Welcome Fragrance) and Hall of Impression (*yìn táng*), and local points to bleed with a three-edged needle. For marked damp-heat, add SP-9 (*yīn líng quán*, Yin Mound Spring), and ST-36 (*zú sān lǐ*, Leg Three Li). For lung wind, add LU-5 (*chǐ zé*, Cubit Marsh), and LU-11 (*shào shāng*, Lesser Shang). [26: 479] [27: 495] [61: 365] [46: 594, 597, 650] [4: 130]

drool 涎 *xián*: One of the five humors. Drool and spittle are together known as DROOL-SPITTLE or SPITTLE HUMOR, which keep the mouth moist and help digestion. Drool is said to spring from the cheeks, and to flow out from the corners of the mouth during sleep. Spittle is said to spring from under the tongue, and to be spat out of the mouth. When the spleen and stomach are normal, there is ample liquid; there is harmony of mouth, there is no dryness of mouth or thirst, and food is flavorsome. In spleen-stomach vacuity cold, cold drool wells upward and there is a bland taste in the mouth and nausea. In intense stomach fire, drool is scant and the mouth is dry. Spleen-stomach damp-heat or worm accumulations, wind stroke, or epilepsy can cause drooling or foaming at the corners of the mouth. Compare PHLEGM-DROOL. [26: 486] [27: 74] [36: 98]

drooling 流涎 *liú xián*: Flowing of drool from the mouth; attributed to spleen heat or spleen-stomach vacuity cold disturbing normal bearing. [26: 486]

drooling from the corner of the mouth during sleep 睡时口角流涎 *shuì shí kǒu jiǎo liú xián*: Flowing of drool from the angles of the mouth during sleep; a sign of spleen vacuity or stomach heat. In infants this may be a sign of intestinal worms. Drooling from one side of the mouth is associated with deviated mouth and facial paralysis.

drool is the humor of the spleen 涎为脾液 *xián wéi pí yè*: The spleen opens at the mouth; hence, drool is the humor of the spleen. [27: 61]

drool-spittle 涎唾 *xián tuò*: See SPITTLE.

drooping of the upper eyelid 上胞下垂 *shàng bāo xià chuí*: Drooping of usually one but sometimes two eyelids, in severe cases, causing the patient to hold the head back to see properly. If not congenital, it is attributable to spleen vacuity causing disharmony of the network vessels allowing wind to settle in the eyelid. MED Supplement the spleen and boost qi; dispel wind and free the network vessels. Use Center-Supplementing Qi-Boosting Decoction (*bǔ zhōng yì qì tāng*) or Ginseng Construction-Nourishing Decoction (*rén shēn yǎng róng tāng*) with judicious addition of silkworm (*bái jiāng cán*), scorpion (*quán xiē*), red peony (*chì sháo yào*), and cyathula (*chuān niú xī*). ACU Needle with supplementation at BL-20 (*pí shū*, Spleen Transport), and ST-36 (*zú sān lǐ*, Leg Three Li), and with drainage at BL-1 (*jīng míng*, Bright Eyes), BL-2 (*zǎn zhú*, Bamboo Gathering), GB-1 (*tóng zǐ liáo*, Pupil Bone-Hole), TB-23 (*sī zhú kōng*, Silk Bamboo Hole), GB-15 (*tóu lín qì*, (Head) Overlooking Tears), GB-20 (*fēng chí*, Wind Pool), LI-4 (*hé gǔ*, Union Valley), and GB-14 (*yáng bái*, Yang White) joining Fish's Lumbus (*yú yāo*). [26: 58] [27: 402] [97: 30] [4: 126]

drowsiness after eating 食后困顿 *shí hòu kùn dùn*: Desire to sleep occurring after eating, or, in severe cases, before the end of meal. It occurs in spleen qi vacuity with fatigue, lack of strength, withered-yellow facial complexion, poor appetite,

abdominal distention after eating, unsolid stool, and a pale enlarged tongue. It results from phlegm-damp encumbering the spleen with heaviness of the head and body, glomus and oppression in the chest and stomach duct, small intake of food, sloppy stool, sticky unpleasant sensation in the mouth, fat body, a white slimy tongue fur, and a soggy moderate pulse. [92: No. 195]

drug 药 *yào*: MEDICINAL.

drum distention 鼓 *gǔ*, 鼓胀 *gǔ zhàng*, 臌 *gǔ*, 臌胀 *gǔ zhàng*: **1.** Severe abdominal distention. Drum distention is also called ABDOMINAL DISTENTION, SIMPLE DRUM, and SPIDER DRUM (the spider having a rotund body and thin limbs) when swelling of the limbs is absent, as is usually the case. Drum distention is associated with a somber yellow coloration of the skin, and prominent green-blue veins (caput medusae). Causes include: a) emotional frustration (anger damaging the liver); b) fondness of liquor and sweet fatty food; c) glomus lump; d) enduring illness; e) water toxin qi bind (mentioned in *The Origin and Indicators of Disease* (*zhū bìng yuán hòu lùn*), now understood as blood fluke infestation). Two major pathomechanisms operate. *Spleen disease affecting the liver:* Fondness of liquor and sweet fatty food causes damage to the spleen and prevents it from transforming damp turbidity so that damp-heat brews. The damp-heat then obstructs qi dynamic, causing liver depression. On the one hand, prolonged liver depression can cause blood stasis; on the other, it can cause liver qi to invade the spleen and the stomach, impairing movement and transformation of water-damp. Spleen vacuity and water-damp exacerbate each other, spleen qi vacuity gives way to spleen yang vacuity, which finally leads to dual vacuity of the spleen and kidney with inhibited urination that prevents the discharge of fluids. Drum distention thus arises as a result of qi stagnation, blood stasis, and water collecting in the abdomen. *Liver and spleen disease affecting the kidney:* Spleen vacuity deprives the kidney of nourishment, causing insufficiency of kidney yang and inhibited bladder qi transformation. Debilitation of the life gate fire (kidney yang) exacerbates spleen yang vacuity. Liver depression transforms into heat to damage yin causing liver-kidney yin vacuity. Damp-heat can similarly damage yin. In former times, distinction was made between QI DRUM, BLOOD DRUM, WATER DRUM, and WORM DRUM. However, modern texts suggest that no clearly defined line can be drawn between the first three. Distinctions are now made between: qi stagnation and damp obstruction; water-damp encumbering the spleen; brewing damp-heat; liver-spleen blood stasis; spleen-kidney yang vacuity; liver-kidney yin vacuity. WMC ascites due to cirrhosis, abdominal tumors, or tubercular peritonitis. **Qi stagnation and damp obstruction** causing distention that is not hard to the touch, associated with reduced eating with a tendency to bloating, belching, short voidings of scant urine, a white slimy tongue fur, and a stringlike pulse. MED Course the liver and rectify qi; move dampness and dissipate the fullness. Use Bupleurum Liver-Coursing Powder (*chái hú shū gān sǎn*) or Stomach-Calming Poria (Hoelen) Five Decoction (*wèi líng tāng*). ACU Base treatment for drum distention mainly on ST, CV, and PC. Main points (applicable to all patterns): ST-25 (*tiān shū*, Celestial Pivot), CV-6 (*qì hǎi*, Sea of Qi), PC-6 (*nèi guān*, Inner Pass), and ST-36 (*zú sān lǐ*, Leg Three Li). For qi stagnation and damp obstruction, add LR-3 (*tài chōng*, Supreme Surge), SP-6 (*sān yīn jiāo*, Three Yin Intersection), BL-18 (*gān shū*, Liver Transport), BL-20 (*pí shū*, Spleen Transport), SP-9 (*yīn líng quán*, Yin Mound Spring), and CV-12 (*zhōng wǎn*, Center Stomach Duct), needling with drainage. **Water-damp encumbering the spleen** drum distention is marked by enlargement, fullness, and distention. To the touch, it feels like a bag of water, which reflects the amassment of water due to devitalized spleen yang. Stomach duct glomus and abdominal fullness is relieved slightly by heat, which indicates cold contending with the water. Scant urine, sloppy stool, swelling of the face and lower limbs reflects water evil encumbering the spleen and damage to kidney yang. A white slimy tongue fur and a moderate pulse reflect exuberant dampness and debilitation of yang. If the abdomen is large as an urn and the limbs are thin as brushwood from shedding of the major masses of the flesh, this is a sign of debilitation of spleen yang, which indicates a poor prognosis. MED Warm the center and rectify the spleen; move qi and disinhibit water. Use Spleen-Firming Beverage (*shí pí yǐn*). ACU Use the main points given above, and add BL-20 (*pí shū*, Spleen Transport), CV-12 (*zhōng wǎn*, Center Stomach Duct), LR-13 (*zhāng mén*, Camphorwood Gate), and SP-9 (*yīn líng quán*, Yin Mound Spring), needling with even supplementation and drainage and adding moxa. **Brewing damp-heat** drum distention is marked by fullness and hardness with a tensed sense of propping in the stomach duct and abdomen. The abdomen feels scorching hot. Other signs include vexation and thirst, bitter taste in the mouth, thirst without desire to drink, constipation or sloppy stool, rough voidings of reddish urine, yellowing of the skin, red tongue with grayish or blackish yellow slimy tongue fur, and a rapid stringlike pulse. MED Treat by clearing heat and disinhibiting dampness and by offensive precipitation to expel water. Use Center Fullness Separating and Dispersing Pill (*zhōng mǎn fēn xiāo wán*) combined with Capillaris Decoction (*yīn chén hāo*

tāng). Alternatively use Boats and Carts Pill (*zhōu chē (jū) wán*). ACU Use the main points given above and add BL-19 (*dǎn shū*, Gallbladder Transport), LR-3 (*tài chōng*, Supreme Surge), GB-34 (*yáng líng quán*, Yang Mound Spring), LI-11 (*qū chí*, Pool at the Bend), SP-6 (*sān yīn jiāo*, Three Yin Intersection), SP-9 (*yīn líng quán*, Yin Mound Spring), and GV-9 (*zhì yáng*, Extremity of Yang); needle with drainage. **Liver-spleen blood stasis** drum distention is characterized by enlargement, hardness and fullness, prominent green-blue veins on the abdomen, stabbing pain in the ribside and abdomen, dull blackish complexion, blood moles on the head, neck, chest, and arms, and red marks on the hands, purple-brown lips, thirst without desire to swallow fluids, black stool, purple-red tongue possibly with purple macules, and a fine rough or scallion-stalk pulse. MED Quicken the blood and transform stasis; move qi and disinhibit water. Use Construction-Regulating Beverage (*tiáo yíng yǐn*). ACU Use the main points given above and add SP-10 (*xuè hǎi*, Sea of Blood), LR-3 (*tài chōng*, Supreme Surge), LI-4 (*hé gǔ*, Union Valley), SP-6 (*sān yīn jiāo*, Three Yin Intersection), and GB-34 (*yáng líng quán*, Yang Mound Spring), needling with even supplementation and drainage or pricking to bleed. **Spleen-kidney yang vacuity** drum distention causes enlargement with distention and discomfort that becomes more pronounced in the evening. It is accompanied by oppression in the stomach duct, torpid intake, lassitude of spirit, fear of cold, swelling of the lower limbs, short voidings of scant urine, withered-yellow or bright white facial complexion, pale enlarged purple tongue, and forceful stringlike sunken pulse. MED Warm and supplement the spleen and kidney; promote qi transformation and move water. Use Aconite Center-Rectifying Decoction (*fù zǐ lǐ zhōng tāng*) combined with Poria (Hoelen) Five Powder (*wǔ líng sǎn*) or Life Saver Kidney Qi Pill (*jì shēng shèn qì wán*). ACU Use the main points given above, and add BL-20 (*pí shū*, Spleen Transport), BL-23 (*shèn shū*, Kidney Transport), CV-12 (*zhōng wǎn*, Center Stomach Duct), GV-4 (*mìng mén*, Life Gate), KI-3 (*tài xī*, Great Ravine), and CV-3 (*zhōng jí*, Central Pole), needling with supplementation and adding moxa. **Liver-kidney yin vacuity** causes enlargement, distention, fullness and discomfort, in severe cases with prominent green-blue vessels. Other signs include short voidings of scant urine, vexation and insomnia, periodic bleeding gums or nosebleed in some cases, dry mouth, red-crimson tongue with little liquid, and a thin rapid stringlike pulse. MED Enrich the liver and kidney; cool the blood and transform stasis. Use Six-Ingredient Rehmannia Pill (*liù wèi dì huáng wán*) or All-the-Way-Through Brew (*yī guàn jiān*) combined with Infradiaphragmatic

Stasis-Expelling Decoction (*gé xià zhú yū tāng*).
ACU Use the main points given above and add
BL-23 (*shèn shū*, Kidney Transport), BL-18 (*gān
shū*, Liver Transport), BL-17 (*gé shū*, Diaphragm
Transport), CV-4 (*guān yuán*, Pass Head), KI-3
(*tài xī*, Great Ravine), LR-3 (*tài chōng*, Supreme
Surge), KI-6 (*zhào hǎi*, Shining Sea), KI-2 (*rán gǔ*,
Blazing Valley), and SP-10 (*xuè hǎi*, Sea of Blood),
needling with supplementation. See entries listed
below. Compare GU DISTENTION. **2.** QI DISTEN-
TION. [80: 415] [106: 466] [26: 775] [113: 12, 14,
19] [46: 594–597, 602] [37: 379]

Drum Distention

VACUITY DISTENTION (*xū zhàng*)

REPLETION DISTENTION (*shí zhàng*)

COLD DISTENTION (*hán zhàng*)

HEAT DISTENTION (*rè zhàng*)

FOOD DISTENTION (*shí zhàng*)

QI DISTENTION (*qì zhàng*)

WORM DRUM (*chóng gǔ*)

BLOOD DRUM (*xuè gǔ*)

QI DRUM (*qì gǔ*)

WATER DRUM (*shuǐ gǔ*)

GU DISTENTION (*gǔ zhàng*)

SIMPLE ABDOMINAL DISTENTION (*dān fù zhàng*)

---

drumskin pulse 革脉 *gé mài*: A pulse that is
floating and beats against the palpating fingers. A
drumskin pulse is hard on the outside and empty
in the middle like the skin of a drum. It signifies
blood collapse and loss of essence. *On Cold Damage* (*shāng hán lùn*) states, "Contending cold and
vacuity is called drumskin." It is similar to and,
according to some, identical with the *scallion-stalk
pulse*. [26: 411]

dry 干 *gān*, 燥 *zào*: Lacking in moisture (e.g., dry
tongue); characterized by absence of moisture (e.g.,
dry cholera). See DRYNESS.

dry blood consumption 干血痨 *gān xuè láo*: A
disease recorded in *On Blood Patterns* (*xuè zhèng
lùn*) that in signs and treatment corresponds to
what is mentioned in *Essential Prescriptions of the
Golden Coffer* (*jīn guì yào lüè*) as "dry blood."
Dry blood consumption is mostly seen in women.
It results from long steaming of vacuity heat and
internal binding of dry blood with stasis and stagnation, stemming from damage by the five taxations. When, in enduring conditions, static blood
is not eliminated, new blood is engendered with
difficulty, and liquid and blood fail to create luxuriance in the outer body. Signs include absence of
menstruation, markedly emaciated body, no desire
for food and drink, steaming bone tidal heat [ef-
fusion], encrusted skin, and dull black complexion.
MED Quicken the blood and move stasis; clear accumulated heat. Use Rhubarb and Wingless Cock-

roach Pill (*dà huáng zhè chóng wán*). After this,
nourish and harmonize the blood with Tangkuei
Blood-Supplementing Decoction (*dāng guī bǔ xuè
tāng*) and Four Agents Decoction (*sì wù tāng*). [26:
597]

dry bound stool 大便干结 *dà biàn gān jié*, 大便
燥结 *dà biàn zào jié*: See CONSTIPATION.

dry cholera 干霍乱 *gān huò luàn*: Synonym:
intestinal-gripping sand (*shā*). Blockage of the
stomach and intestines by foul turbidity due to dietary irregularity or contraction of mountain forest miasma and characterized by desire but failure to vomit and desire but failure to "drain,"
gripping abdominal pain, vexation and oppression,
and, in severe cases, blue-green facial complexion,
cold limbs, sweating, and hidden pulse. The chief
characteristic of cholera is simultaneous vomiting
and diarrhea. Dry cholera differs in that the patient wants to vomit but cannot, and has the same
urge to defecate as experienced in diarrhea; hence
the name "dry cholera." Since it is also characterized by gripping abdominal pain, it is also
called "intestinal-gripping sand" (see SAND (*shā*)).
MED Disinhibit qi and diffuse congestion; repel
turbidity and foulness. Use formulas such as Liquid
Storax Pill (*sū hé xiāng wán*), Jade Pivot Elixir (*yù
shū dān*), and Agastache/Patchouli Qi-Righting
Powder (*huò xiāng zhèng qì sǎn*). ACU Prick
BL-40 (*wěi zhōng*, Bend Center) and the Twelve
Well Points (*shí èr jǐng xué*) to bleed, and moxa
CV-8 (*shén què*, Spirit Gate Tower) and CV-11
(*jiàn lǐ*, Interior Strengthening); then needle CV-11
(*jiàn lǐ*, Interior Strengthening), CV-12 (*zhōng
wǎn*, Center Stomach Duct), BL-22 (*sān jiāo shū*,
Triple Burner Transport), LI-4 (*hé gǔ*, Union Valley), LR-3 (*tài chōng*, Supreme Surge), and TB-1
(*guān chōng*, Passage Hub). In addition, one can
wet one's hand and beat the patient's knees and
wrists until purple-black speckles appear, which
can then be pricked to drain the malign blood. [26:
598]

dry eyes 目干涩 *mù gān sè*: Lack of fluid to ensure the smooth movement of the eyelids, usually
attributable to insufficiency of lung yin with vacuity fire flaming upward, to liver-kidney yin development or to insufficiency of liver blood. MED Treat
by nourishing blood and clearing heat, enriching
the liver and kidney, or by supplementing the liver
and nourishing the blood, depending on the cause.
[26: 201]

dry fall 干陷 *gān xiàn*: A disease pattern arising
when a headed flat-abscess (*jū*) fails to suppurate
and attributed to the failure of right qi to overcome the evil. In such patterns, the flat-abscess
(*jū*) has a dark dull appearance, and is associated
with mild or distending pain. The base of the sore
is flat and purple in color, and the head is dry and

ulcerated. Other signs include heat effusion and slight aversion to cold, spontaneous sweating, lassitude of spirit, rapid vacuous pulse, and, in severe cases, cold of the limbs and a faint pulse. MED Treat by supplementing qi and nourishing the blood and by drawing toxin and outthrusting the evil, assisted by clearing the heart and quieting the spirit. Internal Expression Toxin-Dispersing Powder (*tuō lǐ xiāo dú sǎn*) plus bovine bezoar (*niú huáng*) and amber (*hǔ pò*) is an appropriate formula. WMC toxemia. See FALL PATTERN; HEADED FLAT-ABSCESS. [26: 598] [96: 135]

dry formula 燥剂 *zào jì*: One of the TEN FORMULA TYPES. Dry [medicinals] can eliminate dampness. Formulas predominantly containing such medicinals are called dry formulas. For example, Five-Peel Beverage (*wǔ pí yǐn*), containing mulberry root bark (*sāng bái pí*), tangerine peel (*chén pí*), ginger skin (*jiāng pí*), areca husk (*dà fù pí*), and poria skin (*fú líng pí*), is used to treat swelling of the limbs, fullness in the stomach duct and abdomen, panting, and inhibited urination. Stomach-Calming Powder (*píng wèi sǎn*) is also a dry formula. [27: 306] [97: 653]

dry hair 发枯 *fà kū*: A condition in which the hair lacks moisture and sheen; attributed to kidney vacuity and blood heat with yin-blood failing to nourish the hair. MED Treat by enriching yin and nourishing, assisted by clearing heat. Variants of Four Agents Decoction (*sì wù tāng*) combined with Six-Ingredient Rehmannia Pill (*liù wèi dì huáng wán*) may be used. [26: 869]

drying dampness 燥湿 *zào shī*: A method of treatment used to eliminate center burner dampness with dry bitter medicinals. See DRYING DAMPNESS WITH WARMTH AND BITTERNESS; DRYING DAMPNESS WITH COLD AND BITTERNESS. [26: 932]

drying dampness and harmonizing the center 燥湿和中 *zào shī hé zhong*: DRYING DAMPNESS AND HARMONIZING THE STOMACH.

drying dampness and harmonizing the stomach 燥湿和胃 *zào shī hé wèi*: Synonym: *drying dampness and harmonizing the center*. A method of treatment used to treat damp turbidity obstructing the spleen and causing spleen-stomach disharmony manifesting in glomus and fullness in the stomach duct and abdomen, belching and swallowing of upflowing acid, vomiting and diarrhea, reduced eating and fatigue, a bland taste in the mouth, and thick slimy tongue fur. MED Drying dampness and harmonizing the center makes use of warm acrid dampness-drying, aromatic turbidity-transforming, and heat-clearing dampness-transforming medicinals such as atractylodes (*cāng zhú*), magnolia bark (*hòu pò*), agastache/patchouli (*huò xiāng*), and car-

damom (*bái dòu kòu*). Representative formulas include Stomach-Calming Powder (*píng wèi sǎn*) and Agastache/Patchouli Qi-Righting Powder (*huò xiāng zhèng qì sǎn*). [16: 480]

drying dampness and transforming phlegm 燥湿化痰 *zào rè huà tán*: Synonym: *fortifying the spleen and transforming phlegm*. A method of treatment used to address damp phlegm arising when devitalization of spleen yang results in impairment of normal movement and transformation, characterized by white easily expectorated phlegm, oppression in the chest and nausea, slimy glossy white tongue, and in some cases dizziness and heart palpitations. MED Dampness-drying phlegm-transforming formulas include Two Matured Ingredients Decoction (*èr chén tāng*) plus ovate atractylodes (*bái zhú*) or atractylodes (*cāng zhú*), or Six Gentlemen Decoction (*liù jūn zǐ tāng*). ACU Base treatment mainly on ST and CV. Main points: Select CV-12 (*zhōng wǎn*, Center Stomach Duct), ST-36 (*zú sān lǐ*, Leg Three Li), and ST-40 (*fēng lóng*, Bountiful Bulge); needle with even supplementation and drainage and add moxa. Selection of points according to signs: For oppression in the chest, add CV-17 (*shān zhōng*, Chest Center), CV-22 (*tiān tú*, Celestial Chimney), and LI-4 (*hé gǔ*, Union Valley). For nausea, PC-6 (*nèi guān*, Inner Pass), ST-25 (*tiān shū*, Celestial Pivot), and CV-6 (*qì hǎi*, Sea of Qi). For dizzy head, add ST-8 (*tóu wéi*, Head Corner) and ST-41 (*jiě xī*, Ravine Divide). For heart palpitations, add HT-7 (*shén mén*, Spirit Gate), PC-6 (*nèi guān*, Inner Pass), BL-15 (*xīn shū*, Heart Transport), and CV-6 (*qì hǎi*, Sea of Qi). [26: 932]

drying dampness with cold and bitterness 苦寒燥湿 *kǔ hán zào shī*: A method of treatment used to eliminate damp-heat causing gastrointestinal damp-heat signs such as abdominal pain, abdominal distention, thin hot putrid-smelling stool, and a yellow slimy tongue fur. Commonly used cold bitter dampness-drying medicinals include coptis (*huáng lián*), scutellaria (*huáng qín*), phellodendron (*huáng bǎi*), bitter orange (*zhǐ ké*), and polyporus (*zhū líng*). [26: 432]

drying dampness with warmth and bitterness 苦温燥湿 *kǔ wēn zào shī*: A method of treatment used to eliminate cold-damp with bitter warm medicinals. Drying dampness with warmth and bitterness is used to treat cold-damp patterns characterized by signs such as oppression in the chest, nausea, retching and vomiting, abdominal distention, thin clear stool, and white slimy tongue. MED Commonly used warm bitter dampness-drying medicinals include magnolia bark (*hòu pò*), atractylodes (*cāng zhú*), pinellia (*bàn xià*), and cardamom (*bái dòu kòu*). Formulas include Stomach-Calming Powder (*píng wèi sǎn*) and

Priceless Qi-Righting Powder (*bù huàn jīn zhèng qì sǎn*). [26: 432]

dry leg qi 干脚气 *gān jiǎo qì*: LEG QI characterized by the absence of water swelling. Dry leg qi arises when yin vacuity internal heat, damp-heat, and wind-toxin transforming into heat damage construction-blood, depriving the sinews of nourishment, causing lack of strength, pain, numbness, hypertonicity, and withering of the lower leg, accompanied by reduced food intake, hot reddish urine, red tongue, and rapid stringlike pulse. ⌐WMC¬ beriberi (attributed to vitamin B₁ deficiency). ⌐MED¬ Diffuse congestion and transform dampness; harmonize construction and clear heat. Use medicinals such as atractylodes (*cāng zhú*), ovate atractylodes (*bái zhú*), anemarrhena (*zhī mǔ*), phellodendron (*huáng bǎi*), tangkuei (*dāng guī*), white peony (*bái sháo yào*), dried/fresh rehmannia (*shēng dì huáng*), chaenomeles (*mù guā*), areca (*bīng láng*), notopterygium (*qiāng huó*), duhuo (*dú huó*), mutong (*mù tōng*), northern fangji (*hàn zhōng fáng jǐ*), achyranthes (*niú xī*), licorice (*gān cǎo*), and ginger (*jiāng*). ⌐ACU¬ Base treatment mainly on SP, KI, and GB. Select SP-10 (*xuè hǎi*, Sea of Blood), SP-6 (*sān yīn jiāo*, Three Yin Intersection), KI-3 (*tài xī*, Great Ravine), KI-6 (*zhào hǎi*, Shining Sea), ST-36 (*zú sān lǐ*, Leg Three Li), GB-34 (*yáng líng quán*, Yang Mound Spring), and GB-39 (*xuán zhōng*, Suspended Bell); needle with supplementation. Selection of points according to signs: For cramps, add BL-57 (*chéng shān*, Mountain Support). For lumbar pain, add BL-40 (*wěi zhōng*, Bend Center). For swollen knees, GB-33 (*xī yáng guān*, Knee Yang Joint) and GB-31 (*fēng shì*, Wind Market). [26: 598] [46: 669]

dry lichen 干癣 *gān xiǎn*: From *The Origin and Indicators of Disease* (*zhū bìng yuán hòu lùn*). LICHEN (*xiǎn*) that is characterized by clearly circumscribed thickening of the skin fissuring, and itching that causes scaling, and that is attributed to wind-damp settling in the skin. ⌐WMC¬ chronic eczema; neurodermatitis. ⌐MED¬ Apply Coptis Powder (*huáng lián sǎn*), which comprises alum (*bái fán*) and coptis (*huáng lián*). Alternatively, use Chinese Wolfsbane Paste (*láng dú gāo*). A further alternative is sulfur (*shí liú huáng*) ground to a powder and applied mixed with vinegar. [26: 599]

dry lips 唇燥 *chún zào*, 唇干 *chún gān*: Synonym: *parched lips*. Lack of moisture in the lips, in severe cases with cracking. Dry lips may be due to the dryness evil, external evils passing into the interior, or effulgent yin vacuity fire. See also CRACKED LIPS. [6: 126]

dry [medicinals] can eliminate dampness 燥可去湿 *zào kě qù shī*: Dry medicinals can be used to treat internally exuberant damp turbidity causing

glomus in the chest and abdominal fullness. An example of this is the use of Stomach-Calming Powder (*píng wèi sǎn*) to treat distention and fullness in the stomach duct and abdomen with fatigue, aversion to food, harmony of mouth, absence of thirst, and a thick white slimy tongue. See DRY FORMULA. [27: 306] [26: 931]

dry miliaria 枯痦 *kū péi*: Miliaria whose vesicles are white in color and contain no fluid; an unfavorable sign. See MILIARIA ALBA. [6: 118] [27: 370]

dry mouth 口干 *kǒu gān*, 口燥 *kǒu zào*: A lack of fluid in the mouth, usually, but not necessarily, associated with THIRST, which is the desire to drink. Dry mouth with no desire to drink is observed in depletion of essence-blood with vacuous yang floating upward. [92: No. 88]

dryness 燥 *zào*: Synonym: *dryness qi*. **1.** The opposite of moisture. **2.** One of the SIX QI; dryness as an environmental phenomenon and a potential cause of disease, associated with the autumn in China. **3.** One of the SIX EXCESSES; dryness as an environmental qi causing disease. **4.** A state of the body resulting from contraction of dryness in the environment. Signs include dry nostrils, nosebleed, dry mouth, dry cracked lips, dry "tickly" or sore throat, dry cough with little or no phlegm, rough dry skin, and dry tongue with relatively little liquid. Distinction is made between COOL DRYNESS and WARM DRYNESS. **5.** A state of the body arising from depletion of yin-humor and presenting signs similar to those created by the environmental qi dryness. [6: 106]

dryness damage cough 伤燥咳嗽 *shāng zào ké sòu*: A COUGH arising when externally contracted dryness damages lung qi, and mostly manifesting as a dryness-heat pattern. See DRYNESS-HEAT COUGH. [26: 810]

dryness evil 燥邪 *zào xié*: DRYNESS as a disease-causing entity.

dryness evil invading the lung 燥邪犯肺 *zào xié fàn fèi*: Synonym: *dryness qi damaging the lung*. Damage by the dryness evil, usually in autumn. Dryness is one of the six excesses. In autumn, the weather (in China) is dry, and dry air entering the lung can cause damage to the liquid of the lung. The chief signs are dry cough without phlegm or with scant sticky phlegm that is not easily expectorated. Other signs include dry lips, tongue, pharynx, and nose. In some case, there is generalized heat [effusion] and aversion to cold, or chest pain and expectoration of blood. The tongue is red with yellow or white fur. The pulse is rapid. **Analysis:** When dryness evil damages lung liquid, the lung is deprived of moisture, and diffusion and depuration break down, hence the dry cough without phlegm or with scant sticky phlegm that is not easily expectorated. "When dryness prevails, there is aridity," hence the dry lips, tongue, pharynx, and nose. Lung qi reaches the skin and [body] hair, and when the lung is assailed by dryness, heat effusion and aversion to cold are observed together. If the dryness evil transforms into fire and scorches the network vessels of the lung, there is chest pain and expectoration of blood. Dryness evil damages liquid, and when liquid is damaged, yang becomes hyperactive. Hence the tongue is usually red. When dryness evil assails the exterior, the tongue fur is usually white; when it assails the lung, the tongue fur is usually yellow. Dryness-heat damaging the lung makes the pulse rapid. MED Clear dryness and moisten the lung; suppress cough and transform phlegm. Dryness-Clearing Lung-Rescuing Decoction (*qīng zào jiù fèi tāng*) or Mulberry Leaf and Apricot Kernel Decoction (*sāng xìng tāng*). ACU Base treatment mainly on LU, LI, and KI. Select BL-13 (*fèi shū*, Lung Transport), LU-5 (*chǐ zé*, Cubit Marsh), LU-7 (*liè quē*, Broken Sequence), and LI-4 (*hé gǔ*, Union Valley). Needle with drainage and supplement KI-6 (*zhào hǎi*, Shining Sea). For generalized heat [effusion] and aversion to cold, drain BL-12 (*fēng mén*, Wind Gate), GB-20 (*fēng chí*, Wind Pool), and BL-11 (*dà zhù*, Great Shuttle). **Comparison**: *Wind-heat invading the lung*: Dryness evil invading the lung is characterized by cough without phlegm or with scant phlegm and by dry lips, tongue, pharynx, and nose. Wind-heat invading the lung is marked by pronounced heat effusion and mild aversion to cold. *Lung yin vacuity*: Cough and scant sticky phlegm that is not easily expectorated are observed in both dryness evil invading the lung and in lung yin vacuity. However, lung yin vacuity has effulgent yin vacuity fire signs such as postmeridian tidal heat [effusion], and vexing heat in the five hearts. Dryness evil is marked by exterior signs such as aversion to cold with heat effusion. See AUTUMN DRYNESS. [116: 70] [57: 78][26: 931] [37: 272] [46: 650, 652]

dryness-fire 燥火 *zào huǒ*: DRYNESS-HEAT.

dryness-fire dizziness 燥火眩晕 *zào huǒ xuàn yūn*: DIZZINESS attributed to contraction of DRYNESS-HEAT, characterized by spinning head and black vision, and accompanied by generalized heat [effusion], vexation and agitation, thirst with intake of fluid, unquiet sleep, reddish urine, and an agitated racing pulse. MED Clear fire and moisten dryness. Use Bupleurum Liver-Clearing Beverage (*chái hú qīng gān yǐn*) or Bamboo Leaf and Gypsum Decoction (*zhú yè shí gāo tāng*). ACU Base treatment mainly on GV, LI, PC, and HT. Select GV-20 (*bǎi huì*, Hundred Convergences), LI-4 (*hé gǔ*, Union Valley), LI-11 (*qū chí*, Pool at the Bend), TB-2 (*yè mén*, Humor Gate), PC-7 (*dà líng*, Great Mound), LR-2 (*xíng jiān*, Moving Be-

tween), HT-8 (*shào fǔ*, Lesser Mansion), KI-3 (*tài xī*, Great Ravine), SP-6 (*sān yīn jiāo*, Three Yin Intersection), and HT-7 (*shén mén*, Spirit Gate); needle with drainage. [26: 931] [113: 166, 20, 18, 166]

dryness-heat 燥热 *zào rè*: Synonym: *dryness-fire*. A condition that arises when externally contracted DRYNESS QI (COOL DRYNESS) damages the fluids and transforms into HEAT or FIRE. Dryness-heat is characterized by swelling of the gums, tinnitus, cough, expectoration of blood, or nosebleed. See DRYNESS. [26: 932]

dryness-heat cough 燥热咳嗽 *zào rè ké sòu*: COUGH attributed to damage to lung liquid by wind-heat or dryness qi and characterized by absence of phlegm or scant sticky phlegm, ungratifying expectoration, dry nose and throat, and, in severe cases, by pain in the chest and rib-side, and in some cases by exterior signs such as physical cold and generalized heat [effusion]. MED Clear the lung and moisten dryness with formulas such as Mulberry Leaf and Apricot Kernel Decoction (*sāng xìng tāng*). ACU Base treatment mainly on LU, LI, and KI. Select BL-13 (*fèi shū*, Lung Transport), LU-5 (*chǐ zé*, Cubit Marsh), LU-7 (*liè quē*, Broken Sequence), and LI-4 (*hé gǔ*, Union Valley). Needle with drainage and supplement KI-6 (*zhào hǎi*, Shining Sea). If the cause is wind-heat, add LI-11 (*qū chí*, Pool at the Bend) and GV-14 (*dà zhuī*, Great Hammer) and drain them. [26: 932] [37: 272] [37: 272] [46: 652]

dryness-heat damaging the lung 燥热伤肺 *zào rè shāng fèi*: Synonym: *dryness-heat invading the lung*. DRYNESS-HEAT evil wearing lung liquid and making lung qi unable to diffuse and downbear. Dryness-heat damaging the lung is characterized by dry cough without phlegm or with scant sticky phlegm, red tongue with little liquid, a dry thin white tongue fur, and a fine rapid floating pulse that may be large at the left inch position. These signs are often accompanied by tidal heat [effusion], headache, and constipation. MED Diffuse with lightness and moisten dryness. Compare AUTUMN DRYNESS. [25: 345]

dryness-heat invading the lung 燥热犯肺 *zào rè fàn fèi*: DRYNESS-HEAT DAMAGING THE LUNG.

dryness-heat wilting 燥热痿 *zào rè wěi*: WILTING (*wěi*) that arises when DRYNESS-HEAT damages liquid and the blood, depriving the sinews of nourishment. Dryness-heat wilting is characterized by limpness of the extremities preventing normal movement and is attended by signs such as dry skin and hair, dry mouth, and parched lips. MED Clear heat and moisten dryness; enrich yin and nourish the blood. Use formulas such as Dryness-Clearing Lung-Rescuing Decoction (*qīng zào jiù fèi tāng*). ACU Use the general points given under WILTING, and add GV-14 (*dà zhuī*, Great Hammer), LI-11 (*qū chí*, Pool at the Bend), PC-7 (*dà líng*, Great Mound), and KI-6 (*zhào hǎi*, Shining Sea). Needle with drainage. [26: 932]

dryness phlegm 燥痰 *zào tán*: Synonym: *qi phlegm*. A PHLEGM pattern attributable to lung dryness due either to contraction of DRYNESS EVIL or to lung (or lung-kidney) yin vacuity, and characterized by scant white phlegm or phlegm like grains of rice that is difficult to expectorate, and a withered-white complexion, parched skin, dry mouth, tongue, throat, and nose, cough and hasty panting. The phlegm may be flecked with blood. MED Clear the heat and moisten dryness. For dryness evil, use Mulberry Leaf and Apricot Kernel Decoction (*sāng xìng tāng*) for mild cases and Dryness-Clearing Lung-Rescuing Decoction (*qīng zào jiù fèi tāng*) for more severe cases. Fritillaria and Trichosanthes Powder (*bèi mǔ guā lóu sǎn*) can also be used. For lung yin depletion, use Yin-Nourishing Lung-Clearing Decoction (*yǎng yīn qīng fèi tāng*). For lung-kidney yin depletion, use variations of Six-Ingredient Rehmannia Pill (*liù wèi dì huáng wán*). ACU Base treatment mainly on LU and KI. Drain BL-13 (*fèi shū*, Lung Transport), CV-17 (*shān zhōng*, Chest Center), LU-5 (*chǐ zé*, Cubit Marsh), LI-11 (*qū chí*, Pool at the Bend), and CV-22 (*tiān tú*, Celestial Chimney); and supplement KI-6 (*zhào hǎi*, Shining Sea). For pronounced lung or (lung-kidney) depletion, supplement BL-23 (*shèn shū*, Kidney Transport), BL-43 (*gāo huāng shū*, Gao-Huang Transport), KI-3 (*tài xī*, Great Ravine), TB-2 (*yè mén*, Humor Gate), and SP-6 (*sān yīn jiāo*, Three Yin Intersection), and drain KI-1 (*yǒng quán*, Gushing Spring), HT-8 (*shào fǔ*, Lesser Mansion), and LU-11 (*shào shāng*, Lesser Shang). For blood-flecked phlegm, drain LU-10 (*yú jì*, Fish Border) and LU-6 (*kǒng zuì*, Collection Hole). Compare HEAT PHLEGM. [26: 932] [46: 653] [37: 272]

dryness qi 燥气 *zào qì*: DRYNESS.

dryness qi damaging the lung 燥气伤肺 *zào qì shāng fèi*: DRYNESS EVIL INVADING THE LUNG.

dryness tetany 燥痉 *zào jìng*: TETANY (*jìng*) caused by DRYNESS scorching the fluids. Dryness tetany is seen in advanced stages of febrile disease when exuberant heat has damaged liquid and begun to deprive the sinews of nourishment, thereby transforming into dryness and stirring wind. Dryness tetany is characterized by heat effusion, spasm of the limbs, dry mouth and throat, and dry skin. MED Treat first with Purple Snow Elixir (*zǐ xuě dān*) to open the orifices and settle tetany, and then with Pulse-Restorative Decoction (*fù mài tāng*) to nourish yin with sweet moist medicinals. ACU Base treatment mainly on GV and LR. Needle with drainage at GV-20 (*bǎi huì*, Hundred Con-

vergences), GV-14 (*dà zhuī*, Great Hammer), LI-11 (*qū chí*, Pool at the Bend), GV-16 (*fēng fǔ*, Wind Mansion), LR-3 (*tài chōng*, Supreme Surge), KI-3 (*tài xī*, Great Ravine), and GV-26 (*shuǐ gōu*, Water Trough), and prick the Ten Diffusing Points (*shí xuān*) to bleed in order to clear heat, extinguish wind, and settle tetany. Then needle with supplementation at KI-6 (*zhào hǎi*, Shining Sea), KI-2 (*rán gǔ*, Blazing Valley), TB-2 (*yè mén*, Humor Gate), and SP-6 (*sān yīn jiāo*, Three Yin Intersection) to nourish yin and increase humor. [26: 932] [46: 733]

dry pharynx 咽干 *yān gān*: See DRY THROAT.

dry retching 干呕 *gān ǒu*: Going through the motions of vomiting without bringing up food, despite possible foaming drool. Dry retching is attributed to stomach vacuity counterflow qi or stomach heat. **Stomach vacuity** is observed in patients weak from enduring disease or after vomiting and diarrhea has damaged stomach qi. It is associated with dull stomach duct pain and no thought of food and drink. The pain comes at set times and likes warmth and pressure. Other signs include shortage of qi and laziness to speak, faint low voice, and withered-yellow facial complexion. The tongue is pale with thin white fur. The pulse is weak and vacuous. MED Use Tangerine Peel and Bamboo Shavings Decoction (*jú pí zhú rú tāng*). ACU Base treatment on alarm and lower uniting points of ST, and on PC, SP, and back transporting points. Select CV-12 (*zhōng wǎn*, Center Stomach Duct), ST-36 (*zú sān lǐ*, Leg Three Li), PC-6 (*nèi guān*, Inner Pass), BL-20 (*pí shū*, Spleen Transport), BL-21 (*wèi shū*, Stomach Transport), LR-13 (*zhāng mén*, Camphorwood Gate), SP-4 (*gōng sūn*, Yellow Emperor), and SP-6 (*sān yīn jiāo*, Three Yin Intersection); needle with supplementation. **Stomach cold** dry retching is marked by a low weak sound with occasional ejection of small amounts of foamy drool. In stomach repletion cold patterns, there is cold pain in the stomach duct and abdomen, white tongue fur, and a stringlike sunken pulse. In vacuity patterns, there is glomus and fullness below the heart, no desire to eat, and sloppy stool, shortness of breath and laziness, bland taste in the mouth without thirst, a pale tongue with white fur, fine and weak pulse. MED Treat repletion cold with dissipating cold by warming the center and dissipating cold and by harmonizing the stomach and downbearing counterflow. Use Pinellia and Dried Ginger Powder (*bàn xià gān jiāng sǎn*). For ejection of small amounts of foamy drool and dizziness, use variations of Evodia Decoction (*wú zhū yú tāng*). Treat vacuity patterns by supplementing the spleen and boosting the stomach, and by downbearing counterflow and quieting the center. Use Center-Rectifying Decoction (*lǐ zhōng tāng*) plus clove (*dīng xiāng*), poria (*fú líng*), and pinellia (*bàn xià*). ACU See COLD VOMITING. **Stomach heat** causes frequent, sonorous retching with glomus and blockage below the heart, bitter taste in the mouth, and heart vexation. Repletion heat patterns are observed when externally contracted evil passes from the exterior to the interior, settle in the yang brightness (*yáng míng*), transform into heat, which contends with qi and impairs harmonious downbearing. These are characterized by abdominal pain and fullness with constipation, and thirst with desire to drink, a red tongue with dry yellow fur, and a large replete pulse. Vacuity heat patterns occur when either residual heat in heat (febrile) disease or inappropriate use of dry medicinals damage stomach yin and impair the harmonious downbear of stomach qi. These are marked by a red tongue with scant fur, and a rapid fine pulse. MED Treat repletion patterns by clearing heat and freeing the bowels, and by harmonizing the stomach and downbearing counterflow. Use variations of Stomach-Regulating Qi-Coordinating Decoction (*tiáo wèi chéng qì tāng*). Treat vacuity heat by nourishing the stomach and engendering liquid, and by harmonizing and downbearing center qi. Use Bamboo Leaf and Gypsum Decoction (*zhú yè shí gāo tāng*). ACU See HEAT VOMITING. **Liver depression** causes dry retching when depressed liver qi runs cross counterflow and invades the stomach, causing disharmony of stomach qi. The dry retching is characterized by a low sound and occurs intermittently in relation to emotional disturbance. Accompanying signs include vexation and oppression in the chest and rib-side, torpid intake, a pale red tongue with thin white fur, and a fine stringlike pulse. MED Soothe the liver and rectify qi; harmonize the stomach and downbear counterflow. Use variations of Four-Seven Decoction (*sì qī tāng*). ACU Base treatment mainly on ST, LR, and GB. Select CV-12 (*zhōng wǎn*, Center Stomach Duct), CV-13 (*shàng wǎn*, Upper Stomach Duct), PC-6 (*nèi guān*, Inner Pass), ST-36 (*zú sān lǐ*, Leg Three Li), LR-3 (*tài chōng*, Supreme Surge), SP-6 (*sān yīn jiāo*, Three Yin Intersection), and GB-34 (*yáng líng quán*, Yang Mound Spring); needle with even supplementation and drainage or with drainage. **Food stagnation** is the result of dietary irregularities, excessive consumption of liquor and rich foods, and is characterized by dry retching with the malodor of food, desire to but inability to vomit, glomus in the chest, aversion to food, distention and fullness in the stomach duct and abdomen, foul-smelling stool, a thick slimy tongue fur, and a slippery stringlike pulse. MED Harmonize the stomach and rectify qi; disperse food and abduct stagnation. Use Harmony-Preserving Pill (*bǎo hé wán*). ACU Base treatment on ST and CV. Select CV-12

(*zhōng wǎn*, Center Stomach Duct), CV-10 (*xià wǎn*, Lower Stomach Duct), PC-6 (*nèi guān*, Inner Pass), ST-25 (*tiān shū*, Celestial Pivot), CV-6 (*qì hǎi*, Sea of Qi), ST-36 (*zú sān lǐ*, Leg Three Li), and Li Inner Court (*lǐ nèi tíng*); needle with drainage. [26: 598] [92: No. 189] [46: 659, 660, 662]

dry rib-side pain 干胁痛 *gān xié tòng*: Rib-side pain due to liver-kidney qi blood vacuity. Dry rib-side pain is usually attributable to excesses of drink and sex, causing damage to the liver and kidney and depletion of qi and blood, depriving the channels and network vessels of nourishment. It is characterized by persistent pain in one particular spot. In addition, there are signs of "vacuity turning into detriment." MED Treat by greatly supplementing qi and blood and by nourishing the liver and kidney. Formulas such as Eight Agents Decoction (*bā wù tāng*), Liver-Supplementing Powder (*bǔ gān sǎn*), or Six-Ingredient Rehmannia Pill (*liù wèi dì huáng wán*). ACU Base treatment mainly on LR, KI, SP, and back transport points. Select BL-18 (*gān shū*, Liver Transport), BL-23 (*shèn shū*, Kidney Transport), LR-14 (*qī mén*, Cycle Gate), LR-3 (*tài chōng*, Supreme Surge), SP-6 (*sān yīn jiāo*, Three Yin Intersection), and ST-36 (*zú sān lǐ*, Leg Three Li); needle with supplementation. [26: 597]

dry stool in the stomach 胃中燥矢 *wèi zhōng zào shǐ*: Dry stool in the intestines caused by internal binding of repletion heat and scorching of the fluids by evil heat. *On Cold Damage* (*shāng hán lùn*) says, "In yang brightness (*yáng míng*) disease with delirious speech, tidal heat [effusion], and inability to eat, there must be five or six pellets of dry stool in the stomach. The "stomach" here refers to the intestines. "Dry stool in the stomach" refers repletion heat binding in the intestines with heat scorching the fluids. [27: 366]

dry teeth 齿燥 *chǐ zào*, 牙齿干燥 *yá chǐ gān zào*: Dry-looking, lusterless teeth, especially the two front teeth. If the teeth are grimy and there is bad breath, this sign is ascribed to exuberant stomach fire and major damage to fluids. In enduring sickness, front teeth that are "dry as old bones" are a sign of critical damage to kidney yin. [27: 184] [97: 342] [26: 887] [6: 126]

dry throat 喉咽干燥 *hóu yān gān zào*, 嗌干 *yì gān*, 嗌燥 *yì zào*: Lack of moisture in the throat, associated with or without a desire to drink. Dry throat occurs in both vacuity and repletion patterns: Repletion patterns include wind-heat assailing the lung, dryness-heat damaging the lung, exuberant spleen-stomach heat, and depressed liver-gallbladder heat. Vacuity patterns include lung yin vacuity and kidney yin vacuity. **Wind-heat assailing the lung** can cause a dry throat with a burning sensation, or soreness and itching, and a desire to drink. Other signs of externally contracted wind-heat are present, e.g., heat effusion, aversion to cold, headache, nasal congestion, and red swollen throat. The tongue is red with a thin white or thin yellow fur. The pulse is floating and rapid. [MED] Treat by clearing and diffusing lung heat using Mulberry Leaf and Chrysanthemum Beverage (*sāng jú yǐn*). [ACU] For all repletion patterns, select Sea Source (*hǎi quán*), TB-2 (*yè mén*, Humor Gate), SP-6 (*sān yīn jiāo*, Three Yin Intersection), and KI-6 (*zhào hǎi*, Shining Sea) as the main points, and needle with even supplementation and drainage; prick LU-11 (*shào shāng*, Lesser Shang) to bleed. For wind-heat assailing the lung, drain GV-14 (*dà zhuī*, Great Hammer), BL-13 (*fèi shū*, Lung Transport), GB-20 (*fēng chí*, Wind Pool), TB-5 (*wài guān*, Outer Pass), LI-11 (*qū chí*, Pool at the Bend), and LI-4 (*hé gǔ*, Union Valley). **Dryness-heat damaging the lung** causes a dry throat and nose, dry cough without phlegm or with scant sticky phlegm that is not easily expectorated. These signs are often accompanied by chest pain, heat effusion, headache, generalized pain and discomfort. The tongue is red with thin white fur. The pulse is floating, fine, and rapid. [MED] Clear the lung and moisten dryness with variations of Mulberry Leaf and Apricot Kernel Decoction (*sāng xìng tāng*). [ACU] Use the main points given above, and drain BL-13 (*fèi shū*, Lung Transport), CV-17 (*shān zhōng*, Chest Center), LU-5 (*chǐ zé*, Cubit Marsh), LI-11 (*qū chí*, Pool at the Bend), and CV-22 (*tiān tú*, Celestial Chimney). **Exuberant spleen-stomach heat** causes dry throat and mouth with vexation and thirst, and desire to drink. Other signs include bad breath, scorching stomach duct pain, acid upflow, clamoring stomach, dry stool, and yellow urine. The tongue is red with yellow fur. The pulse is slippery and rapid. [MED] Clear spleen-stomach fire using Stomach-Clearing Powder (*qīng wèi sǎn*). [ACU] Use the main points given above, and drain ST-44 (*nèi tíng*, Inner Court), LI-4 (*hé gǔ*, Union Valley), LU-5 (*chǐ zé*, Cubit Marsh), and LI-1 (*shāng yáng*, Shang Yang). **Depressed liver-gallbladder damp-heat** causes a dry throat with bitter taste in the mouth, dizzy vision, fullness and oppression in the chest and rib-side, no desire to drink, vexation, frequent retching, and alternating heat [effusion] and [aversion to] cold. The tongue is red with a thin yellow tongue fur. The pulse is stringlike and fine. [MED] Clear the liver and drain fire using Tangkuei, Gentian, and Aloe Pill (*dāng guī lóng huì wán*). [ACU] Use the main points given above, and drain LR-3 (*tài chōng*, Supreme Surge), PC-6 (*nèi guān*, Inner Pass), GB-34 (*yáng líng quán*, Yang Mound Spring), LR-2 (*xíng jiān*, Moving Between), and GB-43 (*xiá xī*, Pinched Ravine). **Lung yin vacuity** causes a dry itchy throat with

dry cough without phlegm or with scant sticky phlegm. The voice is hoarse and the nose is dry with snivel. The tongue is red with scant fur, and the pulse is fine. [MED] Enrich lung yin. Use Lily Bulb Metal-Securing Decoction (*bǎi hé gù jīn tāng*) or Yin-Nourishing Lung-Clearing Decoction (*yǎng yīn qīng fèi tāng*). [ACU] For all vacuity patterns, select TB-2 (*yè mén*, Humor Gate), SP-6 (*sān yīn jiāo*, Three Yin Intersection), KI-6 (*zhào hǎi*, Shining Sea), KI-2 (*rán gǔ*, Blazing Valley), and KI-3 (*tài xī*, Great Ravine), as the main points, needling with even supplementation and drainage or with supplementation. If vacuity fire is pronounced and dryness is accompanied by soreness, prick LU-11 (*shào shāng*, Lesser Shang) to bleed. For lung yin vacuity, supplement BL-13 (*fèi shū*, Lung Transport) and BL-43 (*gāo huāng shū*, Gao-Huang Transport), and drain LU-5 (*chǐ zé*, Cubit Marsh). **Liver-kidney yin vacuity** causes dryness of the mouth, throat, and root of the tongue with deafness, tinnitus, dizzy head and eyes, limp aching lumbus and knees, seminal emission, and insomnia. The tongue is red. The pulse is fine and rapid. [MED] Supplement the kidney and nourish yin. Use Six-Ingredient Rehmannia Pill (*liù wèi dì huáng wán*). [ACU] For kidney yin vacuity, use the main point for vacuity given above, and supplement BL-23 (*shèn shū*, Kidney Transport), and drain LR-2 (*xíng jiān*, Moving Between) and LU-10 (*yú jì*, Fish Border). [26: 788] [92: No. 447] [113: 20] [37: 470] [46: 595, 596, 664, 725, 727] [57: 73]

dry tongue fur 舌苔干燥 *shé tāi gān zào*, 苔燥 *tāi zào*: A tongue fur that lacks moisture. A dry tongue fur is usually a heat sign. A tongue that looks dry, and feels dry and rough, or even prickly to the touch, described as a *rough tongue fur*, is mainly seen in externally contracted heat (febrile) diseases and indicates damage to humor by exuberant heat. A slightly dry and slightly slimy tongue fur associated with thirst without desire to drink arises when center phlegm-damp obstruction prevents the fluid from reaching the upper body. [6: 123]

dual clearing of both qi and construction 气营两清 *qì yíng liǎng qīng*: CLEARING BOTH QI AND CONSTRUCTION.

dual disease of qi and construction 气营同病 *qì yíng tóng bìng*: QI AND CONSTRUCTION BOTH ABLAZE. [26: 546]

dual disease of the interior and exterior 表里同病 *biǎo lǐ tóng bìng*: Interior and exterior patterns occurring simultaneously when a) cold evil invades both the exterior and interior, creating exterior signs such as aversion to cold, heat effusion, headache, and aching bones, and interior signs such as abdominal pain and diarrhea, or when b) an evil that initially produces an exterior pattern subsequently enters the interior, creating an interior pattern before the exterior pattern is resolved. Two other conditions may be viewed as dual interior-exterior patterns, though by convention they are differently labeled: a "NEW CONTRACTION," which involves the superimposition of an exterior pattern resulting from contraction of one or more of the six excesses on a pre-existing interior pattern; and "food damage complication," where a food damage pattern develops during a pre-existing externally contracted disease manifesting in an exterior pattern. [6: 152] [27: 211] [97: 326]

dual resolution of both exterior and interior 表里双解 biǎo lǐ shuāng jiě: See RESOLVING BOTH EXTERIOR AND INTERIOR.

dual supplementation of qi and blood 气血双补 qì xuè shuāng bǔ: See SUPPLEMENTING BOTH QI AND BLOOD.

dual vacuity of heart qi and blood 心气血两虚 xīn qì xuè liǎng xū, 心气血俱虚 xīn qì xuè jù xū: Insufficiency of qi and blood depriving the heart of nourishment and making heart spirit fail to keep to its abode. Dual vacuity of heart qi and blood stems from constitution weakness, insufficiency of the source of transformation, or enduring illness that damages blood and wears qi. The chief signs are heart palpitations, shortness of breath, insomnia and profuse dreaming, dizzy head and vision, and a somber white or withered-yellow facial complexion. Other signs include lassitude of spirit and lack of strength, spontaneous sweating, shortage of qi and laziness to speak, pale lips and nails, and lusterless hair. The tongue is pale and tender. The pulse is fine and weak, or fine and rapid. Alternatively, it is skipping, bound, or intermittent. **Analysis:** When heart qi is vacuous, its propelling power is weak; when heart blood is vacuous, the heart is deprived of nourishment. Hence, there are heart palpitations. When heart qi is insufficient, the circulation of ancestral qi is weak, hence there is oppression in the chest and shortness of breath. Since exertion causes wear on qi, it exacerbates these signs. When qi and blood are both vacuous, the heart spirit is deprived of nourishment, hence there is insomnia and profuse dreaming. When heart qi is vacuous, it fails to contain the humor of the heart (sweat), hence the spontaneous sweating. When blood is vacuous, it fails to ascend to nourish the head, face, and brain, hence the lusterless withered-yellow or pale white complexion, pale lips, dizziness, and forgetfulness. [MED] Supplement qi and nourish the blood. Use Eight-Gem Decoction (bā zhēn tāng) or Sagacious Cure Decoction (shèng yù tāng). [ACU] Base treatment mainly on back transport points, HT, PC, and CV. Select BL-15 (xīn shū, Heart Transport), CV-14 (jù què, Great Tower Gate), CV-6 (qì hǎi, Sea of Qi), BL-17 (gé shū, Diaphragm Transport), BL-20 (pí shū, Spleen Transport), PC-6 (nèi guān, Inner Pass), HT-7 (shén mén, Spirit Gate), ST-36 (zú sān lǐ, Leg Three Li), and SP-6 (sān yīn jiāo, Three Yin Intersection); needle with supplementation and moxa. [116: 41] [57: 48] [37: 332, 335] [46: 586, 648]

dual vacuity of heart qi and yin 心气阴两虚 xīn qì yīn liǎng xū: Insufficiency of heart qi that makes the heart beat without force, combined with depletion of heart yin with vacuity heat arising internally. The chief signs are heart palpitations and shortness of breath exacerbated by exertion, insomnia and profuse dreaming, lassitude of spirit and lack of strength, vexing heat in the five hearts, and white face with red cheeks. Other signs include forgetfulness, spontaneous or night sweating, low faint voice, dry mouth and throat, and low fever. The tongue is pale and tender with little liquid. The tongue fur is white, and in some cases, scant. The pulse is fine or fine and rapid. **Analysis:** When heart qi and yin are depleted, the heart is depleted, hence the heart palpitations or fearful throbbing, oppression in the chest and shortness of breath exacerbated by exertion, shortage of qi and lack of strength, and exhaustion of essence-spirit. When the spirit is deprived of nourishment, there is insomnia, profuse dreaming, and forgetfulness. When qi is vacuous, the spirit is deprived of nourishment, hence a frequent desire to sleep. When the fleshy exterior is not kept sound, there is spontaneous sweating and sweating at the slightest exertion. When heart qi is insufficient, its power to move the blood is weakened, and the blood stagnates in the vessels of the heart. When heart yin is insufficient, vacuity fire harasses the inner body, hence there is heart vexation, heat in the hearts of the palms and soles, and, in severe cases, tidal heat [effusion] and night sweating. When yin-liquid is depleted, the throat is dry. When qi vacuity is prominent, the tongue is pale and peeled bare; when yin vacuity is prominent, the tongue is red with little or no fur. [MED] Supplement the heart, supplement qi, and nourish yin. Use Honey-Fried Licorice Decoction (zhì gān cǎo tāng). [ACU] Base treatment mainly on back transport point, HT, PC, and CV. Select BL-15 (xīn shū, Heart Transport), CV-14 (jù què, Great Tower Gate), CV-6 (qì hǎi, Sea of Qi), BL-20 (pí shū, Spleen Transport), PC-6 (nèi guān, Inner Pass), HT-7 (shén mén, Spirit Gate), and SP-6 (sān yīn jiāo, Three Yin Intersection); needle with supplementation. [57: 49] [116: 39] [37: 332, 335] [46: 586, 648]

dual vacuity of heart yin and yang 心阴阳两虚 xīn yīn yáng liǎng xū: Insufficiency of both heart yin and heart yang. The chief signs are heart palpitations and fearful throbbing, oppression in the chest and shortness of breath exacerbated by exertion, physical cold and cold limbs, heart vexation, and heat in the hearts of the palms and soles. Other signs include emaciation, shortage of qi and laziness to speak, fatigue and lack of strength, dizziness, spontaneous or night sweating, and sweating at the slightest exertion. In some cases there may be postmeridian tidal heat [effusion], reddening of the cheeks, sleeplessness, or forgetfulness. The tongue is pale and peeled. The pulse is skipping or intermittent, or faint, fine, and rapid. Analysis: A chief sign of all heart patterns is heart palpitations. Heart yang vacuity is a development of heart qi vacuity. When heart qi is insufficient, there is shortness of breath exacerbated by exertion, and fatigue and lack of strength. When yang is vacuous, the body is deprived of warmth and the fleshy exterior becomes insecure and unsound, hence the physical cold and cold limbs and spontaneous sweating. When yin is vacuous, vacuity heat arises internally, hence the heat in the hearts of the palms and soles, tidal heat [effusion], night sweating, and reddening of the cheeks. When vacuity fire harasses the heart and disquiets the heart spirit, there is heart vexation and sleeplessness. Insufficiency of heart yin deprives the brain of nourishment, hence the dizziness and forgetfulness. When heart yin and yang are both debilitated and fail to warm and nourish, there is fatigue and lack of strength, shortage of qi and laziness to speak, and emaciation. The tongue and pulses also reflect both the heart yin and heart yang vacuity. MED Enrich yin and warm yang; nourish the heart and quiet the spirit. Use Honey-Fried Licorice Decoction (*zhì gān cǎo tāng*). ACU Base treatment mainly on back transport points, HT, PC, and CV. Select BL-15 (*xīn shū*, Heart Transport), CV-14 (*jù què*, Great Tower Gate), CV-4 (*guān yuán*, Pass Head), CV-6 (*qì hǎi*, Sea of Qi), BL-20 (*pí shū*, Spleen Transport), PC-6 (*nèi guān*, Inner Pass), HT-7 (*shén mén*, Spirit Gate), and SP-6 (*sān yīn jiāo*, Three Yin Intersection); needle with supplementation and large amounts of moxa. [116: 43] [37: 332, 335] [46: 586, 648]

dual vacuity of kidney yin and yang 肾阴阳两虚 *shèn yīn yáng liǎng xū*: Insufficiency of both kidney yin and kidney yang, characterized by limb aching lumbus and knees and dizziness, together with signs of vacuity cold and vacuity heat such as physical cold, and a sensation of internal heat. Other signs include lack of strength, tinnitus, dry throat and mouth, liking for warm drinks, long voidings of clear urine, menstrual irregularities, vaginal discharge, and infertility in women, and seminal emission, impotence, and sterility in men. The tonge is is enlarged and slightly red with a thin tongue fur. The pulse is fine and forceless, especially at the cubits. MED Warm and supplement kidney yang; enrich and supplement kidney

yin. A representative formula is Left-Restoring [Kidney Yin] Pill (*zuǒ guī wán*) combined with Right-Restoring [Life Gate] Pill (*yòu guī wán*). MED Base treatment mainly on back transport points, GV, and KI. Select GV-4 (*mìng mén*, Life Gate)ⓜ, BL-23 (*shèn shū*, Kidney Transport)ⓜ, CV-4 (*guān yuán*, Pass Head)ⓜ, KI-3 (*tài xī*, Great Ravine)ⓜ, BL-52 (*zhì shì*, Will Chamber), KI-6 (*zhào hǎi*, Shining Sea), KI-1 (*yǒng quán*, Gushing Spring), and SP-6 (*sān yīn jiāo*, Three Yin Intersection); needle with supplementation. Selection of points according to signs: For dizziness, add GV-20 (*bǎi huì*, Hundred Convergences), GV-16 (*fēng fǔ*, Wind Mansion), and GB-39 (*xuán zhōng*, Suspended Bell). For tinnitus, add TB-17 (*yì fēng*, Wind Screen), GB-2 (*tīng huì*, Auditory Convergence), and TB-3 (*zhōng zhǔ*, Central Islet). For dry pharynx and mouth, add KI-2 (*rán gǔ*, Blazing Valley), TB-2 (*yè mén*, Humor Gate), and Gold Liquid and Jade Humor (*jīn jīn yù yè*). For lumbar pain, add GV-3 (*yāo yáng guān*, Lumbar Yang Pass), BL-40 (*wěi zhōng*, Bend Center), and BL-60 (*kūn lún*, Kunlun Mountains). For seminal emission, add KI-12 (*dà hè*, Great Manifestation), CV-6 (*qì hǎi*, Sea of Qi), HT-7 (*shén mén*, Spirit Gate), and ST-36 (*zú sān lǐ*, Leg Three Li). For menstrual irregularities, KI-5 (*shuǐ quán*, Water Spring) and CV-6 (*qì hǎi*, Sea of Qi). For vaginal discharge, add GB-26 (*dài mài*, Girdling Vessel), BL-30 (*bái huán shū*, White Ring Transport), and BL-32 (*cì liáo*, Second Bone-Hole). [116: 119] [46: 588, 596, 602, 618, 653, 677, 723] [113: 14, 18, 20, 131]

dual vacuity of lung qi and yin 肺气阴两虚 *fèi qì yīn liǎng xū*: See LUNG QI VACUITY; LUNG YIN VACUITY.

dual vacuity of qi and blood 气血俱虚 *qì xuè jù xū*: The simultaneous occurrence of qi and blood vacuity. Because "blood is the mother of qi," blood vacuity causes qi vacuity. Thus, blood vacuity patients often display qi vacuity signs such as shortness of breath and lack of strength. Dual vacuity is treated by dual supplementation of qi and blood, and since "qi engenders blood," the accent is placed on supplementing qi. Thus, the condition Western medicine identifies as anemia is characterized by classic blood vacuity signs such as lusterless facial complexion, pale-colored nails, dizzy head, and heart palpitations, as well as qi vacuity signs such as shortness of breath and lack of strength. Dual vacuity of qi and blood may also develop from failure of vacuous qi to contain the blood. In such cases, the resulting persistent bleeding gives rise to such signs as fatigue and lack of strength, pale tongue, and a soft, soggy pulse. Qi failing to contain the blood is second only to blood heat as a cause of bleeding. MED Supplement both qi and the blood using formulas such as Eight-Gem Decoction (*bā zhēn tāng*) and Tangkuei Blood-Supplementing Decoction (*dāng guī bǔ xuè tāng*). In the latter formula, astragalus (*huáng qí*) should exceed the tangkuei (*dāng guī*) in quantity to place emphasis on supplementing qi. For qi failing to contain the blood, heavy doses of qi-boosting medicinals such as codonopsis (*dǎng shēn*), astragalus (*huáng qí*), and licorice (*gān cǎo*) are combined with small amounts of blood-supplementing medicinals such as tangkuei (*dāng guī*), cooked rehmannia (*shú dì huáng*), and ass hide glue (*ē jiāo*) in variations of Spleen-Returning Decoction (*guī pí tāng*) or Center-Supplementing Qi-Boosting Decoction (*bǔ zhōng yì qì tāng*). ACU Dual vacuity of qi and blood is treated by combining points that supplement both qi and the blood, points that supplement qi, and points that supplement the blood. Base treatment mainly on CV, SP, LU, LR, and back transport points. To supplement both qi and the blood, select ST-36 (*zú sān lǐ*, Leg Three Li), BL-20 (*pí shū*, Spleen Transport), and BL-21 (*wèi shū*, Stomach Transport); needle with supplementation and add moxa. The following points can be used to supplement qi: CV-6 (*qì hǎi*, Sea of Qi), BL-13 (*fèi shū*, Lung Transport), BL-43 (*gāo huāng shū*, Gao-Huang Transport), LU-9 (*tài yuān*, Great Abyss), CV-4 (*guān yuán*, Pass Head), and CV-12 (*zhōng wǎn*, Center Stomach Duct); needle with supplementation and add moxa. The following can be used to supplement the blood: LR-3 (*tài chōng*, Supreme Surge), SP-6 (*sān yīn jiāo*, Three Yin Intersection), BL-17 (*gé shū*, Diaphragm Transport), and LR-13 (*zhāng mén*, Camphorwood Gate). For qi failing to contain the blood, use SP-1 (*yǐn bái*, Hidden White), ST-36 (*zú sān lǐ*, Leg Three Li), CV-4 (*guān yuán*, Pass Head), CV-6 (*qì hǎi*, Sea of Qi), GV-14 (*dà zhuī*, Great Hammer), and GV-20 (*bǎi huì*, Hundred Convergences); needle with supplementation and use large amounts of moxa. [26: 537] [6: 168] [46: 594] [113: 18]

dual vacuity of qi and yin 气阴两虚 *qì yīn liǎng xū*: A pattern of both qi vacuity and yin vacuity commonly occurring in febrile disease. It includes qi vacuity signs such as fatigued spirit and lack of strength, faint low voice, sweating, shortness of breath, torpid intake, and sloppy stool, and yin vacuity signs such as dry mouth, sore throat, vexing heat in the five hearts, postmeridian tidal heat [effusion], and night sweating. It occurs in the following circumstances: (1) Warm heat disease causing wear on the fluids giving rise to a vacuity desertion trend characterized by great sweating, hasty panting, vexation and thirst, pale red or dry crimson tongue, a large diffuse or fine rapid pulse. (2) Advanced-stage warm heat disease and miscellaneous internal damage disease in which depletion of true yin and major damage to original

qi causes lassitude of spirit and physical fatigue, shortage of qi and laziness to speak, dry mouth and pharynx, low fever or tidal heat [effusion] or vexing heat in the five hearts, spontaneous sweating, night sweating, red tongue with scant fur, and a large vacuous or rapid vacuous pulse. (3) Evil lodged in the qi aspect in warm disease causing unthorough sweating that eventually damages qi and humor and and gives rise to the appearance of white miliaria that is dry, white, and sheenless. In addition, dual vacuity of qi and yin is also observed in certain consumptive diseases. MED Boost qi and bank up the origin; enrich yin and downbear fire. Use Pulse-Engendering Powder (*shēng mài sǎn*) or Dryness-Clearing Lung-Rescuing Decoction (*qīng zào jiù fèi tāng*). ACU Base treatment mainly on CV, back transport points, ST, SP, and KI. Select CV-6 (*qì hǎi*, Sea of Qi), ST-36 (*zú sān lǐ*, Leg Three Li), BL-20 (*pí shū*, Spleen Transport), BL-21 (*wèi shū*, Stomach Transport), SP-3 (*tài bái*, Supreme White), and LU-9 (*tài yuān*, Great Abyss) to supplement qi. Select SP-6 (*sān yīn jiāo*, Three Yin Intersection), KI-6 (*zhào hǎi*, Shining Sea), KI-2 (*rán gǔ*, Blazing Valley), and KI-3 (*tài xī*, Great Ravine) to supplement yin. Needle with supplementation at all points. [26: 539] [57: 27] [46: 594] [113: 20]

dual vacuity of stomach qi and yin 胃气阴两虚 *wèi qì yīn liǎng xū*: See STOMACH VACUITY.

dual vacuity of the heart and lung 心肺两虚 *xīn fèi liǎng xū*: See HEART-LUNG QI VACUITY; HEART-LUNG YIN VACUITY; HEART-LUNG YANG VACUITY.

dual vacuity of the heart and spleen 心脾两虚 *xīn pí liǎng xu*: A disease pattern characterized by signs of heart blood vacuity and spleen qi vacuity. Dual vacuity of the heart and spleen arises through excessive thought and anxiety, excessive taxation damage (overwork), enduring illness and improper nourishment, and loss of blood. The chief signs are heart palpitations or fearful throbbing, insomnia and forgetfulness, reduced eating, fatigue, abdominal distention, and sloppy stool. Other signs include withered-yellow facial complexion, and dizzy and flowery vision. In some cases, there may be purple macules under the skin. In women, there may be menstrual irregularities, menstrual block, or flooding and spotting. The tongue is pale and tender. The pulse is fine and forceless. The heart and spleen are closely related. The spleen is the source of qi and blood formation, and also manages the blood. When spleen qi is weak, blood production is insufficient, or blood management breaks down and blood spills out of the vessels. Either case may cause heart blood depletion. The heart governs the blood and vessels. When the blood is abundant, qi is plentiful; when blood is vacuous, qi becomes weak. When heart blood is insufficient and the means to produce qi are lacking, then spleen qi also becomes vacuous. Insufficiency of heart blood deprives the heart of nourishment and causes heart palpitations or fearful throbbing. When the heart spirit is disquieted, and fails to keep to its abode, there is insomnia and profuse dreaming. Insufficiency of the blood depriving the head and eyes of nourishment causes dizziness and forgetfulness; when depriving the skin of nourishment, the facial complexion becomes withered-yellow and lusterless. Spleen qi vacuity with impaired movement and transformation causes poor appetite, abdominal distention, and sloppy stool. Qi vacuity with a generalized reduction in physiological function causes lack of strength and lassitude of spirit. Spleen qi vacuity with no power to contain the blood causes chronic bleeding. Insufficiency of qi and blood causes a pale tender tongue, and a weak fine pulse. WMC anemia; purpura; dysfunctional metrorrhagia. MED Supplement the heart and spleen. Use Spleen-Returning Decoction (*guī pí tāng*). ACU Base treatment mainly on back transport points, HT, SP, and CV. Select BL-15 (*xīn shū*, Heart Transport), BL-20 (*pí shū*, Spleen Transport), BL-17 (*gé shū*, Diaphragm Transport), CV-6 (*qì hǎi*, Sea of Qi), HT-7 (*shén mén*, Spirit Gate), ST-36 (*zú sān lǐ*, Leg Three Li), SP-10 (*xuè hǎi*, Sea of Blood), and SP-6 (*sān yīn jiāo*, Three Yin Intersection); needle with supplementation and add moxa. **Comparison:** Dual vacuity of the heart and spleen, heart-spleen blood vacuity, heart-spleen qi vacuity, and heart-spleen yang vacuity are four distinct patterns involving the same two viscera. Heart palpitations occurs in all of them. Dual vacuity of the heart and spleen and heart-spleen blood vacuity are both marked by heart palpitations, insomnia, and profuse dreaming. Dual vacuity of the heart and spleen is a combination of heart blood vacuity with spleen qi vacuity, and is marked by spleen qi vacuity signs such as abdominal distention and sloppy stool. It therefore differs from heart-spleen blood vacuity, which is a combination of heart blood vacuity and "spleen blood vacuity" (actually spleen qi vacuity and insufficient formation of qi and blood), in which abdominal signs are absent. Heart-spleen qi vacuity is characterized by heart palpitations, spontaneous sweating, shortness of breath, reduced eating, abdominal distention, pale enlarged tongue, and a vacuous pulse, whereas heart blood vacuity is marked by reduced sleep, vexation and agitation, profuse dreaming, pale lips, and a fine pulse. Heart-spleen yang vacuity is similar to heart-spleen qi vacuity, but is more severe and characterized by pronounced exterior cold signs. [57: 93] [27: 149] [27: 148] [97: 121] [37: 351] [46: 585, 586]

dual vacuity of the liver and spleen 肝脾两虚 *gān pí liǎng xū*: A disease pattern of spleen vacuity and liver blood vacuity. The main signs are dizzy head and flowery vision, torpid intake and sloppy stool. Other signs may include numbness of the limbs, dry eyes, pale white lips, fatigue and lack of strength, lusterless nails, pale white or withered-yellow facial complexion, abdominal distention after eating, and scant pale menstrual flow. The tongue is pale white and lusterless. The pulse is fine and weak or fine and soggy. **Analysis:** The liver governs the blood and free coursing. The spleen manages the blood, governs movement and transformation, and is the source of formation of blood and qi. When splenic movement is strong, blood is engendered and does not stray from the vessels, so that liver has blood to store. Dual vacuity of the liver and spleen can arise when the spleen is vacuous, and either the source of qi and blood is reduced or the spleen fails to manage blood. When liver blood is insufficient, it cannot ascend to nourish the head and eyes, hence dizzy head, flowery vision, dry eyes, pale white or withered-yellow facial complexion, and pale white lips. When liver blood is insufficient, the sinews are deprived of nourishment, hence the numbness of the limbs and lusterless nails. When splenic movement is impaired, there is distention after eating. When spleen qi is insufficient, the body is inadequately nourished, so there is fatigue and lack of strength. When blood and qi are depleted, the menstrual flow is scant and pale. The lusterless pale white tongue and the soggy fine pulse are also signs of qi blood depletion. MED Boost the liver and fortify the spleen. Use Eight-Gem Decoction (*bā zhēn tāng*). ACU Base treatment mainly on back transport points, LR, SP, and CV. Select BL-18 (*gān shū*, Liver Transport), BL-20 (*pí shū*, Spleen Transport), BL-17 (*gé shū*, Diaphragm Transport), CV-6 (*qì hǎi*, Sea of Qi), ST-36 (*zú sān lǐ*, Leg Three Li), LR-13 (*zhāng mén*, Camphorwood Gate), LR-3 (*tài chōng*, Supreme Surge), and GB-41 (*zú lín qì*, Foot Overlooking Tears); needle with supplementation and moxa. [116: 147] [46: 585, 589]

dual vacuity of the lung and kidney 肺肾两虚 *fèi shèn liǎng xū*: Simultaneous vacuity of both the lung and kidney. Distinction is made between lung-kidney yin vacuity and lung qi vacuity with kidney yang vacuity. Lung-kidney yin vacuity is characterized by cough, night sweating, vexing heat in the five hearts, tidal heat [effusion], and seminal emission. Lung qi vacuity with kidney yang vacuity is characterized by cough, shortness of breath, spontaneous sweating, fear of cold, cold limbs, and in some cases swelling. MED For lung-kidney yin vacuity, use Lily Bulb Metal-Securing Decoction (*bǎi hé gù jīn tāng*) or Ophiopogon and

Rehmannia Pill (*mài wèi dì huáng wán*). For lung qi vacuity with kidney yang vacuity, use Golden Coffer Kidney Qi Pill (*jīn guì shèn qì wán*) combined with Lung-Supplementing Decoction (*bǔ fèi tāng*). ACU For lung-kidney yin vacuity, base treatment mainly on back transport points, LU, and KI. Select BL-13 (*fèi shū*, Lung Transport), BL-23 (*shèn shū*, Kidney Transport), BL-43 (*gāo huāng shū*, Gao-Huang Transport), LU-5 (*chǐ zé*, Cubit Marsh), KI-3 (*tài xī*, Great Ravine), and KI-6 (*zhào hǎi*, Shining Sea); needle with supplementation. For lung qi vacuity with kidney yang vacuity, base treatment mainly on back transport points, LU, KI, and CV. Select BL-13 (*fèi shū*, Lung Transport), BL-23 (*shèn shū*, Kidney Transport), BL-43 (*gāo huāng shū*, Gao-Huang Transport), GV-4 (*mìng mén*, Life Gate), CV-6 (*qì hǎi*, Sea of Qi), CV-4 (*guān yuán*, Pass Head), LU-9 (*tài yuān*, Great Abyss), KI-3 (*tài xī*, Great Ravine), and ST-36 (*zú sān lǐ*, Leg Three Li); needle with supplementation and large amounts of moxa. [26: 449] [46: 584, 587, 653, 655] [37: 273, 279, 280]

dual vacuity of the spleen and lung 脾肺两 虚 *pí fèi liǎng xū*: Synonym: *spleen-lung vacuity*; *spleen-lung qi vacuity*. Vacuity of both spleen and lung with signs of spleen vacuity such as reduced food intake, sloppy stool, and abdominal distention, and signs of lung vacuity such as shortness of breath, cough, copious phlegm and spontaneous sweating. MED Bank up earth to engender metal. Use Six Gentlemen Decoction (*liù jūn zǐ tāng*) or variations of Ginseng, Poria (Hoelen), and Ovate Atractylodes Powder (*shēn líng bái zhú sǎn*). ACU Base treatment mainly on back transport points, LU, SP, and CV. Select BL-13 (*fèi shū*, Lung Transport), BL-20 (*pí shū*, Spleen Transport), BL-43 (*gāo huāng shū*, Gao-Huang Transport), CV-12 (*zhōng wǎn*, Center Stomach Duct), LR-13 (*zhāng mén*, Camphorwood Gate), LU-9 (*tài yuān*, Great Abyss), SP-3 (*tài bái*, Supreme White), CV-6 (*qì hǎi*, Sea of Qi), and ST-36 (*zú sān lǐ*, Leg Three Li); needle with supplementation and large amounts of moxa. [46: 584, 585, 594] [26: 747] [57: 104]

dual vacuity of yin and yang 阴阳两虚 *yīn yáng liǎng xū*: Vacuity of the yin and yang of the bowels and viscera, especially of kidney yin and kidney yang or vacuity of qi and blood. It arises through the mechanism of detriment to yin affecting yang, detriment to yang affecting yin, or detriment to both yin and yang. Yin or yang vacuity may be more pronounced depending on the pathomechanism involved. The main signs are fear of cold and cold limbs, fatigue and lack of strength, shortage of qi and laziness to speak, spontaneous sweating and night sweating, postmeridian tidal heat [effusion], and vexing heat in the five hearts. Other signs include dullness of essence-spirit, emaciation, heart palpitations and insomnia, and dizzy head and vision. The tongue is enlarged and tender. The pulse is fine, rapid, and forceless. MED Enrich yin and assist yang. Use Golden Coffer Kidney Qi Pill (*jīn guì shèn qì wán*). [26: 622] [57: 24]

duck's slop 鹜溏 *wù táng*, 鸭溏 *yā táng*: From *Elementary Questions* (*sù wèn, zhì zhēn yào dà lùn*). Diarrhea with sloppy stool resembling duck's droppings; generally forms part of a cold-damp pattern resulting from spleen dampness and cold in the large intestine and includes other signs such as clear urine and a slow sunken pulse. ◇ Chin 鸭 *yā*, domestic duck; 溏 *táng*, slop, semiliquid. Eng *slop*, dung, slime, pulp. [27: 364] [97: 466] [26: 983]

dull pain 隐痛 *yǐn tòng*: An unpronounced, usually continuous pain; attributable to insufficiency of qi and blood. See PAIN. [29: 190]

dulu 嘟嚕 *dū lū*: An earthenware pot of varying size used for calcining materials. See CALCINATION. [82: 65]

dwelling place 府 *fǔ*: See HOUSE.

dysentery 痢疾 *lì jí*: A disease characterized by abdominal pain, tenesmus, and stool containing pus and blood (described as mucoid and bloody stool in Western medicine). Dysentery usually occurs in hot weather and arises when gastrointestinal vacuity and eating raw, cold, or unclean food allow damp-heat or other evils to brew in the intestines. It takes the form of vacuity or repletion. Depending on the cause, distinction is made between summerheat dysentery, damp-heat dysentery, cold dysentery, and heat dysentery. Depending on the nature of the stool, distinction is made between RED DYSENTERY (blood in the stool), WHITE DYSENTERY (pus in the stool), and RED AND WHITE DYSENTERY (stool containing pus and blood). Depending on the condition of the patient and stage of the disease, distinction is made between EPIDEMIC DYSENTERY; FOOD-DENYING DYSENTERY, INTERMITTENT DYSENTERY, ENDURING DYSENTERY, and VACUITY DYSENTERY. MED Repletion patterns are treated by clearing heat and transforming dampness, cooling the blood and resolving toxin, and dispersing accumulation and abducting stagnation. Vacuity patterns are treated by supplementing the center and boosting qi and promoting astriction and stemming desertion. ◇ Chin 痢 *lì* is composed of 利 *lì*, uninhibited, with the illness signifier 疒 *chuáng*. In earlier texts, it was used in the less specific sense of "diarrhea" (uninhibited movement of the bowels). Eng from Gk. *dys*, bad, abnormal + *enter(on)*, intestine + *ia*, noun suffix. [26: 673] [97: 588] [27: 360]

dysphagia-occlusion 噎膈 *yē gé*: A disease characterized by sensation of blockage on swallowing, difficulty in getting food and drink down, and, in some cases, immediate vomiting of ingested food. The Chinese term is a compound of *yē* meaning difficulty in swallowing (dysphagia), and *gé* meaning blockage preventing food from going down (occlusion). Dysphagia and occlusion may occur independently. Dysphagia most commonly but not necessarily develops into occlusion. There are four principal patterns: phlegm and qi obstructing each other, liquid depletion and heat bind, static blood binding internally, and qi vacuity and yang debilitation. **Phlegm and qi obstructing each other** arises when anxiety and thought cause qi to bind and engender phlegm, so that the two contend with each other and obstruct the gullet. The main signs are difficulty in swallowing with glomus and fullness in the chest and diaphragm. Relief experienced when the patient is emotionally calm reflects the early stages when qi is binding. Dry mouth and throat reflect depressed heat damaging liquid or binding qi preventing the upward supply of fluids. A tongue that tends to be red, a thin slimy tongue fur, and a fine slippery stringlike pulse are signs of depressed qi and obstructing phlegm with depressed heat damaging liquid. MED Rectify qi and relieve depression; transform phlegm and moisten dryness. Use Diaphragm-Arousing Powder (*qǐ gé sǎn*). ACU Base treatment mainly on back transporting points, CV, ST, LR, and GB. Select BL-20 (*pí shū*, Spleen Transport), BL-21 (*wèi shū*, Stomach Transport), CV-22 (*tiān tú*, Celestial Chimney), CV-17 (*shān zhōng*, Chest Center), CV-12 (*zhōng wǎn*, Center Stomach Duct), ST-21 (*liáng mén*, Beam Gate), BL-18 (*gān shū*, Liver Transport), LR-2 (*xíng jiān*, Moving Between), and GB-34 (*yáng líng quán*, Yang Mound Spring); needle with drainage. **Liquid depletion and heat bind** is characterized by roughness and pain on swallowing. Solid foods are harder to swallow than liquids. There is emaciation, dry mouth, dry bound stool, vexing heat in the five hearts, a red dry tongue that may be fissured, and a rapid fine stringlike pulse. It arises when stomach liquid is depleted and the gullet is deprived of nourishment. Vexing heat in the five hearts and emaciation reflect insufficiency of stomach liquid with increasing kidney yin depression and yin vacuity internal heat. The tongue and pulse reflect severe liquid depletion and pronounced heat. MED Enrich the fluids. Use Five Juices Center-Quieting Beverage (*wǔ zhī ān zhōng yǐn*). ACU Base treatment mainly on back transporting points, CV, ST, and KI. Select BL-23 (*shèn shū*, Kidney Transport), BL-17 (*gé shū*, Diaphragm Transport), SP-6 (*sān yīn jiāo*, Three Yin Intersection), KI-2 (*rán gǔ*, Blazing Valley), KI-6 (*zhào hǎi*, Shining Sea), ST-44 (*nèi tíng*, Inner Court), LI-4 (*hé gǔ*, Union Valley), CV-17 (*shān zhōng*, Chest Center), and CV-12 (*zhōng wǎn*, Center Stomach Duct); needle

with drainage. For dry bound stool, drain SP-14 (*fù jié*, Abdominal Bind), and ST-37 (*shàng jù xū*, Upper Great Hollow). **Static blood binding internally** is characterized by pain, with difficulty in swallowing both solids and liquids. Stool is like sheep's droppings, scant and hard. In some cases there is vomiting of matter like the juice of rice bean (*chì xiǎo dòu*). There is emaciation, dry skin, red tongue with little liquid (may be green-blue or purple), and a rough fine pulse. The stool reflects enduring disease that has damaged yin. The vomiting of matter like red bean juice indicates damage to network vessels. Prolonged inability to swallow food leads to exhaustion of the source of engendering transformation (reduced food assimilation), which causes emaciation and dry skin. The tongue and pulse reflect depletion of yin-blood and static blood binding internally. MED Enrich yin and nourish the blood; break the bind and move stasis. Use Dark-Gate–Freeing Decoction (*tōng yōu tāng*). ACU Base treatment mainly on back transport points, SP, and LR. Select BL-17 (*gé shū*, Diaphragm Transport), BL-18 (*gān shū*, Liver Transport), BL-46 (*gé guān*, Diaphragm Pass), CV-17 (*shān zhōng*, Chest Center), CV-12 (*zhōng wǎn*, Center Stomach Duct), LR-3 (*tài chōng*, Supreme Surge), SP-10 (*xuè hǎi*, Sea of Blood), and SP-6 (*sān yīn jiāo*, Three Yin Intersection); needle with drainage. **Qi vacuity and yang debilitation** causes inability to swallow food with bright white facial complexion, exhaustion of essence-spirit, physical cold, shortness of breath, ejection of clear drool, puffy face, swollen feet, abdominal distention, pale tongue with white fur, and a weak fine or fine sunken pulse. This pattern arises, in severe cases, when detriment to yin affects yang. Ejection of clear drool and devitalized essence-spirit reflects an inability to get food down. The puffy face, swollen feet, and abdominal distention reflects spleen-kidney debilitation. The bright white facial complexion, physical cold and shortness of breath, as well as the tongue and pulse are signs of debilitation of original yang. MED Warm and supplement the spleen and kidney. To warm the spleen use Qi-Supplementing Spleen-Moving Decoction (*bǔ qì yùn pí tāng*); to warm the kidney, use Right-Restoring [Life Gate] Pill (*yòu guī wán*). ACU Base treatment mainly on back transporting points, CV, SP, and ST. Select BL-23 (*shèn shū*, Kidney Transport), BL-20 (*pí shū*, Spleen Transport), BL-21 (*wèi shū*, Stomach Transport), CV-6 (*qì hǎi*, Sea of Qi), BL-17 (*gé shū*, Diaphragm Transport), ST-36 (*zú sān lǐ*, Leg Three Li), SP-4 (*gōng sūn*, Yellow Emperor), KI-3 (*tài xī*, Great Ravine), and Central Eminence (*zhōng kuí*); needle with supplementation and add moxa. For pronounced yang vacuity, moxa GV-4 (*mìng mén*, Life Gate). **Comparison:** Dysphagia-occlusion is similar to STOMACH REFLUX, PLUM-PIT QI, and BLOCK AND REPULSION. Both dysphagia-occlusion and *stomach reflux* are characterized by vomiting of ingested food. Dysphagia-occlusion is largely associated with yin vacuity and heat, and is characterized principally by difficulty in swallowing and blockage preventing downflow that causes food to be brought up in small amounts. Stomach reflux is largely ascribed to yang vacuity with cold and is characterized by no difficulty in getting food down, and by vomiting of ingested food after a long period, usually described as "vomiting in the morning of food ingested in the evening, and vomiting in the evening of food ingested in the morning." Dysphagia-occlusion is also similar to *plum pit qi*.

However, while the former is associated with a palpable blockage of the gullet, plum pit qi is associated only with a feeling of blockage that is caused by qi counterflow and phlegm blockage (formless or intangible evil) that does not cause difficulty in swallowing food. *Block and repulsion* is also similar, but is associated with urinary and fecal blockage. Dysphagia-occlusion is the result of factors such as seven-affect internal damage, intemperate eating and drinking, sexual taxation, and debilitation of essence in old age. [106: 202–205] [80: 275] [92: 198] [26: 888] [27: 410] [97: 637] [37: 300] [46: 670]

dyspnea 喘 *chuǎn*: PANTING.

E

ear 耳 *ěr*: Organ of hearing; orifice of the kidney. The ear's hearing ability depends on the state of essence, marrow, qi, and blood. **Diagnosis:** Ear diseases are largely related to the kidney, but may also be related to the heart, liver, and spleen. The hand greater yang (*tài yáng*) small intestine channel, foot greater yang (*tài yáng*) bladder channel, and hand lesser yang (*shào yáng*) triple burner channel all pass through the region of the ear. The withering of the auricles and shrinking of the lobes in the course of enduring or severe illness is a sign of qi and blood depletion and impending expiration of kidney qi. In recent years, extensive research into ear acupuncture has shown that some diseases of the bowels and viscera are reflected by changes in ear point reactivity. See DISEASES OF THE EAR. [26: 246]

ear acupuncture 耳针 *ěr zhēn*, 耳针疗法 *ěr zhēn liǎo fǎ*: A method of treatment that involves the needling of specific points of the ear. In a wider sense, it also includes massage, medicinal injections, and application of pressure to seeds or metal balls at specific points. When needling ear points, the needle is inserted and rotated for a few seconds. The needle may be retained for 30–60 minutes, during which time the needle may be rotated at intervals. Needles may also be implanted. Ear acupuncture has broad applications. The action of each point is usually indicated by the name. Points named after organs or parts of the body are used to treat diseases of those organs or parts. For example, the anus point is used to treat itching anus, splitting of the anus, hemorrhoids, and prolapse of the rectum; the toe, heel, ankle, and knee points are used to treat pain and stiffness in those areas. Points named after diseases or therapeutic actions treat those diseases or have those therapeutic actions. Thus, the allergy point treats allergies, whereas the panting-calming point relieves coughing and panting. A small number of points are named by their position on the auricle. These include helix points 1–6, which all treat disease of the tonsils and the apex point, which abates heat, reduces inflammation, lowers blood pressure, and resuscitates. Some ear points can be used in acupuncture anesthesia. [26: 248]

ear gate 耳门 *ěr mén*: **1.** The tonguelike projection in front of the ear. WMC tragus. **2.** TB-21 (*ěr mén*, Ear Gate), which is located at the tragus. [27: 63]

earlier heaven 先天 *xiān tiān*: What is received from the parents at an individual's conception; the congenital constitution. Earlier heaven is understood to be governed by the kidney, in opposition to later heaven (or the acquired constitution) governed by the spleen. ◇ Chin 先 *xiān*, first, earlier; 天 *tiān*, heaven, i.e., that upon which life depends. [97: 212] [26: 65]

ear lock 锐发 *ruì fà*: The lock of hair in front of the ear. [27: 63]

early morning diarrhea 晨泄 *chén xiè*: See FIFTH-WATCH DIARRHEA.

ear mushroom 耳菌 *ěr jùn*, 耳蕈 *ěr xùn*: Synonym: *ear pile*. A growth on the ear, bulbous in form and attached to the body by a thinner stem. An ear mushroom may be associated with slight pain, and pressure may cause pain stretching to the vertex of the head. It gradually grows in time and may block the ear hole or hang out of it. It can cause hearing impairment. It is attributed to congealing and gathering of liver and kidney channel fire toxin. WMC benign neoplasm of the ear. MED Clear the liver and drain fire using Gardenia Liver-Clearing Decoction (*zhī zǐ qīng gān tāng*). Sal Ammoniac Powder (*náo shā sǎn*) can be applied topically. [26: 250] [27: 494]

ear pain 耳痛 *ěr tòng*: Pain within the ear, usually associated with reduced hearing ability. Ear pain patterns are identified by attending signs. The main patterns are liver-gallbladder wind-heat, wind with damp-heat, vacuity fire, and qi-blood stasis obstruction. **Liver-gallbladder wind-heat** ear pain is attended by itching. Concurrence of intense triple burner and ministerial fire is characterized by swelling and distention. MED Treat by coursing wind and clearing heat with formulas such as Diaphragm-Cooling Powder (*liáng gé sǎn*). Intense triple burner and ministerial fire is treated by clearing and discharging liver, gallbladder, and triple burner fire, using formulas like Gentian Liver-Draining Decoction (*lóng dǎn xiè gān tāng*). ACU Base treatment mainly on GB, TB, and LI. Select GB-20 (*fēng chí*, Wind Pool), TB-5 (*wài guān*, Outer Pass), TB-17 (*yì fēng*, Wind Screen), GB-2 (*tīng huì*, Auditory Convergence), LI-4 (*hé gǔ*, Union Valley), GV-14 (*dà zhuī*, Great Hammer), and GB-34 (*yáng líng quán*, Yang Mound Spring); needle with drainage. For concurrent intense triple burner and ministerial fire, add TB-3 (*zhōng zhǔ*, Central Islet) and prick TB-1 (*guān chōng,* Passage Hub) to bleed. **Wind evil with damp-heat** causes pain accompanied by erosion and watery discharge. MED Dispel wind, eliminate dampness, and clear heat with formulas such as Sweet Dew Toxin-Dispersing Elixir (*gān lù xiāo dú dān*), minus cardamom (*bái dòu kòu*) and agastache/patchouli (*huò xiāng*) plus large gentian (*qín jiāo*), ledebouriella (*fáng fēng*), and silkworm (*bái jiāng cán*). ACU Base treatment mainly on GB, TB, LI, SP, and ST. Select GB-20 (*fēng chí,* Wind Pool), TB-5 (*wài guān,* Outer Pass), TB-17 (*yì fēng,* Wind Screen), SI-19 (*tīng gōng,* Auditory Palace), TB-3 (*zhōng zhǔ,* Central Islet), LI-11 (*qū chí,* Pool at the Bend), LI-4 (*hé gǔ,* Union Valley), ST-36 (*zú sān lǐ,* Leg Three Li), SP-9 (*yīn líng quán,* Yin Mound Spring), and GB-34 (*yáng líng quán,* Yang Mound Spring); needle with drainage. **Vacuity fire** ear pain is characterized by mild pain and dizziness upon standing up after crouching. MED Nourish the blood and enrich yin with Anemarrhena, Phellodendron, and Rehmannia Pill (*zhī bǎi dì huáng wán*). ACU Base treatment mainly on KI and TB. Select BL-23 (*shèn shū,* Kidney Transport), KI-3 (*tài xī,* Great Ravine), TB-17 (*yì fēng,* Wind Screen), TB-21 (*ěr mén,* Ear Gate), and TB-3 (*zhōng zhǔ,* Central Islet); needle with even supplementation and drainage. **Qi-blood stasis obstruction** is characterized by a pulling pain in the ear with clouded head and tinnitus, thin tongue fur, dark tongue, and a fine rough pulse. MED Clear and drain liver heat; quicken the network vessels and free the orifices. Use Gentian Liver-Draining Decoction (*lóng dǎn xiè gān tāng*) combined with Four Agents Decoction (*sì wù tāng*). ACU Base treatment mainly on TB, LR, and SP. Select TB-17 (*yì fēng,* Wind Screen), TB-3 (*zhōng zhǔ,* Central Islet), SP-10 (*xuè hǎi,* Sea of Blood), LR-3 (*tài chōng,* Supreme Surge), and SP-6 (*sān yīn jiāo,* Three Yin Intersection) as the main points. For gallbladder heat evil, add GB-2 (*tīng huì,* Auditory Convergence), GB-43 (*xiá xī,* Pinched Ravine), and LR-2 (*xíng jiān,* Moving Between), needling with drainage. For external injury with congealing qi and blood, add TB-21 (*ěr mén,* Ear Gate) and LI-4 (*hé gǔ,* Union Valley); needle with even supplementation and drainage and if necessary prick to bleed with a three-edged needle. [26: 250] [50: 503] [46: 595, 618, 723] [113: 486] [13: 699]

ear pile 耳痔 *ěr zhì*: EAR MUSHROOM.

earth 土 *tǔ*: In the doctrine of the five phases, the phase associated with the season of long summer, the spleen (and stomach), the flavor sweetness, and the color yellow. [6: 28]

earth engenders the myriad things 土生万物 *tǔ shēng wàn wù*: The earth produces plant life on which man and animals feed. In the body, spleen belongs to earth; it extracts the essence of grain and water (nutrients in foodstuffs) that nurtures the whole body. [27: 13] [97: 27]

earth failing to dam water 土不制水 *tǔ bù zhì shuǐ*: In the five phases, the spleen belongs to earth and the kidney belongs to water. Normally, the spleen restrains the fluids and ensures their normal movement and transformation, thereby preventing diseases characterized by the flooding of water. When spleen-earth is weak, it fails to restrain water-damp, causing water swelling or phlegm-rheum. NB: Water in this context refers to fluid in the body rather than to the kidney, the viscus belonging to water in the doctrine of the five phases. [27: 13] [97: 27]

earth level 地部 *dì bù*: The lower third of the insertion range of a needle, i.e., the lower third of the distance between the surface of the body and the point of deepest insertion. See HEAVEN, HUMAN, AND EARTH.

earth likes warmth and dryness 土喜温燥 *tǔ xǐ wēn zào*: Earth needs fresh water to produce crops, but if inadequately drained, it remains permanently damp and soggy, and therefore less productive. Its production is greatly increased by warmth. Similarly, the spleen, the viscus that corresponds to earth in the body, needs liquid as well as solid food (water and grain) to supply the body with nutrients (essence of grain and water). However, impairment of the splenic movement and transformation can give rise to water-damp in the body with inhibited urination, water swelling, and phlegm-rheum; conversely, exuberant water-damp and ingestion of raw and cold food places an added burden on the spleen's movement and transformation function. Through five-phase correspondences, "earth likes warmth and dryness" sums up these physiological and pathological characteristics. [27: 13] [97: 27]

earth rampart 地廓 *dì kuò*: See EIGHT RAMPARTS. [27: 500]

Eastern Jin 东晋 *dōng jìn*: The name of a dynasty (A.D. 317–420).

Eastern (Later) 东汉 *dōng hàn*: The name of a dynasty (A.D. 25–220).

Eastern medicine 东医 *dōng yī*: Chinese medicine as it is known in Korea and Japan. [27: 514]

Eastern Wei 东魏 *dōng wèi*: The name of a dynasty (A.D. 534–550).

Eastern Zhou 东周 *dōng zhōu*: The name of a dynasty (770–256 B.C.).

eclampsia 妊娠痫症 *rèn shēn xián zhèng*, 子痫 *zǐ xián*: See EPILEPSY OF PREGNANCY. [26: 341]

efflux 滑 *huá*: Denotes uncontrollable loss of urine, and especially stool or semen. The term occurs in the phrases "seminal efflux," "efflux desertion" (see DESERTION), and "efflux diarrhea" (see DIAR-RHEA). See also EXUBERANCE AND DEBILITATION.

efflux desertion 滑脱 *huá tuō*: See DESERTION.

efflux diarrhea 滑泄 *huá xiè*: Diarrhea with loss of voluntary continence; results when enduring diarrhea causes qi fall. The diarrhea is uncontrollable and may occur in the day or night without regularity. Other signs include reduced intake of food and drink, reversal cold of the limbs, sometimes swelling of the limbs, physical cold and shortness of breath, emaciation, and in some cases heat. Distinction is made between cold and heat. **Cold efflux** is efflux characterized by pronounced cold signs. ⌑MED⌑ Use Five Pillars Powder (*bā zhù sǎn*). ⌑ACU⌑ Base treatment mainly on GV, LU, CV, ST, and SP. Select GV-20 (*bǎi huì*, Hundred Convergences), CV-12 (*zhōng wǎn*, Center Stomach Duct), CV-6 (*qì hǎi*, Sea of Qi), CV-4 (*guān yuán*, Pass Head), ST-25 (*tiān shū*, Celestial Pivot), CV-9 (*shuǐ fēn*, Water Divide), ST-21 (*liáng mén*, Beam Gate), and SP-6 (*sān yīn jiāo*, Three Yin Intersection); needle with supplementation and large amounts of moxa. Perform moxibustion on salt or ginger at CV-8 (*shén què*, Spirit Gate Tower). **Heat efflux** is efflux characterized by pronounced heat signs. ⌑MED⌑ Use Intestine-Securing Pill (*gù cháng wán*) or Chebule Powder (*hē zǐ sǎn*). ⌑ACU⌑ Base treatment mainly on GV, CV, ST, and SP. Select GV-20 (*bǎi huì*, Hundred Convergences), GV-14 (*dà zhuī*, Great Hammer), CV-12 (*zhōng wǎn*, Center Stomach Duct), ST-21 (*liáng mén*, Beam Gate), ST-25 (*tiān shū*, Celestial Pivot), ST-36 (*zú sān lǐ*, Leg Three Li), LI-11 (*qū chí*, Pool at the Bend), ST-44 (*nèi tíng*, Inner Court), SP-6 (*sān yīn jiāo*, Three Yin Intersection), and ST-37 (*shàng jù xū*, Upper Great Hollow); needle with even supplementation and drainage. Moxa CV-12 (*zhōng wǎn*, Center Stomach Duct). See also EFFLUX. [26: 759] [97: 584] [46: 665] [113: 89] [37: 323]

effulgent 旺 *wàng*: Exuberant (of heat or fire). See HEAT.

effulgent gallbladder fire 胆火旺盛 *dǎn huǒ wàng shèng*: See GALLBLADDER HEAT.

effulgent heart fire 心火旺 *xīn huǒ wàng*: See HEART FIRE.

effulgent heart-liver fire 心肝火旺 *xīn gān huǒ wàng*: A disease pattern characterized by signs of both liver fire and heart fire. The chief signs are sleeplessness, distention and fullness in the chest and rib-side, and generalized heat [effusion]. Other signs include red face, red eyes, bitter taste in the mouth, yellow urine, dry stool, vexation, agitation, and irascibility. In some cases there is mania or blood ejection or spontaneous external bleeding. The tongue is red with dry yellow fur. The pulse is stringlike, rapid, and forceful. ⌑MED⌑ Clear the liver, drain fire, and quiet the heart. Use Coptis Toxin-Resolving Decoction (*huáng lián jiě dú tāng*). **Comparison:** Effulgent heart-liver fire is similar to *liver fire flaming upward*. Both have heat effusion, red eyes, thirst, yellow urine, and dry stool. Effulgent heart-liver fire differs by the additional presence of signs of heart fire flaming upward such as insomnia, mania, and blood ejection or spontaneous external bleeding. [116: 135]

effulgent life gate fire 命门火旺 *mìng mén huǒ wàng*: HYPERACTIVE KIDNEY FIRE.

effulgent liver yang 肝阳偏旺 *gān yáng piān wàng*: See ASCENDANT HYPERACTIVITY OF LIVER YANG.

effulgent yin depletion fire 阴亏火旺 *yīn kuī huǒ wàng*: EFFULGENT YIN VACUITY FIRE.

effulgent yin vacuity fire 阴虚火旺 *yīn xū huǒ wàng*: Synonym: *exuberant yin vacuity fire*. A strong fire that arises from yin vacuity according to the principle that when yin is vacuous, heat develops internally. Effulgent yin vacuity fire is characterized by vexation, agitation, and irascibility, reddening of the cheeks, dry mouth and sore throat, and excessive libido. ⌑ACU⌑ Needle with supplementation at BL-23 (*shèn shū*, Kidney Transport), KI-3 (*tài xī*, Great Ravine), and SP-6 (*sān yīn jiāo*, Three Yin Intersection), and with drainage at KI-6 (*zhào hǎi*, Shining Sea), KI-2 (*rán gǔ*, Blazing Valley), BL-17 (*gé shū*, Diaphragm Transport), ST-36 (*zú sān lǐ*, Leg Three Li), ST-44 (*nèi tíng*, Inner Court), and HT-7 (*shén mén*, Spirit Gate). If there is effulgent fire, prick HT-8 (*shào fǔ*, Lesser Mansion) to bleed. Compare YIN VACUITY WITH YANG HYPERACTIVITY. [26: 619] [27: 128] [97: 235]

effuse 发 *fā*: To move outward, as sweat through the interstices; to induce such movement. For example, "effuse the exterior" means to induce sweating so that evils located in the exterior can escape.

effusing sweat 发汗 *fā hàn*: SWEATING[2]

effusion 发 *fā*: **1.** The act of effusing; see EFFUSE. **2.** A large severe WELLING-ABSCESS (*yōng*) or FLAT-ABSCESS (*jū*), e.g., *effusion of the back*. ◇ Chin 发 *fā*, emit, issue, present an appearance. [27: 168]

effusion of the back 发背 *fā bèi*: A HEADED FLAT-ABSCESS of the back, usually on the governing (*dū*) vessel or bladder channel and attributable to stagnation in the channels and blockage of qi and blood stemming either from fire toxin brewing internally or exuberant yin vacuity fire. Distinction is made between effusions of different locations. Effusions of the upper back are located at BL-10 (*tiān zhù*, Celestial Pillar); effusions of the middle of the back are located at GV-8 (*jīn suō*, Sinew Contraction); effusions of the lower back are located at GV-4 (*mìng mén*, Life Gate); reachable sores of the upper back are located at BL-13 (*fèi* *shū*, Lung Transport); reachable sores of the middle of the back are located at BL-43 (*gāo huāng shū*, Gao-Huang Transport); reachable sores of the lower back are located at BL-23 (*shèn shū*, Kidney Transport) and BL-51 (*huāng mén*, Huang Gate). See also REACHABLE SORE; WELLING-ABSCESS. ◇ Chin 发 *fā*, effuse; 背 *bèi*, back. [26: 718] [27: 458] [97: 169] [61: 89]

effusion of the brain 发脑 *fā nǎo*: A HEADED FLAT-ABSCESS located on the pillow bone (occipital bone) or in the region of GB-20 (*fēng chí*, Wind Pool). [26: 719]

effusion of the breast 乳发 *rǔ fā*, 发乳 *fā rǔ*: *Synonym: shell-bursting mammary welling-abscess (yōng).* A severe MAMMARY WELLING-ABSCESS that putrefies after bursting, quickly spreads, and easily gives rise to the development of fistulae. WMC cellulitis of the breast; necrotic cellulitis of the breast. [26: 378] [96: 63]

eggplant disease 茄子疾 *qié zi jí*: YIN PROTRUSION.

eggplant yin 阴茄 *yīn qié*: YIN PROTRUSION.

eight extraordinary vessels 奇经八脉 *qí jīng bā mài*: *Synonym: extraordinary vessels.* Any of the eight vessels that do not home to any organs, have no interior-exterior relationships, and whose function is to supplement the insufficiencies of the other channels. The eight extraordinary vessels are the governing (*dū*), controlling (*rèn*), thoroughfare (*chōng*), girdling (*dài*), yang linking (*yáng wéi*), yin linking (*yīn wéi*), yang springing (*yáng qiāo*), and yin springing (*yīn qiāo*) vessels. ◇ Chin 奇 *qí*, extraordinary, strange, wondrous; 经 *jīng*, channel; 八 *bā*, eight; 脉 *mài*, vessel, pulse; line, range. [27: 85] [97: 329]

eight meeting points 八会穴 *bā huì xué*: A set of eight points, each of which treats diseases of one of eight physiological entities: the viscera, bowels, qi, blood, sinews, marrow, vessels, and bones (see Table 3). Application: The meeting points are used to treat a general category of disease and are combined with others to address the specific needs of a patient. For example, BL-17 (*gé shū*, Diaphragm Transport), the meeting point of the blood, can be combined with SP-1 (*yǐn bái*, Hidden White) and LR-1 (*dà dūn*, Large Pile) to treat flooding and spotting, and GB-34 (*yáng líng quán*, Yang Mound Spring), the meeting point of the sinews, can be coupled with local points in the treatment of sprains and strains in any part of the body. [27: 101] [97: 11]

3.	Eight Meeting Points
Viscera	LR-13 (*zhāng mén*, Camphorwood Gate)
Bowels	CV-12 (*zhōng wǎn*, Central Stomach Duct)
Qi	CV-17 (*dàn zhōng*, Chest Center)
Blood	BL-17 (*gé shū*, Diaphragm Transport)
Sinews	GB-34 (*yáng líng quán*, Yang Mound Spring)
Vessels	LU-9 (*tài yuān*, Great Abyss)
Bone	BL-11 (*dà zhù*, Great Shuttle)
Marrow	GB-39 (*jué gǔ*, Severed Bone)

eight methods 八法 *bā fǎ*: A classification of medicinal treatment methods by Cheng Zhong-Ling of the Qing Dynasty under the eight rubrics SWEATING, EJECTION, PRECIPITATION, HARMONIZATION, WARMING, CLEARING, SUPPLEMENTATION, and DISPERSION. [27: 246] [97: 10]

eight-principle pattern identification 八纲辨证 *bā gāng biàn zhèng*: *Synonym: eight principles.* Identification of disease patterns by eight fundamental principles, namely interior and exterior, cold and heat, vacuity and repletion, and yin and yang. Interior and exterior are the principles of depth of the disease; cold and heat are the nature of disease; vacuity and repletion are the weakness of right qi and strength of evil qi. Yin and yang, which embrace the other six principles, are general categories of disease. Interior, cold, and vacuity are yin, whereas exterior, heat, and repletion are yang. Each principle is associated with specific signs. By matching the patient's signs to them, it is possible to determine the depth and nature of the disease, and the relative strength of the forces that resist disease and those that cause it. Eight-principle pattern identification is a preliminary organization of examination data: treatment should be determined only when other methods of pattern identification have provided a more detailed picture of the patient's condition. [6: 127]

eight principles 八纲 *bā gāng*: See EIGHT-PRINCIPLE PATTERN IDENTIFICATION. ◇ Chin 八 *bā*, eight; 纲 *gāng*, headrope of fishing net, guideline, principle. [26: 25] [27: 205] [97: 11]

eight ramparts 八廓 *bā kuò*: Eight divisions of the eye; the water, wind, heaven, earth, fire, thunder, marsh, and mountain ramparts. These have correspondences with the *five wheels.* The water rampart is the pupil, corresponding to water wheel.

The wind rampart is the black of the eye, corresponding to the wind wheel. The heaven rampart corresponds to the qi wheel. The earth rampart corresponds to the flesh wheel. The fire, thunder, marsh, and mountain ramparts (the upper and lower parts of the inner and outer canthi respectively), correspond to the blood wheel. In former times, the eight ramparts were applied in diagnosis; however, there was disagreement about their diagnostic significance. [27: 500] [97: 11]

eight signs of fright wind 惊风八候 *jīng fēng bā hòu*: Eight traditionally recognized signs of fright wind are: convulsions, pulling, tremor, grabbing, arching, drawing, piercing, looking. See the list below. Since fright wind patterns vary in their manifestations, the eight signs are not necessarily all present at the same time, e.g., jerking of the limbs sometimes is unaccompanied by rigidity of the body or arched-back rigidity. [27: 433]

Eight Signs of Fright Wind

Convulsions (搐 *chù*): spasmodic flexing of the elbow

Pulling (掣 *chè*): drawing together of the shoulders

Tremor (颤 *chàn*): trembling of the arms and legs

Grabbing (搦 *nuò*): clenching of the fist or alternating tensing and slackening of the fingers

Arching (反 *fǎn*): arching of the back (arched-back rigidity, opisthotonos)

Drawing (引 *yǐn*): stretching backward of the arms as if drawing a bow

Piercing (窜 *cuàn*): forward staring of the eyes

Looking (视 *shì*): squinting and exposure of the whites of the eyes

eject 吐 *tù*: **1.** To spontaneously expel matter from the digestive or respiratory tract through the mouth. **2.** To induce expulsion of harmful matter from the digestive tract, throat, or lungs through the mouth. See EJECTION.

ejection 吐法 *tù fǎ*, 涌吐法 *yǒng tù fǎ*: One of the EIGHT METHODS. A method of treatment that involves induction of vomiting, either by medicinals or by mechanical means (e.g., tickling the throat with a feather) in order to expel collected phlegm or lodged food. In clinical practice, ejection is used when phlegm-drool obstructs the throat and hampers breathing or when, after voracious eating, food stagnates in the stomach, causing distention, fullness, and pain. This method may also be used to treat poisoning, provided treatment is administered swiftly after ingestion of the toxic substance. Ejection medicinals include melon stalk (*guā dì*), veratrum (*lí lú*), chalcanthite (*dǎn fán*), gleditsia (*zào jiá*), and salt. Commonly used formulas include the powerful Melon Stalk Powder (*guā*

dì sǎn) and less powerful Ginseng Tops Beverage (*shēn lú yǐn*). Ejection is generally contraindicated in pregnancy and must be used with care in weak patients. [50: 531] [27: 281] [97: 185] [70: 35] [60: 296]

Ejection Medicinals

瓜蒂 (*guā dì*) melon stalk (Cucumeris Melonis Pedicellus)

常山 (*cháng shān*) dichroa (Dichroae Radix)

蜀漆 (*shǔ qī*) dichroa leaf (Dichroae Folium)

胆矾 (*dǎn fán*) chalcanthite (Chalcanthitum)

藜芦 (*lí lú*) veratrum (Veratri Radix et Rhizoma)

人参芦 (*rén shēn lú*) ginseng top (Ginseng Rhizoma)

皂荚 (*zào jiá*) gleditsia (Gleditsiae Fructus)

ejection of foamy drool 吐涎沫 *tǔ xián mò*: Copious drooling or vomiting of foamy drool, attributable to rheum evil. MED Warm and transform using formulas such as Minor Green-Blue Dragon Decoction (*xiǎo qīng lóng tāng*), Poria (Hoelen) Five Powder (*wǔ líng sǎn*), or Evodia Decoction (*wú zhū yú tāng*). Compare VOMITING OF PHLEGM-DROOL and PHLEGM-DROOL CONGESTION. [26: 258] [50: 532]

eject phlegm-drool 吐痰涎 *tù tán xián*: To induce the ejection of harmful substances from the throat and chest by emesis. Ejection of phlegm-drool is used in three conditions: (1) For THROAT WIND, THROAT MOTH, or THROAT IMPEDIMENT caused by exuberant phlegm obstructing the throat, use Realgar Toxin-Resolving Pill (*xióng huáng jiě dú wán*). (2) For WIND STROKE phlegm reversal characterized by phlegm-drool congesting the diaphragm and throat, causing a rasping sound, and comatose states, use Drool-Thinning Powder (*xī xián sǎn*). (3) For phlegm stagnating in the chest and diaphragm, use Sagacious Powder (*rú shèng sǎn*). [70: 40–50] [94: 67]

elbow taxation 肘劳 *zhǒu láo*: *Synonym: tennis elbow.* Pain and weakness in the elbow joint, developing gradually, without any history of obvious injury. The pain sometimes stretches down the lower arm or up to the shoulder. Elbow taxation is exacerbated by rotating movement of the lower arm such as are performed when wringing a flannel. There is no obvious swelling, and despite the pain there is no impeded movement of the joints, although there is a pressure point at the humeral epicondyle. It arises through constant rotation of the lower arm and flexing of the wrist and elbow. It affects people such as carpenters, plumbers, electricians, and tennis players. Unlike sprains, which involve sudden damage to muscles and sinews, tennis elbow develops gradually through a combination of repeated strain and external contraction of wind and cold, which concentrate in the elbow joint. The condition is thus one of taxation damage to qi and blood or wind-cold contracting the vessels and sinew channels. WMC external humeral epicondylitis; radiohumeral bursitis; radiohumeral epicondylitis. ACU Base treatment mainly on local points, selecting LI-11 (*qū chí*, Pool at the Bend), LI-10 (*shǒu sān lǐ*, Arm Three Li), LI-4 (*hé gǔ*, Union Valley), and the ouch point Tip of the Elbow (*zhǒu jiān*); needle with drainage and add moxa. Tapping with a cutaneous needle until blood appears and cupping are methods that may be used. [46: 718]

electroacupuncture 电针疗法 *diàn zhēn liáo fǎ*, 电针 *diàn zhēn*: A method of acupuncture in which an electrical current is applied to needles inserted in the body in order to produce a combined needle and electrical stimulus. Electroacupuncture was first reported after the Communist Party assumed power in China, and over recent years has come to be widely used. Method: Select two suitable acupuncture points, insert needles, and obtain qi. Then wire the needles to the electrical stimulator, and apply a stimulus of appropriate intensity and duration. Then turn off the electrical stimulus and remove the needles. Electroacupuncture can be used in regular body acupuncture, ear acupuncture, head acupuncture, facial acupuncture, and for anesthesia. In patients suffering from heart disease, it is important not to allow the current to pass through the region of the heart. [50: 408] [27: 329]

elevated scar 肉疙瘩 *ròu gē da*: A scar from a wound, burn, or surgical incision that protrudes from the flesh, is pink or deep red in color, uneven, smooth, hairless, and sometimes associated with pain or itching (especially in hot weather). MED Treat by topical application of Black Cloth Paste (*hēi bù gāo*). [26: 261]

eliminate 除 *chú*: See DRAIN.

eliminating depression and stale water 去宛陈莝 *qù yù chén cuò*: From *Elementary Questions* (*sù wèn, tāng yè láo lǐ lùn*). A method of treatment used to address stagnation and old fluid accumulations with medicinals such as kansui (*gān suì*) and morning glory (*qiān niú zǐ*). See EXPELLING WATER. ◇ Chin 去 *qù*, eliminate; 宛, read as *yù*, is the same as 郁 *yù*, depression; 陈 *chén*, old; 莝 *cuò*, old; cut straw. [27: 258]

eliminating fire toxin 去火毒 *qù huǒ dú*: A method of treatment used to remove irritants from medicinal plasters. Plasters applied to the skin immediately after preparation can cause irritation to the skin that in mild cases results in itching and, in severe cases, in blistering and erosion. This irrita-

tion is traditionally attributed to "fire toxin." Fire toxin is removed by one of two methods: storing for long time out of direct sunlight; and soaking in cool water for several days. The latter method is more practical. [27: 325]

eliminating (great) heat with warmth and sweetness 甘温除（大）热 *gān wēn chú (dà) rè*: A method of treatment used to address generalized heat [effusion] with medicinals warm in nature and sweet in flavor. Eliminating heat with warmth and sweetness includes, for example, treating qi vacuity heat marked by generalized heat [effusion], sweating, thirst with desire for warm drinks, shortage of qi and laziness to speak, tender-soft pale tongue, and a large vacuous pulse, using Center-Supplementing Qi-Boosting Decoction (*bǔ zhōng yì qì tāng*). It also includes treating postpartum or taxation fatigue heat effusion marked by hot flesh, red face, vexation and thirst with desire for liquids, pale red tongue, and a large floating vacuous pulse, using Tangkuei Blood-Supplementing Decoction (*dāng guī bǔ xuè tāng*). [26: 186]

eliminating phlegm and opening the orifices 除痰开窍 *chú tán kāi qiào*: TRANSFORMING PHLEGM AND OPENING THE ORIFICES.

eliminating stasis and engendering the new 去瘀生新 *qù yū shēng xīn*: See DISPELLING STASIS AND QUICKENING THE BLOOD.

elixir 丹 *dān*: Originally, any formula containing cinnabar or other minerals; by extension, a formula containing drastic or harsh agents used in small quantities, e.g., Purple Snow Elixir (*zǐ xuě dān*) and Supreme Jewel Elixir (*zhì bǎo dān*). Elixirs applied externally are powder preparations of sublimated or otherwise refined minerals such as mercury (*shuǐ yín*) and sulfur (*shí liú huáng*). Examples include white downborne elixir (*bái jiàng dān*) and red upborne elixir (*hóng shēng*). (See MAGIC MEDICINE.) Those used internally include powder preparations such as Purple Snow Elixir (*zǐ xuě dān*), pill preparations such as Supreme Jewel Elixir (*zhì bǎo dān*) and Five Grains Return-of-Spring Elixir (*wǔ lì huí chūn dān*), and lozenges such as Scourge-Repelling Elixir (*bì wēn dān*). Jade Pivot Elixir (*yù shū dān*) prepared in pill or lozenge form is suitable for both internal and external use. [27: 312] [97: 112]

emaciation 形体消瘦 *xíng tǐ xiāo shòu*, 形体瘦削 *xíng tǐ shòu xuē*, 消瘦 *xiāo shòu*: Synonym: *shedding of the flesh and loss of bulk*. Marked thinning of the body, usually accompanied by other signs of disease. Emaciation appears in a variety of illnesses that present as vacuity or repletion patterns (emaciation is not only a vacuity sign). **Spleen-stomach qi vacuity:** Emaciation due to spleen-stomach qi vacuity is accompanied by poor appetite, distention after eating, sloppy stool, fatigue and lack of strength, shortage of qi and laziness to speak, withered-yellow facial complexion, pale tongue with white fur, and a weak vacuous pulse. MED Fortify the spleen and boost qi. Use Four Gentlemen Decoction (*sì jūn zǐ tāng*) with added medicinals. **Qi-blood vacuity:** Emaciation is accompanied by a withered-yellow lusterless complexion, shortage of qi and laziness to speak, dizziness, heart palpitations, insomnia, pale tongue with thin fur, and a weak fine pulse. MED Boost qi and nourish the blood. Use Eight-Gem Decoction (*bā zhēn tāng*). **Insufficiency of lung yin:** Emaciation due to insufficiency of lung yin is accompanied by cough with scant phlegm that may be flecked with blood (in some cases there may be expectoration of pure blood), dry mouth and throat, tidal heat [effusion] and night sweating, postmeridian reddening of the cheeks, vexing heat in the five hearts, red tongue with little liquid, and a fine rapid pulse. MED Insufficiency of lung yin is treated by nourishing yin and clearing the lung with Lily Bulb Metal-Securing Decoction (*bǎi hé gù jīn tāng*). **Intense stomach heat:** Emaciation due to intense stomach heat is associated with thirst with desire for fluids, increased eating and rapid hungering, heart vexation, bad breath, short voidings of reddish urine, dry bound stool, dry yellow tongue fur, and a forceful rapid stringlike pulse. MED Clear the stomach and drain fire. Use Jade Lady Brew (*yù nǚ jiān*). **Exuberant liver fire:** Emaciation due to exuberant liver fire is accompanied by vexation and agitation, impatience and irascibility, dizzy head and vision, scorching pain in the rib-side, bitter taste in the mouth, red eyes, short voidings of reddish urine, dry bound stool, red tongue with yellow fur, and a stringlike rapid pulse. MED Clear the liver and drain fire. Use Gentian Liver-Draining Decoction (*lóng dǎn xiè gān tāng*) and variations. **Worm accumulation:** Emaciation due to worm accumulation is associated with withered-yellow facial complexion, clamoring stomach, intermittent umbilical pain, poor appetite, predilection for strange foods, sloppy stool, pale tongue with white fur, and a forceless weak pulse. MED Quiet and expel worms. Use Worm-Transforming Pill (*huà chóng wán*). [92: No. 29]

emergency precipitation to preserve yin 急下存阴 *jí xià cún yīn*: A method of treatment involving the use of one of the Qi-Coordinating Decoctions (*chéng qì tāng*) to free stool, discharge heat, and eliminate dryness binds, in order to preserve fluids and prevent development of TETANIC REVERSAL. Emergency precipitation to preserve yin is one form of RAKING THE FIREWOOD FROM BENEATH THE CAULDRON and is used in acute febrile diseases with signs of repletion heat vigorous heat [effusion], vexation and thirst, constipation, dry

yellow tongue fur or black tongue fur with prickles, a forceful sunken replete pulse. [50: 1142]

emesis 吐法 *tù fǎ*: See EJECTION.

emolliating the liver 柔肝 *róu gān*: *Synonyms: nourish the liver; nourish the blood and emolliate the liver.* To treat liver yin vacuity (or insufficiency of liver blood), characterized by loss of visual acuity, dry eyes, night blindness, periodic dizzy head and tinnitus, and pale nails, or poor sleep, profuse dreaming, dry mouth with lack of fluid, and a fine, weak pulse. NB: The liver is described as the "unyielding" viscus; hence the method of treating liver yin vacuity is called emolliation. MED Commonly used liver-emolliating medicinals include tangkuei (*dāng guī*), white peony (*bái sháo yào*), rehmannia (*dì huáng*), flowery knotweed (*hé shǒu wū*), lycium berry (*gǒu qǐ zǐ*), eclipta (*mò hàn lián*), and mulberry (*sāng shèn*). *Systematized Patterns with Clear-Cut Treatments* (*lèi zhèng zhì cái*) states, "The liver is the unyielding viscus, in charge of free coursing. It calls for the use of softness, not hardness, of harmonizing, not quelling." For this reason, emolliating the liver is the standard method of supplementing the liver. ◇ Chin 柔 *róu* is rendered as "emolliate" rather than soften to reduce the danger of misconstruing the term as denoting a treatment for cirrhosis (hardening) of the liver. Eng L. *e(x)*, out; *mollire*, soften. [27: 264] [50: 1196]

emotion 情志 *qíng zhì*: Affect or mind.

empirical formula 验方 *yàn fāng*: A formula that has been empirically shown to be effective for a particular condition. [26: 1000]

empirical points 经验穴 *jīng yàn xué*: An acupuncture point that has been empirically shown to be effective for a particular condition. See SELECTION OF PATHOCONDITION POINTS.

empowering 相使 *xiāng shǐ*: See SEVEN RELATIONS.

emptiness below the heart 心下空虚 *xīn xià kōng xū*: A subjective feeling of emptiness in the area just below the breastbone.

emptiness of the sea of blood 血海空虚 *xuè hǎi kōng xū*: The "sea of blood" can refer either to thoroughfare (*chōng*) vessel or to the liver. In "emptiness of the sea of blood," it appears to refer to the thoroughfare (*chōng*) vessel, which with the controlling (*rèn*) vessel starts in the uterus, percolates into all the yang channels, and irrigates all the essences, and intersects with all the yin channels, thereby helping to maintain the ability of qi and blood to nourish the whole body. Emptiness of the sea of blood is impairment of this capacity, as observed in BLOOD DESERTION. [46: 74] [26: 282]

emptiness of the sea of marrow 髓海空虚 *suǐ hǎi kōng xū*: A kidney vacuity pattern in which the kidney's function of engendering marrow is affected and characterized by dizziness, slowness of thought, forgetfulness, etc. See KIDNEY ENGENDERS BONE AND MARROW. [6: 193]

emptiness of the thoroughfare and controlling vessels 冲任空虚 *chōng rèn kōng xū*: DAMAGE TO THE THOROUGHFARE AND CONTROLLING VESSELS.

empty pain 空痛 *kōng tòng*: A pain associated with a feeling of emptiness and lightness; attributable to yin vacuity, yang vacuity, blood vacuity, or dual vacuity of yin and yang. See PAIN. [29: 190]

empty pain in the head 头脑空痛 *tóu nǎo kōng tòng*: Pain and an empty sensation in the head, associated with kidney vacuity.

encirclement needling 围针法 *wéi zhēn fǎ*: An acupuncture method involving the insertion of needles around a disease site, for example around a boil, angling the tips toward the center of the area.

encrusted skin 肌肤甲错 *jī fū jiǎ cuò*, 甲错 *jiǎ cuò*: Synonym: *snake body*; *snake scales*; *toad skin*. Dry rough scaly hardened skin. It usually observed in emaciated patients with abdominal fullness and inability to eat. **Blood vacuity and wind-dryness:** The skin gradually turns gray, dry, rough, and scaly like the skin of a snake, lizard, or even crocodile. The scales are dense, dirty looking or gray white, and elevated at the edges. The scales are separated by white furrows that create a reticular appearance. Blood vacuity wind-dryness encrusted skin is most pronounced on the extensor side of the limbs, but can cover the whole body, although it rarely invades the face. It may be temporarily relieved in summer and worsens in winter. Occasionally there is itching and the skin may split at the joints, causing soreness. It is associated with dry mouth and pharynx, reduced sweating, pale tongue with little liquid and with white fur, and a forceless fine sunken pulse. This form of encrusted skin traditionally called *snake body*, *snake scales*, and *snake skin*. MED Nourish the blood and moisten the skin; enrich yin and engender liquid. Use Blood-Nourishing Skin-Moistening Beverage (*yǎng xuè rùn fū yǐn*). **Blood heat and wind-dryness:** This form of encrusted skin starts with dry hard papules the size of millet seeds, transpierced by fine hairs, prickly to the touch, and gradually coalescing. It usually occurs on the extensor side of the elbows and knees, and can spread over the whole body. The skin is dry and sloughs, and there is keratosis and splitting of the palms and soles, thickening of the nails, and mild itching. The tongue is red and the pulse is fine and rapid. MED Clear heat and cool the blood; disperse wind and moisten dryness. Use Blood-Cooling Dryness-Moistening Beverage (*liáng xuè rùn zào yǐn*). **Damp-heat obstructing the network vessels:** This form of encrusted skin usually occurs on the nape and neck, behind the ears, forehead and face, and around the nose, and can spread to down the limbs and the medial line of the chest and back. Sometimes there is a clear hemilateral distribution. It is severe in summer and mild in winter, and associated with itching. It starts with hard follicular papules that are prickly to the touch, without change in skin color. As it advances, there appear oily gray-brown scabs, which darken over the years and coalesce to take on a warty appearance. There is often malodor. The tongue is red with stasis speckles with a slimy yellow fur. The pulse is slippery and rapid. MED Clear heat and eliminate dampness; quicken the blood and free the network vessels. Use Dampness-Eliminating Stomach-Calming Poria (Hoelen) Five Decoction (*chú shī wèi líng tāng*), swallowing Rhubarb and Wingless Cockroach Pill (*dà huáng zhè chóng wán*) with it. **Nondistribution of fluids:** The skin is generally rough. Dense cornifying follicular papules appear on the nape, trunk, elbows, and knees, giving the appearance of toad skin that is hard and prickly to the touch. This form of encrusted skin is often associated with dry eyes and clouded, flowery vision. Around hair follicles on the abdomen, lumbus, and buttocks are brown cornified plates, attached at their center and raised at the edges. The condition is more severe in winter than in summer. The tongue is pale with little liquid. The pulse is sunken, fine, and forceless. MED Assist the spleen and nourish the stomach; nourish the blood and moisten dryness. Use Supplemented Atractylodes Paste (*jiā wèi cāng zhú gāo*). ◇ Chin 肌 *jī*, flesh; 肤 *fū*, skin; 甲 *jiǎ*, armor, scales, fingernail or toenail; 错 *cuò*, crossed, uneven, irregular, wrong. In *Essential Prescriptions of the Golden Coffer* (*jīn guì yào lüè*), the term took the form of 甲错, in which 甲 has been interpreted as denoting the skin, although, by primary uses (shell, nail), it clearly connotes something hard. [26: 272] [27: 432] [97: 214] [92: No. 425] [50: 600] [49: 528]

encumbrance 困 *kùn*: Describes the effect of dampness on the spleen. See EXUBERANCE AND DEBILITATION.

end addition 后下 *hòu xià*: An act or instance of adding at the end. See ADD AT END.

enduring 久 *jiǔ*: Chronic or persistent; indicates duration, not degree, of acuteness.

enduring cough 久咳 *jiǔ ké*: From *Elementary Questions* (*sù wèn, ké lùn*). COUGH that persists for an extended period. Enduring cough with copious phlegm is usually due to spleen vacuity engendering phlegm. Enduring cough with scant phlegm is usually attributed to insufficiency of lung yin with depressed lung fire. See SPLEEN COUGH; LUNG VACUITY COUGH; FIRE COUGH. [26: 81]

enduring diarrhea 久泄 *jiŭ xiè*: Chronic or persistent diarrhea.

enduring diarrhea efflux desertion 久泄滑脱 *jiŭ xiè huá tuō*: Desertion due to fluid loss through persistent diarrhea.

enduring dysentery 久痢 *jiŭ lì*: Dysentery that persists for a long period. Enduring dysentery is associated with spleen-kidney depletion and insufficiency of center qi. Signs include sticky and bloody stools, dull pain in the abdomen, vain straining associated in severe cases with prolapse of the rectum, emaciation, lassitude of spirit and lack of strength, and poor appetite. MED For spleen vacuity fall with prolapse of the rectum, use Center-Supplementing Qi-Boosting Decoction (*bŭ zhōng yì qì tāng*). For insecurity of kidney qi, use variations of Mantis Egg-Case Powder (*sāng piāo xiāo sǎn*). For depletion of yin-blood with residual damp-heat, nourish the blood and clear heat with Carriage-Halting Pill (*zhù chē wán*). For spleen-kidney yang vacuity with gradual efflux desertion, warm, supplement, and astringe with Peach Blossom Decoction (*táo huā tāng*) or Pure Yang True Man Viscus-Nourishing Decoction (*chún yáng zhēn rén yǎng zàng tāng*). ACU Base treatment on ST, CV, and back transport points. Main points: ST-25 (*tiān shū*, Celestial Pivot), ST-37 (*shàng jù xū*, Upper Great Hollow), CV-12 (*zhōng wǎn*, Center Stomach Duct), BL-20 (*pí shū*, Spleen Transport), BL-21 (*wèi shū*, Stomach Transport), ST-36 (*zú sān lǐ*, Leg Three Li), CV-4 (*guān yuán*, Pass Head), and CV-6 (*qì hǎi*, Sea of Qi); needle with supplementation and add moxa. Selection of points according to pattern: For spleen vacuity fall with prolapse of the rectum, add GV-1 (*cháng qiáng*, Long Strong) and GV-20 (*bǎi huì*, Hundred Convergences)ⓜ. For insecurity of kidney qi, add BL-23 (*shèn shū*, Kidney Transport), KI-3 (*tài xī*, Great Ravine), and KI-7 (*fù liū*, Recover Flow). For depletion of yin-blood with residual damp-heat, supplement SP-6 (*sān yīn jiāo*, Three Yin Intersection), SP-10 (*xuè hǎi*, Sea of Blood), and KI-6 (*zhào hǎi*, Shining Sea), and drain LI-11 (*qū chí*, Pool at the Bend) and LI-4 (*hé gǔ*, Union Valley). For spleen-kidney yang vacuity, moxa LR-13 (*zhāng mén*, Camphorwood Gate), and GV-4 (*mìng mén*, Life Gate). CROSS MOXA may also be used. See DYSENTERY. [26: 81] [27: 362] [46: 667] [113: 97, 100]

enduring malaria 久疟 *jiŭ nüè*: MALARIA that persists for a long time. Enduring malaria is attributed to dual depletion of qi and blood and spleen-stomach vacuity cold. MED Supplement qi and nourish the blood; warm yang and disperse

yin. Use formulas such as Center-Supplementing Qi-Boosting Decoction (*bŭ zhōng yì qì tāng*), Ginseng Construction-Nourishing Decoction (*rén shēn yǎng róng tāng*), Cinnamon Bark and Aconite Eight-Ingredient Pill (*guì fù bā wèi wán*), and Flowery Knotweed and Ginseng Beverage (*hé rén yǐn*). ACU Base treatment mainly on GV and greater yang (*tài yáng*) points. Drain GV-14 (*dà zhuī*, Great Hammer), PC-5 (*jiān shǐ*, Intermediary Courier), and SI-3 (*hòu xī*, Back Ravine); supplement BL-20 (*pí shū*, Spleen Transport)ⓜ and GV-9 (*zhì yáng*, Extremity of Yang)ⓜ. [26: 82] [46: 649] [113: 169]

enduring pain entering the network vessels 久痛入络 *jiŭ tòng rù luò*: Stubborn wind-cold-damp IMPEDIMENT (*bì*) causing blood stasis. Enduring pain entering the network vessels is treated by dispelling stasis and freeing the channels. [6: 262]

engender 生 *shēng*: **1.** To cause, give rise to. **2.** To benefit (as in the engendering sequence of the five phases). **3.** To produce, or stimulate the production (of fluids, etc.), in methods of supplementation.

engendering 相生 *xiāng shēng*: The sequence in which the five phases and their corresponding phenomena have a nurturing effect on each other, i.e., wood (liver) → fire (heart) → earth (spleen) → metal (lung) → water (kidney) → wood (liver). This reflects the way in which spring gives way to summer, summer gives way to long summer, etc. [6: 29] [27: 9] [97: 386]

engendering flesh 生肌 *shēng jī*: A method of treatment used to promote the regrowth of damaged skin and flesh.

engendering liquid 生津 *shēng jīn*: *Synonym: nourishing the fluids.* A method of treatment used to address damage to liquid in febrile disease, manifesting in heat effusion, dry mouth and thirst, red tongue, and dry lips etc., with medicinals such as scrophularia (*xuán shēn*), ophiopogon (*mài mén dōng*), dried/fresh rehmannia (*shēng dì huáng*), and dendrobium (*shí hú*). ACU Select Gold Liquid and Jade Humor (*jīn jīn yù yè*), Sea Source (*hǎi quán*), TB-2 (*yè mén*, Humor Gate), KI-6 (*zhào hǎi*, Shining Sea), SP-6 (*sān yīn jiāo*, Three Yin Intersection), KI-2 (*rán gǔ*, Blazing Valley), and KI-3 (*tài xī*, Great Ravine) to nourish yin and increase humor. [27: 253] [113: 20]

enlarged tongue 舌胖 *shé pàng*: A tongue that is swollen to a size slightly larger than normal, most clearly indicated by dental impressions on the margin. An enlarged tongue indicates qi vacuity or the presence of water-damp (dampness, phlegm-rheum). An enlarged tongue that is pale in color, with a white, glossy fur, indicates qi vacuity. With a slimy tongue fur, it usually indicates dampness or damp-heat. An enlarged tongue is markedly different from a red sore swollen tongue, which characterizes an intense heat evil or heart fire flaming upward. [6: 120] [27: 130]

enrich 滋 *zī*: See SUPPLEMENT. [26: 757]

enriching and moistening with cold sweet medicinals 甘寒滋润 *gān hán zī rùn*: A method of treatment used to address insufficiency of liver and kidney fluids such as in liver-kidney yin depletion with vacuity fire flaming upward characterized by dry sore throat, cough and panting with blood-flecked phlegm, vexing heat in the heart of the palms and soles, red tongue with scant fur, and a find rapid pulse. [MED] Cold sweet enriching moistening medicinals include dried/fresh rehmannia (*shēng dì huáng*), cooked rehmannia (*shú dì huáng*), ophiopogon (*mài mén dōng*), Sichuan fritillaria (*chuān bèi mǔ*), lily bulb (*bǎi hé*), tangkuei (*dāng guī*), white peony (*bái sháo yào*), raw licorice (*shēng gān cǎo*), scrophularia (*xuán shēn*), and platycodon (*jié gěng*). [27: 269] [97: 137]

enriching (and nourishing) stomach yin 滋养胃阴 *zī yǎng wèi yīn*: Synonym: *nourishing the stomach*. A method of treatment used to address stomach yin vacuity patterns characterized by hunger with small food intake, discomfort in the stomach duct, dry mouth and parched lips, constipation, red tongue with scant fur, and a rapid fine tongue fur. [MED] Agents that enrich stomach yin include glehnia (*běi shā shēn*), ophiopogon (*mài mén dōng*), dendrobium (*shí hú*), and Solomon's seal (*yù zhú*). [ACU] Base treatment mainly on ST, SP, and back transport points. Select BL-20 (*pí shū*, Spleen Transport), BL-21 (*wèi shū*, Stomach Transport), ST-36 (*zú sān lǐ*, Leg Three Li), KI-6 (*zhào hǎi*, Shining Sea), SP-6 (*sān yīn jiāo*, Three Yin Intersection), and ST-44 (*nèi tíng*, Inner Court); needle with supplementation. [27: 279] [97: 584] [46: 659, 660] [37: 296]

enriching (and nourishing) the liver and kidney 滋养肝肾 *zī yǎng gān shèn*: **1.** A method of treatment used to address liver-kidney yin vacuity characterized by dizziness, upbearing fire flush, flowery vision, tinnitus, aching lumbus, dry throat, unquiet sleep, possibly night sweating, yellow urine, red tongue with scant fur, and a fine stringlike pulse. [MED] Use Lycium Berry, Chrysanthemum, and Rehmannia Pill (*qǐ jú dì huáng wán*). [ACU] Base treatment mainly on CV, back transport points, KI, and LR. Select CV-4 (*guān yuán*, Pass Head), BL-23 (*shèn shū*, Kidney Transport), BL-18 (*gān shū*, Liver Transport), SP-6 (*sān yīn jiāo*, Three Yin Intersection), KI-3 (*tài xī*, Great Ravine), KI-2 (*rán gǔ*, Blazing Valley), and LR-3 (*tài chōng*, Supreme Surge). Needle with supplementation and add moxa. **2.** A method of treatment used to nourish liver yin by enriching kidney

yin, i.e., to *enrich water to nourish wood*. [27: 264] [97: 584]

enriching (and supplementing) the liver and kidney 滋补肝肾 *zī bǔ gān shèn*: ENRICHING (AND NOURISHING) THE LIVER AND KIDNEY.

enriching water to moisten wood 滋水涵木 *zī shuǐ hán mù*: A method of treatment used to nourish kidney yin in order to moisten liver yin. In the five phases, wood is engendered by water, hence the liver yin can be supplemented by enriching kidney yin. Enriching water to moisten wood is applied in the treatment of kidney yin depletion with liver yin vacuity, and superabundant liver fire characterized by dizziness, dry eyes, tinnitus, reddening of the cheeks, dry mouth, vexing heat in the five hearts, aching lumbus and limp knees, seminal emission, menstrual irregularities, red tongue with scant fur, and a fine stringlike rapid pulse. [MED] Agents that enrich water to moisten wood include rehmannia (*dì huáng*), cornus (*shān zhū yú*), lycium berry (*gǒu qǐ zǐ*), scrophularia (*xuán shēn*), tortoise plastron (*guī bǎn*), ligustrum (*nǚ zhēn zǐ*), and flowery knotweed (*hé shǒu wū*). [ACU] Base treatment mainly on GB, LR, KI, and SP. Needle with drainage at GV-20 (*bǎi huì*, Hundred Convergences), GB-20 (*fēng chí*, Wind Pool), LR-3 (*tài chōng*, Supreme Surge), and GB-43 (*xiá xī*, Pinched Ravine), and with supplementation at BL-23 (*shèn shū*, Kidney Transport), BL-18 (*gān shū*, Liver Transport), BL-17 (*gé shū*, Diaphragm Transport), KI-6 (*zhào hǎi*, Shining Sea), KI-3 (*tài xī*, Great Ravine), and SP-6 (*sān yīn jiāo*, Three Yin Intersection). [27: 264] [97: 583]

enriching yin 滋阴 *zī yīn*: SUPPLEMENTING YIN.

enriching yin and boosting qi 滋阴益气 *zī yīn yì qì*: A method of supplementing both yin and qi in the treatment of DUAL VACUITY OF QI AND YIN. Commonly used yin-enriching qi-boosting medicinals include codonopsis (*dǎng shēn*), pseudostellaria (*tài zǐ shēn*), ophiopogon (*mài mén dōng*), adenophora/glehnia (*shā shēn*), American ginseng (*xī yáng shēn*), dendrobium (*shí hú*), dried/fresh rehmannia (*shēng dì huáng*), dioscorea (*shān yào*), lycium berry (*gǒu qǐ zǐ*), cornus (*shān zhū yú*), lycium root bark (*dì gǔ pí*), schisandra (*wǔ wèi zǐ*), and turtle shell (*biē jiǎ*). Representative formulas include Pulse-Engendering Powder (*shēng mài sǎn*), Ginseng Root-Securing Pill (*rén shēn gù běn wán*), and Ginseng and Astragalus Powder (*rén shēn huáng qí sǎn*). [57: 27]

enriching yin and clearing heat 滋阴清热 *zī yīn qīng rè*: A method of treatment used to address effulgent yin vacuity fire characterized by steaming bones, tidal heat [effusion], and night sweating. [MED] Yin-enriching heat-clearing formulas include Large Gentian and Turtle Shell Powder (*qín* *jiāo biē jiǎ sǎn*) and Tangkuei Six Yellows Decoction (*dāng guī liù huáng tāng*). This method differs from that of clearing vacuity heat by a greater emphasis on enriching yin. ACU Base treatment mainly on KI. Select SP-6 (*sān yīn jiāo*, Three Yin Intersection), KI-6 (*zhào hǎi*, Shining Sea), KI-3 (*tài xī*, Great Ravine), KI-2 (*rán gǔ*, Blazing Valley), and LR-2 (*xíng jiān*, Moving Between). Needle with even supplemenation and drainage or with supplementation. For tidal heat [effusion], add LU-5 (*chǐ zé*, Cubit Marsh) and LU-10 (*yú jì*, Fish Border). For night sweating, add HT-6 (*yīn xī*, Yin Cleft). See CLEARING VACUITY HEAT. [44: 431] [46: 596]

enriching yin and coursing the liver 滋阴疏肝 *zī yīn shū gān*: HARMONIZING THE LIVER.

enriching yin and disinhibiting dampness 滋阴利湿 *zī yīn lì shī*: A method of treatment used to address damage to yin by damp-heat with thirst and intake of fluids, inhibited urination, heart vexation, insomnia, and, in some cases, cough, vomiting, and nausea. MED A commonly used yin-enriching dampness-disinhibiting formula is Polyporus Decoction (*zhū líng tāng*). [27: 261]

enriching yin and downbearing fire 滋阴降火 *zī yīn jiàng huǒ*: A method of treatment used to address depletion of kidney yin and hyperactivity of kidney fire. MED Treatment is based on kidney-enriching essence-boosting medicinals, and assisted by fire-downbearing yin-firming medicinals such as anemarrhena (*zhī mǔ*), phellodendron (*huáng bǎi*), and moutan (*mǔ dān pí*). Sometimes cornus (*shān zhū yú*), calcined dragon bone (*duàn lóng gǔ*), and calcined oyster shell (*duàn mǔ lì*) are also used. A commonly used yin-enriching fire-downbearing formula is Anemarrhena and Phellodendron Eight-Ingredient Pill (*zhī bǎi bā wèi wán*). ACU See EFFULGENT YIN VACUITY FIRE. [50: 1570] [25: 311]

enriching yin and extinguishing wind 滋阴熄风 *zī yīn xī fēng*: A method of treatment used to address wind stirring from yin vacuity due to damage to true yin by heat in febrile disease, characterized by unpronounced but persistent heat effusion, heat in the hearts of the soles and palms, red facial complexion, vacuity vexation and insomnia, flusteredness and lassitude, tinnitus, wriggling movement or convulsions of the extremities, dry crimson tongue with little fur, and a rapid vacuous pulse. MED Enriching yin and extinguishing wind makes use of medicinals such as rehmannia (*dì huáng*), white peony (*bái sháo yào*), ophiopogon (*mài mén dōng*), egg yolk (*jī zǐ huáng*), tortoise plastron (*guī bǎn*), turtle shell (*biē jiǎ*), oyster shell (*mǔ lì*), and uncaria (*gōu téng*). A representative formula is Major Wind-Stabilizing Pill (*dà dìng fēng zhū*). ACU Base treatment mainly on KI, SP, GB, and LR. Needle with supplementation at SP-6 (*sān yīn*

jiāo, Three Yin Intersection), KI-6 (*zhào hǎi*, Shining Sea), KI-3 (*tài xī*, Great Ravine), and KI-1 (*yǒng quán*, Gushing Spring) and with drainage at GV-20 (*bǎi huì*, Hundred Convergences), GB-20 (*fēng chí*, Wind Pool), LR-3 (*tài chōng*, Supreme Surge), and GB-43 (*xiá xī*, Pinched Ravine). See EXTINGUISHING WIND. [26: 758]

enriching yin and moistening dryness 滋阴润燥 *zī yīn rùn zào*: NOURISHING YIN AND MOISTENING DRYNESS. [26: 758]

enriching yin and resolving the exterior 滋阴解表 *zī yīn jiě biǎo*: Synonym: *nourishing yin and resolving the exterior*. A method of treatment used to enrich yin and promote sweating to resolve an exterior pattern in patients suffering from a yin vacuity that would otherwise rule out sweating on the grounds that it would worsen the vacuity condition further. MED Combine yin-enriching medicinals such as dried/fresh rehmannia (*shēng dì huáng*), Solomon's seal (*yù zhú*), and ophiopogon (*mài mén dōng*) with exterior-resolving medicinals such as fermented soybean (*dàn dòu chǐ*), pueraria (*gé gēn*), perilla leaf (*zǐ sū yè*), scallion white (*cōng bái*), and mint (*bò hé*). A commonly used yin-enriching exterior-resolving formula is Solomon's Seal Variant Decoction (*jiā jiǎn wēi ruí tāng*). ACU Use the points given under RESOLVING THE EXTERIOR and add KI-3 (*tài xī*, Great Ravine) and KI-6 (*zhào hǎi*, Shining Sea), to enrich yin. [26: 758]

enriching yin and supplementing the kidney 滋阴补肾 *zī yīn bǔ shèn*: See SUPPLEMENTING YIN.

enriching yin, calming the liver, and subduing yang 滋阴平肝潜阳 *zī yīn píng gān qián yáng*: FOSTERING YIN AND SUBDUING YANG.

enriching yin to restrain fire 滋阴制火 *zī yīn zhì huǒ*: INVIGORATING THE GOVERNOR OF WATER TO RESTRAIN THE BRILLIANCE OF YANG.

enter the interior 入里 *rù lǐ*: Synonym: *pass into the interior*. (Of evils) to move into the interior. See EXUBERANCE AND DEBILITATION; INTERIOR PATTERN.

enuresis 遗尿 *yí niào*, 遗溺 *yí niào*: 1. Involuntary loss of urine. See URINARY INCONTINENCE. 2. Involuntary loss of urine during sleep, mostly observed in children; commonly referred to as bedwetting. Enuresis is attributable to bad eating habits (excessive eating and drinking) or fatigue due to excessive play, reducing the ability to waken from sleep to urinate. It may also be due to vacuity cold of the lower origin with insecurity of kidney qi, or to spleen-lung qi vacuity affecting regulation of the waterways. MED Stream-Reducing Pill (*suō quán wán*) and Mantis Egg-Case Powder (*sāng piāo xiāo sǎn*) are good general formulas. For vacuity cold of the lower origin, use Chinese

Leek Seed Pill (*jiā jiǔ zǐ wán*) or Oyster Shell Pill (*mǔ lì wán*), which consists of oyster shell (*mǔ lì*) and halloysite (*chì shí zhī*). Spleen-lung qi vacuity can be treated with Center-Supplementing Qi-Boosting Decoction (*bǔ zhōng yì qì tāng*). In addition to treatment, cultivate proper habits in the child. ACU For vacuity cold of the lower origin, base treatment mainly on CV and back transport points. Select CV-4 (*guān yuán*, Pass Head), CV-3 (*zhōng jí*, Central Pole), BL-23 (*shèn shū*, Kidney Transport), BL-28 (*páng guāng shū*, Bladder Transport), and KI-3 (*tài xī*, Great Ravine); needle with supplementation and add moxa. Selection of points according to signs: For frequent enuresis, add moxa at LR-1 (*dà dūn*, Large Pile). For heavy sleep, add GV-20 (*bǎi huì*, Hundred Convergences) and HT-7 (*shén mén*, Spirit Gate). For spleen-lung qi vacuity, base treatment mainly on CV, LU, SP, and ST. Select CV-6 (*qì hǎi*, Sea of Qi), LU-9 (*tài yuān*, Great Abyss), SP-6 (*sān yīn jiāo*, Three Yin Intersection), and ST-36 (*zú sān lǐ*, Leg Three Li); needle with supplementation and add moxa. Selection of points according to signs: For sloppy stool, add BL-20 (*pí shū*, Spleen Transport) and BL-23 (*shèn shū*, Kidney Transport). For frequent urination, add GV-20 (*bǎi huì*, Hundred Convergences) and BL-32 (*cì liáo*, Second Bone-Hole). See URINE. [26: 917] [27: 426]

enuresis in pregnancy 妊娠遗尿 *rèn shēn yí niào*: Enuresis during pregnancy; attributed to a) blood vacuity in pregnancy causing heat in the bladder; b) spleen-lung qi vacuity placing strain on the bladder; or c) liver-kidney yin vacuity with heat harassing the bladder; **Blood vacuity heat in the bladder** is characterized by heart vexation and reddish urine. MED Nourish the blood and clear heat. Use Moutan and Gardenia Free Wanderer Powder (*dān zhī xiāo yáo sǎn*) or make a powder of baiwei (*bái wēi*) and white peony (*bái sháo yào*). **Spleen-lung qi vacuity** causes enuresis with sagging distention in the lesser abdomen. MED Supplement the spleen and lung. Use Center-Supplementing Qi-Boosting Decoction (*bǔ zhōng yì qì tāng*) plus alpinia (*yì zhì rén*) and mantis egg-case (*sāng piāo xiāo*). **Liver-kidney yin vacuity** causes enuresis with lassitude of spirit and dizzy head, and limp aching lumbus and knees. MED Enrich the liver and kidney. Use Six-Ingredient Rehmannia Pill (*liù wèi dì huáng wán*), possibly combined with Mantis Egg-Case Powder (*sāng piāo xiāo sǎn*). [26: 341]

epidemic cough 疫咳 *yì ké*: WHOOPING COUGH.

epidemic disease 疫 *yì*: A transmissible disease that affects many members of a community. See SCOURGE EPIDEMIC.

epidemic dysentery 疫痢 *yì lì*: *Synonyms: seasonal epidemic dysentery; epidemic toxin dysentery.* Severe contagious dysentery attributed to overexuberant epidemic toxin congesting the intestines and damaging qi and the blood. Epidemic dysentery is characterized by acute signs such as high fever, headache, vexation and agitation, thirst, severe abdominal pain, and passing of blood and pus in the stool. The tongue is red or crimson and the pulse is slippery and rapid. The stool usually contains purplish red, often watery blood. In severe cases, there may be coma and tetanic reversal, or critical signs of vacuity desertion such as reversal cold of the limbs and hasty panting. WMC toxic dysentery. MED Clear heat and cool the blood. Use formulas such as Pulsatilla Decoction (*bái tóu wēng tāng*), Rhinoceros Horn and Rehmannia Decoction (*xī jiǎo dì huáng tāng*), or Purple Snow Elixir (*zǐ xuě dān*). [26: 402] [27: 361] [97: 462]

epidemic malaria 疫疟 *yì nüè*: A contagious form of malaria occurring in specific areas. Epidemic malaria is characterized by aversion to cold alternating with baking heat [effusion] and copious sweating and by thirst and oppression in the chest. When damp-heat signs are pronounced, there is thirst without desire to drink and incomplete sweating. In severe cases, there may be clouded spirit. MED Repel foulness and eliminate dampness. Use Membrane-Source–Opening Beverage (*dá yuán yǐn*) or Priceless Qi-Righting Powder (*bù huàn jīn zhèng qì sǎn*). For pronounced damp-heat, treat by clearing heat and transforming dampness with Sweet Dew Toxin-Dispersing Elixir (*gān lù xiāo dú dān*). For high fever and clouded spirit, use Purple Snow Elixir (*zǐ xuě dān*). [26: 402] [27: 358] [97: 462]

epidemic pestilence 疫疠 *yì lì*: SEASONAL QI.

epidemic pestilential qi 疫疠之气 *yì lì zhī qì*: PESTILENTIAL QI. [29: 568]

epidemic throat sand 疫喉痧 *yì hóu shā*: *Synonyms: cinnabar sand; putrefying throat sand.* A disease occurring in winter and spring, characterized by red sore swollen throat, ulceration of the THROAT NODES, and generalized sand (*shā*) speckles. Epidemic throat sand is attributed to seasonal epidemic pestilential toxin that enters the lung and stomach via the mouth and nose. In the throat there is a spreading putrid white membrane that is easily wiped away. The soreness may be so acute as to make the swallowing of soup or water difficult. There is pronounced heat effusion and aversion to cold with body pains. Sand speckles appear dimly all over the body, and develop to a bright scarlet color forming brocade-like patterns. If the speckles are small and diffuse, the condition is called *sand*; if coalescing into clouds, it is called *cinnabar*. The sand speckles may disappear when pressed by the fingers and return when pressure is released.

They spread swiftly from the neck over the chest and back, and then the limbs finally to cover the whole body. Only the face and forehead are unaffected. The area around the mouth is somber white and free of speckles. The tongue is red like meat, and smooth but for fine protruding granules that cover it, giving it the appearance of a red bayberry. An initially white fur gradually becomes thick and slimy. The eruption brings abatement of heat effusion and gives way to the sloughing of the bran-like scales. WMC scarlet fever. MED In the initial stage, treat by outthrusting toxin with coolness and acridity using variations of Lonicera and Forsythia Powder (*yín qiào săn*). In the mid-stage, discharge heat and resolve toxin with Construction-Cooling Qi-Clearing Decoction (*liáng yíng qīng qì tāng*). In the final stages, enrich yin and nourish humor with Yin-Nourishing Lung-Clearing Decoction (*yăng yīn qīng fèi tāng*). Avoid using warm acrid exterior resolution or premature use of cold bitter draining precipitants. Patients should be isolated. [26: 402] [27: 499] [97: 426]

epidemic toxin dysentery 疫毒痢 *yì dú lì*: EPIDEMIC DYSENTERY.

epilepsy 痫 *xián*, 癫痫 *diān xián*, 羊痫风 *yáng xián fēng*: A disease characterized by brief episodes (fits) of temporary loss of spirit, white complexion, fixity of the eyes, or sudden clouding collapse, foaming at the mouth, upward-staring eyes, clenched jaw, and convulsions of the limbs, and in some cases, squealing like a goat or pig. After an episode, the patient experiences fatigue and then returns to normal. Epilepsy is attributed to fear and fright or emotional imbalance, dietary intemperance, and taxation damaging the liver, spleen, and kidney channels and causing wind-phlegm to be carried upward by qi. The congenital aspect of the disease was understood early since in *The Inner Canon* (*nèi jīng*) it is also referred to as "fetal disease" (*tāi bìng*). MED Epilepsy is usually a repletion pattern, but repeated episodes can lead to vacuity of right. Treatment at the time of fits takes the form of sweeping phlegm and diffusing the orifices, extinguishing wind and settling epilepsy, using formulas such as Fit-Settling Pill (*dìng xián wán*). Treatment between fits (remission period) takes the form of supplementing the spleen and kidney, using Four Gentlemen Decoction (*sì jūn zĭ tāng*), Major Origin-Supplementing Brew (*dà bŭ yuán jiān*), or Placenta Pill (*hé chē wán*). ACU In fits, base treatment mainly on CV, GV, LR, PC, and SP. Select GV-26 (*shuĭ gōu*, Water Trough), KI-1 (*yŏng quán*, Gushing Spring), GV-16 (*fēng fŭ*, Wind Mansion), CV-15 (*jiū wěi*, Turtledove Tail), PC-6 (*nèi guān*, Inner Pass), LI-4 (*hé gŭ*, Union Valley), LR-3 (*tài chōng*, Supreme Surge), SP-6 (*sān yīn jiāo*, Three Yin Intersection), ST-40 (*fēng lóng*, Bountiful Bulge), SI-3 (*hòu*

xī, Back Ravine), and BL-62 (*shēn mài*, Extending Vessel); needle with drainage. Between fits, base treatment mainly on HT, SP, ST, and LR. Select HT-7 (*shén mén*, Spirit Gate), SP-6 (*sān yīn jiāo*, Three Yin Intersection), LR-3 (*tài chōng*, Supreme Surge), ST-40 (*fēng lóng*, Bountiful Bulge), Alert Spirit Quartet (*sì shén cōng*), GV-8 (*jīn suō*, Sinew Contraction), GB-34 (*yáng líng quán*, Yang Mound Spring), BL-62 (*shēn mài*, Extending Vessel), KI-6 (*zhào hăi*, Shining Sea), and GV-20 (*băi huì*, Hundred Convergences); needle with supplementation and moxa if necessary or use catgut embedding. [26: 1005, 929] [46: 640] [37: 345] [27: 394] [97: 660]

epilepsy of pregnancy 子痫 *zĭ xián*: *Synonyms: pregnancy wind tetany; child wind*. From *The Origin and Indicators of Disease* (*zhū bìng yuán hòu lùn*). A disease of pregnancy characterized by fits. It occurs in patients usually suffering from liver-kidney yin vacuity when yin-blood vacuity is exacerbated by pregnancy. When yin is vacuous, yang is hyperactive. This causes liver wind harassing the inner body, and vacuity fire flaming upward that stirs heart fire. Wind and fire fan each other, causing signs such as sudden collapse unconsciousness, and convulsions of the limbs. The patient soon comes around, but then another fit usually starts. WMC eclampsia. MED Enrich yin and subdue yang; calm the liver and extinguish wind. Use Antelope Horn Powder (*líng yáng jiăo săn*) or Gastrodia and Uncaria Beverage (*tiān má gōu téng yĭn*). For exuberant phlegm-drool congestion with phlegm rale in the throat, and hanging eyes and clenched jaw, clear heat and sweep phlegm by adding dried bamboo sap (*zhú lì*) and bile arisaema (*dăn xīng*) to the above formula. ACU For persistent convulsions and coma, acupuncture can be used to revive the patient. For convulsions, needle LI-11 (*qū chí*, Pool at the Bend), BL-57 (*chéng shān*, Mountain Support), and LR-3 (*tài chōng*, Supreme Surge). For coma, needle GV-26 (*rén zhōng*, Human Center), PC-6 (*nèi guān*, Inner Pass), GV-20 (*băi huì*, Hundred Convergences), GB-20 (*fēng chí*, Wind Pool), and KI-1 (*yŏng quán*, Gushing Spring). For clenched jaw, use ST-7 (*xià guān*, Below the Joint) and ST-6 (*jiá chē*, Cheek Carriage). [26: 57]

epilepsy pattern 痫证 *xián zhèng*: See EPILEPSY.

episode 发作 *fā zuò*: *Synonym: attack*. An occurrence of recurrent pathological state.

eroding foot 脚丫糜烂 *jiăo yā mí làn*: FOOT QI SORE.

erosion 糜烂 *mí làn*: See ULCERATION.

eructation 嗳气 *ài qì*, 噫气 *yì qì*: BELCHING.

essence 精 *jīng*: That which is responsible for growth, development, and reproduction, and determines the strength of the constitution, and is manifest physically in the male in the form of semen. Essence is composed of earlier heaven essence (congenital essence), which is inherited from the parents and constantly supplemented by later heaven essence (acquired essence) produced from food by the stomach and spleen. Later heaven essence is considered to be the same as, or a derivative of, the essence of grain and water from which qi, blood, and fluids are also produced. Essence is often referred to as essential qi, and because it is stored by the kidney, it is also called kidney essential qi. Its functions can be deduced from the following passage from the first chapter of *Elementary Questions* (*sù wèn*): "[In the male] at the age of two eights [i.e., sixteen], kidney qi is exuberant, the "heavenly tenth" (*tiān guǐ*) arrives, essential qi flows forth, yin and yang are in harmony, and [he] can beget offspring... At the age of seven eights [i.e., fifty-six] the "heavenly tenth" (*tiān guǐ*) is exhausted, essence diminishes, the kidney grows weak, and the body loses its tone; at eight eights, the teeth and hair fall out. [In the female] at the age of two sevens, the "heavenly tenth" (*tiān guǐ*) arrives, the controlling vessel flows, and the thoroughfare vessel fills, the menses come according to their times, and [she] can bear offspring... At seven sevens, the controlling vessel empties, the thoroughfare vessel weakens, the "heavenly tenth" is exhausted, the passages of the earth are cut, the body deteriorates, and she can no longer bear children." This quotation shows how the natural development of the individual from birth to death and reproductive capacity are explained in terms of kidney essential qi. Pathologies of essence include congenital insufficiency, late or improper maturation, premature senility, or sexual and reproductive dysfunctions. [27: 75] [97: 626]

essence and blood are of the same source 精血同源 *jīng xuè tóng yuán*: Essence and blood share a common source, are similar in nature, and often suffer from insufficiency simultaneously. Blood is derived from the essence of grain and water (acquired essence) and congenital essence is partly derived from acquired essence. Both essence and blood are yin in nature. The blood is stored by the liver, and essence is stored by the kidney. Insufficiency of essence-blood is commonly observed, and is treated by nourishing the liver and supplementing the kidney. [27: 75]

essence-blood 精血 *jīng xuè*: Blood and essence seen as one. See ESSENCE AND BLOOD ARE OF THE SAME SOURCE. [27: 75] [97: 627]

essence chamber 精室 *jīng shì*, 精房 *jīng fáng*: **1.** LIFE GATE. *The Classic of Difficult Issues* (*nàn jīng, 36*) states, "The life gate is the abode of essence and spirit and to which source qi is connected. In the male, it stores essence; in the fe-

male, it ties [around] the uterus." **2.** *Synonyms: house of essence*; *palace of essence*. Specifically (and more commonly), the place where semen is stored. [50: 1672]

essence gate 精关 *jīng guān*: The barrier that regulates the discharge of semen. The Chinese term *jīng* means essence and its physical manifestation, semen. The "essence gate" is not clearly defined as an anatomical structure. Zhang Jie-Bin (Ming, 1563–1640) described a "gate that is felt to open on ejaculation," which is now often called the essence gate. Signs such as seminal efflux, seminal emission, and premature ejaculation are attributed to "insecurity of the essence gate" due to kidney disease. See LIFE GATE. [36: 102]

essence-marrow depletion 精髓虚亏 *jīng suǐ xū kuī*: See INSUFFICIENCY OF KIDNEY ESSENCE.

essence of grain and water 水谷之精微 *shuǐ gǔ zhī jīng wēi*: The nutrients contained in food (grain and water). [27: 21] [97: 132]

essence-spirit 精神 *jīng shén*: ESSENCE and SPIRIT considered together; the manifestation of the life force. NB: The expression 精神 *jīng shén* as colloquially used in Chinese is roughly the equivalent of the English 'energy' (colloquial sense) or 'vitality'. It is also come to be used in a modern psychology as the equivalent of the English 'mind'. [27: 82] [97: 627]

essence turbidity 精浊 *jīng zhuó*: A persistent discharge from the urethra like rice water (water that rice has been washed in) or like flower and water paste. Essence turbidity may be associated with itching or pain in the urethra, and, in severe cases, the pain is like the cutting of a knife or like a burning fire. The urine remains clear. Essence turbidity is attributable to a) excesses of drinking and sex causing obstruction by "wasted essence" (old semen), b) kidney essence depletion with frenetic stirring of the ministerial fire causing discharge of wasted essence with fire, or c) damp-heat flowing down in the essence chamber. A white discharge is called WHITE TURBIDITY, whereas discharge containing blood is called RED TURBIDITY. When persistent, both forms manifest as vacuity patterns. Red turbidity is a sign of more pronounced vacuity with effulgent ministerial fire. MED Burning pain in the urethra calls for action focusing on the fire, using Firewood-Raking Beverage (*chōu xīn yǐn*) or Anti-Turbidity Root-Securing Pill (*zhì zhuó gù běn wán*). Essence turbidity due to damp-heat flowing into the essence chamber with frequent urination is treated by percolating disinhibition with Poria (Hoelen) Five Powder (*wǔ líng sǎn*) combined with Origin-Boosting Powder (*yì yuán sǎn*). When essence turbidity persists for a long period and the burning pain subsides, treatment should focus on quieting the heart and securing the kidney by using Origin-Securing Brew (*mì yuán jiān*) or Cuscuta Seed Pill (*tù sī zǐ wán*) and variations. For debilitation of the life gate fire, use formulas such as Right-Restoring [Life Gate] Pill (*yòu guī wán*) or Cinnamon Bark and Aconite Eight-Ingredient Pill (*guì fù bā wèi wán*). ACU For effulgent fire with pronounced burning sensation on urination, base treatment mainly on KI and HT. Select KI-3 (*tài xī*, Great Ravine), KI-6 (*zhào hǎi*, Shining Sea), KI-2 (*rán gǔ*, Blazing Valley), HT-8 (*shào fǔ*, Lesser Mansion), and SP-6 (*sān yīn jiāo*, Three Yin Intersection), needling with even supplementation and drainage. For damp-heat flowing into the essence chamber, base treatment mainly on CV and SP. Select CV-3 (*zhōng jí*, Central Pole), BL-28 (*páng guāng shū*, Bladder Transport), SP-9 (*yīn líng quán*, Yin Mound Spring), SP-6 (*sān yīn jiāo*, Three Yin Intersection), and CV-4 (*guān yuán*, Pass Head), needling with even supplementation and drainage. For enduring conditions without scorching pain, calm the heart and secure the kidney. Base treatment mainly on BL, CV, and KI. Select CV-4 (*guān yuán*, Pass Head), BL-23 (*shèn shū*, Kidney Transport), KI-3 (*tài xī*, Great Ravine), BL-15 (*xīn shū*, Heart Transport), HT-7 (*shén mén*, Spirit Gate), and SP-6 (*sān yīn jiāo*, Three Yin Intersection); needle with supplementation. For debilitation of the life gate fire, base treatment mainly on GV and KI. Select CV-4 (*guān yuán*, Pass Head), BL-23 (*shèn shū*, Kidney Transport), GV-4 (*mìng mén*, Life Gate), and KI-3 (*tài xī*, Great Ravine), needling with supplementation and adding moxa. [26: 832]

essential qi 精气 *jīng qì*: Any essential element of the body (blood, qi, fluid, essence); specifically, the acquired essence and the essence stored by the viscera and indissociable from the essential qi that is stored by the kidney and used in reproduction. See KIDNEY STORES ESSENCE. [27: 75] [97: 627]

ethereal soul 魂 *hún*: A nonphysical aspect of the human being, said to be stored by the liver, as distinct from *pò*, the corporeal soul, said to be stored by the lung. *The Magic Pivot* (*líng shū*) states, "That which goes hither and thither with the spirit is called the ethereal soul." It also says, "The liver stores the blood, and the blood houses the ethereal soul." When the liver fails to store the blood or liver blood is insufficient, there are signs such as sleep walking and sleep talking. This condition is sometimes called the "ethereal soul failing to be stored." [26: 833]

evacuate vacuity and replenish repletion 虚虚实实 *xū xū shí shí*: To exacerbate vacuity and exacerbate repletion. Two basic principles of treatment are "vacuity is treated by supplementing" and "repletion is treated by draining." If vacuity and repletion are misidentified and the opposite

principle of treatment is applied, the result is evacuation of vacuity or replenishment of repletion, in either case an exacerbation of the condition.

even supplementation and drainage 平补平泻 *píng bǔ píng xiè*: Synonym: *neutral supplementation and drainage (obs)*. **1.** From *Wondrous Response Canon* (*shén yìng jīng*). An acupuncture technique in which drainage is followed by supplementation. **2.** A method of manipulation that neither supplements nor drains, and is intended only to obtain qi. Method: After insertion, lifting and thrusting is performed with even lifts and thrusts and/or rotation is performed with even strength in both directions with a medium arc. When qi is obtained the needle is either extracted or retained. NEEDLE POUNDING falls within the scope of NEUTRAL SUPPLEMENTATION AND DRAINAGE. Application: This method is used for patterns in which neither vacuity nor repletion signs are prevalent or for vacuity-repletion complexes such as is often the case in joint pain. It is also suitable for repletion patterns in patients with weak constitutions. See NEEDLE MANIPULATION. [27: 106] [97: 65] [50: 396] [101: 106]

everted-flower hemorrhoids 翻花痔 *fān huā zhì*: Enduring hemorrhoids failing to heal that hang out of the anus and have an unsmooth surface giving the appearance of a flower past its bloom, with outward turned petals; hence the name. Defecation is associated with precipitation of blood and the insufferable pain. See HEMORRHOIDS. [27: 483] [97: 656]

evil 邪 *xié*: Synonyms: *evil qi*; *disease evil*; *pathogen (obs)*. Any entity from outside or from within that threatens health. Evils include SIX EXCESSES, which are the SIX QI, wind, cold, fire, summerheat, dampness, and dryness, in their capacity to cause disease. They also include the warm evils spoken of by the warm heat school, and the various kinds of TOXIN. Evils further include wind, cold, fire, dampness, and dryness arising within the body, and disease-causing products of the body, static blood and phlegm. "Evil" stands in opposition to "right," the force that maintains health. Since evil actively fights right or summons activity of right to eliminate it, it is often called *evil qi*. *Elementary Questions* (*sù wèn*, *píng rè bìng lùn*) states, "For evil to encroach, the qi must be vacuous." Evils may be classified as yin and yang. Wind, fire, summerheat, and dryness are yang, whereas cold and dampness are yin. They interact with the body in accordance with the laws of yin and yang. Yang evils damage yin, and yin evils damage yang. Thus, in treatment, the principle of dispelling evil under specific circumstances is combined with that of supporting right, i.e., supplementing yang qi in the presence of a yin evil, and supplementing yin in the presence of a yang evil. For example, heat evil is treated by clearing, but when it causes damage to fluids, the method of engendering liquid is used. See also the FIVE EVILS. [26: 312]

evil heat 邪热 *xié rè*: Heat in opposition to right qi. *Evil heat* is essentially the same in meaning as *heat evil*. [27: 124] [97: 177]

evil lodged in the pericardium 邪恋心包 *xié liàn xīn bāo*: Coma and FRIGHT REVERSAL persisting for several days. Evil lodged in the pericardium is usually attributable to phlegm combined with evils and is treated by transforming phlegm and clearing the orifices. [26: 313] [27: 149] [97: 313]

evil lodged in the triple burner 邪留三焦 *xié liú sān jiāo*: **1.** An externally contracted heat (febrile) disease pattern of damp-heat lingering lodged in the qi aspect of the triple burner, characterized by cough, oppression in the chest, abdominal distention, sloppy stool, and inhibited urination. **2.** Any evil harassing the triple burner, disturbing normal qi transformation there, and causing signs of water metabolism disturbances, such as oppression in the chest, lower abdominal urgency, and inhibited urination. [26: 312] [27: 166] [97: 178]

evil qi 邪气 *xié qì*: An evil or evils as an active force. See EVIL; QI. [27: 177]

evil repletion 邪实 *xié shí*: Repletion due to the presence of evil.

evils harm the empty orifices 邪害空窍 *xié hài kōng qiào*: External evils entering the body easily cause diseases of the empty orifices, i.e., the mouth, nose, ears, and eyes. [26: 312] [27: 110] [97: 178]

excess 淫 *yín*, 淫气 *yín qì*: Any of the six qi (wind, cold, fire, summerheat, dampness, and dryness) in excess. ◇ Chin *yín*, excessive, spreading, wanton.

excess among the five minds 五志过极 *wǔ zhì guò jí*: A potentially evil excess of one or more of the five minds (basic mental/emotional activities) (joy, anger, anxiety, thought, fear). See FIVE MINDS FORMING FIRE; MIND; INTERNAL DAMAGE BY THE SEVEN AFFECTS.

excessive wearing of heart construction 心营 过耗 *xīn yíng guò hào*: Excessive wear on heart yin. Damage to yin by enduring heat effusion in externally contracted heat (febrile) disease or by effulgent yin vacuity fire in TAXATION DETRIMENT. Excessive wearing of heart construction is characterized by emaciation, night heat effusion, heat vexation, tendency to sweat, crimson tongue, and a rapid fine pulse. [26: 95]

excrescence 胬肉 *nǔ ròu*: EXCRESCENCE. See EXCRESCENCE CREEPING OVER THE EYE. [26: 654] [27: 503]

excrescence creeping over the eye 胬肉攀睛 *nǔ ròu pān jīng*: A gray-white fleshy growth at the canthus that progressively grows over the eye, in severe cases partially affecting vision. Excrescence creeping over the eye arises when heat congesting in the heart and lung channel cause qi stagnation and blood stasis. It may also result from effulgent yin vacuity fire. WMC pterygium. MED Course wind and clear heat; enrich and downbear fire; free the network vessels and dissipate stasis. Use Anemarrhena, Phellodendron, and Rehmannia Pill (*zhī bǎi dì huáng wán*) plus red peony (*chì sháo yào*) and carthamus (*hóng huā*). Obstruction-Abrading Spirit Light Paste (*mó zhàng líng guāng gāo*) can be applied topically. ACU Base treatment mainly on local eye points, GB, and LR. Select BL-1 (*jīng míng*, Bright Eyes), GB-20 (*fēng chí*, Wind Pool), and LR-14 (*qī mén*, Cycle Gate); needle with drainage. Prick Greater Yang (*tài yáng*) to bleed. [26: 654]

exhaust 竭 *jié*, 衰竭 *shuāi jié*: Deplete critically. See EXUBERANCE AND DEBILITATION.

exhaustion of the lower origin 下元虚惫 *xià yuán xū bèi*: Synonym: *vacuity of the true origin in the lower body*. Severe kidney depletion, especially kidney yang depletion. [27: 164]

exhaustion of yin and desertion of yang 阴竭 阳脱 *yīn jié yáng tuō*: Severe yin and yang vacuity. See DESERTION. [26: 624] [27: 130] [97: 236]

expectoration of blood 咯血 *kǎ xuè*: The bringing up of blood from the chest. The term has two meanings: (1) *Confucian Filiality* (*rú mén shì qīn*) describes this pattern as the expectoration of a blood clot or fresh blood preceded by a sensation of fishy-smelling blood in the throat. Expectoration of blood is mostly attributable to effulgent yin vacuity fire or lung dryness-heat. MED Enrich yin and downbear fire. Use Adenophora/Glehnia and Ophiopogon Decoction (*shā shēn mài dōng tāng*), Mulberry Leaf and Apricot Kernel Decoction (*sāng xìng tāng*), or Six-Ingredient Rehmannia Pill (*liù wèi dì huáng wán*). (2) In some books, such as *On Blood Patterns* (*xuè zhèng lùn*), this term refers to expectoration of phlegm streaked with threads of blood, which arises when effulgent heart channel fire disquiets the blood vessels. MED Clear the heart. Expectoration of blood calls for careful correlation of all signs. ◇ See EXPECTORATION OF PHLEGM. [26: 435] [27: 420] [97: 402] [19: 2576]

expectoration of phlegm 咯痰 *kǎ tán*: Bringing up phlegm from the lung by coughing.

¹**expel** 驱 *qū*, 逐 *zhú*, 追 *zhuī*, 排 *pái*: To promote the elimination from the body (of cold, phlegm, pus, static blood, stones, water, wind, worms). See following entries.

²**expel** 排托 *pái tuō*: EXPELLING PUS AND EXPRESSING TOXIN.

expelling cold accumulations 攻逐寒积 *zhú hán*: A method of treatment used to address stagnation and accumulation patterns characterized by abdominal distention, abdominal pain, constipation, a thick slimy tongue fur, or moist tongue with white fur and absence of thirst call for this method of treatment. Other signs may include by aversion to cold, cold limbs, and thirst with a desire for warm fluids. The method of expelling cold accumulations treats external cold contractions with pre-existing food accumulations. MED The basic medicinal is generally rhubarb (*dà huáng*), which is used with warm and hot agents such as aconite (*fù zǐ*), dried ginger (*gān jiāng*), and cinnamon bark (*ròu guì*). Warm agents with a powerful draining precipitant action such as croton (*bā dòu*) may be prescribed, but in clinical practice few cases warrant their use. A representative formulas is Spleen-Warming Decoction (*wēn pí tāng*).

expelling cold and opening the orifices 逐寒开窍 *zhu hán kāi qiào*: Synonym: *warm opening*. To treat cold-damp phlegm turbidity obstructing the pericardium with coma by means of formulas such as Liquid Storax Pill (*sū hé xiāng wán*). This method is used, for example, in the treatment of wind stroke with clouding collapse, unconsciousness, green-blue or white complexion, cold limbs and a sunken pulse. See OPENING THE ORIFICES. [26: 606] [27: 276] [97: 464]

expelling phlegm 逐痰 *zhú tán*: To eliminate phlegm forcefully.

expelling pus 排脓 *pái nóng*: To promote suppuration to help a sore run its natural course. See EXPELLING PUS AND EXPRESSING TOXIN.

expelling pus and expressing toxin 排脓托毒 *pái nóng tuō dú*: EXPRESSING TOXIN AND OUTTHRUSTING PUS. See INTERNAL EXPRESSION.

expelling stasis 逐瘀 *zhú yū*: A method of treatment used to address blood amassment and internal static blood binds. It includes: (1) internal static blood bind characterized by abdominal pain and distention (sometimes with palpable lumps), black stool, scant menstrual flow, black menstrual flow, heat effusion, and, in severe cases, manic states, and constipation; (2) menstrual block or scant menstrual flow, black menstrual flow and irregular menses resulting from the presence of static blood; (3) uterine concretions and gatherings with malign discharge; (4) the condition identified by Western medicine as extrauterine pregnancy. MED The principal medicinals used are blood breakers and draining precipitants such as rhubarb (*dà huáng*), mirabilite (*máng xiāo*), wingless cockroach (*zhè chóng*), peach kernel (*táo rén*), carthamus (*hóng huā*), sparganium (*sān léng*), zedoary (*é zhú*), and pangolin scales (*chuān shān jiǎ*). Peach Kernel Qi-Coordinating Decoction (*táo hé chéng qì tāng*) is used for recent static blood formations, and Dead-On Pill (*dǐ dàng wán*) is used for old formations. In recent times, extrauterine pregnancy has been treated by the method of expelling static blood, using Engendering Transformation Decoction (*shēng huà tāng*) with the addition of rhubarb (*dà huáng*) and mirabilite (*máng xiāo*), or combined with Nine Pains Pill (*jiǔ tòng wán*). [6: 253]

expelling stones 排石 *pái shí*: A method of treatment used to cause gallstones or urinary stones to be passed out of the body through the stool or urine respectively. Before the modern era, Chinese medicine medicine knew of urinary stones (see STONE STRANGURY), but did not know of gallstones. The term 排石 *pái shí* comes from Western medicine (排石药 *pái shí yào* translating the English 'lithogogue'), and is now used to describe Chinese medical treatments for gallstones or urinary calculus. Formulas whose names contain the term 'expelling stones', such as Biliary Calculus Decoction (*dǎn dào pái shí tāng*), are modern creations. [64: 1288] [60: 235]

expelling water 逐水 *zhú shuǐ*: A method of treatment used to eliminate by precipitation yang water repletion patterns such as severe hydrothorax and ascites, characterized by urinary and fecal stoppage, abdominothoracic fullness inhibiting respiration, and a forceful replete pulse. This method may be used where the evil is strong, yet right qi is still resilient enough to withstand attack. In modern clinical practice, it is mainly used to treat what Western medicine identifies as ascites due to cirrhosis of the liver. Commonly used water-expelling medicinals are kansui (*gān suì*), genkwa (*yuán huā*), euphorbia/knoxia (*dà jǐ*), and morning glory (*qiān niú zǐ*). Ten Jujubes Decoction (*shí zǎo tāng*) and Boats and Carts Pill (*zhōu chē (jū) wán*) drain abdominal water, whereas Drool-Controlling Elixir (*kòng xián dān*) is used to drain hydrothorax. ACU Base treatment mainly on CV and back transport points. Select CV-9 (*shuǐ fēn*, Water Divide), BL-22 (*sān jiāo shū*, Triple Burner Transport), LI-4 (*hé gǔ*, Union Valley), LU-7 (*liè quē*, Broken Sequence), LI-6 (*piān lì*, Veering Passageway), and SP-9 (*yīn líng quán*, Yin Mound Spring); needle with drainage. [6: 252] [26: 606] [27: 258] [97: 464] [46: 676] [113: 183]

expelling worms 驱虫 *qū chóng*: Synonym: *killing worms*. A method of treatment used to cause the elimination of worms (especially in the intestines). Commonly used worm-expelling medicinals are listed below.

Worm-Expelling Medicinals (1)

使君子 (*shǐ jūn zǐ*) quisqualis (Quisqualis Fructus)

苦楝皮 (kǔ liàn pí) chinaberry (root) bark (Meliae Cortex (Radicis))

槟榔 (bīng láng) areca (Arecae Semen)

大腹皮 (dà fù pí) areca husk (Arecae Pericarpium)

南瓜子 (nán guā zǐ) pumpkin seed (Cucurbitae Semen)

雷丸 (léi wán) omphalia (Omphalia)

鹤虱 (hè shī) carpesium seed (Carpesii Fructus)

榧子 (fěi zǐ) torreya (Torreyae Semen)

芜荑 (wú yí) elm cake (Ulmi Fructus Praeparatio)

贯众 (guàn zhòng) aspidium (Aspidii Rhizoma)

Modern research has shown that certain traditional medicinals have the power to expel different parasites recognized in modern medicine.

Worm-Expelling Medicinals (2)

Roundworm (Ascaris)

使君子 (shǐ jūn zǐ) quisqualis (Quisqualis Fructus)

苦楝根皮 (kǔ liàn gēn pí) chinaberry root bark (Meliae Radicis Cortex)

川楝子 (chuān liàn zǐ) toosendan (Toosendan Fructus)

山道年蒿 (shān dào nián hāo) Levant wormseed flower and leaf (Artemisiae Cinae Flos et Folium)

榧子 (fěi zǐ) torreya (Torreyae Semen)

Pinworm (oxyurid)

百部 (bǎi bù) stemona (Stemonae Radix)

贯众 (guàn zhòng) aspidium (Aspidii Rhizoma)

鹤虱 (hè shī) carpesium seed (Carpesii Fructus)

雷丸 (léi wán) omphalia (Omphalia)

大蒜 (dà suàn) garlic (Allii Sativi Bulbus)

石榴皮 (shí liú pí) pomegranate rind (Granati Pericarpium)

鸦胆子 (yā dǎn zǐ) brucea (Bruceae Fructus)

Tapeworm (taenia)

槟榔 (bīng láng) areca (Arecae Semen)

南瓜子 (nán guā zǐ) pumpkin seed (Cucurbitae Semen)

仙鹤草根芽 (xiān hè cǎo gēn yá) agrimony root sprout (Agrimoniae Rhizoma Pullulatum)

雷丸 (léi wán) omphalia (Omphalia)

贯众 (guàn zhòng) aspidium (Aspidii Rhizoma)

Hookworm (ancylostomum)

槟榔 (bīng láng) areca (Arecae Semen)

雷丸 (léi wán) omphalia (Omphalia)

榧子 (fěi zǐ) torreya (Torreyae Semen)

苦楝根皮 (kǔ liàn gēn pí) chinaberry root bark (Meliae Radicis Cortex)

石榴皮 (shí liú pí) pomegranate rind (Granati Pericarpium)

Fasciolopsis

槟榔 (bīng láng) areca (Arecae Semen)

榧子 (fěi zǐ) torreya (Torreyae Semen)

ACU The main acupuncture point for expelling worms is Hundred Worm Nest (bǎi chóng wō), in the inside of the thigh, three body-inches up from the kneecap. For roundworm, for example, this point can be combined with BL-20 (pí shū, Spleen Transport), BL-25 (dà cháng shū, Large Intestine Transport), ST-4 (dì cāng, Earth Granary), SP-15 (dà hèng, Great Horizontal), LI-4 (hé gǔ, Union Valley), and ST-36 (zú sān lǐ, Leg Three Li). [50: 861] [97: 323] [37: 320] [16: 571]

expiration sweating 绝汗 jué hàn: *Synonym: desertion sweating.* Sweating in critical conditions where separation of yin and yang is imminent. Expiration of qi is characterized by putting forth of pearly sweat that sticks to the body and does not run. Dissipation of qi is marked by putting forth of oily sweat, and incessant panting. Extreme vacuity is marked by incessant cold sweating. MED Return yang and stem desertion with medicinals such as ginseng (rén shēn), aconite (fù zǐ), dragon bone (lóng gǔ), and oyster shell (mǔ lì). [26: 754] [27: 290] [97: 445]

expire 绝 jué: To come to an end; to be critically exhausted.

expressing toxin and outthrusting pus 托毒透脓 tuō dú tòu nóng: *Synonym: expelling pus and expressing toxin.* An INTERNAL EXPRESSION method applied when right qi is exuberant. See INTERNAL EXPRESSION.

expression 托法 tuō fǎ: INTERNAL EXPRESSION [26: 143]

extended tongue 伸舌 shēn shé: *Synonym: protracted tongue.* A tongue that is habitually extended out of the mouth and cannot be retracted. An extended tongue that feels scorching hot accompanied by unclear spirit-mind reflects phlegm-heat evil harassing the heart spirit affecting the "sprout of the heart" (the tongue). MED Clear the heart and transform phlegm. A limp, numb, extended tongue is usually a sign of qi vacuity. Compare PROTRUSION AND WORRYING OF THE TONGUE. [26: 337]

exterior 表 biǎo: The outer part of the body as opposed to the interior; includes the *fleshy exterior* (i.e., the skin and exterior muscles of the head, limbs and trunk) and *bowels*, which are the organs of the exterior through which the essence of grain and water (nutrients in food) are absorbed and waste is expelled. See EXTERIOR AND INTERIOR. ◇ Chin 表 biǎo, surface, exterior. [97: 325]

exterior and interior 表里 biǎo lǐ: The outer part of the body and the inner part of the body; two of the EIGHT PRINCIPLES. The skin and the [body] hair, the flesh, and the superficial channels are exterior. The bone marrow, the bowels and viscera, etc., are considered as interior. Exterior and interior are two of eight principles of pattern identification, by which the depth of penetration of external evils is determined. External evils usually pass through the exterior before penetrating the interior; hence their presence makes exterior-interior pattern identification a necessity. Internal damage miscellaneous diseases originate within the body and invariably manifest as interior patterns, so that the need for interior-exterior pattern identification is of little significance. In the cold damage and warm disease theories, exterior and interior have specific definitions. In cold damage, there are two definitions: a) the yang channels are exterior and the yin channels are interior, b) among the yang channels, greater yang (*tài yáng*) is exterior, whereas yang brightness (*yáng míng*) is interior, with lesser yang (*shào yáng*) as "half exterior half interior." In warm disease triple burner pattern identification, the upper burner is exterior, whereas the middle and lower burners are interior. [26: 356]

exterior cold 表寒 *biǎo hán*: Exterior cold patterns are characterized by pronounced cold signs with a distinct aversion to cold. The pulse is tight and floating, and the tongue fur is thin, white, and moist. "When cold prevails there is pain," and in exterior cold patterns headache and generalized pain and heaviness are also pronounced. Runny nose with clear snivel (nasal mucus), and expectoration of clear thin phlegm are common signs. Exterior cold patterns are generally caused by contraction of wind-cold evil. [MED] Exterior cold patterns are treated with warm acrid exterior-resolving medicinals. The most commonly used are ephedra (*má huáng*), cinnamon twig (*guì zhī*), notopterygium (*qiāng huó*), perilla leaf (*zǐ sū yè*), schizonepeta (*jīng jiè*), and ledebouriella (*fáng fēng*). Formulas include Ephedra Decoction (*má huáng tāng*) and Schizonepeta and Ledebouriella Toxin-Vanquishing Powder (*jīng fáng bài dú sǎn*). [ACU] Base treatment mainly on LI, LU, and BL. Select BL-13 (*fèi shū*, Lung Transport), GB-20 (*fēng chí*, Wind Pool), BL-12 (*fēng mén*, Wind Gate), LU-7 (*liè quē*, Broken Sequence), LI-4 (*hé gǔ*, Union Valley), KI-7 (*fù liū*, Recover Flow), and BL-11 (*dà zhù*, Great Shuttle); needle with drainage and moxa can be used. [46: 595, 650, 652] [113: 18] [6: 150]

exterior cold and interior heat 表寒里热 *biǎo hán lǐ rè*: A pattern of cold in the exterior and heat in the interior arising when external evil passes into the interior and transforms into heat before the exterior cold has resolved. It can also arise in a condition of internal heat when cold evil is contracted. Exterior cold and interior heat patterns are characterized by aversion to cold, heat effusion, absence of sweating, and generalized pain. These signs may

be accompanied by vexation and agitation, thirst, and constipation. [26: 356]

exterior heat 表热 *biǎo rè*: Exterior heat patterns are characterized by pronounced heat signs, such as a red sore pharynx and a relatively red tongue with dry fur. In addition to the regular external signs, the pulse is floating and rapid. Other signs include cough and the production of thick white or yellow phlegm. Most exterior heat patterns are attributable to contraction of wind-heat evil. Note that identification of exterior heat patterns is based on assessment of heat and cold "signs" rather than the actual body temperature. Heat effusion as a sign does not necessarily correspond to heat in the sense of the eight principles. [MED] Exterior heat patterns are treated with cool acrid exterior-resolving medicinals such as mint (*bò hé*), arctium (*niú bàng zǐ*), fermented soybean (*dàn dòu chǐ*), and mulberry leaf (*sāng yè*). Formulas include Lonicera and Forsythia Powder (*yín qiào sǎn*) and Mulberry Leaf and Chrysanthemum Beverage (*sāng jú yǐn*). [ACU] Base treatment mainly on LU, LI, and PC. Select BL-13 (*fèi shū*, Lung Transport), GB-20 (*fēng chí*, Wind Pool), TB-5 (*wài guān*, Outer Pass), LU-10 (*yú jì*, Fish Border), LU-5 (*chǐ zé*, Cubit Marsh), LI-4 (*hé gǔ*, Union Valley), LI-11 (*qū chí*, Pool at the Bend), and GV-14 (*dà zhuī*, Great Hammer); needle with drainage. For red sore pharynx, prick LU-11 (*shào shāng*, Lesser Shang) and LI-1 (*shāng yáng*, Shang Yang) to bleed with a three-edged needle. [6: 150] [46: 595, 651, 653] [113: 18]

exterior heat and interior cold 表热里寒 *biǎo rè lǐ hán*: A condition of heat in the exterior with cold in the interior arising on contraction of wind-heat in patients ordinarily suffering from spleen-stomach vacuity cold. Signs include heat effusion without sweating, sore throat and cough, sloppy diarrhea, long clear voidings of urine, pale enlarged tongue, slightly yellow turbid tongue fur, and a moderate floating pulse. [26: 357]

exterior heat passing into the interior 表热传里 *biǎo rè chuán lǐ*: HEAT EVIL PASSING INTO THE INTERIOR.

exterior pattern 表证 *biǎo zhèng*: The manifestation of disease in the exterior of the body, caused by any of the SIX EXCESSES entering the body's exterior. Exterior pattern is characterized by sudden onset and by aversion to cold (or the milder aversion to wind), heat effusion, headache, a thin tongue fur, and a floating pulse. Other possible signs are headache, nasal congestion, and aching pain in the limbs and joints. Exterior patterns vary according to the offending evil and its strength in relation to that of right qi. Wind accompanied by cold or heat is the most common cause; summerheat, dampness, and dryness are less common.

Distinction is made between EXTERIOR COLD, EXTERIOR HEAT, EXTERIOR VACUITY, and EXTERIOR REPLETION. Exterior patterns are treated by sweating to expel the evil from the body. [27: 208] [97: 325]

exterior repletion 表实 *biǎo shí*: Exterior patterns without sweating are exterior repletion patterns. In most cases, exterior repletion patterns are exterior cold patterns caused by contraction of exuberant cold evil that obstructs defense qi and blocks the interstices, and manifesting in a tight floating pulse. MED Treat with strong sweat-effusing warm acrid exterior-resolving medicinals. The classical formula is Ephedra Decoction (*má huáng tāng*). ACU Base treatment mainly on LI, LU, and BL. Select BL-13 (*fèi shū*, Lung Transport), BL-12 (*fēng mén*, Wind Gate), LU-7 (*liè què*, Broken Sequence), BL-64 (*jīng gǔ*, Capital Bone), LI-4 (*hé gǔ*, Union Valley), KI-7 (*fù liū*, Recover Flow), and BL-11 (*dà zhù*, Great Shuttle); needle with drainage and moxa can be used. The last three points are used to effuse sweat and resolve the exterior. [6: 150] [46: 650, 652] [113: 18] [75: 63]

exterior repletion and interior vacuity 表实里虚 *biǎo shí lǐ xū*: A pattern arising either when patients ordinarily suffering from heart, spleen, or kidney vacuity contract external evil, or when external contractions manifesting as exterior cold are wrongly treated by offensive attack. Signs include heat effusion and aversion to cold without sweating with lassitude of spirit, shortness of breath, torpid intake, fatigued limbs, heart palpitations, lumbar pain, a white tongue fur, and a floating pulse. [26: 357]

exterior resolution 解表 *jiě biǎo*: See RESOLVING THE EXTERIOR.

exterior vacuity 表虚 *biǎo xū*: Exterior patterns with persistent sweating and heat effusion. Exterior vacuity results from construction-defense disharmony in which the body's resistance to external evils is lowered and, despite sweating, fails to expel the evil. Such conditions are reflected in a moderate (i.e., not tight) floating pulse. MED Exterior patterns with sweating should be treated with formulas that have a sweat-effusing effect. A persistent exterior pattern with sweating characterized by pronounced exterior vacuity signs such as a moderate floating pulse and a thin moist tongue fur should be treated with Cinnamon Twig Decoction (*guì zhī tāng*). This formula harmonizes construction and defense. ACU Base treatment mainly on LU, LI, and BL. Select BL-13 (*fèi shū*, Lung Transport), GB-20 (*fēng chí*, Wind Pool), LU-7 (*liè què*, Broken Sequence), BL-64 (*jīng gǔ*, Capital Bone), ST-36 (*zú sān lǐ*, Leg Three Li), LI-4 (*hé gǔ*, Union Valley), and SI-3 (*hòu xī*, Back

Ravine); needle with even supplementation and drainage. The last two points are used to check sweating and secure the exterior. [6: 150] [113: 18] [46: 650, 652] [113: 18] [75: 47] [46: 602, 653, 655]

exterior vacuity and interior repletion 表虚里实 *biǎo xū lǐ shí*: A condition arising a) when patients with constitutional insufficiency of defense qi contract evil, and evil heat binds in the interior; b) when patients suffering from heat brewing in the stomach and intestines and abiding food contract wind evil; or c) when exterior patterns are not treated properly and interior repletion is treated by sweating. Such a condition is characterized by exterior vacuity signs such as aversion to wind and sweating, and by interior repletion signs such as abdominal pain, constipation, and thick yellow tongue fur. [26: 356]

external 外 *wài*: Located or originating outside (the body), as in *external evil*.

external blowing 外吹 *wài chuī*: Synonym: *external blowing mammary welling-abscess*. A post-partum MAMMARY WELLING-ABSCESS, so called on account of the belief that it arose when, after breast-feeding, the infant slept soundly in the mother's bosom and its cool breath invaded the breast. Compare INTERNAL BLOWING. ◇ Chin 外 *wài*, external, outer; 吹 *chuī*, blow. So called because it was originally attributed to external wind blowing on the breast or the breath of the infant. [26: 211] [27: 460]

external blowing mammary welling-abscess 外吹乳痈 *wài chuī rǔ yōng*: EXTERNAL BLOWING.

external cause 外因 *wài yīn*: One of the THREE CAUSES [OF DISEASE]; any evil that assails the body from outside. External causes are the SIX EXCESSES (and WARM EVIL). [27: 106] [97: 157]

external cold 外寒 *wài hán*: **1.** Externally contracted cold evil, characterized by signs such as aversion to cold, heat effusion, absence of sweating, headache, generalized pain, and a tight floating pulse, which develop when cold evil assails the exterior and prevents the normal diffusion and outthrust of yang qi. **2.** Insufficiency of yang qi at the surface of the body, marked by physical cold and fear of cold. *Elementary Questions* (*sù wèn, tiáo jīng lùn*) states, "When yang is vacuous, there is external cold." [26: 212]

external cold invading the stomach 外寒犯胃 *wài hán fàn wèi*: See STOMACH REPLETION COLD. [116: 95]

external contraction 外感 *wài gǎn*: Contraction of external evil; a condition resulting from contraction of external evil. [27: 110] [97: 158]

external contraction lumbar pain 外感腰痛 *wài gǎn yāo tòng*: Lumbar pain attributed to external evil invading the channels and network vessels. External contraction lumbar pain usually forms a repletion pattern and is treated by dispelling the evil and freeing the network vessels. See WIND-DAMP LUMBAR PAIN; COLD-DAMP LUMBAR PAIN; DAMP-HEAT LUMBAR PAIN. See also LUMBAR PAIN. [26: 213]

external contraction sleeplessness 外感不得 卧 *wài gǎn bù dé wò*: Insomnia due to contraction of the external evils. External contraction sleeplessness is observed in exterior heat, internal heat, half exterior and half interior heat, qi-aspect heat, blood-aspect heat, residual heat, and excessive sweating or precipitation. See SLEEPLESSNESS. [50: 456]

external contraction stomach duct pain 外 感胃脘痛 *wài gǎn wèi wǎn (guǎn) tòng*: Pain in the stomach due to contraction of external evils such as cold evil or damp-heat. Cold patterns usually occur in people suffering from preexisting center qi cold; heat patterns usually occur in patients with accumulated internal heat. **Cold evil** invades the stomach in sudden cold weather and invariably congeals and binds with phlegm-rheum and food accumulations, thereby obstructing qi dynamic. Such patterns are characterized by fulminant pain, glomus and oppression below the heart, aversion to cold and reversal cold, clear uninhibited urine and stool, ejection of cold drool, tight floating or stringlike sunken pulse. MED Warm and dissipate with formulas such as Five Accumulations Powder (*wǔ jī sǎn*). ACU Base treatment mainly on alarm and uniting points of ST, PC, SP, LI, and LU. Select CV-12 (*zhōng wǎn*, Center Stomach Duct), ST-36 (*zú sān lǐ*, Leg Three Li), PC-6 (*nèi guān*, Inner Pass), SP-4 (*gōng sūn*, Yellow Emperor), LI-4 (*hé gǔ*, Union Valley), and LU-7 (*liè quē*, Broken Sequence); needle with drainage and add moxa. Selection of points according to associated evil: For phlegm-rheum, add ST-40 (*fēng lóng*, Bountiful Bulge), ST-25 (*tiān shū*, Celestial Pivot), and CV-6 (*qì hǎi*, Sea of Qi). For food accumulation, add CV-10 (*xià wǎn*, Lower Stomach Duct), Li Inner Court (*lǐ nèi tíng*), and CV-21 (*xuán jī*, Jade Swivel). For pronounced pain, add ST-34 (*liáng qiū*, Beam Hill). For pronounced qi stagnation, add CV-17 (*shān zhōng*, Chest Center). **Damp-heat** invades the stomach in sudden hot weather, giving rise to sudden gripping pain. Although the extremities may be cold, there is copious sweating from the forehead, and although there may be aversion to cold, there are clear heat signs such as dry mouth and tongue, yellow or red urine, and a rapid pulse. MED Clear and resolve with variations of Center-Clearing Decoction (*qīng zhōng tāng*). ACU Base treatment mainly on alarm and uniting points of ST, PC, SP, LU, and LI. Select CV-12 (*zhōng wǎn*, Center Stomach Duct), ST-36 (*zú sān lǐ*, Leg Three Li), PC-6 (*nèi guān*, Inner Pass), SP-4 (*gōng sūn*, Yellow Em-

peror), LI-11 (*qū chí*, Pool at the Bend), SP-9 (*yīn líng quán*, Yin Mound Spring), ST-45 (*lì duì*, Severe Mouth), and ST-44 (*nèi tíng*, Inner Court); needle with drainage. For dry mouth and tongue, add Gold Liquid and Jade Humor (*jīn jīn yù yè*), and KI-6 (*zhào hǎi*, Shining Sea) See STOMACH DUCT PAIN. [26: 213] [50: 457] [46: 660] [37: 311]

external evil 外邪 *wài xié*: Evil invading the body from outside. See EVIL. [27: 107] [97: 157]

external injury 外伤 *wài shāng*: Synonym: *trauma*. Any damage to the body from outside; includes KNOCKS AND FALLS, INCISED WOUNDS, BURNS AND SCALDS, and snake bites. Most external injuries involve damage to the skin and flesh, the sinews and bone, and the qi and blood. Knocks and falls include most BONE FRACTURES and sinew damage. Incised wounds primarily lead to BLOOD SPILLAGE; BURNS AND SCALDS cause damage to the skin and flesh and damage to yin. [27: 119] [97: 157]

external injury lumbar pain 外伤腰痛 *wài shāng yāo tòng*: Lumbar pain due to external injury preventing bending and stretching and turning, and even pain when breathing. See STATIC BLOOD LUMBAR PAIN. [37: 391]

external kidney 外肾 *wài shèn*: Scrotum or the male genitals. [97: 158]

externally contracted heat (febrile) disease 外 感热病 *wài gǎn rè bìng*: Any disease caused by influences originating outside the body, characterized by heat effusion and a usually rapid stage-by-stage progression. The earliest extant compilation dealing with external heat (febrile) diseases, *On Cold Damage* (*shāng hán lùn*), written in the Han Dynasty, identifies and treats diseases according to their location among the six channels. Further accumulation of experience and developments in medical thought in the ages that followed culminated in the doctrine of warm diseases. *On Warm Heat* (*wēn rè lùn*) and *Systematized Identification of Warm Diseases* (*wēn bìng tiáo biàn*) are two works of the Qing Dynasty that further synthesized the laws governing the origin and development of external heat diseases into the system known as four-aspect pattern identification and treatment. As a result of these latter-day developments there have emerged two separate schools of thought, the "cold damage" school and the "warm diseases" school. [6: 222]

externally contracted heat (febrile) disease pattern identification 外感热病辨证 *wài gǎn rè bìng biàn zhèng*: Identification of sign patterns of external heat (febrile) disease. It includes DISEASE-EVIL PATTERN IDENTIFICATION, SIX-CHANNEL PATTERN IDENTIFICATION, and FOUR-ASPECT PATTERN IDENTIFICATION. Despite differences between these methods of pattern identification, certain general guidelines are common to both. Disease of external origin are usually (but not always) characterized by heat effusion and stage-by-stage development (initial stage, exuberant heat effusion stage, and recovery stage). Externally contracted heat diseases bear two main characteristics: heat effusion and stage-by-stage development. Heat effusion results from the fierce struggle between right qi and the evil, and is the essential characteristic of externally contracted heat diseases. Its progress reflects the changing relationship between right qi and evil qi. For example, high fever reflects the strong reaction of an undamaged right qi to a highly toxic evil. The heat effusion will gradually subside as right qi overcomes the evil. A remittent heat effusion or persistent heat effusion sets in when the evil has weakened, but has not been fully eradicated and right qi has suffered damage. Absence of initial-stage heat effusion, or even a sudden drop in body temperature, are signs of yang collapse resulting from the presence of a highly toxic evil and extreme vacuity of right. Externally contracted heat diseases usually develop through three stages: the initial stage, the exuberant heat effusion stage, and the recovery stage. These three stages reflect the changing relationship between the evil and right. In the initial stage, the struggle between the evil and right has still not reached its height, so that the heat effusion is less severe than in the exuberant heat effusion stage. As the struggle becomes more intense, the disease moves into the exuberant heat effusion stage; signs are most pronounced, indicating that the disease has reached its climax. It is at this crucial stage that deterioration or improvement is decided. If right defeats evil, the disease passes into the recovery stage. If it fails to do so, the patient's condition deteriorates, possibly leading to death. Of course, recovery may come about at any point during the progression of a disease if evil qi weakens and right qi strengthens, either spontaneously or by appropriate treatment. Similarly, deterioration or relapse may occur at any time if evil qi strengthens and right qi weakens, either spontaneously or by inappropriate treatment. Most incidences of externally contracted heat disease are characterized by the above-mentioned three stages. [6: 222]

external medicine 外科 *wài kē*: The branch of medicine that deals with sores, knocks and falls, and bone fractures. For a list of external medical diseases, see DISEASE. ◊ Chin 外 *wài*, outside, external; 科 *kē*, department. Note that term is used in Western medicine as the equivalent of the English "surgery." [27: 298] [96]

external obstruction 外障 *wài zhàng*: Any disease of the eyelids, canthi, white of the eye or black of the eye. External obstructions include red sore swollen eyes (e.g., fire eye), erosion, tearing, eye discharge, or dryness of the eyes, eye screens and membranes, and excrescences of the canthi. They may be attended by subjective sensations such as pain, itching, dryness, and aversion to light. They are mostly attributable to invasion of the six excesses or depressed heat or phlegm-fire in the inner body, or to external injury. In some cases, they may be attributable to liver-kidney vacuity with vacuity fire flaming upward or spleen qi vacuity. Compare INTERNAL OBSTRUCTION. [26: 214] [27: 508] [97: 158]

external welling-abscess 外痈 *wài yōng*: A WELLING-ABSCESS in the exterior of the body. External welling-abscesses are characterized by clearly circumscribed redness, swelling, heat, and pain; they are easily dispersed, easily form pus and rupture, and easily heal. [WMC] cellulitis; acute abscesses. [MED] Oral: In the early stages, disperse wind and clear heat, quicken the blood and move stasis using Immortal Formula Life-Giving Beverage (*xiān fāng huó mìng yǐn*). Upper body welling-abscesses are largely attributable to wind-heat and can be treated by Arctium Flesh-Resolving Decoction (*niú bàng jiě jī tāng*); lower body welling-abscesses are largely attributable to damp-heat, and can be treated with Fish Poison Yam Toxin-Transforming Decoction (*bì xiè huà dú tāng*). If there is a concurrent exterior pattern, Schizonepeta and Ledebouriella Toxin-Vanquishing Powder (*jīng fáng bài dú sǎn*) can be used to resolve the exterior and dissipate evil. For repletion heat interior patterns, Internal Coursing Coptis Decoction (*nèi shū huáng lián tāng*) can be used. Welling-abscesses that are slow to suppurate can be treated with Pus-Outthrusting Powder (*tòu nóng sǎn*). Excessive discharge of pus can be treated by supplementing blood and qi. Topical: In the early stages, clear heat and disperse swelling with Golden Yellow Powder (*jīn huáng sǎn*), Jade Dew Powder (*yù lù sǎn*), or Tai Yi Plaster (*tài yī gāo*). After pus has formed, the welling-abscess should be cut open and Five-to-Five Elixir (*wǔ wǔ dān*) or Nine-to-One Elixir (*jiǔ yī dān*) should be applied to raise pus and dispel putridity. When the discharge of pus ceases, use Flesh-Engendering Powder (*shēng jī sǎn*) or Flesh-Engendering Jade and Red Paste (*shēng jī yù hóng gāo*) to engender flesh and promote closure. See WELLING-ABSCESS.[1] [26: 214] [27: 458] [97: 158]

extinguishing wind 熄风 *xī fēng*: *Synonym: calming and extinguishing internal wind.* Any method of treatment used to eliminate internal wind. Extinguishing wind includes the methods listed below. [27: 267] [26: 833] [97: 632] [50: 1671]

Extinguishing Wind

ENRICHING YIN AND EXTINGUISHING WIND (*zī yīn xī fēng*)

CALMING THE LIVER AND EXTINGUISHING WIND (*píng gān xī fēng*)

DRAINING FIRE AND EXTINGUISHING WIND (*xiè huǒ xī fēng*)

HARMONIZING THE BLOOD AND EXTINGUISHING WIND (*hé xuè xī fēng*)

---

extinguishing wind and transforming phlegm 熄风化痰 *xī fēng huà tán*: CONTROLLING WIND AND TRANSFORMING PHLEGM.

extraordinary organ 奇恒之腑 *qí héng zhī fǔ*: Any of a class of organs comprising the brain, the marrow, the bones, the vessels, the uterus, and the gallbladder, distinguished from the bowels on the grounds that they do not decompose food and convey waste and from the viscera on the grounds they do not produce and store essence. The gallbladder is an exception, because it is classed both as a bowel and as an extraordinary organ. It is considered a bowel because it plays a role in the processing and conveyance of food, and stands in interior-exterior relationship with its paired viscus, the liver. However, the bile that it produces is regarded as a "clear fluid" rather than as waste; hence it is also classed among the extraordinary organs. [27: 24] [97: 329]

extraordinary vessel 奇经 *qí jīng*: See EIGHT EXTRAORDINARY VESSELS.

extreme heat engendering cold 热极生寒 *rè jí shēng hán*: Transmutation of heat into cold. Heat is yang, whereas cold is yin. Since yin and yang are mutually transmutable, heat can give way to cold, as the heat of summer gives way to the cold of winter. In the body, damage to yin by extreme heat can cause yang desertion characterized by counterflow cold of the limbs with great sweating, and a faint pulse on the verge of expiration. Similarly, heat lying deep in the body can cause SEVERE HEAT AND SEVERE REVERSAL. [26: 875] [27: 134]

extreme heat engendering wind 热极生风 *rè jí shēng fēng*: Synonym: *exuberant heat stirring wind*. See LIVER WIND STIRRING INTERNALLY.

exuberance 盛 *shèng*: Vigor and abundance. Describes both yin and yang entities.

exuberance and debilitation 盛衰 *shèng shuāi*: Exuberance denotes vigor and profusion; debilitation denotes weakness and scarcity. Both describe strength or weakness of organs or physiological elements (qi, blood, fluid, essence), but in the main, exuberance qualifies evils. **1.** Exuberant evils, physiological elements, and yin-yang aspects of the organs are often described in terms of the way in which they affect the parts of the organism.

Invasion (犯 *fàn*) and **assailment** (袭 *xí*) both describe the intrusion of an exuberant evil into the body; invasion also describes intrusion of the qi of one bowel or viscus into another, e.g., liver qi invading the stomach. **Fettering** (束 *shù*) denotes the inhibitive effect of an external evil on the lung or exterior. **Encumbrance** (困 *kùn*) refers to the inhibitive effect of dampness (or damp-heat) on the splenic function of moving water-damp (often manifesting as heavy cumbersome limbs). **Congealing** (凝 *níng*) is an attribute of dampness, but often describes the dampening effect of cold on the movement of blood or qi. **Clouding** (蒙 *méng*) and (蔽 *bì*) and **confounding** (迷 *mí*) both denote the effect of phlegm on the orifices of the heart resulting in essence-spirit (mental) derangement or coma. **Harassment** (扰 *rǎo*) describes the effect of heat or phlegm causing dizziness or essence-spirit (mental) derangement. **Flood** (泛 *fàn*) denotes water accumulations due to kidney yang vacuity. **Shooting** (射 *shè*) and **intimidation** (凌 *líng*) describe the effect of water flood on the lung and heart respectively. **Upsurge** (上冲 *shàng chōng*) describes the upward movement of qi, as in the sensation associated with RUNNING PIGLET or in the pathomechanism associated with UPSURGING YELLOW HUMOR. **Bind** (结 *jié*) suggests intensification or concentration when applied to qi, affects, or evils, and also describes the substantial hardening produced as a result (e.g., phlegm nodes). **Contention** (相搏 *xiāng bó*) describes the mutually inhibitive effect as of phlegm and qi that results in the binding of the two to produce scrofula, phlegm nodes, etc. **Mutual fanning** (相煽 *xiāng shàn*) frequently describes the interaction of wind and fire. **Stirring** (动 *dòng*) describes the development of wind, either as a result of blood vacuity or of liver fire flaming upward (repletion); it also describes the effect of exuberant heat on the blood, causing frenetic blood. Terms describing the effect of heat may be found under HEAT. See also TRANSFORMATION. **2.** Terms related to debilitation describe the degree and nature of weakness. **Debilitation** (衰 *shuāi*) itself is a general word, but is often applied to severe conditions. **Devitalization** (不振 *bù zhèn*) usually describes a weakened state of the essence-spirit, i.e., lack of mental or general vigor; in the context of spleen yang, it describes a relatively severe weakness. **Insecurity** (不固 *bù gù*) denotes failure to retain sweat, stool, or essence, or to resist invading evils. **Downward fall** (下陷 *xià xiàn*) is the downward movement of vacuous qi manifesting in the form of prolapse of the rectum and fecal incontinence or prolapse of the uterus. Both insecurity and downward fall are results of debilitation. **Detriment** (损 *sǔn*) describes the reductive effect of damaging influences. **Despoliation** (夺 *duó*) is sudden or harsh detriment to body elements. **Wearing** (耗 *hào*) denotes gradual detriment. **Taxation** is severe, usually gradual detriment to the organs, often in diseases Western medicine would describe as consumptive. **Depletion** (亏 *kuī*) and **exhaustion** (竭 *jié*) describe severe, usually gradual reduction, the former usually being applied to kidney essence, and the latter to the blood, fluids, or essence. **Collapse** (亡 *wáng*) denotes critical insufficiency of yin, yang, blood, or fluids. **Desertion** (脱 *tuō*) is similar to collapse, but also implies the resultant loss to the body; it is also particularly associated with loss of physiological elements, and hence is often used in conjunction with the term **efflux** (滑 *huá*), which denotes loss of liquids or blood. **Floating** (浮 *fú*) sometimes describes extreme yang vacuity characterized by vacuity heat signs in the upper body or outer body, and also describes exterior repletion heat in initial-stage externally contracted heat (febrile) diseases. **Expiration** (绝 *jué*) refers to a critical weakness, usually of organ functions, which portends death.

exuberant fire tormenting metal 火盛刑金 *huǒ shèng xíng jīn*: **1.** Liver fire affecting the lung. See WOOD FIRE TORMENTING METAL. **2.** Heart fire or fire-heat affecting the lung. Heart fire can damage lung yin, giving rise to panting and cough with phlegm-streaked blood; an intense heat evil becoming depressed in the lung or phlegm-heat obstructing the lung can give rise to high fever, hasty rapid breathing, flaring nostrils, and in severe cases coughing of blood. [26: 97]

exuberant heart fire 心火盛 *xīn huǒ shèng*: HYPERACTIVE HEART FIRE.

exuberant heart qi 心气盛 *xīn qì shèng*: Heart vexation, insomnia, laughing while dreaming in intense heart fire patterns. [27: 148] [97: 119]

exuberant heart-stomach fire 心胃火盛 *xīn wèi huǒ shèng*: Synonym: *heart-stomach repletion fire*. A disease pattern arising when, in intense heart fire, evil heat invades the stomach. The chief signs are vexation and insomnia, red face, thirst, mouth sores, scorching pain in the stomach duct, swallowing of upflowing acid, and swift digestion and rapid hungering. Other signs include mania and delirious speech, red urine with inhibited voidings and stinging pain, bloody urine, immediate vomiting of ingested food, bad breath, bleeding gums, sore swollen gums, and constipation. The tongue is red with yellow fur. The pulse is slippery and rapid. MED Clear the heart and quiet the spirit; drain fire and harmonize the stomach. Heart-Draining Decoction (*xiè xīn tāng*) or Red-Abducting Powder (*dǎo chì sǎn*). ACU Base treatment mainly on PC, HT, and ST. Use the main points under EXUBERANT HEART FIRE, and add ST-44 (*nèi tíng*, Inner Court), ST-36 (*zú sān lǐ*, Leg Three Li), and

LI-4 (*hé gǔ*, Union Valley); needle with drainage. Selection of points according to signs: For stomach duct pain, add CV-12 (*zhōng wǎn*, Center Stomach Duct), ST-45 (*lì duì*, Severe Mouth), and TB-6 (*zhī gōu*, Branch Ditch). For swallowing of upflowing acid, add BL-18 (*gān shū*, Liver Transport) and GB-40 (*qiū xū*, Hill Ruins). For bloody urine, add CV-4 (*guān yuán*, Pass Head). For vomiting, add CV-12 (*zhōng wǎn*, Center Stomach Duct) and PC-6 (*nèi guān*, Inner Pass). For bad breath, add CV-24 (*chéng jiāng*, Sauce Receptacle). For bleeding gums, add ST-45 (*lì duì*, Severe Mouth) and ST-6 (*jiá chē*, Cheek Carriage). For treatment of other signs, see EXUBERANT HEART FIRE. [57: 96] [46: 596, 659, 670, 725, 740] [113: 18, 154, 216] [37: 311, 349]

exuberant heart qi 心气盛 *xīn qì shèng*: Synonym: *exuberant heart yang*; *heart qi repletion*. The heart governs the blood and vessels and stores the spirit, and exuberant heart qi manifests in disease patterns of the spirit mind and of the blood and vessels. *The Magic Pivot* (*líng shū*) states, "When heart qi is exuberant, there is dreaming and a tendency to laughing and fear." *The Origin and Indicators of Disease* (*zhū bìng yuán hòu lùn*) states, "When heart qi is exuberant, making the spirit superabundant, there is pain in the chest, propping fullness in the rib-side, pain under the rib-side, pain in the anterior chest, back, shoulder blade, armpit, or pain in the inside of the arm, and incessant joy and laughing; this is repletion of heart qi." TRT Clear the heart and drain fire. [50: 340] [97: 119]

exuberant heart yang 心阳盛 *xīn yáng shèng*: EXUBERANT HEART QI. [50: 340] [97: 119]

exuberant heat stirring wind 热盛动风 *rè shèng dòng fēng*: See EXTREME HEAT ENGENDERING WIND.

exuberant internal yin cold 阴盛内寒 *yīn shèng nèi hán*: See EXUBERANT YIN. [26: 619] [27: 129] [97: 236]

exuberant lung-stomach heat 肺胃热盛 *fèi wèi rè shèng*: In warm disease, a qi-aspect heat pattern manifesting in classic signs of wind warmth: high fever, cough, rapid breathing, thirst, and yellow tongue fur. MED The main formula treating exuberant lung-stomach heat is Supplemented Ephedra, Apricot Kernel, Gypsum, and Licorice Decoction (*jiā wèi má xìng shí gān tāng*), which clears heat and diffuses the lung. This formula may be combined with heat-clearing phlegm-transforming formulas such as Minor Chest Bind Decoction (*xiǎo xiàn xiōng tāng*) and further supplemented with heat-clearing toxin-resolving medicinals such as lonicera (*jīn yín huā*), forsythia (*lián qiào*), scutellaria (*huáng qín*), and gardenia (*shān zhī zǐ*). ACU Base treatment mainly on

LU, ST, and LI. Select LU-10 (*yú jì,* Fish Border), LU-5 (*chǐ zé,* Cubit Marsh), LI-11 (*qū chí,* Pool at the Bend), ST-44 (*nèi tíng,* Inner Court), ST-36 (*zú sān lǐ,* Leg Three Li), and LI-4 (*hé gǔ,* Union Valley); needle with drainage. Prick LU-11 (*shào shāng,* Lesser Shang) or LI-1 (*shāng yáng,* Shang Yang) to bleed. See QI-ASPECT PATTERN. [6: 233] [46: 650, 652]

exuberant qi-aspect heat 热盛气分 *rè shèng qì fèn*: Intense heat in the qi aspect, characterized by vigorous heat [effusion] without aversion to cold, red facial complexion, vexation, great sweating and great thirst, dry yellow tongue fur, and a large surging pulse. [26: 873] [27: 134] [97: 455]

exuberant stomach heat 胃热壅盛 *wèi rè yōng shèng*: *Synonym: intense stomach heat.* Severe heat in the stomach characterized by vexing thirst with desire for cold drinks, bad breath, putrefying mouth and lips, painful swollen gums, burning sensation in the stomach duct and abdomen, short voidings of yellow urine, constipation, and a red tongue with a thick yellow fur. Occurring in externally contracted heat (febrile) disease, constipation is more common, and, in severe cases, it is accompanied by clouded spirit, delirious speech, and manic agitation. MED Use Stomach-Clearing Powder (*qīng wèi sǎn*) or Jade Lady Brew (*yù nǚ jiān*). For externally contracted heat (febrile) disease, use Qi-Coordinating Decoctions (*chéng qì tāng*). ACU Base treatment mainly on ST and LI. Select ST-44 (*nèi tíng,* Inner Court), ST-36 (*zú sān lǐ,* Leg Three Li), and LI-4 (*hé gǔ,* Union Valley); needle with drainage. For constipation, add LI-11 (*qū chí,* Pool at the Bend), ST-37 (*shàng jù xū,* Upper Great Hollow), and TB-6 (*zhī gōu,* Branch Ditch). [26: 440] [27: 157] [97: 399] [46: 596] [113: 102]

exuberant yang 阳盛 *yáng shèng*: A surfeit of yang heat, especially exuberant evil heat and exuberant right qi characterized by vigorous heat [effusion], absence of sweating, rough breathing, vexation and agitation, and thirst. This situation is described in *Elementary Questions* (*sù wèn*) in the following the words: "when yang is exuberant there is external heat." [26: 714] [27: 128] [97: 714]

exuberant yang damages yin 阳盛阴伤 *yáng shèng yīn shāng*: In the ebb and flow of yin and yang, excessively exuberant yang heat invariably harms yin-liquid. Exuberant qi-aspect heat is treated by engendering liquid with cold sweet medicinals; gastrointestinal heat bind is treated by swift precipitation to preserve yin; exuberant construction-blood heat is treated by clearing construction and nourishing yin, supported if necessary by cooling the blood and resolving toxin. Preventing damage to yin is an important principle in the treatment of all patterns of excessively exuberant yang heat. [26: 715] [27: 128] [97: 241]

exuberant yang qi 阳气盛 *yáng qì shèng*: **1.** Excessively strong yang qi manifesting in a heat pattern. **2.** Strong yang qi. *The Magic Pivot* (*líng shū*) states, "When yin qi is wasted, and yang qi is exuberant, there is sleep in the day." [26: 714]

exuberant yang repelling yin 阳盛格阴 *yáng shèng gé yīn*: A manifestation of extreme heat resembling cold arising when, in a disease that is fundamentally one of heat, the evil lies deep in the interior, blocks yang qi, and prevents it from reaching the exterior, causing false cold signs such as reversal cold of the limbs, a sunken hidden pulse, and inability to take cold medicines. The patient will feel vexation and heat in the heart [region], the abdomen feels scorching hot to the touch, reflecting the fundamental nature of the disease. However, the rest of the body is cold, and the patient does not wish to be covered. The exuberant heat (exuberant yang) thus holds the yin cold in the exterior at bay. [26: 714] [27: 129] [97: 241]

exuberant yin 阴盛 *yīn shèng*: *Synonym: exuberant internal yin cold.* Exuberant yin causes debilitation of yang and the appearance of internal cold signs such as REVERSE-FLOW, phlegm-rheum, and water qi. *Elementary Questions* (*sù wèntiáo jīng lùn*) states, "WHEN YIN IS EXUBERANT, THERE IS INTERNAL COLD." [27: 128] [97: 232]

exuberant yin repelling yang 阴盛格阳 *yīn shèng gé yáng*: *Synonyms: repelled yang.* A disease pattern in which exuberant internal cold forces yang qi to the outer body, causing signs of true internal cold and false external heat. False external heat signs include floating heat effusion, thirst, agitation of the extremities and a large surging pulse. However, despite heat effusion, the patient likes to keep well wrapped up; despite thirst, he does not drink much, likes hot drinks, or rinses his mouth without wishing to swallow. Despite agitation, the spirit-mind is clear. Although the pulse is large and surging, it is forceless under pressure. Hence the heat signs are false. [26: 619]

exuberant yin vacuity fire 阴虚火盛 *yīn xū huǒ shèng*: EFFULGENT YIN VACUITY FIRE.

eye 眼睛 *yǎn jīng*, 眼 *yǎn*, 目 *mù*: Organ of vision; governed by the liver (see LIVER OPENS AT THE EYES). Parts of the eye are given in the list of entries below.

Parts of the Eye

FIVE WHEELS (*wǔ lún*)

EIGHT RAMPARTS (*bā kuò*)

CANTHUS (*zì*)

EYELID (*yǎn jiǎn*)

EYELID RIM (*yǎn xián*)

EYE NEST (*mù kē*)

IRIS (*jīng lián*)
DARK OF THE EYE (*hēi jīng*)
WHITE OF THE EYE (*bái jīng*)
PUPIL SPIRIT (*tóng shén*)
SPIRIT JELLY (*shén gāo*)
EYE TIE (*yǎn xì*)

Diagnosis: Observing the eyes most often involves observing the spirit. Since the "essence of the bowels and viscera flows up into the eyes," the eyes reflect the state of the bowels and viscera to some extent. Furthermore, the eyes connect through to the brain, which is referred to as the sea of marrow, and "the essence of marrow is in the pupils." Therefore, the pupils, marrow, and essence are considered to be closely related; and the pupils are considered to reflect marrow and essence. In practical diagnosis, if the pupils are normal in enduring or severe illnesses, the disease is considered to be still curable. Conversely, if patients have lusterless eyes, and tend to keep their eyes shut, taking no interest in the world, or if the spirit of their eyes has an abnormal appearance, the condition is critical. If the eyes are turned upward or sideways, or look fixedly ahead, the condition is one of LIVER WIND STIRRING INTERNALLY. Dilation of the pupils may, in severe illness, be a sign of approaching death. Reddening of the eyes, often with copious discharge that occurs as part of a broader pattern, usually indicates externally contracted wind-heat, heart fire, or liver fire. See RED EYES.

Eye Signs

CLOUDED VISION (*mù hūn*)
FLOWERY VISION (*mù huā*)
DRY EYES (*mù gān sè*)
EYE PAIN (*mù tòng*)
EYE DISCHARGE (*yǎn chī*)
ITCHY EYES (*mù yǎng*)
AVERSION TO LIGHT (*wù guāng xiū míng*)
YELLOWING OF THE EYES (*mù huáng*)
TEARING ON EXPOSURE TO WIND (*yíng fēng liú lèi*)

Lusterless eyes indicate a dual vacuity of blood and qi. Swollen and painful darks of the eyes (corneae) are generally associated with liver fire. Yellowing of the whites of the eyes (sclerae) indicate jaundice, which most often signifies damp-heat, and in rare cases, cold-damp. Dark rings around the eyes indicate kidney vacuity, whereas green-blue or purple rings indicate intraorbital bleeding. Sunken eyes indicate a severe condition of damage to liquid and humor desertion. Slight puffiness around the eyes indicates incipient water swelling. However, senile debilitation of kidney qi may be characterized by slackening and puffiness of the lower lids,

though in most cases this does not constitute a sign of disease. Bulging of the eyes is usually caused by binding phlegm-fire depression. For diseases of they eye, see the entries listed below. [27: 27] [97: 150] [26: 199]

Eye diseases

ULCERATION OF THE EYELID RIM (*yǎn xián chì làn*)
STY (*zhēn yǎn*)
PEPPERCORN SORE (*jiāo chuāng*)
MILLET SORES (*sù chuāng*)
PHLEGM NODE OF THE EYELID (*yǎn bāo tán hé*)
INGROWN EYELASH (*quán máo dǎo jié*)
UPPER EYELID DROOP (*shàng bāo xià chuí*)
WIND-FIRE EYE (*fēng huǒ yǎn*)
EXCRESCENCE CREEPING OVER THE EYE (*nǔ ròu pān jīng*)
FIRE GAN (*huǒ gān*)
BLOOD FLYING TO THE EYE (*mù fēi xuè*)
EYE SCREEN (*mù yì*)
EXTERNAL OBSTRUCTION (*wài zhàng*)
INTERNAL OBSTRUCTION (*nèi zhàng*)
  GREEN-BLUE WIND INTERNAL OBSTRUCTION (*qīng fēng nèi zhàng*)
RED AUREOLA SURROUNDING THE DARK OF THE EYE (*wū lún chì yūn*)
RED VESSELS INVADING THE EYE (*chì mài qīn jīng*)
RED BLOOD THREADS (*hóng chì xuè sī*)
TANGLED RED THREAD-LIKE VESSELS (*chì sī qiú mài*)
CLEAR-EYE BLINDNESS (*qīng máng*)
SUDDEN BLINDNESS (*bào máng*)
NIGHT BLINDNESS (*yè máng*)
NEARSIGHTEDNESS (*néng jìn qiè yuǎn*)
FARSIGHTEDNESS (*néng yuǎn qiè jìn*)
MURKY EYE OBSTRUCTION (*hùn jīng zhàng*)
CHILD EYE GAN (*xiǎo ér gān yǎn*)

---

eyebrow bone 眉棱骨 *méi léng gǔ*: The bone that forms the prominence of the eyebrow. WMC superciliary arch. ◇ Chin 眉 *méi*, eyebrow; 棱 *léng*, ridge; 骨 *gǔ*, bone. [27: 446]

eyebrow bone pain 眉棱骨痛 *méi léng gǔ tòng*: Pain felt in the eyebrow bone. It is mostly attributable to external contraction of wind-heat and phlegm damp lying depressed in the inner body. It is often seen together with yang brightness (*yáng míng*) headache and lesser yang (*shào yáng*) headache. MED Dispel wind, clear fire, and flush phlegm. *Incisive Light on the Source of Miscellaneous Disease* (*zá bìng yuán liú xī zhú*) suggests a formula containing ledebouriella (*fáng fēng*), notopterygium (*qiāng huó*), scutellaria (*huáng qín*), and licorice (*gān cǎo*). Alternatively, use variations of Phlegm-Abducting Decoction (*dǎo tán tāng*). ACU Main points: BL-2 (*zǎn zhú*, Bamboo Gathering), LI-4 (*hé gǔ*, Union Valley), GV-24 (*shén tíng*, Spirit Court), ST-8 (*tóu wéi*, Head Corner), and ST-41 (*jiě xī*, Ravine Divide); needle with drainage. To dispel wind and clear fire, add GB-20 (*fēng chí*, Wind Pool), TB-5 (*wài guān*, Outer Pass), and GV-14 (*dà zhuī*, Great Hammer). To flush phlegm, add ST-36 (*zú sān lǐ*, Leg Three Li) and ST-40 (*fēng lóng*, Bountiful Bulge). [27: 446] [26: 427] [46: 595, 597, 623] [4: 140]

eye discharge 眼眵 *yǎn chī*: Thick sticky turbid substance collecting around the canthi and eyelid rims in eye diseases such as wind-fire eye.

eye gan 疳眼 *gān yǎn*: CHILD EYE GAN.

eyelid 眼睑 *yǎn jiǎn*, 目胞 *mù bāo*: *Synonym: retainer.* Either of the two movable protective folds, which, when closed, cover the anterior surface of the eyeball. They eyelid is the FLESH WHEEL in the context of the FIVE WHEELS. [27: 66]

eyelid rim 眼弦 *yǎn xián*, 目弦 *mù xián*, 弦 *xián*: The edge of the eyelid (palpebral margin) from which the eyelashes grow. [27: 66] [26: 200] [97: 517]

eyelid vacuous as a ball 胞虚如球 *bāo xū rú qiú*: SPLEEN VACUOUS AS A BALL.

eye nest 目窠 *mù kē*: The eye socket and eyelids. [27: 66]

eye pain 目痛 *mù tòng*: Any pain of the eye. Pain in the eye during the day is a yang pattern; pain during the night is a yin pattern. Pain accompanied by vexation and oppression indicates qi repletion; pain accompanied by aversion to cold indicates qi vacuity. Intermittent dull pain indicates stirring of yin vacuity fire; pain like the pricking of a needle, that continues unabated indicates fire evil. Pain accompanied by dryness signifies wearing of the fluids or water depletion and blood vacuity. Red sore eyes with copious sticky discharge indicate wind-heat congestion. Mild redness and soreness with inhibited stool and urine indicates repletion fire blazing internally. Pain that refuses pressure and likes cold compresses indicates repletion, whereas pain that likes pressure and hot compresses indicates vacuity. [26: 201]

eye screen 目翳 *mù yì*, 翳 *yì*: **1.** Any external obstruction involving murky opacity or deformation of the black of the eye, or any scarring of this area left after disease, e.g., CONGEALED-FAT SCREEN. Screens may occur in repletion patterns of liver wind-heat and vacuity patterns of liver-kidney depletion and effulgent vacuity fire. Repletion patterns are treated by coursing wind and clearing heat, resolving toxin and draining the liver. Vacuity patterns are treated by enriching the liver and kidney, and nourishing yin and clearing heat. In addition, screens may arise through TRUE EYE DAMAGE in external injury. **2.** Any internal or external obstruction that blocks the line of vision, including internal eye screens, such as *round eye screens.* See INTERNAL OBSTRUCTION; EXTERNAL OBSTRUCTION. [26: 934]

eye tie 目系 *mù xì*, 眼系 *yǎn xì*: That which connects the eye to the brain. *The Magic Pivot (líng shū dà huò lùn)* states, "... evils strike the nape and, encountering vacuity of the body, they enter deeply, following the eye tie into the brain. When they enter the brain, the brain spins. When the brain spins, it causes tension in the eye tie. When the eye tie is tense, the [vision of the] eye becomes dizzy and spins." WMC optic nerve and surrounding structure. [27: 12] [97: 74]

F

¹**face** 面 *miàn*, 颜 *yán*: The anterior aspect of the head including the eyes, nose, cheeks, lips, and chin. Inspecting various aspects of the face is important in diagnosis. See INSPECTION; FACIAL COMPLEXION. Conditions affecting the face include *mole* (BLACK MOLE, BLOOD MOLE); ACNE; DRINKER'S NOSE; DEVIATED MOUTH AND EYES; TOAD HEAD SCOURGE; FACIAL PAIN. [27: 63]

²**face** 廉 *lián*: Surface or aspect.

facial complexion 面色 *miàn sè*: The color and sheen of the skin of the face, especially as a reflection of health or sickness. The state of blood and qi is intimately related to the facial complexion. *The Magic Pivot* (*líng shū, xié qì zàng fǔ bìng yīn piān*) states, "The qi and blood of the twelve primary channels and the three-hundred and sixty-five network vessels [all the channels of the body] ascend to the face." This statement emphasizes the importance of the complexion as a reflection of the general state of health. The color of the complexion is analyzed in terms of the five colors—blue-green, red, yellow, white, and black. When applied to the human complexion, they take on a relative significance. Thus, two people who have vastly different complexions when healthy, may both be described as having an "white" complexion when suffering from a certain disease, even though the actual color is different. "White" here refers to a relative paling compared with the normal complexion. (NB: that the color names are retained in translation because of possible five-phase associations with the bowels and viscera that might be lost with more idiomatic translations such as "pale" for white, or "sallow" for yellow.) Basic morbid facial complexions and their significance are as follows: **White:** White complexions usually indicate cold or vacuity. A bright white (very white) complexion with facial vacuity edema generally indicates yang qi vacuity and occurs after massive bleeding, in chronic nephritis, or in wheezing panting patterns. A lusterless pale white complexion (a complexion slightly paler than normal), together with general and facial emaciation, normally points to blood vacuity. *The Magic Pivot* (*líng shū, jué qì piān*) states, "Blood desertion is characterized by a white complexion that is perished and sheenless." The sudden appearance of a somber white complexion (white tinged with blue-green) in acute diseases is usually attributable to fulminant yang qi desertion and is seen in various forms of shock. However, somber white may

also be observed in cases of external wind-cold diseases characterized by aversion to cold, shivering, and severe abdominal pain due to interior cold. **Green-blue:** Blue-green or bluish complexions are principally associated with wind-cold, blood stasis, pain, and qi block patterns. Child fright-wind and epilepsy are characterized by a dark blue-green complexion. A grayish blue-green complexion with blue-green-purple lips is associated with inner body blood stasis and impaired flow of qi and blood, and occurs in diseases classified in Western medicine as cirrhosis of the liver and cardiac failure. In severe wind-cold headaches and abdominal pain due to interior cold, impeded flow of yang qi may be reflected in a bluish somber white complexion. In cases of lung qi block, a dark blue-green-purple complexion may result from obstructed flow of blood and qi. This corresponds to conditions such as pulmogenic heart disease and asphyxia in Western medicine. **Red:** Red complexions generally occur in heat patterns, with distinction being made between vacuity heat and repletion heat. Externally contracted wind-heat may be characterized by a red face and red eyes. Interior repletion heat patterns are characterized by tidal reddening of the face, excessive sweating, thirst, constipation, and other signs of repletion heat. A somber white complexion with tidal reddening of the cheeks in the afternoon indicates effulgent yin vacuity fire. In severe illnesses characterized by cold sweating, reversal cold in the limbs, and a somber white complexion with reddening of the cheeks that appear as if smeared with oil paint indicates "upcast yang" or overfloating of vacuous yang, i.e., it is a critical sign of imminent outward desertion of yang qi. In addition, in some severe or enduring illnesses, signs such as those described in *The Magic Pivot* (*líng shū, wǔ sè piān*) may appear: "If red, thumb-sized flushes appear on the cheeks, although there may be slight improvement, death will ensue promptly." **Yellow:** Yellow is associated with dampness and vacuity. Yellowing of the whites of the eyes (sclerae) and generalized yellowing of the skin indicate jaundice. A vivid yellow indicates damp-heat and is known as yang yellow. A dark yellow color points to cold-damp, and is known as yin jaundice. Yang yellow is seen mostly in cases described in Western medicine as acute icteric infectious hepatitis, acute cholecystitis, cholelithiasis, and toxic hepatitis; yin yellow occurs in cirrhosis of the liver and cancer of the head of the pancreas. A pale yellow skin that is dry and puffy, accompanied by pale lips but no yellowing of whites of the eyes (sclerae), is referred to as withered-yellow, which is a vacuity yellow. The condition characterized by this complexion is sometimes called YELLOW SWELLING, and is normally caused by excessive loss of blood or depletion of blood and qi after major illnesses, or by spleen-stomach damage resulting from intestinal parasites. It may be seen in diseases known in Western medicine as ankylostomiasis (hookworm disease), anemia, and malnutrition due to poor assimilation. **Black:** Black is associated with kidney vacuity and blood stasis. A soot-black complexion, dark gray complexion, or purple-black complexion may occur in enduring diseases, patterns characterized by kidney essence depletion, or in static blood accumulation patterns. In Western medicine, a soot-black complexion may be seen in chronic hyperadrenocorticalism, or in the final stages of cirrhosis of the liver. A dark gray complexion may be seen in chronic kidney dysfunction, and a purple-black complexion may occur in chronic heart-lung dysfunctions. A black complexion indicates intractable or severe illness. *Essential Prescriptions of the Golden Coffer* (*jīn guì yào lüè*) states that "black jaundice" is associated with kidney vacuity and blood stasis, and usually indicates that the condition is hard to cure. See TEN-PRINCIPLE INSPECTION OF THE COMPLEXION. [6: 116] [26: 423]

facial pain 面痛 *miàn tòng*: Pain in any part of the face. Facial pain usually occurs in episodes and is acute. Patterns include wind-heat, wind-cold, liver depression transforming into fire, and blood stagnation and blood stasis. **Wind-heat** possibly with phlegm is marked by periodic pain that may be burning or stabbing, associated with a sensation of heat and exacerbated by heat. It usually affects one side of the face, and occasionally the upper or lower half of the face. Wind-heat may be complicated by phlegm obstructing the network vessels, in which case there may also be dizziness, oppression in the chest, and numbness of the limbs. MED Course wind and dissipate heat; flush phlegm and quicken the network vessels. Use Facial Pain No.1 Formula (*miàn tòng yī hào fāng*). ACU Base treatment mainly on yang brightness (*yáng míng*) and reverting yin (*jué yīn*). Main points: ST-2 (*sì bái*, Four Whites), ST-7 (*xià guān*, Below the Joint), Greater Yang (*tài yáng*), LI-4 (*hé gǔ*, Union Valley), and LR-3 (*tài chōng*, Supreme Surge). For wind-heat, add GB-20 (*fēng chí*, Wind Pool), TB-5 (*wài guān*, Outer Pass), and GV-14 (*dà zhuī*, Great Hammer), needling with drainage. Selection of points according to sign: 1) For forehead pain, add BL-2 (*zǎn zhú*, Bamboo Gathering), GB-14 (*yáng bái*, Yang White), ST-8 (*tóu wéi*, Head Corner), and SI-3 (*hòu xī*,

Back Ravine). 2) For upper jaw pain, add SI-18 (*quán liáo*, Cheek Bone-Hole), ST-2 (*sì bái*, Four Whites), GB-3 (*shàng guān*, Upper Gate), and LI-20 (*yíng xiāng*, Welcome Fragrance). 3) For the lower jaw, add CV-24 (*chéng jiāng*, Sauce Receptacle), ST-6 (*jiá chē*, Cheek Carriage), TB-17 (*yì fēng*, Wind Screen), and ST-44 (*nèi tíng*, Inner Court). **Wind-cold** causes severe pain that refuses cold. During bouts of pain the complexion may turn a somber white. If the wind-cold is complicated by phlegm obstructing the network vessels, further signs include puffiness of the face and heavy head as if swathed (bag-over-the-head sensation). MED Course wind and dissipate cold; flush phlegm and free the network vessels. Use Facial Pain No.2 Formula (*miàn tòng èr hào fāng*). ACU To the basic points, add GB-20 (*fēng chí*, Wind Pool), TB-5 (*wài guān*, Outer Pass), and GV-16 (*fēng fǔ*, Wind Mansion), needling with drainage and adding moxa. **Liver depression transforming into fire** is another cause of facial pain that is easily distinguished from the wind-heat pattern by rib-side pain, irascibility, sighing, and unquiet sleep. MED Clear the liver and drain fire; flush phlegm and quicken the network vessels. Facial Pain No.3 Formula (*miàn tòng sān hào fāng*). ACU To the basic points, add SP-6 (*sān yīn jiāo*, Three Yin Intersection), GB-34 (*yáng líng quán*, Yang Mound Spring), LR-2 (*xíng jiān*, Moving Between), and PC-8 (*láo gōng*, Palace of Toil), needling with drainage. **Blood vacuity and blood stasis** is marked by severe continual pain of fixed location. There are general signs of qi vacuity such as shortage of qi, faint low voice, laziness to speak, and stasis speckles on the tongue. MED Supplement qi and quicken the blood; transform stasis and free the network vessels. Facial Pain No.4 Formula (*miàn tòng sì hào fāng*). ACU To the basic points, add ST-36 (*zú sān lǐ*, Leg Three Li), SP-6 (*sān yīn jiāo*, Three Yin Intersection), CV-6 (*qì hǎi*, Sea of Qi), and PC-6 (*nèi guān*, Inner Pass), needling with supplementation and adding moxa. [92: No. 74] [46: 624, 595]

facial prominence 顀 *zhuō*: The region below the eye. ◇ Chin The character 顀 is composed of 出 *chū*, go out (stick out); with the signifier 頁 *yè*, head, and many be interpreted to mean a prominent point on the head. [48: 320]

failure of the interlocking bones to open 交骨不开 *jiāo gǔ bù kāi*: The absence of movement of bone preventing childbirth. The meaning of the term depends on the interpretation given to the "interlocking bones." (1) Taking the interlocking bones to be the two parts of what modern medicine calls the pubis, the ancients believed that they were normally closed, but would open to allow child delivery. They also believed that poor nutrition in pregnancy, causing original qi vacuity and preventing qi and blood from reaching the area, could account for their failure to open. (2) Taking the interlocking bones to mean the sacrococcygeal joint, failure of the interlocking bones to open means the failure of the sacrococcygeal joint to move the lower opening of the pelvis to facilitate delivery. This can be treated with Bone-Opening Powder (*kāi gǔ sǎn*). [26: 237] [97: 221]

failure to acclimatize to a new environment 水土不服 *shuǐ tǔ bù fú*: Problems such as poor appetite, abdominal distention, abdominal pain, diarrhea, and menstrual irregularities attributed to moving to a new environment. Such conditions usually disappear in a short time. ◇ Chin 水 *shuǐ*, water; 土 *tǔ*, earth; 不 *bù*, not; 服 *fú*, give in to, adapt to, obey, serve. Failure to adapt to water and earth. [26: 150] [27: 122] [97: 132]

failure to rise 不起 *bù qǐ*, 不举 *bù jǔ*: IMPOTENCE.

faint 晕倒 *yūn dǎo*, 晕厥 *yūn jué*: To lose consciousness.

faint pulse 微脉 *wēi mài*: A pulse so fine and weak that it is barely perceptible. It indicates vacuity desertion or qi and blood vacuity. WMC The fine pulse is observed in shock or chronic disease. [6: 143] [26: 811]

faint pulse verging on expiration 脉微欲绝 *mài wēi yù jué*: See FAINT PULSE.

falling curtain screen 垂帘翳 *chuí lián yì*: A disease characterized by fine thread-like vessels on the upper margin of the dark of the eye that appear to fall like a curtain over the eye and that in severe cases cover the pupil. Falling curtain screen is associated with tearing and aversion to light, dryness and pain, and obstructed vision. WMC trachomatous corneal pannus. MED Course wind and clear heat; calm the liver and abate screens. Use Abalone Shell Powder (*shí jué míng sǎn*) as oral medication and Spirifer Fossil Elixir (*shí yàn dān*) applied topically. ACU Select BL-2 (*zǎn zhú*, Bamboo Gathering), BL-1 (*jīng míng*, Bright Eyes), GB-1 (*tóng zǐ liáo*, Pupil Bone-Hole), GB-20 (*fēng chí*, Wind Pool), GB-41 (*zú lín qì*, Foot Overlooking Tears), Thumb Bone Hollow (*dà gǔ kōng*), Little Finger Bone Hollow (*xiǎo gǔ kōng*), BL-18 (*gān shū*, Liver Transport), and BL-19 (*dǎn shū*, Gallbladder Transport); needle with drainage. [26: 304] [37: 468]

fall pattern 陷证 *xiàn zhèng*: A disease pattern in which sore-toxin attacks the inner body. Distinction is made between FIRE FALL, DRY FALL, and VACUITY FALL. WMC toxemia. See also INWARD FALL. [26: 616]

false spiritedness 假神 *jiǎ shén*: False signs of vitality suddenly appearing in patients suffering from enduring and severe illness. Such signs, which include sudden garrulousness, improvement in appetite and facial complexion, are the "last radiance of the setting sun" or the "last flicker of the candle," boding imminent death. [27: 115]

farsightedness 能远怯近 *néng yuǎn qiè jìn*: Ability to see distant but not close objects clearly, usually without any visible changes within the eye. Farsightedness is attributed to insufficiency of yin and superabundance of yang, or to congenital causes. WMC hyperopia; in the elderly, presbyopia. MED Enrich yin and brighten the eyes with formulas such as Lycium Berry, Chrysanthemum, and Rehmannia Pill (*qǐ jú dì huáng wán*). [26: 562]

fat heat gan 肥热疳 *féi rè gān*: See COLD-HEAT GAN.

fat gan 肥疳 *féi gān*: See COLD-HEAT GAN.

fatigue 疲倦 *pí juàn*, 倦怠 *juàn dài*: Synonym: *fatigue and lack of strength*. Tiredness and lack of strength. Fatigue is observed in dual vacuity of qi and blood, spleen vacuity with damp encumbrance, and damage to qi by summerheat-heat. [92: No. 30]

fatigue and lack of strength 倦怠乏力 *juàn dài fá lì*: FATIGUE.

fatigued cumbersome limbs 四肢困倦 *sì zhī kùn juàn*: Limbs that lack in strength and feel unwieldy. A sign of dampness and spleen vacuity.

fatigued limbs and lack of strength 肢倦乏力 *zhī juàn fá lì*: Weakness of the extremities. A sign of spleen vacuity.

fatigued spirit and lack of strength 神疲乏力 *shén pí fá lì*: See LASSITUDE OF SPIRIT AND LACK OF STRENGTH.

fat meat, fine grain, and strong flavors 膏梁厚味 *gāo liáng hòu wèi*: Rich food. Eating of fat meat, fine grain, and strong flavors over a long period can engender internal heat and cause sores. [27: 121]

fat qi 肥气 *féi qì*: From *The Magic Pivot* (*líng shū, xié qi zang fǔ bìng xíng*). One of the FIVE ACCUMULATIONS. Lump glomus under the rib-side like an upturned cup, attributed to liver qi depression and congealing static blood. In *The Classic of Difficult Issues* (*nàn jīng*), it is said to be the liver accumulation (one of the five accumulations), and is described as being a glomus lump under the rib-side, like an upturned cup, and having a head and a foot. When the disease is persistent, malaria or cough may arise. MED Treat with Fat Qi Pill (*féi qì wán*). [27: 415] [97: 355]

fat sore 肥疮 *féi chuāng*: Synonym: *sand-heap perverse crop*. A scalp disease characterized by yellow scabs. Fat sores start with small papules or pustules like millet grains that exude yellow water after rupture to gradually form sulfur-colored platelike scabs transpierced by hairs. Falling of the scabs reveals an eroded wound, which when it finally heals leaves a scar. Fat sores are itchy and have a strange smell similar to that of rat's urine. They are attributed to spleen-stomach damp-heat sweltering the scalp or to contact infection. [WMC] favus (also known as honeycomb ringworm and formerly known by the term tinea favosa). [MED] Wash with a decoction of scallions or sophora twigs (*huái zhī*) and remove the scabs. Apply Fat Oil Paste (*féi yóu gāo*). It may help to pluck the affected area of hair. [26: 384] [27: 473] [97: 355]

fatty tumor 脂瘤 *zhī liú*: Synonym: *mealy tumor*. A TUMOR (a growth on the outside of the body) that is round, soft, and of varying size. A fatty tumor is found mostly on the head and face or back. It can be ruptured to produce a substance like bean curd dregs. It is treated mainly by external medical methods. [26: 548]

favorable measles pattern 麻疹顺证 *má zhěn shùn zhèng*: The manifestation of measles in patients with abundant right qi and mild evil toxin. A favorable measles pattern is characterized by mild heat effusion, cough without hasty breathing, and clear spirit qi (i.e., clear head) throughout the whole course of the disease. Heat effusion runs for three or four days before papules erupt on the head and face, spreading to the chest, back, and limbs. The papules are even and a lustrous red. Apart from possible cough, there should be no other signs. The eruption reaches the full extent of its development in three days, after which it slowly disappears, during which time the heat effusion and cough abate and the appetite returns. [26: 588]

favorable pattern (**sign**) 顺证 *shùn zhèng*: A normal pattern occurring in a disease that bodes a good outcome. In measles, for example, red papules or speckles that are bright red and evenly distributed and associated with heat effusion, no complications, clear mind, and gradual return of the appetite constitutes a favorable pattern. Compare UNFAVORABLE PATTERN (SIGN). [27: 227]

[1]**fear** 恐 *kǒng*: One of the FIVE MINDS (mental and emotional activities); associated with the kidney.

[2]**fear** 相畏 *xiāng wèi*: See SEVEN RELATIONS.

fear causes qi to precipitate 恐则气下 *kǒng zé qì xià*: Fear can damage kidney qi, causing urinary incontinence, seminal emission, and efflux diarrhea. [27: 145] [97: 462]

fearful throbbing 怔忡 *zhēng chōng*: Severe heart palpitations that is not brought on by emotional stimulus. Fearful throbbing is so called because its severity itself causes alarm. See HEART PALPITATIONS. ◇ Chin 怔 *zhēng*, fear, terror; 忡 *chōng*, anxiety, heavy-heartedness. [26: 351]

fear of cold 怕冷 *pà lěng*: AVERSION TO COLD.

fear of wind 怕风 *pà fēng*: AVERSION TO WIND.

febrile disease 热病 *rè bìng*: HEAT DISEASE.[1] [26: 872]

fecal block 便闭 *biàn bì*, 大便闭 *dà biàn bì*: See CONSTIPATION; BLOCK; QI BLOCK.

fecal incontinence 大便失禁 *dà biàn shī jìn*: Involuntary loss of stool. Fecal incontinence is attributable to spleen-kidney yang vacuity, qi vacuity fall, or exuberant heat toxin. **Spleen-kidney yang vacuity** causes prolonged diarrhea with frequent defecation the makes the anus incapable of containment, so that there is periodic discharge of slimy stool. Other signs include physical cold and fear of cold, lack of warmth in the limbs, reduced eating, abdominal distention, aching lumbus, tinnitus, and long voidings of clear urine. The tongue is pale and enlarged with white, possibly glossy, fur. The pulse is sunken and fine. [MED] Treat by warming and supplementing the spleen and kidney, assisted by promoting astriction and stemming desertion. Use Six Pillars Beverage (*liù zhù yǐn*) with cinnamon bark (*ròu guì*), dried ginger (*gān jiāng*), and halloysite (*chì shí zhī*). [ACU] Base treatment mainly on CV, GV, and back transport points. Select BL-25 (*dà cháng shū*, Large Intestine Transport), BL-20 (*pí shū*, Spleen Transport), BL-23 (*shèn shū*, Kidney Transport), GV-4 (*mìng mén*, Life Gate), ⓜ CV-4 (*guān yuán*, Pass Head), ⓜ CV-12 (*zhōng wǎn*, Center Stomach Duct), LR-13 (*zhāng mén*, Camphorwood Gate), ST-25 (*tiān shū*, Celestial Pivot), and ST-36 (*zú sān lǐ*, Leg Three Li); needle with supplementation and moxa. CROSS MOXA can be applied. **Qi vacuity fall** causes involuntary passing of stool of which the patient is unaware at the time. In severe cases, there is prolapse of the rectum. Other signs include emaciation, dullness of essence-spirit, poor appetite, oppression in the stomach duct after eating, heart palpitations and shortness of breath, shortage of qi and laziness to speak, faint low voice, and a bright white facial complexion. The tongue is pale and enlarged with dental impressions on the margins. The pulse is sunken, fine, and forceless. [MED] Supplement the center and boost qi; raise the fall and stem desertion. Use Pure Yang True Man Viscus-Nourishing Decoction (*chún yáng zhēn rén yǎng zàng tāng*) plus astragalus (*huáng qí*), and dried ginger (*gān jiāng*). [ACU] Base treatment mainly on GV and BL. Select GV-20 (*bǎi huì*, Hundred Convergences), BL-25 (*dà cháng shū*, Large Intestine Transport), GV-1 (*cháng qiáng*, Long Strong), BL-57 (*chéng shān*, Mountain Support), ST-36 (*zú sān lǐ*, Leg Three Li), SP-6 (*sān yīn jiāo*, Three Yin Intersection), and CV-6 (*qì hǎi*, Sea of Qi); needle with supplementation and moxa. **Intense heat toxin** causing fecal incontinence is observed in epidemic toxin dysentery. This disease begins rapidly and is characterized by diarrhea that contains pus and bright purple blood or that is like blood water. Other signs include high fever, vexation and agitation, and thirst. In severe cases, there is TETANIC REVERSAL and clouded spirit with involuntary discharge of stool. The tongue is red with yellow fur. The pulse is surging and rapid or slippery and rapid. MED Clear heat and resolve toxin; cool construction and open the orifices. Use Coptis Toxin-Resolving Decoction (*huáng lián jiě dú tāng*) combined with Pulsatilla Decoction (*bái tóu wēng tāng*). For orifice block with clouded spirit, use Peaceful Palace Bovine Bezoar Pill (*ān gōng niú huáng wán*) or Supreme Jewel Elixir (*zhì bǎo dān*). ACU Base treatment mainly on LI and ST. Select LI-4 (*hé gǔ*, Union Valley), ST-25 (*tiān shū*, Celestial Pivot), ST-37 (*shàng jù xū*, Upper Great Hollow), ST-44 (*nèi tíng*, Inner Court), LI-11 (*qū chí*, Pool at the Bend), and GV-14 (*dà zhuī*, Great Hammer), needling with drainage; prick the Ten Diffusing Points (*shí xuān*) to bleed. See EFFLUX DIARRHEA. [92: No. 216] [46: 665, 671] [113: 88, 106] [4: 138]

fecal qi 矢气 *shǐ qì*: FLATUS.

fecal stoppage 大便不通 *dà biàn bù tōng*: See CONSTIPATION.

feeble-mindedness 痴呆 *chī dāi*: DEMENTIA.

feeding accumulation 乳食积滞 *rǔ shí jī zhì*: A disease of the stomach and intestines in infants due to milk damage or food damage. **Simple suckling accumulation** arises when the infant cries urgently for food and begins feeding while still crying or when feeding problems arise in spleen-stomach vacuity. In such cases, other signs include heart vexation, poor sleep, hot breath, the sour smell of milk in the mouth, vomiting of undigested milk, and diarrhea or constipation. MED Treat by dispersing milk and harmonizing the stomach for Harmony-Preserving Pill (*bǎo hé wán*). ACU Base treatment mainly on SP and ST. Select CV-10 (*xià wǎn*, Lower Stomach Duct), ST-36 (*zú sān lǐ*, Leg Three Li), and SP-5 (*shāng qiū*, Shang Hill). Apply shallow needling without needling retention; do not use moxa. Add BL-20 (*pí shū*, Spleen Transport), BL-21 (*wèi shū*, Stomach Transport), SP-4 (*gōng sūn*, Yellow Emperor), and LR-13 (*zhāng mén*, Camphorwood Gate), needle with supplementation and moxa for spleen-stomach vacuity. **Milk damage and food damage accumulation** is characterized by the inability to taste ingested foods, poor stomach intake, glomus in the stomach duct and abdominal distention. In some cases there may be tidal or low fever, and if the condition continues the child may become emaciated. MED The tip is treated by dispersing accumulation and abducting stagnation, whereas

the root is treated by regulating the stomach and spleen. Harmony-Preserving Pill (*bǎo hé wán*) or Stomach-Calming Powder (*píng wèi sǎn*) may be used initially and subsequently replaced with Spleen-Arousing Pill (*qǐ pí wán*) or Ginseng, Poria (Hoelen), and Ovate Atractylodes Powder (*shēn líng bái zhú sǎn*). ACU Base treatment mainly on CV and ST. Select CV-10 (*xià wǎn*, Lower Stomach Duct), ST-25 (*tiān shū*, Celestial Pivot), CV-6 (*qì hǎi*, Sea of Qi), ST-36 (*zú sān lǐ*, Leg Three Li), Li Inner Court (*lǐ nèi tíng*), and CV-21 (*xuán jī*, Jade Swivel); needle with drainage. Add GV-14 (*dà zhuī*, Great Hammer) for tidal heat [effusion]. SPINE PINCHING also provides a useful complement to medicinal therapy. [26: 378] [46: 662, 702] [113: 336]

feel the pulse 切脉 *qiè mài*: See PULSE EXAMINATION. [26: 109]

female malaria 牝疟 *pìn nüè*: From *Essential Prescriptions of the Golden Coffer* (*jīn guì yào lüè, nüè bìng mài zhèng bìng zhì*). MALARIA in patients with yang vacuity with the malarial evil lying in the lesser yin (*shào yīn*) channel, characterized by pronounced shivering with little or no heat effusion, pale white complexion, and regular episodes. MED Outthrust the evil with warm acrid medicinals using Bupleurum, Cinnamon Twig, and Dried Ginger Decoction (*chái hú guì jiāng tāng*) plus dichroa leaf (*shǔ qī*). ACU Base treatment mainly on GV, hand and foot greater yang (*tài yáng*) channels, and KI. Select GV-14 (*dà zhuī*, Great Hammer), SI-3 (*hòu xī*, Back Ravine), PC-5 (*jiān shǐ*, Intermediary Courier), GV-13 (*táo dào*, Kiln Path), GB-39 (*jué gǔ*, Severed Bone), KI-3 (*tài xī*, Great Ravine), and KI-4 (*dà zhōng*, Large Goblet); needle with drainage and add moxa. For principles of treatment, see MALARIA. ◇ Chin 牝 *pìn*, female; 疟 *nüè*, malaria. Apparently so-called because of the preponderance of cold (yin, female) signs. [26: 272] [27: 359] [97: 217] [113: 172] [46: 650]

femur 髀骨 *bì gǔ*: The bone of the upper leg. Also called *thigh bone*.

fen 分 *fēn*: **1.** Synonym: *candareen*. A unit of weight now equal to one hundredth of a *liang*, now equal to 0.3125 g. See tables 21 and 23, page 717. **2.** A unit of length equal to tenth of a body-inch, or *cun*. [27: 111]

fetal 胎 *tāi*: Of or related to the fetus or the prenatal period.

fetal emaciation 胎瘦 *tāi shòu*: FETAL FEEBLENESS.

fetal epilepsy 胎痫 *tāi xián*: EPILEPSY occurring within a hundred days of birth. [27: 434]

fetal feebleness 胎弱 *tāi ruò*: Synonyms: *fetal emaciation*; *fetal timidity*. Any condition of qi or blood vacuity from birth, characterized by thin weak skin, lack of hair, physical cold and cold limbs, yellow facial complexion and emaciated flesh, inhibited bending and stretching of the sinews, and limp aching lumbus. MED Supplement qi and blood; enrich the liver and kidney. Use Perfect Major Supplementation Decoction (*shí quán dà bǔ tāng*) and Six-Ingredient Rehmannia Pill (*liù wèi dì huáng wán*) or their variations. [26: 454] [27: 426] [97: 410]

fetal fright 胎惊 *tāi jīng*: Fright wind in neonates other than umbilical wind, characterized by episodes of FRIGHT REVERSAL, loss of consciousness, convulsions of the extremities, and spasm of the face. Fetal fright was traditionally attributed to poor nutrition or emotional disturbances during pregnancy. [27: 433]

fetal grime 胎垢 *tāi gòu*: Continued occurrence of menses during pregnancy; apparently has no negative effect on the child. [27: 448]

fetal heat 胎热 *tāi rè*: **1.** A pathocondition in neonates resulting from contraction of heat in the uterus, attributed to the mother eating acrid hot foods or to a heat disease that was not properly cleared and resolved, and characterized by open eyes, red face, puffy swelling of the eyelids, continual crying, reddish urine, and thick stool. MED Clear heat and resolve toxin. Use Major Forsythia Beverage (*dà lián qiào yǐn*) or Stomach-Clearing Powder (*qīng wèi sǎn*). **2.** Loss of eye brightness (visual acuity) with inability to see lights and fires, headache, dizziness, swelling of the cheeks and chin, attributed to liver channel heat toxin attacking upward as a result of excessive consumption of fried food and acrid hot-spicy foods and firy liquor. during pregnancy [26: 456] [50: 1132] [27: 436] [97: 410]

fetal heat cinnabar toxin 胎热丹毒 *tāi rè dān dú*: Synonym: *red wandering wind*. A form of INFANTILE CINNABAR TOXIN characterized by red smooth swollen patches on the head, trunk, and limbs. Fetal heat cinnabar toxin is attributed to deep-lying internal fetal toxin contending with the blood and exacerbated by wind. In some cases, warm clothing and the internal heat of breast milk may encourage the evil. Spreading from the abdomen and the back to the limbs is favorable; moving from the limbs to the abdomen and the back and to the scrotum is unfavorable. MED Oral: In the initial stages use Cimicifuga and Pueraria Decoction (*shēng má gé gēn tāng*) followed by Wind-Expelling Powder (*qū fēng sǎn*). In severe cases, use Major Forsythia Beverage (*dà lián qiào yǐn*). If the patient has abdominal distention and does not take milk, toxic qi has entered the interior. In such cases, use Purple Snow Powder (*zǐ xuě sǎn*). Topical: Four Colors Powder (*sì sè sǎn*). [50: 1136]

fetal jaundice 胎疸 *tāi dǎn*, 胎黄 *tāi huáng*: Yellowing of skin in neonates attributed to damp-heat in the mother during pregnancy or to congenital insufficiency of original qi, that in mild cases disappears without treatment. **Damp-heat** causing severe fetal jaundice is characterized by a golden coloring of the skin accompanied by vigorous heat [effusion], constipation, and reddish urine. MED Clear heat and transform dampness. Use Gardenia and Phellodendron Decoction (*zhī zǐ bǎi pí tāng*) or Capillaris Decoction (*yīn chén hāo tāng*) with additions. **Congenital insufficiency of original qi**, spleen qi vacuity, and nontransformation of cold-damp cause fetal jaundice characterized by a dark yellow lusterless complexion, cold limbs, and sloppy stool. MED Warm the spleen and transform dampness. Use Center-Rectifying Decoction (*lǐ zhōng tāng*) plus capillaris (*yīn chén hāo*). [26: 455] [27: 435] [97: 410]

fetal lichen 胎癣 *tāi xiǎn*: SUCKLING LICHEN.

fetal mounting 胎疝 *tāi shàn*: Swelling of the scrotum in neonates. [27: 436] [97: 409]

fetal obesity 胎肥 *tāi féi*: A condition of fatness at birth. The neonate suffering from fetal obesity is fat at birth and has pinkish eyes. After the first month, he begins to lose weight. Additional signs are vexing heat in the five hearts, difficult defecation, and drooling. Fetal obesity is attributed to stomach heat in the mother. [26: 46]

fetal origin 胎元 *tāi yuán*: **1.** The fetus. **2.** The original qi of the mother used to nourish the fetus. AFTERBIRTH. [27: 336] [97: 409]

fetal qi 胎气 *tāi qì*: **1.** The essential qi received by the fetus from the mother. The development of the fetus is depending upon fetal qi. If fetal qi is insufficient, the child will suffer from developmental diseases and a weak body. Hence, a child unable to stand and walk at the age of four or five is said to suffer from insufficiency of fetal qi. **2.** The ability of the fetus to affect the health of the mother, e.g., *upward forcing of fetal qi,* and specifically, certain diseases of pregnancy, e.g., puffing of the face during pregnancy, or abdominal pain during pregnancy. [26: 454] [97: 409]

fetal qi forcing upward 胎气上逼 *tāi qì shàng bī*: Synonym: *upward forcing of fetal qi*. Stirring of the fetus with qi counterflow, usually attributable to qi-blood disharmony stemming from illness or general weakness in the mother. [27: 447]

fetal redness 胎赤 *tāi chì*: **1.** A condition of neonates characterized by redness of the skin that gives the appearance of having been smeared with cinnabar and attributed to contraction of heat toxin in the uterus. **2.** Ulceration of the eyelid in infants; FETAL WIND. [27: 435] [97: 409]

fetal spotting 胎漏 *tāi lòu*: Passing of blood via the vagina in pregnancy. Fetal spotting is usually caused by qi-blood vacuity, kidney vacuity, or blood heat causing insecurity of the thoroughfare (*chōng*) and controlling (*rèn*) vessels and preventing the containment of blood that nourishes the fetus. It may take the form of periodic bleeding in small amounts, or spotting according to the times of the period. **Qi vacuity** patterns are characterized by shortage of qi and laziness to speak. MED Supplement qi and quiet the fetus with Origin-Lifting Brew (*jǔ yuán jiān*). ACU Base treatment mainly on GV, CV, and SP. Select GV-20 (*bǎi huì*, Hundred Convergences), CV-4 (*guān yuán*, Pass Head), ST-36 (*zú sān lǐ*, Leg Three Li), CV-6 (*qì hǎi*, Sea of Qi), and SP-6 (*sān yīn jiāo*, Three Yin Intersection); needle with supplementation and moxa. **Blood vacuity** patterns are characterized by pale yellow facial complexion, as well as fatigue and lack of strength. MED Supplement the blood and quiet the fetus with Fetal Origin Beverage (*tāi yuán yǐn*). ACU Base treatment mainly on CV, SP, and back transport points. Select CV-4 (*guān yuán*, Pass Head), ST-36 (*zú sān lǐ*, Leg Three Li), SP-6 (*sān yīn jiāo*, Three Yin Intersection), BL-20 (*pí shū*, Spleen Transport), and BL-21 (*wèi shū*, Stomach Transport); needle with supplementation and moxa. **Kidney vacuity** patterns are characterized by dizzy head, tinnitus, and frequent urination. MED Secure the kidney and quiet the fetus with Fetal Longevity Pill (*shòu tāi wán*). ACU Base treatment mainly on CV, SP, and KI. Select CV-4 (*guān yuán*, Pass Head), CV-6 (*qì hǎi*, Sea of Qi), SP-6 (*sān yīn jiāo*, Three Yin Intersection), BL-23 (*shèn shū*, Kidney Transport), KI-3 (*tài xī*, Great Ravine), KI-7 (*fù liū*, Recover Flow), and GV-4 (*mìng mén*, Life Gate); needle with supplementation and moxa. **Blood heat** patterns are characterized by dry mouth and pharynx, and vexation. MED Clear heat, cool the blood, and quiet the fetus with Yin-Safeguarding Brew (*bǎo yīn jiān*). ACU Base treatment mainly on CV and SP. Select CV-6 (*qì hǎi*, Sea of Qi), CV-3 (*zhōng jí*, Central Pole), SP-6 (*sān yīn jiāo*, Three Yin Intersection), SP-1 (*yǐn bái*, Hidden White), SP-10 (*xuè hǎi*, Sea of Blood), and KI-2 (*rán gǔ*, Blazing Valley); needle with drainage. In repletion pattern fetal spotting, a draining needle stimulus should be applied with care. The needle sensation must be increased gradually from weak to strong, and draining should not be performed until the patient has become accustomed to it. [26: 455] [27: 449] [97: 410] [46: 594, 688] [113: 289] [37: 426] [59: 107]

fetal timidity 胎怯 *tāi qiè*: FETAL FEEBLENESS.

fetal toxin 胎毒 *tāi dú*: Boils, pox, or other sores in infants traditionally attributed to heat toxin in the mother, but understood by Western medicine to be attributable to infection after birth. [27: 123] [97: 410]

fetal water 胎水 *tāi shuǐ*: A condition of abdominal fullness, swelling, and distention associated with panting in the sixth and seventh month of pregnancy. [27: 448]

fetal wind 胎风 *tāi fēng*: A condition of neonates characterized by generalized heat [effusion] and redness of the skin like that produced by a burn. Fetal wind is attributed to spleen-stomach heat accumulation in the mother due to excessive consumption of acrid hot foods during pregnancy. [26: 454] [27: 443] [97: 409]

fetid water snail 臭田螺 *chòu tián luó*: FOOT QI SORE.

fetter 束 *shù*: To inhibit the normal action (of a part of the body). Describes the inhibitive effect of evils, especially on the exterior of the body or the lung. See EXUBERANCE AND DEBILITATION.

fetus 胎 *tāi*: The child in the womb.

fever 发热 *fā rè*, 热 *rè*: HEAT EFFUSION.

fifteen network vessels 十五络 *shí wǔ luò*: See NETWORK VESSEL. [26: 7]

fifth-watch cough 五更嗽 *wǔ gēng (jīng) sòu*: COUGH occurring or becoming more severe just before daybreak (4–6 a.m.) A few coughs just before daybreak usually indicate phlegm-fire. Cough before daybreak with copious phlegm usually indicates spleen vacuity. A daytime cough that is worse in the early morning indicates food accumulation in the stomach. MED Treat phlegm-fire patterns with Two Matured Ingredients Decoction (*èr chén tāng*) plus scutellaria (*huáng qín*), platycodon (*jié gěng*), and mulberry root bark (*sāng bái pí*). Spleen vacuity patterns are treated with Six Gentlemen Decoction (*liù jūn zǐ tāng*) plus blast-fried ginger (*páo jiāng*). For food accumulation patterns see FOOD COUGH. [26: 117]

fifth-watch diarrhea 五更泄 *wǔ gēng (jīng) xiè*: Synonym: *early morning diarrhea*. Described in *Prolonging Life and Preserving the Origin* (*shòu shì bǎo yuán, xiè xiè*). Diarrhea before daybreak. Fifth-watch diarrhea is usually caused by kidney vacuity; hence the term is often considered synonymous with KIDNEY DIARRHEA. Strictly speaking, however, fifth-watch diarrhea may also be caused by food accumulation, liquor accumulation, and liver fire. **Food accumulation** causes attacks of pain before daybreak relieved slightly by diarrhea. The pulse is sunken and slippery. MED Use variations of Harmony-Preserving Pill (*bǎo hé wán*). **Liquor accumulation** fifth-watch diarrhea is heralded by pain before daybreak and is characterized by yellow foamy diarrhea, reddish urine or urine like rice water, and a rapid surging or rapid wiry pulse. MED Sichuan Coptis and Bitter Orange Decoction (*chuān lián zhǐ ké tāng*). **Liver fire** fifth-watch diarrhea is characterized by continual pain in the chest and rib-side that reaches

into the lesser abdomen, and is associated with reduced sleep. Before daybreak, there is pain in the
left lower abdomen with a desire to go to the toi-
let, that is is relieved by defecation. The pulse
is stringlike and rapid. MED Use Gentian Liver-
Draining Decoction (*lóng dǎn xiè gān tāng*). See
KIDNEY DIARRHEA; DIARRHEA. [26: 117] [27: 264]
[97: 51]

fifty-year-old's shoulder 五十肩 *wǔ shí jiān*:
LEAKY SHOULDER WIND. [46: 631]

filiform needle 毫针 *háo zhēn*: One of the NINE
NEEDLES of ancient China that has been developed
into a variety of fine needles of varying length most
commonly used in performing acupuncture today.
The filiform needle is now generally made from a
stainless steel wire that is sharpened at one end
and has a thin wire of copper, stainless steel, or silver wrapped around its opposite end as a handle.
Stainless steel is chosen for the body of the needle
because of its flexibility, strength, and resistance
to oxidation. Though silver and gold also resist
oxidation, they are expensive, and are relatively
soft metals. Thus, they are used only in specific
systems of practice when their pliability does not
impede treatment. Filiform needles range in size
from 15 mm to 150 mm in length and 0.22 mm to
0.30 mm (30 to 34 gauge) in diameter. [27: 332]
[26: 582] [46: 455]

fine pulse 细脉 *xì mài*: Synonym: *small pulse*. A
pulse that feels like a well-defined fine thread under
the fingers. The fine pulse indicates dual vacuity of
qi and blood, or of yin and yang, and in particular
points to blood and yin vacuity. [6: 142] [27: 195]

finger-press needle insertion 指切进针法 *zhǐ
qiè jìn zhēn fǎ*: Synonym: *nail-press needle insertion*. Two-handed needle insertion technique involving the application of pressure with a single
nail. Method: (1) Press either the thumbnail, or
the nail of the index finger of the left hand, onto
the skin surface over the point. (2) Holding the
handle of the needle with right thumb and forefinger, support the needle tip against the finger nail.
(3) Keeping the needle next to the nail, insert it
through the skin with a quick, firm downward motion. Application: The single-finger press is used
to insert needles 2" or less in length. It is also
employed in areas near to a palpable pulse: the
pressing finger covers the pulse and the needle is
inserted next to it, thus protecting the blood vessel
from injury during insertion. This method, though
used in China, does not meet Western standards of
a clean field because the needle comes into contact
with the thumbnail. [46: 460]

finger standard 指寸法 *zhǐ cùn fǎ*: From *A
Thousand Gold Pieces Prescriptions* (*qiān jīn yào
fāng*). Finger measurements as a standard for calculating the body-inch. The finger standard in-

cludes the MIDDLE FINGER BODY-INCH (the length
of the phalange of the middle finger), THUMB
BODY-INCH (the distance between the two transverse creases), and HAND STANDARD (the breath
of the hand measured at the middle joints of the
fingers). See BODY-INCH. [26: 420]

finger vein examination 诊指纹 *zhěn zhǐ wén*:
INFANT'S FINGER EXAMINATION.

fire 火 *huǒ*: **1.** Flames and heat from burning matter. **2.** One of the FIVE PHASES; the phase with
which summer, south, red, the heart, and joy are
associated. **3.** In physiology, a transmutation of
yang qi explained as a vital force, e.g., sovereign
fire, ministerial fire, and lesser fire. **4.** One of the
SIX QI; hot weather. See HEAT. **5.** One of the
SIX EXCESSES, which when invading the body, can
causes the following signs: (1) Pronounced generalized or local signs of heat, such as high fever,
aversion to heat, desire for coolness, flushed complexion, reddening of the eyes, reddish urine, red
tongue, yellow fur, rapid pulse, or, in sore patterns, redness, heat, pain, and swelling. (2) Thick,
sticky excreta, such as thick snivel (nasal mucus),
thick yellow phlegm, sour watery vomitus, murky
urine, blood and pus in the stool, acute diarrhea,
or foul-smelling stools, often with a burning sensation on discharge. For this reason *Elementary
Questions* (*sù wèn*) states, "Turbid water is associated with heat," and "all sour retching and vomiting, fulminant downpour, and lower body distress are ascribed to heat." (3) Damage to the
fluids characterized by a dry tongue with little liquid, thirst with desire for cold fluids, and dry hard
stool. (4) Bleeding, and maculopapular eruptions
that occur when the fire evil scorches the blood and
causes frenetic blood movement. (5) Disturbances
of the spirit and vision as *Elementary Questions*
(*sù wèn*) states, "All heat with visual distortion
is ascribed to fire," and "excessive agitation and
mania are associated with fire." **6.** A pathological state that is either caused by fire as one of the
six excesses, and classified as heat among the eight
principles, or any similar pathological state arising from the transformation of other evils, from
the transformation of yang qi, or from yin vacuity. **6a.** The transformation of yang qi due to affect damage (emotional disturbance) or the transformation of exterior evils as they enter the interior causes repletion fire. This condition is characterized by high fever, headache, red eyes, bitter taste in the mouth, dry mouth, thirst with desire for cold drinks, vexation and agitation, rib-side
pain, abdominal pain that refuses pressure, constipation, red tongue with dry yellow fur and sometimes prickles, and a rapid replete pulse. In severe
cases, there is blood ejection or spontaneous external bleeding, or maculopapular eruptions. The
most common repletion fire patterns are gastroin-

testinal repletion fire or liver-gallbladder repletion fire. **6b.** Depletion of yin humor and yin-yang imbalance in the organs causes vacuity fire, which is characterized by mild heat signs, tidal reddening of the face, vexing heat in the five hearts, steaming bone taxation heat [effusion], vexation and insomnia, night sweating, short voidings of reddish urine, dry mouth and throat, red tongue with scant fur, or a bare red tongue without fur, and a forceless rapid fine pulse. Compare HEAT. [6: 104] [26: 95] [29: 325] [36: 209, 280]

fire and water aid each other 水火相济 *shuǐ huǒ xiāng jì*: Heart fire and kidney water balance each other. In the doctrine of the five phases, the heart belongs to fire and the kidney belongs to water, and each restrains the other. Compare FIRE AND WATER FAILING TO AID EACH OTHER. [27: 14] [26: 150] [27: 14] [97: 132]

fire and water failing to aid each other 水火不济 *shuǐ huǒ bù jì*: A failure in the relationship between heart fire and kidney water arising either when kidney water is insufficient and fails to complement heart fire or heart fire moves frenetically and damages kidney yin. Signs such as vexation, insomnia, and seminal emission are observed. See FIRE AND WATER AID EACH OTHER. Compare NONINTERACTION OF THE HEART AND KIDNEY; DEPLETED WATER AND EFFULGENT FIRE. [27: 14] [50: 358]

fire and water processing 水火制 *shuǐ huǒ zhì*, 水火共制 *huǒ shuǐ gòng zhì*: Fire and water treatment involves treatment with both fire and water, sometimes with the use of adjuvants. The main forms are: STEAMING; BOILING; DOUBLE-BOILING; DISTILLATION; SCALDING. See PROCESSING OF MEDICINALS. [11: 20] [74: 10]

fire by nature flames upward 火性上炎 *huǒ xìng shàng yán*: Fire is characterized by rising flames, and diseases in the body attributed to fire are associated with upper body heat signs. Distinction is made between repletion and vacuity fire. Repletion fire includes fire heat damaging the lung, which causes panting and cough, coughing of blood, and nosebleed, and fire distressing the heart spirit, which manifests as headache, vomiting, clouded spirit, and delirious raving. Vacuity fire, which is yang hyperactivity due to yin vacuity stemming from depletion of essence blood, manifests as vexation and agitation, sore throat, hoarse voice, bleeding gums, and tinnitus. Most of these signs reflect the upward flaming nature of fire. [26: 96]

fire cinnabar 火丹 *huǒ dān*: CINNABAR TOXIN. [26: 96] [27: 471] [97: 122]

fire cinnabar leg 火丹脚 *huǒ dān jiǎo*: Synonyms: *fire flow*; *lower limb fire flow*. Cinnabar toxin affecting the legs. See CINNABAR TOXIN.

fire cough 火咳 *huǒ ké*, 火嗽 *huǒ sòu*: COUGH due to fire evil damaging the lung. Fire cough is characterized by cough with scant phlegm that may be streaked with blood, vexation thirst, red facial complexion, chest and rib-side pain, and constipation. Distinction is made between repletion and vacuity. **Repletion** fire cough is characterized by a surging rapid or stringlike rapid pulse. MED Repletion fire cough is treated by clearing the lung and draining fire using White-Draining Powder (*xiè bái sǎn*) or Diaphragm-Cooling Powder (*liáng gé sǎn*). ACU Base treatment mainly on LU and LI. Select BL-13 (*fèi shū*, Lung Transport), LU-10 (*yú jì*, Fish Border), LI-11 (*qū chí*, Pool at the Bend), GV-14 (*dà zhuī*, Great Hammer), and GV-12 (*shēn zhù*, Body Pillar); needle with drainage. Prick LU-11 (*shào shāng*, Lesser Shang) to bleed. **Vacuity** fire cough is characterized by a red tongue with scant fur and a forceless rapid fine pulse. MED Vacuity fire cough is treated by enriching yin and downbearing fire, using formulas such as Yin-Enriching Clearing Transforming Pill (*zī yīn qīng huà wán*). ACU Base treatment mainly on LU and KI. Select BL-13 (*fèi shū*, Lung Transport), BL-43 (*gāo huāng shū*, GaoHuang Transport), LU-5 (*chǐ zé*, Cubit Marsh), KI-3 (*tài xī*, Great Ravine), and KI-6 (*zhào hǎi*, Shining Sea); needle with supplementation. [26: 96]

fire cup 火罐 *huǒ guàn*: A cup-like instrument used in fire cupping. See CUPPING. [26: 98]

fire cupping 火罐 *huǒ guàn*: See CUPPING.

fire depression 火郁 *huǒ yù*: See HEAT DEPRESSION. [25: 73] [44: 104]

fire depression cough 火郁嗽 *huǒ yù sòu*: Synonym: *taxation cough*. COUGH due to fire depression. Zhu Dan-Xi considered taxation cough to be caused by fire depression. In *Dan Xi's Experiential Methods* (*dān xī xīn fǎ*) he states, "Taxation cough is fire depression cough. Use chebule (*hē zǐ*) to treat lung qi. Fire causing extreme damage and becoming depressed causes distention, fullness, and sleeplessness. Chebule's sour bitter flavor promotes contraction and downbears fire. It is assisted by pumice (*hǎi fú shí*) soaked in child's urine (*tóng biàn*), cyperus (*xiāng fù zǐ*), trichosanthes (*guā lóu*), indigo (*qīng dài*), apricot kernel (*xìng rén*), and pinellia leaven (*bàn xià qū*); blend with fresh ginger (*shēng jiāng*) and honey (*mì*) [to make pills, which are] sucked in the mouth." ACU Base treatment mainly on LU, KI, PC, and LR. Select BL-13 (*fèi shū*, Lung Transport), LU-5 (*chǐ zé*, Cubit Marsh), KI-6 (*zhào hǎi*, Shining Sea), PC-6 (*nèi guān*, Inner Pass), LR-3 (*tài chōng*, Supreme Surge), and SP-6 (*sān yīn jiāo*, Three Yin Intersection); needle with drainage and prick LU-11 (*shào shāng*, Lesser Shang) and PC-8 (*láo gōng*, Palace of Toil) to bleed. See TAXATION COUGH. [26: 98] [18: Vol 2, 1149] [46: 646, 652]

fire depression panting 火郁喘 *huǒ yù chuǎn*: PANTING attributable to fire depression obstructing the lung and preventing the diffusion of lung qi. Fire depression panting is characterized by hasty rapid panting, oppressed and confused spirit-affect, reversal cold of the limbs, and a sunken hidden pulse. MED Diffuse depressed heat. Use Free Wanderer Powder (*xiāo yáo sǎn*) combined with Left-Running Metal Pill (*zuǒ jīn wán*). ACU Base treatment mainly on LU and LR. Select Panting Stabilizer (*dìng chuǎn*), LU-7 (*liè quē*, Broken Sequence), LU-5 (*chǐ zé*, Cubit Marsh), CV-17 (*shān zhōng*, Chest Center), PC-6 (*nèi guān*, Inner Pass), LR-3 (*tài chōng*, Supreme Surge), SP-6 (*sān yīn jiāo*, Three Yin Intersection), BL-18 (*gān shū*, Liver Transport), and GB-34 (*yáng líng quán*, Yang Mound Spring). Needle with drainage. For exuberant fire evil, prick PC-8 (*láo gōng*, Palace of Toil) and LU-11 (*shào shāng*, Lesser Shang) to bleed. [26: 98]

fire diarrhea 火泄 *huǒ xiè*, 火泻 *huǒ xiè*: HEAT DIARRHEA. [26: 96]

fire eye 火眼 *huǒ yǎn*: WIND-FIRE EYE.

fire failing to engender earth 火不生土 *huǒ bù shēng tǔ*: Kidney yang failing to warm the spleen. Earth represents the spleen, whereas fire represents kidney yang (not the heart). In kidney yang vacuity (insufficiency of the life gate fire), the spleen is deprived of warmth and its ability to transform food water-damp is affected. Hence, there are signs of spleen-kidney yang vacuity such as such as cold limp lumbus and knees, nontransformation of food, inhibited urination, swelling, and fifth-watch diarrhea. See SPLEEN-KIDNEY YANG VACUITY. [27: 13]

fire fall 火陷 *huǒ xiàn*: Transmission of the heat toxin from FLAT-ABSCESS (*jū*) of the head to construction-blood. In its exuberant heat toxin stage, a flat-abscess of the head becomes dark purple in color, pus ceases to flow from the open head, and the opening becomes dry. The base of the flat-abscess becomes broad and diffuse. At this stage, the heat toxin enters the construction blood, causing vigorous heat [effusion], thirst, heart vexation, agitation, delirious speech, constipation, reddish urine, a crimson tongue, and a rapid pulse. MED Clear construction, cool the blood, and resolve toxin. Use Construction-Clearing Decoction (*qīng yíng tāng*), Rhinoceros Horn and Rehmannia Decoction (*xī jiǎo dì huáng tāng*), or Coptis Toxin-Resolving Decoction (*huáng lián jiě dú tāng*). If necessary, Peaceful Palace Bovine Bezoar Pill (*ān gōng niú huáng wán*) or Purple Snow Elixir (*zǐ xuě dān*) may also be used to open the orifices. For topical treatment, see HEADED FLAT-ABSCESS.

WMC toxemia. See FALL PATTERN. [26: 97] [27: 458] [97: 122] [96: 135]

fire flow 流火 *liú huǒ*: Synonym: *fire cinnabar leg*. Cinnabar toxin affecting the legs. See CINNABAR TOXIN. [27: 471] [97: 482]

fire formation 化火 *huà huǒ*: See TRANSFORMATION INTO FIRE.

fire gan 火疳 *huǒ gān*: A red granule, like a pomegranate seed in shape, bulging forward from deep within the white of the eye, and growing gradually larger. Fire gan is associated with redness, pain, tearing, aversion to light, and unclear vision. In some cases, it can affect the pupil, leading to loss of sight. In the latter stages, pain and redness abate to leave purple-blue or blue-gray patches. MED Clear heat and resolve toxin; clear the blood and dissipate binds. Use formulas such as Heart-Washing Powder (*xǐ xīn sǎn*). Formulas containing biles may be applied topically. See GAN. [26: 96] [27: 502] [97: 122]

fire-girdle sore 火带疮 *huǒ dài chuāng*: GIRDLING FIRE CINNABAR.

fire headache 火头痛 *huǒ tóu tòng*: Synonym: *fire heat headache*. HEADACHE characterized by throbbing or distending pain reaching into the tooth bed (the jaw) or from in front of the ear to within the ear, and attended by heat vexation, thirst, constipation, and a large surging pulse. Fire headache is attributed to yang brightness (*yáng míng*) fire surging upward. WMC vascular headache, otogenic headache, odontogenic headache. MED Clear heat and drain fire, using White Tiger Decoction (*bái hǔ tāng*) or Jade Lady Brew (*yù nǚ jiān*). ACU Base treatment mainly on ST and LI. Select ST-8 (*tóu wéi*, Head Corner), ST-44 (*nèi tíng*, Inner Court), ST-36 (*zú sān lǐ*, Leg Three Li), LI-4 (*hé gǔ*, Union Valley), and KI-6 (*zhào hǎi*, Shining Sea); needle with drainage. [26: 98]

fire heart pain 火心痛 *huǒ xīn tòng*: HEAT HEART PAIN. [26: 95]

fire heat 火热 *huǒ rè*: Heat produced by fire.

fire heat headache 火热头痛 *huǒ rè tóu tòng*: FIRE HEADACHE. [26: 98]

fire needle 火针 *huǒ zhēn*: A needle 3–4" long with a pointed tip and a handle made of horn, bamboo, or wood. Fire needle is used in fire needling. [26: 97] [27: 382] [97: 122]

fire needling 火针 *huǒ zhēn*, 火针疗法 *huǒ zhēn liáo fǎ*: A method of acupuncture involving the swift pricking of the skin with a red hot needle. Fire needling is used in the treatment of welling-abscess (*yōng*), scrofula, stubborn lichen (*xiǎn*), and impediment (*bì*) pain. This method corresponds to *red-hot needling* among the *nine needling methods*. [26: 97]

fire panting 火喘 *huǒ chuǎn*: **1.** *Synonym: lung-stomach flaming fire panting.* PANTING due to lung-stomach flaming fire arising when repletion fire in the stomach surges up into the lung, and characterized by periodic panting that is relieved by eating, and resumes after eating. [MED] Clear fire and flush phlegm using White Tiger Decoction (*bái hǔ tāng*) or Phlegm-Abducting Decoction (*dǎo tán tāng*). [ACU] Base treatment mainly on LU, ST, LI, and CV. Select LU-1 (*zhōng fǔ*, Central Treasury), BL-13 (*fèi shū*, Lung Transport), Panting Stabilizer (*dìng chuǎn*), LU-5 (*chǐ zé*, Cubit Marsh), LU-7 (*liè quē*, Broken Sequence), ST-44 (*nèi tíng*, Inner Court), LI-4 (*hé gǔ*, Union Valley), and ST-40 (*fēng lóng*, Bountiful Bulge); needle with drainage. For exuberant fire evil, add LU-11 (*shào shāng*, Lesser Shang), pricking to bleed. **2.** PANTING due to ascent of thoroughfare (*chōng*) vessel fire. [MED] Discharge thoroughfare vessel fire with Kidney-Enriching Gate-Opening Pill (*zī shèn tōng guān wán*). [26: 97] [113: 63, 66]

fire phlegm 火痰 *huǒ tán*: **1.** Heat phlegm. **2.** Externally contracted dryness phlegm. **3.** A pattern of phlegm lodged in the stomach duct with clamoring stomach, rising phlegm, vomiting and retching, swallowing of upflowing acid, and baking heat in the head and face. [26: 98]

fire processing 火制 *huǒ zhì*: Processing medicinals by the application of heat. Fire processing methods involve either direct or indirect contact of the materials with a heat source, sometimes with adjuvants. Care is required in controlling time and temperature, and the quantity of any additive used; excessively high temperatures can cause undesirable changes in a medicinal's characteristics. The most common forms of fire processing are the various forms of STIR-FRYING and MIX-FRYING. Less commonly used methods are ROASTING and STONE-BAKING. [74: 5] [11: 17]

fire rampart 火廓 *huǒ kuò*: See EIGHT RAMPARTS. [26: 24] [27: 500] [97: 123]

fire stroke 火中 *huǒ zhòng*: A condition similar to wind stroke, characterized by sudden clouding collapse (clouding of consciousness and collapse), loss of consciousness, inability to speak, deviated eyes and mouth, red facial complexion, vexation and agitation, and constipation. Fire stroke is usually attributed to fulminant heart fire harassing the heart spirit, or less commonly to kidney yin vacuity with vacuity fire flaming upward. [MED] For fulminant heart fire harassing the heart spirit, clear the heart and drain fire; free the orifices and quiet the spirit. Use formulas such as Bovine Bezoar Heart-Clearing Pill (*niú huáng qīng xīn wán*) or Diaphragm-Cooling Powder (*liáng gé sǎn*). For kidney yin vacuity with vacuity fire flam-

ing upward, enrich water to constrain fire. Use Six-Ingredient Rehmannia Pill (*liù wèi dì huáng wán*). If there is copious phlegm, use variations of Fritillaria and Trichosanthes Powder (*bèi mǔ guā lóu sǎn*). [ACU] Base treatment mainly on GV, LI, hand and foot reverting yin (*jué yīn*) PC/LR, and HT. Main points: GV-26 (*shuǐ gōu*, Water Trough), GV-20 (*bǎi huì*, Hundred Convergences), PC-9 (*zhōng chōng*, Central Hub), LI-4 (*hé gǔ*, Union Valley), LR-2 (*xíng jiān*, Moving Between), PC-6 (*nèi guān*, Inner Pass), KI-1 (*yǒng quán*, Gushing Spring), and GB-34 (*yáng líng quán*, Yang Mound Spring); needle with drainage. Prick HT-8 (*shào fǔ*, Lesser Mansion) to bleed. Selection of points according to patterns: For fulminant heart fire, add PC-8 (*láo gōng*, Palace of Toil) and HT-7 (*shén mén*, Spirit Gate), and needle with drainage. For vacuity fire flaming upward, add KI-3 (*tài xī*, Great Ravine), KI-6 (*zhào hǎi*, Shining Sea), and KI-2 (*rán gǔ*, Blazing Valley), and needle with even supplementation and drainage. For copious phlegm, add ST-40 (*fēng lóng*, Bountiful Bulge), and CV-12 (*zhōng wǎn*, Center Stomach Duct), and needle with drainage. [26: 95] [50: 329] [14: 54] [113: 22] [46: 596, 615]

fire supplementation and fire drainage 火补 火泻 *huǒ bǔ huǒ xiè*: See MOXIBUSTION SUPPLEMENTING AND DRAINING. [26: 97]

fire wind damage 火伤风 *huǒ shāng fēng*: A condition characterized by dry cough without phlegm, dry mouth, sore pharynx and a dry red tongue. [MED] Clear and dissipate wind-fire using formulas such as Mulberry Leaf and Chrysanthemum Beverage (*sāng jú yǐn*) and Licorice and Platycodon Decoction (*gān jié tāng*). [ACU] Base treatment mainly on LU, GB, and LI. Select GB-20 (*fēng chí*, Wind Pool), TB-5 (*wài guān*, Outer Pass), LU-5 (*chǐ zé*, Cubit Marsh), LI-4 (*hé gǔ*, Union Valley), LI-11 (*qū chí*, Pool at the Bend), and GV-14 (*dà zhuī*, Great Hammer); needle with drainage, and prick LU-11 (*shào shāng*, Lesser Shang) to bleed. [26: 98]

firm pulse 牢脉 *láo mài*: *Synonym: confined pulse* (*obs*). A forceful sunken pulse that feels "tied to the bone"; hence its name. It is associated with cold pain. In clinical practice, the name *firm pulse* is rarely used. Instead it is called a stringlike sunken pulse or a sunken full pulse. [6: 140] [27: 195] [97: 311]

first yang [channel] 一阳 *yì yáng*: Lesser yang (*shào yáng*). [27: 90]

first yin [channel] 一阴 *yì yīn*: Reverting yin (*jué yīn*). [27: 90]

fish 鱼 *yú*: The fleshy part of the hand below the base of the thumb, so named because it resembles a fish's belly. [WMC] thenar (eminence). [27: 74]

fish mouth 鱼口 *yú kǒu*: **1.** A bubo sore that has burst and fails to heal. **2.** A bubo sore on the left side of the body, as distinct a from BIAN TOXIN SORE, which is one on the right. [27: 487] [97: 360] [61: 259]

fish network vessels 鱼络 *yú luò*: The network vessels of the fish's margin. Congestion of blood in the fish network vessels is an indication of yang brightness (*yáng míng*) disease. *The Magic Pivot* (*líng shū, xié qì zàng fǔ bìng xíng*) states, "Fish network [flushed with] blood indicate yang brightness disease." *The Magic Pivot* (*líng shū, lùn jí zhěn chǐ*) states, "Green-blue blood vessels on the white flesh of the fish means cold in the stomach." [26: 649] [81: 583]

fish's margin 鱼际 *yú jì*: The boundary between the red (tanned) and white flesh on the fish (thenar eminence). [27: 74] [50: 964] [81: 583]

fishy smell 腥味 *xīng wèi*: The smell characteristic of fish or blood.

fissured tongue 舌裂 *shé liè*: A tongue bearing deep longitudinal furrows or creases. The fissures vary in depth and position. Occurring in conjunction with a dry tongue, they indicate fluid vacuity. They may also occur in exuberant heat patterns, in conjunction with a crimson tongue. [6: 121]

fistula 漏疮 *lòu chuāng*: See ANAL FISTULA.

five accumulations 五积 *wǔ jī*: Substantial lumps in the chest or abdomen, each associated with one viscus. See DEEP-LYING BEAM; FAT QI; GLOMUS QI; RUSHING RESPIRATION; RUNNING PIGLET. See Table 4. [26: 125] [27: 415]

4.	The Five Acumulations
Deep-lying beam	Heart accumulation
Fat qi	Liver accumulation
Glomus qi	Spleen accumulation
Rushing respiration	Lung accumulation
Running piglet	Kidney accumulation

five aversions 五恶 *wǔ wù*: AVERSIONS OF THE FIVE VISCERA. [27: 62]

five colors 五色 *wǔ sè*: Green-blue, red, yellow, white, and black, associated in in the doctrine of the five phases with the liver, heart, spleen, lung, and kidney respectively. See DISEASE CORRESPONDENCES OF THE FIVE COLORS. [26: 115] [27: 173] [97: 44]

Five Dynasties 五代 *wǔ dài*: Name of a dynastic period (A.D. 907–960)

five entries 五入 *wǔ rù*: FIVE FLAVOR ENTRIES.

five evils 五邪 *wǔ xié*: **1.** *The Classic of Difficult Issues* (*nàn jīng, 49*) states, "There is wind stroke, summerheat damage, food, drink and taxation fatigue, cold damage, and dampness damage. These are called the five evils." **2.** Vacuity evil, repletion evil, bandit evil, mild evil, regular evil. *The Clas-*

sic of Difficult Issues (*nàn jīng, 50*) states, "That coming from behind is vacuity evil; that coming from ahead is repletion evil; that coming from the restraining phase is bandit evil; that coming from the restrained phase is mild evil; that causing disease of self is regular evil." Behind refers to the mother organ, ahead is the child organ, and self is the affected organ itself. **3.** In *Essential Prescriptions of the Golden Coffer* (*jīn guì yào lüè, zàng fǔ jīng luò xiān hòu bìng mài zhèng*), wind, cold, dampness, fog, and food damage are referred to as the five evils. [26: 117] [27: 108] [97: 43]

five-flavor entries 五味所入 *wǔ wèi suǒ rù*: Synonym: *five entries*. The viscera entered, i.e., acted upon, by sour, bitter, sweet, acrid, and salty agents. *Elementary Questions* (*sù wèn*) states, "The five-flavor entries are: sourness enters the liver; bitterness enters the heart; sweetness enters the spleen; acridity enters the lung; saltiness enters the kidney." Thus, for example, sour medicinals may be used to treat, or conduct the action of other medicinals to treat, disease of the liver or of liver channel. [27: 62]

five flavors 五味 *wǔ wèi*: Acridity, sourness, sweetness, bitterness, and saltiness. Medicinals or foodstuffs of different flavors have different actions. Acridity can dissipate and move; sourness can contract and astringe; sweetness can supplement and relax (i.e., relieve pain and tension); bitterness can drain and dry; saltiness can soften hardness and induce moist precipitation. These actions are explained by modern pharmacy as follows: Acrid medicinals contain volatile oils; sour medicinals contain organic acids; sweet medicinals contain sugars; bitter medicinals contain biological alkalis, glycosides, or bitter substances. In addition to the five flavors, there is a sixth, blandness, which has a water-disinhibiting action. According to *Elementary Questions* (*sù wèn*), the flavors can be classified as yin and yang: "Acrid and sweet effusing (i.e., diaphoretic) and dissipating medicinals are yang; sour and bitter upwelling (i.e., emetic) and discharging (i.e., draining) medicinals are yin; salty upwelling and discharging medicinals are yin; bland percolating and discharging medicinals are yang." According to *The Comprehensive Herbal Foundation* (*běn cǎo gāng mù*), there is a relationship between flavor and *bearing*: "no sour or salty medicinals bear upward; no sweet or acrid ones bear downward. No cold medicinals float; no hot ones sink." [27: 316] [26: 119]

five gan 五疳 *wǔ gān*: Any of the gan patterns associated with disease of one of the five viscera. See GAN OF THE HEART; GAN OF THE LIVER; GAN OF THE SPLEEN; GAN OF THE LUNG; GAN OF THE KIDNEY. [27: 434] [27: 434] [97: 49]

five governings 五主 *wǔ zhǔ*: See GOVERNINGS OF THE FIVE VISCERA.

five hearts 五心 *wǔ xīn*: The soles of the feet, the palms of the hand, and the center of the chest.

five humors 五液 *wǔ yì*: Sweat, snivel (nasal mucus), tears, drool, and spittle. See FIVE VISCERA FORM HUMORS.

five impediments 五痹 *wǔ bì*: **1.** From *Elementary Questions* (*sù wèn, bì lùn*). Sinew, vessel, flesh, skin, and bone impediment. **2.** From *Central Treasury Canon* (*zhōng zàng jīng, bì lùn*). Sinew, bone, blood, flesh, and qi impediment (*bì*). **3.** From *Central Treasury Canon* (*zhōng zàng jīng, bì lùn*). Wind, cold, dampness, heat, and qi impediment (*bì*). [26: 122]

Five Impediments

Elementary Questions (*sù wèn, bì lùn*)
  sinew impediment (*jīn bì*)
  vessel impediment (*mài bì*)
  flesh impediment (*ròu bì*)
  skin impediment (*pí bì*)
  bone impediment (*gǔ bì*)

Central Treasury Canon (*zhōng zàng jīng, bì lùn*)
  sinew impediment (*jīn bì*)
  bone impediment (*gǔ bì*)
  blood impediment (*xuè bì*)
  flesh impediment (*ròu bì*)
  qi impediment (*qì bì*)

Central Treasury Canon (*zhōng zàng jīng, bì lùn*)
  wind impediment (*fēng bì*)
  cold impediment (*hán bì*)
  damp impediment (*shī bì*)
  heat impediment (*rè bì*)
  qi impediment (*qì bì*)

---

five limpnesses 五软 *wǔ ruǎn*: Five signs of poor development in infants. Softness of the head, limpness of the neck, limpness of the hands and feet, limpness of the flesh, and limpness of the mouth. Compare FIVE SLOWNESSES; FETAL FEEBLENESS. [27: 436] [27: 432]

five minds 五志 *wǔ zhì*: Joy, anger, anxiety, thought, fear. These are five basic forms of mental and emotional activity, which in excess can cause disease. See MIND; EXCESS AMONG THE FIVE MINDS; INTERNAL DAMAGE BY THE SEVEN AFFECTS. [27: 61] [97: 44]

five minds forming fire 五志化火 *wǔ zhì huà huǒ*: Excess of one or more of the five minds (joy, anger, anxiety, thought, and fear) causing fire signs such as vexation and agitation, irascibility, dizziness, insomnia, bitter taste in the mouth, rib-side pain, panting and cough, and blood ejection. In modern medicine, lasting mental or emotional activity causes nervous excitement or depression, which affects normal functions of the body. In Chinese medicine, the five minds or seven affects are seen to cause disturbances of qi and depletion of the true yin of the bowels and viscera, causing heat signs. [26: 117] [27: 118]

five movements and six qi 五运六气 *wǔ yùn liù qì*: See DOCTRINE OF PERIODS AND QI. [26: 122]

five odors 五臭 *wǔ xiù*: Animal odor, burnt odor, fragrant odor, fishy odor, and putrid odor. [26: 121]

five offices 五官 *wǔ guān*: **1.** The nose, eyes, lips, tongue, and ears. *The Magic Pivot* (*líng shū, wǔ yuè wǔ shǐ piān*) states, "The nose is the office of the lung, the eyes are the office of the liver, the lips are the office of the spleen, the tongue is the office of the heart, and the ears are the office of the lung." **2.** Five diagnostic correspondences of colors and positions to disease. The liver governs green-blue; the heart, red; the spleen, yellow; the lung, white; the kidney, black. Disease of the liver is characterized by green-blue eyes; disease of the spleen is characterized by yellowing of the lips; disease of the heart is characterized by a short curled tongue and reddening of the cheeks; disease of the lung is characterized by flaring nostrils; kidney disease is characterized by blackening of the eye sockets, or black coloration of the cheeks, forehead, and face. *The Magic Pivot* (*líng shū, wǔ sè piān*) also states, "Green-blue or black is pain; yellow or red is heat; white is cold. These are the five offices." [27: 27] [97: 47]

five periods and six qi 五运六气 *wǔ yùn liù qì*: FIVE MOVEMENTS AND SIX QI. See DOCTRINE OF PERIODS AND QI. [26: 122]

five phases 五行 *wǔ xíng*: Wood, fire, earth, metal, and water. The five phases, like yin and yang, are categories of quality and relationship. The ancient Chinese saw phenomena within the universe as the products of the movement and mutation of five entities: wood, fire, earth, metal, and water. These represent qualities that relate to each other in specific ways. Other groups of five phenomena that have like qualities and relate to each other in analogous ways are said to belong to the five phases. See Tables 5 and 6. "*Wood is the bending and the straightening.*" It grows upward and spreads outward; it has the characteristics of growth, upward effusion, orderly reaching, and uninhibitedness. It is associated with spring, the time of growth at the beginning of the cycle of the seasons, and with the east, the position at which the sun rises to herald the new day. It is associated with the green of new leaves and the sour taste of unripe fruit. "*Fire is the flaming upward,*" having the quality of heat and upward motion. It is associated with summer, when the heat of the sun reaches its peak, and with the south, the position toward which (in the northern hemisphere) the sun moves as it approaches the time when it gives off its greatest heat. It is related to the red and to bitterness. *"Earth is the sowing and reaping,"* representing the planting and harvesting of crops and the bringing forth of phenomena. It is associated with the long summer, the season in which the momentum of summer heat ripens the crops. Long summer is the intermediate season between summer and fall, and is related to the central position. Earth is yellow in color (the Chinese word includes brown) and is associated with the sweetness of ripened fruit. *"Metal is the working of change,"* having the qualities of purification, elimination, and reform. Metal implements help man cut grain and slaughter animals, thereby working the changes that ensure his survival. This notion is akin to that of autumn, the season when the first frosts kill life and purify nature. Metal is also associated with West, the position at which the sun sets, and with the white color of frost and with the purifying action of acrid-smelling things. *"Water is the moistening and descending to low places,"* having the qualities of moistening, downward movement, and coldness. Water is associated with winter, the season in which nature preserves itself until the spring, and with the north, where the sun hides in the daily cycle. It is also associated with the blackness of night and with saltiness, the taste of sea water. In medicine, the five viscera are each associated with one of the five phases: *Liver-wood:* The liver controls the movement of qi around the body; it spreads qi just as the trees spread their branches. Hence *The Inner Canon* (*nèi jīng*) says that the liver "thrives by orderly reaching." Also, just as trees and other plants sprout upward in spring, so liver yang tends to stir upward. *Heart-fire:* The heart has the function of propelling qi and blood to warm and nourish the whole body. It is like a fire that drives the body just as the fiery heat of summer makes nature flourish. *Spleen-earth:* The spleen is ascribed the function of assimilating nutrients from ingested foods, expressed in traditional terms as "moving and transforming the essence of grain and water" (i.e., food). It is the source of qi and blood that nourish and drive the body, just as earth brings forth the crops in long summer. *Lung-metal:* The lung draws in fresh air, and is ascribed the function of working change on the fluids by turning them into red blood. It is also given the function of controlling the downward movement of fluids to the kidney and bladder, so that it is responsible for the purifying removal of waste fluids. Thus, the lung has qualities that correspond to the purifying frost of autumn. *Kidney-water:* The kidney is the low place to which the fluids of the body flow.

In addition to this, the kidney stores essence, just as nature preserves itself in winter dormancy. The phenomena associated with each of the five phases not only bear qualitative similarities to each other, but also relate to other phenomena associated with the same phase in like fashion. Just as water engenders wood, so winter gives way to spring, and the kidney nourishes the liver. More about five-phase relationships under ENGENDERING, RESTRAINING, REBELLION, and OVERWHELMING. ◇ Chin 五 *wǔ*, five; 行 *xíng*, move, movement. **Eng** *phase*, Gk. *phanein*, show, appear. The term is often rendered "five elements," however, the term "element," as used in Greek philosophy, means a constituent of the material world. The Chinese *xíng* are a system whereby phenomena and their interrelationships are classified, and the term, which literally means "movement," reflects the changes occurring in the yearly cycle on which the five-phase associations are largely built. The English "phase," originally meant the different aspects presented by the moon, and derived from "phasis," the first appearance of the new moon. [6: 28] [27: 80] [97: 43]

5. Five Phases in Nature				
Wood	Fire	Earth	Metal	Water
Sour	Bitter	Sweet	Acrid	Salty
Green-blue	Red	Yellow	White	Black
Birth	Growth	Transformation	Withdrawal	Storage
Wind	Summer-heat	Dampness	Dryness	Cold
East	South	Center	West	North
Spring	Summer	Long summer	Autumn	Winter
Wind	Summer-heat	Dampness	Dryness	Cold

6. Five Phases in Man				
Wood	Fire	Earth	Metal	Water
Liver	Heart	Spleen	Lung	Kidney
Gall-bladder	Small intestine	Stomach	Large intestine	Bladder
Eyes	Tongue	Mouth	Nose	Ears
Sinew	Vessels	Flesh	Skin & body hair	Bone
Anger	Joy	Thought	Sorrow	Fear
Nails	Complexion	Lips	Body hair	Hair
Tears	Sweat	Drool	Snivel	Spittle
Stringlike	Surging	Moderate	Downy	Stone-like
Shouting	Laughing	Singing	Wailing	Moaning
Ethereal soul	Spirit	Ideation	Animal soul	Mind

Five Pillar Points 五柱穴 *wŭ zhù xué*: Five points: CV-12 (*zhōng wăn*, Center Stomach Duct), CV-14 (*jù què*, Great Tower Gate), CV-10 (*xià wăn*, Lower Stomach Duct), and bilateral ST-21 (*liáng mén*, Beam Gate), (CV-12 is two body-inches from each of the other points), which are poled to treat spleen vacuity diarrhea and cold-damp diarrhea. NB: CV-12 is four body-inches above the umbilicus and is two inches from each of the other points. Compare CROSS MOXA. [78: 94]

five proprieties 五宜 *wŭ yí*: The dietary requirements of the five viscera. [27: 318]

five slownesses 五迟 *wŭ chí*: Five forms of retardation in the development of infants: slowness to stand; slowness to walk; slowness to grow hair; slowness to teethe; slowness to speak. Compare FIVE LIMPNESSES. [27: 436] [97: 45]

five stranguries 五淋 *wŭ lín*: Stone, qi, unctuous, taxation, and blood strangury. The general features of strangury are urinary frequency and urgency and difficult voiding, as well as dribbling incontinence. STONE STRANGURY, UNCTUOUS STRANGURY, and BLOOD STRANGURY, which are characterized respectively by calculus, milky urine, and bloody urine, are mostly caused by damp-heat in the lower burner. QI STRANGURY takes two forms: if characterized by distention and pain in the lower abdomen stretching into the scrotum, inhibited urination and pain after urination, it is the result of bladder qi stagnation; if characterized by pain and distention in the lower abdomen and dribble after urination, it is the result of spleen-kidney qi vacuity. TAXATION STRANGURY is strangury brought on by overexertion and is characterized by dull pain in the urethra after voiding and by fatigued limbs. Often developing

from other forms of strangury, it is a manifestation of spleen qi and/or kidney yang vacuity. [27: 425] [97: 50]

five taxations 五劳 *wŭ láo*: **1.** *Elementary Questions* (*sù wèn, xuān míng wŭ qì*). Damage by the five taxations: prolonged vision damages the blood; prolonged lying damages qi; prolonged sitting damages the flesh; prolonged standing damages the bones; and prolonged walking damages the sinews. **2.** Visceral taxation damage, i.e., lung taxation, liver taxation, heart taxation, spleen taxation, and kidney taxation. [26: 121] [27: 118] [97: 44]

five taxations and seven damages 五劳七伤 *wŭ láo qī shāng*: See FIVE TAXATIONS; SEVEN DAMAGES.

five transport points 五俞穴 *wŭ shū xué*, 五输穴 *wŭ shū xué*, 五腧穴 *wŭ shū xué*: Any of a series of five points below the elbows or knees on each of the twelve channels. The five points are the well, brook (spring), stream, channel (river), and uniting points, which each have five-phase correspondences that differ from the yang to the yin channels. On the lung channel, for example, LU-11 (*shào shāng*, Lesser Shang) is the well point corresponding to wood; LU-10 (*yú jì*, Fish Border) is the brook point corresponding to fire; LU-9 (*tài yuān*, Great Abyss) is the stream point corresponding to earth; LU-8 (*jīng qú*, Channel Ditch) is the channel point corresponding to metal. The points of the other channels are presented in Table 7. The names well, brook, stream, channel, and uniting reflect the nature of the flow of qi at each of these points. The ancient Chinese likened the flow of qi in the channels to the flow of water from its source in the mountains to its home in the sea. At the well points, which are located at the ends of the digits, the qi is shallow and meek. At the brook points, on the hands and feet, the qi has a gushing quality. At the channel points in the area of the wrist and ankle, the qi is described as being like water pouring downward from a shallow place to a deeper one. At the river points on the forearm and lower leg, the qi has developed into a powerful flow. At the uniting points at the knees and elbows, the qi goes deep into the body to unite with its home organ, just as a river flows into the sea. These names are only intended to describe the nature of the qi at each of the five points; they are not intended to indicate the direction of the flow of qi. On the yang channels of the foot and the yin channels of the arm, the image of the five transport points suggests that qi is moving counter to its actual direction. Application: The transport points are used in different ways clinically. They can be used in the treatment of certain conditions or at certain times of the year. They can also be used in a way that applies to five-phase relationships.

7. Transport Points of Yin Channels				
Well Wood	Spring Fire	Stream Earth	Channel Metal	Uniting Water
LU-11	LU-10	LU-9	LU-8	LU-5
PC-9	PC-8	PC-7	PC-5	PC-3
HT-9	HT-8	HT-7	HT-4	HT-3
SP-1	SP-2	SP-3	SP-5	SP-9
LR-1	LR-2	LR-3	LR-4	LR-8
KI-1	KI-2	KI-3	KI-7	KI-10

Transport Points of Yang Channels				
Well Metal	Spring Water	Stream Wood	River Fire	Uniting Earth
LI-9	LI-8	LI-7	LI-4	LI-3
TB-1	TB-2	TB-3	TB-6	TB-10
SI-1	SI-2	SI-3	SI-5	SI-8
ST-45	ST-44	ST-43	ST-42	ST-36
GB-44	GB-43	GB-38	GB-40	GB-34
BL-67	BL-66	BL-65	BL-60	BL-40

(1) Employment according to type of condition: Clinical experience recorded in modern literature shows that the well points are most effective for conditions characterized by clouded spirit, the spring points are best for externally contracted heat (febrile) diseases, the stream points treat pain in the joints, the channel (river) points treat cough and panting, whereas the uniting points treat bowel patterns. These indications partly agree with what the classics say. (2) Employment according to the seasons: The text and commentaries of *The Classic of Difficult Issues* (*nàn jīng*) suggest the following: In the spring and summer months yang qi rises and the qi in the body flows on the exterior. Superficial needling is appropriate during this period, so well and spring points are often employed. In the autumn and winter months yang qi sinks downward and the qi of the body is relatively deep. During this time, it is appropriate to needle deeply, so river and uniting points are often applied. Accordingly, the texts prescribes

the well points in spring, the spring points in summer, the river points in autumn, and the uniting points in winter. This conflicts with *The Inner Canon* (*nèi jīng*), which prescribes the spring points in spring, the river points in summer, the uniting points in fall, and the well points in winter. (3) Employment according to five-phase correspondences: The transport points can be used in a way that applies the five-phase correspondences of the transport points in relation to the five-phase correspondences of the channel, in accordance with the principles that vacuity is treated by supplementing the mother and repletion is treated by draining the child. In this context, the mother and child may be the mother or child transport points either on the affected channel or on the mother or child channels. Thus, shortness of breath and copious sweat forming part of a vacuity pattern of the lung (metal) channel can be treated by supplementing either the earth point of the lung channel (earth engenders, i.e., is mother of metal) or the earth point of the spleen (earth) channel. Thus, lung vacuity can be treated either by supplementing LU-9 or SP-3. Acute cough and panting, which forms a lung repletion pattern, can be treated by draining the water point (LU-5) of the lung channel (water is engendered by, i.e., is the child of metal) or by draining the water point of the water channel (KI-10). ◊ Chin 五 *wǔ*, five; 俞 *shū*, transport, shunt; 穴 *xué*, cave, hole. More at TRANSPORT POINT. [46: 145] [26: 120] [50: 202] [37: 103]

five unmanlinesses 五不男 *wǔ bù nán*: Five forms of male sterility: 天 (*tiān*) "heaven" (congenital eunuchism); 漏 (*lòu*) "leak" (seminal discharge); 犍 (*jiān*) "gelding" (castration); 怯 (*qiè*) "timidity" (impotence); and 痀 (*ē*) "freakishness" (hermaphroditism). [26: 114] [27: 428] [97: 51]

five unwomanlinesses 五不女 *wǔ bù nǚ*: Five forms of female infertility: 螺 (*luó*) "snail" (deformity of vagina); 纹 (*wén*) constricted vagina; 鼓 (*gǔ*) "drum" (imperforate hymen); 角 (*jiǎo*) "horn" (excessively developed clitoris); 脉 (*mài*) "vessel" (infertility due to lifelong absence of menses or to menstrual irregularity, or flooding and vaginal discharge). [26: 114] [27: 455] [97: 51] [50: 196]

five viscera 五脏 *wǔ zàng*: The heart, lung, spleen, liver, and kidney. Each viscus has a five-phase ascription by which they are sometimes referred: heart-fire, lung-metal, spleen-earth, liver-wood, and kidney-water. See BOWELS AND VISCERA. [27: 16]

five viscera and six bowels cough 五脏六腑咳 *wǔ zàng liù fǔ ké*: From *Elementary Questions* (*sù wèn, ké lùn*). Cough associated with disease in the various organs (HEART COUGH, SPLEEN COUGH, etc.). Although cough is essentially associated with disease of the lung, other organs may be involved. Other organs can affect the lung, and enduring cough can affect the function of other organs. Thus, *heart cough* means cough due to disease not only in the heart but also in the lung. [27: 379]

five viscera form humors 五脏化液 *wǔ zàng huà yè*: The heart, lung, liver, spleen and kidney are each related to the production of sweat, snivel, tears, drool, and spittle, respectively. *Elementary Questions* (*sù wèn, xuān míng wǔ qì piān*) states, "The five viscera form the humors; the heart forms sweat, the lung forms snivel, the liver forms tears, the spleen forms drool, and the kidney forms spittle." Zhang Zhi-Cong commented on this saying, "The five viscera receive the liquid of grain and water, which pour out to the external orifices to form the five humors." [26: 126] [27: 61] [97: 56]

five voices 五声 *wǔ shēng*: The five qualities of the voice, each having a five-phase ascription: shouting (liver-wood), laughing (heart-fire), singing (spleen-earth), wailing (lung-metal), and groaning (kidney-water). These are each associated with a viscus through the five phases. [27: 9] [97: 45]

five waters 五水 *wǔ shuǐ*: From *Essential Prescriptions of the Golden Coffer* (*jīn guì yào lüè, shuǐ qì bìng mài zhèng bìng zhì*). WATER SWELLING manifesting in different ways depending on which viscus it affects. **Heart water** is characterized by a heavy body and shortage of qi, heart vexation and sleeplessness, and swelling of the lower yin. **Liver water** is characterized by distention, fullness, and pain beneath the rib-side and in the abdomen preventing the patient from turning sides, and by urine that is sometimes copious and sometimes scant. **Spleen water** is characterized by abdominal fullness and difficult urination, and by heavy cumbersome limbs. **Lung water** is characterized by inhibited breathing, heavy body, difficult urination, and duck's slop stool. **Kidney water** is marked by lumbar pain, difficult urination, enlarged abdomen and swollen umbilicus, by exudation of water-damp from the lower yin, cold lower extremities, and emaciated face and body. [27: 419]

five wheels 五轮 *wǔ lún*: The flesh wheel, blood wheel, qi wheel, wind wheel, and water wheel. The **flesh wheel** is comprised of the upper and lower eyelid, and belongs to the spleen, which governs the flesh and stands in interior-exterior relationship with the stomach. Diseases affecting the flesh wheel are often related to the spleen and stomach. The **blood wheel** is the inner and outer canthus, and belongs to the heart, which commands the blood and stands in interior-exterior relationship with the small intestine. Disease affecting the blood wheel are often associated with the heart and small intestine. The **qi wheel** is the white of the eye (sclera), and belongs to the lung, which governs qi and stands in interior-exterior relationship with the large intestine. Disease of the qi wheel is often ascribed to the lung and the large intestine. The **wind wheel** is associated with the dark of the eye, and belongs to the liver, which is the viscus of wind and wood and stands in interior-exterior relationship with gallbladder. Disease of the wind wheel is often associated with the liver and gallbladder. The **water wheel** is the pupil, and belongs to the kidney, which governs water and stands in interior-exterior relationship to the bladder. Disease of the water wheel is often associated with the kidney and bladder. The correspondences of the five wheels are characteristic of Chinese medicine, but should not be applied too rigidly. [26: 124]

fixed impediment 着痹 *zhuó bì*: IMPEDIMENT (*bì*) due to a prevalence of dampness, and characterized by a feeling of heaviness that keeps the patient "fixed" to the spot, i.e., hampers movement. See DAMP IMPEDIMENT. [27: 500] [97: 46]

flailing of the arms and legs 扬手踯足 *yáng shǒu zhí zú*, 手舞足蹈 *shǒu wǔ zú dào*: Wild uncontrollable movement of the limbs. A sign of severe AGITATION.

flaking 镑 *bàng*: A method of processing thin flakes that are planed off from hard medicinals such as rhinoceros horn (*xī jiǎo*) and antelope horn (*líng yáng jiǎo*) with a "flaking knife." [26: 963]

flame upward 上炎 *shàng yán*: An attribute of fire that it flames upward. Disease patterns such as liver fire flaming upward are characterized by severe headache, red complexion, reddening of the eyes, and dry mouth. See HEAT.

flare-tip abscess 燸疽 *biāo jū*: TIP-ABSCESS.

flaring nostrils 鼻煽 *bí shān*: Dilatation of the nostrils on inhalation; a sign associated with rapid breathing due to lung heat. [6: 126]

flash-cupping 闪罐 *shǎn guàn*: A method of cupping whereby the cup is swiftly removed after application and repeatedly reapplied until the required degree of reddening or static blood appears. This method is used for local pain or numbness or for impaired functions. See CUPPING. [27: 346] [26: 515]

flat-abscess 疽 *jū*: *Synonym: ju (obs)*. **1.** HEADLESS FLAT-ABSCESS. A deep malign suppuration in the flesh, sinew, and even the bone, attributed to toxic evil obstructing qi and the blood. **2.** HEADED FLAT-ABSCESS. Prior to the Song Dynasty, the term *jū* meant only headless flat-abscess. From Song Dynasty, it came to be used to denote certain superficial sores. For this reason, the terms HEADED FLAT-ABSCESS and HEADLESS

FLAT-ABSCESS became current to distinguish the two. ◇ Chin 疽 *jū* is composed of the 疒 *chuáng*, the illness signifier and 且 *qiě*, a ritual offerings table, as phonetic (and possibly a semantic) element. The character is explained in medical texts as meaning the same as 阻 *zǔ*, obstruct or impede, and 沮 which has a number of meanings distinguished in modern Mandarin by pronunciation: 沮 *jū*, name of various rivers; 沮 *jù*, wet, moist; marsh, swamp; 阻 *zǔ*, obstruct, thwart, defeat, wasted. *Orthodox External Medicine* (*wài kē zhèng zōng, yōng jū mén*) states, "疽 (flat-abscess) means 沮 (marsh, swamp)." The notion of "marsh" or "swamp" connotes an accumulation of water due to lack of drainage, an image that continually recurs in Chinese medicine. The fact that a major feature of 疽 is that it is flat, placing it in opposition to 痈, which is raised, possibly makes the notion of the "marsh" as a broad accumulation of water in low-lying land doubly pertinent to understanding how 疽 was originally conceived and why it was so named. [26: 490] [27: 463] [97: 491] [48: 150]

flat-abscess of the brain 脑疽 *náo jū*: See MOUTH-LEVEL NAPE FLAT-ABSCESS.

flatus 矢气 *shǐ qì*: Synonym: *fecal qi*. Qi (i.e., gas) discharged through the anus. See PASSING OF FLATUS. ◇ Chin 矢 *shǐ*, arrow, and by transference, an oath; used as a euphemistic substitute for 屎 *shǐ*, excrement; 气 *qì*, gas, vapor, qi. The qi (gas) of excrement. [27: 168] [97: 163]

flavor 味 *wèi*: See FIVE FLAVORS.

flesh 肉 *ròu*, 肌 *jī*: **1.** The soft parts of the body other than the viscera and skin. WMC The flesh is governed by the spleen and reflects the state of the spleen. Emaciation, whatever disease it occurs in, is attributed to spleen vacuity. See SPLEEN GOVERNS THE FLESH. Diseases associated with the flesh include FLESH WILTING and FLESH IMPEDIMENT. **2.** The soft parts of the body other than viscera, including the skin. For example, parts of the body such as the back of the hands and arms that easily tan are called the red flesh in contradistinction to the inner surface, which is called the white flesh. ◇ Chin 肉 *ròu* originally portrayed meating hanging from a rack, suggesting that the word was first applied to animal flesh as meat for human consumption. 肌 *ròu*, which has 肉 (月) as its signifier, denotes flesh as an anatomical entity. In the context of the human body, the two characters are identical in meaning, and often occur together in the compound 肌肉 *jī ròu*, also denoting flesh. This combination is now used in Western medicine in the specific sense of muscle (red flesh).

flesh divide 肉分 *ròu fēn*: Any furrow or grain of the flesh. The major divides are the partings between major masses of flesh (muscles), while the minor divides are partings between smaller masses of flesh. [50: 542] [27: 31]

flesh goiter 肉瘿 *ròu yǐng*: A disease manifesting in single or multiple swellings of the neck below the skin that have the appearance of upturned cups, soft and spongy to the touch, that never rupture, and that may be associated with sweating, oppression in the chest and heart palpitations. Flesh goiter is attributed to binding depression damaging the spleen preventing the normal movement of spleen qi. WMC thyroid tumor; tuberculous goiter. MED Treat by opening depression and transforming phlegm, assisted by softening hardness. Use Sargassum Jade Flask Decoction (*hǎi zǎo yù hú tāng*) as oral medication, and apply Harmonious Yang Decongealing Plaster (*yáng hé jiě níng gāo*) mixed with Cinnamon Twig and Musk Powder (*guì shè sǎn*). ACU Base treatment mainly on CV, GB, TB, and ST. Select TB-13 (*nào huì*, Upper Arm Convergence), LR-3 (*tài chōng*, Supreme Surge), TB-6 (*zhī gōu*, Branch Ditch), CV-12 (*zhōng wǎn*, Center Stomach Duct), ST-36 (*zú sān lǐ*, Leg Three Li), ST-40 (*fēng lóng*, Bountiful Bulge), CV-22 (*tiān tú*, Celestial Chimney), SI-17 (*tiān róng*, Celestial Countenance), and LI-17 (*tiān dǐng*, Celestial Tripod); needle with even supplementation and drainage. For thyroid enlargement, add Qi Goiter (*qì yǐng*) and the paravertebrals of the neck (3–5). Selection of points according to signs: For copious sweat, add HT-6 (*yīn xī*, Yin Cleft). For heart palpitations, add HT-7 (*shén mén*, Spirit Gate). For oppression in the chest, add PC-6 (*nèi guān*, Inner Pass) and CV-17 (*shān zhōng*, Chest Center). [26: 262] [27: 476] [97: 182] [113: 387] [37: 446]

flesh impediment 肌痹 *jī bì*, 肉痹 *ròu bì*: An IMPEDIMENT (*bì*) pattern characterized by pain in the flesh that may be accompanied by sweating, limp wilting limbs, numbness of the skin, and clouded essence-spirit. Flesh impediment is usually attributed to damage by cold-damp, but distinction is made between repletion and vacuity patterns. WMC dermatomyositis. MED Repletion patterns are treated with Five Impediments Decoction (*wǔ bì tāng*) and vacuity patterns are treated with Wondrous Effect Astragalus Decoction (*shén xiào huáng qí tāng*). ACU For repletion patterns, base treatment mainly on CV, ST, SP, and GV. Select BL-23 (*shèn shū*, Kidney Transport), GV-4 (*mìng mén*, Life Gate), CV-4 (*guān yuán*, Pass Head), ST-36 (*zú sān lǐ*, Leg Three Li), SP-9 (*yīn líng quán*, Yin Mound Spring), and SP-5 (*shāng qiū*, Shang Hill); needle with drainage and large amounts of moxa. For vacuity patterns, base treatment mainly on CV, ST, SP, and GV. Select BL-23 (*shèn shū*, Kidney Transport), BL-20 (*pí shū*, Spleen Transport), GV-4 (*mìng* *mén,* Life Gate), CV-4 (*guān yuán,* Pass Head), ST-36 (*zú sān lǐ,* Leg Three Li), LI-10 (*shǒu sān lǐ,* Arm Three Li), SP-9 (*yīn líng quán,* Yin Mound Spring), SP-5 (*shāng qiū,* Shang Hill), and SP-6 (*sān yīn jiāo,* Three Yin Intersection); needle with supplementation and large amounts of moxa. [26: 262] [27: 404] [97: 182] [46: 628,638] [37: 364]

flesh tumor 肉瘤 *ròu liú:* A swelling on the surface of the body that is initially the size of a peach and gradually grows to the size of a fist, has a broad root, is firm but supple, and is associated with no change in skin color or signs of heat or cold. A flesh tumor is attributed to binding depression of spleen qi stemming from damage to the spleen by thought and anxiety. MED Fortify the spleen and boost qi; open depression and transform phlegm. Use variations of Spleen-Returning Decoction (*guī pí tāng*). WMC myofibroma; lipoma. [26: 262]

flesh wheel 肉轮 *ròu lún:* One of the FIVE WHEELS; the eyelid. The flesh wheel is related to the spleen, and diseases affecting it are mostly attributed to disease of the spleen and stomach. [26: 262] [27: 500, 866] [97: 182]

flesh wilting 肉痿 *ròu wěi:* Synonym: *spleen wilting.* WILTING (*wěi*) attributed to spleen qi heat depriving the flesh of nutrition or to dampness damaging the spleen and affecting the flesh, and characterized by numbness of the flesh and, in severe cases, inability to move the limbs. MED Clear heat and disinhibit dampness; fortify the spleen and harmonize the stomach. Use variations of Gardenia and Coptis Two Matured Ingredients Decoction (*zhī lián èr chén tāng*). ACU Base treatment on back transport points, CV, ST, and SP. Select BL-20 (*pí shū,* Spleen Transport), CV-12 (*zhōng wǎn,* Center Stomach Duct), ST-36 (*zú sān lǐ,* Leg Three Li), SP-9 (*yīn líng quán,* Yin Mound Spring), PC-6 (*nèi guān,* Inner Pass), SP-6 (*sān yīn jiāo,* Three Yin Intersection), and KI-7 (*fù liū,* Recover Flow). Needle with even supplementation and drainage. [26: 262] [27: 402] [97: 182] [113: 242] [46: 638]

fleshy exterior 肌表 *jī biǎo:* The exterior of the body comprised of the skin and flesh and the face, neck, back, abdomen, and limbs.

fleshy protuberance before the ear 耳前起肉 *ěr qián qǐ ròu:* Synonyms: *ear gate; shelter; pearl of the ear.* The tongue-like projection in front of the ear. WMC tragus.

flicking stone pulse 弹石脉 *tán shí mài:* See SEVEN STRANGE PULSES. [27: 199] [27: 199]

floating 浮 *fú:* Location in or tendency to move or carry toward the upper or outer body. The word floating occurs in the terms: FLOATING HEAT EFFUSION; FLOATING HEAT; FLOATING PULSE; FLOATING-RED FACIAL COMPLEXION; VACUOUS YANG FLOATING UPWARD; UPFLOATER. See also *floating and sunken complexions* under TEN-PRINCIPLE INSPECTION OF THE COMPLEXION.

floating heat 浮热 *fú rè:* Exterior heat at the onset of externally contracted heat (febrile) disease. Compare FLOATING HEAT EFFUSION. [97: 483]

floating heat [effusion] 浮热 *fú rè:* Heat felt at the surface of the body on initial palpation but quickly felt no longer. A floating heat effusion is a false heat sign observed in EXUBERANT YIN REPELLING YANG. Compare FLOATING HEAT. [27: 129] [97: 483]

floating pulse 浮脉 *fú mài:* The floating pulse is pronounced at the superficial level but vacuous at the deep level. Described as being "like wood floating on water," it is felt as soon as the fingers touch the skin, but it becomes markedly less perceptible when further pressure is applied, as a piece of floating wood escapes from the finger when pressed down in water. Although classically associated with exterior patterns, the floating pulse may be indistinct in patients of heavy build, with weak constitutions, or those suffering from severe water swelling, even when an exterior pattern is present. A floating pulse may also occur in enduring illnesses or after a major loss of blood, indicating a critical insufficiency of right qi rather than an exterior pattern. In these cases, it differs slightly from the floating pulse occurring in externally contracted disease. Being slightly less pronounced at the superficial level, and markedly less pronounced at the deep level, it is sometimes referred to as a vacuous floating pulse. **Similar pulses:** A large floating pulse without foundation is known as a *scattered pulse,* which is large at the superficial level, but because of its lack of force, ceases to be felt as soon as the slightest pressure is applied. It indicates the dissipation of qi and blood, and the impending expiration of the essential qi of the organs. It is usually attended by other critical signs. A floating pulse that is empty in the middle is known as a *scallion-stalk pulse,* which is mostly seen in patients suffering from heavy blood loss. [6: 139] [27: 193] [97: 483]

floating-red facial complexion 面色浮红 *miàn sè fú hóng:* Tidal reddening of the face marked by pale red patches like dabs of rouge that constantly change location; observed in UPCAST YANG patterns. [27: 129]

flood 泛 *fàn:* Describes the behavior of excess fluid in the body, as in the term "kidney vacuity water flood," which denotes water swelling caused by kidney vacuity. See EXUBERANCE AND DEBILITATION.

flooding 崩中 *bēng zhōng:* See FLOODING AND SPOTTING. [27: 433]

flooding and spotting 崩漏 *bēng lòu:* Any abnormal discharge of blood via the vagina. Flooding (*bēng*) is heavy menstrual flow or abnormal bleeding via the vagina (uterine bleeding); spotting (*lòu*), lit. "leaking" in Chinese, is a slight, often continual discharge of blood via the vagina. If the flow is deep red and clotted, it is usually a sign of heat. Since each may give way to the other, they are commonly referred to together. Flooding and spotting usually occur in puberty or at menopause. It is attributed to insecurity of the thoroughfare (*chōng*) and controlling (*rèn*) vessels, which may stem from a variety of causes. WMC metrorrhagia (uterine bleeding). See entries listed below and the following entries. ◊ Chin 崩 *bēng*, collapse, landslide; 漏 *lòu*, leak, trickle. [26: 642] [27: 433]

Flooding and Spotting

BLOOD HEAT FLOODING AND SPOTTING (*xuè rè bēng lòu*)

QI VACUITY FLOODING AND SPOTTING (*qì xū bēng lòu*)

LIVER-KIDNEY YIN VACUITY FLOODING AND SPOTTING (*gān shèn yīn xū bēng lòu*)

BLOOD STASIS FLOODING AND SPOTTING (*xuè yū bēng lòu*)

QI DEPRESSION FLOODING (*qì yù xuè bēng*)

POSTPARTUM FLOODING (*chǎn hòu xuè bēng*)

flooding with abdominal pain 血崩腹痛 *xuè bēng fù tòng*: FLOODING AND SPOTTING (abnormal discharge of blood via the vagina) with abdominal pain is attributed either to blood stasis or blood vacuity. MED If due to blood stasis, the abdominal pain refuses pressure and is relieved by the passing of clots. Move stasis and relieve pain with formulas such as Sudden Smile Powder (*shī xiào sǎn*). If due to blood vacuity, it is characterized by abdominal pain that likes warmth and pressure and is treated by nourishing the blood and stanching bleeding with Ass Hide Glue and Mugwort Four Agents Decoction (*jiāo ài sì wù tāng*). ACU For blood stasis, base treatment mainly on CV, SP, ST, and LR. Select CV-6 (*qì hǎi*, Sea of Qi), SP-6 (*sān yīn jiāo*, Three Yin Intersection), SP-1 (*yǐn bái*, Hidden White), SP-10 (*xuè hǎi*, Sea of Blood), SP-8 (*dì jī*, Earth's Crux), ST-30 (*qì chōng*, Qi Thoroughfare), LR-3 (*tài chōng*, Supreme Surge), ST-36 (*zú sān lǐ*, Leg Three Li), and ST-25 (*tiān shū*, Celestial Pivot), needle with even supplementation and drainage. For blood vacuity, base treatment mainly on CV and SP, select CV-4 (*guān yuán*, Pass Head), SP-6 (*sān yīn jiāo*, Three Yin Intersection), BL-20 (*pí shū*, Spleen Transport), BL-17 (*gé shū*, Diaphragm Transport), ST-36 (*zú sān lǐ*, Leg Three Li), CV-12 (*zhōng wǎn*, Center Stomach Duct), and needle with supplementation. See FLOODING AND SPOTTING. [26: 281] [46: 688] [37: 319] [59: 15]

flooding with clouding vision 血崩昏暗 *xuè bēng hūn àn*: Abnormal discharge of blood from the uterus attended by clouding of vision. Excessive blood loss through flooding and spotting causing the heart and liver to be deprived of nourishment and thereby causing clouding of vision and, in severe cases, sudden collapse and unconsciousness. MED Supplement the blood and stanch bleeding. Use Root-Securing Flood-Stanching Decoction (*gù běn zhǐ bēng tāng*). ACU To supplement the blood and stanch bleeding, base treatment mainly on GV, CV, and SP. Select GV-20 (*bǎi huì*, Hundred Convergences), CV-6 (*qì hǎi*, Sea of Qi), CV-4 (*guān yuán*, Pass Head), SP-6 (*sān yīn jiāo*, Three Yin Intersection), SP-10 (*xuè hǎi*, Sea of Blood), ST-36 (*zú sān lǐ*, Leg Three Li), BL-20 (*pí shū*, Spleen Transport), SP-1 (*yǐn bái*, Hidden White), and SP-2 (*dà dū*, Great Metropolis); needle with supplementation and large amounts of moxa. To treat blood desertion patterns, base treatment mainly on CV and GV. Select GV-26 (*shuǐ gōu*, Water Trough), GV-25 (*sù liáo*, White Bone-Hole), PC-6 (*nèi guān*, Inner Pass), GV-20 (*bǎi huì*, Hundred Convergences), CV-4 (*guān yuán*, Pass Head), and KI-1 (*yǒng quán*, Gushing Spring); needle with supplementation or direct moxa. Apply moxa on salt or ginger at CV-8 (*shén què*, Spirit Gate Tower). [26: 281] [46: 731]

flowery vision 目花 *mù huā*: A general term embracing various kinds of visual disturbances such as blurring, distortion, floaters, nearsightedness, etc. See CLOUDED VISION. ◊ Chin 目 *mù*, eye; 花 *huā*, flower.

flowing phlegm 流痰 *liú tán*: A chronic destructive condition of the joints characterized by the formation of pus that can "flow," or spread, to other parts, and that after rupture discharges like thin phlegm. Flowing phlegm is nowadays considered to be a form of HEADLESS FLAT-ABSCESS. It is most commonly observed in children and adolescents often found to have a history of consumption (pulmonary tuberculosis), and affects most commonly the hip bone or spine and less commonly the knee, ankle, shoulder, elbow, or wrist. Flowing phlegm is named differently according to location. Flowing phlegm of the spine is called *tortoise's-back phlegm*, whereas that of the hip is called *Jumping Round phlegm* after GB-30 (*huán tiào*, Jumping Round). It arises in patients suffering from insufficiency of the congenital constitution or from kidney yin depletion in enduring illness, when external evils exploit a vacuity and enter the body and cause phlegm turbidity to gather and congeal. It may be brought on by disharmony of qi and blood stemming from knocks and falls. The condition begins with slight local swelling associated with distention but without redness, heat, or marked pain. The swelling gradually spreads, becomes painful, and suppurates, and the surrounding flesh becomes atrophied. In an advanced stage, effulgent yin depletion fire may cause postmeridian heat effusion, night sweating, encumbered body and lack of strength, and reduced food intake. Following rupture, clear thin pus is discharged, the flesh is purple, the mouth of the sore is depressed, does not close easily, and the cavity is like a tunnel. In the initial stage, it is treated by supplementing the liver and kidney, warming the channels and transforming phlegm using formulas like Harmonious Yang Decoction (*yáng hé tāng*). In the middle stage, treatment aims to support right and expel toxin. In the advanced stage after suppuration and rupture, emphasis is placed on supporting right to help the sore to close. Patients with signs of dual depletion of qi and blood can be given Ginseng Construction-Nourishing Decoction (*rén shēn yǎng róng tāng*), whereas those with signs of effulgent yin depletion can be given Major Yin Supplementation Pill (*dà bǔ yīn wán*). If there is tunneling, Thousand Gold Pieces Powder (*qiān jīn sǎn*) can be applied topically. ⌐WMC⌐ tuberculosis of the bone or joints. See HEADLESS FLAT-ABSCESS; FLAT-ABSCESS; SORE. [26: 478]

flowing rheum 流饮 *liú yǐn*: **1.** PHLEGM-RHEUM in the narrow sense. **2.** Phlegm-rheum that flows from place to place, having no fixed location. ⌐MED⌐ Use Three Flowers Spirit Protection Pill (*sān huā shén yòu wán*). [26: 478]

fluctuating generalized heat [effusion] 身热起伏 *shēn rè qǐ fú*: A generalized heat [effusion] characterized by alternating periods of abatement and of increase; observed for example in damp-heat lodged in the qi aspect.

fluid collapse 亡津液 *wáng jīn yè*: A severe form of DAMAGE TO FLUIDS. [26: 27] [27: 207]

fluids 津液 *jīn yè*: All the fluids of the human body, comprising *liquid* (*jīn*), thinner fluids, and *humor* (*yè*), thicker turbid ones. The term "fluids" embraces all the normal fluid substances of the human body. The term refers to fluids actually flowing within the human body and to sweat, saliva, stomach juices, urine, and other fluids secreted by or discharged from the body. The main functions of fluids are to keep the bowels and viscera, the flesh, the skin, the hair, and the orifices adequately moistened, to lubricate the joints, and to nourish the brain, marrow, and bones. Though referring to a single entity, "fluids" is often differentiated into two basic forms, liquid and humor, to highlight specific characteristics. Liquid refers to fluid that is relatively thin, mobile, and yang in quality, whereas humor denotes thicker, less mobile yin fluid. Liquid is mostly found in the surface of the flesh and in the mucous membranes, moisturizing the flesh, skin, and hair and keeping the eyes,

ears, mouth, nose, and other orifices moistened. Sweat and urine are both produced from these fluids. Humor is located primarily in the bowels and viscera, the brain, and the bones and is responsible for lubricating the joints and also partially responsible for moistening the skin. Despite the distinction, liquid and humor form a single entity and are mutually convertible. This distinction is most often made in pathology as in cases of damage to liquid or humor desertion. The term "yin humor" is sometimes used synonymously with humor, emphasizing its yin nature (thick, heavy, and relatively immobile). It may also loosely denote all the nutritious fluids of the body and, as such, is used in contradistinction to yang qi. The formation, distribution, and discharge of fluids involve complex processes in which the lung, spleen, kidney, stomach, small intestine, large intestine, bladder, and other organs play major roles. *Elementary Questions* (*sù wèn, jīng mài bié lùn*) gives the following description: "Drink (饮 *yǐn*, imbibed fluid) enters the stomach, where it is churned and its essential qi is strained off. This is then carried to the spleen and further distributed by spleen qi. It passes up to the lung which ensures regular flow through the waterways down to the bladder. In this way, water essence is distributed to the four parts, by passing through the five channels." Fluid processing begins in the stomach where the essential qi (the useful part) of the fluids is absorbed. The spleen then carries this essential qi up to the lung to be distributed among the other organs. The statement appearing in *Elementary Questions* (*sù wèn, tài yīn yáng míng lùn*) that the spleen "moves the fluids of the stomach" highlights the active role of the spleen in assimilation of fluids. The lung, by governing diffusion and depurative downbearing, ensures the regular flow of water through the waterways. The kidney's function is to "distill" fluid, bearing the clear up and the turbid down. It plays a part in distributing fluids around the entire body and is responsible for transforming surplus and waste fluid into urine, which is discharged through the bladder. The intestines are also involved in the absorption of fluids; the small intestine separates the clear from the turbid and the large intestine conveys the waste material downward while further absorbing fluid. *The Magic Pivot* (*líng shū, jīng mài piàn*) comments: "The small intestine governs humor," and "the large intestine governs liquid." Thus, assimilation and initial conveyance of fluids are dependent on the stomach's intake function and the spleen's function of moving and transforming the "essence" contained in food. The distribution of fluids around the body, including moisturization of the flesh, skin, and [body] hair, is dependent on the lung's function of ensuring diffusion and depurative downbearing. The transformation of fluids into sweat is also dependent on this function. For these reasons, the lung is said to be the "upper source of water" and to ensure regular flow through the waterways. The kidney plays the most important role in the formation and replacement of fluids since the roles of the stomach, the spleen, and the lung are dependent on the warming and activating function of kidney qi. More importantly, the production and discharge of urine and normal replacement of fluids in the body is intimately related to kidney qi transformation. This is why it is said: "The kidney governs the water of the whole body." Finally, because the lung, spleen, stomach, and kidney are located in all three burners, the term "triple burner" is often used to denote the waterways and the formation, movement, and discharge of fluids is attributed to the triple burner qi transformation. *Elementary Questions* (*sù wèn, líng lán mì diǎn lùn*) states, "The triple burner holds the office of the sluices; it manifests as the waterways." See also FIVE HUMORS. Pathologies of the fluids include DAMAGE TO LIQUID and HUMOR DESERTION. [6: 45] [27: 76] [97: 435]

flush 涤 *dí*, 荡涤 *dàng dí*: Forceful elimination (of evils). See FLUSHING PHLEGM. [26: 823]

flushing phlegm 涤痰 *dí tán*: *Synonym: flushing stubborn phlegm.* A method of treatment used to eliminate stubborn phlegm or phlegm-rheum. [MED] Phlegm-flushing medicinals include chlorite/mica (*méng shí*), niter (*xiāo shí*), bile arisaema (*dǎn xīng*), bamboo sugar (*tiān zhú huáng*), and aquilaria (*chén xiāng*). Phlegm-rheum gathering in the rib-side with cough causing rib-side pain and expectoration of phlegm with a glossy tongue fur and stringlike sunken pulse is treated by the method of flushing phlegm with Ten Jujubes Decoction (*shí zǎo tāng*). Old phlegm in repletion heat patterns causing mania and withdrawal patterns, thick phlegm, constipation, a thick yellow slimy tongue fur, and a forceful rapid slippery pulse can be flushed with Chlorite/Mica Phlegm-Rolling Pill (*méng shí gǔn tán wán*). Thick copious phlegm with cough and qi ascent can be flushed with gleditsia (*zào jiá*) that has been subjected to nature-preservative burning taken with a decoction of jujubes. Many phlegm-flushing medicinals are drastic and harsh in action, and should be used with care in vacuity. They are contraindicated in pregnancy or expectoration of blood. [27: 272] [97: 486] [25: 265]

flushing stubborn phlegm 荡涤顽痰 *dàng dí wán tán*: See FLUSHING PHLEGM. [26: 823]

flusteredness 心慌 *xīn huāng*: A state of mental discomposure, confusion, and fear. Flusteredness is a sign of HEART DISEASE.

flying corpse 飞尸 *fēi shī*: CONSUMPTION.

flying flag wind 悬旗风 *xuán qí fēng*, 悬旗风 *xuán qí fēng*: A condition marked by redness, swelling, and hardening of the uvula, so called because the uvula appears conspicuous like a flag in the throat. The uvula is cherry red with a purple blood blister at the tip. Movement of the tongue is inhibited, eating and swallowing are difficult. There is vexation and oppression in the chest and a surging floating pulse. Flying flag wind is caused by phlegm heat in the stomach and liver channels binding in the throat or excessive consumption of hot spicy food causing lung-stomach heat to accumulate and fume up into the throat. [MED] Clear and drain heat toxin with Coptis Toxin-Resolving Decoction (*huáng lián jiě dú tāng*) plus forsythia (*lián qiào*), dandelion (*pú gōng yīng*), arctium (*niú bàng zǐ*), isatis root (*bǎn lán gēn*), and pueraria (*gé gēn*). For external treatment, lance to drain blood and toxin, and use a mouthwash of decocted lonicera (*jīn yín huā*) and licorice (*gān cǎo*). Compare FLYING THROAT. [26: 986] [17: 290] [27: 496] [97: 519]

flying gates 飞门 *fēi mén*: The lips. [27: 30]

flying throat 飞扬喉 *fēi yáng hóu*: A large blood blister hanging from the palate; attributed to latent heat in the bowels and viscera surging upward. Flying throat is the same as flying flag wind, but springs from the palate rather than the uvula. [MED] Clear heat and drain fire; cool the blood and resolve toxin. Use Coptis Toxin-Resolving Decoction (*huáng lián jiě dú tāng*). Compare FLYING FLAG WIND. [17: 290]

folk medicinal 民间药 *mín jiān yào*: Any medicinal that is used in folk medicine as distinct from orthodox Chinese medicine. See MEDICINAL.

fontanel 囟 *xìn*: Either of two gaps between the bones of the skull that close between the age of 6 months and two years, especially the larger one. The larger fontanel, the "fontanel gate" or "forehead fontanel" (called anterior fontanel in Western medicine) is located just in front of the vertex; the smaller one, called "pillow fontanel" (called the posterior fontanel in Western medicine), is on the back of the head. The main diseases associated with the fontanels are UNUNITED SKULL (nonclosure of the fontanels), BULGING FONTANEL, and DEPRESSED FONTANEL. ◇ Chin 囟 *xìn* is a pictographic representation of the skull with nose and sutures. Eng from MF. fontanele, a little spring or fountain. [26: 287] [27: 63] [97: 213]

fontanel gate 囟门 *xìn mén*: The anterior fontanel. See FONTANEL.

food 食 *shí*, 饮食 *yǐn shí*, 水谷 *shuǐ gǔ*: 1. *Synonym: grain and water.* Items of sustenance that enter the body by the mouth. In Chinese medical texts, food is often referred to as *grain and water*, as in the term *nontransformation of grain and wa-*

ter. **2.** Abbreviation for diseases caused by food such as FOOD DAMAGE and FOOD ACCUMULATION etc., see QI, BLOOD, PHLEGM, AND FOOD PATTERN IDENTIFICATION.

food accumulation 食积 *shí jī*: Stagnation and accumulation of food attributable to spleen-stomach movement and transformation failure and characterized by fullness and oppression in the chest and stomach duct, in some cases with hardness or glomus lump, abdominal pain that refuses pressure, hard stool, reduced food intake, putrid belching, and swallowing of upflowing acid. MED If the signs are all of repletion, use accumulation-attacking medicinals such as rhubarb (*dà huáng*) and morning glory (*qiān niú zǐ*). If stagnation is in the early stage, or if accumulation has formed but the patient's constitution is weak, use Harmony-Preserving Pill (*bǎo hé wán*). For spleen vacuity, Six Gentlemen Decoction (*liù jūn zǐ tāng*) may also be included in the treatment. ACU Base treatment mainly on CV, ST, and GV. Main points: Li Inner Court (*lǐ nèi tíng*), CV-21 (*xuán jī*, Jade Swivel), CV-12 (*zhōng wǎn*, Center Stomach Duct), CV-6 (*qì hǎi*, Sea of Qi), ST-25 (*tiān shū*, Celestial Pivot), and ST-36 (*zú sān lǐ*, Leg Three Li). For repletion, needle with drainage. For early-stage stagnation or weak constitution, needle with drainage and add moxa. For spleen vacuity, add BL-20 (*pí shū*, Spleen Transport) and BL-21 (*wèi shū*, Stomach Transport), needle with drainage and add moxa. Selection of points according to signs: For glomus lump, apply large amounts of moxa at Glomus Root (*pǐ gēn*). For hard stool, add ST-37 (*shàng jù xū*, Upper Great Hollow), BL-25 (*dà cháng shū*, Large Intestine Transport), and TB-6 (*zhī gōu*, Branch Ditch). For putrid belching and swallowing of upflowing acid, add GB-40 (*qiū xū*, Hill Ruins) and SP-4 (*gōng sūn*, Yellow Emperor). Compare FOOD DAMAGE, ABIDING FOOD, and FOOD STAGNATION. [6: 215] [26: 471] [27: 412] [97: 45] [25: 228] [14: 104] [46: 662] [113: 18, 102, 223]

food accumulation abdominal pain 食积腹痛 *shí jī fù tòng*: ABDOMINAL PAIN due to dietary irregularities, spleen vacuity, and food stagnating in the stomach and intestines. Food accumulation abdominal pain does not like pressure, and is accompanied by distention and fullness, aversion to food, belching, swallowing of upflowing acid, and constipation. Severe pain may be accompanied by the urge to defecate and may be relieved by defecation. The tongue fur is slimy. The pulse is string-like, and possibly sunken and slippery. MED Rectify qi and harmonize the center; disperse food and abduct stagnation. Use formulas such as Harmony-Preserving Pill (*bǎo hé wán*) and Unripe Bitter Orange Stagnation-Abducting Pill (*zhǐ shí dǎo zhì wán*). ACU Base treatment mainly on CV and

ST. Select CV-10 (*xià wǎn*, Lower Stomach Duct), ST-25 (*tiān shū*, Celestial Pivot), ST-21 (*liáng mén*, Beam Gate), Li Inner Court (*lǐ nèi tíng*), CV-6 (*qì hǎi*, Sea of Qi), ST-36 (*zú sān lǐ*, Leg Three Li), and CV-21 (*xuán jī*, Jade Swivel); needle with drainage. For pronounced pain, add ST-34 (*liáng qiū*, Beam Hill). [26: 472] [46: 662] [37: 320]

food accumulation cough 食积咳嗽 *shí jī ké sòu*: FOOD COUGH.

food accumulation phlegm cough 食积痰嗽 *shí jī tán sòu*: FOOD COUGH.

food accumulation rib-side pain 食积胁痛 *shí jī xié tòng*: RIB-SIDE PAIN arising when dietary irregularities cause food stagnation and congestion of qi dynamic. The rib-side pain is associated with distention and glomus in the stomach duct and abdomen, oppression in the chest, nausea, and no thought of food. In some cases, there is a sausage-shaped protuberance under the ribs. MED Treat by abductive dispersion to eliminate the accumulation using formulas like Harmony-Preserving Pill (*bǎo hé wán*) and variations. ACU Base treatment mainly on CV, ST, PC, LR, and GB. Select Li Inner Court (*lǐ nèi tíng*), CV-10 (*xià wǎn*, Lower Stomach Duct), ST-25 (*tiān shū*, Celestial Pivot), CV-6 (*qì hǎi*, Sea of Qi), ST-36 (*zú sān lǐ*, Leg Three Li), LR-14 (*qī mén*, Cycle Gate), PC-6 (*nèi guān*, Inner Pass), LR-3 (*tài chōng*, Supreme Surge), and GB-34 (*yáng líng quán*, Yang Mound Spring). Needle with drainage. [26: 472] [50: 1119] [46: 662, 636]

food accumulation vomiting 食积呕吐 *shí jī ǒu tù*: Synonym: *food vomiting*. VOMITING due to food accumulation arising when affect damage, external contraction of evil qi, or dietary irregularities cause damage to the spleen and impair the normal transformation of food. Vomiting is accompanied by fullness and oppression (in severe cases, pain and distention) in the stomach duct and abdomen, putrid belching, aversion to food, immediate vomiting of ingested foods, or vomiting in the evening of food ingested in the morning, turbid slimy tongue fur, and a slippery string-like pulse. MED Disperse food and transform accumulation; fortify the spleen and harmonize the stomach. Formulas include Harmony-Preserving Pill (*bǎo hé wán*). ACU Base treatment on alarm and lower uniting points of ST, and on PC and CV. Select CV-12 (*zhōng wǎn*, Center Stomach Duct), ST-36 (*zú sān lǐ*, Leg Three Li), PC-6 (*nèi guān*, Inner Pass), CV-10 (*xià wǎn*, Lower Stomach Duct), Li Inner Court (*lǐ nèi tíng*), and CV-21 (*xuán jī*, Jade Swivel); needle with drainage and add moxa. [26: 471] [46: 639] [113: 72]

food cough 食咳 *shí ké*: Synonyms: *food accumulation cough*; *food accumulation phlegm cough*. Food accumulation engendering phlegm and causing phlegm-qi to surge upward. Signs include cough with copious phlegm that is pronounced at dawn. There may be oppression in the chest and abdominal distention. Other signs include sour belching, nausea, sloppy stool, and a slippery sunken pulse. MED Transform phlegm and disperse the accumulation. Use formulas such as Two Matured Ingredients Decoction (*èr chén tāng*) combined with Stomach-Calming Powder (*píng wèi sǎn*), Three-Seed Filial Devotion Decoction (*sān zǐ yǎng qīn tāng*), and Five Accumulations Powder (*wǔ jī sǎn*). If there is lung fire and phlegm heat with a sunken rapid and slippery pulse, treatment should also be directed toward clearing lung fire. For this latter case, use formulas such as Anemarrhena and Fritillaria Cough-Quieting Decoction (*èr mǔ níng sòu tāng*). ACU Base treat mainly CV, SP, ST, and LU. Select CV-12 (*zhōng wǎn*, Center Stomach Duct), ST-25 (*tiān shū*, Celestial Pivot), CV-6 (*qì hǎi*, Sea of Qi), ST-36 (*zú sān lǐ*, Leg Three Li), ST-40 (*fēng lóng*, Bountiful Bulge), LI-4 (*hé gǔ*, Union Valley), Li Inner Court (*lǐ nèi tíng*), LU-9 (*tài yuān*, Great Abyss), and SP-3 (*tài bái*, Supreme White). Needle with drainage and moxa if appropriate. For lung fire and phlegm heat, add PC-1 (*tiān chí*, Celestial Pool), LI-11 (*qū chí*, Pool at the Bend), and prick LU-11 (*shào shāng*, Lesser Shang) to bleed (and do not use moxa). [26: 470]

food damage 伤食 *shāng shí*: Described in *Dan Xi's Experiential Methods* (*dān xī xīn fǎ*). Any disease pattern of damage to stomach and spleen by food. Food damage is caused by voracious eating or spleen-stomach vacuity. *Elementary Questions* (*sù wèn*) states, "Overeating causes damage to the stomach and intestines." It is characterized by aversion to food, nausea and vomiting, belching, putrid-smelling vomitus and qi, swallowing of upflowing acid, painful bloating of the abdomen, diarrhea or constipation, foul-smelling stool and flatus, and relief from pain and distention after defecation or passing of flatus. The tongue fur is slimy and either thick or yellow. In food damage, when food accumulation remains untransformed for days, the resulting condition is called ABIDING FOOD. MED Treat by dispersing food and abducting stagnation, usually referred to as "abductive dispersion." Commonly used medicinals include medicated leaven (*shén qū*), crataegus (*shān zhā*), barley sprout (*mài yá*), radish seed (*lái fú zǐ*), gizzard lining (*jī nèi jīn*), unripe bitter orange (*zhǐ shí*), and areca (*bīng láng*). Formulas such as the preparatory Harmony-Preserving Pill (*bǎo hé wán*) are frequently used. ACU Base treatment mainly on CV and ST. Select CV-12 (*zhōng wǎn*, Center Stomach Duct), CV-10 (*xià wǎn*, Lower Stomach Duct), ST-25 (*tiān shū*, Celestial Pivot), CV-6 (*qì hǎi*, Sea of Qi), and ST-36 (*zú sān lǐ*, Leg Three Li) as the main points. For voracious eating, add

Li Inner Court (*lǐ nèi tíng*) and ST-37 (*shàng jù xū*, Upper Great Hollow); needle all points with drainage. For spleen-stomach vacuity, add BL-20 (*pí shū*, Spleen Transport), BL-21 (*wèi shū*, Stomach Transport), CV-4 (*guān yuán*, Pass Head), and SP-4 (*gōng sūn*, Yellow Emperor); needle all points with supplementation, adding moxa. Selection of points according to signs: For constipation, add BL-25 (*dà cháng shū*, Large Intestine Transport). For diarrhea, add PC-6 (*nèi guān*, Inner Pass). For glomus and oppression, add SP-4 (*gōng sūn*, Yellow Emperor). For putrid belching and swallowing of upflowing acid, add GB-40 (*qiū xū*, Hill Ruins) and GB-34 (*yáng líng quán*, Yang Mound Spring). Compare ABIDING FOOD, FOOD STAGNATION, and FOOD ACCUMULATION. [26: 804] [27: 352] [97: 198] [25: 118] [46: 662] [13: 328] [113: 223]

food damage diarrhea 伤食泻 *shāng shí xiè*: Synonym: *food diarrhea*. Diarrhea due to food damage, i.e., food poisoning, excessive consumption of alcohol or fatty and spicy foods, or ingestion of food that is too hot or too cold in temperature, or by voracious eating. Food damage diarrhea includes some forms of stomach, large intestinal, and small intestinal diarrhea. It is not clearly distinguished from spleen diarrhea in the case of diarrhea caused by fatty foods. Diarrhea due to excesses in respect to general dietary norms is classed as food damage diarrhea; if due to organ diseases, e.g., vacuity or dampness, it is classed as spleen diarrhea. See also DIARRHEA. MED Disperse food and harmonize the stomach with Harmony-Preserving Pill (*bǎo hé wán*). For vacuity, use variations of Center-Ordering Decoction (*zhì zhōng tāng*). ACU Base treatment mainly on CV and ST. Select CV-12 (*zhōng wǎn*, Center Stomach Duct), CV-10 (*xià wǎn*, Lower Stomach Duct), BL-20 (*pí shū*, Spleen Transport), ST-25 (*tiān shū*, Celestial Pivot), ST-36 (*zú sān lǐ*, Leg Three Li), PC-6 (*nèi guān*, Inner Pass), and Li Inner Court (*lǐ nèi tíng*); needle with drainage. For vacuity, add moxa. [6: 215] [26: 805] [97: 415] [46: 662] [13: 328] [113: 223]

food damage headache 伤食头痛 *shāng shí tóu tòng*: HEADACHE attributed to food stagnating in the stomach. Food damage headache is attended by glomus and fullness in the chest and diaphragm, putrid belching, swallowing of upflowing acid, aversion to food, and a slippery replete pulse. In some cases there may be generalized heat [effusion]. See HEADACHE. MED Disperse food and abduct stagnation using formulas such as Saussurea, Amomum, Unripe Bitter Orange, and Ovate Atractylodes Pill (*xiāng shā zhǐ zhú wán*), Center-Ordering Decoction (*zhì zhōng tāng*), or Harmony-Preserving Pill (*bǎo hé wán*) and variations. ACU Base treatment mainly on ST and LI. Select ST-8 (*tóu wéi*, Head Corner), Greater

Yang (*tài yáng*), CV-12 (*zhōng wǎn*, Center Stomach Duct), PC-6 (*nèi guān*, Inner Pass), ST-25 (*tiān shū*, Celestial Pivot), ST-36 (*zú sān lǐ*, Leg Three Li), LI-4 (*hé gǔ*, Union Valley), and Li Inner Court (*lǐ nèi tíng*) and needle with drainage. For selection of points according to affected area, see HEADACHE. [26: 805] [46: 662] [25: 118] [46: 662, 622] [13: 328] [113: 223]

food-denying dysentery 噤口痢 *jìn kǒu lì*: Dysentery characterized by poor appetite and vomiting of anything ingested. [MED] Use Food Denial Powder (*kāi jìn sǎn*). [ACU] Base treatment on ST and LI. Select LI-4 (*hé gǔ*, Union Valley), ST-25 (*tiān shū*, Celestial Pivot), ST-37 (*shàng jù xū*, Upper Great Hollow), CV-12 (*zhōng wǎn*, Center Stomach Duct), PC-6 (*nèi guān*, Inner Pass), LR-13 (*zhāng mén*, Camphorwood Gate), and ST-44 (*nèi tíng*, Inner Court), and needle with drainage. For enduring dysentery, add BL-20 (*pí shū*, Spleen Transport), CV-4 (*guān yuán*, Pass Head), CV-6 (*qì hǎi*, Sea of Qi), ST-36 (*zú sān lǐ*, Leg Three Li), and ST-21 (*liáng mén*, Beam Gate); needle with supplementation and add moxa. [27: 362] [97: 644] [113: 96] [46: 667]

food depression 食郁 *shí yù*: Nondispersion of food due to inhibited qi dynamic; characterized by bloating of the stomach duct and abdomen, belching of sour putrid qi, inability to eat, abnormal stool, and, in severe cases, jaundice, glomus lump, and drum distention; usually associated with a tight slippery pulse. [MED] Treat by abductive dispersion and disinhibiting the center, using formulas such as Food Depression Decoction (*shí yù tāng*) or Harmony-Preserving Pill (*bǎo hé wán*). [ACU] Base treatment mainly on CV, ST, PC, LR, and SP. Select CV-10 (*xià wǎn*, Lower Stomach Duct), CV-12 (*zhōng wǎn*, Center Stomach Duct), ST-36 (*zú sān lǐ*, Leg Three Li), ST-25 (*tiān shū*, Celestial Pivot), PC-6 (*nèi guān*, Inner Pass), LR-3 (*tài chōng*, Supreme Surge), GB-34 (*yáng líng quán*, Yang Mound Spring), and SP-6 (*sān yīn jiāo*, Three Yin Intersection); needle with drainage. [26: 472] [46: 646, 662]

food diarrhea 食泄 *shí xiè*: FOOD DAMAGE DIARRHEA.

food distention 食胀 *shí zhàng*: Distention attributable to nontransformation of food stemming from excessive consumption of raw cold foods such as gourds and fruits or irregular eating, and marked by hard distended abdomen with pain in severe cases, belching, and acid upflow. A distinction is made between cold and heat. **Cold:** Cold patterns are usually characterized by uninhibited stool and inability to eat, whereas heat patterns are characterized by dry bound stool. [MED] Cold patterns are treated by warming the center and abductive dispersion using Stomach-Calming Po-

ria (Hoelen) Five Decoction (*wèi líng tāng*) plus crataegus (*shān zhā*) and barley sprout (*mài yá*). In severe cases, use Center-Rectifying Decoction (*lǐ zhōng tāng*) plus clove (*dīng xiāng*), magnolia bark (*hòu pò*), and aconite (*fù zǐ*). [ACU] Base treatment on the CV, ST, and PC. Select CV-10 (*xià wǎn*, Lower Stomach Duct), ST-25 (*tiān shū*, Celestial Pivot), CV-6 (*qì hǎi*, Sea of Qi), PC-6 (*nèi guān*, Inner Pass), ST-36 (*zú sān lǐ*, Leg Three Li), ST-21 (*liáng mén*, Beam Gate), and KI-13 (*qì xué*, Qi Point); needle with drainage and add moxa. **Heat:** Heat patterns characterized by dry stool should be treated by abductive dispersion and clearing transformation using formulas such as Harmony-Preserving Pill (*bǎo hé wán*) or Saussurea and Areca Pill (*mù xiāng bīng láng wán*). [ACU] As for cold patterns, but without moxa. [26: 470] [46: 685]

food gan 食疳 *shí gān*: SPLEEN GAN.

food malaria 食疟 *shí nüè*: A kind of malaria described in *A Unified Treatise on Diseases, Patterns, and Remedies According to the Three Causes* (*sān yīn jí yī bìng zhèng fāng lùn*) as follows: "When the patient has [alternating aversion to] cold and heat [effusion], rapid hungering and inability to eat, propping fullness after eating, and tense painful abdomen, occurring at day intervals, this is called stomach malaria. When none of the six bowels except the stomach has malaria, this is commonly called food malaria. Other forms of malaria with dietary irregularities can mutate into this pattern. *Zhang's Clear View of Medicine* (*zhāng shì yī tōng, nüè*) states, "Food malaria is attributable to dietary irregularities that engender phlegm in the center stomach duct, which is exacerbated by wind qi; hence there is rapid hungering and inability to eat, and propping fullness after eating, enlarged abdomen, and frequent retching. Repletion is treated by Two Matured Ingredients Decoction (*èr chén tāng*) plus bitter orange (*zhǐ ké*) and tsaoko (*cǎo guǒ*). When it is due to irregular eating or excessive physical exertion, persists for a long time, and is associated with a vacuous pulse, use Center-Rectifying Decoction (*lǐ zhōng tāng*) plus unripe bitter orange (*zhǐ shí*) and unripe tangerine peel (*qīng pí*). When the patient ordinarily suffers from yin vacuity taxation, or when malaria has turned into taxation, then the formula should contain cinnamon twig (*guì zhī*), ginger (*jiāng*), and jujube (*dà zǎo*); winddispelling phlegm-sweeping medicinals cannot be used alone. If the exterior evil is exuberant, Minor Center-Fortifying Decoction (*xiǎo jiàn zhōng tāng*) or Astragalus Center-Fortifying Decoction (*huáng qí jiàn zhōng tāng*) can be used as the main treatment, followed by Six-Ingredient Pill (*liù wèi wán*), with all ingredients used raw, plus cinnamon twig (*guì zhī*) and turtle shell (*biē jiǎ*). [22: 254] [50: 1115]

food-phlegm 食痰 *shí tán*: Food stagnation or accumulation in combination with phlegm as a cause of disease. Compare FOOD DAMAGE and FOOD ACCUMULATION. See also QI, BLOOD, PHLEGM, AND FOOD PATTERN IDENTIFICATION. [3: 78,81]

food reversal 食厥 *shí jué*: A REVERSAL pattern resulting from voracious eating and drinking when contraction of wind-cold or depression and anger stir and cause qi to rise counterflow, blocking the clear orifices. The signs are CLOUDING REVERSAL, asphyxiation, abdominal distention and fullness, and a slippery replete pulse in patients who have overeaten. [26: 470] [27: 401]

food stagnating in the stomach duct 食滞胃脘 *shí zhì wèi wǎn* (*guǎn*): Food accumulating in the stomach after overeating affects splenic movement and transformation, marked by distention and stomach duct pain, putrid belching, retching and vomiting, thick slimy tongue fur, and a slippery pulse. WMC indigestion; gastritis. See FOOD STAGNATION. [26: 471] [27: 158] [97: 417] [29: 424]

food stagnation 食滞 *shí zhì*: 1. Food stagnating and collecting in the stomach and intestines. The term *food stagnation* is essentially the same as FOOD DAMAGE (the one term describing the condition and the other describing the cause). Compare FOOD ACCUMULATION, FOOD DAMAGE, ABIDING FOOD, FOOD STAGNATION STOMACH DUCT PAIN, and FOOD STROKE. 2. Feeding irregularities in infants causing damage to the spleen and stomach, and causing food to collect in the stomach and intestines. It is characterized by warm head and hot abdomen, belching and bloating, poor appetite, abdominal distention and fullness with pain that refuses pressure, vomiting of sour putrid matter, and in some cases by stool that has the smell of rotten eggs. See FEEDING ACCUMULATION. [27: 120] [97: 416]

food stagnation stomach duct pain 食滞脘痛 *shí zhì wǎn* (*guǎn*) *tòng*: Stomach duct pain due to food stagnation. Food stagnation stomach duct pain is attributed to excessive consumption of raw or cold foods or to dietary irregularities impairing splenic movement and transformation. Signs other than stomach pain include putrid belching, swallowing of upflowing acid, distention and oppression in the stomach duct and abdomen relieved by vomiting, and a slippery replete pulse. MED Disperse accumulation and abduct stagnation using Harmony-Preserving Pill (*bǎo hé wán*) or Saussurea, Amomum, Unripe Bitter Orange, and Ovate Atractylodes Pill (*xiāng shā zhǐ zhú wán*). ACU Base treatment mainly on alarm and uniting points of ST, PC, SP, and CV. Select CV-12 (*zhōng wǎn*, Center Stomach Duct),

ST-36 (*zú sān lǐ*, Leg Three Li), PC-6 (*nèi guān*, Inner Pass), ST-25 (*tiān shū*, Celestial Pivot), SP-4 (*gōng sūn*, Yellow Emperor), ST-21 (*liáng mén*, Beam Gate), CV-6 (*qì hǎi*, Sea of Qi), and CV-21 (*xuán jī*, Jade Swivel); needle with drainage and, if necessary, add moxa. For pronounced pain, add ST-34 (*liáng qiū*, Beam Hill). [26: 471] [46: 662] [37: 320] [46: 660]

food stroke 食中 *shí zhòng*: A form of WIND-LIKE STROKE, arising when excessive liquor consumption and overeating with contraction of wind-cold or severe anger cause food to stagnate in the center, hampering the movement of stomach qi and preventing normal upbearing and downbearing. Signs include sudden clouding collapse, inability to speak, inability to move the limbs, and fullness and oppression in the chest and diaphragm. MED First make the patient drink a decoction of ginger and salt and apply mechanical ejection. Then use formulas to course evil and transform stagnation, and to rectify qi and harmonize the stomach, such as Agastache/Patchouli Qi-Righting Powder (*huò xiāng zhèng qì sǎn*), Wondrous Atractylodes Powder (*shén zhú sǎn*), and Stomach-Calming Powder (*píng wèi sǎn*). ACU Base treatment mainly on GV, LI, hand and foot reverting yin (*jué yīn*) PC/LR, CV, and ST. Select GV-26 (*shuǐ gōu*, Water Trough), GV-20 (*bǎi huì*, Hundred Convergences), PC-9 (*zhōng chōng*, Central Hub), CV-12 (*zhōng wǎn*, Center Stomach Duct), LI-4 (*hé gǔ*, Union Valley), LR-2 (*xíng jiān*, Moving Between), BL-21 (*wèi shū*, Stomach Transport), ST-25 (*tiān shū*, Celestial Pivot), CV-21 (*xuán jī*, Jade Swivel), and ST-36 (*zú sān lǐ*, Leg Three Li); needle with drainage. Selection of points according to causes: If attributable to contraction of wind-cold, add GB-20 (*fēng chí*, Wind Pool), TB-5 (*wài guān*, Outer Pass), and LU-7 (*liè quē*, Broken Sequence). When attributable to anger, add BL-18 (*gān shū*, Liver Transport), LR-3 (*tài chōng*, Supreme Surge), PC-6 (*nèi guān*, Inner Pass), and SP-6 (*sān yīn jiāo*, Three Yin Intersection). [26: 470]

food taxation gan yellowing 食劳疳黄 *shí láo gān huáng*: YELLOW SWELLING.

food vomiting 食呕 *shí ǒu*: FOOD ACCUMULATION VOMITING. [26: 471]

foot damp qi 脚湿气 *jiǎo shī qì*: See FOOT QI SORE.

foot greater yang bladder channel 足太阳膀胱经 *zú tài yáng páng guāng jīng*: Abbreviation: BL. One of the TWELVE CHANNELS; the channel that internally homes to the bladder, nets the kidney, and links with the brain, and whose external pathway starts above the eye, runs over the head, either side of the spine down the nape and back, over the buttocks and down to the back of the knee. **Pathway:** The foot greater yang (*tài yàng*) bladder channel starts at the inner canthus of the eye, travels upwards over the forehead, intersecting the governing (*dū*) vessel at GV-24 (*shén tíng*, Spirit Court) and the leg lesser yin (*shào yīn*) gallbladder channel at GB-15 (*tóu lín qì*, (Head) Overlooking Tears). It travels on up to the vertex and again meets the governing *dū* vessel GV-20 (*bǎi huì*, Hundred Convergences). A branch separates at the vertex and goes down to the area just above the ear, meeting the foot lesser yang *shào yáng* gallbladder channel at GB-7 (*qū bìn*, Temporal Hairline Curve), GB-8 (*shuài gǔ*, Valley Lead), GB-10 (*fú bái*, Floating White), GB-11 (*tóu qiào yīn*, Head Orifice Yin), and GB-12 (*wán gǔ*, Completion Bone). A vertical branch enters the brain from the vertex to meet the governing vessel at GB-12 (*wán gǔ*, Completion Bone), and reemerges to run down the nape of the neck and the muscles of the medial aspect of the scapula, meeting the governing vessel again at GV-14 (*dà zhuī*, Great Hammer) and GV-13 (*táo dào*, Kiln Path). It continues downward, parallel to the spine, to the lumbar region. Here, the channel submerges, following the paravertebral muscles, and nets the kidney before homing to the bladder. A branch separates in the lumbar region and runs down the buttocks and the posterior midline of the thighs to the popliteal fossa behind the knee. A further branch separates from the main channel at the nape of the neck, descending lateral to the paravertebral branch mentioned above, along the medial border of the scapula and down to the gluteal region where it crosses the buttocks and intersects with the gallbladder channel at GB-30 (*huán tiào*, Jumping Round). It then passes down the posterolateral aspect of the thigh to meet the other branch of the same channel in the popliteal fossa. The channel continues downward through the gastrocnemius muscle, emerges posterior to the lateral malleolus, and then runs along the lateral margin of the fifth metatarsal bone, crossing its tuberosity, to the lateral tip of the little toe at BL-67 (*zhì yīn*, Reaching Yin). **Signs:** Signs associated with the exterior course of the channel are: heat effusion and aversion to cold, headache, stiff neck, pain in the lumbar spine, nasal congestion, eye pain and tearing; pain in the posterior thigh, popliteal region, gastrocnemius, and foot. Signs associated with the internal course of the channel are: lower abdominal pain and distention, inhibited urination, urinary block and enuresis; mental disorders; and arched-back rigidity. [6: 63] [27: 87] [97: 273]

foot greater yin spleen channel 足太阴脾经 *zú tài yīn pí jīng*: **Abbreviation:** SP. One of the TWELVE CHANNELS; the channel that homes to the spleen, nets the stomach, and links with the root of the tongue, and whose external pathway

starts at the large toe and runs along the inside of the foot, and up the inside of the leg, up the abdomen to end at the side of the chest. **Pathway:** The foot greater yin (*tài yīn*) spleen channel starts on the medial tip of the great toe and runs up the medial aspect of the foot along the border of the light and dark skin. It then passes in front of the medial malleolus and up the posterior side of the leg along the posterior margin of the tibia. Here, it crosses and runs anterior to the foot reverting yin (*jué yīn*) liver channel, passing medial to the knee and running up the anteromedial aspect of the thigh. It penetrates the abdomen and intersects with the controlling (*rèn*) vessel at CV-3 (*zhōng jí*, Central Pole) and CV-4 (*guān yuán*, Pass Head) before homing to the spleen and netting the stomach. It continues upward, passes through the diaphragm to intersect with the foot lesser yang (*shào yáng*) gallbladder channel at GB-24 (*rì yuè*, Sun and Moon) and the foot reverting yin (*jué yīn*) liver channel at LR-14 (*qī mén*, Cycle Gate), ascends to the side of the esophagus, crosses the hand greater yin (*tài yīn*) lung channel at LU-1 (*zhōng fǔ*, Central Treasury), and finally proceeds up to the root of the tongue to disperse over the tongue's lower surface. A branch breaks off in the area of the stomach, crossing the diaphragm to transport qi to the heart. **Signs:** Signs associated with the exterior course of the channel are: heaviness in the head or body, weak wilting limbs; generalized heat EFFUSION; pain in the posterior mandibular region and the lower cheek, and motor impairment of the tongue; cold along the inside of the thigh and knee, or swelling of the legs and feet. Signs associated with the internal course of the channel are: pain in the stomach duct and sloppy diarrhea or stool containing untransformed food, rumbling intestines, retching and nausea, abdominal lump glomus, reduced food intake, jaundice, and inhibited urination. [6: 57] [27: 87] [50: 760] [97: 270]

foot lesser yang gallbladder channel 足少阳胆经 *zú shào yáng dǎn jīng*: **Abbreviation:** GB. One of the TWELVE CHANNELS; the channel that internally homes to the gallbladder and nets the liver, and whose external pathway starts at the side of the head, traverses the ear, passes forward over the ear, and then zigzags over the side of the head, passes down the neck, over the shoulders, down the side of the chest, and down the outer face of the legs to end at the tip of the fourth toe. **Pathway:** The foot lesser yang (*shào yáng*) gallbladder channel starts from the outer canthus of the eye, traverses the temple to LI-19 (*hé liáo*, Grain Bone-Hole), then rises to the corner of the forehead where it intersects with the foot yang brightness (*yáng míng*) stomach channel at ST-8 (*tóu wéi*, Head Corner). Descending behind the ear, it passes down the neck in front of the hand lesser yang (*shào yáng*) triple burner channel and meets the hand greater yang (*tài yáng*) small intestine channel at SI-17 (*tiān róng,* Celestial Countenance). After reaching the shoulder, it turns back and runs behind the triple burner channel to intersect the governing vessel at GV-14 (*dà zhuī,* Great Hammer). It then moves parallel with the shoulderline outwards to intersect with the hand greater yang (*tài yáng*) small intestine channel at SI-12 (*bǐng fēng,* Grasping the Wind), before crossing over to ST-12 (*quē pén,* Empty Basin) in the supraclavicular fossa. A branch separates from the main channel behind the ear and passes the hand lesser yang (*shào yáng*) triple burner channel at TB-17 (*yì fēng,* Wind Screen) before entering the ear. It emerges in front of the ear meeting SI-19 (*tīng gōng,* Auditory Palace) on the hand greater yang (*tài yáng*) small intestine channel and ST-7 (*xià guān,* Below the Joint) on the foot yang brightness (*yáng míng*) stomach channel before terminating at the outer canthus of the eye. Another branch separates from the outer canthus and runs downwards to ST-5 (*dà yíng,* Great Reception) on the mandible. Turning upwards, it crosses the hand lesser yang (*shào yáng*) triple burner channel and ascends to the infraorbital region before traveling down the cheek into the neck where it joins the main channel again at ST-12 (*quē pén,* Empty Basin) in the supraclavicular fossa. From here it submerges in the chest, meets PC-1 (*tiān chí,* Celestial Pool) of the hand reverting yin (*jué yīn*) pericardium channel, and passes through the diaphragm before netting the liver and homing to the gallbladder. It then follows the inside of the false ribs to emerge in the qi street in the inguinal region where it skirts round the genitals and submerges into the hip at GB-30 (*huán tiào,* Jumping Round). Yet another branch separates from the main channel at the supraclavicular fossa at ST-12 (*quē pén,* Empty Basin), descending into the axilla and running down the lateral aspect of the thorax. It intersects the foot reverting yin (*jué yīn*) liver channel at LR-13 (*zhāng mén,* Camphorwood Gate) before turning back to the sacral region to cross the foot greater yang (*tài yáng*) bladder channel at BL-31 (*shàng liáo,* Upper Bone-Hole) and BL-34 (*xià liáo,* Lower Bone-Hole). From here it passes laterally over to GB-30 (*huán tiào,* Jumping Round) on the hip joint, descending down the lateral aspect of the thigh and knee, and passing along the anterior aspect of the fibula to its lower extremity. It crosses in front of the lateral malleolus, and runs over the dorsum of the foot, traveling between the fourth and fifth metatarsal bones before terminating at the lateral side of the tip of the fourth toe at GB-44 (*zú qiào yīn,* Foot Orifice Yin). Another branch separates on the dorsum of the foot at GB-41 (*zú lín qì,* Foot Overlooking Tears)

and runs between the first and second metatarsal bones to the end of the great toe, crossing under the toenail to join with the foot reverting yin (*jué yīn*) liver channel at LR-1 (*dà dūn,* Large Pile). **Signs:** Signs associated with the external course of the channel are: alternating heat [effusion] and [aversion to] cold; headache; malaria; gray facial complexion; eye pain; pain under the chin; subaxillary swelling; scrofula; deafness; and pain in the lateral aspect of the buttocks and in the thigh, knee, and fibula. Signs associated with the internal course of the channel are: rib-side pain, vomiting, bitter taste in the mouth, and chest pain. [27: 62] [6: 59] [50: 760] [97: 271]

foot lesser yin kidney channel 足少阴肾经 *zú shào yīn shèn jīng:* **Abbreviation:** KI. One of the TWELVE CHANNELS; the channel that internally homes to the kidney, nets the bladder, and links with the spine, liver, diaphragm, throat, root of the tongue, the lung, heart, and thoracic cavity, and whose external pathway starts at the small toe, passes over the sole of the foot, passes around the inner ankle body, rises up the inside of the leg, passes over the abdomen, to end in the chest. **Pathway:** The foot lesser yin (*shào yīn*) kidney channel starts on the underside of the little toe, crosses the sole of the foot obliquely to emerge out of the arch of the foot under the navicular tuberosity at KI-2 (*rán gǔ,* Blazing Valley). It then proceeds posterior to the medial malleolus and continues into the heel. From here, it travels up the rear medial aspect of the lower leg to intersect with the foot greater yin (*tài yīn*) spleen channel at SP-6 (*sān yīn jiāo,* Three Yin Intersection). Traveling up through the gastrocnemius muscle, it ascends across the medial aspect of the popliteal fossa and the posteromedial aspect of the thigh to the base of the spine where it meets the governing vessel at GV-1 (*cháng qiáng,* Long Strong). It continues up the interior of the spinal column to home to the kidney, after which it turns downwards to net the bladder and intersect with the controlling (*rèn*) vessel at CV-4 (*guān yuán,* Pass Head) and CV-3 (*zhōng jí,* Central Pole). A branch ascends from the kidney, goes directly to the liver, crosses the diaphragm, enters the lung, and follows the throat up to the root of the tongue. A further branch separates in the lung, links through to the heart, and disperses in the chest. **Signs:** Signs associated with the external course of the channel are: lumbar pain, counterflow cold of the legs, weak wilting legs, dry mouth, sore pharynx, and pain in the lateral gluteal region and in the posterior aspect of the thigh; there may also be pain in the soles of the feet. Signs associated with the internal course of the channel are: dizziness, facial swelling, blurred vision, gray facial complexion, shortness of breath, short, rapid breathing, somnolence or vexation, enduring diarrhea, sloppy stool, or dry stool evacuated with difficulty. There may also be abdominal distention, nausea and vomiting, or impotence. [27: 87] [6: 59] [50: 758] [97: 271]

foot qi sore 脚气疮 *jiǎo qì chuāng: Synonym: foot damp qi; fetid water snail; eroding foot; foot rot; Hongkong foot.* A condition of the toes attributed to damp-heat pouring downward and contact with damp toxin characterized in the initial stage by water vesicles and itching between the toes and in later stages by scaling, crusting, and erosion. Foot qi sores may also give off a strange smell, which accounts for the alternate name "fetid water snail." They are common in people who live or work in damp or wet environments, and are prevalent in hot humid climates (as is reflected in the now popular name 香港脚 (*xiāng gǎng jiǎo*), Hongkong foot). Foot qi sores are are attributed to spleen-stomach channel damp-heat pouring downward. [WMC] tinea pedis; athlete's foot. [MED] Oral: Use Fish Poison Yam Dampness-Percolating Decoction (*bì xiè shèn shī tāng*). If painful and swollen, it can be treated with Coptis Toxin-Resolving Decoction (*huáng lián jiě dú tāng*). Topical: Apply Six-to-One Powder (*liù yī sǎn*) or calcined alum (*kū fán*). Vinegar Soaking Formula (*cù pào fāng*) may also be used (see GOOSE-FOOT WIND). [ACU] Pole ouch points (*ā shì xué*), 30–60 minutes a day, and needle with drainage at Eight Winds (*bā fēng*), ST-36 (*zú sān lǐ*, Leg Three Li), and BL-60 (*kūn lún*, Kunlun Mountains). Selection of points according to pattern: For pronounced damp-heat pouring downward, add SP-9 (*yīn líng quán*, Yin Mound Spring) and GB-41 (*zú lín qì*, Foot Overlooking Tears). NB: Another form of foot qi sore, also called foot lichen (*jiǎo xiǎn*), is characterized by dryness and itching, thickening, peeling, and in cold weather cracking of the skin. [50: 1406] [26: 648] [96: 262] [42: 157]

foot reverting yin liver channel 足厥阴肝经 *zú jué yīn gān jīng: Abbreviation: LR.* One of the TWELVE CHANNELS; the channel that homes internally to the liver, nets the gallbladder, and links the genitals, stomach, diaphragm, throat, and eyes and whose external pathway starts at the large toe and rises up the inside of the leg, skirts the genitals, passes over the stomach, and ends at the side of the chest. **Pathway:** The foot reverting yin (*jué yīn*) liver channel starts on the dorsum of the great toe and runs up the foot between the first and second metatarsal bones to a point one body-inch in front of the medial malleolus. It then proceeds upward to SP-6 (*sān yīn jiāo*, Three Yin Intersection), where it intersects with the foot greater yin (*tài yīn*) spleen channel. Continuing up the medial aspect of the leg, it recrosses the foot greater yin (*tài yīn*) spleen channel eight body-inches above the medial malleolus, thereafter running posterior to

that channel over the knee and thigh. Once again it crosses the foot greater yin (*tài yīn*) spleen channel at SP-12 (*chōng mén*, Surging Gate) and SP-13 (*fǔ shè*, Bowel Abode), and then skirts around the genitals and penetrates the lower abdomen where it meets the controlling (*rèn*) vessel at CV-2 (*qū gǔ*, Curved Bone), CV-3 (*zhōng jí*, Central Pole), and CV-4 (*guān yuán*, Pass Head). It ascends, moving toward the lateral aspect of the trunk to home to the liver and then nets the gallbladder. Continuing its upward course through the diaphragm, it disperses over the rib-side, then runs up to the neck posterior to the pharynx, enters the nasopharynx, and meets the tissues surrounding the eyes. The channel finally runs up the forehead to meet the governing vessel at the vertex. A branch breaks off below the eye and runs through the cheeks to contour the inside of the lips. Another branch separates from the liver, passes through the diaphragm, and enters the lung. **Signs:** Signs associated with the external course of the channel are: headache, dizziness, blurred vision, tinnitus, and heat effusion. Signs associated with the internal course of the channel are: fullness, distention, and pain in the rib-side with lump glomus, fullness and oppression in the chest and stomach duct, abdominal pain, vomiting, jaundice, swill diarrhea, lower abdominal pain, mounting qi (*shàn qì*), enuresis, urinary block, and yellow urine. [6: 59] [27: 88] [97: 272]

foot rot 烂脚 *làn jiǎo*, 烂脚丫 *làn jiǎo yā:* FOOT DAMP QI.

foot yang brightness malaria 足阳明疟 *zú yáng míng nüè:* MALARIA in the foot yang brightness (*yáng míng*) channel. *Elementary Questions (sù wèn, cì nüè piān)* states, "Foot yang brightness (*yáng míng*) malaria causes the person first to be cold as if sprinkled with water; when the cold is pronounced, the heat effusion comes; when the heat effusion goes, sweating comes. [The patient] likes to see sunlight, moonlight, and fire qi and gains gratification from them. [For this], needle the yang brightness on the instep." [MED] Use a large packet of Bamboo Leaf and Gypsum Decoction (*zhú yè shí gāo tāng*). [50: 756] [9: 471]

foot yang brightness stomach channel 足阳明胃经 *zú yáng míng wèi jīng: Abbreviation: ST.* One of the TWELVE CHANNELS; the channel that homes to the stomach and nets the spleen, and whose external pathway starts at the side of the nose, crosses the side of the head, face and neck, runs down the chest, through the nipples, over the abdomen, and down the outer anterolateral face of the leg to end at tip of the second toe. **Pathway:** The foot yang brightness (*yáng míng*) stomach channel starts at the side of the nose, and then ascends to the inner canthus of the eye to intersect the foot greater yang (*tài yáng*) bladder channel at BL-1 (*jīng míng*, Bright Eyes). It then descends parallel to the nose, penetrates the maxilla into the upper gum and joins the governing vessel at GV-24 (*shén tíng*, Spirit Court) in the philtrum. It skirts back along the upper and lower lips to join the controlling (*rèn*) vessel at CV-24 (*chéng jiāng*, Sauce Receptacle) in the mentolabial groove on the chin. From this point, it runs along the mandible to the point ST-5 (*dà yíng*, Great Reception) and rounds the angle of the mandible to ST-6 (*jiá chē*, Cheek Carriage). It proceeds upward in front of the ear, intersects with the foot lesser yang (*shào yáng*) gallbladder channel at GB-3 (*shàng guān*, Upper Gate), and continues along the hairline, intersecting the foot lesser yang (*shào yáng*) channel again at GB-6 (*xuán lí*, Suspended Tuft), from where it crosses to the middle of the forehead to intersect with the governing vessel at GV-24 (*shén tíng*, Spirit Court). A branch separates at ST-5 (*dà yíng*, Great Reception), runs down the throat to the point ST-9 (*rén yíng*, Man's Prognosis), and then continues down to the supraclavicular fossa. From here it crosses through to the back to intersect the governing vessel at GV-14 (*dà zhuī*, Great Hammer), and then descends internally, crossing the diaphragm and intersecting with the controlling (*rèn*) vessel internally at CV-13 (*shàng wǎn*, Upper Stomach Duct), and CV-12 (*zhōng wǎn*, Center Stomach Duct), before homing to the stomach and netting the spleen. Another branch separates at ST-12 (*quē pén*, Empty Basin), runs down the surface of the trunk along the mammillary line, and continues downward, passing beside the umbilicus to enter the qi street (the inguinal region) at ST-30 (*qì chōng*, Qi Thoroughfare). Yet another branch starts in the area of the pylorus, descending internally to join the branch just described at ST-30 (*qì chōng*, Qi Thoroughfare) in the inguinal region. It emerges here and runs down to ST-31 (*bì guān*, Thigh Joint) on the anterior aspect of the thigh. It travels down the thigh to the high point above the knee at ST-32 (*fú tù*, Crouching Rabbit), and on down to the patella, then proceeds downward along the lateral side of the tibia to ST-42 (*chōng yáng*, Surging Yang) on the dorsum of the foot, finally terminating at the lateral side of the tip of the second toe. A branch separates at ST-36 (*zú sān lǐ*, Leg Three Li), three body-inches below the knee and runs down lateral and parallel to the main branch, terminating on the lateral side of the middle toe. Yet another branch breaks off from the main branch on the dorsum of the foot at ST-42 (*chōng yáng*, Surging Yang), terminating on the medial side of the great toe where it nets the spleen channel at SP-1 (*yǐn bái*, Hidden White). **Signs**: Signs along the external course of the channel are: high fever, malaria, red face, sweating,

clouded spirit and delirious speech, manic agitation, aversion to cold, pain in the eyes, dry nose and nosebleed, lip and mouth sores, sore larynx, swelling in the neck, deviated mouth, chest pain, and cold or pain, redness, and swelling in the lower limbs. Signs along the internal course of the channel are: pronounced abdominal distention and fullness, and water swelling, vexation and discomfort while active or recumbent, and mania and withdrawal. There may also be swift digestion and rapid hungering, and yellow urine. [6: 59] [27: 86] [97: 272]

forceful 有力 *yǒu lì*: Strong, powerful. The term forceful is most commonly used in the pulse examination to describe any pulse that beats with force. See PULSE CONDITION.

forceless 无力 *wú lì*: Weak, lacking in strength. The term forceless is most commonly used in the pulse examination to describe any pulse that beats without force. See PULSE CONDITION. **NB**: The same Chinese term is rendered in other contexts as LACK OF STRENGTH.

forehead 额 *é*, 额颅 *é lú*, 颜 *yán*: The part of the head below the front hairline and above the brow. [26: 947]

forehead fontanel 额囟 *é xìn*: FONTANEL GATE.

forgetfulness 健忘 *jiàn wàng*: *Synonym: poor memory.* Tendency to forget matters. Forgetfulness occurs most commonly in vacuity patterns such as depletion of kidney essence and insufficiency of the heart and spleen, but also in repletion patterns such as affect damage and phlegm turbidity harassing the upper body. **Depletion of kidney essence** observed in advancing age or after debilitating sickness causes forgetfulness with aching lumbus and weak legs, dizzy head and tinnitus, and in some cases seminal emission and premature ejaculation, and is accompanied by heat signs such as vexing heat in the five hearts, red tongue, and rapid fine pulse. ⌈MED⌉ Supplement the kidney and boost essence using Six-Ingredient Rehmannia Pill (*liù wèi dì huáng wán*) plus spiny jujube (*suān zǎo rén*), schisandra (*wǔ wèi zǐ*), polygala (*yuǎn zhì*), and acorus (*shí chāng pú*). If there is also kidney yang vacuity, deerhorn glue (*lù jiǎo jiāo*), cistanche (*ròu cōng róng*), morinda (*bā jǐ tiān*), star anise (*bā jiǎo huí xiāng*), and placenta (*zǐ hé chē*) may be added. ⌈ACU⌉ Base treatment mainly on back transport points and KI. Select BL-23 (*shèn shū*, Kidney Transport), BL-15 (*xīn shū*, Heart Transport), CV-4 (*guān yuán*, Pass Head), KI-4 (*dà zhōng*, Large Goblet), KI-3 (*tài xī*, Great Ravine), and BL-52 (*zhì shì*, Will Chamber); needle with supplementation. **Insufficiency of the heart and spleen** often stems from excessive thinking and is accompanied by lassitude of spirit, reduced food intake, and heart palpitations. ⌈MED⌉ Supplement the heart and spleen using Spleen-Returning Decoction (*guī pí tāng*). ACU Base treatment mainly on back transport, CV, HT, and SP. Select BL-15 (*xīn shū*, Heart Transport), CV-14 (*jù què*, Great Tower Gate), BL-20 (*pí shū*, Spleen Transport), BL-17 (*gé shū*, Diaphragm Transport), CV-6 (*qì hǎi*, Sea of Qi), ST-36 (*zú sān lǐ*, Leg Three Li), HT-5 (*tōng lǐ*, Connecting Li), and SP-6 (*sān yīn jiāo*, Three Yin Intersection); needle with supplementation and moxa. **Affect damage** involves the liver. Here, forgetfulness is accompanied by susceptibility to fright and fear. MED Course the liver, resolve depression, and free the network vessels using Bupleurum Liver-Coursing Powder (*chái hú shū gān sǎn*) plus curcuma (*yù jīn*) and acorus (*shí chāng pú*). ACU Base treatment mainly on the back transport points, HT, PC, and LR. Select BL-15 (*xīn shū*, Heart Transport), BL-18 (*gān shū*, Liver Transport), PC-6 (*nèi guān*, Inner Pass), LR-3 (*tài chōng*, Supreme Surge), SP-6 (*sān yīn jiāo*, Three Yin Intersection), HT-7 (*shén mén*, Spirit Gate), and HT-5 (*tōng lǐ*, Connecting Li); needle with even supplementation and drainage. **Phlegm turbidity harassing the upper body** causes forgetfulness with dizziness together with signs such as oppression in the chest, nausea, and vomiting. MED Downbear counterflow, transform phlegm, and open the orifices using Gallbladder-Warming Decoction (*wēn dǎn tāng*) again with the addition of acorus (*shí chāng pú*) and curcuma (*yù jīn*). ACU Base treatment mainly on ST. Select ST-8 (*tóu wéi*, Head Corner), CV-12 (*zhōng wǎn*, Center Stomach Duct), PC-6 (*nèi guān*, Inner Pass), CV-17 (*shān zhōng*, Chest Center), ST-41 (*jiě xī*, Ravine Divide), and ST-40 (*fēng lóng*, Bountiful Bulge); needle with even supplementation and drainage. ◇ Chin 健 *jiàn*, constant, healthy; 忘 *wàng*, forgetting. [26: 651] [92: No. 51] [97: 479] [46: 618, 622, 647] [37: 349]

formation 化 *huà*: See TRANSFORMATION.

formula 方剂 *fāng jì*, 方 *fāng*: A remedy; a medicinal recipe or prescription, giving the ingredients often with their weights or proportions. [26: 89]

fortify 健 *jiàn*: See SUPPLEMENT.

fortifying the center 健中 *jiàn zhōng*: To fortify the spleen and stomach. See FORTIFYING THE SPLEEN; FORTIFYING THE STOMACH.

fortifying the spleen 健脾 *jiàn pí*: Synonym: *boosting the spleen*. A method of treatment used to address impaired splenic movement and transformation, characterized by a withered yellow facial complexion, lack of strength in the limbs, reduced appetite, stomach duct pain that likes pressure or is relieved by eating, sloppy stool, a pale tongue with white fur, and a soggy weak pulse. MED Spleen-fortifying medicinals include codonopsis (*dǎng shēn*), ovate atractylodes (*bái*

zhú), poria (*fú líng*), dioscorea (*shān yào*), and coix (*yì yǐ rén*). A commonly used formula is Four Gentlemen Decoction (*sì jūn zǐ tāng*). ACU Base treatment mainly on back transport points, CV, ST, and SP. Select BL-20 (*pí shū*, Spleen Transport), BL-21 (*wèi shū*, Stomach Transport), ST-36 (*zú sān lǐ*, Leg Three Li), CV-12 (*zhōng wǎn*, Center Stomach Duct), and SP-6 (*sān yīn jiāo*, Three Yin Intersection), and needle and moxa. See SPLEEN QI VACUITY; SPLENIC MOVEMENT AND TRANSFORMATION FAILURE. Compare MOVING THE SPLEEN. [27: 262]

fortifying the spleen and boosting qi 健脾益气 *jiàn pí yì qì*: Synonym: *fortifying the spleen and supplementing qi*. A method of treatment used to address qi vacuity and splenic movement and transformation failure, characterized by bright white facial complexion, faint voice, reduced food intake, sloppy stool, lack of strength in the limbs, and moderate weak or soft fine pulse. MED A classic spleen-fortifying qi-boosting formula is Four Gentlemen Decoction (*sì jūn zǐ tāng*). In this formula, ginseng (*rén shēn*) and licorice (*gān cǎo*) boost qi, whereas ovate atractylodes (*bái zhú*), and poria (*fú líng*) fortify the spleen. In Spleen-Returning Decoction (*guī pí tāng*), astragalus (*huáng qí*), and ginseng (*rén shēn*) are used to fortify the spleen and boost qi. ACU Use the points under FORTIFYING THE SPLEEN, and add CV-6 (*qì hǎi*, Sea of Qi), and SP-3 (*tài bái*, Supreme White); needle with supplementation and moxa. Compare SUPPLEMENTING THE SPLEEN AND BOOSTING QI. [43: 162] [46: 594]

fortifying the spleen and coursing the liver 健脾疏肝 *jiàn pí shū gān*: Synonym: *banking up earth and repressing wood*. A method of treatment used to address binding depression of liver qi causing impaired splenic movement characterized by rib-side pain and distention, no thought of food or drink, abdominal distention and rumbling intestines, thin stool, white slimy tongue, and a stringlike pulse. MED Liver-coursing medicinals such as bupleurum (*chái hú*), unripe tangerine peel (*qīng pí*), saussurea (*mù xiāng*), and Buddha's hand flower (*fó shǒu huā*) are combined with spleen-fortifying medicinals such as ovate atractylodes (*bái zhú*), poria (*fú líng*), coix (*yì yǐ rén*), and dioscorea (*shān yào*). Spleen-fortifying liver-coursing formulas include Free Wanderer Powder (*xiāo yáo sǎn*) or Saussurea and Amomum Six Gentlemen Decoction (*xiāng shā liù jūn zǐ tāng*) plus alpinia (*yì zhì rén*), magnolia bark (*hòu pò*), and medicated leaven (*shén qū*). ACU Base treatment mainly on ST, SP, CV, and LR. Needle with drainage at LR-14 (*qī mén*, Cycle Gate) and LR-3 (*tài chōng*, Supreme Surge), and with supplementation at BL-20 (*pí shū*, Spleen Transport), BL-21 (*wèi shū*, Stomach Transport), ST-36 (*zú sān lǐ*,

Leg Three Li), CV-12 (*zhōng wǎn*, Center Stomach Duct), and SP-6 (*sān yīn jiāo*, Three Yin Intersection). [26: 652] [27: 263] [97: 479]

fortifying the spleen and disinhibiting dampness 健脾利湿 *jiàn pí lì shī*: FORTIFYING THE SPLEEN AND DISINHIBITING WATER.

fortifying the spleen and disinhibiting water 健脾利水 *jiàn pí lì shuǐ*: Synonyms: *fortifying the spleen and disinhibiting dampness*; *fortifying the spleen and percolating dampness*. A method of treatment used to address water-damp due to the spleen failing dam water manifesting in generalized swelling, oppression in the stomach duct and reduced food intake, abdominal distention, and sloppy stool. MED A classic spleen-fortifying water-disinhibiting formula is Poria (Hoelen) Five Powder (*wǔ líng sǎn*), among whose ingredients ovate atractylodes (*bái zhú*) and poria (*fú líng*) fortify the spleen, and polyporus (*zhū líng*) and alisma (*zé xiè*) disinhibit water. ACU Base treatment mainly on CV, back transport points, and SP. Select BL-20 (*pí shū*, Spleen Transport), CV-6 (*qì hǎi*, Sea of Qi), ST-36 (*zú sān lǐ*, Leg Three Li), SP-9 (*yīn líng quán*, Yin Mound Spring), BL-23 (*shèn shū*, Kidney Transport), CV-9 (*shuǐ fēn*, Water Divide), and BL-22 (*sān jiāo shū*, Triple Burner Transport); needle with supplementation and moxa. [80: 515] [46: 676]

fortifying the spleen and harmonizing the stomach 健脾和胃 *jiàn pí hé wèi*: Synonym: *harmonizing the stomach and spleen*. A method of treatment used to enhance splenic movement and transformation and treat glomus and fullness. MED A representative spleen-fortifying stomach harmonizing formula is Unripe Bitter Orange and Glomus-Dispersing Pill (*zhǐ shí xiāo pǐ wán*). Spleen-Fortifying Pill (*jiàn pí wán*) and Sudden Smile Pill (*shī xiào wán*) also possess a spleen-fortifying stomach-harmonizing action. ACU Base treatment mainly on back transport points, CV, SP, and ST. Select BL-20 (*pí shū*, Spleen Transport), BL-21 (*wèi shū*, Stomach Transport), CV-12 (*zhōng wǎn*, Center Stomach Duct), ST-36 (*zú sān lǐ*, Leg Three Li), ST-25 (*tiān shū*, Celestial Pivot), CV-6 (*qì hǎi*, Sea of Qi), PC-6 (*nèi guān*, Inner Pass), and SP-6 (*sān yīn jiāo*, Three Yin Intersection); needle with supplementation and moxa. [46: 602]

fortifying the spleen and percolating dampness 健脾渗湿 *jiàn pí shèn shī*: FORTIFYING THE SPLEEN AND DISINHIBITING WATER.

fortifying the spleen and transforming phlegm 健脾化痰 *jiàn pí huà tán*: DRYING DAMPNESS AND TRANSFORMING PHLEGM.

fortifying the spleen, warming the kidney, and transforming phlegm 健脾温肾化痰 *jiàn pí wēn shèn huà tán*: A method of treatment used to address spleen-kidney yang vacuity with lung cold and phlegm obstruction characterized by physical cold and cold limbs, cold aching back and lumbus, cough with copious phlegm, enuresis accompanying acute cough, white tongue fur, and a slow sunken pulse. MED A representative spleen-fortifying kidney-warming phlegm-transforming formula is Phlegm-Rheum Pill (*tán yìn wán*). ACU Base treatment mainly on back transport points, SP, ST, LU, and KI. Select BL-20 (*pí shū*, Spleen Transport), BL-23 (*shèn shū*, Kidney Transport), BL-13 (*fèi shū*, Lung Transport), SP-3 (*tài bái*, Supreme White), GV-4 (*mìng mén*, Life Gate), KI-7 (*fù liū*, Recover Flow), LI-4 (*hé gǔ*, Union Valley), ST-40 (*fēng lóng*, Bountiful Bulge), ST-36 (*zú sān lǐ*, Leg Three Li), and LU-9 (*tài yuān*, Great Abyss); needle with supplementation and moxa. [115: 243] [46: 585, 587, 653]

fortifying the stomach 健胃 *jiàn wèi*: A method of treatment used to improve the stomach's governing of intake and decomposition of food. Since stomach qi is normal when it bears downward freely, fortifying the stomach often involves the downbearing and qi. MED Commonly used stomach-fortifying medicinals include clove (*dīng xiāng*), cardamom (*bái dòu kòu*), amomum (*shā rén*), magnolia bark (*hòu pò*), and tangerine peel (*chén pí*). For damp turbidity complication, aromatic dampness-transforming medicinals can be added. For food stagnation complication, food-dispersing stagnation-abducting medicinals can also be added. For qi vacuity complication, spleen-fortifying qi-boosting medicinals can be added. ACU Base treatment mainly on transport and alarm points of the stomach, and other ST points. Select BL-21 (*wèi shū*, Stomach Transport), CV-12 (*zhōng wǎn*, Center Stomach Duct), and ST-36 (*zú sān lǐ*, Leg Three Li); needle with supplementation and add moxa. For phlegm turbidity, add LI-4 (*hé gǔ*, Union Valley), and ST-40 (*fēng lóng*, Bountiful Bulge). For stagnation add ST-25 (*tiān shū*, Celestial Pivot), ST-21 (*liáng mén*, Beam Gate), PC-6 (*nèi guān*, Inner Pass), CV-6 (*qì hǎi*, Sea of Qi), Li Inner Court (*lǐ nèi tíng*), and CV-21 (*xuán jī*, Jade Swivel). For qi vacuity, add BL-20 (*pí shū*, Spleen Transport), CV-6 (*qì hǎi*, Sea of Qi), and CV-4 (*guān yuán*, Pass Head), [26: 652] [46: 586, 660] [113: 12]

forward-staring eyes 直视 *zhí shì*: A condition in which the eyes look forward fixedly and are spiritless. Forward-staring eyes accompany unclear affect-mind in conditions such as wind stroke, fright wind, and epilepsy, and are mostly attributed to liver wind stirring internally. [27: 398]

foster 育 *yù*: Supplement (especially yin). See SUPPLEMENT.

fostering yin 育阴 *yù yīn*: SUPPLEMENTING YIN.

fostering yin and subduing yang 育阴潜阳 *yù yīn qián yáng*: Synonym: *enriching yin, calming the liver, and subduing yang*. A method of treatment used to address liver-kidney yin vacuity with ascendant liver yang characterized by headache, dizziness, tinnitus or deafness, vexation and agitation, irascibility, baking heat in the head and face, dry mouth and throat, insomnia and profuse dreaming, a red tongue, and a rapid string-like fine pulse. ⌐MED⌐ Medicinals that enrich the liver and kidney yin such as cooked rehmannia (*shú dì huáng*), lycium berry (*gǒu qǐ zǐ*), and eclipta (*mò hàn lián*) are combined with yang-subduing medicinals such as crude oyster shell (*shēng mǔ lì*), crude dragon bone (*shēng lóng gǔ*), crude abalone shell (*shēng shí jué míng*), and loadstone (*cí shí*). To these may also be added liver-calming medicinals such as uncaria (*gōu téng*), chrysanthemum (*jú huā*), and gastrodia (*tiān má*) to perform the triple action of enriching yin, calming the liver, and subduing yang. ⌐ACU⌐ Base treatment mainly on KI, LR, GB, and PC. Needle with supplementation at BL-23 (*shèn shū*, Kidney Transport), BL-18 (*gān shū*, Liver Transport), KI-3 (*tài xī*, Great Ravine), LR-3 (*tài chōng*, Supreme Surge), and SP-6 (*sān yīn jiāo*, Three Yin Intersection), and with drainage at GV-20 (*bǎi huì*, Hundred Convergences), GB-20 (*fēng chí*, Wind Pool), PC-6 (*nèi guān*, Inner Pass), LI-11 (*qū chí*, Pool at the Bend), and KI-1 (*yǒng quán*, Gushing Spring). [26: 439] [46: 596] [37: 338]

foul smell 秽臭 *huì chòu*: The smell of filth, as distinct from fishy, animal, or putrid smells.

foul turbidity 秽浊 *huì zhuó*: Damp turbidity, mountain forest miasma, or foul-smelling excreta. The term "foul," used in the sense of filthy or dirty, describes color and smell; "turbidity," means dirty, thick, and heavy, and describes evils such as phlegm and dampness that have an obstructive effect of evils on clear, light yang qi. See also DAMP TURBIDITY; FOUL SMELL. [97: 528]

four-aspect pattern identification 卫气营血辨证 *wèi qì yíng xuè biàn zhèng*: Identification of disease pattern according to the four aspects: defense (*wèi*), qi, construction (*yíng*), and blood. According to doctrine of warm diseases, warm evils invade the body to first affect defense, and then progress, unless halted by right qi or treatment, through the other aspects. When disease affects defense, sweat-effusing treatment may be given. Only when it reaches the qi aspect can qi-clearing treatment be prescribed. When it enters construction, treatment involves outthrusting heat to the qi aspect. Finally, when it reaches blood and causes depletion and frenetic movement, blood cooling and dissipation is prescribed. [6: 232]

four aspects 卫气营血 *wèi qì yíng xuè*: See DEFENSE, QI, CONSTRUCTION, AND BLOOD.

four bends wind 四弯风 *sì wān fēng*: A skin disease most common in children, affecting the elbows, backs of the knees, ankles, etc. (the "bends"), and characterized by roughening and thickening of the skin, itching, and exudation when the skin is scratched open. ⌐WMC⌐ ectopic eczema. ⌐MED⌐ Dispel wind and percolate dampness. Oral: Mysterious Three Pill (*sān miào wán*). Topical: Indigo Powder (*qīng dài sǎn*). In persistent cases, use kochia (*dì fū zǐ*), cnidium seed (*shé chuáng zǐ*), zanthoxylum (*huā jiāo*), flavescent sophora (*kǔ shēn*), and alum (*bái fán*). See DAMP SORES. [26: 207]

four command points 四总穴 *sì zǒng xué*: Points ST-36 (*zú sān lǐ*, Leg Three Li), BL-40 (*wěi zhōng*, Bend Center), LU-7 (*liè quē*, Broken Sequence), and LI-4 (*hé gǔ*, Union Valley), which "command" the body and are used to treat ailments that affect those particular sections. ST-36 is the command point of the abdomen, and treats diarrhea, constipation and abdominal pain and distention. BL-40 is the command point of the back and lumbus, and treats pain in those parts. LI-4 is the command point of the face and mouth and is useful for treating such diseases as toothache, swollen cheeks, nosebleed and headache. LU-7 is the command point of the head and nape, and treats headache and stiffness of the nape. Command points are often combined with points more specific to the disease being treated. For example, treatment of lumbar pain might pair BL-40, the command point of the back, with local points such as BL-23 and BL-30. [26: 207]

four examinations 四诊 *sì zhěn*: The four examinations, INSPECTION, LISTENING AND SMELLING, INQUIRY, and PALPATION, provide the raw data for diagnosis. Correlation of data from all four examinations is essential for complete diagnosis. The four examinations are followed by PATTERN IDENTIFICATION. [6: 144] [27: 169] [97: 148]

four extremities 四极 *sì jí*: The limbs.

four gates 四关 *sì guān*: **1.** The elbow and knee joints. **2.** The shoulder, elbow, hip, and knee joints. **3.** Of the five transport points, the four that lie below the elbow and knee. **4.** From *The Great Compendium of Acupuncture and Moxibustion* (*zhēn jiǔ dà chéng*). The two source points of the hand yang brightness (*yáng míng*) channel, LI-4 (*hé gǔ*, Union Valley), and two source points of the foot reverting yin (*jué yīn*) channel, LR-2 (*xíng jiān*, Moving Between). **Application**: The four gates treat liver yang headache, dizziness, insomnia, and epilepsy. *Song to Elucidate Mysteries* (*biāo yōu fù*) also suggests: "For cold or head impediment (*bì*) pain, just open the four gates." [50: 411] [27: 73] [97: 148] [46: 34]

four greatnesses 四大 *sì dà*: The four signs of yang brightness channel patterns, i.e., great heat [effusion], great sweating, great vexing thirst, and a large floating pulse. ◇ Chin 四 *sì*, four; 大 *dà*, large, great. [6: 226]

four natures 四性 *sì xìng*: FOUR QI. [26: 203]

four patterns of fright wind 惊风四证 *jīng fēng sì zhèng*: Fright patterns, wind patterns, phlegm patterns, and heat patterns occurring in fright wind. Fright, externally contracted wind evil, exuberant phlegm and extreme heat are the causes of fright wind that may be seen in different combinations in different patients. Each of the four patterns is characterized by a prevalence of one the four causes. [26: 1002]

four qi 四气 *sì qì*: Synonym: *four natures*. The four natures of medicinals, cold, heat, warmth, and coolness. Cold medicinals are ones effective in treating heat patterns, whereas hot medicinals are those effective in treating cold patterns. Warm and cool medicinals are medicinals with mild hot or cold natures. In addition, there is also a balanced nature whose nature is neither predominantly hot nor cold. [26: 205] [27: 314] [97: 140]

four rheums 四饮 *sì yǐn*: PHLEGM-RHEUM; SUSPENDED RHEUM; SPILLAGE RHEUM; PROPPING RHEUM.

four seas 四海 *sì hǎi*: The SEA OF MARROW, SEA OF BLOOD, SEA OF QI, and SEA OF GRAIN AND WATER. *The Magic Pivot* (*líng shū, hǎi lùn*) states, "People have four seas... the sea of marrow, the sea of blood, the sea of qi, and the sea of grain and water." "The stomach is the sea of grain and water... The thoroughfare (*chōng*) vessel is the sea of the twelve channels... Chest center is the sea of qi... The brain is the sea of marrow." The four seas can be regulated at specific points on the body: the sea of marrow at GV-20 (*bǎi huì*, Hundred Convergences) and GV-16 (*fēng fǔ*, Wind Mansion); the sea of qi above and below the pillar bone (collar bone) and at ST-9 (*rén yíng*, Man's Prognosis); the sea of grain and water at ST-30 (*qì chōng*, Qi Thoroughfare), and ST-36 (*zú sān lǐ*, Leg Three Li); and the sea of blood at BL-11 (*dà zhù*, Great Shuttle), ST-37 (*shàng jù xū*, Upper Great Hollow), and ST-39 (*xià jù xū*, Lower Great Hollow). [50: 411] [26: 205] [46: 107]

fourteen-channel point 十四经穴 *shí sì jīng xué*, 十四经经穴 *shí sì jīng jīng xué*: CHANNEL POINT. [26: 8] [27: 99]

fourteen channels 十四经 *shí sì jīng*: From *Elaboration of the Fourteen Channels* (*shí sì jīng fā huī*). The TWELVE CHANNELS plus the thoroughfare (*chōng*) and controlling (*rèn*) vessels. [26: 8]

foxy mounting 狐疝 *hú shàn*: Synonym: *vulpine mounting*. Protrusion of the small intestine into the scrotum. The intestine retracts periodically of its own accord, and can be drawn back in by the patient himself in lying posture. MED Use Qi-Abducting Decoction (*dǎo qì tāng*). ACU Base treatment mainly on CV, ST, and the three yin channels of the foot. CV-4 (*guān yuán*, Pass Head), Qi Gate (*qì mén*), ST-29 (*guī lái*, Return), ST-36 (*zú sān lǐ*, Leg Three Li), KI-6 (*zhào hǎi*, Shining Sea), LR-1 (*dà dūn*, Large Pile), and Moxibustion Triangle (*sān jiǎo jiǔ*); needle with supplementation and add moxa. Selection of points according to signs: For acute lesser-abdominal pain, add SP-6 (*sān yīn jiāo*, Three Yin Intersection) and LR-3 (*tài chōng*, Supreme Surge). For lesser-abdominal pain with painful distention of the scrotum, add CV-6 (*qì hǎi*, Sea of Qi) and LR-8 (*qū quán*, Spring at the Bend). ◇ Chin 狐 *hú*, fox; 疝 *shàn*, mounting disease. The name derives from the sly, unpredictable way in which the intestine slides in and out of the scrotum, resembling the way in which a fox slyly slips in and out of its lair. [26: 388] [27: 429] [97: 361] [46: 681] [113: 192]

foxy odor 狐臭 *hú chòu*: Synonym: *armpit odor*; *body odor*. An unpleasant body odor noted especially in the armpits, but sometimes also at the nipples, umbilicus, genitals, and anus. Foxy odor is attributed to damp-heat brewing internally or heredity. Many sufferers also have oily ears. MED It can be treated by topical application of calcined alum (*kū fán*), or Litharge Powder (*mì tuó sēng sǎn*) plus calcined alum, or longan pit (*lóng yǎn hé*) and (black) pepper (*hú jiāo*) in the ratio of 20 to 50. See also SWEATING ARMPITS. [26: 388] [27: 486] [97: 361]

freckle 雀斑 *què bān*: A small brown patch on the skin. Freckles arise when kidney-water fails to nourish the upper body and fire stagnates and binds into macules. MED Take Supplemented Six-Ingredient Rehmannia Pill (*jiā wèi liù wèi dì huáng wán*) and dab and wash with Jade Countenance Pill (*yù róng wán*). ◇ Chin 雀 *què*, sparrow; 斑 *bān*, patch, macule. [61: 366]

free 通 *tōng*: To enhance normal activity and/or remove obstructions. Terms of similar meaning include: **move** (行 *xíng*), to promote normal movement (e.g., move qi); **disinhibit** (利 *lì*), to promote movement and elimination (e.g., disinhibit water, disinhibit dampness; disinhibit the joints); **drain** (泻 *xiè*, and **discharge** (泄 *xiè*, to promote elimination of evils (e.g., drain fire) or parts affected by them (e.g., drain the heart); **diffuse** (宣 *xuān*), to promote general or outward spreading movement of a body part or its qi (e.g., diffuse the lung); **outthrust** (透 *tòu*), to promote the movement of evils out through the body's exterior (e.g., outthrust heat) or promote the ability of a body part to allow the elimination of evils (e.g., outthrust the exterior); **downbear** (降 *jiàng*), promote the downward movement of qi, evils, etc. (e.g., downbear qi); **precipitate** (下 *xià*), to promote the downward movement of evils, especially through the digestive tract (see PRECIPITATION); **disperse** (消 *xiāo*), to promote the disintegration of evils (e.g., disperse food, disperse phlegm); **rectify** (理 *lǐ*) and **normalize** (顺 *shùn*), to the restore orderly movement of qi, especially liver qi (e.g., normalize qi, rectify qi, rectify the liver); **course** (疏 *shū*), to free body parts or evils affecting them (e.g., course the channels, course the liver, course the exterior, course wind); **soothe** (舒 *shū*), to promote normal action, thereby eliminating pain, soreness, or tension (e.g., soothe the liver, soothe the sinews); **loosen** (宽 *kuān*), to relieve tension or oppression (e.g., loosen the chest); **open** (开 *kāi*), promote movement into, out of, or through a body part (e.g., open the stomach, open the orifices). See the following entries.

freeing blocks 通闭 *tōng bì*: OPENING THE ORIFICES.

freeing formula 通剂 *tōng jì*: One of the TEN FORMULA TYPES. A formula whose main action is performed by freeing and disinhibiting medicinals. See FREEING [MEDICINALS] CAN ELIMINATE STAGNATION. [27: 305] [97: 499]

freeing [medicinals] can eliminate stagnation 通可去滞 *tōng kě qù zhì*: Freeing and disinhibiting medicinals can eliminate various forms of stagnation. For example, rice-paper plant pith (*tōng cǎo*), vaccaria (*wáng bù liú xíng*), and rhaponticum/echinops (*lòu lú*) can be used to free milk in female patients suffering from postpartum qi and blood stagnation. Clematis (*wēi líng xiān*) and fangji (*fáng jǐ*) can treat damp impediment (*bì*) due stagnation of dampness characterized by heavy aching limbs. See FREEING FORMULA. [26: 612] [97: 499]

freeing menstruation 通经 *tōng jīng*: Synonym: *promoting menstruation*. A method of treatment used to restore normal menstruation in the treatment of MENSTRUAL BLOCK. Distinction is made between vacuity and repletion forms of menstrual block. **Qi-blood vacuity** patterns are marked by menstrual block, dizzy head and flowery vision, tinnitus, heart palpitations, shortness of breath and lack of strength, pale tongue without fur, and a fine sunken pulse. MED Use tangkuei (*dāng guī*), white peony (*bái sháo yào*), ligusticum (*chuān xiōng*), codonopsis (*dǎng shēn*), ovate atractylodes (*bái zhú*), licorice (*gan cǎo*), and salvia (*dān shēn*) to supplement qi and nourish the blood. ACU Base treatment on CV and back transport

points. Select CV-4 (*guān yuán*, Pass Head), CV-6 (*qì hǎi*, Sea of Qi), BL-18 (*gān shū*, Liver Transport), BL-23 (*shèn shū*, Kidney Transport), BL-17 (*gé shū*, Diaphragm Transport), BL-20 (*pí shū*, Spleen Transport), ST-36 (*zú sān lǐ*, Leg Three Li), SP-6 (*sān yīn jiāo*, Three Yin Intersection), and the Four Flowers (*sì huā*). Needle with supplementation and add moxa. **Qi stagnation and blood stasis** patterns are marked by menstrual block with mental depression, rashness, impatience, irascibility, oppression in the chest and rib-side pain, distending pain in the smaller abdomen, dark purple tongue margins possibly with purple speckles, and a stringlike or rough pulse. MED Use medicinals such as tangkuei (*dāng guī*), ligusticum (*chuān xiōng*), red peony (*chì sháo yào*), peach kernel (*táo rén*), carthamus (*hóng huā*), cyperus (*xiāng fù zǐ*), and corydalis (*yán hú suǒ*) to move qi and quicken the blood. ACU Base treatment on CV, SP and LR, selecting CV-3 (*zhōng jí*, Central Pole), SP-8 (*dì jī*, Earth's Crux), Li Inner Court (*lǐ nèi tíng*), SP-10 (*xuè hǎi*, Sea of Blood), LI-4 (*hé gǔ*, Union Valley), PC-6 (*nèi guān*, Inner Pass), BL-18 (*gān shū*, Liver Transport), LR-3 (*tài chōng*, Supreme Surge), and SP-6 (*sān yīn jiāo*, Three Yin Intersection); needle with even supplementation and drainage, and add moxa. [26: 614] [46: 686] [50: 1325]

freeing milk 通乳 *tōng rǔ*: Synonym: *promoting lactaction*. A method of treatment used to promote the flow of breast milk after delivery. Freeing milk takes one of two forms. **Supplementing qi and blood:** This is used to treat patients with qi and blood vacuity and little or no milk, but without distention or pain in the breasts. General signs include pale complexion and nails, pale tongue without fur, and a fine vacuous pulse. MED Agents used include codonopsis (*dǎng shēn*), astragalus (*huáng qí*), tangkuei (*dāng guī*), ophiopogon (*mài mén dōng*), platycodon (*jié gěng*), vaccaria (*wáng bù liú xíng*), and rice-paper plant pith (*tōng cǎo*). ACU Base treatment mainly on ST and LR. Select CV-17 (*shān zhōng*, Chest Center), ST-18 (*rǔ gēn*, Breast Root), SI-1 (*shào zé*, Lesser Marsh), BL-20 (*pí shū*, Spleen Transport), and ST-36 (*zú sān lǐ*, Leg Three Li); needle with supplementation. Moxa can also be added. If due to excessive blood loss in childbirth, add BL-18 (*gān shū*, Liver Transport) and BL-17 (*gé shū*, Diaphragm Transport). **Moving qi and freeing the network vessels:** This is used to treat qi stagnation and breast milk stoppage with distention and fullness of the breasts, thin tongue fur, and stringlike pulse. MED Agents used include tangkuei (*dāng guī*), ligusticum (*chuān xiōng*), bupleurum (*chái hú*), cyperus (*xiāng fù zǐ*), pangolin scales (*chuān shān jiǎ*), and vaccaria (*wáng bù liú xíng*). ACU Base treatment mainly on

ST, LR, and PC. CV-17 (*shān zhōng*, Chest Center), ST-18 (*rǔ gēn*, Breast Root), SI-1 (*shào zé*, Lesser Marsh), PC-6 (*nèi guān*, Inner Pass), LR-14 (*qī mén*, Cycle Gate), and LR-3 (*tài chōng*, Supreme Surge); needle with even supplementation and drainage. [26: 803] [46: 693] [113: 319]

freeing qi 通气 *tōng qì*: MOVING QI.

freeing the channels 通经 *tōng jīng*: **1.** A method of treatment used to address obstructed channels. **2.** PROMOTING MENSTRUATION. [26: 614] [27: 508] [97: 499]

freeing the channels and quickening the network vessels 通经活络 *tōng jīng huó luò*: A method of treatment used to relieve obstruction channels and network vessels by evils.

freeing the network vessels 通络 *tōng luò*: A method of treatment used to relieve obstruction network vessels by evils.

freeing the orifices 通窍 *tōng qiào*: OPENING THE ORIFICES. Also used for orifices other than those of the heart, e.g., the nose (e.g., freeing the orifices of the nose).

freeing the vessels 通脉 *tōng mài*: **1.** A method of treatment used to warm and free yang qi to revive the pulse beat. For example, in lesser yin (*shào yīn*) disease with diarrhea, there is true cold in the inner body characterized by cold limbs and a faint pulse on the verge of expiration, and false heat in the outer body marked by absence of aversion to cold and a floating red complexion. Cold is the true nature of the disease and it repels yang outward causing absence of aversion to cold, whereas yang also floats upward to cause an UPCAST YANG floating red complexion. MED Use Vessel-Freeing Counterflow Cold Decoction (*tōng mài sì nì tāng*), in which licorice (*gān cǎo*), aconite (*fù zǐ*), and dried ginger (*gān jiāng*) return yang and stem desertion, and scallion white with root (*lián xū cōng bái*) frees yang qi. The formula as a whole warms and frees yang qi to restore strength to the pulse. ACU Base treatment mainly on LU, PC, and BL. Select LU-9 (*tài yuān*, Great Abyss), PC-6 (*nèi guān*, Inner Pass), BL-15 (*xīn shū*, Heart Transport), BL-17 (*gé shū*, Diaphragm Transport), BL-14 (*jué yīn shū*, Reverting Yin Transport), ST-36 (*zú sān lǐ*, Leg Three Li), and LI-4 (*hé gǔ*, Union Valley); needle with supplementation. For the lesser yin disease example, CV-4 (*guān yuán*, Pass Head), BL-20 (*pí shū*, Spleen Transport), BL-23 (*shèn shū*, Kidney Transport), and KI-7 (*fù liū*, Recover Flow); needle with supplementation and add moxa. **2.** To boost qi and supplement the blood to treat scant breast milk. See FREEING MILK. [27: 279] [113: 19]

freeing the waterways 宣通水道 *xuān tōng shuǐ dào*: A method of treatment used to open lung qi and disinhibit dampness. Freeing the waterways is used in the treatment of cough and panting with water swelling affecting the upper body and particularly the face, inhibited urination with dark yellow urine, glossy white tongue fur, a slippery floating pulse, and in some cases heat effusion and aversion to cold. MED Agents that free the waterways include ephedra (*má huáng*), cinnamon twig (*guì zhī*), duckweed (*fú píng*), poria with skin (*lián pí fú líng*), apricot kernel (*xìng rén*), and mulberry root bark (*sāng bái pí*). ACU Base treatment mainly on back transport points, LU, SP, CV, and ST. Select BL-13 (*fèi shū*, Lung Transport), BL-20 (*pí shū*, Spleen Transport), BL-23 (*shèn shū*, Kidney Transport), BL-22 (*sān jiāo shū*, Triple Burner Transport), Panting Stabilizer (*dìng chuǎn*), LU-9 (*tài yuān*, Great Abyss), SP-3 (*tài bái*, Supreme White), CV-9 (*shuǐ fēn*, Water Divide), CV-6 (*qì hǎi*, Sea of Qi), ST-36 (*zú sān lǐ*, Leg Three Li), and SP-9 (*yīn líng quán*, Yin Mound Spring); needle with supplementation and add moxa. [26: 397]

freeing yang 通阳 *tōng yáng*: A method of treatment used to address stoppage of yang qi due to cold-damp obstruction or congealing phlegm and stasis obstruction. Examples of freeing yang include: a) treating CHEST IMPEDIMENT (*xiōng bì*) due to phlegm turbidity obstruction with Trichosanthes, Chinese Chive, and White Liquor Decoction (*guā lóu xiè bái bái jiǔ tāng*); b) treating dampness obstructing the triple burner in damp warm disease using Three Kernels Decoction (*sān rén tāng*); c) treating phlegm turbidity and stasis obstructing chest yang causing gripping heart pain (angina pectoris) using Liquid Storax Pill (*sū hé xiāng wán*) or Sudden Smile Powder (*shī xiào sǎn*); or d) treating counterflow reversal cold of the limbs with Tangkuei Counterflow Cold Decoction (*dāng guī sì nì tāng*). [26: 613] [27: 277] [97: 499]

free-rib pain 季肋痛 *jì xié tòng*: Pain in the region of the FREE RIBS. Free-rib pain is mostly attributed to liver vacuity. It occurs in liver qi vacuity as a continual pain together with signs such as gallbladder timidity and susceptibility to fright, blurred vision, and tinnitus. In liver blood vacuity, the pain is dull or marked by a feeling of hypertonicity, and is associated with frequent heat vexation, dry mouth, dizzy head and flowery vision, and red tongue. It may also be caused by kidney vacuity. WMC hypochondriac pain. MED Treat liver qi vacuity with Four Gentlemen Decoction (*sì jūn zǐ tāng*) combined with Mume Pill (*wū méi wán*). Treat liver blood vacuity with All-the-Way-Through Brew (*yī guàn jiān*). Kidney vacuity can be treated with variations of Eight-Ingredient Rehmannia Pill (*bā wèi dì huáng wán*). See also RIB-SIDE PAIN. [26: 281]

free ribs 季肋 *jì lè*, 季胁 *jì xié*: *Synonym: soft ribs.* [WMC] The costal cartilage of the 11th and 12th ribs. ◇ Chin 季 *jì* small; end, tip. 肋 *lè* rib. [26: 381] [27: 69] [97: 141] [19: 3796]

frenetic blood heat 血热妄行 *xuè rè wàng xíng*: *Synonym: frenetic movement of hot blood.* Excessive movement of the blood due to blood heat manifesting in the form of bleeding or maculopapular eruptions. See BLOOD HEAT.

frenetic movement 妄行 *wàng xíng*: Pathological movement or activity of the blood manifesting in the form of bleeding or maculopapular eruptions; when due to blood heat, as is usually the case, it is also referred to as frenetic blood heat. See BLOOD HEAT.

frenetic movement of hot blood 血热妄行 *xuè rè wàng xíng*: See FRENETIC BLOOD HEAT.

frenzied sesame seed pulse 麻促脉 *má cù mài*: See TEN STRANGE PULSES. [27: 199]

frequent sighing 善太息 *shàn tài xī*: See SIGHING.

frequent urination 小便频数 *xiǎo biàn pín shuò*, 小便数 *xiǎo biàn shuò*, 尿频 *niào pín*: Increased frequency of urination, most commonly due to bladder heat or kidney (yin or yang) vacuity. **Bladder damp-heat:** Frequent urination due to bladder damp-heat is accompanied by urinary urgency, scorching pain on urination, and short voidings of yellow murky urine. [MED] Clear and disinhibit damp-heat. Use Eight Corrections Powder (*bā zhèng sǎn*). [ACU] Base treatment mainly on CV, SP, and ST. Select CV-3 (*zhōng jí*, Central Pole), LR-2 (*xíng jiān*, Moving Between), SP-6 (*sān yīn jiāo*, Three Yin Intersection), SP-9 (*yīn líng quán*, Yin Mound Spring), BL-28 (*páng guāng shū*, Bladder Transport), and ST-36 (*zú sān lǐ*, Leg Three Li); needle with drainage. **Kidney yang vacuity:** Frequent urination due to vacuous kidney yang failing to retain urine is accompanied by copious clear urine. Other signs include lack of warmth in the extremities, dizziness, tinnitus, limp aching lumbus and knees, and an enlarged pale tongue. [MED] Warm and supplement kidney yang. Use Eight-Ingredient Pill (*bā wèi wán*) plus psoralea (*bǔ gǔ zhī*), velvet deerhorn (*lù róng*), mantis egg-case (*sāng piāo xiāo*), and rubus (*fù pén zǐ*). [ACU] Base treatment mainly on CV, back transport points, GV, and KI. Select CV-6 (*qì hǎi*, Sea of Qi), SP-6 (*sān yīn jiāo*, Three Yin Intersection), CV-3 (*zhōng jí*, Central Pole), BL-23 (*shèn shū*, Kidney Transport), KI-3 (*tài xī*, Great Ravine), GV-4 (*mìng mén*, Life Gate), and CV-4 (*guān yuán*, Pass Head), needling with supplementation and adding moxa. **Kidney yin vacuity:** Frequent urination due to yin vacuity heat is characterized by pale yellow urine, and accompanied by dizziness, tinnitus, steaming bone tax-

ation heat [effusion], vacuity vexation, and night sweating. Although, like the bladder damp-heat pattern, it is a heat pattern, kidney yin vacuity is not associated with burning pain, urinary urgency, and the yellow or reddish urine observed in damp-heat. [MED] Enrich kidney yin. Use Six-Ingredient Rehmannia Pill (*liù wèi dì huáng wán*) and variations. [ACU] Base treatment mainly on CV, KI, and SP. Select CV-3 (*zhōng jí*, Central Pole), CV-6 (*qì hǎi*, Sea of Qi), SP-6 (*sān yīn jiāo*, Three Yin Intersection), SP-9 (*yīn líng quán*, Yin Mound Spring), BL-23 (*shèn shū*, Kidney Transport), KI-3 (*tài xī*, Great Ravine), KI-6 (*zhào hǎi*, Shining Sea), and KI-2 (*rán gǔ*, Blazing Valley); needle with even supplementation and drainage or with supplementation. **Binding depression of liver qi:** Frequent urination due to binding depression of liver qi in women is characterized by frequent urination with urgency, scant voidings, and a feeling of distention in the lower abdomen. [MED] Use Free Wanderer Powder (*xiāo yáo sǎn*) plus plantago seed (*chē qián zǐ*). In pregnancy, frequent short voiding with scant urine indicates fetal pressure and is attributable to qi vacuity. Frequent urination with thick unctuous urine combined with great thirst with intake of fluid, and swift digestion and rapid hungering is a sign of *dispersion-thirst*. Frequent urination with pain on voiding indicates *strangury*. [ACU] Base treatment mainly on CV, SP, and LR. Select CV-3 (*zhōng jí*, Central Pole), CV-6 (*qì hǎi*, Sea of Qi), SP-6 (*sān yīn jiāo*, Three Yin Intersection), LR-3 (*tài chōng*, Supreme Surge), PC-6 (*nèi guān*, Inner Pass), TB-6 (*zhī gōu*, Branch Ditch), and GB-34 (*yáng líng quán*, Yang Mound Spring); needle with drainage or with even supplementation and drainage. [26: 75] [92: No. 225] [42: 200] [14: 180] [4: 101] [46: 588, 597, 646]

fright 惊 *jīng*: **1.** One of the SEVEN AFFECTS. See LIVER GOVERNS FRIGHT. **2.** Conditions of spasm understood by analogy to fright. *Elementary Questions* (*sù wèn*) states that liver disease is associated with fright. The liver is the viscus of wind and wood; it governs the sinews. The liver is associated with wood in the five phases, and just as trees (wood) are swayed by the wind, so the liver can be stirred by internal wind. ARCHED-BACK RIGIDITY and CONVULSIONS are seen as shaking and bending the body by wind. Fright, like wind, causes spasm, since the sinews (muscles) of a person subjected to a frightening stimulus will tense. For this reason fright is associated with liver-wood. Wind and fright both manifest as hypertonicity of sinews, which are governed by the liver. See FRIGHT WIND.

fright causes derangement of qi 惊则气乱 *jīng zé qì luàn*: Fright and other strong emotional stimuli can upset normal qi dynamic, and throw qi and blood into disorder, causing disquietude of the heart spirit and even mental derangement. [26: 1001] [27: 145]

fright convulsions 惊搐 *jīng chù*: Convulsions associated with fright wind. [27: 145]

fright epilepsy 惊痫 *jīng xián*: **1.** Epilepsy caused by fright. **2.** Fright wind (in Tang and Song medical records). [26: 1003]

fright heat [effusion] 惊热 *jīng rè*: A disease pattern in children characterized by heat effusion and susceptibility to fright. Fright heat [effusion] is a generalized, but not high fever associated with a green-blue complexion, sweating, vexation and agitation, and susceptibility to fright in the night. It arises by heat engendering fright or fright engendering heat, but in either case is associated with internal heat in the heart and liver channels. [MED] Clear heat and drain fire with Red-Abducting Powder (*dǎo chì sǎn*) plus chrysanthemum (*jú huā*), uncaria (*gōu téng*), and coptis (*huáng lián*). [26: 1002]

fright mania 惊狂 *jīng kuáng*: Susceptibility to fright and manic derangement. [118: 235] [50: 1429]

fright palpitations 惊悸 *jīng jì*: HEART PALPITATIONS brought on by fright or heart palpitations associated with fear and susceptibility to fright. Fright palpitations is observed in heart-gallbladder qi vacuity, heart blood vacuity, effulgent yin vacuity fire, blood stasis, water-rheum, and phlegm fire patterns. [MED] Treat heart-gallbladder qi vacuity with Neutral Supplementing Heart-Settling Elixir (*píng bǔ zhèn xīn dān*) combined with Loadstone and Cinnabar Pill (*cí zhū wán*). Alternatively, use Gallbladder-Warming Decoction (*wēn dǎn tāng*) or Spiny Jujube Decoction (*suān zǎo rén tāng*). Treat heart blood vacuity with Spirit-Quieting Mind-Stabilizing Pill (*ān shén dìng zhì wán*) plus amber (*hǔ pò*), loadstone (*cí shí*), cinnabar (*zhū shā*), mix-fried licorice (*gān cǎo*), biota seed (*bǎi zǐ rén*), schisandra (*wǔ wèi zǐ*), and spiny jujube (*suān zǎo rén*). Treat effulgent yin vacuity fire with Coptis and Ass Hide Glue Decoction (*huáng lián ē jiāo tāng*) combined with Anemarrhena, Phellodendron, and Rehmannia Pill (*zhī bǎi dì huáng wán*) plus spiny jujube (*suān zǎo rén*), mother-of-pearl (*zhēn zhū mǔ*), and oyster shell (*mǔ lì*). Treat blood stasis with House of Blood Stasis-Expelling Decoction (*xuè fǔ zhú yū tāng*). Treat water-rheum with Poria (Hoelen), Cinnamon Twig, Ovate Atractylodes, and Licorice Decoction (*líng guì zhú gān tāng*) plus pinellia (*bàn xià*), tangerine peel (*chén pí*), fresh ginger (*shēng jiāng*), polyporus (*zhū líng*), alisma (*zé xiè*), dragon bone (*lóng gǔ*), and oyster shell (*mǔ lì*). To treat phlegm-fire, use Coptis Gallbladder-Warming Decoction (*huáng lián wēn dǎn tāng*) plus gardenia

(*shān zhī zǐ*), scutellaria (*huáng qín*), fritillaria (*bèi mǔ*), trichosanthes (*guā lóu*), spiny jujube (*suān zǎo rén*), mother-of-pearl (*zhēn zhū mǔ*), oyster shell (*mǔ lì*), and abalone shell (*shí jué míng*). [ACU] Base treatment mainly on HT and LR. Main points: HT-7 (*shén mén*, Spirit Gate), PC-6 (*nèi guān*, Inner Pass), BL-15 (*xīn shū*, Heart Transport). For heart-gallbladder qi vacuity, add BL-19 (*dǎn shū*, Gallbladder Transport), GB-34 (*yáng líng quán*, Yang Mound Spring), and ST-36 (*zú sān lǐ*, Leg Three Li); needle with supplementation. For insufficiency of heart blood, add ST-36 (*zú sān lǐ*, Leg Three Li), SP-6 (*sān yīn jiāo*, Three Yin Intersection), and HT-5 (*tōng lǐ*, Connecting Li), needling with supplementation. For effulgent yin vacuity fire, add BL-14 (*jué yīn shū*, Reverting Yin Transport), BL-23 (*shèn shū*, Kidney Transport), and KI-3 (*tài xī*, Great Ravine), needling with even supplementation and drainage. For blood stasis, add CV-17 (*shān zhōng*, Chest Center), BL-17 (*gé shū*, Diaphragm Transport), SP-10 (*xuè hǎi*, Sea of Blood), and LR-3 (*tài chōng*, Supreme Surge), needling with even supplementation and drainage. For water-rheum collecting internally, add CV-17 (*shān zhōng*, Chest Center), CV-6 (*qì hǎi*, Sea of Qi), CV-12 (*zhōng wǎn*, Center Stomach Duct), and ST-36 (*zú sān lǐ*, Leg Three Li), needling with even supplementation and drainage. For phlegm-fire stirring internally, add LU-5 (*chǐ zé*, Cubit Marsh), PC-6 (*nèi guān*, Inner Pass), and ST-40 (*fēng lóng*, Bountiful Bulge), needling with drainage. See HEART PALPITATIONS and FEARFUL THROBBING. [26: 1002] [46: 648] [113: 148]

fright reversal 惊厥 *jīng jué*: Synonym: *child fright reversal*. **1.** Sudden loss of consciousness occurring when strong emotional stimulus disrupts the flow of qi and blood. **2.** The signs associated with FRIGHT WIND. [27: 433]

fright wind 惊风 *jīng fēng*: Synonym: *child fright wind*; *infantile convulsions*. A disease of infants and children, characterized by convulsions and loss of consciousness. Fright wind is equivalent to TETANY in adults. Distinction is made between acute and chronic forms. [WMC] infantile convulsions. See ACUTE FRIGHT WIND; CHRONIC FRIGHT WIND; EIGHT SIGNS OF FRIGHT WIND; FOUR PATTERNS OF FRIGHT WIND. ◇ Chin 惊 *jīng*, fright; 风 *fēng*, wind. Wind, especially liver wind, can cause various forms of spasm (hypertonicity of the sinews, tetany, tugging and slackening, arched-back rigidity). Wind as a natural phenomenon bends, sways, and contorts trees (wood), and as an evil, it affects the sinews, which are governed by liver-wood. Fright is a natural response that manifests physically in the form of tension or jerking of the sinews, and hence is analogous to wind in its effects on the body. Fright wind is so called because in some instances it is thought to be caused by fright, and also by analogy of manifestations. See FRIGHT. [26: 1001] [27: 432]

frog rale in the throat 喉中有水鸡声 *hóu zhōng yǒu shuǐ jī shēng*: A continuous high-pitched rale produced by phlegm blocking the respiratory tract, so named because of its similarity to the croaking of frogs (in chorus). Frog rale in the throat is characteristic of wheezing patterns. *The Orthodox Tradition of Medicine* (*yī xué zhèng zhuàn*) states, "Hasty panting with frog rale in the throat is called "wheezing." WMC Occurs in diseases classified in Western medicine as asthma and asthmatic bronchitis. See PHLEGM RALE. [27: 185] [58: 126]

front teeth 板齿 *bǎn chǐ*: The two upper front teeth. See DRY FRONT TEETH. [26: 362]

frost 霜 *shuāng*: A powder produced by frosting. See FROSTING.

frostbite 冻疮 *dòng chuāng*: Severe damage to the skin and flesh that arises when cold and wind cause qi and blood to congeal and stagnate. Frostbite usually affects the hands and feet and the ears. The affected areas present a somber white complexion that gradually turns purple-red and forms macules, burning sensation, itching, and numbness and, in severe cases, rupture and the development of sores that heal with difficulty. Frostbite can be prevented by adequate clothing and physical movement. MED Warm yang and dispel cold; regulate construction and defense. Oral: Tangkuei Counterflow Cold Decoction (*dāng guī sì nì tāng*). Topical: Red Spirit Wine (*hóng líng jiǔ*) or boil ginger and chillies to make a wash. For open sores, apply Flesh-Engendering Jade and Red Paste (*shēng jī yù hóng gāo*). ACU Localized frostbite: Base treatment mainly on ouch points and local points. Method: Prick the surrounding area, then apply moxa to quicken the blood and free the network vessels, and to warm the vessels and dissipate cold. Selection of points according to affected area: For the back of the hand, select LI-4 (*hé gǔ*, Union Valley), Eight Evils (*bā xié*), and TB-4 (*yáng chí*, Yang Pool). For back (upper face) of the foot, select BL-60 (*kūn lún*, Kunlun Mountains), LR-2 (*xíng jiān*, Moving Between), and GB-41 (*zú lín qì*, Foot Overlooking Tears); needle with even supplementation and drainage and add moxa. Generalized frost bite: Main points: GV-14 (*dà zhuī*, Great Hammer), GV-26 (*rén zhōng*, Human Center), and KI-1 (*yǒng quán*, Gushing Spring); needle with supplementation. For generalized frostbite with shock, select GV-20 (*bǎi huì*, Hundred Convergences), ST-36 (*zú sān lǐ*, Leg Three Li), and pole CV-8 (*shén què*, Spirit Gate Tower), CV-6 (*qì hǎi*, Sea of Qi), and CV-4 (*guān yuán*, Pass Head); needle with supplementation and add moxa. West-

ern medical treatment may be necessary. [50: 805–6] [96: 419] [27: 485] [97: 304]

frosting 制霜 *zhì shuāng*: The production of a fine crisp powder by methods other than simple grinding is known as frosting. The following methods exist: (1) One method is the defatting and grinding of seeds. The seeds are first sun-dried or stir-fried, the husks are removed, and the kernels are pounded to an almost paste-like consistency. The materials are sandwiched between layers of paper, and then sun-dried, baked, or pressed, so that the paper absorbs the oil. The paper is repeatedly changed until the materials are light, loose and no longer stick together. Medicinals processed in this way include croton frost (*bā dòu shuāng*) and trichosanthes seed frost (*guā lóu rén shuāng*). (2) Another method, used to treat certain gourds, is efflorescence. For example, watermelon (*xī guā*) is frosted by gouging out a small lump to form a hole in which a small amount of mirabilite (*máng xiāo*) is placed. The lump is then replaced, and the watermelon is hung up to air. The mirabilite (*máng xiāo*) comes out and effloresces, so that a fine, white frost forms on the surface of the watermelon, which when brushed off is ready to use. (3) The production of persimmon frost (*shì shuāng*) represents a third method of frosting: dried persimmon (*shì bǐng*) is exposed to the sun in the day and to the dew at night and then is covered to allow the skin to saccharify and form a frost. [27: 326] [82: 60]

fullness 满 *mǎn*: A subjective sensation of expansion and pressure, which may or may not be associated with objectively perceptible distention.

fullness and distention in the heart [region] and abdomen during pregnancy 妊娠心腹胀满 *rèn shēn xīn fù zhàng mǎn*: A disease pattern attributed to contraction of cold or food damage in women usually suffering from vacuity cold, causing congestion of stomach qi internal obstruction. Fullness is often accompanied by oppression in the stomach duct and no thought of food. Where cold contraction is a factor, there is pronounced distention after eating that likes warmth and pressure, and treatment takes the form of warming the center and dissipating cold with formulas such as Saussurea and Amomum Six Gentlemen Decoction (*xiāng shā liù jūn zǐ tāng*). Where there is food damage, there is painful distention after eating, putrid belching, and swallowing of upflowing acid, and treatment takes the form of dispersing food and transforming stasis using formula such as Harmony-Preserving Pill (*bǎo hé wán*). [26: 341] [97: 340]

fullness and oppression in the chest and diaphragm 胸膈满闷 *xiōng gé mǎn mèn*: A subjective feeling of stifling fullness in the lower part of the chest. Fullness and oppression in the chest and diaphragm is associated with phlegm.

fullness below the heart 心下满 *xīn xià mǎn*: Fullness in the stomach duct, sometimes associated with counterflow qi ascent. [27: 377] [97: 119]

fullness in the chest 胸满 *xiōng mǎn*: Synonym: *thoracic fullness*. From *Elementary Questions* (*sù wèn*). A bloated feeling in the chest. *The Golden Mirror of Medicine* (*yī zōng jīn jiàn*) comments as follows: "In exterior repletion without sweating, oppression in the chest and panting is wind-cold oppression in the chest. In interior repletion with rough urination, oppression in the chest with heat vexation is heat congestion oppression in the chest. In [conditions of] swelling of the eyes and face, oppression in the chest and panting that prevents the patient from lying down, is oppression in the chest due to collecting rheum. In [conditions of] inhibited breathing, oppression in the chest relieved by sighing is qi stagnation oppression in the chest.... In the absence of heat effusion, aversion to cold or other disease, if there is only oppression in the chest and wilted lips, green-blue tongue, dry mouth with desire only to wash the mouth with water but not to swallow, this is blood stasis oppression in the chest." These different forms are treated by resolving the exterior, draining heat, transforming rheum, moving qi, and quickening the blood. [26: 550] [27: 470]

fullness of pregnancy 子满 *zǐ mǎn*: Swelling, distention, panting and fullness in pregnancy. Fullness of pregnancy arises in women normally suffering from spleen-kidney yang vacuity with internal water-damp evil when in the sixth or seventh month of pregnancy the growing fetus affects the upward and downward bearing of qi dynamic and disturbs movement and transformation, so that water-damp gathers and spreads to cause generalized swelling with abdominal distention, panting and fullness. ⟨MED⟩ Warm yang and fortify the spleen; rectify qi and move water. Use Poria (Hoelen) Five Powder (*wǔ líng sǎn*) plus tingli (*tíng lì zǐ*). Alternatively, use Carp Soup (*lǐ yú tāng*). [26: 56]

full physique with vacuous qi 形盛气虚 *xíng shèng qì xū*: Obesity with soft muscles, shortage of qi, lack of strength, and lack of vitality indicating yang qi vacuity. [6: 116]

fulminant 暴 *bào*: Sudden and violent.

fulminant clouding 暴昏 *bào hūn*: Sudden stupor or loss of consciousness.

fulminant desertion 暴脱 *bào tuō*: The manifestation of critical depletion of qi, blood, yin, or yang occurring suddenly as a result of major blood loss, sweating, diarrhea, or wind stroke, as distinct from VACUITY DESERTION, which occurs after gradual

debilitation in enduring sickness. ⟨WMC⟩ shock. See DESERTION. [27: 218]

fulminant desertion of heart qi 心气暴脱 *xīn qì bào tuō*: Vacuity desertion of heart qi and debilitation of original qi after enduring illness has caused insufficiency of heart qi in elderly patients with debilitated visceral qi when new factors bring on sudden worsening that damages yang and wear qi. The chief signs are unclear spirit-mind, dripping great sweat, and reversal cold of the limbs. Other signs include heart palpitations or fearful throbbing, stifling oppression in the heart and chest, green-blue or purple lips, bright white facial complexion, faint low voice, and weak breathing. The tongue is either pale or green-blue or purple. The pulse is faint and verging on expiration. ⟨MED⟩ Return yang and stem counterflow. Ginseng and Aconite Decoction (*shēn fù tāng*), or Ginseng, Aconite, Dragon Bone, and Oyster Shell Decoction (*shēn fù lóng mǔ tāng*). ⟨ACU⟩ Base treatment mainly on CV, GV, and HT. Select BL-15 (*xīn shū*, Heart Transport), CV-14 (*jù què*, Great Tower Gate), GV-26 (*rén zhōng*, Human Center), GV-25 (*sù liáo*, White Bone-Hole), PC-6 (*nèi guān*, Inner Pass), GV-20 (*bǎi huì*, Hundred Convergences), CV-8 (*shén què*, Spirit Gate Tower)⟨m⟩, CV-4 (*guān yuán*, Pass Head), KI-1 (*yǒng quán*, Gushing Spring), and HT-7 (*shén mén*, Spirit Gate); needle with supplementation and moxa, or just moxa. **Analysis**: Fulminant desertion of heart yang is a development of heart yang vacuity and heart vessel stasis obstruction. When heart yang lacks power, there is heart palpitations or fearful throbbing, oppression in the chest, and shortness of breath, which are exacerbated by movement. When phlegm-stasis obstructs the vessels of the heart, the principle that "when there is stoppage, there is pain" comes into play, hence the stifling oppression and pain in the heart and chest. Fulminant desertion of heart yang causes liquid to drain with qi, hence the cold dripping sweat. As qi deserts outward, the body is deprived of warmth, hence the reversal cold of the limbs, aversion to cold, and liking for warmth. Heart yang's sudden failure makes it powerless to move blood to nourish the upper body, hence the somber white complexion and pale tongue. When blood flows sluggishly, then the lips turn green-blue or purple, the face becomes dark and stagnant, and the tongue becomes pale purple, possibly with stasis macules. The outward desertion of yang qi causes a major drainage of ancestral qi, hence breathing becomes weak and faint. As yang deserts and qi dissipates, the spirit looses its governing, and the spirit-mind becomes hazy and, in severe cases, comatose. With the rapid outward desertion of yang qi, the pulse becomes rapid and forceless. When yang qi reaches the verge of expiration, the pulse becomes faint and verging on expiration. Periodic discontinuity in vessel qi is reflected in a bound, skipping, or intermittent pulse. [57: 47] [116: 45] [46: 731] [37: 336]

fulminant downpour 暴注 *bào zhù*: Acute abdominal pain, with sudden bouts of diarrhea characterized by a forceful stream of watery stool or explosive defecation. [27: 365] [97: 635]

fulminant flooding 暴崩 *bào bēng*: Sudden bleeding via the vagina unassociated with menstruation. Fulminant flooding arises when sudden anger damages the liver or knocks or falls damage the thoroughfare (*chōng*) and controlling (*rèn*) vessels, and thus cause frenetic movement of the blood. MED Stanch bleeding with Ten Cinders Powder (*shí huī sǎn*), as well as with Pure Ginseng Decoction (*dú shēn tāng*). When the bleeding has subsided, treat according to pattern identification for FLOODING AND SPOTTING. ACU (1) Emergency management to stop the bleeding: Base treatment mainly on CV and SP. Select GV-20 (*bǎi huì*, Hundred Convergences), CV-6 (*qì hǎi*, Sea of Qi), CV-4 (*guān yuán*, Pass Head), SP-6 (*sān yīn jiāo*, Three Yin Intersection), SP-10 (*xuè hǎi*, Sea of Blood), SP-1 (*yǐn bái*, Hidden White), and SP-2 (*dà dū*, Great Metropolis), needling with supplementation. (2) When bleeding subsides, treat according to pattern: For sudden anger damaging the liver, add to the above points LR-3 (*tài chōng*, Supreme Surge), PC-6 (*nèi guān*, Inner Pass), LR-13 (*zhāng mén*, Camphorwood Gate), TB-6 (*zhī gōu*, Branch Ditch), and BL-18 (*gān shū*, Liver Transport), needling with drainage. For knocks, falls or sprains damaging the PV and CV, add SP-8 (*dì jī*, Earth's Crux), ST-30 (*qì chōng*, Qi Thoroughfare), SP-12 (*chōng mén*, Surging Gate), and LR-2 (*xíng jiān*, Moving Between), needling with even supplementation and drainage. [26: 889]

fulminant reversal 暴厥 *bào jué*: From *Elementary Questions* (*sù wèn, dà qí lùn*). An ancient disease name denoting sudden collapse and loss of consciousness with a pulse that is agitated and racing as if it were panting. See REVERSAL PATTERN. Compare SUDDEN REVERSAL. [27: 400]

fulminant seasonal cough 时行暴咳 *shí xíng bào ké*: SEASONAL COUGH.

fume 薰 *xūn*: Of heat evil, to affect organs or parts of the body, e.g., spleen damp-heat fuming up into the lung.

G

gallbladder 胆 *dǎn*: The bowel that stands in interior-exterior relationship with the liver. The gallbladder's main function is to secrete bile, which is formed from an excess of liver qi. The gallbladder is also a curious organ since its bile is considered to be "clear fluid" rather than waste. A bitter taste in the mouth may be a sign of gallbladder disease. It is also said that the GALLBLADDER GOVERNS DECISION, which means that the ability to maintain balanced judgment in the face of adversity is attributed to the gallbladder. When gallbladder qi is weak and timid, there are signs such as lack of courage and decision, timidity, doubt and suspicion, and frequent sighing. The "gallbladder governs decision" can be interpreted in modern terms to mean that certain aspects of the nervous system are traditionally ascribed in Chinese medicine to the gallbladder. More at GALLBLADDER DISEASE. [26: 944] [27: 21] [97: 411]

gallbladder channel 胆经 *dǎn jīng*: FOOT LESSER YANG GALLBLADDER CHANNEL. [26: 945]

gallbladder cough 胆咳 *dǎn ké*: COUGH with vomiting of bile or green-colored bitter tasting water. [26: 944]

Gallbladder Disease Patterns

Simple patterns
GALLBLADDER VACUITY (*dǎn xū*)

INSUFFICIENCY OF GALLBLADDER QI (*dǎn xū bù zú*)

GALLBLADDER HEAT (*dǎn rè*)

GALLBLADDER REPLETION (*dǎn shí*)

DEPRESSED GALLBLADDER AND HARASSING PHLEGM (*dǎn yù tán rǎo*)

Complex patterns
HEART VACUITY AND GALLBLADDER TIMIDITY (*xīn xū dǎn què*)

LIVER-GALLBLADDER DAMP-HEAT (*gān dǎn shī rè*)

---

gallbladder disease 胆病 *dǎn bìng*: Any morbidity of the gallbladder. The most common morbidities of the gallbladder are GALLBLADDER HEAT (or exuberant gallbladder fire), constrained emotions causing inhibition of gallbladder qi, and GALLBLADDER VACUITY. Gallbladder disease manifests headache, dizziness, tinnitus, and profuse dreaming. It may also manifest as alternating heat [effusion] and [aversion to] cold, bitter taste in the mouth, retching of bitter fluid, yellow eyes, rib-side pain, and qi fullness in the abdomen and inability to eat, or as dizziness, blurred vision, insomnia, susceptibility to fright and fear, and sighing. [MED] Depending on the pattern, treat by draining the gallbladder and clearing heat or by warming the gallbladder and calming the spirit. See GALLBLADDER HEAT and GALLBLADDER VACUITY [26: 945]

gallbladder distention 胆胀 *dǎn zhàng*: **1.** Pain and distention below the rib-side, with bitter taste in the mouth, and sighing. Gallbladder distention is usually the result of cold evil affecting the gallbladder. [MED] Use medicinals such as bupleurum (*chái hú*), curcuma (*yù jīn*), tangerine peel (*chén pí*), tangkuei (*dāng guī*), poria (*fú líng*), gardenia husk (*shān zhī pí*), tribulus (*cì jí lí*), bitter orange (*zhǐ ké*), and silk tree flower (*hé huān huā*). [ACU] Base treatment mainly on back transport points, LR, GB, TB, PC, and SP. Select BL-19 (*dǎn shū*, Gallbladder Transport) BL-20 (*pí shū*, Spleen Transport) TB-6 (*zhī gōu*, Branch Ditch), PC-6 (*nèi guān*, Inner Pass), LR-3 (*tài chōng*, Supreme Surge), LR-14 (*qī mén*, Cycle Gate), SP-6 (*sān yīn jiāo*, Three Yin Intersection), CV-6 (*qì hǎi*, Sea of Qi), and GB-34 (*yáng líng quán*, Yang Mound Spring). Needle with even supplementation and drainage, adding moxa. **2.** A DISTENTION pattern with the above-mentioned signs. [MED] Add gallbladder channel medicinals such as bupleurum (*chái hú*), unripe tangerine peel (*qīng pí*), and forsythia (*lián qiào*) to the formula that addresses the main distention pattern. [ACU] Add to the above points ST-25 (*tiān shū*, Celestial Pivot), and ST-36 (*zú sān lǐ*, Leg Three Li), needling with drainage and adding moxa. [26: 945] [46: 636]

gallbladder fire sleeplessness 胆火不得卧 *dǎn huǒ bù dé wò*: See SLEEPLESSNESS. [26: 944]

gallbladder governs decision 胆主决断 *dǎn zhǔ jué duàn*: The ability to maintain balanced judgment in the face of adversity is attributed to the gallbladder. Strong gallbladder qi ensures greater invulnerability to such stimuli. When gallbladder qi is weak and timid, fear and fright may lead to disease. See GALLBLADDER VACUITY AND QI TIMIDITY. [27: 43] [97: 412]

gallbladder heat 胆热 *dǎn rè*: Heat in the gallbladder arising when evil heat invades the gallbladder channel, causing depression of channel qi. The main signs of gallbladder heat are headache on both sides of the head, pain in the canthi, dizziness, tinnitus, bitter taste in the mouth, dry throat, fullness and pain in the chest and rib-side, and alternating heat [effusion] and [aversion to] cold. Other signs include vomiting of bitter water, vexation and agitation, and irascibility, as well as insomnia. In some cases, there is jaundice. The tongue is red with yellow fur. The pulse is stringlike, rapid, and forceful. ⟨MED⟩ Clear heat and disinhibit the gallbladder. Use Sweet Wormwood and Scutellaria Gallbladder-Clearing Decoction (*hāo qín qīng dǎn tāng*). ⟨ACU⟩ Base treatment mainly on GB and LR. Select GB-24 (*rì yuè*, Sun and Moon), LR-14 (*qī mén*, Cycle Gate), PC-6 (*nèi guān*, Inner Pass), LR-3 (*tài chōng*, Supreme Surge), GB-34 (*yáng líng quán*, Yang Mound Spring), LR-2 (*xíng jiān*, Moving Between), and GB-43 (*xiá xī*, Pinched Ravine); needle with drainage. Selection of points according to signs: For headache add GB-20 (*fēng chí*, Wind Pool), and GB-4 (*hàn yàn*, Forehead Fullness). For fullness and pain in the chest, add CV-17 (*shān zhōng*, Chest Center). For fullness and pain in the rib-side, add TB-6 (*zhī gōu*, Branch Ditch). For alternating heat [effusion] and [aversion to] cold, add GV-14 (*dà zhuī*, Great Hammer). Analysis: The gallbladder channel is the lesser yang (*shào yáng*) channel, which starts at the outer canthus, skirts around the ear, and spreads over the chest. Gallbladder heat is especially associated with signs on this part of the pathway. Signs associated with the gallbladder include alternating heat [effusion] and [aversion to] cold, bitter taste in the mouth, dry throat, and dizzy vision. The gallbladder stands in exterior-interior relationship with the liver, and gallbladder heat patterns are associated with the liver signs. [27: 154] [97: 410] [46: 590, 596, 602] [57: 114]

gallbladder heat profuse sleeping 胆热多睡 *dǎn rè duō shuì*: Increased sleep due to gallbladder repletion heat with phlegm in the chest and diaphragm. Gallbladder heat profuse sleeping is characterized by long periods of sleep between which the patient occasionally gets up. Other signs include ungratifying thought, head clouded and oppressed as though drunken, vexation and congestion in the heart and chest, bitter taste in the mouth, and heavy clouded head and vision. ⟨MED⟩ Clear the gallbladder and discharge heat. Use Root Poria Powder (*fú shén sǎn*). ⟨ACU⟩ Base treatment mainly on back transport points, HT, SP, LR, GB, and ST. Select BL-19 (*dǎn shū*, Gallbladder Transport), BL-18 (*gān shū*, Liver Transport), BL-15 (*xīn shū*, Heart Transport), HT-7 (*shén mén*, Spirit Gate), SP-6 (*sān yīn jiāo*, Three Yin Intersection), LR-3 (*tài chōng*, Supreme Surge), GB-34 (*yáng líng quán*, Yang Mound Spring), GB-43 (*xiá xī*, Pinched Ravine), LI-11 (*qū chí*, Pool at the Bend), KI-6 (*zhào hǎi*,

Shining Sea), and ST-40 (*fēng lóng*, Bountiful Bulge). Needle with drainage. [26: 945]

gallbladder holds the office of justice, from which decision emanates 胆者，中正之官，决断出焉 *dǎn zhě, zhōng zhèng zhī guān, jué duàn chū yān*: See GALLBLADDER GOVERNS DECISION. [27: 43]

gallbladder jaundice 胆黄 *dǎn huáng*: JAUNDICE (yellowing of the skin and eyes) that arises when gallbladder qi is damaged by great fright or fear or through injury from fighting. Gallbladder jaundice is characterized by a greenish-yellow coloring of the skin, and is accompanied by qi fullness or hardness in the chest, no thought of food or drink, and clouded head and fatigue. ⟨MED⟩ Treat by supplementing qi with warm sweet medicinals, stemming desertion with sour constraining medicinals, assisted by quieting the spirit with heavy settlers. ⟨ACU⟩ Base treatment mainly on back transport points, ST, SP, and HT. Select BL-20 (*pí shū*, Spleen Transport), BL-19 (*dǎn shū*, Gallbladder Transport), BL-15 (*xīn shū*, Heart Transport), ST-36 (*zú sān lǐ*, Leg Three Li), SP-6 (*sān yīn jiāo*, Three Yin Intersection), HT-7 (*shén mén*, Spirit Gate), PC-6 (*nèi guān*, Inner Pass), and GB-34 (*yáng líng quán*, Yang Mound Spring); needle with supplementation and, if appropriate, add moxa. Selection of points according to signs: For qi fullness and hardness in the chest, add CV-17 (*shān zhōng*, Chest Center), CV-12 (*zhōng wǎn*, Center Stomach Duct), and CV-6 (*qì hǎi*, Sea of Qi). For no thought of food and drink, add CV-12 (*zhōng wǎn*, Center Stomach Duct) and ST-25 (*tiān shū*, Celestial Pivot). See YIN JAUNDICE. [26: 945]

gallbladder lacking decisiveness 胆无决断 *dǎn wú jué duàn*: Failure of the gallbladder's function of governing decision-making. See GALLBLADDER GOVERNS DECISION.

gallbladder pure heat 胆瘅 *dǎn dān*: A disease manifesting as bitter taste in the mouth and arising when depressed heat in the gallbladder that fails to be discharged by free coursing flows upward into the mouth. *Elementary Questions* (*sù wèn, qí bìng lùn*). "When there is illness marked by bitter taste in the mouth... the disease is called 'gallbladder pure heat'." ⟨MED⟩ Use formulas such as Gentian Liver-Draining Decoction (*lóng dǎn xiè gān tāng*). [97: 413] [26: 946]

gallbladder qi vacuity 胆气虚 *dǎn qì xū*: GALLBLADDER VACUITY.

gallbladder qi vacuity and timidity 胆气虚怯 *dǎn qì xū qiè*: INSUFFICIENCY OF GALLBLADDER QI.

gallbladder qi vacuity cold 胆气虚寒 *dǎn qì xū hán*: GALLBLADDER VACUITY.

gallbladder repletion 胆实 *dǎn shí*: Inhibited gallbladder qi characterized by fullness and oppression in the chest and stomach duct, pain and distention in the rib-side, dry mouth with bitter taste, pain in the sides of the forehead and region of the outer canthus. [27: 154] [27: 411]

gallbladder timidity 胆怯 *dǎn qiè*: Synonym: *gallbladder timidity and susceptibility to fright*. Fear in the heart with no courage to face people. This is poorly distinguished from HEART VACUITY AND GALLBLADDER TIMIDITY. [50: 1121]

gallbladder timidity and susceptibility to fright 胆怯易惊 *dǎn qiè yì jīng*: GALLBLADDER TIMIDITY.

gallbladder vacuity 胆虚 *dǎn xū*: Synonyms: *gallbladder vacuity and qi timidity*; *insufficiency of gallbladder qi*; *gallbladder qi vacuity*; *gallbladder qi vacuity cold*. A pattern of gallbladder vacuity and failure of the decision-making capacity. The chief signs are anxiety and indecision, clouded vision, tinnitus and poor hearing, dizzy head, "timid gallbladder" (lack of courage) and susceptibility to fright. Other signs include lassitude of spirit, insomnia, sighing, distention and fullness under the rib-side, and sloppy diarrhea. The tongue fur is thin, white, and glossy. The pulse is stringlike, fine, and slow. *The Pulse Canon* (*mài jīng*) gives a somewhat different list of signs: "In gallbladder vacuity... dizziness, REVERSAL, wilting, inability to the shake the toes, crippling, inability to sit but not stand, sudden collapse, yellow eyes, seminal emission, and blurred vision." **Analysis**: The gallbladder governs decision. When this function is impaired, there is anxiety and indecision. The eyes, ears, and rib-side lie on the pathway of the gallbladder channel; gallbladder vacuity is associated with clouded vision, tinnitus, and distention and fullness under the rib-side, and frequent sighing. With the liver, the gallbladder shares signs such as distention and pain in the chest and rib-side, sighing, and a stringlike pulse. MED Boost qi and warm the gallbladder. Use Ten-Ingredient Gallbladder-Warming Decoction (*shí wèi wēn dǎn tāng*). ACU Base treatment mainly on back transport points, GB, and HT. Select BL-19 (*dǎn shū*, Gallbladder Transport), BL-15 (*xīn shū*, Heart Transport), GB-34 (*yáng líng quán*, Yang Mound Spring), GB-40 (*qiū xū*, Hill Ruins), HT-7 (*shén mén*, Spirit Gate), PC-6 (*nèi guān*, Inner Pass), and ST-36 (*zú sān lǐ*, Leg Three Li); needle with supplementation and moxa. See also GALLBLADDER GOVERNS DECISION. Compare DISQUIETING OF HEART QI. [27: 154] [57: 113] [50: 1122] [46: 590, 645, 648]

gallbladder vacuity and qi timidity 胆虚气怯 *dǎn xū qì qiè*: GALLBLADDER VACUITY.

gallbladder vacuity sleeplessness 胆虚不得眠 *dǎn xū bù dé mián*: SLEEPLESSNESS (insomnia) due to gallbladder vacuity and the presence of evils causing disquietude of the spirit. Gallbladder vacuity insomnia is characterized by waking with a sudden fright or start after falling asleep and is accompanied by heart vexation, heart palpitations, and disquieted spirit. MED Warm the gallbladder using Gallbladder-Warming Decoction (*wēn dǎn tāng*) or ground stir-fried spiny jujube (*suān zǎo rén*) taken with wine. ACU Base treatment mainly on HT, GB, and LR. Select Alert Spirit Quartet (*sì shén cōng*), HT-7 (*shén mén*, Spirit Gate), SP-6 (*sān yīn jiāo*, Three Yin Intersection), BL-15 (*xīn shū*, Heart Transport), BL-19 (*dǎn shū*, Gallbladder Transport), BL-14 (*jué yīn shū*, Reverting Yin Transport), GB-34 (*yáng líng quán*, Yang Mound Spring), and GB-40 (*qiū xū*, Hill Ruins); needle with supplementation. [26: 945]

gallbladder wind toxin qi 胆风毒气 *dǎn fēng dú qì*: Wind-toxin qi invading the gallbladder and causing clouded head and profuse sleeping. [26: 944]

galloping gan 走马疳 *zǒu mǎ gān*: GALLOPING GAN OF THE TEETH AND GUMS.

galloping gan of the teeth and gums 走马牙疳 *zǒu mǎ yá gān*: Synonym: *galloping gan*. Rapidly developing gan of the teeth and gums. Galloping gan of the gums begins with soreness, reddening, swelling, and hardening of the edges of the gum, in severe cases with whitening and putrefaction of the gums. The white color of the gum can easily turn black, and exude a purple-black bloody discharge that is accompanied by a foul smell. The ulcerated area is sore and slightly itchy. If the ulceration is deep, the wings of the nose and surrounding area assume a green-blue or brown color. In the worst cases, the lips are affected, the teeth may drop out, the ulceration may pierce the cheeks, and the bridge of the nose may collapse. MED Clear heat, resolve toxin, and dispel putridity, using Aloe Gan-Dispersing Beverage (*lú huì xiāo gān yǐn*). For spleen vacuity, Ginseng and Poria Gruel *rén shēn fú líng zhōu*, which consists of ginseng (*rén shēn*) and poria (*fú líng*) ground to a powder and cooked as a gruel, may also be taken with the formula. ◇ Chin 走马 *zǒu mǎ*, running or galloping horse; describes the rapid development of the condition. [26: 301] [27: 266] [50: 689]

gan 疳 *gān*: Synonym: *gan pattern, gan disease*. **1.** A disease of infancy or childhood characterized by emaciation, dry hair, heat effusion of varying degree, abdominal distention with visible superficial veins, yellow face and emaciated flesh, and loss of essence-spirit vitality. Pathomechanically, it essentially involves dryness of the fluids due to damage to spleen and stomach owing to dietary factors, evils, and in particular, worms. Other viscera besides the spleen may be affected, hence there are the *five gan* (i.e., GAN OF THE HEART,

GAN OF THE LUNG, GAN OF THE LIVER, GAN OF THE SPLEEN, and GAN OF THE KIDNEY). Gan disease is also labeled differently according to the specific area affected, e.g., GAN OF THE BRAIN and GAN OF THE SPINE. Signs specifically attributed to gan include GAN DIARRHEA, GAN DYSENTERY, GAN HEAT EFFUSION, GAN SWELLING AND DISTENTION, and GAN THIRST. [WMC] malnutrition; chronic indigestion; parasite infestation. **2.** Various kinds of ulcerations and sores, e.g., CHILD EYE GAN, GAN OF THE TEETH AND GUMS, FIRE GAN, LOWER BODY GAN, and GAN OF THE NOSE. [26: 488] [97: 486] [17: 125]

gan accumulation 疳积 *gān jī*: **1.** Gan of the spleen. **2.** Gan pattern. [26: 489]

gan consumption 疳痨 *gān láo*: A severe form of gan of the lung, characterized by bright white complexion, steaming bone tidal heat [effusion], postmeridian reddening of both cheeks caused by spleen-lung vacuity, lassitude of essence-spirit, periodic dry cough and throat diseases, and night sweating. Traditionally, conditions of this nature were considered as consumption in patients over fifteen years of age and gan in patients under fifteen years of age. [WMC] pulmonary tuberculosis. [MED] Chinese medicine treats gan consumption by boosting qi and fostering yin, and by supplementing the lung and nourishing the spleen. Representative formulas include Adenophora/Glehnia and Ophiopogon Decoction (*shā shēn mài dōng tāng*) or Turtle Shell Powder (*biē jiǎ sǎn*), which can be varied according to need. [ACU] Base treatment mainly on LU, SP, ST, KI, and back transport points. Select LU-9 (*tài yuān*, Great Abyss), BL-13 (*fèi shū*, Lung Transport), BL-20 (*pí shū*, Spleen Transport), BL-43 (*gāo huāng shū*, Gao-Huang Transport), CV-10 (*xià wǎn*, Lower Stomach Duct), ST-36 (*zú sān lǐ*, Leg Three Li), SP-5 (*shāng qiū*, Shang Hill), Four Seams (*sì fèng*), SP-6 (*sān yīn jiāo*, Three Yin Intersection), and KI-3 (*tài xī*, Great Ravine); needle with supplementation. Selection of points according to signs: For steaming bone tidal heat [effusion], add KI-6 (*zhào hǎi*, Shining Sea), KI-2 (*rán gǔ*, Blazing Valley), LU-5 (*chǐ zé*, Cubit Marsh), and LU-10 (*yú jì*, Fish Border). For cough and sore pharynx, add LU-5 (*chǐ zé*, Cubit Marsh), and prick LU-11 (*shào shāng*, Lesser Shang) to bleed. For night sweating, add HT-6 (*yīn xī*, Yin Cleft) [26: 489] [27: 386] [27: 283]

gan diarrhea 疳泻 *gān xiè*: Gan disease with diarrhea. Diarrhea is a common phenomenon in gan disease, and is related to morbidity of the stomach and spleen. [MED] Support the spleen and harmonize the stomach. Use formulas devised to take account of the root and tip of the disease, such as Ginseng, Poria (Hoelen), and Ovate Atractylodes

Powder (*shēn líng bái zhú sǎn*) varied according to signs. [ACU] Base treatment mainly on SP and ST. Select CV-10 (*xià wǎn*, Lower Stomach Duct), ST-36 (*zú sān lǐ*, Leg Three Li), SP-5 (*shāng qiū*, Shang Hill), Four Seams (*sì fèng*), CV-12 (*zhōng wǎn*, Center Stomach Duct), LR-13 (*zhāng mén*, Camphorwood Gate), BL-20 (*pí shū*, Spleen Transport), and BL-21 (*wèi shū*, Stomach Transport). Needle with supplementation and add moxa. [26: 489]

gan disease 疳疾 *gān jí*: See GAN. [26: 488]

gan disease ascending to the eye 疳疾上目 *gān jí shàng mù*: See GAN; CHILD EYE GAN. [26: 488]

gan dysentery 疳痢 *gān lì*: Gan disease complicated by dysentery. Gan dysentery is usually caused by unclean food. Treatment should take account of the guiding principle "in acute conditions treat the tip; in moderate (i.e., chronic) diseases treat the root" and "acting in accordance with personal factors." See CHILD DYSENTERY. [26: 488]

gan heat effusion 疳热 *gān rè*: Gan disease with HEAT EFFUSION. Gan disease is related to insufficiency of the fluids, and hence one common sign is heat effusion. The fever may be high or low, enduring or short-lived. There may be morning heat effusion abating in the evening, night heat effusion abating in the daytime, hot head without hot body, or tidal heat [effusion] in the five hearts. Since gan disease can manifest in different patterns, the heat effusion is explained and treated in different ways. [26: 488]

gan of the bone 骨疳 *gǔ gān*: GAN OF THE KIDNEY. [26: 529]

gan of the brain 脑疳 *nǎo gān*: Sores of the head or dryness of the hair in gan disease. Gan of the brain is at root attributable to insufficiency of qi and blood. Although it is called gan of the brain, it is not to be confused with other diseases involving the brain proper. ◇ Chin 脑 *nǎo*, brain; 疳 *gān*, gan. [26: 800]

gan of the heart 心疳 *xīn gān*: One of the FIVE GAN; a pattern of depressed heat in the heart channel attributed to breast-feeding difficulties. Gan of the heart is characterized by generalized heat [effusion], yellow face with reddening of the cheeks, mouth and tongue sores, vexing oppression in the chest and diaphragm, thirst and desire for cold drinks, dysentery with stool containing pus and blood, night sweating, grinding of teeth, and susceptibility to fright. [MED] Clear the heart and drain fire using formulas such as Heart-Draining Red-Abducting Decoction (*xiè xīn dǎo chì tāng*). [26: 92] [27: 434] [97: 118]

gan of the kidney 肾疳 *shèn gān*: Synonym: *gan of the bone*. One of the FIVE GAN; a pattern of deep-lying heat attributed to breast-feeding difficulties or to insufficiency of kidney qi. Gan of the kidney is characterized by emaciation, blackish complexion, gum sores, upper body heat and lower body cold, heat effusion and aversion to cold, vomiting, reduced suckling, efflux diarrhea with prolapse of the anus in severe cases, ulceration of the anus, often together with signs of insufficiency of kidney qi such nonclosure of the fontanels, slowness to teethe, and slowness to walk. MED Enrich the kidney and supplement the spleen using Six-Ingredient Rehmannia Pill (*liù wèi dì huáng wán*) supplemented with other medicinals. [26: 689] [27: 435] [97: 337]

gan of the liver 肝疳 *gān gān*: Synonyms: *wind gan*; *gan of the sinew*. One of the FIVE GAN; a pattern of heat invading the liver channel owing to breast-feeding problems; characterized by emaciation, abdominal distention, green-yellow face, dysentery with frequent defecation and stool containing blood or mucus, shaking of the head and rubbing of the eyes, night blindness, and reluctance to open the eyes. MED Clear the liver and drain heat with Bupleurum Liver-Clearing Beverage (*chái hú qīng gān yǐn*). [26: 330] [27: 434] [97: 284]

gan of the lung 肺疳 *fèi gān*: One of the FIVE GAN; a pattern of damage to the lung by depressed heat usually stemming from breast-feeding problems. Gan of the lung is characterized by cough, inhibited throat, copious snivel making the child cry, abdominal distention, diarrhea with stool like rice water, reduced suckling, fishy smell in the mouth, dry skin, and emaciated limbs. In some cases, sores under the nose, vigorous heat [effusion], and AB-HORRENCE OF COLD are observed. MED Clear the lung and drain heat using formulas such as White-Draining Powder (*xiè bái sǎn*) supplemented with other medicinals. [26: 447] [27: 434] [97: 350]

gan of the mouth 口疳 *kǒu gān*: Gan disease with sores of the mouth. Gan of the mouth is attributed to damp-heat brewing internally and insufficiency of liver yin. MED Clear heat and disinhibit dampness using Indigo Powder (*qīng dài sǎn*) and variations taken orally. [26: 61] [27: 435] [97: 31]

gan of the nose 鼻疳 *bí gān*: A disease characterized by redness, itching, and sores of the nose spreading to the lips associated with copious yellow snivel (nasal mucus), dry skin and hair, dry skin, and tidal heat [effusion] in the extremities. Gan of the nose is attributed to accumulated upper burner heat scorching and congesting in the lung. In some cases, attributable to damp-heat heat, the sides of the nose are purple, ulcerated, exude pus, and are itchy but not painful. MED Clear heat and cool the blood with formulas such as Five Happinesses Toxin-Transforming Elixir (*wǔ fú huà dú dān*). Damp-heat is treated by clearing heat and

disinhibiting dampness with Red-Abducting Powder (*dǎo chì sǎn*) plus gardenia (*shān zhī zǐ*) and alisma (*zé xiè*). Indigo Powder (*qīng dài sǎn*) can be applied topically. [26: 853] [17: 125]

gan of the sinew 筋疳 *jīn gān*: GAN OF THE LIVER.

gan of the spine 脊疳 *jǐ gān*: Gan disease with emaciation of the back and protrusion of the bones of the spine. [26: 561]

gan of the spleen 脾疳 *pí gān*: Synonym: *gan accumulation*. One of the FIVE GAN; a condition characterized by a yellow facial complexion, emaciation, ability to take food with rapid hungering, stool sometimes hard sometimes thin, unquiet sleep, copious sweating, grinding of the teeth, and tendency to lie face downward. Spleen gan is attributed to enduring food accumulation and stagnation and spleen-stomach vacuity and malnutrition stemming from breast-feeding difficulties; hence the alternate name *gan accumulation*. MED In the early stages, it can be treated by regulating the spleen and stomach using formulas such as Harmony-Preserving Pill (*bǎo hé wán*). In advanced stages, there are pronounced signs of gan accumulation such as withered-yellow facial complexion, congestion and oppression in the chest and diaphragm, distention and enlargement of the abdomen, reduced suckling, persistent diarrhea with sour-smelling stool, lassitude of spirit and lack of strength, laziness to speak and reduced physical movement. This can be treated by dispersing gan (accumulation) and fortifying the spleen using formulas such as Chubby Child Pill (*féi ér wán*) and Ginseng, Poria (Hoelen), and Ovate Atractylodes Powder (*shēn líng bái zhú sǎn*). [26: 748] [27: 434]

gan of the teeth and gums 牙疳 *yá gān*: A condition of red swollen gums, in severe cases with putrefaction, suppuration, and ulceration, and bleeding. See WIND-HEAT GAN OF THE TEETH AND GUMS; GREEN-LEG GAN OF THE TEETH AND GUMS; GALLOPING GAN OF THE TEETH AND GUMS. [26: 132] [97: 75]

gan pattern 疳证 *gān zhèng*: See GAN.

gan sore 疳疮 *gān chuāng*: LOWER BODY GAN. [26: 488] [97: 487]

gan swelling and distention 疳肿胀 *gān zhǒng zhàng*: Gan disease with swelling and distention. Gan swelling and distention is caused by nondiffusion of lung qi, splenic movement and transformation failure, and kidney vacuity. MED If swelling and distention of the abdomen is accompanied by signs such as qi counter cough and panting, glomus and oppression in the chest and diaphragm, treatment should aim to diffuse the lung and dispel dampness, using Imperial Garden Qi-Evening Powder (*yù yuàn yún qì sǎn*). If kidney qi is insufficient and is unable to dam water causing swelling of the limbs, treatment should focus on disinhibiting water and harmonizing the spleen using formulas such as Five-Peel Beverage (*wŭ pí yĭn*) or Polyporus Powder (*zhū líng sǎn*). [26: 488]

gan thirst 疳渴 *gān kě*: Gan disease with thirst and desire for fluids. Gan thirst is usually caused by stomach heat or insufficiency of the fluids. MED Stomach heat should be treated by clearing heat and harmonizing the stomach, whereas insufficiency of the fluids should be treated by boosting qi and engendering liquid. Formulas such as Sweet Dew Beverage (*gān lù yĭn*) plus gypsum (*shí gāo*) and anemarrhena (*zhī mŭ*) to clear heat, or Pulse-Engendering Powder (*shēng mài sǎn*) supplemented with additional qi-boosting yin-nourishing medicinals may be used. ACU Base treatment mainly on SP and ST. Main points: CV-10 (*xià wǎn*, Lower Stomach Duct), ST-36 (*zú sān lĭ*, Leg Three Li), SP-5 (*shāng qiū*, Shang Hill), Four Seams (*sì fèng*), and SP-6 (*sān yīn jiāo*, Three Yin Intersection). For stomach heat, add ST-44 (*nèi tíng*, Inner Court) and LI-4 (*hé gŭ*, Union Valley); needle with drainage. For insufficiency of the fluids, add TB-2 (*yè mén*, Humor Gate), KI-6 (*zhào hăi*, Shining Sea), and KI-3 (*tài xī*, Great Ravine), needling with supplementation. [26: 488]

gan toxin eye 疳毒眼 *gān dú yăn*: CHILD EYE GAN.

gao 膏 *gāo*: The region below the heart. See GAO-HUANG. [50: 1666]

gao-huang 膏肓 *gāo huāng*: The region below the heart and above the diaphragm. When a disease is said to have entered the gao-huang, it is difficult to cure. [50: 1666]

gaping gums 牙宣 *yá xuān*, 牙龈宣露 *yá yín xuān lù*: Exposure of the roots of the teeth, often associated swelling, bleeding, putrefaction, etc. Gaping gums are usually caused by stomach channel heat accumulation, but especially in the elderly it may be the result of insufficiency of kidney qi. WMC periodontitis; gingival atrophy. **Stomach channel heat accumulation:** When gaping gums is due to stomach heat, they start with swelling of the gums, and as the roots of the teeth become exposed, the gums may bleed, putrefy and suppurate. Associated signs include bad breath, thirst, desire for cool drinks, constipation, slippery rapid pulse, and a thick yellow tongue fur. MED Stomach heat patterns are treated by clearing the stomach and draining fire with formulas such as Stomach-Clearing Powder (*qīng wèi sǎn*) or Jade Lady Brew (*yù nǚ jiān*). ACU Base treatment mainly on ST and LI. Select ST-44 (*nèi tíng*, Inner Court), LI-4 (*hé gŭ*, Union Valley), LI-11 (*qū chí*, Pool at the Bend), and SP-10 (*xuè hăi*, Sea of Blood), needling with drainage. Also bleed the gums between the teeth. **Insufficiency of kidney qi:** When due to insufficiency of kidney qi, gaping gums usually appear after loosening of the teeth. MED Insufficiency of kidney qi is treated by banking up the kidney origin with variations of Six-Ingredient Rehmannia Pill (*liù wèi dì huáng wán*). ACU Base treatment mainly on KI and LI. Select BL-23 (*shèn shū*, Kidney Transport), KI-3 (*tài xī*, Great Ravine), CV-4 (*guān yuán*, Pass Head), and LI-11 (*qū chí*, Pool at the Bend); needle with supplementation and moxa. See GUM. ◇ Chin 牙 *yá*, tooth, teeth; 宣 *xuān*, announce, disclose, reveal, spread abroad, gape. [26: 132] [92: No. 131] [46: 595, 725] [37: 310, 474] [4: 128]

gaping mouth and raised shoulders 张口抬肩 *zhāng kǒu tái jiān*: A sign of severe panting in which the patient opens his mouth wide and lifts his shoulders in order to facilitate respiration. [26: 609]

gastric 胃 *wèi*: Of or relating to the stomach.

gastric disharmony 胃不和 *wèi bù hé*: DISHARMONY OF STOMACH QI.

gastric dispersion 胃消 *wèi xiāo*: STOMACH DISPERSION.

gastric harmonization 和胃 *hé wèi*: HARMONIZING THE STOMACH.

gastric juices 胃汁 *wèi zhī*: STOMACH YIN.

gastric pain 胃痛 *wèi tòng*: STOMACH PAIN.

gastric stagnation 胃滞 *wèi zhì*: STOMACH QI STAGNATION.

gastro- 胃 *wèi*: A combining form meaning "stomach," used in combinations such as *gastrointestinal*, of or pertaining to the stomach and/or intestines.

gastrointestinal accumulation 肠胃积滞 *cháng wèi jī zhì*: Accumulation of food in the stomach and intestines. **Comparison:** Gastrointestinal accumulation shares the basic characteristics of FOOD DAMAGE (aversion to food, nausea, vomiting or belching (with putrid smelling vomitus or gas), diarrhea or constipation, foul-smelling stool and flatus, relief from pain and distention after defecation or the passing of flatus. However, gastrointestinal accumulation is usually more severe than most cases of food damage, especially with the addition of palpable accumulation lumps in the abdomen, painful distention that refuses pressure, diarrhea with ungratifying defecation, or tenesmus. Causes include excessive consumption, especially of cold, raw, fried, rich, or fatty foods, and ingestion of unclean foodstuffs. MED Use offensive precipitation in accordance with the principle that "lodging is treated by attack." Both abductive dispersers and offensive precipitants are used. Commonly used formulas include Minor Qi-Coordinating Decoction (*xiǎo chéng qì tāng*), Unripe Bitter Orange Stagnation-Abducting Pill (*zhǐ shí dǎo zhì wán*), and Saussurea and Areca Pill (*mù xiāng bīng láng wán*). [6: 215]

gastrointestinal disharmony 肠胃不和 *cháng wèi bù hé*: Any disturbance of the function of the stomach and/or intestine; characterized by any of a variety of signs such as glomus and fullness, nausea, vomiting, belching, hiccough, diarrhea, constipation, etc. Gastrointestinal disharmony is attributable to pathologies of the stomach, spleen, intestines, liver, kidney, and lung.

gastrointestinal harmonization 调和肠胃 *tiáo hé cháng wèi*: See HARMONIZING THE STOMACH AND INTESTINES. [6: 234]

gastrointestinal heat bind 热结肠胃 *rè jié cháng wèi*: HEAT BINDING IN THE STOMACH AND INTESTINES.

gastrointestinal qi distention 胃肠胀气 *wèi cháng zhàng qì*: See QI DISTENTION.

gate tower 阙 *què*: The glabella, or region between the eyebrows. [27: 63]

gathering 聚 *jù*: A type of abdominal lump. See CONCRETIONS, CONGLOMERATIONS, ACCUMULATIONS, AND GATHERINGS.

gathering place of the ancestral sinews 宗筋所聚 *zōng jīn suǒ jù*: The anterior yin; the penis. See ANCESTRAL SINEW. [27: 35]

gathering place of the ancestral vessels 宗脉所聚 *zōng mài suǒ jù*: The ears or eyes. [27: 94]

gathering qi 宗气 *zōng qì*: ANCESTRAL QI. [26: 342]

GB 胆 *dǎn*, 足少阳胆经 *zú shào yáng dǎn jīng*: Abbreviation for the gallbladder or foot lesser yang (*shào yáng*) gallbladder channel.

gelatin 胶 *jiāo*: GLUE.

generalized heat [effusion] 身热 *shēn rè*: Synonym: *hot body*. A condition in which the whole of the body is is hot. See HEAT EFFUSION. ◇ Chin 身 *shēn*, body; 热 *rè*, heat. 'Body' here is taken to mean the whole body. In some contexts, it appears to mean the trunk as opposed to the head, e.g., 头热身不热 *tóu rè shēn bù rè*, hot head without hot body (see GAN DYSENTERY). [50: 777]

generalized heaviness 身重 *shēn zhòng*: HEAVY BODY.

generalized impediment 周痹 *zhōu bì*: Generalized wandering pain, heaviness, and numbness due to wind-cold-damp evil invading the blood vessels. [81: 111]

generalized pain 身痛 *shēn tòng*, 周身痛 *zhōu shēn tòng*: Pain felt in all four limbs, the back, and the lumbus. It may occur in externally contracted disease or when enduring disease causes damage to qi and blood. Generalized aching accompanied by heat effusion and aversion to cold generally occurs in exterior patterns such as wind-cold fettering the

exterior, or damp in the FLESHY EXTERIOR. [29: 193]

generalized slimy tongue fur 揩苔 *kěn tāi*: See SLIMY TONGUE FUR. ◇ Chin 揩 *kěn*, take by force, extort, despoil. [6: 123]

genital cold 阴寒 *yīn hán*: Synonym: *yin cold*. A subjective feeling of cold in the anterior yin (i.e., the external genitals). Genital cold occurs in patterns of vacuity cold of the lower origin, liver channel damp-heat, and damp phlegm pouring downward. **Vacuity cold of the lower origin** with congealing of cold qi gives rise to genital cold accompanied by impotence in males and by cold in the abdomen and impaired fertility in women. MED Warm the kidney and dissipate cold. Use Golden Coffer Kidney Qi Pill (*jīn guì shèn qì wán*). ACU Base treatment mainly on CV and the three yin channels of the foot. Select CV-4 (*guān yuán*, Pass Head), SP-6 (*sān yīn jiāo*, Three Yin Intersection), CV-3 (*zhōng jí*, Central Pole), BL-23 (*shèn shū*, Kidney Transport), CV-6 (*qì hǎi*, Sea of Qi), and GV-4 (*mìng mén*, Life Gate); needle with supplementation and add moxa. **Liver channel damp-heat** can cause coldness of the anterior yin, testicles, and sacrum and coccyx, aversion to cold and liking for warmth, watery sweating of the genitals, limp wilting anterior yin (impotence), and dribble after voiding. Genital cold due to liver channel damp-heat was first recorded in *Zhang's Clear View of Medicine* (*zhāng shì yī tōng*), and is mentioned in some modern texts. The logic of how damp-heat can cause genital cold is obscure. MED Clear heat and transform dampness with Bupleurum Dampness-Overcoming Decoction (*chái hú shèng shī tāng*). ACU Base treatment mainly on SP, LR, and GB. Select LR-2 (*xíng jiān*, Moving Between), GB-43 (*xiá xī*, Pinched Ravine), GB-34 (*yáng líng quán*, Yang Mound Spring), SP-9 (*yīn líng quán*, Yin Mound Spring), LI-4 (*hé gǔ*, Union Valley), SI-3 (*hòu xī*, Back Ravine), and KI-7 (*fù liū*, Recover Flow); needle with drainage. **Damp phlegm pouring downward** causes genital cold in obese females. Genital cold in women accompanied by itching and continuous vaginal discharge is due to cold-damp. MED Dry dampness and abduct phlegm with Two Matured Ingredients Decoction (*èr chén tāng*) plus atractylodes (*cāng zhú*), ovate atractylodes (*bái zhú*), notopterygium (*qiāng huó*), and ledebouriella (*fáng fēng*). Cold-damp with itching and vaginal discharge is treated by inserting Cnidium Seed Powder (*shé chuáng zǐ sǎn*) in the vagina. ACU Base treatment mainly on CV and ST. Select CV-12 (*zhōng wǎn*, Center Stomach Duct), BL-20 (*pí shū*, Spleen Transport), CV-6 (*qì hǎi*, Sea of Qi), ST-36 (*zú sān lǐ*, Leg Three Li), and ST-40 (*fēng lóng*, Bountiful Bulge); needle with drainage. For cold-damp, base treatment mainly on ST and SP. Select ST-36 (*zú sān lǐ*, Leg Three Li), SP-9 (*yīn líng quán*, Yin Mound Spring), and LI-4 (*hé gǔ*, Union Valley); needle with drainage and large amounts of moxa. Selection of points according to signs: For genital itch, add CV-3 (*zhōng jí*, Central Pole), BL-34 (*xià liáo*, Lower Bone-Hole), and SP-6 (*sān yīn jiāo*, Three Yin Intersection). For continuous vaginal discharge, add GB-26 (*dài mài*, Girdling Vessel), BL-30 (*bái huán shū*, White Ring Transport), CV-6 (*qì hǎi*, Sea of Qi), SP-6 (*sān yīn jiāo*, Three Yin Intersection), SP-12 (*chōng mén*, Surging Gate), and ST-30 (*qì chōng*, Qi Thoroughfare). [26: 621] [50: 657] [56: 71] [42: 198] [46: 679] [97: 232]

genital erosion 阴蚀 *yīn shí*: Synonym: *invisible worm sore of the genitals*. From *The Divine Husbandman's Herbal Foundation Canon* (*shén nóng běn cǎo jīng*). Erosion of the genitals arising when affect-mind depressed fire damages the liver and spleen, causing damp-heat to pour downward to the lower body, where it lies depressed and steams, thereby engendering worms. Genital erosion is characterized by ulceration of the external genitals exuding pus and blood, possibly with itching and soreness, swelling, and sagging sensation. It is usually associated with red and white vaginal discharge and dribbling urination. MED Clear heat, disinhibit dampness, and kill worms. Use Fish Poison Yam Dampness-Percolating Decoction (*bì xiè shèn shī tāng*). Decoct Itch-Soothing Decoction (*tā yǎng tāng*) as a steam-wash. [97: 231] [27: 454] [26: 624]

genital sweating 阴汗 *yīn hàn*: See YIN SWEATING. [26: 617]

ghost gate 鬼门 *guǐ mén*: Sweat pore. [26: 558]

ghost talk 鬼言 *guǐ yán*: Speaking as if possessed by a ghost. ◇ Chin 鬼 *guǐ*, ghost; 言 *yán*, talk, speech.

ginkgo poisoning 白果中毒 *bái guǒ zhòng dú*: A condition resulting from excessive consumption of raw ginkgo nuts and characterized by heat effusion, vomiting, diarrhea, FRIGHT REVERSAL, convulsions, rigidity of the limbs, green-blue or purple skin complexion, weak chaotic pulse, and in severe cases, coma and death. MED Take a decoction of 30 g licorice (*gān cǎo*) or 30–60 g ginkgo husk (*bái guǒ ké*). [26: 223] [126: 656]

girdling fire cinnabar 缠腰火丹 *chán yāo huǒ dān*: Synonym: *girdling snake cinnabar*; *fire-girdle sore*. A sore on one side of the chest, rib-side, or abdomen characterized initially by pain and reddening of the skin and in advanced stages by blisters containing clear fluid in a long belt formation. It usually starts with a stabbing pain, slight heat effusion, and fatigue, developing from one side of the trunk, and gradually turning from a bright to a turbid red color. It is attributed to wind-fire

in the heart and liver channels, or to spleen-lung channel damp-heat. It usually only affects one side of the body. In older patients, it can last 1–2 months, or even longer. WMC herpes zoster (shingles). MED Clear heat, disinhibit dampness, and resolve toxin. In the early stages, with burning pain and itching, take Gentian Liver-Draining Decoction (*lóng dǎn xiè gān tāng*); if there are blisters, ulceration, and exudation, and severe pain, take Dampness-Eliminating Stomach-Calming Poria (Hoelen) Five Decoction (*chú shī wèi líng tāng*), and apply powdered realgar (*xióng huáng*) blended with the juice pressed from Chinese leek (*jiǔ cài*). ACU Base treatment mainly on points surrounding the affected area, LI, LR, and SP. Select LI-11 (*qū chí*, Pool at the Bend), SP-10 (*xuè hǎi*, Sea of Blood), TB-5 (*wài guān*, Outer Pass), LR-3 (*tài chōng*, Supreme Surge), SP-6 (*sān yīn jiāo*, Three Yin Intersection), and points surrounding the affected area; needle with drainage and retain the needles for 30 minutes. Treat twice a day. Selection of points according to patterns: For wind-fire in the heart and liver channels, add HT-8 (*shào fǔ*, Lesser Mansion), PC-8 (*láo gōng*, Palace of Toil), GB-43 (*xiá xī*, Pinched Ravine), and LR-2 (*xíng jiān*, Moving Between). For spleen-lung channel damp-heat, add ST-44 (*nèi tíng*, Inner Court), SP-9 (*yīn líng quán*, Yin Mound Spring), and LI-4 (*hé gǔ*, Union Valley). Selection of points according to affected area: For the rib-side, add LI-4 (*hé gǔ*, Union Valley), TB-6 (*zhī gōu*, Branch Ditch) and GB-34 (*yáng líng quán*, Yang Mound Spring). For anywhere above the waist, add TB-6 (*zhī gōu*, Branch Ditch), and PC-6 (*nèi guān*, Inner Pass). For anywhere below the waist, add SP-9 (*yīn líng quán*, Yin Mound Spring). Ear acupuncture: Lung (*fèi*), Heart (*xīn*), Spleen (*pí*), Liver (*gān*), Spirit Gate (*shén mén*), and Sympathetic (*jiāo gǎn*). If heat is pronounced, add Gallbladder (*dǎn*); if dampness is pronounced, add Stomach (*wèi*). Choose 2–3 points at at time; apply a strong stimulus and retain needles for 20–30 minutes. Treat 1–2 times a day. ◇ Chin 缠 *chán*, wrap around; 腰 *yāo*, waist, lumbus; 火 *huǒ*, fire; 丹 *dān*, cinnabar. [50: 1646] [26: 998, 97] [113: 450] [46: 708] [37: 448]

girdling snake cinnabar 缠腰蛇丹 *chán yāo shé dān*: GIRDLING FIRE CINNABAR.

girdling vessel 带脉 *dài mài*: Abbreviation: GIV. One of the EIGHT EXTRAORDINARY VESSELS; the vessel that encircles the body at the waste. **Pathway**: Starting below the lateral tip of the tenth rib, the girdling vessel encircles the trunk like a belt, dipping down into the lower abdominal region anteriorly, and running across the lumbar region posteriorly. The girdling vessel has no points of its own, but it intersects with three points on the foot lesser yang (*shào yáng*) gallbladder channel, GB-26 (*dài mài*, Girdling Vessel), GB-27 (*wǔ shū*, Fifth Pivot), and GB-28 (*wéi dào*, Linking Path). Some books also give LR-13 (*zhāng mén*, Camphorwood Gate). Functions: This channel serves to bind up all the channels running up and down the trunk, thus regulating the balance between upward and downward flow of qi in the body. Signs: (White) vaginal discharge, prolapse of the uterus, abdominal distention and fullness, limp lumbus. ◇ Chin 带 *dài*, belt, girdle, strap (see also VAGINAL DISCHARGE); *mài*, vessel. [6: 69] [27: 89] [97: 392]

GIV 带脉 *dài mài*: Abbreviation for the girdling vessel.

glabella 印堂 *yìn táng*, 阙 *què*, 阙中 *què zhōng*: The region between the eyebrows. Also called the *gate tower; middle gate tower.* [27: 63]

glans penis 阴头 *yīn tóu*: YIN HEAD. ◇ Chin 阴 *yīn*, yin (opposite of yang); 头 *tóu*, head. Eng from L. *glans*, akin to Gk. *balanos*, acorn; L. *penis*, (of the) penis; literally "acorn of the penis."

glomus 痞 *pǐ*: A localized subjective feeling of fullness and blockage. In the chest (GLOMUS IN THE CHEST), it can be associated with a feeling of oppression in severe cases; hence the terms fullness in the chest, distention in the chest, glomus in the chest, and oppression in the chest are largely synonymous. In the abdomen, glomus is the sensation of a lump that cannot be detected by palpation. HARD GLOMUS BELOW THE HEART, which can be subjectively felt and objectively palpated, is a sign of evil heat with water collecting in the stomach. Any palpable abdominal mass is referred to as GLOMUS LUMP, although in texts predating *On Cold Damage* (*shāng hán lùn*), these were referred to as *glomus*. Lump glomus in traditional literature are labeled differently, according to shape, behavior, and pathomechanism; see CONCRETIONS, CONGLOMERATIONS, ACCUMULATIONS, AND GATHERINGS; DEEP-LYING BEAM; STRINGS AND AGGREGATIONS; INQUIRY; PALPATION. ◇ Chin The character 痞 *pǐ* is made up of the illness signifier with the character 否, which when pronounced *pǐ* means blocked. Earlier dictionaries such as *Explanation of Characters* (说文解字 *shuō wén*) say it means pain. Eng from L. *glomus*, a ball-shaped mass; *pl.* glomi. [26: 672] [27: 377] [97: 587]

glomus below the heart 心下痞 *xīn xià pǐ*: Feeling of fullness and oppression, and sensation of blockage below the heart, i.e., in the stomach duct. See GLOMUS. [27: 377] [97: 118]

glomus blockage 痞塞 *pǐ sè*: GLOMUS with a sensation of blockage. See GLOMUS.

glomus in the chest 胸痞 *xiōng pǐ*: Synonym: *thoracic glomus*. A localized feeling of fullness in the chest, often associated with oppression. Glomus in the chest is observed in PULMONARY

WELLING-ABSCESS (*fèi yōng*), EXTERNAL CONTRACTION, HEART IMPEDIMENT, and LIVER QI DEPRESSION. In pulmonary welling-abscess, it is a manifestation of lung qi congestion and is associated with dull pain and ejection of turbid, fishy-smelling phlegm or pus and blood. In externally contracted wind-cold or wind-heat that has entered the interior before the exterior pattern of heat effusion and aversion to cold has been resolved it also indicates lung qi congestion. In heart impediment, characterized by dull pain radiating into the shoulder and arm and attacks of gripping heart pain (angina pectoris), glomus in the chest is caused by blood stasis, which can further be observed from stasis speckles on the tongue and interrupted (结代 *jié dài*) pulses. Finally, glomus in the chest can be a manifestation of liver qi depression, always readily identifiable by its classic signs—sighing, ribside distention, menstrual irregularities, and irascibility. ACU CV-12 (*zhōng wǎn*, Center Stomach Duct), and PC-6 (*nèi guān*, Inner Pass), can be selected to treat glomus in the chest. Points may be added on the basis of pattern identification. [27: 377] [97: 470]

glomus lump 痞块 *pǐ kuài*: Any palpable abdominal mass. These are classified in ancient literature as CONCRETIONS, CONGLOMERATIONS, ACCUMULATIONS, AND GATHERINGS, sometimes being given more specific names as STRINGS AND AGGREGATIONS or DEEP-LYING BEAM. The presence of a glomus lump invariably heralds pronounced abdominal distention. WMC tumor or enlargement of an organ. [27: 34] [27: 417]

glomus qi 痞气 *pǐ qì*: **1.** One of the FIVE ACCUMULATIONS, the accumulation of the spleen; a prominent mass in the stomach duct shaped like an upturned dish, accompanied by emaciation of the flesh and lack of strength in the limbs, and if persistent, may also be associated with jaundice. Glomus qi is attributable to spleen vacuity and qi depression causing glomus blockage and binding accumulation. MED Treat by fortifying the spleen and dissipating stagnation. Use Glomus Qi Pill (*pǐ qì wán*) from *Three Causes Formulary* (*sān yīn fāng*), which contains aconite main tuber (*chuān wū tóu*), aconite (*fù zǐ*), halloysite (*chì shí zhī*), zanthoxylum (*huā jiāo*), dried ginger (*gān jiāng*), and shaved cinnamon bark (*guì xīn*). **2.** Fullness and discomfort in the anterior chest, mostly arising after inappropriate precipitation cold damage when the disease evil fails to disperse and turbid qi gathers and binds. MED Use Pinellia Heart-Draining Decoction (*bàn xià xiè xīn tāng*) or Unripe Bitter Orange Center-Rectifying Pill (*zhǐ shí lǐ zhōng wán*) and variations. [26: 672] [27: 415] [97: 587]

glossy scalp wind 油风 *yóu fēng*: *Synonym:* *demon-licked head*. A disease of sudden onset marked by dryness and falling of the hair in patches leaving the scalp red, smooth, and lustrous, with or without itching. WMC alopecia areata (pelade). MED Nourish the blood and dispel wind. Oral: Wondrous Response True-Nourishing Elixir (*shén yìng yǎng zhēn dān*). Topical: Rub slices of fresh ginger (*shēng jiāng*) on the affected area. For persistent conditions, perform tapping with a seven-star needle once a day. [26: 345] [61: 368]

glossy tongue fur 滑苔 *huá tāi*: A moist shiny tongue fur. A glossy thin white tongue fur is a sign of cold or cold-damp. A glossy thick white tongue fur is a sign of internally exuberant damp turbidity. A glossy sticky white tongue fur indicates phlegm-damp. A glossy thin yellow tongue fur indicates damp-heat, or an external evil starting to transform into heat and enter the interior before damaging the fluids. A glossy thick yellow tongue fur indicates severe damp-heat or phlegm-heat. [6: 123]

glue 胶 *jiāo*: The reduced extract of boiled skins, bone, shells or horns. Glues are hard and even somewhat brittle at normal temperature, their gluey quality only becoming fully apparent when heated. Most are supplementing medicinals. Examples include ass hide glue (*ē jiāo*), tiger bone glue (*hǔ gǔ jiāo*), turtle shell glue (*biē jiǎ jiāo*), tortoise plastron glue (*guī bǎn jiāo*), and deerhorn glue (*lù jiǎo jiāo*). [27: 313]

going alone 单行 *dān xíng*: See SEVEN RELATIONS.

goiter 瘿 *yǐng*: Swelling at the front and sides of the neck that moves up and down as the patient swallows. Goiter largely corresponds in Western medicine to enlargement of the thyroid gland. Records of it in Chinese literature first appeared in the 3rd century B.C. The disease is mentioned in *Zhuang Zi*, and in *Lü's Spring and Autumn* (吕氏春秋 *lǚ shì chūn qiū, jìn shù piān*). The latter text states, "In places of light [轻] water, there is much baldness and many people with goiters," which indicates that a connection between goiter, environmental factors, and baldness had been observed. In *A Thousand Gold Pieces Prescriptions for Emergencies* (*bèi jí qiān jīn yào fāng*) by Sun Si-Miao (A.D. 581–682) of the Tang Dynasty, many formulas contain kelp (*kūn bù*), sargassum (*hǎi zǎo*), and pig's thyroid gland (*zhū yè*), now all known to be rich in iodine, deficiency of which is now known to be a major cause. *A Unified Treatise on Diseases, Patterns, and Remedies According to the Three Causes* (*sān yīn jí yī bìng zhèng fāng lùn*) of the Song classifies goiter into five kinds, stone, flesh, sinew, blood, and qi goiter. **Stone goiter** is marked by hard, fixed lumps in the neck that feel uneven to the touch. It is accompanied by irascibility, profuse sweating, oppression in the chest, and heart palpitations. In advanced cases, the wind-pipe, gullet, and vocal chords are all subjected to pressure. Stone goiter is attributed to qi depression, damp phlegm, and static blood congealing and stagnating. WMC tumor of thyroid. MED Transform phlegm and relieve depression; move stasis and soften hardness. Use Sargassum Jade Flask Decoction (*hǎi zǎo yù hú tāng*). Topical: Apply Harmonious Yang Decongealing Plaster (*yáng hé jiě níng gāo*) and dab on powdered asafetida (*ē wèi*). **Flesh goiter** is characterized by single or multiple lumps like upturned cups, whose skin color is normal, and that are soft and spongy or firm like steamed bread. This goiter never ruptures. It may be accompanied by rash temperament, profuse sweating, heart palpitations, and oppression in the chest, and is attributed to binding depression damaging the spleen and preventing spleen qi from moving. WMC thyroid adenoma and tubercular enlargement of the thyroid gland. MED Treat by relieving depression and transforming phlegm, assisted by softening hardness. Use Sargassum Jade Flask Decoction (*hǎi zǎo yù hú tāng*). Topical: Apply Harmonious Yang Decongealing Plaster (*yáng hé jiě níng gāo*) and dab on Cinnamon Bark and Musk Powder (*guì shè sǎn*), which comprises ephedra (*má huáng*), asarum (*xì xīn*), cinnamon bark (*ròu guì*), small gleditsia (*zhū yá zào*), raw pinellia (*shēng bàn xià*), raw arisaema (*shēng nán xīng*), musk (*shè xiāng*), and borneol (*bīng piàn*). **Sinew goiter** is characterized by a hard lump with green-blue veins [lit. sinews] knotted like worms. It is attributed to anger qi damaging the liver with effulgent fire and dryness of the blood. MED Clear the liver and resolve depression; nourish the blood and soothe the sinews (veins). Use Liver-Clearing Aloe Pill (*qīng gān lú huì wán*). **Blood goiter** is characterized by lumps on the neck with a purple-red coloration of the skin and entangled red thread-like vessels. It is attributed to fulminant liver fire causing the blood to boil and further complicated by contending external evils. WMC hemangioma of the neck. MED Enrich yin and repress fire; nourish the blood and transform stasis. Use Scutellaria and Coptis Two Matured Ingredients Decoction (*qín lián èr chén tāng*) or combine sargassum (*hǎi zǎo*), clamshell powder (*hǎi gé fěn*), kelp (*kūn bù*), alisma (*zé xiè*), pig's thyroid gland (*zhū yè*), scutellaria (*huáng qín*), and coptis (*huáng lián*), with Four Agents Decoction (*sì wù tāng*). **Qi goiter** is a large lump on the neck, of normal skin coloration. It is soft to the touch and varies in size according with joyful or angry moods. It is attributed to affect-mind depression or to "water and earth" (local environmental) factors. WMC endemic goiter. |MED| Rectify qi and resolve depression; transform phlegm and soften hardness; fortify the spleen and eliminate dampness. Use variations of Depression-Overcoming Pill (*yuè jú wán*), Four Seas Depression-Soothing Pill (*sì hǎi shū yù wán*), or Sargassum Jade Flask Decoction (*hǎi zǎo yù hú tāng*). Analysis of goiter varies considerably. One modern analysis makes a fourfold distinction: qi depression and phlegm obstruction; phlegm bind and blood stasis; exuberant liver fire; and heart-liver yin vacuity. **Qi depression and phlegm obstruction** can cause diffuse symmetrical lumps at the front of the neck that are soft to the touch and have smooth skin. These are accompanied by oppression in the chest, sighing, and scurrying pain in the chest and rib-side. |MED| Rectify qi and soothe depression; transform phlegm and disperse goiter. Use Four Seas Depression-Soothing Pill (*sì hǎi shū yù wán*). **Phlegm bind and blood stasis** causes goiter characterized by persistent lumps that are hard and noded. There is oppression in the chest, poor intake of food, and stasis speckles or macules on the tongue. |MED| Rectify qi and transform phlegm; quicken the blood and disperse goiter. Use Sargassum Jade Flask Decoction (*hǎi zǎo yù hú tāng*). **Exuberant liver fire** gives rise to soft smooth lumps with heat vexation, profuse sweating, rashness and impatience, baking heat in the face, bitter taste in the mouth, protruding eyeballs, tremors of the extremities, red tongue with yellow fur, and rapid stringlike pulse. |MED| Clear the liver and discharge fire; calm the liver and extinguish wind. Use Gardenia Liver-Clearing Decoction (*zhī zǐ qīng gān tāng*). **Heart-liver yin vacuity** gives rise to soft smooth lumps accompanied by heart palpitations, heart vexation, reduced sleep, dry eyes, dizzy vision, tremor of the hands, emaciation and lack of strength, and a rapid fine stringlike pulse. |MED| Enrich and nourish yin-essence; quiet the heart and emolliate the liver. Use Celestial Emperor Heart-Supplementing Elixir (*tiān wáng bǔ xīn dān*) or All-the-Way-Through Brew (*yī guàn jiān*). [26: 995, 197, 262, 287, 741, 546] [27: 307] [97: 373] [80: 481]

goose-claw wind 鹅爪风 *é zhǎo (zhuǎ) fēng*: ASHEN NAIL. [26: 965]

goose-foot wind 鹅掌风 *é zhǎng fēng*: A skin disease of the hand characterized by vesicles, itching, and thickening of the skin. Goose-foot wind is caused by wind toxin or dampness invading the skin. In the initial stages, it is characterized by small vesicles and itching. Later, the white skin sheds. When it persists for long periods, the skin becomes thick and rough and tends to crack, especially in winter, and, in severe cases, the nails may thicken, turn gray, and crack. |WMC| tinea manus and eczema rhagadiforme. |MED| Use Vinegar Soaking Formula (*cù pào fāng*). This formula

is is made by soaking schizonepeta (*jīng jiè*), ledebouriella (*fáng fēng*), lycium root bark (*dì gǔ pí*), carthamus (*hóng huā*), gleditsia (*zào jiá*), hydnocarpus (*dà fēng zǐ*), and alum (*bái fán*) in vinegar for three or four days. The formula is applied by soaking the affected parts for half and hour each evening (each batch can be used for two weeks). |ACU| Base treatment mainly on LI, SI, and PC. Select LI-4 (*hé gǔ*, Union Valley), SI-3 (*hòu xī*, Back Ravine), PC-8 (*láo gōng*, Palace of Toil), HT-8 (*shào fǔ*, Lesser Mansion), PC-7 (*dà líng*, Great Mound), LI-11 (*qū chí*, Pool at the Bend), and Eight Evils (*bā xié*). Needle with drainage. [26: 965] [37: 450] [42: 157] [61: 347] [96: 261]

goose-mouth sore 鹅口疮 *é kǒu chuāng*: Synonym: *snow mouth*. A mouth disease in the newborn, caused by accumulated heat in the spleen and heart channels and characterized by ulceration of the mouth, white scales all over the tongue, sore mouth and tongue, and, in severe cases, vexation and agitation. This disease is one form of *fetal heat*. [26: 694] [27: 499] [97: 567] [61: 395]

gourd tongue 匏舌 *páo shé*: PHLEGM POUCH.

govern 主 *zhǔ*: To control or be closely associated with. Early texts commonly use political government as a source of metaphors to express physiological activity and relationships. For example, *The Inner Canon* (*nèi jīng*) states, "The stomach and spleen hold the office of the granaries; they manage the five flavors [i.e., food]." Thus, "the stomach governs intake [of food]" and "the spleen governs movement and transformation of the essence of grain and water." ◇ Chin 主 *zhǔ*, lord, governor; to govern; main; mainly associated with.

governing complexion 主色 *zhǔ sè*: See RIGHT COMPLEXION.

governings of the five viscera 五脏所主 *wǔ zàng suǒ zhǔ*: Synonym: *five governings*. The specific parts of the body governed by the viscera. The heart governs the vessels; the lung governs the skin and [body] hair; the liver governs the sinew; the spleen governs the flesh; the kidney governs the bone. Note that the flesh overlaps the category of the sinews, and therefore these are not strict anatomical categories. See SINEW. [26: 126] [27: 61] [97: 56]

governing vessel 督脉 *dū mài*: Abbreviation: GV. One of the EIGHT EXTRAORDINARY VESSELS; a vessel whose main pathway ascends the spine, and whose main function is regulate the yang channels. Pathway: The governing vessel has four courses. According to *The Magic Pivot* (*líng shū*), the main course of this vessel originates in the pelvic cavity. Emerging in the perineum at CV-1 (*huì yīn*, Meeting of Yin), it then passes posteriorly to GV-1 (*cháng qiáng*, Long Strong) at the tip of the coccyx. From this point, it ascends along the spine to GV-16 (*fēng fǔ*, Wind Mansion) in the nape of the neck. It enters the brain and ascends to the vertex, emerging at GV-20 (*bǎi huì*, Hundred Convergences) and continuing forward along the midline to the forehead, running down the nose and across the philtrum to terminate in the upper gum. The second channel starts in the lower abdomen and runs down through the genitals into the perineal region. From here it passes through the tip of the coccyx, where it diverts into the gluteal region. Here it intersects both the leg lesser yin (*shào yīn*) kidney channel and the leg greater yang *tài yáng* bladder channel before returning to the spinal column. It then travels up the spine and links through to the kidney. A third path starts at the same two bilateral points as the foot greater yang (*tài yáng*) bladder channel at the inner canthi of the eyes. The branches rise up over the forehead to meet at the vertex. The channel then enters the brain and splits into two channels that descend along opposite sides of the spine to the waist, to join with the kidney. The fourth path starts in the lower abdomen, travels up past the navel, continues upward to join with the heart, then enters the throat, crosses the cheek, splits into two and rounds the lips, and runs up the cheek to the center of the infraorbital region. Functions: The governing vessel is the sea of the yang channels. All six yang channels converge at the point GV-14 (*dà zhuī*, Great Hammer). The governing vessel has a regulating effect on the yang channels, so it is said that it governs all the yang channels of the body. The governing vessel homes to the brain and nets the kidney. The kidney engenders marrow and the brain is known as the "sea of marrow." Therefore, the governing vessel reflects the physiology and pathology of the brain and the spinal fluid, as well as their relationship with the reproductive organs. Signs: Arched-back rigidity, pain and stiffness in the back, child fright reversal, heavy-headedness, hemorrhoids, infertility, malaria, mania and withdrawal, and visceral agitation (mental disorders). [6: 68] [97: 601]

governor 主 *zhǔ*: The (organ) that governs.

grain and water 水谷 *shuǐ gǔ*: Food.

grandchild network vessel 孙络 *sūn luò*: Synonym: *grandchild vessel*. Any of the finer network vessels. *The Magic Pivot* (*líng shū*) states, "The channels are in the interior; the lateral branches are the network vessels; the branches of the network vessels are the grandchildren." See NETWORK VESSEL. [27: 95] [97: 244]

grandchild vessel 孙脉 *sūn mài*: GRANDCHILD NETWORK VESSEL. [26: 518]

grand cleft 巨分 *jù fēn*: The depression between the nose and the upper lip. In Western medicine, this is called the nasolabial groove or sulcus na-

solabialis. ◇ Chin 巨 *jù*, giant, large; 分 *fēn* cleft, divide. [27: 64] [97: 76]

grande piqûre 巨刺 *jù cì*: GREAT NEEDLING.

grating 锉, 剉 *cuò*: Some hard, bony materials such as antelope horn (*líng yáng jiǎo*), and rhinoceros horn (*xī jiǎo*) are grated in small particles using a steel rasp. [82: 32]

graying of the hair 发白 *fà bái*: Partial or complete whitening of the hair in youth or middle age; attributable to liver-kidney depletion and insufficiency of yin-blood depriving the hair of nourishment. MED Enrich the liver and kidney; boost qi and nourish the blood. Use Flowery Knotweed Life-Extending Elixir (*shǒu wū yán shòu dān*) or a decoction of pure flowery knotweed (*hé shǒu wū*). Mulberry Paste (*sāng shèn zǐ gāo*) can be taken as a regular drink. [26: 869]

greater abdomen 大腹 *dà fù*: The part of the abdomen above the umbilicus. WMC upper abdomen. [27: 68]

greater yang 太阳 *tài yáng*: **1.** The hand greater yang (*tài yáng*) small intestine and foot greater yang (*tài yáng*) bladder channels. Greater yang is the exuberance of yang qi. The greater yang channels are the most exterior of all the yang channels, and are most susceptible to contraction of external evils; hence it is said that "greater yang governs openness." **2.** TEMPLE. [26: 130] [27: 68]

greater yang bowel disease 太阳腑病 *tài yáng fǔ bìng*: In six-channel pattern identification, disease of the bladder. Greater yang bowel patterns arise when evil passes into the bladder, which is the bowel of the greater yang. Distinction is traditionally made between water amassment and blood amassment patterns. Blood amassment is characterized by smaller-abdominal pain and distention, and manic states. It is distinguished from the water amassment by uninhibited urination. However, according to *Medical Insights* (*yī xué xīn wù*), the Poria (Hoelen) Five Powder (*wǔ líng sǎn*) pattern of water amassment is the only greater yang bowel pattern, whereas blood amassment is a lower burner pattern because the pathology is not located in the bladder. MED Water amassment is treated by freeing yang and disinhibiting water with Poria (Hoelen) Five Powder (*wǔ líng sǎn*), whereas blood amassment is treated by moving blood and dispelling stasis with Peach Kernel Qi-Coordinating Decoction (*táo hé chéng qì tāng*). See COLD DAMAGE WATER AMASSMENT PATTERN and COLD DAMAGE BLOOD AMASSMENT PATTERN. [26: 131] [27: 219] [97: 61] [6: 225]

greater yang channel 太阳经 *tài yáng jīng*: See GREATER YANG.

greater yang channel disease 太阳经病 *tài yáng jīng bìng*: Synonym: *greater yang exterior pattern*. Disease characterized by aversion to cold or wind, headache, and a floating pulse. *On Cold Damage (shāng hán lùn)* states, "In disease of greater yang, the pulse is floating, the head and nape are rigid and painful, and there is aversion to cold." Usually there is heat effusion. Other possible signs include generalized pain, together with tension and stiffness in the neck and back. This pattern is seen in many initial-stage externally contracted heat (febrile) diseases, and in terms of eight-principle pattern identification, it is an exterior cold pattern. According to the doctrine of cold damage, externally contracted heat (febrile) diseases are mostly attributable to contraction of wind-cold evil, which first affects the yang channels. Of the yang channels, the greater yang is the first to be affected; consequently, it is said to govern the exterior of the body. The greater yang channel passes through the head and neck, so that when its qi is depressed by an invading wind-cold evil, stiffness and pain occur in this region. Aversion to cold or wind and heat effusion are the pathological reactions of a body whose right qi (construction and defense) is struggling to resist evil qi. The floating pulse reflects disease in the exterior. Although *On Cold Damage* makes no reference to the tongue or its fur, it is important to note that in most cases the tongue fur is thin, white, and moist. Differentiation between vacuity and repletion of the exterior is of crucial importance in identifying greater yang diseases. Judgment rests largely on the following factors: the presence or absence of aversion to cold or wind; whether the floating pulse is tight or moderate; and most crucially, the presence or absence of sweating. Exterior vacuity patterns involve sweating. They most commonly occur where, owing to construction-defense disharmony, the interstices are unsound and allow sweat to flow, whereas resistance is inadequate to expel the evil. In exterior repletion patterns, which occur when cold evil invades greater yang, sweating does not occur since the evil impedes construction qi, leading to blockage of the interstices. MED The principal method used to treat greater yang (*tài yáng*) diseases is sweating, i.e., exterior resolution. Its effect is to free defense qi, open the interstices, and expel the evil from the body through sweating. Greater yang (*tài yáng*) diseases characterized by the cold evil present in the exterior are treated by resolving the exterior with warm acrid medicinals (warm acrid exterior resolution). Greater yang exterior repletion patterns—pathomechanically explained as obstruction of defense qi by an external evil leading to blockage of the interstices—are treated by promoting diffusion and dissipating the evil using Ephedra Decoction (*má huáng tāng*), which effuses sweat (i.e., is diaphoretic). Exterior vacuity patterns, pathomechanically explained as construction-defense disharmony preventing expulsion

of the evil, are primarily treated by harmonizing construction and defense, using Cinnamon Twig Decoction (*guì zhī tāng*), which resolves the flesh. Ephedra Decoction, containing both ephedra (*má huáng*) and cinnamon twig (*guì zhī*), dissipates the evil. Cinnamon-Twig Decoction, containing cinnamon twig (*guì zhī*) and white peony (*bái sháo yào*), is designed to harmonize construction and defense as a prerequisite for expulsion of the evil. Both Ephedra Decoction and Cinnamon Twig Decoction are frequently varied. A number of important formulas are derived from Ephedra Decoction. For example, Major Green-Blue Dragon Decoction (*dà qīng lóng tāng*) treats patterns comprising signs such as agitation and absence of sweating, which arise when exterior cold, failing resolution by sweating (diaphoresis), becomes depressed and transforms into heat. Minor Green-Blue Dragon Decoction (*xiǎo qīng lóng tāng*) is used for dual patterns of exterior cold and interior rheum, where exterior signs such as aversion to cold, heat effusion, and absence of thirst are accompanied by pronounced cough and panting. Ephedra, Apricot Kernel, Gypsum, and Licorice Decoction (*má xìng gān shí tāng*), a variant of Ephedra Decoction, treats heat brewing in the lung with heat effusion, thirst, cough, and panting. Cinnamon Twig Decoction (*guì zhī tāng*) may be varied depending on the signs. For instance, pueraria (*gé gēn*) may be added when signs include stiffness in the neck and back, whereas magnolia bark (*hòu pò*) and apricot kernel (*xìng rén*) may be added for the treatment of patterns that include panting. Most patterns treated by Cinnamon-Twig Decoction, Ephedra Decoction, and their variations fall within the scope of greater yang (*tài yáng*) disease. [27: 219] [97: 61] [6: 225] [26: 130]

greater yang disease 太阳病 *tài yáng bìng*: Any of a number of diseases affecting greater yang (*tài yáng*). **Greater yang channel disease:** Disease of the greater yang (*tài yáng*) channels forming Cinnamon Twig Decoction (*guì zhī tāng*) or Ephedra Decoction (*má huáng tāng*) patterns. Greater yang disease patterns are exterior patterns that are observed before the evil passes into the interior. Thus urine and stool are generally not affected, and there is no thirst. GREATER YANG CHANNEL DISEASE. **Greater yang bowel patterns:** Greater yang patterns arise when evil enters the bladder or bladder region. They include greater yang water amassment and greater yang blood amassment. Water amassment is characterized by a floating pulse, heat effusion, thirst with inhibited urination, lesser-abdominal fullness, and in some cases immediate vomiting of ingested fluids, the principal feature being inhibited urination. GREATER YANG BOWEL DISEASE. [27: 219] [97: 61] [6: 225] [26: 130]

greater yang exterior pattern 太阳表证 *tài yáng biǎo zhèng*: GREATER YANG CHANNEL DISEASE.

greater yang headache 太阳头痛 *tài yáng tóu tòng*: **1.** Headache occurring in greater yang (*tài yáng*) disease in cold damage, attended by stiffness of the neck and accompanied by aversion to cold, heat effusion, and floating pulse. MED Classically, greater yang headache without sweating is treated with Ephedra Decoction (*má huáng tāng*), whereas with sweating it is treated with Cinnamon Twig Decoction (*guì zhī tāng*). It can also be treated with formulas containing ligusticum (*chuān xiōng*), notopterygium (*qiāng huó*), duhuo (*dú huó*), and ephedra (*má huáng*). ACU Select GB-20 (*fēng chí*, Wind Pool), GV-16 (*fēng fǔ*, Wind Mansion), ST-8 (*tóu wéi*, Head Corner), TB-5 (*wài guān*, Outer Pass), LI-4 (*hé gǔ*, Union Valley), GB-12 (*wán gǔ*, Completion Bone), and BL-64 (*jīng gǔ*, Capital Bone). **2.** Headache characterized by pain on the path of the greater yang (*tài yáng*) channel, i.e., one that runs over the vertex and that is associated with stiffness of the neck, back, and lumbus. MED Formulas used to treat it often contain notopterygium (*qiāng huó*) and ephedra (*má huáng*), which act as conductors. ACU Select BL-10 (*tiān zhù*, Celestial Pillar), GV-14 (*dà zhuī*, Great Hammer), SI-3 (*hòu xī*, Back Ravine), and BL-60 (*kūn lún*, Kunlun Mountains). See HEADACHE. [26: 131] [113: 9] [4: 154] [71: 23]

greater yin 太阴 *tài yīn*: The hand greater yin (*tài yīn*) lung and foot greater yin (*tài yīn*) spleen channels. Greater yin is characterized by an exuberance of yin qi. Among the yin channels, the greater yin are the most closely associated with the exterior; hence it is said that "greater yin governs opening." [27: 91]

greater yin channel 太阴经 *tài yīn jīng*: See GREATER YIN.

greater yin disease 太阴病 *tài yīn bìng*: Greater yin disease is characterized by abdominal fullness with periodic pain, vomiting, diarrhea, nonmovement of ingested food, absence of thirst, and a weak, moderate pulse. The pathomechanism of greater yin disease is failure of movement and transformation of the food, resulting from devitalization of spleen yang, and manifesting as vomiting and diarrhea. The abdominal distention is explained by spleen vacuity qi stagnation, whereas the abdominal pain results from vacuity cold. Although it rarely occurs naturally in the progression of externally contracted heat (febrile) diseases, it may arise when incorrect treatment of yang diseases, such as inappropriate precipitation in greater yang (*tài yáng*) and lesser yang (*shào yáng*) disease, or excessive use of cold and cool freeing precipitants in yang brightness (*yáng míng*)

disease, damages spleen yang. It may also occur when, owing to a regular spleen qi vacuity, cold evil enters the greater yin directly. This is known as a direct strike on greater yin. Like the yang brightness bowel pattern, greater yin disease is a digestive tract disease, but presents as vacuity rather than as repletion. It is characterized by vomiting, diarrhea, absence of thirst, vacuity fullness and pain, and a weak, moderate pulse, whereas yang brightness bowel patterns are identified by the presence of constipation, thirst, great repletion and fullness, and a sunken replete pulse. It is said, "Greater yin disease is associated with vacuity, and yang brightness disease is associated with repletion." MED Since greater yin (*tài yīn*) disease is attributable to damage to spleen yang by cold, it is treated by warming the center and dissipating cold, and by restoring the correct and fortifying the spleen. The principal formula is Center-Rectifying Pill (*lǐ zhōng wán*). Where interior cold is pronounced, Aconite Center-Rectifying Decoction (*fù zǐ lǐ zhōng tāng*) is used, which is the same formula with the addition of aconite (*fù zǐ*). [26: 130] [27: 219] [97: 62]

greater yin headache 太阴头痛 *tài yīn tóu tòng*: HEADACHE attributed to phlegm-damp encumbering the spleen and preventing the normal upbearing of clear yang. Greater yin headache is characteristically attended by heavy-headedness, copious phlegm, generalized heaviness, and in some cases abdominal pain and fullness, and is associated with a moderate sunken pulse. MED Dry dampness and transform phlegm using Atractylodes Dampness-Eliminating Decoction (*cāng zhú chú shī tāng*). ACU Base treatment mainly on CV and ST. Select ST-8 (*tóu wéi*, Head Corner), Greater Yang (*tài yáng*), CV-12 (*zhōng wǎn*, Center Stomach Duct), ST-36 (*zú sān lǐ*, Leg Three Li), LI-4 (*hé gǔ*, Union Valley), and ST-40 (*fēng lóng*, Bountiful Bulge); needle with drainage. For abdominal pain and fullness, add ST-25 (*tiān shū*, Celestial Pivot), CV-6 (*qì hǎi*, Sea of Qi), and PC-6 (*nèi guān*, Inner Pass). See HEADACHE. [26: 130]

great heat [effusion] 大热 *dà rè*: High fever in either exterior or interior patterns. For example, *On Cold Damage* (*shāng hán lùn, tài yáng bìng mài zhèng bìng zhì shàng piān*) states, "If there is sweating and panting and absence of great heat [effusion], one can give Ephedra, Apricot Kernel, Licorice, and Gypsum Decoction (*má huáng xìng rén gān cǎo shí gāo tāng*). [51: 109] [6: 226]

great heat in the qi aspect 气分大热 *qì fèn dà rè*: The equivalent in doctrine of warm diseases of the yang brightness (*yáng míng*) channel pattern in the doctrine of cold damage. See QI-ASPECT PATTERN; YANG BRIGHTNESS CHANNEL PATTERN. [6: 234]

great needling 巨刺 *jù cì*: Synonym: *grande piqûre*. One of the NINE NEEDLING METHODS; an acupuncture method involving the deep needling of channel points on the side of the body opposite to the side affected. It is normally used to treat disease of the channels. Compare CROSS NEEDLING, which involves the shallow needling of network vessels on the opposite side of the body. See also SELECTION OF CONTRALATERAL POINTS. [26: 184]

great network vessel of the spleen 脾之大络 *pí zhī dà luò*: A large network vessel that branches off directly from the spleen, issues at SP-21 (*dà bāo,* Great Embracement), and disperses over the chest and rib-side. [26: 748] [27: 95] [97: 561]

great network vessel of the stomach 胃之大络 *wèi zhī dà luò*: A large network vessel that branches direct from the stomach, passes up the stomach, traverses the diaphragm, and after connecting with the lung, turns outward to exit below the left breast, at the apical pulse (*xū lǐ*), roughly corresponding to ST-18 (*rǔ gēn,* Breast Root). [26: 437]

great numbing wind 大麻风 *dà má fēng*: PESTILENTIAL WIND.

great qi 大气 *dà qì*: The qi of the environment, air. [97: 20]

great respiration 太息 *tài xī*: **1.** Periodic extended exhalation to relieve oppression in the chest. In normal people one inhalation and one exhalation forms "one respiration" equal to four beats of the pulse. When every fourth respiration is a deep inhalation equal to five beats of the pulse, this is called "intermittent great respiration." **2.** SIGHING. [50: 214] [92: 54] [81: 148]

great seminal discharge 精液大泄 *jīng yè dà xiè*: Continuous seminal efflux; the most severe form of *seminal loss.*

¹**great sweating** 大汗 *dà hàn*: The flow of sweat in large amounts. Great sweating in yang collapse is called DESERTION SWEATING; great sweating due to inappropriate sweating (diaphoresis) is called LEAKING SWEAT. See both these entries and SWEATING. [26: 43]

²**great sweating** 大汗出 *dà hàn chū*: One of the FOUR GREATNESSES associated with yang brightness (*yáng míng*) channel patterns. See SWEATING. [6: 226]

great vexing thirst 大烦渴 *dà fán kě*: One of the FOUR GREATNESSES associated with yang brightness (*yáng míng*) channel patterns. [6: 226]

great wind 大风 *dà fēng*: PESTILENTIAL WIND.

green-blue 青 *qīng*: Green, blue, or greenish blue. This color is classically described as "the color of new shoots of grass," but in context of the complexion, for example, it is more often than not a color that would be more naturally described in English as blue.

green-blue face 面青 *miàn qīng*: GREEN-BLUE FACIAL COMPLEXION.

green-blue facial complexion 面色青 *miàn sè qīng*: Synonym: *green-blue face.* A sign of wind-cold, blood stasis, pain, and qi-block patterns. Child fright wind and epilepsy are characterized by a somber green-blue complexion. A grayish green-blue complexion with green-blue or purple lips is associated with internal blood stasis and impaired flow of qi and blood, and occurs in diseases classified in Western medicine as cirrhosis of the liver and cardiac failure. In severe wind-cold headaches and abdominal pain due to interior cold, impeded flow of yang qi may be reflected in a bluish somber white complexion. In cases of blocked lung qi, a dark green-blue or purple complexion may result from obstructed flow of blood and qi. This corresponds to conditions such as pulmogenic heart diseases and asphyxia in Western medicine. [6: 117] [92: No. 72]

green-blue vaginal discharge 青带 *qīng dài*: See LIVER CHANNEL DAMP-HEAT VAGINAL DISCHARGE; DAMP TOXIN VAGINAL DISCHARGE. [27: 445] [97: 324]

green-blue wind 青风 *qīng fēng*: GREEN-BLUE WIND INTERNAL OBSTRUCTION. [26: 353] [27: 506] [97: 324]

green-blue wind internal obstruction 青风内障 *qīng fēng nèi zhàng*: Synonym: *green-blue wind.* A disease of the eye in which the pupil takes on a green-blue color and is sometimes dilated, accompanied by a faint red areola surrounding the dark of the eye (ciliary congestion). Green-blue wind internal obstruction is accompanied by mild distention in the head, mild aversion to light and tearing, and gradual decrease in visual acuity. If appropriate treatment is not given, it can turn into GREEN WIND INTERNAL OBSTRUCTION. It is caused by liver-kidney yin vacuity with wind-fire harassing the upper body. MED Nourish yin and clear heat; calm the liver and extinguish wind. Use formulas like Green Wind Antelope Horn Beverage (*lù fēng líng yáng yǐn*). [26: 352]

green herbs 青草 *qīng cǎo*: Fresh medicinal plant products, usually picked in the wild. See HERBAL MEDICINAL.

green-leg gan of the teeth and gums 青腿牙疳 *qīng tuǐ yá gān*: Gan of the teeth and gums accompanied by green-blue swelling of the lower limbs. Green-leg gan of the teeth and gums is attributed to cold-damp qi stagnating in the channels, causing inhibited flow of qi and blood, and resulting in stasis in the lower body. With depressed heat in the stomach and intestines, heat toxin surges upward to scorch the teeth and gums, causing sore swollen gums, and gradual ulceration, putrefaction, and bleeding. In severe cases, the ulceration can pierce the cheek and spread to the lips, whereas the green-blue coloring of the legs forms into pronounced cloud-like patches the color of eggplants, with painful hard swelling of the sinews and flesh that makes walking difficult. WMC scurvy. MED Dissipate cold, quicken the network vessels, and resolve toxin. Use formulas such as Network-Quickening Qi Flow Beverage (*huó luò liú qì yǐn*). See GAN OF THE TEETH AND GUMS. [26: 354]

green water pouring into the eye 绿水灌珠 *lǜ shuǐ guàn zhū*: GREEN WIND INTERNAL OBSTRUCTION.

green wind 绿风 *lǜ fēng*: GREEN WIND INTERNAL OBSTRUCTION. [26: 858] [27: 506] [97: 539]

green wind internal obstruction 绿风内障 *lǜ fēng nèi zhàng*: Synonyms: *green wind*; *green water pouring into the eye*. A disease of the eye in which the pupil becomes turbid and light green in color, causing loss of visual acuity and giving lights the appearance of being surrounded by a rainbow-like halo. Other signs include distended pain stretching into the eye sockets, forehead, nose and jaw, nausea and vomiting, and faint red areola surrounding the dark of the eye (ciliary congestion). Green wind internal obstruction is caused by liver-gallbladder wind-fire harassing the upper body, or hyperactivity of yang due to yin vacuity and disharmony of the qi and blood. WMC glaucoma. MED Clear heat, calm the liver, and extinguish wind. Use Green Wind Antelope Horn Beverage (*lǜ fēng líng yáng yǐn*) and variations. Alternatively, it can be treated by enriching water and moistening wood with Eye Brightener Rehmannia Pill (*míng mù dì huáng wán*) and variations. See also YELLOW WIND INTERNAL OBSTRUCTION. [26: 885]

grimy 垢 *gòu*: Dirty, turbid, and unclean (in appearance); applied to tongue fur and facial complexion. See TONGUE FUR and GRIMY FACE.

grimy face 面垢 *miàn gòu*: From *On Cold Damage* (*shāng hán lùn*). A facial complexion that looks dirty as if covered with dust and grime that cannot be washed away. Grimy face is usually attributed to contraction of summerheat evil, stomach heat sweltering upward, or to internal accumulation and stagnation. [26: 424] [27: 716] [97: 385]

grimy tongue fur 苔垢 *tāi gòu*: A dirty-looking tongue coating. It indicates, on the one hand, the presence of turbid evils such as turbid damp and turbid phlegm, and on the other, stomach qi vacuity. In stomach qi vacuity attention must be paid to safeguarding stomach qi when dispelling the evil. [27: 449] [6: 123]

grinding 研 *yán*, 研末 *yán mò*, 磨 *mó*: Reduction to powder in pestle and mortar. Cinnabar (*zhū shā*) and pearl (*zhēn zhū*) are processed in this way.

grinding of the teeth 啮齿 *niè chǐ*, 嚼齿 *niè chǐ*, 齘齿 *xiè chǐ*, 齿齘 *chǐ xiè*, 嘎牙 *gā yá*, 咬牙 *yǎo yá*: Synonym: *bruxism*. Involuntary grinding of the teeth, especially in sleep. In children, it is a sign of stomach heat, intestinal parasites, or gan accumulation. [97: 521]

gripping pain 绞痛 *jiǎo tòng*: A pain over a large area that feels as if the affected area is being wrung or gouged. Gripping pain is attributable to tangible evils or congealing cold, and is observed in heart pain due to heart blood stasis obstruction, smaller abdominal or lumbar pain due to stone strangury, or stomach duct pain and abdomen in ROUNDWORM REVERSAL. See PAIN. [29: 190]

gripping pain in the abdomen 腹中绞痛 *fù zhōng jiǎo tòng*: Acute wringing or cutting pain over a large area of the abdomen. Gripping pain in the abdomen observed in ROUNDWORM REVERSAL and heat cholera. See GRIPPING PAIN.

groin 鼠蹊 *shǔ xī*: The depression between the lower abdomen and the thigh. [97: 231]

groping in the air and pulling at invisible strings 撮空理线 *cuō kōng lǐ xiàn*: See PICKING AT BEDCLOTHES.

grossness 臃肿 *yōng zhǒng*: Severe obesity.

gu 蛊 *gǔ*: **1.** Toxin of poisonous *chóng* (insects, reptiles, etc.) damaging the liver and spleen and causing blockage of the network vessels and manifesting in the form of drum distention (gu distention). **2.** Sexual taxation in males. **3.** Lesser-abdominal heat pain with white turbid urine. **4.** Poison derived from insects used in ancient times to harm others, as mentioned in the *Zhou Book of Rites* (周礼 *zhōu lǐ*). [26: 1003] [27: 414] [97: 516] [130: 46–50]

gua-sha 刮痧 *guā shā*: Synonym: *sand scraping*. A method of treating repletion heat SAND (*shā*) distention patterns whereby the skin on the back, limbs, and other parts of the body is lubricated and then scraped with a ceramic spoon, the edge of a rice bowl, or similar object (purpose-made scrapers are available). Method: The area to be treated is first lubricated with oil such as sesame oil, or nowadays often petroleum jelly (Vaseline). The area is scraped until the red papules become fully visible and coalesce. Gua-sha is usually applied to the back. Here, the area either side of the spine is scraped, working from shoulders downward. The papules may then be pricked with a three-edged needle to drain blackish purple blood and allow the the sand toxin to escape. For the head, forehead, elbows, wrists, legs, and knees, etc., flax yarn or hair dipped in sesame oil can be used. Soft parts of the abdomen may be rubbed with salt. More at SAND (*shā*). [26: 381] [50: 924]

gu distention 蛊胀 *gǔ zhàng*: **1.** DRUM DISTENTION. **2.** DRUM DISTENTION due to gu toxin. **3.** Simple abdominal distention. [26: 1003]

gum 龈 *yín*, 牙龈 *yá yín*, 牙齗 *yá yín*: The flesh surrounding the teeth. The upper gum belongs to the foot yang brightness (*yáng míng*) stomach channel, whereas the lower gum belongs to the hand yang brightness large intestine channel. Gum problems include: SPONTANEOUS BLEEDING OF THE GUMS; GAPING GUMS; GAN OF THE TEETH AND GUMS; GALLOPING GAN OF THE TEETH AND GUMS; BONE TROUGH WIND. Patterns in which gum problems may occur include EXUBERANT STOMACH HEAT; KIDNEY YIN VACUITY; SPLEEN FAILING TO MANAGE THE BLOOD; UPCAST YANG; COLD ENVELOPING FIRE; DRYNESS-HEAT.

gurgling intestines 肠鸣漉漉 *cháng míng lù lù*: Severe rumbling intestines.

gu toxin 蛊毒 *gǔ dú*: Ancient disease name denoting various severe conditions that have been equated with scrub typhus, chronic blood fluke infestation, severe hepatitis, cirrhosis of the liver, and severe bacillary or amebic dysentery of modern medicine. [26: 1003] [27: 122] [97: 517]

GV 督脉 *dū mài*: Abbreviation for the governing (*dū*) vessel.

gynecological diseases 妇科疾病 *fù kē jí bìng*: See WOMEN'S DISEASES.

H

habitual miscarriage 滑胎 *huá tāi*, 数坠胎 *shù zhuì tāi*: Miscarriage successively occurring three times or more. Habitual miscarriage is attributable to qi vacuity, kidney vacuity, blood heat, blood vacuity, or external injury. MED Treat with pills of ground eucommia (*dù zhòng*), dipsacus (*xù duàn*), dioscorea (*shān yào*), and glutinous rice (*nuò mǐ*) blended with jujube paste (*zǎo ní*). This formula can be taken as soon as pregnancy is suspected, and may be discontinued when the danger period is over. See BLOOD HEAT HABITUAL MISCARRIAGE; BLOOD VACUITY HABITUAL MISCARRIAGE; KIDNEY VACUITY HABITUAL MISCARRIAGE; QI VACUITY HABITUAL MISCARRIAGE. [26: 759] [27: 449] [97: 585]

hacking of blood 咳血 *kà xuè*, 咯血 *kǎ xuè*: Expectoration of blood in short frequent coughs. Compare EXPECTORATION OF BLOOD.

hair 发 *fà*, 头发 *tóu fà*: The filamentous outgrowth from the scalp. The hair [of the head] is the external bloom of the kidney and is the surplus of the blood. *Elementary Questions* (*sù wèn, shàng gǔ tiān zhēn lùn*) states "... When kidney qi is replete, the hair grows and the teeth change..." "... When kidney qi is debilitated, the hair falls and the teeth desiccate." Diseases of the hair include DRY HAIR; GRAYING OF THE HAIR; HAIR LOSS. [26: 869]

hair loss 发落 *fà luò*: Falling out of the hair. The hair [of the head] is the external bloom of the kidney and is the surplus of the blood. Hair loss is attributed to kidney vacuity or blood vacuity depriving the hair of nourishment. It commonly is commonly the result of illness, childbirth, or malnutrition. The hair becomes sparse and sheenless, and may lighten in color (turning yellowish brown in Chinese people). In severe cases, the loss of hair may be complete. MED Enrich the kidney and nourish the blood using Four Agents Decoction (*sì wù tāng*), Six-Ingredient Rehmannia Pill (*liù wèi dì huáng wán*), or Flowery Knotweed Life-Extending Elixir (*shǒu wū yán shòu dān*). [26: 869]

hair needling 毛刺 *máo cì*: One of the nine needling methods; shallow needling of the skin with a short fine filiform needle. [27: 335]

hair [of the head] is the surplus of the blood 发为血之馀 *fà wéi xuè zhī yú*: The hair is related to liver blood. The ancient Chinese observed that (Chinese) hair is black and bears a sheen when qi and blood are exuberant in youth, and loses its color and sheen with increasing kidney qi vacuity of advancing years, for which reason it is said that the KIDNEY, ITS BLOOM IS IN THE HAIR [OF THE HEAD]. Since "the liver and kidney are of the same source," and "the liver stores the blood," the health of the hair is understood to be related not only to the kidney but also to the liver. NB: The skin and [body] hair are governed by the lung. [26: 869] [27: 42]

half-body numbness 半身麻木 *bàn shēn má mù*: Numbness of half of the body, either the left or right side or upper or lower part. **Left body numbness** is due to vacuity of the blood in qi. MED Spleen-Returning Decoction (*guī pí tāng*). ACU Base treatment mainly on back transport points and CV. Select BL-20 (*pí shū*, Spleen Transport), BL-17 (*gé shū*, Diaphragm Transport), CV-6 (*qì hǎi*, Sea of Qi), ST-36 (*zú sān lǐ*, Leg Three Li), SP-6 (*sān yīn jiāo*, Three Yin Intersection), and LR-3 (*tài chōng*, Supreme Surge); needle with supplementation. **Right body numbness** is due to vacuity of the qi in blood. MED Use Astragalus Center-Fortifying Decoction (*huáng qí jiàn zhōng tāng*). ACU Base treatment mainly on back transport points and CV. Select BL-20 (*pí shū*, Spleen Transport), BL-21 (*wèi shū*, Stomach Transport), CV-6 (*qì hǎi*, Sea of Qi), BL-43 (*gāo huāng shū*, Gao-Huang Transport), ST-36 (*zú sān lǐ*, Leg Three Li), SP-3 (*tài bái*, Supreme White), LU-9 (*tài yuān*, Great Abyss), and SP-6 (*sān yīn jiāo*, Three Yin Intersection); needle with supplementation and add moxa. **Upper body numbness** is caused by clear yang failing to bear upward, and is treated with Center-Supplementing Qi-Boosting Decoction (*bǔ zhōng yì qì tāng*). ACU Base treatment mainly on GV and CV. Select GV-20 (*bǎi huì*, Hundred Convergences), CV-6 (*qì hǎi*, Sea of Qi), CV-4 (*guān yuán*, Pass Head), and ST-36 (*zú sān lǐ*, Leg Three Li); needle with supplementation and add moxa. **Numbness and limpness up to the knees** is caused by stomach damp phlegm and dead blood obstruction. MED Use Four Agents Decoction (*sì wù tāng*) plus ginseng (*rén shēn*), cyathula (*chuān niú xī*), and coix (*yì yǐ rén*). ACU Base treatment mainly on CV, ST, SP, and LR. Select CV-12 (*zhōng wǎn*, Center Stomach Duct), ST-36 (*zú sān lǐ*, Leg Three Li), ST-40 (*fēng lóng*, Bountiful Bulge), SP-10 (*xuè hǎi*, Sea of Blood), LR-3 (*tài chōng*, Supreme Surge), and SP-6 (*sān yīn jiāo*, Three Yin Intersection); needle with even supplementation and drainage. For selection of points according to specific affected areas, see HEMIPLEGIA. [26: 174] [46: 595, 597, 615]

half exterior half interior pattern 半表半里证 *bàn biǎo bàn lǐ zhèng*: MIDSTAGE PATTERN.

hall of impression 印堂 *yìn táng*: The region between the eyebrows. ⌈WMC⌉ glabella. [27: 63]

Han 汉 *hàn*: Name of a dynasty (206 B.C.–A.D. 220).

hand greater yang small intestine channel 手太阳小肠经 *shǒu tài yáng xiǎo cháng jīng*: Abbreviation: SI. One of the TWELVE CHANNELS; the channel that homes to the small intestine, nets the heart, and links with the stomach and nose, and whose external pathway runs from the end of the little finger up the posterior extensor aspect of the upper limb, over the should blade, up the neck, over the face, to terminate in the ear. **Pathway:** The small intestine channel starts on the outside edge of the little finger tip and travels along the ulnar side of the hand to the wrist, emerging at the ulnar styloid process. Continuing up the posterior aspect of the ulna, it passes between the olecranon of the ulna and the medial epicondyle of the humerus on the medial side of the elbow. It then runs up the posteromedial side of the upper arm, emerging behind the shoulder joint and circling around the superior and inferior fossae of the scapula. At the top of the shoulder, it intersects the foot greater yang (*tài yáng*) bladder channel at BL-36 (*chéng fú*, Support) and BL-11 (*dà zhù*, Great Shuttle), connecting with the governing (*dū*) vessel at GV-14 (*dà zhuī*, Great Hammer) before turning downward into the supraclavicular fossa. Here it submerges at ST-12 (*quē pén*, Empty Basin), nets the the heart, and follows the esophagus down through the diaphragm to the stomach. It then intersects with the controlling (*rèn*) vessel internally at CV-13 (*shàng wǎn*, Upper Stomach Duct) and CV-12 (*zhōng wǎn*, Center Stomach Duct) before homing to the small intestine. A branch separates from the channel at ST-12 (*quē pén*, Empty Basin) and runs up the neck to the cheek. The channel then travels to the outer canthus of the eye where it meets the foot lesser yang (*shào yáng*) gallbladder channel at GB-1 (*tóng zǐ liáo*, Pupil Bone-Hole), and then turns back across the temple to enter the ear at SI-1 (*shào zé*, Lesser Marsh). Another branch breaks off from the former branch on the mandible, rises to the infraorbital region, and continues to the inner canthus where it meets the foot greater yang (*tài yáng*) bladder channel at BL-1, then crosses horizontally to the zygomatic region. *The Magic Pivot* (*líng shū*) claims that another branch descends internally from the small intestine to emerge at SI-9, the lower uniting point of the small intestine.

Signs: Signs associated with the external course of the channel are: erosion of the glossal and oral mucosa, pain in the cheeks, sore pharynx, tearing, stiffness of the neck, pain on the lateral aspect of the shoulder and upper arm. Signs associated with the internal course of the channel are: lower abdominal pain and distention with the pain stretching around to the lumbus; lower abdominal pain radiating into the testicles; diarrhea; stomach pain with dry feces, and constipation. [6: 56] [97: 107]

hand greater yin lung channel 手太阴肺经 *shǒu tài yīn fèi jīng*: Abbreviation: LU. One of the TWELVE CHANNELS; the channel that homes to the lung, nets the large intestine, links with the stomach and throat, and whole external pathways runs from the superorlateral aspect of the chest down the anterior flexor aspect of the upper limb, to the end of the the thumb. **Pathway:** The lung channel starts in the region of the stomach in the center burner and descends to connect with the large intestine. It then returns upward through the cardiac orifice, passes through the diaphragm, and homes to the lung. Continuing its ascendant path, it passes through the respiratory tract into the throat, then veers downward, following the clavicle to enter the axilla. From here, the channel runs down the anterior aspect of the upper arm, lateral to the heart and pericardium channels, traverses the cubital fossa, and continues along the anterior aspect of the forearm to the radial styloid process of the wrist. It crosses the radial pulse, traverses the thenar eminence, and travels along the radial side of the thumb to its tip. A branch leaves the main pathway proximal to the wrist, passes round to the dorsum of the hand, and then runs down the inside of the index finger to its tip. **Signs:** Signs associated with the external course of the channel are: heat effusion and aversion to cold (with or without sweating), nasal congestion, headache, pain in the supraclavicular fossa, chest, shoulders, and back, and cold pain along the channel on the arm. Signs associated with the internal course of the channel are: cough, wheezing and panting, rapid breathing, fullness and oppression in the chest, expectoration of phlegm-drool, dry throat, change in urine color, heart vexation, spitting of blood, and heat in the palms. Other possible signs include fullness and distention in the abdomen and sloppy stool diarrhea. [6: 50] [27: 86] [97: 105]

hand lesser yang triple burner channel 手少阳三焦经 *shǒu shào yáng sān jiāo jīng*: Abbreviation: TB. One of the TWELVE CHANNELS; the channel that homes to the triple burner, nets the pericardiac network, and links with the ear and eye, and whose external pathway starts at the end of the ring finger, ascends the medial line of the extensor aspect line of the upper limb, across the shoulder, up the side of the neck, across the region of the ear to the eye. **Pathway:** The triple burner channel starts at the ulnar side of the tip of the fourth finger and travels up between the fourth and fifth metacarpal bones on the dorsum of the hand to the outside of the wrist. Proceeding up the posterior midline of the forearm between the radius and the ulna, it runs over the olecranon process of the elbow, and then travels up the posterior midline of the upper arm to the shoulder. Here, the channel meets the hand greater yang (*tài yáng*) small intestine channel at SI-12 (*bǐng fēng*, Grasping the Wind) and then runs over to the back to meet the governing (*dū*) vessel at GV-14 (*dà zhuī*, Great Hammer). It crosses back over the shoulder to intersect the foot lesser yang (*shào yáng*) gallbladder channel at GB-21 (*jiān jǐng*, Shoulder Well) before running into the supraclavicular fossa, penetrating internally at ST-12 (*quē pén*, Empty Basin) and traveling into the mid-chest region to meet the controlling (*rèn*) vessel at CV-17 (*shān zhōng*, Chest Center), where it links with the pericardium. It then descends internally, homing through each of the three burners successively. A branch breaks off from the mid-chest region at CV-17 (*shān zhōng*, Chest Center), rises to emerge in the supraclavicular fossa, then runs up the neck and behind the ear to intersect with the foot lesser yang (*shào yáng*) gallbladder channel at GB-6 (*xuán lí*, Suspended Tuft) and GB-14 (*yáng bái*, Yang White) on the forehead, before winding down around the cheek to return to the infraorbital region where it meets the hand greater yang (*tài yáng*) small intestine channel at SI-18 (*quán liáo*, Cheek Bone-Hole). Another branch separates behind the ear, enters the ear to reemerge in front of it, and intersects with the hand greater yang (*tài yáng*) small intestine channel at SI-19 (*tīng gōng*, Auditory Palace). It then crosses in front of the foot lesser yang (*shào yáng*) gallbladder channel at GB-3 (*shàng guān*, Upper Gate) and runs along the zygoma to terminate at the outer canthus at TB-23 (*sī zhú kōng*, Silk Bamboo Hole). *The Magic Pivot* (*líng shū*) adds that an internal branch descends from the triple burner to emerge at its lower uniting point, BL-53 (*bāo huāng*, Bladder Huang). **Signs:** Signs associated with the external course of the channel are: sore throat, pain in the cheeks, red eyes and pain, deafness; pain behind the ears and on the posterior aspect of the shoulder and upper arm. Signs associated with the internal course of the channel are: abdominal distention and fullness, or hardness and fullness in the lower abdomen; urinary frequency and distress, vacuity edema of the skin, water swelling, and enuresis. [6: 45] [27: 88] [97: 107]

hand lesser yin heart channel 手少阴心经 *shǒu shào yīn xīn jīng*: Abbreviation: HT. One of the TWELVE CHANNELS; the channel that homes to the heart, nets the small intestine, and links with the throat and eyes, and whose external pathway runs from the the armpit, down the posterior flexor aspect of the upper limb, to the end of the little finger. **Pathway:** The heart channel starts in the heart, and emerges through the blood vessels surrounding this organ. Traveling downward, it passes through the diaphragm to connect to the small intestine. Another branch separates from the heart, traveling upward along the side of the esophagus to meet the tissues surrounding the eye. A further channel separates from the heart and travels directly up into the lung, and then veers downward to emerge below the axilla. It travels down the medial aspect of the upper arm, medial to the hand greater yin (*tài yīn*) lung and hand reverting yin (*jué yīn*) pericardium channels, and passes over the antecubital fossa. It continues down the anteromedial margin of the forearm to the capitate bone on the wrist, traveling along the radial side of the fifth metacarpal bone to terminate at the tip of the little finger. **Signs:** Signs associated with the external course of the channel are: generalized heat EFFUSION, headache, eye pain, pain in the chest and back muscles, dry throat, thirst with the urge to drink, and hot or painful palms; reversal coldof the limbs; or pain in the scapular region and/or the medial aspect of the forearm. Signs associated with the internal course of the channel are: heart pain, fullness and pain in the chest and rib-side, pain in the hypochondriac region; heart vexation; rapid breathing, discomfort in lying posture, dizziness with fainting spells; and mental diseases. [6: 53] [27: 87] [97: 105]

hand reverting yin pericardium channel 手厥阴心包经 *shǒu jué yīn xīn bāo jīng*: Abbreviation: PC. One of the TWELVE CHANNELS; the channel that homes to the pericardiac network, nets the triple burner, and links with the diaphragm, and whose external pathway starts on the lateral aspect of the chest, runs through the armpit, down the midline of the extensor aspect of the upper limb, to the tip of the middle finger. **Pathway:** The foot reverting yin (*jué yīn*) pericardium channel starts in the chest, where it homes to the pericardium. Descending through the diaphragm into the abdomen, it connects successively to the upper, middle, and lower burners. A branch runs out horizontally from the center of the chest, emerges at the rib-side three body-inches below the anterior axillary fold, and then skirts around the axilla to the upper arm. The channel runs down the midline of the ventral aspect of the upper arm between the hand greater yin (*tài yīn*) lung channel and the hand lesser yin (*shào yīn*) heart channel, crosses the center of the cubital fossa and then proceeds down the forearm between the tendons of the palmaris longus and flexor carpi radialis muscles. It travels through the palm and along the ulnar aspect of the middle finger until it reaches the tip. Another branch separates in the palm and proceeds along the lateral aspect of the fourth finger to its tip. Signs: Signs associated with the external course of the channel are: stiffness of the neck, spasm in the limbs, red facial complexion, pain in the eyes, subaxillary swelling, hypertonicity of the elbow and arm inhibiting movement, and hot palms. Signs associated with the internal course of the channel are: delirious speech, CLOUDING REVERSAL, heart vexation, fullness and oppression in the chest and rib-side, heart palpitations, heart pain, constant laughing. [27: 86] [46: 58] [97: 108]

hand standard 一夫法 *yì fū fǎ*: From *A Thousand Gold Pieces Prescriptions* (*qiān jīn yào fāng*). The breadth of the hand at the creases of the middle joints when the fingers rest together, taken as a standard for calculating three body-inches. See BODY-INCH. [26: 1]

hand yang brightness large intestine channel 手阳明大肠经 *shǒu yáng míng dà cháng jīng*: Abbreviation: LI. One of the TWELVE CHANNELS. Pathway: The hand yang brightness (*yáng míng*) large intestine channel begins at the radial side of the tip of the index finger and proceeds upward between the first and second metacarpal bones of the hand and between the tendons of the extensor pollicis longus and brevis muscles at the wrist. It continues along the radial margin of the forearm to the radial margin of the lateral aspect of the elbow, then up the lateral aspect of the upper arm and over the shoulder joint. After intersecting the hand greater yang (*tài yáng*) channel at SI-12 (*bǐng fēng*, Grasping the Wind), the channel rises to just below the spinous process of the seventh cervical vertebra, and intersects with the governing (*dū*) vessel at GV-14 (*dà zhuī*, Great Hammer), where all six yang regular channels meet. It then travels straight into the supraclavicular fossa to ST-12, from where it connects through to the lung, passes through the diaphragm, and homes to the large intestine. A branch separates from the main channel at ST-12 (*quē pén*, Empty Basin) in the supraclavicular fossa, passes up the neck, and traverses the cheek before entering the lower gum. From here it skirts around the lips, passes the foot yang brightness (*yáng míng*) channel at ST-4 (*dì cāng*, Earth Granary), and then meets the same channel coming from the other side of the body at the philtrum. It then continues around the nostril of the opposite side to terminate at the side of the nose. In other words, right and left channels cross over at the philtrum and run for the last short stretch on the opposite side of the body from which they originated. *The Magic Pivot* (*líng shū*) describes yet another branch that separates from the

main channel at ST-12 (*quē pén*, Empty Basin), descends past ST-13 (*qì hù*, Qi Door) and penetrates the lung, passes through the diaphragm, homes to the large intestine, and descends to the lower limb to emerge at ST-37 (*shàng jù xū*, Upper Great Hollow), which is the lower uniting point of the large intestine. Signs: Signs associated with the external course of the channel are: heat effusion, parched dry mouth and thirst, sore throat, nosebleed, toothache, red sore eyes, swelling of the neck, palpable red swelling and inhibited bending and stretching of the fingers. There may also be pain, sensation of cold, or painful and palpably hot, red swelling in the region of the shoulder and upper arm. Signs associated with the internal course of the channel are: lower abdominal pain, wandering abdominal pain, rumbling intestines, sloppy stool, and excretion of thick, slimy yellow matter. There may also be rapid panting respiration. [6: 56] [27: 86] [97: 107] [44: 29]

harass 扰 *rǎo*: Trouble, worry, torment (as by phlegm and phlegm fire). "Harass" occurs in the terms PHLEGM-FIRE HARASSING THE HEART and PHLEGM TURBIDITY HARASSING THE UPPER BODY. See EXUBERANCE AND DEBILITATION. [27: 377] [97: 118]

hard glomus below the heart 心下痞硬 *xīn xià pǐ yìng*: Blockage and fullness below the heart (i.e., the pit of the stomach) with palpable hardness. Hard glomus between the stomach arises when evil heat causes obstruction in the stomach duct. [WMC] Hard glomus below the heart is commonly observed in acute gastroenteritis with indigestion. See GLOMUS. [27: 377]

hard glomus in the chest 胸中痞硬 *xiōng zhōng pǐ yìng*: From *On Cold Damage* (*shāng hán lùn*). Hard fullness and sense of blockage in the chest. Hard glomus in the chest is attributable to phlegm-drool obstructing the diaphragm and cold evil congesting the upper body. If there are signs of qi surging up into the throat and labored breathing, it can be treated by ejection with Melon Stalk Powder (*guā dì sǎn*) according to the principle of "what is high is brought up." See GLOMUS. [26: 548] [27: 377] [50: 1273]

hardness 坚 *jiān*: Any hard swelling or mass, treated by the method of softening.

hard tetany 刚痉 *gāng jìng*, 刚痓 *gāng cì* (*jìng*): A TETANY pattern characterized by heat effusion, absence of sweating, aversion to cold, rigidity of the neck, shaking heat, clenched jaw, and hypertonicity or convulsions of the extremities (in severe cases, arched-back rigidity), and a tight stringlike pulse. [MED] Use Duhuo and Pueraria Decoction (*dú huó gé gēn tāng*). Compare SOFT TETANY; YANG TETANY. [26: 528] [27: 373]

harelip 兔唇 *tù chún*: A congenitally cleft lip. Surgical treatment of this deformity was recorded in the Jin dynasty (A.D. 265–420). [26: 386]

harmonious flow of qi and blood 气血冲和 *qì xuè chōng hé*: Coordinated action and free movement of qi and the blood. Qi and blood are mutually dependent. Qi relies on the blood for nourishment, and the blood relies on qi for propulsion. Hence, it is traditionally said that QI IS THE COMMANDER OF THE BLOOD and BLOOD IS THE MOTHER OF QI. Harmonious flow of qi and blood is the maintenance of balance and harmony in this relationship. [26: 537]

harmonization 和法 *hé fǎ*, 和解法 *hé jiě fǎ*: One of the EIGHT METHODS. A method of adjusting functions within the human body, that is used when an evil is at midstage penetration or there is disharmony between qi and blood or between the organs, and such methods as sweating (diaphoresis), ejection, precipitation, warming, clearing, dispersion, and supplementation cannot be applied. The main forms of harmonization are listed below. [97: 359] [6: 254]

Harmonization

HARMONIZING LESSER YANG (*hé jiě shào yáng*)
RECTIFYING QI AND HARMONIZE CONSTRUCTION (*lǐ qì hé yíng*)
HARMONIZING THE LIVER AND STOMACH (*tiáo hé gān wèi*)
HARMONIZING THE LIVER AND SPLEEN (*tiáo hé gān pí*)
HARMONIZING THE STOMACH AND INTESTINES (*tiáo hé cháng wèi*)
INTERRUPTING MALARIA (*jié nüè*)

---

harmonize 和 *hé*, 和解 *hé jiě*, 调和 *tiáo hé*: To coordinate one element of the body with the rest of the body, e.g., HARMONIZING THE STOMACH and HARMONIZING THE LIVER, or coordinate two elements of the body, e.g., HARMONIZING THE LIVER AND STOMACH; HARMONIZING THE LIVER AND SPLEEN; HARMONIZING THE SPLEEN AND STOMACH; HARMONIZING THE STOMACH AND INTESTINES; HARMONIZING THE EXTERIOR AND INTERIOR (usually called HARMONIZING LESSER YANG); HARMONIZING CONSTRUCTION AND DEFENSE. All of these fall within the range of HARMONIZATION, with the exception of harmonizing construction and defense, which falls in the category of exterior resolution. See HARMONIZATION. [27: 249] [97: 495]

harmonizing construction and defense 调和营卫 *tiáo hé yíng wèi*: A method of treatment used to address construction-defense disharmony characterized by heat effusion, sweating, aversion to cold, noise in the nose, dry retching, and a weak floating pulse. [MED] The major formula for harmonizing construction-defense disharmony is Cinnamon Twig Decoction (*guì zhī tāng*), in which cinnamon twig (*guì zhī*) resolves the flesh and dispels wind, whereas peony (*sháo yào*) constrains yin, thereby bringing construction into harmony. [ACU] Base treatment mainly on GB, BL, SI, and ST. Needle with drainage at GB-20 (*fēng chí*, Wind Pool), GV-16 (*fēng fǔ*, Wind Mansion), GV-14 (*dà zhuī*, Great Hammer), and BL-64 (*jīng gǔ*, Capital Bone); needle with even supplementation and drainage at BL-62 (*shēn mài*, Extending Vessel), SI-3 (*hòu xī*, Back Ravine), and ST-36 (*zú sān lǐ*, Leg Three Li). See CONSTRUCTION-DEFENSE DISHARMONY. [26: 862] [75: 47]

harmonizing lesser yang 和解少阳 *hé jiě shào yáng*: Synonym: *harmonizing the exterior and interior*; *harmonizing midstage patterns*. A method of treatment used to resolve the exterior and harmonize the interior to treat lesser yang (*shào yáng*) midstage patterns in externally contracted heat (febrile) diseases, which are characterized by alternating heat EFFUSION and [aversion to] cold, oppression and fullness in the chest and rib-side region, bitter taste in the mouth and dry pharynx, and nausea and vomiting. [MED] The main medicinals used to harmonize lesser yang are bupleurum (*chái hú*) or sweet wormwood (*qīng hāo*), which outthrust exterior evils, combined with scutellaria (*huáng qín*), which clears interior heat. These are further combined with center-harmonizing medicinals such as pinellia (*bàn xià*), fresh ginger (*shēng jiāng*), licorice (*gān cǎo*), and jujube (*dà zǎo*). Vacuity of right qi may justify the judicious addition of medicinals such as codonopsis (*dǎng shēn*). Minor Bupleurum Decoction (*xiǎo chái hú tāng*), which in modern clinical practice is usually prescribed without ginseng (*rén shēn*), licorice (*gān cǎo*), and jujube (*dà zǎo*), is the standard decoction for clearing lesser yang (*shào yáng*) liver-gallbladder heat. Midstage patterns involving abdominal pain and distention and other yang brightness (*yáng míng*) bowel repletion signs may be treated with Major Bupleurum Decoction (*dà chái hú tāng*) or other formulas that contain draining precipitants such as rhubarb (*dà huáng*), mirabilite (*máng xiāo*), and unripe bitter orange (*zhǐ shí*). [ACU] Base treatment mainly on GB, TB, LR, and PC. Select GB-20 (*fēng chí*, Wind Pool), TB-5 (*wài guān*, Outer Pass), TB-4 (*yáng chí*, Yang Pool), PC-6 (*nèi guān*, Inner Pass), GB-40 (*qiū xū*, Hill Ruins), and LR-5 (*lǐ gōu*, Woodworm Canal); needle with even supplementation and drainage. [26: 382] [27: 259] [97: 359] [75: 209]

harmonizing midstage patterns 和解半表半里 *hé jiě bàn biǎo bàn lǐ*: HARMONIZING LESSER YANG.

harmonizing the blood and extinguishing wind 和血熄风 *hé xuè xī fēng*: A method of treatment used to treat liver wind stirring internally in patients with blood vacuity from damage to yin-blood in febrile disease characterized by parched lips and dry tongue, hypertonicity of the sinews, wriggling of the extremities, dizziness, and a rapid fine pulse. [MED] Commonly used blood-harmonizing wind-extinguishing medicinals include ass hide glue (*ē jiāo*), dried/fresh rehmannia (*shēng dì huáng*), raw white peony (*shēng bái sháo yào*), egg yolk (*jī zǐ huáng*), crude oyster shell (*shēng mǔ lì*), mix-fried licorice (*gān cǎo*), root poria (*fú shén*), and star jasmine stem (*luò shí téng*). See EXTINGUISHING WIND. [ACU] Base treatment mainly on back transport points, and points of the three yin channels of the foot and GB. Needle with supplementation at BL-20 (*pí shū*, Spleen Transport), BL-18 (*gān shū*, Liver Transport), BL-17 (*gé shū*, Diaphragm Transport), SP-6 (*sān yīn jiāo*, Three Yin Intersection), KI-6 (*zhào hǎi*, Shining Sea), and LR-8 (*qū quán*, Spring at the Bend), and with drainage at GV-20 (*bǎi huì*, Hundred Convergences), GB-20 (*fēng chí*, Wind Pool), LR-3 (*tài chōng*, Supreme Surge), and KI-1 (*yǒng quán*, Gushing Spring). See EXTINGUISHING WIND. [26: 382] [27: 268] [97: 359] [46: 596]

harmonizing the center 和中 *hé zhōng*: HARMONIZING THE STOMACH. [26: 382]

harmonizing the exterior and interior 和解表里 *hé jiě biǎo lǐ*: HARMONIZING LESSER YANG.

harmonizing the liver 和肝 *hé gān*: Synonym: *enriching yin and coursing the liver*. A method of treatment used to free the movement of liver qi using yin-enriching and liver-coursing medicinals in the treatment of liver-kidney yin vacuity with qi stagnation characterized by scurrying pain in the chest and rib-side, abdominal distention, no fluid on the tongue, dry throat, thin weak or vacuous stringlike pulse. [MED] A representative liver-harmonizing formula is All-the-Way-Through Brew (*yī guàn jiān*), comprising glehnia (*běi shā shēn*), ophiopogon (*mài mén dōng*), tangkuei body (*dāng guī shēn*), dried rehmannia (*gān dì huáng*), lycium berry (*gǒu qǐ zǐ*), and toosendan (*chuān liàn zǐ*), adding coptis (*huáng lián*) stir-fried in wine for dry mouth and bitter taste in the mouth. [ACU] Base treatment mainly on back transport points, KI, and LR. Select BL-18 (*gān shū*, Liver Transport), BL-23 (*shèn shū*, Kidney Transport), KI-3 (*tài xī*, Great Ravine), PC-6 (*nèi guān*, Inner Pass), LR-3 (*tài chōng*, Supreme Surge), SP-6 (*sān yīn jiāo*, Three Yin Intersection), and GB-34 (*yáng líng quán*, Yang Mound Spring); needle with supplementation. [27: 265] [46: 646]

harmonizing the liver and spleen 调和肝脾 *tiáo hé gān pí*: Synonym: *liver-spleen harmoniza-*

tion. A method of treatment used to address liver-spleen disharmony attributed to liver qi depression and impaired spleen movement and transformation and marked by such as abdominal distention, abdominal pain, rumbling intestines, and diarrhea, which occur in episodes association with emotional depression. [MED] Liver-coursing medicinals such as bupleurum (*chái hú*) and white peony (*bái sháo yào*) are combined with spleen-fortifying medicinals such as ovate atractylodes (*bái zhú*), poria (*fú líng*), and tangerine peel (*chén pí*). Formulas include Pain and Diarrhea Formula (*tòng xiè yào fāng*) and Free Wanderer Powder (*xiāo yáo sǎn*). [ACU] Base treatment mainly on back transport points, SP, and ST. Needle with supplementation at BL-20 (*pí shū*, Spleen Transport), CV-12 (*zhōng wǎn*, Center Stomach Duct), LR-13 (*zhāng mén*, Camphorwood Gate), ST-36 (*zú sān lǐ*, Leg Three Li), SP-3 (*tài bái*, Supreme White), and SP-6 (*sān yīn jiāo*, Three Yin Intersection), and with drainage or with even supplementation and drainage at BL-18 (*gān shū*, Liver Transport), LR-14 (*qī mén*, Cycle Gate), PC-6 (*nèi guān*, Inner Pass), LR-3 (*tài chōng*, Supreme Surge), and GB-34 (*yáng líng quán*, Yang Mound Spring). [27: 259] [97: 494] [46: 602, 646] [37: 318, 324]

harmonizing the liver and stomach 调和肝胃 *tiáo hé gān wèi*: A method of treatment used to address disharmony between the liver and stomach from impaired liver free coursing and stomach qi downbearing, characterized by the classic liver sign of distending pain in the chest and rib-side, and by stomach signs such as pain, fullness, and distention in the stomach duct, poor appetite, belching, vomiting of sour matter, or retching and nausea. [MED] Liver-coursing medicinals such as evodia (*wú zhū yú*) and perilla (*zǐ sū*) are used in combination with stomach-harmonizing medicinals such as pinellia (*bàn xià*) or fresh ginger (*shēng jiāng*), or with stomach heat-clearing medicinals such as coptis (*huáng lián*) and bamboo shavings (*zhú rú*). The emphasis may be variously placed on coursing the liver, harmonizing the stomach, or clearing the stomach, depending on the nature of the pattern. Four-Seven Decoction (*sì qī tāng*) is prescribed for conditions with prominent depression of liver qi, whereas Left-Restoring [Kidney Yin] Pill (*zuǒ guī wán*) are used to treat patterns in which impaired harmonious downflow of stomach qi is prominent. [ACU] Base treatment mainly on ST, LR, and PC. Needle with supplementation at BL-21 (*wèi shū*, Stomach Transport), CV-12 (*zhōng wǎn*, Center Stomach Duct), ST-36 (*zú sān lǐ*, Leg Three Li), ST-25 (*tiān shū*, Celestial Pivot), and SP-6 (*sān yīn jiāo*, Three Yin Intersection), and with drainage or with even supplementation and drainage at BL-18 (*gān shū*, Liver Transport), PC-6 (*nèi guān*, Inner Pass), LR-3 (*tài chōng,* Supreme Surge), LR-14 (*qī mén,* Cycle Gate), ST-25 (*tiān shū,* Celestial Pivot), and GB-34 (*yáng líng quán,* Yang Mound Spring). [27: 260] [46: 602, 646] [37: 314, 324] [46: 578]

harmonizing the spleen and stomach 调和脾胃 *tiáo hé pí wèi*: FORTIFYING THE SPLEEN AND HARMONIZING THE STOMACH.

harmonizing the stomach 和胃 *hé wèi*: Synonym: *harmonizing the center.* A method of treatment used to address stomach qi disharmony characterized by distention and oppression in the stomach duct, belching, vomiting of sour fluid, and pale tongue with white fur. MED Stomach-harmonizing medicinals include tangerine peel (*chén pí*), ginger pinellia (*jiāng bàn xià*), saussurea (*mù xiāng*), and amomum (*shā rén*). Use formulas such as Stomach-Calming Powder (*píng wèi sǎn*). ACU Base treatment mainly on ST and PC. Select ST-36 (*zú sān lǐ,* Leg Three Li), PC-6 (*nèi guān,* Inner Pass), CV-12 (*zhōng wǎn,* Center Stomach Duct), ST-25 (*tiān shū,* Celestial Pivot), and CV-6 (*qì hǎi,* Sea of Qi). Needle with even supplementation and drainage. [26: 382] [97: 359] [46: 602, 578]

harmonizing the stomach and checking vomiting 和胃止呕 *hé wèi zhǐ ǒu*: See CHECKING VOMITING; HARMONIZING THE STOMACH.

harmonizing the stomach and downbearing qi 和胃降气 *hè wèi jiàng qì*: See HARMONIZING THE STOMACH.

harmonizing the stomach and intestines 调和肠胃 *tiáo hé cháng wèi*: A method of treatment used to address gastrointestinal disharmony with disrupted upbearing and downbearing and cold-heat complexes presenting with glomus and fullness below the heart, vomiting, rumbling intestines, and diarrhea. MED Cold bitter medicinals such as coptis (*huáng lián*) and scutellaria (*huáng qín*) are used with warm acrid medicinals such as dried ginger (*gān jiāng*) and pinellia (*bàn xià*). The cold bitter medicinals drain heat, while the acrid medicinals dissipate glomus, and together have the effect of harmonizing the center burner and restoring normal upbearing and downbearing. A representative formula for harmonizing the stomach and intestines is Pinellia Heart-Draining Decoction (*bàn xià xiè xīn tāng*). ACU Base treatment on CV and ST. Select CV-12 (*zhōng wǎn,* Center Stomach Duct), ST-25 (*tiān shū,* Celestial Pivot), CV-6 (*qì hǎi,* Sea of Qi), ST-36 (*zú sān lǐ,* Leg Three Li), and PC-6 (*nèi guān,* Inner Pass). Needle with even supplementation and drainage. [6: 256]

harmonizing the stomach and rectifying qi 和胃理气 *hé wèi lǐ qì*: Synonym: *rectifying qi and harmonizing the stomach.* A method of treatment used to address qi and phlegm-damp stag-

nating in the stomach duct, characterized by distention and oppression in the stomach duct, swallowing of upflowing acid, vomiting of sour fluid, and belching. MED Commonly used stomach-harmonizing qi-rectifying medicinals include unripe bitter orange (*zhǐ shí*), tangerine peel (*chén pí*), ginger pinellia (*jiāng bàn xià*), bamboo shavings (*zhú rú*), and calcined ark shell (*duàn wǎ léng zǐ*). ACU Base treatment mainly on ST, PC, CV, and SP. Main points: ST-36 (*zú sān lǐ,* Leg Three Li), PC-6 (*nèi guān,* Inner Pass), and ST-25 (*tiān shū,* Celestial Pivot); needle with even supplementation and drainage. For qi stagnation, drain CV-6 (*qì hǎi,* Sea of Qi) and LR-3 (*tài chōng,* Supreme Surge). For phlegm evil, add CV-12 (*zhōng wǎn,* Center Stomach Duct), ST-40 (*fēng lóng,* Bountiful Bulge), and LI-4 (*hé gǔ,* Union Valley), adding moxa. For dampness evil, add SP-9 (*yīn líng quán,* Yin Mound Spring) and LI-4 (*hé gǔ,* Union Valley) and moxa. [26: 382] [97: 359]

harmonizing the stomach and resolving liquor 和胃解醒 *hé wèi jiě chéng*: HARMONIZING THE STOMACH AND RESTORING SOBERNESS.

harmonizing the stomach and restoring soberness 和胃醒酒 *hé wèi xǐng jiǔ*: A method of treatment used to dispel the effects of liquor and relieve the nausea, vomiting, and retching that it causes. MED A representative stomach-harmonizing soberness-restoring formula is Pueraria Flower Liquor-Resolving Decoction (*gé huā jiě chéng tāng*).

harmonizing the stomach and transforming phlegm 和胃化痰 *hé wèi huà tán*: A method of treatment used to address cough with copious phlegm, oppression in the chest, nausea and vomiting, dizziness, insomnia, and heart palpitations. MED Use phlegm-transforming medicinals such as pinellia (*bàn xià*), tangerine peel (*chén pí*), and poria (*fú líng*). Damp turbidity harassing the upper body, characterized by dizziness and headache, is treated with ovate atractylodes (*bái zhú*) and gastrodia (*tiān má*). When manifesting as insomnia and heart palpitations, unripe bitter orange (*zhǐ shí*) and bamboo shavings (*zhú rú*) are often added. A representative formula is Two Matured Ingredients Decoction (*èr chén tāng*). ACU Base treatment mainly on LU, ST, CV, and back transport points. Select BL-13 (*fèi shū,* Lung Transport), LU-9 (*tài yuān,* Great Abyss), LI-4 (*hé gǔ,* Union Valley), ST-36 (*zú sān lǐ,* Leg Three Li), CV-12 (*zhōng wǎn,* Center Stomach Duct), BL-20 (*pí shū,* Spleen Transport), BL-21 (*wèi shū,* Stomach Transport) and ST-40 (*fēng lóng,* Bountiful Bulge). Needle with even supplementation and drainage. See DRYING DAMPNESS AND TRANSFORMING PHLEGM. [46: 586, 597, 653]

harmony of mouth 口中和 *kǒu zhōng hé*: A normal taste in the mouth and absence of dryness and thirst or sliminess. Harmony of mouth is observed in healthy individuals, and in patients suffering from mild disease. See TASTE IN THE MOUTH. [27: 187] [97: 31]

hasty breathing 气促 *qì cù*: Rapid breathing with short breaths. See SHORTNESS OF BREATH; PANTING. [50: 274]

hasty panting 喘促 *chuǎn cù*: See PANTING.

hauling the boat upstream 逆流挽舟 *nì liú wǎn zhōu*: A method of treatment used to address DYSENTERY due to externally contracted evil complicated by dampness, which, in addition to the main signs of dysentery (tenesmus and the passing of blood and stool), is marked by exterior signs such as aversion to cold, heat effusion, headache, generalized pain, and absence of sweating. The method of hauling the boat upstream is so named because it treats conditions of inward fall from the exterior by bringing the evil back out of the interior like hauling a boat upstream. MED Use Ginseng Toxin-Vanquishing Powder (*rén shēn bài dú sǎn*). This formula courses the exterior and eliminates dampness. It combines a dissipating action with a freeing action so that it resolves the exterior and eliminates the interior stagnation. This formula is very dry and acrid, and should only be used when the classic signs present. [26: 495] [27: 251] [97: 440] [46: 667] [75: 62]

head 头 *tóu*: The uppermost part of the body that contains the brain, and houses the FIVE OFFICES (nose, eyes, lips, tongue, and ears), which partly overlap with the SEVEN ORIFICES, the two eyes, two ears, two nostrils, and the mouth. The head is the confluence of the yang channels and the dwelling place of bright essence. See FACE; FACIAL COMPLEXION; EAR; NOSE; MOUTH; HAIR; SPIRIT; TONGUE; THROAT; TEETH. Diseases affecting the head are listed under DISEASE. [26: 906]

headache 头痛 *tóu tòng*, 头疼 *tóu téng*: Pain in the head. The head is the confluence of yang, and the brain is the house of clear essence. Distinction is also made between MEDIAL HEADACHE and HEMILATERAL HEADACHE, although the term headache usually refers to medial headache. The qi and blood of the five viscera and six bowels ascend to the head. Headache may be attributable to the six excesses or to internal damage, and arises by pathomechanisms such as obstruction of yang qi, lodging of turbid evil in the upper body, ascendant liver yang, and essence-marrow or qi-blood depletion, etc. The nature, severity, and duration of headaches are all important factors in diagnosis. New headaches (headaches of recent onset) often indicate external disease. Distinction is also made according to the exact location of the pain.

The location of the headache can show which channel is affected, and hence which channel should be treated. **Greater yang** (*tài yáng*) **headache:** Pain reaches from the head down the neck and back. **Yang brightness** (*yáng míng*) **headache:** Pain in the anterior forehead, sometimes stretching down to the eyebrow bone (superciliary arch). **Lesser yang** (*shào yáng*) **headache:** Pain on the sides of the head or in the temporal region. **Greater yin** (*tài yīn*) **headache:** Pain and heaviness in the head accompanied by abdominal fullness and spontaneous sweating. **Lesser yin** (*shào yīn*) **headache:** Pain stretching into the teeth and deep into the brain. **Reverting yin** (*jué yīn*) **headache:** Pain at the vertex stretching to the corners of the forehead, accompanied by a subjective feeling of counterflow qi ascent with retching in severe cases.

Headache

External contraction
COMMON COLD HEADACHE (*gǎn mào tóu tòng*)
WIND-COLD HEADACHE (*fēng hán tóu tòng*)
WIND-HEAT HEADACHE (*fēng rè tóu tòng*)
WIND-DAMP HEADACHE (*fēng shī tóu tòng*)

Internal damage
QI VACUITY HEADACHE (*qì xū tóu tòng*)
YANG VACUITY HEADACHE (*yáng xū tóu tòng*)
BLOOD VACUITY HEADACHE (*xuè xū tóu tòng*)
YIN VACUITY HEADACHE (*yīn xū tóu tòng*)
LIVER YANG HEADACHE (*gān yáng tóu tòng*)
FOOD DAMAGE HEADACHE (*shāng shí tóu tòng*)
LIQUOR DAMAGE HEADACHE (*shāng jiǔ tóu tòng*)

Six-Channel
GREATER YANG HEADACHE (*tài yáng tóu tòng*)
YANG BRIGHTNESS HEADACHE (*yáng míng tóu tòng*)
LESSER YANG HEADACHE (*shào yáng tóu tòng*)
GREATER YIN HEADACHE (*tài yīn tóu tòng*)
LESSER YIN HEADACHE (*shào yīn tóu tòng*)
REVERTING YIN HEADACHE (*jué yīn tóu tòng*)

Miscellaneous
TRUE HEADACHE (*zhēn tóu tòng*)
HEAD WIND (*tóu fēng*)
HEMILATERAL HEADACHE (*piān tóu tòng*)
THUNDER HEAD WIND (*léi tóu fēng*)
BRAIN WIND (*nǎo fēng*)
VERTEX HEADACHE (*diān dǐng tóu tòng*)

ACU Select points given under individual types and add the following points according to the location of pain. For frontal headache, add GV-23 (*shàng xīng*, Upper Star), GB-14 (*yáng bái*, Yang White), and ST-41 (*jiě xī*, Ravine Divide). For hemilateral headache, add Greater Yang (*tài yáng*), GB-8 (*shuài gǔ*, Valley Lead), and TB-5 (*wài guān*, Outer Pass). For posterior headache, add BL-10 (*tiān zhù*, Celestial Pillar), BL-9 (*yù zhěn*, Jade Pillow), and BL-65 (*shù gǔ*, Bundle Bone). For vertex headache, add GV-20 (*bǎi huì*, Hundred Convergences), Alert Spirit Quartet (*sì shén cōng*), and LR-3 (*tài chōng*, Supreme Surge). For eyebrow pain, add BL-2 (*zǎn zhú*, Bamboo Gathering). and Fish's Lumbus (*yú yāo*). [26: 909] [27: 391] [97: 165]

headache and stiff painful nape 头项强痛 *tóu xiàng qiáng tòng*: A condition usually caused by obstruction of the channels by an externally contracted evils (the six excesses), usually forming exterior patterns. Occurring in enduring disease, it is a sign of wind-damp impediment (*bì*). MED Treat exterior patterns by effusing and dissipating exterior resolution. Treat wind-damp impediment by dispelling wind-damp and freeing the channels and network vessels. ACU Select GV-16 (*fēng fǔ*, Wind Mansion), GB-20 (*fēng chí*, Wind Pool), LI-4 (*hé gǔ*, Union Valley), LU-7 (*liè quē*, Broken Sequence), and ST-8 (*tóu wéi*, Head Corner). Needle with drainage. [26: 910] [97: 165]

headache with pulling sensation 头痛如掣 *tóu tòng rú chè*: Synonym: *iron-band headache*. HEADACHE characterized by pressure or tension as though the head were squeezed by a tight iron band. Headache with pulling sensation is observed in LIVER WIND STIRRING INTERNALLY. [6: 188]

headed flat-abscess 有头疽 *yǒu tóu jū*: Synonym: *flat-abscess*. A yang-type sore on the surface of the body. A headed flat-abscess is characterized in the initial stage by single or multiple white sores the size of millet seeds. Headed flat-abscesses may be named according to its location, e.g., EFFUSION OF THE BRAIN or EFFUSION OF THE BACK. They are caused by external contraction of wind-damp fire toxin, or damp-heat fire toxin brewing in the interior causing accumulation of heat in the viscera, construction-defense disharmony, and evil causing blockage in the flesh and skin. Distinction is made between vacuity and repletion. **Repletion:** Repletion patterns are characterized by local redness and heat, a large swelling with one or several white heads, pain that in severe cases is acute, generalized heat [effusion], thirst, constipation, reddish urine, a surging rapid pulse, and a red tongue with yellow fur. MED Clear heat and course wind; resolve toxin and quicken the blood. Immortal Formula Life-Giving Beverage (*xiān fāng huó mìng yǐn*) or Coptis Toxin-Resolving Decoction (*huáng lián jiě dú tāng*) can be taken as oral medication; Golden Yellow Powder (*jīn huáng sǎn*) can be applied topically. If, after bursting, the putrid flesh does not disappear, Five-to-Five Elixir (*wǔ wǔ dān*) can be used. If, after elimination of the putrid flesh, a bright red wound is left, Flesh-Engendering Powder (*shēng jī sǎn*)

or Flesh-Engendering Jade and Red Paste (*shēng jī yù hóng gāo*) can be prescribed. **Vacuity:** The sore is flat with a diffuse root, dark and dull in color, only mildly painful at onset; it is slow to suppurate and exudes clear thin pus, and is associated with lassitude of spirit and reduced food intake, lusterless complexion, a forceless rapid pulse, and crimson or pale tongue. MED Treatment differs depending on whether yin vacuity or dual vacuity of qi and blood is more pronounced. For yin vacuity, use Bamboo Leaf and Astragalus Decoction (*zhú yè huáng qí tāng*) from *The Golden Mirror of Medicine* (*yī zōng jīn jiàn*), which consists of ginseng (*rén shēn*), raw astragalus (*shēng huáng qí*), gypsum (*shí gāo*), pinellia (*bàn xià*), ophiopogon (*mài mén dōng*), white peony (*bái sháo yào*), licorice (*gān cǎo*), ligusticum (*chuān xiōng*), tangkuei (*dāng guī*), scutellaria (*huáng qín*), dried/fresh rehmannia (*shēng dì huáng*), and bitter bamboo leaf (*kǔ zhú yè*). For qi-blood vacuity, use Internal Expression Toxin-Dispersing Powder (*tuō lǐ xiāo dú sǎn*). If a headed flat-abscess is not treated or is mistreated, the toxic evil may fall inward to form a FALL PATTERN. [26: 255]

head fire cinnabar 抱头火丹 *bào tóu huǒ dān*: Cinnabar toxin affecting the head. See CINNABAR TOXIN. [97: 334]

head heavy as if swathed 头重如裹 *tóu zhòng rú guǒ*: Heavy-headedness characterized by a feeling of encumbrance, as though the head were swathed in cloth or bandages. See HEAVY-HEADEDNESS. ◇ Chin 头 *tóu*, head; 重 *zhòng*, heavy; 如 *rú*, like, as if; 裹 *guǒ*, bandage(d), wrap(ped). [6: 132]

headless flat-abscess 无头疽 *wú tóu jū*: A yin sore growing between sinew and bone or deep in the flesh. A headless flat-abscesses are attributed to the inward fall of toxin, congealing cold and stagnant qi, and are characterized by diffuse swelling and dull skin coloring. They are persistent, take a long time to burst and a long time to heal, and can cause rotting of the sinew and flesh. MED Warm the channels and dissipate cold; quicken the blood and transform stasis. Take Harmonious Yang Decoction (*yáng hé tāng*), Awake to Dispersion Pill (*xǐng xiāo wán*), or Minor Golden Elixir (*xiǎo jīn dān*) orally and apply Harmonious Yang Decongealing Plaster (*yáng hé jiě níng gāo*) topically. The headless flat-abscess includes BONE FLAT-ABSCESS and FLOWING PHLEGM. See also FLAT-ABSCESS; SORE. [26: 744]

head marrow 头髓 *tóu suǐ*: BRAIN.

head wind 头风 *tóu fēng*: **1.** Persistent remittent, usually intense headache attributed to wind-cold or wind-heat invasion and obstruction of the channels by phlegm or static blood. Head wind may be accompanied by various other signs such as eye pain and loss of vision, runny nose, nausea, or dizziness, numbness of the head, or stiffness of the neck. [MED] Treat mainly by dispelling wind and freeing the network vessels, adding cold-dispelling, fire-clearing, phlegm-transforming, and stasis-expelling action as needed. Formulas used include Wind-Dispersing Powder (*xiāo fēng sǎn*), Ligusticum and Asarum Phlegm-Abducting Decoction (*xiōng xīn dǎo tán tāng*) and House of Blood Stasis-Expelling Decoction (*xuè fǔ zhú yū tāng*) and variations. Head wind on one side of the head is called HEMILATERAL HEAD WIND, whereas head wind of the temples with pain penetrating into the brain is called BRAIN-SQUEEZING WIND. Furthermore, PHLEGM REVERSAL HEADACHE, KIDNEY REVERSAL HEADACHE, and DAMP-HEAT HEADACHE can also be considered as a head wind when they have persisted over prolonged periods. [WMC] Head wind is often observed in what modern medicine calls glaucoma, migraine, vascular headache, rhinitis, paranasal sinusitis, brain tumors, and nervous headache. [ACU] Base treatment mainly on points of the three yang channels, GV, and LU. Main points: GB-20 (*fēng chí*, Wind Pool), GV-20 (*bǎi huì*, Hundred Convergences), Greater Yang (*tài yáng*), LI-4 (*hé gǔ*, Union Valley), LU-7 (*liè quē*, Broken Sequence), and SI-3 (*hòu xī*, Back Ravine). Selection of points according to causes: For wind-cold, add GV-16 (*fēng fǔ*, Wind Mansion) and TB-5 (*wài guān*, Outer Pass), and needle with even supplementation and drainage and add moxa. For wind-heat, add GV-14 (*dà zhuī*, Great Hammer) and LI-11 (*qū chí*, Pool at the Bend), needling with even supplementation and drainage. For phlegm depression and blood stasis, add ouch points (*ā shì xué*), ST-40 (*fēng lóng*, Bountiful Bulge), CV-12 (*zhōng wǎn*, Center Stomach Duct), SP-9 (*yīn líng quán*, Yin Mound Spring), SP-6 (*sān yīn jiāo*, Three Yin Intersection), and BL-17 (*gé shū*, Diaphragm Transport), needling with drainage and, if appropriate, add moxa. Selection of points according to signs: For eye pain, add BL-2 (*zǎn zhú*, Bamboo Gathering) and GV-23 (*shàng xīng*, Upper Star). For runny nose with malodorous snivel, add LI-20 (*yíng xiāng*, Welcome Fragrance) and GV-26 (*shuǐ gōu*, Water Trough). For nausea, add ST-36 (*zú sān lǐ*, Leg Three Li) and PC-6 (*nèi guān*, Inner Pass). For tinnitus, add TB-17 (*yì fēng*, Wind Screen), TB-3 (*zhōng zhǔ*, Central Islet), TB-21 (*ěr mén*, Ear Gate), and SI-19 (*tīng gōng*, Auditory Palace). For hemilateral head wind, add Greater Yang (*tài yáng*) joining GB-8 (*shuài gǔ*, Valley Lead). For brain-squeezing wind, add GV-22 (*xìn huì*, Fontanel Meeting), KI-3 (*tài xī*, Great Ravine), and GV-23 (*shàng xīng*, Upper Star). For selection of points according to affected area, see HEADACHE. **2.** Any condition characterized by the contraction of wind evil in the head

and that causes headache, dizziness, deviated eyes and mouth, itching and scaling of the scalp, etc. [26: 906] [27: 392] [97: 164]

head-wind white scaling 头风白屑 *tóu fēng bái xiè*: WHITE SCALING WIND.

hearing impairment 重听 *zhòng tīng*: Poor hearing with incorrect perception of sounds. See DEAFNESS. [26: 443]

heart 心 *xīn*: **1.** Abbreviation: HT. The organ located in the chest, and surrounded by the pericardium. The heart governs the blood and vessels, stores the spirit, and opens at the tongue. Its associated channel connects with the small intestine, which is its corresponding exterior organ. It belongs to fire in the five phases. The heart's principal functions are summed up in the phrases the HEART GOVERNS THE BLOOD AND VESSELS and the HEART STORES THE SPIRIT, i.e., the heart is responsible for moving the blood around the body and is the seat of consciousness and mental vitality. The importance of the heart and spirit is emphasized in *The Magic Pivot* (*líng shū*), where it states, "The heart is governor of the five viscera and the six bowels, and is the abode of the spirit," and in *Elementary Questions* (*sù wèn, líng lán mì diǎn lùn*), which states, "heart holds the office of monarch, whence the spirit light emanates." The HEART GOVERNS THE TONGUE, (or the *heart is the sprout of the tongue*) i.e., some diseases are reflected in reddening of the tip of the tongue. The HEART GOVERNS SPEECH, i.e., clear speech is only possible when the heart spirit is unclouded. Finally, the HEART GOVERNS SWEAT and HEART, ITS BLOOM IS IN THE FACE. For the main disease patterns of the heart, see HEART DISEASE. **2.** The heart [region], i.e., the upper stomach duct (the upper part of the stomach and lower section of the esophagus). ◇ Chin The character 心 *xīn* is a pictographic representation of the heart. [26: 89] [27: 17] [97: 116]

heart accumulation 心积 *xīn jī*: DEEP-LYING BEAM. [26: 94]

heart and kidney interact 心肾相交 *xīn shèn xiāng jiāo*: The heart and kidney balance and complement each other. The heart is in the upper burner, and belongs to fire. The kidney is in the lower burner and belongs to water. The yang in the heart descends to the kidney to warm and nourish kidney yang. The yin of the kidney ascends to the heart, and nourishes heart yin. Under normal circumstances, heart fire and kidney water interact in this way and maintain a balance. This is referred to as the heart and kidney interacting, or fire and water aiding each other. Kidney yin depletion or intense heart fire can upset this balance, causing signs such as heart vexation, fearful throbbing, and insomnia, a pattern referred to as noninteraction of the heart and kidney. [27: 121]

heart and small intestine stand in interior-exterior relationship 心与小肠相表里 *xīn yǔ xiǎo cháng xiāng biǎo lǐ*: See HEART IS CONNECTED WITH THE SMALL INTESTINE. [26: 94]

heart blood 心血 *xīn xuè*: See HEART QI AND HEART BLOOD.

heart blood vacuity 心血虚 *xīn xuè xū*: The manifestation of insufficiency of HEART BLOOD; a disease pattern characterized by disquieting of the heart spirit and yin-blood insufficiency. It may occur when fire forming as a result of excess among the five minds (emotions) damages yin, or when enduring illness causes damaging wear on yin-blood. Heart blood vacuity is often accompanied by signs of spleen vacuity, and the combined pattern is known as HEART-SPLEEN BLOOD VACUITY. The chief signs of heart blood vacuity are heart palpitations or fearful throbbing, insomnia, profuse dreaming, and forgetfulness. Other signs include dizziness, a lusterless withered-yellow or pale white complexion, pale lips, and night sweating. The tongue is pale white. The pulse is fine and weak or fine and rapid. **Analysis:** The heart stores the spirit and governs the blood and vessels. When heart blood is insufficient, it fails to nourish the heart, hence the heart palpitations or fearful throbbing. When blood fails to nourish the heart, the spirit does not keep to its abode, hence the insomnia and profuse dreaming. When blood fails to nourish the brain, there is dizziness and forgetfulness. When blood does not ascend to nourish to the face, lips, and tongue, there is a lusterless withered-yellow or pale white facial complexion, and pale lips and tongue. When heart blood is insufficient, the vessels are not full, and the pulse is fine and weak. Blood vacuity means that the whole body is improperly nourished. Through the body's self-regulating action, the heart can try to compensate for this by speeding up, hence the forceless fine rapid pulse. Blood failing to nourish the heart causes spirit qi to float astray, giving rise to night sweating. WMC nutritional disturbance, neurosis, tachycardia, arrhythmia, anemia, and hyperthyroidism. MED Nourish the blood and quiet the spirit. Use Four Agents Decoction (*sì wù tāng*). ACU Base treatment mainly on back transport points, HT, PC, and CV. Select BL-15 (*xīn shū*, Heart Transport), BL-17 (*gé shū*, Diaphragm Transport), CV-14 (*jù què*, Great Tower Gate), SP-6 (*sān yīn jiāo*, Three Yin Intersection), CV-6 (*qì hǎi*, Sea of Qi), HT-7 (*shén mén*, Spirit Gate), and PC-6 (*nèi guān*, Inner Pass); needle with supplementation and moxa. [27: 146] [97: 120] [6: 172] [37: 332, 347] [46: 586, 648]

heart blood vacuity sleeplessness 心血虚不得卧 *xīn xuè xū bù dé wò*: Internal damage SLEEPLESSNESS resulting from wear on heart blood by excessive thinking. Heart blood vacuity insomnia is characterized by awakening with fright during the night and is associated with vexing heat in the five hearts, dry mouth and tongue, and rapid fine pulse. MED Use formulas such as Celestial Emperor Heart-Supplementing Elixir (*tiān wáng bǔ xīn dān*). ACU Base treatment mainly on HT, back transport points, and the three yin channels of the foot. Select Alert Spirit Quartet (*sì shén cōng*), HT-7 (*shén mén*, Spirit Gate), SP-6 (*sān yīn jiāo*, Three Yin Intersection), BL-15 (*xīn shū*, Heart Transport), BL-20 (*pí shū*, Spleen Transport), BL-17 (*gé shū*, Diaphragm Transport), and LR-3 (*tài chōng*, Supreme Surge). Needle with supplementation. See SLEEPLESSNESS. [26: 91]

heart channel 心经 *xīn jīng*: HAND LESSER YIN HEART CHANNEL. [26: 95]

heart channel cough 心经咳嗽 *xīn jīng ké sòu*: HEART COUGH. [26: 95]

heart construction 心营 *xīn yíng*: HEART YIN. See EXCESSIVE WEARING OF HEART CONSTRUCTION.

heart cough 心咳 *xīn ké*: *Synonym: heart channel cough.* COUGH accompanied by pain in the heart, swollen throat. MED Use Platycodon Decoction (*jié gěng tāng*) or Diaphragm-Cooling Powder (*liáng gé sǎn*) minus rhubarb (*dà huáng*) and mirabilite (*máng xiāo*) and plus coptis (*huáng lián*) and bamboo leaf (lophatherum) (*dàn zhú yè*). ACU Base treatment mainly on LU, PC, CV, and HT. Select BL-13 (*fèi shū*, Lung Transport), LU-5 (*chǐ zé*, Cubit Marsh), CV-17 (*shān zhōng*, Chest Center), PC-6 (*nèi guān*, Inner Pass) CV-14 (*jù què*, Great Tower Gate), LU-1 (*zhōng fǔ*, Central Treasury), LI-4 (*hé gǔ*, Union Valley), and PC-8 (*láo gōng*, Palace of Toil); needle with drainage, and prick LU-11 (*shào shāng*, Lesser Shang) and HT-8 (*shào fǔ*, Lesser Mansion) to bleed. [97: 117] [26: 96] [27: 379]

heart-covering bone 蔽心骨 *bì xīn gǔ*: The bone that covers the heart (see HEART[1,2]), i.e., TURTLEDOVE'S TAIL (xiphoid process) or the BREASTBONE (sternum) as a whole. [27: 68] [97: 620]

heart disease 心病 *xīn bìng*: A disease of the heart. The main functions of the heart are to govern the blood and vessels and to govern the spirit; hence heart disease manifests primarily in signs such as heart palpitations or fearful throbbing, heart pain, oppression in the chest and shortness of breath on the one hand, and signs such as forgetfulness, abstraction (absence of mind), flusteredness, insomnia, and susceptibility to fright on the other. Heart disease patterns are listed below.

Heart disease patterns

Simple patterns

   HEART QI VACUITY (*xīn qì xū*)

   HEART YANG VACUITY (*xīn yáng xū*)

   HEART BLOOD VACUITY (*xīn xuè xū*)

   HEART YIN VACUITY (*xīn yīn xū*)

   DUAL VACUITY OF HEART QI AND BLOOD (*xīn qì xuè liǎng xū*)

   DUAL VACUITY OF HEART YIN AND YANG (*xīn yīn yáng liǎng xū*)

   FULMINANT DESERTION OF HEART YANG (*xīn yáng bào tuō*)

   HEART HEAT (*xīn rè*)

   HEART FIRE (*xīn huǒ*)

   HYPERACTIVE HEART FIRE (*xīn huǒ kàng shèng*)

   INTENSE INTERNAL HEART FIRE (*xīn huǒ nèi chì*)

   HEART FIRE FLAMING UPWARD (*xīn huǒ shàng yán*)

   HEART IMPEDIMENT (*xīn bì*)

   HEART VESSEL STASIS OBSTRUCTION (*xīn mài bì zǔ*)

   NONINTERACTION OF THE HEART AND KIDNEY (*xīn shèn bù jiāo*)

   PHLEGM FIRE HARASSING THE HEART (*tán huǒ rǎo xin*)

   PHLEGM CONFOUNDING THE ORIFICES OF THE HEART (*tán mí xīn qiào*)

   WATER QI INTIMIDATING THE HEART (*shuǐ qì níng xīn*)

Combined patterns

   HEART-LUNG QI VACUITY (*xīn fèi qì xū*)

   HEART-LUNG YANG VACUITY (*xīn fèi yáng xū*)

   HEART-LUNG YIN VACUITY (*xīn fèi yīn xū*)

   DUAL VACUITY OF THE HEART AND SPLEEN (*xīn pí liǎng xū*)

   HEART-SPLEEN QI VACUITY (*xīn pí qì xū*)

   HEART-SPLEEN BLOOD VACUITY (*xīn pí xuè xū*)

   HEART-SPLEEN YANG VACUITY (*xīn pí yáng xū*)

   HEART-LIVER BLOOD VACUITY (*xīn gān xuè xū*)

   EXUBERANT HEART-LIVER FIRE (*xīn gān huǒ wàng*)

   HEART-KIDNEY QI VACUITY (*xīn shèn qì xū*)

   HEART-KIDNEY YANG VACUITY (*xīn shèn yáng xū*)

   NONINTERACTION OF THE HEART AND KIDNEY (*xīn shèn bù jiāo*)

   HEART-KIDNEY YIN VACUITY (*xīn shèn yīn xū*)

   HEART-KIDNEY QI VACUITY (*xīn shèn qì xū*)

   EXUBERANT HEART-STOMACH FIRE (*xīn wèi huǒ shèng*)

Of these, the most important basic patterns are heart blood vacuity, heart yin vacuity, heart qi vacuity, heart yang vacuity, heart fire, and phlegm confounding the orifices of the heart. **Heart blood vacuity** manifests general signs of heart disease such as heart palpitations or fearful throb-bing, insomnia, and profuse dreaming, together with signs of blood vacuity including a lusterless white or withered-yellow facial complexion, pale lips, and a fine weak pulse. **Heart yin vacuity** shares with heart blood vacuity the same general signs of heart disease (heart palpitations or fear-ful throbbing, insomnia, profuse dreaming), but is marked by yin vacuity signs such as vexing heat in the five hearts, tidal heat [effusion], night sweating, red tongue with scant fur, and a fine rapid pulse. **Heart qi vacuity** in addition general heart signs heart palpitations or fearful throbbing, manifests in signs of insufficiency of heart qi such as oppres-sion in the chest and shortness of breath exacer-bated by exercise, together with general qi vacuity signs such as lassitude of spirit and lack of strength, a white face, and spontaneous sweating. In some cases, there may be pain in the chest. **Heart yang vacuity** is like heart qi vacuity in that it manifests in heart palpitations or fearful throbbing, oppres-sion in the chest and shortness of breath, as well as lassitude of spirit and lack of strength, but is marked by pronounced cold signs such as physical cold and cold limbs. In severe cases, critical heart yang vacuity gives way to desertion, manifesting in dripping sweat, reversal cold of the limbs, stupor, and faint pulse on the verge of expiration. **Heart fire** includes principally two patterns: HYPERAC-TIVE HEART FIRE characterized by heart vexation, or, in severe cases, manic agitation and deliri-ous speech or incessant laughing, and HEART FIRE FLAMING UPWARD characterized by tongue sores. **Phlegm confounding the orifices of the heart** occurs in several different diseases, and manifests in a) mental depression and dementia (withdrawal disease); b) clouded spirit-mind seeming both con-scious and unconscious (damp warmth); c) sudden clouding collapse, unconsciousness, phlegm-drool foaming at the mouth, and convulsions of the limbs (epilepsy). $\boxed{\text{WMC}}$ cardiovascular diseases, nervous and mental disorders, and conditions involving ero-sion of the tip of the tongue. [26: 92]

heart dispersion 消心 *xiāo xīn*: CENTER DISPER-SION. [26: 480]

heart distention 心胀 *xīn zhàng*: A condition at-tributable to insufficiency of heart yang or cold evil invading the heart, characterized by heart vexation, shortness of breath, and unquiet sleep. $\boxed{\text{MED}}$ Heart distention can be treated with medic-inals such as amber (*hǔ pò*), salvia (*dān shēn*), cinnabar (*zhū shā*), root poria (*fú shén*), biota seed (*bǎi zǐ rén*), aquilaria (*chén xiāng*), unripe tangerine peel (*qīng pí*), curcuma (*yù jīn*), jun-cus (*dēng xīn cǎo*), and ginger skin (*jiāng pí*). If heart distention occurs in combination with dis-tention disease, heart channel medicinals such as coptis (*huáng lián*) and asarum (*xì xīn*) can be added to the formula addressing the distention.

ACU Base treatment mainly on back transport points and CV. Select BL-15 (*xīn shū*, Heart Transport), CV-14 (*jù què*, Great Tower Gate), CV-17 (*shān zhōng*, Chest Center), PC-6 (*nèi guān*, Inner Pass), CV-4 (*guān yuán*, Pass Head), and GV-4 (*mìng mén*, Life Gate); needle with even supplementation and drainage and moxa. [26: 94] [37: 333]

heart fire 心火 *xīn huǒ*: **1.** *Synonym: sovereign fire.* The heart as an active force. **2.** Pathological fire in the heart forming either vacuity or repletion patterns. See HEART FIRE FLAMING UPWARD; INTENSE HEART FIRE; HYPERACTIVE HEART FIRE. [97: 117] [26: 90]

heart-fire 心火 *xīn huǒ*: The heart viewed as belonging to fire in the doctrine of the five phases. [26: 90]

heart fire deflagrating internally 心火内焚 *xīn huǒ nèi fén*: INTENSE INTERNAL HEART FIRE.

heart fire flaming upward 心火上炎 *xīn huǒ shàng yán*: *Synonym: upflaming heart fire.* A VACUITY or REPLETION pattern of the heart characterized by upper body signs. Signs mainly associated with heart fire flaming upward include reddening of the tip of the tongue, vexation, cracking of the tongue, and erosion of the oral and glossal mucosa. The pulse is rapid. Heart fire flaming upward is the result of hyperactive heart fire or heart yin vacuity. It may occur with liver fire in effulgent heart-liver fire, which is a repletion pattern, or with kidney yin vacuity in noninteraction between the heart and kidney, which is an effulgent yin vacuity fire pattern. Sometimes, heart fire may spread to the small intestine. Signs associated with effulgent heart-liver fire include headache, reddening of the eyes, agitation, and irascibility, in addition to the general signs of heart fire flaming upward. Noninteraction between the heart and kidney is characterized by vexation, insomnia, and occasionally by dryness of the pharynx and mouth, upbearing fire flush, a red, mirror tongue, and a fine, rapid pulse. Heart fire spreading to the small intestine is characterized by painful dribbling urination with reddish urine. MED Clear heat and drain fire. Use coptis (*huáng lián*), lotus embryo (*lián zǐ xīn*), forsythia (*lián qiào*), licorice (*gān cǎo*), raw licorice (*shēng gān cǎo*), bamboo leaf (lophatherum) (*dàn zhú yè*), mutong (*mù tōng*), and juncus (*dēng xīn cǎo*). Formulas that treat heart fire flaming upward include variations of Heart-Draining Decoction (*xiè xīn tāng*) combined with Red-Abducting Powder (*dǎo chì sǎn*) to abduct heart fire downward. Noninteraction of the heart and kidney can be treated with Coptis and Ass Hide Glue Decoction (*huáng lián ē jiāo tāng*) supplemented with medicinals that quiet heart and spirit. Where signs of effulgent heart-liver fire are pronounced, heart-

clearing fire-draining can be used with the judicious addition of liver-clearing medicinals such as moutan (*mǔ dān pí*), gardenia (*shān zhī zǐ*), large gentian (*qín jiāo*), and mulberry twig (*sāng zhī*). Heat spreading from the heart to the small intestine can be treated with Red-Abducting Powder (*dǎo chì sǎn*), which abducts the heat downward and out through the bowels. ACU Base treatment mainly on HT, PC, and GV. PC-8 (*láo gōng*, Palace of Toil), HT-8 (*shào fǔ*, Lesser Mansion), PC-9 (*zhōng chōng*, Central Hub), HT-9 (*shào chōng*, Lesser Surge), and GV-26 (*shuǐ gōu*, Water Trough) can all be used to treat heart fire flaming upward. Select two or three of these points and needle with drainage or prick to bleed with a three-edged needle. Selection of points according to concurrent patterns: For effulgent heart-liver fire, add LR-2 (*xíng jiān*, Moving Between), GB-43 (*xiá xī*, Pinched Ravine), and GB-34 (*yáng líng quán*, Yang Mound Spring), needling with drainage. For noninteraction of the heart and kidney, add BL-15 (*xīn shū*, Heart Transport), BL-23 (*shèn shū*, Kidney Transport), KI-3 (*tài xī*, Great Ravine), HT-7 (*shén mén*, Spirit Gate), and SP-6 (*sān yīn jiāo*, Three Yin Intersection), needling with supplementation. For heart fire spreading to the small intestine, add CV-4 (*guān yuán*, Pass Head), ST-39 (*xià jù xū*, Lower Great Hollow), and SI-2 (*qián gǔ*, Front Valley), needling with drainage. Compare EXUBERANT HEART FIRE; HEART HEAT; STIRRING OF THE MINISTERIAL FIRE. [6: 172] [27: 148] [97: 120] [46: 586, 596]

heart (fire) spreading heat to the small intestine 心（火）移热于小肠 *xīn (huǒ) yí rè yú xiǎo cháng*: Effulgent HEART FIRE affecting the SMALL INTESTINE's function of separating the clear and the turbid. The heart and small intestine stand in interior-exterior relationship to each other. When there is effulgent heart fire, the heart can pass on the heat to the small intestine, causing short voidings of reddish urine, burning pain on urination, or blood in the urine, urinary diseases often being associated with the small intestine (see SMALL INTESTINE). This pattern is the principal manifestation of the interior-exterior relationship between the heart and the small intestine (see HEART CONNECTS WITH THE SMALL INTESTINE). MED Use Red-Abducting Powder (*dǎo chì sǎn*). ACU Base treatment mainly on HT, and its alarm and lower uniting points. Select PC-8 (*láo gōng*, Palace of Toil), HT-8 (*shào fǔ*, Lesser Mansion), CV-4 (*guān yuán*, Pass Head), ST-39 (*xià jù xū*, Lower Great Hollow), and SI-2 (*qián gǔ*, Front Valley); needle with drainage. [26: 93] [6: 172]

heart forms sweat 心为汗 *xīn wéi hàn*: From *Elementary Questions* (*sù wèn, xuān míng wǔ qì piān*). Sweat comes from the blood, which is ruled by the heart; hence it is said that the heart forms sweat. Same in meaning as *sweat is the humor of the heart.* See HEART GOVERNS SWEAT. [27: 147]

heart-gallbladder vacuity timidity 心胆虚怯 *xīn dǎn xū qiè:* HEART VACUITY AND GALLBLADDER TIMIDITY.

heart governs speech 心主言 *xīn zhǔ yán:* The heart spirit determines the clarity of speech. When heat enters the pericardium, the outer protection of the heart, one sign is delirious speech. See HEART GOVERNS THE TONGUE. [26: 91] [27: 38] [97: 119]

heart governs sweat 心主汗 *xīn zhǔ hàn:* "Sweat is the humor of the heart," i.e., it is one of the five humors (sweat, snivel, tears, drool, spittle) and is associated with the heart. In clinical practice, sweating is often observed in heart patterns, e.g., in heart yin vacuity with heart fire harassing the inner body, in heart yang vacuity with insecurity of defense yang, and in heart qi heat. Oily sweat is associated with debilitation of heart qi. Conversely, sweating can affect the heart, since excessive sweating can damage heart qi and lead to yang collapse. The heart governs the blood, which is closely related to sweat. Excessive sweating can damage the blood, and blood vacuity reduces the source of sweat. Hence it is said, "WHEN BLOOD IS DESPOLIATED, THERE IS NO SWEAT; WHEN SWEAT IS DESPOLIATED, THERE IS NO BLOOD." [26: 90]

heart governs the blood and vessels 心主血脉 *xīn zhǔ xuè mài:* All the blood and vessels of the body are subordinate to the heart. *Elementary Questions (sù wèn, wǔ zàng shēng chéng piān)* states, "All blood belongs to the heart." *Elementary Questions (sù wèn, wěi lùn)* says, "The heart governs the blood and vessels of the whole body." In Wang Bing's annotations of *Elementary Questions (sù wèn, wǔ zàng shēng chéng piān)*, we find the statement "The liver stores the blood, and the heart moves it; when a person moves, blood moves through all the channels, whereas when he rests, the blood returns to the liver." This statement shows with greater clarity than the original statements of *The Inner Canon (nèi jīng)* that the speed of the heartbeat was understood to be related to exertion. It would also appear to indicate that heart was understood to pump (move) the blood around the body, although the modern notion of blood circulation is not implicit here. Note that although the blood is "governed" by the heart, it is intimately related to the liver and the spleen. [6: 79] [26: 90] [27: 37] [97: 119]

heart governs the spirit light 心主神明 *xīn zhǔ shén míng:* HEART STORES THE SPIRIT.

heart governs the tongue 心主舌 *xīn zhǔ shé:* *The Magic Pivot (líng shū)* states, "Heart qi flows through to the tongue; when the heart is in harmony, the tongue can distinguish the five flavors." When the heart and spirit are healthy, the tongue can move normally and speech is fluent. When the heart spirit is unclear, as when the heart (or pericardium) is affected by an evil, the tongue becomes sluggish or develops a tremor and speech is impeded. Sufficiency of heart blood is reflected in a fresh vital appearance of the tongue, whereas heart blood vacuity is reflected in a pale dull tongue. In heart yin vacuity or effulgent heart fire, the tip (or the whole body) of the tongue is red, prickly, or eroded. Stagnation of the heart blood is characterized by a purple tongue with dark blood stasis speckles. For these reasons, it is also said that the "tongue is the sprout of the heart" and the "heart opens at the tongue." Despite the special relationship between the heart and tongue, the condition of all the other organs, particularly the spleen, is reflected in the state of the tongue and its fur. [6: 80] [26: 90]

heart governs the vessels 心主脉 *xīn zhǔ mài:* See HEART GOVERNS THE BLOOD AND VESSELS.

heart, its bloom is in the face 心，其华在面 *xīn, qí huá zài miàn:* The health of the heart is reflected in the face. The heart governs all the blood vessels of the body, ensuring that blood reaches all parts of the body. The face is particularly rich in blood vessels, and reflects the state of qi and blood, and the organs. [27: 37]

heart heat 心热 *xīn rè: Synonym: heart qi heat.* Any externally contracted heat (febrile) disease pattern of the heart, manifesting in a red facial complexion, heat vexation in the heart, unquiet sleep, and reddish urine. In some cases there may be manic delirious speech, blood ejection, or spontaneous external bleeding. [27: 148] [97: 118] [50: 337]

heart heat susceptibility to fright 心热多惊 *xīn rè duō jīng:* A condition of DREAM TALKING, vexation, oppression and fright crying in infants and children that is attributable to depressed heat causing congestion and stagnation in the bowels and viscera and disharmony of qi and blood. Heart heat susceptibility to fright is characterized by dream talking, vexation and oppression, and crying from fright. MED Clear heat and settle fright using variations of Red-Abducting Powder (*dǎo chì sǎn*) with Bovine Bezoar Heart-Clearing Pill (*niú huáng qīng xīn wán*). ACU Base treatment mainly on HT and PC. Select HT-7 (*shén mén,* Spirit Gate), PC-6 (*nèi guān,* Inner Pass), BL-15 (*xīn shū,* Heart Transport), PC-8 (*láo gōng,* Palace of Toil), HT-8 (*shào fǔ,* Lesser Mansion), and HT-9 (*shào chōng,* Lesser Surge). Needle with drainage or prick to bleed. [26: 94] [27: 149] [46: 596]

heart holds the office of monarch, whence the spirit light emanates 心者，君主之官也，神明出焉 *xīn zhě, jūn zhǔ zhī guān yě, shén míng chū* *yān*: From *Elementary Questions* (*sù wèn, líng lán mì diǎn lùn*). The heart is to the body as the monarch is to the nation; it is the seat of the spirit. *The Inner Canon* (*nèi jīng*) describes the functions of the internal organs by analogy to government. Just as the monarch leads the nation and embodies its consciousness, so the heart is considered to be the seat of consciousness in the body. By a similar metaphor, it is sometimes referred to as the "palace." See HEART STORES THE SPIRIT.

heart impediment 心痹 *xīn bì*: A disease of the heart characterized by pain and suffocating oppression and caused by stasis obstruction of the heart vessels. *Elementary Questions* (*sù wèn*) states, "Heart impediment is stoppage in the vessels..." The stoppage may actually be due to either a) an inadequate warming and propulsion of the blood as a result of insufficiency of yang qi or b) an obstruction of the heart vessels by static blood forming when internal phlegm turbidity impedes blood flow. Signs of heart impediment include dull pain and oppression in the area anterior to the heart, which is attributed to impaired yang qi perfusion or obstruction of the network vessels by phlegm stasis (blood stasis resulting from the presence of phlegm). Attacks are characterized by gripping pain in the heart (angina pectoris), green-blue or purple complexion, cold limbs, and a faint fine pulse verging on expiration, indicating severe obstruction of heart qi and heart yang. Heart palpitations, fearful throbbing, fatigued spirit, and shortness of breath are general signs of heart qi vacuity between attacks. WMC coronary or other heart disease. MED Nourish the heart and dispel the evil, quicken the blood and free the vessels. Use Heart-Supplementing Elixir (*bǔ xīn dān*) or a combination of Pulse-Engendering Powder (*shēng mài sǎn*) and Spleen-Returning Decoction (*guī pí tāng*). If obstruction is pronounced, use Coronary No.2 (*guàn xīn èr hào*) to quicken the blood, rectify qi, and transform stasis. ACU Base treatment mainly on CV, back transport points, HT, PC, and SP. Select BL-15 (*xīn shū*, Heart Transport), BL-20 (*pí shū*, Spleen Transport), BL-17 (*gé shū*, Diaphragm Transport), BL-14 (*jué yīn shū*, Reverting Yin Transport), CV-14 (*jù què*, Great Tower Gate), CV-6 (*qì hǎi*, Sea of Qi), CV-17 (*shān zhōng*, Chest Center), HT-7 (*shén mén*, Spirit Gate), PC-6 (*nèi guān*, Inner Pass), PC-4 (*xī mén*, Cleft Gate), SP-6 (*sān yīn jiāo*, Three Yin Intersection), and ST-36 (*zú sān lǐ*, Leg Three Li). Needle with even supplementation and drainage. Compare CHEST IMPEDIMENT. [26: 94] [27: 405] [97: 118] [42: 125] [15: 201] [37: 332]

heart is averse to heat 心恶热 *xīn wù rè*: The heart is vulnerable to heat. The heart is the fire viscus; it governs the blood and vessels. When heat is pronounced, heart blood is easily damaged.

Also, the heart governs the spirit light; high fever is often accompanied by clouded spirit, delirious speech, and mania. This is why the heart is averse to heat. [27: 61] [97: 20]

heart is connected with the small intestine 心合小肠 *xīn hé xiǎo cháng*: The heart stands in exterior-interior relationship with the small intestine, the heart being interior and the small intestine exterior. The heart channel connects with the small intestine, and the small intestine channel connects with the heart. This relationship is manifest in heart heat spreading to the small intestine, which is characterized by bloody urine. [27: 38] [97: 121]

heart is connected with the vessels 心合脉 *xīn hé mài*: Phrase from *Elementary Questions* (*sù wèn*). See HEART GOVERNS THE BLOOD AND VESSELS. [26: 91]

heart-kidney qi vacuity 心肾气虚 *xīn shèn qì xū*: A disease pattern characterized by signs of both HEART QI VACUITY and KIDNEY QI VACUITY. The chief signs of heart-kidney qi vacuity are heart palpitations, seminal efflux, and premature ejaculation. Other signs include shortness of breath, spontaneous sweating, limp aching lumbus, reduced visual acuity, bright white facial complexion, and fatigue and lack of strength. Urinary signs include incontinence, dribble after voiding, or frequent voidings of clear urine. **Analysis:** The heart governs the blood and vessels. Heart qi vacuity reduces the pumping action of the heart, causing heart palpitations. Sweat is the humor of the heart, and when heart qi is vacuous and fails to contain sweat, sweat flows out, hence spontaneous sweating. The kidney stores essence and controls the two yin. Kidney qi vacuity gives rise to "insecurity of the essence gate" (control over discharge of semen), hence there is seminal efflux and premature ejaculation. When kidney qi is vacuous, there is urinary incontinence, dribble after voiding, or frequent voidings of clear urine. Furthermore, the kidney opens at the ears, and when kidney qi is vacuous, hearing acuity is reduced. The lumbus is the house of the kidney; when kidney qi is vacuous, there is limp aching lumbus. When heart and qi is vacuous, there is a generalized weakening of functions that manifests as fatigue and lack of strength and a white facial complexion. The pale enlarged tongue with white fur, and the forceless vacuous pulse are also qi vacuity signs. MED Boost qi and nourish the heart; supplement the kidney and secure essence. Golden Coffer Kidney Qi Pill (*jīn guì shèn qì wán*) with additions. ACU Base treatment mainly on back transport points, HT, KI, and CV. Select BL-15 (*xīn shū*, Heart Transport), BL-23 (*shèn shū*, Kidney Transport), CV-14 (*jù què*, Great Tower Gate), CV-4 (*guān yuán*, Pass

Head), KI-3 (*tài xī*, Great Ravine), BL-52 (*zhì shì*, Will Chamber), PC-6 (*nèi guān*, Inner Pass), and HT-7 (*shén mén*, Spirit Gate); needle with supplementation and add moxa. [26: 149] [116: 140] [46: 648, 678] [37: 384]

heart-kidney yang vacuity 心肾阳虚 *xīn shèn yáng xū*: A disease pattern characterized by signs of both HEART YANG VACUITY and KIDNEY YANG VACUITY. The chief signs are heart palpitations and scant urine. Others include stifling oppression in the heart and chest, green-blue or purple lips, fear of cold and cold limbs, inhibited urination, jerking sinews and twitching flesh, and puffy swelling of the limbs. The tongue is pale with a glossy white fur. The pulse is sunken and faint. Analysis: When heart yang is insufficient, its power to move the blood is weak, hence the heart palpitations and stifling oppression in the heart and chest. When kidney yang is insufficient, qi transformation is inhibited, hence the inhibited urination and puffy swelling of the limbs. When water is retained, clear yang fails to rise, hence there is dizziness. When the sinews are deprived of nourishment, there is jerking of the sinews and twitching of the flesh. "When yang is vacuous, there is external cold," hence the aversion to cold and cold limbs. The pale tongue with glossy white tongue fur, and the sunken pulse also also yang vacuity signs. MED Warm yang and dissipate cold; disinhibit water and disperse yin. Use True Warrior Decoction (*zhēn wǔ tāng*). ACU Base treatment mainly on back transport points, HT, KI, and CV. Select BL-15 (*xīn shū*, Heart Transport), BL-23 (*shèn shū*, Kidney Transport), CV-14 (*jù què*, Great Tower Gate), CV-17 (*shān zhōng*, Chest Center), GV-4 (*mìng mén*, Life Gate), CV-4 (*guān yuán*, Pass Head), PC-6 (*nèi guān*, Inner Pass), HT-7 (*shén mén*, Spirit Gate), KI-3 (*tài xī*, Great Ravine), and KI-7 (*fù liū*, Recover Flow); needle with supplementation and amounts of moxa. Comparison: *Heart-kidney qi vacuity:* Heart-kidney yang vacuity is a development of heart-kidney qi vacuity. It shares the same signs, and differs by being more severe and by the additional presence of yang vacuity external cold. See HEART YANG VACUITY and KIDNEY YANG VACUITY. [6: 171] [57: 94] [116: 137] [46: 648] [37: 386, 387]

heart-kidney yin vacuity 心肾阴虚 *xīn shèn yīn xū*: A condition characterized by signs of HEART YIN VACUITY and KIDNEY YIN VACUITY. The main signs of heart-kidney yin vacuity are heart palpitations or fearful throbbing, and seminal emission. Other signs include insomnia, forgetfulness, heart vexation, aching lumbus, loosening of the teeth, yellow urine, dry stool, and night sweating. The tongue is red with scant fur. The pulse is fine and rapid. Analysis: The kidney stores essence; when yin-essence is vacuous it fails to restrain

yang, hence there is night sweating and seminal emission. Insufficiency of kidney essence causes lumbar pain. Insufficiency of bone and marrow causes loosening of the teeth. The heart governs the vessels; when heart blood is vacuous, the heart spirit is not stored and nourished, hence the heart vexation, insomnia, and forgetfulness. When the blood fails to nourish the heart, there are palpitations. When heart and kidney yin are vacuous, fluids are insufficient, hence the yellow urine and dry stool. The red tongue with scant fur and the rapid fine pulse are signs of effulgent yin vacuity fire. MED Enrich the kidney and nourish the heart; downbear fire and quiet the spirit. Use Celestial Emperor Heart-Supplementing Elixir (*tiān wáng bǔ xīn dān*). ACU Base treatment mainly on back transport points, HT, KI, and CV. Select BL-15 (*xīn shū*, Heart Transport), BL-23 (*shèn shū*, Kidney Transport), BL-17 (*gé shū*, Diaphragm Transport), CV-14 (*jù què*, Great Tower Gate), PC-6 (*nèi guān*, Inner Pass), HT-7 (*shén mén*, Spirit Gate), KI-3 (*tài xī*, Great Ravine), BL-52 (*zhì shì*, Will Chamber), and SP-6 (*sān yīn jiāo*, Three Yin Intersection); needle with supplementation. See HEART YIN VACUITY; KIDNEY YIN VACUITY. [116: 139] [46: 648] [37: 332, 386]

heart-level effusion 对心发 *duì xīn fā*: An EFFUSION OF THE BACK, at the level of the heart. See ²EFFUSION. [26: 93]

heart-liver blood vacuity 心肝血虚 *xīn gān xuè xū*: A condition characterized by signs of LIVER BLOOD VACUITY and HEART BLOOD VACUITY arising when a) insufficient blood production, b) excessive loss of blood, c) construction-yin depletion in enduring disease, or d) damage to yin in heat (febrile) disease causes the heart to have nothing to govern and the liver to have nothing store. The main signs are heart palpitations and fearful throbbing, forgetfulness, insomnia possibly with profuse dreaming, dizzy head and clouded vision, and numbness of the limbs. Other signs include pale white facial complexion, susceptibility to fright, hypertonicity of the sinews, night blindness, and lusterless nails. The tongue is pale, and the pulse is fine and forceless. MED Supplement heart blood and nourish liver blood. Use Four Agents Decoction (*sì wù tāng*) or Liver-Supplementing Decoction (*bǔ gān tāng*). ACU Base treatment mainly on back transport points, HT, LR, SP, and CV. Select BL-15 (*xīn shū*, Heart Transport), BL-18 (*gān shū*, Liver Transport), BL-17 (*gé shū*, Diaphragm Transport), LR-3 (*tài chōng*, Supreme Surge), SP-6 (*sān yīn jiāo*, Three Yin Intersection), ST-36 (*zú sān lǐ*, Leg Three Li), HT-7 (*shén mén*, Spirit Gate), PC-6 (*nèi guān*, Inner Pass), and KI-3 (*tài xī*, Great Ravine); needle with supplementation and moxa. [46: 586, 648] [57: 91] [37: 348]

heart-lung qi vacuity 心肺气虚 *xīn fèi qì xū*: A disease pattern arising when enduring cough and panting causes LUNG VACUITY that affects the heart, or when INSUFFICIENCY OF HEART QI causes LUNG QI VACUITY. The chief signs are heart palpitations, shortness of breath, cough, and panting on exertion. Other signs include pale white lusterless facial complexion, lassitude of spirit with lack of strength, coughing of thin clear phlegm, stifling oppression in the heart and chest, low timid voice, and spontaneous sweating. The tongue is pale with thin white fur. The pulse is fine and weak. MED Supplement the heart and lung. Four Gentlemen Decoction (*sì jūn zǐ tāng*) plus astragalus (*huáng qí*) and dioscorea (*shān yào*), or use Origin-Preserving Decoction (*bǎo yuán tāng*) plus calcined dragon bone (*duàn lóng gǔ*), aster (*zǐ wǎn*), and tussilago (*kuǎn dōng huā*). ACU Base treatment mainly on back transport points, CV, and LU. Select BL-15 (*xīn shū*, Heart Transport), BL-13 (*fèi shū*, Lung Transport), CV-14 (*jù què*, Great Tower Gate), BL-43 (*gāo huāng shū*, Gao-Huang Transport), CV-4 (*guān yuán*, Pass Head), CV-6 (*qì hǎi*, Sea of Qi), LU-9 (*tài yuān*, Great Abyss), and ST-36 (*zú sān lǐ*, Leg Three Li); needle with supplementation and moxa. [57: 92] [6: 171] [116: 123] [57: 92] [37: 282] [46: 594, 655]

heart-lung yang vacuity 心肺阳虚 *xīn fèi yáng xū*: A disease pattern characterized by signs of both HEART YANG VACUITY and LUNG YANG VACUITY. The main signs are stifling oppression and pain in the heart and chest. Other signs include heart palpitations, forceless cough and panting, fear of cold, lack of warmth in the hands and feet, and dark purple lips. The tongue is dark in color and enlarged. The tongue fur is white and glossy. The pulse is sunken, slow, and forceless. Analysis: The lung inhabits the upper burner and governs the qi of the whole body. The heart governs the vessels. Hence, when the yang of the chest is devitalized, causing qi stagnation and blood stasis, there is stifling oppression and pain in the heart and chest. When heart yang is vacuous, its pumping power is reduced; hence there are heart palpitations. Lung qi vacuity gives rise to forceless cough and panting; insufficiency of yang qi causes fear of cold, cold limbs, and green-blue or purple lips. The dark, enlarged tongue with white glossy fur and the forceless slow sunken pulse are all indications of yang vacuity. MED Boost qi and assist yang; loosen the chest and relieve pain. Use Origin-Preserving Decoction (*bǎo yuán tāng*). ACU Base treatment mainly on back transport points, CV, GV, and LU. Select BL-15 (*xīn shū*, Heart Transport), BL-13 (*fèi shū*, Lung Transport), CV-14 (*jù què*, Great Tower Gate), LU-9 (*tài yuān*, Great Abyss), CV-6 (*qì hǎi*, Sea of Qi), CV-4 (*guān yuán*, Pass Head), GV-4 (*mìng mén*, Life Gate), and

ST-36 (*zú sān lǐ*, Leg Three Li); needle with supplementation and large amounts of moxa. [116: 126] [37: 274, 280] [46: 594]

heart-lung yin vacuity 心肺阴虚 *xīn fèi yīn xū*: A disease pattern characterized by signs of both HEART YIN VACUITY and LUNG YIN VACUITY. The chief signs are dry cough, heart palpitations, and tidal heat [effusion]. Other signs include cough with scant sticky phlegm that is not easy to expectorate, heart vexation, reduced sleep, profuse dreaming, dry lips, dry throat, scant urine, postmeridian tidal heat [effusion], vexing heat in the five hearts, and night sweating. The tongue is red and dry with scant fur. The pulse is fine and rapid. Lung yin vacuity with fire that scorches the liquid causes counterflow qi and dry cough or cough with scant sticky phlegm that is difficult to expectorate. Heart yin vacuity with blood failing to nourish the heart and depriving the spirit of nourishment explains the reduced sleep and sleeplessness. The dry lips, dry throat, scant urine, postmeridian tidal heat [effusion], vexing heat in the five hearts, and night sweating are all signs of effulgent yin vacuity fire. Yin vacuity explains the dry scant tongue fur and fine pulse; vacuity fire flaming upward explains the red tongue and rapid pulse. MED Enrich vacuity and downbear fire; moisten the lung and quiet the spirit. Use variations of Aster Decoction (*zǐ wǎn tāng*). ACU Base treatment mainly on back transport points, HT, LU, and KI. Select BL-15 (*xīn shū*, Heart Transport), BL-13 (*fèi shū*, Lung Transport), BL-17 (*gé shū*, Diaphragm Transport), BL-43 (*gāo huāng shū*, Gao-Huang Transport), LU-5 (*chǐ zé*, Cubit Marsh), SP-6 (*sān yīn jiāo*, Three Yin Intersection), PC-6 (*nèi guān*, Inner Pass), HT-7 (*shén mén*, Spirit Gate), KI-3 (*tài xī*, Great Ravine), and KI-6 (*zhào hǎi*, Shining Sea); needle with supplementation. [37: 279, 335] [46: 648, 653] [116: 124]

heart mounting 心疝 *xīn shàn*: A MOUNTING (*shàn*) pattern of abdominal pain with a bulge in the abdomen and a subjective sensation of qi surging up from the umbilicus to the heart. Heart mounting is attributed to cold affecting the heart channel. MED Warm the channels and dissipate cold; harmonize the blood and relieve pain. ACU Base treatment on back transport points, HT, PC, and ST. Select BL-15 (*xīn shū*, Heart Transport), BL-20 (*pí shū*, Spleen Transport), HT-7 (*shén mén*, Spirit Gate), PC-6 (*nèi guān*, Inner Pass), ST-36 (*zú sān lǐ*, Leg Three Li), and ST-25 (*tiān shū*, Celestial Pivot); needle with supplementation and add moxa. [26: 92] [27: 431] [97: 117]

heart opens at the tongue 心开窍于舌 *xīn kāi qiào yú shé*: Synonym: *tongue is the sprout of the heart*. See HEART GOVERNS THE TONGUE.

heart pain 心痛 *xīn tòng*, 心疼 *xīn téng*: **1.** Pain in the heart itself. WMC cardiodynia; angina pectoris. Heart pain includes the TRUE HEART PAIN spoken of in *The Magic Pivot* (*líng shū*), the COMING AND GOING HEART PAIN and INFLUX HEART PAIN spoken of in *A Thousand Gold Pieces Prescriptions* (*qiān jīn yào fāng*). **2.** Pain in the pit of the stomach or heart [region]. WMC cardialgia. [26: 93]

heart pain stretching to the back 心痛彻背 *xīn tòng chè bèi*: HEART PAIN with pain also felt in the back; a sign of HEART IMPEDIMENT. [26: 93]

heart palpitations 心悸 *xīn jì*: Rapid throbbing of the heart. Distinction is made between *fright palpitations* ('heart palpitations' in the narrow sense) and *fearful throbbing*. Fright palpitations are brought on by fright or emotional stimulus, and are therefore clearly paroxysmal in nature. They occurs in both vacuity and repletion patterns. In Western medicine, they are often found to be a nervous disorder. Fearful throbbing occurs continually, and although it is associated with a feeling of fear, it is not brought on by emotional stimulus. It is more severe than fright palpitations, and is experienced as a violent throbbing felt not only in the chest, but even as low as the umbilical region. It is observed in patients in a poor state of health and always forms part of vacuity patterns. From the Western medical perspective, it is usually the manifestation of organic rather than nervous disease. In some older books the terms "fright palpitations" and "fearful throbbing" were used interchangeably. Heart palpitations occur in a wide variety of patterns and combinations of patterns. The basic patterns include heart-gallbladder vacuity timidity; dual vacuity of the heart and spleen; effulgent yin vacuity fire; insufficiency of heart qi; insufficiency of heart yang; dual vacuity of qi and yin; water-rheum intimidating the heart; blood stasis obstruction; phlegm-fire harassing the heart. **Heart-gallbladder vacuity timidity** arises when the heart fails to store the spirit and the gallbladder lacks decisiveness. There is a tendency to fear and fright which brings on heart palpitations. Other signs include reduced sleep and profuse dreaming, thin white tongue fur, and a stirred rapid pulse or a vacuous stringlike pulse. MED Calm fright and stabilize the mind; nourish the heart and quiet the spirit. Spirit-Quieting Mind-Stabilizing Pill (*ān shén dìng zhì wán*) is an appropriate formula. ACU Base treatment mainly on HT, PC, GB, and back transport points. Select HT-7 (*shén mén*, Spirit Gate), PC-6 (*nèi guān*, Inner Pass), BL-15 (*xīn shū*, Heart Transport), BL-19 (*dǎn shū*, Gallbladder Transport), GB-34 (*yáng líng quán*, Yang Mound Spring), and ST-36 (*zú sān lǐ*, Leg Three Li); needle with supplementation. **Dual vacuity of the heart and spleen** manifests in heart pal-

pitations or fearful throbbing by causing insufficiency of heart blood that deprives the heart of nourishment. Other signs include lassitude of spirit and shortness of breath, forgetfulness, insomnia, dizzy head and vision, lusterless complexion, spontaneous sweating, pale red tongue, and a fine weak pulse. MED Supplement the blood and nourish the heart; boost qi and quiet the spirit. Use Spleen-Returning Decoction (*guī pí tāng*). ACU Base treatment mainly on HT, SP, ST, and back transport points. Main points: HT-7 (*shén mén*, Spirit Gate), PC-6 (*nèi guān*, Inner Pass), and BL-15 (*xīn shū*, Heart Transport). Add HT-5 (*tōng lǐ*, Connecting Li), BL-17 (*gé shū*, Diaphragm Transport), ST-36 (*zú sān lǐ*, Leg Three Li), and SP-6 (*sān yīn jiāo*, Three Yin Intersection), to engender heart blood. Add BL-20 (*pí shū*, Spleen Transport), and CV-12 (*zhōng wǎn*, Center Stomach Duct) for dual vacuity of heart and spleen. Needle with supplementation and use moxa on the back transport points. For insomnia, add ST-45 (*lì duì*, Severe Mouth). For shortness of breath, add BL-13 (*fèi shū*, Lung Transport). **Effulgent yin vacuity fire** arises in kidney yin vacuity when "water fails to help fire" and prevents the stirring of heart fire (noninteraction of the heart and kidney), or when "water fails to restrain fire" and the ministerial fire becomes hyperactive and harasses the heart spirit. This condition occurs in patients who do a great deal of mental work. Heart palpitations are accompanied by vexation, heat in the hearts of the palms and soles, reduced sleep and profuse dreaming, dizzy head and vision, tinnitus, upbearing fire flush, lumbar pain, red tongue with thin yellow fur, and a fine rapid pulse. MED Enrich yin and clear fire; nourish the heart and quiet the spirit. Use formulas like Coptis and Ass Hide Glue Decoction (*huáng lián ē jiāo tāng*). ACU Base treatment mainly on HT, PC, KI, and back transport points. Select HT-7 (*shén mén*, Spirit Gate), PC-4 (*xī mén*, Cleft Gate), BL-15 (*xīn shū*, Heart Transport), BL-23 (*shèn shū*, Kidney Transport), BL-14 (*jué yīn shū*, Reverting Yin Transport), KI-3 (*tài xī*, Great Ravine), KI-6 (*zhào hǎi*, Shining Sea), and SP-6 (*sān yīn jiāo*, Three Yin Intersection). Needle with even supplementation and drainage. **Insufficiency of heart qi** is the result of constitutional vacuity, degeneration of health with old age, or enduring illness. It gives rise to heart palpitations by causing feeble movement of blood that deprives the heart of nourishment. In such cases, heart palpitations or fearful throbbing is accompanied by lassitude of spirit and lack of strength, lusterless complexion, spontaneous sweating, laziness to speak, clouded or dizzy head, pale tongue with white fur, and a fine weak or moderate sunken pulse. MED Nourish the heart and boost qi; quiet the spirit and stabilize mind. A representative formula is Four Gentlemen Panting Decoction (*chuǎn sì jūn zǐ tāng*). ACU Base treatment mainly on HT, PC, CV, and back transport points. Select HT-7 (*shén mén*, Spirit Gate), PC-6 (*nèi guān*, Inner Pass), BL-15 (*xīn shū*, Heart Transport), CV-6 (*qì hǎi*, Sea of Qi), CV-4 (*guān yuán*, Pass Head), and ST-36 (*zú sān lǐ*, Leg Three Li). Needle with supplementation and use moxa. **Insufficiency of heart yang** shares the same causes as insufficiency of heart qi and differs by the further presence of cold signs. Heart palpitations are exacerbated by physical movement and is accompanied by physical cold and cold limbs, a somber white facial complexion, oppression in the chest and shortness of breath, a pale tongue with white fur, a forceless sunken fine or vacuous weak pulse. MED Warm and supplement heart yang; quiet the spirit and stabilize mind. A representative formula is Cinnamon Twig, Licorice, Dragon Bone, and Oyster Shell Decoction (*guì zhī gān cǎo lóng gǔ mǔ lì tāng*). ACU Base treatment mainly on HT, PC, CV, and back transport points. Select HT-7 (*shén mén*, Spirit Gate), BL-15 (*xīn shū*, Heart Transport), CV-14 (*jù què*, Great Tower Gate), PC-6 (*nèi guān*, Inner Pass), and GV-4 (*mìng mén*, Life Gate); needle with supplementation and add moxa. **Dual vacuity of qi and yin** causes heart palpitations or fearful throbbing accompanied by reddening of the cheeks, coughing of blood-flecked phlegm, oppression in the chest, shortness of breath, lusterless complexion, spontaneous or night sweating, red tongue with little fur, and a rapid fine pulse that may be irregular. MED Treat by boosting qi and nourishing the heart and by enriching yin blood. A representative formula is Honey-Fried Licorice Decoction (*zhì gān cǎo tāng*). ACU Base treatment mainly on HT, PC, CV, and back transport points. Select HT-7 (*shén mén*, Spirit Gate), PC-6 (*nèi guān*, Inner Pass), BL-15 (*xīn shū*, Heart Transport), CV-14 (*jù què*, Great Tower Gate), CV-6 (*qì hǎi*, Sea of Qi), ST-36 (*zú sān lǐ*, Leg Three Li), and SP-6 (*sān yīn jiāo*, Three Yin Intersection). Needle with supplementation. If vacuity fire signs are not pronounced, moxa can also be used. For spontaneous or night sweating, add LI-4 (*hé gǔ*, Union Valley), SI-3 (*hòu xī*, Back Ravine), and HT-6 (*yīn xī*, Yin Cleft). For coughing of blood and oppression in the chest, add LU-5 (*chǐ zé*, Cubit Marsh) and BL-13 (*fèi shū*, Lung Transport). For pronounced vacuity fire, add HT-8 (*shào fǔ*, Lesser Mansion), needling with drainage. **Water-rheum (water qi) intimidating the heart** has its root in spleen-kidney yang vacuity and is associated with signs of impaired movement of water such as short voidings of scant urine and swelling of the lower limbs. In addition to these signs, heart palpitations are accompanied by glomus and full-

ness in the chest and stomach duct, thirst with no desire to drink, physical cold and cold limbs, dizziness, vomiting and ejection of drool, pale tongue with glossy fur, and a slippery stringlike pulse or a slippery fine sunken pulse. MED Supplement yang, promote qi transformation, and move water. A representative formula is Poria (Hoelen), Cinnamon Twig, Ovate Atractylodes, and Licorice Decoction (*líng guì zhú gān tāng*). ACU Base treatment mainly on ST, HT, PC, CV, and back transport points. Select HT-7 (*shén mén*, Spirit Gate), PC-6 (*nèi guān*, Inner Pass), BL-15 (*xīn shū*, Heart Transport), BL-22 (*sān jiāo shū*, Triple Burner Transport), BL-20 (*pí shū*, Spleen Transport), CV-17 (*shān zhōng*, Chest Center), ST-36 (*zú sān lǐ*, Leg Three Li), and ST-40 (*fēng lóng*, Bountiful Bulge). Needle with supplementation. **Heart blood stasis obstruction** is traceable to binding depression of liver qi and lung qi congestion, and spleen, kidney, and lung vacuity. In such patterns, heart palpitations are accompanied by periodic heart pain like the stabbing of a needle. Other signs include oppression in the chest, green-blue or purple nails, a tongue that is purple in color or bears stasis speckles, and a rough or interrupted pulse. MED Quicken the blood and transform stasis; rectify qi and free the network vessels. A representative formula is Peach Kernel and Carthamus Brew (*táo rén hóng huā jiān*). ACU Base treatment mainly on HT, PC, SP, LR, and back transport points. Select BL-15 (*xīn shū*, Heart Transport), HT-7 (*shén mén*, Spirit Gate), PC-6 (*nèi guān*, Inner Pass), CV-17 (*shān zhōng*, Chest Center), BL-17 (*gé shū*, Diaphragm Transport), SP-10 (*xuè hǎi*, Sea of Blood), LI-4 (*hé gǔ*, Union Valley), and LR-3 (*tài chōng*, Supreme Surge); needle with even supplementation and drainage. **Phlegm-fire harassing the heart** causes heart palpitations induced by fright, accompanied by oppression in the chest, vexation and agitation, profuse nightmares, and dry mouth with bitter taste. Other signs include insomnia, constipation, yellow or reddish urine, slimy yellow tongue fur, and a slippery stringlike pulse. MED Clear heat and transform phlegm; quiet the heart spirit. A representative formula is Coptis Gallbladder-Warming Decoction (*huáng lián wēn dǎn tāng*). ACU Base treatment mainly on ST, HT, PC, GB, and back transport points. Select HT-7 (*shén mén*, Spirit Gate), PC-6 (*nèi guān*, Inner Pass), BL-15 (*xīn shū*, Heart Transport), ST-40 (*fēng lóng*, Bountiful Bulge), GB-34 (*yáng líng quán*, Yang Mound Spring), and LU-5 (*chǐ zé*, Cubit Marsh); needle with drainage. For oppression in the chest, add CV-17 (*shān zhōng*, Chest Center). For vexation, add PC-5 (*jiān shǐ*, Intermediary Courier). For insomnia, nightmares, and profuse dreaming, add ST-45 (*lì duì*, Severe Mouth). See also BLOOD VACUITY

HEART PALPITATIONS; QI VACUITY HEART PAL-
PITATIONS; COLLECTING RHEUM HEART PALPITA-
TIONS; QI STAGNATION BLOOD STASIS HEART PAL-
PITATIONS; STIRRING HEART PALPITATIONS. [80:
197] [26: 93] [92: No. 180]

heart pulse is surging 心脉洪 *xīn mài hóng*:
A SURGING PULSE is associated with HEART DIS-
EASE and the season summer. *Elementary Ques-*
tions (sù wèn) states, "The heart pulse is hook-
like." *The Classic of Difficult Issues (nàn jīng,*
15) states, "The summer pulse is hook-like." The
hook-like pulse is now usually referred to as the
surging pulse. See SURGING PULSE. [9: 336] [131:
200] [9: 336]

heart qi 心气 *xīn qì*: See HEART QI AND HEART
BLOOD.

heart qi and heart blood 心气、心血 *xīn qì xīn*
xuè: Heart qi and heart blood form part of the
blood and qi of the whole body, and are the basis
for the physiological activity of the heart. When
heart qi and heart blood are abundant, the heartbeat is regular, the pulse is moderate and forceful,
and the complexion is healthy and lustrous. Insufficiency of heart qi and depletion of heart blood are
characterized by a lusterless complexion, heart palpitations, and a slow, rapid or interrupted (结代
jié dài) pulse. Heart blood and heart qi are greatly
interdependent. Insufficiency of heart qi may lead
to blood stagnation characterized by a green-blue
or purple complexion and lack of warmth in the extremities. Heart blood depletion leads to impairment of the blood's nourishing function. It may
also deprive heart qi of support, causing dizziness,
fatigued spirit, shortness of breath, and copious
sweat. [6: 80]

heart qi heat 心气热 *xīn qì rè*: HEART HEAT.

heart qi repletion 心气实 *xīn qì shí*: EXUBERANT
HEART QI.

heart qi vacuity 心气虚 *xīn qì xū*: The manifestation of insufficiency of heart qi; a disease pattern
characterized by heart palpitations, shortness of
breath, fatigue, and lack of strength, reflecting general qi vacuity and inhibited movement of blood.
Heart qi vacuity usually appears in gradually developing, enduring illness. Pathomechanisms include: (1) insufficiency of ancestral qi preventing it
from adequately penetrating the heart and vessels
and driving respiration; (2) water qi intimidating
the heart, which results from kidney yang vacuity; (3) wind-cold-damp impediment (*bì*) settling
in the heart; (4) damp turbidity or static blood
obstructing the heart and vessels; (5) acute forms
of heart qi vacuity resulting from fulminant desertion of yang qi. Heart qi vacuity may occur with
lung qi vacuity, the resulting condition being referred to as *heart-lung qi vacuity*. Heart qi vacuity
may also present with cold-damp, damp turbidity,

and static blood complications. The chief signs of
heart qi vacuity are heart palpitations or fearful
throbbing and shortness of breath exacerbated by
exertion, and fatigue and lack of strength. Other
signs include oppression in the chest, white face,
and spontaneous sweating. In some cases, there
may be sleeplessness or profuse sleep, forgetfulness,
chest pain, tendency to sorrow and weepiness, abstraction, convulsions, and susceptibility to fright.
The pulse is weak and fine, or interrupted (bound,
skipping, or intermittent). WMC cardiac failure,
angina pectoris, arrhythmia, general asthenia, and
neurosis. **Analysis:** When heart qi is insufficient, its
propelling action is weakened, hence heart palpitations or fearful throbbing. When heart qi is vacuous, the circulation of ancestral qi is weak, hence
oppression in the chest and shortness of breath.
Exertion causes wear on qi and therefore exacerbates these signs. When qi is vacuous, external
defense is insecure, hence the shortage of qi, laziness to speak, fatigue, and spontaneous sweating.
When heart qi is vacuous, either the heart spirit
is deprived of nourishment and there is profuse
sleeping, or there is nothing to quiet the spirit and
stabilize the mind, so that there is sleeplessness,
forgetfulness, susceptibility to fright, abstraction,
or tendency to sorrow and weepiness. Qi vacuity
engenders phlegm, deprives the sinews of nourishment, hence convulsions. When heart qi is insufficient and fails to commend the blood, the blood
stagnates in the heart vessels, giving rise to pain;
failing to make blood ascend to the face, it gives
rise to white face and pale tongue; failing to propel
the blood, it gives rise to an intermittent or bound
pulse. When heart qi is vacuous, it cannot move
the blood to nourish the whole body, and through
the body's self-regulation function, it may attempt
to compensate by speeding up propulsion, causing
a rapid pulse, or if vessel qi is discontinuous, a skipping pulse (rapid irregularly interrupted pulse).
MED Heart qi vacuity is treated by supplementing
heart qi with medicinals such as mix-fried licorice
(*zhì gān cǎo*), astragalus (*huáng qí*), codonopsis
(*dǎng shēn*), and ginseng (*rén shēn*). Appropriate formulas include Honey-Fried Licorice Decoction (*zhì gān cǎo tāng*) and Heart-Nourishing Decoction (*yǎng xīn tāng*). ACU Base treatment
mainly on HT, back transport points, and CV. Select BL-15 (*xīn shū*, Heart Transport), CV-14 (*jù*
què, Great Tower Gate), HT-7 (*shén mén*, Spirit
Gate), CV-4 (*guān yuán*, Pass Head), CV-6 (*qì hǎi*,
Sea of Qi), BL-20 (*pí shū*, Spleen Transport), and
ST-36 (*zú sān lǐ*, Leg Three Li); needle with supplementation and add moxa. [116: 31] [6: 170] [37:
282] [46: 594, 655]

heart qi vacuity sleeplessness 心气虚不得卧
xīn qì xū bù dé wò: An internal damage SLEEP-
LESSNESS pattern attributed to HEART QI VACU-

ITY and the heart spirit failing to contain itself and characterized by unquiet sleep, sudden waking from sleep, heart palpitations, lassitude of spirit and lack of strength, desire for heat and aversion to cold, and a forceless pulse that may be slow. MED Boost qi and nourish the heart using formulas like Ginseng Construction-Nourishing Decoction (*rén shēn yǎng róng tāng*) and Spleen-Returning Decoction (*guī pí tāng*). ACU Base treatment mainly on HT and back transport points. Select Alert Spirit Quartet (*sì shén cōng*), HT-7 (*shén mén*, Spirit Gate), SP-6 (*sān yīn jiāo*, Three Yin Intersection), BL-15 (*xīn shū*, Heart Transport), BL-20 (*pí shū*, Spleen Transport), ST-36 (*zú sān lǐ*, Leg Three Li), and CV-6 (*qì hǎi*, Sea of Qi). Needle with supplementation. See SLEEPLESSNESS. [26: 91]

heart [region] and abdomen 心腹 *xīn fù*: The heart [region] (the pit of the stomach, and the abdomen as a whole).

heart spirit 心神 *xīn shén*: The spirit that is governed by the heart. See HEART STORES THE SPIRIT.

heart spirit failing to contain itself 心神失守 *xīn shén shī shǒu*: SPIRIT FAILING TO KEEP TO ITS ABODE. [27: 371]

heart-spleen blood vacuity 心脾血虚 *xīn pí xuè xū*: A disease pattern of HEART BLOOD VACUITY and SPLEEN VACUITY (splenic transformation failure and the spleen failing to manage the blood). The main signs are heart palpitations and insomnia. Other signs may include fearful throbbing, forgetfulness, profuse dreaming, lusterless complexion, pale lips, and pale scant menstrual flow. The tongue is pale with scant fur. The pulse is fine, bound or intermittent. **Analysis:** The heart governs the blood and stores the spirit. The spleen is the source of qi and blood formation and stores reflection. Heart-spleen blood vacuity deprives the spirit of nourishment, hence there is heart palpitations, insomnia, fearful throbbing, and forgetfulness. Blood vacuity deprives the face of nourishment, hence the complexion is lusterless. Insufficiency of the blood means less blood for menstruation, hence the menstrual flow is scant and pale. MED Boost qi and supplement the blood; fortify the spleen and quiet the heart. Use Spleen-Returning Decoction (*guī pí tāng*). Compare DUAL VACUITY OF THE HEART AND SPLEEN; HEART-SPLEEN QI VACUITY. ACU Base treatment mainly on back transport points, HT, SP, and CV. Select BL-15 (*xīn shū*, Heart Transport), BL-20 (*pí shū*, Spleen Transport), BL-17 (*gé shū*, Diaphragm Transport), PC-6 (*nèi guān*, Inner Pass), HT-7 (*shén mén*, Spirit Gate), ST-36 (*zú sān lǐ*, Leg Three Li), SP-10 (*xuè hǎi*, Sea of Blood), and SP-6 (*sān yīn jiāo*, Three Yin Intersection); needle with

supplementation and moxa. [46: 585, 586] [116: 130] [37: 332, 342,]

heart-spleen qi vacuity 心脾气虚 *xīn pí qì xū*: A disease pattern of SPLEEN QI VACUITY and HEART QI VACUITY. The main signs are heart palpitations, reduced eating, and abdominal distention. Other signs include white facial complexion, spontaneous sweating, fatigue and lack of strength, and shortness of breath with rapid breathing on exertion. The tongue is pale with a white fur. The pulse is forceless and vacuous. **Analysis:** When heart qi is vacuous, the heart's pumping action is weak, hence there are heart palpitations. When spleen qi is vacuous, movement and transformation breaks down, hence there is reduced eating and abdominal distention. In heart-spleen qi vacuity physiological functions are lowered, hence there is spontaneous sweating and shortness of breath with rapid breathing on exertion. When the source of qi and blood is reduced, the patient becomes improperly nourished, hence fatigue and lack of strength. MED Supplement the heart and spleen. Use Ginseng Spleen-Returning Pill (*rén shēn guī pí wán*). ACU Base treatment mainly on back transport points, HT, SP, and CV. Select BL-15 (*xīn shū*, Heart Transport), BL-20 (*pí shū*, Spleen Transport), CV-14 (*jù què*, Great Tower Gate), CV-4 (*guān yuán*, Pass Head), CV-6 (*qì hǎi*, Sea of Qi), PC-6 (*nèi guān*, Inner Pass), HT-7 (*shén mén*, Spirit Gate), ST-36 (*zú sān lǐ*, Leg Three Li), SP-3 (*tài bái*, Supreme White), and LR-13 (*zhāng mén*, Camphorwood Gate); needle with supplementation and moxa. Compare DUAL VACUITY OF THE HEART AND SPLEEN. [116: 129] [37: 332, 351] [46: 594]

heart-spleen vacuity 心脾两虚 *xīn pí liǎng xū*: DUAL VACUITY OF THE HEART AND SPLEEN.

heart-spleen yang vacuity 心脾阳虚 *xīn pí yáng xū*: A disease pattern characterized by HEART YANG VACUITY and SPLEEN YANG VACUITY signs. The chief signs are stifling oppression and pain in the heart and chest and thin sloppy stool. Other signs include heart palpitations, reduced eating, rumbling intestines, somber white facial complexion, shortage of qi and laziness to speak, spontaneous sweating, lassitude of spirit, somnolence, and physical cold and cold limbs. The tongue is pale or dark and purple; the tongue fur is white; and the pulse is weak. **Analysis:** When heart yang is insufficient, heart qi is depleted, hence the heart palpitations, spontaneous sweating, lassitude of spirit, and somnolence. When yang qi is too weak to move the blood, stasis obstruction of the heart vessels develops and qi dynamic stagnates, hence the stifling oppression and pain in the heart and chest. Spleen yang vacuity develops from spleen qi vacuity. Spleen qi vacuity causing impaired movement and transformation of grain and water accounts for the reduced eating and for the internal collection of water-damp that manifests in rumbling intestines and sloppy stool diarrhea. Yang vacuity deprives the limbs of warmth, hence the physical cold and cold limbs. The somber white facial complexion, shortage of qi and laziness to speak, spontaneous sweating, pale or dark purple tongue with white fur, and the weak pulse, are all indications of heart-spleen yang vacuity. MED Assist yang and boost qi; fortify the spleen and nourish the heart. Use Origin-Preserving Decoction (*bǎo yuán tāng*) plus tangkuei (*dāng guī*), ovate atractylodes (*bái zhú*), tangerine peel (*chén pí*), and schisandra (*wǔ wèi zǐ*). For pronounced yang vacuity, add aconite (*fù zǐ*) and dried ginger (*gān jiāng*). ACU Base treatment mainly on back transport points, HT, SP, and CV. Select BL-15 (*xīn shū*, Heart Transport), BL-20 (*pí shū*, Spleen Transport), BL-17 (*gé shū*, Diaphragm Transport), CV-4 (*guān yuán*, Pass Head), CV-6 (*qì hǎi*, Sea of Qi), GV-4 (*mìng mén*, Life Gate), PC-6 (*nèi guān*, Inner Pass), HT-7 (*shén mén*, Spirit Gate), CV-12 (*zhōng wǎn*, Center Stomach Duct), ST-36 (*zú sān lǐ*, Leg Three Li), and LR-13 (*zhāng mén*, Camphorwood Gate); needle with supplementation and large amounts of moxa. Compare DUAL VACUITY OF THE HEART AND SPLEEN. [116: 132] [37: 280] [46: 665]

heart-stomach repletion fire 心胃实火 *xīn wèi shí huǒ*: EXUBERANT HEART-STOMACH FIRE.

heart stores the spirit 心藏神 *xīn cáng shén*: *Synonym: heart governs the spirit light*. This phrase comes from *Elementary Questions* (*sù wèn*). The heart is the seat of consciousness and mental function. If the heart fulfills its functions normally and blood and qi are abundant, the mind is lucid, alert, and responsive to the environment. If, however, the heart is diseased, the heart spirit may be disquieted, causing signs such as heart vexation, susceptibility to fright palpitations (heart palpitations due to emotional stimulus), diminished sleep, or profuse dreaming. In severe cases, there may be signs either of loss of sensibility, such as clouding sleep (hypersomnia) or coma, or of mental diseases, delirious speech, or manic agitation. [26: f95] [27: 37] [97: 120]

heart sweating 心汗 *xīn hàn*: SWEATING in the heart [region], i.e., in the pit of the stomach (scrobiculus cordis). Heart sweating is associated with damage to the heart and spleen by anxiety, thought, fright, or fear. MED Supplement the heart and spleen; constrain the spirit and boost qi. Use formulas such as Pulse-Engendering Powder (*shēng mài sǎn*), Spleen-Returning Decoction (*guī pí tāng*), or Heart-Supplementing Elixir (*bǔ xīn dān*). ACU Base treatment on back trans-

port points, HT, LI, and SI. Select BL-20 (*pí shū*, Spleen Transport), BL-15 (*xīn shū*, Heart Transport), HT-7 (*shén mén*, Spirit Gate), LI-4 (*hé gǔ*, Union Valley), SI-3 (*hòu xī*, Back Ravine), and HT-6 (*yīn xī*, Yin Cleft). Needle with supplementation. [26: 90] [27: 252] [97: 309] [46: 602]

heart tie 心系 *xīn xì*: The large blood vessels communicating directly with the heart. WMC includes the aorta, pulmonary artery, pulmonary veins, superior vena cava, and inferior vena cava. [27: 94] [97: 117]

heart vacuity 心虚 *xīn xū*: HEART QI VACUITY, HEART YANG VACUITY, HEART BLOOD VACUITY, or HEART YIN VACUITY; characterized by heart palpitations or fearful throbbing, insomnia, and dizziness. Heart qi vacuity is characterized by general qi vacuity signs such as fatigue, shortness of breath, spontaneous sweating, a pale enlarged tongue, and heart-specific qi vacuity signs such as interrupted pulses (结代 *jié dài*), and pain in the heart itself. Heart yang vacuity is the same as heart qi vacuity, but is differentiated by the addition of pronounced cold signs such as somber white complexion and blue lips, reversal cold of the limbs, and, in severe cases, vacuity desertion signs such as clouded spirit, fine pulse on the verge of expiration, and great sweating. Heart blood vacuity is characterized by general blood vacuity signs such as pale lusterless complexion, pale tongue, and fine pulse, together with general heart vacuity signs. See HEART QI VACUITY; HEART BLOOD VACUITY; HEART YIN VACUITY; HEART YANG VACUITY. [27: 147] [97: 116]

heart vacuity and gallbladder timidity 心虚胆怯 *xīn xū dǎn qiè*: *Synonym: heart-gallbladder vacuity timidity*. A feeling of emptiness in the heart and susceptibility to fright and fear. Vacuous heart and timid gallbladder usually occurs in insufficiency of heart blood and heart qi debilitation, and is partly related to mental factors. WMC observed in anemia and neurosis. MED Nourish the heart and quiet the spirit, or warm the gallbladder and quiet the spirit. Compare GALLBLADDER VACUITY. [26: 93] [27: 148] [97: 121] [50: 343]

heart vessel obstruction 心脉痹阻 *xīn mài bì zǔ*: A disease pattern characterized by stifling oppression and pain in the heart and chest that arises when HEART QI VACUITY or HEART YANG VACUITY allow phlegm and blood stasis to cause obstruction of the heart vessels. The chief signs are stifling oppression and pain (sometimes stabbing) in the heart and chest that may stretch to the shoulder, back, or inner arm, as well as heart palpitations and fearful throbbing, and panting. There may be attacks of cutting or stabbing pain, in severe cases with CLOUDING REVERSAL. Other signs include dark, stagnant green-blue or purple facial complexion, green-blue or purple lips, lassitude of spirit and lack of strength, shortage of qi and laziness to speak, fear of cold and cold limbs, glomus lump under the rib-side, water swelling, drum distention (ascites), and expectoration of blood. The tongue is pale green-blue sometimes with stasis speckles or macules. The pulse is sunken and slow or sunken and rough. It may also be skipping, bound, or intermittent. Analysis: When the yang qi of the heart is debilitated, its propelling action is weak, so that blood stasis develops (heart blood stasis obstruction); hence heart palpitations or fearful throbbing. The LUNG FACES THE HUNDRED VESSELS, and when blood becomes stagnant in the lung, lung qi is inhibited and ascends counterflow, causing oppression in the chest and panting with inability to lie down. Static blood damaging the network vessels of the lung causes expectoration of blood. The liver stores blood, and when blood stagnates in the liver, a glomus lump develops. When blood flow is inhibited, the facial complexion and lips become green-blue or purple. Inhibited blood flow can also cause water disease such as drum distention (ascites) and water swelling. Yang vacuity is reflected in lassitude of spirit and lack of strength, shortage of qi, and laziness to speak. When fluids are not distributed normally, they can gather to form phlegm. When phlegm turbidity and static blood obstruct the vessels of the heart and the whole body, the principle that "when there is stoppage, there is pain" comes into play, hence periodic stifling oppression and pain in the heart and chest. The pain can travel along the hand lesser yin (*shào yīn*) heart channel to the shoulder or inner arm. Blood stasis is classically reflected in stabbing pain, while phlegm turbidity obstruction is characterized by oppression and pain. When stasis and phlegm occur together, there is oppression and pain in the anterior chest, with periodic stabbing pain. Qi stagnation is reflected in distending pain. When cold evil suddenly enters the body and settles in the vessels of the heart, the vessels become hypertonic, thus exacerbating the stasis obstruction. When this happens, there is sudden excruciating pain. The pulses all reflect the inhibitive action of blood stasis on vessel qi. MED Warm yang and boost qi; dispel phlegm and expel stasis. Use Peach Kernel and Carthamus Brew (*táo rén hóng huā jiān*), House of Blood Stasis-Expelling Decoction (*xuè fǔ zhú yū tāng*), or Trichosanthes, Chinese Chive, and White Liquor Decoction (*guā lóu xiè bái bái jiǔ tāng*). ACU Base treatment mainly on back transport points, CV, SP, and LR. Select BL-15 (*xīn shū*, Heart Transport), BL-17 (*gé shū*, Diaphragm Transport), CV-14 (*jù què*, Great Tower Gate), CV-17 (*shān zhōng*, Chest Center), PC-6 (*nèi guān*, Inner Pass), SP-10 (*xuè hǎi*, Sea of Blood), SP-6 (*sān yīn jiāo*, Three Yin Intersec-

tion), and LR-3 (*tài chōng*, Supreme Surge); needle with drainage and add moxa. [46: 595] [37: 334] [57: 51] [116: 53]

heart vexation 烦热 *fán rè*: Synonym: *heart vexation* (*obs*). A feeling of unrest or irritability that focuses in the heart region. Vexation is commonly observed in either vacuity or repletion heat. In severe cases, it is associated with agitation, i.e., increased physical movement. See VEXATION AND AGITATION; HEAT VEXATION; HEAT VEXATION IN THE CHEST; ANGUISH; VACUITY VEXATION. [27: 372]

heart water 心水 *xīn shuǐ*: One of the FIVE WATERS spoken of in *Essential Prescriptions of the Golden Coffer* (*jīn guì yào lüè*), characterized by generalized swelling and shortage of qi, vexation and agitation with inability to rest, and swelling of the lower yin. [27: 419] [97: 116]

heart wilting 心痿 *xīn wěi*: VESSEL WILTING.

heart worm disease 心虫病 *xīn chóng bìng*: See ROUNDWORM. [26: 94]

heart yang 心阳 *xīn yáng*: See HEART YIN AND HEART YANG.

heart yang vacuity 心阳虚 *xīn yáng xū*: Synonym: *devitalization of heart yang*. HEART QI VACUITY with pronounced cold signs and blood stasis signs. The chief signs are heart palpitations, shortness of breath, stifling oppression and possibly pain in the chest exacerbated by exertion, as well as aversion to cold and cold limbs. Other signs include lassitude of spirit and lack of strength, shortage of qi and laziness to speak, spontaneous sweating, and bright white or dark stagnant complexion. In some cases, there may be profuse sleeping. The tongue is pale and soft, or pale green-blue. The pulse is slow, possibly faint, or rapid and forceless. It may be skipping, bound, or intermittent. Heart yang vacuity often occurs in conjunction with kidney yang vacuity, the combined pattern being referred to as HEART-KIDNEY YANG VACUITY, in which physical cold and cold limbs are more pronounced, and are accompanied by kidney yang vacuity signs such as scant urine or water swelling. Analysis: Heart yang vacuity is a development of heart qi vacuity. When heart yang is depleted, its propelling action is weak, hence the heart palpitations or fearful throbbing. When blood moves sluggishly, it stagnates and obstructs the heart vessels, hence there is heart pain. When heart yang is insufficient, the yang of the chest is devitalized and does not circulate properly, hence there is oppression in the chest and shortness of breath. Exertion causes wear on qi and hence exacerbates the heart palpitations and oppression in the chest. When yang qi is vacuous, the spirit is deprived of nourishment, hence the lassitude of spirit and profuse sleeping; at the same time, the body is deprived of warmth, hence the physical cold and cold limbs. Yang vacuity makes external defense insecure, hence spontaneous sweating, shortage of qi, and laziness to speak. Failure to make the blood ascend to the head and face and to transform water-damp gives rise to a bright white facial complexion and a pale soft enlarged tongue. If the movement of blood is sluggish, the facial complexion may be dark and stagnant, and the tongue pale green-blue. Inability to propel the blood also accounts for the slow, faint, bound, and intermittent pulses. If vacuous yang "gallops outward" (makes an outward show of force), the pulse may be rapid, and if vessel qi is discontinuous, it can be skipping (rapid and irregularly interrupted). MED Warm and supplement heart yang. Use Origin-Preserving Decoction (*bǎo yuán tāng*) or Cinnamon Twig, Licorice, Dragon Bone, and Oyster Shell Decoction (*guì zhī gān cǎo lóng gǔ mǔ lì tāng*). ACU Base treatment mainly on back transport points, HT, and CV. Select BL-15 (*xīn shū*, Heart Transport), CV-14 (*jù què*, Great Tower Gate), CV-17 (*shān zhōng*, Chest Center), CV-4 (*guān yuán*, Pass Head), CV-6 (*qì hǎi*, Sea of Qi), GV-4 (*mìng mén*, Life Gate), PC-6 (*nèi guān*, Inner Pass), and HT-7 (*shén mén*, Spirit Gate), needle with supplementation and moxa. For blood stasis signs, add BL-17 (*gé shū*, Diaphragm Transport), SP-10 (*xuè hǎi*, Sea of Blood), LR-3 (*tài chōng*, Supreme Surge), and SP-6 (*sān yīn jiāo*, Three Yin Intersection); needle with even supplementation and drainage. **Comparison:** *Heart qi vacuity:* Heart yang vacuity is similar to heart qi vacuity. Both share heart palpitations or fearful throbbing, oppression in the chest and shortness of breath exacerbated by exertion, and lassitude of spirit and lack of strength. Either may be associated with heart pain. Heart yang vacuity is associated with cold signs such as fear of cold and cold limbs, which are not observed in heart qi vacuity. Furthermore, because heart yang vacuity is more severe than heart qi vacuity, the propelling action of qi is weaker, and blood stasis signs are more pronounced. Thus the heart palpitations, fearful throbbing, oppression in the chest, shortness of breath, and heart pain are more marked. The dark stagnant complexion and pale green-blue tongue are not observed in qi vacuity. *Fulminant desertion of heart yang:* Heart yang qi vacuity must also be distinguished from fulminant desertion of heart yang. Heart yang qi vacuity is a chronic condition of heart palpitations or fearful throbbing, oppression in the chest, shortness of breath, aversion to cold, and cold limbs. Fulminant desertion of heart yang is a critical development of heart yang vacuity, characterized by a somber white complexion, dripping cold sweat, reversal cold of the limbs, a faint pulse on the verge of expiration, and, in se-

vere cases, coma. *Dual vacuity of heart yin and yang* shares the cold signs of heart yang vacuity, and is further marked by yin vacuity signs such as emaciation, heart vexation, tidal heat [effusion], night sweating, dry throat lacking liquid, heat effusion and spontaneous sweating at the slightest exertion, peeling tongue fur, and faint fine rapid pulse. [27: 147] [97: 120] [37: 280] [46: 595]

heart yin 心阴 *xīn yīn*: Synonym: *heart construction.* See HEART YIN AND HEART YANG.

heart yin and heart yang 心阴、心阳 *xīn yīn, xīn yáng*: Heart yin and heart yang refer to the complementary aspects of the heart's functions. Heart yang refers to a strong heartbeat, smooth blood flow, and the lively, expansive aspect of mental activity. Heart yin refers to a regular, moderate heartbeat and the calm, passive aspect of mental activity. Yin and yang complement and counterbalance each other, ensuring that the heart beats forcefully and regularly, and performs all its normal functions. An essential prerequisite of normal function is an abundance of heart blood and exuberance of heart qi. Insufficiency of heart blood or heart qi may debilitate heart yin or yang. Since "when yang is vacuous, there is cold," and "when yin is vacuous, there is heat," such cases present with signs not only of qi or blood vacuity, but also of vacuity cold and vacuity heat. [6: 80]

heart yin vacuity 心阴虚 *xīn yīn xū*: The manifestation of insufficiency of heart yin, characterized chiefly by heart palpitations, heart vexation, insomnia, and profuse dreaming. Other signs include vexing heat in the five hearts, postmeridian tidal heat [effusion], reddening of the cheeks, night sweating, dry mouth and throat, and forgetfulness. The tongue is red with little liquid and little or no fur. The pulse is fine and rapid. Heart yin vacuity regularly occurs in conjunction with kidney yin, the combined pattern being called HEART-KIDNEY YIN VACUITY. **Analysis:** When heart yin is depleted, the heart is deprived of nourishment, hence the heart palpitations. At the same time, there is effulgent yin vacuity fire, which harasses the spirit, causing heart vexation, insomnia, and profuse dreaming. Vacuity fire also causes tidal heat [effusion], night sweating, vexing heat in the five hearts, and reddening of the cheeks. It also accounts for the red tongue with little liquid, and the fine rapid pulse. When yin liquid is depleted, the mouth and throat are dry. MED Enrich yin and quiet the spirit. Use Heart-Supplementing Elixir (*bǔ xīn dān*) or Cinnabar Spirit-Quieting Pill (*zhū shā ān shén wán*). ACU Base treatment mainly on back transport points, HT, PC, and CV. Select BL-15 (*xīn shū*, Heart Transport), BL-20 (*pí shū*, Spleen Transport), BL-17 (*gé shū*, Diaphragm Transport), PC-6 (*nèi guān*, Inner Pass), HT-7 (*shén mén*, Spirit Gate), SP-6 (*sān yīn jiāo*, Three Yin Intersection), KI-3 (*tài xī*, Great Ravine), and KI-6 (*zhào hǎi*, Shining Sea), needling with supplementation. For night sweating add HT-6 (*yīn xī*, Yin Cleft), and SI-3 (*hòu xī*, Back Ravine). **Comparison:** *Heart blood vacuity:* Both heart yin vacuity and heart blood vacuity share heart palpitations or fearful throbbing, insomnia, and profuse dreaming. Heart blood vacuity is marked by a lusterless white or withered-yellow facial complexion, pale lips, and a fine weak pulse. There are no heat signs. Heart yin vacuity arises from insufficiency of yin humor and vacuity fire. Hence in addition to heart palpitations and insomnia, there are pronounced heat signs such as heart vexation, vexing heat in the five hearts, tidal heat [effusion], night sweating, red tongue with scant fur, and a fine rapid pulse. *Dual vacuity of heart qi and yin:* Heart yin vacuity shares with dual vacuity of heart qi and yin signs of insufficiency of heart yin such as heart palpitations, insomnia, vexing heat in the five hearts, tidal heat [effusion], and night sweating. In addition to these signs, dual vacuity of heart qi and yin is marked by signs of insufficiency of heart qi such as oppression in the chest and shortness of breath exacerbated by exertion, shortage of qi and laziness to speak, lassitude of spirit, and lack of strength. These latter signs are absent in heart yin vacuity. *Dual vacuity of heart yin and yang:* Heart yin vacuity and and dual vacuity of heart yin and yang are both marked by heart palpitations, heart vexation, insomnia, profuse dreaming, and heat in the heart of the palms and soles. Dual vacuity of heart yin and yang is marked by signs of yang vacuity such as listlessness of essence-spirit, oppression in the chest, shortness of breath, physical cold and cold limbs, shortage of qi and laziness to speak, fatigue, and lack of strength. These latter signs are absent in kidney yin vacuity. *Heart-lung yin vacuity:* Heart yin vacuity shares with heart-lung yin vacuity signs of insufficiency of heart yin and effulgent yin vacuity fire, such as heart palpitations, heart vexation, insomnia, profuse dreaming, vexing heat in the five hearts, tidal heat [effusion], night sweating, reddening of the cheeks, a red tongue with scant fur, and a rapid fine pulse. Heart-lung yin vacuity is marked by the addition of signs of of lung yin vacuity and impaired depurative downbearing, such as dry cough without phlegm or with scant sticky phlegm, in severe cases with pain in the chest and expectoration of blood. These latter signs are absent in heart yin vacuity. *Heart-kidney yin vacuity:* Heart yin vacuity and heart-kidney yin vacuity both share heart palpitations, insomnia, vexing heat in the five hearts, tidal heat [effusion], night sweating, red tongue with little fur, and a rapid fine pulse. Heart-kidney vacuity in ad-

dition to these signs is marked by signs of frenetic stirring of the ministerial fire such as limp aching lumbus and knees, excessive libido, persistent erection, seminal emission, and in women, dreaming of intercourse. [26: 93] [27: 148] [97: 120] [116: 37] [37: 332, 335] [46: 602, 648]

heat 热 *rè*: **1.** The opposite of cold. Heat is the manifestation of the sun and fire. Hot weather (and artificially heated environments) cause sweating, and without an adequate increase in fluid intake, thirst. There may be vexation and other discomforts naturally attributed to heat by the individual. In the healthy individual, these natural responses abate on exposure to cooler temperatures. **2.** The external evils FIRE and SUMMERHEAT manifesting in the body in pathological signs such as high fever, fear of heat, desire for coolness, thirst, red face, red eyes, reddish urine, red tongue with yellow fire, and rapid pulse. Fire and summerheat are two of the SIX EXCESSES. They result from exposure to heat in the environment or to spells of weather that are abnormally hot for the season. **3.** Any condition manifesting in signs similar to those of fire and summerheat that are the result of a) yin vacuity or b) the transformation of either external evils passing into the interior or of the transformation of yang qi as a result of affect damage (physiologically disruptive effects of emotional and mental states). See FIRE. **4.** One of eight parameters under which any of the above pathological conditions are classified. The terms that describe the action of heat in the body that produces heat patterns include: **blaze** (燔 *fán*), to burn vigorously (e.g., qi and construction both ablaze); **deflagrate** (焚 *fén*), to burn intensely (e.g., heart fire deflagrating internally); **effulgent** (旺 *wàng*), burning brightly (e.g., effulgent yin vacuity fire); **steam** (蒸 *zhēng*), to rise gently upward or out to the surface (e.g., steaming bones); **flame upward** (上炎 *shàng yán*), (of fire) to rise like a flame to produce upper body signs. (e.g., liver fire flaming upward); **scorch** (灼 *zhuó*), to damage slightly by burning (e.g., evil heat scorching the network vessels); **condense** (炼 *liàn*), reduce fluids (producing phlegm). **5.** Heat effusion or subjective sensations of heat that may or may not be classified as heat among the eight principles. **6.** One of the FOUR NATURES (heat, cold, warmth, coolness) of medicinals, used in the treatment of cold patterns. **NB:** The term 'heat' is distinguished from 'fire',' 'summerheat', and 'warmth' as follows. 'Fire' in the context of the six excesses means heat in the broad sense, but may also denote intense heat as opposed to the milder form, warmth. Heat occurring between the summer solstice and the autumn equinox is called 'summerheat', in contrast to 'fire' and 'heat', which usually denote heat occurring at other times of the year. 'Heat' and 'fire' may also denote states arising within the body as a result of transformation of other evils or of yang qi. In this context, 'fire' denotes more intense forms of heat, as in 'extreme heat transforming into fire' and 'damp depression transforming into fire', and specifically denotes heat that manifests in upper body signs, e.g., 'liver fire flaming upward' and 'heart fire'. [26: 870] [97: 488]

heat bind 热结 *rè jié*: Synonym: *yang bind*. HEAT gathering and binding in a particular location. When heat binds in the stomach and intestines, there is dry bound stool, and a sunken replete pulse; in severe cases, there may be tidal heat [effusion] and delirious speech. See YANG BRIGHTNESS DISEASE. When heat binds in the blood aspect, a blood amassment pattern emerges. *Systematized Identification of Warm Diseases* (*wēn bìng tiáo biàn*) states, "Heat bind with circumfluence is not a stoppage of qi. There is no need for unripe bitter orange (*zhǐ shí*) and magnolia bark (*hòu pò*); simply use mirabilite (*máng xiāo*) to enter yin and resolve the heat bind." According to *On Cold Damage* (*shāng hán lùn*), in greater yang (*tài yáng*) heat that fails to resolve, heat binds in the bladder, and the patient becomes manic, and passes blood. If blood is passed, the patient will recover. ACU For gastrointestinal heat bind, see HEAT CONSTIPATION. See YANG BRIGHTNESS BOWEL PATTERN; QI-ASPECT PATTERN; HEAT CONSTIPATION; COLD DAMAGE BLOOD AMASSMENT PATTERN. [26: 874] [27: 127] [97: 150]

heat binding in the bladder 热结膀胱 *rè jié páng guāng*: Synonym: *bladder heat bind*. A repletion pattern of contention between blood and heat. Heat binding in the bladder develops when greater yang (*tài yáng*) disease fails to resolve, transforms into heat, and enters the interior. The heat then binds in the bladder causing hard fullness of the lower abdomen, uninhibited urination, heat effusion without aversion to cold, and manic mental states. [26: 874] [27: 166] [97: 455]

heat binding in the stomach and intestines 热结肠胃 *rè jié cháng wèi*: Synonym: *gastrointestinal heat bind*. See HEAT BIND. [26: 874]

heat bind with circumfluence 热结旁流 *rè jié páng liú*: Hard stool in the intestines, allowing looser stool to pass around it, manifesting in constipation followed by foul-smelling diarrhea. It is associated with abdominal fullness and distention with pain that refuses pressure, a red tongue with thick dry yellow, possibly gray fur with prickles, a sunken replete rapid pulse. In some cases, there may be vexation and agitation, clouded spirit, and delirious raving. *On Warm Epidemics* (*wēn yì lùn*) states: "Heat bind with circumfluence, is due to stomach domain repletion with internal heat con-

gestion. There is first constipation, and then diarrhea that is pure fetid water completely without feces, three or four, or up to ten times a day. The appropriate treatment is Major Qi-Coordinating Decoction (*dà chéng qì tāng*). When bound stool appears, the diarrhea will stop. If taking the decoction fails to produce bound stool, and there is diarrhea with fetid water and the ingested decoction, this is because the evil in the large intestinal is exuberant, causing it to fail to perform the office of conveyance. Thus, one knows that the evil is still present, and the illness will not be alleviated. [In such cases,] it is appropriate to precipitate again." See yang brightness (*yáng míng*) bowel patterns. [97: 454] [50: 1241]

heat block 热闭 *rè bì*: A pathology in which heat evil congests in the bowels and viscera and in the channels and network vessels, blocking normal movement out of the body. When in measles, for example, the heat toxin is not thrust outward to produce a MACULOPAPULAR ERUPTION but instead falls inward to block the lung and cause cough and hasty panting, the resulting condition is described as an internal heat toxin block. When in strangury patterns heat hampers bladder function causing painful rough (disfluent) urination, the condition is often described as a bladder heat block. See BLOCK. [26: 873] [97: 450]

heat-block tetanic reversal 热闭痉厥 *rè bì jìng jué*: CLOUDED SPIRIT and TETANY (pronounced spasm) due to an evil blocked in the interior. It occurs, for example, in CHILD FRIGHT WIND occurring in high fever. See BLOCK.

heat chest bind 热结胸 *rè jié xiōng*: HEAT REPLETION CHEST BIND. [26: 874]

heat cholera 热霍乱 *rè huò luàn*: Synonym: *heat qi cholera*. CHOLERA arising when obstruction of center burner after internal damage by rich food or external contraction of summerheat-heat or damp-heat. In addition to the principal signs of cholera (simultaneous vomiting and diarrhea), there is gripping pain in the abdomen, hot malodorous stool, oppression in the chest, heart vexation, heat effusion, thirst, yellow or reddish urine, a yellow slimy tongue fur, and a rapid surging or rapid sunken pulse. MED Clear heat and transform dampness; repel foulness and drain turbidity. Use Coptis and Magnolia Bark Beverage (*lián pò yǐn*) or Coptis and Elsholtzia Powder (*huáng lián xiāng rú sǎn*). ACU Base treatment mainly on LI, ST, SP, and PC. Select LI-4 (*hé gǔ*, Union Valley), ST-25 (*tiān shū*, Celestial Pivot), ST-37 (*shàng jù xū*, Upper Great Hollow), ST-36 (*zú sān lǐ*, Leg Three Li), LI-11 (*qū chí*, Pool at the Bend), ST-44 (*nèi tíng*, Inner Court), SP-9 (*yīn líng quán*, Yin Mound Spring), PC-6 (*nèi guān*, Inner Pass), and PC-7 (*dà líng*, Great Mound); needle with drainage. [26: 876]

heat constipation 热秘 *rè bì*: CONSTIPATION due to heat binding in the large intestine (see HEAT BIND). Heat constipation is accompanied by generalized heat [effusion], red facial complexion, aversion to heat and desire for coolness, mouth and tongue sores, dry mouth and parched lips, yellow or reddish urine, yellow tongue fur, and a rapid replete pulse. MED Treat by clearing heat and draining precipitation using Diaphragm-Cooling Powder (*liáng gé sǎn*), Three Yellows Bitter Orange and Ovate Atractylodes Pill (*sān huáng zhǐ zhú wán*), or Saussurea and Areca Pill (*mù xiāng bīng láng wán*). ACU Base treatment mainly on the alarm, back transport, and lower uniting points of LI, and on ST and LI. Select BL-25 (*dà cháng shū*, Large Intestine Transport), ST-25 (*tiān shū*, Celestial Pivot), ST-37 (*shàng jù xū*, Upper Great Hollow), LI-4 (*hé gǔ*, Union Valley), LI-11 (*qū chí*, Pool at the Bend), ST-44 (*nèi tíng*, Inner Court), SP-14 (*fù jié*, Abdominal Bind), and KI-6 (*zhào hǎi*, Shining Sea); needle with drainage. [26: 873] [97: 450] [46: 670] [37: 326] [113: 102]

heat cough 热嗽 *rè sòu*: COUGH attributed to depressed heat damaging the lung. Heat cough is treated in different ways depending on the quantity of phlegm. **Scant yellow phlegm:** Heat cough is usually associated with scant thick sticky yellow phlegm that takes repeated coughing to expectorate and that may be flecked with blood, and attended by a dry sore throat, hot breath issuing from the nose, and sometimes heat effusion. MED Clear heat and moisten the lung using formulas such as Coptis Phlegm-Transforming Beverage (*huáng lián huà tán yǐn*). ACU Base treatment on LU and LI. Select BL-13 (*fèi shū*, Lung Transport), LI-11 (*qū chí*, Pool at the Bend), LI-4 (*hé gǔ*, Union Valley), LU-10 (*yú jì*, Fish Border), LU-5 (*chǐ zé*, Cubit Marsh), and GV-14 (*dà zhuī*, Great Hammer); needle with drainage. Prick LU-11 (*shào shāng*, Lesser Shang) to bleed. **Copious yellow phlegm:** In some cases, heat cough is associated with copious yellow phlegm with a fishy smell, accompanied by fullness and oppression in the chest and stomach duct, heat vexation, red facial complexion, and rapid pulse. MED Treat by clearing heat and sweeping phlegm with formulas such as Minor Chest Bind Decoction (*xiǎo xiàn xiōng tāng*) or Scutellaria and Pinellia Pill (*qín bàn wán*). ACU Base treatment on LU and LI. Select BL-13 (*fèi shū*, Lung Transport), LI-11 (*qū chí*, Pool at the Bend), LI-4 (*hé gǔ*, Union Valley), LU-10 (*yú jì*, Fish Border), LU-5 (*chǐ zé*, Cubit Marsh), ST-40 (*fēng lóng*, Bountiful Bulge), CV-22 (*tiān tú*, Celestial Chimney), and CV-17 (*shān zhōng*, Chest Center). Needle with drainage. [26: 876]

heat damages qi 热伤气 *rè shāng qì*: Heat and summerheat cause the interstices to open and let sweat flow, thereby damaging liquid and wearing qi. See, for example, SUMMERHEAT-HEAT. [26: 875]

heat damaging the network vessels of the lung 热伤肺络 *rè shāng fèi luò*: Heat in the lung causing bloody expectorate. Both repletion heat and vacuity heat can damage the network vessels of the lung. **Repletion heat:** Repletion heat is observed in diseases of recent onset. It is attributable to depressed evils transforming into heat and is characterized by expectoration of copious amounts of blood, heat effusion, red facial complexion, red tongue with yellow fur, and slippery rapid pulse. MED White-Draining Powder (*xiè bái sǎn*) combined with Indigo and Clamshell Powder (*dài gé sǎn*) plus imperata (*bái máo gēn*), lotus root node (*ǒu jié*), eclipta (*mò hàn lián*), and dried/fresh rehmannia (*shēng dì huáng*). ACU Base treatment mainly on LU, LI, and PC. Drain LU-10 (*yú jì*, Fish Border), PC-8 (*láo gōng*, Palace of Toil), BL-13 (*fèi shū*, Lung Transport), and LI-11 (*qū chí*, Pool at the Bend), and prick LU-11 (*shào shāng*, Lesser Shang), and LI-1 (*shāng yáng*, Shang Yang) to bleed. **Vacuity heat:** Vacuity heat is observed in patients suffering from chronic disease or depletion of lung-kidney yin when vacuity fire scorches the lung, and is characterized by expectoration of scant amounts of blood or merely blood-flecked phlegm, periodic low fever, postmeridian tidal heat [effusion], flushing of the cheeks, pale red tongue, and rapid fine pulse. MED Lily Bulb Lung-Securing Decoction (*bǎi hé gù fèi tāng*). Add imperata (*bái máo gēn*), lotus root node (*ǒu jié*), eclipta (*mò hàn lián*), and dried/fresh rehmannia (*shēng dì huáng*) to stanch bleeding and add sweet wormwood (*qīng hāo*), turtle shell (*biē jiǎ*), lycium root bark (*dì gǔ pí*), and baiwei (*bái wēi*), to clear vacuity heat. ACU Base treatment mainly on LU and KI. Drain LU-5 (*chǐ zé*, Cubit Marsh), LU-6 (*kǒng zuì*, Collection Hole), LU-10 (*yú jì*, Fish Border), and Hundred Taxations (*bǎi láo*), and supplement KI-2 (*rán gǔ*, Blazing Valley), and KI-3 (*tài xī*, Great Ravine). [46: 650, 652] [26: 875] [27: 161] [97: 454]

heat damaging the sinews 热伤筋脉 *rè shāng jīn mài*: High or enduring heat effusion scorches construction-yin, depriving the sinews of nourishment and thereby causing hypertonicity of the limbs, wilting (*wěi*) and limpness, or paralysis. [26: 875] [27: 136] [97: 454]

heat damaging the spirit light 热伤神明 *rè shāng shén míng*: Heat causing spirit-mind signs such as CLOUDED SPIRIT, mania etc. Heat damaging the spirit light is most commonly observed in heat entering the pericardium in warm disease. [26: 875] [27: 149] [97: 454]

heat depression 热郁 *rè yù*: A condition that arises when any persistent depression (damp depression, qi depression, etc.) transforms into heat, and that is characterized by clouded head and dizzy vision, thirst with desire for fluid, dry lips and tongue, yellow or reddish urine, and a rapid sunken pulse. Sometimes the flesh is scorching hot to the touch. Qi depression is the underlying cause of all of the six depressions, and is attributed to constrained affect-mind causing binding depression of liver qi. Whatever other forms of depression liver qi depression causes, it can always transform into heat. ⃞MED Use Heat Depression Decoction (*rè yù tāng*). [26: 877] [27: 136]

heat diarrhea 热泻 *rè xiè*, 热泄 *rè xiè*: *Synonym: fire diarrhea.* DIARRHEA caused by heat distressing the stomach and intestines. Heat diarrhea patterns are marked by abdominal pain and rumbling intestines. Pain comes in bouts with diarrhea. The stool is thick and sticky, or watery, or containing untransformed food. Other signs include burning pain in the anus, tenesmus, thirst with desire for cold drinks, and rough voidings of reddish urine. ⃞WMC ⃞MED Clear heat and drain fire with formulas such as Scutellaria Decoction (*huáng qín tāng*), Pueraria, Scutellaria, and Coptis Decoction (*gé gēn qín lián tāng*), or Saussurea and Coptis Pill (*xiāng lián wán*) ⃞ACU Base treatment mainly on CV, ST, and SP. Select CV-12 (*zhōng wǎn*, Center Stomach Duct), ST-25 (*tiān shū*, Celestial Pivot), ST-36 (*zú sān lǐ*, Leg Three Li), LI-11 (*qū chí*, Pool at the Bend), ST-44 (*nèi tíng*, Inner Court), SP-9 (*yīn líng quán*, Yin Mound Spring), SP-6 (*sān yīn jiāo*, Three Yin Intersection), and ST-37 (*shàng jù xū*, Upper Great Hollow); needle with drainage. For qi vacuity with heat, add BL-20 (*pí shū*, Spleen Transport) and SP-6 (*sān yīn jiāo*, Three Yin Intersection). [26: 876] [50: 1236] [27: 263] [97: 450]

heat disease 热病 *rè bìng*: **1.** *Synonym: febrile disease.* Any disease characterized by heat effusion (fever), caused by externally contracted evil. Compare HEAT DISEASE. See EXTERNALLY CONTRACTED HEAT (FEBRILE) DISEASE; COLD DAMAGE; WARM DISEASE. **2.** Febrile disease in summer caused by latent qi. [26: 872]

heat distention 热胀 *rè zhàng*: DISTENTION arising when damage by liquor and rich food causes damp-heat to brew in the center or when depressed qi transforms into fire. Heat distention is characterized by abdominal fullness and distention, dry bound stool, yellow or reddish urine, and a rapid surging pulse. In some cases there is heat effusion. ⃞MED Drain fire and dry dampness using Center Fullness Separating and Dispersing Pill (*zhōng mǎn fēn xiāo wán*) or Tangkuei, Gentian, and Aloe

Pill (*dāng guī lóng huì wán*). ⃞ACU Base treatment mainly on ST, CV, PC, SP, and LI. Select ST-25 (*tiān shū*, Celestial Pivot), CV-6 (*qì hǎi*, Sea of Qi), PC-6 (*nèi guān*, Inner Pass), ST-36 (*zú sān lǐ*, Leg Three Li), LI-4 (*hé gǔ*, Union Valley), LI-11 (*qū chí*, Pool at the Bend), ST-44 (*nèi tíng*, Inner Court), SP-9 (*yīn líng quán*, Yin Mound Spring), and SP-6 (*sān yīn jiāo*, Three Yin Intersection); needle with drainage. [26: 874] [46: 597, 602]

heat distressing the large intestine 热迫大肠 *rè pò dà cháng*: Impairment of the large intestine's governing of conveyance and transformation manifesting in abdominal pain, diarrhea with malodorous yellow stool, burning pain in the anus, short voidings of yellow urine, dry yellow tongue fur, and a slippery rapid pulse. [26: 872] [27: 163] [97: 454]

heat dysentery 热痢 *rè lì*: DYSENTERY forming a heat pattern. Heat dysentery is usually attributable to exuberant heat in the intestines causing accumulation and stagnation. It is characterized by the general signs of dysentery (abdominal pain, tenesmus, and red and white stool) in addition to generalized heat [effusion], vexation and thirst with intake of fluid, hot reddish urine, slimy yellow tongue fur, and a forceful rapid slippery pulse. ⃞MED Clear heat, cool the blood, and resolve toxin. Use formulas such as Pulsatilla Decoction (*bái tóu wēng tāng*). ⃞ACU Base treatment on ST and LI. Select LI-4 (*hé gǔ*, Union Valley), ST-25 (*tiān shū*, Celestial Pivot), ST-37 (*shàng jù xū*, Upper Great Hollow), LI-11 (*qū chí*, Pool at the Bend), ST-44 (*nèi tíng*, Inner Court), and GV-14 (*dà zhuī*, Great Hammer); needle with drainage. [26: 873]

heat effusion 发热 *fā rè*, 热 *rè*: *Synonym: fever.* Abnormal bodily heat that can be detected by palpation or that is experienced subjectively; fever. Heat effusion occurring with aversion to cold or aversion to wind at the onset of illness indicates external evils invading the FLESHY EXTERIOR. If the aversion to cold is more pronounced than the heat effusion, the pattern is one of wind-cold. Pronounced heat effusion with only aversion to wind suggests wind-heat. Heat effusion without aversion to cold occurs in various patterns. Distinction is made between vigorous heat [effusion], tidal heat [effusion], vexing heat in the five hearts, steaming bone tidal heat [effusion], baking heat [effusion], and unsurfaced heat. **Vigorous heat [effusion]**, a persistent high fever without aversion to cold, occurs as external evil passes from the exterior into the interior of the body. **Tidal heat [effusion]**, heat effusion that recurs at regular intervals, usually every afternoon, is in most cases due to internal heat from yin vacuity. Because the heat effusion feels as though it is radiating out from the innermost part of the body, it is also called *steaming* *bone tidal heat [effusion]*. See also POSTMERIDIAN TIDAL HEAT [EFFUSION] and LATE AFTERNOON TIDAL HEAT [EFFUSION]. **Baking heat** EFFUSION is the steady heat effusion that is associated with damage to yin, and attended by heart vexation, insomnia, and oppressive feverishness. **Vexing heat in the five hearts** refers to heat in the center of the soles and palms, and the center of the chest. It is usually a sign of yin or blood vacuity but may also occur when evils are deep-lying in the yin aspect or when fire becomes depressed. **Unsurfaced heat effusion** is caused by dampness trapping hidden heat so that the heat can only be felt after longer palpation. **High fever**, heat effusion as shown by a high reading on the thermometer, is a modern medical term now often used in Chinese medical literature. See also GAN HEAT EFFUSION; QI VACUITY HEAT EFFUSION; HOT BACK; HOT HEAD. ◇ Chin 发 *fā*, emit, put forth, effuse; 热 *rè*, heat. Chinese has no unique term for the notion of a hot state of the body that corresponds to the English 'fever' (Eng from the L. *febris*, related to *fovere*, to warm or keep warm), it expresses the idea as 'giving off heat'. In describing different types of fever (see examples above), 发 is often dropped. As a result, the notion of fever is poorly distinguished in the terminology from heat as a cause of disease or a morbid state. Although there is a conceptual distinction between fever and heat, as seen the observation that mild fever may be occur in wind-cold patterns, the borderline between the two in other contexts is not always clear. Consequently, 身热不外扬 *shēn rè bù wài yáng*, for example, could be rendered as 'unsurfaced fever' or 'unsurfaced heat'. Furthermore, the concept of (发) 热 is wider than that of fever in that it denotes palpable body heat or heat sensations (as in yin vacuity) that are not normally described in English as fever either in the colloquial or in the modern medical sense of the word. At the risk of obscuring a familiar concept with an unfamiliar expression, the term 'heat effusion' is here introduced. The word effusion is enclosed in brackets where it does not appear, yet is implicit in the Chinese. The word 'fever' is retained in terms of Western medical origin, e.g., high fever. [26: 719] [27: 356]

heat [effusion] and [aversion to] cold 恶寒发热 *wù hán fā rè*, 寒热 *hán rè*: See the separate entries HEAT EFFUSION; AVERSION TO COLD.

heat entering construction-blood 热入营血 *rè rù yíng xuè*: In warm disease, heat evil entering the construction aspect or blood aspect. See CONSTRUCTION-ASPECT PATTERN; BLOOD-ASPECT PATTERN; CLEARING CONSTRUCTION; COOLING THE BLOOD. [84: 37]

heat entering the blood aspect 热入血分 *rè rù xuè fèn*: HEAT EVIL invading the blood aspect in warm heat disease. Heat entering the blood aspect easily causes wear on the blood and causes it to move frenetically. Signs include heat effusion becoming more pronounced at night, clouded spirit, agitation, or convulsions, patches and macules, bleeding, and a deep crimson tongue. *On Warm Heat* (*wēn rè lùn*) says that "Entry into the blood poses the danger of wear on the blood and stirring of the blood. It calls for cooling and dissipating blood." See BLOOD-ASPECT PATTERN. [26: 871] [27: 136] [97: 452]

heat entering the blood chamber 热入血室 *rè rù xuè shì*: EVIL HEAT exploiting vacuity during menstruation or after childbirth to enter the blood chamber (thoroughfare (*chōng*) vessel and uterus) to contend with the blood. Heat entering the blood chamber is characterized by hard fullness in the lower abdomen or chest and rib-side, alternating heat [effusion] and [aversion to] cold, and nonsensical talk at night. MED Treat with Minor Bupleurum Decoction (*xiǎo chái hú tāng*). ACU Base treatment on GB, LR, and SP. Select GB-20 (*fēng chí*, Wind Pool), LR-3 (*tài chōng*, Supreme Surge), LR-14 (*qī mén*, Cycle Gate), CV-6 (*qì hǎi*, Sea of Qi), SP-6 (*sān yīn jiāo*, Three Yin Intersection), BL-17 (*gé shū*, Diaphragm Transport), SP-10 (*xuè hǎi*, Sea of Blood), and SP-8 (*dì jī*, Earth's Crux); needle with drainage. *On Cold Damage* (*shāng hán lùn*) says: "For heat entering the blood chamber, LR-14 (*qī mén*, Cycle Gate) must be needled." [26: 871] [27: 136] [97: 452]

heat entering the pericardium 热入心包 *rè rù xīn bāo*: A warm heat disease pattern characterized by high fever, clouded spirit, delirious speech, reversal cold of the limbs, and convulsions. See PERICARDIAC PATTERN. [27: 149] [97: 452]

heat epilepsy 热痫 *rè xián*: EPILEPSY due to accumulated heat. Heat epilepsy occurs in infants when feeding damages the stomach, heat accumulates in the stomach and gives rise to wind phlegm. It is characterized by drawing together of mouth and eye, jerking of the limbs, rigid lumbus and back, arched rigidity of the neck, foaming at the mouth, sound in the nose, vigorous heat [effusion], and crying. MED Abate heat effusion and eliminate epilepsy using formulas such as Uncaria Beverage (*gōu téng yǐn*) and variations. ACU Use the general points given for fits under EPILEPSY, and needle GV-14 (*dà zhuī*, Great Hammer), ST-44 (*nèi tíng*, Inner Court), and ST-45 (*lì duì*, Severe Mouth). Prick Twelve Well Points (*shí èr jǐng xué*) to bleed. [26: 876]

heat evil 热邪 *rè xié*: HEAT as a disease-causing agent, causing repletion patterns that are hot and yang in nature with signs such as heat effusion, rough breathing, redness and swelling, burning pain, and constipation. Compare EVIL HEAT. [26: 872] [27: 214] [97: 448]

heat evil congesting the lung 热邪壅肺 *rè xié yōng fèi*: Synonym: *heat evil obstructing the lung.* HEAT EVIL upsetting lung function. Heat evil congesting the lung is characterized by heat effusion, cough with thick yellow sticky phlegm possibly streaked with blood, a tongue that is red at the tip and margins with a dry yellow fur, and a rapid surging or rapid stringlike pulse. In severe cases, there may be hasty rapid breathing and chest and rib-side pain. This condition is more severe than the more common WIND EVIL INVADING THE LUNG, and is attributed to phlegm-heat that arises when external evils invade the lung, where they then lie depressed and transform into heat, which damages the liquid of the lung and condenses it to form phlegm that obstructs the network vessels of the lung. WMC bronchitis; pneumonia; concurrent infections in emphysema and in bronchial asthma. MED Clear and drain lung heat with White-Draining Powder (*xiè bái sǎn*). ACU Base treatment mainly on LU and LI. Select BL-13 (*fèi shū*, Lung Transport), LU-7 (*liè quē*, Broken Sequence), LU-5 (*chǐ zé*, Cubit Marsh), LI-4 (*hé gǔ*, Union Valley), LI-11 (*qū chí*, Pool at the Bend), LU-10 (*yú jì*, Fish Border), GV-14 (*dà zhuī*, Great Hammer), and ST-40 (*fēng lóng*, Bountiful Bulge); needle with drainage, and prick LU-11 (*shào shāng*, Lesser Shang) to bleed. [26: 872] [27: 160] [97: 453] [37: 274, 283] [46: 653]

heat evil obstructing the lung 热邪阻肺 *rè xié zǔ fèi*: HEAT EVIL CONGESTING THE LUNG.

heat evil passing into the interior 热邪传里 *rè xié chuán lǐ*: Synonym: *exterior heat passing into the interior.* Externally contracted evil moving from the exterior of the body into the interior, marked by the disappearance of aversion to wind or cold, increase in heat effusion, reddening of the eyes, oppression in the chest, vexation and agitation, thirst with intake of fluid, constipation, red tongue with yellow fur, a rapid pulse, and in severe cases delirious speech. [26: 872]

heat formation 化热 *huà rè*: See TRANSFORMATION INTO HEAT.

heat gan 热疳 *rè gān*: See COLD-HEAT GAN. [26: 872] [27: 453] [97: 450]

heat heart pain 热心痛 *rè xīn tòng*: Synonyms: *heat reversal heart pain; fire heart pain.* HEART PAIN attributed to depressed heat that may arise when summerheat toxin enters the heart or after continual consumption of hot medicinals or hot food. Heat heart pain is characterized by intermittent burning stomach duct pain that fears heat and likes cold, sometimes accompanied by red or yellow face and eyes, generalized heat effusion, vex-

ation and agitation, heat in the palms and soles, and hard stool. MED Resolve depression and drain heat with Toosendan Powder (*jīn líng zǐ sǎn*) or, in severe cases, Major Qi-Coordinating Decoction (*dà chéng qì tāng*). See REVERSAL HEART PAIN. [26: 871]

heat hiccough 热呃 *rè è*: HICCOUGH attributed to stomach fire ascending counterflow or depressed phlegm-fire. Heat hiccough is a forceful hiccough accompanied by red facial complexion, vexation and thirst, dry mouth and dry tongue, yellow tongue fur, and a rapid large surging pulse. MED Harmonize the stomach and downbear fire using formulas such as Tangerine Peel and Bamboo Shavings Decoction (*jú pí zhú rú tāng*) or Stomach-Quieting Beverage (*ān wèi yǐn*). For patterns with constipation, use Diaphragm-Cooling Powder (*liáng gé sǎn*), whereas for phlegm-fire in the stomach use Pinellia and Scutellaria Pill (*bàn huáng wán*). ACU Base treatment mainly on ST, LR, and PC. Main points: BL-17 (*gé shū*, Diaphragm Transport), CV-17 (*shān zhōng*, Chest Center), PC-6 (*nèi guān*, Inner Pass), ST-36 (*zú sān lǐ*, Leg Three Li), CV-14 (*jù què*, Great Tower Gate), ST-25 (*tiān shū*, Celestial Pivot), and LR-3 (*tài chōng*, Supreme Surge). Selection of points according to pattern: For stomach fire ascending counterflow, add ST-44 (*nèi tíng*, Inner Court) and LI-4 (*hé gǔ*, Union Valley), and needle with drainage. For depressed phlegm fire, add ST-40 (*fēng lóng*, Bountiful Bulge). For constipation, add TB-6 (*zhī gōu*, Branch Ditch), and needle with drainage. See HICCOUGH. [26: 872] [80: 302] [113: 76] [46: 596, 602] [37: 307]

heat impediment 热痹 *rè bì*: **1.** An IMPEDIMENT (*bì*) pattern attributed either to heat toxin pouring into the joints or externally contracted wind-cold-damp evil contending with internally brewing heat. It is characterized by hot red swollen painful joints sometimes accompanied by heat effusion and thirst. WMC rheumatic arthritis; rheumatoid arthritis; gout. MED Clear heat and dispel dampness; diffuse impediment and relieve pain. Use formulas such as Cinnamon Twig, Peony, and Anemarrhena Decoction (*guì zhī sháo yào zhī mǔ tāng*). ACU Main points: GV-14 (*dà zhuī*, Great Hammer), LI-4 (*hé gǔ*, Union Valley), and LI-11 (*qū chí*, Pool at the Bend). Needle to a shallow depth and drain, or use cutaneous needle. For selection of points according to affected area, see IMPEDIMENT (*bì*). **2.** VESSEL IMPEDIMENT. [26: 875] [97: 450]

heat in the (heart of the) palms and soles 手足心热 *shǒu zú xīn rè*: Feeling of heat in the palms and soles.

heat in the stomach 胃中热 *wèi zhōng rè*: See STOMACH HEAT. [27: 157]

heat is treated with cold 热者寒之 *rè zhě hán zhī*: From *Elementary Questions* (*sù wèn, zhì zhēn yào dà lùn*). Cold and cool medicinals are used for heat patterns. Heat patterns include exterior heat, internal heat, vacuity heat, and repletion heat. Exterior heat forming a repletion pattern is treated by RESOLVING THE EXTERIOR WITH COOLNESS AND ACRIDITY, while interior heat is treated by CLEARING. Vacuity heat is treated by ENRICHING YIN to abate heat or by ELIMINATING GREATE HEAT WITH SWEETNESS AND WARMTH. [27: 239]

heat malaria 热疟 *rè nüè*: MALARIA characterized by pronounced heat effusion and mild aversion to cold. *Universal Aid Formulary* (*pǔ jì fāng, zhū nüè mén*) states, "Evil in the yang brightness (*yáng míng*) channel is heat malaria, which is treated mainly by precipitation." See FOOT YANG BRIGHTNESS MALARIA. [50: 1236]

heat night crying 热夜啼 *rè yè tí*: Crying in infants and children attributed to fetal heat, fright heat, or wind-heat. Heat night crying is associated with supine posture, copious tearing, red facial complexion reddish urine, generalized heat [effusion] (possibly with sweating), and hot breath. The crying is exacerbated by heat and light. MED Clear the heart and quiet the spirit using Red-Abducting Powder (*dǎo chì sǎn*) plus coptis (*huáng lián*). ACU Base treatment mainly on HT, GV, LI, SI, and empirical points. Needle with drainage at BL-15 (*xīn shū*, Heart Transport), HT-8 (*shào fǔ*, Lesser Mansion), HT-7 (*shén mén*, Spirit Gate), GV-14 (*dà zhuī*, Great Hammer), and LI-4 (*hé gǔ*, Union Valley), and with even supplementation and drainage at Quiet Sleep (*ān mián*), Hall of Impression (*yìn táng*), and SI-3 (*hòu xī*, Back Ravine). [26: 872]

heat panting 热喘 *rè chuǎn*: PANTING attributed to intense lung heat. Heat panting arises when heat scorches the lung and prevents the normal downward movement of water, causing phlegm-fire to congest and obstruct the airways. It is associated with copious thick phlegm, heat vexation, and fullness in the chest. MED Clear the lung, drain heat, and flush phlegm. Use formulas such as Fire-Draining Lung-Clearing Decoction (*xiè huǒ qīng fèi tāng*). Contraction of cold when there is heat in the lung and accumulated phlegm in the center can also give rise to a panting pattern sometimes referred to as "cold-enveloping-heat panting," which is treated by diffusing depressed heat with formulas such as Ephedra Panting-Stabilizing Decoction (*má huáng dìng chuǎn tāng*). ACU Base treatment mainly on LU, LI, ST, and SP. Select Panting Stabilizer (*dìng chuǎn*), LU-5 (*chǐ zé*, Cubit Marsh), LU-7 (*liè quē*, Broken Sequence), LI-4 (*hé gǔ*, Union Valley), ST-40 (*fēng lóng*, Bountiful Bulge), and SP-2 (*dà dū*, Great Metropolis),

needling with drainage. Prick LU-11 (*shào shāng*, Lesser Shang) to bleed. For coughing of blood, add LU-6 (*kǒng zuì*, Collection Hole), and LU-10 (*yú jì*, Fish Border), needling with drainage. For panting from cold enveloping heat, add BL-12 (*fēng mén*, Wind Gate) and BL-13 (*fèi shū*, Lung Transport). [26: 874]

heat pattern 热证 *rè zhèng*: Any sign or signs indicating the presence of heat. Heat patterns arise when a yang evil invades the body or when yin humor becomes insufficient. Thus, heat patterns are caused by a surfeit of yang or a deficit of yin, and form repletion heat or vacuity heat patterns. **Repletion heat:** Repletion heat patterns are characterized by red complexion, reddening of the eyes, vigorous heat [effusion], agitation, thirst, desire for cold fluids, hard stool, short voidings of reddish urine, a red or crimson tongue with a yellow fur, and rapid pulse or a rapid large surging pulse. MED Repletion heat is treated by clearing, according to the principle that heat is treated with cold. Heat-clearing fire-draining medicinals such as gypsum (*shí gāo*), anemarrhena (*zhī mǔ*), coptis (*huáng lián*), and rhubarb (*dà huáng*) are commonly used. Heat-clearing toxin-resolving medicinals are useful in specific cases. Formulas frequently used to treat repletion heat patterns include White Tiger Decoction (*bái hǔ tāng*) and Heart-Draining Decoction (*xiè xīn tāng*). In treating vacuity heat, nourishing yin is of greater importance than clearing heat. Medicinals frequently used include sweet wormwood (*qīng hāo*), baiwei (*bái wēi*), lanceolate stellaria (*yín chái hú*), lycium root bark (*dì gǔ pí*), anemarrhena (*zhī mǔ*), and phellodendron (*huáng bǎi*). Sweet Wormwood and Turtle Shell Decoction (*qīng hāo biē jiǎ tāng*) is a commonly used vacuity-heat–clearing formula. See also SUPPLEMENTING YIN. ACU PC-8 (*láo gōng*, Palace of Toil), HT-8 (*shào fǔ*, Lesser Mansion), PC-9 (*zhōng chōng*, Central Hub), HT-9 (*shào chōng*, Lesser Surge), and GV-26 (*shuǐ gōu*, Water Trough) can be used to treat heart fire; LU-10 (*yú jì*, Fish Border), LU-5 (*chǐ zé*, Cubit Marsh), LI-11 (*qū chí*, Pool at the Bend), LU-11 (*shào shāng*, Lesser Shang), and LI-1 (*shāng yáng*, Shang Yang) can be selected to treat lung heat; LR-2 (*xíng jiān*, Moving Between), GB-43 (*xiá xī*, Pinched Ravine), and GB-34 (*yáng líng quán*, Yang Mound Spring) can be selected to treat liver-gallbladder fire; ST-44 (*nèi tíng*, Inner Court), ST-36 (*zú sān lǐ*, Leg Three Li), LI-4 (*hé gǔ*, Union Valley), and ST-45 (*lì duì*, Severe Mouth) can be selected to treat stomach fire (heat); ST-25 (*tiān shū*, Celestial Pivot), LI-4 (*hé gǔ*, Union Valley), ST-36 (*zú sān lǐ*, Leg Three Li), and ST-44 (*nèi tíng*, Inner Court) can be selected to treat large intestine fire (heat); HT-8 (*shào fǔ*, Lesser Mansion), ST-39 (*xià jù xū*, Lower Great Hollow), and SI-2 (*qián gǔ*, Front Valley) can be selected to treat small intestine fire (heat); CV-3 (*zhōng jí,* Central Pole), SP-9 (*yīn líng quán,* Yin Mound Spring), and SP-6 (*sān yīn jiāo,* Three Yin Intersection) can be selected to treat exuberant bladder heat; needle with drainage or prick to bleed. **Vacuity heat:** Vacuity heat patterns are marked by vexing heat in the five hearts (palms, soles and chest), steaming bone tidal heat [effusion], dry throat and mouth, smooth bare red tongue (mirror tongue), and a thin, rapid pulse. MED Medicinals frequently used for clearing vacuity heat include sweet wormwood (*qīng hāo*), baiwei (*bái wēi*), lanceolate stellaria (*yín chái hú*), lycium root bark (*dì gǔ pí*), anemarrhena (*zhī mǔ*), and phellodendron (*huáng bǎi*). Sweet Wormwood and Turtle Shell Decoction (*qīng hāo biē jiǎ tāng*) is a formula commonly used for clearing vacuity heat. ACU KI-6 (*zhào hǎi,* Shining Sea), KI-2 (*rán gǔ,* Blazing Valley), KI-1 (*yǒng quán,* Gushing Spring), HT-8 (*shào fǔ,* Lesser Mansion), and HT-7 (*shén mén,* Spirit Gate) can be selected to treat kidney vacuity with fire stirring; ST-36 (*zú sān lǐ,* Leg Three Li), SP-6 (*sān yīn jiāo,* Three Yin Intersection), SP-3 (*tài bái,* Supreme White), and BL-20 (*pí shū,* Spleen Transport) can be selected to treat spleen-stomach vacuity fire; BL-13 (*fèi shū,* Lung Transport), BL-43 (*gāo huāng shū,* Gao-Huang Transport), ST-36 (*zú sān lǐ,* Leg Three Li), SP-6 (*sān yīn jiāo,* Three Yin Intersection), KI-3 (*tài xī,* Great Ravine), KI-6 (*zhào hǎi,* Shining Sea), and KI-2 (*rán gǔ,* Blazing Valley) can be used to treat lung taxation vacuity heat; use both supplementation and drainage to address the vacuity and the heat respectively. [6: 152] [27: 212] [46: 596, 656]

heat phlegm 热痰 *rè tán*: **1.** A phlegm pattern characterized by cough with thick sticky yellow or white phlegm that is difficult to expectorate and by rapid breathing. General signs include heat effusion, dry mouth, sore swollen throat, red tongue with yellow fur, and slippery rapid pulse, all of which indicate heat. In internal damage miscellaneous disease, repeated incidence of heat phlegm signs often gives rise to PHLEGM-FIRE. This occurs when phlegm heat failing to clear brews internally and Transforms into fire. **Comparison:** Heat phlegm should be distinguished from DRYNESS PHLEGM. Dryness phlegm is caused by dryness evil or lung (or lung-kidney) yin vacuity, and is characterized by scant phlegm that is difficult to expectorate, and signs of yin humor depletion such as dry mouth, tongue, throat, and nose. In contrast, heat phlegm is characterized by thick yellow or white phlegm, rapid breathing, and pronounced heat signs. Dryness phlegm is either vacuity or repletion; heat phlegm is always a repletion pattern. WMC Heat phlegm usually falls within the scope of acute inflammatory respiratory dis-

eases (or acute attacks in chronic conditions) in Western medicine. MED Clear heat and resolve toxin; transform phlegm. Commonly used medicinals include scutellaria (*huáng qín*), lonicera (*jīn yín huā*), dandelion (*pú gōng yīng*), houttuynia (*yú xīng cǎo*), mulberry root bark (*sāng bái pí*), tingli (*tíng lì zǐ*), Sichuan fritillaria (*chuān bèi mǔ*), trichosanthes (*guā lóu*), dried bamboo sap (*zhú lì*), fresh phragmites (*xiān lú gēn*), and wax gourd seed (*dōng guā zǐ*). Formulas include Lonicera and Phragmites Mixture (*yín wěi hé jì*) and its variations. ACU Base treatment mainly on LU, LI, and back transport points. Select BL-13 (*fèi shū,* Lung Transport), LU-5 (*chǐ zé,* Cubit Marsh), GV-14 (*dà zhuī,* Great Hammer), LI-11 (*qū chí,* Pool at the Bend), LI-4 (*hé gǔ,* Union Valley), ST-40 (*fēng lóng,* Bountiful Bulge), and CV-22 (*tiān tú,* Celestial Chimney); needle with drainage. For sore swollen throat, drain LU-11 (*shào shāng,* Lesser Shang) or prick to bleed. **2.** A disease pattern arising in patients suffering from phlegm disease, when eating hot spicy foods and rich fried or roasted meats, using excessively thick clothing or bedclothes, and from heat evil due to hot weather triggers panting, expectoration, cough, and spitting. **3.** Phlegm-heat confounding the heart arising when phlegm and heat contend with each other, gather and bind. It is characterized by turbid thick gluey yellow phlegm that is sometimes flecked with blood and that is difficult to expectorate, and by a surging pulse, red face, heat vexation and heart pain, frequent laughing, mania and withdrawal, clamoring stomach, anguish, fearful throbbing, and dry mouth and lips. MED Clear the heart, drain fire, and abduct phlegm. Use Qi-Clearing Phlegm-Transforming Pill (*qīng qì huà tán wán*) or Chlorite/Mica Phlegm-Rolling Pill (*méng shí gǔn tán wán*). ACU Base treatment mainly on GV, HT, ST, and PC. Select GV-26 (*shuǐ gōu,* Water Trough), BL-15 (*xīn shū,* Heart Transport), ST-36 (*zú sān lǐ,* Leg Three Li), ST-40 (*fēng lóng,* Bountiful Bulge), ST-44 (*nèi tíng,* Inner Court), HT-7 (*shén mén,* Spirit Gate), PC-7 (*dà líng,* Great Mound), and PC-5 (*jiān shǐ,* Intermediary Courier); needle with drainage. **4.** FIRE PHLEGM. [6: 218] [26: 875] [22: 283] [97: 452] [37: 272, 353] [46: 652]

heat qi cholera 热气霍乱 *rè qì huò luàn*: HEAT CHOLERA. [26: 873]

heat repletion chest bind 热实结胸 *rè shí jié xiōng*: Synonym: *heat chest bind*. A CHEST BINDattern (painful hard fullness in the center and abdomen) accompanied by heat effusion, heart vexation, anguish, clouding and oppression, dry mouth, constipation, and a slippery sunken pulse. MED Open binds and discharge heat using Three Yellows Heart-Draining Decoction (*sān huáng xiè xīn tāng*) or Major Chest Bind Decoction (*dà xiàn* *xiōng tāng*). ACU See MAJOR CHEST BIND. [26: 875]

heat reversal 热厥 *rè jué*: A REVERSAL PATTERN that occurs in generalized heat [effusion] and headache and that is attributable to overexuberant evil depressing yang qi and preventing its warming force from reaching the extremities. Its features are clouded spirit, reversal cold of the limbs, and a sunken or hidden pulse that is slippery under pressure. There may be aversion to heat, thirst with desire for fluids, flailing of the arms and legs, vexation and agitation, insomnia, scorching (palpable) heat in the chest and abdomen, constipation and reddish urine. MED Diffuse depressed heat. Use Counterflow Cold Powder (*sì nì sǎn*) for mild patterns and White Tiger Decoction (*bái hǔ tāng*), Major Qi-Coordinating Decoction (*dà chéng qì tāng*), or Diaphragm-Cooling Powder (*liáng gé sǎn*) for severe patterns. ACU Base treatment mainly on ST, LI, and KI. Select LI-4 (*hé gǔ*, Union Valley), LI-11 (*qū chí*, Pool at the Bend), GV-14 (*dà zhuī*, Great Hammer), KI-3 (*tài xī*, Great Ravine), ST-44 (*nèi tíng*, Inner Court), ST-43 (*xiàn gǔ*, Sunken Valley), and KI-1 (*yǒng quán*, Gushing Spring). Needle with drainage, and prick the Ten Diffusing Points (*shí xuān*) to bleed. See REVERSAL PATTERN; YANG REVERSAL. [26: 874] [27: 401] [97: 45] [37: 401] [42: 181]

heat reversal heart pain 热厥心痛 *rè jué xīn tòng*: See HEAT HEART PAIN. [26: 874]

heat scorching kidney yin 热灼肾阴 *rè zhuó shèn yīn*: Damage to kidney yin by evil heat, usually occurring in advanced stages of warm heat disease and characterized by low fever, scorching (palpable) heat in the hearts of the palms and soles, dry mouth and teeth, deafness, dry smooth emaciated crimson tongue, and a rapid fine or rapid vacuous pulse. Since the teeth are the surplus of the bones, which are governed by the kidney, and since the kidney opens at the ears, dry teeth and deafness are kidney signs. MED Use variations of Pulse-Restorative Decoction (*fù mài tāng*). ACU Drain points such as LI-4 (*hé gǔ*, Union Valley), LI-11 (*qū chí*, Pool at the Bend), LU-11 (*shào shāng*, Lesser Shang), LI-1 (*shāng yáng*, Shang Yang), ST-44 (*nèi tíng*, Inner Court), and LR-2 (*xíng jiān*, Moving Between) to drain the heat, and needle with supplementation at KI-6 (*zhào hǎi*, Shining Sea), KI-2 (*rán gǔ*, Blazing Valley), KI-3 (*tài xī*, Great Ravine), and BL-23 (*shèn shū*, Kidney Transport) to supplement kidney yin. [26: 872] [50: 1240] [27: 165] [97: 454] [83: 117] [46: 596]

heat sore 热疮 *rè chuāng*: A sore on the lips, at the corners of the mouth, or around the nose, composed of a cluster of vesicles the size and shape of millet seeds or rice beans and containing fluid that is initially clear and progressively turbid. A heat sore, which may be associated with itching or burning pain, usually clears within a week, but easily occurs again. It is attributable to externally contracted heat or upward steaming lung-stomach heat. MED Clear heat and dissipate wind. Use formulas such as Magnolia Flower Lung-Clearing Powder (*xīn yí qīng fèi sǎn*) as oral medication and applying Coptis Paste (*huáng lián gāo*) topically. ACU Base treatment mainly on LI, LR, ST, and LU. Select LI-4 (*hé gǔ*, Union Valley), LI-11 (*qū chí*, Pool at the Bend), ST-44 (*nèi tíng*, Inner Court), ST-36 (*zú sān lǐ*, Leg Three Li), LR-2 (*xíng jiān*, Moving Between), and LU-5 (*chǐ zé*, Cubit Marsh); needle with drainage. Prick LU-11 (*shào shāng*, Lesser Shang) and ST-45 (*lì duì*, Severe Mouth) to bleed. [26: 876] [27: 472] [97: 450] [4: 129–30] [14: 186–7]

heat strangury 热淋 *rè lín*: **1.** STRANGURY attributable to damp-heat brewing in the lower burner. Heat strangury is characterized by the general features of strangury (urinary urgency with frequent difficult and painful voidings), as well as by reddish urine. Other possible signs include alternating heat [effusion] and [aversion to] cold, lumbar pain, and smaller-abdominal distention and pain. MED Clear heat and disinhibit dampness using formulas such as Eight Corrections Powder (*bā zhèng sǎn*), Red-Abducting Powder (*dǎo chì sǎn*), or Five Stranguries Powder (*wǔ lín sǎn*). ACU Base treatment mainly on the three yin channels of the foot and alarm and back transport points of BL (CV-3 and BL-28). Select BL-28 (*páng guāng shū*, Bladder Transport), CV-3 (*zhōng jí*, Central Pole), SP-9 (*yīn líng quán*, Yin Mound Spring), LR-2 (*xíng jiān*, Moving Between), KI-3 (*tài xī*, Great Ravine), LR-8 (*qū quán*, Spring at the Bend), SP-6 (*sān yīn jiāo*, Three Yin Intersection), LI-4 (*hé gǔ*, Union Valley), and TB-5 (*wài guān*, Outer Pass). Needle with drainage. **2.** A general term for strangury patterns. [26: 873] [46: 674] [27: 426] [97: 450]

heat stroke 热中 *rè zhòng*: **1.** From *Elementary Questions* (*sù wèn, fēng lún*). A disease characterized by reddening of the eyes, arising when wind evil invades the stomach, which is linked to the eyes by channel. **2.** A qi vacuity and effulgent fire pattern attributable to damage to the spleen through dietary irregularities or taxation fatigue and characterized by generalized heat [effusion], heart vexation, panting, headache, aversion to cold, and in some cases thirst. The pulse is large and floating (and forceless). MED Use Center-Supplementing Qi-Boosting Decoction (*bǔ zhōng yì qì tāng*). [26: 871]

heat sweating 热汗 *rè hàn*: YANG SWEATING.

heat tearing 热泪 *rè lèi*: TEARING (lacrimation) that is attributable to invasion of wind-heat, to intense liver-lung heat, to flaming yin vacuity fire, or to foreign bodies entering the eye, and that is associated with a hot sensation. Heat tearing may be further associated with aversion to light, swelling of the eyes, and a red facial complexion. It is often observed in external obstructions of the eye. Methods of treatment include coursing wind, clearing heat, nourishing yin, calming the liver, cooling the blood, and dispelling stasis, depending upon the cause. If a foreign body is the cause, this should be removed by washing. [26: 873]

heat toxin 热毒 *rè dú*: **1.** TOXIN that arises from depression of fire-heat disease evil and that gives rise to various external medical diseases such as WELLING-ABSCESS (*yōng*), CLOVE SORES (*dīng chuāng*), CINNABAR TOXIN (*dān dú*), etc. Compare DAMP TOXIN. **2.** Warm toxin. [26: 872] [27: 115, 456]

heat toxin precipitation of blood 热毒下血 *rè dú xià xuè*: Discharging blood from the anus, attributable to heat toxin brewing in the large intestine and causing frenetic movement of the blood. Heat toxin precipitation of blood is characterized by bright red bloody stool, abdominal pain, burning pain in the anus, and dry mouth and tongue. MED Clear heat and resolve toxin; cool the blood and stanch bleeding. Use Coptis Pill (*huáng lián wán*) and Blood-Cooling Rehmannia Decoction (*liáng xuè dì huáng tāng*). ACU Base treatment mainly on BL, ST, and LI. Select ST-25 (*tiān shū*, Celestial Pivot), BL-25 (*dà cháng shū*, Large Intestine Transport), ST-37 (*shàng jù xū*, Upper Great Hollow), GV-1 (*cháng qiáng*, Long Strong), BL-57 (*chéng shān*, Mountain Support), BL-32 (*cì liáo*, Second Bone-Hole), SP-6 (*sān yīn jiāo*, Three Yin Intersection), LR-3 (*tài chōng*, Supreme Surge), and PC-8 (*láo gōng*, Palace of Toil); needle with drainage. [26: 872]

heat vexation 烦热 *fán rè*: From *Elementary Questions* (*sù wèn, zhì zhēn yào dà lùn*). HEART VEXATION accompanied by heat effusion, or agitation with a subjective feeling of heat and oppression. In externally contracted heat (febrile) disease, heat vexation appearing in exterior patterns indicates that evil heat is not being discharged, whereas its appearance in interior patterns indicates exuberant repletion heat; in interior patterns with fecal stoppage and lesser-abdominal pain, it is caused by dry stool binding internally. In internal damage miscellaneous disease, it is caused by effulgent liver fire or effulgent yin vacuity fire. Compare HEAT VEXATION IN THE CHEST. [26: 772] [27: 357] [97: 497] [50: 1272]

heat vexation in the chest 胸中烦热 *xiōng zhōng fán rè*: From *Elementary Questions* (*sù wèn, zhì zhēn yào dà lùn*). A feeling of oppression, anguish, unease, and heat in the chest. Heat vexa-

tion in the chest is usually attributable to internal heat, but can also occur in external contractions. **Hyperactive heart fire:** Heat vexation in the chest attributable to hyperactivity of heart fire is associated with erosion of the mouth and tongue, thirst, and reddish urine. MED Clear heat and disinhibit urine. Use Red-Abducting Powder (*dǎo chì sǎn*). **Blood vacuity with flaming fire** gives rise to heat vexation in the chest with anxiety and insomnia. MED Clear heat and eliminate vexation; nurture yin and quiet the spirit. Use Coptis, Ass Hide Glue, and Egg Yolk Decoction (*huáng lián ē jiāo jī zǐ huáng tāng*). Heat vexation in the chest with heat in the hearts of the palms and soles is called VEXING HEAT IN THE FIVE HEARTS. **Externally contracted heat (febrile) disease:** Heat vexation in the chest may occur in exterior patterns or after they have abated. MED In exterior patterns, course the exterior and clear heat with Gardenia and Fermented Soybean Decoction (*zhī zǐ chǐ tāng*). For residual heat after the exterior pattern has been resolved, use Bamboo Leaf and Gypsum Decoction (*zhú yè shí gāo tāng*). Heat vexation in the chest occurring in pregnancy is called VEXATION OF PREGNANCY. ◇ Chin 烦 *fán*, vexation; 热 *rè*, heat. [26: 548]

heat vomiting 热呕 *rè ǒu*: VOMITING attributable to accumulated spleen-stomach heat or heat evil invading the stomach. Heat vomiting is characterized by immediate vomiting of ingested food or even violent vomiting often just at the sight of food. It is accompanied by red facial complexion, heart vexation, thirst, constipation, yellow or reddish urine, and a rapid surging pulse. WMC Heat vomiting is observed in acute gastritis, cholecystitis, pancreatitis, or hepatitis. MED Clear heat and drain fire; harmonize the stomach and check vomiting. Use formulas such as Minor Bupleurum Decoction (*xiǎo chái hú tāng*), Bamboo Shavings Decoction (*zhú rú tāng*), or Rhubarb and Licorice Decoction (*dà huáng gān cǎo tāng*). ACU Base treatment mainly on ST, LI, and CV. Select CV-12 (*zhōng wǎn*, Center Stomach Duct), PC-6 (*nèi guān*, Inner Pass), ST-36 (*zú sān lǐ*, Leg Three Li), LI-4 (*hé gǔ*, Union Valley), LI-11 (*qū chí*, Pool at the Bend), and ST-44 (*nèi tíng*, Inner Court); needle with drainage. For incessant vomiting, prick Gold Liquid and Jade Humor (*jīn jīn yù yè*) or PC-8 (*láo gōng*, Palace of Toil) to bleed. [26: 876] [97: 448]

heat wheezing 热哮 *rè xiāo*: WHEEZING due to accumulated phlegm-heat causing congestion and counterflow of lung qi. Heat wheezing is characterized by rough rapid panting, phlegm rale in the throat, raised chest, cough with thick yellow phlegm, vexation and oppression in the chest and diaphragm, red facial complexion, spontaneous sweating, thirst with intake of fluid, red tongue with slimy yellow tongue fur, and a slippery rapid pulse. In some cases, there may also be exterior signs, as when patients suffering from accumulated internal heat contract external cold, which is a pattern of cold enveloping heat. MED Diffuse the lung and clear heat; dispel phlegm and stabilize panting. Use formulas such as Panting-Stabilizing Decoction (*dìng chuǎn tāng*) or Mulberry Root Bark Decoction (*sāng bái pí tāng*). For cold enveloping heat, treatment should aim to dissipate cold in order to resolve depressed heat, using Spleen-Effusing Decoction Plus Pinellia (*yuè bì jiā bàn xià tāng*). ACU Base treatment mainly on LU, LI, and ST. Select LU-7 (*liè quē*, Broken Sequence), LU-5 (*chǐ zé*, Cubit Marsh), LI-4 (*hé gǔ*, Union Valley), LU-11 (*shào shāng*, Lesser Shang), Panting Stabilizer (*dìng chuǎn*), ST-40 (*fēng lóng*, Bountiful Bulge), CV-17 (*shān zhōng*, Chest Center), LI-11 (*qū chí*, Pool at the Bend), and GV-14 (*dà zhuī*, Great Hammer); needle with drainage. Selection of points according to signs: For cold enveloping heat, add BL-13 (*fèi shū*, Lung Transport) and BL-12 (*fēng mén*, Wind Gate). For vexation and oppression in the chest and diaphragm, add LU-10 (*yú jì*, Fish Border) and PC-7 (*dà líng*, Great Mound). For thirst with intake of fluid, add KI-6 (*zhào hǎi*, Shining Sea), and KI-3 (*tài xī*, Great Ravine). [26: 873] [27: 383] [97: 450] [46: 654]

heaven 天 *tiān*: The sky or heavens; the highest cosmic principle or force. The Chinese concept of heaven includes not only the physical sky or space covering the earth, but also weather and the seasons, and the notion of Nature and the forces and laws that govern it. [97: 57]

heaven and man are mutually responsive 天人相应 *tiān rén xiāng yìng*: Man and his natural environment bear certain similarities to each other and are interactive. This principle has multiple facets: (1) the correspondence between the phases (metal, wood, water, fire, and earth) and the organs of the five viscera (lung, liver, kidney, heart, and spleen); (2) naïve correspondences such as "heaven has the sun and moon; man has two eyes"; (3) correspondence in the DOCTRINE OF PERIODS AND QI and its practical application of the MIDDAY-MIDNIGHT POINT SELECTION; (4) the guideline applied in the treatment and prevention of disease of "acting in accordance with seasonal, geographical, and personal factors." See FIVE PHASES; HOLISM. [26: 102] [27: 107] [97: 60]

heaven-borne blisters 天泡疮 *tiān pào chuāng*: A disease characterized by blisters. WMC pemphigus. Two types are identified. (1) A disease of sudden onset occurring in summer or autumn, marked by blisters on the head, limbs, and body, easily affecting children. The blisters are clearly demarcated and have shiny skin. They are white at the tip and red at the root. When ruptured, they exude fluid and spread quickly, and are infectious. This form of heaven-borne blisters arise when summerheat-damp invades the lung channel and lies depressed in the skin. MED Clear heat and disinhibit dampness. Use formulas such as Coptis Toxin-Resolving Decoction (*huáng lián jiě dú tāng*). (2) A nonseasonal disease slow in development and which is not infectious, marked by thin-walled blisters of different sizes that are red at the root and which exude fluid when they burst. It is accompanied by general signs such as prolonged heat effusion, oppression in the chest, and torpid stomach. In persistent cases, there may be yin vacuity signs such as steaming bone tidal heat [effusion], smooth bare red tongue, and rapid fine pulse. MED Use Spleen-Clearing Dampness-Eliminating Beverage (*qīng pí chú shī yǐn*). If there is damage to yin, use Stomach-Boosting Decoction (*yì wèi tāng*). Topical: Wash with licorice (*gān cǎo*) water. ◇ Chin 天 *tiān*, heaven; weather; season; nature; 泡 *pào*, blister; 疮 *chuāng*, sore. [26: 103] [96: 257] [61: 362] [92: No. 511]

heaven current 天行 *tiān xíng*: Synonyms: seasonal qi; seasonal current. A disease prevalent in a particular place at a particular time, marked by the similar signs in both young and old; an epidemic. Distinction is made between cold and heat. A heavenly current of a cold nature is called a SEASONAL COLD EPIDEMIC, whereas one of a hot nature is called HEAVEN-CURRENT WARM EPIDEMIC. [26: 103] [27: 347]

heaven-current cough 天行嗽 *tiān xíng sòu*: SEASONAL COUGH.

heaven-current red eye 天行赤眼 *tiān xíng chì yán*: Compare WIND-FIRE EYE. [26: 103]

heaven-current warm epidemic 天行温疫 *tiān xíng wēn yì*: SCOURGE EPIDEMIC. [26: 103] [27: 347]

heaven, human, and earth 天人地 *tiān rén dì*: Three interrelated concepts of Chinese cosmology. In acupuncture, 'heaven', 'human', and 'earth' denote shallow, medium, and deep levels of insertion respectively. See BURNING MOUNTAIN FIRE METHOD and HEAVEN-PENETRATING COOLING METHOD for examples.

heaven, human, and earth supplementation and drainage 天人地三才补泻 *tiān rén dì sān cái bǔ xiè*, 三才补泻 *sān cái bǔ xiè* ¡heaven, human, and earth¿: A method of needling that involves a three-stage insertion to achieve supplementation and a three-stage withdrawal to achieve drainage. Method: Supplementation is achieved by inserting the needle to a shallow depth (heaven), advancing to a middle depth (human), and then further advancing to the deepest level (earth). The needle is then removed in a single movement.

Drainage is achieved by first inserting the needle to the deepest level, and then withdrawing to the mid-level, and finally to the shallow level before removal. [27: 341]

heaven level 天部 *tiān bù*: The upper third of the insertion depth of a needle, i.e., the upper third of the distance between the surface of the body and the level of deepest insertion. See HEAVEN, HUMAN, AND EARTH.

8.	Heavenly Stems & Earthly Branches			
The Heavenly Stems		The Earthly Branches		
甲 *jiǎ*	S1	子 *zǐ*	B1
乙 *yǐ*	S2	丑 *chǒu*	B2
丙 *bǐng*	S3	寅 *yín*	B3
丁 *dīng*	S4	卯 *mǎo*	B4
戊 *wù*	S5	辰 *chén*	B5
己 *jǐ*	S6	巳 *sì*	B6
庚 *gēng*	S7	午 *wǔ*	B7
辛 *xīn*	S8	未 *wèi*	B7
壬 *rén*	S9	申 *shēn*	B9
癸 *guǐ*	S10	酉 *yǒu*	B10
		戌 *xū*	B11
		亥 *hài*	B12

heavenly stems and earthly branches 天干地支 *tiān gān dì zhī*: A double series of signs used in combination to designate years, months, days, and hours. See Table 8.

heavenly tenth 天癸 *tiān guǐ*: Synonym: *tian-gui*. **1.** That upon which development of the human body, sexual function, and in women the ability to produce offspring depends. *Elementary Questions* (*sù wèn, shàng gǔ tiān zhēn lùn*) states, "[In the male] at the age of two eights [i.e., sixteen] kidney qi is exuberant, "heavenly tenth" (*tiān guǐ*) arrives, essential qi flows forth, yin and yang are in harmony, and [he] can beget offspring... At the age of seven eights [i.e., fifty-six] the "heavenly tenth" is exhausted, essence diminishes, the kidney grows weak, and the body loses its tone; at eight eights, the teeth and hair fall out. [In the female] at the age of two sevens, the heavenly tenth arrives, the controlling (*rèn*) vessel flows, and the thoroughfare (*chōng*) vessel fills, the menses come according to their times, and [she] can bear offspring... At seven sevens, the controlling (*rèn*) vessel empties, the thoroughfare (*chōng*) vessel weakens, the heavenly tenth is exhausted, the passages of the earth are cut, the body deteriorates, and she can no longer bear children." These statements indicate that the arrival of the heavenly tenth corresponds to the point at which reproductive maturity is reached, and its "exhaustion" to the point at which reproductive function disappears. They further appear to indicate that the heavenly tenth is a product (material or functional) of the "exu-

berant kidney qi," "kidney qi" being most clearly understood in this context as the essential qi of the kidney. The term *tiān guǐ* is composed of *guǐ*, meaning the tenth heavenly stem (S10) preceded by the *tiān*, heaven. According to one interpretation, heaven denotes earlier heaven (congenital constitution), whereas *guǐ* denotes "yin water" (as in the combination 壬癸 (*rén guǐ*), yin and yang water), by which *tiān guǐ* would be the "yin water of earlier heaven," i.e., kidney yin or original yin. However, this interpretation is difficult to reconcile with the association of *tiān guǐ* with kidney qi in the cited passage. **2.** Original yin. **3.** Menstruation. ◇ Chin 天 *tiān*, heaven; 癸 *guǐ* tenth heavenly stem. [36: 103] [27: 439] [97: 59]

heaven-penetrating cooling method 透天凉 *tòu tiān liáng*: A draining needle manipulation method that combines the lifting and thrusting, slow and quick, and open and closed techniques. The heaven-penetrating cooling method is used to treat heat pathoconditions such as HEAT IMPEDIMENT, WELLING-ABSCESS SWELLING, and STEAMING BONE. Method: (1) Determine the depth to which the needle will be inserted, and divide this depth into heaven, human, and earth levels. (2) Ask the patient to inhale deeply and slowly. (Steps 2 through 6 are performed during inhalation.) (3) Thrust slowly and lift quickly at the earth level six times. Insert the needle to the earth level six times. (4) Bring the needle up to the human level. Thrust slowly and lift quickly at the human level six times. (5) Bring the needle up to the heaven level. Thrust the needle slowly and lift the needle quickly at this level six times. (6) Repeat steps 3 through 5. (7) Ask the patient to exhale, and withdraw the needle quickly, leaving the point uncovered. [46: 471–2]

heaven rampart 天廓 *tiān kuò*: See EIGHT RAMPARTS. [26: 24]

heaviness 重 *zhòng*, 沉重 *chén zhòng*: The state of being heavy. See HEAVY.

heavy 重 *zhòng*, 沉重 *chén zhòng*: Greater weight or a feeling of greater weight than normal or average.

heavy body 身重 *shēn zhòng*, 身体沉重 *shēn tǐ chén zhòng*: Synonym: *generalized heaviness*. A sensation of heaviness with inhibited physical movement. Heavy body is due to dampness in the fleshy exterior arising through exposure to external dampness, wind contending with water, or yang vacuity water flood. **Dampness in the fleshy exterior** arises through exposure to external dampness, and is characterized by heavy body and generalized pain with difficulty in turning side. There is heat effusion and aversion to cold, headache and distention in the head as if the head were swathed, oppression in the chest, torpid intake, a thin white slimy tongue fur, and a moderate soggy pulse. MED Promote sweating and dispel dampness, using Notopterygium Dampness-Overcoming Decoction (*qiāng huó shèng shī tāng*). **Wind contending with water** arises when external wind fetters the lung and affects qi transformation. The heavy body it causes is less marked than in the previous pattern, and there is swelling of the eyes and face. Attending signs include fear of wind and cold, heat effusion, headache, aching joints, cough, sore throats, scant urine, a thin white tongue fur, and a pulse that is floating. MED Diffuse the lung and disinhibit water using Spleen-Effusing Decoction Plus Ovate Atractylodes (*yuè bì jiā zhú tāng*). **Yang vacuity water flood** gives rise to heavy body when qi transformation is weakened owing to spleen-kidney yang vacuity. Heavy body in this case is not associated with pain. In addition, there is puffy swelling of the slower limbs that pits when pressure is applied, a withered-yellow of somber white lusterless complexion, torpid intake, sloppy stool, lassitude of spirit and cold limbs, heavy aching lumbus, short voidings of scant urine, a pale enlarged tongue with a white slimy fur, and a pulse that is sunken, fine and moderate. MED Spleen-Firming Beverage (*shí pí yǐn*) or True Warrior Decoction (*zhēn wǔ tāng*). [92: No. 20] [26: 338]

heavy cumbersome head and body 头身困重 *tóu shēn kūn zhòng*: See HEAVY BODY; HEAVY-HEADEDNESS.

heavy cumbersome limbs 肢体困重 *zhī tǐ kūn zhòng*: Limbs that feel heavy and difficult to move; a sign of dampness.

heavy formula 重剂 *zhòng jì*: One of the TEN FORMULA TYPES; a formula comprising medicinals that are heavy in weight. Heavy [medicinals] can eliminate timidity, i.e., they are effective for various conditions involving susceptibility to fear and fright. An example of a heavy formula is Loadstone and Cinnabar Pill (*cí zhū wán*), which contains loadstone (*cí shí*), cinnabar (*zhū shā*), and medicated leaven (*shén qū*). [27: 306] [97: 419]

heavy-headedness 头重 *tóu zhòng*: Feeling of heaviness in the head, sometimes combined with dizziness. Heavy-headedness can be caused by wind-damp, damp-heat, phlegm-damp, or insufficiency of center qi. **Wind-damp** heavy-headedness is accompanied by headache, HEAD HEAVY AS IF SWATHED (bag-over-the-head sensation), exacerbation in rainy yin-type weather, nasal congestion, a heavy cumbersome, aching body, oppression in the chest, thin slimy tongue fur, and floating moderate or soggy pulse. MED Dispel wind and overcome dampness with Notopterygium Dampness-Overcoming Decoction (*qiāng huó*

shèng shī tāng), and if there is a stomach complication, add magnolia bark (*hòu pò*), atractylodes (*cāng zhú*), and pinellia (*bàn xià*) to rectify qi. ACU Base treatment mainly on triple-yang channel points, GV and ST. Select GB-20 (*fēng chí*, Wind Pool), GV-16 (*fēng fǔ*, Wind Mansion), GV-20 (*bǎi huì*, Hundred Convergences), Greater Yang (*tài yáng*), LI-4 (*hé gǔ*, Union Valley), SI-3 (*hòu xī*, Back Ravine), SP-9 (*yīn líng quán*, Yin Mound Spring), and ST-8 (*tóu wéi*, Head Corner); needle with drainage. **Damp-heat** heavy-headedness is accompanied by a painful distention (feeling of pressure in the head) that worsens at noon, red face, generalized heat [effusion], vexation, oppression in the chest, no desire for food and drink, dark yellow urine, yellow slimy tongue fur, and a slippery rapid or soggy rapid pulse. MED Clear heat and transform dampness using Clear Sky Paste (*qīng kōng gāo*). ACU Base treatment mainly on ST and LI. Select Greater Yang (*tài yáng*), LI-4 (*hé gǔ*, Union Valley), LI-11 (*qū chí*, Pool at the Bend), ST-36 (*zú sān lǐ*, Leg Three Li), and SP-9 (*yīn líng quán*, Yin Mound Spring); needle with drainage. **Phlegm-damp** heavy-headedness is worst in the morning on rising and is accompanied by dizziness, tinnitus, somnolence, glomus and oppression in the chest and stomach duct, nausea and drool ejection, white slimy tongue fur, and a soggy slippery pulse. MED Dry dampness and transform phlegm with formulas such as Pinellia, Ovate Atractylodes, and Gastrodia Decoction (*bàn xià bái zhú tiān má tāng*). ACU Base treatment mainly on CV, GB, ST, and LI. Select GV-20 (*bǎi huì*, Hundred Convergences), GB-20 (*fēng chí*, Wind Pool), PC-6 (*nèi guān*, Inner Pass), LI-4 (*hé gǔ*, Union Valley), CV-12 (*zhōng wǎn*, Center Stomach Duct), ST-36 (*zú san lǐ*, Leg Three Li), ST-40 (*fēng lóng*, Bountiful Bulge), ST-8 (*tóu wéi*, Head Corner), Greater Yang (*tài yáng*), and SP-9 (*yīn líng quán*, Yin Mound Spring); needling with drainage. **Insufficiency of center qi** heavy-headedness is characterized by fuzzy-headedness or empty-headedness and dizziness, and is accompanied by lusterless complexion, fatigued spirit and lack of strength, reduced food intake, sloppy stool, pale tongue with dental impressions, and forceless moderate pulse. MED Use Center-Supplementing Qi-Boosting Decoction (*bǔ zhōng yì qì tāng*) to upbear clear yang. ACU Base treatment mainly on CV and ST. Select GV-20 (*bǎi huì*, Hundred Convergences), CV-12 (*zhōng wǎn*, Center Stomach Duct), CV-6 (*qì hǎi*, Sea of Qi), CV-4 (*guān yuán*, Pass Head), ST-36 (*zú sān lǐ*, Leg Three Li), and SP-3 (*tài bái*, Supreme White); needle with supplementation and add moxa. [92: No. 61] [26: 906] [27: 393] [97: 165] [46: 621] [37: 361] [113: 163, 202]

heavy [medicinals] can eliminate timidity 重可去怯 *zhòng kě qù qiè*: Medicinals that are heavy in substance like loadstone (*cí shí*) and cinnabar (*zhū shā*) have a settling and quieting action that makes them effective for the treatment of mental derangement, fright and fear, and forgetfulness. [97: 419]

heavy pain 重痛 *zhòng tòng*: A pain, often an aching pain, associated with a sensation of heaviness; attributed to internal or external dampness. See PAIN. [29: 190]

heavy settler 重镇药 *zhòng zhèn yào*: Any mineral or shell product used, for example, to quiet the spirit in patterns characterized by heart palpitations and manic agitation. See QUIETING THE SPIRIT WITH HEAVY SETTLERS.

heel bone 跟骨 *gēn gǔ*: The bone in the heel of the foot. WMC calcaneus. [27: 72]

heel pain 足跟痛 *zú gēn tòng*, 脚跟痛 *jiǎo gēn tòng*: Pain in either or both heels that is usually unassociated with swelling yet makes walking difficult. Heel pain is a sign of kidney vacuity. If associated with intermittent heat in the lower leg, it is due kidney yin vacuity. If associated with inability to stand for long periods it is due to kidney yang vacuity sign. In some cases, dampness may collect in the heel causing local swelling. Damp-heat may also be observed. MED Kidney yin vacuity is treated by supplementing the kidney and enriching yin with Six-Ingredient Rehmannia Pill (*liù wèi dì huáng wán*) or Four Agents Decoction (*sì wù tāng*) and variations. Kidney yang vacuity is treated by supplementing the kidney and warming yang, using Cinnamon Bark and Aconite Eight-Ingredient Pill (*guì fù bā wèi wán*). For swelling due to dampness, use Statesman Shi's Wine-Steeped Formula (*shǐ guó gōng jìn jiǔ fāng*). For damp-heat, use Anemarrhena and Phellodendron Eight-Ingredient Pill (*zhī bǎi bā wèi wán*). ACU Base treatment mainly on KI, BL, and PC. Main points: KI-3 (*tài xī*, Great Ravine) joined to BL-60 (*kūn lún*, Kunlun Mountains), KI-6 (*zhào hǎi*, Shining Sea), BL-62 (*shēn mài*, Extending Vessel), and PC-7 (*dà líng*, Great Mound); needle with supplementation. For kidney yin vacuity, add BL-23 (*shèn shū*, Kidney Transport), BL-52 (*zhì shì*, Will Chamber), and SP-6 (*sān yīn jiāo*, Three Yin Intersection); needle with supplementation. For kidney yang vacuity, add BL-23 (*shèn shū*, Kidney Transport), GV-4 (*mìng mén*, Life Gate), CV-4 (*guān yuán*, Pass Head), and KI-7 (*fù liū*, Recover Flow); needle with supplementation and add moxa. For dampness, add SP-9 (*yīn líng quán*, Yin Mound Spring), and ST-36 (*zú sān lǐ*, Leg Three Li), needling with even supplementation and drainage, and, if appropriate, adding moxa. For damp-heat, SP-9 (*yīn líng quán*, Yin Mound

Spring), LI-11 (*qū chí*, Pool at the Bend), ST-44 (*nèi tíng*, Inner Court), and SP-6 (*sān yīn jiāo*, Three Yin Intersection), needling with drainage. [26: 322] [97: 269] [46: 587, 596] [37: 440]

helix 耳轮 *ěr lún*: The outer rim of the auricle. [26: 251] [27: 67]

hematuria 尿血 *niào xuè*: BLOODY URINE.

hemilateral headache 偏头痛 *piān tóu tòng*, 头偏痛 *tóu piān tòng*: **1.** HEMILATERAL HEAD WIND. **2.** Any headache on one side or one part of the head, as opposed to MEDIAL HEADACHE (the more common type). [26: 651]

hemilateral head wind 偏头风 *piān tóu fēng*: Synonym: *hemilateral headache; side head wind*. Pain in the temple or the corner of the head, either on the left side or the right, or switching from one to the other. Pain may stretch into the eye, and enduring pain may affect vision. In some cases, there are other accompanying signs such as nausea and vomiting. Hemilateral head wind is attributed to wind evil assailing the lesser yang (*shào yáng*) or liver vacuity and binding depression of phlegm-fire. In former times, it was believed that pain on the left was attributable to wind or blood, or to exuberant blood vacuity fire, whereas pain in the right was due to phlegm or heat, or to qi vacuity complicated by phlegm. MED Dispel wind and free the network vessels; soothe the liver and sweep phlegm; or supplement the liver and nourish the blood. Use Clear Sky Paste (*qīng kōng gāo*) or Hemilateral Headache Decoction (*sàn piān tāng*). ACU Base treatment mainly on GB, LR, ST, SP, and back transport points. Main points: GB-20 (*fēng chí*, Wind Pool), GV-20 (*bǎi huì*, Hundred Convergences), Greater Yang (*tài yáng*), joining GB-8 (*shuài gǔ*, Valley Lead), TB-3 (*zhōng zhǔ*, Central Islet), and GB-34 (*yáng líng quán*, Yang Mound Spring); needle with drainage. To soothe the liver and sweep phlegm, add PC-6 (*nèi guān*, Inner Pass), LR-3 (*tài chōng*, Supreme Surge), SP-6 (*sān yīn jiāo*, Three Yin Intersection), ST-40 (*fēng lóng*, Bountiful Bulge), and ST-36 (*zú sān lǐ*, Leg Three Li), needling with even supplementation and drainage; if there is phlegm-fire, prick Greater Yang (*tài yáng*) to bleed, and needle LI-4 (*hé gǔ*, Union Valley) and ST-44 (*nèi tíng*, Inner Court) to drain. To supplement the liver and nourish the blood, add BL-18 (*gān shū*, Liver Transport), BL-17 (*gé shū*, Diaphragm Transport), and BL-20 (*pí shū*, Spleen Transport), and needle with supplementation. See HEAD WIND; HEADACHE. [26: 651] [97: 525]

hemilateral sagging 偏坠 *piān zhuì*: SAGGING OF ONE TESTICLE.

hemilateral sweating 偏沮 *piān jù*: Sweating on one side of the body; observed in wind stroke. *Elementary Questions* (*sù wèn, shēng qì tōng tiān lùn*) states, "Hemilateral sweating causes hemilateral withering." The healthy side of the body sweats, whereas the affected side is dry. [27: 398]

hemilateral wind 偏风 *piān fēng*: HEMILATERAL WITHERING.

hemilateral withering 偏枯 *piān kū*: Synonym: *hemilateral wind*. Hemiplegia with gradual emaciation. See HEMIPLEGIA. [26: 650] [27: 397] [97: 524]

hemiplegia 半身不遂 *bàn shēn bù suì*, 半身不随 *bàn shēn bù suí*: Paralysis of one half of the body. Hemiplegia is the result of wind stroke, and is observed in all wind stroke visceral patterns, bowel patterns, and channel patterns usually in conjunction with deviated eyes and mouth. It is traditionally attributed to a) debilitation of construction and defense, vacuity of the vessels, and evil qi (wind, cold, dampness, phlegm, or static blood) exploiting the vacuity and entering; b) qi vacuity; or c) kidney vacuity with insufficiency of essential qi. MED Nourish the blood and dispel wind; warm the channels and free the network vessels; boost qi and quicken the blood; supplement the kidney and boost essence. Applicable formulas include the following: Large Gentian Decoction (*dà qín jiāo tāng*), Major Network-Quickening Elixir (*dà huó luò dān*), Yang-Supplementing Five-Returning Decoction (*bǔ yáng huán wǔ tāng*), Eight-Gem Decoction (*bā zhēn tāng*), and Rehmannia Drink (*dì huáng yǐn zi*). ACU Base treatment mainly on points of the hand and foot yang brightness (*yáng míng*) LI and ST, supported by points of the greater yang (*tài yáng*) and lesser yang (*shào yáng*). Main points: LI-15 (*jiān yú*, Shoulder Bone), LI-11 (*qū chí*, Pool at the Bend), LI-4 (*hé gǔ*, Union Valley), TB-5 (*wài guān*, Outer Pass), GB-30 (*huán tiào*, Jumping Round), GB-34 (*yáng líng quán*, Yang Mound Spring), ST-36 (*zú sān lǐ*, Leg Three Li), ST-42 (*chōng yáng*, Surging Yang), and BL-60 (*kūn lún*, Kunlun Mountains). In the early stages, needle both sides. One of the following three methods can be used. (1) First drain the unaffected side, then supplement the affected side. (2) Needle or moxa the two sides alternately. (3) Needle only the affected side, using a medium stimulus. In enduring cases, apply moxa on both sides to supplement. Selection of points according to affected area: For paralysis of the upper limbs, add TB-14 (*jiān liáo*, Shoulder Bone-Hole), TB-4 (*yáng chí*, Yang Pool), and SI-3 (*hòu xī*, Back Ravine). For paralysis of the lower limbs, add GB-31 (*fēng shì*, Wind Market), ST-33 (*yīn shì*, Yin Market), and GB-39 (*xuán zhōng*, Suspended Bell). For hypertonicity of the elbow, add PC-3 (*qū zé*, Marsh at the Bend) and LU-5 (*chǐ zé*, Cubit Marsh). For hypertonicity of the wrist, add PC-7 (*dà líng*, Great Mound). For hypertonicity of

the knee, add LR-8 (*qū quán*, Spring at the Bend), KI-10 (*yīn gǔ*, Yin Valley). For hypertonicity of the ankle, add KI-3 (*tài xī*, Great Ravine) and KI-6 (*zhào hǎi*, Shining Sea). For hypertonicity of the fingers, add Eight Evils (*bā xié*), and SI-3 (*hòu xī*, Back Ravine) joining PC-8 (*láo gōng*, Palace of Toil). For hypertonicity of the toes, add Eight Winds (*bā fēng*) and KI-1 (*yǒng quán*, Gushing Spring). For deviation of the mouth, add TB-17 (*yì fēng*, Wind Screen), ST-4 (*dì cāng*, Earth Granary), ST-6 (*jiá chē*, Cheek Carriage), BL-2 (*zǎn zhú*, Bamboo Gathering), and ST-2 (*sì bái*, Four Whites). For stiff tongue and sluggish speech, add CV-23 (*lián quán*, Ridge Spring), Gold Liquid and Jade Humor (*jīn jīn yù yè*), and HT-5 (*tōng lǐ*, Connecting Li). See WIND STROKE; hemilateral withering. ◇ Chin 半 *bàn*, half; 身 *shēn*, body; 不 *bù*, not; 遂 *suì*, follow (conscious direction). [26: 174] [27: 397] [97: 164] [46: 616]

hemorrhoid 痔 *zhì*, 痔疮 *zhì chuāng*: Synonym: *pile*. A protuberance on the inside or outside of the anus, often accompanied by constipation and the passage of fresh blood. A Western medical distinction between internal, external, and mixed hemorrhoids, often seen in modern literature. In traditional medicine, a broad distinction is made between repletion and vacuity. **Vacuity** patterns arise when long sitting or standing or walking, enduring dysentery or diarrhea, constipation and straining, or pregnancy cause general depletion and center qi fall that causes loosening of the sinews and vessels. The hemorrhoids usually hang out of the anus and cannot be retracted; they are accompanied by a sensation of sagging distention in the anus. Attending signs may include shortness of breath, laziness to speak, reduced food intake, lack of strength, pale tongue, and weak pulse. MED Treat with Center-Supplementing Qi-Boosting Decoction (*bǔ zhōng yì qì tāng*). If there is bleeding, use Spleen-Returning Decoction (*guī pí tāng*). If there is constipation, use Straitened Spleen Hemp Seed Pill (*pí yuē má rén wán*). ACU Base treatment mainly on BL and empirical points. Main points for hemorrhoids: BL-32 (*cì liáo*, Second Bone-Hole), GV-1 (*cháng qiáng*, Long Strong), BL-35 (*huì yáng*, Meeting of Yang), BL-57 (*chéng shān*, Mountain Support), and Two Whites (*èr bái*); needle with supplementation and add moxa. To address the vacuity, add GV-20 (*bǎi huì*, Hundred Convergences), and CV-8 (*shén què*, Spirit Gate Tower), and apply moxa. Selection of points according signs: For bloody stool, add SP-6 (*sān yīn jiāo*, Three Yin Intersection), SP-1 (*yǐn bái*, Hidden White), ST-36 (*zú sān lǐ*, Leg Three Li), and CV-4 (*guān yuán*, Pass Head). For constipation, add BL-25 (*dà cháng shū*, Large Intestine Transport), ST-25 (*tiān shū*, Celestial Pivot), TB-6 (*zhī gōu*, Branch Ditch), and CV-4 (*guān yuán*, Pass Head). **Repletion** patterns arise when dietary irregularities such as excessive consumption of hot acrid foods, enduring constipation, or wind, dampness, dryness, or heat external contractions either cause congestion of qi and blood and engender wind and transform into dryness, or give rise to damp-heat stagnation and turbid qi and static blood pouring down to the anus. Attending signs include thirst, constipation, reddish urine, red tongue and yellow fur, and slippery rapid pulse. MED Congestion of qi and blood engendering wind and transforming into dryness is treated by clearing heat and cooling the blood and by moistening dryness and coursing wind. Use Blood-Cooling Rehmannia Decoction (*liáng xuè dì huáng tāng*). Treat damp-heat by clearing heat and disinhibiting dampness with Pig's Intestines and Coptis Pill (*zàng lián wán*). If there is constipation, use Major Qi-Coordinating Decoction (*dà chéng qì tāng*). ACU Use the same main points for hemorrhoids as given above, but needle with drainage. To clear heat and cool the blood, and moisten dryness and course wind, add GB-20 (*fēng chí*, Wind Pool), LR-3 (*tài chōng*, Supreme Surge), SP-6 (*sān yīn jiāo*, Three Yin Intersection), KI-6 (*zhào hǎi*, Shining Sea), KI-3 (*tài xī*, Great Ravine), and ST-44 (*nèi tíng*, Inner Court), needling with drainage. To clear heat and disinhibit dampness, add SP-5 (*shāng qiū*, Shang Hill) and SP-6 (*sān yīn jiāo*, Three Yin Intersection), needling with drainage. Selection of points according to signs: For sore swollen anus, add BL-54 (*zhì biān*, Sequential Limit), BL-2 (*zǎn zhú*, Bamboo Gathering), and BL-58 (*fēi yáng*, Taking Flight). For red sore, add PC-8 (*láo gōng*, Palace of Toil). For bloody stool, add LU-6 (*kǒng zuì*, Collection Hole) and SP-6 (*sān yīn jiāo*, Three Yin Intersection). For constipation, add BL-25 (*dà cháng shū*, Large Intestine Transport), ST-25 (*tiān shū*, Celestial Pivot), TB-6 (*zhī gōu*, Branch Ditch), LI-4 (*hé gǔ*, Union Valley), and LI-11 (*qū chí*, Pool at the Bend). Other methods of treating hemorrhoids include HEMORRHOID DESICCATION and HEMORRHOID POINT PICKING. For severe cases, modern surgical ligature replaces the traditional treatments. See also EVERTED-FLOWER HEMORRHOIDS. [26: 585] [27: 482] [97: 538] [46: 714] [46: 596] [61: 237]

hemorrhoid desiccation 枯痔法 *kū zhì fǎ*: A method of treating advanced-stage internal hemorrhoids using a powder medicine such as Alum Hemorrhoid-Desiccating Powder (*kū zhì sǎn*) or Three-Shot Gun (*sān pǐn yī tiáo qiāng*) to erode away the hemorrhoids and make them dry up and slough off. Because of the danger of arsenic poisoning, this method is no longer widely used. It should not be applied to patients with anemia, hyperten-

sion, cirrhosis of the liver, or active tuberculosis. [26: 414] [27: 296] [97: 387]

hemorrhoid point picking 挑痔 *tiāo zhì*, 挑治痔法 *tiāo zhì zhì fǎ*, 挑痔疗法 *tiāo zhì liáo fǎ*: Picking of points on the back to treat hemorrhoids. Patients with hemorrhoids are often found to have *hemorrhoid points*, i.e., small tiny papular protuberances on the back (from vertebra C_7 down to $L_{4/5}$). These are of a white, red, or brown coloration that does not fade when pressed. **Method**: Choose papules close to the spine and at as low a position on the back or lumbus as possible. Use a thick needle to pick open the papule, and then pick out ten or so of the fibers visible within the rupture. Apply a dressing. [26: 421] [46: 716]

hen cough 鸡咳 *jī ké*: WHOOPING COUGH.

heralding speckle 报点 *bào diǎn*: A speckle that forewarns of macular eruption. In measles, for example, faint red speckles may appear at the hairline two or three days before the eruption actually occurs. [26: 682]

heralding tip 报标 *bào biāo*: HERALDING SPECKLE. [26: 682] [27: 314] [97: 137]

herbal foundation 本草 *běn cǎo*: Synonym: ben-cao; pen-ts'ao. **1.** Collectively, the items used in Chinese medicinal remedies, so called because herbs constitute the majority; materia medica. **2.** Any traditional work consisting of a systematic listing of Chinese medicinals with illustrations, e.g., *The Divine Husbandman's Herbal Foundation Canon* (*shén nóng běn cǎo jīng*), *The Comprehensive Herbal Foundation* (*běn cǎo gāng mù*), and *The Essential Herbal Foundation* (*běn cǎo bèi yào*). ◇ Chin 本 *běn*, stock, stem, root, base; 草 *cǎo*, herb, grass. The term means "basic herbs," herbs comprising the majority of Chinese medicinals. *Bencao* is the Pinyin transliteration, and *pen-ts'ao* is the older Wade-Giles transcription. [26: 188] [27: 314]

herbal medicinal 草药 *cǎo yào*: Any medicinal herb that is used locally and scantly or not mentioned in literature. Such herbs are often referred to as "GREEN HERBS" when sold fresh. See MEDICINAL. [27: 314] [97: 338]

heron cough 鹭鸶咳 *lù sī ké*: WHOOPING COUGH.

hiccough 呃逆 *è nì*: Counterflow upsurge of stomach qi causing a continual series of sudden short sounds produced by a jerking of the stomach. Hiccough may be caused by excessive consumption of raw or cold or hot spicy foods, or cold bitter or warm dry medicines. It may also be caused by emotional stimulus, or by stomach vacuity cold in enduring or severe disease. Distinction is made between COLD HICCOUGH; HEAT HICCOUGH; VACUITY HICCOUGH; REPLETION HICCOUGH; STASIS HICCOUGH; PHLEGM HICCOUGH; QI HICCOUGH. [26: 317] [27: 410] [97: 377] [50: 764]

hidden pulse 伏脉 *fú mài*: A pulse even deeper than the sunken pulse, considerable pressure being needed to feel it. It is associated with fulminant desertion of yang qi and deep-lying cold, and generally appears in conjunction with severe vomiting, diarrhea, and pain. [27: 195] [97: 205]

high-altitude wind sparrow-vision internal obstruction 高风雀目内障 *gāo fēng què mù nèi zhàng*: A condition that starts with poor vision in dark places, and subsequently, reduced visual acuity in the daytime, narrowing of the field of vision, and in severe cases clear-eye blindness. If the pupil turns golden yellow with time, the condition is called *yellow wind*. WMC pigmentary degeneration of retina. MED Enrich the liver and kidney and supplement qi and the blood with formulas such as Right-Restoring [Life Gate] Pill (*yòu guī wán*) or Center-Supplementing Qi-Boosting Decoction (*bǔ zhōng yì qì tāng*) with judicious addition of chlorite/mica (*méng shí*), bat's droppings (*yè míng shā*), atractylodes (*cāng zhú*), and fresh pig's liver (*zhū gān*). ACU Base treatment mainly on back transport points, KI, LR, SI, and BL. Select BL-18 (*gān shū*, Liver Transport), BL-23 (*shèn shū*, Kidney Transport), LR-2 (*xíng jiān*, Moving Between), BL-1 (*jīng míng*, Bright Eyes), GB-37 (*guāng míng*, Bright Light), SI-6 (*yǎng lǎo*, Nursing the Aged), GV-4 (*mìng mén*, Life Gate), KI-3 (*tài xī*, Great Ravine), and CV-4 (*guān yuán*, Pass Head); needle with supplementation and add moxa. ◇ Chin 高风 *gāo fēng*, literally "high wind," refers to a wind high up (in the upper part of the body). [26: 487] [27: 505] [97: 492] [37: 466]

hip bone 胯骨 *kuà gǔ*, 跨骨 *kuà gǔ*, 骻骨 *kuà gǔ*, 髁骨 *kē gǔ*: The bone that can be felt on either side of the body just below the umbilicus. WMC ilium. [26: 1008] [27: 70] [97: 473]

hoarse voice 声音嘶哑 *shēng yīn sī yǎ*, 嘶嗄 *sī shà*: A harsh, husky, muffled, faltering, or forced voice; attributable to wind-cold, wind-heat, heat evil invading the lung, lung-kidney yin vacuity, or blood stasis and phlegm. WMC dysphonia. **Wind-cold** hoarse voice is associated with an itchy throat, swollen larynx, cough, heat effusion, aversion to cold, thin white tongue fur, and a tight floating pulse. MED Course wind and dissipate cold; diffuse the lung and restore the voice. Use Rough and Ready Three Decoction (*sān ào tāng*). ACU Base treatment mainly on GV, LU, and LI. Select GB-20 (*fēng chí*, Wind Pool), BL-13 (*fèi shū*, Lung Transport), LU-8 (*jīng qú*, Channel Ditch), LI-4 (*hé gǔ*, Union Valley), CV-22 (*tiān tú*, Celestial Chimney), and CV-23 (*lián quán*, Ridge Spring); needle with even supplementation and drainage and, if appropriate, moxa. **Wind-heat** hoarse voice is accompanied by sore throat with burning sensation, heat effusion, aversion to cold,

cough with yellow phlegm, thin yellow tongue fur, and a rapid floating pulse. MED Course wind and clear heat; diffuse the lung and restore the voice. Use Mulberry Leaf and Chrysanthemum Beverage (*sāng jú yǐn*). ACU Base treatment mainly on GV, LU, and LI. Select GB-20 (*fēng chí*, Wind Pool), GV-14 (*dà zhuī*, Great Hammer), LU-7 (*liè quē*, Broken Sequence), LU-5 (*chǐ zé*, Cubit Marsh), LI-4 (*hé gǔ*, Union Valley), LI-11 (*qū chí*, Pool at the Bend), and CV-23 (*lián quán*, Ridge Spring); needle with drainage and prick LU-11 (*shào shāng*, Lesser Shang) to bleed. **Heat (dryness-heat) evil** invading the lung causes a hoarse voice accompanied by red sore swollen throat with a sense of blockage, thick phlegm, oppression in the chest, dry stool and reddish urine, red tongue with sticky yellow fur, and a slippery rapid pulse. MED Treat with Dryness-Clearing Lung-Rescuing Decoction (*qīng zào jiù fèi tāng*). ACU Base treatment mainly on back transport points, LU, and KI. Select BL-13 (*fèi shū*, Lung Transport), LU-5 (*chǐ zé*, Cubit Marsh), LI-11 (*qū chí*, Pool at the Bend), LU-10 (*yú jì*, Fish Border), LI-18 (*fú tú*, Protuberance Assistant), and KI-6 (*zhào hǎi*, Shining Sea); needle with drainage and prick LU-11 (*shào shāng*, Lesser Shang) to bleed. **Lung-kidney yin vacuity** hoarse voice is an long-standing condition associated with dry sore itchy throat, sticky phlegm, red tongue with scant fur, and a fine rapid pulse. MED Enrich the lung and kidney; clear heat and restore the voice. Use Lily Bulb Lung-Securing Decoction (*bǎi hé gù fèi tāng*) or Six-Ingredient Rehmannia Pill (*liù wèi dì huáng wán*). ACU Base treatment mainly on back transport points, LU, and KI. Select BL-13 (*fèi shū*, Lung Transport), BL-23 (*shèn shū*, Kidney Transport), BL-43 (*gāo huāng shū*, Gao-Huang Transport), GB-25 (*jīng mén*, Capital Gate), KI-6 (*zhào hǎi*, Shining Sea), KI-3 (*tài xī*, Great Ravine), SP-6 (*sān yīn jiāo*, Three Yin Intersection), GV-15 (*yǎ mén*, Mute's Gate), and CV-23 (*lián quán*, Ridge Spring); needle with supplementation. **Blood stasis and phlegm** hoarse voice is also a long-standing condition that may gradually worsen; it is accompanied by a sore dry throat possibly with visible nodes or lumps; the tongue is purple with thin fur, and the pulse is fine and stringlike. MED Treat with borax (*péng shā*), pumice (*hǎi fú shí*), sterculia (*pàng dà hǎi*), chebule (*hē zǐ*), shancigu (*shān cí gū*), bolbostemma (*tǔ bèi mǔ*), tangerine pip (*jú hé*), and litchee pit (*lì zhī hé*). ACU Base treatment mainly on back transport points, SP, ST, and LR. Select BL-17 (*gé shū*, Diaphragm Transport), SP-10 (*xuè hǎi*, Sea of Blood), SP-6 (*sān yīn jiāo*, Three Yin Intersection), LR-3 (*tài chōng*, Supreme Surge), BL-20 (*pí shū*, Spleen Transport), CV-12 (*zhōng wǎn*, Center Stomach Duct), ST-36 (*zú sān lǐ*, Leg Three Li), ST-40 (*fēng lóng*, Bountiful Bulge),

CV-22 (*tiān tú*, Celestial Chimney), and CV-23 (*lián quán*, Ridge Spring); needle with even supplementation and drainage. Compare LOSS OF VOICE; SUDDEN LOSS OF VOICE. See also THROAT LICHEN (*xiǎn*). ◇ Chin 声 *shēng*, voice; 音 *yīn*, sound; 嘶 *sī*, hoarse; neigh; 哑 *yǎ*, mute, silent. [92: No. 450] [37: 285]

holism 整体观 *zhěng tǐ guān*, 整体观念 *zhěng tǐ guān niàn*: The philosophical notion that phenomena are more than the sum of their component parts; in medicine, the application of this principle, involving the treatment of the whole person rather than isolated signs or diseases. Chinese medicine is considered holistic on the grounds of a perceived emphasis on the relationship between the human being and the environment and the relationship of the parts of the body to the whole in contrast to the emphasis of Western medicine on analysis and detail, in which a global view of the individual and his or her environment is partially lost. Holism is also seen in the universal correspondences of yin-yang and the five phases. [26: 910] [27: 320] [97: 644]

home 属 *shǔ*: Of channels, to meet the organs to which they belong, e.g., the foot greater yin (*tài yīn*) lung channel homes to the lung. [6: 50]

honey pill 蜜丸 *mì wán*: Medicinal preparation consisting of powdered medicinals bound together with a small quantity of honey, and formed into round spheres, usually up to 0.5 cm in diameter. [97: 629]

Hongkong foot 香港脚 *xiāng gǎng jiǎo*: A popular modern name for FOOT DAMP QI.

hooking and cutting 钩割法 *gōu gē fǎ*: A surgical method of treating the eyes whereby diseased tissue is lifted up with a hook and removed with a knife. [125: 95]

hot 热 *rè*: *adj.* **1.** Of or relating to heat. See HEAT. **2.** Of a nature tending to create heat and reduce cold, e.g., hot agent. See FOUR NATURES.

hot back 背热 *bèi rè*: Palpable heat or feeling of heat in the back. A hot back is a sign of lung heat or yin vacuity. **Lung heat** may be associated with effusion of heat from the back, which gets worse after noon, together with a dry mouth, cough, coughing of yellow phlegm, distending pain in the chest and back, constipation, red complexion, yellow tongue fur, and a rapid pulse. MED Clear and downbear lung fire with Family Secret White-Draining Powder (*jiā mì xiè bái sǎn*). ACU Base treatment mainly on GV, LU, and LI. Select GV-14 (*dà zhuī*, Great Hammer), BL-13 (*fèi shū*, Lung Transport), LU-5 (*chǐ zé*, Cubit Marsh), LU-10 (*yú jì*, Fish Border), LI-11 (*qū chí*, Pool at the Bend), ST-44 (*nèi tíng*, Inner Court), and ST-36 (*zú sān lǐ*, Leg Three Li); needle with drainage. **Yin vacuity** may be associated a feeling of heat in the back

that gets worse at night, associated with aching pain in the back and lumbus, heat in the hearts of the hands and feet, night sweating, red tongue with little fur, and a rapid fine pulse. MED Enrich yin and clear heat with Anemarrhena, Phellodendron, and Rehmannia Pill (*zhī bǎi dì huáng wán*). Heat in the back at night that abates in the daytime with no other signs is seen in yin vacuity of the elderly. Washing in warm water can reduce the discomfort. ACU Base treatment mainly on KI, BL, and GV. Supplement BL-23 (*shèn shū*, Kidney Transport), KI-3 (*tài xī*, Great Ravine), KI-6 (*zhào hǎi*, Shining Sea), KI-2 (*rán gǔ*, Blazing Valley), and drain GV-14 (*dà zhuī*, Great Hammer), BL-40 (*wěi zhōng*, Bend Center), and LR-2 (*xíng jiān*, Moving Between). Alternatively, needle all points with even supplementation and drainage. [92: No. 163] [46: 596] [37: 274]

hot body 身热 *shēn rè*: GENERALIZED HEAT [EFFUSION].

hot formula 热剂 *rè jì*: One of the TWELVE FORMULA TYPES. Heat can eliminate cold; hence hot formulas treat cold patterns. For example, Counterflow Cold Decoction (*sì nì tāng*), which contains dried ginger (*gān jiāng*), aconite (*fù zǐ*), and licorice (*gān cǎo*), treats aversion to cold, counterflow cold of the limbs, curled-up lying posture, watery diarrhea containing untransformed food, absence of thirst, and a forceless deep fine pulse. [27: 307] [27: 307] [97: 448]

hot head 头热 *tóu rè*: From *Essential Prescriptions of the Golden Coffer* (*jīn guì yào lüè*). A feeling of heat in the head. A hot head is usually attributable to yin vacuity with upbearing fire, or liver wind or liver yang harassing the upper body, and is often associated with redness of the checks and baking heat [effusion] that can be palpated. MED Enrich yin and downbear fire; calm the liver and subdue yang. Use Gastrodia and Uncaria Beverage (*tiān má gōu téng yǐn*) or Uncaria Powder (*gōu téng sǎn*). ACU Base treatment mainly on back transport points, and points of the three yin channels of the foot, HT, and GB. Main points: BL-23 (*shèn shū*, Kidney Transport), BL-18 (*gān shū*, Liver Transport), KI-3 (*tài xī*, Great Ravine), KI-6 (*zhào hǎi*, Shining Sea), and SP-6 (*sān yīn jiāo*, Three Yin Intersection); needle with supplementation. Selection of points according to patterns: For upbearing vacuity fire, prick HT-8 (*shào fǔ*, Lesser Mansion) and KI-1 (*yǒng quán*, Gushing Spring) to bleed. For liver wind and liver yang harassing the upper body, add GB-20 (*fēng chí*, Wind Pool), GV-20 (*bǎi huì*, Hundred Convergences), BL-17 (*gé shū*, Diaphragm Transport), LR-3 (*tài chōng*, Supreme Surge), and GB-43 (*xiá xī*, Pinched Ravine); needle with drainage. [26: 910] [27: 165]

hot [medicinals] can eliminate cold 热可去寒 *rè kě qù han*: Medicinals that are hot in nature such as dried ginger (*gān jiāng*) and aconite (*fù zǐ*) can treat cold patterns. See HOT FORMULA. [27: 307] [26: 873]

hot pack [method] 熨法 *yùn fǎ*, 热熨 *rè yùn*: A method of treatment in which a cloth bag containing medicinals that have been warmed, usually by stir-frying, is applied to the body to relieve pain. The hot pack method is used to treat wind-cold-damp impediment, cold pain in the stomach duct and abdomen. For example, stomach qi pain can be treated with a hot pack of stir-fried tangerine leaves. Salt, sand, or earth can also be used. Care should be taken not to burn the patient. [27: 293]

hot tears 泪热 *lèi rè*: Discharge of hot tear fluid; observed, for example, in WIND-FIRE EYE.

house 府 *fǔ*: Synonym: *mansion*. Place of dwelling or activity. See following entries for examples. It should be noted that this term in ancient Chinese was undifferentiated from the term rendered in the present text as BOWEL.

house of bright essence 精明之府 *jīng míng zhī fǔ*: The head. [27: 35] [97: 627]

house of essence 精府 *jīng fǔ*: ESSENCE CHAMBER[2].

house of the blood 血之府 *xuè zhī fǔ*: The vessels. [27: 34] [97: 189]

house of the kidney 肾之府 *shèn zhī fǔ*: The lumbus. [27: 34] [97: 338]

house of the marrow 髓之府 *suǐ zhī fǔ*: The bones. [27: 35] [97: 660]

house of the original spirit 元神之府 *yuán shén zhī fǔ*: The brain. [26: 101] [27: 34] [97: 42]

house of the sinews 筋之府 *jīn zhī fǔ*: The knees. The knee is an area in which many large sinews converge, and is the location of GB-34 (*yáng líng quán*, Yang Mound Spring), the meeting point of the sinews. Limpness of the sinews affecting the knees is observed especially in insufficiency of the kidney and liver. [26: 740] [27: 34] [97: 566]

HT 心 *xīn*, 手少阴心经 *shǒu shào yīn xīn jīng*: Abbreviation for the heart or hand lesser yin (*shào yīn*) heart channel.

huang 肓 *huāng*: **1.** The region below the heart and above the diaphragm. See GAO-HUANG. **2.** HUANG MEMBRANE. [50: 803]

huang membrane 肓膜 *huāng mó*: The fatty membrane below the heart and above the diaphragm. [50: 803]

Hua Tuo's paravertebral points 华佗夹脊穴 *huá tuó jiá jǐ xué*: A group of points, named after the famous 3rd century B.C. (Eastern Han) physician Hua Tuo, located along either side of the spine about 0.5 body-inches lateral to the lower end of the spinous process of each vertebra. Their functions are similar to those of the governing (*dū*) vessel and transport points between which they are located. They are notably used for diseases of the back and lumbus. Although Hua Tuo's points do not include points beside the cervical vertebrae, in modern clinical practice, however, cervical paravertebral points are used effectively in the treatment of neck diseases. The extended group may be referred to simply as paravertebral points. [27: 103]

human center 人中 *rén zhōng*: **1.** The philtrum. **2.** GV-26, which is located in the philtrum. [26: 18] [27: 66] [97: 12]

human-center clove sore 人中疔 *rén zhōng dīng*: A CLOVE SORE at the human center (philtrum). A human-center clove sore starts as a small lump like a small bean. It is hard, swollen, and painful, and is attended by general signs. It should not be squeezed for fear of encouraging a process of spread and exacerbation known as "running yellow" (see CLOVE SORE RUNNING YELLOW). Similar sores may occur in the sauce receptacle (the groove between the lip and chin) or at the corners of the mouth, known as *sauce receptacle clove sore* and *tiger's-whiskers clove sore* respectively. [27: 468]

human level 人部 *rén bù*: The middle third of the insertion range of a needle, i.e., the middle third of the distance between the surface of the body and the point of deepest insertion. See HEAVEN, HUMAN, AND EARTH.

humor 液 *yè*: Any fluid in the human body, and specifically a thicker fluid in contrast to "liquid." See FIVE HUMORS; FLUIDS. [27: 76] [97: 533]

humor desertion 脱液 *tuō yè*: See DAMAGE TO YIN.

humor-increasing moist precipitation 增液润下 *zēng yè rùn xià*: See MOIST PRECIPITATION. [27: 256] [27: 256] [97: 633]

hunchback 龟背 *guī bèi*: TORTOISE BACK. [27: 436] [97: 293]

hundred-day cough 百日咳 *bǎi rì ké*, 百晬咳 *bǎi zuì ké*, 百晬嗽 *bǎi zuì sòu*: WHOOPING COUGH.

hyperactive heart fire 心火亢盛 *xīn huǒ kàng shèng*: Synonym: *intense heart fire; exuberant heart fire*. A heart disease pattern characterized by signs such as heat vexation, insomnia, and mouth sores, arising when the six excesses lie depressed in the inner body and transform into fire, when the patient is given to excessive consumption of hot acrid foods or warm supplementing medicinals, or when affect-mind causes transformation into fire. The main signs, heart vexation, insomnia, and mouth sores, are accompanied by red face, thirst, yellow urine, dry stool, blood ejection and spontaneous external bleeding, manic agitation and delirious speech, heat effusion, and skin sores that are red, swollen, and painful. The tongue is red or red at the tip. The tongue fur is yellow. The pulse is rapid. **Analysis:** The heart stores the spirit and opens at the tongue. Its bloom is in the face. When heart fire is exuberant, it harasses the spirit. The resulting condition of disquieted heart spirit is characterized by heart vexation, insomnia, and, in severe cases, manic agitation and delirious speech. When heart fire flames upward, signs such as red face, red tongue, and painful ulcerating mouth sores are observed. When exuberant heat damages liquid, there is thirst, yellow urine, and dry stool. When heat congests, blood stasis develops, hence sores on the skin. When heat damages the blood network vessels and causes frenetic movement of the blood, there is blood ejection and spontaneous external bleeding. Exuberant heat is also reflected in the yellow tongue fur and the rapid pulse. MED Clear the heart and drain fire. Use Heart-Draining Decoction (*xiè xīn tāng*) or Palace-Clearing Decoction (*qīng gōng tāng*). ACU Base treatment mainly on PC and HT. Select PC-8 (*láo gōng*, Palace of Toil), HT-8 (*shào fǔ*, Lesser Mansion), and CV-14 (*jù què*, Great Tower Gate), needling with drainage and prick PC-9 (*zhōng chōng*, Central Hub), and HT-9 (*shào chōng*, Lesser Surge) to bleed. Selection of points according to signs: For mouth sores, add KI-2 (*rán gǔ*, Blazing Valley). For vexation and agitation, add KI-1 (*yǒng quán*, Gushing Spring), and PC-5 (*jiān shǐ*, Intermediary Courier). For insomnia, add HT-7 (*shén mén*, Spirit Gate), BL-15 (*xīn shū*, Heart Transport), and HT-5 (*tōng lǐ*, Connecting Li). For thirst, add TB-2 (*yè mén*, Humor Gate), CV-23 (*lián quán*, Ridge Spring), KI-6 (*zhào hǎi*, Shining Sea), and SP-6 (*sān yīn jiāo*, Three Yin Intersection). For dry stool, add LI-4 (*hé gǔ*, Union Valley), LI-11 (*qū chí*, Pool at the Bend), ST-37 (*shàng jù xū*, Upper Great Hollow), and TB-6 (*zhī gōu*, Branch Ditch). For blood ejection, add ST-44 (*nèi tíng*, Inner Court), and PC-4

(*xī mén*, Cleft Gate). Compare HEART FIRE FLAMING UPWARD, INTENSE INTERNAL HEART FIRE, and HEART HEAT. [57: 50] [26: 90] [116: 47] [50: 342] [46: 596, 670, 740] [113: 18, 154] [37: 349]

hyperactive kidney fire 肾火偏亢 *shèn huǒ piān kàng*: effulgent life gate fire. Effulgent yin vacuity with fire causing discharge of semen. The kidney is a yin viscus that stores fire and water (true yin and true yang), which must remain in balance if the body is to remain healthy. Depletion of kidney-water or liver-yin vacuity can give rise to hyperactive kidney fire, which manifests in the form of excessive libido, seminal emission, and premature ejaculation. MED Use Anemarrhena, Phellodendron, and Rehmannia Pill (*zhī bǎi dì huáng wán*). ACU Base treatment mainly on KI. Select BL-23 (*shèn shū*, Kidney Transport), KI-3 (*tài xī*, Great Ravine), KI-6 (*zhào hǎi*, Shining Sea), BL-52 (*zhì shì*, Will Chamber), SP-6 (*sān yīn jiāo*, Three Yin Intersection), and LR-3 (*tài chōng*, Supreme Surge); needle with even supplementation and drainage. For seminal emission and premature ejaculation, add BL-15 (*xīn shū*, Heart Transport), HT-7 (*shén mén*, Spirit Gate), and PC-6 (*nèi guān*, Inner Pass). [26: 687] [27: 164] [97: 339] [46: 588] [37: 384, 388]

hyperactivity 亢 *kàng*: In the doctrine of yin and yang, pronounced strengthening and prevalence of yang.

hypersomnia 昏睡 *hūn shuì*: CLOUDING SLEEP.

hypertonicity 拘急 *jū jí*, 拘挛 *jū luán*: Stiffness and tension in the limbs inhibiting normal bending and stretching. Hypertonicity is usually attributable to wind, and occurs, for example, in impediment (*bì*). See TENSION OF THE SINEWS. [27: 374] [97: 334]

hypertonicity of the limbs 四肢拘急 *sì zhī mài jū jí*: See HYPERTONICITY.

hypertonicity of the sinews 筋脉拘急 *jīn mài jū jí*: See TENSION OF THE SINEWS.

identifying patterns and administering treatment 辨证施治 *biàn zhèng shī zhì*: See DETERMINING TREATMENT BY PATTERNS IDENTIFIED.

identifying patterns and determining treatment 辨证论治 *biàn zhèng lùn zhì*: See DETERMINING TREATMENT BY PATTERNS IDENTIFIED.

identifying patterns and seeking the causes 辨证求因 *biàn zhèng qiú yīn*: SEEK THE CAUSE FROM PATTERNS IDENTIFIED. [26: 899]

illness 病 *bìng*: DISEASE.

immediate vomiting of ingested fluids 水入则吐 *shuǐ rù zé tù*: Vomiting of fluids very soon after ingestion; a sign of water-damp collecting internally.

immediate vomiting of ingested food 食入即吐 *shí rù jí tù*: Vomiting of food very soon after eating. Immediate vomiting of ingested food is observed in heat vomiting, food accumulation vomiting, phlegm vomiting, and dysphagia-occlusion (*yē gé*).

impact injury 碰撞损伤 *pèng zhuàng sǔn shāng*: KNOCKS AND FALLS.

impaired depurative downbearing of the lung 肺失肃降 *fèi shī sù jiàng*, 肺失清肃 *fèi shī qīng sù*: A pathomechanism involving a disturbance of the lung's functions of governing depurative downbearing and regulation of the waterways. The lung governs the qi of the whole body. If, for any reason, lung qi is inhibited, there may be signs such as cough, nasal congestion, and counterflow qi, and if the movement and distribution of water is affected, causing inhibited urination, puffy swelling and panting and cough may be observed. See LUNG DISEASE. [50: 954] [6: 175] [46: 652] [113: 18, 51]

impaired harmonious downbearing of the stomach 胃失和降 *wèi shī hé jiàng*: NONDOWNBEARING OF STOMACH QI.

impaired lung depuration 肺失清肃 *fèi shī qīng sù*: Poor depurative downbearing. The lung governs depurative downbearing, i.e., its qi is clean in nature and cleansing in action, and it moves downward and governs regulation of the waterways. Impaired lung depuration is reflected in panting counterflow, cough, and inhibited urination. [27: 159] [97: 352]

impaired pulmonary depuration 肺失清肃 *fèi shī qīng sù*: IMPAIRED LUNG DEPURATION.

impairment of gastric harmony and downbearing 胃失和降 *wèi shī hé jiàng*: NONDOWNBEARING OF STOMACH QI.

impairment of splenic movement and transformation 脾失健运 *pí shī jiàn yùn*: SPLENIC MOVEMENT AND TRANSFORMATION FAILURE.

impediment 痹 *bì*: *Synonym: bi (obs); obturation (obs).* **1.** Blockage, as in THROAT IMPEDIMENT. **2.** *Synonym: wind-cold-damp impediment.* Blockage of the channels arising when wind, cold, and dampness invade the FLESHY EXTERIOR and the joints, and manifesting in signs such as joint pain, sinew and bone pain, and heaviness or numbness of the limbs. *Elementary Questions (sù wèn, bì lùn)* states, "When wind, cold, and damp evils concur and combine, they give rise to impediment." Distinction is made between three pattern types, each of which corresponds to a prevalence of one of three evils: **wind impediment** (or moving impediment) characterized by wandering pain and attributed to a prevalence of wind; **cold impediment** (or painful impediment) associated with acute pain and attributed to a prevalence of cold; and **damp impediment** (or fixed impediment) characterized by heaviness and attributed to a prevalence of dampness. A fourth type, **heat impediment** occurs when the three evils transform into heat. Impediment is readily complicated by qi vacuity and blood vacuity. See BLOOD IMPEDIMENT; BLOOD VACUITY IMPEDIMENT; QI VACUITY IMPEDIMENT. Other specific forms of bi include JOINT-RUNNING WIND (*lì jié fēng*); GENERALIZED IMPEDIMENT; FLESH IMPEDIMENT; SKIN IMPEDIMENT; SINEW IMPEDIMENT; BONE IMPEDIMENT; VESSEL IMPEDIMENT. ⟦WMC⟧ arthritis; sciatica; spondylosis. ⟦ACU⟧ Base treatment on points chosen according to patterns, local points, and points on the affected channel, supporting them with ouch points (*ā shì xué*). The main points are chosen according to the prevalence of wind, cold, dampness, heat, and complications; see WIND IMPEDIMENT, COLD IMPEDIMENT, DAMP IMPEDIMENT, and HEAT IMPEDIMENT. In addition to these, choose from the following points according to the affected area: Shoulder: LI-15 (*jiān yú*, Shoulder Bone), TB-14 (*jiān liáo*, Shoulder Bone-Hole), SI-10 (*nào shū*, Upper Arm Transport), LI-4 (*hé gǔ*, Union Valley), TB-5 (*wài guān*, Outer Pass), and SI-3 (*hòu xī*, Back Ravine). Elbow: LI-11 (*qū chí*, Pool at the Bend), LU-5 (*chǐ zé*, Cubit Marsh), TB-10 (*tiān jǐng*, Celestial Well), LI-4 (*hé gǔ*, Union Valley), and TB-5 (*wài guān*, Outer Pass). Wrist: TB-4 (*yáng chí*, Yang Pool), TB-5 (*wài guān*, Outer Pass), and LI-5 (*yáng xī*, Yang Ravine). SI-4 (*wàn gǔ*, Wrist Bone). Spine: GV-26 (*shuǐ gōu*, Water Trough), GV-12 (*shēn zhù*, Body Pillar), GV-4 (*mìng mén*, Life Gate), and GV-3 (*yāo yáng guān*, Lumbar Yang Pass). Thigh: GB-30 (*huán tiào*, Jumping Round), GB-29 (*jū liáo*, Squatting Bone-Hole), GB-39 (*xuán zhōng*, Suspended Bell), GB-34 (*yáng líng quán*, Yang Mound Spring), and BL-40 (*wěi zhōng*, Bend Center). Knee: Eye of the Knee (*xī yǎn*), ST-34 (*liáng qiū*, Beam Hill), GB-34 (*yáng líng quán*, Yang Mound Spring), SP-9 (*yīn líng quán*, Yin Mound Spring), and GB-33 (*xī yáng guān*, Knee Yang Joint). Ankle: BL-62 (*shēn mài*, Extending Vessel), KI-6 (*zhào hǎi*, Shining Sea), BL-60 (*kūn lún*, Kunlun Mountains), GB-40 (*qiū xū*, Hill Ruins), and ST-41 (*jiě xī*, Ravine Divide) **3.** Blockage affecting the bowels and viscera that may or may not be related to wind-cold-damp impediment. See HEART IMPEDIMENT; LIVER IMPEDIMENT; SPLEEN IMPEDIMENT; LUNG IMPEDIMENT; KIDNEY IMPEDIMENT; BLADDER IMPEDIMENT. [26: 769] [46: 629]

impediment pattern 痹证 *bì zhèng*: See IMPEDIMENT.

impediments of the five viscera 五脏痹 *wǔ zàng bì*: Synonym: *visceral impediment*. Forms of IMPEDIMENT (*bì*) that develop when sinew impediment, vessel impediment, bone impediment, and skin impediment, etc., through repeated contraction of cold, wind and dampness, begin to affect the associated viscus. They may also be caused by qi and blood vacuity, essence depletion, or nonmovement of yang qi permitting evil qi to enter and gather in the chest and abdomen. [27: 36] [97: 47]

imperial physician 御医 *yù yī*: A healer employed to treat the emperor and members of the court. [27: 516]

impotence 阳痿 *yáng wěi*,-阴痿 *yīn wěi*: Synonym: *yang wilt*; *yin wilt*; *yang rising failure*; *failure to rise*; *loss of yin organ use*. Inability to perform coitus from failure to achieve or maintain a full erection. Impotence is caused by debilitation of the life gate fire, liver-kidney vacuity fire, heart-spleen vacuity, binding depression of liver qi, liver channel damp-heat pouring downward, spleen-stomach of damp-heat, or fright damaging the kidney. **Debilitation of the life gate fire** causing impotence is identified by genital cold, lumbar pain, limp knees, tinnitus, hair loss, loosening of the teeth, fear of cold, cold limbs, emaciated body, shortness of breath and lack of strength, dizziness, bright white facial complexion, pale enlarged tongue possibly with dental impressions, and a fine slow sunken weak pulse. MED Warm

and supplement the kidney with Right-Restoring [Life Gate] Pill (*yòu guī wán*) or Procreation Elixir (*zàn yù dān*). ACU Select CV-4 (*guān yuán*, Pass Head), SP-6 (*sān yīn jiāo*, Three Yin Intersection), BL-23 (*shèn shū*, Kidney Transport), GV-4 (*mìng mén*, Life Gate), and KI-3 (*tài xī*, Great Ravine); needle with supplementation and add moxa. Selection of points according to signs: For seminal emission and seminal efflux, add CV-6 (*qì hǎi*, Sea of Qi) and BL-52 (*jīng gōng*, Palace of Essence). For dizzy head and tinnitus, add GV-20 (*bǎi huì*, Hundred Convergences), GB-2 (*tīng huì*, Auditory Convergence), and TB-3 (*zhōng zhǔ*, Central Islet). **Liver-kidney vacuity fire** impotence arises when damage to liver-kidney yin causes frenetic movement of kidney fire. It is accompanied by premature ejaculation, seminal emission or efflux, vexation and thirst, red tongue, and rapid fine pulse. MED Enrich yin and downbear fire. Use Anemarrhena and Phellodendron Eight-Ingredient Pill (*zhī bǎi bā wèi wán*) or Major Yin Supplementation Pill (*dà bǔ yīn wán*). ACU Needle with supplementation at CV-4 (*guān yuán*, Pass Head), SP-6 (*sān yīn jiāo*, Three Yin Intersection), BL-23 (*shèn shū*, Kidney Transport), BL-18 (*gān shū*, Liver Transport), and KI-3 (*tài xī*, Great Ravine), and with drainage at KI-2 (*rán gǔ*, Blazing Valley), KI-6 (*zhào hǎi*, Shining Sea), LR-3 (*tài chōng*, Supreme Surge), GB-34 (*yáng líng quán*, Yang Mound Spring), HT-8 (*shào fǔ*, Lesser Mansion), and HT-7 (*shén mén*, Spirit Gate). **Heart-spleen vacuity** impotence is associated with signs of heart-spleen qi vacuity such as heart palpitations, shortness of breath, spontaneous sweating, emaciation, fatigued spirit and lack of strength, reduced food intake, distention of the stomach duct, sloppy stool, pale tongue, and a fine pulse, or with signs of heart-spleen blood vacuity such as heart palpitations or fearful throbbing, susceptibility to fright, profuse dreaming, loss of sleep, bright white facial complexion, emaciated body and fatigued spirit, pale tongue, and a fine pulse. In clinical practice, heart-spleen qi vacuity and heart-spleen blood vacuity are not clearly differentiated. MED Nourish the heart and spleen with Spleen-Returning Decoction (*guī pí tāng*) or Major Origin-Supplementing Brew (*dà bǔ yuán jiān*) and variations. ACU Select BL-15 (*xīn shū*, Heart Transport), BL-20 (*pí shū*, Spleen Transport), BL-23 (*shèn shū*, Kidney Transport), LR-6 (*zhōng dū*, Central Metropolis), ST-36 (*zú sān lǐ*, Leg Three Li), and SP-6 (*sān yīn jiāo*, Three Yin Intersection); needle with supplementation and add moxa. Selection of points according to signs: For seminal emission and seminal efflux, add the points mentioned above. For heart palpitations and insomnia, add HT-7 (*shén mén*, Spirit Gate) and PC-6 (*nèi guān*, Inner Pass). For dizzy head and vision, add

ST-36 (*zú sān lǐ*, Leg Three Li), and BL-17 (*gé shū*, Diaphragm Transport), and apply moxa at GV-20 (*bǎi huì*, Hundred Convergences). **Binding depression of liver qi** patterns arise when affect-mind dissatisfaction cause binding and depression of qi and disturb the liver's free coursing. Impotence occurring in such patterns is accompanied by the classic signs of binding depression of liver qi such as oppression in the chest, frequent sighing, rib-side distention, bitter taste in the mouth, and a dry throat that may feel as though it is blocked by a foreign body. The tongue is thin and white, while the pulse is sunken. MED Course the liver and resolve depression. Use Depression-Freeing Decoction (*dá yù tāng*) plus complanate astragalus seed (*shā yuàn zǐ*) and psoralea (*bǔ gǔ zhī*). Alternatively, use Counterflow Cold Powder (*sì nì sǎn*) plus psoralea (*bǔ gǔ zhī*) and mistletoe (*sāng jì shēng*). ACU Select CV-3 (*zhōng jí*, Central Pole), CV-2 (*qū gǔ*, Curved Bone), PC-6 (*nèi guān*, Inner Pass), LR-3 (*tài chōng*, Supreme Surge), SP-6 (*sān yīn jiāo*, Three Yin Intersection), BL-18 (*gān shū*, Liver Transport), BL-17 (*gé shū*, Diaphragm Transport), and ST-36 (*zú sān lǐ*, Leg Three Li); needle with even supplementation and drainage or with drainage. **Liver channel damp-heat pouring downward** patterns develop when mind-affect depression causes binding depression of liver qi that prevents fluids from being transformed and allows damp turbidity to arise, which in time transforms into heat and obstructs qi dynamic. In this case, impotence takes the form of an insufficient erection. Other signs include dampness or itching of the scrotum, reddish urine with pain on urination, and a dry mouth with a bitter taste. There are signs of binding depression of liver qi and liver channel signs such as rashness, impatience, and irascibility, rib-side pain, lesser-abdominal pain, and distending pain in the testicles. MED Clear heat and disinhibit dampness with Gentian Liver-Draining Decoction (*lóng dǎn xiè gān tāng*) or Tangkuei, Gentian, and Aloe Pill (*dāng guī lóng huì wán*). ACU Select LR-8 (*qū quán*, Spring at the Bend), CV-1 (*huì yīn*, Meeting of Yin), BL-18 (*gān shū*, Liver Transport), GB-34 (*yáng líng quán*, Yang Mound Spring), LR-2 (*xíng jiān*, Moving Between), SP-9 (*yīn líng quán*, Yin Mound Spring), KI-7 (*fù liū*, Recover Flow), and SP-6 (*sān yīn jiāo*, Three Yin Intersection). Needle with drainage. **Spleen-stomach damp-heat** patterns are attributable to damp-turbidity brewing internally and transforming into heat. This pathomechanism develops from dietary irregularities or from a liking for strong liquor and rich food in obese patients who get little exercise. Externally contracted damp-heat may also be a factor. The main signs are impotence with weak libido, torpid intake, nausea and vomiting, sticky

mouth with sweet flavor, and oppression and fullness in the chest and heavy limbs. The tongue fur is yellow and slimy or white and slimy, while the tongue is red. The pulse is slippery and rapid. MED Diffuse the center burner; transform dampness and clear heat. Use Three Kernels Decoction (*sān rén tāng*) or Sweet Dew Toxin-Dispersing Elixir (*gān lù xiāo dú dān*). ACU Select CV-4 (*guān yuán*, Pass Head), SP-6 (*sān yīn jiāo*, Three Yin Intersection), CV-3 (*zhōng jí*, Central Pole), SP-9 (*yīn líng quán*, Yin Mound Spring), BL-31 through BL-34 (*bā liáo*, Eight Bone-Holes), KI-7 (*fù liū*, Recover Flow), LR-8 (*qū quán*, Spring at the Bend), and ST-36 (*zú sān lǐ*, Leg Three Li); needle with drainage. **Fear and fright damaging the kidney** causes impotence that is characterized by failure to achieve an erection only in sexual contact and that is associated with general susceptibility to fright, suspicion, and apprehension. The tongue and pulse in such cases may be normal. MED Quiet the spirit and stabilize the mind using Mind-Stabilizing Pill (*dìng zhì wán*). ACU Select GV-1 (*cháng qiáng*, Long Strong), HT-7 (*shén mén*, Spirit Gate), CV-14 (*jù què*, Great Tower Gate), BL-19 (*dǎn shū*, Gallbladder Transport), BL-23 (*shèn shū*, Kidney Transport), and GB-34 (*yáng líng quán*, Yang Mound Spring); needle with supplementation. **Phlegm-stasis** can be responsible for a poor or unlasting erection with limp aching lower limbs. Other signs include dizziness, tinnitus, distention and pain in the smaller abdomen and testicles, and dry sparse yellowed pubic hair, dull tongue with stasis macules and slimy tongue fur, and a hard but forceless or interrupted (结代 *jié dài*) wrist pulse with a faint instep yang pulse. Phlegm-stasis impotence is rarely discussed in traditional literature, and its appearance in modern literature seems to be based on Western medical recognition that impotence can be the result of arteriosclerosis, hyperlipemia, hypertension, and obesity. MED Treat by quickening the blood, dispelling stasis, and transforming phlegm, assisted by boosting qi and supplementing the kidney. Use Rejuvenation Elixir (*huán shào dān*) or House of Blood Stasis-Expelling Decoction (*xuè fǔ zhú yū tāng*). ACU Main points: CV-1 (*huì yīn*, Meeting of Yin), CV-2 (*qū gǔ*, Curved Bone), and LR-12 (*jí mài*, Urgent Pulse). Supporting points: ST-40 (*fēng lóng*, Bountiful Bulge), CV-6 (*qì hǎi*, Sea of Qi), BL-15 (*xīn shū*, Heart Transport), BL-17 (*gé shū*, Diaphragm Transport), BL-23 (*shèn shū*, Kidney Transport), GV-4 (*mìng mén*, Life Gate), and BL-31 through BL-34 (*bā liáo*, Eight Bone-Holes). First tap BL-15, BL-17, BL-23, GV-4, and Eight Bone-Holes. Then needle ST-40 making the needle sensation travel upward rather than downward. Then needle CV-1, and after obtaining qi, twirl and remove needle without retaining. Needle CV-2, CV-6, and LR-12, with drainage, retaining the needles for ten minutes. Finally, after needling, moxa CV-6. Treat once every two days in 12-session courses. At least two courses are necessary. NB: Impotence is not easy to cure when, as is most commonly the case, it forms a vacuity pattern. In the treatment of vacuity impotence, success has been attained in recent years by the use of *chóng* products such as in Agelena and Hornet's Nest Pill (*zhī fēng wán*), which comprises agelena (*cǎo zhī zhū*), hornet's nest (*lù fēng fáng*), cooked rehmannia (*shú dì huáng*), placenta (*zǐ hé chē*), epimedium (*yín yáng huò*), and cistanche (*ròu cōng róng*). ◊ Chin 阳 *yáng*, yang, the opposite of yin; 痿 *wěi*, wilt, droop. Here, as is often the case, yang refers to the male member. In *The Inner Canon* (*nèi jīng*), it was called *yīn wěi*, "yin wilt," yin denoting, as it commonly does, the "private parts." [56: 21] [26: 716] [92: No. 238] [27: 427] [97: 239] [113: 136] [46: 679] [42: 198] [46: 602] [113: 136] [37: 385]

inability to eat 不食 *bù shí*: Failure to take normal, adequate, or any sustenance. See REDUCED FOOD INTAKE.

inability to get food down 食不下 *shí bù xià*: Difficulty in swallowing food or difficult passage of food to the stomach; a sign of DYSPHAGIA-OCCLUSION.

inability to recognize people 不知人 *bù zhī rén*: LOSS OF CONSCIOUSNESS. ◊ Chin 不 *bù*, not; 知 *zhī*, know; 人 *rén*, person. [27: 386] [97: 490]

inability to suckle 不能吮乳 *bù néng shǔn rǔ*: Inability of the child to take milk.

in acute conditions treat the tip 急则治标 *jí zé zhì biāo*: Treat secondary manifestations when these are acute. For example, the sudden appearance of sore swollen throat preventing swallowing (tip) in patients suffering from yin vacuity fever (root) is an acute condition requiring immediate attention. In severe cases, swelling of the throat can cause life-threatening asphyxiation, hence its treatment is more urgent than that of the root. Compare IN MODERATE (CHRONIC) CONDITIONS TREAT THE TIP. See also ROOT AND TIP. [27: 234]

inch 寸 *cùn*: **1.** A unit of measure equal to a tenth of a cubit (*chǐ*.) **2.** BODY-INCH. **3.** Of the three positions of the wrist pulse, the one furthest from the elbow. See WRIST PULSE. [27: 188] [97: 28]

inch opening 寸口 *cùn kǒu*: See WRIST PULSE.

inch whiteworm 寸白虫 *cùn bái chóng*: Synonym: *spleen worm disease*; *white worm disease*. From *The Origin and Indicators of Disease* (*zhū bìng yuán hòu lùn*). One of the NINE WORM DISEASES. A worm disease attributed to eating raw or improperly cooked pork or other meat and characterized by abdominal pain, abdominal disten-

tion, and diarrhea with the passing of white segments (proglottids). Inch whiteworm is so called because the worm is passed in short segments. WMC tapeworm infestation (cestodiasis, taeniasis). MED Treat by expelling worms until the head segment (scolex) is passed. Use medicinals such as areca (*bīng láng*), pumpkin seed (*nán guā zǐ*), agrimony (*xiān hè cǎo*), and pomegranate rind (*shí liú pí*). [26: 41] [27: 189]

incised wound 金创 *jīn chuāng*, 金疮 *jīn chuāng*: A cut in the flesh made with a knife blade or similar object. Incised wounds in mild cases are associated with pain, bleeding and damage to the skin and flesh. In severe cases, there is damage to sinew with persistent bleeding and severe pain. Massive bleeding can cause somber white complexion, dizziness, black vision, and scallion-stalk or faint fine pulse. Minor cuts can be treated with Sagacious Incised Wound Powder (*rú shèng jīn dāo sǎn*) or Litharge Paste (*tuó sēng gāo*) and appropriately wrapped. Nowadays, major cuts are stitched, and massive bleeding is treated by transfusion. [26: 394] [27: 119] [61: 332]

incised-wound tetany 金疮风 *jīn chuāng fēng*: LOCKJAW.

increase 增 *zēng*: See SUPPLEMENTATION.

increased eating with rapid hungering 多食易饥 *dū shí yì jī*, 多食善饥 *dū shí shàn jī*: SWIFT DIGESTION WITH RAPID HUNGERING. [92: No. 194]

increasing food intake 进食 *jìn shí*, 纳食 *nà shí*: OPENING THE STOMACH.

increasing humor 增液 *zēng yè*: See INCREASING WATER TO MOVE THE SHIP.

increasing water to move the ship 增水行舟 *zēng shuǐ xíng zhōu*: Synonym: *refloating the grounded ship*. A method of MOIST PRECIPITATION applied in warm disease to treat constipation due to heat bind and desiccation of humor and presenting as half vacuity, half repletion patterns. MED Increasing water to move the ship involves large doses Humor-Increasing Decoction (*zēng yè tāng*), which contains large amounts of scrophularia (*xuán shēn*), dried/fresh rehmannia (*shēng dì huáng*), and ophiopogon (*mài mén dōng*), which boost the fluids and eliminate the heat bind by facilitating the passage of stool. In cases of pronounced repletion heat, this formula can be supplemented with rhubarb (*dà huáng*) and mirabilite (*máng xiāo*), thus forming Humor-Increasing Qi-Coordinating Decoction (*zēng yè chéng qì tāng*). ACU Base treatment mainly on alarm, back transport, and lower uniting points of LI, and on LI and ST. Select BL-25 (*dà cháng shū*, Large Intestine Transport), ST-25 (*tiān shū*, Celestial Pivot), ST-37 (*shàng jù xū*, Upper Great Hollow), LI-4 (*hé gǔ*, Union Valley), LI-11 (*qū chí*, Pool at the Bend), SP-14 (*fù jié*, Abdominal Bind), ST-44 (*nèi tíng*,

Inner Court), and KI-6 (*zhào hǎi*, Shining Sea); needle with drainage. [6: 254] [46: 670] [113: 102] [37: 326]

incrusted skin 肌肤甲错 *jī fū jiǎ cuò*, 甲错 *jiǎ cuò*: ENCRUSTED SKIN.

indication 主治 *zhǔ zhì*: Usually plural. The diseases or signs for which a medicinal or formula should be described.

indirect moxibustion 间接灸 *jiān jiē jiǔ*: Moxibustion performed on an insulating material such as crushed garlic or a slice of ginger that spreads the heat and reduces its intensity, as well as protecting skin from burning. See the entries listed below. [27: 343] [97: 309]

Indirect Moxibustion

MOXIBUSTION ON GARLIC (*gé suàn jiǔ*)
MOXIBUSTION ON SALT (*gé yán jiǔ*)
MOXIBUSTION ON GINGER (*gé jiāng jiǔ*)
MOXIBUSTION ON CAKE (*gé bǐng jiǔ*)
  MOXIBUSTION ON ACONITE CAKE (*fù bǐng jiǔ*)
  MOXIBUSTION ON FERMENTED BEAN CAKE (*chǐ bǐng jiǔ*)
  MOXIBUSTION ON PEPPER CAKE (*jiāo bǐng jiǔ*)

indistinct vision 视瞻昏渺 *shì zhān hūn miǎo*: Unclear vision. *The Level-Line of Pattern Identification and Treatment* (*zhèng zhì zhǔn shéng*) speaks of "indistinct vision without any internal or external eye signs." This is observed in various internal obstructions. [125: 275] [27: 505] [97: 374]

ineffectiveness of the yin organ 阴器不用 *yīn qì bù yòng*: IMPOTENCE.

infant 小儿 *xiǎo ér*: Newborn or young child. In examining infants, special attention is paid to the head. A head that is unusually small or large generally indicates depletion of kidney essence or an insufficiency of the congenital constitution that may be accompanied by water-rheum. A depressed fontanel indicates yin humor depletion, whereas a bulging fontanel indicates acute or chronic fright-wind (see FONANTEL). Failure of the cranial sutures to close and the inability to keep the head upright indicate an insufficiency of kidney essence and bone marrow vacuity. An uncontrollable shaking of the head indicates a wind disease. In infants, the difficulty of performing the pulse examination calls for the use of one finger instead of three, or its replacement with the finger examination. See INFANT'S FINGER EXAMINATION; CHILDREN'S DISEASES.

infantile cinnabar toxin 小儿丹毒 *xiǎo ér dān dú*: CINNABAR TOXIN occurring in infants. WMC erysipelas and other inflammatory diseases. [50: 131]

infants' and children's diseases 小儿疾病 *xiǎo ér jí bìng*: CHILDREN'S DISEASES.

infant's finger examination 小儿指诊 *xiǎo ér zhǐ zhěn*: Synonym: FINGER VEIN EXAMINATION. A diagnostic method based on observation of the veins in the fingers of children, developed by Wang Chao of the Tang Dynasty, and further refined by Chen Fu-Zheng in *The Young Child Compendium* (*yòu yòu jí chéng*). The examination of the finger veins has considerable clinical value in diagnosing children below the age of three, before natural thickening of the skin makes the veins indistinct. The finger examination provides supplementary diagnostic data that is particularly useful in judging the severity of disease. It also helps to compensate for difficulties of pulse examination due to the infant's very short radial pulse, which must be taken with only one finger, and to disturbances of the pulse that result from the distress commonly experienced by infants in unfamiliar surroundings. The greater yin (*tài yīn*) lung channel runs from the chest through the inch, bar, and cubit, and through the FISH'S MARGIN (thenar eminence) to the tip of the thumb. The veins of the inner side of the index finger lie on a branch that separates from the main channel at a point proximal to the wrist, and provide diagnostic data that accords with that of the radial pulse. The finger is divided into three segments, known as *bars*. The first segment, from the metacarpophalangeal joint to the proximal interphalangeal joint is known as the *wind bar*. The second, from the proximal interphalangeal joint to the distal interphalangeal joint, is known as the *qi bar*. The final segment, from the distal interphalangeal joint to the fingertip, is called the *life bar*. The examination should be conducted with the child facing a good light source (sunlight being preferable to electric light). The practitioner holds the child's index finger in his left hand, and rubs it several times with the right hand from the life bar down to the wind bar, to enable the veins to stand out more clearly. In healthy infants, the veins appear as dimly visible, pale purple, or reddish-brown lines. Generally, they are only visible in the wind bar. In sickness, the color and degree of fullness of the veins may undergo change. The depth, color, paleness, stagnation, and length are examined. **Depth:** Veins that are particularly distinct and close to the surface indicate an exterior pattern. An external evil is assailing the exterior, and right qi is trying to resist, hence qi and the blood tend toward the surface. Veins that appear deep and only dimly visible indicate the presence of an evil in the interior. **Color:** Bright red usually indicates wind-cold. Purple-red indicates interior heat; pale yellow indicates spleen vacuity; purple black reflects depression in the blood network vessels and indicates a severe or critical condition. A green-blue coloring is observed in fright wind and pain patterns. Black generally indicates blood stasis.

Pale veins are a vacuity sign. **Stagnation:** Veins of a stagnant complexion (i.e., visually discernible impairment of blood flow) are associated with repletion patterns such as phlegm-damp, food stagnation, or binding depression of evil heat. **Length:** The longer the visible veins, the more severe the disease. If the veins are distinct only in the wind bar, the condition is relatively mild. If they are also distinct in the qi bar, the condition is more severe. The infant's life may be in jeopardy if veins become distinct in the life bar (hence its name). Extension of visible veins through all the bars to the fingertip is the mark of a critical condition. In external contractions, visible veins confined to the wind bar indicate invasion of the network vessels. If they extend into the qi bar and are deeper in color, the evil has entered the channels. Extension into the life bar marks penetration into the bowels and viscera. [6: 119] [27: 176] [44: 648] FINGER VEIN EXAMINATION.

infant's gate 子门 *zǐ mén:* The mouth of the uterus. WMC *Orificium uteri.*

infant's-pillow pain 儿枕痛 *ér zhěn tòng: Synonym: mother's blood lump.* Postpartum lower abdominal pain caused by static blood. This pattern may stem from incomplete elimination of the LOCHIA or wind-cold exploiting vacuity to invade the uterine vessels causing a collection of static blood. Both patterns involve stasis, but their pathomechanisms differ. **Incomplete elimination of the lochia:** Infant's-pillow pain stemming from incomplete elimination of the LOCHIA is characterized by hardness and pain in the lower abdomen that refuses pressure or a palpable lump combined with RETENTION OF THE LOCHIA. MED Quicken the blood and eliminate stasis. Use Bind-Dissipating Pain-Relieving Decoction (*sàn jié dìng téng tāng*). ACU Base treatment mainly on CV, SP, and ST. Main points: CV-4 (*guān yuán,* Pass Head), CV-6 (*qì hǎi,* Sea of Qi), SP-6 (*sān yīn jiāo,* Three Yin Intersection), CV-3 (*zhōng jí,* Central Pole), and SP-10 (*xuè hǎi,* Sea of Blood). For incomplete elimination of the LOCHIA, add LR-8 (*qū quán,* Spring at the Bend) and LR-3 (*tài chōng,* Supreme Surge), needling with even supplemenation and drainage and adding moxa. **Wind-cold:** Invasion of wind-cold is characterized by cold pain in the lower abdomen that likes warmth, accompanied by a white green-blue or white complexion, lack of warmth in the limbs and stagnant inhibited flow of LOCHIA. MED Warm the channels, dissipate cold, and dispel stasis. Use Engendering Transformation Decoction (*shēng huà tāng*). ACU To the main points given above, add ST-25 (*tiān shū,* Celestial Pivot), ST-36 (*zú sān lǐ,* Leg Three Li), ST-29 (*guī lái,* Return), and SP-8 (*dì jī,* Earth's Crux), needling with even supplementation and drainage and adding moxa. Compare

POSTPARTUM ABDOMINAL PAIN. ◊ Chin 儿 *ér,* infant, child; 枕 *zhěn,* pillow; 痛 *tòng,* pain; probably from the association of the pain with an abdominal mass imagined to be the pillow on which the infant's head lay. [26: 386] [27: 542]

infertility 不孕 *bù yùn: Synonym: being without child; breaking lineage.* Inability to become pregnant between menarche and menopause. In clinical practice, a woman who fails to become pregnant within three years of normal conjugal life without the use of contraception is considered infertile. Discounting male factors, Chinese medicine recognizes congenital factors (see FIVE UNWOMANLINESSES) and acquired factors. Infertility that can be treated is attributed to a variety of causes. See KIDNEY VACUITY INFERTILITY; LIVER DEPRESSION INFERTILITY; BLOOD VACUITY INFERTILITY; PHLEGM-DAMP INFERTILITY; KIDNEY VACUITY INFERTILITY; UTERINE COLD INFERTILITY; BLOOD STASIS INFERTILITY. ◊ Chin 不 *bù,* not; 孕 *yùn,* (getting) pregnant. [26: 126] [92: No. 401] [27: 545] [97: 64]

infixation 疰 *zhù: Synonym: influx.* Term used in disease names indicating infection and permanent lodging. Examples include *worm infixation, toxin infixation* (both old names for pulmonary consumption), and *summer infixation.* ◊ Chin 疰 is composed of the illness signifier 疒 with 主 *zhǔ,* which may have been included purely for its phonetic value, or, as has been suggested, also for its semantic value. As an abbreviation of 住 *zhù,* to lodge, it has been suggested that it reflects how the disease becomes permanently lodged in the body. As an abbreviated form of 注 *zhù,* to flow, it might reflect how the evil flows into the body; and indeed the character 注 is used interchangeably with 疰 (see INFLUX). Note that these characters are akin to 蛀 *zhù,* to be eroded by worms. [26: 487] [48: 254]

influx 注 *zhù:* INFIXATION. Occurs in disease names such as *demonic influx, cadaverous influx,* and *taxation influx,* all denoting *pulmonary consumption.* See INFIXATION. [48: 151]

influx heart pain 注心痛 *zhù xīn tòng:* Sudden heart pain with dark green-blue face and eyes, clouded spirit and delirious speech, and a pulse now large, now small, different at both hands as if belonging to two different people. MED Free yang and move qi; quicken the blood and transform stasis. Use Liquid Storax Pill (*sū hé xiāng wán*), Coronary Liquid Storax Pill (*guān xīn sū hé wán*) or Salvia Beverage (*dān shēn yǐn*). See HEART PAIN. [26: 343] [27: 502]

ingrown eyelash 拳毛倒睫 *quán máo dào jié,* 拳毛倒插 *quán máo dào chā,* 倒睫拳毛 *dào jié quán máo:* An eyelash that rubs against the eyeball, usually as the result of a improperly treated peppercorn or ulceration of the eyelid rim. The eyelash should be removed. [26: 552] [92: No. 465]

inhibited bladder qi transformation 膀胱气化 不利 *páng guāng qì huà bù lì:* See BLADDER QI TRANSFORMATION FAILURE.

inhibited menstruation 月经不利 *yuè jīng bù lì,* 月水不利 *yuè shuǐ bù lì,* 经行不利 *jīng xíng bù lì:* See SCANT MENSTRUATION.

inhibited qi dynamic 气机不利 *qì jī bù lì:* Reduced activity of qi that disrupts the normal upbearing of the clear and downbearing of the turbid, and manifesting in signs such as hiccough, cough and panting, glomus and oppression in the chest and stomach duct, abdominal distention, abdominal pain, and disease of stool and urine. [26: 545] [27: 143] [97: 95]

inhibited urination 小便不利 *xiǎo biàn bù lì:* Difficult voiding of scant urine. Inhibited urination is ascribed to nondiffusion of lung qi, devitalization of spleen yang, debilitation of kidney yang, internal damp-heat obstruction, or qi stagnation with damp obstruction. These patterns all involve reduced flow of urine to the bladder due to yang qi vacuity or the presence of evil qi. In addition, there are yin vacuity patterns, which, according to some, should not strictly be considered as inhibited urination patterns because they are essentially attributable to depletion of fluids. **Nondiffusion of lung qi** inhibited urination results from invasion of wind evil (wind-cold or wind-heat) and is associated with swelling of the eyelids gradually giving way to generalized water swelling, heavy aching limbs, heat effusion, fear of wind, cough and hasty panting, sometimes sore throat, thin white tongue fur, and a tight floating or rapid floating pulse. MED Diffuse the lung and move water with formulas such as Spleen-Effusing Decoction (*yuè bì tāng*). ACU Base treatment mainly on alarm and back transport points of BL, and on LU and LI. Select LU-5 (*chǐ zé,* Cubit Marsh), LI-11 (*qū chí,* Pool at the Bend), LI-4 (*hé gǔ,* Union Valley), CV-3 (*zhōng jí,* Central Pole), BL-13 (*fèi shū,* Lung Transport), BL-28 (*páng guāng shū,* Bladder Transport), and BL-22 (*sān jiāo shū,* Triple Burner Transport); needle with drainage. Selection of points according to signs: For water swelling, add CV-9 (*shuǐ fēn,* Water Divide), CV-6 (*qì hǎi,* Sea of Qi), ST-36 (*zú sān lǐ,* Leg Three Li), GV-26 (*rén zhōng,* Human Center), and LI-6 (*piān lì,* Veering Passageway). For heat effusion and fear of wind, add GB-20 (*fēng chí,* Wind Pool), TB-5 (*wài guān,* Outer Pass), and GV-14 (*dà zhuī,* Great Hammer). For cough and panting, add LU-7 (*liè quē,* Broken Sequence). For sore swollen throat, prick LU-11 (*shào shāng,* Lesser Shang) to bleed. **Devitalization of spleen yang** can cause inhibited urination associated with water swelling that

is more severe below the waist, lassitude of spirit and physical fatigue, withered-yellow facial complexion, head heavy as if swathed, heavy cumbersome limbs, distention and fullness in the stomach duct and abdomen, reduced food intake, sloppy stool, lack of warmth in the extremities, pale enlarged tongue, glossy white tongue fur, and a forceless slow sunken pulse. MED Warm and move spleen yang; promote the qi transformation and move water. Use Spleen-Firming Beverage (*shí pí yǐn*) and variations. ACU Base treatment mainly on back transport points, SP, and ST. Select BL-20 (*pí shū,* Spleen Transport), BL-23 (*shèn shū,* Kidney Transport), BL-22 (*sān jiāo shū,* Triple Burner Transport), SP-6 (*sān yīn jiāo,* Three Yin Intersection), ST-36 (*zú sān lǐ,* Leg Three Li), and CV-4 (*guān yuán,* Pass Head); needle with supplementation and add moxa. Selection of points according to signs: For generalized swelling, add CV-9 (*shuǐ fēn,* Water Divide), CV-6 (*qì hǎi,* Sea of Qi), ST-36 (*zú sān lǐ,* Leg Three Li), and SP-9 (*yīn líng quán,* Yin Mound Spring). For heavy-headedness, add ST-8 (*tóu wéi,* Head Corner) and Greater Yang (*tài yáng*). For distention and fullness in the stomach duct and abdomen, add PC-6 (*nèi guān,* Inner Pass), ST-25 (*tiān shū,* Celestial Pivot), and CV-6 (*qì hǎi,* Sea of Qi). For sloppy stool, add CV-12 (*zhōng wǎn,* Center Stomach Duct), LR-13 (*zhāng mén,* Camphorwood Gate), and ST-25 (*tiān shū,* Celestial Pivot). **Kidney yang vacuity** inhibited urination is associated with water swelling that is more pronounced below the waist, bright white facial complexion, panting, cough, and phlegm rale, heart palpitations and hasty breathing, physical cold and cold limbs, cold heavy aching lumbus and knees, pale enlarged tongue with dental impression, glossy white tongue fur, and a sunken weak cubit pulse. MED Warm the kidney and assist yang; promote qi transformation and move water. Use True Warrior Decoction (*zhēn wǔ tāng*). ACU Base treatment mainly on back transport points, GV, CV, KI, and SP. Select BL-23 (*shèn shū,* Kidney Transport), GV-4 (*mìng mén,* Life Gate), CV-4 (*guān yuán,* Pass Head), CV-6 (*qì hǎi,* Sea of Qi), BL-20 (*pí shū,* Spleen Transport), BL-22 (*sān jiāo shū,* Triple Burner Transport), KI-10 (*yīn gǔ,* Yin Valley), and SP-6 (*sān yīn jiāo,* Three Yin Intersection); needle with supplementation and add moxa. Selection of points according to signs: For generalized swelling, see above. For panting, cough, and phlegm rale, add BL-13 (*fèi shū,* Lung Transport), LU-9 (*tài yuān,* Great Abyss), ST-40 (*fēng lóng,* Bountiful Bulge), and LI-4 (*hé gǔ,* Union Valley). For heart palpitations and hasty breathing, add BL-15 (*xīn shū,* Heart Transport), CV-14 (*jù què,* Great Tower Gate), and HT-7 (*shén mén,* Spirit Gate). For cold heavy aching lumbus, add GV-3 (*yāo yáng guān,* Lumbar

Yang Pass) and BL-40 (*wěi zhōng*, Bend Center). **Internal damp-heat obstruction** causes inhibited urination associated with heart vexation, desire to vomit, bitter taste in the mouth with sticky slimy sensation, thirst without desire to drink, torpid intake and abdominal distention, constipation or sloppy and grimy stool, red tongue with yellow fur, and a soggy rapid pulse. MED Treat by clearing heat and disinhibiting dampness, and offensively expelling water-damp, with formulas such as Coursing and Piercing Drink (*shū záo yǐn zi*). ACU Base treatment mainly on alarm and back transport points of BL, and on SP. Select CV-3 (*zhōng jí*, Central Pole), BL-28 (*páng guāng shū*, Bladder Transport), SP-6 (*sān yīn jiāo*, Three Yin Intersection), SP-9 (*yīn líng quán*, Yin Mound Spring), and KI-7 (*fù liū*, Recover Flow); needle with drainage. Selection of points according to signs: For thirst, add TB-2 (*yè mén*, Humor Gate), and KI-6 (*zhào hǎi*, Shining Sea). For torpid intake and abdominal distention, add ST-44 (*nèi tíng*, Inner Court), PC-6 (*nèi guān*, Inner Pass), and ST-25 (*tiān shū*, Celestial Pivot). For constipation, add, LI-4 (*hé gǔ*, Union Valley), LI-11 (*qū chí*, Pool at the Bend), TB-6 (*zhī gōu*, Branch Ditch), and ST-37 (*shàng jù xū*, Upper Great Hollow). For sloppy grimy stool, add ST-25 (*tiān shū*, Celestial Pivot), and ST-37 (*shàng jù xū*, Upper Great Hollow). **Qi stagnation with damp obstruction** causes inhibited urination accompanied by bitter taste in the mouth, dry pharynx, constrained feeling in the chest and rib-side, reduced food intake, belching, swallowing of upflowing acid, and abdominal distention after eating, in severe cases with enlargement of the abdomen but with no hardness under pressure. The tongue is red with a thin yellow fur, and the pulse is stringlike. MED Course the liver and resolve depression; move qi and disinhibit water. Use Bupleurum Liver-Coursing Powder (*chái hú shū gān sǎn*) combined with Stomach-Calming Poria (Hoelen) Five Decoction (*wèi líng tāng*). ACU Base treatment mainly on alarm and back transport points of BL, and on LR, GB, PC, and SP. Select CV-3 (*zhōng jí*, Central Pole), BL-28 (*páng guāng shū*, Bladder Transport), LR-3 (*tài chōng*, Supreme Surge), GB-34 (*yáng líng quán*, Yang Mound Spring), PC-6 (*nèi guān*, Inner Pass), ST-36 (*zú sān lǐ*, Leg Three Li), SP-6 (*sān yīn jiāo*, Three Yin Intersection), and SP-9 (*yīn líng quán*, Yin Mound Spring); needle with drainage. Selection of points according to signs: For discomfort in the chest and ribs, add LR-14 (*qī mén*, Cycle Gate) and GB-24 (*rì yuè*, Sun and Moon). For belching and swallowing of upflowing acid, add CV-17 (*shān zhōng*, Chest Center) and CV-6 (*qì hǎi*, Sea of Qi). For abdominal distention after eating, add CV-12 (*zhōng wǎn*, Center Stomach Duct), CV-10 (*xià wǎn*, Lower

Stomach Duct), ST-25 (*tiān shū*, Celestial Pivot), and CV-6 (*qì hǎi*, Sea of Qi). **Yin vacuity** can also cause inhibited urination associated with short voidings of yellow urine, dizziness, tinnitus, heart vexation, bitter taste in the mouth, dry pharynx, vexing heat in the five hearts, limp aching lumbus and knees, in some cases repeated episodes of water swelling, red tongue with scant fur, and fine rapid pulse. MED Treat by enriching the liver and kidney, and by disinhibiting urine. Use Life Saver Kidney Qi Pill (*jì shēng shèn qì wán*). ACU Base treatment mainly on back transport points and KI. Select BL-23 (*shèn shū*, Kidney Transport), BL-22 (*sān jiāo shū*, Triple Burner Transport), CV-4 (*guān yuán*, Pass Head), KI-10 (*yīn gǔ*, Yin Valley), SP-6 (*sān yīn jiāo*, Three Yin Intersection), KI-3 (*tài xī*, Great Ravine), and KI-7 (*fù liū*, Recover Flow); needle with supplementation. Selection of points according to signs: For heart vexation, add HT-7 (*shén mén*, Spirit Gate) and HT-5 (*tōng lǐ*, Connecting Li). For dry pharynx, add KI-6 (*zhào hǎi*, Shining Sea) and TB-2 (*yè mén*, Humor Gate). For limp aching lumbus and knees, GV-3 (*yāo yáng guān*, Lumbar Yang Pass) and BL-40 (*wěi zhōng*, Bend Center). Inhibited urination due to exhaustion of yin liquid through excessive promotion of sweating, ejection, or precipitation is treated exclusively by nourishing yin and increasing humor, and hence goes beyond the scope of inhibited urination proper. See DRIBBLING URINARY BLOCK; STRANGURY-TURBIDITY; SHIFTED BLADDER; WATER SWELLING. [92: No. 223] [26: 75] [14: 124] [113: 19] [37: 380] [46: 672–3]

inhibited urination in pregnancy 妊娠小便不利 *rèn shēn xiǎo biàn bù lì*: From *The Origin and Indicators of Disease* (*zhū bìng yuán hòu lùn*). Difficult voiding of scant urine during pregnancy. Inhibited urination in pregnancy is attributed to accumulated heat in the small intestine and heat binding in the bladder, obstructing qi transformation. It may also be due to spleen-lung qi vacuity and impaired regulation of the waterways, preventing normal downward transportation to the bladder. **Accumulated heat in the small intestine** causes inhibited urination with thirst, heart vexation, and reddish urine. MED Clear heat and move water. Use Eight Corrections Powder (*bā zhèng sǎn*). **Spleen-lung qi vacuity** is characterized by heart palpitations, shortness of breath, and lassitude of spirit and lack of strength. MED Supplement the spleen and lung with variations of Center-Supplementing Qi-Boosting Decoction (*bǔ zhōng yì qì tāng*). [26: 340]

inhibition 不利 *bù lì*: Disfluency (of qi, fluids, or dampness) or difficulty (of physical movement, urination, and speech). Methods of treating such conditions are often described as *disinhibition*. See STOPPAGE. [92: No. 223] [27: 143] [97: 95]

inhibition of lung qi 肺气不利 *fèi qì bù lì*: Any disturbance of depurative downbearing of lung qi and the lung's governing of the waterways. The lung governs the qi of the whole body and governs the regulation of the waterways. The appearance of cough or nasal congestion on the one hand, or inhibited urination or water swelling on the other are signs of inhibition of lung qi. Compare NON-DIFFUSION OF LUNG QI. [26: 448] [27: 159] [97: 352]

initial-stage qi-aspect heat 气分初热 *qì fèn chū rè*: A warm disease pattern arising when evil first enters the qi aspect. The main signs include generalized heat EFFUSION, thirst, heart vexation, anguish, and mixed yellow and white tongue fur. Initial-stage qi-aspect heat is treated with Gardenia and Fermented Soybean Decoction (*zhī zǐ chǐ tāng*) to clear heat and outthrust evils. The main formula treating exuberant lung-stomach heat is Supplemented Ephedra, Apricot Kernel, Gypsum, and Licorice Decoction (*jiā wèi má xìng shí gān tāng*), which clears heat and diffuses the lung. This formula may be combined with heat-clearing phlegm-transforming formulas such as Minor Chest Bind Decoction (*xiǎo xiàn xiōng tāng*) and further supplemented with heat-clearing toxin-resolving medicinals such as lonicera (*jīn yín huā*), forsythia (*lián qiào*), scutellaria (*huáng qín*), and gardenia (*shān zhī zǐ*). [26: 233]

injection fluid 注射剂 *zhù shè jì*, 注射液 *zhù shè yì*: Intramuscular or acupoint injection fluids are made either by distillation or decoction followed by complex filtering procedures.

in moderate (chronic) conditions treat root 缓则治本 *huǎn zé zhì běn*: Treat the root of disease when there are no secondary manifestations that are more pressing Compare IN ACUTE CONDITIONS TREAT THE TIP. See also ROOT AND TIP. [27: 234]

inner body 内 *nèi*: The inner part of the body; synonymous with interior, but used especially in the context of deep-lying and internal disease. *interior*.

inner canthus 大眦 *dà zì*: The inner angle of the eye. [27: 65]

innominate toxin swelling 无名肿毒 *wú míng zhǒng dú*: Localized pain and swelling that suddenly appears on any part of the body. *The Great Compendium of External Medicine* (*wài kē dà chéng*) states, "... not a welling-abscess (*yōng*), not a flat-abscess (*jū*), not a sore, not lichen (*xiǎn*), resembling a malign sore in form, either healing or worsening; it is called an innominate toxin swelling." It is caused by wind, cold, or heat lodging in the channels. When due to wind evil, there is neither head nor root. When due to qi contending with the blood, there is a head but no root.

When due to wind-cold, the swelling is hard and white. When due to heat toxin, the swelling is red and hot. [MED] For exterior patterns, treat by dissipation, using Schizonepeta and Ledebouriella Toxin-Vanquishing Powder (*jīng fáng bài dú sǎn*). For interior patterns, treat by precipitation with formulas such as Internal Coursing Coptis Decoction (*nèi shū huáng lián tāng*). See TOXIN; TOXIN SWELLING. ◇ Chin 无 *wú*, no; 名 *míng*, name; 肿 *zhǒng*, swelling; 毒 *dú*, toxin. [26: 743] [27: 471] [97: 66] [92: No. 388] [50: 179]

inquiry 问诊 *wèn zhěn*: One of the *four examinations*; examination by questioning the patient or those attending him. According Zhang Jing-Yue (Ming, 1563–1640), inquiry should be based on ten questions: 1. Heat effusion and aversion to cold. 2. Sweating. 3. Head and body. 4. Stool and urine. 5. Food and drink. 6. Chest. 7. Deafness. 8. Thirst. 9. Identifying yin and yang from the pulse and complexion. 10. Noting any odors or abnormalities of the spirit. The first eight of these items, actually the only ones that are essentially part of inquiry, are still to this day considered to apply. To those eight, can be added hearing and vision, sleep, previous disease, emotional problems, and diseases specific to women and men. **Cold and heat:** The practitioner should inquire whether the patient suffers from sensations of cold or heat. Heat and cold can sometimes be felt, but sometimes not. The term "HEAT EFFUSION" generally denotes heat that can be felt, but in some case refers to what the patient experiences. AVERSION TO COLD is a patient's subjective feeling of cold; in the patient suffering from aversion to cold, heat effusion may sometimes be detected by an observer palpating the skin. This combination of heat effusion and aversion to cold is a typical indication of the onset of external diseases. The prominence of aversion to cold indicates the presence of external wind-cold; a milder aversion to cold, often called AVERSION TO WIND, with a more pronounced heat effusion indicates wind-heat. ALTERNATING HEAT [EFFUSION] AND [AVERSION TO] COLD is usually seen in midstage penetration patterns, such as malaria. An unabating high fever without aversion to cold indicates that the disease has already entered the interior. A persistent but remittent high fever, unabated by sweating, with intermittent aversion to cold, indicates that the evil is intense and the condition is relatively severe. LATE AFTERNOON TIDAL HEAT [EFFUSION], a persistent high fever that peaks from about 3 to 5 p.m., is principally associated with gastrointestinal heat bind. Persistent heat effusion accompanied by signs of dampness evil indicates lingering damp-heat. A low fever (often little more than hot palms and soles and flushed cheeks) that occurs in the afternoon or evening, and abates after night or morning sweating, is known as STEAMING BONE TIDAL HEAT [EFFUSION], and is attributable to yin vacuity. Heat effusion that is present during the day and rises at night indicates a relatively severe condition. If the patient feels hot and vexed, but has a normal or slightly high body temperature, the condition is generally found to be heat in the bowels and viscera. An irregularly intermittent low fever with lassitude and weakness usually indicates qi vacuity. Aversion to cold usually accompanies heat effusion, but occurring alone, it is a sign of yang vacuity. Often resulting from a sudden drop in body temperature, such a condition demands special attention since it may indicate vacuity desertion due to collapse of yang. A fluctuating generalized heat [effusion], i.e., one characterized by alternating reduction and increase, indicates damp-heat lodged in the qi aspect. An unsurfaced heat, i.e., one that can only be felt by extended palpation, indicates dampness and heat binding together, with the former preventing the latter from being easily detected at the surface of the body. SHIVERING is pronounced trembling due to cold. In malaria, it comes at regular intervals and is followed by high fever; in other febrile diseases, shivering is a sign of exuberant interior heat preventing yang qi from effusing to the exterior. As aversion to cold, it may also be the sign of pronounced yang vacuity. **Sweating:** Sweat is produced from the fluids and blood, and is said to be formed by the heart (see HEART FORMS SWEAT). Normal secretion is regulated by construction and particularly by defense. Abnormal secretion, therefore, reflects the state of the fluids and blood, as well as that of construction and defense. Excessive sweating during the daytime or sweating at the slightest physical exertion is termed SPONTANEOUS SWEATING. This most often occurs in patients suffering from qi vacuity or yang vacuity and is an indication of vacuous defense qi and a slackening of the interstices. Sweating during the night is termed NIGHT SWEATING and generally occurs in patients suffering from yin vacuity. It indicates yin vacuity internal heat and insecurity of construction qi. Heat effusion with dry skin and absence of sweating may occur either in depletion of blood and fluids, or in external disease when the exterior is assailed by an evil, depressing defense qi and blocking the interstices. Correlation with other signs is necessary to ensure a right diagnosis. Sweating provides a valuable indicator of the patient's condition. OILY SWEAT streaming constantly from the skin indicates yang collapse vacuity desertion, and is a severe condition. If, as a result of sweating, the body temperature drops and the pulse stabilizes, right qi is dispelling the evil from the body. A much less common sign of evil expulsion is SHIVER SWEATING. This refers to a shivering bout followed

by sweating that reduces a persistent high fever. Sweating fails to abate heat effusion in two cases: a) in exterior patterns with construction-defense disharmony preventing the expulsion of an exterior evil, characterized by continuing, intermittent, but not severe heat effusion with aversion to wind, and spontaneous sweating; b) in great qi-aspect heat patterns where high fever and great sweating are accompanied by aversion to heat and great vexation and thirst. **Head:** Inquiry about the head entails asking about headache, dizziness, and heavy-headedness. The head contains the brain marrow and is an area where the channels are highly concentrated. Most of the regular and irregular channels, in particular the yang channels, pass through the head. HEADACHE is among the most common signs of disease, occurring in both external diseases and internal damage. The nature, severity, and duration of headaches are all important factors in diagnosis. Headache of recent onset usually indicates external disease. Enduring headache indicates internal damage. Severe headaches usually form part of repletion patterns, whereas dull headaches are generally associated with vacuity. If the pain is exacerbated by exposure to wind and cold, the patient is likely to be suffering from a wind-cold disease. Exacerbation by warmth generally indicates ascendant hyperactivity of liver yang. A headache accompanied by heavy-headedness, known as a HEAD HEAVY AS IF SWATHED (bag-over-the-head sensation), is generally attributable to phlegm-damp clouding the upper body. Frontal headaches are often associated with the yang brightness (*yáng míng*) channel; pain in the temporal area is generally associated with the lesser yang (*shào yáng*) channel; pain in the back of the head and neck is associated with the greater yang (*tài yáng*) channel; and pain at the vertex is generally associated with the reverting yin (*jué yīn*) channel. DIZZINESS, which in some literature includes a vague distinction between DIZZY HEAD and DIZZY VISION, may be associated with liver yang, wind-phlegm, and vacuity diseases. **Hearing and vision:** The ears are the orifices of the kidney, and vacuity of kidney essential qi may cause TINNITUS (ringing in the ears) and DEAFNESS. Because the ears are located on the path of the lesser yang (*shào yáng*) channel, disease affecting the lesser yang (*shào yáng*) may lead to deafness. Loss of hearing may also occur in warm disease repletion patterns where evil qi clouds the clear orifices. Loss of hearing acuity and deafness, occurring in some chronic diseases, generally are part of qi or kidney vacuity patterns. Gradual loss of hearing in old age is due to vacuity. Tinnitus and deafness fundamentally have identical meaning in pattern identification. The eyes are the orifices of the liver. DIZZY VISION and FLOWERY VISION are generally associated with liver fire or ascendant hyperactivity of liver yang, and liver-kidney essence-blood depletion. Loss of visual acuity and dry eyes are usually attributable to liver-kidney insufficiency. **Body:** Inquiry about the body involves asking the patient about pain, discomfort, lumps, or similar irregular phenomena in the trunk or limbs. Generalized aching accompanied by heat effusion and aversion to cold generally occurs in exterior patterns. Pain of specific location, or wandering pain in the joints, generally indicates an impediment (*bì*) pattern. Insufficiency of qi and blood with blood failing to nourish the sinews may cause relatively mild aching and numbness in the sinews and bones. Heavy body and fatigued limbs usually indicates damp encumbrance. **Urination:** Asking about the patient's urine is indispensable part of the inquiry examination. Urine provides a valuable indicator of repletion, vacuity, cold, and heat. It is produced from fluids and its production and voiding depend on qi transformation; hence urination can provide useful information about the state of the fluids and qi transformation. URINARY INCONTINENCE, the total loss of control over voidings is most commonly a sign of severe qi vacuity or wind stroke desertion patterns. ENURESIS, also called *bedwetting* especially when observed in children, as is most commonly the case, is due to bad sleeping and waking habits, spleen-lung qi vacuity affecting regulation of the waterways, or insecurity of kidney qi. LONG VOIDINGS OF CLEAR URINE and in particular PROFUSE URINATION AT NIGHT (nocturia) indicate vacuous kidney yang failing to perform its containing function. SHORT VOIDINGS OF REDDISH URINE, when not due to inadequate replacement of fluids lost through sweating in hot weather, indicate repletion heat. INHIBITED URINATION is any reduction of urine volume or difficulty in discharge of urine attributed to qi vacuity or the presence of evil resulting in inhibition of the qi transformation. SHIFTED BLADDER is a specific form of inhibited urination characterized by frequent short voidings of scant urine, which arises in pregnancy due to pressure on movement of the bladder. STRANGURY inhibited urination with frequency and stinging pain on voiding, sometimes with the passing of stones or blood. BLOODY URINE conventionally refers to the presence of bloody urine in patterns other than strangury, and is attributed either to insufficiency of kidney yin with effulgent heart-liver fire spreading to the small intestine or to dual depletion of the spleen and kidney preventing the blood from being contained. **Stool:** Stool changes are largely attributable to morbidity of the spleen, stomach, and intestines, but may also be associated with liver and kidney dysfunction. CONSTIPATION and hard, dry stool are mainly attributable to heat and

repletion, although cold and vacuity are not uncommon causes. Constipation with fullness, distention, and pain in the abdomen occurring in externally contracted heat (febrile) disease is a result of gastrointestinal heat bind repletion pattern of heat constipation. Constipation marked by dry hard stool without pronounced abdominal distention is a vacuity pattern attributed to insufficiency of intestinal humor due to blood and fluid depletion. Vacuity constipation includes cold constipation, which involves difficult defecation experienced by the elderly as a result of yang vacuity affecting movement and transformation of food. DIARRHEA and sloppy stool occur in vacuity, repletion, cold, and heat patterns. Fulminant diarrhea usually indicates repletion. Enduring diarrhea generally indicates vacuity, or a vacuity-repletion complex. Diarrhea characterized by frequent evacuation of small amounts of stool with tenesmus and a burning sensation indicates damp-heat in the large intestine. ABDOMINAL PAIN is observed in vacuity and repletion patterns. Abdominal pain followed, and relieved, by diarrhea is most often attributable to food accumulations. Bouts of diarrhea with abdominal pain that is unrelieved by defecation are brought on by emotional stimuli. This is due to liver-spleen disharmony. Diarrhea occurring shortly after eating indicates spleen-stomach qi vacuity. Diarrhea each day before dawn is known as EARLY MORNING DIARRHEA and is attributable to spleen-kidney yang vacuity. Diarrhea with loss of the voluntary control over bowel movements, sometimes accompanied by prolapse of the rectum, is known as INTESTINAL VACUITY EFFLUX DESERTION, and is attributed to vacuity cold or to center qi fall. **Diet:** Dietary considerations are categorized in three parts: thirst and fluid intake; food intake and digestion; and taste in the mouth. (1) Thirst and fluid intake: Inquiry about thirst and fluid intake provides a valuable indicator of heat and cold. Absence of thirst, or intake of warm fluids in small amounts, indicates a cold pattern. Thirst with little or no desire to drink, or immediate vomiting of ingested fluids, indicates water-damp collecting internally and impaired upbearing of fluids. Thirst with a preference for cold fluids and severe thirst with large fluid intake are signs of heat. Thirst unallayed by a large fluid intake, together with a high increase in urine volume, indicates dispersion-thirst. (2) Food intake and digestion: Information concerning the patient's intake of solid foods is particularly valuable in prognosis. Maintenance of a good appetite and digestion in spite of long or severe illness shows that the stomach qi has not expired and the patient's prospects for recovery are good. Hence it is said, "If sustenance is taken, the body thrives." Persistent poor appetite may affect the prospects for recovery. Most illnesses characterized by a reduced food intake, distention, and oppression after eating are traceable to spleen-stomach vacuity or inner body damp-heat obstruction. A normal appetite with indigestion signifies a strong stomach and a weak spleen. Increased eating with rapid hungering and clamoring stomach after eating indicates stomach heat. Stomach pain slightly relieved by eating signals a vacuity. Predilection for rich and fatty foods increases susceptibility to phlegm-damp. A perverted appetite indicates worm accumulations. (3) Taste in the mouth: Taste changes are of corroborative value in pattern identification. If the taste in the mouth is unaffected by illness, the mouth is said to be in harmony. This indicates that there is no heat in the interior. A bitter taste in the mouth is a sign of heat, and usually indicates stomach heat, liver heat, or liver-gallbladder damp-heat. A sweet or bland taste or slimy sensation in the mouth indicates damp obstruction or spleen vacuity with dampness. A sour putrid taste is usually attributable to food stagnation. Intermittent acid upflow usually indicates stomach heat, or invasion of the stomach by liver fire. **Chest and abdomen:** All the major organs, with the exception of the brain, are located within the chest and abdomen. Most diseases of the bowels and viscera are therefore reflected by pain or discomfort in this region. Inquiry thus involves identifying possible glomus, fullness, distention, and pain, and determining the presence of cold or heat and vacuity or repletion. GLOMUS and FULLNESS possibly with pain, and accompanied by coughing and copious phlegm indicates CHEST IMPEDIMENT (*xiōng bì*) or a cold-rheum pattern. If the same signs are accompanied by vexation heat, thirst, and slimy tongue fur, the pattern is one of phlegm-heat. A feeling of oppression in the chest with weak breathing indicates vacuity. RIB-SIDE PAIN AND DISTENTION indicates either binding depression of liver qi or liver-gallbladder damp-heat. Both of these are readily identifiable by the correlation of other signs. Lancinating pain and oppression around the heart, with ashen complexion, and dripping cold sweat, is termed TRUE HEART PAIN and is a critical condition. ABDOMINAL PAIN occurs in vacuity and repletion patterns. When the pain likes pressure, it is ascribed to vacuity; if it refuses pressure, it is ascribed to repletion. Pain soothed by the application of heat is attributable to cold. Stabbing or lancinating pain of specific location indicates accumulation of static blood forming an INTERNAL WELLING-ABSCESS (*nèi yōng*). Remittent scurrying pain of nonspecific location is usually qi pain. Intermittent scurrying pain in the umbilical region may indicate a WORM ACCUMULATION. ABDOMINAL DISTENTION relieved by the passing of flatus or belching is usually related to qi stagna-

tion or food accumulation; it is often further characterized by torpid intake. Continued distention without relief, together with hard stools, indicates repletion. Periodically abating vacuity distention combined with sloppy stool form a vacuity pattern. *Essential Prescriptions of the Golden Coffer* (*jīn guì yào lüè*) describes the former as "abdominal fullness with little or no relief," and the latter as "abdominal fullness recurring after periods of relief." **Sleep:** Sleep disturbances include insomnia, somnolence, and clouding sleep. SLEEPLESSNESS (insomnia), the inability to gain a full night's rest, is observed in a number patterns. When marked by reduced and unquiet sleep, profuse dreaming, heart palpitations, and susceptibility to fright and fear, it is attributable to insufficiency of heart blood, disquieting of the heart spirit, or liver blood insufficiency. When characterized by heart vexation and interior heat, initial insomnia, or, in severe cases, nightlong sleeplessness, it is attributable to effulgent yin vacuity fire. Persistent, severe insomnia with signs of both heart fire and kidney vacuity indicate noninteraction of the heart and kidney. Insomnia due to phlegm-fire harassing the upper body, spleen-stomach vacuity, or indigestion, is loosely termed UNQUIET SLEEP DUE TO STOMACH DISHARMONY. SOMNOLENCE, pronounced drowsiness and tendency to sleep for long periods, occurs most notably in external diseases such as heat entering the pericardium or phlegm clouding the orifices of the heart. It may also be a sign of debilitation of yang qi, which is referred to in *On Cold Damage* (*shāng hán lùn*), where it states, "When the lesser yin (*shào yīn*) is affected by disease... there is desire only for sleep." Patients suffering from yang vacuity may fall asleep almost instantly, but readily awaken. This condition is distinguished from the former by the absence of heat signs. CLOUDING SLEEP, equivalent to hypersomnia in Western medicine, occurs in heat entering the pericardium. **Old Illnesses:** Old illness includes both long-standing illnesses and previous illnesses. Information about the patient's history of illness is important when judging new conditions. (1) Presence of long-standing ailments: The practitioner should ask patients whether they were already suffering from any long-standing complaint when the present condition arose. Liver fire and liver yang disease is a predisposing factor for stirring of internal wind and sudden wind strokes. Enduring diarrhea or water swelling frequently indicates spleen-kidney yang vacuity. Patients ordinarily suffering from phlegm-rheum may be found to have insufficiency of lung, spleen, and kidney qi transformation. (2) Previous treatment and its implications for medication: Patients should be questioned about previous treatment and its effects. If, for example, a condition was previously identified as a heat pattern, yet treatment with cold or cool medicinals produced no marked effect, either the pattern was wrongly identified, or the diagnosis was right but the formula chosen was inappropriate. Possibly, the formula was simply not strong enough. Reappraisal in the light of presenting signs should pinpoint the error. **Attitudes, emotions, lifestyle, and working environment:** People who are taciturn and melancholy by nature are more prone than others to binding depression of liver qi. Impulsiveness, rashness, and impatience are predisposing factors for liver fire flaming upward and upstirring of liver yang. Predilection for cold, raw, and fatty foods, and smoking may cause phlegm-damp. Attention should be paid to the diseases commonly associated with the patient's occupation; for example, the occupational diseases of outdoor manual laborers include low back pain and aching legs, and cold-damp bi. **Women:** Menstruation and childbearing are associated not only with the uterus, but also the heart, the liver, the spleen, and kidney, as well as the thoroughfare (*chōng*) and controlling (*rèn*) vessels. Information concerning menstruation, pregnancy, and childbirth is therefore relevant in many nongynecological diseases. The practitioner should ask about menstruation, history of pregnancy and childbirth, and future plans with regard to having children. When inquiring about menstrual history, attention should be paid to the length of the menstrual period (premature or delayed arrival of periods), flow, color (light red, red, purple), and the consistency (thin, thick, clotted) of the discharge. Any abnormalities in these are called MENSTRUAL IRREGULARITIES. ADVANCED MENSTRUATION (i.e., premature arrival of periods) with a heavy flow and a thick red discharge, generally indicates blood heat. DELAYED MENSTRUATION (i.e., late periods) with reduced flow and a light-colored discharge generally implies blood vacuity. A heavy flow with a thin pale discharge indicates qi vacuity. Purple discharge with clots indicates blood stasis. MENSTRUATION AT IRREGULAR INTERVALS (i.e., periods sometimes early sometimes late) is due to binding depression of liver qi, spleen vacuity, or kidney vacuity. A clotted flow indicates binding depression of liver qi, a pale thin flow indicates either spleen or kidney vacuity. A scant pale thin flow indicates kidney vacuity, while a copious flow indicates spleen vacuity (blood management failure). Excessive childbearing frequently leads to depletion of the thoroughfare (*chōng*) and controlling (*rèn*) vessels. Women with histories of miscarriage and difficult deliveries may be suffering from nongynecological diseases such as insufficiency of qi and blood or liver-kidney depletion. Information concerning menstruation and pregnancy is vitally important in selecting medication for nongynecolog-

ical diseases, since in pregnancy qi-breaking and blood-quickening medicinals and needling of SP-6 (*sān yīn jiāo*, Three Yin Intersection), GB-21 (*jiān jǐng*, Shoulder Well), and any points on the lower abdomen can cause miscarriage. VAGINAL DISCHARGE many be normal if scant and white. A copious clear white discharge without malodor is called white vaginal discharge and is caused by cold-damp pouring downward with spleen vacuity. A foul-smelling copious thick yellow discharge is called yellow vaginal discharge and is due to damp-heat pouring downward. **Men:** Problems specific to men include notably SEMINAL EMISSION, IMPOTENCE, and PREMATURE EJACULATION which are broadly attributed to kidney vacuity. **Children:** For infants and children, general inquiry about their development is important for assessing the state of their kidney essential qi and spleen-stomach function. When infants are breast-fed, inquiry about lactation may be pertinent. [6: 130] [97: 227]

insects in the ear 虫入耳 *chóng rù ěr*, 百虫入耳 *bǎi chóng rù ěr*: Insects that have found their way into the ear should be removed as quickly as possible. Drip oil, scallion juice (*cōng zhī*), garlic juice (*suàn zhī*), or alcohol into the affected ear, and remove the insect, taking care not to damage the ear drum. [26: 255]

insecurity 不固 *bù gù*: Failure to secure or be secured; vulnerability (to invasion by evils or loss of essential elements). The word "insecurity" occurs in the term "insecurity of defense qi," which denotes weakness of defense qi and a consequent loosening of the interstices, laying the body open to invasion by external evils. It also occurs in "insecurity of kidney qi," which denotes impairment of the kidney's function of storing essence, and is characterized by seminal emission, seminal efflux, and premature ejaculation, or urinary frequency, enuresis, and incontinence.

insecurity of bladder qi 胕气不固 *pāo qì bù gù*: Weakness of bladder qi failing to retain urine (often stemming from kidney yang vacuity) and manifesting as urinary incontinence or enuresis. [27: 165] [97: 524]

insecurity of defense qi 卫气不固 *wèi qì bù gù*: INSECURITY OF EXTERIOR QI.

insecurity of defensive yang 卫阳不固 *wèi yáng bù gù*: INSECURITY OF EXTERIOR QI.

insecurity of exterior qi 表气不固 *biǎo qì bù gù*: Synonym: *insecurity of defense qi; insecurity of the defensive exterior; insecurity of defensive yang*. Vacuity of the yang qi that defends the body. Yang qi vacuity manifests in fear of cold, and because it causes looseness of the interstices (sweat pores), there is spontaneous sweating. *Elementary Questions* (*sù wèn*) states, "Yang protects the outer body and thereby assures security." Insecurity of exterior qi is a failure of this function. [26: 356] [27: 132] [97: 326]

insecurity of heart qi 心气不固 *xīn qì bù gù*: *Synonym: noncontraction of heart qi.* A condition in which the heart spirit floats astray, characterized by dissipated spirit, forgetfulness, susceptibility to fright, heart palpitations, spontaneous sweating or sweating at the slightest exertion. [26: 92]

insecurity of kidney qi 肾气不固 *shèn qì bù gù*: *Synonym: insecurity of the lower origin.* Breakdown of the kidney's governing of opening and closing or storing of essence that manifests in urinary disturbances, such as frequent and long voidings of clear urine, incontinence, enuresis, and dribbling urination, or disturbances of the reproductive function such as seminal emission, seminal efflux, and premature ejaculation. Insecurity of kidney qi results from debilitation of kidney qi in old age or maldevelopment of kidney qi in youth, or from damage through sexual intemperance or early marriage (early commencement of sexual activity). It is usually, therefore, accompanied by signs of general kidney vacuity such as fatigued spirit, lumbar back pain, limpness of the knees, a tongue that tends to be pale, and a fine weak pulse. Mild cold signs are also observed. Furthermore, stirring fetus due to kidney vacuity may also be considered as a manifestation of insecurity of kidney qi (see STIRRING FETUS). MED Secure the kidney and astringe essence. Combine general qi-supplementing medicinals with medicinals that astringe essence and check enuresis such as Cherokee rose fruit (*jīn yīng zǐ*), euryale (*qiàn shí*), dragon bone (*lóng gǔ*), oyster shell (*mǔ lì*), tribulus (*cì jí lí*), lotus stamen (*lián xū*), dioscorea (*shān yào*), and mantis egg-case (*sāng piāo xiāo*). Use Golden Lock Essence-Securing Pill (*jīn suǒ gù jīng wán*) to treat seminal emission, and Stream-Reducing Pill (*suō quán wán*) to treat copious urine with urinary frequency or incontinence in the aged. Use Mantis Egg-Case Powder (*sāng piāo xiāo sǎn*) for enuresis in children. ACU Base treatment mainly on KI, CV, and back transport points. Select CV-4 (*guān yuán*, Pass Head), BL-23 (*shèn shū*, Kidney Transport), BL-52 (*zhì shì*, Will Chamber), KI-3 (*tài xī*, Great Ravine), KI-7 (*fù liū*, Recover Flow), GV-4 (*mìng mén*, Life Gate), SP-6 (*sān yīn jiāo*, Three Yin Intersection), and ST-36 (*zú sān lǐ*, Leg Three Li); needle with supplementation and moxa. Selection of points according to signs: For enuresis, add CV-3 (*zhōng jí*, Central Pole) and BL-28 (*páng guāng shū*, Bladder Transport). For dribbling urination, add BL-20 (*pí shū*, Spleen Transport), BL-28 (*páng guāng shū*, Bladder Transport), CV-3 (*zhōng jí*, Central Pole), and SP-9 (*yīn líng quán*, Yin Mound Spring). For seminal emission, add BL-15 (*xīn shū*, Heart Transport), PC-6 (*nèi*

guān, Inner Pass), and HT-7 (*shén mén*, Spirit Gate). For seminal efflux, add CV-3 (*zhōng jí*, Central Pole), CV-2 (*qū gǔ*, Curved Bone), and KI-12 (*dà hè*, Great Manifestation). [6: 193] [27: 165] [97: 339] [46: 674, 678] [37: 372, 378] [113: 130]

insecurity of the defensive exterior 卫表不固 *wèi biǎo bù gù*: INSECURITY OF EXTERIOR QI.

insecurity of the essence gate 精关不固 *jīng guān bù gù*: Inability to withhold semen manifesting in signs such as seminal emission, seminal efflux, and premature ejaculation. See ESSENCE GATE.

insecurity of the lower origin 下元不固 *xià yuán bù gù*: INSECURITY OF KIDNEY QI.

insecurity of the thoroughfare and controlling vessels 冲任不固 *chōng rèn bù gù*: Damage to the thoroughfare (*chōng*) and controlling (*rèn*) vessels with dual vacuity of qi and blood, causing flooding and spotting, miscarriage, or vaginal discharge. [26: 895] [27: 146]

insensitive impediment 顽痹 *wán bì*: A condition of numbness of the skin and flesh with inability to sense pain or itching, and sometimes aching pain in the extremities. [22: 270]

insensitivity of the flesh 肌肉不仁 *jī ròu bù rén*: Inability to experience pain, itching, cold or heat in the flesh. *Elementary Questions* (*sù wèn, wěi lùn*) states, "When spleen qi is hot, then the stomach is dry, there is thirst and insensitivity of the flesh. This develops into flesh wilting." *The Clear Rationale of Cold Damage* (*shāng hán míng lǐ lùn, bù rén*) states, "Insensitive means not lithe, not knowing itching, not knowing pain, not knowing cold, and not knowing heat. Any bending and stretching, moxibustion and acupuncture treatment is not felt. This is called insensitivity, which arises when evil qi is congested, right is qi blocked and hidden by evil qi that lies depressed and fails to effuse, and when construction and defense qi are vacuous and scant, and cannot move freely." See WILTING; IMPEDIMENT; and WIND STROKE. [50: 600]

insensitivity of the skin 肌肤不仁 *jī fū bù rén*: Numbness of the skin. *Essential Prescriptions of the Golden Coffer* (*jīn guì yào lüè, zhòng fēng lì jié bìng mài zhèng bìng zhì*) states, "When evil is in the network vessels, there is insensitivity of the skin." See NUMBNESS AND TINGLING OF THE SKIN. ◇ Chin 肌肤 *jī fū*, skin, flesh; 不仁 *bù rén*, not human, callous, insensitive. [50: 600] [26: 272]

insomnia 失眠 *shī mián*: SLEEPLESSNESS.

inspection 望诊 *wàng zhěn*: *Synonym: visual examination; looking examination.* One of the FOUR EXAMINATIONS; looking at the patient and his phlegm, urine, and stool for diagnostic information. In inspection, attention is paid to the spirit, general physical appearance, and any part of the body where there is discomfort. Special attention focuses on the complexion and tongue, which are important indicators of the bowels and viscera. Inspection theoretically covers products discharged from the body (stool, urine, vomitus, phlegm), although, in practice, information concerning these matters is gleaned through inquiry. See SPIRIT; ¹BEARING; FACIAL COMPLEXION; INFANT'S FINGER EXAMINATION; TONGUE; TONGUE FUR; HEAD; STOOL; URINE. See also SAND VEINS; FISH NETWORK VESSELS. [27: 170] [6: 114]

instep yang pulse 跗阳脉 *fū yáng mài*: One of the three positions and nine indicators. A pulse 1.5 body-inches in front of ST-41 (*jiě xī*, Ravine Divide) on the upper side of the foot. The instep pulse lies on the foot yang brightness (*yáng míng*) stomach channel, and indicates the state of the stomach and spleen. [27: 189]

insufficiency 不足 *bù zú*: Lack (of substance) or incompleteness (of function); opposite of *superabundance*. Compare VACUITY AND REPLETION. See also EXUBERANCE AND DEBILITATION.

insufficiency of center qi 中气不足 *zhōng qì bù zú*: Synonym: *spleen-stomach qi vacuity*. Weakness of the spleen and stomach qi in the center burner with movement and transformation failure. Signs include yellow facial complexion with little luster, pale or dull lips, poor appetite, abdominal distention after eating, dizziness, low voice, shortness of breath, fatigue with lack of strength, sloppy stool, tender-soft tongue with thick fur, and a vacuous pulse. In some cases, there is stomach pain that likes pressure. MED Supplement the center and boost qi, using Center-Supplementing Qi-Boosting Decoction (*bǔ zhōng yì qì tāng*). ACU Base treatment mainly on back transports, CV, SP, and ST. Select BL-20 (*pí shū*, Spleen Transport), BL-21 (*wèi shū*, Stomach Transport), CV-12 (*zhōng wǎn*, Center Stomach Duct), ST-36 (*zú sān lǐ*, Leg Three Li), CV-4 (*guān yuán*, Pass Head), and CV-6 (*qì hǎi*, Sea of Qi); needle with supplementation and add moxa. See SPLEEN QI VACUITY; STOMACH QI VACUITY. [50: 237] [27: 155] [46: 594] [43: 162, 271] [14: 171]

insufficiency of center yang 中阳不足 *zhōng yáng bù zú*: SPLEEN-STOMACH YANG VACUITY.

insufficiency of essence-blood 精血不足 *jīng xuè bù zú*: Synonym: *liver-kidney essence-blood depletion*. A combined pattern of INSUFFICIENCY OF KIDNEY ESSENCE and LIVER BLOOD VACUITY. MED Nourish the liver and supplement the kidney. Six-Ingredient Rehmannia Decoction (*liù wèi dì huáng tāng*) plus tangkuei (*dāng guī*), white peony (*bái sháo yào*), ligusticum (*chuān xiōng*), spiny jujube (*suān zǎo rén*), and flowery knotweed (*hé shǒu wū*). [50: 1671]

insufficiency of fluids 津液不足 *jīn yè bù zú*: Reduction of body fluids (see *fluids*) as a result of vigorous heat [effusion] with great sweating, profuse urination, vomiting, and diarrhea. It may also result from misappropriate use of sweat-effusing medicinals, water-disinhibiting medicinals, draining precipitant medicinals, or warm dry medicinals. Distinction is made between the mild form, DAMAGE TO LIQUID, and the severe form, DAMAGE TO YIN (humor desertion). [6: 46]

insufficiency of gallbladder qi 胆气不足 *dǎn qì bù zú*: Synonyms: *gallbladder vacuity and qi timidity*; *gallbladder qi vacuity*; *gallbladder vacuity*. A pattern arising after illness as a result of dysfunction among the internal organs. Signs include vacuity vexation, insomnia, susceptibility to fright, bitter taste in the mouth, doubt and suspicious, and frequent sighing. It is treated by warming the gallbladder and quieting the spirit. [50: 1123]

insufficiency of heart blood 心血不足 *xīn xuè bù zú*: See HEART BLOOD VACUITY.

insufficiency of heart construction 心营不足 *xīn yíng bù zú*: INSUFFICIENCY OF HEART YIN.

insufficiency of heart qi 心气不足 *xīn qì bù zú*: See HEART QI VACUITY.

insufficiency of heart yin 心阴不足 *xīn yīn bù zú*: Synonym: *insufficiency of heart construction*. See HEART YIN VACUITY.

insufficiency of kidney essence 肾精不足 *shèn jīng bù zú*: A disease pattern resulting from enduring illness or improper development during the fetal stage. Insufficiency of kidney essence differs from kidney yin and yang vacuity in that vacuity signs are accompanied by neither cold nor heat signs of any marked degree. The kidney governs the bones and engenders marrow, and the brain is the sea of marrow. Only when kidney essential qi is abundant can the bone, marrow, and brain fulfill their functions. Insufficiency of kidney essence may thus lead to signs of essence-marrow depletion and sea-of-marrow vacuity, such as impairment of intellectual function, osteodystrophy, and deficiency of the reproductive function. Insufficiency of kidney essence is generally characterized by dizziness, tinnitus, limp aching lumbus and knees, deficient reproductive function, loss of head hair, and loosening of the teeth. Insufficiency of essence-marrow or sea-of-marrow vacuity manifests in different ways according to age. In children, it can result in retarded growth and development, short stature, sluggishness of physical movement, low intelligence, weak bones, or retarded closure of the fontanels. In adults, it may lead to premature senility, or weakness in the legs, difficulty in walking, dullness of essence-spirit, and slowness of physical movement. MED "Insufficiency of essence is treated by supplementation with flavor." Commonly used medicinals include: placenta (*zǐ hé chē*), deerhorn (*lù jiǎo*) tortoise plastron (*guī bǎn*), eucommia (*dù zhòng*), lycium berry (*gǒu qǐ zǐ*), cistanche (*ròu cōng róng*), morinda (*bā jǐ tiān*), cynomorium (*suǒ yáng*), cornus (*shān zhū yú*), cuscuta (*tù sī zǐ*), and cooked rehmannia (*shú dì huáng*). Formulas include Left-Restoring [Kidney Yin] Pill (*zuǒ guī wán*) and powdered placenta (*zǐ hé chē*). Where cold signs are present, Right-Restoring [Life Gate] Pill (*yòu guī wán*) may be used to replenish essence and warm the kidney. The presence of heat signs calls for Placenta Great Creation Pill (*hé chē dà zào wán*), which enriches the kidney and boosts essence. ACU Base treatment mainly on KI and back transport points. Select BL-23 (*shèn shū*, Kidney Transport), BL-52 (*jīng gōng*, Palace of Essence), KI-3 (*tài xī*, Great Ravine), SP-6 (*sān yīn jiāo*, Three Yin Intersection), and GB-39 (*jué gǔ*, Severed Bone); needle with supplementation. [37: 386] [6: 193]

insufficiency of kidney water 肾水不足 *shèn shuǐ bù zú*: See KIDNEY YIN VACUITY. [26: 687]

insufficiency of kidney yin 肾阴不足 *shèn yīn bù zú*: See KIDNEY YIN VACUITY.

insufficiency of liver blood 肝血不足 *gān xuè bù zú*: See LIVER BLOOD VACUITY.

insufficiency of liver blood rib-side pain 肝血不足胁痛 *gān xuè bù zú xié tòng*: Rib-side pain characterized by continuous dull pain and accompanied by dizzy head and vision, lusterless complexion, menstrual irregularities, pale red tongue with scant fur, and a fine rapid pulse. MED Treat with All-the-Way-Through Brew (*yī guàn jiān*) plus adenophora/glehnia (*shā shēn*), ophiopogon (*mài mén dōng*), tangkuei (*dāng guī*), white peony (*bái sháo yào*), dried/fresh rehmannia (*shēng dì huáng*), lycium berry (*gǒu qǐ zǐ*), toosendan (*chuān liàn zǐ*), and silk tree flower (*hé huān huā*), ACU Base treatment mainly on back transport points, LR and SP. Select BL-18 (*gān shū*, Liver Transport), BL-23 (*shèn shū*, Kidney Transport), BL-20 (*pí shū*, Spleen Transport) LR-14 (*qī mén*, Cycle Gate), LR-2 (*xíng jiān*, Moving Between), GB-34 (*yáng líng quán*, Yang Mound Spring), SP-6 (*sān yīn jiāo*, Three Yin Intersection), and ST-36 (*zú sān lǐ*, Leg Three Li); needle with supplementation. For dizzy head and vision, add GV-20 (*bǎi huì*, Hundred Convergences) and GB-20 (*fēng chí*, Wind Pool). [46: 636]

insufficiency of liver qi 肝气不足 *gān qì bù zú*: See LIVER QI VACUITY.

insufficiency of liver yin 肝阴不足 *gān yīn bù zú*: See LIVER YIN VACUITY.

insufficiency of spleen qi 脾气不足 *pí qì bù zú*: See SPLEEN QI VACUITY.

insufficiency of spirit qi 神气不足 *shén qì bù zú*: Lack of spirit or vigor. See SPIRIT QI.

insufficiency of stomach yin 胃阴不足 *wèi yīn bù zú*: Synonym: *stomach yin depletion.* See STOMACH YIN VACUITY.

insufficiency of the brain marrow 脑髓不足 *nǎo suǐ bù zú*: *The Magic Pivot* (*líng shū*, *hǎi lùn*) says, when the brain is insufficient, the brain turns and the ears ring. [26: 127]

insufficiency of the life fire 命火不足 *mìng huǒ bù zú*: See KIDNEY YANG VACUITY.

insufficiency of the true origin 真元不足 *zhēn yuán bù zú*: See KIDNEY YANG VACUITY.

insufficiency of true yang 真阳不足 *zhēn yáng bù zú*: See KIDNEY YANG VACUITY.

insufficiency of true yin 真阴不足 *zhēn yīn bù zú*: See KIDNEY YIN VACUITY.

insufflate 嗅 *xiù*, 吹 *chuī*: To blow (into the nose, throat, or ear). See INSUFFLATION. [27: 295] [97: 277]

insufflation 吹药 *chuī yào*: A topical powder for ear, nose, throat, and mouth diseases that is blown into the nose, traditionally through rolled up paper, fine bamboo tubes or straws. A sore swollen throat with qi block in children, for example, can be treated by insufflating ground raw licorice (*shēng gān cǎo*) and impure mirabilite (*pò xiāo*) (Throat Insufflation Powder (*chuī hóu sǎn*)) into the throat. Chronic paranasal sinusitis can be treated by insufflating powdered calcined yellow croaker's otolith (*yú nǎo shí*) into the nose. Common cold with nasal congestion can be treated by insufflating powdered centipeda (*é bù shí cǎo*) into the nose. See NASAL INSUFFLATION. [27: 295] [97: 277]

intense heart fire 心火炽盛 *xīn huǒ chì shèng*: HYPERACTIVE HEART FIRE.

intense heat 炽 *chì*: Heat stronger than exuberant heat.

intense internal heart fire 心火内炽 *xīn huǒ nèi chì*: Synonym: *heart fire deflagrating internally.* A pattern characterized by heart vexation, insomnia, fearful throbbing, and, in severe cases, manic agitation, delirious speech, and incessant laughing. Treat by clearing heat and draining fire, assisted by nourishing the heart and quieting the spirit. Use Cinnabar Spirit-Quieting Pill (*zhū shā ān shén wán*) plus scutellaria (*huáng qín*), gardenia (*shān zhī zǐ*), and forsythia (*lián qiáo*). [26: 90] [80: 220] [50: 342]

intense stomach fire 胃火炽盛 *wèi huǒ chì shèng*: See EXUBERANT STOMACH HEAT.

intercourse bleeding 交接出血 *jiāo jiē chū xuè*, 交结出血 *jiāo jié chū xuè*: Bleeding during or after intercourse. Intercourse bleeding is usually attributed to frenetic liver fire preventing blood storage and a vacuous spleen failing to contain the blood. MED Regulate and supplement the kidney and spleen. Use formulas such as Center-Supplementing Qi-Boosting Decoction (*bǔ zhōng yì qì tāng*) or Spleen-Returning Decoction (*guī pí tāng*) plus oven earth (*fú lóng gān*). A local examination should be performed to see if there is any lesion. [97: 221]

interdependence of yin and yang 阴阳相互依存 *yīn yáng xiāng hù yī cún*: See YIN AND YANG ARE ROOTED IN EACH OTHER.

interior 里 *lǐ*: The inner part of the body as opposed to the exterior, especially the bowels and viscera. See EXTERIOR AND INTERIOR. Compare INTERNAL.

interior attack does not shun cold 攻里不远寒 *gōng lǐ bù yuǎn hán*: From *Elementary Questions* (*sù wèn, liù yuán zhèng jì lùn*). Heat accumulated in the interior cannot be eliminated unless cold precipitants are used. Cold in the abdomen giving rise to cold constipation can also be treated with cold precipitants provided these are suitably combined with other medicinals. Cold constipation can be treated with Rhubarb and Aconite Decoction (*dà huáng fù zǐ tāng*), which consists of rhubarb (*dà huáng*), aconite (*xián fù zǐ*), and asarum (*xì xīn*). Rhubab is cold and bitter, while aconite is greatly acrid and hot and asarum is warm and acrid. These medicinals combined together to form a WARM PRECIPITATION formula. [27: 244]

interior cold 里寒 *lǐ hán*: Cold patterns of the bowels and viscera attributable to insufficiency of yang qi or external cold passing to the interior and characterized by cold limbs and aversion to cold, somber white complexion, cold aching lumbus and knees, sloppy stool and diarrhea, long voidings of clear urine, pale tongue with glossy white fur, and a sunken slow or faint fine pulse. [97: 151] [27: 209]

interior heat 里热 *lǐ rè*: Any heat pattern arising when external evils enter the interior and transform into heat, or when internal depression engenders heat, usually taking the form of gastrointestinal or lung-stomach repletion heat or depressed liver-gallbladder heat. Interior heat is characterized by heat effusion, aversion to heat rather than cold, thirst with intake of fluid, vexation and agitation or vexation with bitter taste in the mouth, short voiding of reddish urine, red tongue with yellow fur, and a rapid surging or forceful rapid string-like pulse. [26: 762] [27: 209] [6: 151]

interior of the chest 胸中 *xiōng zhōng*: The chest cavity. *The Magic Pivot* (*líng shū, jīng mài*) states, "The kidney foot lesser yin (*shào yīn*) vessel... A branch goes out to the pericardium from the lung, and enters the interior of the chest. *Elementary Questions* (*sù wèn, sù wèn zhì zhen yào dà lùn*)

states, "When there is trouble in the interior of the chest, the throat becomes blocked and there is coughing." In *The Classified Canon* (*lèi jīng*), Zhang Jing-Yue annotates this line, saying: "The interior of the chest is the location of the lung." [26: 548]

interior pattern 里证 *lǐ zhèng*: Any disease pattern that indicates disease of the interior. (1) Any disease of the internal organs, in contradistinction to externally contracted heat (febrile) disease, e.g., liver disease characterized by dizziness, rib-side pain; heart disease characterized by heart palpitations or fearful throbbing; spleen disease characterized by abdominal distention and diarrhea; and kidney disease characterized by lumbar pain and seminal emission. (2) In externally contracted heat (febrile) disease, an interior pattern arises when an evil that has caused an exterior pattern passes into the interior. Rarely, external evils may strike the interior directly; in most cases, they pass through the exterior. Hence febrile disease interior patterns are identified when aversion to wind or cold—which may or may not be accompanied by heat effusion or sweating—gives way to high fever or tidal heat [effusion], vexation and agitation, thirst, clouded spirit, abdominal pain or distention, diarrhea or constipation, short voidings of reddish urine or inhibited urination, dry yellow tongue fur, and a rapid sunken pulse. See also INTERIOR COLD; INTERIOR HEAT; INTERIOR REPLETION; INTERIOR VACUITY. [26: 762] [27: 208] [6: 11]

interior repletion 里实 *lǐ shí*: 1. Any disease pattern resulting from external evil transforming into heat and entering the interior to bind in the stomach and intestines and thereby causing vigorous heat [effusion], vexation and thirst, abdominal pain and constipation (bowel repletion pattern). 2. Binding depression of qi and blood, gathering of phlegm, food stagnation, and worm accumulation. [27: 210] [6: 151]

interior vacuity 里虚 *lǐ xū*: Any pattern that arises when the yin, yang, qi, or blood or one or more of the bowels and viscera is debilitated, and that is marked by shortage of qi, laziness to speak, heart palpitations, lassitude of the spirit, dizziness, cloudy vision, decreased food intake, fatigued limbs, aching lumbus and limp knees, insomnia, dream emission, pale tongue fur, and weak vacuous pulse. [50: 745] [27: 209] [6: 151]

interlocking bones 交骨 *jiāo gǔ*: The joint between the coccyx and sacrum. [27: 69] [97: 221]

intermittent dysentery 休息痢 *xiū xī lì*: From *The Origin and Indicators of Disease* (*zhū bìng yuán hòu lùn*). Dysentery that goes on for months and years, continually starting and stopping; hence the name. Intermittent dysentery usually arises from inappropriate treatment or stems from such factors as qi-blood vacuity or insufficiency of the spleen and kidney, causing right vacuity and lingering evil, whereby damp-heat lies latent in the stomach and intestines. During periods of remission, the only signs that remain are lassitude of spirit and lack of strength, poor appetite, emaciation, and lack of warmth in the extremities. **Episodes:** MED Treat by clearing heat and transforming dampness; if necessary, complement with supplementing qi and blood or warming the spleen and kidney. Use formulas such as Saussurea and Coptis Pill (*xiāng lián wán*) or Carriage-Halting Pill (*zhù chē wán*) and variations. ACU Base treatment on ST and LI. Needle with drainage at LI-4 (*hé gǔ*, Union Valley), ST-25 (*tiān shū*, Celestial Pivot), ST-37 (*shàng jù xū*, Upper Great Hollow), and ST-44 (*nèi tíng*, Inner Court), and with supplementation at BL-20 (*pí shū*, Spleen Transport), BL-21 (*wèi shū*, Stomach Transport), and CV-4 (*guān yuán*, Pass Head). **Remission:** MED Fortify the spleen and stomach; supplement qi and blood. Use Center-Supplementing Qi-Boosting Decoction (*bǔ zhōng yì qì tāng*) or Eight-Gem Decoction (*bā zhēn tāng*) and variations. For kidney vacuity, use Four Spirits Pill (*sì shén wán*). ACU Base treatment on CV, ST, and back transport points. Select CV-12 (*zhōng wǎn*, Center Stomach Duct), CV-4 (*guān yuán*, Pass Head), ST-36 (*zú sān lǐ*, Leg Three Li), LR-13 (*zhāng mén*, Camphorwood Gate), BL-20 (*pí shū*, Spleen Transport), and BL-21 (*wèi shū*, Stomach Transport). Needle with supplementation and add moxa. For kidney vacuity, add BL-23 (*shèn shū*, Kidney Transport), KI-3 (*tài xī*, Great Ravine), and GV-4 (*mìng mén*, Life Gate). See DYSENTERY. [26: 273] [27: 362] [97: 207] [113: 97] [46: 667]

intermittent only, without stomach 但代无胃 *dàn dài wú wèi*: See PULSE BEREFT OF STOMACH QI.

intermittent pulse 代脉 *dài mài*: Synonym: *regularly interrupted pulse*. A moderate weak pulse that pauses at regular intervals. It indicates debilitation of the visceral qi and is seen in heart disease, fear and fright, and severe knocks and falls. See PULSE CONDITION; SPLEEN PULSE IS MODERATE. [50: 427] [6: 142]

internal 内 *nèi*: Located or arising within the body, especially of diseases due to excesses of the seven affects (internal damage) and evils resembling their external counterparts (e.g., internal wind, internal dampness). Compare INTERIOR.

internal block 内闭 *nèi bì*: See BLOCK.

internal block clouding reversal 内闭昏厥 *nèi bì hūn jué*: CLOUDING REVERSAL (clouding of consciousness due to abnormal qi flow) in internal block patterns in which evil is trapped in the interior. See BLOCK.

internal blowing 内吹 *nèi chuī*: Synonym: *internal blowing mammary welling-abscess*. A MAMMARY WELLING-ABSCESS (*rǔ yōng*) occurring during pregnancy, attributable to effulgent fetal qi and depressed heat evil. It heals with difficulty after birth and special attention is needed to preserve the fetus. See MAMMARY WELLING-ABSCESS. Compare EXTERNAL BLOWING. ◇ Chin 内 *nèi*, internal, inner; 吹 *chuī*, blow. So called because it was originally attributed to wind blowing on the breast from inside the body due to movement of the fetus. [26: 143] [27: 460] [67: 338]

internal blowing mammary welling-abscess 内吹乳痈 *nèi chuī rǔ yōng*: INTERNAL BLOWING.

internal cause [of disease] 内因 *nèi yīn*: One of the THREE CAUSES OF DISEASE; the seven affects—joy, anger, anxiety, thought, grief, fear, and fright—as causes of disease. The seven affects are normal responses of the individual, but when excessively intense or persistent, they can disturb the yin-yang and qi-blood balance and cause diseases of the bowels and viscera. This is known as *internal damage* or *affect damage*. Internal causes are not to be confused with evils that arise internally. (Internal fire and internal wind, for example, may be the result of affect damage, but they can also develop from insufficiency or from transformation of external evils, which are not internal causes.) Internal damage to the heart and spirit is characterized by heart palpitations or fearful throbbing, forgetfulness, and insomnia, or by abstraction, sorrow or anxiety with tendency to weep, and visceral agitation with frequent stretching and yawning. It may also take the form of fulminant exuberance of heart fire, characterized by manic agitation or mental derangement. Internal damage to the liver manifests as binding depression of liver qi characterized by mental depression, irascibility, pain in the rib-side, belching, and plum-pit qi. In women, this condition may cause swelling of the breasts, painful distention in the lower abdomen, and menstrual irregularities. Affect-mind disturbance that damages both the heart and spleen takes the form of disquieting of the heart spirit and impairment of spleen-stomach movement and transformation. This is characterized by attacks of abdominal pain, together with retching and nausea; or rumbling intestines and diarrhea. Other patterns include glomus and oppression in the chest and stomach duct, little thought of food and drink, and menstrual block. If the spleen fails to manage the blood, flooding and spotting may also occur. Mental and emotional factors have a distinct bearing on physical health. In treating internal damage conditions, a dual approach is necessary. Patients must be encouraged to deal with their emotional problems, while a proper physical analysis should be made of the state of yin and yang, blood and qi, and the organs. See THREE CAUSES. [6: 106] [26: 143] [27: 106] [97: 83]

internal cold 内寒 *nèi hán*: Cold arising from within when yang qi is debilitated and cannot warm the body. Internal cold affects the movement and transformation of water humor and causes the retention of turbid yin. When yang is vacuous, yin is exuberant, and when yin is exuberant, there is internal cold. The spleen governs the movement and transformation of water-damp. The kidney governs the regulation of water-humor, and kidney yang is the root of the yang qi of the whole body. This pattern is therefore essentially one of spleen-kidney yang vacuity. Its clinical characteristics are vomiting and diarrhea, abdominal pain, and counterflow cold of the limbs, in some cases with water swelling and phlegm-rheum, etc. The patient's snivel, phlegm, drool and spittle, and urine are clear and cold, while his stool is thin. This reflects the statement in *Elementary Questions* (*sù wèn, zhì zhēn yào dà lùn*), "All disease with watery humors that are clear, pure, and cold is ascribed to cold." Internal cold is the opposite of external cold, i.e., cold entering the body from outside. These two forms of cold are to some degree mutually conducive. For example, individuals whose yang qi is weak are especially vulnerable to external cold evil; and damage to the body's yang qi by cold can cause internal cold. [26: 145] [6: 104]

internal damage 内伤 *nèi shāng*: **1.** Any detrimental effect on bowel and visceral qi produced by intemperance of the seven affects (mental and emotional problems) or excesses of hunger, satiety, taxation fatigue, and sexual activity. **2.** Any disease pattern resulting from such causes. [27: 117] [97: 83] [26: 145]

internal damage by the seven affects 内伤七情 *nèi shāng qī qíng*, 七情内伤 *qī qíng nèi shāng*: Synonym: *affect damage*. Damage to yin, yang, qi, and blood, etc., by excesses of the seven affects (joy, anger, anxiety, thought, sorrow, fear, and fright). Powerful or lasting emotions and certain mental activities can damage yin, yang, qi, blood, and eventually the bowels and viscera. *Elementary Questions* (*sù wèn*) describes the effect of six of the affects specifically on qi. See JOY CAUSES QI TO SLACKEN; ANGER CAUSES QI TO RISE; THOUGHT CAUSES QI TO BIND; SORROW CAUSES QI TO DISPERSE; FRIGHT CAUSES DERANGEMENT OF QI; FEAR CAUSES QI TO PRECIPITATE; EXCESS AMONG THE FIVE MINDS. See also AFFECT.

internal damage headache 内伤头痛 *nèi shāng tóu tòng*: HEADACHE due to internal damage to the bowels and viscera or qi and blood, or to the presence of phlegm-damp or stasis, i.e., not due to external causes. Internal damage headaches develop gradually, are periodic, and are accompanied by other signs of insufficiency of bowels and visceral qi or internal evils. See entries listed below. See also HEADACHE. [26: 146]

Internal Damage Headache

QI VACUITY HEADACHE (*qì xū tóu tòng*)
BLOOD VACUITY HEADACHE (*xuè xū tóu tòng*)
YIN VACUITY HEADACHE (*yīn xū tóu tòng*)
YANG VACUITY HEADACHE (*yáng xū tóu tòng*)
KIDNEY VACUITY HEADACHE (*shèn xū tóu tòng*)
STATIC BLOOD HEADACHE (*yū xuè tóu tòng*)
PHLEGM-DAMP HEADACHE (*tán shī tóu tòng*)
PHLEGM REVERSAL HEADACHE (*tán jué tóu tòng*)
PHLEGM FIRE HEADACHE (*tán huǒ tóu tòng*)
FOOD DAMAGE HEADACHE (*shāng shí tóu tòng*)
LIQUOR DAMAGE HEADACHE (*shāng jiǔ tóu tòng*)
LIVER YANG HEADACHE (*gān yáng tóu tòng*)
GREATER YIN HEADACHE (*tài yīn tóu tòng*)
LESSER YIN HEADACHE (*shào yīn tóu tòng*)

internal damage lumbar pain 内伤腰痛 *nèi shāng yāo tòng*: Lumbar pain due to liver, spleen, or kidney vacuity, to damp phlegm or static blood, or else to internal injury. MED Treat by supplementing the spleen and kidney, possibly assisted by nourishing the liver, with the addition of dampness-drying, phlegm-transforming, blood-quickening, and stasis-transforming medicinals as necessary. See LUMBAR PAIN; KIDNEY VACUITY LUMBAR PAIN; VACUITY-TAXATION LUMBAR PAIN; DAMP PHLEGM LUMBAR PAIN; BLOOD STASIS LUMBAR PAIN. [26: 146]

internal damage miscellaneous diseases 内伤杂病 *nèi shāng zá bìng*: Synonym: *miscellaneous diseases*. Various diseases due to internal damage, i.e., to causes other than externally contracted heat (febrile) diseases.

internal damage sleeplessness 内伤不得卧 *nèi shāng bù dé wò*: From *Pathoconditions, Causes, Pulses, and Treatments* (*zhèng yīn mài zhì*). Sleeplessness due to internal damage by liver fire, gallbladder fire, lung congestion, stomach disharmony, heart blood vacuity, heart qi vacuity, etc. For example, in the case of lung congestion, panting and cough with shoulders leaning forward can be exacerbated by lying down. See SLEEPLESSNESS and the entries listed below. [26: 145] [80:] [50: 251]

Internal Damage Sleeplessness

LIVER FIRE SLEEPLESSNESS (*gān huǒ bù dé wò*)
GALLBLADDER FIRE SLEEPLESSNESS (*dǎn huǒ bù dé wò*)
STOMACH DISHARMONY SLEEPLESSNESS (*wèi bù hé bù dé wò*)
HEART BLOOD VACUITY SLEEPLESSNESS (*xīn xuè xū bù dé wò*)

HEART QI VACUITY SLEEPLESSNESS (*xīn qì xū bù dé wò*)

LUNG CONGESTION SLEEPLESSNESS (*fèi yōng bù dé wò*)

internal damage stomach duct pain 内伤胃 脘痛 *nèi shāng wèi wǎn (guǎn) tòng*: Pain in the stomach due to a variety of internal damage factors including accumulated cold, accumulated heat, spleen-stomach vacuity cold, yin vacuity, food accumulation, phlegm-rheum, qi depression (qi stagnation), blood stasis, and worm accumulation. **Accumulated cold** stomach duct pain is attributed to insufficiency of stomach yang and damage by cold drinks causing yin cold to congeal and bind, and is characterized by stomach duct pain that refuses cold and is accompanied by counterflow cold of the extremities, uninhibited clear stool and urine (clean untransformed stool and clear urine), ejection of foamy drool, and a slow pulse. MED Warm the center and dissipate cold with formulas such as Lesser Galangal and Cyperus Pill (*liáng fù wán*) or Tsaoko Pill (*dòu kòu wán*). ACU Base treatment mainly on alarm and uniting points of ST, PC, and SP. Main points: CV-12 (*zhōng wǎn*, Center Stomach Duct), ST-36 (*zú sān lǐ*, Leg Three Li), PC-6 (*nèi guān*, Inner Pass), SP-4 (*gōng sūn*, Yellow Emperor). CV-6 (*qì hǎi*, Sea of Qi) and ST-25 (*tiān shū*, Celestial Pivot), needling with even supplementation and drainage and large amounts of moxa. Also, perform moxibustion on salt or ginger at CV-8 (*shén què*, Spirit Gate Tower). **Accumulated heat** stomach duct pain is due to intense stomach heat or affect-mind binding depression gradually causing fire formation and is characterized by a urgent pain with scorching hot feeling in the stomach duct, thirst, dry lips, generalized heat [effusion] and red face, constipation and copious sweating, rapid pulse, and in some cases vexation, agitation, and irascibility, and is treated by clearing heat and abduction with formulas like Center-Clearing Decoction (*qīng zhōng tāng*), Liver-Transforming Brew (*huà gān jiān*) and Stomach-Regulating Qi-Coordinating Decoction (*tiáo wèi chéng qì tāng*). ACU Use the main points given above. For intense stomach heat, add ST-44 (*nèi tíng*, Inner Court), ST-45 (*lì duì*, Severe Mouth), TB-6 (*zhī gōu*, Branch Ditch), and PC-6 (*nèi guān*, Inner Pass), needling with drainage. For heat accumulation due to affect-mind binding depression transforming into heat, add LR-3 (*tài chōng*, Supreme Surge), LR-14 (*qī mén*, Cycle Gate), GB-34 (*yáng líng quán*, Yang Mound Spring), and SP-6 (*sān yīn jiāo*, Three Yin Intersection), needling with drainage. **Spleen-stomach vacuity cold** stomach duct pain is characterized by stomach pain that is worse on an empty stomach and slightly relieved

by eating, warmth, and pressure, and accompanied by fatigued limbs and lack of strength, reduced food intake, sloppy stool, forceless fine sunken pulse. MED Supplement the spleen and warm yang; use formulas such as Astragalus Center-Fortifying Decoction (*huáng qí jiàn zhōng tāng*) or Center-Rectifying Pill (*lǐ zhōng wán*). If there is spleen-kidney vacuity with failure to contain blood manifesting in the form of blood ejection or bloody stool, Yellow Earth Decoction (*huáng tǔ tāng*) can be used. ACU Base treatment mainly on back transport points, CV, ST, and SP. Main points: BL-20 (*pí shū*, Spleen Transport), BL-21 (*wèi shū*, Stomach Transport), CV-12 (*zhōng wǎn*, Center Stomach Duct), CV-6 (*qì hǎi*, Sea of Qi), LR-13 (*zhāng mén*, Camphorwood Gate), ST-36 (*zú sān lǐ*, Leg Three Li), and SP-6 (*sān yīn jiāo*, Three Yin Intersection), needling with supplementation and adding moxa. For spleen-kidney depletion and failure to contain blood, add BL-23 (*shèn shū*, Kidney Transport), CV-4 (*guān yuán*, Pass Head), KI-3 (*tài xī*, Great Ravine), SP-10 (*xuè hǎi*, Sea of Blood), and PC-4 (*xī mén*, Cleft Gate), needling with supplementation and adding moxa. **Yin vacuity** stomach duct pain is heat pain caused by yin vacuity, and is characterized by clamoring stomach and rapid hungering, dry mouth with little liquid, difficult defecation, red tongue fur (possibly with peeling fur), and a rapid fine string-like pulse, and can be treated with Six-Ingredient Rehmannia Pill (*liù wèi dì huáng wán*) or All-the-Way-Through Brew (*yī guàn jiān*). ACU Needle with even supplementation and drainage at main points given under spleen-stomach vacuity cold above. For yin vacuity heat pain, add KI-6 (*zhào hǎi*, Shining Sea), ST-44 (*nèi tíng*, Inner Court), and PC-6 (*nèi guān*, Inner Pass), needling with drainage. See FOOD STAGNATION STOMACH DUCT PAIN; PHLEGM-RHEUM STOMACH DUCT PAIN; QI DEPRESSION STOMACH DUCT PAIN; STATIC BLOOD STOMACH DUCT PAIN; ROUNDWORM STOMACH DUCT PAIN; LIVER-STOMACH QI PAIN; STOMACH QI PAIN; STOMACH DUCT PAIN. [26: 146] [46: 660] [37: 311] [113: 216]

internal dampness 内湿 *nèi shī*: Dampness that arises when the spleen is vacuous and fails to move and transform fluids, and that is characterized by poor appetite, diarrhea, abdominal distention, scant urine, yellow face, puffy swelling, a pale tongue with glossy fur, and a moderate soggy pulse. Since the spleen action of moving and transforming the fluids relies on the warming action of kidney yang, internal dampness is often observed in patients with spleen-kidney yang vacuity. Internal dampness and external dampness are mutually conducive. Spleen vacuity makes the body vulnerable to external dampness but also may spontaneously cause internal dampness. External dampness entering the body may easily damage the spleen, causing internal dampness. See DAMPNESS. [27: 112] [97: 84]

internal dispersion 内消 *nèi xiāo*: One of the three main methods of treating sores. It involves the use of dispersing and dissipating medicinals to eliminate sores in the initial stage prior to suppuration. It includes the following forms: **Exterior resolution:** In the initial stage of sores (first seven days), prior to suppuration or damage to right qi, the appearance of exterior signs (aversion to cold, heat effusion) call for the use of exterior-resolving medicinals to discharge the sore toxin through sweating. Heat patterns are treated by cool acrid exterior resolution with formulas such as Toad Venom Pill (*chán sū wán*), whereas cold patterns are treated by warm acrid exterior resolution, using formulas such as Unlimited Efficacy Elixir (*wàn líng dān*). Such treatment should be applied with care in case of severe right qi vacuity. **Freeing the interior:** In the initial or middle stage of sores, when there is exuberant heat toxin brewing in the interior, sores can be dispersed by draining precipitants that expel the toxins from the bowels and viscera. A commonly used interior-freeing formula is Internal Coursing Coptis Decoction (*nèi shū huáng lián tāng*). If there is effulgent yin vacuity fire depriving the stomach and intestines of moisture, Intestine-Moistening Decoction (*rùn cháng tāng*) should be used. **Clearing heat and resolving toxin:** Most sores are attributable to heat, and heat clearing medicinals are used in the initial stage, suppurative stage, and post-rupture stage wherever there are signs of repletion heat and fire toxin causing redness, swelling, heat, pain, or discharge of thick pus accompanied by general signs such as heat effusion, vexation and agitation, thirst, rapid pulse, red or crimson tongue with a yellow fur, and, in severe cases, even clouded spirit and delirious speech. Distinction is made between heat in the qi aspect, which is treated by cold bitter fire draining with formulas such as Coptis Toxin-Resolving Decoction (*huáng lián jiě dú tāng*), and heat in the construction aspect, which is treated by cooling the blood and clearing heat with Rhinoceros Horn and Rehmannia Decoction (*xī jiǎo dì huáng tāng*). **Warming the channels and freeing the network vessels:** Yin cold sore patterns at any stage of development are treated by warming the channels and freeing the network vessels using oral formulas such as Harmonious Yang Decoction (*yáng hé tāng*) and Duhuo and Mistletoe Decoction (*dú huó jì shēng tāng*) and topical formulas such as Harmonious Yang Decongealing Plaster (*yáng hé jiě níng gāo*). **Moving qi:** Initial-stage sores often involve qi stagnation and blood stasis. On the basis of the principles that "qi is the commander

of the blood," and "when qi moves, blood moves," moving qi can be used alone or in combination with other methods to treat initial-stage stores. An appropriate qi-moving formula is Free Wanderer Powder (*xiāo yáo sǎn*). **Moving stasis and harmonizing construction:** Swelling and pain due to blood stasis can often be relieved by regulating construction-blood. The method of moving stasis and harmonizing construction can be used alone or in combination with other methods. An appropriate formula is Blood-Quickening Stasis-Dissipating Decoction (*huó xuè sàn yū tāng*). [26: 144, 864] [27: 288] [97: 84]

internal dryness 内燥 *nèi zào*: Depletion of the bodily fluids and yin blood not attributable to dryness evil. Internal dryness is not caused by any evil, either external or internal, but by an insufficiency of blood and fluids. These conditions are usually called damage to fluids, damaged yin, or exhaustion of the blood and fluids. [27: 114] [97: 85]

internal expression 内托 *nèi tuō: Synonym: expression.* Pushing (toxin) outward from within; one of the three main methods of treating sores (see SORE). It involves the use of qi and blood-supplementing medicinals to support right qi, express the toxin, and prevent it from falling inward. It includes two forms: **Expressing toxin and outthrusting pus:** This method is used for midstage sores when toxin is exuberant, but right qi has not yet been damaged, and the sore has still not burst. The treatment uses medicinals such as astragalus (*huáng qí*), tangkuei (*dāng guī*), ligusticum (*chuān xiōng*), pangolin scales (*chuān shān jiǎ*), angelica (*bái zhǐ*), and gleditsia thorn (*zào jiǎo cì*). **Supplemental expression:** This method is used when right qi vacuity prevents the expulsion of toxin so that the sore becomes flat with a broad root, and either fails to burst or bursts to produce only a thin scant discharge without abatement of swelling and accompanied by generalized heat [effusion], devitalized essence-spirit, yellow facial complexion, and a forceless rapid pulse. It makes use of medicinals such as astragalus (*huáng qí*), ovate atractylodes (*bái zhú*), poria (*fú líng*), codonopsis (*dǎng shēn*), mix-fried licorice (*gān cǎo*), tangkuei (*dāng guī*), white peony (*bái sháo yào*), gleditsia thorn (*zào jiǎo cì*), angelica (*bái zhǐ*), lonicera (*jīn yín huā*), forsythia (*lián qiào*), platycodon (*jié gěng*), and tangerine peel (*chén pí*). ◇ Chin 内 *nèi*, internal; 托 *tuō*, hold up, support. Gently pushing out (toxin) by internally acting medicinals. [26: 143] [27: 289] [27: 289]

internal fire (heat) 内火（热） *nèi huǒ (rè):* Fire (or heat) arising within the body due to internal factors (affect damage), transformation of externally contracted evils, or insufficiency of yin-humor. Internal fire or heat may form a repletion or vacuity pattern. **Repletion fire** (heat) may arise internally as a result of an imbalance between yin and yang or excesses of the five minds. For example, liver fire, resulting from transformation of liver qi depression, manifests in red eyes, dry mouth, sudden deafness or tinnitus, vomiting of sour or bitter fluid, dry stool, and slippery, stringlike pulse. The red eyes and the stringlike pulse are clear indicators of repletion. **Vacuity fire** (vacuity heat) arises internally from yin vacuity, or in some cases (e.g., effulgent heart fire due to heart yin vacuity) from excesses of the five minds. Vacuity heat differs from repletion heat in the following ways: (1) Signs of yin vacuity are present. (2) The fire and heat signs are less pronounced than in repletion heat, the most common being vexation and a red, dry, or mirror tongue. (3) Generally, there is no high fever. (4) Thirst, if present, is generally not severe. (5) The pulse is generally rapid but forceless. [6: 105] [36: 280–281]

internal food damage tetany 内伤饮食痉 *nèi shāng yǐn shí jìng*: TETANY (arched-back rigidity, clenched jaw, convulsions, etc.) resulting from food stagnation causing damage to the stomach and spleen. Internal food damage tetany occurs after vomiting or diarrhea and is characterized by TETANIC REVERSAL (tetany and clouding of consciousness due to abnormal qi flow) and is accompanied by lassitude of the spirit, and pale white complexion; it is attributable to spleen-stomach yang vacuity and exhaustion of fluids. MED Warm and move spleen yang using Center-Rectifying Decoction (*lǐ zhōng tāng*) plus clove (*dīng xiāng*), cinnamon bark (*ròu guì*), nutmeg (*ròu dòu kòu*), and chebule (*hē zǐ*). ACU Base treatment mainly on back transport points, SP, ST, and LR. Select BL-20 (*pí shū*, Spleen Transport), BL-21 (*wèi shū*, Stomach Transport), CV-10 (*xià wǎn*, Lower Stomach Duct), ST-25 (*tiān shū*, Celestial Pivot), ST-36 (*zú sān lǐ*, Leg Three Li), Li Inner Court (*lǐ nèi tíng*), GV-20 (*bǎi huì*, Hundred Convergences), GV-16 (*fēng fǔ*, Wind Mansion), LR-3 (*tài chōng*, Supreme Surge), and GV-8 (*jīn suō*, Sinew Contraction); needle with supplementation and add moxa. [26: 146] [46: 662, 733]

internal heat 内热 *nèi rè*: **1.** Heat signs due to excessive wear on yin humor, such as tidal heat [effusion], night heat effusion, vexing heat in the five hearts, night heat effusion, vexation and thirst, dry bound stool, short voidings of reddish urine, red tongue with scant fur, and a fine rapid pulse. *Elementary Questions* (*sù wèn, tiáo jīng lùn*) states, "When yin is vacuous, there is internal heat." **2.** Evil heat entering the interior, characterized by red face and eyes, heart vexation, heat effusion, thirst with a liking for cold drinks, constipation,

short voidings of reddish urine, red tongue with dry yellow tongue fur, and a rapid sunken pulse. In severe cases, there is clouded spirit and delirious raving. [26: 147]

internal injury 内伤 *nèi shāng*, 内损 *nèi sǔn*: Damage to the bowels and viscera and other deep structures of the head, chest, and abdomen through knocks and falls, lifting heavy weights, or spraining. Mild swelling and distention with pain of unfixed location indicates damage to qi. Pronounced pain with red, green-blue, or purple coloration of the skin, and spillage of blood from the vessels, and signs such as heat effusion and shivering, retching of blood, bloody stool, blood urine, or coughing of blood indicate damage to the blood. Acute pain in the chest, ribs, or abdomen, with CLOUDING REVERSAL, blood ejection, and bloody stool indicate damage to bowels and viscera. MED When necessary, internal injury is now treated by modern surgical techniques. Damage to qi is treated with Origin-Restoring Qi-Freeing Powder (*fù yuán tōng qì sǎn*). For damage to the blood and the organs, use Peach Kernel and Carthamus Four Agents Decoction (*táo hóng sì wù tāng*). For injury to the middle or lower part of the trunk, use Peach Kernel Qi-Coordinating Decoction (*táo hé chéng qì tāng*). [26: 145]

internal obstruction 内障 *nèi zhàng*: Any of a number of diseases of the spirit pupil and inner eye manifesting in poor vision. Internal obstructions mostly occur in vacuity patterns and are most commonly attributable to insufficiency of the liver and kidney or dual depletion of qi and blood. Other causes include effulgent yin vacuity fire, qi stagnation and blood stasis, wind-fire and phlegm-damp harassing the clear orifices, and external injury. Signs include subjective sensations like *mouches volantes*, black floaters, lights and flames appearing to be surrounded rainbow-like halos, clouded vision, night blindness, or sudden blindness. Very often there are no visible objective signs, although the pupil may be dilated or contracted, deformed, or abnormal in color. Internal obstructions include GREEN-BLUE WIND INTERNAL OBSTRUCTION and GREEN WIND INTERNAL OBSTRUCTION (corresponding to glaucoma). Compare EXTERNAL OBSTRUCTION. [27: 508] [26: 147] [27: 508] [97: 85]

internal phlegm turbidity block 痰浊内闭 *tán zhuó nèi bì*: Synonym: *phlegm block*. **1.** Any BLOCK PATTERN either attributed by phlegm turbidity invariably associated with wind or heat or arising from other causes and causing phlegm turbidity signs. **2.** A block pattern developing from damp-heat in warm heat disease. See BLOCK. [26: 767]

internal welling-abscess 内痈 *nèi yōng*: A suppuration within the chest or abdomen affecting the organs. See LIVER WELLING-ABSCESS; INTESTINAL WELLING-ABSCESS; PULMONARY WELLING-ABSCESS; WELLING-ABSCESS OF THE STOMACH DUCT; WELLING-ABSCESS.

internal welling-abscess of the stomach duct 胃脘内痈 *wèi wǎn (guǎn) nèi yōng*: See WELLING-ABSCESS OF THE STOMACH DUCT[1].

internal wind 内风 *nèi fēng*: **1.** An ancient term denoting a disease arising in sexual taxation with sweating when wind evil invades. **2.** Liver wind. In the early phase of Chinse medicine, all wind was believed to be of external origin. However, subsequent theories posited that certain signs such as dizziness, tremor, and convulsions previously attributed to the invasion of external wind were due to a "wind" arising internally due to a yin-yang imbalance. See LIVER WIND STIRRING INTERNALLY. [26: 144, 627] [27: 111] [97: 84]

interrupting malaria 截疟 *jié nüè*: A method of treating MALARIA applied two to three hours before an episode to prevent its arrival. Interrupting malaria makes used of medicinals such as dichroa (*cháng shān*), areca (*bīng láng*), tsaoko (*cǎo guǒ*), and ginger pinellia (*jiāng bàn xià*), and formulas such as Malaria-Interrupting Seven-Jewel Beverage (*jié nüè qī bǎo yǐn*) or Spleen-Clearing Beverage (*qīng pí yǐn*), or by needling points such GV-14 (*dà zhuī*, Great Hammer), SI-3 (*hòu xī*, Back Ravine), and PC-5 (*jiān shǐ*, Intermediary Courier), needling with drainage. See MALARIA. [50: 1648] [46: 649]

intersection point 交会穴 *jiāo huì xué*: Any point at which two or more channels intersect. Intersection points have the ability to transmit a stimulus through both or all channels that intersect at the point. Application: Intersection points are used to treat disease affecting two or more of the intersecting channels. SP-6 (*sān yīn jiāo*, Three Yin Intersection), for example, is often used to treat diseases that affect any or all of the three yin channels of the foot because it is the intersection point of the liver, spleen, and kidney. Genitourinary diseases can be treated with point formulas that include CV-3 (*zhōng jí*, Central Pole) because that point is the intersection point of the three leg yin channels and the controlling vessel, all of which are intimately connected with the genitourinary region. [26: 237]

interstice 腠理 *còu lǐ*: An anatomical entity of unclear identity, explained in modern dictionaries as being the "grain" of the skin, flesh, and organs or the connective tissue in the skin and flesh. *Elementary Questions* (*sù wèn*), "Clear yang effuses through the interstices." Usage of the term suggests that the interstices correspond to the sweat ducts in Western medicine. See SWEATING. [26: 794]

interstices of the flesh 肉腠 *ròu còu*, 肌腠 *jī còu*: The interstices located in the flesh. See INTERSTICE. [26: 262, 272] [27: 31] [97: 604]

intestinal afflux 肠澼 *cháng pì*: **1.** (In ancient texts) dysentery. **2.** BLOOD ARROW; bloody stool due to intestinal stasis. ◇ Chin 肠 *cháng*, intestine; 澼 *pì*, stagnation or accumulation of water. [26: 797]

intestinal aggregation 肠癖 *cháng pì*: *Synonym: blood arrow*. A disease characterized by the spurting of blood from the anus, described in *The Gateway to Medicine* (*yī xué rù mén*) as "enduring swill diarrhea stemming originally from wind damage invasion of the stomach and allowing damp toxin to form an aggregation and to pour into the large intestine to contend with the lesser yin, giving rise to what is called 'intestinal aggregation', known popularly as 'blood arrow' because of the forceful issue of blood like an arrow that shoots far." MED Use Blood-Cooling Rehmannia Decoction (*liáng xuè dì huáng tāng*) plus saussurea (*mù xiāng*) and areca (*bīng láng*). For pronounced signs of damp toxin, use Center-Supplementing Qi-Boosting Decoction (*bǔ zhōng yì qì tāng*) minus bupleurum (*chái hú*) and tangerine peel (*chén pí*), plus scutellaria (*huáng qín*), coptis (*huáng lián*), ligusticum (*chuān xiōng*), charred sophora fruit (*huái jiāo tàn*), and bitter orange (*zhǐ ké*). ◇ Chin *cháng*, intestine; 癖 *pì* is composed of 疒 *chuáng*, the illness signifier and 辟 *pì*, a homophone borrowed to represent the sound. Chinese medical sources say that 癖 is the same as 澼, stagnate, accumulate. [26: 797] [97: 290]

intestinal dryness constipation 肠燥便秘 *cháng zào biàn bì*: See INTESTINAL HUMOR DEPLETION.

intestinal dryness with difficult defecation 肠燥便艰 *cháng zào biàn jiān*: See LARGE INTESTINAL HUMOR DEPLETION.

intestinal humor depletion 肠液亏耗 *cháng yè kuī hào*: See LARGE INTESTINAL HUMOR DEPLETION.

intestinal impediment 肠痹 *cháng bì*: IMPEDIMENT (*bì*) disease affecting the large and small intestine causing thirst with desire for fluids, inhibited urination, and diarrhea. Owing to obstruction of the large and small intestine qi, the waterways suffer blockage, so that waste is not transformed and the clear and the turbid are not separated.

intestinal vacuity efflux desertion 肠虚滑脱 *cháng xū huá tuō*: Enduring diarrhea culminating in reduced uplift of yang qi manifesting in persistent diarrhea with periodic fecal incontinence or prolapse of the rectum resulting from bowel movements. Generally there is dull abdominal pain, general physical debilitation, and vacuity cold signs. MED Astringe the intestines and stem desertion. Commonly used medicinals include halloysite (*chì shí zhī*), limonite (*yǔ yú liáng*), pomegranate rind (*shí liú pí*), chebule (*hē zǐ*), nutmeg (*ròu dòu kòu*), and poppy husk (*yīng sù ké*). Formulas include Major Peach Blossom Decoction (*dà táo huā tāng*) and True Man Viscus-Nourishing Decoction (*zhēn rén yǎng zàng tāng*). Although intestinal insecurity is treated mainly by astringing the intestines and checking diarrhea, qi-rectifying medicinals such as saussurea (*mù xiāng*), bitter orange (*zhǐ ké*), and tangerine peel (*chén pí*) are added to prevent stagnation. Upraising medicinals, qi-supplementing medicinals, and yang-warming medicinals may also be employed. ACU Base treatment mainly on back transport points, SP, ST, and CV. Select BL-20 (*pí shū*, Spleen Transport), BL-23 (*shèn shū*, Kidney Transport), CV-4 (*guān yuán*, Pass Head), CV-12 (*zhōng wǎn*, Center Stomach Duct), LR-13 (*zhāng mén*, Camphorwood Gate), ST-25 (*tiān shū*, Celestial Pivot), ST-36 (*zú sān lǐ*, Leg Three Li), GV-20 (*bǎi huì*, Hundred Convergences), CV-6 (*qì hǎi*, Sea of Qi), and SP-6 (*sān yīn jiāo*, Three Yin Intersection); needle with supplementation and moxa. For prolapse of rectum, add BL-25 (*dà cháng shū*, Large Intestine Transport), GV-1 (*cháng qiáng*, Long Strong), and BL-57 (*chéng shān*, Mountain Support). [46: 665, 671] [37: 320] [6: 182]

intestinal welling-abscess 肠痈 *cháng yōng*: WELLING-ABSCESS (*yōng*) of the intestine; attributed to congealing blood that stems from damp-heat or from general qi and blood stagnation. WMC appendicitis, periappendicular abscess. Intestinal welling-abscess was first mentioned in *Elementary Questions* (*sù wèn*), which attributed it to lesser yang (*shào yáng*) reverse flow and claimed it to be uncurable and fatal. Zhang Ji (2nd–3rd centuries A.D.), in *On Cold Damage and Miscellaneous Diseases* (*shāng hán zá bìng lùn*), described the presuppurative and suppurative stages in detail and prescribed treatments. *Essential Prescriptions of the Golden Coffer* (*jīn guì yào lüè*) gives his description as follows: "Intestinal welling-abscess [is marked by] swollen glomus in the lesser abdomen that is painful when pressed and like strangury although though urine is normal, and [by] periodic heat effusion and spontaneous sweating followed by aversion to cold. If the pulse is slow and tight, pus has not yet formed, and it can be treated by precipitation, which should be manifest in blood [in the stool]. If the pulse is surging and rapid, pus has formed; precipitation cannot be administered. Rhubarb and Moutan Decoction (*dà huáng mǔ dān pí tāng*) is the main treatment." Distinction is made between large intestinal welling-abscess and small intestinal welling-abscess on the basis of the location of pain. If the pain is in the vicinity of ST-25 (*tiān shū*, Celestial

Pivot), it is called a *large intestinal welling-abscess*, whereas if in the vicinity of CV-4 (*guān yuán*, Pass Head), it is called a *small intestinal welling-abscess*. Any intestinal welling-abscess that makes it difficult to the stretch out the right leg is called a *leg-flexing intestinal welling-abscess*. However, these distinctions are now considered to have little clinical significance. The first perceptible sign of large intestinal welling-abscess is abdominal pain that gradually localizes on the right side. The pain is of fixed location and refuses pressure, and is accompanied by coughing or sneezing. The right leg may flex and be difficult to stretch out. There is aversion to cold and heat effusion, with nausea and vomiting, constipation (or diarrhea in some cases), and reddish urine. The tongue fur is thin, slimy and yellow. The pulse is rapid and forceful. As the condition advances, the abdomen becomes tensed and tender, and in some cases a lump may be felt. As vigorous heat [effusion] develops, the pulse becomes surging and rapid. MED Treat with medicinals such as Rhubarb and Moutan Decoction (*dà huáng mǔ dān pí tāng*). If tenderness is less pronounced, the facial complexion is somber white, and the pulse fine and weak, the condition (recognized in Western medicine as chronic appendicitis) can be treated with Coix, Aconite, and Baijiang Powder (*yì yǐ fù zǐ bài jiàng sǎn*). ACU Base treatment mainly on ST and LI. ST-25 (*tiān shū*, Celestial Pivot), ST-37 (*shàng jù xū*, Upper Great Hollow), Appendix Point (*lán wěi xué*), and LI-4 (*hé gǔ*, Union Valley). Needle with drainage, and retain the needles for 40–60 minutes. Treatments should be given once or twice a day, and, in severe cases, every four hours. Selection of points according to signs: For heat effusion, add GV-14 (*dà zhuī*, Great Hammer) and LI-11 (*qū chí*, Pool at the Bend). For pain around the umbilicus or tense abdominal skin, add CV-6 (*qì hǎi*, Sea of Qi) and SP-14 (*fù jié*, Abdominal Bind). For nausea and vomiting, add PC-6 (*nèi guān*, Inner Pass) and ST-36 (*zú sān lǐ*, Leg Three Li). [26: 797] [27: 461] [97: 289] [46: 713] [96: 458] [61: 224]

intestinal wind 肠风 *cháng fēng*: **1.** Bleeding hemorrhoids. See HEMORRHOIDS. **2.** Bloody stool resulting from TAXATION DETRIMENT to the bowels and viscera, disharmony of qi and blood, and wind-cold and heat toxin contending in the large intestine. **3.** Precipitation of blood before the passage of stool; proximal bleeding. It is attributed either to external wind entering and settling or to internal wind exploiting the lower body. MED For external wind, use Sophora Fruit Pill (*huái jiǎo wán*). For internal wind, use Stomach Wind Decoction (*wèi fēng tāng*). For constitutional vacuity, use Ginseng Stomach Wind Decoction (*rén shēn wèi fēng tāng*). For dampness complication, with bloody stool like the juice of adzuki beans, or purplish-black, use Yang-Upbearing Dampness-Eliminating Ledebouriella Decoction (*shēng yáng chú shī fáng fēng tāng*), which contains ledebouriella (*fáng fēng*), atractylodes (*cāng zhú*), ovate atractylodes (*bái zhú*), scutellaria (*huáng qín*), peony (*sháo yào*), and fresh ginger (*shēng jiāng*). ACU Base treatment mainly on ST, BL, LI, and SP. Select ST-37 (*shàng jù xū*, Upper Great Hollow), BL-57 (*chéng shān*, Mountain Support), GV-1 (*cháng qiáng*, Long Strong), LI-4 (*hé gǔ*, Union Valley), LI-11 (*qū chí*, Pool at the Bend), SP-10 (*xuè hǎi*, Sea of Blood), and SP-6 (*sān yīn jiāo*, Three Yin Intersection); needle with drainage. Selection of points according to pattern: For external wind, add GB-20 (*fēng chí*, Wind Pool) and TB-5 (*wài guān*, Outer Pass). For internal wind, add GB-20 (*fēng chí*, Wind Pool), LR-3 (*tài chōng*, Supreme Surge), KI-6 (*zhào hǎi*, Shining Sea), and KI-1 (*yǒng quán*, Gushing Spring). For constitutional vacuity, add CV-4 (*guān yuán*, Pass Head), BL-20 (*pí shū*, Spleen Transport), and SP-3 (*tài bái*, Supreme White), and use moxa. For dampness complication, add SP-9 (*yīn líng quán*, Yin Mound Spring), ST-36 (*zú sān lǐ*, Leg Three Li), and LR-2 (*xíng jiān*, Moving Between), and use moxa. [26: 796] [46: 739] [113: 111-113] [37: 329]

intestinal wind bleeding 肠风下血 *cháng fēng xià xuè*, 肠风便血 *cháng fēng biàn xuè*: See INTESTINAL WIND.³

intestine 肠 *cháng*: Either of the two intestines. See LARGE INTESTINE; SMALL INTESTINE.

intestine-gripping sand 绞肠痧 *jiǎo cháng shā*: DRY CHOLERA.

intimidate 凌 *líng*: To threaten. "Intimidate" describes the harmful effects of water qi, as in the expression "water qi intimidating the heart," a pattern in which water qi developing as a result of spleen-kidney yang vacuity collects above the diaphragm hampering heart yang, and characterized by heart palpitations and hasty breathing.

intradermal needle 皮内针 *pí nèi zhēn*: A small needle, such as the wheat-grain and thumb-tack needles, implanted in the skin for extended periods. See NEEDLE IMPLANTATION. [27: 330] [97: 170]

invade 犯 *fàn*: To intrude. Describes, for example, evils entering the body, and liver qi entering the stomach.

invasion of the lung by a warm evil 温邪犯肺 *wēn xié fàn fèi*: See WARM EVIL INVADING THE LUNG.

inverted menstruation 倒经 *dào jīng*: COUNTERFLOW MENSTRUATION.

invigorate 壮 *zhuàng*: See SUPPLEMENTATION.

invigorating fire 壮火 *zhuàng huǒ*: See INVIGORATING YANG.

invigorating the governor of water to restrain the brilliance of yang 壮水之主以制阳光 *zhuàng shuǐ zhī zhǔ yǐ zhì yáng guāng*: A comment by Wang Bing of the Tang dynasty on the line in *Elementary Questions* (*sù wèn*) that reads "Wherever cold [is applied], but heat [remains], treat the yin." The implication of this comment is that wherever the use of cold or cool medicinals to treat heat patterns produces no effect or makes the heat worse, the heat pattern is one of yin vacuity with hyperactive yang, i.e., a condition essentially of yin vacuity that is treated by enriching kidney yin (the true water of the kidney viscus). According to this principle, insufficiency of kidney yin with yin vacuity flaming upward causing dizzy head and vision, aching lumbus and limp legs, dry throat, and steaming bone with aching pain is treated with Six-Ingredient Rehmannia Pill (*liù wèi dì huáng wán*). Invigorating the governor of water to restrain the brilliance of yang is now often called *invigorating water to restrain yang*, *enriching water to restrain fire*, or *enriching yin to moisten yang*. [27: 328]

invigorating water to restrain yang 壮水制阳 *zhuàng shuǐ zhì yáng*: See INVIGORATING THE GOVERNOR OF WATER TO RESTRAIN THE BRILLIANCE OF YANG. [27: 238]

invigorating yang 壮阳 *zhuàng yáng*: Synonym: *invigorating fire*. A method of treatment used to strengthen the yang qi of the body with warming and supplementing medicinals. Invigorating yang usually refers to strengthening the yang qi of the heart and kidney, and especially the latter. See SUPPLEMENTATION. [27: 281] [97: 223]

invisible gan worms 疳蟹 *gān nì*: GAN OF THE NOSE. [26: 489]

invisible worm 蟹 *nì*: A disease attributed to erosion by worms. ◇ Chin 蟹 *nì*, probably from 匿 *nì*, hidden, concealed. [26: 100]

invisible worm sore 蟹疮 *nì chuāng*: See GENITAL EROSION.

invisible worm sore of the nose 鼻蟹疮 *bí nì chuāng*: A heat sore in the area of the nostrils caused by wind-heat lodged in the lung channel, or by a continually runny nose, or developing from a heat sore. Invisible worm sores of the nose are most commonly observed in children, and are characterized by a purple coloration, ulceration, a thick exudate, and itching without pain. WMC eczema of the nose. MED Take Bovine Bezoar Upper-Body-Clearing Pill (*niú huáng shàng qīng wán*) and apply clamshell powder (*gé fěn*), indigo (*qīng dài*), gypsum (*shí gāo*), calomel (*qīng fěn*), and phellodendron (*huáng bǎi*) topically. [26: 857] [50: 1662]

invisible worm sore of the genitals 阴蜃 *yīn nì*: See GENITAL EROSION. [26: 626]

inward fall 内陷 *nèi xiàn*: Passage (of evils) into the inner body, due to exuberance of the evil or vacuity of right. For example, when measles is erupting, if the measles toxin is especially strong, or if the wind-cold is contracted, right qi cannot resist, and the evil "falls inward." When this happens, the measles papules suddenly disappear, the face becomes white, and breathing becomes rapid and hasty. Inward fall is also observed in patients suffering from welling-abscess (*yōng*) and sores when the sore-toxin falls inward and enters construction blood, i.e., it starts to affect the whole body in a process corresponding to what Western medicine describes in terms of the development of toxemia (see FALL PATTERN). Distinction is made between FIRE FALL, DRY FALL, and VACUITY FALL. Compare RUNNING YELLOW. ◇ Chin 内 *nèi*, inward; 陷 *xiàn*, collapse, slump, fall. [27: 133] [97: 84] [96: 133] [50: 245]

irascibility 易怒 *yì nù*: Proneness to anger. Anger is the mind of the liver, and irascibility is seen in patterns such as ascendant liver yang, binding depression of liver qi, and five minds forming fire.

iris 黄仁 *huáng rén*, 睛帘 *jīng lián*, 虹彩 *hóng cǎi*: The colored part of the eye between the white of the eye and the pupil that expands and contracts. The iris corresponds to the WIND WHEEL among the five wheels. [26: 694] [27: 65] [97: 503]

iron-band headache 头痛如掣 *tóu tòng rú chè*: HEADACHE WITH PULLING SENSATION.

itching 瘙痒 *sào yǎng*: An irritation relieved, at least temporarily, by scratching. Itching over extensive areas of the body is a sign of wind or blood diseases. If it refuses heat and is accompanied by general heat signs, it is attributable to blood heat, which generally occurs in young people. If it is more pronounced in the autumn and winter and is accompanied by a lusterless complexion, heart palpitations, insomnia, dizziness or flowery vision, it is a sign of blood vacuity, which is more common among the elderly. If scratching gives rises to vesicles that emit a watery discharge, the pattern is one of wind-damp. Itching on the face, chest, neck, and hands, that refuses cold and likes warmth, and accompanied by a tight or moderate floating pulse is a sign of wind-cold. [92: No. 408] [6: 103] [48: 414]

itchy ear 耳痒 *ěr yǎng*: Irritation of the ears, attributed to liver wind and that may be attended by thickening of the skin due to continual scratching. MED Secure the kidney and clear the liver; eliminate wind and relieve itch. For topical treatment, steep wine or sesame oil in zanthoxylum (*huā jiāo*) and apply as ear drops. ACU Base treatment mainly on GB, LR, and KI. Select GB-20 (*fēng chí*, Wind Pool), TB-17 (*yì fēng*, Wind Screen), LR-3 (*tài chōng*, Supreme Surge), SP-6 (*sān yīn jiāo*, Three Yin Intersection), KI-3 (*tài xī*, Great Ravine), KI-1 (*yǒng quán*, Gushing Spring), and GB-2 (*tīng huì*, Auditory Convergence); needle with even supplementation and drainage. [97: 174] [26: 251] [46: 596]

itchy eyes 目痒 *mù yǎng*: Irritation of the eyes, attributed to wind-fire, damp-heat, blood vacuity engendering wind, or to abatement of an evil and restoration of right after enduring disease. **Wind-heat:** Itch due to wind-heat is a pronounced itch with scorching sensation, slight fear of light, tearing, and a scant stringy discharge. MED If heat signs are mild, use Wind-Expelling One Zi Powder (*qū fēng yī zì sǎn*); if pronounced, use Lonicera and Forsythia Powder (*yín qiào sǎn*). ACU Base treatment mainly on GB and LI. Select GB-20 (*fēng chí*, Wind Pool), TB-5 (*wài guān*, Outer Pass), LI-4 (*hé gǔ*, Union Valley), LI-11 (*qū chí*, Pool at the Bend), GB-1 (*tóng zǐ liáo*, Pupil Bone-Hole), GB-41 (*zú lín qì*, Foot Overlooking Tears), and Greater Yang (*tài yáng*); needle with drainage. **Damp-heat** causes itchy eyes with red ulcerated eyelid rims, and tears and copious eye discharge. In some cases, there are large grain-like lumps inside the eyelids with itching like wriggling worms. MED Clear heat and eliminate dampness with variations of Three Yellows Decoction (*sān huáng tāng*). ACU Base treatment mainly on LI, ST, SP, and BL. Select LI-11 (*qū chí*, Pool at the Bend), LI-4 (*hé gǔ*, Union Valley), ST-36 (*zú sān lǐ*, Leg Three Li), SP-9 (*yīn líng quán*, Yin Mound Spring), Greater Yang (*tài yáng*), BL-1 (*jīng míng*, Bright Eyes), and GV-23 (*shàng xīng*, Upper Star); needle with drainage. **Blood vacuity:** Itchy eyes due to blood vacuity engendering wind is characterized by mild itching of both eyes that is temporarily relieved by rubbing, dryness and discomfort of the eyes, a facial complexion with little lust, a pale tongue, and a fine stringlike pulse. MED Nourish the blood and dispel wind with Four Agents Decoction (*sì wù tāng*) plus schizonepeta spike (*jīng jiè suì*) and tribulus (*cì jí lí*). ACU Base treatment mainly on GB, LR, SP, and ST. Select GB-20 (*fēng chí*, Wind Pool), LR-3 (*tài chōng*, Supreme Surge), BL-20 (*pí shū*, Spleen Transport), ST-36 (*zú sān lǐ*, Leg Three Li), SP-6 (*sān yīn jiāo*, Three Yin Intersection), KI-6 (*zhào hǎi*, Shining Sea), LR-8 (*qū quán*, Spring at the Bend), GB-1 (*tóng zǐ liáo*, Pupil Bone-Hole), GB-41 (*zú lín qì*, Foot Overlooking Tears), and Greater Yang (*tài yáng*); neddle with even supplementation and drainage. **Abatement of evil:** Itching eyes due to abatement of an evil and restoration of right after enduring illness requires no particular treatment. Itching is also associated with the PEPPERCORN SORE and

ULCERATION OF THE EYELID RIM. [26: 201] [97: 150] [92: No. 454] [125: 82] [46: 596, 720] [37: 485]

itchy throat 喉痒 *hóu yǎng*: Irritation in the throat, sometimes associated with swelling and soreness. Itchy throat is attributed to scorching yin vacuity fire depriving the throat of nourishment or to stomach fire fuming the lung. MED Treat variously by the methods of enriching yin and down-bearing fire, disinhibiting the throat, clearing the stomach, and resolving toxin. [26: 733]

itinerant healer 走方医 *zǒu fāng yī*: *Synonym: bell healer*. A doctor that roams from place to place, ringing a bell to attract customers, and usually offering herbal or simple cures passed on orally from master to student. [27: 516]

J

jade doors 玉户 *yù hù*: YIN DOOR. [97: 136]

jade gates 玉门 *yù mén*: YIN DOOR. [97: 136]

jade pillow bone 玉枕骨 *yù zhěn gǔ*: PILLOW BONE. [27: 63]

jade stem 玉茎 *yù jīng*: PENIS. [97: 136]

Jaundice

YANG JAUNDICE (*yáng huáng*)

YIN JAUNDICE (*yīn huáng*)

ACUTE JAUNDICE (*jí huáng*)

SCOURGE JAUNDICE (*wēn huáng*)

VACUITY JAUNDICE (*xū huáng*)

GALLBLADDER JAUNDICE (*dǎng huáng*)

FIVE JAUNDICES (*wǔ dǎn*)

GRAIN JAUNDICE (*gǔ dǎn*)

LIQUOR JAUNDICE (*jiǔ dǎn*)

BLACK JAUNDICE (*hēi dǎn*)

YELLOW SWEAT (*huáng hàn*)

DAMP-HEAT JAUNDICE (*shī rè huáng dǎn*)

BLOOD AMASSMENT JAUNDICE (*xuè xū huáng dǎn*)

jaundice 黄疸 *huáng dǎn*: A condition characterized by the three classic signs of yellow skin, yellow eyes, and yellow urine, i.e., generalized YELLOWING of the body, yellowing of the whites of the eyes (sclera), and darker-than-normal urine. Jaundice arises when contraction of seasonal evils or dietary irregularities cause damp-heat or cold-damp to obstruct the center burner, and prevents bile from flowing according to its normal course. For different jaundice patterns, see entries listed below. NB: Theories about of the cause of jaundice have varied over the centuries. *The Inner Canon (nèi jīng)* established the notion that it was due damp-heat and hence largely associated with the spleen. Subsequent generations of physicians elaborated various specific pathomechanisms without changing this basic understanding. In the Jin-Yuan period, the distinction between yin jaundice and yang jaundice gained widespread acceptance. In the Ming dynasty, Zhang Jing-Yue proposed the term 胆黄 *dǎn huáng*, "gallbladder jaundice," claiming that the disease arose when damage to gallbladder qi caused bile to discharge, i.e., leak from the gallbladder and flow to the skin. In the Qing Dynasty, Shen Jin-Ao also observed a contagious form of jaundice that he called "heaven-current epidemic scourge," which he nevertheless believed to be attributable to damp-heat. In *A Clinical Guide with*

Case Histories (lín zhèng zhǐ nán yī àn) of 1766, the theories of damp-heat and gallbladder involvement are combined. ◇ Chin 黄 *huáng*, yellow; 疸 *dǎn*, jaundice. The *huáng* was added to prevent confusion arising from homophones of *dǎn*. Eng *jaundice* from Old French *jaunice* (modern *jaunisse*), *jaune*, yellow, + *ice*, noun suffix. [26: 697] [27: 366] [97: 504] [80: 391]

jaw corner 頜 *hé*: The part of the face below the ear. [27: 65]

jerking sinews and twitching flesh 筋惕肉䐃 *jīn tì ròu rùn (shùn)*: From *On Cold Damage (shāng hán lùn, biàn tài yáng bìng zhèng bìng zhì)*. Spasmodic jerking of the sinew and flesh. **Insufficiency of blood and liquid:** Jerking sinews and twitching flesh mostly arises when copious sweating damages yang, causing blood vacuity and wear on liquid that deprives the sinews of nourishment. MED Use Four Agents Decoction (*sì wù tāng*). **Damage to yang:** Less commonly the cause is damage to yang by cold-damp in cold damage, preventing water qi transformation. MED Use True Warrior Decoction (*zhēn wǔ tāng*). [26: 741] [27: 375] [92: No. 340] [50:]

Jin 晋 *jìn*: The name of a dynasty (A.D. 265–420).

Jin 金 *jīn*: The name of a Tartar dynasty (A.D. 1115–1234).

jin 斤 *jīn*: *Synonym: catty.* A unit of measure divided into 16 liang, and now roughly equal to 500 g. See tables 21 and 23, page 717.

joining points 透穴 *tòu xué*: See POINT JOINING.

joint 骨节 *gǔ jié*, 关节 *guān jié*: A joining point of two bones. [26: 976]

joint pain 骨节疼痛 *gǔ jié téng tòng*: Pain in any joint. Enduring joint pain is observed in impediment (*bì*) patterns. Joint pain of limited duration is observed in some externally contracted febrile disease patterns such as wind-cold exterior patterns and qi-aspect heat. Joint pain may also attend certain sores such as streaming sores and red bayberry sores. [26: 383]

joint-running wind 历节风 *lì jié fēng*, 历节 *lì jié*: *Synonyms: white tiger joint-running wind; pain wind.* A disease described in *Essential Prescriptions of the Golden Coffer (jīn guì yào lüè)*, characterized by redness and swelling of the joints, with acute pain and difficulty bending and stretching. Joint-running wind is attributed to transformation of wind-cold-damp into heat in patients suffering from liver-kidney vacuity, and falls within the scope of IMPEDIMENT (*bì*). ◇ Chin 厉 *lì*, pass through, go around, pervade; 节 *jié*, joint; 风 *fēng*, wind. So called because it is a condition that runs through, i.e., pervades, many joints. [26: 914] [27: 407] [97: 77]

jowl 颐 *yí*: The lower part of the cheek. [26: 911] [27: 64] [97: 598]

jowl effusion 发颐 *fā yí*: A sore of the lower cheek arising in cold damage or warm disease when residual toxin congests locally before the cessation of sweating or before full eruption of papules. It begins with generalized heat [effusion] and aversion to cold and a nodelike swelling on one cheek that is slightly warm and painful. The swelling grows and spreads to the ear and the pain increases. Finally, the swelling ruptures and discharges foul-smelling pus. In severe cases, there is swollen pharynx and congesting phlegm that makes swallowing difficult. WMC osteomyletis of the mandible, alveolar abscess. MED In the initial stage, treat by clearing heat and resolving toxin assisted by dissipating the exterior, using formulas such as Universal Aid Toxin-Dispersing Beverage (*pǔ jì xiāo dú yǐn*) as oral medication and applying Golden Yellow Paste (*jīn huáng gāo*) topically. In the suppurative stage, treat by INTERNAL EXPRESSION to outthrust the toxin using Pus-Outthrusting Powder (*tòu nóng sǎn*). [26: 720] [27: 369] [97: 169]

joy 喜 *xǐ*: One of the FIVE MINDS; associated with the heart.

joy causes qi to slacken 喜则气缓 *xǐ zé qì huǎn*: Unconstrained emotions ensure the disinhibited flow of qi. However, excessive joy leads to a dissipation of essence-spirit, and a weakening of heart qi that manifests in heart palpitations, insomnia, and mental diseases. [26: 683] [27: 145] [97: 543]

judging the inside from the outside 从外测内 *cóng wài cèi nèi*: Judging the internal state of the body by external manifestations. [27: 169]

juice 汁 *zhī*: **1.** The extractable fluid from any part of a plant. **2.** The fluid produced when medicinal materials are boiled in water.

Jumping-Round flowing phlegm 环跳流痰 *huán tiào liú tán*: Flowing phlegm in the region of GB-30 (*huán tiào*, Jumping Round). See FLOWING PHLEGM. [26: 933]

K

kampo 汉方 *hàn fāng*: The form of Chinese medicine practiced in Japan. ◇ Chin 汉 *hàn*, China, Han; 方 *fāng*, formula, remedy. Eng *kampo*, from *kan pō*, the Japanese pronunciation of the Chinese characters.

KI 肾 *shèn*, 足少阴肾经 *zú shào yīn shèn jīng*: The kidney or foot lesser yin kidney channel.

kidney 肾 *shèn*: Either of the two viscera located in the small of the back, on either side of the spine; the two kidneys as a single functional unit. The kidney is in the interior, and its exterior correspondence is the bladder, with which it is connected by channels. In the five phases, it belongs to water. The kidney governs water, stores essence, governs reproduction, is the root of early heaven, governs the bone and engenders the marrow, has its blood in the hair of the head, opens at the ears and at the two yin. A principal function of the kidney is to turn fluids into urine for discharge by the bladder. Hence, *The Inner Canon* (*nèi jīng*) states that the KIDNEY GOVERNS WATER. Another major function is expressed in the phrase the KIDNEY STORES ESSENCE. In a narrow sense, essence is equivalent to the modern notions of male and female gametes that come together in reproduction. In a broader sense, the essential qi of the kidney is responsible not only for reproductive capacity but also for the growth, development, and aging of the body. For this reason, it is also said that the KIDNEY IS THE ROOT OF EARLIER HEAVEN, i.e., the basis of the congenital constitution. The statement "the KIDNEY GOVERNS THE BONES AND ENGENDERS MARROW" can also be seen to describe a manifestation of kidney essential qi whose health is reflected in the development of firm, strong bones in youth and whose degeneration is reflected in the increasing brittleness in age. See also the TEETH ARE THE SURPLUS OF THE BONE. The statement "the KIDNEY, ITS BLOOM IS IN THE HAIR [OF THE HEAD]" reflects the observation that the hair is an indicator of age. The kidney's governing of water corresponds to its role in water metabolism recognized in modern medicine; its role of storing essence corresponds to genetic functions, which modern medicine does not ascribe to the kidney. A partial explanation for why the reproductive as well as the urination functions were ascribed to the kidney may be seen in the observation that the external organs of reproduction are combined with those or urination, as reflected in the phrase "the KIDNEY OPENS AT THE TWO YIN" (the anus and genitals). The statement "the KIDNEY OPENS AT THE EARS" reflects the observation that tinnitus and deafness are intimately related to the state of the kidney. The kidney relates to the other organs as follows. **Kidney and heart:** The HEART AND KIDNEY INTERACT. The heart is located in the upper burner and the kidney in the lower burner. Physiologically, the heart connects with the lower burner through the kidney and the kidney connects with the upper burner through the heart. The two viscera are interdependent and counterbalance each other. If this relationship is upset, the resulting condition is known as noninteraction of the heart and kidney, characterized by insomnia, profuse dreaming, lumbar pain, and dream emissions. **Kidney and lung:** The LUNG IS THE GOVERNOR OF QI and KIDNEY IS THE ROOT OF QI. The lung controls breathing and governs the qi of the whole body. However, lung qi must combine with the essential qi of the kidney to produce true qi. Thus, it is said in *Jing-Yue's Complete Compendium* (*jīng yuè quán shū*), "The lung is the governor of qi and the kidney is the root of qi." Although breathing is the function of the lung, it is nevertheless in one aspect dependent on the kidney. Only when kidney qi is sufficient can respiratory qi be constrained. Hence it is said, "The kidney governs the absorption of qi." If kidney essential qi is insufficient, it is incapable of ensuring the absorption of qi through the lung. This results in respiratory insufficiency characterized by shortness of breath and rapid breathing at the slightest exertion. Such conditions are termed "kidney failing to absorb qi" (qi absorption failure) and "qi not descending to the root." Sun Si-Miao's *A Thousand Gold Pieces Prescriptions* (*qiān jīn yào fāng*) states, "Kidney disease ... will result in qi vacuity and diminished respiratory qi." The only effective treatment for such cases is the method of supplementing the kidney to improve qi absorption. **Kidney and liver:** The LIVER STORES THE BLOOD and the KIDNEY STORES ESSENCE; the LIVER GOVERNS FREE COURSING; the KIDNEY GOVERNS STORAGE. The liver and the kidney are intimately related. The two viscera have manifold connections through the channels, and physiologically they are mutually engendering and counterbalancing. In clinical practice, the kidney and the liver are often treated together. The relationship between them may be divided into two broad aspects: the liver stores blood and the kidney stores essence. Kidney essence and liver blood are mutually engendering, for which reason it is said, "The liver and kidney are of the same source." Depletion of kidney essence and insufficiency of liver blood may both lead to what is known as dual vacuity of liver and kidney yin. Conversely, hyperactivity of liver yang and liver fire are not only detrimental to liver blood, but may also, at a further stage of development, damage kidney essence. Hence, therapy often involves both nourishing the liver and enriching the kidney. The liver's governing of free coursing and the kidney's governing of storage are interdependent, mutually counterbalancing functions of the liver and kidney. Disturbance of these functions may bring on such diseases as advanced menstruation, profuse menstruation, menstrual block, and seminal emission, which are frequently eliminated by combined treatment of the two. **Kidney and spleen:** The kidney's relationship to the spleen is seen in its influence of kidney yang over spleen-stomach movement and transformation. Kidney yang, also known as "life gate fire," represents a motive force in the digestive process. Insufficiency of kidney yang (debilitation of life gate fire) leads to impairment of the digestive function. This is known as spleen-kidney yang vacuity and is characterized by cold and pain in the abdomen, persistent diarrhea, early morning diarrhea, nontransformation of food, and water swelling. ◇ Chin The lower part of the character 肾 *shèn* is flesh signifier 肉 *ròu* in its abbreviated form 月. The upper part is said to be an abbreviated form of 坚 *jiān*, meaning firm, and in this context denoting the firmness of the flesh in the lumbar region. [6: 93] [26: 691] [27: 52] [97: 336]

kidney accumulation 肾积 *shèn jī*: RUNNING PIGLET. [26: 693]

kidney channel 肾经 *shèn jīng*: FOOT LESSER YIN KIDNEY CHANNEL. [26: 693]

kidney channel cough 肾经咳嗽 *shèn jīng ké sòu*: KIDNEY COUGH. [26: 693]

kidney channel malaria 肾经疟 *shèn jīng nüè*: WARM MALARIA.

kidney cough 肾咳 *shèn ké*: *kidney channel cough*. COUGH occurring in bouts that cause lumbar pain, and, in severe cases, coughing of spittle and drool. If caused by contraction of cold evil, it can be treated with Ephedra, Aconite, and Asarum Decoction (*má huáng fù zǐ xì xīn tāng*). If due to desiccation of kidney yin, it can be treated with Root-Securing Pill (*gù běn wán*) or Metropolis Qi Pill (*dū qì wán*) plus ginseng (*rén shēn*) and ophiopogon (*mài mén dōng*). [26: 688] [27: 380] [97: 337]

kidney depletion 肾亏 *shèn kuī*: See KIDNEY VACUITY. [26: 693] [27: 164]

kidney diarrhea 肾泄 *shèn xiè*: Persistent diarrhea that occurs in the early morning and is heralded by rumbling intestines. It may be characterized by throughflux diarrhea with clear watery stool, nontransformation of food, or ungratifying defecation that resembles dysentery, but is not dysentery. Other signs include fear of cold in the abdomen, periodic cold of the lumbus and knees, soot-black complexion, pale tongue with white fur, and a fine sunken pulse. The main cause is kidney yang vacuity and insufficiency of the life gate fire, causing a reduction in the supply of warmth and nourishment to spleen and stomach. MED Warm and supplement the life gate. Swallow Kidney-Quieting Pill (*ān shèn wán*), Rousing Spirit Elixir (*zhèn líng dān*), or Four Spirits Pill (*sì shén wán*) with Major Seven Qi Decoction (*dà qī qì tāng*). ACU Base treatment mainly on back transport points, CV, GV, and ST. Select BL-23 (*shèn shū*, Kidney Transport), CV-4 (*guān yuán*, Pass Head), GV-4 (*mìng mén*, Life Gate), BL-20 (*pí shū*, Spleen Transport), CV-12 (*zhōng wǎn*, Center Stomach Duct), LR-13 (*zhāng mén*, Camphorwood Gate), ST-25 (*tiān shū*, Celestial Pivot), and ST-36 (*zú sān lǐ*, Leg Three Li); needle with supplementation and add moxa. See FIFTH-WATCH DIARRHEA. [27: 364] [97: 337]

kidney disease 肾病 *shèn bìng*: Any disease of the kidney. Kidney disease usually takes the form of vacuity, and even repletion patterns are mostly root vacuity and tip repletion patterns. Kidney disease is manifests in a) disturbances in sexual functions (infertility, sterility, impotence, seminal emission) b) developmental deficiencies and early aging, c) urinary disturbances, d) deafness, e) limp aching lumbus and knees. Kidney disease patterns include the following:

Kidney Disease Patterns

Simple patterns
KIDNEY QI VACUITY (*shèn qī xū*)
KIDNEY YANG VACUITY (*shèn yáng xū*)
INSECURITY OF KIDNEY QI (*shèn qì bù gù*)
KIDNEY VACUITY WATER FLOOD (*shèn xū shuǐ fàn*)
INSUFFICIENCY OF KIDNEY ESSENCE (*shèn jīng bù zú*)
KIDNEY YIN VACUITY (*shèn yīn xū*)

Complex patterns
DUAL VACUITY OF KIDNEY YIN AND YANG (*shèn yīn yáng liǎng xū*)
KIDNEY FAILING TO ABSORB QI (*shèn bù nà qì*)
LIVER-KIDNEY YIN VACUITY (*gān shèn yīn xū*)
HEART-KIDNEY YIN VACUITY (*xīn shèn yīn xū*)
NONINTERACTION OF THE HEART AND KIDNEY (*xīn shèn bù jiāo*)
LUNG-KIDNEY YIN VACUITY (*fèi shèn yīn xū*)

SPLEEN-KIDNEY YANG VACUITY (*pí shèn yáng xū*)
HEART-KIDNEY YANG VACUITY (*xīn shèn yáng xū*)

The main basic patterns are kidney qi vacuity, kidney yang vacuity, insecurity of kidney qi, kidney failing to absorb qi, kidney vacuity water flood, and kidney yin vacuity. **Kidney qi vacuity** is due to insufficiency of earlier heaven, taxation damage, or enduring illness affecting the kidney, and is characterized by limp aching lumbus and knees and devitalized essence-spirit exacerbated by overexertion. Other signs include dizziness, deafness, and tinnitus. Kidney yang vacuity and kidney failing to absorb qi share with insecurity of kidney qi such signs as limp aching lumbus and knees, dizziness, deafness, and tinnitus. **Kidney yang vacuity** is a development of kidney qi vacuity, characterized by additional cold signs such as fear of cold and cold limbs. Other possible manifestations are impotence and fifth-watch diarrhea. **Insecurity of kidney qi** is specific form of kidney vacuity, in which failure of the storage function gives rise to seminal emission and/or premature ejaculation, profuse urination at night and/or enuresis, clear thin vaginal discharge, or stirring fetus, in addition to basic kidney vacuity signs. KIDNEY FAILING TO ABSORB QI is usually a complex pattern of kidney-lung qi vacuity that arises when lung vacuity affects the kidney and that is characterized by vacuity panting. **Kidney vacuity water flood** is characterized by generalized swelling and scant urine with general kidney qi vacuity signs such as aching lumbus and physical cold. **Insufficiency of kidney essence** in infants and children manifests in RETARDED CLOSURE OF THE FONTANELS and poor development; in adult life, it manifests in the regression of sexual function (loss of libido, sterility in men and infertility in women), and mental faculties (forgetfulness, dementia), hair loss, loosening of the teeth, and weakness of the bone. These signs are combined with others that suggest an emphasis on kidney yin or kidney yang vacuity. **Kidney yin vacuity** is characterized by reddening of the cheeks, tidal heat [effusion], dry mouth, and sore throat. Since kidney yin and kidney yang are the root of the yin and yang of all the viscera, dual patterns are commonly encountered. See DUAL VACUITY OF KIDNEY YIN AND YANG. See the entries listed below. [26: 689]

kidney dispersion 肾消 *shèn xiāo*: **1.** LOWER DISPERSION. **2.** Thirst without large fluid intake, swelling of the legs, impotence, and frequent urination. [26: 689] [27: 165] [97: 340]

kidney distention 肾胀 *shèn zhàng*: ABDOMINAL FULLNESS stretching to the back with hip and lumbar pain. MED Warm the channels and dissipate cold using Channel-Warming (Menses-Warming) Decoction (*wēn jīng tāng*). In distention disease,

these signs can be treated by adding kidney channel medicinals such as duhuo (*dú huó*), anemarrhena (*zhī mǔ*), asarum (*xì xīn*), and cinnamon bark (*ròu guì*) to the formula treating the main pattern. [26: 693]

kidney engenders bone and marrow 肾生骨髓 *shèn shēng gǔ suǐ*: The Inner Canon (*nèi jīng*) says that "the kidney engenders bone and marrow," "governs the bones," and "its fullness is in the bone." The growth, development, and healing of the bones depends on the nourishment and activation provided by kidney essential qi. Insufficiency of kidney essential qi may result in RETARDED CLOSURE OF THE FONTANELS and soft bones in infants. It may also lead to marrow vacuity characterized by wilting (*wěi*) legs that prevent the patient from walking, or pain or stiffness of the lower lumbar spine preventing the patient from lying either prone or supine. Furthermore, the teeth are the surplus of the bones. In clinical practice, slow growth of teeth in children and the premature loosening and loss of teeth in adults are found to be due to insufficiency of kidney essential qi. Hence, some tooth diseases are vacuity patterns that can be treated through the kidney. Because the kidney governs the bones and engenders marrow, and the brain is known as the "sea of marrow," a close link can be seen between the kidney and the brain. Insufficiency of kidney essential qi may lead to emptiness of the sea of marrow, manifesting as dizziness, slowness of thought, or forgetfulness, all of which can be treated as kidney complaints. [26: 688] [6: 94] [27: 53] [97: 340]

kidney essence 肾精 *shèn jīng*: The reproductive essence of the kidney; falls within the scope of KIDNEY YIN. [26: 693]

kidney failing to absorb qi 肾气 *shèn bù nà qì*: Synonym: *vacuous kidney failing to absorb qi*. Kidney qi vacuity preventing the absorption of lung qi (air breathed in). The kidney failing to absorb qi is characterized by shortness of breath, panting, rapid breathing at the slightest movement, spontaneous sweating, and a forceless fine pulse or a vacuous floating pulse without root. WMC chronic cardiopulmonary failure. See SUPPLEMENTING THE KIDNEY TO PROMOTE QI ABSORPTION for treatment. [26: 687] [97: 339]

kidney fixity 肾着 *shèn zhuó*: Cold pain and heaviness in the lumbar region that prevents normal turning and exacerbated by yin-type (dull wet) weather; it is attributable to kidney vacuity cold-damp becoming "fixed" in the inner body. MED Use Kidney Fixity Decoction (*shèn zhuó tāng*) or Lumbus-Lightening Decoction (*qīng yāo tāng*). ACU Base treatment mainly on GV, KI, BL, and SP. Select BL-23 (*shèn shū*, Kidney Transport), GV-3 (*yāo yáng guān*, Lumbar Yang Pass),

KI-3 (*tài xī*, Great Ravine), BL-40 (*wěi zhōng*, Bend Center), ouch points (*ā shì xué*), GV-4 (*mìng mén*, Life Gate), and SP-9 (*yīn líng quán*, Yin Mound Spring); needle with drainage and use large amounts of moxa. [26: 692] [27: 61] [46: 596, 633] [37: 389]

kidney forms spittle 肾为唾 *shèn wéi tuò*: From *Elementary Questions* (*sù wèn, xuān míng wǔ qì piān*). Same in meaning as SPITTLE IS THE HUMOR OF THE KIDNEY.

kidney gan 肾疳 *shèn gān*: **1.** A GAN pattern characterized by marked emaciation, bleeding gums or ulcerated gums, periodic heat effusion and aversion to cold, copious sweating, and a lack of strength in the limbs; it is attributed to deep-lying heat in the bowels and viscera that results from excessive consumption of sweet fatty foods or intemperate eating and that damages the fluids and in time causes desiccation of kidney yin. It is commonly observed in children suffering from insufficiency of earlier heaven and poor constitution and may accompany ununited skull, crane's-knee wind, and the five slowness. MED Enrich the kidney and supplement the spleen. Use Six-Ingredient Rehmannia Pill (*liù wèi dì huáng wán*). **2.** PURULENT EAR. [50: 905] [26: 689] [27: 435] [97: 337]

kidney governs agility 肾主伎巧 *shèn zhǔ jì qiǎo*: Mental and physical agility are dependent upon kidney qi being abundant, and marrow and essence being plentiful. See KIDNEY HOLDS THE OFFICE OF LABOR, WHENCE AGILITY EMANATES. [27: 54] [97: 339]

kidney governs earlier heaven 肾主先天 *shèn zhǔ xiān tiān*: The kidney is associated with congenital matters (earlier heaven meaning prior to birth). Nonclosure of the fontanels and the FIVE SLOWNESSES (slowness to stand, slowness to walk, slowness to speak, slowness to grow hair, and slowness to teethe) are treated by supplementing the kidney. [27: 54] [97: 339]

kidney governs fear 肾主恐 *shèn zhǔ kǒng*: The kidney is related to fear. In regard to the correspondences between the five phases and five minds (five mental states or emotion), *Elementary Questions* (*sù wèn, yīn yáng yìng xiàng dà lùn*) says that water "is fear among the five minds." In the traditional understand, the essential qi of all five viscera is dependent on the kidney, and that insufficiency of kidney channel qi or kidney water could cause liver, heart, and stomach disease with fear figuring among the signs. More importantly, when kidney water is ample, liver blood is sufficient and the gallbladder (which governs decision) is vigorous; insufficiency of kidney water can cause insufficiency of liver blood and weakness of the gallbladder, which can manifest in the tendency to experience fear. Fear is not only the result of illness, but

may cause it: "fear causes qi to precipitate" and damages kidney essence. Fear can damage kidney qi, causing urinary incontinence, seminal emission, and efflux diarrhea. The terms *fear* and *fright* denote distinct concepts. Compare FRIGHT. See FIVE MINDS. [27: 56] [26: 691] [27: 53]

kidney governs hibernation 肾主蛰 *shèn zhǔ zhé*: [50: 903] From *Elementary Questions* (*sù wèn, liù jié zàng xiàng lùn*), "The kidney governs hibernation, is the root of storage, and the place of essence." In the doctrine of the five phases, the kidney is associated with water phase, and in turn with winter. Winter is the time when animals hibernate and the forces of nature become dormant. [50: 903]

kidney governs opening and closing 肾主开阖 *shèn zhǔ kāi hé*: Kidney qi governing the storage and release of urine in the bladder. See KIDNEY GOVERNS WATER. [27: 53]

kidney governs qi absorption 肾主纳气 *shèn zhǔ nà qì*: The lung's ability to absorb qi partly depends on the kidney. If kidney essential qi is insufficient, it is incapable of ensuring the absorption of qi through the lung. This results in respiratory insufficiency characterized by shortness of breath and rapid breathing at the slightest exertion. Such conditions are termed KIDNEY FAILING TO ABSORB QI, or *qi not homing to the root*. See SUPPLEMENTING THE KIDNEY TO PROMOTE QI ABSORPTION for treatment. "The kidney governs qi absorption" means essentially the same as the "KIDNEY IS THE ROOT OF QI." [26: 2688] [27: 53]

kidney governs reproduction 肾主生殖 *shèn zhǔ shēng zhí*: Reproduction is a function of the kidney. Growth, development, and reproduction rely on the essential qi stored by the kidney. Kidney essential qi is derived from the reproductive essence of the parents (congenital essence), out of which the fetus develops. After birth, kidney essential qi is gradually nurtured by the essence of food (acquired essence) and reaches fullness in puberty; women menstruate (and ovulate) according to the monthly cycle, and men are able to produce semen. [6: 94] [27: 54] [97: 339]

kidney governs storage 肾主闭藏 *shèn zhǔ bì cáng*: The kidney ensures the retention of urine and semen (essence). Breakdown of this function manifests as seminal emission, premature ejaculation, enuresis, and long voidings of clear urine. [36: 100] [6: 93]

kidney governs the bones and engenders marrow 肾主骨，生髓 *shèn zhǔ gǔ, shēng suǐ*: See KIDNEY ENGENDERS BONE AND MARROW.

kidney governs the ears 肾主耳 *shèn zhǔ ěr*: See KIDNEY OPENS AT THE EARS. [26: 687]

kidney governs water 肾主水 *shèn zhǔ shuǐ*: The kidney "distills fluids," regulates their distribution, and discharges waste water, thereby maintaining normal water metabolism in the body. For this reason, the kidney is said to govern water. Body fluids are derived from fluids taken in by the stomach. Through the spleen's movement and transformation and the lung's regulation of the waterways, they are distributed throughout the body, and waste water is carried down to the bladder before being discharged. The QI TRANSFORMATION of the kidney plays a vital role in this. This is why it is said that the kidney governs water. Impairment of this action due to kidney yang vacuity can either cause disorders of fluid metabolism such as scant urine or water swelling or water containment failure, characterized by long voidings of clear urine or profuse urination at night. The function of the bladder is to store and discharge urine and is closely related to the kidney. Storage relies on the retentive power of kidney qi, while discharge relies on the power of the kidney to permit flow. This is known as the "opening and closing" function of the kidney that controls the flow of urine down to the bladder, and enables the bladder to store up to a certain amount of urine before permitting its discharge. *Elementary Questions* (*sù wèn, líng lán mì diǎn lùn*) says, "The bladder... stores fluid, and by qi transformation discharges it." In reality, "qi transformation" referred to here is a function of the kidney. According to *Elementary Questions* (*sù wèn, xuān míng wǔ qì piān*), "Inhibition of the bladder manifests as dribbling urinary block, and its failure to ensure containment, as enuresis." Pathologies associated with the bladder include DRIBBLING URINARY BLOCK, DRIBBLE AFTER VOIDING, FREQUENT URINATION, URINARY URGENCY, PAINFUL URINATION, ENURESIS, or URINARY INCONTINENCE, which in the absence of disease of the bladder itself are generally attributed to disease of the kidney. [27: 53] [97: 338]

kidney holds the office of labor, whence agility emanates 肾者，作强之官，伎巧出焉 *shèn zhě, zuò qiáng zhī guān, jì qiǎo chū yān*: From *Elementary Questions* (*sù wèn, líng lán mì diǎn lùn*). See KIDNEY GOVERNS AGILITY. [27: 54]

kidney impediment 肾痹 *shèn bì*: An IMPEDIMENT (*bì*) pattern arising from persistent bone impediment that fails to heal with subsequent contraction of external evil, from bone damage due to long walking, or from sexual taxation. Kidney impediment is characterized by the inability to straighten the lumbus and back; this produces a stoop, lumbar pain, hypertonicity of the lower limbs, and seminal emission. MED Boost the kidney and dispel evils using Five Impediments Decoction (*wǔ bì tāng*) plus duhuo (*dú huó*), quilled cinnamon (*guān guì*), eucommia (*dù zhòng*), achyranthes (*niú xī*), astragalus (*huáng qí*), and fish

poison yam (*bì xiè*). ACU See BONE IMPEDIMENT. [26: 693] [27: 406] [27: 406] [97: 337]

kidney is averse to dryness 肾恶燥 *shèn wù zào*: The kidney is vulnerable to dryness. The kidney governs water, stores essence, and engenders bone and marrow. Dryness damages the fluids of the body and wears kidney essence, and severe depletion of kidney yin can lead to desiccation of bone and marrow. See BONE WILTING (*wěi*). [26: 692]

kidney is connected with the bladder 肾合膀胱 *shèn hé páng guāng*: The kidney stands in interior-exterior relationship with the bladder. The kidney channel connects with the bladder and the bladder channel connects with the kidney. The kidney governs water within the body, and the bladder (essentially by the action of kidney qi) governs the "opening and closing," i.e., the release and temporary storage of urine. [27: 56] [97: 339]

kidney is on the left and the life [gate] is on right 左肾右命 *zuǒ shèn yòu mìng*: See LIFE GATE. [27: 57] [97: 145]

kidney is the gate of the stomach 肾者胃之关 *shèn zhě wèi zhī guān*: The kidney opens at the two yin (anus and genitals), and controls the discharge of urine and to some extent the stool through its function of governing water. Hence it is the lower gate through which grain and water entering the stomach must pass to leave the body. NB: According to one modern interpretation, 胃 is understood to be 谓, making the phrase read as "the kidney is the so-called gate." [9: 756]

kidney is the root of earlier heaven 肾为先天之本 *shèn wéi xiān tiān zhī běn*: The kidney is the basis of the congenital constitution. Reproduction, growth, development, and aging in which the congenital constitution ("earlier heaven") are reflected are related to the state of kidney qi. [27: 55]

kidney is the root of qi 肾为气之本 *shèn wéi qì zhī běn*: The root of qi is an epithet given to the kidney because it governs qi absorption. See KIDNEY GOVERNS QI ABSORPTION.

kidney is the water viscus; it governs fluids 肾者水脏，主津液 *shèn zhě shuǐ zàng, zhǔ jīn yè*: The kidney is ascribed to water in the five phases and plays a major role in fluid metabolism. See KIDNEY GOVERNS WATER; VISCUS OF FIRE AND WATER.

kidney, its bloom is in the hair [of the head] 肾，其华在发 *shèn, qí huá zài fà*: This line, from *Elementary Questions* (*sù wèn*) is interpreted to mean that the general condition of the hair, hair growth, and hair loss are all associated with the strength of the kidney essential qi. Loss of hair in old age is one sign of debilitation of essential qi. However, the hair also relies on the nourishing action of the blood, so it is also said, "the hair [of the head] is the surplus of the blood." [27: 55]

kidney, its fullness is in the bone 肾，其充在骨 *shèn, qí chōng zài gǔ*: See KIDNEY ENGENDERS BONE AND MARROW.

kidney opens at the ears 肾开窍於耳 *shèn kāi qiào yú ěr*: Synonym: *kidney governs the ears.* From *Elementary Questions* (*sù wèn, jīn guì zhen yán lùn*). The kidney determines hearing ability. The kidney is said to open at the ears since only when kidney qi is abundant is hearing acute. *The Magic Pivot* (*líng shū*) states, "The kidney qi reaches the ears, and if the kidney is in harmony, the ears perceive the five sounds." The ears are connected with the brain, the "sea of marrow," which is dependent upon the kidney for nourishment. Insufficiency of kidney essential qi causes tinnitus (ringing in the ears) and hearing impairment. Debilitation of essential qi in old age often leads to deafness. *The Magic Pivot* (*líng shū, hǎi lùn*) states, "When the sea of marrow is insufficient, the brain spins and the ears ring." [27: 55]

kidney opens at the two yin 肾开窍於二阴 *shèn kāi qiào yú èr yīn*: The kidney opens at the "two yin," i.e., the "posterior yin," which refers to the anus, and the "anterior yin," which refers to the genital organs. These organs are located in the lower burner, and their function is associated with kidney qi, so that they are referred to as the outer orifices of the kidney. This relationship is also reflected in various diseases. For example, kidney vacuity may lead to changes in urination and defecation such as scant urine, long voidings of clear urine, incontinence and enduring diarrhea, or fecal incontinence. The reproductive system may also be affected, causing impotence, premature ejaculation, or seminal emission. [27: 55]

kidney panting 肾喘 *shèn chuǎn*: PANTING caused by kidney evil interfering with the lung, occurring when water gathers in the kidney channel, ascends counterflow and seizes the lung. Kidney panting takes the form of qi counterflow and rapid panting, inability to lie flat, cough, and vomiting. ⎡MED⎤ Depurate the lung and downbear qi; warm the kidney and disinhibit water. Use White-Draining Powder (*xiè bái sǎn*) or True Warrior Decoction (*zhēn wǔ tāng*). [26: 693]

kidney pulse is sunken 肾脉沉 *shèn mài chén*: The sunken pulse is associated with the kidney and the season winter. *Elementary Questions* (*sù wèn, xuān míng wǔ qì piān*) says, "The kidney pulse is stonelike." *The Classic of Difficult Issues* (*nàn jīng, 15*) "The winter pulse is stonelike." A stonelike pulse is now usually referred to as a sunken pulse. See FLOATING PULSE. [9: 336] [131: 200]

kidney qi 肾气 *shèn qì*: The qi engendered by kidney essence; the functional activity of the kidney. *Elementary Questions* (*sù wèn, shàng gǔ tiān zhēn lùn*) states, "[In the male] at the age of two eights [i.e., sixteen], kidney qi is exuberant, the reproductive function matures, essential qi flows forth, yin and yang are in harmony, and [he] can beget offspring..." *The Magic Pivot* (*líng shū, mài dù piān*) states, "Kidney qi flows through to the ears; when the kidney is in harmony, the ears can hear the five sounds." The term kidney qi often specifically denotes the kidney's governing of storage. Thus insecurity of kidney qi denotes insufficiency of kidney qi manifesting in urinary disturbances such as frequent and long voidings of clear urine, or incontinence, enuresis, and dribbling, and disturbances of the reproductive function such as seminal emission, seminal efflux, and premature ejaculation. [97: 339] [50: 904]

kidney qi flows to the ears 肾气通于耳 *shèn qì tōng yú ěr*: From *The Magic Pivot* (*líng shū*): "Kidney qi flows to the ears, and if the kidney is in harmony, the ear perceives the five sounds." See KIDNEY OPENS AT THE EARS. [27: 55]

kidney qi vacuity 肾气虚 *shèn qì xū*: Debilitation of of original qi in the kidney due to insufficiency of earlier heaven, taxation damage, or enduring illness affecting the kidney, and characterized by limp aching lumbus and knees and devitalized essence-spirit exacerbated by overexertion. Other signs include dizziness, lack of strength, deafness, tinnitus, heel pain, loose teeth and hair loss, seminal efflux, premature ejaculation, vaginal discharge, and flooding and spotting. The tongue is pale and enlarged; the pulse is fine and weak, especially at the cubit. ⎡MED⎤ Supplement and boost kidney qi. Use Left-Restoring [Kidney Yin] Pill (*zuǒ guī wán*). Treatment can be varied according to signs. Where continuous aching pain in the lumbus and knees is the main sign, accompanied by limpness of the legs and knees, exacerbated by exertion and relieved by rest, Left-Restoring [Kidney Yin] Pill (*zuǒ guī wán*) can be combined with Young Maid Pill (*qīng é wán*). Where deafness or tinnitus is the main sign, accompanied by dizziness, lack of strength, and aching lumbus, use Deafness Left-Benefiting Loadstone Pill (*ěr lóng zuǒ cí wán*). Where dizziness and lassitude of spirit are the main signs, accompanied by aching lumbus and tinnitus, use Left-Restoring [Kidney Yin] Pill (*zuǒ guī wán*) plus codonopsis (*dǎng shēn*) and astragalus (*huáng qí*). ⎡ACU⎤ Base treatment mainly on BL, KI, GV, CV. Select BL-23 (*shèn shū*, Kidney Transport), GV-4 (*mìng mén*, Life Gate), CV-4 (*guān yuán*, Pass Head), CV-6 (*qì hǎi*, Sea of Qi), ST-36 (*zú sān lǐ*, Leg Three Li), and KI-3 (*tài xī*, Great Ravine); needle with supplementation. Selection of points according to signs: For dizziness, add GV-20 (*bǎi huì*, Hundred Convergences), GV-16 (*fēng fǔ*, Wind Mansion), and GB-39 (*xuán zhōng*, Suspended Bell). For deafness or tinnitus, add TB-17 (*yì fēng*, Wind Screen),

GB-2 (*tīng huì*, Auditory Convergence), SI-19 (*tīng gōng*, Auditory Palace), and TB-3 (*zhōng zhǔ*, Central Islet). For limp aching lumbus and knees, add GV-3 (*yāo yáng guān*, Lumbar Yang Pass), BL-40 (*wěi zhōng*, Bend Center), GB-34 (*yáng líng quán*, Yang Mound Spring), GB-39 (*xuán zhōng*, Suspended Bell), and BL-60 (*kūn lún*, Kunlun Mountains). For seminal emission, add KI-12 (*dà hè*, Great Manifestation), and HT-7 (*shén mén*, Spirit Gate). For heel pain, add PC-7 (*dà líng*, Great Mound), BL-62 (*shēn mài*, Extending Vessel), and BL-60 (*kūn lún*, Kunlun Mountains). For vaginal discharge, add GB-26 (*dài mài*, Girdling Vessel), BL-30 (*bái huán shū*, White Ring Transport), BL-32 (*cì liáo*, Second Bone-Hole), and SP-6 (*sān yīn jiāo*, Three Yin Intersection), [116: 108] [91: 153] [46: 588, 677, 690] [37: 383, 439, 479]

kidney qi wandering wind 肾气游风 *shèn qì yóu fēng*: Red swollen cloud-like patches on the lower limbs attributable to kidney fire brewing internally and externally contracted wind evil lying depressed in the skin. This is one form of RED WANDERING CINNABAR. MED Clear heat and course wind; drain fire and resolve toxin. Use Double Resolution Sage-Inspired Powder (*shuāng jiě tōng shèng sǎn*) as oral medicinal and apply mixed with powdered phellodendron (*huáng bǎi mò*). [26: 690]

kidney reversal headache 肾厥头痛 *shèn jué tóu tòng*: HEADACHE due to reverse flow of kidney qi in patterns of lower body vacuity and upper body repletion. Kidney reversal headache is characterized by an unbearable vertex headache, accompanied by counterflow cold of the limbs, glomus and oppression in the chest and stomach duct, copious phlegm, and stringlike pulse. MED Warm the kidney to promote qi absorption. Use formulas such as True Jade Pill (*yù zhēn wán*), Return Again Elixir (*lái fù dān*), or Galenite Elixir (*hēi xí dān*). [26: 692]

kidney rock 肾岩 *shèn yán*: A sore on or close to the yin head (glans penis) that begins either as a hard painful itchy node exuding watery fluid and subsequently rupturing to form a flat open sore, or grows into a cauliflower shape; in either case in advanced stage, it is accompanied by a stone-like hard swelling in the groin. General signs include lethargic body and torpid spirit. In severe cases, the penis rots away and the patient's life is threatened. It is attributed to binding depression of the fire that arises when liver-kidney depletion or excessive anxiety, thought, depression and anger give rise to exuberant ministerial fire and liver channel blood dryness. WMC carcinoma of the penis. MED In the initial stage, treat by enriching yin and downbearing fire, and supplementing the liver and kidney with formulas such as Anemarrhena and Phellodendron Eight-Ingredient Pill (*zhī bǎi*

bā wèi wán) or Major Yin Supplementation Pill (*dà bǔ yīn wán*). In advanced stages, characterized by dual depletion of qi and blood, treat by supplementing qi and nourishing the blood. Peach Blossom Powder (*táo huā sǎn*) may be applied topically. See ROCK. ◊ Chin 肾 *shèn*, kidney; 言 *yán*, rock. [26: 688] [27: 481] [97: 336]

kidney sac 肾囊 *shèn náng*: SCROTUM.

kidney sac wind 肾囊风 *shèn náng fēng*: SCROTAL WIND.

kidney stands in interior-exterior relationship with the bladder 肾与膀胱相表里 *shèn yǔ páng guāng xiāng biǎo lǐ*: The kidney is in the interior, whereas the bladder is in the exterior. The two are closely related. The kidney drains waste fluids from the body, and passes them to the bladder, which regulates their passage out of the body. Storage relies on the retentive power of kidney qi, whereas discharge relies on the power of the kidney to permit flow. The "opening and closing" of the bladder is thus seen as a function of the kidney. [27: 57]

kidney stores essence 肾藏精 *shèn cáng jīng*: Growth, development, and reproduction rely on the essential qi stored by the kidney. Kidney essential qi is derived from the reproductive essence of the parents (congenital essence), out of which the embryo develops. After birth, it is gradually nurtured by the essence of food (acquired essence) and reaches fullness in puberty, when men are able to produce semen and women begin menstruating—important signs of the reproductive function coming to maturity. In old age, the kidney essential qi weakens, so that the reproductive function gradually fades away, and the body degenerates. *Elementary Questions* (*sù wèn, shàng gǔ tiān zhēn lùn*) states, "[In the male] at the age of two eights [i.e., sixteen] kidney qi is exuberant, the "heavenly tenth" (*tiān guǐ*) arrives, essential qi flows forth, yin and yang are in harmony, and [he] can beget offspring... At the age of seven eights [i.e., fifty-six] heavenly tenth is exhausted, essence diminishes, the kidney grows weak, and the body loses its tone; at eight eights, the teeth and hair fall out. [In the female] at the age of two sevens, heavenly tenth arrives, the controlling (*rèn*) vessel flows, and the thoroughfare vessel fills, the menses come according to their times, and [she] can bear offspring... At seven sevens, the controlling (*rèn*) vessel empties, the thoroughfare vessel weakens, heavenly tenth is exhausted, the passages of the Earth are cut, the body deteriorates, and she can no longer bear children." In this quotation, (*tiān guǐ*) is explained as meaning viability of the reproductive function. See HEAVENLY TENTH. [27: 52] [97: 339]

kidney stores mind 肾藏志 *shèn cáng zhì*: The kidney stores will, spirit, and/or memory. This phrase comes from *Elementary Questions (sù wèn, tiáo jīng lùn)*. The character 志 (*zhì*), meaning mind(-power), will, or emotion, was also used in the sense of memory or record (later distinguished as 誌, but no longer in the PRC's modern simplified script). See MIND. [27: 55] [27: 52] [97: 339]

kidney vacuity 肾虚 *shèn xū*: Any vacuity pattern of the kidney (INSUFFICIENCY OF KIDNEY ESSENCE, KIDNEY YIN VACUITY, KIDNEY YANG VACUITY, INSECURITY OF KIDNEY QI) most commonly characterized by devitalized essence-spirit, dizzy head and tinnitus, forgetfulness and insomnia, aching lumbus and limp legs, seminal emission, premature ejaculation, and impotence. See also KIDNEY DISEASE. [26: 690]

kidney vacuity deafness 肾虚耳聋 *shèn xū ěr lóng*: DEAFNESS due to kidney vacuity. MED Supplement kidney qi. Use Six-Ingredient Pill (*liù wèi wán*) plus powdered phellodendron (*huáng bǎi mò*), anemarrhena (*zhī mǔ*), polygala (*yuǎn zhì*), and acorus (*shí chāng pú*). See DEAFNESS. [50: 910]

kidney vacuity delayed menstruation 肾虚经行后期 *shèn xū jīng xíng hòu qī*: DELAYED MENSTRUATION (arrival of menstrual periods eight days or more later than the expected time) due to kidney vacuity arising when congenital insufficiency, early marriage, excessive childbirth, or sexual intemperance causes damage to kidney qi and lead to depletion of essence-blood and insufficiency of the thoroughfare (*chōng*) and controlling (*rèn*) vessels, preventing the uterus from filling on time. The flow is scant and is accompanied by a dizzy head and tinnitus, and limp aching lumbus and knees. MED Supplement the kidney and nourish yin. Use Yin-Securing Brew (*gù yīn jiān*) plus cinnamon bark (*ròu guì*) or Six-Ingredient Rehmannia Pill (*liù wèi dì huáng wán*). ACU Base treatment mainly on CV and the three yin channels of the foot. Select CV-6 (*qì hǎi*, Sea of Qi), KI-13 (*qì xué*, Qi Point), SP-6 (*sān yīn jiāo*, Three Yin Intersection), BL-23 (*shèn shū*, Kidney Transport), CV-4 (*guān yuán*, Pass Head), KI-3 (*tài xī*, Great Ravine), and KI-6 (*zhào hǎi*, Shining Sea); needle with supplementation. [26: 691]

kidney vacuity dizziness 肾虚眩晕 *shèn xū xuàn yūn*: DIZZINESS due to insufficiency of kidney essence depriving the brain marrow of nourishment. Kidney vacuity dizziness is dizzy head with tinnitus, lassitude of the spirit, forgetfulness, and aching lumbus and weak legs. If the condition is one of kidney yang vacuity, signs include cold limbs and fear of cold, pale tongue, and a weak fine pulse, and is treated by supplementing the kidney and warming yang with Right-Restoring [Life

Gate] Pill (*yòu guī wán*) or Golden Coffer Kidney Qi Pill (*jīn guì shèn qì wán*). If kidney yin vacuity is prominent, signs include heart vexation, red tongue, and rapid fine pulse, and is treated by enriching yin and supplementing the kidney using Left-Restoring [Kidney Yin] Pill (*zuǒ guī wán*) or Anemarrhena and Phellodendron Eight-Ingredient Pill (*zhī bǎi bā wèi wán*). ACU Base treatment on KI, GV, and back transport points. Select GV-20 (*bǎi huì*, Hundred Convergences), GV-16 (*fēng fǔ*, Wind Mansion), BL-23 (*shèn shū*, Kidney Transport), GB-39 (*xuán zhōng*, Suspended Bell), and KI-3 (*tài xī*, Great Ravine). If yin vacuity is prominent, add KI-6 (*zhào hǎi*, Shining Sea), KI-1 (*yǒng quán*, Gushing Spring), and HT-7 (*shén mén*, Spirit Gate); if yang vacuity is prominent, add GV-4 (*mìng mén*, Life Gate) and CV-4 (*guān yuán*, Pass Head), needling with supplementation and adding moxa. [26: 691] [46: 619]

kidney vacuity habitual miscarriage 肾虚滑胎 *shèn xū huá tāi*: HABITUAL MISCARRIAGE due to kidney vacuity. Kidney vacuity habitual miscarriage is accompanied by aching lumbus, sagging in the smaller abdomen, dizzy head and tinnitus, limp aching knees, and in some cases vaginal bleeding. MED Supplement the kidney and quiet the fetus using Fetal Longevity Pill (*shòu tāi wán*), to which charred mugwort (*ài yè tàn*) and charred eucommia (*dù zhòng tàn*) may be added for pronounced bleeding. ACU Base treatment mainly on CV and KI. Select BL-23 (*shèn shū*, Kidney Transport), KI-3 (*tài xī*, Great Ravine), CV-4 (*guān yuán*, Pass Head), CV-3 (*zhōng jí*, Central Pole), KI-12 (*dà hè*, Great Manifestation), and KI-13 (*qì xué*, Qi Point); moxa every point 15–20 minutes twice a day. See HABITUAL MISCARRIAGE. [26: 691] [59: 107]

kidney vacuity headache 肾虚头痛 *shèn xū tóu tòng*: HEADACHE attributed to kidney vacuity and insufficiency of the sea of marrow. Kidney vacuity headache may be due to kidney yang or kidney yin vacuity. **Kidney yang vacuity** patterns are marked by aversion to cold, lack of warmth in the limbs, white facial complexion, pale tongue and a fine sunken pulse. MED Warm and supplement kidney yang using variations of Right-Restoring [Life Gate] Pill (*yòu guī wán*). ACU Base treatment for both kidney yang vacuity and kidney yin vacuity mainly on back transport points and KI. Main points: GV-20 (*bǎi huì*, Hundred Convergences), GB-19 (*nǎo kōng*, Brain Hollow), BL-2 (*zǎn zhú*, Bamboo Gathering), BL-23 (*shèn shū*, Kidney Transport), KI-3 (*tài xī*, Great Ravine), and GB-39 (*jué gǔ*, Severed Bone). Supplement GV-4 (*mìng mén*, Life Gate), CV-4 (*guān yuán*, Pass Head), and KI-7 (*fù liū*, Recover Flow) to address kidney yang vacuity, and apply moxa. **Kidney yin vacuity** is marked by an empty feeling in the head, dizziness, tinnitus, lack of strength in the lumbus and knees, red tongue, and fine pulse. MED Enrich kidney yin using formulas such as Six-Ingredient Rehmannia Pill (*liù wèi dì huáng wán*) or Major Origin-Supplementing Brew (*dà bǔ yuán jiān*) and variations. ACU Use the main points given above, and add BL-52 (*zhì shì*, Will Chamber), and SP-6 (*sān yīn jiāo*, Three Yin Intersection); needle with supplementation. For selection of points according to affected area, see HEADACHE. [26: 692] [46: 622] [37: 364]

kidney vacuity infertility 肾虚不孕 *shèn xū bù yùn*: Female INFERTILITY arising when insufficiency of kidney qi or damage to kidney qi by enduring sickness or sexual taxation causes depletion of essence-blood that deprives the thoroughfare (*chōng*) and controlling (*rèn*) vessels of nourishment and reduces receptivity to male essence (sperm). Kidney vacuity infertility is associated with lassitude of essence-spirit, dizzy head and tinnitus, aching lumbus and limp legs, and menstrual irregularities. MED Warm the kidney and regulate menstruation; regulate the thoroughfare (*chōng*) and controlling (*rèn*) vessels. Use Unicorn-Rearing Pill (*yù lín zhū*). If insufficiency of kidney yang (physical cold and cold limbs, cold feeling in the smaller abdomen) is prominent, psoralea (*bǔ gǔ zhī*), morinda (*bā jǐ tiān*), cinnamon bark (*ròu guì*), and aconite (*fù zǐ*) can be added. If the emphasis is on insufficiency of kidney yin (reddening of the cheeks and lips, tidal heat [effusion], and night sweating), this formula can be combined with Six-Ingredient Rehmannia Decoction (*liù wèi dì huáng tāng*). ACU For kidney yang vacuity, base treatment on back transport points, GV, CV, KI, and ST. Select BL-23 (*shèn shū*, Kidney Transport), GV-4 (*mìng mén*, Life Gate), CV-4 (*guān yuán*, Pass Head), KI-3 (*tài xī*, Great Ravine), CV-3 (*zhōng jí*, Central Pole), CV-7 (*yīn jiāo*, Yin Intersection), CV-2 (*qū gǔ*, Curved Bone), ST-29 (*guī lái*, Return), and KI-6 (*zhào hǎi*, Shining Sea); needle with supplementation and large amounts of moxa. For kidney yin vacuity, base treatment on back transport point, CV, and KI. Select BL-23 (*shèn shū*, Kidney Transport), CV-4 (*guān yuán*, Pass Head), KI-3 (*tài xī*, Great Ravine), KI-6 (*zhào hǎi*, Shining Sea), KI-2 (*rán gǔ*, Blazing Valley) KI-5 (*shuǐ quán*, Water Spring), ST-13 (*qì hù*, Qi Door), and Infant's Palace (*zǐ gōng*); needle with supplementation. [26: 691] [46: 683] [59: 101]

kidney vacuity lumbar pain 肾虚腰痛 *shèn xū yāo tòng*: LUMBAR PAIN due to kidney vacuity. Limp aching lumbus and knees and lack of strength in the legs exacerbated by exercise and from which rest brings little relief, accompanied by a forceless fine pulse, qi timidity and lack of strength, and clear uninhibited urine together indicate insufficiency of kidney yang. A forceless surging pulse with yellow or reddish urine, and periodic flaming

of vacuity fire indicate insufficiency of kidney yin. MED Supplement the kidney. Mild cases can be treated with Young Maid Pill (*qīng é wán*). More severe cases with signs of essence-blood depletion can be treated with Tangkuei and Rehmannia Beverage (*dāng guī dì huáng yǐn*), Left-Restoring [Kidney Yin] Pill (*zuǒ guī wán*), or Right-Restoring [Life Gate] Pill (*yòu guī wán*). ACU For insufficiency of kidney yang, base treatment mainly on BL and GV. Select BL-23 (*shèn shū*, Kidney Transport), GV-4 (*mìng mén*, Life Gate), GV-3 (*yāo yáng guān*, Lumbar Yang Pass), BL-40 (*wěi zhōng*, Bend Center), ouch points (*ā shì xué*), and CV-4 (*guān yuán*, Pass Head); needle with supplementation and add moxa. For kidney yin vacuity, base treatment mainly on BL and KI. Select BL-23 (*shèn shū*, Kidney Transport), KI-3 (*tài xī*, Great Ravine), BL-52 (*zhì shì*, Will Chamber), BL-40 (*wěi zhōng*, Bend Center), ouch points (*ā shì xué*), and BL-60 (*kūn lún*, Kunlun Mountains); needle with supplementation. For effulgent yin vacuity fire, add KI-6 (*zhào hǎi*, Shining Sea), KI-2 (*rán gǔ*, Blazing Valley), and HT-8 (*shào fǔ*, Lesser Mansion), needling with drainage. [26: 691] [46: 633] [113: 229] [37: 390]

kidney vacuity menstrual block 肾虚经闭 *shèn xū jīng bì*: MENSTRUAL BLOCK (abnormal absence of menses) due to kidney vacuity arising when insufficiency of earlier heaven (congenital deficiencies), early marriage, excessive childbirths, or sexual intemperance cause damage to kidney qi, thereby causing insufficiency of the thoroughfare (*chōng*) and controlling (*rèn*) vessels and uterine blood vacuity. Kidney vacuity menstrual block is associated with dizzy head and tinnitus, limp aching lumbus and knees, and frequent urination. MED Supplement the kidney and nourish the blood using Yin-Securing Brew (*gù yīn jiān*) plus deerhorn glue (*lù jiǎo jiāo*), psoralea (*bǔ gǔ zhī*), and cistanche (*ròu cōng róng*). ACU Base treatment mainly on back transport points, CV, KI, ST, and SP. Select BL-23 (*shèn shū*, Kidney Transport), KI-3 (*tài xī*, Great Ravine), CV-4 (*guān yuán*, Pass Head), KI-2 (*rán gǔ*, Blazing Valley), BL-20 (*pí shū*, Spleen Transport), BL-17 (*gé shū*, Diaphragm Transport), ST-36 (*zú sān lǐ*, Leg Three Li), and SP-6 (*sān yīn jiāo*, Three Yin Intersection); needle with supplementation. For pronounced kidney yang vacuity, use moxa at GV-4 (*mìng mén*, Life Gate) and CV-3 (*zhōng jí*, Central Pole). [26: 691]

kidney vacuity scant menstruation 肾虚月经过少 *shèn xū yuè jīng guò shǎo*: SCANT MENSTRUATION due to kidney vacuity arising when congenital insufficiency, early marriage, excessive childbirth, excessive breast feeding, or sexual intemperance leads to damage to kidney qi, essence-blood depletion, and insufficiency of blood in the thoroughfare (*chōng*) and controlling (*rèn*) vessels and the vessels of the uterus. The flow is scant, thin, and dull red, and is accompanied by dizzy head and tinnitus, and aching lumbus and limp legs. MED Supplement the kidney and nourish the blood with Tangkuei and Rehmannia Beverage (*dāng guī dì huáng yǐn*) plus astragalus (*huáng qí*). ACU Base treatment mainly on KI, SP, LR, and back transport points. Select BL-23 (*shèn shū*, Kidney Transport), BL-17 (*gé shū*, Diaphragm Transport), BL-20 (*pí shū*, Spleen Transport), BL-21 (*wèi shū*, Stomach Transport), KI-3 (*tài xī*, Great Ravine), KI-5 (*shuǐ quán*, Water Spring), LR-3 (*tài chōng*, Supreme Surge), ST-36 (*zú sān lǐ*, Leg Three Li), and SP-6 (*sān yīn jiāo*, Three Yin Intersection). Needle with supplementation. For insufficiency of kidney qi, add CV-4 (*guān yuán*, Pass Head), CV-6 (*qì hǎi*, Sea of Qi), and GV-4 (*mìng mén*, Life Gate), and apply moxa. [26: 691] [46: 683]

kidney vacuity seminal emission 肾虚遗精 *shèn xū yí jīng*: SEMINAL EMISSION due to kidney vacuity exacerbated by hyperactivity of heart yang (noninteraction of the heart and kidney) due to excessive thought and preoccupation or by sexual intemperance. **Hyperactivity of heart yang and kidney yin vacuity:** This pattern is mainly caused by excessive thought and preoccupation and is characterized by frequent seminal emission accompanied by dry mouth and tongue, red face and cheeks, and fatigue. In severe cases, the patient can suffer an emission as soon as he closes his eyes, and may have several emissions in one night. MED Clear the heart and contain essence with formulas such as Heart-Supplementing Elixir (*bǔ xīn dān*) or Six-Ingredient Rehmannia Pill (*liù wèi dì huáng wán*). ACU Base treatment mainly on back transport points, KI, SP, HT, and PC. Needle with supplementation at BL-23 (*shèn shū*, Kidney Transport), KI-3 (*tài xī*, Great Ravine), and SP-6 (*sān yīn jiāo*, Three Yin Intersection) with drainage at BL-15 (*xīn shū*, Heart Transport), HT-7 (*shén mén*, Spirit Gate), PC-8 (*láo gōng*, Palace of Toil), KI-6 (*zhào hǎi*, Shining Sea), PC-6 (*nèi guān*, Inner Pass), and PC-7 (*dà líng*, Great Mound). Selection of points according to signs: For insomnia, add Alert Spirit Quartet (*sì shén cōng*) and Insomnia (*shī mián*). For profuse dreaming, add GB-44 (*zú qiào yīn*, Foot Orifice Yin) and ST-45 (*lì duì*, Severe Mouth). **Depletion of kidney essence and stirring of the ministerial fire:** The signs are weak wilting lumbus and legs, aching pain in the bones, night heat EFFUSION and spontaneous sweating, frequent erection, frequent seminal emission, red tongue and rapid fine pulse. MED Enrich yin and downbear fire; replenish essence with medicinals of strong flavor. Use astringent yin-nourishing medicinals such as cooked

rehmannia (*shú dì huáng*), swim bladder (*yú biào*), lycium berry (*gǒu qǐ zǐ*), goat's kidney (*yáng shèn*), pig's spine marrow (*zhū jǐ suǐ*), and schisandra (*wǔ wèi zǐ*). ACU Base treatment mainly on CV, KI, and back transport points. Needle with supplementation at CV-4 (*guān yuán*, Pass Head), BL-23 (*shèn shū*, Kidney Transport), BL-52 (*zhì shì*, Will Chamber), and KI-3 (*tài xī*, Great Ravine), and with drainage at KI-6 (*zhào hǎi*, Shining Sea), KI-1 (*yǒng quán*, Gushing Spring), and HT-8 (*shào fǔ*, Lesser Mansion). **Exhaustion of the lower origin from sexual intemperance:** This is characterized by seminal efflux, aching lumbus and limp legs, pale tongue, and fine sunken pulse, combined with kidney yang vacuity signs such as fear of cold and cold limbs. MED It can be treated by dual supplementation of yin and water and by warming and containing the life gate, using formulas such as Deerhorn Major Supplementation Decoction (*lù róng dà bǔ tāng*). ACU Base treatment mainly on CV, KI, GV, and back transport points. Select CV-4 (*guān yuán*, Pass Head), BL-23 (*shèn shū*, Kidney Transport), KI-3 (*tài xī*, Great Ravine), GV-4 (*mìng mén*, Life Gate), KI-7 (*fù liū*, Recover Flow), BL-52 (*zhì shì*, Will Chamber), KI-12 (*dà hè*, Great Manifestation), and ST-36 (*zú sān lǐ*, Leg Three Li); needle with supplementation and add moxa. [26: 692] [46: 678]

kidney vacuity tinnitus 肾虚耳鸣 *shèn xū ěr míng*: TINNITUS attributable to kidney vacuity and insufficiency of essential qi and characterized by continuous tinnitus like the sound of the tide or cicadas, or at night like the sound of a battle drum. The patient may also have the sensation of someone blowing in his or her ear producing a peculiar itch. It is treated by supplementing the kidney and boosting qi. TINNITUS. [26: 691]

kidney vacuity toothache 肾虚牙痛 *shèn xū yá tòng*: TOOTHACHE attributable to insufficiency of kidney yin with vacuity fire flaming upward. See TOOTHACHE.

kidney vacuity vaginal discharge 肾虚带下 *shèn xū dài xià*: VAGINAL DISCHARGE due to kidney vacuity arising when early marriage or excessive childbirth damages kidney qi and causes insufficiency of kidney yang, cold-damp pouring downward, and consequent damage to the thoroughfare (*chōng*) vessel and girdling (*dài*) vessel vessel. The discharge is copious, thin, clear, and persistent. Other signs include somber facial complexion, severe lumbar pain, cold sensation in the smaller abdomen, sloppy stool, and long clear voidings of urine. MED Warm yang and supplement the kidney using Internal Supplementation Pill (*nèi bǔ wán*). If the condition persists and forms an efflux desertion pattern, medicinals such as calcined dragon bone (*duàn lóng gǔ*), calcined cuttlefish bone (*duàn wū zéi gǔ*), calcined oyster shell (*duàn mǔ lì*), euryale (*qiàn shí*), and toosendan (*chuān liàn zǐ*) can be added for extra astringent discharge-checking action. For older patients in a weak state of health and with a severe pouring discharge, ginseng (*rén shēn*) and cimicifuga (*shēng má*) can be added to supplement and upraise qi and promote astriction. ACU Base treatment mainly on CV, GIV, SP, BL, and KI. Select GB-26 (*dài mài*, Girdling Vessel), BL-30 (*bái huán shū*, White Ring Transport), CV-6 (*qì hǎi*, Sea of Qi), SP-6 (*sān yīn jiāo*, Three Yin Intersection), CV-4 (*guān yuán*, Pass Head), BL-23 (*shèn shū*, Kidney Transport), KI-3 (*tài xī*, Great Ravine) and BL-32 (*cì liáo*, Second Bone-Hole); needle with supplementation and add moxa. [26: 961]

kidney vacuity water flood 肾虚水泛 *shèn xū shuǐ fàn*: Synonym: *kidney yang vacuity water flood*. WATER SWELLING due to kidney yang depletion that prevents the normal transformation of water-damp. The kidney governs water and stands in interior-exterior relationship with the bladder. If kidney yang is vacuous, it cannot govern water, bladder qi transformation (opening and closing action of the bladder) is inhibited, and urine decreases. At the same time, splenic movement and transformation is deprived of the warming action of kidney yang, so that water gathers to create water swelling that is most pronounced in the lower body and characterized by failure of the flesh to rebound swiftly after pressure is released. Other signs include heavy aching lumbus, cold limbs and fear of cold, pale enlarged tongue, white glossy tongue fur, and a fine sunken pulse. WMC chronic nephritis. MED Use Golden Coffer Kidney Qi Pill (*jīn guì shèn qì wán*). ACU Base treatment mainly on CV, back transport points, and KI. Select CV-9 (*shuǐ fēn*, Water Divide), CV-6 (*qì hǎi*, Sea of Qi), BL-22 (*sān jiāo shū*, Triple Burner Transport), ST-36 (*zú sān lǐ*, Leg Three Li), BL-23 (*shèn shū*, Kidney Transport), BL-20 (*pí shū*, Spleen Transport), GV-4 (*mìng mén*, Life Gate), CV-4 (*guān yuán*, Pass Head), KI-3 (*tài xī*, Great Ravine), and KI-7 (*fù liū*, Recover Flow); needle with supplementation and moxa. Compare HEART-KIDNEY YANG VACUITY. [26: 690] [46: 676]

kidney water 肾水 *shèn shuǐ*: Kidney yin. [26: 687]

kidney-water 肾水 *shèn shuǐ*: The kidney viewed as corresponding to water in the five phases. [26: 687]

kidney water 肾水 *shèn shuǐ*: One of the FIVE WATERS described in *Essential Prescriptions of the Golden Coffer* (*jīn guì yào lüè*). WATER SWELLING in kidney vacuity; characterized by lumbar pain, difficult urination, abdominal distention and swelling around the umbilicus, water-damp

seeping out of the lower yin, cold lower extremities, and facial and general emaciation. *Essential Prescriptions of the Golden Coffer* (*jīn guì yào lüè*) states, "In kidney water, there is enlarged abdomen, lumbar pain, the inability to urinate, dampness of the genitals like the sweaty nose of an ox, counterflow cold of the legs, and thin face." [26: 687] [27: 419] [97: 336]

kidney wheezing 肾哮 *shèn xiāo*: WHEEZING attributed to kidney water intimidating the lung. See WHEEZING. [26: 689]

kidney wilting 肾痿 *shèn wěi*: BONE WILTING. [26: 693]

kidney worm 肾虫 *shèn chóng*: PINWORM. [26: 693]

kidney worm disease 肾虫病 *shèn chóng bìng*: PINWORM DISEASE. [26: 693]

kidney yang 肾阳 *shèn yáng*: See KIDNEY YIN AND KIDNEY YANG.

kidney yang vacuity 肾阳虚 *shèn yáng xū*: The manifestation of debilitation of kidney yang (variously referred to as insufficiency of true yang, insufficiency of the true origin, exhaustion of the lower origin, or debilitation of the life gate fire). Kidney yang is the root of the yang of the entire body, and is related most closely to the yang qi of the spleen, lung, and heart. Kidney yang vacuity may cause, or be caused by, vacuity of the yang qi of these three related viscera. Kidney yang vacuity is characterized by both vacuity and cold signs, such as bright white facial complexion, torpor of essence-spirit, aversion to cold, lack of warmth in the extremities, dizziness, tinnitus, limp aching lumbus and knees, and an enlarged pale tongue. Where the reproductive function is affected, seminal efflux, impotence, sterility or infertility, and menstrual irregularities may be observed. Where the transformative function of kidney qi is impaired, signs include long voidings of copious clear urine, profuse urination at night, or scant urine, urinary block, and water swelling. In severe cases, water-rheum may flood upward, intimidating the heart and shooting into the lung. Such cases are characterized by heart palpitations, rapid panting, and inability to assume a lying posture. Spleen-kidney yang vacuity is characterized by pronounced water swelling or enduring diarrhea, clear-food diarrhea, or by early morning diarrhea. Qi absorption failure, which generally stems from lung qi vacuity, is characterized by rapid breathing at the slightest exertion. Heart-kidney yang debilitation is identified by the presence of heart palpitations, panting, water swelling, and, in severe cases, by reversal cold of the limbs, putting forth of oily sweat, and other critical signs. WMC Simple kidney yang vacuity may be seen in chronic nephritis, general asthenia, and neurasthenia sexualis. Spleen-kidney yang vacuity is associated with chronic nephritis and chronic diarrhea. Qi absorption failure is seen in pulmonary emphysema. Heart-kidney yang debilitation is observed in heart failure. MED "Boosting the source of fire to eliminate the entrenched surfeit of yin" is the method used to treat kidney yang vacuity. Commonly used are medicinals that warm and supplement kidney yang, such as aconite (*fù zǐ*), cinnamon bark (*ròu guì*), fenugreek (*hú lú bā*), psoralea (*bǔ gǔ zhī*), alpinia (*yì zhì rén*), curculigo (*xiān máo*), and epimedium (*yín yáng huò*). Formulas include Cinnamon Bark and Aconite Eight-Ingredient Pill (*guì fù bā wèi wán*), which warms the lower burner and is used for general kidney yang vacuity. Spleen-kidney yang vacuity presenting with enduring, clear-food, or early morning diarrhea may be treated with Four Spirits Pill (*sì shén wán*) and variations, which warm and supplement the spleen and kidney. Where water swelling is pronounced, True Warrior Decoction (*zhēn wǔ tāng*) or Life Saver Kidney Qi Pill (*jì shēng shèn qì wán*) may be used to warm yang and disinhibit water. Qi absorption failure may be treated with combinations including such formulas as Ginseng with Gecko Powder (*shēn jiè sǎn*) or Galenite Elixir (*hēi xí dān*), which warm the kidney and promote qi absorption. Impending desertion due to heart-kidney yang debilitation should be treated with such yang-returning desertion-stemming formulas as Ginseng and Aconite Decoction (*shēn fù tāng*). Kidney yang vacuity occurring in combination with insufficiency of essence-blood may be treated according to the principle that the "essence promotes qi formation"; use formulas that replenish essence and supplement the kidney, such as Right-Restoring [Life Gate] Pill (*yòu guī wán*). MED Moxibustion at GV-4 (*mìng mén*, Life Gate), BL-23 (*shèn shū*, Kidney Transport), CV-4 (*guān yuán*, Pass Head), KI-3 (*tài xī*, Great Ravine), and ST-36 (*zú sān lǐ*, Leg Three Li) helps supplement kidney yang. At SP-9 (*yīn líng quán*, Yin Mound Spring) and CV-9 (*shuǐ fēn*, Water Divide) it will disinhibit water, where severe water swelling is present. Spleen-kidney yang vacuity with cold diarrhea calls for the addition of points such as BL-20 (*pí shū*, Spleen Transport)ⓜ, SP-6 (*sān yīn jiāo*, Three Yin Intersection)ⓜ, BL-25 (*dà cháng shū*, Large Intestine Transport)ⓜ, and ST-25 (*tiān shū*, Celestial Pivot)ⓜ to supplement the spleen and large intestine. Heart-kidney yang vacuity may be treated with the back transport point of the heart, BL-15 (*xīn shū*, Heart Transport)ⓜ, which will supplement the heart, and points such as HT-7 (*shén mén*, Spirit Gate) and PC-6 (*nèi guān*, Inner Pass), which quiet the spirit and heart respectively. [27: 164] [6: 192] [97: 338] [113: 11, 14]

kidney yang vacuity water flood 肾阳虚水泛 *shèn yáng xū shuǐ fàn*: KIDNEY VACUITY WATER FLOOD.

kidney yin 肾阴 *shèn yīn*: See KIDNEY YIN AND KIDNEY YANG.

kidney yin and kidney yang 肾阴、肾阳 *shèn yīn, shèn yáng*: The two opposing, yet complementary aspects of kidney essential qi. Kidney yin and kidney yang are interdependent and mutually counterbalancing. Imbalance between the two is fundamentally attributable to insufficiency of kidney essential qi. When kidney yin or yang vacuity reaches a certain point, it may affect its complement, so that the condition becomes one of dual vacuity of kidney yin and yang (detriment of yin or yang affecting its complement). Kidney yin has a moistening and nourishing effect on all the organs of the body, and when it is vacuous, general signs such as interior heat, dizziness, tinnitus, limpness of the knees and lower back, seminal emission, red tongue, and dry mouth are likely to appear. Owing to the loss of the nourishing effect of the kidney yin, a whole variety of diseases, such as noninteraction of the heart and kidney, ascendant liver yang, liver wind stirring internally, or heart fire flaming upward may develop. If the lung is affected, such signs as dry cough, tidal heat [effusion], upbearing fire, and dry pharynx are observed. Kidney yang warms and activates the other organs. Insufficiency of kidney yang may therefore lead to disturbances of water metabolism and the reproductive function, and may also diminish the activity of the other organs. If kidney yang fails to perform its activating function, signs of heart-kidney yang vacuity such as heart palpitations, a slow pulse, sweating, shortness of breath, and cold of the limbs may be observed. Impaired absorption of qi by the kidney affects the lung, provoking rapid breathing at the slightest exertion. If the spleen is deprived of the warming action of kidney yang, there may be early morning diarrhea or nontransformation of food. Conversely, yin or yang vacuity in other organs may affect kidney yin or yang. For example, liver yin vacuity, ascendant hyperactivity of liver yang, heart yin vacuity, or effulgent heart fire may eventually "sap kidney yin," creating kidney yin vacuity. Often, lung yin vacuity also affects kidney yin, and diarrhea caused by spleen yang vacuity may eventually affect kidney yang, this condition being known as spleen-kidney yang vacuity. Since kidney yin and kidney yang are the root of the yin and yang of all the organs of the body, they may also be referred to as "true yin" or "original yin," and "true yang" or "original yang." [6: 96]

kidney yin depletion 肾阴亏虚 *shèn yīn kuī xū*: See KIDNEY YIN VACUITY.

kidney yin vacuity 肾阴虚 *shèn yīn xū*: Synonym: *insufficiency of kidney water*; *insufficiency of true yin*; *depletion of the lower origin*. The manifestation of insufficiency of kidney yin. Kidney yin is the root of all yin of the body. It is most closely related to the heart, liver, and lung. Thus, kidney yin depletion frequently leads to vacuity of heart, liver, or lung yin. Conversely, persistent yin vacuity in the three related viscera may culminate in depletion of kidney yin. Hence in clinical practice, kidney yin vacuity most commonly occurs in dual vacuity patterns. Kidney yin vacuity is characterized by vacuity and heat signs, and varies greatly in severity. Mild cases are characterized by dizziness, tinnitus, dry pharynx, dry mouth, tidal heat [effusion], lumbar pain, seminal emission, night sweating, and in some cases bleeding gums. The pulse is fine and rapid, and the tongue is distinctly red in color. Severe cases are marked by shedding of flesh and loss of bulk (severe emaciation) and a red mirror tongue. The dual patterns are identified by additional signs. Liver-kidney yin vacuity is characterized by headache, blurred or flowery vision, and loss of visual acuity, as well as irregular menses and sterility. Heart-kidney yin vacuity is characterized by such signs as insomnia, heart palpitations, forgetfulness, and profuse dreaming. Cough, expectoration of blood, and steaming bone tidal heat [effusion] are observed in lung-kidney yin vacuity. |WMC| Liver-kidney yin vacuity is seen in some forms of hypertension, neurosis, and menstrual disorders, whereas heart-kidney yin vacuity may occur in tachycardia, hyperthyroidism, and neurosis. Lung-kidney yin vacuity is seen in pulmonary tuberculosis. |MED| Treat by the principle of "invigorating the governor of water to restrain the brilliance of yang." Commonly used medicinals that enrich kidney yin include: rehmannia (*dì huáng*), tortoise plastron (*guī bǎn*), asparagus (*tiān mén dōng*), turtle shell (*biē jiǎ*), scrophularia (*xuán shēn*), flowery knotweed (*hé shǒu wū*), cornus (*shān zhū yú*), ligustrum (*nǔ zhēn zǐ*), and eclipta (*mò hàn lián*). Six-Ingredient Rehmannia Pill (*liù wèi dì huáng wán*) is the basic formula prescribed. For mild cases, Double Supreme Pill (*èr zhì wán*) may be used. Where effulgent fire signs are prominent, use Anemarrhena, Phellodendron, and Rehmannia Pill (*zhī bǎi dì huáng wán*). For liver-kidney yin vacuity, use Lycium Berry, Chrysanthemum, and Rehmannia Pill (*qǐ jú dì huáng wán*). For heart-kidney yin vacuity, use Celestial Emperor Heart-Supplementing Elixir (*tiān wáng bǔ xīn dān*). For lung-kidney yin vacuity, use Lily Bulb Metal-Securing Decoction (*bǎi hé gù jīn tāng*). Where signs of essence-blood depletion are present, kidney essential qi must also be supplemented. |ACU| Base treatment mainly on back transport points and KI. Select BL-23 (*shèn shū*, Kidney Transport), CV-4 (*guān yuán*, Pass Head), KI-3 (*tài xī*, Great Ravine), BL-52 (*zhì shì*, Will Chamber), KI-6 (*zhào hǎi*, Shining Sea), KI-1 (*yǒng quán*, Gushing Spring), and SP-6 (*sān yīn jiāo*, Three Yin Intersection); needle with supplementation. Selection of points according to signs: For dizziness, add GV-20 (*bǎi huì*, Hundred Convergences), GV-16 (*fēng fǔ*, Wind Mansion), and GB-39 (*xuán zhōng*, Suspended Bell). For tinnitus, add TB-17 (*yì fēng*, Wind Screen), GB-2 (*tīng huì*, Auditory Convergence), and TB-3 (*zhōng zhǔ*, Central Islet). For dry pharynx and mouth, add KI-2 (*rán gǔ*, Blazing Valley), TB-2 (*yè mén*, Humor Gate), and Gold Liquid and Jade Humor (*jīn jīn yù yè*). For tidal heat [effusion], add KI-2 (*rán gǔ*, Blazing Valley), HT-8 (*shào fǔ*, Lesser Mansion), LU-10 (*yú jì*, Fish Border), and PC-5 (*jiān shǐ*, Intermediary Courier). For lumbar pain, add GV-3 (*yāo yáng guān*, Lumbar Yang Pass), BL-40 (*wěi zhōng*, Bend Center), and BL-60 (*kūn lún*, Kunlun Mountains). For seminal emission, add KI-12 (*dà hè*, Great Manifestation), CV-6 (*qì hǎi*, Sea of Qi), HT-7 (*shén mén*, Spirit Gate), and ST-36 (*zú sān lǐ*, Leg Three Li). For night sweating, add SI-3 (*hòu xī*, Back Ravine) and HT-6 (*yīn xī*, Yin Cleft). Selection of points according to concurrent pattern: For liver-kidney yin vacuity, add BL-18 (*gān shū*, Liver Transport) and LR-3 (*tài chōng*, Supreme Surge). For heart-kidney yin vacuity, add BL-15 (*xīn shū*, Heart Transport), BL-17 (*gé shū*, Diaphragm Transport), CV-14 (*jù què*, Great Tower Gate), PC-6 (*nèi guān*, Inner Pass), and HT-7 (*shén mén*, Spirit Gate). For lung-kidney yin vacuity, add BL-13 (*fèi shū*, Lung Transport), BL-43 (*gāo huāng shū*, Gao-Huang Transport), and LU-5 (*chǐ zé*, Cubit Marsh); needle all points with supplementation. [6: 191] [46: 587, 596, 602, 618, 653, 677, 723] [113: 18, 20, 131]

killing 相杀 *xiāng shā*: See SEVEN RELATIONS. [27: 308]

killing worms 杀虫 *shā chóng*: EXPELLING WORMS.

king of face 面王 *miàn wáng*: The bulb or tip of the nose. [27: 66] [97: 385]

king's palace 王宫 *wáng gōng*: MOUNTAIN ROOT. [27: 64] [97: 68]

knee 膝 *xī*: The joint between the upper and lower leg, whose anterior aspect is protected by the kneecap and whose dorsal surface is called the back of the knee (popliteal fossa). The knee is the place at which important sinews converge; hence *Elementary Questions* (*sù wèn*) states, "The knees are the house of the sinew." Limpness of the knees is associated with insufficiency of the liver and kidney, and knee pain is associated with the same and/or with the presence of wind-cold-damp. See HOUSE

OF THE SINEWS; LIMP LUMBUS AND KNEES; KNEE PAIN; CRANE'S-KNEE WIND. [97: 637]

knee joint 骸关 *hái guān*, 膝解 *xī jiě*: See KNEE.

knee pain 膝痛 *xī tòng*: Pain in the knee joint, and the channels and sinews that pass through. *Zhang's Clear View of Medicine* (*zhāng shì yī tōng, xī tòng*) states, "The knees are the house of the sinews... there is no knee pain that is not due to liver-kidney vacuity allowing wind-damp qi to invade." Knee pain is treated primarily by supplementing the liver and boosting the kidney, dispelling evils and freeing the network vessels. Knee pain with ability to bend but not stretch and with swelling usually involves wind-heat. This can be treated with Supplemented Mysterious Two Powder (*jiā wèi èr miào sǎn*) or Mysterious Two Powder (*èr miào sǎn*). If there is yin vacuity, there is heat and pain without swelling. This is treated with Hidden Tiger Pill (*hǔ qián wán*). When dampness flows into the legs and knees, there is impediment and weakness with pain and heaviness. This can be treated with Duhuo and Mistletoe Decoction (*dú huó jì shēng tāng*). For vacuity cold with wind-damp, use Tiger Bone Four Jin Pill (*hǔ gǔ sì jīn wán*). For liver-kidney vacuity heat with limp wilting sinews and bones with tremor and shaking, use Velvet Deerhorn Four Jin Pill (*lù róng sì jīn wán*). The literature states that if there is pain at BL-40 (*wěi zhōng*, Bend Center), the foot greater yang (*tài yáng*) bladder channel is affected; if the pain is on the outer face of the knee, the foot lesser yang (*shào yáng*) gallbladder channel is affected; if the pain is on the inner face, the foot triple yin is affected. See CHANNEL CONDUCTOR for medicinals that can be added in such cases. ACU Select as main points Eye of the Knee (*xī yǎn*), ST-35 (*dú bí*, Calf's Nose), ST-34 (*liáng qiū*, Beam Hill) (*hé dìng*, Crane Top), BL-40 (*wěi zhōng*, Bend Center), and GB-34 (*yáng líng quán*, Yang Mound Spring). For wind-heat, add GB-20 (*fēng chí*, Wind Pool), TB-5 (*wài guān*, Outer Pass), LI-11 (*qū chí*, Pool at the Bend), and LI-4 (*hé gǔ*, Union Valley), needling with drainage. For yin vacuity, supplement BL-23 (*shèn shū*, Kidney Transport), and KI-3 (*tài xī*, Great Ravine), and drain KI-6 (*zhào hǎi*, Shining Sea), and KI-1 (*yǒng quán*, Gushing Spring). For pronounced dampness, ST-36 (*zú sān lǐ*, Leg Three Li), SP-9 (*yīn líng quán*, Yin Mound Spring), and SP-5 (*shāng qiū*, Shang Hill), needling with drainage. For vacuity cold with wind-damp, add GV-4 (*mìng mén*, Life Gate)ⓜ, GB-20 (*fēng chí*, Wind Pool), LI-11 (*qū chí*, Pool at the Bend), ST-36 (*zú sān lǐ*, Leg Three Li), and SP-9 (*yīn líng quán*, Yin Mound Spring), needling with drainage. For pain on the inner face, add LR-8 (*qū quán*, Spring at the Bend), LR-7 (*xī guān*, Knee Joint), and LR-3 (*tài chōng*, Supreme Surge). For pain on the outer face, add GB-33 (*xī yáng guān*, Knee Yang Joint), and GB-43 (*xiá xī*, Pinched Ravine). For pain on the upper part of the knee, add ST-33 (*yīn shì*, Yin Market). See also CRANE'S-KNEE WIND. [26: 891]

knee's eye wind 膝眼风 *xī yǎn fēng*: See CRANE'S-KNEE WIND.

knocks and falls 跌打 *dié dǎ*: **1.** Blows, collisions, collapses, or falls from heights, especially when resulting in injury. **2.** Any injury resulting from knocks and falls. Injuries from knocks and falls include stasis swelling (bruises), cuts and grazes, sprains, bone fractures, dislocations, and damage to the bowels and viscera. MED Dispel stasis, move qi, relieve pain, stanch bleeding, soothe the sinews, and strengthen the bones. Commonly used formulas include Seven Pinches Powder (*qī lí sǎn*), Origin-Restorative Blood-Quickening Decoction (*fù yuán huó xuè tāng*), Sinew-Strengthening Blood-Nourishing Decoction (*zhuàng jīn yǎng xuè tāng*), and Bone-Righting Purple Gold Elixir (*zhèng gǔ zǐ jīn dān*), etc. Fractures and dislocations also require BONE RIGHTING treatment. See also INCISED WOUND; BLOOD STASIS; SPRAIN; BONE FRACTURE; DISLOCATION; INTERNAL INJURY. [26: 641] [97: 557] [61: 329]

L

lack of strength 乏力 *fá lì*, 无力 *wú lì*: A sign of qi vacuity.

lack of strength in the lumbus and knees 腰膝无力 *yāo xī wú lì*: LIMP LUMBUS AND KNEES.

lack of warmth in the extremities 四肢欠温 *sì zhī qiàn wēn*, 四肢不温 *sì zhī bù wēn*: Synonym: *cold extremities*. Mild cold in the extremities; a sign of general yang vacuity. Compare the more severe REVERSAL COLD OF THE EXTREMITIES. [6: 146] [92: No. 145]

lacquer bite 漆咬 *qī yǎo*: LACQUER SORE.

lacquer sore 漆疮 *qī chuāng*: Synonym: *lacquer bite*. A sore attributed to contact with lacquer sudden redness, swelling, heat, and itching, papules and blisters that when ruptured by scratching exude water and leave an eroded wound. In severe cases, if it spreads over the whole body, generalized signs such as physical cold, heat effusion, and headache are observed. WMC dermatitis rhus. Chinese lacquer is produced from *Rhus verniciflua*, which contains urushiol, a drastic skin-sensitizing agent that produces severe dermatitis in some people. MED Use Macule-Transforming Toxin-Resolving Decoction (*huà bān jiě dú tāng*) or Coptis Toxin-Resolving Decoction (*huáng lián jiě dú tāng*) plus lonicera (*jīn yín huā*), cicada molting (*chán tuì*), schizonepeta (*jīng jiè*), and flavescent sophora (*kǔ shēn*). For topical application, use a cooled decoction of equal proportions of spindle tree wings (*guǐ jiàn yǔ*), and raw sanguisorba (*shēng dì yú*), and sprinkle on Indigo Powder (*qīng dài sǎn*). [26: 822] [27: 476] [97: 628] [96: 274] [61: 371]

lacrimation 流泪 *liú lèi*: Also written as lachrymation. TEARING.

lai 癞 *lài*: 1. Leprosy. 2. Synonym: *lai sore*. SCAB (*jiè*) and LICHEN (*xiǎn*) etc., that lead to hair loss on the affected area. [48: 472]

lai great wind 癞大风 *lài dà fēng*: PESTILENTIAL WIND.

lai scalp sore 癞头疮 *lài tóu chuāng*: BALD WHITE SCALP SORE. [26: 989]

lai sore 癞疮 *lài chuāng*: LAI.

large intestinal cold bind 大肠寒结 *dà cháng hán jié*: Constipation due to cold qi in the large intestine and accompanied by dull abdominal pain, bland taste in the mouth, white tongue with scant fur, and a stringlike sunken pulse. MED Warm yang and free the stool. Use Pinellia and Sulfur

Pill (*bàn liú wán*) or Spleen-Warming Decoction (*wēn pí tāng*). For pronounced abdominal cold-pain, add cinnamon bark (*ròu guì*) and saussurea (*mù xiāng*), to warm yang, rectify qi, and relieve pain. If these formulas do not relieve constipation, tangkuei (*dāng guī*) and cistanche (*ròu cōng róng*) can be used to provide an acrid moistening stool-freeing action. ACU Base treatment mainly on alarm, lower uniting, and back transport points of LI, and on CV and SP. Select BL-25 (*dà cháng shū*, Large Intestine Transport), ST-25 (*tiān shū*, Celestial Pivot), ST-37 (*shàng jù xū*, Upper Great Hollow), TB-6 (*zhī gōu*, Branch Ditch), SP-6 (*sān yīn jiāo*, Three Yin Intersection), CV-4 (*guān yuán*, Pass Head)ⓜ, CV-6 (*qì hǎi*, Sea of Qi)ⓜ, and CV-8 (*shén què*, Spirit Gate Tower)ⓜ; needle with supplementation or with even supplementation and drainage, and add large amounts of moxa. [27: 163] [97: 23] [80: 364] [37: 325] [113: 102] [46: 670]

large intestinal cough 大肠咳 *dà cháng ké*: COUGH occurring in bouts that cause involuntary loss of urine. MED Use Center-Supplementing Qi-Boosting Decoction (*bǔ zhōng yì qì tāng*) minus cimicifuga (*shēng má*) and plus platycodon (*jié gěng*). See FIVE VISCERA AND SIX BOWELS COUGH. [27: 380] [97: 22]

large intestinal damp-heat 大肠湿热 *dà cháng shī rè*: Synonym: *damp-heat pouring down into the large intestine*; *downpour of damp-heat into the large intestine*. A disease pattern generally characterized by abdominal pain and diarrhea with ungratifying defecation and foul-smelling stool. An alternative pattern is dysentery characterized by frequent defecation and blood and pus in the stool, abdominal pain, tenesmus, and a burning sensation in the rectum. In both cases, general signs include heat effusion, bitter taste in the mouth, and a slimy yellow tongue fur. WMC colitis, dysentery. MED Clear heat and disinhibit dampness; resolve toxin. Use medicinals such as pulsatilla (*bái tóu wēng*), ash (*qín pí*), coptis (*huáng lián*), scutellaria (*huáng qín*), phellodendron (*huáng bǎi*), sanguisorba (*dì yú*), and purslane (*mǎ chǐ xiàn*). A basic formula is Pulsatilla Decoction (*bái tóu wēng tāng*). ACU Base treatment mainly on LI and ST. Select BL-25 (*dà cháng shū*, Large Intestine Transport), LI-4 (*hé gǔ*, Union Valley), LI-11 (*qū chí*, Pool at the Bend), ST-25 (*tiān shū*, Celestial Pivot), ST-37 (*shàng jù xū*, Upper Great Hollow), and ST-44 (*nèi tíng*, Inner Court); needle with drainage and add moxa. [6: 209] [27: 163] [97: 23] [26: 51] [116: 72] [57: 120]

large intestinal disease 大肠病 *dà cháng bìng*: Any morbidity of the large intestine. Large intestinal disease is attributable to evils such as heat, cold, stagnation, dampness, and wind, or to vacuity. Rumbling intestines or pain around the umbilicus, constipation or diarrhea, bloody stool or tenesmus with blood and pus in the stool, and prolapse of the rectum are signs of large intestinal disease. The main patterns are listed below. [26: 51]

Large Intestinal Disease Patterns

LARGE INTESTINAL VACUITY COLD (*dà cháng xū hán*)

LARGE INTESTINAL HUMOR DEPLETION (*dà cháng yè kuī*)

LARGE INTESTINAL DAMP-HEAT (*dà cháng shī rè*)

LARGE INTESTINAL HEAT BIND (*dà cháng rè jié*)

LARGE INTESTINAL COLD BIND (*dà cháng hán jié*)

large intestinal distention 大肠胀 *dà cháng zhàng*: A DISTENTION pattern described in *The Magic Pivot* (*líng shū, zhàng lùn*) as follows: "Large intestinal distention is rumbling intestines with pain. When cold evil is again contracted in winter, there is swill diarrhea containing untransformed food." Large intestinal distention may also be observed in distention disease patterns. MED Add large intestine channel medicinals such as angelica (*bái zhǐ*), cimicifuga (*shēng má*), scutellaria (*huáng qín*), and gypsum (*shí gāo*) to formulas for treating distention such as Magnolia Bark Center-Warming Decoction (*hòu pò wēn zhōng tāng*) combined with Stomach-Calming Poria (Hoelen) Five Decoction (*wèi líng tāng*) for cold-damp, and Center-Rectifying Decoction (*lǐ zhōng tāng*) or Magnolia Bark, Fresh Ginger, Pinellia, Licorice, and Ginseng Decoction (*hòu pò shēng jiāng bàn xià gān cǎo rén shēn tāng*) for vacuity cold. ACU Base treatment mainly on alarm, back transport, and lower uniting points of LI, and on CV and ST. Select BL-25 (*dà cháng shū*, Large Intestine Transport), ST-25 (*tiān shū*, Celestial Pivot), ST-37 (*shàng jù xū*, Upper Great Hollow), CV-12 (*zhōng wǎn*, Center Stomach Duct), CV-6 (*qì hǎi*, Sea of Qi), PC-6 (*nèi guān*, Inner Pass), and ST-36 (*zú sān lǐ*, Leg Three Li); needle with even supplementation and drainage and moxa. [26: 51] [46: 602]

large intestinal heat bind 大肠热结 *dà cháng rè jié*: EVIL HEAT in the large intestine causing the stool to become dry and hard; characterized by constipation, abdominal pain that refuses pressure, dry yellow tongue fur, and a sunken replete pulse.

Large intestinal heat bind is seen in externally contracted heat (febrile) disease manifesting as yang brightness bowel repletion patterns (corresponding to qi-aspect patterns in the warm disease school). ACU Base treatment mainly on alarm, back transport, and lower uniting points of LI, and on ST and LI. Select BL-25 (*dà cháng shū*, Large Intestine Transport), ST-25 (*tiān shū*, Celestial Pivot), ST-37 (*shàng jù xū*, Upper Great Hollow), LI-4 (*hé gǔ*, Union Valley), LI-11 (*qū chí*, Pool at the Bend), SP-14 (*fù jié*, Abdominal Bind), and KI-6 (*zhào hǎi*, Shining Sea); needle with drainage. [26: 51] [46: 670] [113: 102] [37: 326]

large intestinal humor depletion 大肠液亏 *dà cháng yè kuī*: Synonyms: *intestinal humor depletion; large intestinal liquid depletion; large intestinal yin vacuity dryness bind*. A disease pattern of the large intestine caused by general lack of liquid and blood in the body. Large intestinal humor depletion is observed in postpartum blood vacuity, liquid depletion in the aged, and in enduring and severe diseases. It may also occur in externally contracted heat (febrile) disease prior to replenishment of the fluids. Signs comprise dry hard stool and difficult defecation. Generally, no pronounced abdominal distention or pain is observed. The patient is in a weak state of health. ACU Base treatment mainly on back transport points, SP, ST, and KI. Select BL-17 (*gé shū*, Diaphragm Transport), BL-20 (*pí shū*, Spleen Transport), BL-21 (*wèi shū*, Stomach Transport), BL-25 (*dà cháng shū*, Large Intestine Transport), SP-6 (*sān yīn jiāo*, Three Yin Intersection), ST-36 (*zú sān lǐ*, Leg Three Li), and KI-6 (*zhào hǎi*, Shining Sea); needle with supplementation, and moxa, if necessary. For large intestinal humor depletion occurring in externally contracted heat (febrile) disease, add LI-4 (*hé gǔ*, Union Valley), LI-11 (*qū chí*, Pool at the Bend), and GV-14 (*dà zhuī*, Great Hammer), [26: 51] [27: 163] [37: 328] [46: 670]

large intestinal vacuity 大肠虚 *dà cháng xū*: Large intestinal qi vacuity; characterized by enduring diarrhea, nontransformation of food, pale stool without malodor, rumbling intestines, and prolapse of the anus. It usually takes the form of LARGE INTESTINAL VACUITY COLD. [27: 163] [97: 23]

large intestinal vacuity cold 大肠虚寒 *dà cháng xū hán*: Vacuity cold affecting the large intestine's governing of conveyance. Large intestinal vacuity cold is usually associated with spleen-kidney yang vacuity, and is characterized thin diarrhea, reduced food intake, cold of the limbs, aching lumbus, aversion to cold, thin tongue fur, and a fine sunken pulse. WMC This pattern is often observed in chronic enteritis or chronic dysentery. ACU Base treatment mainly on alarm, back transport, lower uniting points of LI, and on CV and ST. Select BL-25 (*dà cháng shū,* Large Intestine Transport), ST-25 (*tiān shū,* Celestial Pivot), ST-37 (*shàng jù xū,* Upper Great Hollow), CV-12 (*zhōng wǎn,* Center Stomach Duct), LR-13 (*zhāng mén,* Camphorwood Gate), ST-36 (*zú sān lǐ,* Leg Three Li), and CV-6 (*qì hǎi,* Sea of Qi); needle with supplementation and moxa. For spleen-kidney yang vacuity, add BL-20 (*pí shū,* Spleen Transport), BL-23 (*shèn shū,* Kidney Transport), CV-4 (*guān yuán,* Pass Head), and GV-4 (*mìng mén,* Life Gate). **Comparison:** Spleen and stomach and the large and small intestine are all part of the digestive tract. Spleen-stomach yang vacuity and large intestinal vacuity cold are similar, but slightly different. The stomach is the sea of the grain and water; when spleen-stomach yang fail to take in food, decompose, move and transform it, the stool is sloppy and thin and contains undigested food; at the same time there is poor appetite, glomus and oppression in the stomach duct and abdomen after eating, signs that the disease is in the center burner. In large intestinal vacuity cold, by contrast, the disease in the lower burner; diarrhea and rumbling intestines are pronounced, and there may be constipation instead of diarrhea. There is no reduction in appetite and no oppression in the stomach duct after eating. [27: 163] [27: 1163] [97: 23] [57: 123] [91: 196] [46: 666]

large intestinal welling-abscess 大肠痈 *dà cháng yōng:* WELLING-ABSCESS (*yōng*) of the large intestine; an intestinal welling-abscess characterized by pain at ST-25 (*tiān shū,* Celestial Pivot). See INTESTINAL WELLING-ABSCESS. [27: 461]

large intestinal yin vacuity dryness bind 大肠阴虚燥结 *dà cháng yīn xū zào jié:* LARGE INTESTINAL HUMOR DEPLETION.

large intestine 大肠 *dà cháng,* 回肠 *huí cháng:* One of the SIX BOWELS; an organ that stands in exterior-interior relationship with the lung, and whose function is to receive waste passed down from the small intestine and then form it into stool before discharging it from the body. Thus, the large intestine is said to govern transformation and conveyance of waste. Since it absorbs further fluid from the waste, it is also said to govern liquid. Diseases of the large intestine commonly manifest as diarrhea, dry stool, or constipation. See LARGE INTESTINAL DISEASE. [97: 21]

large intestine channel 大肠经 *dà cháng jīng:* HAND YANG BRIGHTNESS LARGE INTESTINE CHANNEL. [26: 51]

large intestine governs conveyance 大肠主传导 *dà cháng zhǔ chuán dǎo:* LARGE INTESTINE HOLDS THE OFFICE OF CONVEYANCE, WHENCE MUTATION EMANATES.

large intestine governs liquid 大肠主津 *dà cháng zhǔ jīn:* The large intestine is said to govern liquid because it absorbs fluid from the food waste to form it into firm stool. [6: 87]

large intestine governs transformation and conveyance of waste 大肠主传化糟粕 *dà cháng zhǔ chuán huà zāo pò:* From *Elementary Questions* (*sù wèn*). The large intestine conveys waste downward and out of the body, transforming it into stool as it does so. See LARGE INTESTINE HOLDS THE OFFICE OF CONVEYANCE, WHENCE MUTATION EMANATES. [27: 52] [97: 24]

large intestine holds the office of conveyance, whence mutation emanates 大肠者，传导之官也，变化出焉 *dà cháng zhě, chuán dǎo zhī guān yě, biàn huà chū yān:* From *Elementary Questions* (*sù wèn, líng lán mì diǎn lùn*). The large intestine takes the waste passed on from the small intestine, and conveys it downward to the anus, further transforming it as it does so. Statements such as *large intestine governs transformation and conveyance of waste* and *large intestine governs conveyance* derive from this. [27: 52]

large pulse 大脉 *dà mài:* A broad pulse, i.e., the opposite of a fine pulse. Compare SURGING PULSE. [27: 196] [97: 21]

laryngeal prominence 结喉 *jié hóu:* Adam's apple.

larynx 喉 *hóu:* The lower part of the throat. WMC laryngeal part of the pharynx. Compare PHARYNX; THROAT. [27: 29]

lassitude of spirit 神疲 *shén pí:* See next entry.

lassitude of spirit and lack of strength 神疲乏力 *shén pí fá lì:* Synonym: *fatigued spirit and lack of strength.* Lack of mental vigor and physical strength. A principal sign of qi vacuity.

last flicker of the lamp 残灯复明 *cán dēng fù míng:* The final flaring of an oil lamp when, after the oil has run out, the flame burns briefly on the wick; a metaphor for the sudden brief regaining of vigor before death in certain critical conditions. See LAST RADIANCE OF THE SETTING SUN.

last radiance of the setting sun 回光反照 *huí guāng fǎn zhào:* A brief brightening of the sky after the sun's descent below the horizon; a metaphor for a sudden brief strengthening of the spirit before death; it means the same as LAST FLICKER OF THE LAMP. See FALSE SPIRITEDNESS.

late afternoon tidal heat [effusion] 日晡（所）潮热 *rì bū (suǒ) cháo rè:* Heat effusion that becomes higher at the Late Afternoon watch, i.e., 3-5 p.m.; one form of POSTMERIDIAN TIDAL HEAT [EFFUSION]. See TIDAL HEAT [EFFUSION]. [26: 135] [27: 365] [97: 89]

late emergence 晚发 *wǎn fā:* Latent qi warm disease. (1) A warm disease attributable to contraction of cold in the winter and emerging in the new year between Pure Brightness (5th solar term) and Summer Solstice (10th solar term). (2) Warm disease attributed to contraction of summerheat-damp in the summer that, after remaining latent in the interior, is made to emerge in the autumn by a newly contracted evil. [26: 635] [27: 355] [97: 520]

latent 伏 *fú*: Present but not visible or active. [48: 79]

latent qi 伏气 *fú qì*: Any evil qi that remains latent in the body and that causes disease after some time. [26: 273]

latent qi warm disease 伏气温病 *fú qì wēn bìng*: Any warm disease attributable to external evil that has lain latent and brewed in the interior for some time or internal heat that is made to emerge by a new contraction. *Elementary Questions (sù wèn, yīn yáng yìng xiàng dà lùn)* mentions such diseases in the following terms: "Damage by cold in winter inevitably gives rise to warm disease in the spring." Latent qi warm disease differs from exterior patterns of initial contractions in that they are associated with pronounced signs of internal heat or transformation into dryness and scorching of yin, and manifest as qi or blood aspect patterns. Signs include a fine rapid pulse or a sunken rapid agitated pulse, a thick slimy tongue fur, or a red tongue without fur, reddish urine, thirst, and heat effusion. MED Clear interior heat, paying attention to the need to safeguard the fluids. See WARM DISEASE; SPRING WARMTH; WARM MALARIA; LATE EMERGENCE. [26: 274] [27: 345] [97: 205]

latent summerheat 伏暑 *fú shǔ*: A disease in the autumn attributable to summerheat-damp evil contracted in the summer lying latent in the body. [26: 275]

Later Han 后汉 *hòu hàn*: The name of a dynasty (A.D. 25–220).

later heaven 后天 *hòu tiān*: That in an individual's makeup which is determined after conception; the acquired constitution. Later heaven is considered to be governed by the spleen and stomach, which as the source of engendering transformation produce from food what is required for the growth of the body and maintenance of its activities. ◇ Chin 后 *hòu*, after, later; 天 *tiān*, heaven, i.e., that upon which life depends. [27: 45]

Later Jin 后晋 *hòu jìn*: The name of a dynasty (936–946 A.D.).

Later Liang 后梁 *hòu liáng*: The name of a dynasty (907–923 A.D.).

Later Tang 后唐 *hòu táng*: The name of a dynasty (923–936 A.D.).

Later Zhou 后周 *hòu zhōu*: The name of a dynasty (951–960 A.D.).

latrine bleeding 圊血 *qīng xuè*: Bloody stool.

laziness to speak 懒言 *lǎn yán*: Reduced frequency of speech and lack of vigor in enunciation reflecting general weakness due to qi vacuity.

leaking roof pulse 屋漏脉 *wū lòu mài*: See SEVEN STRANGE PULSES. [27: 199] [27: 199] [97: 46]

leaking sweat 漏汗 *lòu hàn*: One form of GREAT SWEATING. Great sweating that results from inappropriate sweating treatment. *On Cold Damage (shāng hán lùn, biàn tài yáng bìng mài zhèng bìng zhì)* states, "In greater yang (*tài yáng*) disease, when sweat-effusing treatment causes incessant leaking [of sweat], and causes the patient to have aversion to cold, difficult urination, and slight tension in the four limbs making stretching difficult, this is treated with Cinnamon Twig Decoction (*guì zhī tāng*) plus aconite (*fù zǐ*)." The term sweat leak was subsequently coined from this. Incessant leaking of sweat can lead to external desertion of yang qi and internal desertion of yin humor, causing short scant voidings of urine, hypertonicity, or even jerking sinews and twitching flesh; it is treated by supporting yang and securing the exterior using Cinnamon Twig Decoction Plus Aconite (*guì zhī jiā fù zǐ tāng*) or True Warrior Decoction (*zhēn wǔ tāng*). ACU Base treatment mainly on LI, SI, and BL. Select LI-4 (*hé gǔ*, Union Valley), SI-3 (*hòu xī*, Back Ravine), HT-6 (*yīn xī*, Yin Cleft), BL-13 (*fèi shū*, Lung Transport), GB-20 (*fēng chí*, Wind Pool), BL-64 (*jīng gǔ*, Capital Bone), BL-62 (*shēn mài*, Extending Vessel), and ST-36 (*zú sān lǐ*, Leg Three Li); needle with supplementation and moxa. [26: 823] [46: 602] [113: 18] [75: 47]

leaky shoulder wind 漏肩风 *lòu jiān fēng*: Synonyms: *fifty-year-old's shoulder; frozen shoulder*. Pain and reduced movement in the shoulder. Leaky shoulder wind is attributed to excessive fatigue creating vacuity that wind-cold exploits to enter the body; hence the name "leaky shoulder wind." In accordance with the observation made in *The Inner Canon (nèi jīng)* that cold is associated with contracture and tautness, the wind-cold invades the sinews and vessels, causing qi and blood to stagnate; hence the popular English name "frozen shoulder" accords with the pathomechanism described by the Chinese. Since is most common in people of approximately 50 years old, it is often called fifty-year-olds' shoulder. ACU Base treatment mainly on three yang channels of the hand. Select LI-15 (*jiān yú*, Shoulder Bone), SI-9 (*jiān zhēn*, True Shoulder), LI-14 (*bì nào*, Upper Arm), LI-11 (*qū chí*, Pool at the Bend), LI-4 (*hé gǔ*, Union Valley), and ST-38 (*tiáo kǒu*, Ribbon Opening); needle with drainage. Selection of points according to causes: For prevalence of wind, add GB-20 (*fēng chí*, Wind Pool), TB-5 (*wài guān*, Outer Pass), and LU-7 (*liè quē*, Broken Sequence). For prevalence of cold, add TB-14 (*jiān liáo*, Shoulder Bone-Hole) and SI-10 (*nào shū*, Upper Arm Transport), using warm needle (burning moxa on needles) or moxa on ginger. For prevalence of dampness, add SP-9 (*yīn líng quán*, Yin Mound Spring) and ST-36 (*zú sān lǐ*, Leg Three Li). Selection of points according to location: For pain on the greater yin (*tài yīn*) channel, add LU-5 (*chǐ zé*, Cubit Marsh) and SP-9 (*yīn líng quán*, Yin Mound Spring). For pain on the yang brightness (*yáng míng*) or lesser yang (*shào yáng*), add ST-36 (*zú sān lǐ*, Leg Three Li) and GB-34 (*yáng líng quán*, Yang Mound Spring). For pain on the greater yang (*tài yáng*) channel, add SI-3 (*hòu xī*, Back Ravine) and ST-38 (*tiáo kǒu*, Ribbon Opening) joining BL-57 (*chéng shān*, Mountain Support). ◇ Chin 漏 *lòu*, leak; 肩 *jiān*, shoulder; 风 *fēng*, wind. [46: 631]

lean cold gan 瘦冷疳 *shòu lěng gān*: See COLD-HEAT GAN.

leaven 麹 *qū*, 麴 *qú*: MEDICATED LEAVEN.

leg-flexing intestinal welling-abscess 缩脚肠痈 *suō jiǎo cháng yōng*: An INTESTINAL WELLING-ABSCESS (*cháng yōng*) attended by severe pain causing the patient to keep his leg bent. [27: 461]

leg-flexing streaming sore 缩脚流注 *suō jiǎo liú zhù*: A streaming sore occurring in the iliac fossa and causing hypertonicity of the sinews on the affected side that prevents movement and pain and discomfort that is partly relieved by flexing the leg; hence the name. A lump can be felt in the iliac fossa, which ripples under the fingers when pus has formed. There is no change in skin color. Other signs may include heat effusion, aversion to cold, absence of sweating or presence of slight sweating, and reduced eating. [WMC] abscess of the iliac fossa. See SUMMERHEAT-DAMP STREAMING SORE; STREAMING SORE. [26: 946] [27: 571] [97: 633]

leg-hoisting sand 吊脚痧 *diào jiǎo shā*: CHOLERA CRAMPS. [26: 259]

leg pain 腿痛 *tuǐ tòng*: Pain in the upper or lower leg. Leg pain is mostly attributable to wind-cold-damp and sometimes to damp-heat; less commonly, it is a sign of a DAMP PHLEGM STREAMING SORE. **Wind-cold-damp** leg pain is due to wind-cold-damp with prevalence of cold and manifests in severe pain (sometimes accompanied by numbness and swelling) and aversion to cold and desire for warmth. [MED] Warm and dissipate with Ovate Atractylodes and Aconite Decoction (*bái zhú fù zǐ tāng*). [ACU] Base treatment mainly on CV, SP, ST, and GB. Select GB-20 (*fēng chí*, Wind Pool), BL-23 (*shèn shū*, Kidney Transport), CV-4 (*guān yuán*, Pass Head), ST-36 (*zú sān lǐ*, Leg Three Li), SP-9 (*yīn líng quán*, Yin Mound Spring), and

SP-6 (*sān yīn jiāo*, Three Yin Intersection), according to the area affected, add GB-31 (*fēng shì*, Wind Market), ST-32 (*fú tù*, Crouching Rabbit), BL-40 (*wěi zhōng*, Bend Center), and GB-34 (*yáng líng quán*, Yang Mound Spring), for upper leg, and GB-34 (*yáng líng quán*, Yang Mound Spring), BL-57 (*chéng shān*, Mountain Support), GB-39 (*xuán zhōng*, Suspended Bell), BL-60 (*kūn lún*, Kunlun Mountains), and GB-40 (*qiū xū*, Hill Ruins), for the lower leg; needle with drainage and moxa. For prevalence of cold, warm-needle GV-4 (*mìng mén*, Life Gate), and apply moxa at CV-8 (*shén què*, Spirit Gate Tower). **Damp-heat** leg pain is characterized by pain in either the upper or lower leg often with redness, swelling, and heat, and accompanied by reddish urine. [MED] Clear heat and transform dampness with Tangkuei Pain-Assuaging Decoction (*dāng guī niān tòng tāng*). Wind, cold, dampness or other evils invading in yin vacuity, yang vacuity, or kidney vacuity requires treatment that takes account of the vacuity. [ACU] Base treatment mainly on SP, LI, and ST. Select ST-36 (*zú sān lǐ*, Leg Three Li), ST-41 (*jiě xī*, Ravine Divide), SP-9 (*yīn líng quán*, Yin Mound Spring), LI-11 (*qū chí*, Pool at the Bend), ST-44 (*nèi tíng*, Inner Court), SP-5 (*shāng qiū*, Shang Hill), and GV-14 (*dà zhuī*, Great Hammer); needle with drainage. For selection of points according to the area affected, see wind-cold-damp above. See IMPEDIMENT (*bì*). [26: 851] [46: 597, 629] [37: 364]

leg qi 脚气 *jiǎo qì*: A disease characterized by numbness, pain, limpness, and in some cases any of a variety of possible signs such as hypertonicity or swelling, withering, redness and swelling of the calf, heat effusion, and in advanced stages by abstraction of spirit-mind, heart palpitations, panting, oppression in the chest, nausea and vomiting, and deranged speech. Leg qi arises when externally contracted damp evil and wind toxin or accumulating dampness due to damage by excessive consumption of rich food engenders heat and pours down into the legs. Chest and abdominal signs are attributed to leg qi surging into the heart. [WMC] beriberi (attributed to vitamin B_1 deficiency). [MED] Treat primarily by diffusing congestion and expelling dampness and secondarily by dispelling wind and clearing heat. Formulas such as Cockcrow Powder (*jī míng sǎn*) can be used. Different forms include DAMP LEG QI, DRY LEG QI, COLD-DAMP LEG QI, DAMP PHLEGM LEG QI, and LEG QI SURGING INTO THE HEART. [26: 648] [97: 523]

leg qi attacking the heart 脚气攻心 *jiǎo qì gōng xīn*: LEG QI SURGING INTO THE HEART. [26: 648]

leg qi entering the heart 脚气入心 *jiǎo qì rù xīn*: LEG QI SURGING INTO THE HEART. [26: 648]

leg qi surging into the heart 脚气冲心 *jiǎo qì chōng xīn*: Synonym: *leg qi attacking the heart; leg qi entering the heart.* LEG QI manifesting in heart palpitations, panting, nausea and vomiting, and, in severe cases, by abstraction and deranged speech. Leg qi surging into the heart is attributed to evil toxin ascending to attack the heart and chest. [MED] When attributable to damp toxin attacking upward damaging yang, treat by warming yang and dissipating cold and by expelling dampness and discharging toxin with Evodia Decoction (*wú zhū yú tāng*) plus pinellia (*bàn xià*), aconite (*fù zǐ*), asarum (*xì xīn*), dried ginger (*gān jiāng*), shaved cinnamon bark (*guì xīn*), and licorice (*gān cǎo*). When attributable to damp-fire attacking upward, treat by diffusing congestion and expelling dampness and by cooling the blood and clearing fire with Evodia Decoction (*wú zhū yú tāng*) combined with Bovine Bezoar Heart-Clearing Pill (*niú huáng qīng xīn wán*). [ACU] Base treatment on SP, ST, and PC. Select PC-6 (*nèi guān*, Inner Pass), CV-14 (*jù què*, Great Tower Gate), PC-8 (*láo gōng*, Palace of Toil), ST-36 (*zú sān lǐ*, Leg Three Li), SP-9 (*yīn líng quán*, Yin Mound Spring), KI-1 (*yǒng quán*, Gushing Spring), and LU-5 (*chǐ zé*, Cubit Marsh); needle with drainage. Selection of points according to signs: For heart palpitations, add PC-4 (*xī mén*, Cleft Gate). For panting, add CV-17 (*shān zhōng*, Chest Center) and Panting Stabilizer (*dìng chuǎn*). For vomiting, add CV-12 (*zhōng wǎn*, Center Stomach Duct). For clouded spirit, add GV-26 (*shuǐ gōu*, Water Trough). For vacuity desertion, moxa CV-6 (*qì hǎi*, Sea of Qi) and CV-4 (*guān yuán*, Pass Head). [26: 648] [46: 669]

leprosy 疠风 *lì fēng*, 大麻风 *dà má fēng*, 麻风 *má fēng*, 大风 *dà fēng*, 大风恶疾 *dà fēng è jí*, 癞大风 *lài dà fēng*: PESTILENTIAL WIND. [61: 312]

lesser abdomen 少腹 *shào fù*: **1.** The lateral lower abdomen, i.e., sides of the smaller abdomen. **2.** The smaller abdomen. [27: 58] [97: 87]

lesser-abdominal pain 少腹痛 *shào fù tòng*: **1.** SMALLER-ABDOMINAL PAIN. **2.** Pain in the abdomen below the umbilicus on either the left, right or both sides. It is due to cold stagnating in the liver channel, binding depression of liver qi, large intestinal damp-heat or lower burner vacuity cold. **Cold stagnating in the liver channel** causes lesser-abdominal pain stretching into the testicles. The pain is acute with sagging distention. In some cases the scrotum retracts. The pain is exacerbated by cold and slightly relieved by heat. Other signs include bright white facial complexion, physical cold and cold limbs, a white glossy tongue fur, and a sunken slippery string-like pulse. [MED] Warm and dissipate liver channel cold. Use Tangkuei Counterflow Cold Decoc-

tion (*dāng guī sì nì tāng*) plus evodia (*wú zhū yú*) and fresh ginger (*shēng jiāng*). **Binding depression of liver qi** causes qi stagnation in the lesser abdomen with pain stretching into the testicles. The pain is fluctuating and intermittent, and is brought on by emotional stimulus or excessive exertion. Alternatively, in the lesser abdomen or to the side of the umbilicus there is a lump that gathers and dissipates at irregular intervals and that is associated with periodic acute, even unbearable, distending pain exacerbated by pressure. [MED] Course the liver and rectify qi. Use Bupleurum Liver-Coursing Powder (*chái hú shū gān sǎn*) plus toosendan (*chuān liàn zǐ*), fennel (*huí xiāng*), psoralea (*bǔ gǔ zhī*), and fenugreek (*hú lú bā*). **Large intestinal damp-heat** causing lesser-abdominal pain occurs in dysentery with stool containing pus and blood, tenesmus, and thirst with desire to drink. [MED] Clear heat, disinhibit dampness; quicken the blood and relieve pain. Pulsatilla Decoction (*bái tóu wēng tāng*). **Lower burner vacuity cold** causes continuous lesser abdominal pain, usually more severe on the left side, together with a bright white facial complexion, fatigue and lack of strength, physical cold and fear of cold, and lack of warmth in the extremities. Other signs include vomiting or diarrhea. The tongue is pale with white fur, and the pulse is stringlike and slow. Lower burner vacuity cold, like liver channel qi stagnation, causes cold pain. However, in lower burner qi vacuity, the liver viscus is affected rather than the liver channel, and instead of pain stretching into the testicles, there is vomiting or diarrhea. [MED] Warm and dissipate cold in the liver viscus. Use Evodia Decoction (*wú zhū yú tāng*). [92: No. 203]

lesser fire 少火 *shào huǒ*: From *Elementary Questions* (*sù wèn, yīn yáng yìng xiàng dà lùn*). The healthy fire (i.e., yang qi) of the body that maintains life; it is distinct from *vigorous fire*, which is pathological fire. The lesser fire is probably so named because in a healthy body it is yang contained by yin. [27: 59]

lesser yang 少阳 *shào yáng*: The hand lesser yang (*shào yáng*) triple burner and foot lesser yang gallbladder channels. "Lesser" implies the waning of yang. The lesser yang is between the greater yang (*tài yáng*) and yang brightness (*yáng míng*); hence it is said that the lesser yang is the pivot. The lesser yang has copious qi and scant blood. See OPENING, CLOSING, AND PIVOT. [26: 148] [27: 91] [50: 228]

lesser yang channel 少阳经 *shào yáng jīng*: See LESSER YANG.

lesser yang disease 少阳病 *shào yáng bìng*: Synonym: *midstage pattern.* Disease of the hand lesser yang (*shào yáng*) triple burner and the foot lesser yang (*shào yáng*) gallbladder channels. Because the lesser yang is located between the greater yang (*tài yáng*) and yang brightness (*yáng míng*), lesser yang disease is often referred to as a *midstage disease pattern*. The essential signs are alternating heat [effusion] and [aversion to] cold, chest and rib-side pain and fullness, bitter taste in the mouth, and vomiting. Other signs include no desire for food and drink, heart vexation, desire to vomit, dizzy vision, painful hard glomus under the rib-side, and a stringlike pulse. Lesser yang disease occurs when, owing to debilitation of right qi, an evil invades the body through the interstices and binds in the gallbladder, impeding qi dynamic and disrupting upbearing and downbearing. Bitter fullness in the chest and rib-side is explained by the lesser yang gallbladder channel that traverses this area. Alternating heat effusion and aversion to cold are explained by the struggle between the evil and right. Heart vexation, bitter taste in the mouth, dry pharynx, dizzy vision, as well as vomiting and no desire for food and drink, are the result of gallbladder heat rising counterflow up the channel, disturbing the harmony and downbearing of stomach qi. A stringlike pulse is classically associated with the gallbladder. Lesser yang disease is different from greater yang and yang brightness, lying midway between the two. Greater yang disease can pass to both yang brightness and lesser yang. Lesser yang disease may resolve in an exterior pattern through a constant sweat, or may pass to the yang brightness to form an interior pattern. It may pass to the yin channels, causing vacuity patterns. Consequently, lesser yang disease is commonly termed a midstage pattern. However, it may occur in combination with an exterior pattern characterized by heat effusion, aversion to cold, and vexing pain in the joints of the limbs, or with a yang brightness interior pattern characterized by abdominal fullness and constipation. MED Lesser yang is treated by the method of harmonization and resolution. This involves outthrusting the evil and clearing the interior, and regulating qi dynamic, in accordance with the principle of supporting right and dispelling evil. The chief formula used is Minor Bupleurum Decoction (*xiǎo chái hú tāng*). However, where an exterior pattern is also present, causing a greater yang and lesser yang combination, sweat-effusing action is needed. In such cases, Bupleurum and Cinnamon Twig Decoction (*chái hú guì zhī tāng*) is used. Where an interior pattern is present, forming a lesser yang and yang brightness combination, an appropriate formula is Major Bupleurum Decoction (*dà chái hú tāng*), which possesses an additional precipitant effect. [6: 227] [27: 219] [97: 87]

lesser yang headache 少阳头痛 *shào yáng tóu tòng*: 1. HEADACHE occurring yin lesser yang

(*shào yáng*) disease in cold damage, i.e., attended by alternative heat effusion and aversion to cold, and a rapid stringlike pulse. MED Treat with Minor Bupleurum Decoction (*xiǎo chái hú tāng*) and variations. ACU Select TB-4 (*yáng chí*, Yang Pool), GB-40 (*qiū xū*, Hill Ruins), GB-20 (*fēng chí*, Wind Pool), and GV-16 (*fēng fǔ*, Wind Mansion). 2. HEADACHE on the pathway of the lesser yang (*shào yáng*), i.e., the corners of the head or temples. MED Use formulas with bupleurum (*chái hú*) as the conductor. ACU Select Greater Yang (*tài yáng*), GB-8 (*shuài gǔ*, Valley Lead), TB-2 (*yè mén*, Humor Gate), and GB-43 (*xiá xī*, Pinched Ravine). See HEADACHE. [113: 9] [4: 154]

lesser yin 少阴 *shào yīn*: The hand lesser yin (*shào yīn*) heart and foot lesser yin kidney channels. "Lesser" implies a waning of yin qi. The lesser yin is said to have copious qi and scant blood. The lesser yin is located between the greater yin (*tài yīn*) and reverting yin (*jué yīn*); hence it is said "lesser yin is the pivot." See OPENING, CLOSING, AND PIVOT. [26: 148] [27: 91] [97: 86]

lesser yin channel 少阴经 *shào yīn jīng*: See LESSER YIN.

lesser yin disease 少阴病 *shào yīn bìng*: Disease of the foot lesser yin (*shào yīn*) kidney channel and the hand lesser yin (*shào yīn*) heart channel. Lesser yin disease arises when the heart and kidney are vacuous, and there is a marked drop in resistance to disease. It takes two different forms, vacuity cold and vacuity heat. **Vacuity cold:** Cold evil damages yang qi, and the main form is a vacuity cold pattern that manifests as aversion to cold, curled-up lying posture, somnolence, reversal cold of the limbs, and faint fine pulse. Clear-food diarrhea may occur in some cases. Generally there is no heat effusion, and, in severe cases, the limbs may suffer a drop in temperature, indicated yang collapse vacuity desertion. In *On Cold Damage* (*shāng hán lùn*), the section on lesser yin disease is headed with the statement, "The patient has a faint fine pulse, and desires only to sleep." A faint fine pulse indicates vacuity of qi and blood, and desire only for sleep indicates debilitation of the spirit. These are both signs of general vacuity. Wherever a faint fine pulse occurs, whether in disease of recent onset or enduring disease, thought should be given to the possibility of lesser yin disease. Absence of heat effusion, aversion to cold, curled-up lying posture, and reversal cold of the limbs occurring with such a pulse indicate the presence of exuberant internal cold and the inability of debilitated yang to warm and nourish the skin and muscle and fully permeate the limbs, thereby confirming the presence of lesser yin disease. Clear-food diarrhea is explained by kidney vacuity affecting the spleen (spleen-kidney yang vacuity), causing failure to move and transform food. Great sweating, reversal cold in the limbs, and a faint pulse verging on expiration indicate fulminant desertion of yang qi. MED This type of lesser yin disease pattern is treated by the method of returning yang and stemming counterflow, and the main formula is Counterflow Cold Decoction (*sì nì tāng*), which can be varied to suit different patterns. Where vacuity is predominant, ginseng (*rén shēn*) may be added; where cold is predominant, dried ginger (*gān jiāng*) can be increased in quantity. Where exuberant yin repels yang, pig's bile may be added. Patterns that include signs of water qi may be treated with True Warrior Decoction (*zhēn wǔ tāng*), a standard variant of Counterflow Cold Decoction. **Vacuity heat:** Rarely, a transmuted lesser yin pattern of vacuity heat may be observed. Insufficiency of kidney yin and heart fire flaming upward causes signs such as heart vexation, insomnia, and dry pharynx and mouth. *On Cold Damage* (*shāng hán lùn*) provides little detail concerning this second pattern, although clinical observation shows that a red or crimson tongue, and a rapid pulse that is either fine or vacuous are determining signs. This form of lesser yin disease is treated by enriching yin and clearing heat, the main formula being Coptis and Ass Hide Glue Decoction (*huáng lián ē jiāo tāng*). [6: 228] [27: 219] [97: 87]

lesser yin headache 少阴头痛 *shào yīn tóu tòng*: HEADACHE attributed to cold evil invading the lesser yin (*shào yīn*). Lesser yin headache is attended by cold legs and qi counterflow, heart pain, vexation and oppression, and fine sunken pulse. MED Warm the channels and dispel cold using formulas such as Ephedra, Aconite, and Asarum Decoction (*má huáng fù zǐ xì xīn tāng*) and variations. ACU Base treatment mainly on GV, KI, and CV. Select GV-20 (*bǎi huì*, Hundred Convergences), BL-23 (*shèn shū*, Kidney Transport), CV-4 (*guān yuán*, Pass Head), GV-4 (*mìng mén*, Life Gate), KI-3 (*tài xī*, Great Ravine), and KI-1 (*yǒng quán*, Gushing Spring). Needle with supplementation and add moxa. For heart pain with vexation and oppression, add HT-7 (*shén mén*, Spirit Gate) and BL-15 (*xīn shū*, Heart Transport). See HEADACHE. [26: 148]

LI 大肠 *dà cháng*, 手阳明大肠经 *shǒu yáng míng dà cháng jīng*: The large intestine or large intestine channel.

Liang 梁 *liáng*: The name of a dynasty (502–557 A.D.).

liang 两 *liǎng*: *Synonym:* tael. A unit of weight traditionally equal to one sixteenth of a JIN, now equal to 31.25 g. It is divided into 10 qian and 100 fen. See tables 21 and 23, page 717.

Liao 辽 *liáo*: The name of a dynasty (916–1125 A.D.).

lichen 癣 *xiǎn*: A skin disease characterized by elevation of the skin, serous discharge, scaling, and itching. Lichen is associated with wind, heat, and dampness. Lichen characterized by dryness and scaling of the skin is called DRY LICHEN, whereas lichen that exudes a discharge is called DAMP LICHEN. A number of specific forms exist. An itchy lichen around the nail that causes it to lose its luster and become deformed is ASHEN NAIL. Lichen of the foot characterized by itching and scaling of the skin between the toes is traditionally called FOOT DAMP QI in Chinese medicine; in China, it is now commonly known as *Hong Kong foot*, and in the West as *athlete's foot*. Other forms of lichen include: COIN LICHEN, characterized by clearly circumscribed red macules that often heal from the center; OXHIDE LICHEN, marked by thickening and hardening of the skin, like the skin on the neck of an ox; PINE BARK LICHEN, a scaling lichen that looks like pine bark; SUCKLING LICHEN, a popular lichen in infants affecting the head and face and capable of spreading to other parts of the body; YIN LICHEN is a lichen affecting the anterior and posterior yin, i.e., the anus and genitals, and surrounding areas and attributed to wind-heat-damp invading the skin. Furthermore, PURPLE AND WHITE PATCH WIND, GOOSE-FOOT WIND, BALD SCALP SORE, and FAT SORE are also classified in some modern sources as lichen. ◇ Chin 癣 *xiǎn*, is 藓 *xiǎn*, lichen, moss, with the grass signifier replaced with a sickness classifier to denote a pathological "lichen" on the body. NB: 'Lichen' is here not to be confused with same term as used Western medicine. [96: 258]

Lichen

BLOWN BLOSSOM LICHEN (*chuī huā xiǎn*)
COIN LICHEN (*yuán xiǎn*)
DAMP LICHEN (*shī xiǎn*)
FETAL LICHEN (*tāi xiǎn*)
OXHIDE LICHEN (*niú pí xiǎn*)
PEACH-BLOSSOM LICHEN (*tāo huā xiǎn*)
PINE BARK LICHEN (*sōng pí xiǎn*)
SUCKLING LICHEN (*nǎi xiǎn*)
THROAT LICHEN (*hóu xiǎn*)
WIND LICHEN (*fēng xiǎn*)
YIN LICHEN (*yīn xiǎn*)
YIN VACUITY THROAT LICHEN (*yīn vacuity hóu xiǎn*)

life bar 命关 *mìng guān*: One of the three bars of the finger. See INFANT'S FINGER EXAMINATION. [26: 396]

life fire 命火 *mìng huǒ*: LIFE GATE FIRE.

life gate 命门 *mìng mén*: A physiological entity of disputed morphological identity. The term "life gate" first appears in *The Inner Canon* (*nèi jīng*), where it refers to the eyes. Reference to a "life gate" as an internal organ body first appears in *The Classic of Difficult Issues* (*nàn jīng, 36*), which states, "The two kidneys are not both kidneys. The left one is the kidney, and the right is the life gate." The question of the life gate invited little discussion until the Ming and the Qing, when various different theories were put forward: a) both kidneys contain the life gate; b) the space between the kidneys is the life gate; c) the life gate is the stirring qi between the kidneys; d) the life gate is the root of original qi and the house of fire and water, e) the life gate is the fire of earlier heaven or the true yang of the whole body; f) the life gate is the gate of birth, i.e., in women the BIRTH GATE and in men the ESSENCE GATE. [6: 97] [26: 395] [36: 100–103]

life gate fire 命门之火 *mìng mén zhī huǒ*: Synonym: *life fire*. The basic fire of life; kidney yang. The life gate lives within kidney yin, and is the basis of sexual and reproductive functions. It warms and nourishes the five viscera and six bowels, is intimately involved in growth, development, and aging. The spleen and stomach require the warming action of the life gate fire for the function of movement and transformation to be normal. [26: 396]

lifting and thrusting 提插法 *tí chā fǎ*: A method of needle manipulation whereby after insertion the needle is retracted (but not removed from the body) and then thrust back to the depth of the original insertion. Method: Lift the needle a short distance relative to the depth of the flesh at the point; then thrust back to the original depth. Keep the direction of insertion constant to avoid local pain and residual discomfort after needling. Keep the distance covered by this motion at 0.3–0.5 body-inches. Take care to avoid raising the needle too far and thus withdrawing the needle or thrusting it too deeply and going below the recommended needling depth. Use quick vigorous movements to drain, and gentle slow ones to supplement. According to one theory, a sharp thrust with a gentle lift supplements (as if pushing the qi in), whereas a sharp lift with a gentle thrust drains (as if pulling the qi out). A moderate lift and thrust produces even supplementation and drainage. See LIFTING AND THRUSTING SUPPLEMENTATION AND DRAINAGE. Compare NEEDLE POUNDING. [101: 54] [46: 463]

lifting and thrusting supplementation and drainage 提插补泻 *tí chā bǔ xiè*: A method of achieving supplementation and drainage that involves varying the emphasis on lifting the needle (retracting without extracting) and re-thrusting the needle after insertion. Emphasis on thrusting supplements, whereas emphasis on lifting drains. In other words, vigorous thrusts followed by gentle lifts have a supplementing effect, whereas vigorous lifts followed by gentle thrusts have a draining effect. See NEEDLE MANIPULATION (TECHNIQUE); LIFTING AND THRUSTING; HEAVEN, HUMAN, AND EARTH SUPPLEMENTATION AND DRAINAGE. [27: 341] [97: 547]

light formula 轻剂 *qīng jì*: One of the TEN FORMULA TYPES. A formula containing medicinals that are light in weight. Light [medicinals] can eliminate repletion, i.e., medicinals light in weight can be used to treat exterior repletion patterns. For example, Ephedra Decoction (*má huáng tāng*) treats heat effusion, aversion to cold, headache, generalized pain, lumbar and joint pain, thirst, absence of sweating, panting, and a tight floating pulse. [27: 306] [27: 301] [97: 394]

light [medicinals] can eliminate repletion 轻可去实 *xuān kě qù shí*: Medicinals that are light in weight, such as ephedra (*má huáng*) and pueraria (*gé gēn*) can be used to treat exterior repletion patterns in initial-stage wind-warmth. See LIGHT FORMULA. [26: 837] [97: 394]

light stir-frying 微炒 *wēi chǎo*: Stir-frying of short duration to remove the moisture content of medicinal materials so that they are left dry, at least on the outer surface, but without producing any change in form or medicinal characteristics. [27: 324]

like cold 喜冷 *xǐ lěng*: (Of pain and discomfort) to be relieved by the contact with cold objects or by ingestion of cold drinks. E.g., "thirst with liking for cold things".

like heat 喜热 *xǐ rè*: (Of pain and discomfort) to be relieved by contact with hot objects or by ingestion of hot drinks. E.g., "abdominal pain that likes heat."

like pressure 喜按 *xǐ àn*: (Of pain or discomfort, especially in the chest or abdomen) to be relieved by pressure; as sign of interior vacuity. Examples: "abdominal pain that refuses pressure"; "pain and distention in stomach duct and abdomen that refuses pressure." [50: 1465]

like treatment of unlike disease 异病同治 *yì bìng tóng zhì*: Using a common method of treatment for different diseases (i.e., patterns). For example, vacuity cold diarrhea, prolapse of the rectum, or prolapse of the uterus are different disease (disease patterns), but when attributable to center qi fall, they may all be treated with Center-Supplementing Qi-Boosting Decoction (*bǔ zhōng yì qì tāng*). See DETERMINING TREATMENT ACCORDING TO PATTERNS PRINCIPLE OF TREATMENT.

Compare UNLIKE TREATMENT OF LIKE DISEASE. [27: 231]

liking for cool drinks 喜冷饮 *xǐ lěng yǐn*: A preference for drinking cool or chilled fluids a sign of interior heat. It is treated by clearing heat and engendering liquid. *Elementary Questions* (*sù wèn, nue=4 lun=4*) states, "When yang is exuberant, there is heat in the outer body; when yin is vacuos, there us heat in the inner body. When there is heat in both the inner and out body, there is panting and thirst; hence a desire for cold drinks."

limb 肢 *zhī*: An arm or leg.

limb joint pain 肢节痛 *zhī jié tòng*: Pain in the joints of the limbs. Limb joint pain usually attributable to wind-damp, wind-cold, phlegm-rheum, static blood lodged in the channels and network vessels, or to blood vacuity depriving the sinews of nourishment. It falls largely within the category of IMPEDIMENT (*bì*). [26: 383] [97: 356]

limb reversal 肢厥 *zhī jué*: REVERSAL COLD OF THE EXTREMITIES.

limp aching lumbus and knees 腰膝酸软 *yāo xī suān ruǎn*: Synonym: *aching lumbus and limp knees*. A combined condition of LIMP LUMBUS AND KNEES and ACHING LUMBUS.

limp aching lumbus and legs 腰腿酸软 *yāo tuǐ suān ruǎn*: Synonym: *aching lumbus and limp legs*. Aching pain in the lumbus accompanied by limpness or weakness of the knees that creates difficulty rising to a standing posture, impedes physical movement, and prevents prolonged standing or walking. Essentially the same as LIMP ACHING LUMBUS AND KNEES.

limp hands and enuresis 手撒遗尿 *shǒu sā yí niào*: A sign observed in desertion patterns.

limp lumbus and knees 腰膝软弱 *yāo xī ruǎn ruò*: Synonym: *lack of strength in the lumbus and knees*. Insufficient power in the lumbus and knees to perform normal movements, in severe cases, called *limp* or *weak wilting lumbus and knees*, severely restricting movement. Limpness of the lumbus and knees, especially limpness of the lumbus, often accompanies aching of the lumbus, hence the combined terms *limp aching lumbus and knees* and *aching lumbus and limp knees*. Such conditions are attributed to liver-kidney vacuity, cold-damp, or damp-heat (or combinations of liver-kidney vacuity with cold-damp or damp-heat); they differ from simple aching lumbus, which is mostly due to kidney vacuity. **Liver-kidney vacuity** patterns involve persistent aching lumbus or lumbar pain with cold knees, and may be slightly relieved by rest and exacerbated by taxation. Other signs include cold extremities, fear of cold and desire for warmth, tinnitus, deafness, long voidings of clear urine, frequent urination, sloppy stool or diarrhea, hair loss, loosening of the teeth,

shortness of breath, general fatigue and lassitude of spirit exacerbated by physical strain, pale tongue, and a deep fine pulse. In severe cases, there may be seminal emission and impotence. MED Nourish liver blood and supplement kidney qi using Dipsacus Pill (*xù duàn wán*). ACU Base treatment mainly on BL and GV. Main points for all patterns: BL-23 (*shèn shū*, Kidney Transport), GV-3 (*yāo yáng guān*, Lumbar Yang Pass), BL-40 (*wěi zhōng*, Bend Center), and BL-57 (*chéng shān*, Mountain Support); For liver-kidney vacuity, add BL-18 (*gān shū*, Liver Transport), BL-52 (*zhì shì*, Will Chamber), KI-3 (*tài xī*, Great Ravine), and LR-3 (*tài chōng*, Supreme Surge), needling with supplementation. **Cold-damp** limp aching lumbus and knees is associated with cold, heaviness, or pain, exacerbated by yin-type cold rainy weather and relieved by warmth, and associated with a normal tongue with white fur and a fine sunken pulse that may be moderate. MED Eliminate dampness and free impediment using Dampness-Eliminating Impediment-Alleviating Decoction (*chú shī juān bì tāng*). When the liver and kidney have been damaged in enduring conditions, the method should be to boost the liver and kidney, supplement qi and blood, strengthen the lumbus and knees, and dispel cold-damp using formulas such as Duhuo and Mistletoe Decoction (*dú huó jì shēng tāng*). ACU To the main points given above, add GV-4 (*mìng mén*, Life Gate) and SP-9 (*yīn líng quán*, Yin Mound Spring), needling with even supplementation and drainage and adding moxa. **Damp-heat** patterns are marked by limp wilting lumbus and knees prevent long standing and walking, and in some cases there may be redness and swelling. Other signs include short voidings of reddish urine, constipation, yellow, possibly slimy tongue fur, and a rapid, possibly stringlike pulse. Damp-heat conditions are often observed in wilting (*wěi*) and leg qi patterns. MED Treat repletion pattern with Mysterious Two Pill (*èr miào wán*), Pain-Assuaging Decoction (*niān tòng tāng*), or Tangkuei Pain-Assuaging Decoction (*dāng guī niān tòng tāng*). ACU To the main points given above, add SP-9 (*yīn líng quán*, Yin Mound Spring), LI-11 (*qū chí*, Pool at the Bend), and LI-4 (*hé gǔ*, Union Valley), needling with drainage. BL-40 (*wěi zhōng*, Bend Center) can be pricked to bleed; for damp-heat occurring in vacuity-repletion complexes, needle these points with even supplementation and drainage, and needle BL-23 (*shèn shū*, Kidney Transport), BL-18 (*gān shū*, Liver Transport), BL-60 (*kūn lún*, Kunlun Mountains), and KI-3 (*tài xī*, Great Ravine) with supplementation. [92: No. 167] [46: 596, 633] [37: 388–391] [113: 228–231]

limp tongue 舌痿 *shé wěi*: A tongue that is soft and floppy, moves with difficulty, and cannot be extended. The spleen governs the flesh, and the tongue is flesh. A limp tongue is therefore a manifestation of a debilitated spleen, but it may may occur when wearing of yin humor deprives the sinews of nourishment. In a new disease, a limp tongue is the result of heat scorching yin. In an enduring disease, a limp crimson tongue means that yin depletion has reached an extreme, while a limp white tongue indicates dual vacuity of qi and blood. MED Supplement the center and nourish the blood. Take Center-Supplementing Qi-Boosting Decoction (*bǔ zhōng yì qì tāng*) in the morning and Spleen-Returning Pill (*guī pí wán*) in the evening. [26: 268]

limp wilting lumbus and knees 腰膝痿软 *yāo xī wěi ruǎn*: Synonym: *weak wilting lumbus and knees*. Severe lack of strength in the lumbus and knees. Compare LIMP LUMBUS AND KNEES.

linger 留恋 *liú liàn*: To remain and resist elimination; said of evils and heat effusion.

lip 唇 *chún*, 嘴唇 *zuǐ chún*: Either of the two folds of flesh that form the opening of the mouth, which are normally redder and darker in the color than the surrounding areas of the face. Pale lips indicate a dual vacuity of blood and qi. Green-blue or purple lips are seen in both blood stasis and cold patterns and indicate impaired flow of blood and qi. Parched lips indicate damage to liquid. Gaping corners of the mouth and shrinking of the philtrum signify imminent desertion of right qi. Drooling from the corners of the mouth during sleep generally indicates spleen vacuity or stomach heat. In infants, this may be a sign of intestinal parasites. Drooling from one side of the mouth is associated with deviation of the mouth and facial paralysis. See CRACKED LIPS; LIP WIND; COCOON LIP; HARELIP. See also MOUTH. [27: 28] [97: 511]

lip wind 唇风 *chún fēng*: Synonym: *donkey's-mouth wind*. Redness, soreness, and swelling usually of the lower lip that in time can rupture and exude fluid. In China, it is popularly called "donkey's-mouth wind" because of the distorted appearance it gives the sufferer's mouth. [27: 499] [61: 400]

liquid 津 *jīn*: Synonym: *liquid qi*. The thinner fluids of the human body. See FLUIDS. [48: 210]

liquid failing to bear upward 津不上承 *jīn bù shàng chéng*: Breakdown in the upward supply of fluid to head head, face, nose, throat, mouth, eye, and ears. Liquid failing to bear upward is attributable to damage to fluid in a) externally contracted heat (febrile) disease, b) diseases of the bowels and viscera preventing normal distribution of liquid, c) internal static blood obstruction preventing the ascent of fluids. The main signs are dry mouth and lips, dry tongue with little liquid, sore dry throat, nosebleeds, tinnitus and deafness, and

dry eyes with scant tear fluid. Other signs include dry cough without phlegm, thirst with taking of fluids, dizzy head and flowery vision. The tongue is red or crimson with a dry or peeling yellow fur. The pulse is large or fine and rapid. MED Ophiopogon and Asparagus Decoction (*èr dōng tāng*) or Dryness-Clearing Lung-Rescuing Decoction (*qīng zào jiù fèi tāng*). ACU Base treatment mainly on KI, SP, and LU. Select KI-6 (*zhào hǎi*, Shining Sea), KI-2 (*rán gǔ*, Blazing Valley), SP-6 (*sān yīn jiāo*, Three Yin Intersection), TB-2 (*yè mén*, Humor Gate), Sea Source (*hǎi quán*), and Gold Liquid and Jade Humor (*jīn jīn yù yè*); needle with supplementation or with even supplementation and drainage. If the cause is blood stasis internal obstruction, needle with even supplementation and drainage at BL-17 (*gé shū*, Diaphragm Transport), SP-10 (*xuè hǎi*, Sea of Blood), and LR-3 (*tài chōng*, Supreme Surge). Selection of points according to signs: For dry sore throat, add LI-4 (*hé gǔ*, Union Valley) and KI-7 (*fù liū*, Recover Flow); prick LU-11 (*shào shāng*, Lesser Shang) to bleed. For dry nose and nosebleed, add GV-23 (*shàng xīng*, Upper Star), LI-4 (*hé gǔ*, Union Valley), and LI-20 (*yíng xiāng*, Welcome Fragrance). For tinnitus and deafness, add BL-23 (*shèn shū*, Kidney Transport), TB-17 (*yì fēng*, Wind Screen), GB-2 (*tīng huì*, Auditory Convergence), and TB-3 (*zhōng zhǔ*, Central Islet). For dry cough without phlegm, add BL-13 (*fèi shū*, Lung Transport) and LU-5 (*chǐ zé*, Cubit Marsh). [57: 33] [113: 20] [46: 595, 602, 653] [37: 470, 476, 479]

liquid of the lung 肺津 *fèi jīn*: See LUNG YIN.

liquid qi 津气 *jīn qì*: LIQUID.

liquor damage 伤酒 *shāng jiǔ*: Dizziness, headache, nausea, retching and vomiting, agitation and rashness, or clouding sleep attributable to excessive liquor consumption. Liquor is hot in nature and toxic, and tends to cause heat signs. Liquor damage is treated by harmonizing the stomach and promoting soberness, using such formulas as Amomum Splenic Beverage (*suō pí yǐn*) and Pueraria Flower Liquor-Resolving Decoction (*gé huā jiě chéng tāng*). Long-term intemperate drinking causes damage to the stomach and spleen causing glomus blockage in the chest and diaphragm, reduced food intake, and diarrhea. This is treated by fortifying the spleen and disinhibiting dampness using formulas such as Stomach-Calming Poria (Hoelen) Five Decoction (*wèi líng tāng*) or Poria (Hoelen) Five Powder (*wǔ líng sǎn*). For spleen-kidney vacuity, Stomach Gate Brew (*wèi guān jiān*) can be used. If there is damage to yin-blood marked by tidal heat [effusion] and stirring of the blood, treatment should take the form of cooling the blood and nourishing yin, using formulas such as Clearing Transforming Beverage (*qīng huà* *yīn*). Severe cases of liquor damage can cause concretions and conglomerations, jaundice, and drum distention. [ACU] Base treatment mainly on back transport points, CV, SP, LI, and ST. To harmonize the stomach, select BL-20 (*pí shū*, Spleen Transport), BL-21 (*wèi shū*, Stomach Transport), CV-12 (*zhōng wǎn*, Center Stomach Duct), ST-36 (*zú sān lǐ*, Leg Three Li), ST-25 (*tiān shū*, Celestial Pivot), and SP-6 (*sān yīn jiāo*, Three Yin Intersection), and needle with supplementation. To fortify the spleen and disinhibit dampness, select LR-13 (*zhāng mén*, Camphorwood Gate), PC-6 (*nèi guān*, Inner Pass), CV-6 (*qì hǎi*, Sea of Qi), and SP-9 (*yīn líng quán*, Yin Mound Spring), and needle with supplementation and add moxa. To supplement the spleen and kidney, select BL-23 (*shèn shū*, Kidney Transport), CV-4 (*guān yuán*, Pass Head), KI-3 (*tài xī*, Great Ravine), LR-13 (*zhāng mén*, Camphorwood Gate), and SP-4 (*gōng sūn*, Yellow Emperor), and needle with supplementation. To cool the blood and nourish yin, select BL-17 (*gé shū*, Diaphragm Transport), LR-3 (*tài chōng*, Supreme Surge), SP-10 (*xuè hǎi*, Sea of Blood), KI-6 (*zhào hǎi*, Shining Sea), KI-2 (*rán gǔ*, Blazing Valley), and LR-2 (*xíng jiān*, Moving Between), and needle with even supplementation and drainage. See LIQUOR JAUNDICE; WATER DRUM. [26: 805] [46: 595, 663] [37: 398]

liquor damage headache 伤酒头痛 *shāng jiǔ tóu tòng*: HEADACHE due to excessive consumption of liquor. Liquor damage headache is attended by clouding and dizziness, nausea, retching and vomiting, thirst, rapid pulse, and, in severe cases, clouded spirit. [MED] Harmonize the stomach and resolve liquor using formulas such as Pueraria Flower Liquor-Resolving Decoction (*gé huā jiě chéng tāng*). See HEADACHE. [ACU] Select Hall of Impression (*yìn táng*), BL-2 (*zǎn zhú*, Bamboo Gathering), GB-20 (*fēng chí*, Wind Pool), CV-17 (*shān zhōng*, Chest Center), and ST-36 (*zú sān lǐ*, Leg Three Li). Needle with drainage. [26: 805]

liquor jaundice 酒疸 *jiǔ dǎn*, 酒黄疸 *jiǔ huáng dǎn*: JAUNDICE arising when excessive liquor consumption gives rise to steaming depressed damp-heat that causes bile leakage. Liquor jaundice is characterized by yellowing of the body and eyes with red macules on the face, anguish, heat, and pain in the heart, dry nose, abdominal fullness with no desire to eat, and periodic desire to vomit. [MED] Clear heat and disinhibit damp-heat; resolve liquor toxin. If the pulse is floating and slippery and there is a pronounced desire to vomit, mechanical ejection should be used. If the pulse is sunken and slippery, and there is abdominal fullness and constipation, precipitation should be used. Liquor jaundice can be treated with formulas such as Gardenia and Rhubarb Decoction (*zhī zǐ dà huáng tāng*) from *Essential Prescriptions*

of the Golden Coffer (*jīn guì yào lüè*), and Pueraria Flower Liquor-Resolving Decoction (*gé huā jiě chéng tāng*). [ACU] Base treatment mainly on GB, SP, LI, and ST. Select BL-19 (*dǎn shū*, Gallbladder Transport), GB-34 (*yáng líng quán*, Yang Mound Spring), LR-3 (*tài chōng*, Supreme Surge), SP-9 (*yīn líng quán*, Yin Mound Spring), LI-11 (*qū chí*, Pool at the Bend), ST-44 (*nèi tíng*, Inner Court), SP-6 (*sān yīn jiāo*, Three Yin Intersection), ST-36 (*zú sān lǐ*, Leg Three Li), and GV-9 (*zhì yáng*, Extremity of Yang); needle with drainage. For pronounced heat, add GV-14 (*dà zhuī*, Great Hammer). See also JAUNDICE. [26: 479] [27: 367] [97: 484] [46: 664] [37: 398]

listening and smelling 闻诊 *wén zhěn*: One of the FOUR EXAMINATIONS; examination of the body by listening and smelling. In *The Inner Canon* (*nèi jīng*), the "listening and smelling" examination was limited to listening, and was primarily concerned with the relationship of five notes of the Chinese scale (*jiǎo, zhēng, gōng, shāng, yǔ*) and the five voices (shouting, laughing, singing, crying, and moaning) to the five viscera. In the Han Dynasty, Zhang Ji placed voice, breathing, panting, coughing, vomiting, and hiccough sounds within the listening and smelling examination. Since the Chinese *wén* means both listening and smelling, examination of smells was added to the scope of examination without any need for a change in name. *On Warm Epidemics Expanded* (*guǎng wēn yì lùn*) by Dai Bei-Shan, gives "identification of odors" as one of five main diagnostic methods, emphasizing that special attention should be paid to unusual smells. **Sounds:** Attention is paid to the quality of the patient's voice, spontaneous cries, and coherence of speech, as well as breathing, cough, and hiccough. Changes in quality of voice and breathing are a direct reflection of disease changes in the lung and the state of original qi. Verbal expression and response to questions reflect the state of the SPIRIT. (1) Voice: A faint frail voice with faltering speech, which, in severe cases, hampers comprehension, indicates a vacuity of lung or original qi. *Elementary Questions* (*sù wèn*) states, "If the patient has a faint voice and takes a long time to get his words out, his qi is depleted." This condition is most often seen in damage to the lungs by enduring cough, pneumonia affecting the kidney, or vacuous original qi. A rough turbid voice generally indicates a repletion pattern where the lung has been invaded by an external evil, preventing diffusion of lung qi. This may occur in diseases classified in Western medicine as bronchitis and laryngitis. A hoarse voice or loss of voice indicates lung block when it is associated with repletion signs. It indicates detriment to the lung when accompanied by vacuity signs. Diagnosis is made based on accompanying signs. Groaning, outcries, etc., indicate distention, pain, or oppressive sensations. Their significance must be determined by thorough questioning. *Essential Prescriptions of the Golden Coffer (jīn guì yào lüè)* states, "If the patient tends to keep still and frequently emits cries, he has pain in the joints. If his voice is weak and indistinct, the pain is in the center of the chest and diaphragm. If he can talk clearly without interruption, but keeps his voice low, the pain is in the head." In other words, when the disease is in the joints, movement causes pain. Thus, the patient tends to keep as still as possible, and may utter sounds of pain and discomfort when he moves. When the disease is in the center of the chest and diaphragm, the respiratory tract is constricted, so that the patient's voice is faint and broken. Any attempt to talk only aggravates the pain. In those suffering from headaches, raising the voice causes cranial vibrations that increase pain; however, since the respiratory tract is not affected, the voice is clear and undistorted. (2) Speech: Incoherent expression and response to inquiry indicate diseases of the heart. *Elementary Questions (sù wèn)* states, "Failure to keep clothing and bedclothes adjusted, loss of all sense of propriety in speech, and inability to recognize relatives indicate derangement of the spirit." The pattern may be repletion or vacuity, the former characterized by a vigorous or strident voice, the latter by a low weak voice. Confused, strident speech in externally contracted heat (febrile) diseases is known as delirious speech and most commonly occurs in repletion patterns. MUSSITATION, where the patient talks to himself in a low voice with frequent repetitions, is usually seen in vacuity patterns. SOLILOQUY is talking to oneself, but ceasing when another approaches, and is a sign of a deranged heart-spirit (insanity). (3) Breathing: Disturbances of normal breathing include panting, wheezing, qi ascent, shortness of breath, shortage of qi, and rough breathing. PANTING is hasty, rapid, labored breathing with discontinuity between inhalation and exhalation, in severe cases with gaping mouth, raised shoulders, flaring nostrils, and inability to lie down. It is most commonly due to external evils assailing the lung or to phlegm turbidity obstructing the lung (both repletion), but may also be due to insufficiency of qi and yin of the lung or to the kidney failing to absorb qi (both vacuity patterns). In repletion panting, breathing is rough and the patient feels relief when he breathes out; in vacuity panting he feels relief when he can draw in a long breath. WHEEZING is a whistling phlegm rale in the throat associated with rapid breathing. Since it occurs with panting, it is often called *wheezing and panting*. Distinction is made between cold wheezing and heat wheezing. Cold wheezing is due to yang vacuity with phlegm-rheum collecting internally or

to cold rheum obstructing the lung. Heat wheezing is attributed to effulgent yin vacuity fire or to heat phlegm obstructing the lung. QI ASCENT is rapid breathing with more exhalation than inhalation. It is due to phlegm-rheum obstructing the lung, external evils assailing the lung, or effulgent yin vacuity fire. SHORTNESS OF BREATH is short rapid breathing with discontinuity between breaths. It is like vacuity panting, but there is no raising of the shoulders. It is mostly due to insufficiency of lung qi, but may also arise when water-rheum causes inhibited lung qi. SHORTAGE OF QI is low faint breathing with a lusterless facial complexion, fatigue and laziness to speak, a weak voice, and a tendency to take deep breaths in order to continue speaking. It is usually a sign of insufficiency of yang qi of the whole body. ROUGH BREATHING is breathing that produces a rough sound in the nose, and generally occurs in repletion patterns where the lung has been invaded by an external evil. (4) Cough: Cough and panting with qi ascent, accompanied by a frog rale in the throat, is caused by phlegm in the respiratory tract obstructing the smooth flow of air. This condition is commonly observed in cold-rheum cough and panting patterns. A heavy turbid cough with a gurgling sound of phlegm indicates phlegm turbidity congesting the lung. A dry cough indicates lung dryness or yin vacuity. A faint forceless cough indicates lung qi or lung yin vacuity. Long bouts of continuous coughing that are finished with a sonorous crow and accompanied by pronounced flushing of the face (which may even turn purple in severe cases) indicate whooping cough. (5) Hiccough: Although occasional bouts of hiccough are not abnormal, when occurring in enduring or severe illness, they must be given special attention. Short, relatively high-pitched, forceful hiccoughs indicate repletion heat. Protracted, low-pitched, weak hiccoughs indicate stomach qi ascending counterflow. **Odors:** The smell of the patient's breath and excreta can give some indication of their condition. (1) Breath and body smells: Bad breath is generally attributable to stomach heat. In some cases, however, it is due to stagnation of food in the stomach and intestines or indigestion; in other cases, it is due to gan of the mouth, gan of the teeth and gum, tooth decay, or throat diseases. Belching of sour foul-smelling qi (gas) is due to food damage. In modern medicine, the unusual malodor given off by patients suffering from hepatic coma is known as the hepatic odor. This odor, which may be the same as the "cadaverous odor" referred to in *On Warm Epidemics Expanded (guǎng wēn yì lùn)* is due to exuberant toxic heat in the inner body. (2) Excreta odors: The putrid smell of phlegm, pus, urine, or stool that is thick and turbid indicates damp-heat or toxic heat. The "fishy" smell of thin excreta is usually due to vacuity cold. ◇ Chin 闻 *wén*, listen, smell; 诊 *zhěn*, examine. [6: 128] [27: 184] [97: 444] [29: 164]

little thought of food and drink 饮食少思 *yǐn shí shǎo sī*: See POOR APPETITE.

liver 肝 *gān*: The viscus located on right side beneath the diaphragm. The liver is an interior organ and is connected by channels to the gallbladder, which is its corresponding exterior organ. In the five phases, the liver belongs to wood. The liver stores the blood, governs free coursing, governs the sinews, governs the making of strategies. It opens at the eyes and its bloom is in the nails. It governs fright and is averse to wind. The LIVER STORES THE BLOOD means that the liver can retain blood and regulate the amount of blood flowing throughout the body. The LIVER GOVERNS FREE COURSING means that it makes qi course freely round the body, ensuring normal mental and emotional activity, and secretion and discharge of bile. Impairment of this function leads to BINDING DEPRESSION OF LIVER QI, very often associated with rashness, impatience, and irascibility, for which reason it is often said that the LIVER IS THE UNYIELDING VISCUS. The LIVER GOVERNS THE SINEWS means that the liver maintains the proper movement of the sinews and the joints. The LIVER IS THE ROOT OF RESISTANCE TO FATIGUE, an attribute that rests on the liver's relationship to the sinews. Since according to traditional theory, the NAILS ARE THE SURPLUS OF THE SINEWS, it is also said that the LIVER, ITS BLOOM IS IN THE NAILS. The LIVER OPENS AT THE EYES stresses the important connection between the state of the eyes and the state of the liver. The statement that LIVER GOVERNS THE MAKING OF STRATEGIES comes from a statement in *Elementary Questions* (*sù wèn, líng lán mì diǎn lùn*) "The liver holds the office of general, whence strategies emanate," which means that the ability to make plans is related to the state of the liver. Liver qi depression can cause rashness, impatience, and anger, whereas insufficiency of liver qi manifests in a tendency toward fright (compare GALLBLADDER GOVERNS DECISION). Hence it is also said that ANGER DAMAGES THE LIVER and the LIVER GOVERNS FRIGHT. The notion that the LIVER IS AVERSE TO WIND derives from the liver's five-phase associations with wood. Trees (living wood) are bent and shaken by the wind; likewise various forms of spasm affecting the body are seen to be the result of wind. For example, clenched jaw and arched-back rigidity, which may occur in diseases such as lockjaw are attributed to LIVER WIND STIRRING INTERNALLY. Fright, like wind, causes tensing of the body, and hence some diseases involving liver wind are labeled as fright, e.g., FRIGHT WIND. The liver channel is the foot reverting yin (*jué yīn*) channel, which starts from the great toe, passes up the leg, passes through the genitals and lower abdomen, crosses the rib-side and the throat, connects through to the eyes and then continues on to the vertex of the head. Liver disease often manifests in localized morbidity along the channel pathway. The liver's relationships with the other viscera are as follows. **Liver and heart:** Wang Bing's annotations of *Elementary Questions* (*sù wèn, wǔ zàng shēng chéng piān*) state, "The liver stores the blood, and the heart moves it; when a person moves, blood moves through all the channels, whereas when he rests, the blood returns to the liver." When the body's yin-blood is sufficient, the liver has what it stores and the heart has what it governs, and at the same time heart and liver yang are duly restrained from growing hyperactive. However, if yin-blood is insufficient, the liver has nothing to store and the heart has nothing to govern, and at the same time there is nothing to restrain liver and heart yang. Under such circumstances, a condition of exuberant heart-liver fire can develop. **Liver and kidney:** The liver stores blood, whereas the kidney stores essence. Both depletion of kidney essence and insufficiency of liver blood can give rise to a dual condition of liver-kidney yin vacuity. Conversely, liver fire or hyperactivity of liver yang can damage liver blood, and eventually damage kidney essence, which is treated by nourishing the liver and enriching the kidney. For these reasons, it is said that the LIVER AND KIDNEY ARE OF THE SAME SOURCE. The liver's governing of free coursing and the kidney's governing of storage are interdependent, mutually counterbalancing functions of the liver and kidney. Disturbance of the functions of the two can cause such signs as advanced menstruation, profuse menstruation, menstrual block, and seminal emission, which are frequently addressed by combined treatment of the liver and kidney. **Liver and lung:** The liver governs upbearing, whereas the lung governs downbearing; the liver is the unyielding viscus, whereas the lung is the delicate viscus. When the liver upbearing is too strong and liver downbearing is too weak, liver fire can invade the lung causing *liver fire invading the lung*. **Liver and spleen-stomach:** Healthy spleen and stomach function rely on the free-coursing action of the liver. Liver qi depression can invade the stomach and cause stomach qi disharmony. See LIVER QI INVADING THE STOMACH. ◇ Chin 肝 *gān* is composed of 月, an abbreviated form of 肉 *ròu*, flesh, combined with the phonetic 干 *gān*. [6: 89] [97: 282]

liver accumulation 肝积 *gān jī*: From *The Pulse Canon* (*mài jīng, píng wǔ zàng jī jù mài zhèng*). See FAT QI. [26: 333]

liver and gallbladder stand in interior-exterior relationship 肝与胆相表里 *gān yǔ dǎn* *xiāng biǎo lǐ*: See LIVER IS CONNECTED WITH THE GALLBLADDER. [27: 43]

liver and kidney are mutually engendering 肝肾相生 *gān shèn xiāng shēng*: See LIVER AND KIDNEY ARE OF THE SAME SOURCE. [27: 43]

liver and kidney are of the same source 肝肾同源 *gān shèn tóng yuán*: The liver and kidney are intimately related. The relationship between the two has three aspects: (1) The liver and kidney are mutually engendering, i.e., they nourish and support each other. The liver relies on the nourishment of liver yin to perform its function of free coursing, whereas the regeneration of kidney yin relies upon the free coursing function. (2) The liver stores the blood, whereas the kidney stores essence; blood and essence are both yin; hence "the liver and kidney are of the same source" also reflects the notion that blood and essence are of the same source. (3) The ministerial fire present in both the kidney and the liver is traced to a common source in the life gate. [26: 331] [27: 43] [97: 288]

liver blood 肝血 *gān xuè*: The blood stored by the liver. The notion of liver blood in inseparable from that of liver yin. However, in clinical practice, the term liver blood vacuity is used to label conditions in which signs of yin vacuity and yang hyperactivity are not necessarily present. See LIVER STORES THE BLOOD. [27: 39] [97: 283]

liver blood vacuity 肝血虚 *gān xuè xū*: The manifestation of insufficiency of liver blood. Liver blood vacuity is attributed to either or both of two causes: a) damage to yin-blood in the course of enduring illness, which deprives the liver of blood for storage and of adequate nourishment; and b) continual expectoration of blood, nosebleed, or profuse menstruation due to blood storage failure. In addition to general blood vacuity signs, liver blood vacuity is associated with a variety of patterns: blood failing to nourish the liver, blood failing to nourish the sinews or eyes, and thoroughfare (*chōng*) and controlling (*rèn*) vessel diseases. Signs include dizziness, insomnia, profuse dreaming, flowery vision, blurred vision, inhibited sinew movement, lusterless nails, reduced menstrual flow, or alternating menstrual block and flooding and spotting. In severe cases, the kidney may be affected, resulting in liver-kidney essence-blood depletion, and consequently in such signs as lumbar pain, seminal emission, sterility, menstrual block, emaciation, and tidal heat [effusion], in addition to the above-mentioned signs. MED Since liver blood and kidney essence are mutually engendering, treatment usually involves dual treatment of liver and kidney. The basic method of treatment is supplementing the blood and nourishing the liver. Commonly used medicinals that sup-

plement both liver and kidney include rehmannia (*dì huáng*), white peony (*bái sháo yào*), tangkuei (*dāng guī*), lycium berry (*gǒu qǐ zǐ*), cornus (*shān zhū yú*), ligustrum (*nǚ zhēn zǐ*), eclipta (*mò hàn lián*), mulberry (*sāng shèn*), flowery knotweed (*hé shǒu wū*), tortoise plastron (*guī bǎn*), and turtle shell (*biē jiǎ*). For most simple cases of liver blood insufficiency Liver-Supplementing Decoction (*bǔ gān tāng*) and Four Agents Decoction (*sì wù tāng*) or their variations can be used. For blood failing to nourish the sinews or network vessels, characterized by signs such as numbness in the extremities or impaired locomotion, blood-nourishing and network-freeing medicinals such as millettia (*jī xuè téng*), carthamus (*hóng huā*), mistletoe (*sāng jì shēng*), dipsacus (*xù duàn*), and achyranthes (*niú xī*) are indicated. Blood failing to nourish the head and eyes, marked by loss of visual acuity and dizziness, can be treated with Lycium Berry, Chrysanthemum, and Rehmannia Pill (*qǐ jú dì huáng wán*) or similar formulas. Disharmony of the thoroughfare (*chōng*) and controlling (*rèn*) vessels due to liver blood vacuity can be treated with Black Free Wanderer Powder (*hēi xiāo yáo sǎn*) (Free Wanderer Powder supplemented with cooked rehmannia) and its variations. Depletion of liver-kidney essence-blood is generally treated with such formulas as Left-Restoring [Kidney Yin] Pill (*zuǒ guī wán*) and its variations which supplement kidney essence and nourish liver blood. ACU Base treatment mainly on back transport points, LR, SP, and ST. Select BL-18 (*gān shū*, Liver Transport), BL-20 (*pí shū*, Spleen Transport), BL-17 (*gé shū*, Diaphragm Transport), LR-14 (*qī mén*, Cycle Gate), LR-3 (*tài chōng*, Supreme Surge), SP-6 (*sān yīn jiāo*, Three Yin Intersection), and ST-36 (*zú sān lǐ*, Leg Three Li); needle with supplementation. For liver-kidney essence-blood depletion, add BL-23 (*shèn shū*, Kidney Transport), BL-52 (*zhì shì*, Will Chamber), KI-3 (*tài xī*, Great Ravine), and CV-4 (*guān yuán*, Pass Head), [6: 189] [27: 150] [97: 285] [46: 594, 636]

liver channel 肝经 *gān jīng*: FOOT REVERTING YIN LIVER CHANNEL. [26: 332]

liver channel cough 肝经咳嗽 *gān jīng ké sòu*: LIVER COUGH.

liver channel damp-heat vaginal discharge 肝经湿热带下 *gān jīng shī rè dài xià*: A continual unabating flow of malodorous thick sticky yellow or mixed white and yellow VAGINAL DISCHARGE accompanied by oppression in the chest and distention of the breasts, dizzy head and vision, bitter taste in the mouth, and dry throat. MED Drain the liver, clear heat, and disinhibit dampness. Use Gentian Liver-Draining Decoction (*lóng dǎn xiè gān tāng*) or a decoction of 25 g pulsatilla (*bái tóu wēng*), phellodendron (*huáng bǎi*), and flavescent sophora (*kŭ shēn*). ACU Base treatment mainly on CV, GIV, SP, and LR. Select GB-26 (*dài mài*, Girdling Vessel), BL-30 (*bái huán shū*, White Ring Transport), CV-6 (*qì hăi*, Sea of Qi), SP-6 (*sān yīn jiāo*, Three Yin Intersection), CV-3 (*zhōng jí*, Central Pole), LR-2 (*xíng jiān*, Moving Between), SP-9 (*yīn líng quán*, Yin Mound Spring), and LR-3 (*tài chōng*, Supreme Surge). Needle with drainage. [26: 332]

liver channel repletion fire 肝经实火 *gān jīng shí huǒ*: See LIVER FIRE; LIVER FIRE FLAMING UPWARD. [26: 332]

liver cold 肝寒 *gān hán*: **1.** Insufficiency of the yang qi of the liver causing melancholy, lassitude, lack of stamina, lack of warmth in the limbs, and a sunken fine slow pulse. **2.** Cold evil congealing and stagnating in the liver channel. See COLD STAGNATING IN THE LIVER VESSEL. [27: 151] [97: 284]

liver cough 肝咳 *gān ké*: COUGH causing pain in both rib-sides that in severe cases makes it difficult for the patient to turn onto his or her side. MED Use Bupleurum Drink (*chái hú yǐn zi*) or Green-Blue–Draining Half-and-Half Decoction (*xiè qīng gè bàn tāng*). See FIVE VISCERA AND SIX BOWELS COUGH. [26: 329] [27: 397] [97: 283]

liver counterflow headache 肝逆头痛 *gān nì tóu tòng*: HEADACHE due to counterflow qi ascent of liver qi due to damage to the liver by anger. Liver counterflow headache is one form of LIVER REVERSAL HEADACHE. [27: 392]

liver depression 肝郁 *gān yù*: A pattern resulting from BINDING DEPRESSION OF LIVER QI. [26: 333] [97: 152]

liver depression advanced menstruation 肝郁经行先期 *gān yù jīng xíng xiān qī*: ADVANCED MENSTRUATION (i.e., premature arrival of periods) arising when anger damages the liver, causing liver depression, which transforms into heat, which in turn harasses the thoroughfare (*chōng*) and controlling (*rèn*) vessels, causing frenetic flow of blood. Advanced menstruation due to liver depression is associated with varying quantity of menstrual flow that is either red or purple and sometimes clotted, distention of the breasts, distending pain in the smaller abdomen, vexation and agitation, and irascibility. MED Course the liver, resolve depression, and clear heat. Use Moutan and Gardenia Free Wanderer Powder (*dān zhī xiāo yáo sǎn*). ACU Base treatment on the CV and three yin channels of the foot. Select CV-4 (*guān yuán*, Pass Head), SP-10 (*xuè hăi*, Sea of Blood), LR-3 (*tài chōng*, Supreme Surge), LR-2 (*xíng jiān*, Moving Between), SP-6 (*sān yīn jiāo*, Three Yin Intersection), and SP-8 (*dì jī*, Earth's Crux); needle with drainage. [26: 334] [46: 682]

liver depression and spleen vacuity 肝郁脾虚 *gān yù pí xū*: A form of LIVER-SPLEEN DISHARMONY in which binding depression of the liver qi gives rise to or exacerbates impairment of splenic movement and transformation. Liver depression and spleen vacuity is characterized by rib-side pain, aversion to food, abdominal distention, sloppy stool diarrhea, and fatigued limbs. See BINDING DEPRESSION OF LIVER QI. [26: 334] [27: 151]

liver depression delayed menstruation 肝郁经行后期 *gān yù jīng xíng hòu qī*: DELAYED MENSTRUATION due to liver depression. Menstrual flow is scant and dark, and is accompanied by smaller-abdominal distention, fullness, and pain, mental depression, glomus in the chest relieved slightly by belching, distention and fullness in the chest, rib-side, and breasts, white tongue fur, and stringlike pulse. MED Use Liver-Coursing Depression-Resolving Decoction (*shū gān jiě yù tāng*) ACU Base treatment mainly on CV and the three yin channels of the foot. Select CV-6 (*qì hăi*, Sea of Qi), KI-13 (*qì xué*, Qi Point), SP-6 (*sān yīn jiāo*, Three Yin Intersection), BL-18 (*gān shū*, Liver Transport), LR-3 (*tài chōng*, Supreme Surge), PC-6 (*nèi guān*, Inner Pass), and LR-5 (*lí gōu*, Woodworm Canal); needle with drainage. [46: 683] [67: 75]

liver depression infertility 肝郁不孕 *gān yù bù yùn*: INFERTILITY attributed to liver qi depression. Liver depression infertility is associated with painful distention of the breasts during menstruation, irregular cycle, clots in the menstrual flow, affect-mind depression or rashness, impatience and irascibility, distention and fullness in the chest and rib-side, a dark red tongue, and a stringlike pulse. MED Use Depression-Opening Jade-Planting Decoction (*kāi yù zhòng yù tāng*) or Liver-Coursing Depression-Resolving Decoction (*shū gān jiě yù tāng*). ACU Base treatment on back transport points, LR, CV, and SP. Select BL-18 (*gān shū*, Liver Transport), LR-3 (*tài chōng*, Supreme Surge), Qi Gate (*qì mén*) LR-2 (*xíng jiān*, Moving Between), CV-3 (*zhōng jí*, Central Pole), PC-6 (*nèi guān*, Inner Pass), SP-10 (*xuè hăi*, Sea of Blood), SP-4 (*gōng sūn*, Yellow Emperor), and SP-6 (*sān yīn jiāo*, Three Yin Intersection); needle with drainage. Qi Gate (*qì mén*) is three body-inches below the umbilicus and three body-inches to the side. It is noted for its ability to treat infertility. [37: 416] [59: 101] [67: 395] [46: 431]

liver depression rib-side pain 肝郁胁痛 *gān yù xié tòng*: RIB-SIDE PAIN attributable to binding depression of liver qi, usually stemming from anger, sorrow, or grief. Pain in both rib-sides may be accompanied by GLOMUS BLOCKAGE in the chest and diaphragm, hypertonicity of sinews, heaviness of the lumbus and legs. In severe cases, the pain may be unbearable and stretch into the armpits. The rib-side pain may be accompanied by vexation, agitation, and pronounced irascibility. MED Treat by resolving depression and rectifying qi; complement by discharging depressed fire for depressed qi transforming into fire. Use Toosendan Powder (*jīn líng zǐ sǎn*) or Moutan and Gardenia Free Wanderer Powder (*dān zhī xiāo yáo sǎn*). Compare LIVER QI RIB-SIDE PAIN. ACU See LIVER QI RIB-SIDE PAIN. [26: 333]

liver depression transforming into fire 肝郁化火 *gān yù huà huǒ*: DEPRESSED WOOD TRANSFORMING INTO FIRE.

liver disease 肝病 *gān bìng*: Any disease affecting the liver. Most liver diseases arise through the following pathomechanisms: a) damage by the seven affects upsetting free coursing of the liver and causing binding depression of liver qi, which can transform into fire, causing stasis obstruction of the liver's network vessels; b) insufficiency of yin blood, hyperactivity of liver yang, and liver wind stirring internally; c) damp-heat brewing internally; or d) cold congealing in the liver vessel. Signs of liver disease include rib-side pain and distention, dizzy head or dizzy vision, tinnitus, red eyes, irascibility, or susceptibility to fright and fear, blood ejection and spontaneous external bleeding, numbness of the limbs, convulsions and TETANIC REVERSAL, menstrual irregularities, and mounting qi (*shàn qì*).

Liver Disease Patterns

Simple patterns

BINDING DEPRESSION OF LIVER QI (*gān qì yù jié*)

LIVER FIRE FLAMING UPWARD (*gān huǒ shàng yán*)

ASCENDANT HYPERACTIVITY OF LIVER YANG (*gān yáng shàng kàng*)

LIVER WIND STIRRING INTERNALLY (*gān fēng nèi dòng*)

LIVER BLOOD VACUITY (*gān xuè xū*)

COLD STAGNATING IN THE LIVER VESSEL (*hán zhì gān mài*)

Complex patterns

DUAL VACUITY OF THE LIVER AND SPLEEN (*gān pí liǎng xū*)

HEART-LIVER BLOOD VACUITY (*xīn gān xuè xū*)

LIVER-STOMACH DISHARMONY (*gān wèi bù hé*)

LIVER-SPLEEN DISHARMONY (*gān pí bù hé*)

LIVER QI INVADING THE STOMACH (*gān qì fàn wèi*)

LIVER QI INVADING THE SPLEEN (*gān qì fàn pí*)

SPLEEN DAMPNESS AND LIVER DEPRESSION (*pí shī gān yù*)

LIVER FIRE INVADING THE LUNG (*gān huǒ fàn fèi*)

LIVER-KIDNEY YIN VACUITY (*gān shèn yīn xū*)

LIVER-GALLBLADDER DAMP-HEAT (*gān dǎn shī rè*)

Binding depression of liver qi is impairment of the liver's free coursing function. The main signs are mental depression, oppression in the chest, and frequent sighing. Other signs include vexation, agitation, and irascibility, and distending pain along the liver channel such as in the rib-side, breasts, or lesser abdomen. There may be disquieted sleep or a liking for quiet and rest. Binding depression of liver qi can also manifest as epilepsy, concretions and gatherings under the rib-side, drum distention, reduced food intake, belching, or diarrhea. The tongue body usually shows no change, and the tongue fur is thin and white. The pulse is stringlike. **Ascendant hyperactivity of liver yang** is a yin-yang imbalance, usually kidney yin vacuity preventing yin from restraining yang. The main signs are vexation, agitation, and irascibility, red face, and generalized heat [effusion]. Other signs include headache, dizziness, sudden clouding collapse, insomnia, profuse dreaming, forgetfulness and heart palpitations, or limp aching lumbus and knees. The tongue is red, and the pulse is stringlike and forceful or stringlike, fine, and rapid. **Liver fire flaming upward** is characterized by red face, red eyes, bitter taste in the mouth, dry mouth, as well as vexation, agitation, and irascibility. Other signs include headache, dizziness, tinnitus, deafness, scorching pain in the rib-side, and insomnia and profuse dreaming, blood ejection or spontaneous external bleeding, constipation, and reddish urine. The tongue is red with a yellow fur. The pulse is stringlike and rapid. Ascendant hyperactivity of liver yang and liver flaming flaming upward may both manifest in signs of fire surging upward such as red face and red eyes, headache, and dizziness. Both are characterized by heat signs such as red tongue and a rapid pulse; and both may be exacerbated by affect-mind disturbances. Hyperactivity of liver yang is at root a vacuity pattern, with liver-kidney yin vacuity signs such as limp aching lumbus and knees, dry eyes, and tinnitus. Liver fire flaming upward is a repletion pattern, and manifests in repletions signs such as bitter taste in the mouth, dry mouth, constipation, yellow urine yellow tongue fur, and a forceful rapid pulse. **Liver blood vacuity** is characterized chiefly by dull rib-side pain, dizziness, and dry eyes. Secondary signs include lusterless facial complexion, numbness or hypertonicity of the limbs, shaking of the extremities, dry, thin or brittle nails, and susceptibility to fright and fear. The tongue is pale and pulse is fine. **Liver wind stirring internally** is a development of ascendant hyperactivity of liver yang, blood vacuity, or exuberant heat evil. Liver yang transforming into wind manifests in dizziness that upsets balance, shaking of the head and tremor of the limbs. It may also also manifest in sudden collapse and hemiplegia (WIND STROKE). Blood vacuity engendering wind manifests in tremor of the limbs, twitching of the flesh, hypertonicity of the joints, and numbness of the limbs. Extreme heat engendering wind occurs in high fever and is characterized by convulsions of the limbs, rigidity of the nape and neck, arched by rigidity, and clenched jaw (ACUTE FRIGHT WIND). **Cold stagnating in the liver vessel** is characterized by lesser-abdominal pain, possibly stretching into the testicles, or with retracted testicles. Secondary signs include bright white facial complexion, physical cold and cold limbs, green-blue or pulse lips, long voidings of clear urine, and sloppy stool. **Liver-gallbladder damp-heat** results from impaired free coursing due either to internal damp-heat stemming from excessive consumption of fatty or sweet foods, or to externally contracted damp-heat, and is characterized by alternating heat [effusion] and [aversion to] cold, bitter taste in the mouth, rib-side pain, abdominal pain and distention, nausea and vomiting, aversion to food, yellowing of the skin, and yellow or reddish urine. MED Methods of treating liver disease include: COURSING THE LIVER AND RECTIFYING QI; QUICKENING THE BLOOD; DRAINING THE LIVER; NOURISHING THE BLOOD AND EMOLLIATING THE LIVER; SUBDUING YANG AND EXTINGUISHING WIND; CLEARING HEAT AND TRANSFORMING DAMPNESS. [26: 329]

liver distention 肝胀 *gān zhàng*: **1.** Rib-side fullness and distention with pain stretching into the lower abdomen. Liver distention is usually caused by cold affecting the liver channel and is treated by coursing the liver and dissipating cold. MED Use Liver-Warming Brew (*nuǎn gān jiān*). ACU Base treatment mainly on LR, PC, and CV. Select LR-14 (*qī mén*, Cycle Gate), LR-3 (*tài chōng*, Supreme Surge), PC-6 (*nèi guān*, Inner Pass), GB-34 (*yáng líng quán*, Yang Mound Spring), CV-6 (*qì hǎi*, Sea of Qi), SP-6 (*sān yīn jiāo*, Three Yin Intersection), and LR-1 (*dà dūn*, Large Pile); needle with even supplementation and drainage and moxa. For lower abdominal pain, add GB-40 (*qiū xū*, Hill Ruins), and LR-5 (*lǐ gōu*, Woodworm Canal), **2.** The same signs occurring in distention disease. [26: 332]

liver fire 肝火 *gān huǒ*: A fire pattern developing from excesses of the seven affects, liver yang transforming into fire, or heat or damp-heat brewing in the liver channel. Liver fire is characterized by red facial complexion, red eyes, dizziness, bitter taste in the mouth, rashness, impatience, and irascibility, red tongue margins, and rapid stringlike pulse. When the upper body signs are pronounced, it is called LIVER FIRE FLAMING UPWARD. [27: 151] [26: 328] [97: 282]

liver fire dizziness 肝火眩晕 *gān huǒ xuàn yūn*: DIZZINESS due to depletion of kidney water and upward flaming of liver-gallbladder ministerial fire, and associated with headache, upbearing fire flush, bitter taste in the mouth, red eyes, red tongue, and rapid stringlike pulse. WMC hypertension; cerebral atherosclerosis. MED When effulgent fire is prominent, it is treated by clearing the liver and draining fire with Gentian Liver-Draining Decoction (*lóng dǎn xiè gān tāng*); when yin vacuity is prominent, it is treated by enriching yin and downbearing fire with Anemarrhena and Phellodendron Eight-Ingredient Pill (*zhī bǎi bā wèi wán*). ACU Base treatment on LR, GB, and KI. Main points: GV-20 (*bǎi huì*, Hundred Convergences), GB-20 (*fēng chí*, Wind Pool), LR-3 (*tài chōng*, Supreme Surge), GB-43 (*xiá xī*, Pinched Ravine), KI-3 (*tài xī*, Great Ravine), and SP-6 (*sān yīn jiāo*, Three Yin Intersection); needle with even supplementation and drainage. For effulgent fire, add GB-34 (*yáng líng quán*, Yang Mound Spring) and LR-2 (*xíng jiān*, Moving Between), needling with drainage. For yin vacuity, add KI-6 (*zhào hǎi*, Shining Sea), BL-23 (*shèn shū*, Kidney Transport), and BL-18 (*gān shū*, Liver Transport), needling with supplementation. See DIZZINESS. [26: 328] [46: 618] [113: 14]

liver fire flaming upward 肝火上炎 *gān huǒ shàng yán*: Synonym: *upflaming liver fire*. LIVER FIRE characterized by pronounced upper body signs. Liver fire flaming upward is attributed to liver qi depression transforming into fire, to depressed internal damp-heat evils, or to excessive consumption of sweet and fatty foods or warming and supplementing medicinals. Liver fire flaming upward is characterized by qi and fire rising to the head, and by pronounced heat signs. The main signs are red face, red eyes, bitter taste in the mouth, dry mouth, as well as vexation, agitation, and irascibility. Other signs include scorching pain in the rib-side, headache, dizziness, tinnitus, deafness, insomnia and profuse dreaming, reddish urine, and constipation. In some cases, there is blood ejection or spontaneous external bleeding. The tongue is red with yellow fur. The pulse is stringlike and rapid. **Analysis:** Liver fire flames upward attacking the head and eyes. Hence there is red face and red eyes, headache, dizziness, tinnitus, and deafness. When fire lies depressed in the liver channel, there is scorching pain in the rib-side. When it carries gallbladder qi upward, there is a bitter taste in the mouth and dry mouth. Impairment of liver qi's orderly reaching manifests in vexation, agitation, and irascibility. When depressed heat harasses the inner body, there is insomnia and profuse dreaming. When the blood network vessels are scorched and the blood moves frenetically, there is blood ejection and spontaneous external bleeding. Exuberant fire scorches liquid, hence the constipation and red urine. The red tongue with yellow fur, and the rapid stringlike pulse are signs of intense liver channel repletion fire. ⎡MED⎤ Clear the liver and drain fire. Use Gentian Liver-Draining Decoction (*lóng dǎn xiè gān tāng*) or Tangkuei, Gentian, and Aloe Pill (*dāng guī lóng huì wán*). ⎡ACU⎤ Base treatment mainly on GB and LR. Select LR-3 (*tài chōng*, Supreme Surge), GB-43 (*xiá xī*, Pinched Ravine), LR-2 (*xíng jiān*, Moving Between), GB-34 (*yáng líng quán*, Yang Mound Spring), and TB-6 (*zhī gōu*, Branch Ditch); needle with drainage. [27: 152] [97: 256] [37: 396] [116: 102]

liver fire invading the lung 肝火犯肺 *gān huǒ fàn fèi*: Liver channel qi fire ascending counterflow to invade lung and disturbing the lung's depurative downbearing. Liver fire invading the lung most commonly arises as a result of anger damaging the liver or heat evil invading the inner body. It is often called "wood fire tormenting metal." The chief signs are cough with yellow phlegm, and scorching pain in the chest and rib-side. Other signs include scant sticky phlegm, cough that in severe cases brings ejection of fresh blood, rashness, impatience, and irascibility, dizzy head and red eyes, red face, and a bitter taste in the mouth. In addition, there may be short voidings of red urine and constipation. The tongue is red with dry yellow fur. The pulse is stringlike and rapid or stringlike, fine, and rapid. Analysis: When liver fire invades the lung, it scorches the lung and disturbs depurative downbearing, hence the cough. When fire damages the network vessels of the lung, blood spills out, hence the coughing of fresh blood. When liquid is scorched by fire, it is condensed into phlegm, hence the scant sticky yellow phlegm. When liver channel repletion fire lies depressed, it gives rise to scorching pain in the chest and rib-side, rashness, impatience, and irascibility. When liver fire flames upward, there is dizziness, red eyes, and bitter taste in the mouth. The red tongue with yellow fur and the rapid stringlike pulse are signs of exuberant liver fire scorching lung liquid. ⎡MED⎤ Clear heat and drain fire; moisten the lung and transform phlegm. Use Indigo and Clamshell Pill (*qīng gé wán*) combined with Metal-Clearing Phlegm-Transforming Decoction (*qīng jīn huà tán tāng*). ⎡ACU⎤ Base treatment mainly on LU and LR. Select BL-13 (*fèi shū*, Lung Transport), LU-10 (*yú jì*, Fish Border), LR-2 (*xíng jiān*, Moving Between), and GB-34 (*yáng líng quán*, Yang Mound Spring); needle with drainage. [97: 286] [6: 93] [116: 144]

liver fire sleeplessness 肝火不得卧 *gān huǒ bù dé wò*: From *Pathoconditions, Causes, Pulses, and Treatments* (*zhèng yīn mài zhì*). SLEEPLESSNESS

due to liver fire arising when excessive anxiety and anger damage the liver and cause counterflow of liver qi or when liver blood is damaged and the spirit fails to confine itself. Liver fire sleeplessness is characterized by unquiet sleep, susceptibility to fright, thirst with copious fluid intake, periodic distention in the rib-side, or pain in the lesser abdomen and free ribs reaching into the genitals, and a rapid stringlike pulse. ⎡MED⎤ Course the liver and clear fire using Gentian Liver-Draining Decoction (*lóng dǎn xiè gān tāng*) or Liver-Coursing Powder (*shū gān sǎn*). ⎡ACU⎤ To the main points given under SLEEPLESSNESS, add BL-18 (*gān shū*, Liver Transport), LR-3 (*tài chōng*, Supreme Surge), LR-2 (*xíng jiān*, Moving Between), and PC-7 (*dà líng*, Great Mound), needling with drainage. [26: 328]

liver fixity 肝着 *gān zhuó*: A disease pattern arising when liver qi and blood become stagnant and depressed. Liver fixity is characterized by glomus and oppression in the rib-side, in severe cases with pain and distention. Discomfort may be slightly relieved by massage and pummeling. There may also be a desire for warm drinks. ⎡MED⎤ Move the blood and dissipate stagnation; free yang and quicken the blood. Use Inula Decoction (*xuán fù huā tāng*) plus tangkuei fine root (*dāng guī xū*), peach kernel (*táo rén*), lycopus (*zé lán*), and curcuma (*yù jīn*). ⎡ACU⎤ Base treatment mainly on LR, GB, LI, HT, and ST. Select BL-18 (*gān shū*, Liver Transport), BL-17 (*gé shū*, Diaphragm Transport), LR-3 (*tài chōng*, Supreme Surge), PC-6 (*nèi guān*, Inner Pass), SP-6 (*sān yīn jiāo*, Three Yin Intersection), GB-34 (*yáng líng quán*, Yang Mound Spring), LR-2 (*xíng jiān*, Moving Between), SP-10 (*xuè hǎi*, Sea of Blood), CV-6 (*qì hǎi*, Sea of Qi), and LI-4 (*hé gǔ*, Union Valley); needle with drainage. [26: 332] [27: 416] [97: 284]

liver forms tears 肝为泪 *gān wéi lèi*: From *Elementary Questions* (*sù wèn, xuān míng wǔ qì piān*). Tears flow from the eyes; the liver opens at the eyes; and tears are formed out of liver humor. Hence it is said that the liver forms tears. [50: 785]

liver-gallbladder damp-heat 肝胆湿热 *gān dǎn shī rè*: Synonym: *damp-heat brewing in the liver and gallbladder*. A disease pattern arising when the liver's free coursing is impaired owing either to internal damp-heat stemming from excessive consumption of fatty or sweet foods, or to externally contracted damp-heat. The chief signs are alternating heat [effusion] and [aversion to] cold, bitter taste in the mouth, rib-side pain, abdominal pain, nausea and vomiting, abdominal distention, aversion to food, yellowing of the skin, and yellow or reddish urine. Stool tends to be dry if heat is more pronounced than dampness, and sloppy if dampness is more pronounced than heat. The tongue fur is yellow and slimy. The pulse is rapid and stringlike. WMC Mostly seen in acute icteric hepatitis or biliary tract infections. MED Course the liver and disinhibit bile; clear and drain damp-heat. Use medicinals such as capillaris (*yīn chén hāo*), bupleurum (*chái hú*), curcuma (*yù jīn*), unripe bitter orange (*zhǐ shí*), scutellaria (*huáng qín*), phellodendron (*huáng bǎi*), gardenia (*shān zhī zǐ*), rhubarb (*dà huáng*), gentian (*lóng dǎn*), isatis root (*bǎn lán gēn*), bushy knotweed (*hǔ zhàng*), and hanging stonecrop (*shí zhǐ jiǎ*). Capillaris Decoction (*yīn chén hāo tāng*) is used for damp-heat jaundice. Major Bupleurum Decoction (*dà chái hú tāng*) is mainly used for liver-gallbladder damp-heat characterized by high fever or alternating heat [effusion] and [aversion to] cold, distending pain in the rib-side, severe pain the upper abdomen, bitter taste in the mouth, nausea and vomiting of bitter fluid, constipation, or jaundice. ACU Base treatment mainly on CV and the three yin channels of the foot. Select BL-18 (*gān shū*, Liver Transport), BL-19 (*dǎn shū*, Gallbladder Transport), LR-14 (*qī mén*, Cycle Gate), GB-24 (*rì yuè*, Sun and Moon), LR-3 (*tài chōng*, Supreme Surge), TB-6 (*zhī gōu*, Branch Ditch), GB-34 (*yáng líng quán*, Yang Mound Spring), and SP-9 (*yīn líng quán*, Yin Mound Spring); needle with drainage. Where heat is predominant, add GV-14 (*dà zhuī*, Great Hammer) and LI-11 (*qū chí*, Pool at the Bend). Where dampness is predominant, add SP-6 (*sān yīn jiāo*, Three Yin Intersection) and ST-36 (*zú sān lǐ*, Leg Three Li). [26: 333] [6: 209] [27: 153] [97: 288] [29: 440]

liver governs free coursing 肝主疏泄 *gān zhǔ shū xiè*: The liver, like wood in the five phases, "thrives by orderly reaching." This is seen in the following areas: **Qi dynamic:** The liver's governing of free coursing is reflected in the regularity and smoothness of qi dynamic. When this function is normal, qi dynamic is smooth and regular, so that qi and blood remain in harmony, the channels are kept free, and the organs all function normally. When it is impaired, qi dynamic is disturbed and a whole variety of diseases may arise as a result. If liver qi is depressed in the liver itself and its associated channel, distending pain develops in the chest and rib-side or lesser abdomen or the breasts become painfully swollen. If liver qi invades the stomach, such signs as attacks of pain in the upper abdomen, nausea, vomiting, and belching appear; if liver qi invades the spleen, there is distending pain in the chest, rib-side, and abdomen, with rumbling intestines and diarrhea. In severe cases, qi stagnation may lead to blood stasis and the development of concretions, accumulations, or glomus lump. Transformation of depressed qi into fire may cause wear-

ing of the blood or frenetic blood movement affecting the liver's blood-storing function. **Bile:** The gallbladder is located behind the right lobe of the liver and stores bile. It is physically connected to the liver, interlinked with it through the "homing" and "netting" connections between the channels of the two organs, and stands in interior-exterior relationship with the liver. Production and secretion of bile depends on surplus qi from the liver being channeled into the gallbladder, where it then accumulates and forms into bile. This means that bile secretion and discharge represents an important aspect of the liver's function of governing free coursing. Disruption of free coursing may thus lead to irregularities in bile secretion and discharge, characterized by jaundice, bitter taste in the mouth, vomiting of yellow fluid, distending pain in the rib-side, DISTENTION QI in the abdomen, and reduced food intake. **Emotional factors:** Joy, anger, anxiety, thought, sorrow, fear, and fright are the *seven affects*, which are natural human responses to the environment. Chinese medicine regards the seven affects as capable of influencing the functions of the bowels and viscera. This is called "internal damage by the seven affects" or simply "affect damage." Especially vulnerable is the free coursing function of the liver. Impairment of free coursing can lead not only to disturbances of qi dynamic and secretion and discharge of bile, but also to emotional disturbances such as mental depression, rashness, impatience, and irascibility. These three aspects of free coursing are clearly interrelated. Impairment of qi dynamic may affect either emotional activity or the secretion and discharge of bile. Emotional disturbance may similarly affect qi dynamic. Disturbances of bile secretion and discharge can cause spleen, stomach, and intestinal dysfunction and thereby upset qi dynamic, which in turn may affect normal mental and emotional activity. The three different aspects of free coursing cannot, therefore, be looked at in isolation. Only by a comprehensive approach can this aspect of the liver be fully understood in clinical practice. [6: 89] [27: 40] [97: 287]

liver governs fright 肝主惊 *gān zhǔ jīng*: The liver is vulnerable to shocks such as produced by loud noises, fearful sights, or emotional stimuli. The liver is the "viscus of wind and wood." Wind blows trees and makes them bend and shake. Fright similarly causes the body to become tense and shake. See FRIGHT. [27: 42]

liver governs physical movement 肝主运动 *gān zhǔ yùn dòng*: See LIVER GOVERNS THE SINEWS. [27: 41]

liver governs the eyes 肝主目 *gān zhǔ mù*: The LIVER OPENS AT THE EYES, and its channel is connected with the EYE TIE. Exuberance and debilitation of the essential qi of the kidney can affect visual acuity. *The Magic Pivot* (*líng shū, mài dù*) states, "Liver qi flows through to the eyes; when the liver is in harmony, the eyes can distinguish the five colors." liver fire flaming upward can manifest as red swollen eyes, whereas liver vacuity can give rise to dry eyes and unclear vision. [26: 328] [27: 41]

liver governs the making of strategies 肝主谋 虑 *gān zhǔ móu lǜ*: See LIVER HOLDS THE OFFICE OF GENERAL, WHENCE STRATEGIES EMANATE.

liver governs the sea of blood 肝主血海 *gān zhǔ xuè hǎi*: Wang Bing's annotations of *Elementary Questions* (*sù wèn, wǔ zàng shēng chéng piān*) state, "The liver stores the blood, and the heart moves it; when a person moves, blood moves through all the channels, whereas when he rests, the blood returns to the liver. Why is this so? Because the liver governs the sea of blood." "The liver governs the sea of blood" is therefore understood to mean that the liver stores the blood and has a regulating action on its movement. See LIVER STORES THE BLOOD. [26: 328]

liver governs the sinews 肝主筋 *gān zhǔ jīn*: From *The Magic Pivot* (*líng shū, jiǔ zhēn lùn*). The sinews (tendons, muscles; see SINEW) are dependent on the liver. "The liver governs the sinews" means essentially the same as the "LIVER GOVERNS PHYSICAL MOVEMENT." Only when liver blood is abundant can their nourishing influence reach the sinews and enable them to move normally. If liver blood is insufficient, the resulting failure of the blood to nourish the sinews adequately brings on hypertonicity (tension and stiffness) or numbness in the limbs, with difficulty in bending and stretching. When liver wind stirs internally, tremors, convulsions, and arched-back rigidity are observed. [27: 41] [97: 285]

liver governs upbearing effusion 肝主升发 *gān zhǔ shēng fā*: Liver qi bears upward and outward, like the branches of a tree stretch up and out. When upbearing effusion is overly strong, signs such as headache and dizziness appear. [27: 40] [97: 287]

liver heat 肝热 *gān rè*: Any condition involving heat evil in the liver, or transformation of depressed liver qi into fire. Characteristics include vexation and oppression, bitter taste in the mouth, dry mouth, heat extremities, yellow or reddish urine, and, in severe cases, manic agitation and inability to rest. [27: 151] [97: 283]

liver heat malign obstruction 肝热恶阻 *gān rè è zǔ*: MALIGN OBSTRUCTION (vomiting in pregnancy) arising when blood gathers to nourish the uterus, and thoroughfare (*chōng*) vessel becomes exuberant, and ascends counterflow carrying liver and stomach qi with it. Liver heat malign ob-

struction usually occurs in women who are normally of a rash and impatient disposition. It is characterized by vomiting of sour fluid and sometimes immediate vomiting of ingested food, dizziness, and bitter taste in the mouth. MED Clear the liver and harmonize the stomach; downbear counterflow and check vomiting. Use Gallbladder-Warming Decoction (*wēn dǎn tāng*) minus fresh ginger (*shēng jiāng*) and jujube (*dà zǎo*) and plus scutellaria (*huáng qín*), coptis (*huáng lián*), phragmites (*lú gēn*), and ophiopogon (*mài mén dōng*). ACU Base treatment mainly on CV, PC, ST, and LR. Select CV-12 (*zhōng wǎn*, Center Stomach Duct), PC-6 (*nèi guān*, Inner Pass), SP-4 (*gōng sūn*, Yellow Emperor), ST-36 (*zú sān lǐ*, Leg Three Li), ST-44 (*nèi tíng*, Inner Court) LR-3 (*tài chōng*, Supreme Surge), SP-6 (*sān yīn jiāo*, Three Yin Intersection), and GB-34 (*yáng líng quán*, Yang Mound Spring), and needle with drainage. [26: 333]

liver heat spontaneous sweating 肝热自汗 *gān rè zì hàn*: SPONTANEOUS SWEATING attributable to liver heat, often accompanied by bitter taste in the mouth and profuse sleeping. MED Clear the liver and constrain sweat using Free Wanderer Powder (*xiāo yáo sǎn*) and variations. ACU Base treatment mainly on LR, GB, LI, HT, and ST. Select LI-4 (*hé gǔ*, Union Valley), KI-7 (*fù liū*, Recover Flow), SI-3 (*hòu xī*, Back Ravine), BL-18 (*gān shū*, Liver Transport), LR-3 (*tài chōng*, Supreme Surge), LR-2 (*xíng jiān*, Moving Between), GB-34 (*yáng líng quán*, Yang Mound Spring), and SP-6 (*sān yīn jiāo*, Three Yin Intersection); needle with drainage. [26: 332] [42: 186] [14: 174]

liver holds the office of general, whence strategies emanate 肝者，将军之官，谋虑出 焉 *gān zhě, jiāng jūn zhī guān, móu lǜ chū yān*: Phrase from *Elementary Questions* (*sù wèn, líng lán mì diǎn lùn*). The ability to make plans is dependent upon a healthy liver. Liver qi depression can give rise to ascendant liver yang, and to rashness, impatience, and anger. Insufficiency of liver qi manifests in a tendency toward fright. Both emotional tendencies can prevent the individual from "keeping a cool head" in matters of planning. Compare LIVER IS THE UNYIELDING VISCUS.

liver impediment 肝痹 *gān bì*: An IMPEDIMENT (*bì*) pattern arising when in enduring impediment further contraction of evils or damage to the liver by anger causes binding depression of liver qi. Liver impediment is characterized by fright during sleep at night, thirst with increased fluid intake, frequent urination, rib-side pain, and enlarged abdomen. MED Course the liver and dispel the evil using Five Impediments Decoction (*wǔ bì tāng*) with the addition of spiny jujube (*suān zǎo* *rén*) and bupleurum (*chái hú*) or with Bupleurum Liver-Coursing Powder (*chái hú shū gān sǎn*). For vacuity patterns, use Liver-Supplementing Powder (*bǔ gān sǎn*), whereas for fire patterns, use Green-Blue–Draining Pill (*xiè qīng wán*) or Gentian Liver-Draining Decoction (*lóng dǎn xiè gān tāng*). ACU Base treatment mainly on back transport points, LR, GB, and SP. Select BL-18 (*gān shū*, Liver Transport), LR-3 (*tài chōng*, Supreme Surge), PC-6 (*nèi guān*, Inner Pass), SP-6 (*sān yīn jiāo*, Three Yin Intersection), GB-20 (*fēng chí*, Wind Pool), SP-10 (*xuè hǎi*, Sea of Blood), BL-23 (*shèn shū*, Kidney Transport), GB-34 (*yáng líng quán*, Yang Mound Spring), SP-9 (*yīn líng quán*, Yin Mound Spring), ST-36 (*zú sān lǐ*, Leg Three Li), and SP-5 (*shāng qiū*, Shang Hill); needle with drainage. For vacuity patterns, supplement BL-20 (*pí shū*, Spleen Transport), BL-21 (*wèi shū*, Stomach Transport), and BL-17 (*gé shū*, Diaphragm Transport). For fire patterns, drain LR-2 (*xíng jiān*, Moving Between), GB-43 (*xiá xī*, Pinched Ravine), and TB-6 (*zhī gōu*, Branch Ditch). [26: 332] [27: 405] [97: 284] [46: 596, 629] [37: 396]

liver is averse to wind 肝恶风 *gān wù fēng*: The liver is the viscus of wind and wood; many of the diseases associated with the liver, such as wind stroke, child fright wind, wind-damp, itching, tetanic disease, and epilepsy, all bear characteristics of wind. [27: 42] [97: 285]

liver is connected with the gallbladder 肝合胆 *gān hé dǎn*: The liver stands in interior-exterior relationship with the gallbladder. The liver channel connects with the gallbladder, and the gallbladder channel connects with the liver. Effulgent gallbladder heat and ascendant liver yang can both manifest in rashness, impatience, and tendency to anger. Liver-calming medicinals can also drain gallbladder fire, and medicinals that drain gallbladder fire can also calm the liver. A connection between the liver's association with the ability to plan and the gallbladder's role in judgment is also quite obvious. [27: 43] [97: 284]

liver is connected with the sinews 肝合筋 *gān hé jīn*: See LIVER GOVERNS THE SINEWS. [26: 329]

liver is often in superabundance 肝常有馀 *gān cháng yǒu yú*: From *Dan Xi's Experiential Methods* (*dān xī xīn fǎ*). Children have delicate livers that are susceptible to evils. When externally contracted evils enter the pericardium and give rise to clouded spirit and heart palpitations, heart fire can affect the liver and thereby stir liver wind that manifests in the form of convulsions. Mutual exacerbation of liver wind and heart fire causes damage to true yin and deprives the sinews of nourishment, hence there is vigorous heat [effusion], fright convulsions, clouded spirit and, in severe cases, arched-back rigidity. [26: 330]

liver is the root of resistance to fatigue 肝者，罢极之本 *gān zhě, pí jí zhī běn*: The liver is related to physical stamina. *Elementary Questions* (*sù wèn*) states, "The liver is the root of resistance to fatigue, the abode of the ethereal soul; its bloom is in the nails; its fullness is in the sinews." The sinews depend on nourishment supplied by liver blood, whose health is also reflected in the nails. [26: 887] [27: 41]

liver is the unyielding viscus 肝为刚脏 *gān wéi gāng zàng*: The liver thrives by orderly reaching, and is averse to being repressed or constrained and to hyperactivity [of its yang aspect]. The *unyielding* nature of the liver is mainly seen in liver qi: mental stimulus gives rise to rashness and impatience, and bouts of anger, which is called *excess of liver qi*. Conversely, insufficiency of liver qi gives rise to susceptibility to fright and fear. The liver and gallbladder stand in interior-exterior relationship, and the unyielding nature is a combined manifestation of both organs." See also SINEW. [27: 40] [97: 287]

liver is yin in substance and yang in function 肝，体阴而用阳 *gān, tǐ yīn ér yòng yáng*: The polarity between yin substance and yang function, seen in all the organs to some extent, is most clear in the case of the liver. Liver blood is the substance of the liver, whereas liver qi and liver yang are its function. The liver governs free coursing and houses the ministerial fire. It governs the sinews and physical movement, the most active aspect of the body. It is the "viscus of wind and wood," and is susceptible to stirring of wind and transformation into fire, which often manifest in dynamic signs. [27: 39]

liver, its bloom is in the nails 肝，其华在爪 *gān, qí huá zài zhǎo*: From the line of *Elementary Questions* (*sù wèn, liù liú zàng xiàng lùn*) that states, "The liver... its bloom is in the nails." Bloom means the outward manifestation of glory. The phrase reflects the observation that when liver blood is abundant, the nails are red, lustrous, and healthy. When liver blood is insufficient, the nails are pale in color and brittle. [27: 42]

liver-kidney depletion 肝肾亏损 *gān shèn kuī sǔn*: See LIVER-KIDNEY YIN VACUITY. [27: 153] [97: 288]

liver-kidney depletion menstrual pain 肝肾亏损痛经 *gān shèn kuī sǔn tòng jīng*: MENSTRUAL PAIN due to liver-kidney depletion that occurs when general vacuity, early marriage, or excessive childbirth cause damage to the liver and kidney and depletion of essence-blood, and the resulting thoroughfare (*chōng*) and controlling (*rèn*) vessel blood vacuity deprives the uterine vessels of nourishment. Liver-kidney depletion menstrual pain is characterized by continual unabating menstrual pain that refuses pressure, and is accompanied by dizziness and tinnitus, and limp aching lumbus and knees. MED Regulate and supplement the liver and kidney using formulas such as Liver-Regulating Decoction (*tiáo gān tāng*). ACU Base treatment mainly on CV, back transport points, and KI. Select CV-4 (*guān yuán*, Pass Head), BL-18 (*gān shū*, Liver Transport), BL-23 (*shèn shū*, Kidney Transport), KI-6 (*zhào hǎi*, Shining Sea), and ST-36 (*zú sān lǐ*, Leg Three Li), and needle with supplementation. Selection of points according to signs: For dizziness and tinnitus, add KI-3 (*tài xī*, Great Ravine). For limp aching lumbus and knees, add Lumbar Eye (*yāo yǎn*). [26: 331] [46: 434] [46: 685]

liver-kidney essence-blood depletion 肝肾精血亏损 *gān shèn jīng xuè kuī sǔn*, 肝肾精血亏虚 *gān shèn jīng xuè kuī xū*: INSUFFICIENCY OF ESSENCE-BLOOD.

liver-kidney yin vacuity 肝肾阴虚 *gān shèn yīn xū*: Synonym: *liver-kidney depletion*. A disease pattern comprising signs of both LIVER YIN VACUITY and KIDNEY YIN VACUITY, that may be caused by insufficiency of either liver or kidney yin. Liver-kidney yin vacuity is characterized by dizziness, distention in the head, unclear vision, tinnitus, dry pharynx and dry mouth, vexing heat in the five hearts, seminal emission, insomnia, aching lumbus and knee, red tongue with little fur, and a forceless fine stringlike pulse. MED Use Six-Ingredient Rehmannia Pill (*liù wèi dì huáng wán*) or Left-Restoring [Kidney Yin] Pill (*zuǒ guī wán*). ACU Base treatment mainly on back transport points, KI, and LR. Select BL-23 (*shèn shū*, Kidney Transport), BL-18 (*gān shū*, Liver Transport), KI-3 (*tài xī*, Great Ravine), BL-52 (*zhì shì*, Will Chamber), LR-3 (*tài chōng*, Supreme Surge), and SP-6 (*sān yīn jiāo*, Three Yin Intersection); needle with supplementation. [26: 331] [27: 153] [97: 288]

liver-kidney yin vacuity flooding and spotting 肝肾阴虚崩漏 *gān shèn yīn xū bēng lòu*: FLOODING AND SPOTTING attributed to liver-kidney yin vacuity arising when congenital insufficiency, early marriage, or marriage wears qi and blood, causing liver-kidney yin vacuity which engenders heat that damages the thoroughfare (*chōng*) and controlling (*rèn*) vessels and gives rise to frenetic movement of the blood. The flooding and spotting is characterized by sudden onset and persistent bright red discharge of varying intensity, and is accompanied by dizzy head and tinnitus, limp aching lumbus and weak knees, reddening of the cheeks, heat in the hearts of the palms and souls, and in some cases postmeridian tidal heat [effusion]. MED Enrich the liver and kidney; clear heat and secure the thoroughfare (*chōng*) vessel. Use Rehmannia and Lycium Root Bark Decoction

(*liǎng dì tāng*) or Clear Sea Pill (*qīng hǎi wán*). ACU Base treatment mainly on CV, SP, KI, and LR. Select CV-4 (*guān yuán*, Pass Head), SP-6 (*sān yīn jiāo*, Three Yin Intersection), BL-23 (*shèn shū*, Kidney Transport), BL-18 (*gān shū*, Liver Transport), KI-3 (*tài xī*, Great Ravine), KI-2 (*rán gǔ*, Blazing Valley), KI-10 (*yīn gǔ*, Yin Valley), and LR-3 (*tài chōng*, Supreme Surge); needle with supplementation. [26: 331] [46: 688]

liver lives on the left 肝生于左 *gān shēng yú zuǒ*: From *Elementary Questions* (*sù wèn, jìn cì lùn*). According to the theory that the "upbearing is on the left and downbearing is on the right," so that the place where liver qi moves is the left. [27: 43] [50: 788]

liver opens at the eyes 肝开窍于目 *gān kāi qiào yú mù*: The liver and the eyes are intimately related. The phrase "the liver opens at the eyes" appears in an enumeration of five phase correspondences in *Essential Prescriptions of the Golden Coffer* (*jīn guì yào lüè*). *The Magic Pivot* (*líng shū, mài dù piān*) states, "Liver qi flows to the eyes; when the liver is in harmony, the eyes can identify the five colors," and *Elementary Questions* (*sù wèn, wǔ zàng shēng chéng piān*) states, "The liver receives blood, so there is sight," These lines emphasize that the eyes are dependent on the nourishing action of liver blood. Insufficiency of liver blood may provoke such conditions as night blindness, dry eyes, and blurred vision; liver fire flaming upward can cause reddening of the eyes and painful swelling of the eyes; ascendant liver yang can manifest as dizzy vision; and internal liver wind may cause a sideways or upward squint. NB: Although the eyes are the specific orifice of the liver, the essential qi of all the organs is reflected in them. *The Magic Pivot* (*líng shū*) states, "The essential qi of the five viscera and the six bowels flows up into the eyes and becomes essence." Thus to some degree the eyes are associated with all the organs, and apart from their special relationship with the liver, the heart and the kidney are perhaps the next most closely related. Effulgent heart fire, for instance, is associated with reddening of the eyes, and insufficiency of kidney yin is associated with diminished visual acuity. See EYE. [27: 41]

liver pulse is stringlike 肝脉弦 *gān mài xián*: Liver disease is typically characterized by a stringlike pulse. The stringlike pulse is also associated with the season spring. This is discussed in *Elementary Questions* (*sù wèn, xuān míng wǔ qì piān*) and in *The Classic of Difficult Issues* (*nàn jīng, 15*). See STRINGLIKE PULSE. [9: 336] [131: 200]

liver qi 肝气 *gān qì*: **1.** The qi of the liver. See LIVER GOVERNS FREE COURSING. **2.** A disease characterized by rib-side qi distention and pain, and oppression in the chest. Usually seen in conjunction with digestive problems. [26: 330]

liver qi ascending counterflow 肝气上逆 *fèi qì shàng nì*: Synonym: *counterflow liver qi*. Upsurge of liver qi characterized by dizziness, headache, red facial complexion, tinnitus, deafness, pain and fullness in the chest and rib-side. The pulse is stringlike and forceful. If the stomach is affected, belching, swallowing of upflowing acid, and, in severe cases, retching of blood are observed. [97: 285]

liver qi depression 肝气郁 *gān qì yù*: BINDING DEPRESSION OF LIVER QI.

liver qi flows to the eyes 肝气通于目 *gān qì tōng yú mù*: *The Magic Pivot* (*líng shū*) states, "Liver qi flows to the eyes; when the liver is in harmony, the eyes can identify the five colors." See LIVER OPENS AT THE EYES. [27: 41]

liver qi invading the spleen 肝气犯脾 *gān qì fàn pí*: Synonym: *liver-wood exploiting the spleen*. A form of LIVER-SPLEEN DISHARMONY in which liver free coursing is excessive and liver qi moves cross counterflow and affects the spleen. Liver qi invading the spleen is characterized by headache, irascibility, bitter taste in the mouth, oppression in the chest and rib-side, glomus and fullness after eating, sloppy diarrhea, and a moderate stringlike pulse. This pattern differs from LIVER QI INVADING THE STOMACH by a predominance of spleen signs such as distention and diarrhea. ⬚MED Use Pain and Diarrhea Formula (*tòng xiè yào fāng*) plus corydalis (*yán hú suǒ*) and saussurea (*mù xiāng*). ⬚ACU Base treatment mainly on back transport points, SP, and ST. Needle with supplementation at BL-20 (*pí shū*, Spleen Transport), CV-12 (*zhōng wǎn*, Center Stomach Duct), LR-13 (*zhāng mén*, Camphorwood Gate), ST-36 (*zú sān lǐ*, Leg Three Li), SP-3 (*tài bái*, Supreme White), and SP-6 (*sān yīn jiāo*, Three Yin Intersection); and with drainage or even supplemenation and drainage at BL-18 (*gān shū*, Liver Transport), LR-14 (*qī mén*, Cycle Gate), PC-6 (*nèi guān*, Inner Pass), LR-3 (*tài chōng*, Supreme Surge), and GB-34 (*yáng líng quán*, Yang Mound Spring), [46: 602, 646] [37: 318, 324] [26: 330] [27: 152] [97: 286] [55]

liver qi invading the stomach 肝气犯胃 *gān qì fàn wèi*: Excessive free coursing of liver qi affecting the stomach. Liver qi invading the stomach manifests in stomach signs such as stomach duct pain, vomiting of sour fluid, torpid stagnant stomach intake, aversion to food, abdominal distention, and diarrhea, in addition to liver signs such as dizziness, rib-side pain, irascibility, smaller-abdominal distention, and a stringlike pulse. If the condition persists, it may develop into LIVER-SPLEEN DISHARMONY. This condition differs from LIVER QI INVADING THE SPLEEN by a predominance of stomach signs such as vomiting of sour fluid and tor-

pid intake. ⬚MED Use Bupleurum Liver-Coursing Powder (*chái hú shū gān sǎn*) or Counterflow Cold Powder (*sì nì sǎn*). ⬚ACU Base treatment mainly on ST, LR, and PC. Needle with supplementation at BL-21 (*wèi shū*, Stomach Transport), CV-12 (*zhōng wǎn*, Center Stomach Duct), ST-36 (*zú sān lǐ*, Leg Three Li), ST-25 (*tiān shū*, Celestial Pivot), and SP-6 (*sān yīn jiāo*, Three Yin Intersection); and with drainage or with even supplementation and drainage at BL-18 (*gān shū*, Liver Transport), PC-6 (*nèi guān*, Inner Pass), LR-3 (*tài chōng*, Supreme Surge), LR-14 (*qī mén*, Cycle Gate), and GB-34 (*yáng líng quán*, Yang Mound Spring), [26: 330] [27: 152] [97: 28] [55] [46: 602, 646] [37: 314, 324]

liver qi, liver yang, liver blood, and liver yin 肝气，肝阳，肝血，肝阴 *gān qì, gān yáng, gān xuè, gān yīn*: The four basic aspects of the liver. Liver qi and liver yang, physiologically speaking, form a single entity, but the term liver yin is considerably broader in meaning, including the "essence" referred to in *Elementary Questions* (*sù wèn*), which states, "Food qi enters the stomach and sends essence to the liver." The liver's yang-qi and its yin-blood under normal circumstances are interdependent and mutually counterbalancing. Liver yin and liver blood nourish liver yang qi, and also prevent it from stirring upward excessively, and when they fail to, a condition that easily develops is ascendant liver yang. At the same time, liver yin and liver blood are dependent on the liver qi's function of governing free coursing to be able to nourish the limbs, the sinews and vessels, the eyes, and the thoroughfare (*chōng*) and controlling (*rèn*) vessels. Diseases of the liver are most clearly understood in terms of the duality of yin and yang. The yang qualities of the liver are seen in the phrases "the liver thrives by orderly reaching" and is "prone to upbearing and stirring," for which reasons it is said to be the unyielding viscus. The diseases on the yang side, liver qi depression and ascendant liver yang, can both affect the yin side. Liver qi depression can lead to liver blood stasis or qi can also transform into fire, damaging liver yin and liver blood. Diseases on the yin side can affect the yang side. If liver yin or liver blood are insufficient, the yang qi of the liver is no longer kept in check and bears upward. Two other liver diseases demonstrate the yin-yang duality. Liver fire is the result of a transformation of depressed liver qi or else it occurs when damp-heat becomes depressed internally. Liver fire tends to affect the blood storage function, causing vomiting of blood, nosebleed, and profuse menstruation. The other of the two diseases, liver wind, is regarded as a movement of yang qi due to severe yin-yang or qi-blood imbalance. Ascendant liver yang, liver fire flaming, and insufficiency of liver yin-blood (yin, blood or both) can all give rise to liver wind. [6: 91]

liver qi rib-side pain 肝气胁痛 *gān qì xié tòng*: Pain at the sides of the ribs attributable to constrained affect-mind and consequent disturbance of the liver's governing of free coursing. Liver qi rib-side pain is distending pain in the rib-side associated with oppression in the chest, and reduced food intake. The pain is a periodic scurrying pain of unfixed location, relieved by belching and exacerbated by emotional stimulus. MED Course the liver and rectify qi using formulas such as Bupleurum Liver-Coursing Powder (*chái hú shū gān sǎn*) or Free Wanderer Powder (*xiāo yáo sǎn*). ACU Base treatment mainly on hand and foot reverting yin (*jué yīn*) PC/LR, TB, and GB. Select BL-18 (*gān shū*, Liver Transport), BL-17 (*gé shū*, Diaphragm Transport), LR-14 (*qī mén*, Cycle Gate), PC-6 (*nèi guān*, Inner Pass), TB-6 (*zhī gōu*, Branch Ditch), LR-3 (*tài chōng*, Supreme Surge), GB-34 (*yáng líng quán*, Yang Mound Spring), and ST-36 (*zú sān lǐ*, Leg Three Li). Needle with drainage. [26: 330] [46: 636]

liver qi vacuity 肝气虚 *gān qì xū*: The manifestation of insufficiency of liver qi; characterized by lusterless complexion, pale lips and lack of strength, tinnitus and deafness, and tendency to fright and fear. Liver qi vacuity is often accompanied by signs of liver blood vacuity. [26: 384] [27: 158] [97: 285]

liver receives blood and there is vision 肝受血而能视 *gān shòu xuè ér néng shì*: Visual acuity is related to the state of liver blood. If liver blood is insufficient, the eyes can suffer lack of nourishment, and signs such as dry eyes, blurred vision, or night blindness arise. In liver fire flaming upward, the eyes become red with discharge. Compare LIVER OPENS AT THE EYES. [27: 53]

liver repletion 肝实 *gān shí*: Any repletion pattern of the liver, including LIVER COLD, LIVER HEAT, LIVER FIRE, and LIVER QI. [27: 151] [97: 283]

liver reversal 肝厥 *gān jué*: REVERSAL and upward surging of liver qi, characterized by reversal cold of the extremities, retching and vomiting, and dizziness and clouding as in epilepsy, sometimes with loss of consciousness. The patient usually displays yin vacuity and effulgent liver signs, and the bouts of liver reversal are often brought on by emotional stimulus. [27: 401] [97: 284]

liver reversal headache 肝厥头痛 *gān jué tóu tòng*: Synonym: *reversal headache*. HEADACHE attributed to disturbance of liver qi. Distinction is made between liver counterflow headache and reverting yin (*jué yīn*) headache. **Liver counterflow headache** occurs when anger damages the liver causing liver qi to rise counterflow to the head. The pain is more pronounced on the left side of the head, and there may also be rib-side pain. MED Course the liver and downbear counterflow. Use Aquilaria Qi-Downbearing Decoction (*chén xiāng jiàng qì tāng*), Perilla Seed Qi-Downbearing Decoction (*sū zǐ jiàng qì tāng*), or Minor Bupleurum Decoction (*xiǎo chái hú tāng*). ACU Base treatment mainly on GB, LR, and GV. Select GV-20 (*bǎi huì*, Hundred Convergences), GB-20 (*fēng chí*, Wind Pool), PC-6 (*nèi guān*, Inner Pass), LR-3 (*tài chōng*, Supreme Surge), SP-6 (*sān yīn jiāo*, Three Yin Intersection), ST-36 (*zú sān lǐ*, Leg Three Li), BL-18 (*gān shū*, Liver Transport), and LR-1 (*dà dūn*, Large Pile); needle with drainage. **Reverting yin headache** occurs in patients ordinarily suffering from stomach qi vacuity, when upsurge of liver qi carries with it cold turbidity qi from the stomach. The pain is at the vertex, and is accompanied by reversal cold of the limbs, and vomiting of drool and foam. See REVERTING YIN HEADACHE.[1] [27: 392] [97: 289] [46: 621, 646] [113: 206]

liver-spleen disharmony 肝脾不和 *gān pí bù hé*: A generic term for LIVER QI INVADING THE SPLEEN and LIVER DEPRESSION AND SPLEEN VACUITY. [26: 332]

liver spleen harmonization 调和肝脾 *tiáo hé gān pí*: HARMONIZING THE LIVER AND SPLEEN.

liver-stomach disharmony 肝胃不和 *gān wèi bù hé*: A pattern arising when binding depression of the liver causes imbalance between the liver and spleen and causes counterflow and derangement of stomach qi. Liver-stomach disharmony is characterized by distending pain in both rib-sides, belching, glomus and fullness in the upper abdomen, torpid intake, stomach duct pain, swallowing of upflowing acid, and clamoring stomach. It differs from LIVER-SPLEEN DISHARMONY in the predominance of stomach signs as opposed to spleen signs. MED Course the liver and harmonize the stomach. Use Counterflow Cold Powder (*sì nì sǎn*) combined with Left-Running Metal Pill (*zuǒ jīn wán*). Alternatively, use Bupleurum Liver-Coursing Powder (*chái hú shū gān sǎn*). ACU Base treatment mainly on ST, PC, LR, and SP. Select CV-12 (*zhōng wǎn*, Center Stomach Duct), ST-36 (*zú sān lǐ*, Leg Three Li), PC-6 (*nèi guān*, Inner Pass), SP-4 (*gōng sūn*, Yellow Emperor), LR-3 (*tài chōng*, Supreme Surge), LR-14 (*qī mén*, Cycle Gate), and GB-34 (*yáng líng quán*, Yang Mound Spring); needle with drainage [26: 329] [46: 660] [113: 216]

liver-stomach qi pain 肝胃气痛 *gān wèi qì tòng*: Synonym: *qi depression stomach duct pain*. STOMACH PAIN arising when affect-mind binding depression (mental or emotional imbalance) causes liver qi to invade the stomach. *Systematized Patterns with Clear-Cut Treatments* (*lèi zhèng zhì cái*) states, "When stomach duct pain is due to the liver exploiting the stomach, there is surging qi and rib-side distention. [MED] Restrain the liver with acridity and sourness, using medicinals such as evodia (*wú zhū yú*), white peony (*bái sháo yào*), unripe tangerine peel (*qīng pí*), chaenomeles (*mù guā*), magnolia bark (*hòu pò*), corydalis (*yán hú suŏ*), and kumquat (*jīn jú*)." See QI DEPRESSION STOMACH DUCT PAIN. Compare STOMACH QI PAIN. [26: 329] [97: 288] [50: 789]

liver stores the blood 肝藏血 *gān cáng xuè*: The liver is capable of retaining blood and regulating the amount of blood in the body. The amount of blood in the various parts of the body varies in accordance with physiological needs. During physical exertion, blood is distributed throughout the body, meeting the increased need for nutrients. When the body is at rest or asleep, blood flows back to the liver to be stored. Therefore it is said, "When the body moves, blood flows through the channels, and when the body is at rest, the blood flows back to the liver where it is stored"; and "the legs receive blood and walk, the hands receive blood and grip." When the liver's blood-storing function is disturbed, two possible conditions may arise. In the first case, the storage capacity of the liver is reduced so that there is not enough blood in the body to supply all needs; if the blood does not nourish the eyes, such diseases as flowery vision (blurred or mottled vision), dry eyes, and night blindness may occur; if the blood fails to nourish the sinews, hypertonicity (tension, stiffness) of the sinews gives rise to inhibited bending and stretching; in women, blood may fail to flow into the thoroughfare (*chōng*) and controlling (*rèn*) vessels, causing reduced menstrual flow or menstrual block. In the second case, the blood-storing function of the liver is impaired, causing a tendency toward bleeding, such as profuse menstrual flow, flooding and spotting, and other forms of bleeding, such conditions being known as failure of the liver to store blood (or blood storage failure). [6: 91] [27: 41] [97: 286]

liver stores the ethereal soul 肝藏魂 *gān cáng hún*: The ethereal soul is closely related to the liver. *The Magic Pivot* (*líng shū*) states, "That which goes hither and thither with the spirit is called the ethereal soul." It also says, "The liver stores the blood, and the blood houses the ethereal soul." When the liver fails to store the blood or liver blood is insufficient, there are signs such as profuse dreaming, disquieted spirit, sleep walking, and sleep talking. These signs are regarded as failure of the ethereal soul to be stored. [27: 41] [97: 286]

liver taxation 肝劳 *gān láo*: **1.** A VACUITY DETRIMENT pattern resulting from damage to the liver. *The Origin and Indicators of Disease* (*zhū*

bìng yuán hòu lùn) states, "In liver taxation, the eyes are dry and dark, the mouth tastes bitter, essence-spirit fails to confine itself so that the patient is fearful and cannot sleep alone, and his eyes do not see clearly. *The Great Peace Sagacious Benevolence Formulary* (*tài píng shèng huì fāng*) states, "To treat liver taxation vacuity heat with red, dry eyes, vexation, oppression, tossing and turning, and congesting and stagnant heat qi flaming in the chest, take liver-draining heat-eliminating Bupleurum Powder (*chái hú sǎn*) formula." It also says: "To treat liver taxation with vacuity cold rib-side pain, distention and fullness, rapid breathing, and cloudedness with no thought of food and drink, take Turtle Shell Powder (*biē jiǎ sǎn*) formula." *Enriching the Meaning of the Wine of Medicine* (*yī chún shèng yì*) states, "Liver taxation arises when yang qi moves counterflow and yin qi is depleted, giving rise to generalized heat [effusion], rib-side pain, dizziness and tinnitus, and slackness of the sinews and joints..." **2.** WIND TAXATION. [50: 782] [26: 331]

liver vacuity 肝虚 *gān xū*: Liver qi vacuity or liver blood vacuity. These diseases are characterized by unclear vision, poor hearing, and susceptibility to fright. See LIVER QI VACUITY; LIVER BLOOD VACUITY. [27: 150] [97: 284]

liver vacuity sparrow-vision internal obstruction 肝虚雀目内障 *gān xū què mù nèi zhàng*: See SPARROW VISION.

liver water 肝水 *gān shuǐ*: One of the FIVE WATERS spoken of in *Essential Prescriptions of the Golden Coffer* (*jīn guì yào lüè*). WATER SWELLING in liver disease, characterized by painful distention and fullness in the rib-side preventing the patient from turning over, together with sometimes copious, sometimes scant urine. [97: 282] [27: 419]

liver welling-abscess 肝痈 *gān yōng*: An INTERNAL WELLING-ABSCESS (*yōng*) affecting the liver that rises when liver depression transforms into fire and stagnant qi and static blood gather and concentrate. In some cases, phlegm due to accumulated dampness may be involved. In the initial state, there is dull pain at LR-14 (*qī mén*, Cycle Gate) gradually giving way to distending pain on the right rib-side that refuses pressure, and prevents the patient from lying on the affected side. The pulse is rapid and stringlike, and there is often aversion to cold and heat effusion. The signs gradually become more pronounced, and if proper treatment is not given, suppuration and rupture occur, with ejection and passing of foul-smelling brown pus and blood. [WMC] liver abscess; suppurative cholecystitis, pyogenic cholangitis, and hepatic echinococcosis. [26: 334] [27: 461] [97: 284]

liver wilting 肝痿 *gān wěi*: See SINEW WILTING. [26: 332]

liver wind 肝风 *gān fēng*: LIVER WIND STIRRING INTERNALLY.

liver wind stirring internally 肝风内动 *gān fēng nèi dòng*: Synonym: *liver wind.* Liver disease manifesting in spasm. *A Clinical Guide with Case Histories (lín zhèng zhǐ nán yī àn)* states, "Internal wind is movement of the body's yang qi," and is the result of "depleted stocks of yin in the viscera." Liver wind arises from extreme yin-yang and qi-blood imbalance. Ascendant liver yang, liver fire flaming upward, and insufficiency of liver yin and/or blood may all, in extreme cases, stir liver wind.   The chief signs of liver wind stirring internally are severe dizziness, headache with pulling sensation (iron-band headache), tension and stiffness in the neck, tingling or numbness in the limbs, or twitching of the sinews and flesh. In severe cases, there may be pulling of the face and eyes, trembling lips, tongue, and fingers, inhibited speech, or unsteady gait. In more severe cases, there may be convulsions or tetanic reversal. *Elementary Questions (sù wèn)* states, "All wind with shaking and [visual] dizziness is ascribed to liver." Usually, the pulse is stringlike, the tongue is red, and the tongue fur is dry. **Liver yang transforming into wind** arises when liver-kidney yin depletion makes yin unable to constrain yang, and liver yang becomes hyperactive and stirs wind. The main signs are dizziness that upsets balance, shaking head and trembling of the limbs, sluggish speech or stiff tongue preventing speech.   There may be sudden collapse and unconsciousness leaving the patient with hemiplegia. Secondary signs include headache, rigidity of the neck, numbness of the extremities, and unsteady gait. The tongue is red with white or slimy tongue fur. The pulse is stringlike and forceful. **Analysis:** When depleted, liver-kidney yin fails to subdue liver yang, and in time will engender wind. When wind evil stirs, fire qi floats upward, causing headache, dizziness, and uncontrollable shaking of the head. Rigidity of the neck, shaking of the limbs, and sluggish speech are also signs of wind stirring. Liver-kidney yin vacuity deprives the sinews of nourishment, hence numbness of the extremities. When wind stirs in the upper body and yin is depleted in the lower body, the condition is one of upper body exuberance and lower body vacuity, hence the unsteady gait. In some cases, fulminant stirring of wind yang causes counterflow and derangement of qi and blood, and liver wind carries phlegm upward to cloud the clear orifices, causing sudden clouding collapse and unconsciousness. When wind-phlegm scurries through the channels, qi and blood are deranged, so there is hemiplegia and stiff tongue preventing speech. The red tongue is a sign of yin vacuity. A white tongue indicates that evil has not yet transformed into fire. A slimy tongue fur suggests a phlegm complication. The forceful stringlike pulse indicates wind yang causing harassment. MED Enrich yin, calm the liver, and extinguish wind. Use Liver-Settling Wind-Extinguishing Decoction (*zhèn gān xī fēng tāng*). ACU Base treatment mainly on LR, GB, and KI. Drain GV-20 (*bǎi huì,* Hundred Convergences), GB-20 (*fēng chí,* Wind Pool), and LR-3 (*tài chōng,* Supreme Surge), and supplement SP-6 (*sān yīn jiāo,* Three Yin Intersection), GB-43 (*xiá xī,* Pinched Ravine), KI-3 (*tài xī,* Great Ravine), and KI-1 (*yǒng quán,* Gushing Spring). **Extreme heat engendering wind,** also called *exuberant heat engendering wind,* results from contracting warm heat disease evil or one or more of the six excesses when the evil becomes depressed, transforms into heat, damages construction-blood and the fluids, scorches the liver channel, and deprives the sinews of nourishment. Occurring in children, this pattern is called FRIGHT WIND, and is observed, for example, in what Western medicine calls encephalitis B. The main signs are high fever with thirst, red face and eyes, convulsions, hypertonicity, upward staring eyes, rigidity of the neck and back, and clenched jaw. Other signs include upward-staring eyes, arched-back rigidity, clenched jaw, short inhibited voidings of urine, constipation, and, in severe cases, clouded spirit and delirious speech. The tongue is red or crimson. The pulse is stringlike and rapid. **Analysis:** Extreme heat stirring wind gives rise to convulsions, hypertonicity, rigidity of the neck and back, upward staring eyes, arched-back rigidity, and clenched jaw. When heat passes to the pericardium, it muddles the heart spirit, hence there is clouded deranged spirit, agitation, and mania. When heat is exuberant, liquid is damaged, hence the high fever, and thirst. The red or crimson tongue is a sign of evil heat harassing construction-blood. MED Clear heat, cool the liver, and extinguish wind. Use Antelope Horn and Uncaria Decoction (*líng jiǎo gōu téng tāng*) or Peaceful Palace Bovine Bezoar Pill (*ān gōng niú huáng wán*). ACU Base treatment mainly on GV, GB, LR, PC, and HT. Select GV-20 (*bǎi huì,* Hundred Convergences), GB-20 (*fēng chí,* Wind Pool), LR-3 (*tài chōng,* Supreme Surge), GV-14 (*dà zhuī,* Great Hammer), LI-11 (*qū chí,* Pool at the Bend), PC-8 (*láo gōng,* Palace of Toil), and HT-8 (*shào fǔ,* Lesser Mansion); needle with drainage and prick Twelve Well Points (*shí èr jǐng xué*) to bleed. **Blood vacuity engendering wind:** Insufficiency of liver blood depriving the sinews of nourishment and giving rise to spasm. The chief signs are numbness of the limbs, hypertonicity of the sinews, jerking sinews and twitching flesh, and clouded flowery vision. Other signs include somber white complexion, pale lips and nails, brittle dry nails, and dull rib-side pain. The tongue is pale and the pulse is string-like and fine. **Analysis:** Blood vacuity engendering wind results from excessive loss of blood (acute or chronic hemorrhage) or blood vacuity in enduring disease. When liver blood is insufficient, it cannot ascend to nourish the head and face, hence the dizziness, tinnitus, lusterless complexion, and pale tongue. When the sinews are deprived of the nourishment of construction-blood, the nails (surplus of the sinews) become lusterless. When blood vacuity stirs wind, there is numbness of the limbs, hypertonicity of the sinews, and twitching of the flesh. When blood is scant and fails to fill the vessels, the pulse is fine. MED Nourish the blood and extinguish wind. Use Tremor-Stabilizing Pill (*dìng zhèn wán*). ACU Base treatment mainly on GV, GB, LR, SP, ST, and KI. Drain GV-20 (*bǎi huì*, Hundred Convergences), GB-20 (*fēng chí*, Wind Pool), and LR-3 (*tài chōng*, Supreme Surge), and supplement SP-6 (*sān yīn jiāo*, Three Yin Intersection), ST-36 (*zú sān lǐ*, Leg Three Li), KI-6 (*zhào hǎi*, Shining Sea), BL-20 (*pí shū*, Spleen Transport), and LR-8 (*qū quán*, Spring at the Bend). [57: 59–61] [116: 103–104] [6: 188] [26: 280] [27: 152, 134, 139] [97: 283, 191] [46: 596, 621]

liver-wood 肝木 *gān mù*: The liver viewed as corresponding to wood in the five phases. [27: 152] [97: 286]

liver-wood exploiting the spleen 肝木乘脾 *gān mù chéng pí*: LIVER QI INVADING THE SPLEEN. [26: 328]

liver yang 肝阳 *gān yáng*: **1.** The yang qi of the liver as distinct from liver yin. See LIVER QI, LIVER YANG, LIVER BLOOD, AND LIVER YIN. **2.** Abbreviation for ASCENDANT HYPERACTIVITY OF LIVER YANG, as in the following entries. [26: 331]

liver yang dizziness 肝阳眩晕 *gān yáng xuàn yūn*: DIZZINESS attributable to ascendant liver yang, which generally stems from constrained affect-mind, and gradual wearing of liver yin. The dizziness is intermittent and is accompanied by unquiet sleep, irascibility, and a stringlike pulse. WMC hypertension; cerebral atherosclerosis. MED Calm the liver and subdue yang with variations of Gastrodia and Uncaria Beverage (*tiān má gōu téng yǐn*). Predominance of liver yin, characterized by heart vexation, reduced sleep, and red tongue with scant fur is treated by enriching liver-kidney yin with formulas such as Double Supreme Pill (*èr zhì wán*) or Lycium Berry, Chrysanthemum, and Rehmannia Pill (*qǐ jú dì huáng wán*). Liver yang dizziness with effulgent fire is treated as LIVER FIRE DIZZINESS. ACU Base treatment on LR, GB, and KI. Needle with drainage at GV-20 (*bǎi huì*, Hundred Convergences), GB-20 (*fēng chí*, Wind Pool), LR-3 (*tài chōng*, Supreme Surge), and GB-43 (*xiá xī*, Pinched Ravine), and a supplement-

ing needle stimulus at BL-18 (*gān shū*, Liver Transport), KI-3 (*tài xī*, Great Ravine), and SP-6 (*sān yīn jiāo*, Three Yin Intersection). For vexation and insomnia, add HT-7 (*shén mén*, Spirit Gate) and Alert Spirit Quartet (*sì shén cōng*). [26: 332] [27: 39] [97: 283] [46: 618] [113: 14]

liver yang headache 肝阳头痛 *gān yáng tóu tòng*: HEADACHE attributed to ascendant liver yang. Liver yang headache is identified by the accompanying dizziness, red facial complexion, flowery vision, tinnitus, bitter taste in the mouth, and rapid stringlike pulse. MED Calm the liver and subdue yang with formulas such as Gastrodia and Uncaria Beverage (*tiān má gōu téng yǐn*) or Mother-of-Pearl Pill (*zhēn zhū mǔ wán*). For exuberant liver-gallbladder fire, use formulas such as Gentian Liver-Draining Decoction (*lóng dǎn xiè gān tāng*) or Tangkuei, Gentian, and Aloe Pill (*dāng guī lóng huì wán*). ACU Base treatment mainly on LR, GB, and KI. Select GB-20 (*fēng chí*, Wind Pool), GV-20 (*bǎi huì*, Hundred Convergences), Greater Yang (*tài yáng*), GB-4 (*hàn yàn*, Forehead Fullness), LR-3 (*tài chōng*, Supreme Surge), KI-3 (*tài xī*, Great Ravine), SP-6 (*sān yīn jiāo*, Three Yin Intersection), LR-2 (*xíng jiān*, Moving Between), and GB-43 (*xiá xī*, Pinched Ravine); needle with drainage. For selection of points according to affected area, see HEADACHE. Selection of points according to signs: For headache with dizziness, add BL-18 (*gān shū*, Liver Transport), KI-3 (*tài xī*, Great Ravine), and GB-19 (*nǎo kōng*, Brain Hollow). For vexation and irascibility, add BL-18 (*gān shū*, Liver Transport), and HT-5 (*tōng lǐ*, Connecting Li). For unquiet sleep, add HT-7 (*shén mén*, Spirit Gate). [26: 331] [46: 622] [113: 203,14]

liver yang transforming into fire 肝阳化火 *gān yáng huà huǒ*: A further development of ascending liver yang. When yang is hyperactive, there is heat; and extreme heat engenders wind. See LIVER FIRE. [26: 331]

liver yang transforming into wind 肝阳化风 *gān yáng huà fēng*: Synonym: *reverting yin transforming into wind*. See LIVER WIND STIRRING INTERNALLY. [57: 60]

liver yin 肝阴 *gān yīn*: **1.** Liver blood and the quiescent aspect of liver function. **2.** The liver as a physical entity. See LIVER QI, LIVER YANG, LIVER BLOOD, AND LIVER YIN. [26: 330] [27: 39] [97: 283]

liver yin vacuity 肝阴虚 *gān yīn xū*: The manifestation of insufficiency of liver blood. Liver yin vacuity is attributed to blood failing to nourish the liver and is characterized by dizziness, headache, unclear vision, dry eyes, night blindness, and scant menstrual flow or menstrual block. Insufficiency of liver yin invariably leaves liver yang unsubdued, causing ascendant liver yang, which is characterized by tinnitus or deafness, red facial complexion, numbness and shaking of the limbs, vexation and agitation, insomnia, and according to the findings of modern medicine, high blood pressure. It may also give rise to liver wind stirring internally. ACU Base treatment mainly on back transport points, LR, GB, and KI. Select BL-18 (*gān shū*, Liver Transport), BL-17 (*gé shū*, Diaphragm Transport), BL-20 (*pí shū*, Spleen Transport), LR-3 (*tài chōng*, Supreme Surge), BL-23 (*shèn shū*, Kidney Transport), KI-3 (*tài xī*, Great Ravine), and SP-6 (*sān yīn jiāo*, Three Yin Intersection); needle with supplementation to supplement liver yin and blood. For ascendant liver yang, add GV-20 (*bǎi huì*, Hundred Convergences), GB-20 (*fēng chí*, Wind Pool), GB-43 (*xiá xī*, Pinched Ravine), and KI-1 (*yǒng quán*, Gushing Spring); needle with drainage. [26: 330] [27: 150] [97: 285] [46: 596]

local point 局部穴位 *jú bù xué wèi*: An acupuncture point at the affected area.

lochia 恶露 *è lù*: Liquid discharge from the uterus after childbirth. If it continues in excess of twenty days, the condition is called PERSISTENT FLOW OF THE LOCHIA, which may be due to qi vacuity, blood heat, or blood stasis. If copious and pale in color, it is due to qi vacuity fall; if crimson, thick and copious, it is attributable to frenetic movement of hot blood; if purple in color and accompanied by sharp abdominal pain, it is due to blood stasis. Absence of normal postpartum discharge is called RETENTION OF THE LOCHIA, which is due to blood stasis or qi-blood vacuity. ◇ Chin 恶 *è*, malign; 露 *lù*, dew. [27: 451] [97: 462]

lockjaw 破伤风 *pò shāng fēng*: Synonym: *incised wound tetany*; *tetanus*. Tetany arising when an external injury or mouth sores permits the invasion of wind evil. Lockjaw begins with lack of strength in the limbs, headache, pain in the cheeks, clenched jaw, difficulty in turning the neck, and heat effusion and aversion to cold. Subsequently, there is a spasm of the facial muscles that creates the appearance of a strange grimace, tightly clenched jaw, stiff tongue, drooling, intermittent generalized spasm and arched-back rigidity. The pulse is rapid or tight and stringlike. Finally, speech, swallowing, and breathing all become difficult, and, in the worst cases, the patient dies of asphyxiation. WMC tetanus (lockjaw). MED Dispel wind and resolve tetany with formulas such as True Jade Powder (*yù zhēn sǎn*) or Five-Tigers-Chasing-the-Wind Powder (*wǔ hǔ zhuī fēng sǎn*). ACU Base treatment mainly on GV, BL, ST, and LI. Select GV-14 (*dà zhuī*, Great Hammer), GV-16 (*fēng fǔ*, Wind Mansion), GV-8 (*jīn suō*, Sinew Contraction), GV-3 (*yāo yáng guān*, Lumbar Yang Pass),

ST-7 (*xià guān*, Below the Joint), ST-6 (*jiá chē*, Cheek Carriage), LI-4 (*hé gǔ*, Union Valley), LI-11 (*qū chí*, Pool at the Bend), BL-60 (*kūn lún*, Kunlun Mountains), LR-3 (*tài chōng*, Supreme Surge), and BL-62 (*shēn mài*, Extending Vessel); needle with drainage. Selection of points according to signs: For clenched jaw, add GV-26 (*shuǐ gōu*, Water Trough) and CV-24 (*chéng jiāng*, Sauce Receptacle). For arched-back rigidity, add GV-12 (*shēn zhù*, Body Pillar), SI-3 (*hòu xī*, Back Ravine), and GB-20 (*fēng chí*, Wind Pool). For convulsive spasm of the limbs, add LI-11 (*qū chí*, Pool at the Bend) and GB-34 (*yáng líng quán*, Yang Mound Spring). For hasty breathing, add LU-5 (*chǐ zé*, Cubit Marsh), PC-6 (*nèi guān*, Inner Pass), and CV-17 (*shān zhōng*, Chest Center). ◇ Chin 破 *pò*, break; 伤 *shāng*, damage, injury; 风 *fēng*, wind. A wind (disease) due an injury involving break in the skin. [26: 513] [27: 484] [97: 463] [113: 346] [61: 328] [50: 1231]

lodge 留 *liú*: To rest and remain fixed; said of evils.

lodged rheum 留饮 *liú yǐn*: A form of PHLEGM-RHEUM. Persistent rheum evil that fails to transform. Lodged rheum may occur in different parts of the body. Rheum lodged in the back affecting the upbearing of yang qi in the governing (*dū*) vessel gives rise to COLD BACK. Rheum lodged in the rib-side affects liver-gallbladder qi dynamic and manifests in pain radiating into the empty basin (supraclavicular fossa). Rheum lodged in the chest hampers chest yang and gives rise to shortness of breath and panting. Rheum lodged in the channels and network vessels gives rise to joint-running pain in the limbs. Rheum lodged in the spleen causes swelling of the abdomen and generalized heaviness. Rheum lodged in the kidney causes swelling of the scrotum and lower legs. If center yang is not restored, although old rheum may be temporarily eliminated, new rheum can accumulate again, so that the condition persists. For this reason, treatment should first be to expel rheum and then to fortify the spleen and warm the kidney and to support the right and transform rheum. [26: 560]

¹**long-bout cough** 顿嗽 *dùn sòu*: A disease pattern described in *Account of Medicine* (*yī shù*) as a cough that comes in bouts of ten or more coughs. It is attributed to lung dryness and damage to liquid. MED Nourish yin and moisten the lung with Dryness-Clearing Lung-Rescuing Decoction (*qīng zào jiù fèi tāng*) or Ophiopogon and Asparagus Decoction (*èr dōng tāng*). Compare WHOOPING COUGH. [26: 778]

²**long-bout cough** 顿咳 *dùn ké*: WHOOPING COUGH. [26: 778]

longevity platform bone 寿台骨 *shòu tái gǔ*: COMPLETION BONE.

long pulse 长脉 *cháng mài*: A long pulse is one that can be felt beyond the inch and cubit positions. If runs straight from head to tail, a feels like long stick. A long pulse that is harmonious and moderate is a sign of effulgent center qi. *Elementary Questions* (*sù wèn, mài yào jīng wēi lùn*) states, "If the pulse is long, qi is in order." If the pulse is long, stringlike and hard, and feels like a rope pulled taut, this is a repletion pattern in which evil and right are both exuberant, and is seen in repletion heat binding internally or exuberant heat stirring wind. *The Bin-Hu Sphygmology* (*bīn hú mài xué*) states, "Long governs superabundance; it is seen in qi counterflow and exuberant fire." [26: 358]

long rinsing 漂 *piāo*, 水漂 *shuǐ piāo*: Steeping materials in clean water that is continuously replaced to eliminate toxic constituents, salts, or malodor, or to remove foreign matter. Sargassum (*hǎi zǎo*), cistanche (*ròu cōng róng*), salted aconite (*xián fù zǐ*), and pinellia (*bàn xià*) are processed in this way. See WATER PROCESSING. [27: 323] [27: 323]

long-standing ailment 宿疾 *sù jí*: See ABIDING AILMENT.

long summer 长夏 *cháng xià*: The third month of summer, i.e., the sixth month in the lunar calendar (the last half of July and first half of August). [27: 14]

long voidings of clear urine 小便清长 *xiǎo biàn qīng cháng*: Copious colorless urine that comes in long voidings. Long voidings of clear urine are a sign of vacuous kidney yang failing to perform its containing function, a vacuity cold pattern, or exuberant internal yin cold, a repletion cold pattern. This is in keeping with the law stated in *The Inner Canon* (*nèi jīng*) that "Any disease with watery humors that are clear, pure, and cold is ascribed to cold." See URINE. [6: 127]

longworm disease 长虫病 *cháng chóng bìng*: From *The Origin and Indicators of Disease* (*zhū bìng yuán hòu lùn*). One of the THREE WORM DISEASES; ROUNDWORM DISEASE. [26: 359]

looking examination 望诊 *wàng zhěn*: INSPECTION.

loosening of the teeth 牙齿松动 *yá chǐ sōng dòng*, 牙齿浮动 *yá chǐ fú dòng*: The loosening of the teeth from the tooth bed. The teeth are the surplus of the bone (governed by the kidney), and are nourished by the gums. The hand yang brightness (*yáng míng*) large intestine channel enters the lower teeth, whereas the foot yang brightness stomach channel enters the upper teeth. Loosening of the teeth is related to the kidney and the yang brightness channels. Distinction can be made between yang brightness heat congestion, kidney yin vacuity, and kidney qi vacuity patterns. In yang brightness patterns, it is accompanied by red swollen or gaping gums, bad breath, constipation, and slippery rapid pulse, red tongue, and yellow-white slightly dry slimy tongue fur. In kidney yin vacuity, it may gradually give rise to gaping gums, and is associated with aching lumbus, dizziness, tinnitus, hair loss, and a fine rapid pulse, a thin shrunken tongue, and a pale red tongue with a thin or scant tongue fur. In kidney qi vacuity, it is associated with aching lumbus, dribble after voiding or urinary incontinence, poor hearing, a sunken fine weak pulse, and a pale red tongue with white fur. MED Yang brightness heat congestion is treated by clearing heat and securing the teeth using Stomach-Clearing Powder (*qīng wèi sǎn*) or Sweet Dew Beverage (*gān lù yǐn*). Kidney yin vacuity patterns can be treated by enriching the kidney and securing the teeth with Six-Ingredient Rehmannia Pill (*liù wèi dì huáng wán*) plus drynaria (*gǔ suì bǔ*). [92: No. 128]

loosening the center 宽中 *kuān zhōng*: COURSING DEPRESSION AND RECTIFYING QI.

loosening the chest 宽胸 *kuān xiōng*: COURSING DEPRESSION AND RECTIFYING QI. [27: 270] [97: 496]

loss of bulk and shedding of flesh 破䐃脱肉 *pò jiǒng (jùn) tuō ròu*: SHEDDING OF FLESH AND LOSS OF BULK.

loss of consciousness 不省人事 *bù xǐng rén shì*, 人事不省 *rén shì bù xǐng*: Loss of ability to perceive and know. See SPIRIT. ◇ Chin 不 *bù*, not; 省 *xǐng*, think, reflect; 人 *rén*, person; 事 *shì*, matter. Obliviousness of people and matters.

loss-of-construction 失营 *shī yíng*: LOSS-OF-LUXURIANCE.

loss-of-luxuriance 失荣 *shī róng*: Synonym: *loss-of-construction*. A hard swelling on the neck. It starts with a slight swelling without change in skin color, and slowly grows and becomes hard as rock. Loss-of-luxuriance is firmly fixed and hard to move. In the advanced stage, it becomes covered with purple patches and ulcerates to exude blood and water. At the same time, qi and blood become gradually debilitated and the patient becomes emaciated like a tree that has lost its splendor; hence the name. WMC It includes primary and secondary malign tumors. MED Boost qi and nourish construction, and dissipate hardness. Use Construction-Harmonizing Hardness-Dissipating Pill (*hé róng sàn jiān wán*). After rupture, use Free Wanderer Powder (*xiāo yáo sǎn*) with additional medicinals or Spleen-Returning Decoction (*guī pí tāng*). ◇ Chin 失 *shī*, lose; 荣 *róng*, luxuriance, glory, splendor. The name apparently derives from the general physical debilitation the condition leads to. [27: 481] [97: 162]

loss of speech 言语不能 *yán yǔ bù néng*: Loss of the ability to speak; observed in wind stroke. See SLUGGISH SPEECH; SLUGGISH TONGUE.

loss of voice 失音 *shī yīn*, 失音不语 *shī yīn bù yǔ*, 失声不语 *shī shēng bù yǔ*, 瘖 *yīn*, 瘖不能 言 *yīn bù néng yán*, 瘖病 *yīn bìng*, 喑 *yīn*, 音哑 *yīn yǎ*: Failure of the voice to sound. Distinction is made between vacuity and repletion. **External contraction:** When loss of voice due to externally contracted wind-cold or wind-heat (sometimes exacerbated by food damage), or to obstruction of the qi paths in the latter stages of pregnancy, it is mostly a repletion pattern, as observed in what Western medicine calls laryngitis, and when is sudden in onset, as is usually the case, it is called SUDDEN LOSS OF VOICE. MED Course wind and dissipate cold; diffuse the lung and open the voice. Use Rough and Ready Three Decoction (*sān ào tāng*) ACU For wind-cold, base treatment mainly on GV, LU, and LI. Select GB-20 (*fēng chí*, Wind Pool), BL-13 (*fèi shū*, Lung Transport), LU-8 (*jīng qú*, Channel Ditch), LI-4 (*hé gǔ*, Union Valley), CV-22 (*tiān tú*, Celestial Chimney), and CV-23 (*lián quán*, Ridge Spring); needle with even supplementation and drainage, and for exuberant cold, add moxa. For wind-heat, base treatment mainly on GV and LU. Select GV-14 (*dà zhuī*, Great Hammer), LU-7 (*liè quē*, Broken Sequence), LU-5 (*chǐ zé*, Cubit Marsh), LI-4 (*hé gǔ*, Union Valley), CV-23 (*lián quán*, Ridge Spring), and LU-9 (*tài yuān*, Great Abyss); needle with drainage. **Damage to kidney-lung qi and yin:** Dual damage to the qi and yin of the kidney and lung is a vacuity pattern. MED Moisten the lung and enrich the kidney. Use Lily Bulb Metal-Securing Decoction (*bǎi hé gù jīn tāng*) or Rehmannia Drink (*dì huáng yǐn zǐ*). ACU Base treatment mainly on back transport points, LU, and KI. Select BL-13 (*fèi shū*, Lung Transport), BL-23 (*shèn shū*, Kidney Transport), LU-9 (*tài yuān*, Great Abyss), KI-3 (*tài xī*, Great Ravine), KI-6 (*zhào hǎi*, Shining Sea), SP-6 (*sān yīn jiāo*, Three Yin Intersection), CV-23 (*lián quán*, Ridge Spring), and GV-15 (*yǎ mén*, Mute's Gate); needle with supplementation. See HOARSE VOICE. [26: 827] [27: 185] [97: 162] [37: 285]

loss of voice in measles 麻疹失音 *má zhěn shī yīn*: Loss of voice occurring in measles; usually attributed to heat toxin blocking the clear orifices. MED Moisten the lung and engender liquid; clear and disinhibit the throat. Use medicinals such as scrophularia (*xuán shēn*), ophiopogon (*mài mén dōng*), cutch (*hái ér chá*), arctium (*niú bàng zǐ*), cicada molting (*chán tuì*), platycodon (*jié gěng*), apricot kernel (*xìng rén*), sterculia (*pàng dà hǎi*), belamcanda (*shè gān*), and mint (*bò hé*). See also SORE THROAT IN MEASLES. [26: 587]

lost heart wind 失心风 *shī xīn fēng*: WITHDRAWAL. *The Level-Line of Pattern Identification and Treatment* (*zhèng zhì zhǔn shéng*) states, "Withdrawal disease is popularly called 'lost heart wind'." ◇ Chin 失 *shī*, to lose, fail; 心 *xīn*, heart; 风 *fēng*, wind. Since the heart stores the spirit, "loss of the heart" means roughly "loss of mind," i.e., insanity. See WIND. [26: 209]

lower body 下 *xià*: The lower part of the body (yin) as opposed to the upper body (yang). It sometimes specifically refers to the lower burner.

lower body distress 下迫 *xià pò*: An urgent desire to pass stool with inhibited evacuation. [27: 365]

lower body gan 下疳 *xià gān*: Synonym: *gan sore*. A sore of the penis, yin head (glans penis), foreskin, vagina or labia that starts with as bean-like lump that is neither painful nor ruptures (hard lower body gan) or that starts as a small sore and gradually ruptures (soft low body gan). See RED BAYBERRY SORE. [26: 37, 488] [29: 87] [27: 22] [97: 26] [61: 251]

lower burner 下焦 *xià jiāo*: The part of the triple burner that includes the kidney, bladder, large intestine, and small intestine, in their function of drawing of fluids to be discharged in the form of urine (and the discharge of solid waste through the anus). The intimate relationship between the kidney and the liver means that the latter organ is to some extent considered to be located in the lower burner. More at TRIPLE BURNER. [26: 38]

lower burner damp-heat 下焦湿热 *xià jiāo shī rè*: Synonym: *damp-heat pouring down; downpour of damp-heat*. A disease pattern arising when damp-heat pours down into the lower burner. Lower burner damp-heat includes LARGE INTESTINAL DAMP-HEAT, which manifests in DAMP-HEAT DYSENTERY and DAMP-HEAT DIARRHEA, and includes BLADDER DAMP-HEAT manifesting in *strangury-turbidity* and DRIBBLING URINARY BLOCK. In addition, lower burner damp-heat may take the form of PUDENDAL ITCH, VAGINAL DISCHARGE, LOWER LIMB FIRE FLOW, FOOT QI SORE, DAMP-HEAT SEMINAL EMISSION, and painful swelling of the lower limb joints. [6: 210] [27: 139] [97: 27]

lower burner damp-heat bloody urine 下焦湿 热尿血 *xià jiāo shī rè niào xuè*: BLADDER DAMP-HEAT BLOODY URINE.

lower burner dispersion-thirst 下消 *xià xiāo*: LOWER DISPERSION.

lower burner governs exit 下焦主出 *xià jiāo zhǔ chū*: The functions of the large intestine and bladder in discharging waste from the body. [27: 59]

lower burner heat bind 热结下焦 *rè jié xià jiāo*: Disease characterized by lower abdominal pain and distention and rough painful urination with bloody urine in severe cases. NB: In this context, LOWER BURNER means large and small intestine and bladder. Compare BLADDER HEAT BIND. [27: 136]

lower burner is like a sluice 下焦如渎 *xià jiāo rú dú*: The lower burner represents the function of the intestines in absorbing fluids from food, and those of the kidney and bladder in discharging it in the form of urine. [26: 38] [27: 58] [6: 100]

lower cheek 颐 *yí*: JOWL. [26: 911]

lower dispersion 下消 *xià xiāo*: Synonym: *kidney dispersion*. A dispersion-thirst pattern marked by the passing of twice as much fluid as is drunk, unctuous or greasy urine like strangury-turbidity, and black face and parched ears; attributed to depletion of kidney water and failure of distilling transformation. MED Supplement the kidney and promote astriction with Six-Ingredient Rehmannia Pill (*liù wèi dì huáng wán*), Pancreas-Enriching Beverage (*zī cuì yǐn*), Left-Restoring [Kidney Yin] Beverage (*zuǒ guī yǐn*), or Major Origin-Supplementing Brew (*dà bǔ yuán jiān*). For yin vacuity affecting yang and debilitated fire failing to form qi, and vacuous qi failing to transform fluids, use Cinnamon Bark and Aconite Eight-Ingredient Pill (*guì fù bā wèi wán*), Right-Restoring [Life Gate] Beverage (*yòu guī yǐn*), Origin-Securing Brew (*mì yuán jiān*), or Yin-Securing Brew (*gù yīn jiān*). ACU Base treatment mainly on back transport points, KI, and SP. Select BL-23 (*shèn shū*, Kidney Transport), KI-3 (*tài xī*, Great Ravine), SP-6 (*sān yīn jiāo*, Three Yin Intersection), and KI-6 (*zhào hǎi*, Shining Sea); needle with supplementation. For yin vacuity affecting yang, add GV-4 (*mìng mén*, Life Gate), and CV-4 (*guān yuán*, Pass Head), using moxa. See DISPERSION-THIRST.[1] [26: 37] [27: 426] [97: 25] [37: 393]

lower extreme 下极 *xià jí*: 1. Synonyms: *king's palace*; *mountain root*. The region between the two inner canthi, i.e., the root of the nose. 2. The anus. 3. The perineum. [27: 30] [97: 25]

lower limb fire flow 下肢流火 *xià zhī liú huǒ*: FIRE CINNABAR LEG. [27: 165]

lower orifices 下窍 *xià qiào*: Synonym: *turbid orifices*. The anal and genital orifices. Compare TWO YIN. [27: 27]

lower origin 下元 *xià yuán*: Original qi of the lower burner; the kidney. Usually only referred to in pathology. Insecurity of the lower origin refers to INSECURITY OF KIDNEY QI, depletion of the lower origin to KIDNEY YIN VACUITY, and exhaustion of the lower origin to KIDNEY YANG VACUITY. Compare TRUE ORIGIN.

lower transverse bone 下横骨 *xià héng gǔ*: Synonym: *covering bone*. The bone above the genitals, i.e., the lower anterior part of the innominate bone. WMC The pubic bone. [27: 68] [97: 26]

lower uniting point 下合穴 *xià hé xué*: Any of a group of points located on the lower limbs, used to treat disease of the six bowels. Each organ has a uniting point located on its associated channel in the vicinity of the elbows or knees (LI-11, TB-10, and SI-8, see TRANSPORT POINT). In addition to these, the three bowels associated with the yang channels of the arm each have a uniting point located on one of the yang channels of the foot. The lower uniting points of the small and large intestines are located on the stomach channel at ST-37 (*shàng jù xū*, Upper Great Hollow) and ST-39 (*xià jù xū*, Lower Great Hollow) respectively, whereas that of the triple burner is on the bladder channel at BL-39 (*wěi yáng*, Bend Yang). Each point is used to treat disease of their respective bowel. The lower uniting points of each channel and their indications are as follows: Stomach channel: ST-36 (*zú sān lǐ*, Leg Three Li), poor digestion, stomach duct pain and distention, abdominal pain, constipation, and diarrhea. Large intestine: ST-37 (*shàng jù xū*, Upper Great Hollow), intestinal welling-abscess (*yōng*) (appendicitis), swill diarrhea. Small Intestine: ST-39 (*xià jù xū*, Lower Great Hollow), diarrhea, abdominal pain, and dysentery. Gallbladder: GB-34 (*yáng líng quán*, Yang Mound Spring), bitter taste in mouth, vomiting, and cholecystitis. Bladder: BL-40 (*wěi zhōng*, Bend Center), dribbling urinary block, and enuresis. Triple Burner: BL-39 (*wěi yáng*, Bend Yang), dribbling urinary block, and enuresis. ◇ Chin 下 *xià*, lower, down; 合 *hé*, unite; 穴 *xué*, cave, hole. See UNITING POINT. [26: 36]

lower yin 下阴 *xià yīn*: ANTERIOR YIN. [26: 37] [27: 69]

lozenge 锭 *dìng*: Synonym: *lozenge preparation*. A solid preparation made by blending finely ground medicinals with flour paste and forming them into spindle shapes, cones, or oblongs. If taken orally, lozenges are crushed and swallowed with water. If to be applied topically, they are crushed and mixed with vinegar or sesame oil. [27: 313]

lozenge preparation 锭剂 *dìng jì*: LOZENGE.

LR 肝 *gān*, 足厥阴肝经 *zú jué yīn gān jīng*: Abbreviation for the liver or the foot reverting yin (*jué yīn*) liver channel.

LU 肺 *fèi*, 手太阴肺经 *shǒu tài yīn fèi jīng*: The lung or hand greater yin (*tài yīn*) lung channel.

lubricate the intestines 滑肠 *huá cháng*: MOISTENING THE INTESTINES.

lubricating formula 滑剂 *huá jì*: One of the TEN FORMULA TYPES. Lubricating [medicinals] can eliminate fixity, i.e., they can eliminate tangible binds in the body. For example, Mallow Seed Powder (*kuí zǐ sǎn*), plus moneywort (*jīn qián cǎo*) and lygodium spore (*hǎi jīn shā*) can be used to treat stone strangury with painful urination or complete stoppage of urine. This formula contains the lubricating medicinals mallow seed (*dōng kuí zǐ*) and dwarf elm bark (*yú bái pí*), which help to free the stones. [27: 306] [97: 584]

lubricating [medicinals] can eliminate fixity 滑可去着 *huá kě qù zhuó*: Lubricating medicinals such as mallow seed (*dōng kuí zǐ*) and dwarf elm bark (*yú bái pí*), which are slippery in substance, can be used to treat stone strangury. See LUBRICATING FORMULA. [26: 759]

lumbar and back pain 腰背痛 *yāo bèi tòng*: From *The Magic Pivot* (*líng shū, wǔ lóng jī yè bié*). Lumbar pain spreading into the back. MED For debilitation of kidney qi and wind-damp exploiting the channels and network vessels, Duhuo and Mistletoe Decoction (*dú huó jì shēng tāng*). For prolonged sitting, use Center-Supplementing Qi-Boosting Decoction (*bǔ zhōng yì qì tāng*) or Eight-Gem Decoction (*bā zhēn tāng*). ACU Base treatment mainly on BL, GV, CV, and KI. Main points: BL-23 (*shèn shū*, Kidney Transport), GV-3 (*yāo yáng guān*, Lumbar Yang Pass), BL-40 (*wěi zhōng*, Bend Center), ouch points (*ā shì xué*), CV-4 (*guān yuán*, Pass Head), BL-60 (*kūn lún*, Kunlun Mountains), and BL-37 (*yīn mén*, Gate of Abundance); needle with supplementation and add moxa. Selection of points according to cause: For debilitation of kidney qi and wind-damp exploiting the channels and network vessels, supplement and moxa KI-3 (*tài xī*, Great Ravine), KI-7 (*fù liū*, Recover Flow), and BL-64 (*jīng gǔ*, Capital Bone), and drain GB-20 (*fēng chí*, Wind Pool), GB-31 (*fēng shì*, Wind Market), TB-5 (*wài guān*, Outer Pass), LI-11 (*qū chí*, Pool at the Bend), and SP-9 (*yīn líng quán*, Yin Mound Spring). For prolonged sitting, add BL-20 (*pí shū*, Spleen Transport), BL-21 (*wèi shū*, Stomach Transport), ST-36 (*zú sān lǐ*, Leg Three Li), SP-6 (*sān yīn jiāo*, Three Yin Intersection), and CV-6 (*qì hǎi*, Sea of Qi); needle with supplementation and add moxa. See also BACK PAIN; ACHING LUMBUS; LUMBAR PAIN. [26: 795] [50: 1619] [46: 594, 633] [113: 228] [14: 83]

lumbar pain 腰痛 *yāo tòng*: Pain in the lumbus, on one or either side, or affecting the spine. The lumbus is the house of the kidney, and lumbar pain is commonly associated with kidney problems. Specific causes include TAXATION DETRIMENT, debility in old age, depletion of kidney qi, contraction of external evils, and external injury. External evils and external injury generally cause acute pain that manifests as a repletion pattern. WMC low back pain; lumbago. See EXTERNAL CONTRACTION LUMBAR PAIN; INTERNAL DAMAGE LUMBAR PAIN; EXTERNAL INJURY LUMBAR PAIN; POSTPARTUM LUMBAR PAIN. Compare PAIN IN THE LUMBAR SPINE; ACHING LUMBUS. [26: 795] [92: No. 164]

Lumbar Pain

BLOOD VACUITY LUMBAR PAIN (*xuè xū yāo tòng*)

DAMP-HEAT LUMBAR PAIN (*shī rè yāo tòng*)

DAMPNESS DAMAGE LUMBAR PAIN (*shāng shī yāo tòng*)

DAMP PHLEGM LUMBAR PAIN (*shī tán yāo tòng*)

COLD-DAMP LUMBAR PAIN (*hán shī yāo tòng*)

EXTERNAL CONTRACTION LUMBAR PAIN (*wài gǎn yāo tòng*)

EXTERNAL INJURY LUMBAR PAIN (*wài shāng yāo tòng*)

INTERNAL DAMAGE LUMBAR PAIN (*nèi shāng yāo tòng*)

KIDNEY VACUITY LUMBAR PAIN (*shèn xū yāo tòng*)

POSTPARTUM LUMBAR PAIN (*chǎn hòu yāo tòng*)

QI STAGNATION LUMBAR PAIN (*qì zhì yāo tòng*)

STATIC BLOOD LUMBAR PAIN (*yū xuè yāo tòng*)

VACUITY-TAXATION LUMBAR PAIN (*xū láo yāo tòng*)

WIND-DAMP LUMBAR PAIN (*fēng hán yāo tòng*)

WIND-HEAT LUMBAR PAIN (*fēng rè yāo tòng*)

---

lumbar pain in pregnancy 妊娠腰痛 *rèn shēn yāo tòng*: From *The Origin and Indicators of Disease* (*zhū bìng yuán hòu lùn*). Lumbar pain during pregnancy. Attributable to kidney vacuity, to assailing wind-coldor to wrenching or contusion that causes static blood to obstruct the channels. In severe cases, there may be sagging of the fetus. **kidney vacuity** pregnancy lumbar pain is associated with a limpness and lack of strength and is exacerbation by exertion. MED Warm and supplement kidney yang with Young Maid Pill (*qīng é wán*). **Wind-cold** pregnancy lumbar pain is marked by cold pain that is exacerbated by exposure to cold. MED Expel wind and dissipate cold. Use Four Agents Decoction (*sì wù tāng*) plus mistletoe (*sāng jì shēng*) and ledebouriella (*fáng fēng*). **Wrenching or contusion** gives rise to stabbing pain and to inhibited turning. Blood stasis is marked by pain of fixed location. MED Quicken the blood and relieve pain; supplement the kidney and quiet the fetus. Chew a wallnut and swallow 9 g of psoralea (*bǔ gǔ zhī*) with warmed wine. [26: 341]

lumbus 腰 *yāo*: The loin or low back. The main pathological conditions that affect the lumbus are LUMBAR PAIN, ACHING LUMBUS, and WAIST AS IF GIRTHED WITH ROPE. [27: 69] [97: 602]

lumbus is the house of kidney 腰为肾之府 *yāo wéi shèn zhī fǔ*: The kidneys are located in the lumbar region, and their health can be reflected there. Lumbar pain is a sign of kidney vacuity (either yin or yang) when of gradual onset, dull in quality, and when the area is cold to the touch. [27: 34] [97: 338]

lung 肺 *fèi*: Viscus located in the chest, connecting with the throat, and opening into the nose. *Elementary Questions* (*sù wèn*) states, "The lung is the canopy of the viscera." Hence the appellation "florid canopy," which was coined later. The lung is interior and is connected by its channel to the large intestine, which is the corresponding exterior organ. In the doctrine of the five phases, it belongs to metal. The main functions of the lung are governing qi, regulation of the waterways, and the exterior of the entire body. The LUNG GOVERNS QI means that the lung is responsible for breathing and the production of true qi. *The Inner Canon* (*nèi jīng*) also states that the LUNG OPENS AT THE NOSE means that the nose is the outer orifice of the lung, by which great qi (air) enters the body. Signs such as nasal congestion and flaring nostrils are related directly to lung disease. The LUNG GOVERNS REGULATION OF THE WATERWAYS refers to lung qi's action in regard to water metabolism. The depurative downbearing action of lung qi carries water downward to the bladder and prevents accumulation of water qi in the body. Hence, it is also said that the LUNG GOVERNS MOVEMENT OF WATER and the LUNG IS THE UPPER SOURCE OF WATER. Disturbance of this function can give rise to inhibited urine and water swelling. The LUNG GOVERNS THE SKIN AND [BODY] HAIR means that the lung by its diffusing action nourishes the skin and the hair and protects the exterior against invading evils. Hence, it is also said that the LUNG ENGENDERS THE SKIN AND [BODY] HAIR and the LUNG GOVERNS THE EXTERIOR OF THE ENTIRE BODY. The lung is closely related to the heart, spleen, and the kidney. **Lung and heart:** The HEART GOVERNS THE BLOOD AND VESSELS, whereas the LUNG FACES THE HUNDRED VESSELS. These statements reflect the complementary nature of the heart's function of governing the blood and the lung's function of governing qi, and may reflect the fact now recognized that the blood passes through the lung before being distributed around the body. For this reason, it is also said the LUNG HOLDS THE OFFICE OF ASSISTANT, WHENCE MANAGEMENT AND REGULATION EMANATE. **Lung and spleen:** The SPLEEN IS THE SOURCE OF PHLEGM FORMATION and the LUNG IS THE RECEPTACLE THAT HOLDS PHLEGM. Damp qi arising when spleen qi is vacuous and fails to move and transform fluids properly gathers and forms into phlegm, which then tends to collect in the lung. **Lung and kidney:** The KIDNEY GOVERNS WATER and the LUNG IS THE UPPER SOURCE OF WATER. The lung regulates the waterways, i.e., it controls the movement of water down to the kidney. It therefore supports the kidney's role of governing water. The LUNG GOVERNS QI and the KIDNEY IS THE ROOT OF QI. The lung's ability to ab-

sorb qi is partly dependent on the kidney. If kidney essential qi is insufficient, it is incapable of ensuring the absorption of qi through the lung. This results in respiratory insufficiency characterized by shortness of breath and rapid breathing at the slightest exertion. Because these two viscera are intimately associated with qi and water, it is said that LUNG AND KIDNEY ARE MUTUALLY ENGENDERING. See PULMONARY. [6: 82] [27: 18] [26: 445]

lung accumulation 肺积 *fèi jī*: From *The Pulse Canon* (*mài jīng*). RUSHING RESPIRATION. [26: 450]

lung and kidney are mutually engendering 肺肾相生 *fèi shèn xiāng shēng*: *Synonyms: metal and water are mutually engendering; lung and kidney are of the same source.* The lung and kidney have a beneficial effect on each other. In water metabolism, the KIDNEY GOVERNS WATER (i.e., urine production), whereas the LUNG IS THE UPPER SOURCE OF WATER and GOVERNS REGULATION OF THE WATERWAYS (i.e., downward movement of water to the kidney). Vacuity of either the lung or kidney can cause water swelling. In respiration, the LUNG GOVERNS QI, whereas the KIDNEY GOVERNS QI ABSORPTION. Although breathing is a function of the lung, it can be affected by kidney vacuity. Kidney vacuity preventing qi absorption gives rise to shortness of breath and panting. In the five phases, the lung is ascribed to metal, and the kidney is ascribed to water. Metal and water are mutually engendering. In the engendering sequence, metal engenders water, and according to the principle of disease in the mother (engendering phase) can affect the child (engendered phase), lung qi vacuity can give rise to kidney qi vacuity. Furthermore, according to the principle that disease in the child affects the mother, kidney qi vacuity can give rise to lung vacuity. [26: 449]

lung and kidney are of the same source 肺肾同源 *fèi shèn tóng yuán*: LUNG AND KIDNEY ARE MUTUALLY ENGENDERING.

lung and large intestine stand in interior-exterior relationship 肺与大肠相表里 *fèi yǔ dà cháng xiāng biǎo lǐ*: LUNG IS CONNECTED WITH THE LARGE INTESTINE. [27: 405] [97: 351]

lung block panting and cough 肺闭喘咳 *fèi bì chuǎn ké*: Any condition in which an external evil obstructs the lung, preventing lung qi from diffusing. Lung block panting and cough is characterized by heat effusion, rapid breathing, cough, and, in severe cases, flaring nostrils, somber complexion, and blue lips. It is common among small children, and arises when wind-cold fetters the outer body, when wind warmth invades the lung, or when fire heat distresses the lung (effulgent fire tormenting metal). In wind-cold fettering the outer body, the signs include aversion to cold, headache, absence of sweating, cough, and panting. Wind warmth invading the lung is characterized by mild aversion to cold and strong heat effusion or the absence of aversion to heat effusion. In addition there is sweating, cough, rib-side pain, red tongue with slightly yellow fur. The pattern of fire heat distressing the lung is characterized by high fever, sweating, vexing thirst, rapid panting breathing, and a large surging pulse. ⟦WMC⟧ Pneumonia. [26: 446] [27: 383] [97: 353]

lung channel 肺经 *fèi jīng*: HAND GREATER YIN LUNG CHANNEL.

lung channel cough 肺经咳嗽 *fèi jīng ké sòu*: LUNG COUGH. [26: 450]

lung congestion sleeplessness 肺壅不得卧 *fèi yōng bù dé wò*: From *Pathoconditions, Causes, Pulses, and Treatments* (*zhèng yīn mài zhì*). The tendency to counterflow qi when lying down in patients suffering from panting and cough counterflow ascent with periodic ejection of phlegm-rheum, pain in the right rib-side stretching into the supraclavicular fossa, and in severe cases, panting with raised shoulders. Lung congestion sleeplessness is attributable to metal being tormented by fire, phlegm, dryness or cold. ⟦MED⟧ For heat, use Family Secret White-Draining Powder (*jiā mì xiè bái sǎn*); for phlegm, use Perilla Seed and Apricot Seed Decoction (*sū zǐ xìng zǐ tāng*) plus pinellia (*bàn xià*) and trichosanthes seed (*guā lóu zǐ*); for dryness, use Family Secret Lung-Moistening Beverage (*jiā mì rùn fèi yǐn*); for cold, use Family Secret Lung-Warming Decoction (*jiā mì wēn fèi tāng*). See SLEEPLESSNESS. [50: 212] [?: Vol. 20, p. 73]

lung cough 肺咳 *fèi ké*: *lung channel cough.* Cough with noisy panting, and, in severe cases, coughing of blood. When due to contraction of external cold, it can be treated with Ephedra Decoction (*má huáng tāng*). When attributable to lung vacuity with fire, it can be treated with White-Draining Powder (*xiè bái sǎn*) plus scutellaria (*huáng qín*). ⟦ACU⟧ When due to external cold, see WIND-COLD COUGH. When due to lung vacuity with fire, base treatment mainly on LU, KI, and back transport points. Select BL-13 (*fèi shū*, Lung Transport), BL-43 (*gāo huāng shū*, Gao-Huang Transport), LU-5 (*chǐ zé*, Cubit Marsh), and KI-6 (*zhào hǎi*, Shining Sea); needle with supplementation. Selection of points according to signs: For spitting of blood, add LU-6 (*kǒng zuì*, Collection Hole). See ORGAN COUGH. [26: 447] [27: 380] [97: 350]

lung disease 肺病 *fèi bìng*: Any morbidity of the lung. The lung governs qi and is in charge of breathing, and opens at the nose; hence, disease of the lung can manifest in signs such as cough, rapid breathing, and nasal congestion and runny

nose. Since phlegm easily collects in the lung (*lung is the receptacle that holds phlegm*); hence lung disease often manifests in copious phlegm. Furthermore, the lung governs the voice; hence lung disease can also manifest in hoarse voice or loss of voice. The lung governs diffusion, depurative downbearing, and the regulation of the waterways, and the pathomechanisms of lung disease are often explained in terms of failure of these functions. Contraction of wind-cold or wind-heat causes nondiffusion of lung qi. In the case of wind-cold, for example, this gives rise to signs such as aversion to cold, heat effusion, and nasal congestion and runny nose. External contractions and internal damage can cause impaired downbearing of lung qi, which manifests in cough, copious phlegm, hasty breathing, and distention and oppression in the chest and diaphragm. When regulation of the waterways is affected, puffy swelling and panting and cough are observed.

Lung Disease Patterns

Simple patterns
 LUNG QI VACUITY (*fèi qì xū*)
 LUNG YANG VACUITY (*fèi yáng xū*)
 LUNG YIN VACUITY (*fèi yīn xū*)
 WIND-HEAT INVADING THE LUNG (*fēng rè fàn fèi*)
 WIND-COLD FETTERING THE LUNG (*fēng hán shù fèi*)
 DRYNESS EVIL INVADING THE LUNG (*zào xié fàn fèi*)
 DRYNESS-HEAT DAMAGING THE LUNG (*zào rè shāng fèi*)
 HEAT EVIL CONGESTING THE LUNG (*rè xié yǒng fèi*)
 PHLEGM TURBIDITY OBSTRUCTING THE LUNG (*tán zhuó zǔ fèi*)
 PHLEGM-HEAT OBSTRUCTING THE LUNG (*tán rè zǔ fèi*)
 WATER-COLD SHOOTING INTO THE LUNG (*shuǐ hán shè fèi*)
 NONDIFFUSION OF LUNG QI (*fèi qì bù xuān*)
 IMPAIRED DEPURATIVE DOWNBEARING OF THE LUNG (*fèi shī sù jiàng*)

Combined patterns
 LUNG-KIDNEY YIN VACUITY (*fèi shèn yīn xū*)
 EXUBERANT LUNG-STOMACH HEAT (*fèi wèi rè shèng*)
 KIDNEY FAILING TO ABSORB QI (*shèn bù nà qì*)
 HEART-LUNG QI VACUITY (*xīn fèi qì xū*)
 LIVER FIRE INVADING THE LUNG (*gān huǒ fàn fèi*)

Distinction is made between vacuity and repletion. Vacuity patterns include yin vacuity and qi vacuity. Repletion patterns are caused by external evils invading the lung (wind-heat invading the lung, wind-cold fettering the lung, dryness evil invading the lung) or by phlegm-rheum or heat brewing in the lung (phlegm turbidity obstructing the lung, phlegm-heat congesting the lung). **Lung qi vacuity** is characterized by dry cough with little phlegm, sometimes with expectoration of blood, loss of voice, tidal heat [effusion], and night sweating. **Lung yin vacuity** is characterized by cough with shortness of breath, low faint voice, aversion to wind, spontaneous sweating, and tendency to nasal congestion. **Wind-heat invading the lung** manifests as cough with sticky red phlegm and slight aversion to cold. Other signs may be nasal congestion with thick yellow snivel, dry mouth and sore throat, slight thirst, and generalized heat [effusion]. The tongue is red with thin yellow fur; the pulse is floating and rapid. **Wind-cold fettering the lung** is characterized by cough with aversion to cold. There may also be slight heat effusion, nasal congestion and runny nose, itchy throat, thin white phlegm. The tongue fur is thin and white; the pulse is floating and tight. **Dryness evil invading the lung** is characterized by dry cough without phlegm or by scant sticky phlegm that is not easily expectorated. In severe cases, there is expectoration of blood and chest pain. In addition, the lips, tongue, throat, and nose may be dry. There may be general aversion to cold. **Phlegm turbidity obstructing the lung** is characterized by cough with copious sticky white phlegm that is easily ejected. Other signs include oppression in the chest and in severe cases panting with phlegm rale. The tongue is pale with a slimy white fur; the pulse is slippery. **Phlegm-heat congesting the lung** arises when either external evils invade the lung, where they lie depressed and transform into heat, thus damaging lung liquid and condensing it into phlegm, or when patients suffering from phlegm contract wind-heat so that phlegm and heat bind together to congest the network vessels of the lung. It is characterized by cough and panting, with thick yellow tongue fur, and vigorous heat. Other signs include thirst, vexation and agitation, in severe cases flaring nostrils. Lung disease is treated by various methods; see the list below. NB: It would appear from the above description that "network vessels of the lung" refers not to blood vessels, but rather to the bronchioles. No modern literature to our knowledge discusses this meaning of "network vessels." [26: 447]

Methods of Treating Lung Disease

BOOSTING (AND SUPPLEMENTING) LUNG QI (*bǔ yì fèi qì*)

DIFFUSING THE LUNG (*xuān fèi*)

DIFFUSING THE LUNG AND TRANSFORMING PHLEGM (*xuān fèi huà tán*)

CLEARING HEAT AND TRANSFORMING PHLEGM (*qīng rè huà tán*)

ENRICHING YIN AND DOWNBEARING FIRE (*zī yīn jiàng huǒ*)

MOISTENING THE LUNG AND TRANSFORMING PHLEGM (*rùn fèi huà tán*)

CONSTRAINING THE LUNG AND SUPPRESSING COUGH (*liǎn fèi zhǐ ké*)

WARMING THE LUNG AND TRANSFORMING RHEUM (*wēn fèi huà yǐn*)

NOURISHING YIN AND CLEARING THE LUNG (*yǎng yīn qīng fèi*)

NOURISHING YIN AND MOISTENING DRYNESS (*yǎng yīn rùn zào*)

---

lung dispersion 肺消 *fèi xiāo*: From *Elementary Questions* (*sù wèn, qì jué lun*). UPPER DISPERSION. [26: 447] [27: 423] [97: 351]

lung dryness 肺燥 *fèi zào*: Any pattern of lung dryness. The lung is ascribed to metal, with which the season autumn is associated. The lung is easily damaged by dryness evil in the autumn. See DRYNESS QI DAMAGING THE LUNG. A similar condition may arise through LUNG YIN VACUITY. The basic signs of any lung dryness are cough, expectoration of blood, dry nose, sore throat, hoarse voice, dry mouth, thirst, and a red tongue with white fur. [27: 161] [97: 351]

lung dryness cough 肺燥咳嗽 *fèi zào ké sòu*: Cough without phlegm, or expectoration of blood-streaked phlegm characteristic of LUNG DRYNESS.

lung engenders the skin and [body] hair 肺生皮毛 *fèi shēng pí máo*: From *Elementary Questions* (*sù wèn, yīn yáng yìng xiàng dà lùn*). See LUNG GOVERNS THE SKIN AND [BODY] HAIR.

lung evil rib-side pain 肺邪胁痛 *fèi xié xié tòng*: RIB-SIDE PAIN occurring when the lung is affected by an evil. Patterns in which lung evil rib-side pain may occur include cold evil assailing the lung, water-rheum collecting internally, or evil heat scorching the lung. Lung evil rib-side pain is accompanied by cough, panting, and copious phlegm. In cold patterns, there is ejection of thin foamy phlegm-drool, low fever or absence of fever (heat effusion), and tight stringlike pulse. Heat patterns are characterized by expectoration of fishy smelling phlegm, red facial complexion, intense internal heat, and rapid pulse. [MED] Cold patterns are treated by effusing sweat and expelling rheum with formulas such as Minor Green-Blue Dragon Decoction (*xiǎo qīng lóng tāng*); heat patterns are treated by clearing heat and flushing phlegm with Thousand Gold Pieces Phragmites Decoction (*qiān jīn wěi jīng tāng*). [ACU] For cold patterns, select GB-20 (*fēng chí*,

Wind Pool), BL-12 (*fēng mén*, Wind Gate), LU-7 (*liè quē*, Broken Sequence), LI-4 (*hé gǔ*, Union Valley), TB-5 (*wài guān*, Outer Pass), LR-14 (*qī mén*, Cycle Gate), TB-6 (*zhī gōu*, Branch Ditch), GB-34 (*yáng líng quán*, Yang Mound Spring); needle with drainage, using moxa if necessary. For heat patterns, select GB-20 (*fēng chí*, Wind Pool), GV-14 (*dà zhuī*, Great Hammer), LU-5 (*chǐ zé*, Cubit Marsh), LI-4 (*hé gǔ*, Union Valley), LI-11 (*qū chí*, Pool at the Bend), TB-5 (*wài guān*, Outer Pass), TB-6 (*zhī gōu*, Branch Ditch), GB-34 (*yáng líng quán*, Yang Mound Spring), and LU-11 (*shào shāng*, Lesser Shang); needle with drainage and prick LI-1 (*shāng yáng*, Shang Yang) to bleed. See also WIND-COLD RIB-SIDE PAIN; PHLEGM-RHEUM RIB-SIDE PAIN. [26: 446]

lung faces the hundred vessels 肺朝百脉 *fèi cháo bǎi mài*: *Elementary Questions* (*sù wèn*) states, "Vessel qi flows into the channel, and channel qi returns to the lung; the lung faces the hundred vessels." This means that the blood of the whole body must pass through the lung channel and the lung proper. [26: 449] [27: 49] [97: 354]

lung fire 肺火 *fèi huǒ*: Fire affecting the lung. Distinction is made between repletion and vacuity fire. **Repletion fire** is characterized by cough with pronounced sound and scant phlegm or thick yellow phlegm sometimes flecked with blood, and is accompanied by red tongue with yellow fur, and slippery rapid pulse. MED Use White-Draining Powder (*xiè bái sǎn*). ACU Base treatment mainly on LU and LI. Select LU-10 (*yú jì*, Fish Border), LU-5 (*chǐ zé*, Cubit Marsh), LI-4 (*hé gǔ*, Union Valley), and LI-11 (*qū chí*, Pool at the Bend); needle with drainage and prick LU-11 (*shào shāng*, Lesser Shang), and LI-1 (*shāng yáng*, Shang Yang), to bleed. **Vacuity fire** is seen in enduring cough in yin vacuity patients, and is characterized by a faint cough and accompanied by tidal heat [effusion], night sweating, and a rapid fine pulse. MED Use Lily Bulb Lung-Securing Decoction (*bǎi hé gù fèi tāng*). ACU Base treatment mainly on LU and KI. Select BL-13 (*fèi shū*, Lung Transport), BL-43 (*gāo huāng shū*, Gao-Huang Transport), LU-5 (*chǐ zé*, Cubit Marsh), BL-23 (*shèn shū*, Kidney Transport), and KI-6 (*zhào hǎi*, Shining Sea); needle with supplementation. [27: 161] [27: 161] [97: 349] [46: 596, 653]

lung forms snivel 肺为涕 *fèi wéi tì*: From *Elementary Questions* (*sù wèn, xuān míng wǔ qì piān*) Snivel (nasal mucus) flows from the nose; the nose is the orifice of the lung; hence snivel is the humor of the lung. This phrase is the same as SNIVEL IS THE HUMOR OF THE LUNG. [50: 952] [27: 61]

lung governs depurative downbearing 肺主肃降 *fèi zhǔ sù jiàng*: Under normal circumstances, lung qi bears downward, drawing breath down the windpipe into the lung and keeping the lung clean of phlegm. The compound term "depurative downbearing" reflects the downward movement of qi and its action of maintaining a clean lung. The word 'depurative' further hints at the five-phase association of metal with the notion of the purifying frost of autumn. If this function is fulfilled, air can pass in and out of the lung freely, the respiratory channels are kept free, breathing is even, and fluids descend to the kidney and bladder. When in external contractions or internal damage, evils invade the lung, they can affect normal depurative downbearing and cause cough with copious phlegm, hasty breathing, and distention and oppression in the chest and diaphragm. Enduring cough can also damage lung qi, impairing normal depurative downbearing and causing lung qi to ascend counterflow, giving rise to severe panting. See IMPAIRED DEPURATIVE DOWNBEARING OF THE LUNG. Compare LUNG GOVERNS REGULATION OF THE WATERWAYS and LUNG IS THE RECEPTACLE THAT HOLDS PHLEGM. ◊ Chin 肃 *sù*, purify, purge; solemn; 降 *jiàng*, to descend, cause to descend. [27: 49] [97: 353]

lung governs diffusion 肺主宣散 *fèi zhǔ xuān sàn*: One aspect of LUNG GOVERNS QI. The lung is responsible for ensuring the movement of qi out toward the body surface. Under normal circumstances, lung qi diffuses outward. When external evil (wind-heat, wind-cold) invades the lung, causing cough with scant or copious phlegm, nasal congestion, runny nose, itchy throat, or hoarse voice, usually accompanied by exterior signs. The resulting pattern is called nondiffusion of lung qi. In severe cases of evil heat, there may be high fever with flaring nostrils, rough panting, with thick yellow phlegm, and if external evil stirs existing cold-rheum, there may be foamy white phlegm-drool and a frog rale in the throat. See NONDIFFUSION OF LUNG QI. [27: 49] [97: 352]

lung governs management and regulation 肺主治节 *fèi zhǔ zhì jié*: See LUNG HOLDS THE OFFICE OF ASSISTANT, WHENCE MANAGEMENT AND REGULATION EMANATE. [27: 49] [97: 353]

lung governs movement of water 肺主行水 *fèi zhǔ xíng shuǐ*: See LUNG IS THE UPPER SOURCE OF WATER.

lung governs qi 肺主气 *fèi zhǔ qì*: The lung takes in clear, natural qi and expels turbid qi. "The lung governs qi" denotes the respiratory function and role played by the lung in the production of true qi (*qì*, in Chinese means breath and breathing as well as qi). Lung qi has the functions of ensuring diffusion and depurative downbearing. If these two functions are fulfilled, air can pass in and out of the lung freely, the respiratory tract is kept free, and breathing is even. Nondiffusion of lung qi is characterized by cough possibly accompanied by exterior signs, whereas impairment of depurative downbearing is characterized by cough and panting. *Elementary Questions* (*sù wèn, zhì zhēn yào dà lùn*) states, "All qi rushing and depression is ascribed to the lung." The respiratory function of the lung is further related to the production of true qi. Inhaled air becomes a main constituent of true qi. *The Magic Pivot* (*líng shū*) states, "True qi is derived from air and from food qi, and fills the body." Inhaled air is combined with grain qi (nutrients in food), which are in turn combined with the essential qi of the kidney to form the true qi that nourishes the whole body. Hence it is said in *Elementary Questions* (*sù wèn*), "The lung governs the qi of the whole body" and "all qi belongs to the lung." In addition to impairing respiration, insufficiency of lung qi may also affect the formation of true qi and thereby trigger generalized qi vacuity, characterized by fatigue and weakness, shortness of breath, and spontaneous sweating. Compare LUNG IS THE GOVERNOR OF QI, KIDNEY IS THE ROOT OF QI. ◇ Chin 气 *qi,* breath, vapor, qi. [27: 49]

lung governs regulation of the waterways 肺主通调水道 *fèi zhǔ tōng tiáo shuǐ dào:* Synonym: *lung governs the movement of water.* The spleen, lung, kidney, intestines, and bladder are jointly responsible for regulating water metabolism. The specific role of the lung is called "governing regulation of the waterways," and represents a combination of the two functions of diffusion and depurative downbearing. By the diffusion of lung qi, fluids are distributed throughout the body, particularly to the skin, where they leave the body in the form of sweat. By depurative downbearing, waste water is conveyed down to the kidney and bladder to be discharged from the body. For this reason it is said, "The lung is the upper source of water." If diffusion is impaired, then the interstices will close up, and thereby prevent sweating. If downbearing is impaired, there may be water swelling and inhibited urination or scant urine. [27: 49]

lung governs the exterior of the entire body 肺主一身之表 *fèi zhǔ yī shēn zhī biǎo:* The exterior of the body is related to lung function. When lung qi is vacuous and the FLESHY EXTERIOR is insecure there is a tendency to spontaneous sweating. When defense is weak, the fleshy exterior is vulnerable to wind-cold invasion, which can give rise to cough. See LUNG GOVERNS THE SKIN AND [BODY] HAIR. [27: 56]

lung governs the movement of water 肺主行水 *fèi zhǔ xíng shuǐ:* See LUNG GOVERNS REGULATION OF THE WATERWAYS. [27: 49] [97: 352]

lung governs the nose 肺主鼻 *fèi zhǔ bí:* See LUNG OPENS AT THE NOSE. [26: 446]

lung governs the skin and [body] hair 肺主皮毛 *fèi zhǔ pí máo:* The skin and [body] hair are closely related to lung function. *Elementary Questions* (*sù wèn, yīn yáng yìng xiàng lùn*) states, "The lung engenders the skin and [body] hair," which is explained as meaning that the skin and [body] hair are dependent on the essential qi supplied by the lung. Certain forms of lung vacuity such as LUNG WILTING may be reflected in dry lusterless skin. In a broader sense, the skin and [body] hair represent the exterior of the body as a defense against external evils. Invasion of external evils is associated with disturbance of normal sweating (absence of sweating or profuse sweating). The function of resisting evils and controlling perspiration is also related to the supply of defense qi. *The Magic Pivot* (*líng shū*) states, "Defense qi warms the flesh and flushes the skin; it replenishes the interstices and controls their opening and closing." Its capacity to fulfill these functions is mainly attributable to the diffusion—or gentle outward movement—of lung qi. This is discussed in *The Magic Pivot* (*líng shū*) in the following way: "The upper burner opens, diffuses the five flavors [i.e., foods of the five flavors], nourishes the skin, fills the body, and moistens the hair, just as the dew waters the earth." The sweat pores, referred to in *Elementary Questions* (*sù wèn, shēn qì tōng tiān lùn*) as "qi gates" were believed to have the function of diffusing lung qi. The relationship of the skin and [body] hair to the lung can be seen in disease. Although the lung itself is in the interior, its governing the qi of the whole body and its intimate relationship with defense qi in particular place it on the first line of the body's defense's to external evils. External evils assailing the FLESHY EXTERIOR usually cause lung disease such as sore throat and nasal congestion. When lung qi is vacuous, the fleshy exterior become "insecure," allowing sweat to flow out (spontaneous sweating). NB: The lung is the only viscus to be affected by invasion of external evils manifesting in exterior patterns. ◇ Chin 皮 *pí,* skin, integument; 毛 *máo,* hair, or specifically hair of the body as opposed to that of the head. [27: 50]

lung governs the voice 肺主声 *fèi zhǔ shēng:* The voice is intimately related to the lung. Lung qi powers the vocal chords. Sufficiency of lung qi is reflected in a full clear voice; lung qi vacuity is reflected in a low faint voice. Contraction of external wind-cold causing congestion of lung qi is reflected a hoarse voice. This is called "replete metal failing to sound." Internal damage pulmonary consumption with great damage to lung qi and hoarse voice is called "broken metal failing to sound." [26: 446] [27: 51] [97: 351]

lung heat 肺热 *fèi rè:* Any pattern of lung heat. Signs include red facial complexion, cough with thick phlegm, chest pain, and, in severe cases, hasty breathing, or expectoration of blood. See WARM EVIL INVADING THE LUNG; HEAT DAMAGING THE NETWORK VESSELS OF THE LUNG; EXUBERANT FIRE TORMENTING METAL; EXUBERANT LUNG-STOMACH HEAT. [27: 161] [97: 350]

lung heat cough 肺热咳嗽 *fèi rè ké sòu*: COUGH due to lung heat. [26: 450]

lung heat scorching the lobes 肺热叶焦 *fèi rè yè jiāo*: Long scorching of the lobes of the lung by depressed heat causing WILTING (*wěi*) patterns. *Elementary Questions* (*sù wèn, wěi lùn*) states, "Lung heat scorching the lobes develops into crippling wilt." Lung heat scorching lobes can give rise to two conditions: (1) LUNG WILTING, characterized by coughing up of foamy turbid drool. (2) Wilting of arms and legs characterized by drying of the skin and body hair and withering of the flesh, lack of strength in the limbs. See WILTING. [26: 450] [27: 161] [97: 354]

lung holds the office of assistant, whence management and regulation emanate 肺者，相傅之官也，治节出焉 *fèi zhě, xiàng fù zhī guān yě, zhì jié chū yān*: From *Elementary Questions* (*sù wèn, líng lán mì diǎn lùn*). The heart holds the office of monarch, and the lung is its assistant. The heart governs the blood, whereas the lung governs qi; the lung therefore helps the heart to carry blood to all parts of the body so that they are all nourished. The ability to influence the heart beat by controlling respiration as in qi-gong may be further evidence for this relationship. *The Inner Canon* (*nèi jīng*) expressed the functions of organs in terms of analogy to government. The lung's action of conveying essence to the skin and [body] hair, its connection with defense qi, its role in the production of blood, its regulation of the waterways through all three burners, means that it has a supporting role in many functions within the economy of the body. [27: 49, 616] [26: 416]

lung impediment 肺痹 *fèi bì*: Damage to lung qi from persistent SKIN IMPEDIMENT (*pí bì*) with further contraction of evils or excessive sorrow or grief. Lung impediment is marked by oppression and vexation in the heart and chest, pain in the chest and back, cough with rapid breathing, and in some cases vomiting and nausea. MED Diffuse the lung and dispel evils with Schisandra Decoction (*wǔ wèi zǐ tāng*). If there are lung heat signs, use Family Secret White-Draining Powder (*jiā mì xiè bái sǎn*). For pronounced lung vacuity, use Pulse-Engendering Powder (*shēng mài sǎn*). ACU See SKIN IMPEDIMENT. [26: 450]

lung is averse to cold 肺恶寒 *fèi wù hán*: From *Elementary Questions* (*sù wèn, xuān míng wǔ qì pian*) The lung cannot tolerate excessive cold. The lung governs qi, is connected with the skin and [body] hair in the outer body, and opens at the nose. Cold evil can directly assail the exterior and damage outer defense yang and easily invade the lung channel. The lung also governs qi. When there is cold, qi becomes stagnant. Spleen-stomach vacuity cold can also affect the lung. These statements support the classical statement that the lung is averse to cold. It should nevertheless be noted that the lung is also susceptible to heat. See AVERSIONS OF THE FIVE VISCERA. [26: 449] [27: 51] [97: 352]

lung is connected with the large intestine 肺合大肠 *fèi hé dà cháng*: The lung stands in interior-exterior relationship with the large intestine. The lung channel connects with the large intestine, and the large intestine channel connects with the lung. The lung's depurative downbearing helps the large's intestine's function of conveying and transforming of waste, and vice versa. Panting due to phlegm congestion can be treated with draining precipitants to free lung qi, whereas some types of constipation are best treated by opening the lung. Medicinals that transform phlegm and suppress cough, such as apricot kernel (*xìng rén*) and trichosanthes (*guā lóu*), also have the effect of moistening the intestines. [27: 51] [97: 353]

lung is connected with the skin and [body] hair 肺合皮毛 *fèi hé pí máo*: See LUNG GOVERNS THE SKIN AND [BODY] HAIR.

lung is connected with the skin; its luxuriance is the [body] hair 肺合皮也，其荣毛也 *fèi hé pí yě, qí róng máo yě*: From *Elementary Questions* (*sù wèn, wǔ zàng shēng chéng piān*). See LUNG GOVERNS THE SKIN AND [BODY] HAIR.

lung is often in insufficiency 肺常不足 *fèi cháng bù zú*: The lung tends toward vacuity; a feature of child pathology. Young children have weak bowels and viscera; their physical body and qi are not yet replete; and their yin and yang are still immature. When yin and yang are both frail, resistance to disease is low. Inability to adjust to heat and cold and irregular feeding cause increased susceptibility to invasion of the six excesses or dietary damage. For these reasons, externally contracted disease, and morbidity of the lung and spleen are common in small children. The lung governs qi, and is in charge of breathing; it is connected with the skin and [body] hair. Since the external defense of children is insecure, evils easily enter the ligature of the lung (the nose, throat, and windpipe). Hence, coughs and colds are very common. The spleen and stomach are the root of later heaven (the acquired constitution); they move and transform the grain and water (food) and distribute its essence; hence they are the source of qi and blood formation. Splenic movement and transformation tend to be underdeveloped in children, which makes it difficult to the supply the essence of grain and qi needed for healthy growth and development. Thus children often suffer from dietary damage causing accumulation and stagnation, retching and vomiting, and diarrhea. The lung is dependent on the spleen for nourishment; hence *Elementary Questions* (*sù wèn, yīn yáng yìng xiàng dà lùn*) states, "The spleen engenders flesh, and flesh engenders the lung." When spleen qi is strong, the essence of grain and water flows up into the lung, and so the strength of lung qi relies on the later-heaven qi of the stomach and spleen. [26: 448]

lung is the delicate viscus 肺为娇脏 *fèi wéi jiāo zàng*: Of all the viscera, the lung, which draws in great qi (air) from outside the body, is most susceptible to six excesses, particularly wind, cold, and heat. Contractions of these evils readily cause nondiffusion of lung qi, which can manifest as cough and nasal congestion. [26: 447] [27: 50] [97: 352]

lung is the florid canopy 肺为华盖 *fèi wéi huá gài*: A phrase contained in Yu Shu's annotation on the 32nd difficulty of *The Classic of Difficult Issues* (*nàn jīng*) doubtlessly based on the statements in *The Inner Canon* (*nèi jīng*). *The Magic Pivot* (*líng shū, jiǔ zhēn lùn*) states, "The lung is the canopy of the five viscera and six bowels." *Elementary Questions* (*sù wèn, wěi lùn*) states, "The lung is chief of the viscera, and is the florid canopy of the heart." The lung is the uppermost of all organs in the chest and abdomen, covering the others like a canopy. It is also governs the exterior of the whole body and forms the outer defense of the bowels and viscera. [27: 50] [97: 352] [50: 954]

lung is the governor of qi, kidney is the root of qi 肺为气之主，肾为气之根 *fèi wéi qì zhī zhǔ, shèn wéi qì zhī gēn*: The lung draws in great qi (air) from the environment, but cannot do so unless the essential qi of the kidney is exuberant. See LUNG GOVERNS QI; KIDNEY GOVERNS QI ABSORPTION. [6: 85]

lung is the receptacle that holds phlegm 肺为贮痰之器 *fèi wéi zhù tán zhī qì*: Fluids are passed by the spleen to the lung, which distributes them around the body. Damp-qi arising when spleen qi is vacuous and fails to move and transform the fluids properly gathers to form phlegm, which collects in the lung. Thus the lung is the receptacle that holds phlegm, i.e., the place where it collects. See SPLEEN IS THE SOURCE OF PHLEGM FORMATION. [6: 84]

lung is the upper source of water 肺为水之上源 *fèi wéi shuǐ zhī shàng yuán*: The lung regulates the waterways and governs the movement of water. It is the viscus associated with water in the upper burner, hence the epithet. [27: 49] [97: 353]

lung, its bloom is in the [body] hair 肺，其华在毛 *fèi, qí huá zài máo*: *Elementary Questions*

(*sù wèn, liù jié zàng xiàng lùn*) states, "The lung... its bloom is in the [body] hair." Bloom means external manifestation of health. The health of the lung is reflected in the luxuriance of the skin. This is because the lung governs transportation of essence to the skin and [body] hair. In the extreme state of pulmonary consumption (TB), the skin takes on a perished-looking complexion and the hair becomes dry and lifeless. This is why the lung is said to have its bloom in the skin and [body] hair. See LUNG ENGENDERS SKIN AND [BODY] HAIR. [27: 51]

lung-kidney yin vacuity 肺肾阴虚 *fèi shèn yīn xū*: A condition comprising signs of LUNG YIN VACUITY and KIDNEY YIN VACUITY. Signs of lung yin vacuity include emaciation and marked ill health, dry cough with little phlegm (sometimes streaked with blood), dry mouth and throat, low hoarse voice, and rapid breathing. Signs of kidney yin vacuity include night sweating, lumbar pain, and seminal emission. Lung and kidney yin vacuity is further characterized by reddening of the cheeks and steaming bone tidal heat [effusion], red tongue, and rapid fine pulse. | MED | Enrich and nourish the lung and kidney. Use Lily Bulb Metal-Securing Decoction (*bǎi hé gù jīn tāng*). See LUNG YIN VACUITY; KIDNEY YIN VACUITY; KIDNEY VACUITY; DUAL VACUITY OF THE LUNG AND KIDNEY. [57: 112]

lung-metal 肺金 *fèi jīn*: The lung as belonging to metal in the doctrine of the five phases.

lung mounting 肺疝 *fèi shàn*: Synonym: *pulmonary mounting*. MOUNTING caused by cold evil invading the lung. *Elementary Questions* (*sù wèn, dà qí lùn*) states, "When the lung pulse is sunken and contending, [this] indicates lung mounting." Wang Bing notes this saying "cold contending with the viscera." Signs include distention and pain in the lesser abdomen and testicles and urinary stoppage. [50: 949]

lung opens at the nose 肺开窍于鼻 *fèi kāi qiào yú bí*: The nose is the outer opening of the respiratory tract, through which air enters the lung. *Elementary Questions* (*sù wèn, yīn yáng yìng xiàng dà lùn*) states, "The lung governs the nose." The sense of smell can function normally only if lung qi is in harmony and breathing is smooth. Thus *The Magic Pivot* (*líng shū*) states, "Lung qi flows to the nose; when the lung is in harmony, the nose can perceive fetor and fragrance." In addition, snivel (nasal mucus) is the humor of the lung. Many lung diseases are the result of the contraction of external evils through the nose and mouth, and are reflected in the condition of the nose. For example, colds may be characterized by nasal congestion and a runny nose, attributable to nondiffusion of lung qi and lung qi ascending counterflow, caused by evil heat congestion in the lung frequently leads to rapid breathing and flaring nostrils. Recent treatment of nasal polyps and chronic rhinitis by needling lung points on the ear also demonstrates the principle that the lung opens at the nose. [26: 446] [27: 50] [6: 83]

lung pulse is floating 肺脉浮 *fèi mài fú*: The floating pulse is associated with diseases of the lung and the season autumn. *Elementary Questions* (*sù wèn, xuān míng wǔ qì piān*) says, "The lung pulse is downy." *The Classic of Difficult Issues* (*nàn jīng, 15*) states, "The autumn pulse is downy." A downy pulse is now usually referred to as a floating pulse. See FLOATING PULSE. [9: 336] [131: 200]

lung qi 肺气 *fèi qì*: **1.** The activating force that accounts for lung function. Lung qi includes ANCESTRAL QI. **2.** Breath. [26: 448]

lung qi ascending counterflow 肺气上逆 *fèi qì shàng nì*: Synonym: *counterflow lung qi*. Impaired depurative downbearing of the lung characterized by severe cough and panting. See IMPAIRED DEPURATIVE DOWNBEARING OF THE LUNG. [27: 159] [97: 352]

lung qi block 肺气闭塞 *fèi qì bì sè*: See QI BLOCK.

lung qi flows to the nose 肺气通于鼻 *fèi qì tōng yú bí*: See LUNG OPENS AT THE NOSE.

lung qi vacuity 肺气虚 *fèi qì xū*: A disease pattern most commonly attributable to repeated impairment of lung qi diffusion and downbearing over a long period of time, although it may also be caused by general qi vacuity. The chief signs are forceless cough and panting and shortness of breath. Other signs include a pale white or bright white facial complexion, fatigue and lack of strength, rapid breathing on exertion, spontaneous sweating, susceptibility to the common cold, laziness to speak, and low timid voice. **Analysis:** When qi is vacuous, depurative downbearing is impaired, hence the forceless cough and panting. At the same time the production of ancestral qi is insufficient, hence shortage of qi that causes shortness of breath and rapid breathing on exertion. Qi vacuity is also reflected in laziness to speak, spontaneous sweating, and a pale white or bright white facial complexion. Qi vacuity makes external defense insecure and the interstices unsound, hence the susceptibility to colds. The lung is the upper source of water, and when lung qi is vacuous, the distribution of fluids is impaired, water collects in the lung and ascends counterflow with qi, hence copious thin phlegm. The pale tongue with white fur and the vacuous pulse are also qi vacuity signs. Since lung qi has its root in the kidney, and ancestral qi penetrates the heart and vessels to drive respiration, when lung qi vacuity reaches a certain degree, it can cause HEART-LUNG QI VACUITY, KIDNEY FAILING TO ABSORB QI, or HEART-KIDNEY YANG VACUITY. MED Lung qi vacuity is treated by boosting lung qi with medicinals such as codonopsis (*dǎng shēn*), astragalus (*huáng qí*), licorice (*gān cǎo*), and schisandra (*wǔ wèi zǐ*). A representative formula is Lung-Supplementing Decoction (*bǔ fèi tāng*), to which Jade Wind-Barrier Powder (*yù píng fēng sǎn*) can be added for insecurity of the defensive exterior. Six Gentlemen Decoction (*liù jūn zǐ tāng*) with additions may also be used. ACU Base treatment mainly on back transport points, LU, SP, and CV. Select BL-13 (*fèi shū*, Lung Transport), BL-43 (*gāo huāng shū*, Gao-Huang Transport), LU-9 (*tài yuān*, Great Abyss), BL-20 (*pí shū*, Spleen Transport), SP-3 (*tài bái*, Supreme White), CV-6 (*qì hǎi*, Sea of Qi), and ST-36 (*zú sān lǐ*, Leg Three Li); needle with supplementation and moxa. See also HEART-LUNG QI VACUITY; KIDNEY FAILING TO ABSORB QI. [116: 61] [57: 71] [6: 176] [46: 584, 494, 655]

lung repletion 肺实 *fèi shí*: EVIL REPLETION in the lung channel, attributable to wind-cold, phlegm-heat, phlegm-damp, phlegm-fire, etc. Signs include cough and rough panting, pain and fullness in the chest, phlegm-drool congestion, expectoration of thick yellow phlegm sometimes flecked with blood, and sudden loss of voice. [27: 158] [27: 158] [97: 350]

lung-stomach flaming fire panting 肺胃火炎喘 *fèi wèi huǒ yán chuǎn*: FIRE PANTING.

lung stores the corporeal soul 肺藏魄 *fèi cáng pò*: See CORPOREAL SOUL. [27: 50] [97: 352]

lung taxation 肺劳 *fèi láo*: A vacuity taxation (severe enduring vacuity) pattern attributable to lung vacuity and characterized by dry sore throat, hoarse voice, loss of sense of smell, red facial complexion, oppression in the chest and shortness of breath, cough and ejection of blood, reduced food intake, emaciation and lack of strength, and heat effusion. MED Boost qi and supplement the lung. Use Ginseng Root-Securing Pill (*rén shēn gù běn wán*). ACU Base treatment mainly on LU and KI. Select BL-13 (*fèi shū*, Lung Transport), BL-20 (*pí shū*, Spleen Transport), BL-43 (*gāo huāng shū*, Gao-Huang Transport), LU-9 (*tài yuān*, Great Abyss), LU-5 (*chǐ zé*, Cubit Marsh), KI-3 (*tài xī*, Great Ravine), KI-6 (*zhào hǎi*, Shining Sea), and ST-36 (*zú sān lǐ*, Leg Three Li); needle with supplementation. Selection of points according to signs: For sore dry throat, add TB-2 (*yè mén*, Humor Gate) and prick LU-11 (*shào shāng*, Lesser Shang) to bleed. For hoarse voice, add LI-18 (*fú tú*, Protuberance Assistant) and PC-5 (*jiān shǐ*, Intermediary Courier). For nose failing to smell fragrance (loss of smell), add LI-20 (*yíng xiāng*, Welcome Fragrance) and GV-23 (*shàng xīng*, Upper

Star). For facial swelling, add CV-9 (*shuǐ fēn*, Water Divide) and BL-22 (*sān jiāo shū*, Triple Burner Transport). For oppression in the chest and shortness of breath, add CV-17 (*shān zhōng*, Chest Center) and PC-6 (*nèi guān*, Inner Pass). For cough and blood ejection, add LU-6 (*kǒng zuì*, Collection Hole). [26: 449] [27: 386] [97: 350]

lung tie 肺系 *fèi xì*: **1.** The area where the lung joins the windpipe. **2.** The trachea and larynx. **3.** The wind-pipe (trachea), throat, and nasal passages. [26: 446] [27: 29] [97: 350]

lung vacuity 肺虚 *fèi xū*: From *Elementary Questions* (*sù wèn, zàng qì fǎ shí lùn*). **1.** Any of various disease patterns of insufficiency of the qi, blood, yin, and yang of the lung, attributable to excessive warmth or cold, to enduring disease and weak health, or to enduring cough damaging the lung. Signs include cough, shortness of breath, copious clear thin phlegm, fatigue and laziness to talk, low weak voice, fear of cold, spontaneous sweating. In some cases there is tidal heat [effusion], night sweating, heat in the hearts of the palms and soles, insomnia, postmeridian reddening of the cheeks, dry mouth and pharynx, cough with no phlegm or with blood-flecked phlegm. The tongue is pale and tender-soft or tender-red. The pulse is vacuous or weak or fine and rapid. **2.** LUNG QI VACUITY. [26: 448] [50: 951]

lung vacuity cough 肺虚咳嗽 *fèi xū ké sòu*: COUGH attributable to LUNG VACUITY, usually insufficiency of lung yin, and sometimes lung qi vacuity. **Insufficiency of lung yin** gives rise to a cough associated with scant phlegm sometimes flecked with blood, emaciation, vexation and insomnia, and postmeridian tidal heat [effusion] and reddening of the cheeks. MED Nourish yin and clear the lung; transform phlegm and suppress cough. Use formulas such as Moonlight Pill (*yuè huá wán*). ACU Base treatment mainly on LU and KI. Select BL-13 (*fèi shū*, Lung Transport), BL-43 (*gāo huāng shū*, Gao-Huang Transport), LU-5 (*chǐ zé*, Cubit Marsh), KI-3 (*tài xī*, Great Ravine), and KI-6 (*zhào hǎi*, Shining Sea); needle with supplementation. **Lung qi vacuity** gives rise to cough associated with panting, faint low voice, tendency to sweat, and a forceless soft pulse. MED Qi vacuity patterns are treated with formulas such as Lung-Supplementing Decoction (*bǔ fèi tāng*). ACU Base treatment mainly on back transport points, CV, and LU. Select BL-13 (*fèi shū*, Lung Transport), BL-20 (*pí shū*, Spleen Transport), CV-6 (*qì hǎi*, Sea of Qi), LU-9 (*tài yuān*, Great Abyss), and ST-36 (*zú sān lǐ*, Leg Three Li); needle with supplementation and add moxa. [26: 448] [46: 653] [37: 273–4]

lung vacuity rapid panting 肺虚喘急 *fèi xū chuǎn jí*: PANTING attributable to lung vacuity.

Yin vacuity patterns are mostly due to lung-kidney yin vacuity, whereas yang vacuity patterns are mostly due to dual vacuity of the spleen and lung or spleen-kidney yang vacuity. Signs include panting and inability to catch one's breath, accompanied by yin vacuity or yang vacuity signs. MED Boost qi and supplement the lung. For yin vacuity, use Metropolis Qi Pill (*dū qì wán*); for yang vacuity, use Kidney Qi Pill (*shèn qì wán*) or Placenta Great Creation Pill (*hé chē dà zào wán*). ACU Base treatment mainly on back transport points, LU, KI, SP, and CV. Main points: BL-13 (*fèi shū*, Lung Transport), Panting Stabilizer (*dìng chuǎn*), BL-43 (*gāo huāng shū*, Gao-Huang Transport), LU-9 (*tài yuān*, Great Abyss), and ST-36 (*zú sān lǐ*, Leg Three Li). Selection of points according to pattern: For lung-kidney yin vacuity, add BL-23 (*shèn shū*, Kidney Transport), KI-3 (*tài xī*, Great Ravine), and KI-6 (*zhào hǎi*, Shining Sea), needling with supplementation. For dual vacuity of spleen and lung, add BL-20 (*pí shū*, Spleen Transport), BL-21 (*wèi shū*, Stomach Transport), and SP-3 (*tài bái*, Supreme White), needling with supplementation and adding moxa. For yang vacuity of spleen and kidney, add BL-20 (*pí shū*, Spleen Transport), BL-23 (*shèn shū*, Kidney Transport), GV-4 (*mìng mén*, Life Gate), CV-4 (*guān yuán*, Pass Head), and CV-6 (*qì hǎi*, Sea of Qi), needling with supplementation and using large amounts of moxa. [26: 449]

lung water 肺水 *fèi shuǐ*: One of the FIVE WATERS spoken of in *Essential Prescriptions of the Golden Coffer* (*jīn guì yào lüè*). WATER SWELLING in lung disease characterized by inhibited breathing, generalized swelling with difficult urination, and duck's slop diarrhea. [27: 419] [97: 349]

lung wilting 肺痿 *fèi wěi*, 肺萎 *fèi wěi*: **1.** A chronic condition characterized by a dull-sounding cough, ejection of thick turbid foamy drool, panting at the slightest exertion, dry mouth and pharynx, emaciation, red dry tongue, and a vacuous rapid pulse. In some cases, there may be tidal heat [effusion], and, in severe cases, the skin and hair may become dry. It is attributed to dryness-heat and enduring cough damaging the lung, or damage to fluid due to other disease depriving the lung of moisturization. MED Treat by enriching yin, clearing heat, and moistening the lung, using Ophiopogon Decoction (*mài mén dōng tāng*) or Dryness-Clearing Lung-Rescuing Decoction (*qīng zào jiù fèi tāng*). With ejection of copious clear white foamy drool without cough or thirst and with dizziness, shortness of breath, lassitude of spirit, fear of cold, pale tongue, and a weak vacuous pulse, the condition is one of damage to qi through enduring illness or vacuity cold in the lung, which is treated by warming the lung and boosting qi with variations of Licorice and Dried Ginger

Decoction (*gān cǎo gān jiāng tāng*). ACU Base treatment mainly on LU and KI. Select BL-13 (*fèi shū*, Lung Transport), BL-43 (*gāo huāng shū*, Gao-Huang Transport), LU-5 (*chǐ zé*, Cubit Marsh), LI-11 (*qū chí*, Pool at the Bend), KI-3 (*tài xī*, Great Ravine), KI-6 (*zhào hǎi*, Shining Sea), and SP-6 (*sān yīn jiāo*, Three Yin Intersection); needle with supplementation. For enduring illness damaging qi, add LU-9 (*tài yuān*, Great Abyss), SP-3 (*tài bái*, Supreme White), and ST-36 (*zú sān lǐ*, Leg Three Li), For vacuity cold, add moxa at GV-4 (*mìng mén*, Life Gate), and CV-4 (*guān yuán*, Pass Head), **2.** A form of consumption. **3.** SKIN AND [BODY] HAIR WILTING. *Indispensable Medical Reading* (*yī zōng bì dú*) states, "Lung wilting is skin and [body] hair wilting." ◇ Chin 痿 *wěi* is composed of the illness signifier 疒 with 委 *wěi*, understood here to be a simplification of 萎 *wěi*, wilt, wither. *The Canon of the Golden Coffer and Jade Sheath* (*jīn guì yù hán jīng*) states, "痿 means 萎, as grasses and trees that have become dry and lifeless. [26: 450] [27: 385] [97: 350] [46: 653]

lung wind 肺风 *fèi fēng*: **1.** Any condition created by wind evil affecting the lung. **2.** Skin sores or itching, facial sores, or redness and ulceration of the bulb of the nose. **3.** Severe DRINKER'S NOSE. [26: 447]

lung wind acne 肺风粉刺 *fèi fēng fěn cì*: DRINKER'S NOSE.

lung yang vacuity 肺阳虚 *fèi yáng xū*: A disease pattern that arises when enduring cough damages lung qi, and detriment to qi affects yang, or when lung qi is damaged in patients usually suffering from yang vacuity. Lung yang vacuity is characterized by forceless cough and panting, bright white facial complexion, and physical cold and cold limbs. MED Warm and supplement lung yang. Use Licorice and Dried Ginger Decoction (*gān cǎo gān jiāng tāng*) or Poria (Hoelen), Licorice, Schisandra, Ginger, and Asarum Decoction (*líng gān wǔ wèi jiāng xīn tāng*). ACU Use the same points as for LUNG QI VACUITY, and use large amounts of moxa. [57: 73] [?: 274]

lung yin 肺阴 *fèi yīn*: *pulmonary liquid*; *lung liquid*. The fluids that keep the lung moist. Lung yin is dependent upon the nourishment from the essence of grain and water transmitted upward by the spleen and the moisturization provided by kidney. It stands in complementary opposition to lung qi. Evil heat or dryness qi invading the lung or internal injury to the lung can in time cause damage to lung yin, which manifests as a dry cold, phlegm-flecked blood, tidal heat [effusion], and night sweating. [26: 448] [27: 48] [97: 349] [46: 653]

lung yin vacuity 肺阴虚 *fèi yīn xū*: A disease pattern of lung vacuity with heat signs. Lung yin vacuity is mostly the result of damage caused by long-lingering lung heat, which frequently develops in patients suffering from either general debilitation from an enduring illness or from impaired lung downbearing. It sometimes arises as a result of invasion of the lung by dryness evil. The chief signs are cough without phlegm or with scant sticky phlegm, and tidal heat [effusion]. Other signs include emaciation, dry throat and mouth, postmeridian tidal heat [effusion], vexing heat in the five hearts, and night sweating. Sometimes the phlegm is flecked with blood or or the voice is hoarse. The tongue is red with little liquid. The pulse is rapid and fine. Lung yin vacuity frequently affects kidney yin, resulting in LUNG-KIDNEY YIN VACUITY. WMC Pulmonary tuberculosis. Analysis: When lung yin is insufficient and vacuity fire burns internally, the lung is steamed by the heat and qi dynamic ascends counterflow, hence the cough. When liquid is scorched by heat and condensed to form phlegm, there is scant sticky phlegm. If the heat scorches the network vessels of the lung, the phlegm may be flecked with blood. When lung yin is depleted, the throat and mouth become dry. When the throat is not kept moist by yin liquid, it is sweltered by vacuity fire, hence the voice becomes hoarse. Lung yin vacuity also means that the body is not properly nourished, hence the emaciation. Intense internal vacuity fire gives rise to postmeridian tidal heat [effusion], and vexing heat in the five hearts. When heat harasses construction-yin, there is night sweating, and when vacuity heat flames upward, the cheeks redden. The red tongue with little liquid, and the rapid fine pulse are further signs of effulgent yin vacuity fire. MED Moisten the lung and suppress cough; enrich yin and downbear fire. Use Lily Bulb Metal-Securing Decoction (*bǎi hé gù jīn tāng*). Comparison: *Heart yin vacuity:* Lung yin vacuity and heart yin vacuity share manifestations of effulgent yin vacuity fire such as dry mouth, scant urine, absence of sweating, dry stool, tidal heat [effusion], and night sweating. Lung yin vacuity is marked by cough with scant phlegm that may be flecked with blood, while heart yin vacuity is characterized by heart palpitations and insomnia. *Dryness evil invading the lung:* Lung yin vacuity is like dryness evil invading the lung in that both are characterized by lung dryness signs such as dry cough, dry skin, and dry mouth. However, lung yin vacuity develops slowly and includes signs of effulgent yin vacuity fire, such as tidal heat [effusion] and night sweating. Dryness evil invading the lung is of rapid onset and is marked by the absence of effulgent yin vacuity fire signs. ACU Base treatment mainly on back transport points, LU, and KI. Select BL-13 (*fèi shū*, Lung Transport), BL-43 (*gāo huāng shū*, Gao-Huang Transport), LU-5 (*chǐ zé*, Cubit Marsh), and KI-6 (*zhào hǎi*, Shining Sea);

needle with supplementation. For lung-kidney yin vacuity, add BL-23 (*shèn shū*, Kidney Transport), KI-3 (*tài xī*, Great Ravine), and SP-6 (*sān yīn jiāo*, Three Yin Intersection). [6: 177] [26: 448] [116: 63] [57: 72] [27: 158] [46: 653]

lusterless facial complexion 面色不华 *miàn sè bù huá*: A complexion that lacks color and vital-ity. See WITHERED-YELLOW FACIAL COMPLEXION; WHITE FACIAL COMPLEXION.

lusterless nails 爪甲不荣 *zhǎo jiǎ bù róng*: Dry pale nails lacking sheen. A sign of liver blood vacu-ity. See LIVER, ITS BLOOM IS IN THE NAILS.

luxuriance and witheredness 荣枯 *róng kū*: See TONGUE SPIRIT.

M

mace 钱 *qián*: QIAN.

macule 斑 *bān*: A patch on the skin. See MACU-
LOPAPULAR ERUPTION.

maculopapular eruption 斑疹 *bān zhěn*: Eruption of macules or papules. Macules are colored
(usually red) patches that are unraised above the
surface of the skin and vary in size. Papules are
like grains of millet in shape and size (or may be
larger), raised above the surface of the skin. The
appearance of maculopapular eruptions in externally contracted heat (febrile) diseases indicates
heat penetrating blood-construction. In internal
damage miscellaneous diseases, they usually indicate blood heat. **Externally contracted disease:** The appearance of maculopapular eruptions
in externally contracted heat (febrile) diseases indicates heat penetrating blood-construction. Provided that they are not too dense or widespread,
maculopapular eruptions indicate that right qi is
capable of expelling evil qi from the body. Thus it
is said, "The appearance of macules and papules is
a favorable sign, provided they are not in excess."
The absence of such maculopapular eruptions may
indicate an evil blockage. In excess, they indicate
that the evil is strong. Macules reflect more severe conditions than papules; for example, intense
toxic heat in the blood aspect. Therefore, careful
attention should be paid to them. Maculopapular
eruptions are a favorable sign when red in color,
and an unfavorable sign when dark and stagnant-
looking. Deep red indicates intense heat, whereas
purplish black indicates intense toxic heat in the
blood aspect, a sign that the condition is extremely
serious. A dark blackish color indicates that right
qi is seriously debilitated, and the condition is critical. However, the significance of maculopapular
eruptions can only be judged in correlation with
other signs. *On Warm Heat* (*wēn rè lùn*) states,
"They [macules and papules] must be viewed together with other external signs before a diagnosis can be made." Papules in febrile disease are
sometimes referred to as *sand* (*shā*). **Internal
damage:** Maculopapular eruptions occurring in
internal damage miscellaneous diseases usually indicates blood heat. If they continually appear and
disappear, are purplish red in color, and if signs
of blood heat are absent, maculopapular eruptions
indicate the failure of the qi to contain the blood or
qi vacuity with blood stasis. If the eruptions are
deep-seated and well-defined, the condition is serious. Deep-seated eruptions do not blanch when
pressure is applied. Well-defined eruptions have
clear edges or are characterized by localized tissue
necrosis. If the edges are not well-defined, and the
color fades under pressure, the condition is mild.
[6: 118]

Ma Dan-Yang's twelve heavenly star points
马丹阳天星十二穴 *mǎ dān yáng tiān xīng shí èr
xué*: Twelve points that Ma Dan-Yang, a Song Dynasty physician, considered the most useful in the
treatment of disease. The points were passed on
to his students and appeared later written in song
form. Ma Dan-Yang's twelve heavenly star points
are presented below. [46: 821] [109: 437]

Ma Dan-Yang's Twelve Heavenly Star Points

ST-36 (*zú sān lǐ*, Leg Three Li): distention in the
heart and abdomen, cold in the stomach, rumbling intestines, swollen legs, aching legs, cold
damage emaciation and detriment, and qi gu

ST-44 (*nèi tíng*, Inner Court): reversal (cold) of
the four limbs, liking for quiet and aversion to
noise, dormant papules, sore throat, yawning,
toothache, malaria, and inability to eat

LI-11 (*qū chí*, Pool at the Bend): pain in the elbow, hemilateral wind preventing the arm from
being stretched, slack sinews with inability to
brush the hair, blockage of the throat, persistent
heat effusion, and hemilateral wind lichen and lai

LI-4 (*hé gǔ*, Union Valley): headache, malaria,
tooth decay, nosebleed, clenched jaw with inability to speak

BL-40 (*wěi zhōng*, Bend Center): lumbar pain,
wind impediment (*fēng bì*), inability to stretch
the knee

BL-57 (*chéng shān*, Mountain Support): lumbar pain, hemorrhoids, difficult defecation, leg
qi with swollen knees, cholera with cramps

LR-3 (*tài chōng*, Supreme Surge): fright epilepsy
wind, distention in the throat and region of the
heart,

BL-60 (*kūn lún*, Kunlun Mountains): cramps
and lumbar pain, fulminant panting and fullness
surging into the heart, inability to lift the legs

GB-30 (*huán tiào*, Jumping Round): lumbar pain,
wind-cold-damp impediment (*fēng hán shī bì*)
with pain in the legs stretching into the calves

GB-34 (*yáng líng quán*, Yang Mound Spring):
swelling and numbness of the knees, cold wind
and hemilateral wind, inability to lift the legs

HT-5 (*tōng lǐ*, Connecting Li): inability to speak, anguish and fearful throbbing; in repletion, swelling of the limbs, and red head and cheeks; in vacuity, inability to eat and sudden loss of voice
LU-7 (*liè quē*, Broken Sequence): hemilateral headache, hemilateral wind numbness, phlegm-drool frequently welling upward, clenched jaw

---

magic medicine 灵药 *líng yào*: Either upborne elixir (*shēng dān*) or white downborne elixir (*bái jiàng dān*), which are produced by sublimation. Upborne elixir is, according to one method, made by heating mercury (*shuǐ yín*), niter (*xiāo shí*), and alum (*bái fán*) in a container with a lid sealed on to make yellow and red crystals settle on the lid on cooling (hence "upborne" elixir). Downborne elixir is made by heating cinnabar (*zhū shā*), realgar (*xióng huáng*), mercury (*shuǐ yín*), borax (*péng shā*), niter (*xiāo shí*), salt (*yán*), alum (*bái fán*), and melanterite (*lǜ fán*) in a sealed container to produce crystals in the container rather than the lid (hence "downborne" elixir). [27: 298]

magic root 灵根 *líng gēn*: TONGUE.

main channel 大经 *dà jīng*: Any large channel. [27: 93] [97: 21]

major chest bind 大结胸 *dà jié xiōng*: *Synonym: phlegm-heat chest bind.* A disease pattern arising when inappropriate application of precipitation of an unresolved exterior pattern in greater yang (*tài yáng*) disease causes the heat evil to fall inward and combine with phlegm and water. Major chest bind is characterized by fullness, hardness and pain in the chest, stomach duct, and umbilical region that is too tender to be touched. Other signs include thirst, dry tongue, late afternoon tidal heat [effusion], and tight sunken pulse. Chest bind was first described in *On Cold Damage* (*shāng hán lùn*) MED Expel water and discharge heat. Use Major Chest Bind Decoction (*dà xiàn xiōng tāng*) or Pill. ACU Select GV-12 (*shēn zhù*, Body Pillar), PC-5 (*jiān shǐ*, Intermediary Courier), PC-7 (*dà líng*, Great Mound), CV-12 (*zhōng wǎn*, Center Stomach Duct), CV-17 (*shān zhōng*, Chest Center), PC-6 (*nèi guān*, Inner Pass), ST-25 (*tiān shū*, Celestial Pivot), SP-9 (*yīn líng quán*, Yin Mound Spring), GV-14 (*dà zhuī*, Great Hammer), LI-11 (*qū chí*, Pool at the Bend), and SP-6 (*sān yīn jiāo*, Three Yin Intersection); needle with drainage. See CHEST BIND. [26: 50] [27: 376] [97: 23]

major divide 大分 *dà fēn*: See FLESH DIVIDE.

major reversal 大厥 *dà jué*: From *Elementary Questions* (*sù wèn*). Severe sudden CLOUDING REVERSAL as though the patient had suddenly died. See REVERSAL PATTERNS; WIND STROKE. [50: 76]

major vacuity of original qi 元气大虚 *yuán qì dà xū*: Severe QI VACUITY.

malar flush 面颊潮红 *miàn jiá cháo hóng*: TIDAL REDDENING OF THE CHEEKS.

malaria 疟疾 *nüè jí*: A recurrent disease characterized by shivering, vigorous heat [effusion], and sweating and classically attributed to contraction of summerheat during the hot season, contact with mountain forest miasma, or contraction of cold-damp. Malaria is explained as evil qi latent at midstage (half exterior and half interior). Different forms are distinguished according to signs and causes.

Malaria

Types distinguished by cause and pattern

WIND MALARIA: heat effusion and spontaneous sweating

SUMMERHEAT MALARIA: vigorous heat [effusion], vexation and thirst

DAMP MALARIA: oppression in the chest, upflow nausea, and aching and heaviness in the trunk and limbs

COLD MALARIA: severe aversion to cold followed by mild heat effusion

WARM MALARIA: pronounced heat effusion followed by mild aversion to cold

PURE-HEAT MALARIA: heat effusion without aversion to cold

FEMALE MALARIA: aversion to cold without heat effusion

PHLEGM MALARIA: dizziness, copious phlegm, and coma

Types distinguished by time of episode

TERTIAN MALARIA: attacks every third day
QUARTAN MALARIA: every fourth day
See also TRIPLE-YIN MALARIA.
ENDURING MALARIA: vacuity signs

Types distinguished by triggering cause

TAXATION MALARIA: caused by irregularities of work and rest

FOOD MALARIA: dietary irregularities
MIASMIC MALARIA: caused by miasma
EPIDEMIC MALARIA: epidemic qi

MED The principle of treatment for malaria is as follows: (1) Initial stage: harmonization. (2) Middle stage: interrupting malaria (using medicinals or acupuncture to prevent imminent episodes). (3) Advanced stage: supplementing vacuity. ACU General malaria-terminating treatment is based mainly on GV, PC, and SI. Select GV-14 (*dà zhuī*, Great Hammer), GV-13 (*táo dào*, Kiln Path), PC-5 (*jiān shǐ*, Intermediary Courier), and SI-3 (*hòu xī*, Back Ravine); needle with drainage 2–3 hours before an expected episode. If episodes are not regular, needle 2–3 times a day. Selection of points according to signs: For pronounced heat, add LI-11 (*qū chí*, Pool at the

Bend) and TB-1 (*guān chōng*, Passage Hub). For high fever and clouded spirit, also prick Ten Diffusing Points (*shí xuān*) to bleed. For alternating heat [effusion] and [aversion to] cold, add GV-13 (*táo dào*, Kiln Path) and Lofty Bone (*chóng gǔ*). For enduring malaria, add moxa at BL-20 (*pí shū*, Spleen Transport) and GV-9 (*zhì yáng*, Extremity of Yang). For mother of malaria (palpable lump), add LR-13 (*zhāng mén*, Camphorwood Gate), Glomus Root (*pǐ gēn*), BL-18 (*gān shū*, Liver Transport), and BL-20 (*pí shū*, Spleen Transport). ◇ Chin 虐 *nüè*, 疒 sickness, combined with 虐 *nüè*, torment. A disease that continually torments the patient with repeated heat effusion and aversion to cold. [26: 827] [27: 357] [97: 374]

male malaria 牡疟 *mǔ nüè*: From *Essential Prescriptions of the Golden Coffer* (*jīn guì yào lüè, nüè bìng mài zhèng bìng zhì*). The character 牡 (male) is held to be a mistranscription of 牝 (female). See FEMALE MALARIA. [26: 327] [27: 359] [97: 217]

malign 恶 *è*: Noxious, severe, difficult to cure. Not to be confused with the term "malignant" as used in Western medicine. [48: 265]

malign blood 恶血 *è xuè*: Blood that has spilled out of the vessels and accumulates outside blood vessels and that manifests is the form of STASIS MACULES, STASIS SPECKLES, or BLOOD SWELLING. [27: 461]

malign complexion 恶色 *è sè*: Synonym: *perished complexion*. A dry complexion, showing no sign of "vital qi" (vitality), a critical sign indicating that stomach qi is exhausted and visceral qi is wasted. The complexions described in *Elementary Questions* (*sù wèn, wǔ zàng shēng chéng piān*) as "green-blue as new shoots of grass; yellow like unripe bitter orange; black as cinders; red as coagulated blood; white as dry bones" are all malign complexions. [26: 685] [97: 461]

malign disease of great wind 大风恶疾 *dà fēng è jí*: PESTILENTIAL WIND.

malign flesh 恶肉 *è ròu*: A disease described in *Emergency Standby Remedies* (*zhǒu hòu bèi jí fāng*)n the following terms: "A fleshy growth red as a rice bean, protruding from the body, becoming longer like cow's or mare's teats or like a cock's crest. It should be treated by taking a decoction of rhaponticum/echinops (*lòu lú*) orally, and by cauterizing the malign flesh with a red-hot needle three times a day and applying Cimicifuga Paste (*shēng má gāo*)." WMC verruca; wart; keloma. [26: 685] [97: 461]

malignity stroke 中恶 *zhòng è*: A disease attributed in ancient times to the malign work of demons, and described in *The Level-Line of Pattern Identification and Treatment* (*zhèng zhì zhǔn shéng*) in the following way: "Malignity stroke

patterns are due to catching some unright qi and are characterized by sudden counterflow cold of the limbs, goose pimples, blackish green-blue head and face, essence-spirit failing to confine itself, deranged raving, clenched jaw, spinning head and collapse, and clouding unconsciousness. They are observed in sudden reversal, visiting hostility... or after attending funerals or going into temples or graveyards." (see SUDDEN REVERSAL; VISITING HOSTILITY). MED Liquid Storax Pill (*sū hé xiāng wán*) can be used to revive the patient, and then treat with Stomach-Calming Powder (*píng wèi sǎn*) plus saussurea (*mù xiāng*), cyperus (*xiāng fù zǐ*), ginseng (*rén shēn*), and agastache/patchouli (*huò xiāng*). ACU Base treatment mainly on GV, LI, and hand and foot reverting yin (*jué yīn*) PC/LR. Select GV-26 (*shuǐ gōu*, Water Trough), PC-9 (*zhōng chōng*, Central Hub), LI-4 (*hé gǔ*, Union Valley), GV-20 (*bǎi huì*, Hundred Convergences), LR-2 (*xíng jiān*, Moving Between), PC-6 (*nèi guān*, Inner Pass), and KI-1 (*yǒng quán*, Gushing Spring); needle with drainage. [26: 139] [27: 121] [97: 79]

malign obstruction 恶阻 *è zǔ*: Synonyms: *pregnancy vomiting; aversion to food*.[2] A condition of aversion to food, nausea and vomiting during pregnancy, not considered untoward unless it severely affects food intake. Malign obstruction is the manifestation of impaired harmonious downbearing of stomach qi. WMC emesis gravidarum (morning sickness). See LIVER HEAT MALIGN OBSTRUCTION; PHLEGM STAGNATION MALIGN OBSTRUCTION; STOMACH COLD MALIGN OBSTRUCTION; STOMACH HEAT MALIGN OBSTRUCTION; WEAK STOMACH MALIGN OBSTRUCTION. ◇ Chin 恶 *è*, malign; *zǔ*, obstruction. The character 恶 read as *wù* means to hate, whereas read as *ě* it means nausea, disgust. The compound term is often explained as nausea or aversion to food causing an obstruction, the 恶 is pronounced *è*. [26: 685]

malign sore 恶疮 *è chuāng*: Any sore that is burning hot, swollen, and itchy and that continues to spread after bursting, and fails to heal. [26: 685] [97: 461]

malodor 臭气 *chòu qì*: Any unpleasant or offensive odor. See ANIMAL ODOR; FISHY SMELL; PUTRID SMELL; FOUL SMELL. [48: 284]

malodorous 臭 *chòu*: Giving off a malodor or bad smell. [48: 284]

malposition of fetus 胎不正 *tāi bù zhèng*, 胎位不正 *tāi wèi bù zhèng*: Incorrect position of the fetus in the uterus; attributed to qi stagnation or fright or fear before delivery. MED Soothe qi and abduct stagnation using formulas such as Fetus-Turning Formula (*zhuǎn tāi fāng*). In modern practice, Carefree Pregnancy Formula (*bǎo chǎn* *wú yōu fāng*), originally devised to calm the fetus, has been used successfully to right the position of the fetus. [ACU] Either of the following two methods may be used: (1) Moxibustion: Select bilateral BL-67 (*zhì yīn*, Reaching Yin) points, and pole for 15–20 minutes (7–15 cones), twice each day. (2) Acupuncture and moxibustion: Select bilateral BL-67 (*zhì yīn*, Reaching Yin) points, and needle for 1–2 fen, needling with even supplementation and drainage, and then moxa for 10–15 minutes each day before bed. [26: 453]

mammary aggregation 乳癖 *rǔ pǐ*: A disease of the breast characterized by a swollen lump like a plum or mume or like an egg that is hard and painful, and that moves when pushed. Mammary aggregation is unassociated with cold or heat or skin color. It is arises most commonly when thought damages the spleen and depressed anger damages the liver, causing qi stagnation and congealing phlegm. It may also be due to liver-kidney yin vacuity. [WMC] hyperplasia of the mammary glands, benign tumor the mammary glands. **Binding depression of liver qi** patterns are characterized by dizziness, rib-side distention, oppression in the chest, belching, distending pain in the lesser abdomen, inhibited menstruation, thin tongue fur, and stringlike pulse. [MED] Course the liver and resolve stasis; transform phlegm and dissipate binds. Use Free Wanderer Powder (*xiāo yáo sǎn*) plus curcuma (*yù jīn*), tangerine pip (*jú hé*), prunella (*xià kū cǎo*), and gizzard lining (*jī nèi jīn*). **Liver-kidney yin vacuity** patterns are marked by postmeridian tidal heat [effusion], dull dark complexion, reddening of the cheeks, dizzy head, tinnitus, lumbar and back pain, scant menstrual flow, red tongue, and a fine rapid pulse. [MED] Supplement the liver and kidney with Menses-Stabilizing Decoction (*dìng jīng tāng*) plus Zhejiang fritillaria (*zhè bèi mǔ*), curcuma (*yù jīn*), tangerine pip (*jú hé*), zedoary (*é zhú*), and asparagus (*tiān mén dōng*). [ACU] Base treatment on yang brightness (*yáng míng*), reverting yin (*jué yīn*), and greater yin (*tài yīn*). Main points: ST-15 (*wū yì*, Roof), CV-17 (*shān zhōng*, Chest Center), ST-36 (*zú sān lǐ*, Leg Three Li), and SP-6 (*sān yīn jiāo*, Three Yin Intersection); needle with even supplementation and drainage. Selection of points according to pattern: For binding depression of liver qi, add PC-6 (*nèi guān*, Inner Pass), GB-21 (*jiān jǐng*, Shoulder Well), and LR-3 (*tài chōng*, Supreme Surge). For liver-kidney depletion, add BL-18 (*gān shū*, Liver Transport) and BL-23 (*shèn shū*, Kidney Transport). [26: 379] [46: 712] [67: 346]

mammary chestnut 乳栗 *rǔ lì*: See MAMMARY NODE; MAMMARY ROCK. [26: 378]

mammary consumption 乳痨 *rǔ láo*: A disease of the breast that develops from a MAMMARY NODE

as a result of qi-blood vacuity or unsuccessful treatment. The mammary node gradually becomes as large as a bowl, is hard and painful, and spreads to the rib-side below the armpit. It becomes purple or black in color and can burst to exude in mild cases white fluid that may be malodorous. If the condition persists, postmeridian tidal heat [effusion], cough, red cheeks, marked emaciation and other signs of internal vacuity heat may be observed. [27: 479] [26: 379]

mammary fistula 乳漏 *rǔ lòu*: A fistula on the breast or areola characterized by a tunnel that penetrates deep into the flesh and exudes pus and in some cases milk; usually attributed to an EFFUSION OF THE BREAST, MAMMARY WELLING-ABSCESS, or MAMMARY CONSUMPTION that owing to improper treatment fails to heal. [MED] Treat topically with formulas such as Red Upborne Elixir (*hóng shēng dān*) applied to a medicated thread that is inserted to draw out the pus. When the putridity has gone, Flesh-Engendering Powder (*shēng jī sǎn*) can be used to engender flesh and close the opening. The method of threaded ligation can be used for areolar fistulas. [26: 379] [27: 479] [97: 357]

mammary flat-abscess 乳疽 *rǔ jū*: A yin-pattern suppurative lesion of the breast. A mammary flat-abscess is characterized by a hard, slightly painful lump in the breast, without any change in skin color. The lump gradually grows larger. Suppuration is slow to develop and is accompanied by aversion cold and heat effusion. Rupture gives rise to a discharge of yellow pus and leaves a deep hole in the breast. [27: 461]

mammary gan 乳疳 *rǔ gān*: Breast sores or lumps that have persisted for may years without healing or that have half healed, look like broken lotus receptacles, and are excruciatingly painful. [WMC] adenocarcinoma of the breast, tuberculosis of the breast. Treated in the same way as MAMMARY ROCK. [26: 377]

mammary node 乳核 *rǔ hé*: Synonyms: *node in the breast*; *breast node*; *mammary chestnut*; *mammary phlegm node*. A hard bound lump in the breast, observed in MAMMARY ROCK and MAMMARY CONSUMPTION. [26: 377]

mammary phlegm [node] 乳痰 *rǔ tán*: MAMMARY NODE. [26: 377] [27: 469] [97: 358]

mammary rock 乳岩 *rǔ yán*: Synonym: *mammary chestnut*. A disease of the breast that starts as a hard, painless mammary node the size of a jujube or chestnut with an uneven surface, and that subsequently grows larger and becomes painful. Before bursting, the nipples become sunken and the lump feels like a heap of chestnuts or an upturned bowl and is connected with the skin so that it does not move when pushed. If the head shows through as purple, it will gradually rupture to leave an opening like a rock cave that exudes foul water or blood. WMC adenocarcinoma of the breast. It is attributable to anxiety and thought causing counterflow of liver spleen-qi. Treat by coursing the liver and rectifying qi with formulas such as Free Wanderer Powder (*xiāo yáo săn*). [26: 377] [27: 482] [97: 356] [61: 199]

mammary toxin sore 乳毒 *rŭ dú*: **1.** A boil of the breast unassociated with pregnancy or breast-feeding. **2.** A postpartum MAMMARY WELLING-ABSCESS. [26: 377]

mammary welling-abscess 乳痈 *rŭ yōng*: A WELLING-ABSCESS (*yōng*) on the female breast. It is most common after childbirth, but may occur in the later stages of pregnancy. It is characterized by a redness and swelling in the breast, which if left untreated can suppurate and burst. Severe cases are called EFFUSION OF THE BREAST. At least since the Song, the breath of the infant has been understood as cause of mammary welling-abscesses, and in *The Golden Mirror of Medicine* (*yī zōng jīn jiàn*) the distinction is made between *external blowing* (mammary welling-abscess developing after childbirth) and *internal blowing* (developing before childbirth). WMC acute mastitis. A number of causes exist: (1) Anxiety or anger affecting the normal free coursing of liver qi, or accumulated stomach heat from excessive consumption of rich foods, causing stagnation in the yang brightness channel and disharmony of construction qi; (2) accumulation and stagnation of milk in the breast; (3) contraction of heat toxin through a damaged nipple; (4) contraction of wind evil in postpartum blood vacuity. MED In the initial stage, treat by soothing the liver and clearing the stomach and by promoting lactation and dissipating binds; use formulas such as Trichosanthes and Arctium Decoction (*guā lóu niú bàng tāng*) plus dandelion (*pú gōng yīng*), tangkuei (*dāng guī*), rhaponticum/echinops (*lòu lú*), and red peony (*chì sháo yào*). For pronounced liver depression, use the same formula minus scutellaria (*huáng qín*), gardenia (*shān zhī zĭ*), and lonicera (*jīn yín huā*), plus perilla stem (*zĭ sū gĕng*), and liquidambar fruit (*lù lù tōng*), to course the liver and resolve depression. For pronounced heat toxin, use Immortal Formula Life-Giving Beverage (*xiān fāng huó mìng yĭn*) plus dandelion (*pú gōng yīng*) to clear heat and resolve toxin. Apply Golden Yellow Powder (*jīn huáng săn*) or crushed dandelion (*pú gōng yīng*) topically. ACU Base treatment on yang brightness (*yáng míng*) and reverting yin (*jué yīn*). Select ST-16 (*yīng chuāng*, Breast Window), GB-21 (*jiān jĭng*, Shoulder Well), PC-6 (*nèi guān*, Inner Pass), ST-36 (*zú sān lĭ*, Leg Three Li), LI-11 (*qū chí*, Pool at the Bend), LI-7 (*wēn liū*, Warm Dwelling), and LR-2 (*xíng jiān*, Moving Between); needle with drainage. Mammary

welling-abscess responds to acupuncture best before suppuration. The above formula is therefore mostly used for presuppurative conditions. In addition, the swelling and surrounding area can be tapped with a cutaneous needle to reduce momentum. Medicinal therapy is more effective for the suppurative stage. Selection of points according to signs: For pronounced liver depression, LR-14 (*qī mén*, Cycle Gate) and GB-41 (*zú lín qì*, Foot Overlooking Tears). For pronounced heat toxin, add ST-44 (*nèi tíng*, Inner Court) ST-18 (*rŭ gēn*, Breast Root), and ST-34 (*liáng qiū*, Beam Hill). For inhibited milk flow, add CV-17 (*shān zhōng*, Chest Center), and SI-1 (*shào zé*, Lesser Marsh). For aversion to cold and heat effusion, add LI-4 (*hé gŭ*, Union Valley), and GB-20 (*fēng chí*, Wind Pool). See WELLING-ABSCESS. [26: 380] [67: 337] [46: 710] [37: 448] [113: 365] [27: 459] [97: 357] [61: 199]

mania 狂 *kuáng*: Any pattern characterized by wild behavior, self-aggrandizement, scolding and shouting, smashing objects and beating people, climbing over walls or onto roofs, failure to modify behavior for either family and friends or outsiders, extraordinary strength, tendency not to rest or to eat, red tongue with yellow fur, and a large string-like slippery rapid pulse; attributed to five-mind fire transformation or phlegm clouding the orifices of the heart. MED Flush phlegm and open the orifices; drain fire and attack accumulations. Use formulas such as Iron Flakes Beverage (*shēng tiĕ luò yĭn*), Chlorite/Mica Phlegm-Rolling Pill (*méng shí gŭn tán wán*), or Major Qi-Coordinating Decoction (*dà chéng qì tāng*). ACU Base treatment mainly on PC, LR, HT, and ST. To drain fire and settle the heart, select GV-26 (*shuĭ gōu*, Water Trough), PC-8 (*láo gōng*, Palace of Toil), PC-5 (*jiān shĭ*, Intermediary Courier), HT-7 (*shén mén*, Spirit Gate), HT-8 (*shào fŭ*, Lesser Mansion), and LR-2 (*xíng jiān*, Moving Between), and prick LU-11 (*shào shāng*, Lesser Shang) to bleed. To flush phlegm, quiet the heart, and open the orifices, select BL-15 (*xīn shū*, Heart Transport), ST-40 (*fēng lóng*, Bountiful Bulge), ST-36 (*zú sān lĭ*, Leg Three Li), PC-7 (*dà líng*, Great Mound), GV-20 (*băi huì*, Hundred Convergences), and SP-1 (*yĭn bái*, Hidden White). Needle with drainage at all points. See MANIA AND WITHDRAWAL. [26: 339] [97: 299] [40: 126] [37: 352] [46: 642] [113: 154]

mania and withdrawal 癫狂 *diān kuáng*: Mental derangement. Mania denotes states of excitement characterized by noisy, unruly, and even aggressive behavior, offensive speech, constant singing and laughter, irascibility, springing walls and climbing roofs, and inability to remain tidily dressed. This is a yang pattern of the heart spirit straying outward owing to hyperactivity of yang qi. Withdrawal refers to emotional depression, indifference, deranged speech, taciturnity, and obliviousness of hunger or satiety. It is a yin pattern caused by binding of depressed qi and phlegm or heart-spleen vacuity. See MANIA; WITHDRAWAL. [26: 1005] [27: 393] [97: 660]

mania evil 狂邪 *kuáng xié*: Evil giving rise to mania.

manic agitation 狂躁 *kuáng zào*: Agitation with signs of mania.

manipulation 手法 *shǒu fǎ*: NEEDLE MANIPULATION.

man's prognosis 人迎 *rén yíng*: *Synonym: man's prognosis pulse.* The pulsating vessel at the sides of the neck. This pulse is mentioned under BLOCK AND REPULSION. [27: 189] [26: 19]

man's prognosis pulse 人迎脉 *rén yíng mài*: MAN'S PROGNOSIS. [26: 19]

marsh rampart 泽廓 *zé kuò*: See EIGHT RAMPARTS.

martial flame 武火 *wǔ huǒ*: A fierce flame. Effusing dissipating medicinals are boiled for a short time over a martial flame. Compare CIVIL FLAME. [26: 358]

massage 按摩 *àn mó*: *Synonym: tui-na.* Rubbing, pressing or other manipulation of the body for the treatment and prevention of disease. Massage helps to free the channels and vessels, and also helps to disinhibit the joints. By stimulating the movement of qi and blood, it can regulate the function of the bowels and viscera, and increase resistance to disease. [26: 419] [27: 488] [97: 390]

massive head scourge 大头瘟 *dà tóu wēn*: A disease that results from invasion of the spleen and stomach channels by seasonal wind-warmth toxin and that is characterized by swelling and redness of the head, and sometimes by painful swelling of the throat, and, in severe cases, signs such as deafness, clenched jaw, clouded spirit, and delirious raving. MED Use Universal Aid Toxin-Dispersing Beverage (*pǔ jì xiāo dú yǐn*). [27: 369] [97: 22]

master points of the eight vessels 八脉交会穴 *bā mài jiāo huì xué*: CONFLUENCE POINTS OF THE EIGHT VESSELS.

mealy tumor 粉瘤 *fěn liú*: FATTY TUMOR.

measles 麻疹 *má zhěn*: A transmissible disease affecting mostly children characterized by eruption of papules the shape of sesame seeds. The disease is located in the spleen and lung channels, and can affect other bowels and viscera. Measles is characterized at onset by heat effusion, cough, and copious tearing, and white speckles inside the mouth. After three days of heat effusion, papules appear behind the ears, on the neck, and face, and spread to the limbs. Eruption is complete when the papules reach the legs. During the first millen-

nium, measles was poorly distinguished from other disease characterized by eruptions. In the Song dynasty, both measles and smallpox were popularly called 麻子 *má zǐ* (lit. "semame seeds"), but Pang An-Shi distinguished a mild form from a severe form. The distinction was consolidated in the Ming, when the term 麻疹 *má zhěn* came to be used for mild eruptive diseases. MED In the initial heat effusion stage, treat by diffusing the lung and outthrusting papules with formulas such as Toxin-Diffusing Exterior-Effusing Decoction (*xuān dú fā biǎo tāng*) or Lonicera and Forsythia Powder (*yín qiào sǎn*). After eruption, treat by clearing heat and resolving toxin with puccoon (*zǐ cǎo*), saffron (*zàng hóng huā*), forsythia (*lián qiào*), lonicera (*jīn yín huā*), coptis (*huáng lián*), Zhejiang fritillaria (*zhè bèi mǔ*), loquat leaf (*pí pá yè*), isatis root (*bǎn lán gēn*), bamboo leaf (lophatherum) (*dàn zhú yè*), mutong (*mù tōng*), and licorice (*gān cǎo*). In the recovery stage, when the papules begin to disappear, it can be treated by the method of engendering liquid and nourishing yin combined with that of clearing residual toxin with variations of Adenophora/Glehnia and Ophiopogon Decoction (*shā shēn mài dōng tāng*). See FAVORABLE MEASLES PATTERN; UNFAVORABLE MEASLES PATTERN; CRITICAL MEASLES PATTERN; MEASLES BLOCK PATTERN; MEASLES TOXIN ENTERING CONSTRUCTION; MEASLES TOXIN FALLING INTO THE LUNG; LOSS OF VOICE IN MEASLES; WHITE-FACE SAND. ◇ Chin 麻 *má*, sesame; 疹 *zhěn*, papules, rash. [26: 587] [27: 386] [39: 172–3]

measles block pattern 麻疹闭证 *má zhěn bì zhèng*: Measles failing to erupt with evil toxin blocked in the inner body. A measles block pattern arises when externally contracted wind-cold, intense internal heat, food stagnation, or exuberant phlegm-damp obstruct lung qi and block the interstices, preventing the normal outthrust of measles papules. The signs are the appearance of speckles not followed by full eruption, or the premature disappearance of measles papules. MED The basic method is to diffuse the lung and outthrust papules. This should be variously combined according the particular pattern with one of the following: coursing wind and resolving the exterior; clearing heat and resolving toxin; dispersing food and abducting stagnation; clearing heat and dispelling phlegm. For topical treatment, boil a handful of coriander (*hú suī*) with water and an appropriate amount of liquor to produce a wash that should be applied warm. For qi vacuity reducing the fight against the toxin characterized by pale white papules that fail to erupt fully, white face and green-blue lips, physical fatigue and lassitude of spirit, lack of warmth in the limbs, diarrhea, pale tongue with white fur, and a faint weak pulse, treat by boosting qi and harmonizing the center and by quickening the blood and outthrusting toxin, using Center-Supplementing Qi-Boosting Decoction (*bŭ zhōng yì qì tāng*) plus carthamus (*hóng huā*). See MACULOPAPULAR ERUPTION. [26: 587]

measles toxin entering construction 麻毒入营 *má dú rù yíng*: Measles with heat evil causing intense heat and entering the construction-blood and in some cases the pericardium. Measles toxin entering construction is marked by papules that coalesce and turn dark purple in color, high fever, vexation and thirst, delirious raving, clouded spirit, tetanic reversal, groping in the air, crimson tongue with prickles, and in some cases bleeding from the mouth, nose, and two yin (anus and genital orifices). [MED] Clear construction and cool the blood with Construction-Clearing Decoction (*qīng yíng tāng*) or Scourge-Clearing Toxin-Vanquishing Beverage (*qīng wēn bài dú yĭn*). These formulas can be complemented by Spirit-Like Rhinoceros Horn Elixir (*shén xī dān*). [26: 586]

measles toxin falling into the lung 麻毒陷肺 *má dú xiàn fèi*: Measles in which, after disappearance of papules, contraction of wind evil causes the measles toxin to fall into the lung. The signs are high fever, cough, hasty breathing, phlegm rale, flaring nostrils, and green-blue lips. [MED] Diffuse the lung and outthrust the evil; clear heat and resolve toxin. Use Ephedra, Apricot Kernel, Licorice, and Gypsum Decoction (*má xìng gān shí tāng*) with additions. [WMC] measles pneumonia. If heat is pronounced, add anemarrhena (*zhī mŭ*), scutellaria (*huáng qín*), isatis root (*băn lán gēn*), houttuynia (*yú xīng căo*), lonicera (*jīn yín huā*), and forsythia (*lián qiào*). If cough is pronounced and phlegm copious, add trichosanthes (*guā lóu*), mulberry root bark (*sāng bái pí*), lycium root bark (*dì gŭ pí*), and platycodon (*jié gĕng*). Western medical treatment may also be recommended. [26: 586]

meat-type food damage 伤肉食 *shāng ròu shí*: See FOOD DAMAGE.

mechanical ejection 探吐 *tàn tù*: Provoking vomiting by the introduction of an instrument into the throat in the treatment of poisoning or food stagnation. Mechanical ejection is usually performed by stimulating the throat with a cleaned chicken's or duck's feather. [27: 281] [27: 281]

medial headache 正头痛 *zhèng tóu tòng*: Synonym: *ambilateral headache* (obs). A pain felt on the right and left side of the head; a regular headache as opposed to a hemilateral headache. See HEADACHE. [97: 142]

medicated leaven 麯 *qū*, 麴 *qú*: Abbreviation: leaven. A medicinal preparation made by fermenting powdered medicinals mixed with flour and then dried in cakes. Medicated leavens can be decocted with other medicinals. They enter the stomach

and spleen and help digestion. The most commonly used is medicated leaven (*shén qū*). Others include pinellia leaven (*bàn xià qū*) and aquilaria leaven (*chén xiāng qū*). [27: 313]

medicated thread drainage 药线引流 *yào xiàn yin liú*: An external medical technique whereby a twisted paper coated with or enveloping medicinal powder is introduced into a fistula to assist the removal of pus and toxin, and promote healing. [26: 978] [27: 297] [97: 384]

medication 用药 *yòng yào*: The use of medicinals, including the choice of medicinals, their final preparation, and their administration to the patient.

medicinal 药 *yào*: Synonym: *agent*. Any animal, vegetable, or mineral product that traditionally is powdered, decocted or prepared as a wine or distillate for oral consumption, or prepared as a powder, paste, or wine for topical application. Medicinals include the drugs of the orthodox literary tradition, often widely distributed beyond their production area, which are now known as CHINESE MEDICINALS (*zhōng yào*), as well as locally used HERBAL MEDICINALS (*căo yào*) or FOLK MEDICINALS (*mín jiān yào*) scantily described in premodern literature. The term CHINESE MEDICINALS AND HERBS (*zhōng căo yào*) covers both categories. Chinese medicinals and to lesser extent herbal medicinals too, have properties described in terms of NATURE AND FLAVOR, TOXICITY, CHANNEL ENTRY, and ACTION.

medicinal dew 药露 *yào lù*: DISTILLATE.

medicinal-induced blister moxibustion 药物发泡灸 *yào wù fā pào jiŭ*: Synonym: *cold moxibustion*; *natural moxibustion*. The application of irritants at acupuncture points to produce blistering. Medicinals used include Japanese ranunculus (*máo gèn*), mylabris (*bān máo*), eclipta (*mò hàn lián*), mashed garlic (*suàn ní*), and white mustard (*bái jiè zĭ*). Because this therapy makes use of the burning properties contained in the medicinals, it is also called *natural moxibustion* and because the "burning" action involves no actual combustion, it is also called *cold moxibustion*. Moxibustion with Japanese ranunculus (*máo gèn*) is used to treat malaria and jaundice. The leaves and stem of the plant is crushed and is applied to appropriate acupuncture points for 1–2 hours until a blister appears. Moxibustion with mylabris (*bān máo*) is used to treat joint pain and jaundice. A piece of sticking plaster is pierced and applied to the skin so that the hole aligns with the acupuncture point. Powdered mylabris is then placed in the hole, and another piece of plaster is stuck over it. The dressing is removed as soon as a blister develops. Moxibustion with eclipta (*mò hàn lián*) is used to treat malaria. Fresh eclipta is crushed and applied to acupuncture points for 3–4 hours until a blister appears. Moxibustion with mashed garlic (*suàn ní*) is applied to acupuncture points for 1–3 hours and is used to treat vacuity consumption and baby moth. Moxibustion with white mustard (*bái jiè zǐ*) is used to treat pulmonary consumption, wheezing and panting, and deviation of the eyes and mouth. The white mustard is ground to a powder, mixed with a little fluid, and applied to the acupuncture for 3–4 hours until a blister appears. *cold moxibustion*. [26: 977, 164, 681, 325, 842 222]

medicinal materials 药材 *yào cái*: Basic animal, vegetable, and mineral products that are processed and prepared for consumption or application.

medicinal paste 药膏 *yào gāo*: *Synonym: oil paste*. A preparation made with vegetable oil and bee's wax, and applied topically in the treatment of sores or burns. Medicinal pastes are made by first heating the oil, blending in the wax, and adding the ground medicinals while the mixture is still hot. The paste is ready for use when cool. Some formula stipulates that certain medicinals be added in the form of decocting slices, which are first fried in the oil and the dregs removed before the wax and powdered medicinals are blended in. Aromatic medicinals such as borneol (*bīng piàn*) and camphor (*zhāng nǎo*) are added after the paste has cooled to ensure that they retain their full strength. Nowadays, finely ground materials are often combined with a petroleum jelly (Vaseline) and glycerin base to make *ointment*. See PASTE. [26: 977] [97: 383]

medicinal preparation 剂型 *jì xíng*: The final form in which medicinals (usually the various ingredients of a formula) are administered, taken, or applied. Commonly used preparations are given in the table below. The most common preparation taken orally is the decoction, whereby the natural medicinals are simply boiled by patients themselves or those attending them. Recent technological advances have led to the development of new preparations such as soluble granules, tablets, and injection fluids, which are quicker acting, more effective, more convenient to use, and more accurately dose-controlled. See Table 9. [27: 311]

9. Medicinal Preparations	
Decoction (*tāng*)	Elixir (*dān*)
Beverage (*yǐn*)	Lozenge (*dǐng*)
Drink (*yǐn zǐ*)	Tea (*chá*)
Pill (*wán*)	Tablet (*piàn*)
Powder (*sǎn*)	Distillate (*lù*)
Wine (*jiǔ*)	Glue (*jiāo*)
Paste (*gāo*)	

medicinal roles 主辅佐引 *zhǔ fǔ zuǒ yǐn*, 君臣佐使 *jūn chén zuǒ shǐ*: See SOVEREIGN, MINISTER, ASSISTANT, AND COURIER.

medicinal wine 药酒 *yào jiǔ*: A preparation made by steeping medicinals in liquor. See WINE.

medicinal with an affinity to flesh and blood 血肉有情之品 *xuè ròu yǒu qíng zhī pǐn*: Any medicinal product derived from animal, traditionally considered to be effective by virtue of its affinity to human and flesh and blood.

[1]**medicine** 医学 *yī xué*: The art of healing.

[2]**medicine** 药 *yào*: See MEDICINAL.

meeting of yin 会阴 *huì yīn*: PERINEUM.

meeting point 会穴 *huì xué*: See EIGHT MEETING POINTS.

membrane source 膜原 *mó yuán*: A membrane of the chest or diaphragm not clearly defined. In the doctrine of warm diseases, the term denotes a location between the exterior and interior, so that evil in the membrane source therefore corresponds to MIDSTAGE PATTERNS in the doctrine of cold damage. See SCOURGE EPIDEMIC. [26: 892]

menopause 经断 *jīng duàn*, 经绝 *jīng jué*, 经水断绝 *jīng shuǐ duàn jué*: Normal cessation of menstruation at about the age of forty-nine. Menopause is attributable to debilitation of kidney qi, cessation of the "heavenly tenth" (*tiān guǐ*), and vacuity of the thoroughfare (*chōng*) and controlling (*rèn*) vessels, and the vessels of the uterus. [27: 443] [97: 377] [67: 163]

men's diseases 男生疾病 *nán shēng jí bìng*: *Synonym: andriatic diseases*. Diseases proper to men; diseases that do not affect women. See DISEASE.

menstrual abdominal pain 经行腹痛 *jīng xíng fù tòng*: See MENSTRUAL PAIN. [26: 814]

menstrual block 经闭 *jīng bì*: *Synonym: amenorrhea*. Absence of menstruation. Between menarche and menopause menstruation normally ceases only in pregnancy. Menstrual block is the continuing absence of menstruation after the age of eighteen or the abnormal cessation of menstrual periods for at least three months in women who are neither pregnant nor lactating. Rarely, lifelong absence of menstruation is unaccompanied by impairment of reproductive function. See the entries listed below. ◇ Chin 经 *jīng*, warp, rule, regular, channel (meridian); to pass; 闭 *bì*, close, shut, end. [27: 441] [97: 376]

Menstrual Block

BLOOD DEPLETION MENSTRUAL BLOCK (*xuè kuī jīng bì*)

BLOOD DESICCATION MENSTRUAL BLOCK (*xuè kū jīng bì*)

KIDNEY VACUITY MENSTRUAL BLOCK (*shèn xū jīng bì*)

QI STAGNATION AND BLOOD STASIS MENSTRUAL BLOCK (*qì zhì xuè yū jīng bì*)

CONGEALING COLD-DAMP MENSTRUAL BLOCK (*hán shī níng zhì jīng bì*)

---

menstrual blood 经血 *jīng xuè*: MENSTRUAL FLOW.

menstrual blood ejection 经行吐血 *jīng xíng tù xuè*: One form of COUNTERFLOW MENSTRUATION. Blood ejection occurring at the time of menstruation, sometimes with reduction in menstrual flow. Menstrual blood ejection is mostly attributable to blood heat and upsurge of qi causing frenetic movement of the blood, but may also be the result of upsurge of qi and vacuity fire. The main patterns are intense stomach heat, depressed liver channel fire, and yin vacuity. ⌈WMC⌋ vicarious menstruation. **Intense stomach heat** tends to cause vomiting of copious amounts of blood when periods are about to come or have already started. It is associated with advanced menstruation and copious menstrual flow. Other signs include dry mouth and throat with desire to drink, a red tongue with yellow fur, and a large surging or rapid surging pulse. ⌈MED⌋ Clear and discharge stomach heat and conduct the blood downward. For repletion heat patterns, use Four Agents Decoction (*sì wù tāng*) plus rhubarb (*dà huáng*), coptis (*huáng lián*), and scutellaria (*huáng qín*). For vacuity heat patterns, use Rhinoceros Horn and Rehmannia Decoction (*xī jiǎo dì huáng tāng*). ⌈ACU⌋ Base treatment mainly on CV, ST, LI, and PC. For repletion heat, select CV-13 (*shàng wǎn*, Upper Stomach Duct), ST-44 (*nèi tíng*, Inner Court), LI-11 (*qū chí*, Pool at the Bend), PC-6 (*nèi guān*, Inner Pass), SP-10 (*xuè hǎi*, Sea of Blood), and PC-4 (*xī mén*, Cleft Gate); needle with drainage. For vacuity heat, drain the points for repletion heat and supplement KI-2 (*rán gǔ*, Blazing Valley) and SP-6 (*sān yīn jiāo*, Three Yin Intersection). **Depressed liver channel fire** tends to cause vomiting of copious amounts of bright red blood before or after periods, and is associated with advanced menstruation. There is heart vexation, irascibility, distention and pain in both rib-sides, bitter taste in the mouth, dry throat, clouded head, tinnitus, yellow urine and bound stool, a red tongue with yellow fur, and a rapid stringlike pulse. ⌈MED⌋ Course the liver and resolve heat; conduct blood downward. Use Liver-Clearing Channel-Conducting Decoction (*qīng gān yǐn jīng tāng*), which is composed of tangkuei fine root (*dāng guī xū*), white peony (*bái sháo yào*), dried/fresh rehmannia (*shēng dì huáng*), moutan (*mǔ dān pí*), gardenia (*shān zhī zǐ*), scutellaria (*huáng qín*), toosendan (*chuān liàn zǐ*), madder (*qiàn cǎo gēn*), achyranthes (*niú xī*), licorice (*gān cǎo*), and imperata (*bái máo gēn*). ⌈ACU⌋ Base treatment mainly on CV, ST, and LR. Select LR-3 (*tài chōng*, Supreme Surge); LR-2 (*xíng jiān*, Moving Between), LR-14 (*qī mén*, Cycle Gate), CV-12 (*zhōng wǎn*, Center Stomach Duct), PC-8 (*láo gōng*, Palace of Toil), ST-34 (*liáng qiū*, Beam Hill), BL-18 (*gān shū*, Liver Transport), and BL-17 (*gé shū*, Diaphragm Transport); needle with drainage. **Yin vacuity** tends to cause vomiting of scant bright red blood during or at the end of periods and is associated with scant menstrual flow and, in some cases, advanced menstruation. Other signs include dizziness and tinnitus, heat in the heart of the palms and soles, reddening of the cheeks, tidal heat [effusion], dry cough with scant phlegm, dry throat and thirst, red or crimson tongue with a peeling fur or no fur, and a rapid fine pulse. ⌈MED⌋ Enrich yin and moisten the lung; conduct blood downward. Use formulas such as Menstruation-Normalizing Decoction (*shùn jīng tāng*). ⌈ACU⌋ Base treatment mainly on KI, SP, ST, and LR. Select KI-6 (*zhào hǎi*, Shining Sea), ST-44 (*nèi tíng*, Inner Court), PC-4 (*xī mén*, Cleft Gate), LR-3 (*tài chōng*, Supreme Surge), and SP-6 (*sān yīn jiāo*, Three Yin Intersection); needle with even supplementation and drainage. [26: 813] [50: 1010] [46: 595, 682, 738] [67: 150] [37: 309, 310]

menstrual bloody stool 经行便血 *jīng xíng biàn xuè*: Synonyms: *deviated menstruation*; *crossed menstruation*. Bloody stool during menstruation. Menstrual bloody stool attributed to predilection for hot spicy foods or long-depressed accumulated heat harassing the thoroughfare (*chōng*) and controlling (*rèn*) vessels, causing frenetic movement of the blood. ⌈MED⌋ Clear heat and resolve toxin and regulate qi and blood with polyporus (*zhū líng*), alisma (*zé xiè*), ovate atractylodes (*bái zhú*), red peony (*chì sháo yào*), ass hide glue (*ē jiāo*), tangkuei (*dāng guī*), and ligusticum (*chuān xiōng*). ⌈ACU⌋ Base treatment mainly on LR, back transport points, BL, SP, and ST. Select LR-3 (*tài chōng*, Supreme Surge), LI-11 (*qū chí*, Pool at the Bend), BL-20 (*pí shū*, Spleen Transport), BL-25 (*dà cháng shū*, Large Intestine Transport), GV-1 (*cháng qiáng*, Long Strong), ST-39 (*xià jù xū*, Lower Great Hollow), BL-57 (*chéng shān*, Mountain Support), and SP-6 (*sān yīn jiāo*, Three Yin Intersection); needle with drainage. [26: 814] [27: 441] [97: 379] [46: 682, 739]

menstrual flow 月经 *yuè jīng*: Synonym: *menstrual blood*. The bloody fluid discharged during the menstrual period. See MENSTRUATION. [27: 440]

menstrual heat effusion 经行发热 *jīng xíng fā rè*, 经来发热 *jīng lái fā rè*: Heat effusion during menstruation; attributed to construction-defense disharmony resulting from contraction of external evils, blood heat, or yin vacuity. **Contraction of cold evil** patterns are characterized by heat effusion, aversion to cold, and absence of sweating. ⌈MED⌋ Effuse the exterior and dissipate cold with

Four Agents Decoction (*sì wù tāng*) plus ephedra (*má huáng*). ACU Base treatment mainly on BL, GV, SP, and LR. Select LR-3 (*tài chōng*, Supreme Surge), SP-6 (*sān yīn jiāo*, Three Yin Intersection), ST-36 (*zú sān lǐ*, Leg Three Li), GV-16 (*fēng fǔ*, Wind Mansion), BL-11 (*dà zhù*, Great Shuttle), GV-14 (*dà zhuī*, Great Hammer), and BL-64 (*jīng gǔ*, Capital Bone); needle with drainage and moxa can be added. **Contraction of wind evil** patterns are marked by heat effusion, aversion to cold, and spontaneous sweating. MED Harmonize construction and defense with Four Agents Decoction (*sì wù tāng*) plus cinnamon twig (*guì zhī*). ACU Base treatment mainly on GB, BL, SI, GV, SP, and LR. Select LR-3 (*tài chōng*, Supreme Surge), SP-6 (*sān yīn jiāo*, Three Yin Intersection), ST-36 (*zú sān lǐ*, Leg Three Li), GB-20 (*fēng chí*, Wind Pool), TB-5 (*wài guān*, Outer Pass), GV-14 (*dà zhuī*, Great Hammer), BL-64 (*jīng gǔ*, Capital Bone), and SI-3 (*hòu xī*, Back Ravine); needle with even supplementation and drainage. **Blood heat** patterns are characterized by heat effusion without aversion to cold, and scorching hot flesh. MED Clear heat and cool the blood with Lycium Root Bark Beverage (*dì gǔ pí yǐn*) plus picrorhiza (*hú huáng lián*). ACU Base treatment mainly on the three yin channels of the foot. Select SP-6 (*sān yīn jiāo*, Three Yin Intersection), LR-3 (*tài chōng*, Supreme Surge), SP-10 (*xuè hǎi*, Sea of Blood), KI-2 (*rán gǔ*, Blazing Valley), and LR-2 (*xíng jiān*, Moving Between); needle with drainage. **Yin vacuity** patterns are marked by postmeridian tidal heat [effusion], night sweating, and heat in the hearts of the palms and soles. MED Nourish yin and clear heat with dried/fresh rehmannia (*shēng dì huáng*), tangkuei (*dāng guī*), white peony (*bái sháo yào*), ligusticum (*chuān xiōng*), astragalus (*huáng qí*), and lycium root bark (*dì gǔ pí*). ACU Base treatment mainly on the three yin channels of the foot. Select LR-3 (*tài chōng*, Supreme Surge), KI-3 (*tài xī*, Great Ravine), KI-6 (*zhào hǎi*, Shining Sea), KI-2 (*rán gǔ*, Blazing Valley), KI-1 (*yǒng quán*, Gushing Spring), SP-6 (*sān yīn jiāo*, Three Yin Intersection), and HT-8 (*shào fǔ*, Lesser Mansion); needle with even supplementation and drainage. [75: 46, 62] [26: 814] [46: 595, 596, 682]

menstrual irregularities 月经不调 *yuè jīng bù tiáo*: Abnormalities of the regularity menstrual cycle or of volume, color or consistency of menstrual flow. **Cycle:** Irregularities of the menstrual cycle include ADVANCED MENSTRUATION (shortening of the cycle attributable to blood heat, blood vacuity, qi vacuity, or liver depression), DELAYED MENSTRUATION (lengthening of cycle attributable to blood vacuity, blood cold, kidney vacuity, qi stagnation, or static blood), MENSTRUATION AT IRREGULAR INTERVALS (sometimes short, sometimes long cycles attributable to liver depression or

kidney vacuity), and MENSTRUAL BLOCK (absence of menstruation attributable to blood depletion, blood desiccation, kidney vacuity, qi stagnation and blood stasis, and congealing cold-damp). **Volume:** Irregularities of volume include SCANT MENSTRUATION (attributable to blood vacuity, blood cold, blood stasis, phlegm-damp or kidney vacuity) and PROFUSE MENSTRUATION (attributable to qi vacuity, blood heat, or taxation damage).

Menstrual Irregularities

Cycle
ADVANCED MENSTRUATION (*yuè jīng xiān qī*)
DELAYED MENSTRUATION (*yuè jīng hòu qī*)
MENSTRUATION AT IRREGULAR INTERVALS (*yuè jīng qián hòu bù dìng qī*)

Volume
MENSTRUAL BLOCK (*jīng bì*)
SCANT MENSTRUATION (*yuè jīng guò shǎo*)
PROFUSE MENSTRUATION (*yuè jīng guò duō*)

Color
PALE MENSTRUAL FLOW (*jīng lái sè dàn*)
PURPLE MENSTRUAL FLOW (*jīng lái sè zǐ*)

Consistency
CLOTTED MENSTRUAL FLOW (*jīng lái chéng kuài*)
TOAD EGG MENSES (*jīng rú hā má zǐ*)

Miscellaneous
MENSTRUAL BLOOD EJECTION (*jīng xíng tù xuè*)
MENSTRUAL HEAT EFFUSION (*jīng xíng fā rè*)
MENSTRUAL MANIA (*jīng lái fā kuáng*)
MENSTRUAL PAIN (*tòng jīng*)
MENSTRUAL VOMITING (*jīng lái ǒu tòu*)
MENSTRUAL PUFFY SWELLING (*jīng lái fú zhǒng*)
PREMENSTRUAL BLOODY STOOL (*jīng qián biàn xuè*)
PREMENSTRUAL SYNDROME (*jīng qián jǐn zhāng zòng hé zhèng*)
POSTMENSTRUAL TIDAL HEAT [EFFUSION] (*jīng hòu cháo rè*)
FLOODING AND SPOTTING (*bēng lòu*)

Color: Irregularities of the color of the menstrual flow include any deviation from a dark red flow that is paler at onset and termination. Generally speaking, a bright red flow indicates heat, pale red indicates blood vacuity or cold, whereas purple indicates static blood. See PALE MENSTRUAL FLOW and PURPLE MENSTRUAL FLOW. **Consistency:** Irregularities of consistency include excessively thin or thick consistency and clotting. Generally, thick flow suggests heat, thin flow indicates qi vacuity, and clotting indicates blood stasis. See CLOTTED MENSTRUAL FLOW; TOAD-EGG MENSES. **Miscellaneous:** Discomfort before, during, or after menstruation most commonly includes abdominal pain during menstruation (due to qi stagnation, blood stasis, congealing cold-damp, qi-blood vacuity, or liver-kidney depletion) and distended breasts (due to liver depression and qi stagnation). See the entries listed below. [26: 168] [27: 439] [97: 110]

Miscellaneous Menstrual Pathoconditions

MENSTRUAL BLOOD EJECTION (*jīng xíng tù xuè*)

MENSTRUAL HEAT EFFUSION (*jīng xíng fā rè*)

MENSTRUAL MANIA (*jīng lái fā kuáng*)

MENSTRUAL PAIN (*tòng jīng*)

MENSTRUAL VOMITING (*jīng lái ǒu tù*)

MENSTRUAL SPONTANEOUS EXTERNAL BLEEDING (*jīng xíng nǜ xuè*)

MENSTRUAL PUFFY SWELLING (*jīng lái fú zhǒng*)

PREMENSTRUAL BLOODY STOOL (*jīng qián biàn xuè*)

PREMENSTRUAL SYNDROME (*jīng qián qí jǐn zhāng zòng hé zhèng*)

POSTMENSTRUAL BLOOD EJECTION AND SPONTANEOUS EXTERNAL BLEEDING (*jīng hòu tù nǜ*)

POSTMENSTRUAL TIDAL HEAT [EFFUSION] (*jīng hòu cháo rè*)

FLOODING AND SPOTTING (*bēng lòu*)

---

menstrual mania 经来发狂 *jīng lái fā kuáng*: Mania during menstruation characterized by deranged spirit-mind, hallucination, manic or delirious raving, and in severe cases, loss of consciousness. Menstrual mania attributed to vexation and anger causing counterflow and derangement of liver qi that carries the blood upward to attack the heart. ⃞MED Soothe the liver and quiet the heart with musk (*shè xiāng*), cinnabar (*zhū shā*), licorice (*gān cǎo*), saussurea (*mù xiāng*), ginseng (*rén shēn*), root poria (*fú shén*), platycodon (*jié gěng*), bupleurum (*chái hú*), and polygala (*yuǎn zhì*). ⃞ACU Base treatment mainly on PC, LR, SP, and HT. Select BL-18 (*gān shū*, Liver Transport), BL-15 (*xīn shū*, Heart Transport), PC-6 (*nèi guān*, Inner Pass), LR-3 (*tài chōng*, Supreme Surge), SP-6 (*sān yīn jiāo*, Three Yin Intersection), HT-7 (*shén mén*, Spirit Gate), ST-36 (*zú sān lǐ*, Leg Three Li), GV-26 (*shuǐ gōu*, Water Trough), PC-8 (*láo gōng*, Palace of Toil), HT-8 (*shào fǔ*, Lesser Mansion), and LR-2 (*xíng jiān*, Moving Between); needle with drainage. [26: 815] [46: 643, 646] [37: 352]

menstrual pain 痛经 *tòng jīng*: Synonym: *menstrual abdominal pain*. Smaller-abdominal pain occurring before, during, or after menstruation. There are three main forms: (1) Lesser-abdominal pain that occurs before or during menstruation, that in severe cases radiates into the lumbus, that likes warmth, and that is associated with scant reddish flow with clots, aversion to cold, sloppy stool, a slimy tongue fur and a tight sunken pulse

is a cold-damp pattern. (2) Smaller-abdominal distention and pain before or during menstruation, with distention more pronounced than pain and relieved by the discharge of clots, scant dribbling flow, distention in the breasts and rib-side, a speckled tongue, and a stringlike sunken pulse indicates liver qi depression. (3) Dull post-menstrual pain that likes pressure, accompanied by scant pale flow, aching lumbus and knees, dizziness, and tinnitus, a pale tongue covered with a thin white fur, and a fine sunken pulse indicates liver-kidney depletion. ⃞TRT To treat the tip, regulate the blood and relieve pain; to treat the root, treat according to the pattern identified. Acupuncture treatment for menstrual pain involves rectifying the qi and blood of the thoroughfare (*chōng*) and controlling (*rèn*) vessels on the fundamental principles of "vacuity is treated by supplementation," "repletion is treated by draining," "cold is treated with heat," and "heat is treated with cold." The methods of treatment are: dissipating cold, clearing heat, supplementing vacuity, or draining repletion. These may be combined with stimulation to move qi or quicken the blood. Care must be taken to avoid indiscriminate use of attacking stasis and expelling blood. Sometimes it is necessary to ensure fullness of qi and blood before freeing action can be effective. See the entries listed below. [26: 672] [59: 71] [27: 442] [97: 488]

Menstrual Pain

QI STAGNATION MENSTRUAL PAIN (*qì zhì tòng jīng*)

BLOOD STASIS MENSTRUAL PAIN (*xuè yū tòng jīng*)

CONGEALING COLD-DAMP MENSTRUAL PAIN (*hán shí níng zhì tòng jīng*)

QI-BLOOD VACUITY MENSTRUAL PAIN (*qì xuè xū ruò tòng jīng*)

LIVER-KIDNEY DEPLETION MENSTRUAL PAIN (*gān shèn kuī sǔn tòng jīng*)

---

menstrual puffy swelling 经来浮肿 *jīng lái fú zhǒng*: Swelling during menstruation that results when a vacuous spleen fails to move and transform water, and water spills into the flesh. ⃞MED Regulate the stomach and spleen; move qi and disinhibit water. [26: 815]

menstrual spontaneous external bleeding 经行衄血 *jīng xíng nǜ xuè*: One form of COUNTERFLOW MENSTRUATION. Spontaneous external bleeding during menstruation. Menstrual spontaneous external bleeding attributed to either liver depression transforming into fire or yin vacuity and lung heat, the heat in either case damaging the network vessels and causing the blood to ascend counterflow with it. ⃞WMC vicarious menstruation.

Liver fire invading the lung is characterized by rashness, impatience, and irascibility, headache, rib-side pain, bitter taste in the mouth, dry throat, and heart vexation. ⬚MED Calm the liver and drain heat with Moutan and Gardenia Free Wanderer Powder (*dān zhī xiāo yáo sǎn*) plus curcuma (*yù jīn*). ⬚ACU Base treatment mainly on PC, LR, LU, and SP. Select BL-13 (*fèi shū*, Lung Transport), LU-10 (*yú jì*, Fish Border), LR-3 (*tài chōng*, Supreme Surge), SP-6 (*sān yīn jiāo*, Three Yin Intersection), PC-6 (*nèi guān*, Inner Pass), PC-8 (*láo gōng*, Palace of Toil), GB-34 (*yáng líng quán*, Yang Mound Spring), and LR-2 (*xíng jiān*, Moving Between); needle with drainage. **Yin vacuity lung heat** is marked by postmeridian tidal heat [effusion], cough, reddening of the cheeks, heat in the heart of the palms and soles. ⬚MED Nourish yin and clear heat with Rhinoceros Horn and Rehmannia Decoction (*xī jiǎo dì huáng tāng*). ⬚ACU Base treatment mainly on LU and KI. Drain LU-6 (*kǒng zuì*, Collection Hole), LU-10 (*yú jì*, Fish Border), and Hundred Taxations (*bǎi láo*), and supplement LU-5 (*chǐ zé*, Cubit Marsh), KI-2 (*rán gǔ*, Blazing Valley), KI-3 (*tài xī*, Great Ravine), LR-3 (*tài chōng*, Supreme Surge), and SP-6 (*sān yīn jiāo*, Three Yin Intersection), [26: 814] [46: 628, 737]

menstrual spotting 经漏 *jīng lòu*, 月漏 *juè lòu*: Synonym: *persistent menstrual flow*. From *Secret Treasure of the Orchid Chamber* (*lán shì mì cáng*). Persistent spotting after menstruation should have fully ceased. See FLOODING AND SPOTTING. [50: 1008] [27: 445]

menstrual vomiting 经来呕吐 *jīng lái ǒu tù*: VOMITING during menstruation. Menstrual vomiting is attributable to nontransformation of ingested fluids or food damage, the former being characterized by vomiting of water matter and the latter by stomach pain. ⬚MED Damage by ingested fluids can be treated with clove (*dīng xiāng*), dried ginger (*gān jiāng*), and ovate atractylodes (*bái zhú*) ground to a powder, taking 5 g at a time mixed with rice decoction. Food damage is treated by dispersing food and abducting stagnation with Saussurea and Amomum Six Gentlemen Decoction (*xiāng shā liù jūn zǐ tāng*). [26: 815]

menstruation 月经 *yuè jīng*: Discharge of bloody fluid from the uterus roughly once a month. Menstruation normally starts between the age of 11 and 15, and ceases permanently sometime after the age of 45. Menstruation occurs roughly every 28 days, and each menstrual period lasts for three to five days. Irregularities in the cycle and in the volume, color, and consistency of the flow, are referred to by the general name of MENSTRUAL IRREGULARITIES. ◇ Chin 月 *yuè*, month; 经 *jīng*, warp, channel, rule. [26: 168] [27: 439] [97: 110]

menstruation at irregular intervals 经行先后无定期 *jīng xíng xiān hòu wú dìng qī*, 月经先后无定期 *yuè jīng xiān hòu wú dìng qī*: Synonym: *chaotic menstruation*. Menstruation that is sometimes advanced and sometimes delayed; attributed to liver qi depression, kidney vacuity, or spleen vacuity. **Liver qi depression** gives rise to menstruation at irregular intervals with purplish red clotted menstrual flow that is either copious or scant, mental depression, painful distention of the breasts, and in some cases distention and pain in the smaller abdomen. ⬚MED For liver qi depression, course the liver and resolve depression using Free Wanderer Powder (*xiāo yáo sǎn*), Bupleurum Liver-Coursing Powder (*chái hú shū gān sǎn*) or Menses-Stabilizing Decoction (*dìng jīng tāng*). ⬚ACU Base treatment mainly on CV and the three yin channels of the foot. Main points: CV-4 (*guān yuán*, Pass Head) SP-8 (*dì jī*, Earth's Crux), and SP-6 (*sān yīn jiāo*, Three Yin Intersection). For liver depression, add PC-6 (*nèi guān*, Inner Pass), LR-3 (*tài chōng*, Supreme Surge), BL-18 (*gān shū*, Liver Transport), BL-17 (*gé shū*, Diaphragm Transport), ST-36 (*zú sān lǐ*, Leg Three Li), and CV-3 (*zhōng jí*, Central Pole), needling with even supplementation and drainage. **Kidney vacuity** causes menstruation at irregular intervals with scant thin pale flow, dizziness, tinnitus, limp aching lumbus and knees, profuse urination at night, unsolid stool, and dull facial complexion. ⬚MED Supplement the kidney and warm yang using Yin-Securing Brew (*gù yīn jiān*) plus cinnamon bark (*ròu guì*), aconite (*fù zǐ*), and psoralea (*bǔ gǔ zhī*). Alternatively, use variations of Right-Restoring [Life Gate] Pill (*yòu guī wán*). ⬚ACU To the main points given above, BL-23 (*shèn shū*, Kidney Transport), KI-7 (*fù liū*, Recover Flow), KI-3 (*tài xī*, Great Ravine), and KI-5 (*shuǐ quán*, Water Spring), needling with supplementation. **Spleen vacuity** causes menstruation at irregular intervals with pale scant flow that is either scant or copious, withered-yellow facial complexion, shortage of qi, laziness to speak, and fatigue and emaciation of the limbs, reduced eating and torpid intake, distention and fullness in the stomach duct and abdomen, and thin sloppy stool. ⬚MED Supplement the spleen and boost qi; nourish the blood and regulate menstruation. Use Ginseng, Poria (Hoelen), and Ovate Atractylodes Powder (*shēn líng bái zhú sǎn*) ⬚ACU To the main points given above, add CV-6 (*qì hǎi*, Sea of Qi), BL-20 (*pí shū*, Spleen Transport), and ST-36 (*zú sān lǐ*, Leg Three Li), needling with supplementation. [26: 813] [27: 441] [97: 377] [46: 683] [37: 419]

meridiometer 经络测定仪 *jīng luò cè dìng yí*: A device for measuring cutaneous electrical resistance as a supposed reflection of the flow of qi and blood in the channels.

metal 金 *jīn*: (In the doctrine of the five phases) the phase associated with the season autumn, the lung (and large intestine), the flavor acridity, and the color white. [6: 28]

metal and water engender each other 金水相生 *jīn shuǐ xiāng shēng*: **1.** Lung-metal and kidney-water stand in mother-child relationship to each other. See LUNG AND KIDNEY ARE MUTUALLY ENGENDERING. **2.** COMBINED TREATMENT OF LUNG AND KIDNEY. [26: 391]

metal gan 金疳 *jīn gān*: A disease of the white of the eye (white part of the eye surrounding the iris) attributed to intense lung heat and characterized by the appearance of gray-white blister-like granules surrounded by red threads (visible blood vessels) and associated with dryness and discomfort of the eyes, aversion to light, and tearing. WMC phlyctenular conjunctivitis. MED Clear heat and drain the lung using mulberry root bark (*sāng bái pí*), alisma (*zé xiè*), scrophularia (*xuán shēn*), licorice (*gān cǎo*), ophiopogon (*mài mén dōng*), scutellaria (*huáng qín*), inula flower (*xuán fù huā*), chrysanthemum (*jú huā*), lycium root bark (*dì gǔ pí*), platycodon (*jié gěng*), and white poria (*bái fú líng*). If it persists or continually recurs, it is due to lung dryness and damage to yin, which is treated by nourishing yin and moistening dryness with variations of Yin-Nourishing Lung-Clearing Decoction (*yǎng yīn qīng fèi tāng*). [26: 391] [27: 502] [97: 346]

¹**method of treatment** 疗法 *zhì fǎ*: Any set of therapeutic techniques, e.g., medicinal therapy, acupuncture, acupressure, food therapy. [6: 242]

²**method of treatment** 治法 *zhì fǎ*: Any specific mode of intervention in one or more bodily processes derived from a PRINCIPLE OF TREATMENT, e.g., "supplementing the blood" and "clearing heat and resolving toxin." [6: 246]

miasmic malaria 瘴疟 *zhàng nüè*: A severe form of malaria attributed to contraction of mountain forest miasmic toxin and traditionally observed to occur in southern China. Miasmic malaria occurs in episodes marked by clouded spirit and delirious raving, and hoarse voice. Distinction is made between cold miasma and heat miasma. MED Heat miasma is treated by repelling foulness and eliminating miasma and by clearing heat and safeguarding liquid using Purple Snow Elixir (*zǐ xuě dān*). Cold miasma is treated by repelling foulness and opening the orifices, transforming turbidity and rectifying qi with variations of Priceless Qi-Righting Powder (*bù huàn jīn zhèng qì sǎn*). Liquid Storax Pill (*sū hé xiāng wán*) can also be used. ACU Base treatment mainly on GV, PC, SI, and LR. Select GV-14 (*dà zhuī*, Great Hammer), GV-13 (*táo dào*, Kiln Path), PC-5 (*jiān shǐ*, Intermediary Courier), SI-3 (*hòu xī*, Back Ravine),

ST-40 (*fēng lóng*, Bountiful Bulge), and CV-12 (*zhōng wǎn*, Center Stomach Duct), needling with drainage, and prick GV-26 (*rén zhōng*, Human Center) and LU-11 (*shào shāng*, Lesser Shang) to bleed. For heat miasma, add LI-11 (*qū chí*, Pool at the Bend) and TB-1 (*guān chōng*, Passage Hub). For cold miasma, add moxa. See MALARIA. [26: 901] [27: 359] [97: 648]

midday-midnight point selection 子午流注 *zǐ wǔ liú zhù*: Synonym: *stem and branch point selection*. A method of needling the five transport points that is founded on the notion that state of qi and blood in the various channels and the receptivity of different points varies in time and that involves calculating the most effective needling times in terms of heavenly stems and earthly branches. [26: 54] [26: 54]

middle 中 *zhōng*: See also CENTER.

middle burner 中焦 *zhōng jiāo*: CENTER BURNER.

middle finger body-inch 中指同身寸 *zhōng zhǐ tóng shēn cùn*: From *A Thousand Gold Pieces Prescriptions* (*qiān jīn yào fāng*). Length of the medial phalange of the middle finger (determined as the distance between the transverse creases) as a standard method of calculating one body-inch. See BODY-INCH. [26: 137]

middle gate tower 阙中 *què zhōng*: Synonyms: *hall of impression*; *gate tower*. The glabella, or region between the eyebrows. [27: 63] [97: 614]

mid-nape flat-abscess 项中疽 *xiàng zhōng jū*: MOUTH-LEVEL NAPE FLAT-ABSCESS.

midstage harmonization 和解半表半里 *hé jiě bàn biǎo bàn lǐ*: See HARMONIZING THE EXTERIOR AND INTERIOR.

midstage pattern 半表半里证 *bàn biǎo bàn lǐ zhèng*: Synonym: *half exterior half interior pattern*. A disease pattern occurring when an exterior evil fails to reach the interior and right qi is too weak to fight it. The signs are alternating heat effusion and aversion to cold, [suffering of] chest and rib-side fullness, heart vexation, no desire for food and drink, bitter taste in the mouth, dry pharynx, dizzy vision, and stringlike pulse. The etiology of midstage patterns is considered in detail under lesser yang (*shào yáng*) disease. MED Since these are not exterior patterns, they cannot be treated by sweating. Because the evil has not completely penetrated the interior, the normal procedures for treatment of interior patterns are also excluded. Instead, the method of harmonization is applied. The basic formula is Minor Bupleurum Decoction (*xiǎo chái hú tāng*), which outthrusts exterior evils and clears the interior. ACU Base treatment mainly on TB and GB. Select TB-4 (*yáng chí*, Yang Pool), PC-6 (*nèi guān*, Inner Pass), GB-40 (*qiū xū*, Hill Ruins), and LR-5 (*lǐ gōu*, Woodworm Canal); needle with even supplementation and drainage. [75: 208] [27: 211] [6: 152]

mild conditions are treated by counteraction 微者逆之 *wēi zhě nì zhī*: From *Elementary Questions* (*sù wèn*). Conditions that are not severe are treated by a therapy of opposite nature, e.g., cold is treated with heat, and heat is treated with cold. Counteraction is also referred to as *straight treatment*. [27: 241]

miliaria 痦 *péi*: See MILIARIA ALBA.

miliaria alba 白痦 *bái péi*: Small white vesicles on the skin, often occurring in damp warmth diseases when damp-heat evil becomes depressed in the FLESHY EXTERIOR and fails to thrust outward and discharge. Miliaria alba is usually located on the neck, but may spread down the upper arms and abdomen. It only occurs when there is sweating. Although its appearance usually indicates that the damp-heat is able to escape from the body, it also shows that dampness evil is viscous and resists transformation. For this reason there is recurrent eruption. When miliaria takes the form of clear, plump vesicles, it is known as miliaria crystallina (sudamina) and is a positive sign. If it is dull white and contains no fluid, it is known as *dry miliaria*, and indicates exhaustion of qi and yin. MED Clear heat, eliminate dampness, and promote diffusion and outthrust. Use Misty Decoction (*yīn yūn tāng*). For dry miliaria due to dual vacuity of qi and yin, add ginseng (*rén shēn*), adenophora/glehnia (*shā shēn*), and dendrobium (*shí hú*). [6: 118] [26: 227]

miliaria crystallina 晶痦 *jīng péi*: Miliaria characterized by plump, glossy, damp vesicles; also known as sudamina. See MILIARIA. [27: 270] [6: 370]

milk accumulation 乳积 *rǔ jī*, 乳食积滞 *rǔ shí jī zhì*: A gastrointestinal disease in infants due to damage by milk and other foods. **Simple milk accumulation** arises when in response to persistent crying the mother is overeager to feed the child. Spleen-stomach vacuity may be a factor preventing the child from digesting milk properly. There are signs such as vexation and crying, unquiet sleep, hot breath, smell of sour milk in the mouth, vomiting of undigested milk, and diarrhea or constipation. MED Disperse milk and harmonize the stomach with Harmony-Preserving Pill (*bǎo hé wán*) prepared as a decoction. **Milk and food accumulation** is characterized by poor stomach intake, glomus in the stomach duct and abdominal distention, and in some cases tidal heat [effusion], and gradual emaciation. MED First treat the tip by dispersing accumulations and abducting stagnation with variations of Harmony-Preserving Pill (*bǎo hé wán*) and Stomach-Calming Powder

(*píng wèi sǎn*). Then treat the root by regulating the stomach and spleen with Ginseng, Poria (Hoelen), and Ovate Atractylodes Powder (*shēn líng bái zhú sǎn*). ACU Base treatment for either pattern mainly on CV, ST, and SP. Main points: CV-12 (*zhōng wǎn*, Center Stomach Duct), ST-25 (*tiān shū*, Celestial Pivot), and ST-36 (*zú sān lǐ*, Leg Three Li). For the treatment of simple milk accumulation, add GB-34 (*yáng líng quán*, Yang Mound Spring). Needle with drainage for refusal to take milk; add BL-20 (*pí shū*, Spleen Transport) and CV-6 (*qì hǎi*, Sea of Qi), needling with supplementation and adding moxa for spleen-stomach vacuity. For the treatment of milk and food accumulation, add Li Inner Court (*lǐ nèi tíng*), SP-2 (*dà dū*, Great Metropolis), and ST-41 (*jiě xī*, Ravine Divide), needling with drainage. Massage and spine pinching is also effective. [26: 378]

millet sores 粟疮 *sù chuāng*: **1.** Generalized eruption of papules like grains of millet, that are red in color, itchy, turn into sores when scratched, and over a long period of time can cause damage to the blood and cause the skin to become thick and rough like snake skin. WMC papular eczema; prurigo. MED Course wind and clear heat. Oral: Use Ledebouriella Sage-Inspired Powder (*fáng fēng tōng shèng sǎn*). Topical: Apply *The Golden Mirror of Medicine* (*yī zōng jīn jiàn*) formula Two-Ingredient Toxin-Drawing Powder (*èr wèi bá dú sǎn*), which consists of realgar (*xióng huáng*) and alum (*bái fán*). If itching is severe, use Wind-Dispersing Powder (*xiāo fēng sǎn*). In enduring conditions, when the skin becomes like snake's skin as a result of wear on the blood, take Gleditsia and Flavescent Sophora Pill (*zào jiǎo kǔ shēn wán*). **2.** A soft yellow granulation like a millet seed growing inside the eyelid, causing tearing, itching, and pain. Millet sores of the eye are similar to and often accompanies a peppercorn sore. They are attributable to spleen-stomach damp-heat and external wind toxin congesting in the eyelid. WMC follicular conjunctivitis. MED Clear heat, eliminate dampness, and dispel wind. Wind-Eliminating Spleen-Clearing Beverage (*chú fēng qīng pí yīn*) plus flavescent sophora (*kǔ shēn*), kochia (*dì fū zǐ*), mutong (*mù tōng*), and red peony (*chì sháo yào*). ACU Base treatment mainly on GB, BL, LI, SP, and ST. Select BL-1 (*jīng míng*, Bright Eyes), BL-2 (*zǎn zhú*, Bamboo Gathering), GB-1 (*tóng zǐ liáo*, Pupil Bone-Hole), Greater Yang (*tài yáng*), LI-4 (*hé gǔ*, Union Valley), GB-20 (*fēng chí*, Wind Pool), ST-44 (*nèi tíng*, Inner Court), SP-9 (*yīn líng quán*, Yin Mound Spring), and ST-36 (*zú sān lǐ*, Leg Three Li); needle with drainage. [50: 1480] [26: 686] [27: 503] [46: 595, 597, 702] [73: 619] [15: 396]

mind 志 *zhì*: Synonym: *spirit-mind*. **1.** Will, determination. **2.** capacity to think, feel, and re-

spond. See SPIRIT. **3.** Affect, emotion. See FIVE
MINDS. **4.** Memory; will. See KIDNEY STORES
MIND. ◇ Chin 志 was originally written as 心 *xīn*,
heart, topped not with 士 *shì* as in the modern
form of the graph, but with 㞢 *zhī*, the original form of the form of 之, a graph that in addition to serving as a genitive particle and as a
third person pronoun, also means 'to go'. The
㞢 may merely be a purely phonetic element, but
as a semantic element (to go), the overall composition of the graph would suggest the meaning
of "direction" of the heart. In actuality, *zhì* has
the meaning of a) will or determination, b) presence of mind or concentration power, c) emotion.
In Chinese medicine, meaning b) and c) are the
most common. In sense b), it is similar in meaning to spirit *shén*, with which it is often combined
to form 神志 *shén zhì* spirit-mind. States such
as insomnia, mania, or epilepsy are traditionally
explained in terms such as the "heart failing to
keep to its abode" and "straying." Accordingly,
the treatment of such states is sometimes described
as "stabilize the mind" (i.e., quiet the spirit). In
the sense of "direction of the heart," the character
志 denotes the emotions joy, anger, anxiety, and
fear, and the mental activity thought, which are
associated with the heart, liver, lung, kidney, and
spleen respectively. Finally, in the phrase 肾藏志
shèn cáng zhì, the kidney stores mind, 志 is interpreted either in sense of will, or as equivalent
to 誌 *zhì*, meaning memory, wherein an individual
finds his orientation in time. The consistency of
basic meaning in the character 志 and the possible
existence of double or multiple interpretations in
different contexts explains the consistent rendering with a single English term mind. [48: 107]
[19: 5200, 4300]

Ming 明 *míng*: The name of a dynasty (A.D. 1368–
1644).

minister 臣 *chén*: See SOVEREIGN, MINISTER, AS-
SISTANT, AND COURIER.

ministerial fire 相火 *xiàng huǒ*: A fire in the
body inhabiting the life gate, liver, gallbladder,
and triple burner, and thought to come essentially
from the life gate (to which extent it is indissociable from kidney yang). It stands in complementary
opposition to the sovereign fire, which is the heart
fire. The sovereign and ministerial fires together
warm the bowels and viscera and power activity
in the body. In insufficiency of liver-kidney yin,
the ministerial fire can be hyperactive, giving rise
to a condition known as *stirring of the ministerial
fire,* which is characterized by dizziness, headache,
unclear vision, tinnitus, deafness, irascibility, profuse dreaming, vexing heat in hearts of the palms,
excessive libido, seminal emission, and premature
ejaculation. This condition is the same as vacuity

fire flaming upward due to liver-kidney yin vacuity.
[26: 415] [27: 59] [97: 386]

minor chest bind 小结胸 *xiǎo jié xiōng*: From
On Cold Damage (*shāng hán lùn, biàn tài yáng
bìng mài zhèng bìng zhì*). A pattern of distention and oppression in the stomach duct with pain
when pressure is applied, and a slippery floating
pulse. MED Loosen the chest, disperse phlegm,
open binds, and drain heat with Minor Chest
Bind Decoction (*xiǎo xiàn xiōng tāng*). ACU Select PC-5 (*jiān shǐ*, Intermediary Courier), CV-12
(*zhōng wǎn*, Center Stomach Duct), ST-36 (*zú sān
lǐ*, Leg Three Li), ST-37 (*shàng jù xū*, Upper Great
Hollow), and ST-43 (*xiàn gǔ*, Sunken Valley); needle with drainage. See CHEST BIND. [26: 77] [27:
376] [97: 34]

minor divide 小分 *xiǎo fēn*: See FLESH DIVIDE.

mirror-like tongue 舌面如镜 *shé miàn rú jìng*:
MIRROR TONGUE.

mirror tongue 镜面舌 *jìng miàn shé*: Synonym:
mirror-like tongue. A completely smooth tongue,
free of liquid and fur. It indicates severe yin humor depletion. A smooth red or deep red tongue
indicates damage to yin by intense heat. If pale in
color, a smooth tongue indicates damage to both
qi and yin. [27: 179] [97: 197]

miscarriage 小产 *xiǎo chǎn*, 半产 *bàn chǎn*: Expulsion of a fetus before the normal time after
the third month of pregnancy. Miscarriage is attributed to damage to the thoroughfare (*chōng*)
and controlling (*rèn*) vessels and inability to contain blood and nourish the fetus stemming from
qi-blood vacuity, kidney vacuity, and external injury. See HABITUAL MISCARRIAGE. [27: 449]

miscellaneous disease 杂病 *zá bìng*, 杂症 *zá
zhèng*: Synonym: *internal damage miscellaneous
disease*. Disease other than externally contracted
heat (febrile) disease. [27: 378] [97: 316]

miscellaneous qi 杂气 *zá qì*: PESTILENTIAL QI.
[26: 950]

mix-frying 炙 *zhì*: Stir-frying with liquid adjuvants. The aim of mix-frying is to change medicinal
characteristics, improve effectiveness, improve the
flavor and smell, resolve toxicity, and prevent rotting. Usually, the adjuvant and materials are first
blended, covered and left to stand for a short time
before frying so that the adjuvant soaks well into
the materials. The most commonly used adjuvants
are honey, vinegar, wine, and brine. [97: 359]

mix-frying with brine 盐炙 *yán zhì*: Stir-frying
materials with a salt solution is known as brine
mix-frying. Salt, being cold in nature, clears heat
and cools the blood; being salty in flavor, it enters
the kidney and softens hardness. It can also improve the flavor, and is a preservative. Brine mix-
frying is a common method of processing medicinals that supplement the kidney, secure essence,

treat mounting qi (*shàn qì*), and drain kidney fire, such as psoralea (*bǔ gǔ zhī*), fennel (*huí xiāng*), anemarrhena (*zhī mǔ*), phellodendron (*huáng bǎi*), and alisma (*zé xiè*). [82: 38]

mix-frying with fat 油炙 *yóu zhì*: Stir-frying medicinal materials in oil, or mixing them with fat or oil before stir-frying. Fat-frying, in which sesame seed or sheep fat in usually used, makes materials crisp and easier to crush, and can eliminate toxicity, such as in the case of tiger bone (*hǔ gǔ*) and nux vomica (*mǎ qián zǐ*). Epimedium (*yín yáng huò*) is stir-fried with sheep fat to increase it kidney-warming yang-invigorating action. [82: 44] [100: 129]

mix-frying with ginger 姜炙 *jiāng zhì*: Stir-frying medicinal materials that have been boiled with fresh ginger (*shēng jiāng*). Magnolia bark (*hòu pò*) may be processed in this way. Method: Place the materials with finely sliced fresh ginger in a brass wok, and cover with enough water to submerge the materials 3 cm below the water surface. Bring to the boil and simmer for 2–3 hours. Strain and remove ginger, and reserve the juice. Wind-dry until half dry, and then blend with the remaining juice. Boil off the fluid until dry. Compare STIR-FRYING WITH GINGER JUICE. [82: 40]

mix-frying with honey 蜜炙 *mì zhì*: Stir-frying with honey. Honey is sweet in flavor and balanced in nature. It moderates tension, boosts the origin, moistens the lung and calms cough, resolves toxin, and improves the flavor. It can reduce excessively pronounced qualities of other medicinals, and can harmonize the various medicinals in a formula and improve their effectiveness. Mix-frying with honey helps to moisten the lung and suppress cough, to boost and nourish, and to right the excessively pronounced natures of medicinals such as aster (*zǐ wǎn*) and astragalus (*huáng qí*). Method: The materials are first blended with honey, and then stir-fried in a heated wok, sprinkling water to help the honey to spread evenly. [82: 41]

mix-frying with turtle's blood 鳖血炙 *biē xuè zhì*: Stir-frying medicinal materials over a low flame after they have been mixed with fresh turtle's blood (*biē xuè*). Bupleurum (*chái hú*) is treated in this way to harmonize exterior and interior or to abate vacuity heat and eliminate postmeridian tidal heat [effusion]. [28: 10]

mix-frying with vinegar 醋炙 *cù zhì*: Stir-frying with vinegar. Vinegar is sour, bitter, and slightly warm, hence it can enter the liver channel, promote contraction, and relieve pain. For this reason, mix-frying with vinegar gives agents increased power to enter the blood and promote contraction, and to emolliate the liver and relieve pain. It can also improve flavor and smell. For example, it can remove the unpleasant odor of flying squirrel's

droppings (*wǔ líng zhī*). Vinegar contains acetic acid and therefore acts as a solvent: it can combine with free alkaloids to form soluble salts making active constituents easily extracted through decoction and increasing the speed with which the medicinal takes effect, as in the case of corydalis (*yán hú suǒ*). Agents most commonly vinegar mix-fried are liver-calming and qi-rectifying medicinals such as unripe tangerine peel (*qīng pí*), cyperus (*xiāng fù zǐ*), bupleurum (*chái hú*), and corydalis (*yán hú suǒ*). Method: Herbs are usually treated by first mixing them with vinegar and leaving them to stand. They are then stir-fried over a low flame until they give off their aroma and turn slightly golden in color. They are then removed from the wok and left to cool ready for use. Animal products and shells are put in the wok and heated over a low flame. They are turned constantly while sprinkling the vinegar over them. Stir-frying continues until the materials completely absorb the vinegar, give off their own aroma, and turn slightly golden. In some cases, it continues until a slightly burnt smell is detected. One or more parts vinegar to five parts of materials represents the usual proportion, i.e., around 60 g of vinegar for every 500 g of materials. [82: 35]

mix-frying with wine 酒炙 *jiǔ zhì*: Stir-frying with wine. Usually, yellow wine, such as Shaoxing rice wine, is used, but white grain liquor is also used on occasions. Wine is acrid, sweet, and very hot. It can conduct medicinals upward, reduce the cold nature of medicinals, and can quicken the blood and free the network vessels. Also, wine is an excellent organic solvent: alkaloids and volatile oils all easily dissolve in it. Mix-frying in wine thus helps to release active constituents, thereby increasing the effectiveness of medication. It also serves to removes fishy or putrid smells. Medicinals processed in this way include scutellaria (*huáng qín*), rhubarb (*dà huáng*), and white peony (*bái sháo yào*). Method: Yellow wine is first sprinkled over the materials, which are then left to stand covered for a while to allow the wine to soak in. Afterwards, they are transferred to the wok where they are continuously stirred over a low flame until they turn to a pale yellow and the aroma of the materials can be smelled. Another method is to sprinkle the wine over the materials after they have been heated over a low flame, and continue stir-frying until the aroma of the materials can be smelled. The duration of frying and the size of flame should not be excessive. Smell and color are good guides. Frying should cease before any burnt smell arises and before any change of color occurs inside the materials. The amount of wine used depends on the material. Generally it is 60–90 g for 500 g of materials. [82: 32]

mobile 走而不守 *zǒu ér bù shǒu*, 善走 *shàn zǒu*: (Of medicinals) tending to move. Medicinals that move qi or quicken the blood such as ligusticum (*chuān xiōng*) and tangkuei (*dāng guī*) are frequently described as mobile. Compare MOBILE AND PENETRATING.

mobile and penetrating 走窜 *zǒu cuàn*, 善窜 能走 *shàn cuàn néng zǒu*: (Of medicinals) tending to move and penetrate blockages. Agents that move qi and quicken the blood, free the channels and quicken the network vessels, or free the orifices and free the spirit, such as saussurea (*mù xiāng*), musk (*shè xiāng*), borneol (*bīng piàn*), camphor (*zhāng nǎo*), Chinese chive (*xiè bái*), pangolin scales (*chuān shān jiǎ*), and gleditsia thorn (*zào jiǎo cì*). Such medicinals are generally aromatic, acrid and dissipating, or warm and bitter.

moderate pulse 缓脉 *huǎn mài*: A pulse with four beats per respiration (slightly faster than a slow pulse) and that is soft and harmonious in its form. Construed as a normal pulse, it is even and moderate, and is a sign of the presence of stomach qi; construed as a pathological pulse, it is without strength, and is mostly seen in dampness patterns and in spleen-stomach vacuity. [50: 1588] [122: 165] [27: 194] [97: 593] [93: 262]

moisten 润 *rùn*: See SUPPLEMENTATION.

moistening dryness 润燥 *rùn zào*: Synonym: *clearing dryness*; COOLING DRYNESS. A method of treatment used to eliminate dryness-heat with moist enriching medicinals. See the entries listed below. [27: 269]

Moistening Dryness

MOISTENING DRYNESS BY LIGHT DIFFUSION (*qīng xuān rùn zào*)

ENRICHING AND MOISTENING WITH COLD SWEET MEDICINALS (*gān hán zī rùn*)

CLEARING THE INTESTINES AND MOISTENING DRYNESS (*qīng cháng rùn zào*)

NOURISHING YIN AND MOISTENING DRYNESS (*yǎng yīn rùn zào*)

NOURISHING THE BLOOD AND MOISTENING DRYNESS (*yǎng xuè rùn zào*)

---

moistening dryness and transforming phlegm 润燥化痰 *rùn zào huà tán*: MOISTENING THE LUNG AND TRANSFORMING PHLEGM. [26: 860]

moistening dryness by light diffusion 轻宣润燥 *qīng xuān rùn zào*: A method of treatment used to address dryness-heat damaging the lung characterized by heat effusion, headache, dry cough with scant phlegm, possibly with qi counterflow panting, tongue that is dry and without fur, or dry thin white tongue fur, and that is red at the tip and margins, using formulas such as Mulberry Leaf and Apricot Kernel Decoction (*sāng xìng tāng*). [27: 269] [97: 394]

moistening the intestines 润肠 *rùn cháng*: MOISTENING THE INTESTINES. [126: 265]

moistening the lung 润肺 *rùn fèi*: See MOISTENING THE LUNG AND TRANSFORMING PHLEGM.

moistening the lung and transforming phlegm 润肺化痰 *rùn fèi huà tán*: Synonym: *moistening dryness and transforming phlegm*. A method of treatment used to address externally contracted warm dryness or lung yin vacuity with vacuity fire scorching, causing phlegm that is difficult to expectorate, with dry throat, pain on swallowing, cough, and red tongue with dry yellow fur. MED Lung-moistening phlegm-transforming medicinals include fritillaria (*bèi mǔ*), trichosanthes (*guā lóu*), adenophora/glehnia (*shā shēn*), ophiopogon (*mài mén dōng*), and pear peel (*lí pí*), etc. Formulas include Fritillaria and Trichosanthes Powder (*bèi mǔ guā lóu sǎn*) and Adenophora/Glehnia and Ophiopogon Decoction (*shā shēn mài dōng tāng*). ACU Base treatment mainly on LU and KI. Select BL-13 (*fèi shū*, Lung Transport) and LU-5 (*chǐ zé*, Cubit Marsh). Selection of points according to patterns: For externally contracted warm dryness, add LI-11 (*qū chí*, Pool at the Bend), LI-1 (*shāng yáng*, Shang Yang), and CV-22 (*tiān tú*, Celestial Chimney), needling with drainage. For lung yin vacuity, add KI-3 (*tài xī*, Great Ravine), BL-43 (*gāo huāng shū*, Gao-Huang Transport), and KI-6 (*zhào hǎi*, Shining Sea), needling with supplementation. [26: 860] [27: 271] [37: 272]

moist formula 湿剂 *shī jì*: One of the TEN FORMULA TYPES. A formula containing moist medicinals. Moist [medicinals] can eliminate desiccation. An example of a moist formula is Dryness-Clearing Lung-Rescuing Decoction (*qīng zào jiù fèi tāng*), which contains, among others, moist medicinals such as ophiopogon (*mài mén dōng*), black sesame (*hēi zhī má*), and apricot kernel (*xìng rén*) and treats dryness-heat in the autumn causing cough without phlegm and dry mouth and tongue. [27: 307] [97: 579]

moist [medicinals] can eliminate desiccation 湿可去枯 *shī kě qù kū*: Moist medicinals such as ophiopogon (*mài mén dōng*) and rehmannia (*dì huáng*) are enriching and moistening, and can treat dryness of liquid and blood. See MOIST FORMULA. [97: 581]

moistness, dryness, putridity, and sliminess 润燥腐腻 *rù zào fǔ nì*: Four basic tongue fur qualities. Moistness and dryness indicate the state of the fluids. A moist tongue indicates sufficiency of the fluids, although a thick moist tongue fur indicates the presence of the dampness evil. A dry tongue fur—no matter what its other qualities may be—indicates damage to fluid. Putridity and sliminess reflect the state of the stomach. A putrid tongue fur is a sign of a superabundance of stomach yang qi carrying the turbid qi of the stomach upward. A slimy tongue fur indicates that the yang qi of the stomach is obstructed by damp turbidity, as in phlegm-rheum or food accumulation and stubborn phlegm patterns. See SLIMY TONGUE FUR. [26: 860]

moist precipitation 润下 *rùn xià: moist precipitation* Treating constipation with moist medicinals. Two forms exist: (1) Using moist oily slippery medicinals such as hemp seed (*huǒ má rén*), and honey (*mì*) to treat dry stool in the elderly, habitual constipation, constipation in pregnancy, and postpartum constipation. Intestine-moistening formulas are based on high fat-content seeds such as hemp seed (*huǒ má rén*), apricot kernel (*xìng rén*), trichosanthes seed (*guā lóu zǐ*), and honey (*mì*). Moist oily slippery medicinals that also have an enriching action, such as oily tangkuei (*yóu dāng guī*), fresh flowery knotweed (*xiān shǒu wū*), and apricot kernel (*xìng rén*), are suitable for people with weak constitutions. Representative formulas include Hemp Seed Pill (*má zǐ rén wán*), Intestine-Moistening Pill (*rùn cháng wán*), and Five Kernels Pill (*wǔ rén wán*). Note that constipation in externally contracted heat (febrile) diseases other than yang brightness (*yáng míng*) heat bind patterns can be treated with medicinals possessing both heat-clearing and intestine-moistening action such as trichosanthes (*guā lóu*) and scrophularia (*xuán shēn*). The use in recent years of an orally administered mixture of scallion juice and oil in the treatment of parasitic intestine obstruction is also a form of moist precipitation. (2) To treat intestinal heat bind and desiccated fluid constipation using fluid-enriching medicinals such as scrophularia (*xuán shēn*), ophiopogon (*mài mén dōng*) with the hearts left in, and dried/fresh rehmannia (*shēng dì huáng*). This method is also called HUMOR-INCREASING MOIST PRECIPITATION. [27: 256] [6: 253]

moist tongue fur 苔润 *tāi rùn*: A thin moist tongue fur is normal, and indicates sufficiency of the fluids. If thick it is a sign of dampness. [6: 123]

mole 痣 *zhì*: See BLACK MOLE; BLOOD MOLE.

morbid 病 *bìng*: Indicative of, or caused by, disease. [26: 489]

morbid complexion 病色 *bìng sè*: A complexion indicative of disease. See COMPLEXION; FACIAL COMPLEXION. [26: 489] [27: 173] [97: 487]

morbid prominence 病㿉 *bìng tuí*: Synonym: *yin bulging*. Swelling of both testicles. ⟨MED⟩ Disinhibit qi and soften hardness with Tangerine Pip Pill (*jú hé wán*). [26: 490] [27:]

morbid pulse 病脉 *bìng mài*: A pulse indicative of disease. See PULSE; PULSE CONDITION. [26: 489]

morning sickness 恶阻 *è zǔ*: MALIGN OBSTRUCTION.

mother-of-malaria 疟母 *nüè mǔ*: Lump glomus occurring in enduring malaria; attributed to stubborn phlegm with static blood binding under the rib-side. ⟨WMC⟩ splenomegaly in malaria. ⟨MED⟩ Quicken the blood and free the network vessels; move qi and disperse hardness. Because the underlying condition is one of vacuity, the principle of simultaneous supplementation and attack should be applied. Use Center-Supplementing Qi-Boosting Decoction (*bǔ zhōng yì qì tāng*) plus turtle shell (*biē jiǎ*) or Four Animals Decoction (*sì shòu yǐn*). ⟨ACU⟩ Base treatment mainly on GV, PC, SI, and LR. Select GV-14 (*dà zhuī*, Great Hammer), GV-13 (*táo dào*, Kiln Path), PC-5 (*jiān shǐ*, Intermediary Courier), SI-3 (*hòu xī*, Back Ravine), LR-13 (*zhāng mén*, Camphorwood Gate), Glomus Root (*pǐ gēn*), BL-18 (*gān shū*, Liver Transport), and BL-20 (*pí shū*, Spleen Transport); needle with drainage. See MALARIA. [26: 827] [27: 360] [97: 374]

mother's blood lump 血母块 *xuè mǔ kuài*: INFANT'S-PILLOW PAIN.

mountain forest miasmic qi 山岚瘴气 *shān lán zhàng qì*: Synonym: *mountain forest miasmic toxin*. **1.** A qi (vaporous exhalation) given off by putrescent matter in damp mountain forest areas and held to be one cause of malaria. It is of note that miasma was formerly regarded in the West as a cause of malaria. **2.** MALARIA caused by mountain forest miasmic qi. See MIASMIC MALARIA. [26: 64] [27: 123] [97: 30]

mountain rampart 山廓 *shān kuò*: See EIGHT RAMPARTS.

mountain root 山根 *shān gēn*: Synonym: *lower extreme; king's palace*. The region between the two inner canthi of the eye; the root of the nose. [27: 64] [97: 30]

mounting 疝 *shàn*: shan (*obs*). Any of various diseases characterized by pain or swelling of the abdomen or scrotum. Traditional literature describes many different diseases and patterns labeled as "mounting." Mounting disease can be divided into three categories: (1) *mounting qi (shàn qì).* Conditions characterized by the protrusion of the abdominal contents through the abdominal wall, the inguen, or base of the abdominal cavity, and usually associated with QI PAIN. Terms for such conditions include *small intestinal mounting qi, small intestinal mounting qi pain,* and *foxy mounting.* ⟨WMC⟩ inguinal hernia. (2) Various diseases of the external genitals. ⟨WMC⟩ hydrocele; hematoma of testis; traumatic injury of testis; orchitis. See entries listed below. (3) Certain forms of acute abdominal pain associated with urinary and fecal stoppage. ◊ Chin 疝 *shàn* is composed of 疒 *chuáng*, illness, with 山 *shān*, mountain. [26: 347, 428] [97: 375]

Mounting (*shàn*)

FOXY MOUNTING (*hú shàn*)
COLD MOUNTING (*hán shàn*)
WATER MOUNTING (*shuǐ shàn*)
QI MOUNTING (*qì shàn*)
BULGING MOUNTING (*tuí shàn*)
PROMINENT MOUNTING (*tuí* (*kuí*) *shàn*)
BLOOD MOUNTING (*xuè shàn*)
SINEW MOUNTING (*jīn shàn*)

mounting-conglomeration 疝瘕 *shàn jiǎ*: Synonym: *conglomeration-mounting*. From *Elementary Questions* (*sù wèn, yù jī zhēng cáng lùn*). **1.** Smaller-abdominal heat pain with discharge of white sticky fluid from the urethra; attributed to wind evil transforming into heat and passing to the lower abdomen to bind with dampness. MED Treat with formulas such as Poria (Hoelen) Five Powder (*wǔ líng sǎn*). **2.** A swelling of the abdomen that moves under pressure, and is associated with abdominal pain stretching into the lumbus and back; attributed to wind-cold and binding with qi and blood in the abdomen. MED Treat with medicinals such as fennel (*huí xiāng*), fenugreek (*hú lú bā*), morinda (*bā jǐ tiān*), aconite main tuber (*chuān wū tóu*), toosendan (*chuān liàn zǐ*), and evodia (*wú zhū yú*). [26: 348]

mounting qi 疝气 *shàn qì*: See MOUNTING. [27: 428] [97: 375]

mounting qi pain 疝气痛 *shàn qì tòng*: See MOUNTING.

mouse sores 老鼠疮 *lǎo shǔ chuāng*: SCROFULA.

mouth 口 *kǒu*: The opening through which food passes into the body. The mouth includes the lips, the tongue, teeth, and palate. It is connected with the wind-pipe (trachea) and the gullet (esophagus). The mouth is the outer orifice of the spleen. *The Magic Pivot* (*líng shū, mài dù*) states, "Spleen qi flows through to the mouth; when the spleen is in harmony, the mouth can taste the five grains." The hand yang brightness yang brightness (*yáng míng*) large intestine channel, yang brightness (*yáng míng*) stomach channel, greater yin (*tài yīn*) spleen channel, lesser yin (*shào yīn*) heart channel, lesser yin (*shào yīn*) kidney channel, reverting yin (*jué yīn*) liver channel, the governing (*dū*) vessel, controlling (*rèn*) vessel, and thoroughfare (*chōng*) vessel all pass through the mouth. Diagnosis: The diagnostic significance of the mouth rests largely on the spleen and stomach. The spleen

opens at the mouth; its bloom is in the lips. If the stomach and the spleen are functioning normally, the individual has a good appetite and normal TASTE IN THE MOUTH. In clinical practice, morbidity of the spleen in reflected in the lips, and the TONGUE and the TONGUE FUR are of great significance in diagnosis. See also LIP, SPLEEN OPENS AT THE MOUTH, MOUTH SORE, CLENCHED JAW, and DEVIATED EYES AND MOUTH. [26: 61]

mouth and tongue sores 口舌生疮 *kǒu shé shēng chuāng*: See MOUTH SORE.

mouth-level nape flat-abscess 对口 *duì kǒu*: Synonym: *mid-nape flat-abscess*; *brain flat-abscess*. A FLAT-ABSCESS (*jū*) on the back of the neck, at the level of the mouth. ◊ Chin 对 *duì*, opposite, facing; 口 *kǒu*, mouth. [27: 462] [97: 175]

mouth sore 口疮 *kǒu chuāng*: Synonym: *sore of the mouth and tongue*. A pale yellow or gray-white ulceration appearing singly or multiply on the inside of the mouth (lips, cheeks or palate). A mouth sore is usually oval in shape, surrounded by a red areola, and has a cratered surface. It is associated with scorching pain, affects eating and swallowing, and is recurrent. It is attributed to repletion fire, spleen heat engendering phlegm, or dual vacuity of the spleen and kidney. WMC aphthous stomatitis. **Repletion fire:** Fire in all channels can be reflected in the heart, and heart fire flaming upward into the mouth can engender more sores. MED Drain fire and clear the heart with Red-Abducting Powder (*dǎo chì sǎn*) variations. ACU Base treatment mainly on HT, PC, and CV. Select PC-8 (*láo gōng*, Palace of Toil), HT-8 (*shào fǔ*, Lesser Mansion), GV-26 (*shuǐ gōu*, Water Trough), CV-24 (*chéng jiāng*, Sauce Receptacle), LI-19 (*hé liáo*, Grain Bone-Hole), and LI-4 (*hé gǔ*, Union Valley); needle with drainage, and prick PC-9 (*zhōng chōng*, Central Hub), and HT-9 (*shào chōng*, Lesser Surge) to bleed. **Spleen heat engendering phlegm:** When spleen heat engenders phlegm, fire and phlegm bind and flame up to the mouth, causing mouth sores. MED Clear heat and dispel phlegm with Two Matured Ingredients Decoction (*èr chén tāng*) variations. ACU Base treatment mainly on SP, ST, and CV. Select BL-20 (*pí shū*, Spleen Transport), ST-36 (*zú sān lǐ*, Leg Three Li), SP-3 (*tài bái*, Supreme White), SP-6 (*sān yīn jiāo*, Three Yin Intersection), ST-40 (*fēng lóng*, Bountiful Bulge), ST-44 (*nèi tíng*, Inner Court), LI-4 (*hé gǔ*, Union Valley), CV-24 (*chéng jiāng*, Sauce Receptacle); and LI-19 (*hé liáo*, Grain Bone-Hole), needle with drainage. **Dual vacuity of the spleen and kidney:** Mouth sores may arise when spleen-kidney vacuity is associated with vacuity heat signs and the mouth is deprived of nourishment. MED Supplement the spleen and boost the kidney with variations of Four Gentlemen Decoction (*sì jūn zǐ tāng*) and Six-Ingredient Rehmannia Pill (*liù wèi dì huáng wán*). ACU Base treatment mainly on back transport points, SP, KI, and CV. Select BL-20 (*pí shū*, Spleen Transport), BL-23 (*shèn shū*, Kidney Transport), KI-3 (*tài xī*, Great Ravine), KI-6 (*zhào hǎi*, Shining Sea), KI-1 (*yǒng quán*, Gushing Spring), HT-8 (*shào fǔ*, Lesser Mansion), ST-36 (*zú sān lǐ*, Leg Three Li), SP-6 (*sān yīn jiāo*, Three Yin Intersection), LI-4 (*hé gǔ*, Union Valley), CV-24 (*chéng jiāng*, Sauce Receptacle), and LI-19 (*hé liáo*, Grain Bone-Hole); needle with supplementation. [26: 62] [113: 9] [46: 596]

mouth wash 漱涤 *shù dí*, 含漱 *hán shù*, 漱口 *shù kǒu*: Rinsing the mouth with a medicinal decoction, usually prepared with heat-clearing toxin-resolving medicinals, to remove putridity and pus; the medicinal decoction used for this purpose. For example, mouth sores arising in measles can be treated with a mouth wash of multiflora rose root (*qiáng wēi gēn*). Baby moth (tonsillitis) can be treated with a mouth wash made of 3 g each of mirabilite efflorescence (*fēng huà xiāo*), alum (*bái fán*), and salt (*shí yán*) boiled with a cup of water and first allowed to cool. [50: 1673] [27: 295] [97: 628]

moving impediment 行痹 *xíng bì*: IMPEDIMENT (*bì*) characterized by wandering pain, caused by a prevalence of wind. See WIND IMPEDIMENT. [27: 403] [97: 231]

moving qi 行气 *xíng qì*: Synonyms: *disinhibiting qi*; *freeing qi*. A method of treatment to dissipate qi stagnation in the treatment of distention, oppression, and pain in the chest and abdomen. Moving qi is a form of rectifying qi, and includes COURSING DEPRESSION AND RECTIFYING QI and HARMONIZING THE STOMACH AND RECTIFYING QI. See also QI-MOVING TECHNIQUE. [27: 270] [97: 213] [50: 594]

moving qi rib-side pain 运气胁痛 *yùn qì xié tòng*: Rib-side pain caused by epidemic pestilential qi ("moving qi"). It is of sudden onset, and is associated with fulminant heat effusion and aversion to cold. There is stabbing pain in either or both rib-sides. Other signs include generalized distention and rapid stringlike pulse. If accompanied by REVERSE-FLOW OF THE LIMBS (severe counterflow cold), the condition is dangerous. MED Clear, resolve and outthrust evil. Use Green-Blue–Draining Half-and-Half Decoction (*xiè qīng gè bàn tāng*). [26: 771]

moving the spleen 运脾 *yùn pí*: A method of treatment used to address a spleen encumbered by dampness characterized by distention, inability to taste food, nausea, bland taste and sticky sensation in the mouth, clouded head, fatigued body,

diarrhea, or abdominal distention, swelling of the extremities, scant urine, a white slimy tongue fur, and a soggy pulse, using medicinals such as atractylodes (*cāng zhú*), magnolia bark (*hòu pò*), tangerine peel (*chén pí*), agastache/patchouli (*huò xiāng*), eupatorium (*pèi lán*), cardamom kernel (*kòu rén*), and poria (*fú líng*). ACU Base treatment mainly on CV, SP, and ST. Select BL-20 (*pí shū*, Spleen Transport), CV-12 (*zhōng wǎn*, Center Stomach Duct), ST-25 (*tiān shū*, Celestial Pivot), LR-13 (*zhāng mén*, Camphorwood Gate), SP-9 (*yīn líng quán*, Yin Mound Spring), ST-36 (*zú sān lǐ*, Leg Three Li), and PC-6 (*nèi guān*, Inner Pass); needle with even supplementation and drainage, and, if appropriate, add moxa. Compare FORTIFYING THE SPLEEN. [27: 263] [46: 597, 602]

¹**moxa** 艾叶 *ài yè*: The prepared leaves of mugwort (*ài yè*), used in the technique of moxibustion, and chosen for this because of their yang qualities and their use in Chinese medicinal therapy to treat cold and dampness diseases. High-grade moxa is ivory or white in color. Being composed nearly entirely of leaf wool, it is easily shaped and permits formation of small cones; it also produces minimum smoke and odor. Burning gently, it is the preferred moxa for application directly to the skin (DIRECT MOXIBUSTION). Moxa that has been cleansed less rigorously, and thus contains higher concentrations of leaf particles, is considered lower grade. Gray or gray-green in color, low-grade (crude) moxa is preferred for indirect moxibustion, a process whereby burning moxa is used to heat, rather than cauterize, the skin. Such applications often require large quantities of moxa wool, while not necessitating the special advantages of the higher grade product. ◇ Eng *moxa*, from Jap. *mugusa*, from *moe kusa*, "burning herb," mugwort.

²**moxa** 艾灸 *ài jiǔ*: vb. moxaing, moxaed. To perform moxibustion; to treat with moxibustion.

moxa burner 温灸器 *wēn jiǔ qì*: Any receptacle designed to hold moxa while it is being burned close to the skin. Moxa burners were often traditionally made of brass. While the moxa burns, the warming instrument is moved slowly over the area to be treated until the skin turns red. A piece of cotton cloth (red) is often placed between the instrument and the skin to prevent accidental burns. This method is particularly suitable for the treatment of women, children, infants, and patients who are afraid of being burned. Different areas of the body can be treated in this way using warming instruments available in flat and angular shapes. [46: 495]

moxa cone 艾炷 *ài zhù*: A hand-rolled conical lump of moxa. Large cones are about the size of a broad bean and are used only in indirect moxibustion; medium cones are the size of a soybean; and small cones are the size of a wheat grain. Moxa cones can be burnt on the skin (DIRECT MOXIBUS-TION) or separated from it by garlic, ginger, or salt (INDIRECT MOXIBUSTION). [27: 343]

moxa pole 艾条 *ài tiáo*: *Synonyms: moxa stick; moxa roll.* A roll of rubbed moxa leaves enclosed in paper, forming cylinders about six inches in length and half an inch in diameter. The lighted moxa pole is held about one inch above the point to be warmed, and is moved slowly in a circular motion to spread the heat over a small area. Alternately, the roll may be moved quickly up and down to increase thermal stimulation in what is called the *pecking sparrow method.* Moxa pole therapy can be combined with acupuncture by warming the area around the needle. Moxa pole is generally applied for 3–15 minutes or until the skin turns red. The proper distance must be maintained to avoid reddening the skin too quickly or burning the patient. Moxa pole treatment, or *poling,* is commonly employed to provide mild heat and move qi and blood in a local area; it thus treats wind-damp impediment (*bì*) pain and similar patterns. [27: 344]

moxa roll 艾卷 *ài juǎn*: MOXA POLE.

moxa stick 艾条 *ài tiáo*: MOXA POLE.

moxibustion 灸法 *jiǔ fǎ*: A method of applying a heat stimulus to the body by burning the dried and sifted leaf particles from the herb mugwort (*ài yè*) on or close to the skin, with the aim of freeing qi and blood, coursing qi, dispersing cold, eliminating dampness and warming yang. Moxibustion is divided into two distinct methods; indirect moxibustion and direct moxibustion. **Caution:** (1) Moxibustion should not be performed on persons who are hungry, have just overeaten, or are intoxicated. (2) Most points for which moxibustion is contraindicated are near large blood vessels, on the face, on prominent skin creases, and at or near mucus membranes or sensory organs. Direct moxibustion is especially contraindicated at these sites. (3) Pregnant women should not receive moxibustion on their abdomen or lumbus. (4) If small blisters form as a result of moxibustion, they should be protected and allowed to heal without treatment. Large blisters, however, should be punctured and drained, and in case of infection occurs appropriate dressing should be applied. ◇ Eng from J. *mugusa,* contraction of *moe kusa,* burning herb + -bustion, contraction of combustion, from L. *combustio.* [27: 342] [97: 249]

moxibustion on aconite cake 附饼灸 *fù bǐng jiǔ*: The application of moxibustion using cakes of aconite (*fù zǐ*) as an insulating medium. The cakes are made by grinding the aconite to a powder and mixing it with yellow wine (rice or millet wine) and formed into a dry, crustlike substance about 0.1" thick. The cake crust is perforated and placed on the point and moxa is burnt on top of it. Because aconite is acrid and hot, this method can treat yang vacuity diseases. It is most commonly administered on enduring sores (and boils) to stop suppuration and permit healing. [27: 344]

moxibustion on cake 隔饼灸 *gé bǐng jiǔ*: The application of moxibustion using small cakes made of warm acrid or aromatic medicinals as an insulating medium. **Method:** A cone of moxa is placed on the cake at the spot to be moxaed, and is ignited. [27: 344] [26: 779] [97: 592]

moxibustion on fermented bean cake 豉饼灸 *chǐ bǐng jiǔ*: The application of moxibustion on a round cake of fermented soybean (*dàn dòu chǐ*) as an insulating medium. Moxibustion on fermented bean cake is used for WELLING-ABSCESS (*yōng*), FLAT-ABSCESS (*jū*), and EFFUSION OF BACK (*fā bèi*) that have ruptured but fail to heal and that are dark and blackish in appearance. Moxibustion on fermented bean cake helps the sores to close. [27: 344]

moxibustion on garlic 隔蒜灸 *gén suàn jiǔ*: The application of moxibustion on a thick slice of garlic as an insulating medium. **Method:** A slice of garlic about 0.2" thick that has been perforated with several holes is placed on the site. The moxa is placed on the garlic and ignited with incense, the garlic being changed after four to five cones have been burnt. In general, five to seven burnings constitute one treatment. This method is used to treat vacuity taxation (tuberculosis), toxicity from sores, scrofula, and abdominal accumulation masses. The patient should be informed that this method sometimes causes blisters. [27: 344] [26: 779] [97: 529]

moxibustion on ginger 隔姜灸 *gé jiāng jiǔ*: Burning of moxa cones on ginger as an insulating medium. A slice of ginger about 0.2" thick (slightly thicker than a quarter dollar) is perforated with a sewing needle and placed on the point. Large cones of moxa are burnt on the slice (lifting it from the skin momentarily when the heat exceeds the patient's tolerance) until the skin at the point is moist and red. This method is ideal for central burner vacuity, abdominal fullness, stomach pain, mounting (*shàn*) pain, diarrhea, vomiting, wind-cold impediment (*bì*) pain, wind-cold exterior patterns, and yang vacuity diseases in general. [27: 344] [26: 779]

moxibustion on pepper cake 椒饼灸 *jiāo bǐng jiǔ*: The application of moxibustion on a thin cake of made of white pepper (*bái hú jiāo*) as an insulating medium. The cake is made by blending the pepper with flour and water and forming the mass into cakes, which are then allowed to dry. **Method:** A pinch of Clove and Cinnamon Powder (*dīng guì sǎn*) is placed on the cake at the site to be moxaed.

The moxa cone is placed on top and ignited. Moxibustion on pepper cake is used to treat IMPEDIMENT (*bì*) patterns (chronic rheumatoid arthritis). [27: 344]

moxibustion on salt 隔盐灸 *gén yán jiŭ*: Burning of moxa cones on salt as an insulating medium. Moxibustion on salt is usually performed on the umbilicus. The umbilicus is filled with table salt, and a large cone of moxa is burned on top of the salt. This method is effective for treatment of cold damage yin patterns, cholera, and wind stroke desertion patterns. It can return yang, stem counterflow and stem desertion. [27: 344] [97: 592]

moxibustion supplementing and draining 艾灸补泻 *ài jiŭ bŭ xiè*: Synonym: *fire supplementation and fire drainage*. Using moxibustion to produce supplementing or draining action. Although moxibustion is generally used for its warming and supplementing action, it can also be used for draining. If a moxa cone is lighted and is allowed to burn naturally, the fire becomes stronger and stronger, until it finally burns the skin. This produces a supplementing stimulus that warms yang and supplements vacuity. If the cone is ignited, made to burn quickly by blowing, and removed before it has it burns the skin, this produces as draining stimulus that dispels cold and dissipates binds. [26: 257]

multiple abortion 妊娠数堕胎 *rèn shēn shù duò tāi*: See HABITUAL MISCARRIAGE. [26: 341]

mumps 痄腮 *zhà sāi*: A febrile disease characterized by soft diffuse swelling and tenderness that affects one side of the face or one side after the other. Mumps is attributed to accumulated gastrointestinal heat and depressed liver-gallbladder fire arising after contraction of warm toxin and causing blockage of the lesser yang (*shào yáng*). It is occurs in epidemics in the winter and spring, and chiefly affects children. ⸢MED⸥ Clear heat and resolve toxin using Universal Aid Toxin-Dispersing Beverage (*pŭ jì xiāo dú yĭn*). ⸢ACU⸥ Base treatment mainly on TB, LI, and ST. Select TB-17 (*yì fēng*, Wind Screen), TB-1 (*guān chōng*, Passage Hub), TB-5 (*wài guān*, Outer Pass), ST-6 (*jiá chē*, Cheek Carriage), LI-4 (*hé gŭ*, Union Valley), and ouch points (*ā shì xué*); needle with drainage. Selection of points according to signs: For high fever and delirious speech, add LI-11 (*qū chí*, Pool at the Bend), ST-36 (*zú sān lĭ*, Leg Three Li), and GV-14 (*dà zhuī*, Great Hammer), prick and Twelve Well Points (*shí èr jĭng xué*) to bleed. For painful swelling of the testicles, add LR-3 (*tài chōng*, Supreme Surge), SP-6 (*sān yīn jiāo*, Three Yin Intersection), LR-8 (*qū quán*, Spring at the Bend), and LR-2 (*xíng jiān*, Moving Between). For difficulty in chewing, add ST-7 (*xià guān*, Below the Joint). For vexation and retching, add CV-12

(*zhōng wăn*, Center Stomach Duct). ◇ Chin 痄 *zhà*, composed of 乍 *zhà*, sudden, abrupt, with the illness signifier 疒; *sāi*, the cheek. **Eng** mumps, related to mumpish (sullenly angry, sulky), so called because of the facial expression characteristic of the disease. [113: 361] [26: 490] [27: 369] [97: 491] [61: 373]

murky eye obstruction 混睛障 *hùn jīng zhàng*: Synonym: *qi obstruction*. A turbid gray-white eye screen like ground glass covering the dark of the eye, that in severe cases is dark red with red vessels and with a red aura around the dark of the eye. Murky eye obstruction is also associated with tearing and aversion to light, and is attributable to long-depressed liver channel wind-heat or damp-heat causing damage to yin and causing blood stasis. ⸢WMC⸥ parenchymatous (interstitial) keratitis. ⸢MED⸥ Dispel wind and calm the liver; dissipate stasis and abate screens. Use Rehmannia Powder (*dì huáng săn*) as oral medication and Obstruction-Abrading Spirit Light Paste (*mó zhàng líng guāng gāo*) for topical application. [26: 573] [27: 504] [97: 532]

mussitation 郑声 *zhèng shēng*: The act of mumbling to oneself haltingly and with frequent repetitions. Mussitation is a sign of dissipation of essence-spirit and is observed in yin or yang collapse patterns. Mussitation is similar to DELIRIOUS SPEECH. However, it is marked by a low voice and occurs in severe conditions in the latter stages of disease with shortness of breath, lassitude of spirit, and withered complexion, whereas delirious speech is marked by a strident voice and usually occurs in repletion heat such as yang brightness patterns or heat entering heart construction. [92: No. 46] [27: 868] [97: 373]

mustering point 募穴 *mù xué*: ALARM POINT.

mutation 变化 *biàn huà*: A combined term denoting transmutation (*biàn*) and transformation (*huà*), i.e., all gradual and major change.

mutual contention of wind and dampness 风湿相搏 *fēng shī xiāng bó*: WIND AND DAMPNESS CONTENDING WITH EACH OTHER. [26: 462] [27: 139] [97: 102]

mutual convertibility of yin and yang 阴阳转化 *yīn yáng zhuăn huà*: The ability of yang to change into or give way to yin, and vice versa. When an exuberant heat evil creates a severe yin-yang imbalance by damaging the blood fluids of the body, it "burns itself out," having nothing left to thrive on. As a result, the original pattern of repletion heat converts into vacuity cold. Conversely, when yang qi becomes so insufficient that it can no longer transform the fluids of the body, the fluids become a secondary evil that causes further disturbance in the body by accumulating in the abdomen in the form of DRUM DISTENTION (ascites).

The original vacuity pattern turns into a repletion pattern. This form of conversion is due to failure of the mutual counterbalancing relationship of yin and yang. [6: 25]

mutual engendering of metal and water 金水相生 *jīn shuǐ xiāng shēng*: The treatment of lung-kidney yin vacuity by nourishing lung yin, and mainly by enriching kidney yin. [26: 390]

mutual fanning of wind and fire 风火相煽 *fēng huǒ xiāng shān*: WIND AND FIRE FANNING EACH OTHER. [26: 456] [27: 134] [97: 101]

mutual need 相须 *xiāng xū*: See SEVEN RELATIONS.

mysterious house (mansion) 玄府 *xuán fǔ*: Synonym: *original house (mansion)*. A sweat pore; so called because it is not visible to naked eye. *Elementary Questions* (*sù wèn, jīng lùn*) states, "When the upper burner is inhibited, then the skin becomes tight, the interstices close, the mysterious houses become blocked, and defense qi fails to be discharged; hence there is external heat." [26: 173] [27: 31] [97: 167]

N

nail 指甲 *zhǐ jiǎ*, 爪 *zhǎo* (*zhuǎ*): The horny plate at the end of each finger and toe. See NAILS ARE THE SURPLUS OF THE SINEWS. [48: 31] [26: 171]

nail press needle insertion 爪切进针法 *zhǎo* (*zhuǎ*) *qiè jìn zhēn fǎ*: See FINGER-PRESS NEEDLE INSERTION.

nails are the surplus of the sinews 爪为筋之馀 *zhǎo wéi jīn zhī yú*: Both the nails and the sinews are associated with the liver. When the sinews are healthy, the nails are hard and supple. When the sinews lack strength, the nails are thin and weak. See also LIVER, ITS BLOOM IS IN THE NAILS. ◇ Chin 爪 *zhǎo* (or *zhuǎ*), nail, claw, talon. [27: 42]

nasal congestion 鼻塞 *bí sè*, 鼻塞不通 *bí sāi bù tōng*, 鼻窒 *bí zhì*, 鼻齆 *bí wèng*: Blockage of the nose impairing the sense of smell. Nasal congestion is attributed to nondiffusion of lung qi due to wind-cold or wind-heat. In wind-cold patterns, it is attended by heat effusion, aversion to cold, headache and generalized pain, white tongue fur, and a floating pulse. In wind-heat patterns, it is accompanied by heat effusion, thirst, and runny nose with turbid snivel (nasal mucus). Nasal congestion is also a principal sign of NASAL POLYP. MED Treat wind-cold patterns by coursing wind and dissipating cold with Apricot Kernel and Perilla Powder (*xìng sū sǎn*). Treat wind-heat patterns by coursing wind and clearing heat with Mulberry Leaf and Chrysanthemum Beverage (*sāng jú yǐn*). For external treatment, insufflate powdered gleditsia (*zào jiá*), asarum (*xì xīn*), magnolia flower[1] (*xīn yí*), zanthoxylum (*huā jiāo*), and aconite (*fù zǐ*). ACU Main points: LI-20 (*yíng xiāng*, Welcome Fragrance), LI-4 (*hé gǔ*, Union Valley), GV-23 (*shàng xīng*, Upper Star), and GB-20 (*fēng chí*, Wind Pool). Selection of points according to pattern: For wind-cold, add TB-5 (*wài guān*, Outer Pass) and LU-7 (*liè quē*, Broken Sequence), needling with drainage and adding moxa. For wind-heat, add GV-14 (*dà zhuī*, Great Hammer) and LI-11 (*qū chí*, Pool at the Bend). Needle with drainage and prick LU-11 (*shào shāng*, Lesser Shang) to bleed. [26: 856]

nasal inoculation 鼻苗 *bí miáo*: Inoculation against smallpox by introducing fluid or scab matter from pox sores into the nose of healthy individuals. This discovery was made in the Ming Dynasty between the years 998 and 1022. See SMALLPOX. [26: 852] [97: 622] [27: 513]

nasal insufflation 嗜鼻 *xù bí*, 吹鼻 *chuī bí*: The blowing of powdered medicinals into the nose. For example, chronic paranasal sinusitis (DEEP-SOURCE NASAL CONGESTION) can be treated with an insufflation of calcined and ground otolith (*yú nǎo shí*) together with a little borneol (*bīng piàn*) into the nose. Common cold with nasal congestion can be treated by insufflating finely ground centipeda (*é bù shí cǎo*). [27: 295] [97: 277]

nasal mucus 涕 *tì*: SNIVEL.

nasal orifices 鼻窍 *bí qiào*: The nostrils as ORIFICES.

nasal passages 鼻隧 *bí suì*: The nostrils and nasal cavity. [26: 856] [27: 66] [97: 623]

nasal polyp 鼻瘜肉 *bí xī ròu*: Synonym: *nose pile*. A growth inside the nose, causing blockage of the airways, and, in severe cases, deformation of the nose. Nasal polyps arise when wind, dampness and heat stagnate in the lung channel. MED Magnolia Flower Powder (*xīn yí sǎn*). [27: 495] [97: 623]

natural moxibustion 天灸 *tiān jiǔ*, 自灸 *zì jiǔ*: MEDICINAL-INDUCED BLISTER MOXIBUSTION.

nature and flavor 性味 *xìng wèi*: QI AND FLAVOR.

nature-preservative burning 烧存性 *shāo cún xìng*: NATURE-PRESERVATIVE CALCINATION.

nature-preservative calcination 煅存性 *duàn cún xìng*: See CHAR-FRYING. [27: 409] [97: 461]

nausea 恶心 *ě xīn*: The desire to vomit. Nausea normally portends vomiting; like vomiting, it is a sign of stomach qi ascending counterflow, which can arise in a variety of stomach disorders including stomach vacuity and cold, heat, dampness, phlegm or food stagnation in the stomach. MED Use the method of harmonizing the stomach and rectifying qi. Combine it with warming the center for stomach cold, with draining fire for stomach heat, with drying dampness and transforming phlegm for phlegm-damp, and with abducting dispersion for food stagnation. See VOMITING. Compare UPFLOW NAUSEA. ◇ Chin 恶 *ě*, sickening, in other contexts read as *wù*, aversion, from the *xīn*, heart (or heart [region]). NB: In modern Chinese, the character 恶 has been replaced by 噁 in the sense of sickening and nausea; thus, Western medical literature in Chinese uses the same term for nausea, written as 噁心 *ě xīn*. [26: 684]

nausea and vomiting 恶心呕吐 *ě xīn ǒu tù*: Desire to vomit and actual vomiting. See NAUSEA; VOMITING.

navel 脐 *qí*: UMBILICUS.

nearsightedness 能近怯远 *néng jìn qiè yuǎn*, 不能远视 *bù néng yuǎn shì*: Ability to see close but not distant objects clearly. Nearsightedness is attributed to superabundance of yin and insufficiency of yang, or to congenital causes. [MED] Supplement the liver and kidney using Long Vistas Pill (*zhù jīng wán*) or Mind-Stabilizing Pill (*dìng zhì wán*). [ACU] Base treatment mainly on back transport points and local points. Select BL-1 (*jīng míng,* Bright Eyes), BL-2 (*zǎn zhú,* Bamboo Gathering), ST-1 (*chéng qì,* Tear Container), GB-20 (*fēng chí,* Wind Pool), BL-18 (*gān shū,* Liver Transport), BL-23 (*shèn shū,* Kidney Transport), and GB-37 (*guāng míng,* Bright Light); needle with even supplementation and drainage. For young people, plum-blossom needle therapy can be effective. Base treatment mainly on back of the neck and around the eyes, selecting points such as BL-1 (*jīng míng,* Bright Eyes), ST-1 (*chéng qì,* Tear Container), GB-20 (*fēng chí,* Wind Pool), GV-14 (*dà zhuī,* Great Hammer), and PC-6 (*nèi guān,* Inner Pass). Tap each point 20-30 times with medium force in alternate-day sessions in two-week courses. [26: 562] [46: 729]

neck 颈项 *jǐng xiàng:* The part of the body that joins the head to the trunk. Morbid changes in the neck include GOITER, SCROFULA, PHLEGM NODE, and MOUTH-LEVEL NAPE FLAT-ABSCESS. If these are soft to the touch, the pattern is generally one of binding depression of phlegm and qi. If the nodes are hard to the touch and static, the pattern is one of congealing stagnation of qi and blood. Conspicuous throbbing of the man's prognosis (*rén yíng*) pulse (at the common carotid artery) accompanied by cough, panting, or water swelling, generally indicates heart-lung qi vacuity or heart-kidney yang vacuity. ◊ Chin 颈 *jǐng,* neck; 项 *xiàng,* nape.

neck bone 颈骨 *jǐng gǔ:* The cervical spine.

¹**needle** 针 *zhēn,* 鍼 *zhēn:* n. Any instrument, usually of metal, used to puncture the skin and flesh in acupuncture. The most commonly used type of needle in modern acupuncture is the FILIFORM NEEDLE, which is a modern finer version of the filiform needle that figured among the NINE NEEDLES of antiquity. Other commonly used needles include the PLUM-BLOSSOM NEEDLE and the THREE-EDGED NEEDLE. ◊ Chin 针 *zhēn,* needle, pin. [27: 332]

²**needle** 针 *zhēn,* 鍼 *zhēn,* 刺 *cì:* vb. trans. To puncture with a needle as in acupuncture. vb. intrans. To perform acupuncture. ◊ Chin 针 *zhēn,* to needle; 刺 *cì,* to prick, stab.

needle breakage 折针 *zhé zhēn:* Breaking of an acupuncture needle below the skin; usually occurs with eroded, chipped or otherwise damaged needles in patients who move unduly after needle insertion. Management: Ensure that the patient maintains the same posture and remove the broken needle with pincers if possible. If this is to no avail, surgical intervention may be necessary. [27: 338] [27: 264]

needle-driving method 逼针法 *bī zhēn fǎ:* See QI-MOVING TECHNIQUE. [46: 456]

needle embedding 埋针 *mái zhēn:* NEEDLE IMPLANTATION.

needle extraction 出针 *chū zhēn,* 引针 *yǐn zhēn,* 排针 *pái zhēn,* 拔针 *bá zhēn,* 起针 *qǐ zhēn:* Removing acupuncture needles from the flesh. Needle extraction is performed according to the following guidelines: (1) Rotate the needle slightly as it is withdrawn to prevent its adhesion to body tissues. (2) Withdraw the needle to just below the skin and then retain it at this depth for a few seconds before it is fully withdrawn. This procedure will generally prevent bleeding and reduce post-needling pain. (3) After withdrawing the needle, wipe the point with an alcohol-soaked cotton swab. (4) Withdraw needles inserted in the eye region slowly and carefully. [27: 333] [97: 152]

needle flicking 弹针 *tán zhēn:* A needle manipulation involving the flicking of the handle of an acupuncture needle as a method of obtaining qi. [27: 333] [97: 541]

needle implantation 埋针 *mái zhēn: Synonym: needle embedding.* The embedding or implantation of intradermal needles such as wheat-grain or thumb-tack needles in the skin for extended periods. The needles are retained from 1 to 3 days—shorter periods in warm weather, and longer periods in cold weather. The patient should be encouraged to keep the area of insertion clean to avoid infection. These needles are generally inserted in the back or limbs and treat various types of chronic, stubborn, or painful diseases such as headache, hemilateral headache, back pain, stomach pain, ribs-side pain, sprained ankles, hypertension, wheezing and panting, menstrual irregularities, deviated eyes and mouth, enuresis, frequent urination, and impediment (*bì*). [26: 501]

needle insertion 进针 *jìn zhēn:* The introduction of an acupuncture needle into the body. There are various different insertion techniques, most of which involve the use of both hands. TWO-HANDED NEEDLE INSERTION techniques include FINGER-PRESS NEEDLE INSERTION, SKIN-PINCHING NEEDLE INSERTION, SKIN-SPREADING NEEDLE INSERTION, and TUBE INSERTION. There is also a SINGLE-HANDED NEEDLE INSERTION. Needles may inserted at different angles. See OBLIQUE INSERTION; PERPENDICULAR INSERTION; TRANSVERSE INSERTION. [27: 333]

Needle Insertion

SINGLE-FINGER NEEDLE INSERTION (*jìn zhēn fǎ*)
TWO-FINGER PRESS NEEDLE INSERTION (*jiā chí jìn zhēn fǎ*)
SKIN-PINCHING NEEDLE INSERTION (*zhǐ qiè jìn zhēn fǎ*)
SKIN-SPREADING NEEDLE INSERTION (*shū zhāng jìn zhēn fǎ*)

TUBE INSERTION (*guǎn zhēn jìn zhēn fǎ*)

SINGLE-HANDED NEEDLE INSERTION (*dān shǒu jìn zhēn fǎ*)

---

needle manipulation (technique) 针刺手法 *zhēn cì shǒu fǎ*: Abbreviation: manipulation. Any manual movement of an acupuncture needle. See entries listed below. [27: 333]

Needle Manipulation Techniques

Basic Techniques
NEEDLE ROTATION (*zhuǎn zhēn*)
NEEDLE POUNDING (*dǎo zhēn*)
NEEDLE FLICKING (*tán zhēn*)
NEEDLE TWISTING (*cuō zhēn*)
NEEDLE WAGGLING (*yáo zhēn*)
NEEDLE RETRACTION (*tuì zhēn*)
NEEDLE REMOVAL (*chū zhēn*)
NEEDLE SCRATCHING (*guā zhēn*)
LIFTING AND THRUSTING (*tí chā*)

Simple supplementation and drainage (s & d) techniques
NEUTRAL S & D (*píng bǔ píng xiè*)
DIRECTIONAL S & D (*yíng suì bǔ xiè*)
ROTATING S & D (*niǎn zhuǎn bǔ xiè*)
QUICK AND SLOW S & D (*xú jí bǔ xiè*)
LIFTING AND THRUSTING S & D (*tí chā bǔ xiè*)
RESPIRATORY S & D (*hū xī bǔ xiè*)
OPEN AND CLOSED S & D (*kāi hé bǔ xiè*)
NINE AND SIX S & D (*jiǔ liù bǔ xiè*)

Complex methods
PENETRATING HEAVEN COOLING METHOD (*tòu tiān liáng*)
BURNING MOUNTAIN FIRE METHOD (*shāo shān huǒ*)

---

needle-picking therapy 挑针疗法 *tiāo zhēn liáo fǎ*: PICKING THERAPY.

needle pounding 捣针 *dǎo zhēn*: Synonym: *pounding*. A needle manipulation technique whereby the needle, after insertion, is repeatedly raised and thrust between two levels of the flesh. Needle pounding differs from LIFTING AND THRUSTING by absence of variation in speed between retraction and thrusting and by a shorter span of movement. It produces EVEN SUPPLEMENTATION AND DRAINAGE, whereas lifting and thrusting is normally used to supplement or drain. [27: 333] [97: 456]

needle removal 出针 *chū zhēn*, 引针 *yǐn zhēn*, 排针 *pái zhēn*, 拔针 *bá zhēn*: The removal of an acupuncture needle from the body. Method: One hand is placed close to the needle to hold the site firm, while the other lifts the needle, usually twirling it to facilitate movement. [27: 334]

needle retention 留针 *liú zhēn*: Leaving acupuncture needles in place for a certain time after insertion. In modern practice needles are often left in place for a period ranging from several minutes to two hours depending on the particular condition. This allows for application of other stimulation methods such as warming the needle, electrical stimulation, or intermittent manipulation. Often needles are retained with little or no additional manipulation. Needle retention in general can increase the ability of a point to relieve pain and quiet the spirit. Some specific treatments require needle retention to achieve satisfactory results. For example, treatment of INTESTINAL WELLING-ABSCESS (appendicitis) or panting generally involves the retention of needles for at least half an hour. The patient must be instructed not to move while the needles are in place. Pain resulting from a change in posture can be relieved by withdrawing the needle to a level just beneath the skin, and then reinserting it to its proper depth. [27: 334] [27: 333] [97: 479]

needle retraction 退针 *tuì zhēn*: The lifting of an inserted needle so that the point of the needle approaches but does not leave the skin. [27: 333] [97: 439]

needle rotation 转针 *zhuǎn zhēn*: Synonym: *needle twirling*. A needle manipulation technique whereby, after insertion, the needle is turned in alternating directions by rubbing it between the thumb and index finger. Needle rotation is used during needle insertion and withdrawal to facilitate the vertical movement of the needle, and otherwise to provide supplementation or drainage. See ROTATING SUPPLEMENTATION AND DRAINAGE. [27: 333] [27: 333]

needle scratching 刮法 *guā fǎ*: Scratching the handle of the needle upward or downward with the finger nail after insertion to encourage the obtaining of qi and intensify the needle sensation. [50: 923]

needle sensation 针感 *zhēn gǎn*: The physical sensation felt in response to needling. [97: 292]

needle sickness 晕针 *yūn zhēn*: Sickness induced by acupuncture treatment and characterized by dizziness, vomiting, oppression in the chest, somber white complexion, fixed eyes and torpid spirit, and, in severe cases, cold sweating and reversal cold in the limbs. Needle sickness is usually the result of excessively strong needle manipulation in persons who are unused to acupuncture treatment, are nervous, tired, hungry, or in a weak state of health. Management: Remove all the needles and allow the patient to lie flat. When the patient is fully conscious, he or she can be given a warm drink with cookies. In more severe cases, it may be necessary to needle GV-26 (*rén zhōng*, Human Center) with PC-9 (*zhōng chōng*, Central Hub) or ST-36 (*zú sān lǐ*, Leg Three Li). [26: 789] [27: 338] [97: 467]

needle twirling 捻针 *niǎn zhēn*: NEEDLE ROTATION. [27: 333]

needle twisting 搓针 *cuō zhēn*: Synonym: *unidirectional twirling*. A needle manipulation technique whereby the needle, after being inserted, is twisted in one direction as cotton is twisted to make a thread. This method produces a strong needle sensation. It should be applied gently without excessive force to prevent the needle tip catching on the flesh, which can cause pain. [27: 333]

needle waggling 摇针 *yáo zhēn*: A needle manipulation technique whereby, after insertion of the needle, the acupuncture point is held firmly with one hand, while the body of the needle is moved to and fro with the other hand. [27: 333]

nest of essence 精窠 *jīng kē*: **1.** The place where essential qi is stored. **2.** The eye socket.

net 络 *luò*: Synonym: *connect*. To link; of channels, to link up with the exterior organ corresponding to the governing viscus, e.g., the hand greater yin (*tài yīn*) lung channel "nets" the large intestine. ◇ Chin 络 *luò*, net, connect. Chinese medicine uses many different terms conveying a general idea of connection. Their usage suggests differences in meaning. The character 络 is used to mean the network vessels (variously called collaterals and connecting vessels in English) and reflects how the network vessels links all parts of the whole body in a mesh. In the context of channel-organ connections, it seems to imply a diffuse connection by contrast to homing (属 *shǔ*), which implies a direct connection. Since the channel-network system has not been charted by modern scientific methods, the precise meaning of the term is unclear. [48: 248] [26: 755]

netting and homing 络属 *luò shǔ*: The connection between channels and their associated organs. For example, the foot yang brightness (*yáng míng*) stomach channel "homes" to the stomach and "nets" the large intestine, the organ that stands in exterior-interior relationship with the stomach. See NET. [6: 50]

network point 络穴 *luò xué*: The point at which a network vessel separates from its main channel is the network point of that channel. For example, the network vessel of the hand reverting yin (*jué yīn*) pericardium channel splits from the main channel at PC-6 (*nèi guān*, Inner Pass), thus PC-6 is the network point of the pericardium channel. Each channel that possesses its own points has a network point; thus each of the twelve regular channels and the governing (*dū*) and controlling (*rèn*) vessels have network points. Two network vessels are associated with the spleen: the spleen network vessel, and the great network vessel of the spleen. Each of these has a network point. Hence there are in total fifteen network points. In addition, *Elementary Questions* (*sù wènpíng rén qì xiàng lùn*) also mentions the great network vessel of the stomach, Vacuous Li (*xū lǐ*) as a network point; hence there is also a doctrine of *six-*

teen network vessels and sixteen network points. See the list below. **Application:** (1) Treatment of internally-externally coupled organs: When a viscus and its related bowel are both affected by disease, it is usual to needle the network point of the channel of the more seriously or chronically affected organ. For example, a patient who presents with signs of lung and large intestine disease can be treated by the network point of either the lung or the large intestine, depending on which organ is more seriously involved. This application includes treatment of diseases that display signs along the course of the channels of two organs that stand in interior-exterior relationship. (2) Treatment of network vessel signs specifically associated with the network vessels. Note that each network vessel may present with signs of either repletion or vacuity. The therapeutic principle is to drain repletion and supplement vacuity by employing the appropriate needle technique at the network point. [27: 95] [97: 447] [46: 157]

Network Points

LU-7 (*liè quē*, Broken Sequence)
HT-5 (*tōng lǐ*, Connecting Li)
PC-6 (*nèi guān*, Inner Pass)
LI-6 (*piān lì*, Veering Passageway)
SI-7 (*zhī zhèng*, Branch to the Correct)
TB-5 (*wài guān*, Outer Pass)
ST-40 (*fēng lóng*, Bountiful Bulge)
BL-58 (*fēi yáng*, Taking Flight)
GB-37 (*guāng míng*, Bright Light)
SP-4 (*gōng sūn*, Yellow Emperor)
KI-4 (*dà zhōng*, Large Goblet)
LV-5 (*lǐ gōu*, Woodworm Canal)
CV-15 (*jiū wěi*, Turtledove Tail)
GV-1 (*cháng qiáng*, Long Strong)
SP-21 (*dà bāo*, Great Embracement)
Vacuous Li (虚里 (*xū lǐ*))

network stroke 中络 *zhòng luò*: WIND STROKE in which the evil is in the network vessels. Network stroke is marked by deviated eyes and mouth, and insensitivity of the skin, but not by difficulty of speech or hemiplegia that characterize channel stroke. [26: 140] [27: 397] [97: 779]

network vessel 络脉 *luò mài*: Branches of the channels that enmesh the body. (1) In a broader sense, "network vessel" denotes any of the *fifteen network vessels*, the *network vessels* (in the narrower sense), and *grandchild network vessels*. Fourteen vessels connect the twelve regular channels, and the governing (*dū*) and controlling (*rèn*) vessels. These together with the great network vessel of the spleen constitute the *fifteen network vessels* (also called *diverging network vessels*). (2) In the narrow sense, "network vessel" denotes the branches of the fifteen network vessels, which enmesh the whole body, the smaller branches of which are known as the *grandchild network vessels*. (3) "Network vessel" also denotes any of the small branches of the network vessels in the surface of the body that are more precisely as *superficial network vessels*. Thus NETWORK VESSEL PRICKING means pricking of the superficial network vessels, which in this context are often referred to as *blood network vessels*. Note that while the superficial network vessels are actual blood vessels, other parts of the channel and network vessel system have no clear correspondence to the circulation system described by modern anatomy since the pathways of qi and blood were never clearly distinguished. [26: 755]

network vessel pricking 络刺 *luò cì*: From *The Magic Pivot* (*líng shū, guān zhēn piān*). One of the NINE NEEDLING METHODS. Bloodletting by pricking the small vessels with a three-edged needle. See BLOODLETTING. [27: 334]

neutral cause [of disease] 不内外因 *bù nèi wài yīn*: One of the THREE CAUSES OF DISEASE; includes dietary irregularities, taxation fatigue, falls, and animal and insect bites. See THREE CAUSES. [26: 126]

neutral supplementation and drainage 平补平泻 *píng bǔ píng xiè*: EVEN SUPPLEMENTATION AND DRAINAGE.

new contraction 新感 *xīn gǎn*: Contraction of a new evil that stirs a deep-lying evil in the body. New contractions of warm disease immediately give rise to an exterior pattern of aversion to cold and stir the deep-lying evil to produce signs of internal heat. [26: 761] [27: 110] [97: 613]

new contraction stirring latent evil 新感引动伏邪 *xīn gǎn yǐn dòng fú xié*: See NEW CONTRACTION.

new contraction warm disease 新感温病 *xīn gǎn wēn bìng*: A warm disease that emerges as soon as the evil is contracted, as distinct from LATENT QI WARM DISEASE, which remains latent for some time before emerging. A new contraction may, under circumstances, stir evil present in the body. This is called *new contraction stirring latent evil*. [26: 761]

night blindness 夜盲 *yè máng*: SPARROW VISION.

night cough 夜嗽 *yè sòu*: Cough occurring only at night and not in the day. Night cough is attributable to depletion of kidney yin and yin vacuity fire flaming upward. The cough comes in continual bouts that do not abate until dawn. In some cases there may be bitter mouth and rib-side pain, and poor appetite. [MED] Nourish yin and downbear fire with Yin-Enriching Clearing Transforming Pill (*zī yīn qīng huà wán*) or Six-Ingredient Rehmannia Pill (*liù wèi dì huáng wán*) plus asparagus (*tiān mén dōng*) and ophiopogon (*mài mén dōng*). [ACU] Base treatment mainly on back transport points, LU, and KI. Select BL-13 (*fèi shū*, Lung Transport), BL-43 (*gāo huāng shū*, Gao-Huang Transport), LU-5 (*chǐ zé*, Cubit Marsh),

and KI-6 (*zhào hǎi*, Shining Sea); needle with supplementation or with even supplementation and drainage. [26: 349]

night crying in infants 小儿夜啼 *xiǎo ér yè tí*: Persistent abnormal crying of infants in the night. Night crying is usually attributable either to spleen cold or heart heat. Spleen cold patterns are characterized by green-blue or white complexion, cold limbs, no desire for milk or food, abdominal pain, and bending of the waist when crying. Heart heat patterns are characterized by a red facial complexion, warm hands and abdomen, warm breath, vexation and agitation, aversion to lights and fire, and crying in supine posture. [ACU] Needle with even supplementation and drainage at Quiet Sleep (*ān mián*), Hall of Impression (*yìn táng*), and SI-3 (*hòu xī*, Back Ravine), and apply three cones of moxa at GV-20 (*bǎi huì*, Hundred Convergences). [26: 349] [27: 437]

night sweating 盗汗 *dào hàn*: Synonym: *thief sweating*. Sweating during the night that ceases on awakening and that generally occurs in patients suffering from yin vacuity. Night sweating is attributable to insufficiency of heart blood, yin vacuity internal heat, and spleen vacuity damp encumbrance. **Insufficiency of heart blood** causes night sweating with heart palpitations and reduced sleep, lusterless complexion, shortness of breath and fatigued spirit, pale tongue with thin fur, and a vacuous pulse. [MED] Supplement the blood, nourish the heart, and constrain sweating. Use Spleen-Returning Decoction (*guī pí tāng*) plus dragon bone (*lóng gǔ*), oyster shell (*mǔ lì*), and schisandra (*wǔ wèi zǐ*). [ACU] Base treatment mainly on LI, SI, and HT. The main points for all patterns are as follows: LI-4 (*hé gǔ*, Union Valley), SI-3 (*hòu xī*, Back Ravine), and HT-6 (*yīn xī*, Yin Cleft); needle with even supplementation and drainage. For insufficiency of heart blood, add BL-15 (*xīn shū*, Heart Transport), BL-17 (*gé shū*, Diaphragm Transport), CV-14 (*jù què*, Great Tower Gate), SP-6 (*sān yīn jiāo*, Three Yin Intersection), CV-6 (*qì hǎi*, Sea of Qi), and HT-7 (*shén mén*, Spirit Gate); needle with supplementation and moxa. **Yin vacuity internal heat** causes frequent night sweating with postmeridian tidal heat [effusion], reddening of the cheeks, vexing heat in the five hearts, emaciation, menstrual irregularities in women and dream emission and seminal efflux in men, a red tongue with scant fur, and a rapid fine pulse. [MED] Enrich yin, downbear fire, and constrain sweating. Use Tangkuei Six Yellows Decoction (*dāng guī liù huáng tāng*) plus glutinous rice root (*nuò dào gēn xū*), and light wheat (*fú xiǎo mài*). [ACU] To the main points given above add BL-23 (*shèn shū*, Kidney Transport), KI-3 (*tài xī*, Great Ravine), SP-6 (*sān yīn jiāo*, Three Yin Intersection), KI-6 (*zhào hǎi*, Shining Sea), and KI-2 (*rán gǔ*, Blazing Valley); needle with supplementation or with even supplementation and drainage. **Spleen vacuity damp encumbrance** causes frequent night sweating with headache with swathed sensation, fatigued cumbersome limbs, torpid intake, sliminess in the mouth, thin slimy white tongue fur, pale tongue, and soggy moderate pulse. ☐MED Transform dampness and harmonize the center; free qi dynamic. Use Agastache/Patchouli, Magnolia Bark, Pinellia, and Poria (Hoelen) Decoction (*huò pò xià líng tāng*) minus apricot kernel (*xìng rén*), polyporus (*zhū líng*), litsea (*dòu chǐ jiāng*), fermented soybean (*dàn dòu chǐ*), and alisma (*zé xiè*), plus glutinous rice root (*nuò dào gēn xū*), atractylodes (*cāng zhú*), and tangerine peel (*chén pí*). ☐ACU To the main points add BL-20 (*pí shū*, Spleen Transport), LR-13 (*zhāng mén*, Camphorwood Gate), CV-12 (*zhōng wǎn*, Center Stomach Duct), ST-36 (*zú sān lǐ*, Leg Three Li), SP-9 (*yīn líng quán*, Yin Mound Spring), and PC-6 (*nèi guān*, Inner Pass); needle with even supplementation and drainage. Moxa may also be used. ◇ Chin 盗 *dào*, thief, steal; 汗 *hàn*, sweat, sweating. The term reflects how this kind of sweating occurs unbeknown to the person while sleeping. [27: 389] [97: 539] [50: 1435] [92: No. 12] [113: 18] [37: 332, 347] [46: 586, 597, 602, 648]

nighttime anal itch 夜晚肛痒 *yè wǎn gāng yǎng*: The main sign of PINWORM DISEASE.

nine and six supplementation and drainage 九六补血 *jiǔ liù bǔ xiè*: A method of supplementing and draining in acupuncture that involves lifting, thrusting, and rotation actions performed in sequences of six or nine, and that is based on the yin-yang significance of odd and even numbers. The ancient Chinese believed that yang numbers were odd and belonged to heaven, while yin number were even and belonged to earth, and hence that supplementation could be achieved by sequences of nine, and drainage through sequences of six. For example, to supplement, a sharp thrust and gentle lift or an anticlockwise rotation is performed nine times. Once qi is obtained, another sequence of nine can be performed after a brief interval. One more sequence is then performed to make three sequences and a total of 27 movements of the needle. To drain, a gentle thrust and sharp life or a clockwise rotation is performed six times. If the evil is still exuberant, the sequence is performed again after a short interval. A third sequence then makes 18 movements of the needle. Numerical determination of supplementation and drainage is now no longer considered to be of practical benefit, and the method is now rarely used. [50: 44]

nine needles 九针 *jiǔ zhēn*: Nine ancient kinds of needle. See entries listed below. [27: 332]

The Nine Needles

CHISEL NEEDLE (*chán zhēn*)

ROUND NEEDLE (*yuán zhēn*)
ARROWHEAD NEEDLE (*dī zhēn*)
SHARP-EDGED NEEDLE (*fēng zhēn*)
SHARP ROUND NEEDLE (*yuán lì zhēn*)
SWORD NEEDLE (*pī zhēn*)
FILIFORM NEEDLE (*háo zhēn*)
LONG NEEDLE (*cháng zhēn*)
LARGE NEEDLE (*cháng zhēn*)

nine needles for returning yang 回阳九针 *huí yáng jiǔ zhēn*: Nine points used in the treatment of yang collapse. See the list below.

Nine Needles for Returning Yang

GV-15 (*yǎ mén*, Mute's Gate)
PC-7 (*dà líng*, Great Mound)
SP-6 (*sān yīn jiāo*, Three Yin Intersection)
KI-1 (*yǒng quán*, Gushing Spring)
KI-3 (*tài xī*, Great Ravine)
CV-12 (*zhōng wǎn*, Center Stomach Duct)
GB-30 (*huán tiào*, Jumping Round)
ST-36 (*zú sān lǐ*, Leg Three Li)
LI-4 (*hé gǔ*, Union Valley)

Three of the points, KI-3 (*tài xī*, Great Ravine), LI-4 (*hé gǔ*, Union Valley), and PC-7 (*dà líng*, Great Mound) are also source points. [27: 332] [97: 12]

nine needling methods 九刺 *jiǔ cì*: From *The Magic Pivot* (*líng shū*, *guān zhēn*). Nine ancient methods of needling. See the entries listed below. [26: 16] [27: 334] [97: 13]

The Nine Needling Methods

TRANSPORT NEEDLING (*shū cì*)
DISTANT NEEDLING (*yuǎn cì*)
CHANNEL NEEDLING (*jīng cì*)
NETWORK VESSEL PRICKING (*luò cì*)
PARTING NEEDLING (*fēn cì*)
GREAT DRAINAGE NEEDLING (*dà xiè cì*)
HAIR NEEDLING (*máo cì*)
GREAT NEEDLING (*jù cì*)
RED-HOT NEEDLING (*cuì cì*)

nine orifices 九窍 *jiǔ qiào*: **1.** The two ears, two eyes, two nostrils, mouth, anterior yin (urethra) and posterior yin (anus). **2.** Two ears, two eyes, two nostrils, mouth, tongue, and throat (according to *The Classic of Difficult Issues* (*nàn jīng, 37*). [27: 27] [97: 13] [50: 42]

nineteen fears 十九畏 *shí jiǔ wèi*: Nineteen medicinals standing in a relationship of awe, i.e., a relationship in which one medicinal's toxicity or action is counteracted or reduced by another or others. See the list below. See also SEVEN RELATIONS. [27: 308]

The Nineteen Fears

sulfur (*shí liú huáng*), fears impure mirabilite (*pò xiāo*)

mercury (*shuǐ yín*) fears sublimed arsenic (*pī shuāng*)

Chinese wolfsbane (*láng dú*) fears litharge (*mì tuó sēng*)

croton (*bā dòu*) fears morning glory (*qiān niú zǐ*)

clove (*dīng xiāng*) fears curcuma (*yù jīn*)

tooth niter (*yá xiāo*), fears sparganium (*sān léng*)

aconite main tuber (*chuān wū tóu*) fears wild aconite (*cǎo wū tóu*) and rhinoceros horn (*xī jiǎo*)

ginseng (*rén shēn*) fears flying squirrel's droppings (*wǔ líng zhī*)

cinnamon bark (*ròu guì*) fears halloysite (*chì shí zhī*)

---

nineteen pathomechanisms 病机十九条 *bìng jī shí jiǔ tiáo*: From *Elementary Questions* (*sù wèn, zhì zhēn yào dà lùn*). Nineteen laws associating signs or patterns to certain evils or organs etc. [26: 490] [27: 123] [97: 488]

The Nineteen Pathomechanisms

all wind with shaking and [visual] dizziness is ascribed to the liver 诸风掉眩，皆属于肝 *zhū fēng diào xuàn, jiē shǔ yú gān*

all cold with contracture and tautness is ascribed to the kidney 诸寒收引，皆属于肾 *zhū hán shōu yǐn, jiē shǔ yú shèn*

all qi rushing and depression is ascribed to the lung 诸气膹郁，皆属于肺 *zhū qì fèn yù, jiē shǔ yú fèi*

all dampness with swelling and fullness is ascribed to the spleen 诸湿肿满，皆属于脾 *zhū shī zhǒng mǎn, jiē shǔ yú pí*

all heat with visual distortion and tugging is ascribed to fire 诸热瞀瘛，皆属于火 *zhū rè mào chì, jiē shǔ yú huǒ*

all painful and itching sores are ascribed to the liver 诸痛痒疮，皆属于心 *zhū tòng yǎng chuāng, jiē shǔ yú xīn*

all reversal with constipation or diarrhea is ascribed to the lower body 诸厥固泄，皆属于下 *zhū jué gù xiè, jiē shǔ yú xià*

all wilting (*wěi*), panting, and retching are ascribed to the upper body 诸痿喘呕，皆属于上 *zhū wěi chuǎn ǒu, jiē shǔ yú shàng*

all clenching, shuddering, and chattering [of the jaws] with the seeming loss of the spirit is ascribed to fire 诸禁鼓栗，如丧神守，皆属于火 *zhū jìn gǔ lì, rú sāng shén shǒu, jiē shǔ yú huǒ*

all tetany and rigidity of the neck is ascribed to dampness 诸痉项强，皆属于湿 *zhū jìng xiàng qiáng, jiē shǔ yú shī*

all counterflow upsurging is ascribed to fire 诸逆冲上，皆属于火 *zhū nì chōng shàng, jiē shǔ yú huǒ*

all major abdominal distention is ascribed to heat 诸腹胀大，皆属于热 *zhū fù zhàng dà, jiē shǔ yú rè*

all excessive agitation and mania is ascribed to fire 诸燥狂越，皆属于火 *zhū zào kuáng yuè, jiē shǔ yú huǒ*

all fulminant rigidity is ascribed to wind 诸暴强直，皆属于风 *zhū bào qiáng zhí, jiē shǔ yú fēng*

all diseases with [abdominal] sounds, where tapping makes a drum-like sound, are ascribed to heat 诸病有声，鼓之如鼓，皆属于热 *zhū bìng yǒu shēng, gǔ zhī rú gǔ, jiē shǔ yú rè*

all diseases with aching pain and swelling of the instep, fright and fear are ascribed to fire 诸病胕肿，疼酸惊骇，皆属于火 *zhū bìng fù zhǒng, téng suān jīng hài, jiē shǔ yú huǒ*

all cramp, arched-back rigidity, and turbid watery humors are ascribed to heat 诸转反戾，水液浑浊，皆属于热 *zhū zhuǎn fǎn lì, shuǐ yè hún zhuó, jiē shǔ yú rè*

all disease with watery humors that are clear, pure, and cold are ascribed to cold 诸病水液澄澈清冷，皆属于寒 *zhū bìng shuǐ yè shéng chè qīng lěng, jiē shǔ yú hán*

all sour retching and vomiting, and fulminant downpour with lower body distress are ascribed to heat 诸呕吐酸，暴注下迫，皆属于热 *zhū ǒu tù suān, bào zhù xià pò, jiē shǔ yú rè*

---

nine worm diseases 九虫病 *jiǔ chóng bìng*: From *The Origin and Indicators of Disease* (*zhū bìng yuán hòu lùn*). Latent worm disease; roundworm disease; whiteworm disease; flesh worm disease; lung worm disease; stomach worm disease; weak worm disease; redworm disease; pinworm disease. By and large, worm patterns are attributable to spleen-stomach vacuity, indiscriminate consumption of cold raw or rich sweet fatty foods, and improper cooking. The most important of the worm patterns are ROUNDWORM, INCH WHITEWORM, REDWORM DISEASE, and PINWORM. See also WORM ACCUMULATION. MED Worm patterns are treated by expelling worms, by fortifying the spleen and boosting the stomach, and by dispersing food and abducting stagnation. [26: 18]

nipple 乳头 *rǔ tóu*: The dark-colored protruding head of the breast in the female, and in males in the corresponding position. The nipples belong to the liver and diseases of them are often treated through the liver channel. [26: 379]

nipple moth 乳蛾 *rǔ é*: BABY MOTH.

nipple wind 乳头风 *rǔ tóu fēng*: *Synonym: cracked nipple.* A disease of the nipple or areola characterized by painful fissuring, bleeding, and exudation of sticky fluid and sometimes with scabbing. WMC cracked nipple (fissure of nipple, rhagadia mammae). Nipple wind is attributed to liver fire failing to discharge and liver-stomach damp-heat. It can easily develop into an EXTERNAL BLOWING MAMMARY WELLING-ABSCESS. MED Treat by clearing the liver and draining fire with formulas such as Gentian Liver-Draining Decoction (*lóng dǎn xiè gān tāng*) taken orally and Flesh-Engendering Jade and Red Paste (*shēng jī yù hóng gāo*) applied topically. For damp ulceration, apply an ointment composed of 20% calcined alum (*kū fán*), 10% calomel (*qīng fěn*), 10% gypsum (*shí gāo*), and 60% petroleum jelly (Vaseline). [26: 379] [96: 154]

nocturia 夜间多尿 *yè jiān duō niào*: PROFUSE URINATION AT NIGHT.

node 核 *hé*, 结核 *jié hé*: Any small abnormal lump under the skin that feels like the stone of a fruit. Scrofula, for example, takes the form of numerous subcutaneous nodes. See SCROFULA; PHLEGM NODE. ◊ Chin 核 *hé*, fruit stone, fruit pit; nucleus.

node in the breast 乳中结核 *rǔ zhōng jié hé*: MAMMARY NODE. [97: 385]

no desire for food and drink 不欲饮食 *bù yù yǐn shí*: See POOR APPETITE.

no desire to eat despite hunger 饥不欲食 *jī bù yù shí*, 知饥不食 *zhī jī bù shí*: Poor appetite with hunger. No desire to eat despite hunger occurs in the following situations: With clamoring stomach characterized by scorching heat sensation, red tongue with scant fur, it indicates insufficiency of stomach yin and vacuity fire. In such cases, the lack of desire to eat is explained by the insufficiency, whereas the presence of hunger is explained as result of the vacuity fire. With dizziness, tinnitus, insomnia, forgetfulness, and dry throat and tongue, it is attributed to insufficiency of kidney yin and frenetic movement of the ministerial fire. In advanced stages of febrile disease with lassitude of spirit, lack of strength, and dry tongue with little liquid, it is a sign of insufficiency of stomach yin resulting from qi, blood, and liquid depletion when the evil has abated. See POOR APPETITE.

noisy nose 鼻鸣 *bí míng*: From *On Cold Damage* (*Shāng Hán Lùn*). Wheezing or hissing sound in the nose due to nasal congestion. [51: 26]

nonchannel point 经外奇穴 *jīng wài qí xué*, 经外穴 *jīng wài xué*: Any point not belonging to channel. ◊ Chin 经 *jīng*, channel; 外 *wài*, outside; 奇 *qí*, extraordinary; 穴 *xué*, hole, cave, acupuncture point. [27: 104] [97: 376]

nonclosure of the birth gate 产门不闭 *chǎn mén bù bì*: Synonym: *nonclosure of the jade gate*. Failure of the birth gate (*orificium vaginae*) to resume normal form after giving birth. Nonclosure of the birth gate is attributed to major postpartum qi-blood vacuity preventing normal contraction or

physical damage to the birth gate during delivery. Vacuity patterns are characterized by shortage of qi and laziness to speak, somber white complexion, and spontaneous sweating. They are treated by major supplementation of qi and blood using formulas such as Perfect Major Supplementation Decoction (*shí quán dà bǔ tāng*). Where swelling, pain, and heat because of injury to the birth gate during delivery are the main features, treatment centers on clearing heat and resolving toxin with formulas such as Free Wanderer Powder (*xiāo yáo sǎn*) plus moutan (*mǔ dān pí*), schizonepeta (*jīng jiè*), lonicera (*jīn yín huā*), and forsythia (*lián qiào*). If the swelling has dispersed but the birth gate still fails to close, Center-Supplementing Qi-Boosting Decoction (*bǔ zhōng yì qì tāng*) should be used. In any case, a concentrated decoction of licorice can be used as an external wash. [26: 575] [97: 218]

nonclosure of the fontanel gate 囟门不合 *xìn mén bù hé*: See UNUNITED SKULL.

nonclosure of the fontanels 囟开不合 *xìn kāi bù hé*: UNUNITED SKULL.

nonclosure of the jade gate 玉门不闭 *yù mén bù bì*: NONCLOSURE OF THE BIRTH GATE. [26: 575]

noncontraction of heart qi 心气不收 *xīn qì bù shōu*: See INSECURITY OF HEART QI. [26: 92]

nondiffusion of lung qi 肺气不宣 *fèi qì bù xuān*: Impairment of lung qi diffusion generally attributable to external evils invading the lung or fettering the exterior. The main signs are cough, hoarse voice, nasal congestion and runny nose, usually accompanied by exterior signs such as heat effusion and aversion to cold. Evil heat congesting the lung may be characterized by the additional presence of high fever, flaring nostrils, rough rapid panting, and thick sticky yellow phlegm sometimes finely streaked with blood, accompanied by red or crimson tongue with rough yellow fur, and rapid slippery pulse. If preexisting cold-rheum ascends and invades the lung following contraction of an external evil, such signs as physical cold and cold limbs, cough and panting, white foaming phlegm and a "frog rale" may be observed. Such a pattern also includes somber white complexion, glossy white tongue fur, and stringlike pulse. MED Nondiffusion of lung qi is treated by the basic method of diffusing the lung with acrid dissipating medicinals, which may be combined with that of clearing heat and transforming phlegm or transforming cold-rheum with warm medicinals. Since this pattern occurs when external evils invade the lung, the use of exterior-coursing medicinals help to promote diffusion of lung qi. Hence, medicinals such as ephedra (*má huáng*), platycodon (*jié gěng*), arctium (*niú bàng zǐ*), and Zhejiang fritillaria (*zhè bèi mǔ*) are commonly used because they both diffuse the lung and resolve the exterior. Rough and Ready Three Decoction (*sān ào tāng*) is a basic formula that can be varied according to need. For wind-cold fettering the exterior creating a repletion pattern without sweating, warm acrid exterior-resolving medicinals may be added, whereas for wind-heat invading the lung, it can be combined with Lonicera and Forsythia Powder (*yín qiào sǎn*). Evil heat congesting the lung calls for additional attention for the need to clear the lung, downbear counterflow, and calm panting; it is often treated with formulas such as Ephedra, Apricot Kernel, Gypsum, and Licorice Decoction (*má xìng shí gān tāng*) or Lonicera and Phragmites Mixture (*yín wěi hé jì*). Nondiffusion of lung qi arising after contraction of cold evil in patients with preexisting cold-rheum should be treated by warming the lung and transforming rheum, using Minor Green-Blue Dragon Decoction (*xiǎo qīng lóng tāng*). ACU LU-7 (*liè quē*, Broken Sequence) and LU-1 (*zhōng fǔ*, Central Treasury) diffuse lung qi. CV-17 (*shān zhōng*, Chest Center) downbears counterflow, transforms phlegm, and loosens the chest. These points are combined with BL-13 (*fèi shū*, Lung Transport) when combating an external evil invading the lung. For heat, use GV-14 (*dà zhuī*, Great Hammer) and LU-5 (*chǐ zé*, Cubit Marsh). For wind-cold, use BL-12 (*fēng mén*, Wind Gate), BL-13 (*fèi shū*, Lung Transport), and GB-20 (*fēng chí*, Wind Pool) with moxa. [50: 950][6: 174][27: 159][97: 352]

nondistribution of pulmonary liquid 肺津不布 *fèi jīn bù bù*: Breakdown of the lung's function of distributing liquid, giving rise to panting and cough. The lung receives essential qi sent from the spleen, and works with the heart to distribute essential qi around the body. When the lung is scorched by heat, lung yin is damaged, normal fluid distribution is upset, and the skin and hair are deprived of moisturization. When the lung is fettered by cold, it fails to move liquid, so that water collects to form rheum. The result in either case is the formation of phlegm, which causes panting and cough. [27: 159] [97: 354]

nondownbearing of stomach qi 胃气不降 *wèi qì bù jiàng*: Synonym: *impaired harmonious downbearing of the stomach*. Disturbance of the normal downbearing of stomach qi. Stomach qi normally bears downward carrying food downward to the intestines. Impaired downbearing is characterized by no thought of food and drink, fullness and distention or pain in the stomach. When stomach qi does not bear downward, it ascends counterflow, manifesting as vomiting, belching, and hiccough. See STOMACH QI ASCENDING COUNTERFLOW. [26: 439] [27: 157] [97: 398]

noninteraction of the heart and kidney 心肾不交 *xīn shèn bù jiāo*: Synonym: *breakdown of heart-kidney interaction*. A disorder of the normal relationship between heart yang and kidney yin. Insufficiency of kidney yin or stirring of heart fire may be the cause of the disorder. Signs include heart vexation, insomnia, profuse dreaming, heart palpitations or fearful throbbing, and seminal emission. WMC This pattern is observed in neurotic and weak patients. MED Use Coptis, Ass Hide Glue, and Egg Yolk Decoction (*huáng lián ē jiāo jī zǐ huáng tāng*) or Peaceful Interaction Pill (*jiāo tài wán*). ACU Base treatment mainly on back transport points, HT, and KI. Select BL-15 (*xīn shū*, Heart Transport), BL-23 (*shèn shū*, Kidney Transport), KI-3 (*tài xī*, Great Ravine), KI-1 (*yǒng quán*, Gushing Spring), HT-7 (*shén mén*, Spirit Gate), PC-8 (*láo gōng*, Palace of Toil), PC-7 (*dà líng*, Great Mound), and SP-6 (*sān yīn jiāo*, Three Yin Intersection); needle with even supplementation and drainage, or supplement the kidney and drain the heart. Selection of points according to signs: For insomnia, add Alert Spirit Quartet (*sì shén cōng*). For profuse dreaming, add GB-44 (*zú qiào yīn*, Foot Orifice Yin) and ST-45 (*lì duì*, Severe Mouth). For heart palpitations, add PC-6 (*nèi guān*, Inner Pass). For seminal emission, add PC-7 (*dà líng*, Great Mound). See PROMOTING HEART-KIDNEY INTERACTION. [26: 94] [27: 27] [97: 121] [46: 678] [37: 348] [113: 145]

nonscarring moxibustion 无瘢痕灸 *wú bān hén jiǔ*: A method of direct moxibustion whereby the moxa cone is removed before it burns the skin. Cones are burned until the skin at the point turns red. Take care to avoid accidental scarring when using this technique. Nonscarring moxibustion is less drastic than scarring moxibustion and is used for mild vacuity cold patterns. Some sources state that extinguishing the cone by pressing it to the skin supplements, and that removing it before extinguishing it drains. [27: 244] [97: 66]

nonseparation of grain and water 水谷不别 *shuǐ gǔ bù bié*: Scant urine and thin sloppy stool arising when water-damp collects and fails to pass out in the urine. [26: 132]

nontransformation of food 完谷不化 *wán gǔ bù huà*: Partially digested food in the stool due to impaired digestion. Nontransformation of food most commonly occurs in spleen vacuity, spleen-kidney yang vacuity, large intestinal vacuity, or cold accumulation patterns, but may also be observed in heat diarrhea. See also SWILL DIARRHEA; THROUGHFLUX DIARRHEA. ◊ Chin 完 *wán*, complete, whole, intact, 谷 *gǔ*, grain, 不 *bù*, not, 化 *huà*, transform; literally, "whole grain not transforming," describing how grain and other types of food remain intact in the stool due to incomplete digestion.

nontransformation of grain and water 水谷不化 *shuǐ gǔ bù huà*: NONTRANSFORMATION OF FOOD.

nonupbearing of clear yang (or qi) 清阳（或气）不升 *qīng yáng (qì) bù shēng*: CLEAR YANG FAILING TO BEAR UPWARD.

nonupbearing of spleen qi 脾气不升 *pí qì bù shēng*: Debilitation of spleen qi affecting its normal upbearing; characterized by lusterless facial complexion, dizziness, tendency to sweat, shortness of breath, reduced food intake, fatigue, abdominal distention, sloppy stool, pale tongue with white fur, and moderate vacuous pulse. In some cases, there is flowery or blurred vision, tinnitus, and eating without being able to distinguish flavors. If due to damp turbidity and food stagnation, there may be signs such as clouded heavy head, fatigue, no desire for food, abdominal distention or pain and distention, a thick slimy tongue fur, and a sunken moderate pulse. [26: 748] [27: 156] [97: 561]

noodle-type food damage 伤面食 *shāng miàn shí*: See FOOD DAMAGE.

no pleasure in eating 纳谷不香 *nà gǔ bù xiāng*, 纳谷不馨 *nà gǔ bù xiāng*: See POOR APPETITE.

normalizing qi 顺气 *shùn qì*: DOWNBEARING COUNTERFLOW AND PRECIPITATING QI. [26: 752] [27: 270]

normalizing qi and transforming phlegm 顺气 化痰 *shùn qì huà tán*: A method of treatment used to address phlegm bind and fullness in the chest, cough and counterflow qi, with copious phlegm and food stagnation, using formulas such as Three-Seed Filial Devotion Decoction (*sān zǐ yǎng qīn tāng*) and Qi-Normalizing Phlegm-Abducting Decoction (*shùn qì dǎo tán tāng*). [60: 324, 358]

normal pulse 正常脉 *zhèng cháng mài*: With approximately four beats per respiration, the normal pulse is steady and even. The normal pulse has a threefold significance: (1) Its smoothness and strength indicate the presence of spirit. (2) It is neither sunken nor floating, and the beat rises and falls evenly and effortlessly, indicating the presence of stomach qi. (3) Strength at the deep level indicates the presence of root. See STOMACH, SPIRIT, AND ROOT. [6: 139]

normal tongue fur 正常舌苔 *zhèng cháng shé tāi*: A thin layer of fur on the tongue observed in healthy people and attributed to upward steaming of stomach qi. Any deviation from this may be pathological. [6: 122]

Northern and Southern Dynasties 南北朝 *nán běi cháo*: The name of a dynastic period (A.D. 420–581).

Northern Dynasties 北朝 *běi cháo*: The name of a dynastic period (A.D. 386–534).

Northern Qi 北齐 *běi qí*: The name of a dynasty (A.D. 550–577).

Northern Song 北宋 *běi sòng*: The name of a dynasty (A.D. 960–1127).

Northern Wei 北魏 *běi wèi*: The name of a dynasty (A.D. 386–534).

Northern Zhou 北周 *běi zhōu*: The name of a dynasty (A.D. 557–581).

nose 鼻 *bí*: Synonym: *bright hall*. An organ located in the center of the face, through which great qi (air) enters the lung; the external orifice of the lung. Diagnosis: The nose and "SNIVEL" (nasal mucus) are of diagnostic value. Flaring nostrils are associated with rapid breathing due to lung heat. Dry nostrils indicate lung heat or contraction of dryness evil. A dry parched black nose indicates intense heat toxin. Prominent blood vessels at the root of the nose in infants are a sign of a weak constitution or weakness of the organs. When this occurs during the course of an illness it indicates fright-wind. In patients suffering from measles, extremely scant papules at the sides of the nostrils indicate nondiffusion of lung qi and the incomplete outthrust of evil heat. Snivel is the humor of the lung. Abnormalities of snivel (nasal mucus) indicate either nondiffusion of lung qi due either to the presence of evil or to lung vacuity. NASAL CONGESTION with turbid snivel is observed in external contraction of wind-heat, whereas nasal congestion and runny nose with clear snivel indicates wind-cold invading the lung (common cold). In the latter case, it thickens and turns yellow on recovery. Thin clear snivel and pronounced sneezing indicates SNIVELING NOSE, which roughly corresponds to allergic rhinitis in Western medicine. Foul-smelling turbid yellow snivel accompanied by recurrent headaches indicates DEEP-SOURCE NASAL CONGESTION, which roughly corresponds to paranasal sinusitis. Compare also BRAIN LEAK and BRAIN-GRIPPING SAND. Bleeding from the nose, called NOSEBLEED, is the most common form of SPONTANEOUS EXTERNAL BLEEDING and is observed in lung heat, stomach fire, liver fire, head wind, liquor damage, yin vacuity, repelled yang, and external injury patterns. Growths within the nasal passages, NASAL POLYPS also result in nasal congestion. Diseases of the exterior of the nose include ACNE and DRINKER'S NOSE. Leprosy, often referred to as PESTILENTIAL WIND, may give rise to collapse of the nose. [26: 852] [26: 479] [97: 622]

nose beam 鼻柱 *bí zhù*: Synonym: *nose pillar*; [*region*] *below the lower extreme*. The stem of the nose. [27: 66] [97: 622]

nosebleed 鼻衄 *bí nǜ*: Spontaneous bleeding from the nose. Nosebleed is attributable to lung heat congesting in the upper body, stomach heat steaming upward, effulgent liver fire, head wind, liquor damage, lung-stomach yin vacuity, repelled yang, or external injury. **Lung heat** nosebleed is associated with dry nose and cough with scant phlegm. MED Clear and drain lung heat with Mulberry Leaf and Chrysanthemum Beverage (*sāng jú yǐn*) minus mint (*bò hé*) and platycodon (*jié gěng*) and plus scutellaria (*huáng qín*), gardenia (*shān zhī zǐ*), and imperata flower (*bái máo huā*). ACU Base treatment mainly on GV and LU. Select GV-23 (*shàng xīng*, Upper Star), LI-4 (*hé gǔ*, Union Valley), LU-11 (*shào shāng*, Lesser Shang), GV-16 (*fēng fǔ*, Wind Mansion), and LU-3 (*tiān fǔ*, Celestial Storehouse); needle with drainage. **Stomach fire** nosebleed is associated with dry mouth, bad breath, vexation and thirst with taking of fluids. [MED] Clear heat and drain stomach heat with Jade Lady Brew (*yù nǚ jiān*). [ACU] Base treatment mainly on GV, LI, and ST. Select GV-23 (*shàng xīng*, Upper Star), LI-2 (*èr jiān*, Second Space), ST-44 (*nèi tíng*, Inner Court), ST-45 (*lì duì*, Severe Mouth), CV-12 (*zhōng wǎn*, Center Stomach Duct), and SP-1 (*yǐn bái*, Hidden White); needle with drainage. **Liver fire** nosebleed is associated with headache, dizziness, red eyes, and irascibility. [MED] Clear and drain liver fire with Gentian Liver-Draining Decoction (*lóng dǎn xiè gān tāng*). [ACU] Base treatment mainly on GV, LR, and KI. Select GV-27 (*duì duān*, Extremity of the Mouth), LR-2 (*xíng jiān*, Moving Between), LR-8 (*qū quán*, Spring at the Bend), KI-1 (*yǒng quán*, Gushing Spring), and BL-40 (*wěi zhōng*, Bend Center); needle with drainage. **Head wind** nosebleed is a pouring nosebleed. [MED] Calm the liver, course wind, and stanch bleeding with Peony and Licorice Decoction (*sháo yào gān cǎo tāng*) plus cimicifuga (*shēng má*) and imperata flower (*bái máo huā*). [ACU] Base treatment mainly on GV, GB, LI, and LU. Select GV-23 (*shàng xīng*, Upper Star), GV-16 (*fēng fǔ*, Wind Mansion), GB-20 (*fēng chí*, Wind Pool), LI-4 (*hé gǔ*, Union Valley), LI-19 (*hé liáo*, Grain Bone-Hole), LU-7 (*liè quē*, Broken Sequence), and SI-3 (*hòu xī*, Back Ravine); needle with drainage. **Liquor damage** nosebleed is a persistent nosebleed due to lung-stomach accumulated heat and is associated with yellow tongue fur and rough breathing. [MED] Clear lung and stomach heat, resolve liquor, and stanch bleeding with Bamboo Leaf and Gypsum Decoction (*zhú yè shí gāo tāng*) plus pueraria flower (*gé huā*) and honey tree fruit (*zhǐ jù zǐ*). [ACU] Base treatment mainly on GV, LU, LI, and ST. Select GV-23 (*shàng xīng*, Upper Star), LI-4 (*hé gǔ*, Union Valley), LI-2 (*èr jiān*, Second Space), ST-44 (*nèi tíng*, Inner Court), ST-45 (*lì duì*, Severe Mouth), LU-11 (*shào shāng*, Lesser Shang), GV-16 (*fēng fǔ*, Wind Mansion), ST-36 (*zú sān lǐ*, Leg Three Li), and SP-6 (*sān yīn jiāo*, Three Yin Intersection); needle with drainage. **Yin vacuity** nosebleed, which is due to insufficiency of kidney and lung yin, is accompanied by tidal heat [effusion], night sweating, dizziness, tinnitus, incessant cough, and a fine rapid pulse. [MED] Enrich yin and nourish lung and kidney yin with Anemarrhena, Phellodendron, and Rehmannia Pill (*zhī bǎi dì huáng wán*) plus scrophularia (*xuán shēn*) and eclipta (*mò hàn lián*). [ACU] Base treatment mainly on GV, LU, and KI. Select GV-23 (*shàng xīng*, Upper Star), LI-4 (*hé gǔ*, Union Valley), BL-13 (*fèi shū*, Lung Transport), BL-23 (*shèn shū*, Kidney Transport), BL-43 (*gāo huāng shū*, Gao-Huang Transport), KI-3 (*tài xī*, Great Ravine), and LU-5 (*chǐ zé*, Cubit Marsh);

needle with supplementation. **Repelled yang** nosebleed arises when there is yin vacuity in the lower body and yang floats upward. It is associated with a forceless large floating pulse at all six positions of the wrist with pronounced weakness at the two cubits. [MED] Conduct the fire back to the origin and subdue floating yang. Use Golden Coffer Kidney Qi Pill (*jīn guì shèn qì wán*) plus achyranthes (*niú xī*) and raw tortoise plastron (*shēng guī bǎn*) [ACU] Base treatment mainly on GV, LU, and KI. Needle with drainage at GV-23 (*shàng xīng*, Upper Star), LI-4 (*hé gǔ*, Union Valley), KI-6 (*zhào hǎi*, Shining Sea), KI-1 (*yǒng quán*, Gushing Spring), and HT-8 (*shào fǔ*, Lesser Mansion), and with supplementation at BL-23 (*shèn shū*, Kidney Transport), KI-3 (*tài xī*, Great Ravine), and LR-3 (*tài chōng*, Supreme Surge). For incessant nosebleed, add moxa at GV-22 (*xìn huì*, Fontanel Meeting) and GV-23 (*shàng xīng*, Upper Star). **External injury** nosebleed is treated by stuffing the nose with a wad of gauze soaked in a suitable preparation. See SPONTANEOUS EXTERNAL BLEEDING. [26: 855] [27: 495, 420] [97: 622]

nose pile 鼻痔 *bí zhì*: NASAL POLYP.

nose pillar 鼻梁 *bí liáng*: Synonym: *nose beam*; [region] *below the lower extreme*. The stem of the nose. [27: 66] [97: 623]

no thought of food and drink 不思饮食 *bù sī yǐn shí*: See POOR APPETITE.

not knowing hunger or satiety 不知饥饱 *bù zhī jī bǎo*: See POOR APPETITE.

not to change one's clothes 不更衣 *bù gēng yī*: From *On Cold Damage* (*Shāng Hán Lùn*). An ancient euphemism for constipation. [26: 127] [97: 65]

nourish 养 *yǎng*: See SUPPLEMENTATION.

nourishing the blood 养血 *yǎng xuè*: SUPPLEMENTING THE BLOOD.

nourishing the blood and emolliating the liver 养血柔肝 *yǎng xuè róu gān*: EMOLLIATING THE LIVER. [27: 264]

nourishing the blood and moistening dryness 养血润燥 *yǎng xuè rùn zào*: A method of treatment used to address blood vacuity constipation characterized by dry stool that is difficult to evacuate and that is accompanied by somber white complexion, lack of redness and moisture in the lips and nails, periodic dizziness, heart palpitations, soft pale tongue body, and rapid fine pulse. [MED] Commonly used blood-nourishing dryness-moistening medicinals include tangkuei (*dāng guī*), dried/fresh rehmannia (*shēng dì huáng*), hemp seed (*huǒ má rén*), peach kernel (*táo rén*), and bitter orange (*zhǐ ké*). [ACU] Base treatment mainly on alarm, back transport, and lower uniting points of LI, and on other back transport points. Select BL-25 (*dà cháng shū*, Large Intestine Transport), ST-25 (*tiān shū*, Celestial Pivot), ST-37 (*shàng jù xū*, Upper

Great Hollow), BL-17 (*gé shū*, Diaphragm Transport), BL-20 (*pí shū*, Spleen Transport), BL-21 (*wèi shū*, Stomach Transport), and SP-6 (*sān yīn jiāo*, Three Yin Intersection); needle with supplementation and add moxa. [27: 270] [37: 328] [113: 102] [97: 431]

nourishing the blood and resolving the exterior 养血解表 *yǎng xuè jiě biǎo*: A method of treatment used to address yin-blood depletion with common cold characterized by headache, generalized heat [effusion], slight aversion to cold, absence of sweating, soft-red tongue with little fur, and a rapid soggy pulse. MED A commonly used blood-nourishing exterior-resolving formula is Scallion White Seven-Ingredient Beverage (*cōng bái qī wèi yǐn*). ACU Base treatment mainly on SP, ST, LR, GB, LU, and LI. Needle with supplementation at BL-20 (*pí shū*, Spleen Transport), BL-17 (*gé shū*, Diaphragm Transport), ST-36 (*zú sān lǐ*, Leg Three Li), SP-6 (*sān yīn jiāo*, Three Yin Intersection), and LR-3 (*tài chōng*, Supreme Surge), with drainage at GB-20 (*fēng chí*, Wind Pool), TB-5 (*wài guān*, Outer Pass), LI-4 (*hé gǔ*, Union Valley), and LU-7 (*liè quē*, Broken Sequence). Compare ENRICHING YIN AND RESOLVING THE EXTERIOR. [26: 867] [27: 264]

nourishing the fluids 养津液 *yǎng jīn yè*: See ENGENDERING LIQUID. [27: 253]

nourishing the heart and quieting the spirit 养心安神 *yǎng xīn ān shén*: A method of treatment used to address disquieted heart spirit due to heart blood depletion characterized by heart palpitations, susceptibility to fright, forgetfulness, insomnia, abstraction, profuse dreaming and seminal emission, dry bound stool, mouth and tongue sores, red tongue with scant fur, and a rapid fine pulse. MED A commonly used heart-nourishing spirit-quieting formula is Biota Seed Heart-Nourishing Pill (*bǎi zǐ yǎng xīn wán*). ACU Base treatment mainly on BL-15 (*xīn shū*, Heart Transport), BL-17 (*gé shū*, Diaphragm Transport), BL-20 (*pí shū*, Spleen Transport), HT-7 (*shén mén*, Spirit Gate), HT-8 (*shào fǔ*, Lesser Mansion), PC-4 (*xī mén*, Cleft Gate), SP-6 (*sān yīn jiāo*, Three Yin Intersection), and PC-5 (*jiān shǐ*, Intermediary Courier). See QUIETING THE SPIRIT. [26: 867] [113: 14] [27: 285] [97: 430]

nourishing the liver 养肝 *yǎng gān*: EMOLLIATING THE LIVER. [27: 264]

nourishing the stomach 养胃 *yǎng wèi*: ENRICHING (AND SUPPLEMENTING) STOMACH YIN. [27: 279]

nourishing yin 养阴 *yǎng yīn*: SUPPLEMENTING YIN.

nourishing yin and clearing the lung 养阴清肺 *yǎng yīn qīng fèi*: A method of treatment used to address lung heat and yin vacuity. The method of nourishing yin and clearing the lung is used for two distinct conditions. (1) Yin vacuity sore

throat or diphtheria. MED Use Yin-Nourishing Lung-Clearing Decoction (*yǎng yīn qīng fèi tāng*). ACU Base treatment mainly on KI and LU. Select KI-3 (*tài xī*, Great Ravine), KI-6 (*zhào hǎi*, Shining Sea), and LU-10 (*yú jì*, Fish Border); needle with even supplementation and drainage. Selection of points according to signs: For pronounced swelling and pain, prick LU-11 (*shào shāng*, Lesser Shang) to bleed. (2) Vacuity taxation cough characterized by dry cough with little phlegm occasionally flecked with blood, postmeridian low fever, night sweating, oppression and dull pain in the chest, dry mouth, tongue with red margins and tip, and rapid fine pulse. MED Use Four Yin Brew (*sì yīn jiān*), consisting of dried/fresh rehmannia (*shēng dì huáng*), ophiopogon (*mài mén dōng*), white peony (*bái sháo yào*), lily bulb (*bǎi hé*), adenophora/glehnia (*shā shēn*), and licorice (*gān cǎo*). ACU Base treatment mainly on LU and KI. Select BL-13 (*fèi shū*, Lung Transport), BL-43 (*gāo huāng shū*, Gao-Huang Transport), LU-5 (*chǐ zé*, Cubit Marsh), KI-6 (*zhào hǎi*, Shining Sea), and KI-3 (*tài xī*, Great Ravine); needle with supplementation. [26: 867] [27: 273] [97: 431]

nourishing yin and moistening dryness 养阴润燥 *yǎng yīn rùn zào*: Synonym: *enriching yin and moistening dryness*. A method of treatment used to address damage to lung-stomach yin by dryness, characterized by dry pharynx and thirst, postmeridian generalized heat [effusion], red tongue, a rapid fine pulse, and sometimes cough with scant phlegm, or constipation. MED A commonly used yin-nourishing dryness-moistening formula is Adenophora/Glehnia and Ophiopogon Decoction (*shā shēn mài dōng tāng*). If there is constipation, Humor-Increasing Decoction (*zēng yè tāng*) may be used. ACU Base treatment mainly on back transport points, LU, KI, ST, and SP. Select BL-13 (*fèi shū*, Lung Transport), BL-43 (*gāo huāng shū*, Gao-Huang Transport), LU-5 (*chǐ zé*, Cubit Marsh), KI-6 (*zhào hǎi*, Shining Sea), BL-21 (*wèi shū*, Stomach Transport), ST-36 (*zú sān lǐ*, Leg Three Li), and SP-6 (*sān yīn jiāo*, Three Yin Intersection); needle with supplementation. [26: 868] [27: 269] [97: 431]

nourishing yin and resolving the exterior 养阴解表 *yǎng yīn jiě biǎo*: ENRICHING YIN AND RESOLVING THE EXTERIOR.

numbing wind 麻风 *má fēng*: Leprosy. See PESTILENTIAL WIND.

numbness 木 *mù*: See NUMBNESS AND TINGLING. [26: 272]

numbness and tingling 麻木 *má mù*: Loss of normal sensation in the skin and flesh. Numbness (*mù*) is described as absence of itching or pain that is insensitive to pressure. Tingling (*má*) is classically described as "bugs crawling in the flesh" unrelieved by pressure. See NUMBNESS AND TINGLING OF THE SKIN. ◇ Chin 麻 *má*, hemp, flax, linen (possibly from the feeling that linen produces on the skin); 木 *mù*, wood (probably from its being symbolic of insensitivity). [92: No. 407]

numbness and tingling of the skin 肌肤麻木 *jī fū má mù*, 皮肤麻木 *pí fū má mù*: Loss of normal sensation in the skin. Numbness and tingling are attributable to wind-damp pestilential qi, phlegm-damp obstruction, qi-blood vacuity, or blood stasis. **Wind-damp pestilential qi** numbness is attributed to pestilential qi (wind, dampness, worms) or contact with clothing or belongings or affected people. It is characterized by localized insensitivity to heat, cold, or pain sometimes with red or white macules. Signs include loss of hair, scaling, and in some cases withering of the flesh, loss of eyebrows, and collapse of the nose. See PESTILENTIAL WIND. MED Dispel wind, transform dampness, quicken the blood, and kill worms. Alternate Safeguard Unlimited Efficacy Elixir (*bǎo ān wàn líng dān*) and Wondrous Response Wind-Dispersing Powder (*shén yìng xiāo fēng sǎn*). **Phlegm-damp obstruction** numbness is associated with heaviness in local joints and heaviness of the limbs reducing agility, a soggy moderate pulse, and a white slimy tongue fur. MED Transform phlegm and eliminate dampness; free the channels and quicken the network vessels. An appropriate formula is Two Matured Ingredients Decoction (*èr chén tāng*) minus mume (*wū méi*) and fresh ginger (*shēng jiāng*), and with the addition of loofah (*sī guā luò*), tangerine pith (*jú luò*), liquidambar fruit (*lù lù tōng*), and unripe bitter orange (*zhǐ shí*). **Qi-blood vacuity** numbness is characterized by its episodic nature and its tendency to be exacerbated by exertion and relieved by rest. It is also associated with coolness in the local area, and can be relieved by warmth. There may be periodic sensations of ants crawling through the flesh or even stabbing pain. It usually occurs in menopausal women on the insides of the upper limbs, and may be associated with menstrual irregularities or flooding and spotting. The tongue is pale and the pulse is fine and forceless. MED Supplement qi and nourish the blood; warm yang and free the network vessels. An appropriate formula is Astragalus and Cinnamon Twig Five Agents Decoction (*huáng qí guì zhī wǔ wù tāng*). **Blood stasis** numbness usually occurs in the lumbus or outside of the thighs and arises through impact. MED Quicken the blood and transform stasis; free the channels and network vessels. An appropriate formula is House of Blood Stasis-Expelling Decoction (*xuè fǔ zhú yū tāng*). See also INSENSITIVITY OF THE SKIN. [26: 272] [92: No. 407]

numbness of the tongue 舌麻 *shé má*: A lack of sensation in the tongue. Numbness of the tongue is attributable to liver wind stirring internally, to blood vacuity, or to phlegm obstruction. **Blood vacuity:** A pale numb tongue is accompanied by a somber white or withered-yellow facial complexion, heart palpitations, shortness of breath, insomnia and profuse dreaming, forgetfulness, and a forceless fine pulse. MED Nourish the blood. Use Spleen-Returning Decoction (*guī pí tāng*) plus blast-fried ginger (*páo jiāng*). **Liver wind:** Numbness of the tongue is accompanied by inhibited speech, dizzy head, headache, and rapid fine stringlike pulse. In some cases, there may sudden collapse leaving the patient with hemiplegia (wind stroke). MED Boost yin, calm the liver, and extinguish wind. Gastrodia and Uncaria Beverage (*tiān má gōu téng yǐn*). **Phlegm obstruction:** Phlegm obstruction can manifest in different ways. The main forms are wind-phlegm and phlegm-fire. In wind-phlegm, the tongue is numb and stiff. This is accompanied by dizzy head and vision, and numbness of the limbs. In some cases, there may be sudden collapse leaving the patient with deviated eyes and mouth or hemiplegia. The tongue is white and glossy or yellow and slimy. The pulse is floating and slippery or stringlike and moderate. In phlegm-fire, the tongue is numb and red. The tongue fur is yellow and slimy or else thick yellow and dry. In addition there is dizzy head and vision, tinnitus, bitter taste in the mouth, vexation and agitation, irascibility, ungratifying defecation, and a rapid slippery stringlike pulse. MED For wind-phlegm use Awake-From-Wind Decoction (*shěng fēng tāng*) plus aquilaria (*chén xiāng*). For phlegm-fire, use Gallbladder-Warming Decoction (*wēn dǎn tāng*) plus bile arisaema [root] (*dǎn xīng*), scorpion (*quán xiē*), gastrodia (*tiān má*), and coptis (*huáng lián*). [92: No. 108]

obesity 肥胖 *féi pàng*: Fatness, corpulence. Traditional literature contains little reference to weight control. With the influence of modern medicine, greater attention is being paid to the problem. Obesity is attributed to phlegm-damp or qi vacuity, or as is often the case, a combination of the two. **Phlegm-damp** obesity is characterized by a large appetite with a predilection for sweet or fatty rich foods, glomus and oppression in the chest and stomach duct, copious phlegm, heavy body, fatigue, aversion to heat, enlarged tongue with thick slimy fur, and a forceful slippery stringlike pulse. MED Dispel phlegm and transform dampness using Gallbladder-Warming Decoction (*wēn dǎn tāng*) or Stomach-Calming Powder (*píng wèi sǎn*) with the judicious addition of crataegus (*shān zhā*), radish seed (*lái fú zǐ*), and Six-to-One Powder (*liù yī sǎn*). This treatment should be combined with control of intake of rich food. ACU Base treatment mainly on CV and ST. Select CV-12 (*zhōng wǎn*, Center Stomach Duct), ST-36 (*zú sān lǐ*, Leg Three Li), ST-40 (*fēng lóng*, Bountiful Bulge), ST-25 (*tiān shū*, Celestial Pivot), CV-6 (*qì hǎi*, Sea of Qi), and CV-9 (*shuǐ fēn*, Water Divide); needle with drainage. Selection of points according to area affected: For the shoulder and back, add GV-14 (*dà zhuī*, Great Hammer) and LI-15 (*jiān yú*, Shoulder Bone). For the chest and breasts, add ST-33 (*yīn shì*, Yin Market) and ST-16 (*yīng chuāng*, Breast Window). For the lower abdomen, add ST-28 (*shuǐ dào*, Waterway). For the buttocks and thighs, add GB-30 (*huán tiào*, Jumping Round), GB-31 (*fēng shì*, Wind Market), and SP-10 (*xuè hǎi*, Sea of Blood). **Qi vacuity** obesity is obesity accompanied by shortage of qi and laziness to speak, spontaneous sweating at the slightest movement, vacuity swelling of the face, poor appetite, lassitude of spirit, somnolence, pale tongue with white fur, and a weak fine pulse. MED Supplement qi and fortify the spleen. Use formulas such as Saussurea and Amomum Six Gentlemen Decoction (*xiāng shā liù jūn zǐ tāng*) combined with physical exercise. ACU Base treatment mainly on back transport points, CV, SP, and ST. Select BL-20 (*pí shū*, Spleen Transport), BL-21 (*wèi shū*, Stomach Transport), ST-36 (*zú sān lǐ*, Leg Three Li), CV-12 (*zhōng wǎn*, Center Stomach Duct), LR-13 (*zhāng mén*, Camphorwood Gate), CV-6 (*qì hǎi*, Sea of Qi), and SP-9 (*yīn líng quán*, Yin Mound Spring); needle with supplementation and moxa. [46: 594, 597] [73: 508] [92: No. 28]

obesity infertility 肥胖不孕 *féi pàng bù yùn*: Infertility resulting when phlegm-damp arising internally in obese people becomes lodged in the thoroughfare (*chōng*) and controlling (*rèn*) vessels or when excessive fat congests the uterus and the uterine vessels. Obesity infertility is usually associated with heart palpitations, shortness of breath, and copious vaginal discharge. MED Treat with Palace-Opening Pill (*qǐ gōng wán*), which contains pinellia (*bàn xià*), atractylodes (*cāng zhú*), ligusticum (*chuān xiōng*), tangerine peel (*chén pí*), cyperus (*xiāng fù zǐ*), medicated leaven (*shén qū*), and poria (*fú líng*). ACU Base treatment mainly on CV and ST. Select CV-12 (*zhōng wǎn*, Center Stomach Duct), ST-36 (*zú sān lǐ*, Leg Three Li), ST-40 (*fēng lóng*, Bountiful Bulge), ST-25 (*tiān shū*, Celestial Pivot), CV-6 (*qì hǎi*, Sea of Qi), CV-4 (*guān yuán*, Pass Head), SP-6 (*sān yīn jiāo*, Three Yin Intersection); and KI-13 (*qì xué*, Qi Point); needle with even supplementation and drainage or with supplementation. Selection of points according to signs: For heart palpitations, add BL-15 (*xīn shū*, Heart Transport), and HT-7 (*shén mén*, Spirit Gate). For shortness of breath, add CV-17 (*shān zhōng*, Chest Center), LU-5 (*chǐ zé*, Cubit Marsh), and LI-4 (*hé gǔ*, Union Valley). For copious vaginal discharge, add GB-26 (*dài mài*, Girdling Vessel), BL-30 (*bái huán shū*, White Ring Transport), and SP-9 (*yīn líng quán*, Yin Mound Spring). [26: 384] [46: 364, 597, 690] [59: 90]

oblique insertion 斜刺 *xié cì*: Synonym: *slanted insertion*. Insertion of a needle at roughly 45°. Application: Oblique insertion is appropriate where the flesh is thin or where an internal organ lies beneath the point; hence it is commonly used on the chest and back. Oblique insertion is also used for moving qi in a particular direction. See DIRECTIONAL SUPPLEMENTATION AND DRAINAGE. [27: 528]

oblique-running pulse 斜飞脉 *xié fēi mài*: An anomaly in the position of wrist pulse in which the pulse runs from the cubit position over the posterior pace of the styloid process of the radius toward LI-4 (*hé gǔ*, Union Valley). [26: 644] [27: 189] [97: 528]

obliviousness of hunger and satiety 不知饥饿 *bù zhī jī è*: See POOR APPETITE.

obstruct 阻 *zǔ*: To cause blockage of the airways, interstices, spleen, etc., hampering their normal functioning. Dampness and phlegm are often described as causing obstruction, as in DAMP-NESS OBSTRUCTING THE CENTER BURNER, DAMP-HEAT OBSTRUCTING THE SPLEEN AND STOMACH, PHLEGM OBSTRUCTING THE NETWORK VESSELS OF THE LUNG, and PHLEGM OBSTRUCTING THE ORIFICES OF THE HEART.

obtaining qi 得气 *dé qì:* Causing the acupuncture needle to elicit the sensations associated with the presence of qi at or near the insertion site. These sensations include subjective sensations in the patient and an objective sensation felt by the practitioner's fingers. The subjective sensation experienced by the patient can be described as twinging (*suān*) distention, heaviness, tingling or numbness depending on the point in question and the condition of the patient. This should not be confused with the local sensation of pricking pain that may accompany needle insertion. Obtaining qi is a deeper sensation, duller in nature, and less localized than the sharp pain associated with the stimulation of subcutaneous nerves. The objective sensation felt by the practitioner can be described, to use the metaphor of *Song to Elucidate Mysteries* (*biāo yōu fù*), as a sudden deep tightening that resembles the feeling of a fish biting on a fishing line. As long as the needle moves easily, qi cannot be obtained. Since some patients report the slightest sensation in order to avoid further probing by the acupuncturist, it is better to rely on the subtle objective sensation. Channel-freeing manipulation, needle flicking, and qi-moving manipulation are techniques designed to help obtain qi. [27: 339] [97: 527]

occipital bone 玉枕骨 *yù zhěn gǔ*, 枕骨 *zhěn gǔ:* PILLOW BONE.

offensive bursting 攻溃 *gōng kuì:* The use of powerful pus-outthrusting medicinals such as pangolin scales (*chuān shān jiǎ*) and gleditsia (*zào jiá*) to promote the expulsion of pus and toxin in the treatment of sores.

offensive treatment 攻 *gōng:* ATTACK.[1]

office of assistant 相傅之官 *xiāng fù zhī guān:* See LUNG HOLDS THE OFFICE OF ASSISTANT, WHENCE MANAGEMENT AND REGULATION EMANATE.

office of conveyance 传导之官 *chuán dǎo zhī guān:* See LARGE INTESTINE HOLDS THE OFFICE OF CONVEYANCE, WHENCE MUTATION EMANATES.

office of general 将军之官 *jiāng jūn zhī guān:* LIVER HOLDS THE OFFICE OF GENERAL, WHENCE STRATEGIES EMANATE. [27: 40]

office of justice 中正之官 *zhōng zhèng zhī guān:* See GALLBLADDER HOLDS THE OFFICE OF JUSTICE, FROM WHICH DECISION EMANATES. [27: 43]

office of labor 作强之官 *zuò qiáng zhī guān:* See KIDNEY HOLDS THE OFFICE OF LABOR, WHENCE AGILITY EMANATES. [27: 54]

office of monarch 君主之官 *jūn zhǔ zhī guān:* See HEART HOLDS THE OFFICE OF MONARCH, WHENCE THE SPIRIT LIGHT EMANATES. [27: 37]

office of reception 受盛之官 *shòu chéng zhī guān:* See SMALL INTESTINE HOLDS THE OFFICE OF RECEPTION, WHENCE THE TRANSFORMATION EMANATES. [27: 38]

office of the granaries 仓廪之官 *cāng lǐn zhī guān:* See SPLEEN AND STOMACH HOLD THE OFFICE OF THE GRANARIES, WHENCE THE FIVE FLAVORS EMANATE. [27: 47]

oil paste 油膏 *yóu gāo:* MEDICINAL PASTE.

oily ashen nail 油灰指甲 *yóu huī zhǐ jiǎ:* ASHEN NAIL.

oily sweat 油汗 *yóu hàn:* Synonym: *sticky sweat.* Sticky oily sweat that does not run easily; observed in yang collapse vacuity desertion patterns. Compare EXPIRATION SWEATING. [26: 344-5]

ointment 软膏 *ruǎn gāo:* A modern preparation made by adding finely ground materials to petroleum jelly (Vaseline) or glycerin. See MEDICINAL PASTE.

old phlegm 老痰 *lǎo tán:* A phlegm pattern arising when fire evil fumes in the upper burner, depressing lung qi, and causing fluids to congeal into phlegm that in time becomes gluey. Old phlegm is characterized by phlegm binding in sticky lumps that adhere to the throat and are difficult to cough up or swallow. Other signs include parched body hair, dry pharynx, thirst, cough and hasty panting, and a complexion that is white like the color of withered bones. ⸤MED⸥ Free depression and downbear fire; soften hardness with cold salty medicinals; moisten the lung and disperse phlegm. Use Two Matured Ingredients Decoction (*èr chén tāng*) plus unripe bitter orange (*zhǐ shí*), pumice (*hǎi fú shí*), mirabilite (*máng xiāo*), scutellaria (*huáng qín*), and indigo (*qīng dài*). [26: 240]

open and closed supplementation and drainage 开阖补泻 *kāi hé bǔ xiè:* A method of achieving supplementation and drainage that involves pressing or not pressing the finger (or an alcohol-soaked swab) on the point after needle extraction. Supplementation is achieved by lightly pressing and rubbing the point after needle extraction to close the hole and prevent channel qi from discharging. Draining is achieved by waggling the needle on extraction without pressing to open the hole and allow channel qi to discharge. Alternatively, slow needle extraction after which the point is quickly pressed with the finger supplements, whereas swift needle extraction with slow pressing of the point drains. *Elementary Questions* (*sù wèn, cì zhì lùn*) states, "Needling repletion, open the needle hole with the left hand; needling vacuity, close the needle hole with the left hand." See NEEDLE MANIPULATION. [26: 709] [46: 470]

opening and discharging 开泄 *kāi xiè*: See OPENING WITH ACRIDITY AND DISCHARGING WITH BITTERNESS.

opening blocks 启闭 *qǐ bì*: OPENING THE ORIFICES.

opening, closing, and pivot 开、合、枢 *kāi, hé, shū*: From *Elementary Questions* (*sù wèn, yīn yáng lí hé lùn*). Interior-exterior levels in the channel system. "Opening" means open to the exterior; "closing" means confined in the interior; "pivot" means located between opening and closing. Among the yang channels, greater yang (*tài yáng*) governs opening, yang brightness (*yáng míng*) governs closing, and lesser yang (*shào yáng*) governs the pivot. Among the yin channels, greater yin (*tài yīn*) governs opening, reverting yin (*jué yīn*) governs closing, and lesser yin (*shào yīn*) governs the pivot. [27: 94]

opening the orifices 开窍 *kāi qiào*: Synonyms: *freeing blocks*; *opening blocks*; *freeing the orifices*; *opening the orifices and arousing the spirit*; *opening the orifices and freeing the spirit*. A method of treatment used to address clouded spirit and coma due to evil obstructing the orifices of the heart. Opening the orifices employs acrid aromatic penetrating medicinals which penetrate the heart and free the orifices, repel foulness, and open blocks. Opening the orifices is applied in the treatment of sudden CLOUDING REVERSAL (clouding of consciousness due to abnormal qi flow) in diseases such as fright wind, epilepsy, wind stroke, or angina pectoris, or in coma caused by internal block occurring in externally contracted heat (febrile) disease. Opening the orifices constitutes emergency treatment of the tip. Its principal effect is to resuscitate the patient, and eliminate distention and oppression in the chest and abdomen caused by foul turbidity. Distinctions are made between the following methods: See CLEARING HEAT AND OPENING THE ORIFICES (cool opening); EXPELLING COLD AND OPENING THE ORIFICES (warm opening); TRANSFORMING PHLEGM AND OPENING THE ORIFICES; CLEARING HEAT, TRANSFORMING PHLEGM, AND OPENING THE ORIFICES. In most cases, prescribed medication comes in the form of prepared formulas. Commonly used orifice-opening medicinals are listed below.

Orifice-Opening Medicinals

麝香 (*shè xiāng*) musk (Moschus)
冰片 (*bīng piàn*) borneol (Borneolum)
苏合香 (*sū hé xiāng*) liquid storax (Styrax Liquidus)
石菖蒲 (*shí chāng pú*) acorus (Acori Rhizoma)

[ACU] To open the orifices of the heart, select as the main points GV-26 (*rén zhōng*, Human Center), KI-1 (*yǒng quán*, Gushing Spring), HT-7 (*shén mén*, Spirit Gate), and PC-8 (*láo gōng*, Palace of Toil); apply wide-range lifting and thrusting and twirling, retaining the needles until the patient regains consciousness. Prick PC-9 (*zhōng chōng*, Central Hub) to bleed. Points may be selected from the following for pricking to bleed in order to enhance the orifice-opening spirit-arousing effect: LU-11 (*shào shāng*, Lesser Shang), LI-1 (*shāng yáng*, Shang Yang), TB-1 (*guān chōng*, Passage Hub), HT-9 (*shào chōng*, Lesser Surge), SI-1 (*shào zé*, Lesser Marsh), SP-1 (*yǐn bái*, Hidden White), LR-1 (*dà dūn*, Large Pile), ST-45 (*lì duì*, Severe Mouth), GB-44 (*zú qiào yīn*, Foot Orifice Yin), and BL-67 (*zhì yīn*, Reaching Yin), See FREEING THE ORIFICES. [6: 265] [27: 275] [97: 75] [14: 54] [46: 729]

opening the orifices and arousing the spirit 开窍醒神 *kāi qiào xǐng shén*: *opening the orifices*.

opening the orifices and freeing the spirit 开窍通神 *kāi qiào tōng shén*: *opening the orifices*.

opening the stomach 开胃 *kāi wèi*: Synonyms: *increasing food intake*; *opening the stomach and increasing food intake*. To increase the appetite. The stomach governs [food] intake. This function is related to the spleen, since the spleen "moves the fluids of the stomach." Opening the stomach thus means increasing the stomach's intake of food. Commonly used stomach-opening medicinals include barley sprout (*mài yá*), crataegus (*shān zhā*), rice sprout (*gǔ yá*), and gizzard lining (*jī nèi jīn*). An example of a stomach-opening formula is Peanut Gruel (*luò huā shēng zhōu*). See also AROUSING THE SPLEEN; DISPERSING FOOD AND ABDUCTING STAGNATION; SUPPLEMENTING THE SPLEEN AND BOOSTING QI. [27: 280] [50: 165]

opening the stomach and increasing food intake 开胃进食 *kāi wèi jìn shí*: OPENING THE STOMACH.

opening with acridity and discharging with bitterness 辛开苦泄 *xīn kāi kǔ xiè*: **1.** A method of treatment that uses acrid-flavored medicinals to diffuse exterior evils and bitter-flavor medicines to clear and drain interior heat. If, for example, a patient has a slight aversion to cold, heat effusion, headache, scant sweat, thirst, sore throat, yellow tongue fur, and a rapid floating pulse, the exterior evil can be effused and dissipated with cool acrid medicinals such as mulberry leaf (*sāng yè*), chrysanthemum (*jú huā*), and vitex (*màn jīng zǐ*), whereas the interior heat can be cleared and discharged with isatis leaf (*dà qīng yè*) and bushy sophora (*shān dòu gēn*). **2.** Synonym: *opening with acridity and downbearing with bitterness*. A method of treatment that uses acrid-flavored medicinals to free phlegm-damp in the chest and stomach duct and bitter-flavored medicinals to treat damp-heat in the chest and stomach duct. The two can be used together to treat phlegm-damp-heat obstruction causing glomus and oppression, distention and fullness, and nausea and vomiting. This method makes use of acrid medicinals such as magnolia bark (*hòu pò*), bitter orange (*zhǐ ké*), ginger pinellia (*jiāng bàn xià*), and tangerine peel (*chén pí*), and bitter medicinals such as coptis (*huáng lián*) and scutellaria (*huáng qín*). [27: 249] [25: 167] [6: 250]

opening with acridity and downbearing with bitterness 辛开苦降 *xīn kāi kǔ jiàng*: OPENING WITH ACRIDITY AND DISCHARGING WITH BITTERNESS.²

open mouth and closed eyes 口开目合 *kǒu kāi mù hé*: A sign observed in desertion patterns.

oppression in the chest 胸闷 *xiōng mèn*: Synonym: *thoracic oppression*. Discomfort and vexation in the chest caused by damp-heat or phlegm-damp obstructing the central burner and inhibiting qi. Compare OPPRESSION IN THE HEART AND CHEST and STIFLING OPPRESSION IN THE HEART AND CHEST. [27: 377]

oppression in the heart and chest 心胸郁闷 *xīn xiōng yù mèn*: See OPPRESSION IN THE CHEST.

oral gan 口疳 *kǒu gān*: GAN OF THE MOUTH.

orally taken paste 内服膏剂 *nèi fú gāo jì*: RICH PASTE.

oral putrefaction 口糜 *kǒu mí*: A white mold-like coating covering the tongue and the whole of the surface of the oral cavity, or small patches of mucosal erosion known as erosion spots. Oral putrefaction indicates the development of sweltering damp-heat in patterns of damage to yin by stomach vacuity. This generally occurs in enduring or severe illnesses and indicates complex patterns that are difficult to cure. [6: 124] [27: 499] [97: 31]

organ 脏腑 *zàng fǔ*: The English term organ is used to denote a bowel or viscus. See BOWELS AND VISCERA.

organ cough 五脏六腑咳 *wǔ zàng liù fǔ ké*: FIVE BOWELS AND SIX VISCERA COUGH.

organ fright pattern 脏腑惊证 *zàng fǔ jīng zhèng*: BOWEL AND VISCERAL FRIGHT PATTERN.

organ pattern identification 脏腑辨证 *zàng fǔ biàn zhèng*: BOWEL AND VISCERAL PATTERN IDENTIFICATION.

organ qi 脏腑之气 *zàng fǔ zhī qì*: BOWEL AND VISCERAL QI.

organ stroke 中脏腑 *zhòng zàng fǔ*: BOWEL AND VISCERAL STROKE.

Oriental medicine 东方医学 *dōng fāng yī xué*: Chinese medicine and the medical arts of Korea, Japan, and other Far Eastern lands that developed from it. In China, this term is rarely used.

orifice 窍 *qiào*: Any one of the openings of the body. The *upper orifices* or *clear orifices* are the eyes, ears, nostrils, and mouth, whereas the *lower orifices* or *turbid orifices* are the anal and genital orifices. These are collectively referred to as the *nine orifices*. ◇ Chin 窍 *qiào*, aperture, opening, literally or symbolically in the sense of receptivity and alertness. Eng from L. *orificium*, orifice. [48: 250] [50: 1318]

orifice of the heart 心窍 *xīn qiào*: **1.** The tongue. *Elementary Questions* (*sù wèn*) says, "The heart governs the tongue... its orifice is the tongue." See HEART GOVERNS THE TONGUE. **2.** (Plural in English) The orifices of the heart spirit. Chinese medicine traditionally holds that when the "orifices of the heart" are free and uninhibited, the spirit-mind is clear, and that when the orifices of the heart are blocked, there is clouded spirit, mania, or withdrawal. Although the literal meaning "orifices of the heart" implies that the term denotes a physical entity, the location and nature of the entity is not explained. Thus the term either denotes a speculative entity or is merely a metaphor describing consciousness as a "window" on the outside world. See PHLEGM CONFOUNDING THE ORIFICES OF THE HEART; OPENING THE ORIFICES. [97: 118] [26: 95]

orifice opening 开窍 *kāi qiào*: See OPENING THE ORIFICES.

orifices of the kidney 肾窍 *shèn qiào*: The ears. See KIDNEY OPENS AT THE EARS. [26: 693]

orifices of the lung 肺窍 *fèi qiào*: The nostrils or nose.

origin 元 *yuán*: Beginning; source. In Chinese medicine, "origin" appears in the terms ORIGINAL QI and LOWER ORIGIN (the kidney). It connotes the basis of life. The character 元 is also a synonym of 玄, dark, mysterious. [48: 19]

original house (mansion) 元府 *yuán fǔ*: MYSTERIOUS HOUSE. [26: 101]

original qi 元气 *yuán qì*: **1.** Source qi. **2.** Right qi. NB: This term does not appear in *The Inner Canon* (*nèi jīng*). [26: 101] [97: 42] [27: 78] [25: 32] [48: 19]

original qi vacuity 元气虚弱 *yuán qì xū ruò*: QI VACUITY. [26: 101]

original yang 元阳 *yuán yáng*: Kidney yang seen as the origin of life, standing in complementary opposition to original yang (kidney yin). See KIDNEY YIN AND KIDNEY YANG. [26: 101]

original yin 元阴 *yuán yīn*: Kidney yin seen as the origin of life, standing in complementary opposition to original yin (kidney yang). See KIDNEY YIN AND KIDNEY YANG; HEAVENLY TENTH. [26: 101] [27: 52] [97: 42]

ouch point 阿是穴 *ā shì xué*: *Synonym: a-shi point*. Points that are sensitive to palpation and chosen as sites for acupuncture treatment. These points are most often used to treat disorders in their immediate vicinity, but also treat disorders distant from the point. Ouch points are not necessarily located on the channels. Because their locations vary and reflect the disease and its relationship to the patient, these points are inherently unchartable. ◇ Chin 阿 *ā*, oh!; 是 *shì*, to be. The character combination literally means "ah, that's it!", but is probably influenced by the ahing and hissing that pressure on a tender spot often elicits. [27: 321]

outcrop 胬肉 *nǔ ròu*: EXCRESCENCE. See EXCRESCENCE CREEPING OVER THE EYE.

outer assisting bone 外辅骨 *wài fǔ gǔ*: The smaller bone of the lower leg. [WMC] fibula. [27: 71] [27: 71] [97: 159]

outer body 外 *wài*: The outer part of the body, the exterior.

outer canthus 外眦 *wài zì*, 小眦 *xiǎo zì*, 锐眦 *ruì zì*: The outer angle of the eye. [26: 212]

outpour diarrhea 注泻 *zhù xiè*: WATER DIARRHEA. [97: 367]

outthrust 透 *tòu*: The spontaneous or induced forcing of evils to and through the exterior of the body, including those which provoke maculopapular outthrust (outbreak of rash) on so doing.

outthrusting papules 透疹 *tòu zhěn*: *Synonym: outthrusting the exterior*. A method of treatment used to promote the eruption of macules in the initial stage of measles. [MED] Outthrusting macules makes use of cool acrid exterior-resolving medicinals such as mint (*bò hé*), schizonepeta (*jīng jiè*), forsythia (*lián qiáo*), coriander (*hú suī*), scallion white (*cōng bái*), cicada molting (*chán tuì*), arctium (*niú bàng zǐ*), tamarisk (*chēng liǔ*), pueraria (*gé gēn*), and platycodon (*jié gěng*). Examples of macule-outthrusting formulas include Toxin-Diffusing Exterior-Effusing Decoction (*xuān dú fā biǎo tāng*), Cimicifuga and Pueraria Decoction (*shēng má gé gēn tāng*), and Bamboo Leaf, Tamarisk, and Arctium Decoction (*zhú yè liǔ bàng tāng*). See MEASLES. [27: 248] [97: 475] [50: 1258] [60: 327]

outthrusting macules 透斑 *tòu bān*: A method of treatment used in febrile disease marked by exuberant internal heat to clear heat and cool the blood in order to treat faint macules that have not fully erupted. A representative macule-outthrusting formula is Macule-Transforming Decoction (*huà bān tāng*), which contains crude gypsum (*shēng shí gāo*), anemarrhena (*zhī mǔ*), raw licorice (*shēng gān cǎo*), scrophularia (*xuán shēn*), rhinoceros horn (*xī jiǎo*), and rice. The method known as cooling the blood and transforming macules makes use of the same formula, Macule-Transforming Decoction (*huà bān tāng*), plus moutan (*mǔ dān pí*), dried/fresh rehmannia (*shēng dì huáng*), isatis leaf (*dà qīng yè*), and lonicera (*jīn yín huā*) and minus raw licorice (*shēng gān cǎo*), and rice. [27: 248]

outthrusting the exterior 透表 *tòu biǎo*: OUTTHRUSTING PAPULES.

overcoming dampness 胜湿 *shèng shī*: Dispel dampness, especially when wind medicinals are used. See WIND CAN OVERCOME DAMPNESS.

overwhelming 相乘 *xiāng chéng*: In the doctrine of the five phases, an abnormal exaggeration of restraining, where one of the phases is weakened, causing the phase that under normal circumstances would overcome it to invade and weaken it further. For example, wood normally restrains earth, but if earth is weak, then wood overwhelms it, rendering earth even weaker. In terms of the viscera, this means that the spleen, normally only restrained by the liver, will, if weak, be completely overwhelmed, becoming even weaker. [6: 29] [27: 10] [97: 387]

oxhide lichen 牛皮癣 *niú pí xiǎn*: : An episodic skin disease characterized by thickening and hardening of the skin that gives it the appearance of the skin of an ox's neck. Oxhide lichen starts with itching, the appearance of irregular flat papules, and in some cases browning of the skin. Subsequently, the papules coalesce and the skin becomes dry and hard with sores that weep and that are itchy especially at night. It is attributed to wind-damp-heat toxin depressed in the skin or to insufficiency of construction-blood and blood vacuity engendering wind and depriving the skin of nourishment. It is often associated with emotional disturbances. [WMC] neurodermatitis. . [MED] Quicken the blood and course wind; clear heat and dispel dampness. Oral: Tangkuei Drink (*dāng guī yǐn zi*). Topical: Ill-Wind Oil Paste (*fēng yóu gāo*). [ACU] Select ouch points (*ā shì xué*), BL-17 (*gé shū*, Diaphragm Transport), BL-12 (*fēng mén*, Wind Gate), BL-40 (*wěi zhōng*, Bend Center), LI-4 (*hé gǔ*, Union Valley), LI-11 (*qū chí*, Pool at the Bend), SP-9 (*yīn líng quán*, Yin Mound Spring), and SP-6 (*sān yīn jiāo*, Three Yin Intersection). Needle with drainage. Tap and cup the ouch points to bring out the depressed heat in the blood aspect. The affected area can be needled obliquely from all sides toward the center. For pronounced itching, add Itch Reliever (*zhǐ yǎng*). See LICHEN. [26: 155] [27: 475] [97: 109] [13: 562] [113: 445]

P

pain 痛 *tòng*, 疼 *téng*, 疼痛 *téng tòng*: A more or less localized feeling of discomfort, distress, or agony that is felt as a result of knocks and falls, cuts in the flesh, severe hunger, contact with fire or hot objects, or various ailments of the body. It can affect any part of the body and occurs in both externally contracted disease and internal damage. Pain is a major item of diagnostic information, and its significance depends on its nature and location.

Types of Pain

ACHING PAIN (*suān tòng*)

DISTENDING PAIN (*zhàng tòng*)

DULL PAIN (*yǐn tòng*)

EMPTY PAIN (*kōng tòng*)

COLD PAIN (*lěng tòng*)

GRIPPING PAIN (*jiǎo tòng*)

HEAVY PAIN (*zhòng tòng*)

PULLING PAIN (*chè tòng*)

SCORCHING PAIN (*zhuó tòng*)

SCURRYING PAIN (*cuàn tòng*)

STABBING PAIN (*cì tòng*)

SORENESS (*tòng*)

Aching pain (酸痛 *suān tòng*) is a pain of continuous duration, felt in the sinews and bones. It is attributable to yin vacuity, yang vacuity, or evils such as cold and dampness. An example is aching lumbus. **Distending pain** (胀痛 *zhàng tòng*), or distention and pain, is pain associated with a feeling of expansion or inflation that may or may not be accompanied by visible or palpable enlargement. It may be experienced in the head, eyes, trunk, or limbs. It is essentially the manifestation of depressed qi dynamic. Qi is formless (insubstantial) and likes to move without being obstructed. When cold congealing in the channels, exuberant fire-heat, impairment of organ function, or poor supply of nourishment to the channels and vessels cause inhibition of qi dynamic, qi ceases to flow smoothly and becomes depressed and gathers. Stomach duct pain due to cold stagnating in the center burner, chest and rib-side pain due to binding depression of liver qi, and headache due to ascendant liver yang are forms of distending pain. **Dull pain** (隐痛 *yǐn tòng*) is a muted, usually persistent pain that is generally bearable. It is attributable to insufficiency of qi and blood, or to

yang qi vacuity failing. **Empty pain** (空痛 *kōng tòng*) is pain associated with a feeling of emptiness and lightness, that likes warmth and pressure. It is associated mainly with insufficiency of essence-blood and may be observed in yang vacuity, yin vacuity, blood vacuity, or in dual vacuity of yin and yang. **Cold pain** (冷痛 *lěng tòng*) is pain associated with an icy sensation. If it is in the surface of the body, the coldness can be felt with the hand. Cold pain is usually accompanied by a desire for warm and hot things. It is attributed to internal or external cold congealing in the sinew vessels and obstructing the channels. Cold is a yin evil that is cold in nature; it easily damages yang qi, and causes a loss in warmth of yang qi wherever it becomes lodged. **Gripping pain** (绞痛 *jiǎo tòng*) is an excruciating acute pain that feels as if the affected area were being wrung and twisted or gouged by a knife. It is usually caused by tangible evils obstructing the channels and network vessels or congealing cold depressing normal qi dynamic. Gripping pain is observed in heart pain due to heart blood stasis (CHEST IMPEDIMENT) or lower abdominal or lumbar pain due to stone strangury, stomach duct pain and abdomen due to ROUNDWORM REVERSAL, or in heat cholera. **Heavy pain** (重痛 *zhòng tòng*) is a pain associated with a feeling of heaviness. It causes a tendency to remain in a lying posture and move little. The pain itself is often an aching pain. Heavy pain is attributable to dampness evil—invading the body from outside or arising within it from spleen vacuity—obstructing qi dynamic. Headache with HEAD HEAVY AS IF SWATHED (bag-over-the-head sensation) and heavy aching limbs are examples of heavy pain. **Pulling pain** (掣痛 *chè tòng*) is a pain associated with a sensation of tension or pulling or a pain that stretches into another area. It arises when the sinew vessels are deprived of nourishment or obstructed. For example, when heart blood stasis deprives the sinew network vessels of nourishment, the sinews become hypertonic. This causes the pulling pain characteristic of chest impediment patterns, where pain stretches through to the back. The liver governs the sinews, and when there is heat in the liver channel, scorching of the sinew vessels causes the sinews to become hypertonic, or when liver yin is insufficient, the sinews are deprived of nourishment and similarly become hypertonic. Hence, pulling pain is largely attributed to the liver. It is observed in chest impediment, liver yin vacuity, and liver channel repletion heat. **Scorching pain** (灼痛 *zhuó tòng*) is a hot burning pain. If the pain is on the surface of the body (such as in sores), the heat can actually be felt with the hand. Usually, it is ascribed to fire-heat evils in the channels or to vacuity heat scorching the channels and network vessels; it is associated with a desire for cool and cold things. Examples include scorching pain the both rib-sides due to liver fire invading the network vessels, and scorching stomach duct pain due to insufficiency of stomach yin. Sores due to heat toxin also commonly manifest in scorching pain and swelling. **Scurrying pain** (窜痛 *cuàn tòng*) is one that repeatedly changes location or one whose location is difficult to pinpoint. Its general location and movement are related to channel pathways. It is associated with qi stagnation or with wind evil obstructing the channels. Hence it is often seen in binding depression of the liver qi and in WIND IMPEDIMENT. **Stabbing pain** (刺痛 *cì tòng*) is like the stabbing of a needle or knife and is limited to a small area of fixed location. It is often described as being like the "cutting of a knife," the "stabbing of a knife," or the "piercing of an awl." It arises when the blood, owing to qi vacuity, qi stagnation, blood vacuity, etc., is obstructed and becomes static, thus blocking channel qi. This type of pain is often referred to as STASIS PAIN. **Soreness** (痛 *tòng*) is pain associated with open wounds or with redness and swelling (e.g., of the eyes or throat). The distinction between pain and soreness made in English does not exist in Chinese. The significance of pain in different locations is discussed on the entries listed below. See also QI PAIN; IMPEDIMENT. [29: 190]

Pain by Location

HEADACHE (*tóu tòng*)

EAR PAIN (*ěr tòng*)

EYE PAIN (*mù tòng*)

RED SORE SWOLLEN EYES (*yǎn jīng hóng zhǒng tòng*)

FACIAL PAIN (*miàn tòng*)

TOOTHACHE (*yá tòng*)

CRICK IN THE NECK (*luò zhěn*)

SORE THROAT (*hóu lóng tòng*)

SHOULDER PAIN (*jiān tòng*)

BACK PAIN (*bèi tòng*)

LUMBAR PAIN (*yāo tòng*)

PAIN IN THE LIMBS (*zhī tǐ téng tòng*)

HEEL PAIN (*zú gēn tòng*)

PAIN IN THE HEART OF THE SOLE (*zú xīn tòng*)

SINEW PAIN (*jīn tòng*)

BONE PAIN (*gǔ tòng*)

JOINT PAIN (*gǔ jié tòng*)

GENERALIZED PAIN (*shēn tòng*)

CHEST PAIN (*xiōng tòng*)

HEART PAIN (*xīn tòng*)

TRUE HEART PAIN (*zhēn xīn tòng*)

RIB-SIDE PAIN (*xié tòng*)

STOMACH PAIN (*wèi tòng*)

STOMACH DUCT PAIN (*wèi wǎn (guǎn) tòng*)

ABDOMINAL PAIN (*fù tòng*)

LESSER-ABDOMINAL PAIN (*shào fù tòng*)

PAINFUL URINATION (*niào tòng*)

MENSTRUAL PAIN (*tòng jīng*)

---

pain at the vertex 巅顶痛 *diān dǐng tòng*: VERTEX HEADACHE.

pain below the heart 心下痛 *xīn xià tòng*: Pain in the pit of the stomach. See STOMACH DUCT PAIN. [26: 90]

painful impediment 痛痹 *tòng bì*: COLD IMPEDIMENT.

painful pendulous external kidney 外肾吊痛 *wài shèn diào tòng*: A condition characterized by painful sagging of the scrotum observed in certain mounting (*shàn*) diseases. ACU Traditionally, treatment often involved burning five cones of moxa at the transverse creases of the underside of the middle joint of the great and second toes. An alternative treatment is to needle or moxa LR-1 (*dà dūn*, Large Pile), LR-3 (*tài chōng*, Supreme Surge), ST-30 (*qì chōng*, Qi Thoroughfare), and SP-6 (*sān yīn jiāo*, Three Yin Intersection). [26: 213] [50: 453]

painful swelling of the yin door 阴户肿痛 *yīn hù zhǒng tòng*: Painful swelling of the *orificium vaginae*, sometimes with rough (disfluent) urination, lower abdominal discomfort, and even heat effusion and aversion to cold. It attributed to depressed anger damaging the liver, liver qi invading the spleen, and damp-heat pouring downward. MED Clear heat and disinhibit dampness with variations of Gentian Liver-Draining Decoction (*lóng dǎn xiè gān tāng*) as oral medication, and a combination of cnidium seed (*shé chuáng zǐ*), kochia (*dì fū zǐ*), phellodendron (*huáng bǎi*), ledebouriella (*fáng fēng*), and flavescent sophora (*kǔ shēn*) prepared as a steam-wash. ACU Base treatment mainly on CV, LR, and SP. Select CV-3 (*zhōng jí*, Central Pole) BL-34 (*xià liáo*, Lower Bone-Hole), LR-2 (*xíng jiān*, Moving Between), SP-9 (*yīn líng quán*, Yin Mound Spring), and SP-6 (*sān yīn jiāo*, Three Yin Intersection); needle with drainage. Also, use a moxa pole to smoke (rather than warm) the affected area for pain relief. [26: 616]

painful urination 尿痛 *niào tòng*: A stinging or burning pain in the urethra on urination with difficulty voiding. It is a chief common feature of strangury patterns. See URINE.

pain in the heart of the sole 足心痛 *zú xīn tòng*: Pain in the center of the sole of the foot, at KI-1 (*yǒng quán*, Gushing Spring). It is usually due to kidney vacuity damp fixity and the life gate fire failing to spread warmth, in which case it is associated with heat pain in the ankle bone and treated with Kidney Fixity Decoction (*shèn zhuó tāng*) combined with Eight-Ingredient Pill (*bā wèi wán*). Pain in the heart of the sole may also be attributable to streaming damp phlegm, which is observed in obese people, and is experienced when the patient walks after long sitting or lying. This is treated with Kidney Fixity Decoction (*shèn zhuó tāng*) combined with Mysterious Two Powder (*èr miào sǎn*). ACU Base treatment mainly on BL, KI and ouch points (*ā shì xué*). Main points: BL-62 (*shēn mài*, Extending Vessel), BL-63 (*jīn mén*, Metal Gate), KI-3 (*tài xī*, Great Ravine), and KI-1 (*yǒng quán*, Gushing Spring). For kidney vacuity damp fixity and the life gate fire failing to spread warmth, add BL-23 (*shèn shū*, Kidney Transport), GV-4 (*mìng mén*, Life Gate), KI-3 (*tài xī*, Great Ravine), KI-7 (*fù liū*, Recover Flow), SP-9 (*yīn líng quán*, Yin Mound Spring), and ST-36 (*zú sān lǐ*, Leg Three Li); needle with supplementation and large amounts of moxa, and add KI-6 (*zhào hǎi*, Shining Sea) for ankle pain. For streaming damp phlegm in obese people, add CV-12 (*zhōng wǎn*, Center Stomach Duct), ST-36 (*zú sān lǐ*, Leg Three Li), ST-40 (*fēng lóng*, Bountiful Bulge), and SP-9 (*yīn líng quán*, Yin Mound Spring); needle with even supplementation and drainage and moxa, if appropriate. [50: 754] [26: 647] [113: 432] [46: 597] [37: 440]

pain in the heart [region] and abdomen 心腹痛 *xīn fù tòng*: See ABDOMINAL PAIN; STOMACH DUCT PAIN.

pain in the limbs 四肢痛 *sì zhī tòng*: Pain in one or more of the limbs. Pain in the limbs is usually caused by wind-cold-damp invading the channels and network vessels, the flesh, and the joints, obstructing the movement of qi. *Elementary Questions* (*sù wèn, bì lùn*) states, "When wind, cold, and damp evils concur and combine, they give rise to IMPEDIMENT (*bì*)." Pain in the limbs can also arise as a result of spleen and stomach. The spleen governs the limbs, and spleen vacuity can cause limb pain. The location and nature of pain in the limbs provides useful diagnostic evidence: Pain in the joints and scurrying pain is usually WIND IMPEDIMENT; Acute pain in the joints exacerbated by cold and relieved by warmth is usually COLD IMPEDIMENT; joint pain with heavy cumbersome body usually indicates DAMP IMPEDIMENT; scorching pain in the joints that likes cold, in some cases with redness and swelling, is usually HEAT IMPEDIMENT; dull pain in the heel or lower leg and knee is usually insufficiency of kidney qi. [29: 192]

pain in the lumbar spine 腰脊痛 *yāo jǐ tòng*: Pain in the spinal vertebrae and adjacent areas. It is caused by sprains, collection of static blood, wind-cold-damp evel invading the channels, and taxation damaging the kidney. [50: 1619]

pain in the soles of the foot 足心痛 *zú xīn tòng*: See PAIN IN THE HEART OF THE SOLE.

pain in the umbilical region 脐腹痛 *qí fù tòng*: Pain in the region of the navel; attributed to congealing cold, spleen-kidney yang vacuity, yang brightness heat bind, gastrointestinal qi stagnation, brewing damp-heat, food damage, or roundworm. **Congealing cold** causes sudden acute pain in the umbilical region without respite that is slightly relieved by warmth, and that is accompanied by no thought of food and drink, rumbling intestines, abdominal cold, diarrhea or constipation, and, in severe cases, reversal cold of the extremities. The tongue is pale or green-blue with a moist white fur, and a sunken tight slow pulse. MED Warm the center and dissipate cold; rectify qi and relieve pain. Use Tiantai Lindera Powder (*tiān tái wū yào sǎn*) plus agents such as dried ginger (*gān jiāng*) and cinnamon bark (*ròu guì*). For constipation, variations of Spleen-Warming Decoction (*wēn pí tāng*) can be used. ACU Base treatment mainly on CV, ST, SP, and LI. Main points: CV-12 (*zhōng wǎn*, Center Stomach Duct), ST-25 (*tiān shū*, Celestial Pivot), and ST-36 (*zú sān lǐ*, Leg Three Li). For congealing cold, add SP-4 (*gōng sūn*, Yellow Emperor), CV-8 (*shén què*, Spirit Gate Tower)ⓜ, and CV-4 (*guān yuán*, Pass Head)ⓜ; needle with drainage and add moxa. **Spleen-kidney yang vacuity** causes continual intermittent pain in the umbilical region that like warmth and pressure and that is exacerbated by exposure to cold. This is accompanied by coldlimbs and fear of cold, thin sloppy stool, pale tongue with a thin white fur, and a weak fine sunken pulse. MED Supplement the spleen and kidney; warm yang and relieve pain. Use Aconite Center-Rectifying Pill (*fù zǐ lǐ zhōng wán*) or use Yin-Rectifying Brew (*lǐ yīn jiān*) plus cinnamon bark (*ròu guì*) and white peony (*bái sháo yào*). ACU To the main points given above add BL-23 (*shèn shū*, Kidney Transport), BL-20 (*pí shū*, Spleen Transport), CV-4 (*guān yuán*, Pass Head), CV-6 (*qì hǎi*, Sea of Qi), and GV-4 (*mìng mén*, Life Gate); needle with supplementation and moxa. **Yang brightness heat bind** causes pain in the umbilical region with fullness that refuses pressure. This is accompanied by tidal heat [effusion], STREAMING SWEAT at the extremities, constipation or in some cases watery diarrhea, short voidings of reddish urine, a red tongue with thick dry yellow fur, and a rapid slippery sunken pulse. MED Clear heat and induce draining precipitation. Use Stomach-Regulating Qi-Coordinating

Decoction (*tiáo wèi chéng qì tāng*), Major Qi-Coordinating Decoction (*dà chéng qì tāng*), and Minor Qi-Coordinating Decoction (*xiǎo chéng qì tāng*). ACU To the main points add BL-25 (*dà cháng shū*, Large Intestine Transport), LI-4 (*hé gǔ*, Union Valley), LI-11 (*qū chí*, Pool at the Bend), ST-44 (*nèi tíng*, Inner Court), ST-37 (*shàng jù xū*, Upper Great Hollow), and TB-6 (*zhī gōu*, Branch Ditch); needle with drainage. **Gastrointestinal qi stagnation** causes pain in the umbilical region less severe than the accompanying fullness and relieved by the passing of flatus and worsened by affect-mind ill-being. There is no desire for food and drink, a thin white tongue fur, and slippery stringlike pulse. MED Downbear qi and dissipate binds; regulate the center and relieve pain. Use variations of Five Milled Ingredients Drink (*wǔ mò yǐn zi*). ACU To the main points add CV-17 (*shān zhōng*, Chest Center), PC-6 (*nèi guān*, Inner Pass), CV-6 (*qì hǎi*, Sea of Qi), and LR-3 (*tài chōng*, Supreme Surge); needle with drainage. **Brewing damp-heat** causes pain in the umbilical region and tenesmus in dysentery. The stool is thick, sticky, and foul-smelling and contains pus and blood. In addition, there is bitter taste in the mouth, dry mouth with no desire to drink, a dark red tongue with a thick slimy yellow fur, and a slippery rapid pulse. MED Clear damp-heat and rectify qi and blood to relieve pain. Use variations of Peony Decoction (*sháo yào tāng*). ACU To the main points add LI-4 (*hé gǔ*, Union Valley), LI-11 (*qū chí*, Pool at the Bend), ST-44 (*nèi tíng*, Inner Court), and ST-37 (*shàng jù xū*, Upper Great Hollow); needle with drainage. **Food damage accumulation** can causes pain in the umbilical region relieved by the passing of flatus or by defecation. There is belching, upflow and nausea, no thought of food and drink, and sometimes diarrhea. Stool contains largely undigested food, and is sour-smelling and malodorous. The tongue fur is thick and slimy at the root, and the pulse is slippery. MED Disperse accumulation and abduct stagnation. Use Saussurea and Areca Pill (*mù xiāng bīng láng wán*) or Unripe Bitter Orange Stagnation-Abducting Pill (*zhǐ shí dǎo zhì wán*). ACU To the main points add Li Inner Court (*lǐ nèi tíng*), CV-21 (*xuán jī*, Jade Swivel), CV-10 (*xià wǎn*, Lower Stomach Duct), and CV-6 (*qì hǎi*, Sea of Qi); needle with drainage. **Round worm** can cause intense pain with periods of complete relief. Sometimes an accumulation lump can be observed. Other signs include emaciation, periodic vomiting of clear water. In some cases, there may be grinding of the teeth in sleep, perverted appetite, passage of worms in the stool, or gray patches on the mouth and face. During attacks of pain, the pulse becomes wiry or sunken and hidden. MED Expel and kill roundworm. Use Worm-Transforming

Pill (*huà chóng wán*) or variations. ACU To the main points add SP-4 (*gōng sūn*, Yellow Emperor), BL-20 (*pí shū*, Spleen Transport), Hundred Worm Nest (*bǎi chóng wō*), and ST-4 (*dì cāng*, Earth Granary); needle with drainage. [92: No. 201] [4: 99] [37: 316–320] [46: 662, 735] [113: 102, 217]

pain like the cutting of a knife 痛如刀割 *tòng rú dāo gē*: See STABBING PAIN; PAIN.

pain like the piercing of an awl 痛如锥刺 *tòng rú zhuī cì*: See STABBING PAIN; PAIN.

pain like the stabbing of a knife 痛如刀刺 *tòng rú dāo cì*: See STABBING PAIN; PAIN.

pain wind 痛风 *tòng fēng*: **1.** *Synonym: white tiger joint-running wind.* An IMPEDIMENT (*bì*) pattern characterized by acute pain of unfixed location. See JOINT-RUNNING WIND. **2.** COLD IMPEDIMENT. [26: 672]

palace 宫 *gōng*: The word "palace" is used in names of parts of the body and acupuncture points. It commonly represents the heart, as in the formula name Peaceful Palace Bovine Bezoar Pill (*ān gōng niú huáng wán*). SEE HEART HOLDS THE OFFICE OF MONARCH, WHENCE THE SPIRIT LIGHT EMANATES.

palace of essence 精宫 *jīng gōng*: ESSENCE CHAMBER².

pale menstrual flow 经来色淡 *jīng lái sè dàn*: Menstrual discharge that is paler than normal in color. Pale menstrual flow is attributable to dual vacuity of qi and blood and spleen-kidney yang vacuity preventing normal movement and transformation. MED Supplement qi and blood to regulate menstruation. Use Eight-Gem Decoction (*bā zhēn tāng*) plus astragalus (*huáng qí*), cyperus (*xiāng fù zǐ*), and fresh ginger (*shēng jiāng*). Take Six-Ingredient Rehmannia Pill (*liù wèi dì huáng wán*) on a regular basis. For severe vacuity, dried ginger (*gān jiāng*) and aconite (*fù zǐ*) may also be used. ACU Base treatment mainly on back transport points, CV, SP, ST, and KI. Select BL-17 (*gé shū*, Diaphragm Transport), BL-20 (*pí shū*, Spleen Transport), BL-23 (*shèn shū*, Kidney Transport), CV-6 (*qì hǎi*, Sea of Qi), CV-4 (*guān yuán*, Pass Head), SP-6 (*sān yīn jiāo*, Three Yin Intersection), ST-36 (*zú sān lǐ*, Leg Three Li), KI-3 (*tài xī*, Great Ravine), and GV-4 (*mìng mén*, Life Gate); needle with supplementation and moxa. [26: 815] [46: 594, 683]

pale tongue 舌淡 *shé dàn*: A pale tongue indicates vacuity of qi and blood. A well-moistened pale enlarged tongue with accompanying cold signs indicates yang qi vacuity. [6: 122]

pale white facial complexion 面色淡白 *miàn sè dàn bái*: A colorless complexion. "Pale" denotes the absence of color, whereas "white" is the color associated with the metal among the five phases. Compare SOMBER WHITE FACIAL COM-

PLEXION and BRIGHT WHITE FACIAL COMPLEXION. [6: 116]

palm heart toxin sore 掌心毒 *zhǎng xīn dú*:
A CLOVE SORE in the middle of palm attributed to intense fire toxin in the heart or pericardium channel. A palm heart toxin sore starts with a small macule or papule that subsequently becomes a hard swollen blister with local pain and itching. The sore is deeply rooted. In severe cases, it is shiny and turns black, with severe local pain and swelling. It can fester and cause deep erosion into the sinew and bone. At this stage alternating heat [effusion] and [aversion to] cold and loss of appetite may be observed. In the early stages, it can be treated by lancing the blister, and prescribing Immortal Formula Life-Giving Beverage (*xiān fāng huó mìng yǐn*) plus turmeric (*jiāng huáng*) and cinnamon twig (*guì zhī*). ACU Base treatment mainly on GV, LI, and PC. Select GV-12 (*shēn zhù*, Body Pillar), GV-10 (*líng tái*, Spirit Tower), LI-4 (*hé gǔ*, Union Valley), BL-40 (*wěi zhōng*, Bend Center), and PC-7 (*dà líng*, Great Mound); needle with drainage and prick PC-9 (*zhōng chōng*, Central Hub) to bleed. For alternating heat [effusion] and [aversion to] cold, add GV-14 (*dà zhuī*, Great Hammer), and LI-11 (*qū chí*, Pool at the Bend), See CLOVE SORE. [27: 469] [26: 720] [97: 557] [113: 356] [37: 441]

palm heart wind 掌心风 *zhǎng xīn fēng*: Goosefoot wind limited to the heart of the palm. See GOOSE-FOOT WIND. [27: 475]

palpation 切诊 *qiè zhěn*, 触诊 *chù zhěn*: One of the FOUR EXAMINATIONS; the process of examining the surface of the body by touch to detect the presence of disease. The pulse examination, an essential part of routine examination, is the most common form of palpation. Palpation of other parts of the body is called body palpation. See PULSE EXAMINATION; BODY PALPATION.

palpitation heart pain 悸心痛 *jì xīn tòng*: Synonym: *vacuity heart pain*. Heart pain associated with heart palpitations. Palpitation heart pain is an intermittent pain that likes pressure and heat, and that is exacerbated by hunger. The pulse is vacuous and weak. MED Supplement the heart and spleen using formulas such as Spleen-Returning Decoction (*guī pí tāng*), Astragalus Center-Fortifying Decoction (*huáng qí jiàn zhōng tāng*), and Mysterious Fragrance Powder (*miào xiāng sǎn*). ACU Base treatment mainly on CV, BL, and PC. Select CV-17 (*shān zhōng*, Chest Center), BL-15 (*xīn shū*, Heart Transport), BL-20 (*pí shū*, Spleen Transport), BL-14 (*jué yīn shū*, Reverting Yin Transport), CV-14 (*jù què*, Great Tower Gate), PC-6 (*nèi guān*, Inner Pass), HT-5 (*tōng lǐ*, Connecting Li), PC-4 (*xī mén*, Cleft Gate), ST-36 (*zú sān lǐ*, Leg Three Li), and SP-6 (*sān yīn jiāo*,

Three Yin Intersection); needle with supplementation and moxa. [26: 592] [37: 332, 335] [46: 734]

palpitations 心悸 *xīn jì*: HEART PALPITATIONS; PALPITATIONS BELOW THE HEART.

palpitations below the heart 心下悸 *xīn xià jì*:
1. Palpitations felt in the region below the heart, i.e., in the stomach duct. From *On Cold Damage* (*shāng hán lùn, biàn tài yáng bìng mài zhèng bìng lùn*), "After excessive promotion of sweating, when the person crosses his hands over the heart trying to press the palpitations below the heart, this is treated with Cinnamon Twig and Licorice Decoction (*guì zhī gān cǎo tāng*)." **2.** HEART PALPITATIONS. [26: 90] [27: 147] [97: 118]

panting 喘 *chuǎn*, 气喘 *qì chuǎn*: Hasty, rapid, labored breathing with discontinuity between inhalation and exhalation, in severe cases with gaping mouth, raised shoulders, flaring nostrils, and inability to lie down. When associated with counterflow movement of qi, it is sometimes called *panting counterflow*. When breathing is usually rapid, it is sometimes called *hasty panting*. When in severe cases it is associated with raising of the shoulders and flaring nostrils, it is RAISED-SHOULDER BREATHING. Panting is a manifestation of impaired diffusion and downbearing of lung qi. Since the LUNG IS THE GOVERNOR OF QI and the KIDNEY IS THE ROOT OF QI, panting is associated primarily with disease of the lung and or kidney. Panting occurs in repletion and vacuity. Repletion panting may occur when externally contracted wind-heat or wind-cold invade the lung, when depressed liver qi invades the lung, or when phlegm arising from spleen-lung vacuity obstructs the lung. Vacuity panting occurs in dual vacuity of lung yin and lung qi, and in failure of the kidney to absorb qi. Kidney vacuity with phlegm obstruction and yang vacuity water flood are vacuity-repletion complexes that may also give rise to panting. The difference between vacuity and repletion panting is succinctly elucidated in *Jing-Yue's Complete Compendium* (*jǐng yuè quán shū*) as follows: "In repletion panting, breathing is deep, and inhalation seems to be never-ending. In vacuity panting, breaths are short with a brief halt between inhalation and exhalation. In repletion panting, the chest feels distended, breathing is rough, and the voice is high and strident; the chest swells as if to burst, unable to contain all the breath it draws in, and relief from discomfort only comes with exhalation. In vacuity panting, the patient is distressed and anxious, and his voice is low and faint; he is panicky, feeling as if he is about to stop breathing; he is unable to catch his breath and feels as though the air is not being absorbed by the lungs; the short rapid breaths give the impression of panting [as from exertion] and relief is felt only when a long breath can be drawn."

Comparison: WHEEZING is noisy breathing that sometimes occurs with panting (WHEEZING AND PANTING), but not on its own. *The Orthodox Tradition of Medicine* (*yī xué zhèng zhuàn*) states, "Hasty panting with FROG RALE IN THE THROAT is called "wheezing;" hasty breathing with discontinuity between breaths is panting." WMC dyspnea (classical repletion panting is seen in acute attacks of bronchial asthma, whereas vacuity panting occurs in pulmonary emphysema or dyspnea due to cardiac failure). See COLD PANTING; HEAT PANTING; REPLETION PANTING; VACUITY PANTING. ◇ Chin 喘 *chuǎn,* pant, be out of breath. [6: 129] [29: 164] [97: 553] [58: 126]

panting counterflow 喘逆 *chuǎn nì:* PANTING with counterflow qi. See PANTING.

panting in pregnancy 妊娠喘 *rèn shēn chuǎn:* PANTING during pregnancy. It arises in patients usually suffering from lung qi vacuity, when during pregnancy water qi ascends and exploits the lung, or when externally contracted wind-cold impairs lung qi diffusion. It can also occur in RETENTION OF DEAD FETUS with rushing upsurge, or when fire stirs the fetal origin and causes qi counterflow. The signs include phlegm panting with rapid breathing, and unquiet sleep. **Lung qi vacuity** is characterized by sudden panting accompanied by lack of strength in the limbs. MED Supplement the lung and boost qi with variations of Pulse-Engendering Powder (*shēng mài sǎn*). **Wind-cold** is characterized by heat effusion and aversion to cold. MED Course wind and dissipate cold with Ginseng and Perilla Beverage (*shēn sū yǐn*). **Retention of dead fetus** is characterized by cessation of fetal movement, disappearance of the fetal heart beat, red face and green-blue tongue, and panting that prevents the patient from lying down. MED Make a decoction of peach kernel (*táo rén*), white peony (*bái sháo yào*), moutan (*mǔ dān pí*), cinnamon bark (*ròu guì*), poria (*fú líng*), tangkuei (*dāng guī*), and ligusticum (*chuān xiōng*). **Fire stirring qi counterflow** causes panting with vexation, agitation, and heat effusion. MED Use scutellaria (*huáng qín*) and cyperus (*xiāng fù zǐ*) ground to a powder and mixed with water. [26: 341]

panting with rale 喘鸣 *chuǎn míng:* Wheezing or phlegm panting. [: 1498]

papular wind lumps 风疹块 *fēng zhěn kuài:* See DORMANT PAPULES.

papule 疹 *zhěn:* Any rounded elevation of the skin. Observed in maculopapular eruptions occurring in externally contracted disease, dormant papules, and other skin diseases. See MACULOPAPULAR ERUPTION; DORMANT PAPULES. [27: 370] [97: 491]

paradoxical treatment 反治 *fǎn zhì:* Synonym: *coacting treatment.* The nonroutine principle of treating false signs with medicinals of opposite nature, e.g., treating heat with heat, cold with cold, the stopped by stopping, and flow by promoting flow. Treating cold with cold, for example, means using heavy does of heat-clearing toxin-resolving agents to treat exuberant heat in externally contracted febrile disease presenting with false signs of cold such as aversion to cold or shivering, and cold of the limbs. Compare STRAIGHT TREATMENT. [26: 317] [50: 294] [27: 235] [97: 115]

paralysis 瘫痪 *tān huàn:* Loss of use of the limbs. Paralysis that is not the result of external injury is attributable to liver-kidney depletion and insufficiency of qi and blood with evil qi (e.g., wind, cold, dampness, heat, phlegm, and stasis) entering the channels and network vessels. In severe cases, the limbs becomes wilted and disabled, preventing all movement. In milder cases, although the patient can move his extremities, he cannot perform normal activities without assistance. Paralysis may affect all limbs, individual limbs, only the legs or only the arms, or the arm and leg of one side of the body or the other. Compare WILTING; HEMIPLEGIA. [26: 1005] [97: 639]

paravertebral sinews 膂筋 *lǚ jīn,* 膂 *lǚ:* The sinews that run down either side of the spine. The paravertebral sinews correspond to various different muscles in Western anatomy. [27: 69]

parch 焦 *jiāo:* Describes the burning and drying effect of heat, as in the expression "lung heat parching the lobes."

parched lips 唇焦 *chún jiāo:* See DRY LIPS.

parched teeth 齿焦 *chǐ jiāo:* Dry teeth. Parched teeth are attributed to damage to yin humor. If the teeth are grimy, the condition is due to kidney vacuity and exuberant fire before stomach yin is exhausted; otherwise it is attributable to major damage to stomach liquid, and desiccation of spleen-kidney yin. [97: 342]

partiality for certain foods 偏食 *piān shí:* A special liking or craving for food of a particular flavor or food of excessively strong flavor. *Elementary Questions* (*sù wèn, wǔ zàng shēng chéng piān*) states, "when one eats many salty foods, the vessels congeal and change color; when one eats many bitter foods, the skin becomes desiccated and its hair drops out; when one eats acrid foods to excess, the sinews become tense and the nails desiccated; when on eats too many sour foods, the skin becomes thick and wrinkled and the lips raised; when on eats too many sweet foods, the bones become painful and the hair drops out." Compare PERVERTED APPETITE. [50: 1401]

[1]**pass** 传 *chuán:* To move or be transmitted.

[2]**pass** 关 *guān:* A narrow gap permitting passage, as in THROAT PASS.

passage and transmutation 传变 *chuán biàn:* SHIFT.

passing of flatus 排气 *pái qì*, 失气 *shī qì*: Farting; breaking wind. Seen in ABDOMINAL FULLNESS; QI STAGNATION; GASTROINTESTINAL ACCUMULATION; FOOD DAMAGE; QI DYSENTERY; SMALL INTESTINAL COUGH. ◇ Chin 失 *shī*, let out, lose; 排 *pái*, expel, eliminate; 气 *qì*, air, breath, flatus, qi.

pass into the interior 入里 *rù lǐ*: ENTER THE INTERIOR.

paste 膏 *gāo*: Synonym: *paste preparation.* Any semi-liquid or virtually solid pharmaceutical preparation. Distinction is made between RICH PASTE, which are taken orally, and MEDICINAL PASTE, which are applied topically. Rich pastes are made by reducing decoctions of agents to a thick consistency and then adding honey or rock candy. Medicinal pastes are made by adding powdered agents to heated mixtures of vegetable oil and wax. A PLASTER is a kind of topically applied medicinal paste that has to be softened by heating before being applied. [27: 312] [97: 629]

paste preparation 膏剂 *gāo jì*: PASTE. [26: 826]

pathogen 邪 *xié*: EVIL.

pathomechanism 病机 *bìng jī*: The process by which a disease arises and develops. ⟨WMC⟩ etiology. See NINETEEN PATHOMECHANISMS.

pathway of qi 气道 *qì dào*: Any way or course traversed by qi. ◇ Chin 气 *qì*, qi; 道 *dào*, path, way, Dao.

pattern 证 *zhèng*, 证候 *zhèng hòu*: Synonym: *disease pattern.* A manifestation of human sickness indicating the nature, location, or cause of sickness. For example, the simultaneous presence of heat effusion, aversion to cold, and floating pulse forms an exterior pattern due to an external contraction; vigorous heat effusion, vexation and thirst, red tongue with yellow fur, and constipation constitutes an *interior repletion pattern*; wind stroke with clenched jaw, red face, rough breathing, phlegm-drool congestion, clenched hands, and a slippery stringlike or moderate sunken pulse constitutes a BLOCK PATTERN, whereas weak breathing, reversal cold in the limbs, pearly sweat, open mouth and closed eyes, open hands and enuresis, and faint fine pulse on the verge of expiration or sunken hidden pulse constitutes a DESERTION PATTERN. The concept of pattern is distinct from that of DISEASE (as a specific kind of morbid condition). A disease may take the form of different patterns. Measles, for example, may take the form of a *favorable* or *unfavorable* pattern. A favorable pattern is characterized by a swift forceful eruption, indicating that body is putting up a strong fight against the measles toxin; an unfavorable pattern is characterized by a poor faltering eruption, indicating that the body is offering poor resistance. Treatment of measles varies according to pattern: favor-

able patterns are treated according to the principle of dispelling the evil, whereas unfavorable patterns also require right-supporting action to help the body's fight against the disease. See also SIGN and PATTERN IDENTIFICATION. ◇ Chin 证 *zhèng*, sign, evidence, proof, manifestation. [27: 347] [97: 305]

pattern identification 辨证 *biàn zhèng*: Identification of disease patterns. Pattern identification is the process by which information gathered through four examinations (inspection, smelling and listening, inquiry, and palpation) is classified into different patterns. The first stage in the process is EIGHT-PRINCIPLE PATTERN IDENTIFICATION, in which four-examination data is classified as interior exterior, cold or heat, vacuity or repletion, and yin or yang. Depending on the results obtained, other pattern identification procedures are applied. See entries listed below. See also DETERMINE TREATMENT BY PATTERNS IDENTIFIED. [27: 438] [97: 372] [27: 438] [97: 372]

Pattern Identification

EIGHT PRINCIPLE PATTERN IDENTIFICATION (*bā gāng biàn zhèng*)

QI-BLOOD PATTERN IDENTIFICATION (*qì xuè biàn zhèng*)

ORGAN PATTERN IDENTIFICATION (*zàng fǔ biàn zhèng*)

DISEASE-EVIL PATTERN IDENTIFICATION (*bìng xié biàn zhèng*)

SIX-CHANNEL PATTERN IDENTIFICATION (*liù jīng biàn zhèng*)

FOUR-ASPECT PATTERN IDENTIFICATION (*wèi qì yíng xuè biàn zhèng*)

PC 心包 *xīn bāo*, 手厥阴心包经 *shǒu jué yīn xīn bāo jīng*: The pericardium or hand reverting yin (*jué yīn*) pericardium channel.

peach-blossom lichen 桃花癣 *táo huā xiǎn*: BLOWN BLOSSOM LICHEN. [26: 324]

pearl of the ear 耳珠 *ěr zhū*: Synonym: *ear gate; shelter; fleshy protuberance in front of the ear.* The tongue-like projection in front of the ear. ⟨WMC⟩ tragus.

pecking sparrow pulse 雀啄脉 *què zhuó mài*: See SEVEN STRANGE PULSES. [27: 199]

peeling fur 剥苔 *bō tāi*: A patchy tongue fur interspersed with mirror-like, furless areas. This generally indicates insufficiency of yin humor and vacuous stomach qi. A peeling fur that is nontransforming and slimy indicates a complex pattern of untransformed phlegm-damp and damage to yin humor and stomach qi. A thick slimy fur that suddenly completely peels away indicates major damage to right qi. [27: 183] [97: 481]

peg ribs 橛肋 *jué lè*: FREE RIBS.

penetrating vessel 冲脉 *chōng mài*: THOROUGH-FARE VESSEL.

penis 阴茎 *yīn jīng*: Synonym: *jade stem*. The male organ of copulation and urination. ◊ Chin 阴 *yīn*, yin the complement of yang; 茎 *jīng*, stem (of a plant).

pen-ts'ao 本草 *běn cǎo*: HERBAL FOUNDATION.

peppercorn sore 椒疮 *jiāo chuāng*: A sore growing on the inner surface of the eyelid. A peppercorn sore is attributed to local contraction of wind toxin combining with accumulated heat in the spleen channel to cause stagnation in the network vessels of the eyelid and disharmony between qi and the blood. The sore is small and looks like a zanthoxylum fruit ("Sichuanese peppercorn"). It is associated with roughness and dryness, aversion to light, and tearing. WMC trachoma. MED Dispel wind and clear heat; dissipate stasis and free the network vessels. An appropriate formula is schizonepeta (*jīng jiè*), ledebouriella (*fáng fēng*), red peony (*chì sháo yào*), scrophularia (*xuán shēn*), tangerine peel (*chén pí*), cicada molting (*chán tuì*), atractylodes (*cāng zhú*), dictamnus (*bái xiān pí*), forsythia (*lián qiào*), raw rhubarb (*shēng dà huáng*), magnolia bark (*hòu pò*), licorice (*gān cǎo*), and bitter bamboo leaf (*kǔ zhú yè*). In severe cases, without appropriate treatment, peppercorn sores may cause disease of the eye itself. [27: 503] [97: 548]

percolate 渗 *shèn*: Disinhibit (especially dampness).

percolating dampness 渗湿 *shèn shī*: See DISINHIBITING WATER AND PERCOLATING DAMPNESS.

perfuse 宣通 *xuān tōng*: (Of qi) to spread throughout.

pericardiac network [vessel] 心包络 *xīn bāo luò*: PERICARDIUM.

pericardiac pattern 心包证 *xīn bào zhèng*: Any warm disease arising when warm evils invade the pericardium and manifesting in signs such as clouded spirit, delirious speech and manic agitation, and, in severe cases, by coma. Portending signs are agitation, somnolence, and trembling of the lip of the tongue. Warm evils usually, though not invariably, pass to the construction aspect before gradually falling inward to the pericardium. In some cases, such as that of what Western medicine calls infectious encephalitis B, the evil falls inward directly from the defense aspect without passing through the construction aspect. This is known as anticipated passage to the pericardium. Two main forms are identified. One is known as heat entering the pericardium, which is characterized by heat signs such as red to crimson tongue, and in most cases a burnt-yellow tongue. The other is a phlegm-damp pattern referred to as phlegm turbidity clouding the pericardium, which is marked by a grimy sticky slimy fur that covers what may or may not be a red or crimson tongue. [6: 236]

pericardium 心包 *xīn bāo*: Synonym: *pericardiac network [vessel]*. The outer covering of the heart. It is traditionally held that evils invading the heart first affect the pericardium, so that conditions such as "clouded spirit" (stupor) and delirious mania due to high fever were termed heat entering the pericardium. By contrast, mental derangement due to phlegm-damp was termed phlegm turbidity (the turbid aspect of phlegm) clouding the pericardium. Both these conditions are in reality heart diseases. [27: 17] [97: 119]

pericardium channel 心包经 *xīn bāo jīng*: See HAND REVERTING YIN PERICARDIUM CHANNEL.

pericardium connects with the triple burner 心包络合三焦 *xīn bāo luò hé sān jiāo*: The hand reverting yin (*jué yīn*) and hand lesser yang (*shào yáng*) triple burner channels are connected and stand in exterior-interior relationship with each other. [26: 91]

perineum 会阴 *huì yīn*, 屏翳 *píng yì*, 纂 *cuàn*: Synonyms: *lower extreme*; *meeting of yin*. The area between two yin, i.e., between the external genitals and the anus. ◊ Chin 会 *huì*, meeting; 阴 *yīn*, yin (the complement of yang), dark, private. So called because it is the meeting place of the anterior and posterior yin, i.e., the anus and genitals. [27: 68] [27: 68] [97: 209]

perished complexion 夭色 *yāo sè*: See MALIGN COMPLEXION. ◊ Chin 夭 *yāo*, to die young. [26: 685]

perpendicular insertion 直刺 *zhí cì*: Insertion of acupuncture needles into the flesh at 90° to the surface of the skin. This is the most common type of insertion, and is applied in fleshy areas of the body. [97: 329]

persistent erection 阳强 *yáng qiáng*, 阳强不倒 *yáng qiáng bù dǎo*, 阴强 *yīn qiáng*, 阴挺 *yīn tǐng*, 阴挺长 *yīn tǐng cháng*, 阴强不倒 *yīn qiáng bù dǎo*, 茎强 *jīng qiáng*, 纵挺不收 *zòng tǐng bù shōu*, 挺长 *tǐng cháng*: See YANG RIGIDITY.

persistent flow of lochia 恶露不尽 *è lù bù jìn*, 恶露不断 *è lù bù duàn*: Flow of the LOCHIA in excess of twenty days. Persistent flow of lochia is attributed to qi vacuity, blood heat, or blood stasis. **Qi vacuity** patterns arise when the containing action of qi is weakened so that the thoroughfare (*chōng*) and controlling (*rèn*) vessels become insecure. They are marked by copious pale thin lochia associated with somber white complexion, laziness to speak, and empty sagging of the smaller abdomen. MED Supplement qi and contain the blood with Origin-Lifting Brew (*jǔ yuán jiān*). ACU Base treatment on CV, SP, and ST. Select CV-4 (*guān yuán*, Pass Head), ST-36 (*zú sān lǐ*, Leg Three Li), and SP-6 (*sān yīn jiāo*, Three

Yin Intersection); needle with supplementation and add moxa. **Blood stasis** patterns arise when residual blood has not been eliminated and causes static blood to obstruct the thoroughfare (*chōng*) and controlling (*rèn*) vessels. This pathomechanism is sometimes exacerbated by the contraction of cold. Blood stasis patterns are characterized by ungratifying rough scant flow of dark purple clotted lochia associated with smaller-abdominal pain. ⸏MED⸏ Transform stasis and stanch bleeding with tangkuei (*dāng guī*), ligusticum (*chuān xiōng*), leonurus (*yì mǔ cǎo*), blast-fried ginger (*páo jiāng*), corydalis (*yán hú suǒ*), and carthamus (*hóng huā*). ⸏ACU⸏ Base treatment on CV and SP. Select CV-3 (*zhōng jí*, Central Pole), CV-5 (*shí mén*, Stone Gate), and SP-8 (*dì jī*, Earth's Crux); needle with drainage and, if appropriate, moxa. **Blood heat** patterns arise when wearing of construction-yin causes internal vacuity heat that harasses the thoroughfare (*chōng*) and controlling (*rèn*) vessels and forces blood to flow downward. They are marked by copious red sticky fetid flow associated with tidal reddening of the face, and a rapid fine pulse. ⸏MED⸏ Nourish yin, clear heat, and stanch bleeding with variations of Yin-Safeguarding Brew (*bǎo yīn jiān*). ⸏ACU⸏ Base treatment on CV and the three yin channels of the foot. Select CV-6 (*qì hǎi*, Sea of Qi), CV-3 (*zhōng jí*, Central Pole), SP-10 (*xuè hǎi*, Sea of Blood), LR-6 (*zhōng dū*, Central Metropolis), and KI-10 (*yīn gǔ*, Yin Valley); needle with drainage without moxa. [26: 686] [59: 180] [97: 462]

persistent menstrual flow 月水不斷 *yuè shuǐ bù duàn*, 月水不绝 *yuè shuǐ bù jué*, 经血水不绝 *jīng xuè shuǐ bù jué*: MENSTRUAL SPOTTING.

perverse crop 鬎鬁 *là lì*, 瘌痢 *là lì*, 腊梨 *là lí*: See BALD WHITE SCALP SORE (white perverse crop) and FAT SORE sand heap perverse crop. ◊ Chin 鬎 (*là*), explained as meaning to shave or crop the hair; 鬁 (*lì*), a perverse condition of the hair (利 being explained as 戾, perverse). Both characters have the classifier 髟 (*biāo*), meaning (long flowing) hair.

perverse qi 戾气 *lì qì*: Any qi that causes highly contagious diseases including all warm epidemics and certain external medical diseases. Perverse qi is transmitted through the air or by direct contact. See PESTILENTIAL QI. [50: 997] [26: 349]

perverted appetite 嗜食异物 *shì shí yì wù*: Craving for strange foods. Eating of raw rice or earth in emaciated infants and children with abdominal distention and a lump in the umbilical region that moves when pushed is a sign of worm accumulation. This is as a result of eating unclean food. Craving for sour foods accompanied by absence of menstruation, nausea, and a harmonious slippery rapid pulse in sexually active women is a

sign of pregnancy. Indulgence in sour foods in pregnancy is not considered harmful if kept in moderation, but, in severe cases, it may accompany signs of stomach vacuity, stomach heat, stomach cold, phlegm stagnation, or liver heat that require appropriate treatment. Compare PARTIALITY FOR CERTAIN FOODS. [29: 200]

pestilence 疬 *lì*: **1.** PESTILENTIAL QI. **2.** Epidemic pestilence. Disease caused by pestilential qi; a violent contagious disease. **3.** PESTILENTIAL WIND (leprosy). [97: 374]

pestilential qi 疬气 *lì qì*: Synonyms: *epidemic pestilential qi; perverse qi; toxic qi; abnormal qi; miscellaneous qi*. Any disease evil that is highly contagious. *Elementary Questions* (*sù wèn, liù yuán zhèng jì dà lùn*) states, "When pestilence comes on a large scale, the people tend to die suddenly." It was formerly believed that pestilential qi resulted from abnormal weather conditions such as prolonged drought or extreme heat. [50: 973] [27: 108] [97: 374] [83: 456]

pestilential wind 疬风 *lì fēng*: Synonym: *leprosy; great numbing wind; numbing wind; great wind; malign disease of great wind; lai great wind; pestilence*. A transmissible disease that is characterized by localized numbing and subsequent appearance of red patches which swell and rupture without suppuration and that may spread to other parts of the body, causing loss of the eyes, collapse of the nose, fissuring of the lips, and boring of holes in the soles of the feet. Pestilential wind is attributed to leprosy toxin stagnating in the skin and muscles. ⸏MED⸏ Dispel wind and transform dampness; quicken the blood and kill worms. First use Safeguard Unlimited Efficacy Elixir (*bǎo ān wàn líng dān*) to cause sweating and then use Wondrous Response Wind-Dispersing Powder (*shén yìng xiāo fēng sǎn*). [26: 949] [27: 486] [50: 973] [96: 269]

petalled gums 齿龈结瓣 *chǐ yín jié bàn*: Gums that are patterned by the presence of coagulated blood observed in warm disease when evil causes frenetic movement of the blood and consequence spilling of the blood in the upper body. Distinction is made between purple and yellow petals. **Purple**: Petals that are purple in color or as black as lacquer indicate exuberant yang brightness (*yáng míng*) heat. ⸏MED⸏ Clear the stomach and engender liquid using White Tiger Decoction (*bái hǔ tāng*) or Jade Lady Brew (*yù nǚ jiān*). **Yellow**: Petals that are yellow brown in color indicate exhaustion of kidney yin and ascendant hyperactivity of vacuous yang. ⸏MED⸏ Rescue the kidney and nourish yin using Rhinoceros Horn and Rehmannia Decoction (*xī jiǎo dì huáng tāng*) or Construction-Clearing Decoction (*qīng yíng tāng*). Yellow petals are an unfavorable sign indicating that the disease is difficult to treat. [83: 77] [50: 901] [12: 99]

pharynx 咽 *yān*: The upper part of the throat, distinguished from the LARYNX. ⌐WMC¬ oral part of the pharynx. Compare LARYNX; THROAT. [27: 486] [97: 401]

philtrum 人中 *rén zhōng*: The groove running between the nose and lips. ⌐WMC¬ nasolabial groove (sulcus nasolabialis). [27: 66] [97: 12]

phlegm 痰 *tán*: **1.** A viscid substance traditionally understood to be a product and a cause of disease. Phlegm may gather in the lung, from where it can be expelled by coughing. However, phlegm as referred to in Chinese medicine is wider in meaning than sputum spoken of in Western medicine, and denotes a viscus fluid that can accumulate anywhere in the body causing a variety of diseases such as stroke, epilepsy, scrofula etc., but which in the absence of expectoration are usually characterized by a slimy tongue fur and a slippery or slippery stringlike pulse. Phlegm is a thick turbid substance that is distinguished from a thinner clearer form of accumulated fluid, rheum (饮 *yǐn*), although the term "phlegm" is sometimes use to cover both. Phlegm and rheum may be the result of the impaired movement and transformation of fluids that is associated with morbidity of the lung, spleen, and kidney. Phlegm—but not rheum—may also result from the "boiling" of the fluids by depressed fire. Invasion of the six excesses, affect damage, and damage by food and drink may all affect the dynamic of bowels and visceral qi causing water humor to gather and form phlegm. The two most important of the five viscera in the formation of phlegm are the spleen and lung. Phlegm is the product of a transformation of fluids; most commonly it is the product of congealing water-damp. The spleen normally moves and transforms water-damp, but when its qi is weak or dampness evil is exuberant, the normal movement and transformation of water-damp is impaired, and dampness gathers to form phlegm. For this reason it is said that the SPLEEN IS THE SOURCE OF PHLEGM FORMATION. It is said that "obese people tend to suffer from phlegm." This saying can be explained by the observation that excessive consumption of sweet or fatty rich foods causes spleen dampness to gather (more at OBESITY). The lung is the upper source of water; it governs depurative downbearing and regulation of the waterways. When dampness and phlegm accumulate, these functions can be overloaded, so that phlegm collects in the lung; hence it is said that the LUNG IS THE RECEPTACLE THAT HOLDS PHLEGM. Phlegm may also form in the lung when heat scorches lung liquid. Phlegm, however, appears not only in the lung; it can follow the upbearing and downbearing of qi and arrive at all places. Thus in addition to expectoration of phlegm, it can, depending on the organ or channel affected, cause vomiting

of phlegm-drool, clouded spirit, mania and withdrawal, phlegm rale in the throat, numbness of the limbs, hemiplegia, scrofula, goiter, mammary aggregation, phlegm nodes, plum-pit qi, or dizziness. **Lung:** Phlegm in the lung causes cough, panting, and oppression in the chest. Clear thin phlegm indicates cold, whereas yellow or thick white phlegm indicates heat. Scant phlegm expectorated with difficulty signifies either heat or dryness. Copious phlegm that is easily expectorated indicates dampness. Coughing of fishy-smelling pus and phlegm generally indicates PULMONARY WELLING-ABSCESS in a pattern of toxic heat brewing in the lung. Expectoration of phlegm containing blood (or pure blood without phlegm) is attributed either to dryness-heat, vacuity fire, or lung heat damaging the network vessels; if the blood is purplish black, it indicates a blood stasis complication. Although many lung diseases lead to local collection of phlegm, it is only when the coughing up of phlegm is more pronounced than other signs that the condition is strictly described as a "phlegm pattern." See COLD PHLEGM; HEAT PHLEGM; DRYNESS PHLEGM; PHLEGM-DAMP. See also PHLEGM-RHEUM. **Spleen-stomach:** Phlegm in the spleen and stomach (also called damp-phlegm) causes easily expectorated phlegm often accompanied by abdominal distention, sloppy stool, yellow face, lassitude of spirit, heavy limbs, white slimy tongue fur, and moderate pulse. PHLEGM-RHEUM. Phlegm in the heart is said to cloud the orifices of the heart (consciousness) and is observed in externally contracted febrile disease and other diseases such as wind stroke. See PHLEGM CONFOUNDING THE ORIFICES OF THE HEART. **Liver channel:** Phlegm in the liver channel is phlegm being carried up by wind yang ascending counterflow (ascendant liver yang transforming into wind), causing sudden collapse, phlegm rale in the throat, and convulsions or hemiplegia, as observed in wind stroke or epilepsy. In binding depression of liver qi, liver qi that ascends counterflow can contend with phlegm so it binds in the throat causing a sensation of blockage by some foreign body known as "plum pit qi" or "qi phlegm." **Phlegm ascending to invade the head:** Phlegm-drool ascending counterflow to the head can cause dizziness, hemilateral headache, deviated eyes and mouth, and hair loss. Depressed gallbladder-stomach heat engendering phlegm that ascends counterflow along the channels to harass clear yang causes dizziness, bitter taste in the mouth, tinnitus, vacuity vexation and insomnia, fright palpitations and profuse dreaming. Wind-phlegm surging up into the head can cause hemilateral headache or pain on one side of the face, or twitching of the eyes and mouth. Cold phlegm attacking the upper body gives rise to cold pain in the brain with a desire for warmth and an aversion to cold. **Kidney channel:** Phlegm in the kidney channel is characterized by black complexion, lassitude of spirit, and phlegm with black flecks and a salty taste. **Exterior channels and network vessels:** Phlegm in the channels and network vessels of the exterior can cause numbness, or PHLEGM NODES (lumps of varying sizes under the skin without change of skin color) or breast lumps called MAMMARY AGGREGATION. Phlegm in the neck can cause SCROFULA or GOITER. **Phlegm deep-lying in the sinews and bone:** After contraction of cold-damp evil, the interstices, channels, and network vessels become blocked, and fluid gathers and binds to form phlegm. This phlegm may penetrate the sinew and bone, causing damp phlegm and cold phlegm patterns such as BONE FLAT-ABSCESS, CRANE'S-KNEE PHLEGM, and FLOWING PHLEGM. See entries beginning with PHLEGM and WIND-PHLEGM; COLD PHLEGM; DAMP PHLEGM; HEAT PHLEGM; OLD PHLEGM; DRYNESS PHLEGM; QI PHLEGM. NB: The compound terms of *phlegm* with *heat* and *damp* take the form of both *heat phlegm, damp phlegm* and *phlegm-heat, phlegm-damp*. This difference seems to be only a matter of convention, e.g., *damp phlegm leg qi* but *phlegm-damp headache*. **2.** An abbreviation for FLOWING PHLEGM, as in ANKLE-BORING PHLEGM. [26: 765] [27: 120] [97: 607] [3: 82] [29: 380] [50: 1630]

phlegm accumulation 痰积 *tán jī*: Accumulation of phlegm turbidity in the chest and diaphragm characterized by copious thick phlegm that is difficult to expectorate, dizziness, oppression in the chest with dull pain, and a slippery stringlike pulse. ⟨MED⟩ Open the chest and flush phlegm with formulas such as Phlegm-Abducting Decoction (*dǎo tán tāng*) or Dried Bamboo Sap Phlegm-Moving Pill (*zhú lì yùn tán wán*). When signs are severe, but both body and qi are replete, Drool-Controlling Elixir (*kòng xián dān*) may be used. For phlegm accumulating in the throat, ejection may be considered. ⟨ACU⟩ Base treatment mainly on CV, ST, and PC. Select CV-12 (*zhōng wǎn*, Center Stomach Duct), CV-17 (*shān zhōng*, Chest Center), ST-36 (*zú sān lǐ*, Leg Three Li), ST-40 (*fēng lóng*, Bountiful Bulge), LI-4 (*hé gǔ*, Union Valley), CV-22 (*tiān tú*, Celestial Chimney), CV-6 (*qì hǎi*, Sea of Qi), and PC-6 (*nèi guān*, Inner Pass); needle with drainage and add moxa. Selection of points according to signs: For dizziness, add ST-8 (*tóu wéi*, Head Corner), and ST-41 (*jiě xī*, Ravine Divide). [26: 767] [27: 381] [97: 609] [46: 597, 602, 618]

phlegm accumulation diarrhea 痰积泄泻 *tán jī xiè xiè*: PHLEGM DIARRHEA. [26: 768]

phlegm accumulation vomiting 痰积呕吐 *tán jī ǒu tù*: PHLEGM VOMITING.

phlegm aggregation 痰癖 *tán pì*: Enduring water-rheum transforming into phlegm, which flows into the rib-side causing periodic pain. See RHEUM AGGREGATION. [26: 768] [97: 609]

phlegm and qi binding together 痰气互结 *tán qì hù jié*: Synonym: *phlegm and qi obstructing each other*; *binding depression of phlegm and qi*. Phlegm turbidity being caused to bind in the throat or chest by depressed qi. The main signs are plum-pit qi, glomus and oppression or scurrying pain in the chest and diaphragm, affect-mind depression, rashness, impatience, and irascibility. Other signs include cough with thick phlegm, sighing, and menstrual irregularities. The tongue is thick and slimy. The pulse is stringlike and slippery. See PLUM-PIT QI. [57: 41]

phlegm and qi obstructing each other 痰气交阻 *tán qì jiāo zǔ*: PHLEGM AND QI BINDING TOGETHER. [57: 41]

phlegm block 痰闭 *tán bì*: See INTERNAL PHLEGM TURBIDITY BLOCK. [26: 765]

phlegm clouding the pericardium 痰蒙心包 *tán méng xīn bāo*: See PHLEGM CONFOUNDING THE ORIFICES OF THE HEART. [26: 767]

phlegm confounding the orifices of the heart 痰迷心窍 *tán mí xīn qiào*: Synonym: *phlegm clouding the pericardium*; *phlegm obstructing the orifices of the heart*; *phlegm turbidity clouding the pericardium*. A disease pattern arising when phlegm turbidity causes disturbance of the heart spirit. Phlegm confounding the orifices of the heart occurs in several different diseases. The main signs are a) mental depression and dementia (withdrawal disease); b) clouded spirit-mind seeming both conscious and unconscious (damp warmth); c) sudden clouding collapse, unconsciousness, phlegm-drool foaming at the mouth, and convulsions of the limbs (epilepsy). Other signs include dull stagnant complexion, no thought of food and drink, soliloquy, indifferent expression, irregular behavior, oppression in the chest and copious phlegm, and phlegm rale in the throat. ⟨WMC⟩ schizophrenia; dementia; nervous system infections such as encephalitis B or epidemic encephalitis; epilepsy; cerebrovascular accident. **Withdrawal disease** is marked by mental depression with the gradual appearance of abnormal behavior, feeble-mindedness (dementia), and soliloquy that ceases when others notice. ⟨MED⟩ Flush phlegm and open the orifices. Use Phlegm-Abducting Decoction (*dǎo tán tāng*) with the judicious addition of acorus (*shí chāng pú*), polygala (*yuǎn zhì*), and cyperus (*xiāng fù zǐ*). For patients suffering from insomnia, add stir-fried spiny jujube (*suān zǎo rén*), biota seed (*bǎi zǐ rén*), cinnabar root poria (*zhū fú shén*), dragon bone (*lóng gǔ*), oyster shell (*mǔ lì*), and amber (*hǔ pò*). For copious phlegm, add white mustard (*bái jiè zǐ*), gleditsia (*zào jiá*), and dried bamboo sap (*zhú lì*). For depressed phlegm transforming into heat, use Phlegm-Abducting Decoction (*dǎo tán tāng*) plus bamboo shavings (*zhú rú*), coptis (*huáng lián*), and rhubarb (*dà huáng*), or combined with Alum and Curcuma Pill (*bái jīn wán*). ACU The main points used to sweep phlegm and open the orifice are CV-12 (*zhōng wǎn*, Center Stomach Duct), ST-36 (*zú sān lǐ*, Leg Three Li), ST-40 (*fēng lóng*, Bountiful Bulge), SP-6 (*sān yīn jiāo*, Three Yin Intersection), GV-26 (*rén zhōng*, Human Center), and PC-5 (*jiān shǐ*, Intermediary Courier); needle with drainage. For withdrawal disease, add GV-20 (*bǎi huì*, Hundred Convergences), HT-7 (*shén mén*, Spirit Gate), PC-7 (*dà líng*, Great Mound), and LR-3 (*tài chōng*, Supreme Surge). **Damp warmth** is marked by indifferent expression and clouded spirit. The patient is sometimes conscious and sometimes unconscious, or seems both conscious and unconscious. Sometimes there is delirious speech. Generalized heat [effusion] is present, but not high. MED Flush phlegm and open the orifices. Use Acorus and Curcuma Decoction (*chāng pú yù jīn tāng*) with judicious addition of coix (*yì yǐ rén*), cardamom (*bái dòu kòu*), polyporus (*zhū líng*), poria (*fú líng*), alisma (*zé xiè*), rice-paper plant pith (*tōng cǎo*), eupatorium (*pèi lán*), and coptis (*huáng lián*). ACU To the main point listed above in the treatment for withdrawal disease add PC-6 (*nèi guān*, Inner Pass), LR-3 (*tài chōng*, Supreme Surge), LI-11 (*qū chí*, Pool at the Bend), LI-4 (*hé gǔ*, Union Valley), and SP-9 (*yīn líng quán*, Yin Mound Spring). **Epilepsy** is characterized by a sudden clouding collapse and unconsciousness convulsions of the limbs, phlegm rale in the throat, phlegm-drool foaming at the mouth, and in some cases the emission of a squeal like a goat's or a pig's. The patient soon regains consciousness. MED Treat with Fit-Settling Pill (*dìng xián wán*) with the judicious addition of curcuma (*yù jīn*), white mustard (*bái jiè zǐ*), centipede (*wú gōng*), and mother-of-pearl (*zhēn zhū mǔ*). ACU To the main points listed above, add GV-16 (*fēng fǔ*, Wind Mansion), CV-15 (*jiū wěi*, Turtledove Tail), PC-6 (*nèi guān*, Inner Pass), LI-4 (*hé gǔ*, Union Valley), and LR-3 (*tài chōng*, Supreme Surge). [116: 49] [6: 219] [26: 765] [27: 149] [46: 597, 641, 642] [37: 346]

phlegm congestion seminal emission 痰壅遗精 *tán yōng yí jīng*: Seminal emission attributed to phlegm congestion. Phlegm congestion seminal emission arises when prolonged thought causes qi to bind and produce phlegm, which confounds the orifices and causes disquietude of essence-spirit. MED Abduct phlegm using Polyporus Pill (*zhū líng wán*), which contains polyporus (*zhū líng*) and pinellia (*bàn xià*). ACU Base treatment mainly on back transport points, CV, ST, HT, and SP. Se-

lect BL-15 (*xīn shū*, Heart Transport), BL-20 (*pí shū*, Spleen Transport), BL-23 (*shèn shū*, Kidney Transport), CV-12 (*zhōng wǎn*, Center Stomach Duct), ST-36 (*zú sān lǐ*, Leg Three Li), ST-40 (*fēng lóng*, Bountiful Bulge), HT-7 (*shén mén*, Spirit Gate), SP-6 (*sān yīn jiāo*, Three Yin Intersection), and PC-6 (*nèi guān*, Inner Pass); needle with even supplementation and drainage. See SEMINAL EMISSION; DREAM EMISSION; SEMINAL EFFLUX; DAMP-HEAT SEMINAL EMISSION. [26: 767] [6: 219] [97: 610] [46: 597, 678]

phlegm constipation 痰秘 *tán bì*: Constipation attributed to damp phlegm obstructing the stomach and intestines. Phlegm constipation is associated with glomus and oppression in the chest and rib-side, panting and fullness, dizziness, sweating from the head, and rumbling intestines. MED Transform phlegm and free the bowels using formulas such as Two Matured Ingredients Decoction (*èr chén tāng*) plus unripe bitter orange (*zhǐ shí*), rhubarb (*dà huáng*), white mustard (*bái jiè zǐ*), and dried bamboo sap (*zhú lì*). Severe cases can be treated with Drool-Controlling Elixir (*kòng xián dān*). ACU Base treatment on alarm, back transport, and lower uniting points of LI, and on CV, ST, and SP. Select BL-25 (*dà cháng shū*, Large Intestine Transport), ST-25 (*tiān shū*, Celestial Pivot), ST-37 (*shàng jù xū*, Upper Great Hollow), TB-6 (*zhī gōu*, Branch Ditch), CV-12 (*zhōng wǎn*, Center Stomach Duct), ST-36 (*zú sān lǐ*, Leg Three Li), ST-40 (*fēng lóng*, Bountiful Bulge), and SP-9 (*yīn líng quán*, Yin Mound Spring); needle with drainage. Selection of points according to signs: For glomus and oppression in the chest and rib-side, add CV-17 (*shān zhōng*, Chest Center) and PC-6 (*nèi guān*, Inner Pass). For dizziness, add ST-8 (*tóu wéi*, Head Corner) and ST-41 (*jiě xī*, Ravine Divide). For panting and fullness, Panting Stabilizer (*dìng chuǎn*), and CV-17 (*shān zhōng*, Chest Center). [26: 765] [113: 102] [46: 597, 602, 670]

phlegm cough 痰咳 *tán ké*, 痰嗽 *tán sòu*: COUGH caused by exuberant phlegm. A phlegm cough is a heavy turbid-sounding cough characterized by copious phlegm that is easily expectorated and relieved by expectoration. It is associated with oppression in the chest, reduced food intake, white slimy tongue fur, and a slippery floating pulse. It is attributed to phlegm-damp brewing internally and ascending to affect the lung. WMC This pattern may be observed in chronic bronchitis, pulmonary emphysema, and bronchodilatation. MED Use Two Matured Ingredients Decoction (*èr chén tāng*), add apricot kernel (*xìng rén*), fritillaria (*bèi mǔ*), aster (*zǐ wǎn*), and tussilago (*kuǎn dōng huā*). ACU Base treatment mainly on LU, SP, and ST. Select BL-13 (*fèi shū*, Lung Transport), ST-40 (*fēng lóng*, Bountiful

Bulge), LI-4 (*hé gǔ,* Union Valley), CV-17 (*shān zhōng,* Chest Center), CV-12 (*zhōng wǎn,* Center Stomach Duct), LU-9 (*tài yuān,* Great Abyss), SP-3 (*tài bái,* Supreme White), and ST-36 (*zú sān lǐ,* Leg Three Li); needle with drainage or with even supplementation and drainage, and, if appropriate, add moxa. [46: 597, 653] [27: 378] [97: 609] [50: 1631]

phlegm-damp 痰湿 *tán shī:* Conditions arising when dampness gathers to form phlegm and characterized by signs of both phlegm and dampness. See the following entries. [26: 768] [27: 120]

phlegm-damp cough 痰湿咳嗽 *tán shī ké sòu:* PHLEGM COUGH. [27: 379]

phlegm-damp headache 痰湿头痛 *tán shī tóu tòng:* HEADACHE attributed to phlegm-damp clouding the upper body. Phlegm-damp headache is a headache with heavy head as if swathed, fullness and oppression in the chest and stomach duct, regular bouts of nausea and vomiting producing copious phlegm, white slimy tongue fur, and slippery pulse. MED Transform phlegm and dispel dampness with formulas such as Phlegm-Abducting Decoction (*dǎo tán tāng*) which can be combined with Ligusticum and Asarum Decoction (*xiōng xīn tāng*). ACU Base treatment mainly on CV and ST. Select ST-8 (*tóu wéi,* Head Corner), Greater Yang (*tài yáng,* CV-12 (*zhōng wǎn,* Center Stomach Duct), LI-4 (*hé gǔ,* Union Valley), and ST-40 (*fēng lóng,* Bountiful Bulge); needle with drainage. For fullness and oppression in the chest and stomach duct, add CV-17 (*shān zhōng,* Chest Center), and PC-6 (*nèi guān,* Inner Pass), See HEADACHE. [26: 768]

phlegm-damp infertility 痰湿不孕 *tán shī bù yùn:* Infertility attributed to phlegm-damp affecting the thoroughfare (*chōng*) and controlling (*rèn*) vessels and obstructing the uterine vessels. Phlegm-damp infertility is observed in obese women who indulge in rich foods and is usually associated with copious vaginal discharge and menstrual irregularities. MED Fortify the spleen and dry dampness; transform phlegm. Use formulas like Atractylodes and Cyperus Phlegm-Abducting Pill (*cāng fù dǎo tán wán*). ACU Base treatment mainly on CV, SP, and ST. Select CV-4 (*guān yuán,* Pass Head), BL-20 (*pí shū,* Spleen Transport), CV-12 (*zhōng wǎn,* Center Stomach Duct), CV-6 (*qì hǎi,* Sea of Qi), ST-30 (*qì chōng,* Qi Thoroughfare), SP-6 (*sān yīn jiāo,* Three Yin Intersection), ST-40 (*fēng lóng,* Bountiful Bulge), ST-36 (*zú sān lǐ,* Leg Three Li), and SP-9 (*yīn líng quán,* Yin Mound Spring); needle with supplementation and add moxa. For copious vaginal discharge, add GB-26 (*dài mài,* Girdling Vessel) and BL-30 (*bái huán shū,* White Ring Transport). See INFERTILITY. [46: 680] [59: 101] [26: 768]

phlegm-damp obstructing the lung 痰湿阻肺 *tán shī zǔ fèi:* Disturbance of diffusion and downbearing of lung qi attributed to phlegm-damp congesting the lung. The lung is the receptacle that holds phlegm, whereas the spleen is the source of phlegm formation. When splenic movement is impaired, dampness gathers and forms phlegm, which affects the lung. Phlegm-damp obstructing the lung manifests as cough and panting exacerbated by physical movement, phlegm-drool congestion, thin white phlegm that is easily expectorated, fullness and oppression in the chest and diaphragm, a slimy or glossy white tongue fur and a moderate soggy pulse. WMC This pattern is observed in chronic bronchitis and bronchial asthma. MED Use Two Matured Ingredients Decoction (*èr chén tāng*) combined with Stomach-Calming Powder (*píng wèi sǎn*) and Three-Seed Filial Devotion Decoction (*sān zǐ yǎng qīn tāng*). ACU Base treatment mainly on LU, SP, and ST. Select BL-13 (*fèi shū,* Lung Transport), LU-5 (*chǐ zé,* Cubit Marsh), ST-40 (*fēng lóng,* Bountiful Bulge), CV-22 (*tiān tú,* Celestial Chimney), LI-4 (*hé gǔ,* Union Valley), CV-17 (*shān zhōng,* Chest Center), PC-6 (*nèi guān,* Inner Pass), LU-9 (*tài yuān,* Great Abyss), SP-3 (*tài bái,* Supreme White), and ST-36 (*zú sān lǐ,* Leg Three Li); needle with supplementation and moxa, if appropriate. **Comparison:** PHLEGM TURBIDITY OBSTRUCTING THE LUNG is similar, but associated with thick sticky phlegm. See PHLEGM TURBIDITY. See also PHLEGM OBSTRUCTING THE NETWORK VESSELS OF THE LUNG. [27: 160] [26: 768] [97: 611] [46: 597, 653]

phlegm depression 痰郁 *tán yù:* A phlegm pattern caused by phlegm and qi becoming depressed and bound, and characterized by panting on exertion, cough, oppression in the chest, blockage in the throat, and a pulse that is sunken and slippery. MED Flush phlegm and resolve depression, using Phlegm Depression Decoction (*tán yù tāng*). [26: 768]

phlegm diarrhea 痰泻 *tán xiè:* *Synonym: phlegm accumulation diarrhea.* From *The Gateway to Medicine* (*yī xué rù mén*).
Diarrhea arising when phlegm accumulating in the lung affects the large intestine through interior-exterior relationship between the two organs. Phlegm diarrhea is an intermittent form of diarrhea with the passing of sticky matter like eggwhite, and associated with dizziness and nausea, oppression in the chest and abdominal fullness, and a slippery stringlike pulse. MED Transform phlegm and dispel dampness with a combination of Two Matured Ingredients Decoction (*èr chén tāng*) and Stomach-Calming Powder (*píng wèi sǎn*). For spleen vacuity engendering phlegm, use Bupleurum and Peony Six Gentlemen Decoction (*chái sháo liù jūn zǐ tāng*). ACU Base treatment mainly on

CV, ST, and SP. Select CV-13 (*shàng wăn*, Upper Stomach Duct), CV-12 (*zhōng wăn*, Center Stomach Duct), ST-25 (*tiān shū*, Celestial Pivot), ST-36 (*zú sān lĭ*, Leg Three Li), PC-6 (*nèi guān*, Inner Pass), ST-40 (*fēng lóng*, Bountiful Bulge), SP-9 (*yīn líng quán*, Yin Mound Spring), LU-5 (*chĭ zé*, Cubit Marsh), and LI-4 (*hé gŭ*, Union Valley); needle with drainage and add moxa. For spleen vacuity engendering phlegm, add BL-20 (*pí shū*, Spleen Transport) and LR-13 (*zhāng mén*, Camphorwood Gate), needling with supplementation and adding moxa. [26: 768]

phlegm-drool 痰涎 *tán xián*: Phlegm-rheum, especially thin white, usually copious fluid ejected via the mouth. "Phlegm" refers to thick fluid, whereas "drool" refers to thin fluid. See PHLEGM VOMITING.

phlegm-drool congestion 痰涎壅盛 *tán xián yōng shèng*: Exuberant phlegm-drool impeding respiration. Phlegm-drool congestion is observed in WIND STROKE patterns, BLOCK patterns, PHLEGM-DAMP OBSTRUCTING THE LUNG, PHLEGM EPILEPSY, THROAT WIND, and WELLING-ABSCESS OF THE THROAT.

phlegm epilepsy 痰痫 *tán xián*: Epilepsy attributed to fright or fear in individuals suffering from phlegm-heat. Phlegm epilepsy is characterized by sudden collapse, fright, shouting, phlegm-drool congestion, and phlegm foaming at the mouth. [MED] Dispel phlegm and clear heat with Phlegm-Rolling Pill (*gŭn tán wán*). [ACU] Use the general points for EPILEPSY, and further needle CV-12 (*zhōng wăn*, Center Stomach Duct), and ST-36 (*zú sān lĭ*, Leg Three Li). [26: 768] [46: 640] [37: 345]

phlegm-fire 痰火 *tán huŏ*: **1.** Phlegm in the lung that is made sticky and lumpy by the action of fire. Phlegm-fire is not usually manifest in overt signs, but external contractions and damage by food and drink can bring on episodes of wheezing and panting, with phlegm that is difficult to expectorate, heat vexation and pain in the chest, and dry mouth and lips. **2.** A phlegm node behind the ears or under the armpit having the appearance of rosary beads and being hard and of fixed location. A phlegm-fire is accompanied by a red tongue with yellow fur and a rapid stringlike pulse. It is the result of liver fire and depressed phlegm. [27: 380] [44: 828]

phlegm-fire dizziness 痰火眩晕 *tán huŏ xuàn yūn*: DIZZINESS attributed to phlegm turbidity with fire clouding clear yang in the upper body. The dizziness is associated with heavy distended eyes, and is accompanied by heart vexation, nausea, and upflow and ejection of phlegm-drool, bitter taste in the mouth, reddish urine, slimy yellow tongue fur, and a slippery stringlike pulse.

[MED] Transform phlegm and downbear fire using formulas such as Upper-Body-Clearing Pill (*qīng shàng wán*) or Coptis Gallbladder-Warming Decoction (*huáng lián wēn dăn tāng*). [ACU] Base treatment mainly on ST and LI. Select ST-8 (*tóu wéi*, Head Corner), CV-12 (*zhōng wăn*, Center Stomach Duct), LI-4 (*hé gŭ*, Union Valley), ST-40 (*fēng lóng*, Bountiful Bulge), ST-41 (*jiě xī*, Ravine Divide), HT-8 (*shào fŭ*, Lesser Mansion), PC-7 (*dà líng*, Great Mound), and LR-2 (*xíng jiān*, Moving Between). Needle with drainage or prick to bleed with three-edged needle. See DIZZINESS. [26: 764]

phlegm-fire fearful throbbing 痰火怔忡 *tán huŏ zhēng chōng*: FEARFUL THROBBING (severe heart palpitations) attributed to phlegm-fire, and usually occurring in periodic attacks. [MED] Clear the heart and abduct phlegm using formulas such as Coptis Gallbladder-Warming Decoction (*huáng lián wēn dăn tāng*). See FEARFUL THROBBING; HEART PALPITATIONS. [ACU] Base treatment mainly on HT, PC, back transport points and ST. Select HT-7 (*shén mén*, Spirit Gate), PC-6 (*nèi guān*, Inner Pass), BL-15 (*xīn shū*, Heart Transport), ST-40 (*fēng lóng*, Bountiful Bulge), LU-5 (*chĭ zé*, Cubit Marsh), and ST-44 (*nèi tíng*, Inner Court); needle with drainage. [26: 764] [46: 648]

phlegm-fire harassing the heart 痰火扰心 *tán huŏ răo xīn*: A disease pattern that arises when affect-mind frustration causes qi depression that transforms into fire, which in turn condenses humor into phlegm, and the phlegm and fire bind together and harass the heart spirit. The chief signs are heart palpitations, vexation and sleeplessness or affect-mind abnormalities or manic agitation, or clouded spirit and delirious speech, vigorous heat [effusion], and phlegm rale. Other signs include red face and rough breathing, thirst with liking for cold drinks, oppression in the chest and copious phlegm, coughing of thick yellow phlegm, reddish urine and constipation, incoherent speech, abnormal crying and laughing, beating people and smashing objects, chiding and cursing regardless of who is present, dizziness, and profuse dreaming. The tongue with red with slimy yellow fur. The pulse is slippery and rapid. **Analysis:** Phlegm and fire binding together and harassing the heart spirit can give rise to a variety of different signs. In mild cases, there is disquieted heart spirit with heart palpitations, heart vexation, sleeplessness, and profuse dreaming. In severe cases, the spirit loses its governing, causing incoherent speech, abnormal crying and laughing, manic agitation, and beating people and smashing objects. Phlegm heat blocking the pericardium deranges the heart spirit, hence the clouded spirit and delirious speech. Exuberant fire causes rough breathing. Fire by nature flames upward, hence the red face. When the brain is affected, there is dizziness. Intense evil heat steams out to the outer body, hence there is vigorous heat [effusion]. Phlegm-heat obstructs qi dynamic, hence oppression in the chest and copious phlegm. When phlegm blocks the airways, it is stirred by the breath, causing phlegm rale in the throat. Exuberant heat damages liquid, hence the thirst and liking for cold drinks, and the reddish urine and constipation. The red tongue with slimy yellow fur and the slippery rapid pulse are signs of exuberant internal phlegm-fire. WMC schizophrenia. MED Clear the heart and drain fire; sweep phlegm and open the orifices. Use Chlorite/Mica Phlegm-Rolling Pill (*méng shí gǔn tán wán*), Iron Flakes Beverage (*shēng tiě luò yǐn*), Peaceful Palace Bovine Bezoar Pill (*ān gōng niú huáng wán*), or Gallbladder-Warming Decoction (*wēn dǎn tāng*). ACU Base treatment mainly on HT, PC, ST, and GV. Select BL-15 (*xīn shū*, Heart Transport), HT-7 (*shén mén*, Spirit Gate), PC-6 (*nèi guān*, Inner Pass), GV-26 (*rén zhōng*, Human Center), KI-1 (*yǒng quán*, Gushing Spring), PC-8 (*láo gōng*, Palace of Toil), HT-8 (*shào fǔ*, Lesser Mansion), SP-6 (*sān yīn jiāo*, Three Yin Intersection), ST-40 (*fēng lóng*, Bountiful Bulge), LU-5 (*chǐ zé*, Cubit Marsh), and ST-44 (*nèi tíng*, Inner Court); needle with drainage; PC-9 (*zhōng chōng*, Central Hub) and HT-9 (*shào chōng*, Lesser Surge) can be pricked to bleed. [116: 51] [57: 52] [26: 764] [97: 609] [46: 597, 648]

phlegm-fire headache 痰火头痛 *tán huǒ tóu tòng*: HEADACHE caused by phlegm-fire ascending counterflow. Phlegm-fire headache is a headache with ringing in the brain or a hemilateral headache attended by fullness and oppression in the chest and stomach duct, nausea and vomiting, upflow and ejection of phlegm-drool, heart vexation, irascibility, red face, thirst, constipation, slimy yellow tongue fur, and a slippery surging pulse. MED Transform phlegm and drain fire with formulas like Chlorite/Mica Phlegm-Rolling Pill (*méng shí gǔn tán wán*). ACU Base treatment mainly on CV and ST. Select ST-8 (*tóu wéi*, Head Corner), Greater Yang (*tài yáng*), CV-12 (*zhōng wǎn*, Center Stomach Duct), LI-4 (*hé gǔ*, Union Valley), LI-11 (*qū chí*, Pool at the Bend), ST-40 (*fēng lóng*, Bountiful Bulge), and ST-44 (*nèi tíng*, Inner Court); needle with drainage. For fullness and oppression in the chest and stomach duct, add CV-17 (*shān zhōng*, Chest Center), and PC-6 (*nèi guān*, Inner Pass). For nausea and vomiting, add PC-6 (*nèi guān*, Inner Pass), and SP-4 (*gōng sūn*, Yellow Emperor), [46: 602, 618] See HEADACHE. [26: 764]

phlegm-fire tetany 痰火痉 (痉) *tán huǒ cì (jìng)*: TETANY (*jìng*) (clenched jaw, arched-back rigidity, convulsions) attributed to phlegm-fire congestion. Phlegm-fire tetany is characterized by pulling of the eyes and mouth, tremor, shaking, or convulsive spasm of the extremities, generalized heat [ef-

fusion], cough with copious phlegm, and a rapid surging pulse. MED Clear heat and drain fire; sweep phlegm and resolve tetany. Use formulas such as Dragon-Embracing Pill (*bào lóng wán*). ACU Base treatment mainly on ST, GV, PC, TB and LI. Select ST-36 (*zú sān lǐ*, Leg Three Li), ST-40 (*fēng lóng*, Bountiful Bulge), ST-44 (*nèi tíng*, Inner Court), LR-2 (*xíng jiān*, Moving Between), GV-26 (*shuǐ gōu*, Water Trough), GV-8 (*jīn suō*, Sinew Contraction), PC-6 (*nèi guān*, Inner Pass), TB-5 (*wài guān*, Outer Pass), LI-4 (*hé gǔ*, Union Valley), and LI-11 (*qū chí*, Pool at the Bend); needle with drainage. [26: 764] [42: 188] [46: 597]

phlegm-fire tinnitus 痰火耳鸣 *tán huǒ ěr míng*: See TINNITUS. [26: 764]

phlegm glomus 痰痞 *tán pǐ*: GLOMUS (a localized feeling of fullness and blockage) attributed to congealing and binding of phlegm and qi and arising when water-rheum gathers to form phlegm and blocks the pathways of qi. Phlegm glomus is characterized by fullness, oppression, and blockage in the chest, rib-side pain, vomiting, cold sensation below the heart, and the sound of water on application of pressure. In some cases, there may be heat effusion or numbness of the limbs. MED Rectify qi and transform phlegm with formulas such as Two Matured Ingredients Decoction (*èr chén tāng*) with the addition of amomum (*shā rén*) and bitter orange (*zhǐ ké*). ACU Base treatment mainly on ST, CV, and PC. Select CV-12 (*zhōng wǎn*, Center Stomach Duct), ST-36 (*zú sān lǐ*, Leg Three Li), ST-40 (*fēng lóng*, Bountiful Bulge), PC-6 (*nèi guān*, Inner Pass), CV-17 (*shān zhōng*, Chest Center), and LR-3 (*tài chōng*, Supreme Surge); needle with drainage. [26: 765] [46: 597, 602]

phlegm-heat 痰热 *tán rè*: Phlegm and heat arising when external evils invade, transform into heat, which then combines with existing phlegm or damages liquid and condenses it into phlegm. [44: 838] [50: 1635]

phlegm-heat chest bind 痰热结胸 *tán rè jié xiōng*: MAJOR CHEST BIND. [27: 376]

phlegm-heat congesting the lung 痰热壅肺 *tán rè yōng fèi*: PHLEGM-HEAT OBSTRUCTING THE LUNG.

phlegm-heat obstructing the lung 痰热阻肺 *tán rè zǔ fèi*: Synonym: *phlegm-heat congesting the lung*. A disease pattern arising when phlegm-heat congests the lung and gives rise to panting and cough. External evils that have invaded become depressed in the lung and transform into heat. The heat damages lung liquid and condenses it to form phlegm, which in turn binds with the heat. The resultant combination of phlegm and heat then congests the network vessels of the lung. The chief signs of phlegm-heat obstructing the lung are cough and panting, thick yellow phlegm, and vigorous heat [effusion]. Other signs include thirst, vexation and agitation, flaring nostrils, expectoration of blood, spontaneous external bleeding, oppression in the chest, coughing up of purulent phlegm and blood with fishy smell, dry bound stool, and short voidings of reddish urine. WMC This pattern is observed in acute bronchitis, pneumonia, pulmonary emphysema with infection, and bronchial asthma with infection. **Analysis:** When phlegm heat congests in the lung, it causes lung qi to ascend counterflow, hence cough. The heat condenses humor into phlegm, hence the thick yellow phlegm. When depuration is hampered, there is labored breathing and flaring nostrils. When phlegm-heat scorches yin liquid, there is thirst, short voidings of reddish urine, and dry bound stool. When phlegm-heat harasses the heart spirit, there is vexation and agitation. When it damages the network vessels of the lung, blood spills out, and there is nosebleed or expectoration of blood. When phlegm-heat obstructs the network vessels of the lung, causing qi stagnation and blood congestion, there is oppression in the chest. Bad blood and putrid flesh suppurate, hence the coughing up of fishy-smelling purulent phlegm. The red tongue with yellow slimy fur and the slippery rapid pulse are both signs of phlegm-heat congesting internally. MED Clear and drain phlegm-heat. Use Mulberry Root Bark Decoction (*sāng bái pí tāng*). ACU Base treatment mainly on LU, LI, and ST. Select BL-13 (*fèi shū*, Lung Transport), LU-7 (*liè quē*, Broken Sequence), LI-4 (*hé gǔ*, Union Valley), LI-11 (*qū chí*, Pool at the Bend), CV-17 (*shān zhōng*, Chest Center), LU-5 (*chǐ zé*, Cubit Marsh), ST-40 (*fēng lóng*, Bountiful Bulge), ST-36 (*zú sān lǐ*, Leg Three Li), and KI-6 (*zhào hǎi*, Shining Sea); needle with drainage and prick LU-11 (*shào shāng*, Lesser Shang) and LI-1 (*shāng yáng*, Shang Yang) to bleed. **Comparison:** *Phlegm turbidity obstructing the lung:* Phlegm-heat congesting the lung and phlegm turbidity obstructing the lung involve phlegm obstructing the network vessels of the lung and impaired depurative downbearing of lung qi that cause cough, panting, and rapid breathing. However, phlegm-heat is marked by thick yellow phlegm and vigorous heat [effusion], whereas phlegm turbidity obstructing the lung is characterized by copious white sticky phlegm that is easy to expectorate. *Liver fire invading the lung:* Phlegm-heat congesting the lung and liver fire invading the lung share signs of cough, panting, and generalized heat [effusion]. However, phlegm-lung congesting the lung is marked by thick yellow phlegm that is not easy to expectorate, whereas liver fire invading the lung is characterized by distention and fullness in the chest and rib-side, vexation, agitation and irascibility, as well as red face and eyes.

See PHLEGM OBSTRUCTING THE NETWORK VESSELS OF THE LUNG. [27: 160] [97: 610] [57: 80] [116: 66] [46: 597, 654] [50: 1635]

phlegm hiccough 痰呃 *tán è*: Hiccough attributed to phlegm turbidity obstruction, characterized by the sound of phlegm, and attended by oppression in the chest and inhibited breathing. MED Transform phlegm and move qi using formulas such as Phlegm-Abducting Decoction (*dǎo tán tāng*). If there are signs of phlegm heat, use Pinellia and Scutellaria Pill (*bàn huáng wán*). ACU Base treatment mainly on CV, PC, ST and LR. Select BL-17 (*gé shū*, Diaphragm Transport), CV-17 (*shān zhōng*, Chest Center), PC-6 (*nèi guān*, Inner Pass), CV-6 (*qì hǎi*, Sea of Qi), CV-12 (*zhōng wǎn*, Center Stomach Duct), ST-25 (*tiān shū*, Celestial Pivot), ST-36 (*zú sān lǐ*, Leg Three Li), ST-40 (*fēng lóng*, Bountiful Bulge), and LR-3 (*tài chōng*, Supreme Surge); needle with drainage. See HICCOUGH. Compare HEAT HICCOUGH. [26: 764] [37: 308] [113: 76] [46: 597]

phlegm lodged in the channels 痰留经络 *tán liú jīng luò*: The presence of phlegm in the channels giving rise to goiter, phlegm nodes, and scrofula, all of which are relatively soft to the touch. [6: 219]

phlegm lodged in the chest and rib-side 痰留胸胁 *tán liú xiōng xié*: Phlegm lodged in the chest and rib-side is composed of stubborn phlegm and accumulated rheum that form a soft mass called an "afflux pouch." Phlegm lodged in the chest and rib-side is characterized by pain in the chest and rib-side exacerbated by coughing, panting, and turning over in bed, There is rapid breathing and expectoration of white phlegm and drool. There may also be fullness and distention in the chest and rib-side, swelling of the face, and a string-like sunken pulse. MED Transform rheum and expel phlegm. Commonly used rheum-transforming agents include ephedra (*má huáng*), cinnamon twig (*guì zhī*), asarum (*xì xīn*), dried ginger (*gān jiāng*), aconite (*fù zǐ*), and white mustard (*bái jiè zǐ*). Phlegm-expelling medicinals include tingli (*tíng lì zǐ*), kansui (*gān suì*), euphorbia/knoxia (*dà jǐ*), and morning glory (*qiān niú zǐ*). A commonly used formula is Minor Green-Blue Dragon Decoction (*xiǎo qīng lóng tāng*), which can be combined with Tingli and Jujube Lung-Draining Decoction (*tíng lì dà zǎo xiè fèi tāng*) or Drool-Controlling Elixir (*kòng xián dān*). [6: 220]

phlegm lodged in the limbs 痰留肢体 *tán liú zhī tǐ*: Any condition characterized by numbness and pain in the upper or lower limbs, or in one limb, unaccompanied by any signs of blood vacuity or wind-cold-damp impediment (*bì*), and characterized by a white slimy tongue fur and slippery pulse. MED Pathfinder Poria (Hoelen) Pill (*zhǐ mí* *fú líng wán*) can eliminate phlegm from the channels and network vessels of the limbs. [6: 221]

phlegm malaria 痰疟 *tán nüè*: MALARIA with signs of depressed phlegm. Phlegm malaria is characterized by alternating heat [effusion] and [aversion to] cold with more heat effusion than cold, headache, twitching of the flesh, vomiting of phlegm-drool, and a slippery stringlike pulse. In severe cases, there may be coma and convulsions. WMC cerebral malaria. MED Transform phlegm and eliminate malaria using formulas such as Bupleurum Stomach-Calming Brew (*chái píng jiān*) or Phlegm-Abducting Decoction (*dǎo tán tāng*) and variations. Exuberant heat with abdominal fullness and dry bound stool can be precipitated with Major Bupleurum Decoction (*dà chái hú tāng*). ACU Base treatment mainly on GV, SI, PC, CV, and ST. Select GV-14 (*dà zhuī,* Great Hammer), GV-13 (*táo dào,* Kiln Path), SI-3 (*hòu xī,* Back Ravine), PC-5 (*jiān shǐ,* Intermediary Courier), CV-12 (*zhōng wǎn,* Center Stomach Duct), ST-36 (*zú sān lǐ,* Leg Three Li), and ST-40 (*fēng lóng,* Bountiful Bulge); needle with drainage. For exuberant heat with abdominal fullness and dry bound stool, add ST-44 (*nèi tíng,* Inner Court), ST-25 (*tiān shū,* Celestial Pivot), LI-4 (*hé gǔ,* Union Valley), and LI-11 (*qū chí,* Pool at the Bend), [46: 649, 670] [113: 170] [26: 767] [27: 359] [97: 608]

phlegm node 痰核 *tán hé*: Any lump below the skin that feels soft and slippery under the finger, is associated with no redness, pain, or swelling, and (unlike SCROFULA) does not suppurate. [26: 765] [27: 479] [97: 608]

phlegm node of the eyelid 眼胞痰核 *yǎn bāo tán hé*: A hard lump growing out of the eyelid that is not painful when pressed and moves when pushed. A phlegm node of the eyelid is initially about the size of a rice grain, but gradually grows large to cause swelling and sagging of the eyelid. It is attributed to damp-heat brewing in the spleen and stomach. WMC chalazion. MED Transform phlegm and dissipate binds. Oral: A representative formula is Stomach-Clearing Decoction (*qīng wèi tāng*), which contains gardenia (*shān zhī zǐ*), bitter orange (*zhǐ ké*), perilla seed (*zǐ sū zǐ*), gypsum (*shí gāo*), Sichuan coptis (*chuān huáng lián*), tangerine peel (*chén pí*), forsythia (*lián qiào*), tangkuei tails (*dāng guī wěi*), schizonepeta spike (*jīng jiè suì*), scutellaria (*huáng qín*), ledebouriella (*fáng fēng*), and raw licorice (*shēng gān cǎo*). Topical: Apply raw arisaema (*shēng nán xīng*) ground with vinegar, which can be frequently applied to the affected area. Large nodes are most effectively treated by surgery. A small incision made in the flesh permits the yellow phlegm node to squeezed out. [26: 636]

phlegm obstructing the network vessels of the lung 痰阻肺络 *tán zǔ fèi luò*: Obstruction of the lung by phlegm, occurring when an external evil impairs the lung's function of distributing fluids, and allows fluids to gather to form phlegm. It is characterized by exuberant phlegm, counterflow qi, panting and cough, etc. NB: The term "network vessels of the lung" would appear to mean the bronchioles. See PHLEGM-HEAT OBSTRUCTING THE LUNG; PHLEGM-DAMP OBSTRUCTING THE LUNG. [50: 1634] [26: 764]

phlegm obstructing the orifices of the heart 痰阻心窍 *tán zǔ xīn qiào*: See PHLEGM CONFOUNDING THE ORIFICES OF THE HEART. [26: 765]

phlegm panting 痰喘 *tán chuǎn*: From *Dan Xi's Experiential Methods* (*dān xī xīn fǎ*). Panting attributed to phlegm turbidity congestion the lung, occurring when phlegm-damp brews in the lung and obstructs the airways. Phlegm panting is characterized by hasty breathing with rale, cough, ungratifying expectoration of thick slimy phlegm, and fullness and oppression in the chest. MED Dispel phlegm, downbear qi, and calm panting with formulas such as Two Matured Ingredients Decoction (*èr chén tāng*), Thousand Strings of Cash Decoction (*qiān mín tāng*), Phlegm-Rolling Pill (*gǔn tán wán*), and Perilla Fruit Qi-Downbearing Decoction (*sū zǐ jiàng qì tāng*). ACU Base treatment mainly on LU, ST and CV. CV-12 (*zhōng wǎn,* Center Stomach Duct), ST-36 (*zú sān lǐ,* Leg Three Li), ST-40 (*fēng lóng,* Bountiful Bulge), LU-1 (*zhōng fǔ,* Central Treasury), BL-13 (*fèi shū,* Lung Transport), CV-22 (*tiān tú,* Celestial Chimney), LU-5 (*chǐ zé,* Cubit Marsh), and Panting (*chuǎn xī*) (one body-inch to the side of C₇); needle with drainage. Select [26: 766] [27: 383] [97: 609] [113: 62] [46: 597]

phlegm pattern 痰证 *tán zhèng*: Any pattern caused by phlegm or drool accumulating and lodged within the body. See PHLEGM. [26: 768]

phlegm-pattern spontaneous sweating 痰证自汗 *tán zhèng zì hàn*: Spontaneous sweating attributed to phlegm turbidity causing internal obstruction of yang qi. In such patterns, spontaneous sweating is accompanied by phlegm signs such as dizziness, oppression in the chest, nausea, and ejection of phlegm drool. MED Regulate the center and transform phlegm. Use Fuzhou Ligusticum Decoction (*fǔ xiōng tāng*) or Qi-Rectifying Phlegm-Downbearing Decoction (*lǐ qì jiàng tán tāng*). ACU Base treatment mainly on CV, ST, PC, LI, and SI. Select CV-12 (*zhōng wǎn,* Center Stomach Duct), ST-36 (*zú sān lǐ,* Leg Three Li), ST-40 (*fēng lóng,* Bountiful Bulge), PC-6 (*nèi guān,* Inner Pass), CV-6 (*qì hǎi,* Sea of Qi), LI-4 (*hé gǔ,* Union Valley); and SI-3 (*hòu xī,* Back Ravine); needle with even supplementation and drainage or with drainage, and, if necessary, add moxa. [26: 765] [50: 1634] [113: 18] [46: 597] [14: 174]

phlegm pouch 痰包 *tán bāo*: Synonym: *gourd tongue*. A swelling on the under surface of the tongue shaped like a gourd, smooth and soft to the touch, and yellow in color. Phlegm pouch hampers eating and speech. When it bursts, it exudes a thick sticky phlegm-like substance similar to egg-white, and sometimes like soy-bean dregs. It tends to recur and resist healing. ⃞WMC ranula (sublingual ptyalocele). **Management**: It should be cut open with sharp scissors to allow the pus to drain. Borneol and Borax Powder (*bīng péng sǎn*) should be applied by insufflation, and heat-clearing phlegm-transforming formulas such as Two Matured Ingredients Decoction (*èr chén tāng*) plus coptis (*huáng lián*), scutellaria (*huáng qín*), bamboo shavings (*zhú rú*), and dandelion (*pú gōng yīng*) should be prescribed as oral medication. [26: 764] [27: 184] [97: 604]

phlegm rale 痰鸣 *tán míng*: An abnormal breathing sound produced by the presence of phlegm in the airways. In wheezing panting patterns, a continuous rale that sounds like the croaking of frogs is called *frog rale in the throat*. This is usually a sign of cold rheum due to phlegm-rheum in the inner body and cold evil in the outer body. In conditions of coma or certain blockages of the throat, a phlegm rale is described as having the *rasping sound of a saw*. [27: 185]

phlegm reversal 痰厥 *tán jué*: A REVERSAL pattern arising when exuberant phlegm causes a qi block and reversal cold in the limbs, and, in severe cases, CLOUDING REVERSAL (syncope). ⃞MED Transform phlegm and downbear qi. If oral medication cannot be administered, use mechanical ejection to treat the tip. Then oral medication should be given to clear and downbear or to warm and dissipate, dry dampness, and supplement the spleen and kidney. Oral formulas include Emergency Drool-Thinning Powder (*jí jiù xī xián sǎn*), Six Gentlemen Decoction (*liù jūn zǐ tāng*), and Six Gentlemen Metal and Water Brew (*jīn shuǐ liù jūn jiān*). ⃞ACU Base treatment on CV and ST. Select CV-12 (*zhōng wǎn*, Center Stomach Duct), ST-40 (*fēng lóng*, Bountiful Bulge), CV-15 (*jiū wěi*, Turtledove Tail), CV-22 (*tiān tú*, Celestial Chimney), PC-8 (*láo gōng*, Palace of Toil), and PC-5 (*jiān shǐ*, Intermediary Courier); needle with drainage and add moxa. See REVERSAL PATTERN. [26: 765] [37: 403]

phlegm reversal headache 痰厥头痛 *tán jué tóu tòng*: HEADACHE attributed to phlegm turbidity ascending counterflow. Phlegm reversal headache is a splitting headache associated with dizziness, generalized heaviness, disquieted heart

spirit, topsy-turvy speech, oppression in the chest, nausea, pronounced heart vexation and hasty rapid breathing, upflow of phlegm and drool or clear watery fluid, reversal cold of the limbs, and a slippery stringlike pulse. ⃞MED Transform phlegm and harmonize the center. Use formulas such as Pinellia, Ovate Atractylodes, and Gastrodia Decoction (*bàn xià bái zhú tiān má tāng*) or Ligusticum and Asarum Phlegm-Abducting Decoction (*xiōng xīn dǎo tán tāng*). ⃞ACU Base treatment mainly on CV and ST. Select ST-8 (*tóu wéi*, Head Corner), Greater Yang (*tài yáng*), CV-12 (*zhōng wǎn*, Center Stomach Duct), ST-36 (*zú sān lǐ*, Leg Three Li), ST-40 (*fēng lóng*, Bountiful Bulge), PC-5 (*jiān shǐ*, Intermediary Courier), and SP-9 (*yīn líng quán*, Yin Mound Spring); needle with drainage. See HEADACHE. [37: 364] [26: 765]

phlegm-rheum 痰饮 *tán yǐn*: Accumulation of fluid in the body. "Phlegm" denotes thick pathological fluids, whereas "rheum" denotes thinner pathological fluids. In practice, the term phlegm-rheum has two specific meanings: (1) Any form of rheum (i.e., thin fluid), arising as a result of lung, spleen, or kidney disturbances preventing the normal transportation and transformation of fluid, and treated by warming and supplementing the spleen and kidney to secure the root and by disinhibiting water and expelling rheum to address the branches. See SUSPENDED RHEUM; PROPPING RHEUM; SPILLAGE RHEUM; LODGED RHEUM; DEEP-LYING RHEUM; FLOWING RHEUM. (2) Synonym: *flowing rheum*. One of the FOUR RHEUMS. Rheum lodged in the stomach and intestines. Phlegm-rheum is characterized by sloppy stool, poor appetite, ejection of foamy drool, and emaciation occurring in obese people. In some cases there may be heart palpitations and shortness of breath. ⃞MED Warm yang and transform rheum with formulas such as Poria (Hoelen), Cinnamon Twig, Ovate Atractylodes, and Licorice Decoction (*líng guì zhú gān tāng*) or Golden Coffer Kidney Qi Pill (*jīn guì shèn qì wán*). ⃞ACU Base treatment mainly on CV, ST, BL, and SI. Select CV-12 (*zhōng wǎn*, Center Stomach Duct), ST-36 (*zú sān lǐ*, Leg Three Li), ST-40 (*fēng lóng*, Bountiful Bulge), ST-25 (*tiān shū*, Celestial Pivot), SP-9 (*yīn líng quán*, Yin Mound Spring), BL-64 (*jīng gǔ*, Capital Bone), SI-3 (*hòu xī*, Back Ravine), and BL-62 (*shēn mài*, Extending Vessel); needle with even supplementation and drainage and moxa can be added. Selection of points according signs: For heart palpitations and shortness of breath, add PC-6 (*nèi guān*, Inner Pass), PC-4 (*xī mén*, Cleft Gate), and CV-6 (*qì hǎi*, Sea of Qi). [26: 766] [46: 597, 602] [75: 60]

phlegm-rheum abdominal pain 痰饮腹痛 *tán yǐn fù tòng*: ABDOMINAL PAIN attributed to phlegm-rheum and associated with rumbling intestines, diarrhea with the passage of white glossy foamy matter without malodor, dizzy head, heart palpitations, nausea and vomiting, ejection of foamy drool, white putrid tongue fur, and a slippery rapid pulse. [MED] Fortify the spleen and eliminate phlegm with Two Matured Ingredients Decoction (*èr chén tāng*) plus atractylodes (*cāng zhú*) and magnolia bark (*hòu pò*). [ACU] Base treatment on back transport points, CV, and ST. Select BL-20 (*pí shū*, Spleen Transport), ST-36 (*zú sān lǐ*, Leg Three Li), CV-12 (*zhōng wǎn*, Center Stomach Duct), ST-40 (*fēng lóng*, Bountiful Bulge), and ST-25 (*tiān shū*, Celestial Pivot); needle with even supplementation and drainage. [37: 319] [27: 381] [97: 608]

phlegm-rheum aversion to cold 痰饮恶寒 *tán yǐn wù hán*: Aversion to cold attributed to phlegm in the chest and diaphragm obstructing yang qi. Phlegm-rheum aversion to cold is associated with generalized aversion to cold or aversion to cold in the back, reduced food intake, heavy limbs, slimy tongue fur, and a slippery pulse. [MED] Free yang and transform phlegm with formulas such as Poria (Hoelen), Cinnamon Twig, Ovate Atractylodes, and Licorice Decoction (*líng guì zhú gān tāng*), Pathfinder Poria (Hoelen) Pill (*zhǐ mí fú líng wán*), or Two Matured Ingredients Decoction (*èr chén tāng*). [26: 766]

phlegm-rheum cough 痰饮咳嗽 *tán yǐn ké sòu*: Cough attributed to phlegm-rheum, with cough as the main sign. Cough is a major signs of phlegm-rheum, and is most commonly seen when cold phlegm-rheum evil collects in the lung and stomach. It is associated with expectoration of copious white, sometimes foamy phlegm. [MED] Warm and transform using formulas such as Minor Green-Blue Dragon Decoction Plus Gypsum (*xiǎo qīng lóng jiā shí gāo tāng*) and Poria (Hoelen), Cinnamon Twig, Ovate Atractylodes, and Licorice Decoction (*líng guì zhú gān tāng*). Advanced-stage phlegm-rheum, which damages yang, manifests in additional signs of insufficiency of kidney yang such as coldlimbs and fear of cold, water swelling, and a fine sunken pulse, which calls for additional action to warm yang and disinhibit water, using formulas such as True Warrior Decoction (*zhēn wǔ tāng*) or Kidney Qi Pill (*shèn qì wán*). Phlegm-rheum collecting under the rib-side with cough causing rib-side pain is treated by draining water-rheum with formulas such as Ten Jujubes Decoction (*shí zǎo tāng*). [ACU] Base treatment mainly on LU, SP, and ST. Select BL-13 (*fèi shū*, Lung Transport), CV-12 (*zhōng wǎn*, Center Stomach Duct), ST-40 (*fēng lóng*, Bountiful Bulge), LI-4 (*hé gǔ*, Union Valley), LU-9 (*tài yuān*, Great Abyss), SP-3 (*tài bái*, Supreme White), ST-36 (*zú sān lǐ*, Leg Three Li), and SP-9 (*yīn líng quán*, Yin Mound Spring); needle with drainage or with even supplementation

and drainage. For cold phlegm-rheum evil collecting in the lung and stomach, add large amounts of moxa. See also PHLEGM-RHEUM; PROPPING RHEUM; SUSPENDED RHEUM. [26: 766] [46: 597, 652]

phlegm-rheum dizziness 痰饮眩晕 *tán yǐn xuàn yūn*: DIZZINESS that arises when spleen vacuity allows phlegm-rheum to collect and ascend to cloud the clear orifices. Phlegm-rheum dizziness is attended by heavy-headedness, oppression in the chest, vomiting, copious phlegm, and hasty panting. [MED] Fortify the spleen and transform rheum with formulas such as Two Matured Ingredients Decoction (*èr chén tāng*), Phlegm-Abducting Decoction (*dǎo tán tāng*), or Six Gentlemen Decoction (*liù jūn zǐ tāng*). [ACU] Base treatment mainly on ST and LI. Select ST-8 (*tóu wéi*, Head Corner), CV-12 (*zhōng wǎn*, Center Stomach Duct), ST-36 (*zú sān lǐ*, Leg Three Li), LI-4 (*hé gǔ*, Union Valley), ST-40 (*fēng lóng*, Bountiful Bulge), and ST-41 (*jiě xī*, Ravine Divide); needle with even supplementation and drainage. [26: 766]

phlegm-rheum rapid panting 痰饮喘急 *tán yǐn chuǎn jí*: Rapid panting that arises when phlegm-rheum congests in the lung and causes counterflow ascent of qi. Phlegm-rheum rapid panting is mostly observed in children. [MED] Treat with Perilla Seed and Tingli Phlegm-Rolling Pill (*sū tíng gǔn tán wán*). [ACU] Base treatment mainly on LU, SP, and ST. Select BL-13 (*fèi shū*, Lung Transport), Panting Stabilizer (*dìng chuǎn*), BL-43 (*gāo huāng shū*, Gao-Huang Transport), LU-9 (*tài yuān*, Great Abyss), CV-12 (*zhōng wǎn*, Center Stomach Duct), ST-40 (*fēng lóng*, Bountiful Bulge), ST-36 (*zú sān lǐ*, Leg Three Li), and SP-9 (*yīn líng quán*, Yin Mound Spring); needle with supplementation or with even supplementation and drainage, and, if appropriate, add moxa. [26: 766] [46: 597, 655]

phlegm-rheum rib-side pain 痰饮胁痛 *tán yǐn xié tòng*: COLLECTING RHEUM RIB-SIDE PAIN. [26: 650, 766]

phlegm-rheum stomach duct pain 痰饮胃脘痛 *tán yǐn wèi wǎn (guǎn) tòng*: Stomach pain that arises when impaired spleen-stomach movement and transformation causes water-damp to gather and gradually turn into phlegm-rheum, which collects in the center burner. Phlegm-rheum stomach duct pain is attended by reduced food intake, nausea, vexation and oppression, ejection of foamy phlegm, and a slippery stringlike pulse. There may also be dizziness, heart palpitations and shortness of breath, and gurgling in the abdomen. [MED] Transform rheum and harmonize the stomach. Use formulas such as Dampness-Eliminating Stomach-Calming Poria (Hoelen) Five Decoction (*chú shī wèi líng tāng*) and Two Matured Ingredients Decoction (*èr chén tāng*). For phlegm-fire, use Center-Clearing Decoction (*qīng zhōng tāng*). For rheum pouring into the limbs and channels and causing lumbar, back, and rib-side pain, or pulling pain in the limbs, manifesting in repletion signs only, offensive expulsion should performed with formulas like Minor Stomach Elixir (*xiǎo wèi dān*), Drool-Controlling Elixir (*kòng xián dān*), or Three Flowers Spirit Protection Pill (*sān huā shén yòu wán*). ACU Base treatment mainly on alarm and uniting points of ST, PC, and SP. Select CV-12 (*zhōng wǎn*, Center Stomach Duct), ST-36 (*zú sān lǐ*, Leg Three Li), ST-40 (*fēng lóng*, Bountiful Bulge), PC-6 (*nèi guān*, Inner Pass), SP-4 (*gōng sūn*, Yellow Emperor), ST-25 (*tiān shū*, Celestial Pivot), and CV-6 (*qì hǎi*, Sea of Qi); needle with drainage. See also INTERNAL DAMAGE STOMACH DUCT PAIN. [46: 597, 660] [26: 766]

phlegm-rheum vomiting 痰饮呕吐 *tán yǐn ǒu tù*: See PHLEGM VOMITING. [26: 767]

phlegm scrofula 痰疬 *tán lì*: **1.** SCROFULA attributed to phlegm arising when abnormalities of hunger and satiety and of joy and anger cause impairment of the splenic movement. Phlegm scrofula begins as lumps the size of a mume (Japanese apricot), which may spread all over the body. In time, they become slightly red, and can rupture to heal easily. MED Move qi and sweep phlegm using formulas such as Scutellaria and Coptis Two Matured Ingredients Decoction (*qín lián èr chén tāng*). ACU Base treatment mainly on ST, CV, and TB. Select as main points Ouch points (*ā shì xué*) (i.e., the nodes themselves), Hundred Taxations (*bǎi láo*) and Tip of the Elbow (*zhǒu jiān*) (see SCROFULA for method). To move qi and sweep phlegm, needle with drainage at CV-12 (*zhōng wǎn*, Center Stomach Duct), ST-36 (*zú sān lǐ*, Leg Three Li), ST-40 (*fēng lóng*, Bountiful Bulge), LI-4 (*hé gǔ*, Union Valley), and TB-10 (*tiān jǐng*, Celestial Well). For treatment according to affected area, see SCROFULA. **2.** Scrofula growing on the yang brightness (*yáng míng*) stomach channel on the front of the neck. [26: 768] [46: 597] [37: 445] [113: 383]

phlegm stagnation malign obstruction 痰滞恶阻 *tán zhì è zǔ*: VOMITING arising in pregnancy when spleen-stomach vacuity causes dampness to gather and form into phlegm and when congestion of blood in the channels causes thoroughfare vessel qi to ascend counterflow and carry the phlegm-rheum upward. Phlegm stagnation malign obstruction is characterized by nausea, vomiting of phlegm-drool, fullness in the chest, and poor appetite. MED Sweep phlegm and downbear counterflow using Minor Pinellia Decoction Plus Poria (Hoelen) (*xiǎo bàn xià jiā fú líng tāng*). ACU Base treatment mainly on CV, ST, and PC.

Select CV-12 (*zhōng wǎn*, Center Stomach Duct), PC-6 (*nèi guān*, Inner Pass), ST-36 (*zú sān lǐ*, Leg Three Li), ST-40 (*fēng lóng*, Bountiful Bulge), ST-25 (*tiān shū*, Celestial Pivot), and SP-4 (*gōng sūn*, Yellow Emperor); needle with even supplementation and drainage and add moxa. [26: 767] [59: 117]

phlegm stroke 痰中 *tán zhòng*: *Synonym: dampness stroke.* A pattern similar to wind stroke that arises when dampness engenders phlegm, which in turn engenders heat, which further engenders wind. Phlegm stroke is characterized by sudden dizziness, numbness, collapse and loss of consciousness, rigidity of the root of the tongue, sound of phlegm in the throat, inability to lift the limbs, and a slippery surging pulse. MED Treat chiefly by transforming phlegm and secondarily by extinguishing wind, using formulas such as Phlegm-Abducting Decoction (*dǎo tán tāng*). ACU Base treatment mainly on GV, LI, hand and foot reverting yin (*jué yīn*) PC/LR, ST and SP. Select GV-26 (*shuǐ gōu*, Water Trough), GV-20 (*bǎi huì*, Hundred Convergences), PC-9 (*zhōng chōng*, Central Hub), LI-4 (*hé gǔ*, Union Valley), GB-20 (*fēng chí*, Wind Pool), LR-3 (*tài chōng*, Supreme Surge), LR-2 (*xíng jiān*, Moving Between), ST-40 (*fēng lóng*, Bountiful Bulge), ST-36 (*zú sān lǐ*, Leg Three Li), ST-44 (*nèi tíng*, Inner Court), PC-5 (*jiān shǐ*, Intermediary Courier), and SP-9 (*yīn líng quán*, Yin Mound Spring); needle with drainage. [26: 764]

phlegm turbidity 痰浊 *tán zhuó*: Phlegm as a turbid entity that is obstructive to the clear yang qi of the body. Phlegm turbidity is often said specifically to refer to PHLEGM-DAMP or PHLEGM-RHEUM. However, phlegm turbidity often implies that the phlegm is thick and sticky, while phlegm-damp often implies that the phlegm is thin. [27: 120] [44: 835]

phlegm turbidity clouding the pericardium 痰浊蒙蔽心包 *tán zhuó méng bì xīn bāo*: See PHLEGM CONFOUNDING THE ORIFICES OF THE HEART.

phlegm turbidity harassing the upper body 痰浊上扰 *tán zhuó shàng rǎo*: A disease pattern whose principal sign is dizziness, arising when phlegm turbidity causes internal obstruction in the chest and disturbs clear yang in the upper body. Dizziness is the essential feature of phlegm turbidity harassing the upper body. Hence it is said, "Where no phlegm is present, dizziness does not arise." Disturbance of vision may be so severe as to force the patient to remain in lying posture. Milder cases present as dizzy head, distention in the head, and heavy-headedness. Other signs include insomnia, oppression in the chest, retching and nausea, little thought of food and drink, or nontransformation of ingested food. The tongue fur is slimy in texture and either white or yellow in color. The pulse is slippery, and may also be string-like. Where there is a heat complication, then vexation and bitter taste in the mouth may also be observed. [WMC] Phlegm turbidity harassing the upper body may be observed in otogenic vertigo and hypertension. [6: 218]

phlegm turbidity obstructing the lung 痰浊阻肺 *tán zhuó zǔ fèi*: A disease pattern arising when phlegm turbidity congests the airways and impairs lung qi diffusion and depuration. The main signs are cough with copious sticky white phlegm that is easily ejected. Other signs include oppression in the chest and panting and phlegm rale in severe cases. The tongue is pale with white slimy fur. The pulse is slippery. [MED] Transform phlegm turbidity; depurate the lung and suppress cough. Use Lung-Clearing Beverage (*qīng fèi yǐn*) with additions. **Analysis:** When phlegm turbidity obstructs the lung, lung qi ascends counterflow, hence cough with copious sticky white phlegm that is easily expectorated. Phlegm turbidity is a tangible evil; when it obstructs the lung, it affects the upward, downward, inward and outward movement of qi, hence the oppression in the chest, panting, and phlegm rale. The pale tongue with white slimy fur, and the slippery pulse are both signs of phlegm turbidity causing internal obstruction. **Comparison:** *Yang vacuity water flood:* The main signs of phlegm turbidity obstructing the lung are copious phlegm, cough, and panting. The chief signs of yang vacuity water swelling are water swelling, fear of cold, and cold limbs. Phlegm turbidity obstructing the lung is a repletion pattern. Yang vacuity water swelling is a vacuity pattern complicated by repletion. *Welling-abscess (yōng) of the lung:* Phlegm turbidity obstructing the lung is marked by copious phlegm, cough, and panting. Welling-abscess (*yōng*) of the lung is marked by chest pain, generalized heat [effusion], and expectoration of fishy-smelling pus and blood. The two are easily distinguished. [116: 64] [50: 1635]

phlegm vomiting 痰呕 *tán ǒu*: Synonyms: *vomiting of phlegm-rheum*; *phlegm accumulation vomiting*. VOMITING that arises when disturbance of spleen-stomach movement and transformation causes dampness to form into phlegm, which lodges in the middle stomach duct and ascends counterflow. Phlegm vomiting takes the form of periodic nausea and vomiting of phlegm-drool, gurgling sounds in the stomach, heart palpitations, dizzy head, and flowery vision. If signs include yellow slimy tongue fur, and rapid stringlike pulse, it is attributed phlegm-heat; if signs include a white slimy tongue fur and a slow sunken pulse, it is ascribed to cold rheum. [MED] Clear heat and transform phlegm with Gardenia and Coptis Two

Matured Ingredients Decoction (*zhī lián èr chén tāng*). Cold rheum is treated by warming the stomach and transforming rheum with formulas such as Major Pinellia Decoction (*dà bàn xià tāng*) or Poria (Hoelen), Cinnamon Twig, Ovate Atractylodes, and Licorice Decoction (*líng guì zhú gān tāng*). If the patient vomits after taking the formula, this is a sign of phlegm qi binding in the throat and diaphragm; in such cases use Return Again Elixir (*lái fù dān*), wait for vomiting, and then take Two Matured Ingredients Decoction (*èr chén tāng*) plus amomum (*shā rén*), clove (*dīng xiāng*), and fresh ginger (*shēng jiāng*). [ACU] Base treatment on alarm and lower uniting points of ST, and on CV and PC. Main points: CV-12 (*zhōng wǎn*, Center Stomach Duct), ST-36 (*zú sān lǐ*, Leg Three Li), PC-6 (*nèi guān*, Inner Pass), ST-40 (*fēng lóng*, Bountiful Bulge), and CV-17 (*shān zhōng*, Chest Center). For phlegm-heat, add ST-44 (*nèi tíng*, Inner Court) and LI-11 (*qū chí*, Pool at the Bend); needle with drainage. For cold rheum, add SP-4 (*gōng sūn*, Yellow Emperor) and BL-20 (*pí shū*, Spleen Transport); needle with drainage and add moxa. [26: 767] [46: 659] [113: 19, 72]

phlegm wheezing 痰哮 *tán xiāo*: Wheezing attributed to phlegm turbidity congestion arising from phlegm-fire lying depressed in the inner body or wind-cold fettering the exterior. Phlegm wheezing is characterized by rapid panting, phlegm rale in the throat sounding like the rasping of a saw. [MED] Diffuse the lung and downbear qi; dispel phlegm and clear fire. Use formulas such as Five Tigers Decoction (*wǔ hǔ tāng*). [ACU] Base treatment mainly on LU, CV, and ST. Select BL-13 (*fèi shū*, Lung Transport), BL-12 (*fēng mén*, Wind Gate), LU-7 (*liè quē*, Broken Sequence), LU-5 (*chǐ zé*, Cubit Marsh), Panting Stabilizer (*dìng chuǎn*), CV-22 (*tiān tú*, Celestial Chimney), CV-17 (*shān zhōng*, Chest Center), ST-40 (*fēng lóng*, Bountiful Bulge), CV-12 (*zhōng wǎn*, Center Stomach Duct), and LI-4 (*hé gǔ*, Union Valley); needle with drainage. See WHEEZING. [26: 765]

photophobia 恶光羞明 *wù guāng xiū míng*: AVERSION TO LIGHT.

physical body 形 *xíng*: The physical body in contrast to the *constitutional body*. Examining the physique is an important part of general diagnosis. A well-developed, strong, firm body indicates a strong constitution. Poor development and emaciation indicate a weak constitution. Obesity with soft flesh, lusterless white skin, shortage of qi, lack of strength, and lack of devitalized essence-spirit indicate what is known as a FULL PHYSIQUE WITH VACUOUS QI, implying a physical constitution characterized by a yang qi vacuity. Such conditions are often seen in diseases described by Western medicine as endocrine disturbances, hypothyroidism, and some forms of hypertension. A pale drawn complexion, emaciation, and dry skin indicate insufficiency of yin-blood, generally seen in constitutional yin vacuity. Such conditions occur often in cases of tuberculosis, which has lead to the saying, "The thin are prone to taxation coughs." [27: 266]

physical cold 形寒 *xing hán*: Outwardly manifest signs of cold, e.g., aversion to cold, desire for warm beverages, curled-up lying posture, cold limbs, etc. *Elementary Questions* (*sù wèn, tiáo jīng lùn*) states, "When yang is vacuous, there is external cold." "Physical cold" is what is meant by "external cold." [50: 685]

physical cold and cold limbs 形寒肢冷 *xing hán zhī lěng*: See PHYSICAL COLD.

pi 僻 *pì*: See AGGREGATION. [48: 442]

picking at bedclothes 循衣摸床 *xún yī mō chuáng*: Synonym: *carphology*. An aimless plucking at bedclothes observed in an extreme stage of disease. It occurs notably in extreme yang bright (*yáng míng*) heat with heat effusion and clouded spirit. Compare GROPING IN THE AIR AND PULLING AT INVISIBLE STRINGS. [26: 753] [27: 373] [97: 568] [6: 116]

picking therapy 挑治疗法 *tiāo zhì liáo fǎ*: *root-severing therapy; needle-picking therapy.* A method of treating disease that involves picking subcutaneous fibers with a needle. Picking therapy is a widely used folk remedy that came to be practiced by Chinese medical health-care workers after the so-called liberation. It is performed at specific sites including acupuncture points, and is mostly used to treat hemorrhoids, but is also used for prolapse of the rectum, clove sores (*dīng chuāng*), welling-abscesses (*yōng*) and flat-abscesses (*jū*) acute conjunctivitis (wind-fire eye), sties, profuse menstruation, and chronic prostatitis. BL-25 (*dà cháng shū*, Large Intestine Transport) and BL-32 (*cì liáo*, Second Bone-Hole) are used for hemorrhoids, and GV-14 (*dà zhuī*, Great Hammer) for conjunctivitis. Method: At the selected site, a three-edged needle or large sewing needle is inserted to a depth of 2–3 mm a lifted so as to draw out and sever white fiber from under the skin. The site is then dressed. Treatment may be repeated at the same point 2–3 weeks later. Attention must be paid to hygiene to avoid infection. [26: 421] [50: 1068] [46: 541]

pick to bleed 挑刺放血 *tiāo cì fàng xuè*, 挑刺出血 *tiāo cì chū xuè*: To perform bleeding with a three-edged needle by a brisk darting and flicking action. See BLOODLETTING.

pigeon chest 鸡胸 *jī xiōng*: CHICKEN BREAST.

¹**pile** 痔 *zhì*: **1.** Any protrusion of flesh from any of the nine orifices, e.g., EAR PILE or YIN PILE. **2.** Specifically, HEMORRHOID. [48: 295]

²**pile** 痔疮 *zhì chuāng*: HEMORRHOID.

pill 丸 *wán*, 丸剂 *wán jì*: A medicinal preparation made by mixing finely ground medicinals with a binding medium (usually honey, water, or flour and water paste), and forming them into small round balls. The pill preparation has the advantage of being more convenient for the patient than the decoction, especially when medication has to be taken over a long period of time. The active constituents are absorbed into the body more slowly, but their effect is longer lasting. Pills are therefore most commonly used in the treatment of enduring diseases, and especially concretions and accumulations. They are also used for certain acute patterns since they can be kept at hand ready for occasional use. Pills are taken by swallowing with, or dissolving in water. See MEDICINAL PREPARATION. [27: 312]

pillow bone 枕骨 *zhěn gǔ*: Synonym: *jade pillow bone.* The bone in the lower back part of the skull, so called because the head rests on this part of the head in supine posture. ⌑WMC⌑ occipital bone. [27: 63] [97: 332]

pillow fontanel 枕囟 *zhěn xìn*: The posterior fontanel. See FONTANEL.

pimples 痤疮 *cuó chuāng*: ACNE.

pinch-and-lift needle insertion 提捏进针法 *tí niē jìn zhēn fǎ*: Synonym: *skin-pinching needle insertion.* A two-handed needle insertion technique whereby the needle is inserted while the other hand (pressing hand) pinches and lifts the flesh. Method: (1) While holding the handle of the needle with the thumb and forefinger of the right hand, pinch the skin around the point with the left hand. (2) Rest the tip of the needle lightly on the point, and insert with a quick, firm downward movement. Application: This technique is applied on parts of the body such as the face where the flesh is thin and shallow. See NEEDLE INSERTION. [46: 640]

pine bark lichen 松皮癣 *sōng pí xiǎn*: LICHEN marked by a thickening of the skin that gives the appearance of pine bark. Pine bark lichen is attributed to factors such as invasion of exterior wind-cold, disharmony between construction and defense and between the thoroughfare (*chōng*) and controlling (*rèn*) vessels, and construction-defense depletion. It starts with red macules of various sizes, covered with white scales that slough away to reveal bleeding speckles and cause itching. It occurs on corresponding positions on the outer (yang) aspect of the limbs. See LICHEN. [27: 474] [97: 332]

pinworm 蛲虫 *náo chóng*: See PINWORM DISEASE.

pinworm disease 蛲虫病 *náo chóng bìng*: Synonym: *kidney worm disease.* *The Origin and Indicators of Disease* (*zhū bìng yuán hòu lùn*). One of the THREE WORM DISEASES and one of the *nine worm diseases.* Pinworm disease is most common in infants and children. It is associated with night-time anal itch that can affect sleep, heart vexation, and susceptibility to fright. [MED] Medicinals effective in treating pinworm include stemona (*bǎi bù*), aspidium (*guàn zhòng*), carpesium seed (*hè shī*), omphalia (*léi wán*), garlic (*dà suàn*), morning glory (*qiān niú zǐ*), pomegranate rind (*shí liú pí*), quisqualis (*shǐ jūn zǐ*), and brucea (*yā dǎn zǐ*). For example, rhubarb (*dà huáng*), morning glory (*qiān niú zǐ*), and quisqualis (*shǐ jūn zǐ*) can be used as oral medication, and use fluids of stemona (*bǎi bù*) and garlic (*dà suàn*) as enemas. Worm-Transforming Pill (*huà chóng wán*) can also be used. Pay attention to regular change of clothing to prevent reinfection. [26: 958]

plain stir-frying 清炒 *qīng chǎo*, 单炒 *dān chǎo*: Stir-frying without any adjuvants. It includes LIGHT STIR-FRYING, SCORCH-FRYING, and BLAST-FRYING.

plaster 膏药 *gāo yào*: A topical paste that is mounted on cloth. It is made by slicing or pounding the ingredients and steeping them in sesame seed oil or tung-oil (*tóng yóu*) for 3–5 days. The mixture is then heated to fry the materials until they char. Flowers, leaves, and pericarps that cannot withstand heat should not be included. The materials are strained off, and the oil is returned to the fire, where it is continuously heated and stirred until the smoke given off turns from white to blue-green. When the temperature reaches 250-300°C (at this temperature, when the oil is dropped in water it will stay together in a globule) the fire is turned down, and yellow upborne elixir (*huáng shēng*) or processed galenite (*qiān fěn*) is slowly stirred in. The pot is removed from the fire when all the yellow upborne elixir (*huáng shēng*) has dissolved. It is then sprinkled with water and stirred, and then steeped in cold water to eliminate the fire toxin. Before use it is melted over a small flame or in water so that it can be spread on cloth or animal skin ready for topical application. Plasters are used for sores and wind-damp pain. They are available ready made and mounted on cloth, and require only warming prior to application. [26: 826] [27: 298] [97: 629]

plaster wind 膏药风 *gāo yào fēng*: Redness and swelling, and, in severe cases, blistering, erosion, and weeping of the skin as a result of applying a medicinal plaster, elephant skin plaster, or the like. The affected area may be square or round like the shape of the plaster, and is clearly circumscribed. It is associated with itching or burning sensation, and spreads if scratched. [MED] Use Three Yellows Wash Preparation (*sān huáng xǐ jì*); if there is ulceration, apply Indigo Paste (*qīng dài gāo*). [96: 276]

-plegia 不遂 *bù suì*: A combining form denoting paralysis, e.g., *hemiplegia*.

plum-blossom needle 梅花针 *méi huā zhēn*: *Synonym: seven-star needle.* A cutaneous needle, traditionally made by binding 5 to 7 sewing needles to a bamboo stick, and used to provide a therapeutic stimulus when lightly tapped on the skin. See *cutaneous needle.* [27: 498] [97: 510]

plum-pit qi 梅核气 *méi hé qì*: *Synonym: qi phlegm.* *Synonym:* Dryness and a sensation of a foreign body present in the throat which can be neither swallowed or ejected. The intensity of the signs fluctuates. The main cause is binding depression of liver qi. [WMC] globus hystericus. [MED] Course the liver and rectify qi. Use Bupleurum Liver-Coursing Powder (*chái hú shū gān sǎn*) combined with Inula and Hematite Decoction (*xuán fù huā dài zhě shí tāng*). [ACU] Base treatment mainly on CV, LI, and PC. Select CV-22 (*tiān tú*, Celestial Chimney), CV-17 (*shān zhōng*, Chest Center), LI-4 (*hé gǔ*, Union Valley), and PC-5 (*jiān shǐ*, Intermediary Courier); needle with even supplementation and drainage and add moxa. For depressed qi, add BL-18 (*gān shū*, Liver Transport), LR-2 (*xíng jiān*, Moving Between), and GB-34 (*yáng líng quán*, Yang Mound Spring). Selection of points according to signs: For glomus and oppression in the chest and stomach duct, add PC-6 (*nèi guān*, Inner Pass), CV-12 (*zhōng wǎn*, Center Stomach Duct), and BL-17 (*gé shū*, Diaphragm Transport). For stagnant phlegm in the throat, add ST-40 (*fēng lóng*, Bountiful Bulge), and BL-20 (*pí shū*, Spleen Transport); needle with drainage. For hiccough or nausea, add CV-12 (*zhōng wǎn*, Center Stomach Duct), PC-6 (*nèi guān*, Inner Pass), ST-36 (*zú sān lǐ*, Leg Three Li), and BL-17 (*gé shū*, Diaphragm Transport). [113: 267] [46: 1360]

pock pimples 痤痱 *cuó fèi*: Sores of varying sizes, the larger of which, called pocks (*cuó*), are between the size of a soybean or a jujube, are red, and contain pus and the smaller of which, called pimples (*fèi*), are small vesicles or pustules. Pock pimples are attributed to lung heat and spleen dampness or summer wind-heat toxin in the skin. Pock pimples of the buttocks are called SEAT SORES. [WMC] furunculosis (multiple furuncles). [MED] Take Coptis Toxin-Resolving Decoction (*huáng lián jiě dú tāng*) and decoct purslane (*mǎ chǐ xiàn*) as a wash. [26: 673] [61: 372]

point 穴位 *xué wèi*, 穴道 *xué dào*: Abbreviation for *acupuncture point.* [27: 97]

point combination 配穴 *pèi xué*: Methods of combining points. See the entries listed below.

Point Combination

COMBINING LOCAL AND DISTANT POINTS (*yuǎn jìn pèi xué fǎ*)

COMBINING SOURCE AND NETWORK POINTS (*yuán luò pèi xué fǎ*)

COMBINING TRANSPORT AND ALARM POINTS (*shū mù pèi xué fǎ*)

COMBINING SAME-NAME CHANNEL POINTS (*tóng míng jīng pèi xué fǎ*)

COMBINING TRANSPORT POINTS (*wǔ shū pèi xué fǎ*)

COMBINING UPPER AND LOWER BODY POINTS (*shàng xià pèi xué fǎ*)

COMBINING LEFT AND RIGHT POINTS (*zuǒ yòu pèi xué fǎ*)

---

point joining 透穴 *tòu xué*: To insert an acupuncture needle (usually by transverse insertion) so that it passes through two or more points. For example, ST-4 (*dì cāng*, Earth Granary) joined to ST-6 (*jiá chē*, Cheek Carriage) treats deviation of the mouth; ST-38 (*tiáo kǒu*, Ribbon Opening) joined to BL-57 (*chéng shān*, Mountain Support) treats shoulder pain and inability to lift the shoulder; TB-5 (*wài guān*, Outer Pass) joined to PC-6 (*nèi guān*, Inner Pass), treats elbow and arm pain; GB-40 (*qiū xū*, Hill Ruins) joined to KI-6 (*zhào hǎi*, Shining Sea) treats ankle pain. [26: 645] [27: 331]

point selection 选穴 *xuǎn xué*: Points are selected by four basic methods: SELECTION OF LOCAL POINTS; SELECTION OF DISTANT POINTS; SELECTION OF POINTS ON THE AFFECTED CHANNEL; SELECTION OF PATHOCONDITION POINTS; SELECTION OF SPECIAL GROUP POINTS.

poling 艾条灸 *ài tiáo jiǔ*: Warming with a *moxa pole*.

polyuria 尿多 *niào duō*: Copious urine. See URINE.

poor appetite 食欲不振 *shí yù bù zhèn*, 食欲减退 *shí yù jiǎn tuì*, 胃口不好 *wèi kǒu bù hǎo*: *Synonym: reduced eat; reduced food intake*. A reduced desire to eat. The stomach governs intake and decomposition of grain and water (i.e., food); the spleen governs movement and transformation of grain and water and the distribution of their essence (i.e., nutrients). Appetite is principally related to the spleen and stomach. The stomach and spleen together form the "root of the later heaven," i.e., the basis of the acquired constitution. "The presence of stomach means life; the absence of stomach is death." A good appetite is a sign of health. In disease, a good appetite is a sign of a mild condition, and its return is a sign of recovery. Sudden return of an appetite in critical illness is a last flicker of the candle, and bodes death. Poor appetite is observed in externally contracted disease and internal damage. In most instances of externally contracted disease, it is of relatively short duration and hence of little significance. In internal damage miscellaneous disease, in which the duration of poor appetite can undermine the health of the patient, it commands greater attention. Distinction can be made between three categories of poor appetite: poor appetite without hunger; aversion to food; and no desire to eat despite hunger. **No thought of food and drink:** Simple poor appetite characterized by lack of thought of food and drink and reduced hunger sensation is what is normally meant by "poor appetite." Traditionally, this is often referred to as *no desire for food and drink, no thought of food and drink, obliviousness of hunger and satiety*, or *no pleasure in eating*. It occurs in a number of situations. (1) With distention after eating, diarrhea, emaciation, and lack of strength, poor appetite is ascribed to spleen-stomach qi vacuity arising when the stomach's function of decomposing food and the spleen's function is impaired. (2) Accompanied by oppression in the stomach duct, heavy cumbersome head and body, rumbling intestines, diarrhea, and slimy tongue fur, it is a sign of dampness encumbering the spleen that prevents the normal upbearing of clear yang and causes disharmony of stomach qi. (3) With aversion to oily food and accompanied by yellowing of the body, abdominal distention and glomus in the stomach duct, nausea, fatigue, and scant yellow urine is a sign of spleen-stomach damp-heat causing disharmony of stomach qi. (4) With belching, abdominal distention, rib-side pain, frequent passing of flatus, and sloppy stool, it is a sign of liver-spleen disharmony. (5) With alternating heat [effusion] and [aversion to] cold, [suffering of] chest and rib-side fullness, bitter taste in the mouth, dry throat, and dizzy vision, it is a sign of cold damage lesser yang (*shào yáng*) disease. **Aversion to food:** Aversion to food is sickness at the sight or thought of food and occurs in two situations. (1) Aversion to food is most commonly observed when voracious eating and drinking impairs decomposition, causing food to stagnate in the stomach. Hence, it is said, "Food damage is invariably characterized by aversion to food." (2) Occurring with vomiting, with absence of menstruation, and with a rapid slippery harmonious pulse in sexually active women, aversion to food is a sign of pregnancy vomiting, which is caused by upsurge of thoroughfare (*chōng*) vessel qi causing disharmony of stomach qi. *Poor appetite* differs from aversion to food in that it is associated with a reduced feeling of hunger. **No desire to eat despite hunger:** This is observed in three situations. (1) With clamoring stomach and scorching heat sensation, a red tongue with scant fur, it indicates insufficiency of stomach yin and vacuity fire. In such cases, the lack of desire to eat is explained by the insufficiency, whereas the presence of hunger is explained as result of the vacuity fire. (2) With dizziness, tinnitus, insomnia, forgetfulness, dry throat and tongue, it is attributed to insufficiency of kidney yin and frenetic movement of the ministerial fire. (3) In advanced stages of febrile disease with lassitude of spirit, lack of strength, and dry tongue with little liquid, a poor appetite is a sign of insufficiency of stomach yin resulting from qi, blood, and liquid depletion when the evil has abated. *Synonym:* The term *reduced food intake* is effectively a synonym of poor appetite, denoting its objective consequence. Poor appetite associated with indigestion is also called TORPID INTAKE, in reference to stomach function (see STOMACH GOVERNS INTAKE). [29: 198]

poor memory 健忘 *jiàn wàng*: See FORGETFULNESS.

poor stomach intake 胃纳不佳 *wèi nà bù jiā*: Impairment of the stomach's governing of food intake. The stomach is responsible for the initial intake of food; it governs decomposition of the grain and water (i.e., food), and when emptied of its contents, the desire to eat rises. Poor stomach intake is reduced eating due to impairment of the stomach's function.

posterior headache 后头痛 *hòu tóu tòng*: Pain affecting the back of the head. See GREATER YANG HEADACHE.

posterior yin 后阴 *hòu yīn*: The anus.

postmenstrual blood ejection and spontaneous external bleeding 经后吐衄 *jīng hòu tù nù*: Bleeding from the mouth or nose after menstruation; attributed to residual lung-stomach vacuity heat and blood heat failing to stay within the vessels causing loss of small amounts of fresh-colored blood. MED Clear lung-stomach vacuity heat using either variations of Rhinoceros Horn and Rehmannia Decoction (*xī jiǎo dì huáng tāng*) or Ophiopogon Drink (*mài mén dōng yǐn zi*). [26: 816]

postmeridian tidal heat [effusion] 午后潮热 *wǔ hòu cháo rè*: Tidal heat effusion occurring any time after midday. Postmeridian tidal heat [effusion] is usually a sign of yin vacuity, but a vigorous heat [effusion] that becomes more pronounced at roughly 3-5 p.m., called LATE AFTERNOON TIDAL HEAT [EFFUSION], is associated with yang brightness (*yáng míng*) interior repletion patterns. See TIDAL HEAT [EFFUSION]. [26: 859]

postpartum 产后 *chǎn hòu*: Occurring in the mother after she has given birth.

postpartum abdominal distention and vomiting 产后腹胀呕吐 *chǎn hòu fù zhàng ǒu tù*: Abdominal distention, fullness and oppression with vomiting and retching after childbirth. Postpartum abdominal distention and vomiting is associated with scant LOCHIA, and occurs when wasted blood attacks the spleen and stomach, causing stomach qi to ascend counterflow. MED Quicken the blood and dispel stasis; fortify the spleen and harmonize the stomach. Use variations of Engendering Transformation Decoction (*shēng huà tāng*). ACU Base treatment mainly on CV, ST, SP, and LR. To quicken the blood and dispel stasis, select CV-6 (*qì hǎi*, Sea of Qi), CV-3 (*zhōng jí*, Central Pole), SP-6 (*sān yīn jiāo*, Three Yin Intersection), LR-3 (*tài chōng*, Supreme Surge), and LR-8 (*qū quán*, Spring at the Bend); needle with even supplementation and drainage and add moxa. To fortify the spleen and harmonize the stomach, select CV-12 (*zhōng wǎn*, Center Stomach Duct), PC-6 (*nèi guān*, Inner Pass), ST-36 (*zú sān lǐ*, Leg Three Li), ST-25 (*tiān shū*, Celestial Pivot), BL-20 (*pí shū*, Spleen Transport), and BL-21 (*wèi shū*, Stomach Transport); needle with supplementation and add moxa. [26: 580]

postpartum abdominal pain 产后腹痛 *chǎn hòu fù tòng*: Synonym: *afterpains.* ABDOMINAL PAIN occurring after childbirth, as a result of blood vacuity or blood stasis. **Blood vacuity** patterns are characterized by dull pain that likes warmth and pressure, fatigue, fear of cold, and, in severe cases, heart palpitations and shortness of breath. MED Supplement the blood and boost qi with Abdomen-Quieting Decoction (*cháng níng tāng*). ACU Base treatment mainly on back transport points, CV, and ST. Select BL-20 (*pí shū*, Spleen Transport), BL-17 (*gé shū*, Diaphragm Transport), ST-36 (*zú sān lǐ*, Leg Three Li), CV-6 (*qì hǎi*, Sea of Qi), CV-4 (*guān yuán*, Pass Head), and SP-10 (*xuè hǎi*, Sea of Blood); needle with supplementation. **Blood stasis** patterns are marked by stabbing abdominal pain that refuses pressure, RETENTION OF THE LOCHIA, and dark purple facial complexion. MED Expel stasis and move the blood with Sudden Smile Powder (*shī xiào sǎn*) combined with Engendering Transformation Decoction (*shēng huà tāng*). For blood stasis giving rise to congealing cold with cold pain or gripping pain in the smaller abdomen that likes warmth, and a sunken tight or stringlike sunken pulse, add to this combination fennel (*huí xiāng*) and evodia (*wú zhū yú*). ACU Base treatment mainly on CV, SP, and ST. Select CV-6 (*qì hǎi*, Sea of Qi), SP-6 (*sān yīn jiāo*, Three Yin Intersection), CV-3 (*zhōng jí*, Central Pole), SP-8 (*dì jī*, Earth's Crux), and SP-10 (*xuè hǎi*, Sea of Blood); needle with even supplementation and drainage and add moxa. If there are also signs of congealing cold, add ST-29 (*guī lái*, Return) and ST-25 (*tiān shū*, Celestial Pivot), and add large amounts of moxa. NB: Postpartum abdominal pain caused by congealing static blood and marked by a palpable lump is called INFANT'S-PILLOW PAIN. [26: 580] [50: 615] [59: 173] [37: 434]

postpartum bleeding 产后出血 *chǎn hòu chū xuè*: See POSTPARTUM FLOODING.

postpartum blood dizziness 产后血晕 *chǎn hòu xuè yūn*: Dizzy head and flowery vision occurring after childbirth. Postpartum blood dizziness is often so severe that the patient cannot get up, and is sometimes accompanied by fullness and oppression in the chest, nausea and vomiting, welling of phlegm and rapid breathing, heart vexation, and, in severe cases, clenched jaw, clouded spirit, and loss of consciousness. WMC postpartum syncope, postpartum shock, postpartum amniotic embolism, postpartum vasomotor collapse. Distinction is made between vacuity and repletion patterns. **Vacuity** patterns result from postpartum flooding and spotting causing yin vacuity and sudden collapse. The blood is usually thin. Dizziness comes on suddenly with heart palpitations, heart vexation, oppression and discomfort, and, in severe cases, clouding loss of consciousness. General signs include somber white complexion, closed eyes and open mouth, limp hands and cold limbs, dripping cold sweat, pale tongue without fur, and a faint pulse on the verge of expiration or a large floating pulse. In vacuity patterns, there may also be signs of upflow of phlegm-fire causing sudden dizzy head and flowery vision, nausea and vomiting, fullness and oppression in the chest and heart, and, in severe cases, loss of consciousness. MED Boost qi and stem desertion using Pure Ginseng Decoction (*dú shēn tāng*) or Qi-Supplementing Dizziness-Resolving Decoction (*bǔ qì jiě yūn tāng*). For clouded spirit, cold limbs, and sweating, apply emergency yang-returning counterflow-stemming treatment using Ginseng and Aconite Decoction (*shēn fù tāng*). Treat vacuity with phlegm-fire by supplementing qi and nourishing the blood and by transforming phlegm and quieting the spirit. Use Engendering Transformation Decoction (*shēng huà tāng*) plus ginseng (*rén shēn*), red tangerine peel (*jú hóng*), dried bamboo sap (*zhú lì*), and ginger juice (*jiāng zhī*) taken in small frequent doses. ACU Base treatment mainly on GV, CV, ST, and SP. Select GV-26 (*rén zhōng*, Human Center), GV-20 (*bǎi huì*, Hundred Convergences), PC-6 (*nèi guān*, Inner Pass), SP-6 (*sān yīn jiāo*, Three Yin Intersection), and ST-36 (*zú sān lǐ*, Leg Three Li); needle with supplementation. In addition, moxa CV-6 (*qì hǎi*, Sea of Qi), GV-20 (*bǎi huì*, Hundred Convergences), and ST-36 (*zú sān lǐ*, Leg Three Li). Selection of points according to signs: For incessant postpartum bleeding, add moxa at SP-1 (*yǐn bái*, Hidden White). For heart palpitations, vexation, and oppression, add HT-7 (*shén mén*, Spirit Gate) and BL-15 (*xīn shū*, Heart

Transport). For dripping cold sweat, add HT-6 (*yīn xī*, Yin Cleft) and LI-4 (*hé gǔ*, Union Valley). For cold limbs and reversal dizziness (fainting), add CV-4 (*guān yuán*, Pass Head) and Hall of Impression (*yìn táng*), and perform moxibustion on ginger at CV-8 (*shén què*, Spirit Gate Tower). If there are signs of qi and blood vacuity with upflow of phlegm-fire, needle with drainage at LU-5 (*chǐ zé*, Cubit Marsh), PC-6 (*nèi guān*, Inner Pass), ST-40 (*fēng lóng*, Bountiful Bulge), ST-44 (*nèi tíng*, Inner Court), and HT-7 (*shén mén*, Spirit Gate). **Repletion** patterns are attributable to stasis obstruction and qi block; they arise when postpartum depletion of original qi and vacuity of the uterine vessels, sometimes exacerbated by contraction of cold, cause congealing and stagnation that prevents normal elimination of the LOCHIA and upsets the movement of qi. Signs include retention or scant flow of the lochia, with periodic lesser-abdominal pain that refuses pressure. In severe cases, there is acute fullness below the heart. General signs include rough breathing and hasty panting, clouded spirit and loss of consciousness, clenched jaw and clenched hand, dark purple complexion and purple tongue, and a rough pulse. MED Move the blood and dispel stasis using Life-Clutching Powder (*duó mìng sǎn*). Either add to this formula tangkuei (*dāng guī*), ligusticum (*chuān xiōng*), or combine it with Engendering Transformation Decoction (*shēng huà tāng*) plus ginseng (*rén shēn*), cyathula (*chuān niú xī*), leonurus (*yì mǔ cǎo*), and flying squirrel's droppings (*wǔ líng zhī*). If there is oppression in the chest, add fresh ginger (*shēng jiāng*), and bile arisaema (*dǎn xīng*) to downbear counterflow and transform phlegm. ACU Base treatment mainly on GV, LR, PC, and SP. Select GV-26 (*rén zhōng*, Human Center), KI-1 (*yǒng quán*, Gushing Spring), LR-1 (*dà dūn*, Large Pile), SP-6 (*sān yīn jiāo*, Three Yin Intersection), LR-3 (*tài chōng*, Supreme Surge), PC-6 (*nèi guān*, Inner Pass), and ST-36 (*zú sān lǐ*, Leg Three Li); needle with drainage. Prick GV-20 (*bǎi huì*, Hundred Convergences) and Ten Diffusing Points (*shí xuān*) to bleed. For oppression in the chest, add CV-12 (*zhōng wǎn*, Center Stomach Duct) and CV-17 (*shān zhōng*, Chest Center). For contraction of cold, add GB-20 (*fēng chí*, Wind Pool), TB-5 (*wài guān*, Outer Pass), and LU-7 (*liè quē*, Broken Sequence). [26: 577] [67: 263] [97: 450] [59: 176]

postpartum communicating bowels 产后交肠病 *chǎn hòu jiāo cháng bìng*: WMC postpartum rectovaginal fistula. [26: 576]

postpartum defecation difficulty 产后大便难 *chǎn hòu dà biàn nán*: Constipation arising when loss of blood after childbirth damages the fluids and deprives the intestines of moisture. MED Moisten the intestines and free the stool using honey (*mì*), hemp seed (*huǒ má rén*), and tangkuei (*dāng guī*). Do not use precipitants. ACU Base treatment mainly on ST and SP. Select BL-20 (*pí shū*, Spleen Transport), BL-21 (*wèi shū*, Stomach Transport), BL-25 (*dà cháng shū*, Large Intestine Transport), SP-6 (*sān yīn jiāo*, Three Yin Intersection), ST-36 (*zú sān lǐ*, Leg Three Li), and CV-4 (*guān yuán*, Pass Head); needle with supplementation and moxa if appropriate. [26: 574]

postpartum depression and veiling 产后郁冒 *chǎn hòu yù mào*: 1. From *Essential Prescriptions of the Golden Coffer* (*jīn guì yào lüè*, *fù rén chǎn hòu bìng mài zhèng bìng zhì*). "Depression" means binding depression, constrained qi; "veiling" means clouding of the spirit. Postpartum depression and veiling is a dizziness and visual distortion with feelings of depression and oppression, accompanied by retching and inability to eat, hard stool, and sweating head. MED Treat by resolving both interior and exterior with Minor Bupleurum Decoction (*xiǎo chái hú tāng*). 2. POSTPARTUM BLOOD DIZZINESS. [26: 581]

postpartum diarrhea 产后泄泻 *chǎn hòu xiè xiè*: Diarrhea occurring after delivery owing to nonmovement of the LOCHIA affecting spleen function. Postpartum diarrhea takes the form of incontinent throughflux diarrhea with green-blue, black, and white stool. MED Use Truly Wondrous Powder (*dì qí sǎn*), comprising four or five awns of schizonepeta (*jīng jiè*), burned to cinders in an oil lamp mixed with a pinch of musk (*shè xiāng*) taken with hot water. See DIARRHEA. [26: 577]

postpartum enuresis 产后遗尿 *chǎn hòu yí niào*: Enuresis arising after childbirth from kidney vacuity and insecurity of bladder qi, from qi-blood vacuity, or from damage to the bladder in childbirth. MED Boost the kidney and supplement the center with Center-Supplementing Qi-Boosting Decoction (*bǔ zhōng yì qì tāng*) combined with Mantis Egg-Case Powder (*sāng piāo xiāo sǎn*). Damage to the bladder may require surgery. ACU Base treatment mainly on back transport points. Select BL-23 (*shèn shū*, Kidney Transport), CV-3 (*zhōng jí*, Central Pole), BL-28 (*páng guāng shū*, Bladder Transport), SP-6 (*sān yīn jiāo*, Three Yin Intersection), and BL-22 (*sān jiāo shū*, Triple Burner Transport); needle with supplementation and add moxa. To boost the kidney and supplement the center, add CV-4 (*guān yuán*, Pass Head), GV-4 (*mìng mén*, Life Gate), KI-3 (*tài xī*, Great Ravine), BL-20 (*pí shū*, Spleen Transport), and ST-36 (*zú sān lǐ*, Leg Three Li). If due to damage to the bladder during delivery, add CV-6 (*qì hǎi*, Sea of Qi) and BL-39 (*wěi yáng*, Bend Yang). In China, acupuncture point injection has been used for postpartum enuresis. Points such as CV-3 (*zhōng jí*, Central Pole) and SP-6 (*sān yīn jiāo*, Three Yin In-

tersection) are injected every other day in 10 days courses with 0.2–.5 ml. of 0.5–1.0% procaine. [26: 581]

postpartum failure of the jade door to heal 产后玉户不敛 *chǎn hòu yù hù bù liǎn*: Failure of damage to the birth gate (*orificium vaginae*) in childbirth to heal within a few days. Postpartum failure of the jade gate to heal can be treated with an oral formula such as Perfect Major Supplementation Decoction (*shí quán dà bǔ tāng*) and topically with bletilla (*bái jí*), dragon bone (*lóng gǔ*), hornet's nest (*lù fēng fáng*), chebule (*hē zǐ*), and phellodendron (*huáng bǎi*), ground in equal proportions and applied after washing the affected area with a decoction of perilla leaf (*zǐ sū*). [26: 576]

postpartum fearful throbbing 产后怔忡 *chǎn hòu zhēng chōng*: FEARFUL THROBBING (severe heart palpitations) attributed to excessive blood loss in childbirth depriving the heart of nourishment. MED Harmonize the stomach and spleen; supplement qi and nourish the blood. Use formulas such as Ginseng Construction-Nourishing Decoction (*rén shēn yǎng róng tāng*) and variations. For incomplete elimination of static blood and inhibited flow of the LOCHIA, Engendering Transformation Decoction (*shēng huà tāng*) can be prescribed to eliminate stasis and engender the new. ACU Base treatment mainly on HT, PC, ST, SP, and back transport points. Select HT-7 (*shén mén*, Spirit Gate), PC-6 (*nèi guān*, Inner Pass), BL-15 (*xīn shū*, Heart Transport), BL-20 (*pí shū*, Spleen Transport), ST-36 (*zú sān lǐ*, Leg Three Li), SP-6 (*sān yīn jiāo*, Three Yin Intersection), and HT-5 (*tōng lǐ*, Connecting Li); needle with supplementation. For residual static blood, add LR-3 (*tài chōng*, Supreme Surge), BL-17 (*gé shū*, Diaphragm Transport), LI-4 (*hé gǔ*, Union Valley), and SP-10 (*xuè hǎi*, Sea of Blood). [26: 577]

postpartum heat effusion 产后发热 *chǎn hòu fā rè*: Heat effusion occurring after childbirth; attributed to external contraction, blood vacuity, blood stasis, food stagnation, or contraction of evil toxin. **External contraction** patterns arise when sudden vacuity of qi and blood causes insecurity of the defensive exterior and allows external evils to exploit the vacuity and enter the body. They are characterized by aversion to cold, heat effusion, headache, pain in limbs, absence of sweating, and in some cases cough and runny nose. MED Nourish the blood and dispel wind with formulas such as Schizonepeta and Ledebouriella Toxin-Vanquishing Powder (*jīng fáng bài dú sǎn*). ACU Base treatment mainly on back transport points, ST, SP, GB, TB, and LI. Needle with supplementation at BL-17 (*gé shū*, Diaphragm Transport), BL-20 (*pí shū*, Spleen Transport), ST-36 (*zú sān lǐ*, Leg

Three Li), and SP-6 (*sān yīn jiāo*, Three Yin Intersection), and with drainage at GB-20 (*fēng chí*, Wind Pool), TB-5 (*wài guān*, Outer Pass), GV-14 (*dà zhuī*, Great Hammer), LI-4 (*hé gǔ*, Union Valley), and LI-11 (*qū chí*, Pool at the Bend). **Blood vacuity** postpartum heat effusion arises after loss of blood in childbirth when yin fails to contain yang and vacuity heat arises internally. It is a mild heat effusion attended by dizziness, heart palpitations, or continual unabating abdominal pain. MED Supplement qi and blood and regulate construction and defense. Use variations of Eight-Gem Decoction (*bā zhēn tāng*). If heat effusion is more pronounced after midday, with reddening of the cheeks, thirst with desire for cold drinks, constipation, and yellow urine, treat by nourishing the blood, enriching yin, and clearing heat with All Yin Brew (*yī yīn jiān*). ACU Base treatment mainly on back transport points, CV, and three yin channels of the foot. Main points: BL-17 (*gé shū*, Diaphragm Transport), BL-20 (*pí shū*, Spleen Transport), ST-36 (*zú sān lǐ*, Leg Three Li), SP-6 (*sān yīn jiāo*, Three Yin Intersection), and SP-10 (*xuè hǎi*, Sea of Blood); needle with supplementation. To supplement qi and blood and to regulate construction and defense, add CV-4 (*guān yuán*, Pass Head), CV-6 (*qì hǎi*, Sea of Qi), BL-15 (*xīn shū*, Heart Transport), and CV-12 (*zhōng wǎn*, Center Stomach Duct). To enrich yin and clear heat, and to nourish the blood, add KI-3 (*tài xī*, Great Ravine), KI-6 (*zhào hǎi*, Shining Sea), and KI-7 (*fù liū*, Recover Flow). **Blood stasis** postpartum heat effusion arises when static blood becomes lodged in the channels, causing disharmony of construction and defense. It is characterized by periodic heat effusion and aversion to cold, retention of the lochia or scant purple clotted LOCHIA with a fishy smell and smaller-abdominal pain that refuses pressure. MED Nourish the blood and expel stasis; resolve heat effusion. Use variations of Engendering Transformation Decoction (*shēng huà tāng*). ACU Base treatment mainly on CV, and SP. Select CV-3 (*zhōng jí*, Central Pole), SP-8 (*dì jī*, Earth's Crux), SP-10 (*xuè hǎi*, Sea of Blood), SP-6 (*sān yīn jiāo*, Three Yin Intersection), and ST-30 (*qì chōng*, Qi Thoroughfare); needle with even supplementation and drainage. **Food stagnation** postpartum heat effusion results from eating sweet fatty foods. It is attended by bloating in the chest and diaphragm, putrid belching, swallowing of upflowing acid, torpid intake, or distention and pain in the stomach duct and abdomen. MED Disperse food and abduct stagnation with Special Achievement Powder (*yì gōng sǎn*) supplemented with other agents. ACU Base treatment mainly on CV, ST, and LI. Select CV-12 (*zhōng wǎn*, Center Stomach Duct), ST-25 (*tiān shū*, Celestial Pivot), CV-6 (*qì hǎi*, Sea of Qi), ST-36 (*zú*

sān lǐ, Leg Three Li), Li Inner Court (*lǐ nèi tíng*) LI-4 (*hé gǔ*, Union Valley), and LI-11 (*qū chí*, Pool at the Bend); needle with drainage. **Evil toxin** postpartum heat effusion arises when evil toxin makes a direct strike on the uterus in postpartum qi-blood vacuity, and wages a struggle with right qi that gives rise to high fever, thirst, sweating, and abdominal pain that refuses pressure. In severe cases, there may be clouded spirit, delirious speech and maculopapular eruptions. MED Clear heat and resolve toxin with agents such as lonicera (*jīn yín huā*), forsythia (*lián qiào*), dried/fresh rehmannia (*shēng dì huáng*), trichosanthes root (*tiān huā fěn*), lycium root bark (*dì gǔ pí*), moutan (*mǔ dān pí*), and isatis leaf (*dà qīng yè*). If signs include clouded spirit and delirious speech, use Peaceful Palace Bovine Bezoar Pill (*ān gōng niú huáng wán*) or Purple Snow (*zǐ xuě*). ACU Base treatment mainly on LI, PC, and LR. Select LI-11 (*qū chí*, Pool at the Bend), LI-4 (*hé gǔ*, Union Valley), LR-2 (*xíng jiān*, Moving Between), GB-34 (*yáng líng quán*, Yang Mound Spring), PC-8 (*láo gōng*, Palace of Toil), and BL-40 (*wěi zhōng*, Bend Center); needle with drainage. Prick Ten Diffusing Points (*shí xuān*) to bleed. [26: 579] [27: 450] [37: 418]

postpartum flooding 产后血崩 *chǎn hòu xuè bēng*: Severe bleeding after childbirth. Postpartum flooding is attributable to a) damage to the thoroughfare (*chōng*), controlling (*rèn*), and uterine vessels, b) damage through physical exertion before the channels have returned to normal after childbirth, c) retention of the afterbirth causing obstruction of the thoroughfare, controlling, and uterine vessels, or d) sex too soon after childbirth. For treatment, see FLOODING and RETENTION OF THE AFTERBIRTH. [26: 577]

postpartum food damage 产后伤食 *chǎn hòu shāng shí*: Food damage that occurs as a result of dietary irregularity causing damage to the spleen and stomach after childbirth. Postpartum food damage is characterized by fullness and oppression in the chest and stomach duct, putrid belching and swallowing of upflowing acid, and sour-smelling stool. MED Treat by simultaneous dispersion and supplementation. Use Engendering Transformation Decoction (*shēng huà tāng*) with the addition of abducting dispersion medicinals. For noodle-type food damage, use medicated leaven (*shén qū*) and barley sprout (*mài yá*). For meat-type food damage, add crataegus (*shān zhā*) and amomum (*shā rén*). For damage by raw or cold foods, add evodia (*wú zhū yú*) and cinnamon bark (*ròu guì*). If there is pronounced vacuity, add ginseng (*rén shēn*) and ovate atractylodes (*bái zhú*). ACU Base treatment mainly on CV, ST, and SP. Select CV-12 (*zhōng wǎn*, Center Stomach Duct), CV-10 (*xià wǎn*, Lower Stomach Duct), ST-25 (*tiān shū*, Celestial Pivot), CV-6 (*qì hǎi*, Sea of Qi), ST-36 (*zú sān lǐ*, Leg Three Li), SP-6 (*sān yīn jiāo*, Three Yin Intersection), and Li Inner Court (*lǐ nèi tíng*); needle with even supplementation and drainage. [26: 580]

postpartum fright heart palpitations 产后惊悸 *chǎn hòu jīng jì*: HEART PALPITATIONS after childbirth that is brought on by fright, associated in severe cases with fixity of the eyes and inability to speak. Postpartum fright palpitations are attributed to blood vacuity and insufficiency of heart qi. [MED] Supplement the heart and quiet the spirit using Heart-Nourishing Decoction (*yǎng xīn tāng*). [ACU] Base treatment mainly on HT, PC, back transport points, SP, and ST. Select BL-15 (*xīn shū*, Heart Transport), CV-14 (*jù què*, Great Tower Gate), PC-6 (*nèi guān*, Inner Pass), HT-7 (*shén mén*, Spirit Gate), BL-17 (*gé shū*, Diaphragm Transport), ST-36 (*zú sān lǐ*, Leg Three Li), SP-6 (*sān yīn jiāo*, Three Yin Intersection), and HT-5 (*tōng lǐ*, Connecting Li); needle with supplementation and add moxa. [26: 581]

postpartum generalized pain 产后遍身疼痛 *chǎn hòu piàn shēn téng tòng*: Generalized pain arising after childbirth when a) qi and blood are depleted and fail to move properly, b) RETENTION OF THE LOCHIA gives rise to blood stasis, or c) wind-cold exploits vacuity to enter the body and cause stagnation in the vessels. [MED] For blood vacuity, nourish and quicken the blood with Perfect Major Supplementation Decoction (*shí quán dà bǔ tāng*). For blood stasis, quicken the blood and transform stasis with Four Agents Decoction (*sì wù tāng*) plus large gentian (*qín jiāo*), peach kernel (*táo rén*), myrrh (*mò yào*), and carthamus (*hóng huā*). For wind-cold, characterized by headache, heat effusion, and aversion to cold, nourish the blood and dispel wind with Pain-Chasing Powder (*qū tòng sǎn*). [26: 579]

postpartum glomus and fullness 产后痞满 *chǎn hòu pǐ mǎn*: GLOMUS and fullness that arise in women usually suffering from stomach qi vacuity when dietary irregularities after childbirth cause further damage to the spleen and stomach, impairing harmonious downbearing of the stomach. [MED] Treat by fortifying the spleen and abductive dispersion. Use Special Achievement Powder (*yì gōng sǎn*). [ACU] Base treatment mainly on ST, CV, and PC. Select ST-25 (*tiān shū*, Celestial Pivot), CV-6 (*qì hǎi*, Sea of Qi), PC-6 (*nèi guān*, Inner Pass), ST-36 (*zú sān lǐ*, Leg Three Li), and BL-20 (*pí shū*, Spleen Transport); needle with even supplementation and drainage. [26: 579]

postpartum headache 产后头痛 *chǎn hòu tóu tòng*: Headache occurring after childbirth either as a result of excessive blood loss that deprives the network vessels of the brain of adequate nour-

ishment, or as a result of stagnant LOCHIA ascending the thoroughfare (*chōng*) vessel to the head. **Blood loss** patterns are characterized by a somber white complexion and dull pain in the smaller abdomen. [MED] Supplement the blood with Eight-Gem Decoction (*bā zhēn tāng*). [ACU] Base treatment mainly on GV, ST, and SP. Select GV-20 (*bǎi huì*, Hundred Convergences), BL-15 (*xīn shū*, Heart Transport), BL-17 (*gé shū*, Diaphragm Transport), BL-20 (*pí shū*, Spleen Transport), CV-6 (*qì hǎi*, Sea of Qi), ST-36 (*zú sān lǐ*, Leg Three Li), and SP-6 (*sān yīn jiāo*, Three Yin Intersection); needle with supplementation. **Static blood ascending counterflow** postpartum headache is associated with stabbing pain in the smaller abdomen that refuses pressure. [MED] Quicken the blood and transform stasis with Hand-of-Buddha Powder (*fó shǒu sǎn*). [ACU] Base treatment mainly on LI, SP, and LR. Select LI-4 (*hé gǔ*, Union Valley), BL-17 (*gé shū*, Diaphragm Transport), CV-3 (*zhōng jí*, Central Pole), SP-8 (*dì jī*, Earth's Crux), SP-6 (*sān yīn jiāo*, Three Yin Intersection), SP-10 (*xuè hǎi*, Sea of Blood), and LR-3 (*tài chōng*, Supreme Surge); needle with even supplementation and drainage. **External wind-cold** can cause headache with other common cold signs. [MED] Use formulas that course wind-cold combined with Four Agents Decoction (*sì wù tāng*). [ACU] Base treatment mainly on GV, LU, and SP. Select GV-20 (*bǎi huì*, Hundred Convergences), GV-14 (*dà zhuī*, Great Hammer), GV-16 (*fēng fǔ*, Wind Mansion), GB-20 (*fēng chí*, Wind Pool), LU-7 (*liè quē*, Broken Sequence), SP-6 (*sān yīn jiāo*, Three Yin Intersection), ST-36 (*zú sān lǐ*, Leg Three Li), and LR-3 (*tài chōng*, Supreme Surge); needle with drainage and add moxa. For affected area, see HEADACHE. [26: 580] [46: 621] [37: 361] [113: 202]

postpartum heart pain 产后心痛 *chǎn hòu xīn tòng*: From *The Origin and Indicators of Disease* (*zhū bìng yuán hòu lùn*). Postpartum pericardiac pain or postpartum true heart pain. Postpartum heart pain occurs in patients with abiding cold when major postpartum vacuity causes the blood to congeal and surge into to the network vessel of the heart or the heart channel. Damaging the network vessel of the heart, it is called postpartum pericardiac network [vessel] pain, which is characterized by oppression and pain in the chest and heart with the pain stretching into the back in severe cases. Damaging the heart channel, it is called postpartum true heart pain is attended by purple-black nails and coldextremities. If it occurs in the morning, the patient dies in the evening; if it occurs in the morning, the patient dies in the morning. [MED] Treat pericardiac network [vessel] pain by dissipating cold with formulas such as Great Rock Honey Decoction (*dà yán mì tāng*). Treat postpartum true heart pain with Great Rock Honey Decoction (*dà yán mì tāng*) combined with Sudden Smile Powder (*shī xiào sǎn*). ACU Base treatment mainly on CV, back transport points, PC, and HT. Main points: CV-17 (*shān zhōng*, Chest Center), BL-15 (*xīn shū*, Heart Transport), PC-6 (*nèi guān*, Inner Pass), and CV-14 (*jù què*, Great Tower Gate); needle with drainage. Selection of points according to pattern: For pericardiac pain, add BL-14 (*jué yīn shū*, Reverting Yin Transport), PC-4 (*xī mén*, Cleft Gate), and ST-36 (*zú sān lǐ*, Leg Three Li). For true heart pain, add BL-17 (*gé shū*, Diaphragm Transport), HT-7 (*shén mén*, Spirit Gate), CV-6 (*qì hǎi*, Sea of Qi), and SP-6 (*sān yīn jiāo*, Three Yin Intersection). [26: 575] [50: 610]

postpartum heat [effusion] and [aversion to] cold 产后寒热 *chǎn hòu hán rè*: See POSTPARTUM SUDDEN BOUTS OF HEAT [EFFUSION] AND [AVERSION] TO COLD. [26: 578]

postpartum hypertonicity 产后拘挛 *chǎn hòu jū luán*: Hypertonicity of the sinews that arises either when wind-cold exploits sudden vacuity of qi and blood, and enters the channels and network vessels or when damage to qi and blood through childbirth leads to insufficiency of liver blood depriving the sinews of nourishment. **Wind-cold** hypertonicity is attended by aversion to cold, heat effusion, and sweating or absence of sweating. MED Nourish the blood and dispel wind with Schizonepeta and Ledebouriella Four Agents Decoction (*jīng fáng sì wù tāng*). ACU Base treatment mainly on GB, LI, LU, and three yin channels of the foot. Needle with drainage and moxa at GV-20 (*bǎi huì*, Hundred Convergences), GB-20 (*fēng chí*, Wind Pool), TB-5 (*wài guān*, Outer Pass), LI-4 (*hé gǔ*, Union Valley), LU-7 (*liè quē*, Broken Sequence), and GB-34 (*yáng líng quán*, Yang Mound Spring), and with supplementation and moxa at BL-20 (*pí shū*, Spleen Transport), BL-23 (*shèn shū*, Kidney Transport), ST-36 (*zú sān lǐ*, Leg Three Li), SP-6 (*sān yīn jiāo*, Three Yin Intersection), and KI-6 (*zhào hǎi*, Shining Sea). **Insufficiency of liver blood** is accompanied by clouded head and dizzy vision, no desire to see people, and dryness of the eyes. MED Nourish the blood and emolliate the liver with Four Agents Decoction (*sì wù tāng*) plus uncaria (*gōu téng*) and chaenomeles (*mù guā*). ACU Base treatment mainly on GB, PC, and the three yin channels of the foot. Needle with drainage and moxa at GV-20 (*bǎi huì*, Hundred Convergences), GB-20 (*fēng chí*, Wind Pool), LR-3 (*tài chōng*, Supreme Surge), GB-34 (*yáng líng quán*, Yang Mound Spring), PC-6 (*nèi guān*, Inner Pass), and PC-8 (*láo gōng*, Palace of Toil), and with supplementation and moxa at BL-18 (*gān shū*, Liver Transport), BL-20 (*pí shū*, Spleen Transport), ST-36 (*zú sān lǐ*, Leg Three Li),

SP-6 (*sān yīn jiāo*, Three Yin Intersection), KI-1 (*yǒng quán*, Gushing Spring), and LR-8 (*qū quán*, Spring at the Bend). [26: 577] [50: 610]

postpartum impediment pattern 产后痹证 *chǎn hòu bì zhèng*: An IMPEDIMENT (*bì*) pattern arising when major postpartum vacuity causes insecurity of the interstices allowing wind-cold-damp evils to exploit the vacuity and enter the flesh and channels and give rise to generalized or local joint pain. MED Treat by supporting right and nourishing the blood, assisted by dispelling the evil. Use variations of Schizonepeta and Ledebouriella Four Agents Decoction (*jīng fáng sì wù tāng*). Use of acrid dry agents should be limited in major vacuity of right qi. ACU Base treatment mainly on CV, SP, ST, LR, and GB. To support right and nourish the blood, select BL-20 (*pí shū*, Spleen Transport), BL-17 (*gé shū*, Diaphragm Transport), CV-6 (*qì hǎi*, Sea of Qi), ST-36 (*zú sān lǐ*, Leg Three Li), LR-3 (*tài chōng*, Supreme Surge), and SP-6 (*sān yīn jiāo*, Three Yin Intersection), needling with supplementation and adding moxa. Selection of points according to external evils: For wind evil, needle with drainage at GB-20 (*fēng chí*, Wind Pool), GV-16 (*fēng fǔ*, Wind Mansion), and SP-10 (*xuè hǎi*, Sea of Blood). For cold evil, needle with drainage and moxa at BL-23 (*shèn shū*, Kidney Transport), GV-4 (*mìng mén*, Life Gate), and CV-4 (*guān yuán*, Pass Head). For dampness evil, needle with drainage and moxa at SP-9 (*yīn líng quán*, Yin Mound Spring) and SP-5 (*shāng qiū*, Shang Hill). [26: 579]

postpartum inhibited urination 产后小便不利 *chǎn hòu xiǎo biàn bù lì*: INHIBITED URINATION (difficulty voiding and scant urine) occurring after childbirth. Three pathomechanisms exist: a) damage to qi and blood and spleen-lung qi vacuity causing inhibited flow through the waterways; b) damage to kidney qi through childbirth causing impairment of the qi transformation; c) binding depression of liver qi due to constrained emotions affecting general qi dynamic and supply of warmth to the bladder. **Spleen-lung qi vacuity** signs include listlessness essence-spirit and laziness to speak. MED Treat by supplementing qi and moistening the lung, supported by moving water. Use formulas such as Qi-Supplementing Bladder-Freeing Beverage (*bǔ qì tōng pāo yǐn*). **Kidney vacuity** signs include aching lumbus and knees, forgetfulness, and dark facial complexion. MED Warm yang, promote qi transformation, and move water. Use formulas such as Kidney Qi Pill (*shèn qì wán*). **Stagnant qi dynamic** patterns are characterized emotional depression, distention and pain in the rib-side, and vexation and agitation. MED Treat by rectifying qi and moving stagnation supported by disinhibiting water. Use formulas such Mutong Powder (*mù tōng sǎn*). ACU Moxibustion on crushed scallion mounted on the umbilicus filled with salt. Burn until the pain becomes unbearable. ACU Base treatment mainly on KI, SP, and back transport points. Main points: BL-23 (*shèn shū*, Kidney Transport), BL-22 (*sān jiāo shū*, Triple Burner Transport), CV-4 (*guān yuán*, Pass Head), CV-6 (*qì hǎi*, Sea of Qi), KI-10 (*yīn gǔ*, Yin Valley), and SP-6 (*sān yīn jiāo*, Three Yin Intersection). Selection of points according to pattern: For spleen-lung qi vacuity, add BL-20 (*pí shū*, Spleen Transport), BL-13 (*fèi shū*, Lung Transport), SP-3 (*tài bái*, Supreme White), and LU-9 (*tài yuān*, Great Abyss), needling with supplementation and adding moxa. For kidney vacuity, add GV-4 (*mìng mén*, Life Gate), KI-3 (*tài xī*, Great Ravine), and KI-7 (*fù liū*, Recover Flow), needling with supplementation and moxa, and adding GV-3 (*yāo yáng guān*, Lumbar Yang Pass) for aching lumbus and knees. For stagnant qi dynamic, add PC-6 (*nèi guān*, Inner Pass), LR-3 (*tài chōng*, Supreme Surge), BL-18 (*gān shū*, Liver Transport), ST-36 (*zú sān lǐ*, Leg Three Li), and GB-34 (*yáng líng quán*, Yang Mound Spring), needling with even supplementation and drainage or with drainage and, if appropriate, adding moxa. Alternatively, apply finger pressure at the diuretic point between CV-8 (*shén què*, Spirit Gate Tower) and CV-2 (*qū gǔ*, Curved Bone). [26: 575] [59: 181–191]

postpartum loss of breast milk 产后乳汁自出 *chǎn hòu rǔ zhī zì chū*: Leaking of milk from the breasts after delivery. Postpartum loss of breast milk is attributed either to spleen-stomach qi vacuity preventing breast milk from being contained or to hyperactive liver fire and excessive free coursing action of the liver. **Qi vacuity** patterns are characterized by absence of distention of the breasts, thin milk, and shortness of breath and lack of strength. MED Treat with variations of Perfect Major Supplementation Decoction (*shí quán dà bǔ tāng*). **Liver heat** patterns are characterized by distention of the breasts, thick milk, heart vexation, irascibility, bitter taste in the mouth, and dry throat. MED Calm the liver and clear heat with Moutan and Gardenia Free Wanderer Powder (*dān zhī xiāo yáo sǎn*). [26: 577]

postpartum loss of speech 产后不语 *chǎn hòu bù yǔ*: Loss of speech attributed to a) uneliminated wasted blood accumulating in the heart, b) damage to heart qi during childbirth preventing heart qi from reaching the tongue, or c) phlegm-heat exploiting the heart causing heart qi block. **Bad blood** accumulating in the heart gives rise to postpartum loss of speech with purple-black facial complexion and oppression in the chest. MED Quicken the blood, move stasis, and free heart qi. Use formulas such as Ligusticum and Tangkuei Powder (*xiōng guī sǎn*) combined with Seven-Gem Powder (*qī zhēn sǎn*). **Heart qi vacu-**

ity patterns are characterized by heart palpitations, shortness of breath, and spontaneous sweating. MED Supplement qi and the blood with Eight-Gem Decoction (*bā zhēn tāng*) with additions. **Phlegm-heat** exploiting the heart is characterized by phlegm rales in the throat, hot face, and raised chest. MED Clear phlegm-heat and calm the stomach with formulas such as Two Matured Ingredients Decoction (*èr chén tāng*) plus bile arisaema (*dǎn xīng*) and uncaria (*gōu téng*). Bloodletting can also be performed between the eyebrows. [26: 575]

postpartum loss of voice 产后瘖 *chǎn hòu yīn*: A thready hoarse voice occurring after childbirth. Postpartum loss of voice is attributed to dual vacuity of the heart and kidney, binding depression of spleen qi (spleen qi vacuity and inhibited movement of qi), or dual vacuity of qi and blood. MED When attributed to dual vacuity of the heart and kidney, use Seven-Gem Powder (*qī zhēn sǎn*). When due to binding depression of spleen qi, use Spleen-Returning Decoction (*guī pí tāng*). When due to dual vacuity of qi and blood, use Eight-Gem Decoction (*bā zhēn tāng*). Postpartum loss of voice is not necessarily directly related to childbirth. For other patterns, see LOSS OF VOICE. [26: 580]

postpartum lumbar pain 产后腰痛 *chǎn hòu yāo tòng*: Lumbar pain after childbirth. It may arise a) when childbirth damages the kidney (the lumbus is the house of the kidney) and wasted blood obstructs the girdling (*dài*) vessel, b) when vacuity of true qi is exploited by external evil, or c) when the lumbus is sprained in postpartum vacuity. **Damage to the kidney in childbirth** gives rise to a dull pain associated with tinnitus. MED Strengthen the lumbus and supplement the kidney with Six-Ingredient Rehmannia Pill (*liù wèi dì huáng wán*) plus eucommia (*dù zhòng*) and dipsacus (*xù duàn*). ACU Base treatment mainly on GV, BL, and ouch points (*ā shì xué*). Main points for all patterns: BL-23 (*shèn shū*, Kidney Transport), GV-3 (*yāo yáng guān*, Lumbar Yang Pass), BL-40 (*wěi zhōng*, Bend Center), and ouch points (*ā shì xué*). For damage to kidney through delivery, add GV-4 (*mìng mén*, Life Gate), BL-52 (*zhì shì*, Will Chamber), BL-58 (*fēi yáng*, Taking Flight), and KI-3 (*tài xī*, Great Ravine), needling with supplementation and adding moxa. **External evil** patterns are characterized by exterior signs. MED Use Construction-Nourishing Kidney-Invigorating Decoction (*yǎng róng zhuàng shèn tāng*). ACU Needle with supplementation the main points given above and at BL-17 (*gé shū*, Diaphragm Transport), BL-20 (*pí shū*, Spleen Transport), LR-3 (*tài chōng*, Supreme Surge), and SP-6 (*sān yīn jiāo*, Three Yin Intersection), and needle with drainage at GV-20 (*bǎi huì*, Hundred Convergences), GB-20 (*fēng chí*, Wind

Pool), and TB-5 (*wài guān,* Outer Pass). **Blood stasis** (including wrenching of the lumbus) patterns are characterized by local stabbing distending pain that is exacerbated by the slightest pressure. MED Quicken the blood and transform stasis with Origin-Restoring Qi-Freeing Powder (*fù yuán tōng qì sǎn*). ACU To the main points given above add BL-17 (*gé shū,* Diaphragm Transport), SP-10 (*xuè hǎi,* Sea of Blood), LR-3 (*tài chōng,* Supreme Surge), and GV-26 (*rén zhōng,* Human Center), needling with even supplementation and drainage. [26: 579]

postpartum night sweating 产后盗汗 *chǎn hòu dào hàn:* Night sweating occurring after childbirth. Postpartum night sweating is attributed to sudden vacuity of qi and blood and yin depletion. MED Regulate and supplement qi and blood with complementary action to constrain sweating. Use Perspiration-Checking Powder (*zhǐ hàn sǎn*). ACU Base treatment mainly on HT, LI, ST, and SP. Select HT-6 (*yīn xī,* Yin Cleft), SI-3 (*hòu xī,* Back Ravine), LI-4 (*hé gǔ,* Union Valley), BL-20 (*pí shū,* Spleen Transport), ST-36 (*zú sān lǐ,* Leg Three Li), and SP-6 (*sān yīn jiāo,* Three Yin Intersection); needle with supplementation and add moxa. [26: 579]

postpartum nontransformation of food 产后完谷不化 *chǎn hòu wán gǔ bù huà:* Diarrhea with untransformed food in the stool due to spleen-kidney vacuity exacerbated by childbirth or postpartum taxation fatigue. MED Warm yang, fortify the spleen, and remove stasis. Use Engendering Transformation Decoction (*shēng huà tāng*) plus alpinia (*yì zhì rén*), amomum (*shā rén*), nutmeg (*ròu dòu kòu*), saussurea (*mù xiāng*), bupleurum (*chái hú*), cimicifuga (*shēng má*), tangerine peel (*chén pí*), and codonopsis (*dǎng shēn*). ACU Base treatment mainly on CV, ST, and SP. Select CV-4 (*guān yuán,* Pass Head), CV-6 (*qì hǎi,* Sea of Qi), ST-25 (*tiān shū,* Celestial Pivot), ST-36 (*zú sān lǐ,* Leg Three Li), BL-20 (*pí shū,* Spleen Transport), BL-23 (*shèn shū,* Kidney Transport), and SP-6 (*sān yīn jiāo,* Three Yin Intersection); needle with supplementation and add moxa. [26: 577]

postpartum panting 产后气喘 *chǎn hòu qì chuǎn:* Panting occurring after childbirth. Postpartum panting is attributed to qi-blood vacuity or wasted blood ascending to attack the lung. **Qi-blood vacuity** postpartum panting arises when excessive blood loss causes sudden exhaustion of construction-blood that leaves defense qi ungoverned. It is characterized by rapid breathing and a rootless vacuous floating pulse on both wrists. MED Treat by major supplementation of qi and the blood using Desertion-Stemming Mother-Reviving Decoction (*jiù tuō huó mǔ tāng*) and apply a hot water bottle on the lower abdomen.

Bad blood patterns may result from nonmovement of the LOCHIA with wasted blood ascending to attack the lung. Such patterns are characterized by rough breathing, purple-black facial complexion and RETENTION OF THE LOCHIA. MED Quicken the blood and expel stasis with formulas such as Life-Clutching Elixir (*duó mìng dān*). See PANTING. [26: 578]

postpartum paralysis 产后瘫痪 *chǎn hòu tān huàn:* Hemiplegia, hypertonicity or numbness of the extremities, occurring after childbirth as a result of excessive loss of blood. MED Supplement qi and nourish the blood. Use formulas such as Astragalus and Cinnamon Twig Five Agents Decoction (*huáng qí guì zhī wǔ wù tāng*) or Yang-Supplementing Five-Returning Decoction (*bǔ yáng huán wǔ tāng*). Do not confuse this condition with a wind pattern, since the use of harsh dry wind-dispelling and blood dissipating medicinals can be harmful. [26: 581]

postpartum pericardiac network [vessel] pain 产后心包络痛 *chǎn hòu xīn bāo luò tòng:* From *Good Remedies for Women* (*fù rén liáng fāng*). Pain and oppression in the heart and chest occurring after childbirth, in severe cases reaching into the back. Postpartum pericardiac network [vessel] pain arises in women who ordinarily suffer from abiding cold and who are suffering major vacuity as a result of childbirth, when cold contends with the blood, causes the blood to congeal and fail to move, and to surge into the network vessels of the heart. Dissipate cold in order to warm and free. Use Great Rock Honey Decoction (*dà yán mì tāng*). See POSTPARTUM HEART PAIN. [50: 617]

postpartum puffy swelling 产后浮肿 *chǎn hòu fú zhǒng:* Swelling after childbirth, usually due to qi stagnation. It occurs in women who tend to suffer from mental depression and the resultant inhibition of qi dynamic when childbirth causes disharmony of qi and blood. It is characterized by resilient swelling (rather than pitting edema) of the limbs without any change in the color of the flesh and is associated with oppression in the chest and rib-side distention, as well as with reduced food intake. MED Rectify qi, move stagnation, and disinhibit dampness using Aristolochia Stem Powder (*tiān xiān téng sǎn*) plus fresh ginger (*shēng jiāng*), chaenomeles (*mù guā*), perilla leaf (*zǐ sū yè*), poria (*fú líng*), and areca husk (*dà fù pí*). Postpartum dual vacuity of the spleen and kidney causing water-damp to spill into the limbs is called POSTPARTUM WATER SWELLING; postpartum swelling before wasted blood has ceased to be eliminated is called POSTPARTUM VACUITY SWELLING OF THE LIMBS. [26: 578]

postpartum raving and hallucination 产后妄言妄见 *chǎn hòu wàng yán wàng jiàn:* Rash or irrational talk and/or seeing of unreal phenomena after childbirth; attributed to qi-blood vacuity stemming from excessive blood loss or blood stasis due to nonelimination of malign blood. **Qi-blood vacuity** patterns arise when excessive blood loss after childbirth deprives the heart of nourishment and the spirit of a place to go. In such cases, panting is attended by shortage of qi and laziness to speak, lusterless facial complexion, and spontaneous sweating. MED Boost qi and supplement the blood with formulas such as Construction-Enriching Qi-Boosting Spirit-Returning Decoction (*zī róng yì qì fù shén tāng*). **Blood stasis** patterns arise from nonelimination of malign blood which then attacks the heart. MED Treat with Spirit-Quieting Engendering Transformation Decoction (*ān shén shēng huà tāng*). [26: 576]

postpartum retention of the lochia 产后恶露不下 *chǎn hòu è lù bù xià*: See RETENTION OF THE LOCHIA. [26: 579]

postpartum sore 产后疮疡 *chǎn hòu chuāng yáng*: A sore arising after childbirth as a result of qi-blood depletion. A postpartum sore is treated by INTERNAL EXPRESSION, supporting right qi and expelling the evil, and harmonizing construction and defense. [26: 580]

postpartum streaming sore 产后流注 *chǎn hòu liú zhù*: A STREAMING SORE appearing on the lumbus, arm, wrist, and leg after delivery. It is characterized by a lump and diffuse swelling and attended by fatigue. [26: 578]

postpartum sudden bouts of heat [effusion] and [aversion] to cold 产后乍寒乍热 *chǎn hòu zhà hán zhà rè*: Synonym: *postpartum heat effusion and aversion to cold*. Abrupt changes from cold to heat after childbirth. Postpartum sudden bouts of heat effusion and aversion to cold attributed to disharmony of construction and defense that results either from dual vacuity of qi and blood and disharmony between yin and yang or from stagnation of wasted blood blocking the channels. MED Treat qi-blood vacuity patterns by supplementing qi and the blood, and harmonizing yin and yang; use formulas such as Four Agents Decoction (*sì wù tāng*) minus rehmannia (*dì huáng*) and plus ginseng (*rén shēn*), dried ginger (*gān jiāng*), licorice (*gān cǎo*), and bupleurum (*chái hú*). Treat wasted blood patterns by quickening the blood and freeing the channels; use Life-Clutching Elixir (*duó mìng dān*) or Engendering Transformation Decoction (*shēng huà tāng*) plus Bupleurum and Pueraria Flesh-Resolving Decoction (*chái gé jiě jī tāng*). ◇ Chin 乍寒乍热 *zhà hán zhà rè*, lit. now hot, now cold. [26: 576]

postpartum summerheat stroke 产后中暑 *chǎn hòu zhòng shǔ*: Contraction of summerheat occurring 1–3 days after delivery, when qi and blood have not recovered and summerheat evil exploits the vacuity to enter the flesh, causing sudden expiration of yin qi and congestion of the yang qi that obstructs the channels. Signs include high fever and unclear spirit-mind. MED If there is dizziness and nausea, oppression in the chest, flusteredness, thirst, and great sweating, this is a portent of summerheat stroke, for which Summerheat-Clearing Qi-Boosting Decoction (*qīng shǔ yì qì tāng*) can be prescribed. When heat strikes the interior, there is vexation, thirst, great sweating, red facial complexion, and a large surging pulse; treatment takes the form of engendering liquid and allaying thirst with formulas such as White Tiger Decoction Plus Ginseng (*bái hǔ jiā rén shēn tāng*). When there is intense stomach heat damaging liquid characterized by vexation and thirst, fecal stoppage, macules, treat by flushing stomach heat with formulas such as Jade Spring Powder (*yù quán sǎn*). If heat toxin enters construction and scorches visceral yin, causing delirious speech, unclear spirit-mind, and convulsions of the limbs, somber white complexion, and a fine weak pulse, treat by clearing heat and nourishing yin with variations of Construction-Clearing Decoction (*qīng yíng tāng*) and Pulse-Engendering Powder (*shēng mài sǎn*). ACU Base treatment mainly on PC, LI, ST, HT, KI, and SP. Main points: BL-20 (*pí shū*, Spleen Transport), SP-6 (*sān yīn jiāo*, Three Yin Intersection), PC-6 (*nèi guān*, Inner Pass), LI-4 (*hé gǔ*, Union Valley), ST-36 (*zú sān lǐ*, Leg Three Li), GV-14 (*dà zhuī*, Great Hammer), and LI-11 (*qū chí*, Pool at the Bend); needle with drainage. Selection of points according to pattern: For forewarning signs of summerheat stroke, add GB-20 (*fēng chí*, Wind Pool) and HT-5 (*tōng lǐ*, Connecting Li). For heat striking the interior, add TB-2 (*yè mén*, Humor Gate), KI-6 (*zhào hǎi*, Shining Sea), and KI-2 (*rán gǔ*, Blazing Valley), and prick Gold Liquid and Jade Humor (*jīn jīn yù yè*) to bleed. For intense stomach heat, add ST-44 (*nèi tíng*, Inner Court) and KI-6 (*zhào hǎi*, Shining Sea). For heat toxin entering construction, add PC-3 (*qū zé*, Marsh at the Bend), PC-9 (*zhōng chōng*, Central Hub), HT-9 (*shào chōng*, Lesser Surge), and BL-40 (*wěi zhōng*, Bend Center), and prick Ten Diffusing Points (*shí xuān*) to bleed. [26: 575] [113: 47] [37: 686]

postpartum tetany 产后病痉 *chǎn hòu bìng jìng*: TETANY (*jìng*) characterized by rigidity of the neck, convulsions of the limbs, clenched jaw, and arched-back rigidity, occurring suddenly after childbirth. Postpartum tetany arises when wind exploits the vacuity created by major postpartum yin-blood depletion to invade and stir liver wind, or when excessive sweating causes damage to liquid and blood collapse, which deprives the sinews of nourishment and causes tetany through extreme vacuity engendering wind. Wind patterns are marked by clenched jaw and straight rigid back or arched-back rigidity. These signs come in bouts after shorts intervals with apparent cessation of breathing; blood collapse patterns are marked by spontaneous sweating, dim vision, and clouded spirit. MED For wind patterns, the mouth should be quickly pried open to allow Minor Life-Prolonging Decoction (*xiǎo xù mìng tāng*) or Tetany-Relieving Powder (*zhǐ jìng sǎn*) plus silkworm (*bái jiāng cán*), and mistletoe (*sāng jì shēng*) to be poured in. See also LOCKJAW. For blood patterns, enrich humor and extinguish wind using Major Wind-Stabilizing Pill (*dà dìng fēng zhū*). Postpartum tetany is a critical condition. If convulsions become feeble, and pearly sweat appears on the skin, while the eyes stare upward, the patient should be quickly given Center-Supplementing Qi-Boosting Decoction (*bǔ zhōng yì qì tāng*) with double the amount of ginseng (*rén shēn*), and with the addition of dried ginger (*gān jiāng*) and aconite (*fù zǐ*). ACU Base treatment mainly on back transport points, GV, SP, ST, GB and LR. Select GV-20 (*bǎi huì*, Hundred Convergences), GB-20 (*fēng chí*, Wind Pool), LR-3 (*tài chōng*, Supreme Surge), BL-17 (*gé shū*, Diaphragm Transport), BL-20 (*pí shū*, Spleen Transport), ST-36 (*zú sān lǐ*, Leg Three Li), SP-6 (*sān yīn jiāo*, Three Yin Intersection), BL-57 (*chéng shān*, Mountain Support), GB-34 (*yáng líng quán*, Yang Mound Spring), and GV-8 (*jīn suō*, Sinew Contraction); needle with supplementation and moxa if appropriate. Selection of points according to cause: For contraction of wind evil stirring liver wind, needle with drainage at GV-16 (*fēng fǔ*, Wind Mansion), TB-5 (*wài guān*, Outer Pass), LI-4 (*hé gǔ*, Union Valley), and KI-1 (*yǒng quán*, Gushing Spring). For blood collapse damaging fluids and extreme vacuity engendering wind, add KI-6 (*zhào hǎi*, Shining Sea) and LR-8 (*qū quán*, Spring at the Bend). [26: 578]

postpartum thirst 产后口渴 *chǎn hòu kǒu kě*: Thirst after childbirth, attributed to damage to fluids through loss of blood or profuse sweating or scorching of the fluids by effulgent yin vacuity fire. MED Treat damage to liquid by engendering liquid and allaying thirst with formulas such as Pulse-Engendering Variant Powder (*jiā jiǎn shēng mài sǎn*) varied according to need. Treat effulgent yin vacuity fire with persistent drinking of fluid by enriching yin and downbearing fire and by engendering liquid and allaying thirst. Use formulas such as Four Agents Decoction (*sì wù tāng*) plus anemarrhena (*zhī mǔ*), phellodendron (*huáng bǎi*), poria (*fú líng*), and astragalus (*huáng qí*). ACU Base treatment mainly on TB, SP, back transport points, and KI. Main points: Gold Liquid and Jade Humor (*jīn jīn yù yè*), TB-2 (*yè mén*,

Humor Gate), and SP-6 (*sān yīn jiāo*, Three Yin Intersection). For blood loss or profuse sweating that damages the fluids, add BL-20 (*pí shū*, Spleen Transport), BL-17 (*gé shū*, Diaphragm Transport), CV-6 (*qì hǎi*, Sea of Qi), LI-4 (*hé gǔ*, Union Valley), KI-6 (*zhào hǎi*, Shining Sea), and KI-2 (*rán gǔ*, Blazing Valley), needling with supplementation. For effulgent yin vacuity fire damaging fluids, needle with supplementation at KI-3 (*tài xī*, Great Ravine), and SP-6 (*sān yīn jiāo*, Three Yin Intersection), and with drainage at HT-8 (*shào fǔ*, Lesser Mansion), KI-6 (*zhào hǎi*, Shining Sea), KI-2 (*rán gǔ*, Blazing Valley), and KI-1 (*yǒng quán*, Gushing Spring). [26: 575] [113: 20] [46: 594, 596]

postpartum tugging and slackening 产后瘈瘲 *chǎn hòu chì zhòng*: Alternating tensing and relaxation of the sinews that arises when postpartum blood vacuity deprives the sinews of nourishment. MED Supplement qi and the blood. Use Ginseng Construction-Nourishing Decoction (*rén shēn yǎng róng tāng*) with additions. ACU Base treatment mainly on back transport points, CV, and three yin channels of the foot. Select BL-20 (*pí shū*, Spleen Transport), BL-17 (*gé shū*, Diaphragm Transport), CV-6 (*qì hǎi*, Sea of Qi), SP-10 (*xuè hǎi*, Sea of Blood), ST-36 (*zú sān lǐ*, Leg Three Li), LR-3 (*tài chōng*, Supreme Surge), SP-6 (*sān yīn jiāo*, Three Yin Intersection), KI-6 (*zhào hǎi*, Shining Sea), BL-57 (*chéng shān*, Mountain Support), and GB-34 (*yáng líng quán*, Yang Mound Spring); needle with supplementation and large amounts of moxa. [26: 580]

postpartum vacuity swelling of the limbs 产后四肢虚肿 *chǎn hòu sì zhī xū zhǒng*: A condition characterized by generalized green-blue swelling accompanied by inhibited flow of the LOCHIA. Postpartum vacuity swelling of the limbs arises when wasted blood has not been completely eliminated, and flows into the channels and network vessels. MED Quicken the blood and transform stasis with Channel-Regulating Powder (*tiáo jīng sǎn*). ACU Base treatment mainly on CV, SP, and ST. Select CV-6 (*qì hǎi*, Sea of Qi), CV-3 (*zhōng jí*, Central Pole), SP-6 (*sān yīn jiāo*, Three Yin Intersection), BL-17 (*gé shū*, Diaphragm Transport), SP-10 (*xuè hǎi*, Sea of Blood), ST-36 (*zú sān lǐ*, Leg Three Li), BL-20 (*pí shū*, Spleen Transport), and BL-23 (*shèn shū*, Kidney Transport); needle with even supplementation and drainage. See POSTPARTUM PUFFY SWELLING. [26: 576]

postpartum vacuity vexation 产后虚烦 *chǎn hòu xū fán*: HEART VEXATION arising after childbirth as a result of qi-blood depletion and vacuity fire that harasses the upper body. Postpartum vacuity vexation is heat vexation with shortage of qi, fatigue, fullness and oppression in the chest and diaphragm, and in more severe cases, with insomnia. [MED] Clear heat and eliminate vexation using Bamboo Leaf Decoction (*dàn zhú yè tāng*). If there is pronounced physical agitation, prescribe Tangkuei Blood-Supplementing Decoction (*dāng guī bǔ xuè tāng*). [ACU] Base treatment mainly on HT, back transport points, and three yin channels of the feet. Select BL-15 (*xīn shū*, Heart Transport), BL-23 (*shèn shū*, Kidney Transport), BL-20 (*pí shū*, Spleen Transport), Alert Spirit Quartet (*sì shén cōng*), HT-7 (*shén mén*, Spirit Gate), SP-6 (*sān yīn jiāo*, Three Yin Intersection), KI-6 (*zhào hǎi*, Shining Sea), LI-4 (*hé gǔ*, Union Valley), and LI-11 (*qū chí*, Pool at the Bend); needle with supplementation. If agitation is present, add LR-3 (*tài chōng*, Supreme Surge), SP-10 (*xuè hǎi*, Sea of Blood), and ST-36 (*zú sān lǐ*, Leg Three Li). [26: 578]

postpartum vigorous heat [effusion] 产后壮热 *chǎn hòu zhuàng rè*: High fever after childbirth. Postpartum vigorous heat [effusion] may be due to contraction of an external evil, but it is frequently due to evil toxin directly striking the uterus in postpartum qi and blood vacuity. See POSTPARTUM HEAT EFFUSION. [67: 293] [26: 579]

postpartum vomiting 产后呕吐 *chǎn hòu ǒu tù*: VOMITING after childbirth. Postpartum vomiting is attributed to cold evil that exploits stomach qi vacuity, blood stasis due to scant elimination of the LOCHIA, or phlegm qi swamping the stomach. **Vacuity cold** patterns are characterized by vomiting with reduced food intake, bland taste in the mouth, and sometimes by dull stomach or abdominal pain, [MED] Warm, nourish, and calm the stomach. Use Saussurea and Amomum Six Gentlemen Decoction (*xiāng shā liù jūn zǐ tāng*) or Center-Rectifying Decoction (*lǐ zhōng tāng*) plus agastache/patchouli (*huò xiāng*). **Blood stasis** due to scant elimination of the LOCHIA is characterized by vomiting with abdominal pain, and ungratifying scant discharge of stagnant lochia. [MED] Quicken the blood and dispel stasis with variations of Engendering Transformation Decoction (*shēng huà tāng*). **Phlegm qi flooding the stomach** is characterized by bloating and oppression in the chest and abdomen. [MED] Dispel phlegm and harmonize the stomach; downbear counterflow and check vomiting. Use variations of Two Matured Ingredients Decoction (*èr chén tāng*). [ACU] Base treatment mainly on CV, ST, SP, and LR. Main points: CV-12 (*zhōng wǎn*, Center Stomach Duct), PC-6 (*nèi guān*, Inner Pass), ST-36 (*zú sān lǐ*, Leg Three Li), and ST-25 (*tiān shū*, Celestial Pivot). Selection of points according to pattern: For cold evil exploiting the stomach, add BL-20 (*pí shū*, Spleen Transport), BL-21 (*wèi shū*, Stomach Transport), CV-4 (*guān yuán*, Pass Head), and CV-6 (*qì hǎi*, Sea

of Qi), needling with even supplementation and drainage, and adding moxa. For rough scant flow of LOCHIA, add CV-3 (*zhōng jí*, Central Pole), SP-6 (*sān yīn jiāo*, Three Yin Intersection), LR-3 (*tài chōng*, Supreme Surge), LR-8 (*qū quán*, Spring at the Bend), and BL-17 (*gé shū*, Diaphragm Transport), needle with supplementation and add moxa. For phlegm qi swamping the stomach, add CV-12 (*zhōng wǎn*, Center Stomach Duct) and ST-40 (*fēng lóng*, Bountiful Bulge), needling with drainage and adding moxa. [26: 580]

postpartum water swelling 产后水肿 *chǎn hòu shuǐ zhǒng*: WATER SWELLING occurring after delivery when spleen-kidney vacuity exacerbated by childbirth disturbs the normal distribution of fluids. Postpartum water swelling is characterized by swelling of the extremities and a moist shiny appearance of the skin. [MED] Treat by major supplementation of qi and blood supported by disinhibiting water. Applicable formulas include Eight-Gem Decoction (*bā zhēn tāng*) plus atractylodes (*cāng zhú*) and poria (*fú líng*). If there is distention and fullness, add tangerine peel (*chén pí*), pinellia (*bàn xià*), and cyperus (*xiāng fù zǐ*). For pronounced vacuity, add ginseng (*rén shēn*) and mutong (*mù tōng*). For pronounced heat, add scutellaria (*huáng qín*) and ophiopogon (*mài mén dōng*). [ACU] Base treatment mainly on CV, back transport points, ST, and SP. Select CV-9 (*shuǐ fēn*, Water Divide), CV-6 (*qì hǎi*, Sea of Qi), BL-22 (*sān jiāo shū*, Triple Burner Transport), BL-20 (*pí shū*, Spleen Transport), BL-23 (*shèn shū*, Kidney Transport), BL-17 (*gé shū*, Diaphragm Transport), ST-36 (*zú sān lǐ*, Leg Three Li), SP-6 (*sān yīn jiāo*, Three Yin Intersection), and SP-9 (*yīn líng quán*, Yin Mound Spring); needle with supplementation and add moxa. For distention and fullness, add ST-25 (*tiān shū*, Celestial Pivot) and PC-6 (*nèi guān*, Inner Pass). If heat is present, needle with drainage at LI-4 (*hé gǔ*, Union Valley) and LI-11 (*qū chí*, Pool at the Bend). [26: 576]

postpartum wind-like stroke 产后类中风 *chǎn hòu lèi zhòng fēng*: Wind-like stroke occurring after childbirth. Postpartum wind-like stroke is attributed to fulminant vacuity of qi and blood and characterized by clenched jaw and rigid neck, and hypertonicity of the sinews. [MED] Use Construction-Enriching Network-Quickening Decoction (*zī róng huó luò tāng*) or variations of Engendering Transformation Decoction (*shēng huà tāng*). [ACU] Base treatment mainly on GB, LR, SP, and ST. Select GV-20 (*bǎi huì*, Hundred Convergences), GB-20 (*fēng chí*, Wind Pool), LR-3 (*tài chōng*, Supreme Surge), BL-57 (*chéng shān*, Mountain Support), GB-34 (*yáng líng quán*, Yang Mound Spring), BL-20 (*pí shū*, Spleen Transport), BL-17 (*gé shū*, Diaphragm Transport), ST-36 (*zú sān lǐ*, Leg Three Li), and SP-6 (*sān yīn jiāo*,

Three Yin Intersection); needle with supplementation and add moxa. [26: 581]

postpartum wind stroke 产后中风 *chǎn hòu zhòng fēng*: WIND STROKE occurring after childbirth. Postpartum wind stroke is attributed to sudden vacuity of qi and blood after delivery, with consequent unsoundness of the interstices allowing external evils to exploit the vacuity and enter the body. Conditions that occur when externally contracted wind evil remains unresolved for ten days or more, characterized by slight headache, aversion to cold, periodic heat effusion, oppression below the heart, dry retching and sweating can be treated by harmonizing construction and defense with Cinnamon Twig Decoction (*guì zhī tāng*). Heat effusion, red facial complexion, panting, and headache can be treated with Bamboo Leaf Decoction (*zhú yè tāng*). Externally contracted wind-cold contending with sinews causing hypertonicity of the sinews, clenched jaw, loss of consciousness, and arched-back rigidity can be treated as true wind stroke, using Hua Tuo's Wind-Healing Powder (*huá tuó yù fēng sǎn*), which nowadays can be applied by nasal feed. ACU Base treatment mainly on GB, TB, SP, ST, LI, and LR. Main points: needle with drainage at GV-20 (*bǎi huì*, Hundred Convergences), GB-20 (*fēng chí*, Wind Pool), and TB-5 (*wài guān*, Outer Pass), and with supplementation at BL-20 (*pí shū*, Spleen Transport), BL-17 (*gé shū*, Diaphragm Transport), ST-36 (*zú sān lǐ*, Leg Three Li), and SP-6 (*sān yīn jiāo*, Three Yin Intersection). Selection of points according to pattern: For Cinnamon Twig Decoction (*guì zhī tāng*) patterns, add GV-16 (*fēng fǔ*, Wind Mansion), LI-4 (*hé gǔ*, Union Valley), and LI-11 (*qū chí*, Pool at the Bend), needling with drainage. For Bamboo Leaf Decoction (*zhú yè tāng*) patterns, add GV-14 (*dà zhuī*, Great Hammer), LI-4 (*hé gǔ*, Union Valley), LI-11 (*qū chí*, Pool at the Bend), LU-7 (*liè quē*, Broken Sequence), and LU-5 (*chǐ zé*, Cubit Marsh), needling with drainage. For externally contracted wind-cold contending with the sinews, add GV-26 (*rén zhōng*, Human Center), KI-1 (*yǒng quán*, Gushing Spring), LI-4 (*hé gǔ*, Union Valley), LU-7 (*liè quē*, Broken Sequence), LR-3 (*tài chōng*, Supreme Surge), BL-57 (*chéng shān*, Mountain Support), and GB-34 (*yáng líng quán*, Yang Mound Spring), needling with drainage and adding moxa. Compare POSTPARTUM WIND-LIKE STROKE. See also LOCKJAW. [26: 575]

post-voiding dribble 尿后馀沥 *niào hòu yú lì*: See DRIBBLE AFTER VOIDING.

¹**pounding** 捣 *dǎo*: CRUSHING.

²**pounding** 捣臼 *dǎo jiù*: NEEDLE POUNDING.

powder 散 *sǎn*: POWDER PREPARATION.

powder preparation 散剂 *sǎn jì*: Synonym: *powder*. A medicinal preparation made by grinding medicinal materials finely. Powders are suitable for both internal and external use, and are convenient for the patient. Orally taken powders are more easily absorbed than pills. Materials that cannot be heated, or do not easily dissolve in water are particularly suitable for preparation in powder form. **Method**: The materials are first carefully dried, then blended and ground together. The coarser particles are sifted off and reground until everything has been ground to a uniformly fine powder. High oil content materials such as bitter apricot kernel (*kǔ xìng rén*) or spiny jujube (*suān zǎo rén*) that are not suited to baking are first set aside while the other medicinals are ground. They are then ground together with a part of the preground powder, which absorbs the oil and facilitates the grinding process. Soft sticky agents such as cooked rehmannia (*shú dì huáng*), cornus (*shān zhū yú*), and lycium berry (*gǒu qǐ zǐ*) may also be ground with part of the preground agents, then sun-dried or oven-dried, and finally ground to a fine powder. Agents such as bovine bezoar (*niú huáng*) and borneol (*bīng piàn*), which, being used in such small quantities, may be lost if ground together with the other medicinals, may be ground in a porcelain mortar and added to the other powdered agents. Finally, medicinals such as realgar (*xióng huáng*), sulfur (*shí liú huáng*), and niter (*xiāo shí*) should not be ground since they may catch fire or explode. [27: 312]

pox 痘 *dòu*, 痘疮 *dòu chuāng*: SMALLPOX.

precedence of pulse over signs 舍证从脉 *shě zhèng cóng mài*: A principle that applies when an apparent contradiction exists between the pulse and other signs, and the pulse should be taken as the truer indicator of the condition. For example, in an internal heat block with a rapid sunken pulse and reversal cold of the limbs, the pulse faithfully represents the true condition. The signs only reflect the misleading presence of cold due to the confinement of heat in the interior. In some cases, pulse and signs represent different aspects of the condition. Where, for example, DRUM DISTENTION (ascites) is accompanied by a weak, faint pulse, the signs truly reflect the repletion of evil qi, whereas the pulse truly reflects the vacuity of right qi. In such cases, giving precedence to the pulse or to the signs would involve a decision about treatment priorities (supplementation followed by attack or attack followed by supplementation). [6: 144] [27: 204]

precedence of signs over the pulse 舍脉从证 *shě mài cóng zhèng*: A principle that applies when an apparent contradiction exists between the pulse and other signs, and these other signs should be taken as a truer indicator of the condition. For example, in gastrointestinal heat bind, characterized by abdominal pain that refuses pressure, constipation, and a thick parched yellow tongue fur, the appearance of a slow fine pulse reflects only misleading side-effects of the condition—the interior heat bind impairing qi dynamic and the smooth flow of blood through the vessels. The signs therefore take precedence over the pulse. [6: 144] [27: 204]

precipitate 下 *xià*: To cause expulsion of stool; to eliminate evil through the bowels. See PRECIPITATION.

precipitating depressed upper body fire 下怫 郁于上之火 *xià fú yù yú shàng zhī huǒ*: To treat a) depressed heat in the lung and stomach characterized by sore swollen throat, mouth and tongue sores, painful swollen gums, gaping of the gums, nosebleed, feverish agitation in the chest and diaphragm, constipation, and bad breath; or b) liver fire flaming upward characterized by headache, reddening of the face and eyes, yellow tongue fur, constipation, deafness and tinnitus, heart vexation, and irascibility. MED The chief medicinal in both cases is rhubarb (*dà huáng*). To treat depressed heat in the lung and stomach it is combined with heat-clearing and toxin-resolving medicinals such as charred gardenia (*hēi shān zhī zǐ*), moutan (*mǔ dān pí*), scrophularia (*xuán shēn*), arctium (*niú bàng zǐ*), and native achyranthes (*tǔ niú xī*). To treat liver fire flaming upward, these are combined with liver-draining medicinals such as aloe (*lú huì*), fetid cassia (*jué míng zǐ*), prunella (*xià kū cǎo*), and gentian (*lóng dǎn*). Diaphragm-Cooling Powder (*liáng gé sǎn*) drains the upper and center burners, and is used to treat depressed heat in the lung and stomach. Tangkuei, Gentian, and Aloe Pill (*dāng guī lóng huì wán*) and Toilette Pill (*gēng yī wán*) drain the liver. [6: 252]

precipitating gastrointestinal heat bind 下胃 肠热结 *xià wèi cháng rè jié*: To eliminate yang brightness (*yáng míng*) bowel repletion through PRECIPITATION. Yang brightness (*yáng míng*) bowel repletion is characterized by tidal heat [effusion], abdominal distention that refuses pressure, constipation, old yellow or burnt-yellow tongue fur, or a dry fissured tongue with parched black fur and prickles at the tip and margins, and a forceful slippery sunken pulse. These signs are classically summarized with the words glomus, fullness, dryness, and repletion. In severe cases there may be delirious speech and manic agitation, or diarrhea characterized by foul-smelling stool and burning sensation on defecation, together with fecal impaction (classically referred to as *heat bind with circumfluence*). MED The principal medicinal used in precipitating gastrointestinal heat bind is rhubarb (*dà huáng*), which frees the stool, drains fire, resolves toxin, and flushes the heat bind. It

is often used with mirabilite (*máng xiāo*), which is salty and cold, and which softens hardness and drains heat. Patients with pronounced abdominal pain and distention should be prescribed formulas that also contain unripe bitter orange (*zhǐ shí*) and magnolia bark (*hòu pò*), which loosen the center and break qi, thereby eliminating glomus and fullness. These three medicinals enhance the precipitant effect of rhubarb (*dà huáng*). Commonly used Formulas include Major Qi-Coordinating Decoction (*dà chéng qì tāng*), Minor Qi-Coordinating Decoction (*xiǎo chéng qì tāng*), and Stomach-Regulating Qi-Coordinating Decoction (*tiáo wèi chéng qì tāng*). [6: 251]

precipitating heat toxin 下热毒 *xià rè dú*: To eliminate heat toxin through PRECIPITATION in patterns of externally contracted heat (febrile) disease either with high fever, agitation, clouded spirit, or with heat toxin penetrating the construction aspect with such signs as frenetic blood movement, maculopapular eruptions, bleeding, and intestinal abscesses. MED The main medicinal used is rhubarb (*dà huáng*), which is combined with large quantities of heat-clearing, toxin-resolving, and blood-cooling medicinals such as coptis (*huáng lián*), scutellaria (*huáng qín*), puccoon (*zǐ cǎo*), moutan (*mǔ dān pí*), cooked rehmannia (*shú dì huáng*), isatis leaf (*dà qīng yè*), lonicera (*jīn yín huā*), and dandelion (*pú gōng yīng*). Two commonly used formulas are Heart-Draining Decoction (*xiè xīn tāng*), which primarily drains heat, and Rhubarb and Moutan Decoction (*dà huáng mǔ dān tāng*), which treats INTESTINAL WELLING-ABSCESS with pus-expelling and toxin-resolving medicinals. [6: 251]

precipitating qi 下气 *xià qì*: DOWNBEARING QI. [27: 270] [27: 319] [97: 212]

Precipitation

> COLD PRECIPITATION (*hán xià*)
> WARM PRECIPITATION (*wēn xià*)
> MOIST PRECIPITATION (*rùn xià*)
> EXPELLING WATER (*zhú shuǐ*)

---

precipitation 下法 *xià fǎ*: One of the EIGHT METHODS. The stimulation of fecal flow to expel repletion evils and remove accumulation and stagnation. *The Inner Canon* (*nèi jīng*) states, "Precipitation involves the drawing out [of evils]" and "lodging is treated by attack." Precipitation involves different methods, which can be classified as follows: (1) DRAINING FIRE: a) PRECIPITATING GASTROINTESTINAL HEAT BIND (used to treat yang brightness bowel patterns); b) PRECIPITATING HEAT TOXIN (used to expel evil fire and heat toxin through the bowels); c) PRECIPITATING DEPRESSED UPPER BODY FIRE (used to treat liver fire flaming upward and depressed heat in the lung and stomach). (2) EXPELLING COLD ACCUMULATIONS. (3) EXPELLING WATER. (4) MOISTENING THE INTESTINES. In addition, precipitation may be combined with other methods of treatment such as transforming phlegm, transforming static blood, dispersing food accumulations, and expelling parasites. Precipitation is an important method of expelling evils, and may be used when the evils binding in the interior give rise to interior repletion patterns. In clinical practice, careful evaluation of the relative strength of right qi and the evil is necessary to ensure that a formula appropriate for the patient's condition is chosen. Different forms of precipitation are listed above, and draining precipitation medicinals are listed below. ◇ Chin 下 *xià*, descend, to cause to descend, precipitate. NB: Chinese medicine expresses the idea of discharging fecal matter from the bowels as downward movement, which is one of the four movements (inward, outward, upward, and downward). *Purge*, a natural English equivalent of *xià*, means to cleanse. [6: 251] [27: 459] [97: 26]

Draining Precipitation Medicinals

Attacking precipitants
大黄 (*dà huáng*) rhubarb (Rhei Rhizoma)
生大黄 (*shēng dà huáng*) raw rhubarb (Rhei Rhizoma Crudum)
玄明粉 (*xuán míng fěn*) refined mirabilite (Mirabilitum Depuratum)
朴硝 (*pò xiāo*) impure mirabilite (Mirabilitum Non-Purum)
芒硝 (*máng xiāo*) mirabilite (Mirabilitum)
番泻叶 (*fān xiè yè*) senna (Sennae Folium)
芦荟 (*lú huì*) aloe (Aloe)
巴豆 (*bā dòu*) croton (Crotonis Semen)
巴豆霜 (*bā dòu shuāng*) croton frost (Crotonis Seminis Pulvis)

Moist Precipitants
火麻仁 (*huǒ má rén*) hemp seed (Cannabis Semen)
郁李仁 (*yù lǐ rén*) bush cherry kernel (Pruni Japonicae Semen)

Water-Expelling Medicinals
甘遂 (*gān suì*) kansui (Kansui Radix)
续随子 (*xù suí zǐ*) caper spurge seed (Euphorbiae Lathyridis Semen)
大戟 (*dà jǐ*) euphorbia/knoxia (Euphorbiae seu Knoxiae Radix)
芫花 (*yuán huā*) genkwa (Daphnes Genkwa Flos)
牵牛子 (*qiān niú zǐ*) morning glory (Pharbitidis Semen)
商陆 (*shāng lù*) phytolacca (Phytolaccae Radix)
续随子 (*xù suí zǐ*) caper spurge seed (Euphorbiae Lathyridis Semen)

precipitation of blood 下血 *xià xuè*: Bloody stool, especially when severe. See BLOODY STOOL.

predecoction 先煎 *xiān jiān*: Decocting hard medicinal materials requiring a long boiling time before the other medicinals of the formula are added. medicinals commonly requiring predecoction include minerals and shells such as gypsum (*shí gāo*), hematite (*dài zhě shí*), goose throat stone (*é guān shí*), oyster shell (*mǔ lì*), and turtle shell (*biē jiǎ*). These are crushed and brought to the boil over a fierce flame and are boiled for 10–15 minutes before adding the other ingredients. Raw arisaema (*shēng nán xīng*) and raw wild aconite (*shēng cǎo wū*) can be predecocted to reduce their toxicity. Ephedra (*má huáng*) can be predecocted to prevent it from causing heart vexation. This is done by boiling it for a few seconds, removing the scum and adding more water before the remaining ingredients are added. [27: 319] [50: 547]

predilection for greasy and rich foods 偏嗜油腻厚味 *piān shì yóu nì hòu wèi*: A tendency to eat fatty, sweet, salty, and spicy foods. It increases susceptibility to phlegm-damp. [6: 134]

pregnancy 妊娠 *rèn shēn*, 胎孕 *tāi yùn*, 妊子 *rèn zǐ*, 重身 *zhòng shēn*, 怀娠 *huái shēn*, 怀孕 *huái yùn*: The state of being great with child. For diseases of pregnancy, see entries listed below. See also CONTRAINDICATIONS OF MEDICINALS IN PREGNANCY. [26: 340]

Diseases of Pregnancy

MALIGN OBSTRUCTION (*è zǔ*)
SWELLING OF PREGNANCY (*zǐ zhǒng*)
BRITTLE FOOT (*cuì jiǎo*)
WRINKLY FOOT (*zhòu jiǎo*)
FULLNESS OF PREGNANCY (*zǐ mǎn*)
STRANGURY OF PREGNANCY (*zǐ lín*)
VEXATION OF PREGNANCY (*zǐ fán*)
COUGH OF PREGNANCY (*zǐ sòu*)
HABITUAL MISCARRIAGE (*huá tāi*)
THREATENED MISCARRIAGE (*xiān zhào liú chǎn*)
EPILEPSY OF PREGNANCY (*zǐ xián*)
SHIFTED BLADDER (*zhuǎn bào*)
ABDOMINAL PAIN IN PREGNANCY (*rèn shēn fù tòng*)
DISTENTION AND FULLNESS IN THE HEART [REGION] AND ABDOMEN IN PREGNANCY (*rèn shēn xīn fù zhàng mǎn*)
DIZZINESS IN PREGNANCY (*rèn shēn xuàn yūn*)
ENURESIS IN PREGNANCY (*rèn shēn yí niào*)
LUMBAR PAIN IN PREGNANCY (*rèn shēn yāo tòng*)
PANTING IN PREGNANCY (*rèn shēn chuǎn*)
SORES IN PREGNANCY (*rèn shēn chuāng yáng*)
SWELLING AND DISTENTION IN PREGNANCY (*rèn shēn zhǒng zhàng*)

URINARY STOPPAGE IN PREGNANCY (*rèn shēn xiǎo biàn bù tōng*)

VOMITING IN PREGNANCY (*rèn shēn ǒu tù*)

WIND STROKE IN PREGNANCY (*rèn shēn zhòng fēng*)

WIND TETANY IN PREGNANCY (*rèn shēn fēng jìng*)

---

pregnancy pulse 妊娠脉 *rèn shēn mài*: A pulse characteristic of pregnancy. In pregnancy, the pulse is often slippery and harmonious, or slippery and rapid, beating forcefully against the fingers. *Elementary Questions* (*sù wèn, yīn yáng bié lùn*) states, "Yin contending differently from yang means having a child." *Elementary Questions* (*sù wèn, píng rén qì xiàng lùn*) states, "Women whose hand lesser yin (*shào yīn*) channel is markedly stirring are pregnant." *The Bin-Hu Sphygmology* (*bīn hú mài xué*) states "Slippery and harmonious can decide pregnancy." *The Golden Mirror of Medicine* (*yī zōng jīn jiàn, sì zhěn xīn fǎ yào jué*) states, "Slippery, racing, and scattered indicates that the fetus must be three months; not scattered under pressure can differentiate a five-month [fetus]." [26: 341]

pregnancy qi 子气 *zǐ qì*: Swelling in pregnancy with long voidings of clear urine, arising when spleen-yang vacuity and damage by dampness allow damp qi to brew internally and disturb movement and transformation, so that water-damp collects and flows downward. MED Use variations of Life-for-All Ovate Atractylodes Powder (*quán shēng bái zhú sǎn*). [26: 56]

premature ejaculation 早泄 *zǎo xiè*: Ejaculation shortly after insertion, followed by subsiding erection that prevents further coitus. Premature ejaculation is attributed to hyperactivity of the ministerial fire, to insecurity of kidney qi, to heart-spleen depletion, to liver channel damp-heat, or to binding depression of liver qi. **Hyperactivity of the ministerial fire:** Premature ejaculation can arise when sexual intemperance, excessive masturbation, or enduring sickness affect the kidney causing depletion of kidney yin and exuberance of the ministerial fire. Alternatively, it may arise when wild desire stirs the sovereign fire above and causes the ministerial fire to become hyperactive below. In the former case, kidney yin signs such as limp aching lumbus and vexing heat in the five hearts are pronounced, whereas in the latter there are marked signs of upward flaming fire such as dizziness, headache, red eyes, tinnitus, and baking heat in the face. In either case, premature ejaculation is associated with excessive libido. MED Use Major Yin Supplementation Pill (*dà bǔ yīn wán*) for kidney yin depletion, and Left-Running Metal Pill (*zuǒ jīn wán*) for signs of fire flaming upward. ACU Base treatment on back transport

points and KI. Needle with supplementation at BL-23 (*shèn shū*, Kidney Transport), KI-3 (*tài xī*, Great Ravine), BL-52 (*zhì shì*, Will Chamber), and KI-7 (*fù liū*, Recover Flow), and with drainage at BL-15 (*xīn shū*, Heart Transport), HT-7 (*shén mén*, Spirit Gate), KI-6 (*zhào hǎi*, Shining Sea), and KI-2 (*rán gǔ*, Blazing Valley). **Insecurity of kidney qi:** Premature ejaculation due to insecurity of kidney qi is a kidney qi vacuity pattern. It differs from the exuberant ministerial fire pattern in that it is associated with reduced rather than with increased libido. Other signs include limp aching lumbus and knees, dull dark complexion, frequent urination and, in severe cases, urinary incontinence. MED Boost the kidney and secure essence with Golden Coffer Kidney Qi Pill (*jīn guì shèn qì wán*) plus tribulus (*cì jí lí*), dragon bone (*lóng gǔ*), and oyster shell (*mǔ lì*). Preparatory medicines include Five-Seed Progeny Pill (*wǔ zǐ yǎn zōng wán*) or Golden Lock Essence-Securing Pill (*jīn suǒ gù jīng wán*). ACU Base treatment on CV, back transport points, GV and KI. Select BL-23 (*shèn shū*, Kidney Transport), GV-4 (*mìng mén*, Life Gate), CV-4 (*guān yuán*, Pass Head), CV-6 (*qì hǎi*, Sea of Qi), KI-10 (*yīn gǔ*, Yin Valley), and GB-25 (*jīng mén*, Capital Gate); needle with supplementation and add moxa. **Heart-spleen depletion:** Premature ejaculation due to dual vacuity of the heart and spleen arises from excessive thinking or anxiety, major or enduring sickness, or dietary irregularities causing insufficiency of qi and blood and qi vacuity fall that weakens the power to contain essence. It is accompanied by shortness of breath and lack of strength, and a lusterless complexion. Accompanying signs may include heart palpitations or fearful throbbing, reduced sleep and profuse dreaming, dizziness, forgetfulness, abdominal distention, sloppy stool, reduced food intake, and torpid intake. MED Supplement the spleen and heart with Spleen-Returning Decoction (*guī pí tāng*). Alternatively use Ginseng Construction-Nourishing Decoction (*rén shēn yǎng róng tāng*). ACU Base treatment on back transport points, CV, ST, and SP. Select BL-15 (*xīn shū*, Heart Transport), BL-20 (*pí shū*, Spleen Transport), BL-17 (*gé shū*, Diaphragm Transport), CV-4 (*guān yuán*, Pass Head), CV-6 (*qì hǎi*, Sea of Qi), ST-36 (*zú sān lǐ*, Leg Three Li), and SP-6 (*sān yīn jiāo*, Three Yin Intersection); needle with supplementation and add moxa. **Liver channel damp-heat:** Liver channel damp-heat may arise either when predilection for sweet, fatty, fried, and spicy foods causes damp-heat to arise within or after repeated contraction of damp-heat evil. When it causes stagnation of qi dynamic, it can stir the ministerial fire, which harasses the essence chamber, causing premature ejaculation. In such cases, premature ejaculation is associated with frequent erections. Accompanying signs include bitter taste in the mouth, torpid intake, oppression in the chest and rib-side pain, hot itchy scrotum, and yellow or reddish urine. The tongue fur is yellow and slimy and the pulse is stringlike, slippery and rapid. [MED] Clear heat and drain dampness with Gentian Liver-Draining Decoction (*lóng dǎn xiè gān tāng*). [ACU] Base treatment on back transport points, LR, GB, and SP. Select BL-18 (*gān shū*, Liver Transport), LR-2 (*xíng jiān*, Moving Between), GB-34 (*yáng líng quán*, Yang Mound Spring), LI-11 (*qū chí*, Pool at the Bend), SP-6 (*sān yīn jiāo*, Three Yin Intersection), and SP-9 (*yīn líng quán*, Yin Mound Spring); needle with drainage and add moxa. **Binding depression of liver qi:** Premature ejaculation due to binding depression of liver qi arises when affect-mind dissatisfaction causes depression and binding of qi dynamic; this impairs liver free coursing and affects the kidney's ability to secure essence. The principal accompanying sign is mental depression; other signs include rib-side distention and distending pain in the lesser abdomen, oppression in the chest, sighing, and in some cases dry mouth with bitter taste, reduced sleep and profuse dreaming, thin white tongue fur, and a stringlike pulse. [MED] Course the liver and rectify qi using Bupleurum Liver-Coursing Powder (*chái hú shū gān sǎn*). [ACU] Base treatment on back transport points, PC, LR, and SP. Select BL-18 (*gān shū*, Liver Transport), BL-23 (*shèn shū*, Kidney Transport), PC-6 (*nèi guān*, Inner Pass), LR-14 (*qī mén*, Cycle Gate), LR-3 (*tài chōng*, Supreme Surge), SP-6 (*sān yīn jiāo*, Three Yin Intersection), and ST-36 (*zú sān lǐ*, Leg Three Li); needle with even supplementation and drainage. [56: 40] [27: 427]

premenstrual bloody stool 经前便血 *jīng qián biàn xuè*: Synonym: *deviated menstruation*. The passing of bloody stool that starts before each menstrual period and that ceases by the end of the period. Premenstrual bloody stool arises when consumption of hot acrid blood drying foods causes heat to become depressed in the intestines so that the filling of the uterus with qi and blood before the menstrual period stirs the latent heat in the intestines and causes frenetic movement of the blood. Accompanying signs include red face and dry lips, dry throat and bitter taste in the mouth, thirst and scant thick purple red menstrual flow or, in severe cases, menstrual block. [MED] Use Sanguisorba Powder (*dì yú sǎn*) plus dried/fresh rehmannia (*shēng dì huáng*), red peony (*chì sháo yào*), and mume (*wū méi*). For unpronounced heat, remove coptis (*huáng lián*) and gardenia (*shān zhī zǐ*). For dry bound stool, add hemp seed (*huǒ má rén*) and bush cherry kernel (*yù lǐ rén*). [26: 815]

premenstrual syndrome 经前期紧张综合症 *jīng qián qī jǐn zhāng zōng hé zhèng*: The regu-

lar occurrence about a week before each menstrual period of signs such as vexation, agitation, and irascibility, variously attended by painful distention of the breasts, clouded head and headache or hemilateral headache, fatigue, somnolence, oppression in the chest, sore throat and hoarse voice, abdominal distention and aching lumbus, water swelling, diarrhea, pain in the joints, urticaria, or itchy skin. Signs characteristically abate swiftly with the onset of menstruation. "Premenstrual syndrome" is a term adopted from Western medicine, but in Chinese medicine signs such as irascibility and painful distention of the breasts are classic signs of binding depression of liver qi. Their regular appearance in the menstrual cycle is understood in terms of the liver's free coursing function and the thoroughfare (*chōng*) and controlling (*rèn*) vessels' control over menstruation. Other signs are explained by different mechanisms, e.g., aching lumbus and knees by insufficiency of kidney yin. [MED] For binding depression of liver qi marked by premenstrual irascibility, painful distention of the breasts, dizzy head or headache, and poor appetite, course the liver and resolve depression with variations of Moutan and Gardenia Free Wanderer Powder (*dān zhī xiāo yáo sǎn*). For insufficiency of kidney yin characterized by limp aching lumbus, dry mouth and red cheeks, and night sweating, treat by enriching yin and supplementing the kidney with Six-Ingredient Rehmannia Pill (*liù wèi dì huáng wán*). [ACU] For binding depression of liver qi, base treatment mainly on LR, PC, and SP. Selection PC-6 (*nèi guān*, Inner Pass), SP-6 (*sān yīn jiāo*, Three Yin Intersection), LR-3 (*tài chōng*, Supreme Surge), BL-18 (*gān shū*, Liver Transport), BL-17 (*gé shū*, Diaphragm Transport), ST-36 (*zú sān lǐ*, Leg Three Li), and LI-4 (*hé gǔ*, Union Valley); needle with even supplementation and drainage and add moxa. Selection of points according to signs: For distending pain in the breasts, add CV-17 (*shān zhōng*, Chest Center), and SI-11 (*tiān zōng*, Celestial Gathering). For dizziness and headache, add GB-20 (*fēng chí*, Wind Pool), Greater Yang (*tài yáng*), and GB-43 (*xiá xī*, Pinched Ravine). For poor stomach intake, add CV-12 (*zhōng wǎn*, Center Stomach Duct) and ST-25 (*tiān shū*, Celestial Pivot). For insufficiency of kidney yin, base treatment mainly on KI and SP. Select BL-23 (*shèn shū*, Kidney Transport), KI-3 (*tài xī*, Great Ravine), KI-6 (*zhào hǎi*, Shining Sea), KI-2 (*rán gǔ*, Blazing Valley), and SP-6 (*sān yīn jiāo*, Three Yin Intersection); needle with supplementation. Selection of points according to signs: For limp aching lumbus and knees, add GV-3 (*yāo yáng guān*, Lumbar Yang Pass) and BL-40 (*wěi zhōng*, Bend Center). For dry mouth, add TB-2 (*yè mén*, Humor Gate). For night sweating, add LI-4 (*hé gǔ*, Union Valley) and HT-6 (*yīn xī*, Yin Cleft). [26: 815] [46: 646, 682] [59: 282]

premenstrual vomiting 经前呕吐 *jīng qián ǒu tù*: VOMITING just before menstrual periods. Premenstrual vomiting arises when ingested water fails to be transformed, or when food damage causes stagnation in patients with weak stomachs. In the first case, the vomitus is watery; in the second, there is stomach pain. MED Treat water-rheum by warming the center and transforming rheum with clove (*dīng xiāng*), dried ginger (*gān jiāng*), and ovate atractylodes (*bái zhú*) ground to a powder (5 g at time with water that rice has been boiled in). Treat food damage by dispersing food and abducting stagnation with Saussurea and Amomum Six Gentlemen Decoction (*xiāng shā liù jūn zǐ tāng*). [26: 815]

preparation 制剂 *zhì jì*: See PREPARATION OF MEDICINALS.

preparation of medicinals 制剂 *zhì jì*: Making a medicinal or medicinals of a formula ready for consumption or application; the making of medicinal preparations. Medicinals are prepared in different ways to ensure maximum effectiveness and convenience of storage or use. The preparation of medicinals from PROCESSING OF MEDICINALS, which refers to the treatment of individual medicinals before they are combined in a formula.

prepared 熟 *shóu*: Cooked.

presence of root 有根 *yǒu gēn*: See STOMACH, SPIRIT, AND ROOT.

presence of spirit 有神 *yǒu shén*: See STOMACH, SPIRIT, AND ROOT.

presence of stomach 有胃 *yǒu wèi*: See STOMACH, SPIRIT, AND ROOT.

prevalence 胜 *shèng*: A strengthening of yin or yang. See WAXING AND WANING OF YIN AND YANG.

pricking and cupping 刺血拔罐 *cì xuè bá guàn*, 刺络拔罐 *cì luò bá guàn*: A method of cupping whereby a cup is applied to an area of skin that has been pricked with a cutaneous needle (e.g., a plum blossom needle). This method, which can draw large amounts of blood if the area has been heavily pricked, is used for CINNABAR TOXIN, SPRAIN, or MAMMARY WELLING-ABSCESS. [46: 500]

prickly heat 痱子 *fèi zi*, 痱疮 *féi chuāng*: Synonym: *prickly heat toxin*. A disease characterized by red papules attended with itching and tingling. Prickly heat occurs mostly in hot summer months, and is attributed to brewing summerheat-damp that inhibits sweating. It most commonly affects infants and obese people, and affects the head, neck, abdomen, back, shoulder, and groin. It appears as red papules the size of millet seeds, which quickly turn into water vesicles or pustules,

and are associated with itching and scorching heat. Scratching can cause the development of a *prickly heat toxin* (sore), equivalent to hidradenitis spoken of in Western medicine. MED Treat by taking orally a decoction of forsythia (*lián qiào*), trichosanthes root (*tiān huā fěn*), red peony (*chì sháo yào*), licorice (*gān cǎo*), talcum (*huá shí*), plantago (*chē qián*), lonicera (*jīn yín huā*), alisma (*zé xiè*), and bamboo leaf (lophatherum) (*dàn zhú yè*) or make a soup of mung bean (*lǜ dòu*), with mint (*bò hé*) and sugar added. [26: 769] [97: 612]

prickly heat toxin 痱毒 *féi dú*: PRICKLY HEAT.

prickly tongue 舌上起芒刺 *shé shàng qǐ máng cì*: See PRICKLY TONGUE.

prickly tongue 舌起芒刺 *shé qǐ máng cì*: Synonym: *prickles on the tongue*. Projections on the tongue surface. Prickles often occur with red speckles, and are invariably accompanied by a scorched yellow or black tongue fur. They indicate exuberant heat. They occur in various externally contracted febrile diseases, particularly yang brightness repletion heat patterns, and in conjunction with maculopapular eruptions. The location of the prickles indicates the location of the heat. Located at the tip of the tongue, they indicate heart heat, while located in the center of the tongue they indicate accumulated spleen-stomach heat. WMC hyperplasia or enlargement of the fungiform papillae. [6: 120] [27: 183] [97: 197]

prick to bleed 点刺放血 *diǎn cì fàng xuè*, 点刺出血 *diǎn cì chū xuè*: To prick the skin with a brisk stabbing action to produce a few drops of blood. See BLOODLETTING. [46: 502]

principle of treatment 治则 *zhì zé*: A general rule guiding selection of methods of treatment. A major principle of treatment especial in the modern practice of Chinese medicine is DETERMINING TREATMENT BY PATTERNS IDENTIFIED, by which treatment addresses illness as reflected in clinical signs rather than addressing a single isolated cause. This principle notably includes LIKE TREATMENT OF UNLIKE DISEASE, UNLIKE TREATMENT OF LIKE DISEASE and ACTION ACCORDING TO TIME, PLACE, AND PERSON and is actually reflected in most principles of treatment. However, the most important procedural principle is TREATING DISEASE INVOLVES SEEKING ITS ROOT, i.e., its essential nature and cause. When the root of a disease is determined and hence the nature of the imbalance is understood, the question of TREATING THE ROOT, TREATING THE TIP, or SIMULTANEOUS TREATMENT OF ROOT AND BRANCH is decided by secondary principles that include IN ACUTE CONDITIONS TREAT THE TIP and IN MODERATE CONDITIONS TREAT THE ROOT. Conditions involving evils require a decision on whether to dispel the evil and support right (see DISPELLING EVIL AND

SUPPORTING RIGHT), such as ATTACK FOLLOWED BY SUPPLEMENTATION, SUPPLEMENTATION FOLLOWED BY ATTACK, or SIMULTANEOUS SUPPLEMENTATION AND ATTACK. All disease can be seen in terms of yin and yang and hence all treatment can be viewed in terms of the restoration of the yin-yang balance, which involves either righting of yin and yang surfeits or righting of yin and yang deficits. Furthermore, a distinction is made between STRAIGHT TREATMENT and PARADOXICAL TREATMENT. Most methods of treatment are straight treatment, e.g., HEAT IS TREATED WITH COLD, COLD IS TREATED WITH HEAT, VACUITY IS TREATED BY SUPPLEMENTING, and REPLETION IS TREATED BY DRAINING. Paradoxical treatment includes: TREATING HEAT WITH HEAT and TREATING COLD WITH COLD. Paradoxical treatment is not strictly contrary to straight treatment, since, for example, cold is treated with cold only when the cold signs are false. Finally, principles of treatment include a number of warnings such as AVOID THE MISTAKE OF USING HEAT AGAINST HEAT, AVOID THE MISTAKE OF USING COLD AGAINST COLD, and DO NOT HARM STOMACH QI. [6: 242]

processing 炮制 *páo zhì*, 炮炙 *páo zhì*: See PROCESSING OF MEDICINALS.

processing of medicinals 炮制 *páo zhì*, 炮炙 *páo zhì*: Abbreviation: processing. The processing of medicinal materials by washing, cutting, frying, etc. Many materials may be purchased ready-processed. Apart from some basic forms of preparation such as CRUSHING, GRATING, GRINDING, and CUTTING, most of these processes fall within three categories: fire processing, water processing, and fire and water processing. **Methods:** Water processing includes SOAKING and LONG RINSING. See entries listed below.

Processing of Medicinals

Basic processing
CUTTING (*qiē*)
CRUSHING (*dǎo*)
GRATING (*cuò*)
FLAKING (*bàng*)
GRINDING (*yán*)

Water processing
WASHING (*xǐ*)
COVERED MOISTENING (*mèn rùn*)
SOAKING (*jìn pào*)
LONG RINSING (*piǎo*)
WATER-GRINDING (*shuǐ fēi*)

Fire processing
STIR-FRYING (*chǎo*)
  PLAIN STIR-FRYING (*qīng chǎo*)
    LIGHT STIR-FRYING (*wéi chǎo*)
    SCORCH-FRYING (*chǎo jiāo*)
    BLAST-FRYING (*pāo*)
    CHAR-FRYING (*chǎo tàn*)
  STIR-FRYING WITH ADJUVANTS (*fù liào chǎo*)
    STIR-FRYING WITH CLAMSHELL POWDER (*gé fěn chǎo*)
    STIR-FRYING WITH EARTH (*tǔ chǎo*)
    STIR-FRYING WITH BRAN (*fū chǎo*)
    STIR-FRYING WITH RICE (*mǐ chǎo*)
  MIX-FRYING (*zhì*)
    MIX-FRYING WITH HONEY (*mì zhì*)
    MIX-FRYING WITH BRINE (*yán zhì*)
    MIX-FRYING WITH GINGER (*jiāng zhì*)
    MIX-FRYING WITH VINEGAR (*cù zhì*)
    MIX-FRYING WITH WINE (*jiǔ zhì*)
ROASTING (*wēi*)
STONE-BAKING (*bèi*)
CALCINATION (*duàn*)

Fire and water processing
BOILING (*zhǔ*)
DOUBLE-BOILING (*dùn*)
STEAMING (*zhēng*)
DISTILLING (*lù*)

Other
FROSTING (*zhì shuāng*)

Aims: Processing aims to eliminate or reduce toxicity, enhance action, or alter properties. Elimination or reduction of toxicity: For example, raw pinellia (*shēng bàn xià*) is treated with fresh ginger (*shēng jiāng*), alum (*bái fán*), or licorice (*gān cǎo*) to prevent poisoning and sore throat. The toxicity of kansui (*gān suì*) is reduced by boiling in vinegar. The precipitating action of croton (*bā dòu*) is moderated by removing its oil content. Dichroa (*cháng shān*) is stir-fried with wine to eliminate its emetic side-effect. Enhancement action: Processing can enhance the effectiveness of some agents. For example, when corydalis (*yán hú suǒ*) is treated with vinegar, it has a stronger pain-relieving effect. When tussilago (*kuǎn dōng huā*) is mix-fried with honey, it has a greater lung-moistening cough-suppressing action and checks diarrhea more effectively. Bupleurum (*chái hú*) mix-fried with vinegar has a greater liver-coursing and depression-resolving action. Alteration of properties: Some medicinals have different actions depending on whether or not they are processed. For example, rehmannia (*dì huáng*) is cold in nature and has a blood-cooling action when raw, but is warm in nature and supplements the blood when steamed with wine (Chinese rice wine). Typha pollen (*pú huáng*) moves the blood and resolves stasis when raw, and can check bleeding when stir-fried. The change action is determined by the nature and action of the adjuvant. Processing with wine tends to check a medicinal's cold nature and make it bear upward. Processing with ginger makes it warm, dissipate, and sweep phlegm. Processing with honey sweetens a medicinal, and helps it to moisten dryness and boost the origin. Processing with salt makes a medicinal enter the kidney, makes it move downward and soften hardness. Processing with vinegar makes it enter the liver, and enables it to promote astriction and relieve pain. Processing with earth (oven earth), makes a medicinal fortify the spleen and stomach and harmonize the center. Processing with rice eliminates dryness and nourishes the stomach. Processing with bran eliminates the harshness of a medicinal and prevents it from damaging the stomach. Soaking in black bean and licorice decoction resolves an agent's toxin and enhances its supplementing action. Compare ¹MEDICINAL PREPARATION. [27: 322] [97: 442]

profuse dreaming 多梦 *duō mèng*: Dreaming more often than normal. Profuse dreaming occurs with insomnia in heart-spleen vacuity and noninteraction of the heart and kidney. When patients suffering from susceptibility to fright, emotional instability, heart palpitations or fearful throbbing wake from dreaming with a start, it is a sign of heart and gallbladder qi vacuity. When patients suffering from dizziness, heart palpitations, irascibility, copious phlegm, and oppression in the chest have confused dreams, this is a sign of phlegm-fire. [26: 273]

profuse menstruation 月经过多 *yuè jīng guò duō*: Greater menstrual flow or longer menstrual period than normal. Profuse menstruation is attributed to qi vacuity, blood heat, or taxation fatigue causing insecurity of the thoroughfare (*chōng*) and controlling (*rèn*) vessels. See QI VACUITY PROFUSE MENSTRUATION; BLOOD HEAT PROFUSE MENSTRUATION; TAXATION DAMAGE PROFUSE MENSTRUATION. Compare SCANT MENSTRUATION. [26: 168] [27: 441]

profuse sweating 多汗 *duō hàn*: Sweating in excess of the normal amount. Sweating naturally increases in hot weather, with physical exertion, and the ingestion of warm foods and beverages, and with hot spicy foods. Profuse sweating as a reflection of disease occurs in many different patterns. See SWEATING.

profuse urination at night 夜间多尿 *yè jiān duō niào*: Synonym: *profuse urination at night*. Waking two, three, or more times a night to urinate, and passing in the night a quarter or more of the whole day's urine; a sign of kidney yang debilitation or spleen-kidney yang vacuity. **Kidney yang debilitation:** Profuse urination at night due to kidney yang debilitation is marked by frequent urination, dribble after voiding or even enuresis or incontinence, and is accompanied by tinnitus, hearing impairment, lumbar and back pain, seminal efflux, premature ejaculation, pale

enlarged tongue with thin white fur, and sunken fine weak pulse. ACU Base treatment mainly on back transport points, CV, and SP. Select BL-23 (*shèn shū*, Kidney Transport), BL-28 (*páng guāng shū*, Bladder Transport), CV-3 (*zhōng jí*, Central Pole), CV-4 (*guān yuán*, Pass Head), KI-3 (*tài xī*, Great Ravine), GV-4 (*mìng mén*, Life Gate), and SP-6 (*sān yīn jiāo*, Three Yin Intersection); needle with supplementation and moxa. **Spleen-kidney yang vacuity:** Profuse urination at night due to spleen-kidney yang vacuity is associated with physical cold, cold limbs, physical fatigue and lassitude of spirit, dizziness and tinnitus, limp aching lumbus and knees, reduced food intake, sloppy stool or clear-food diarrhea, frequent urination, pale enlarged tongue with white fur, and sunken weak pulse. MED For debilitation of kidney yang patterns, boost qi and secure the bladder with formulas such as Mantis Egg-Case Powder (*sāng piāo xiāo sǎn*). For spleen-kidney yang vacuity patterns, use warming yang complemented with securing astriction, using formulas such as Bladder-Securing Pill (*gù pāo wán*). ACU Base treatment mainly on BL and CV. Select BL-20 (*pí shū*, Spleen Transport), BL-23 (*shèn shū*, Kidney Transport), BL-28 (*páng guāng shū*, Bladder Transport), CV-3 (*zhōng jí*, Central Pole), CV-4 (*guān yuán*, Pass Head), CV-6 (*qì hǎi*, Sea of Qi), and ST-36 (*zú sān lǐ*, Leg Three Li); needle with supplementation and moxa. For spleen vacuity fall, add GV-20 (*bǎi huì*, Hundred Convergences). [92: No. 228]

prolapse of the rectum 脱肛 *tuō gāng*: Synonym: *anal desertion*. The downward fall of the rectum through the anus. Prolapse of the rectum is most prevalent among the young and the aged, and is the result of center qi fall, a qi vacuity pattern, or of damp-heat in the large intestine. **Center qi fall:** Prolapse of the rectum due to center qi fall occurs when coughing or defecating. The patient has to press the rectum back into place with the hand. The prolapsed part is pale without redness, swelling, or pain. The facial complexion is white and the lips are pale. There is shortness of breath and in some cases cough. The tongue is pale with scant fur, and the pulse is a forceless weak and vacuous. MED Treat by boosting qi and raising the fall with Center-Supplementing Qi-Boosting Decoction (*bǔ zhōng yì qì tāng*). ACU Base treatment mainly on back transport points, GV, and BL. Select GV-20 (*bǎi huì*, Hundred Convergences), BL-25 (*dà cháng shū*, Large Intestine Transport), GV-1 (*cháng qiáng*, Long Strong), and BL-57 (*chéng shān*, Mountain Support); needle with supplementation and add moxa. Selection of points according to cause: When prolapse of the anus results from enduring diarrhea or dysentery, add ST-36 (*zú sān lǐ*, Leg Three Li), SP-6 (*sān yīn jiāo*, Three Yin Intersection), and

CV-6 (*qì hǎi*, Sea of Qi). When due to excessive childbirth in women, add BL-23 (*shèn shū*, Kidney Transport), CV-6 (*qì hǎi*, Sea of Qi), and SP-6 (*sān yīn jiāo*, Three Yin Intersection). **Kidney yang vacuity:** Prolapse of the rectum with clouded head, flowery vision, forgetfulness, fifth-watch sloppy diarrhea, and in some cases seminal emission and impotence is due to kidney yang vacuity. Other signs include limp aching lumbus and knees, generalized fear of cold, and frequent urination. The tongue is enlarged and tender-soft; the pulse is sunken and fine. [MED] Combine boosting qi, lifting, and securing with powerful warming and supplementing of kidney yang. Use Cinnamon Bark and Aconite Eight-Ingredient Pill (*guì fù bā wèi wán*) plus codonopsis (*dǎng shēn*), astragalus (*huáng qí*), cimicifuga (*shēng má*), bupleurum (*chái hú*), chebule (*hē zǐ*), and sumac gallnut (*wǔ bèi zǐ*). [ACU] Base treatment mainly on GV, CV, and back transport points. Select GV-20 (*bǎi huì*, Hundred Convergences), BL-25 (*dà cháng shū*, Large Intestine Transport), GV-1 (*cháng qiáng*, Long Strong), BL-57 (*chéng shān*, Mountain Support), BL-23 (*shèn shū*, Kidney Transport), GV-4 (*mìng mén*, Life Gate), CV-4 (*guān yuán*, Pass Head), and KI-3 (*tài xī*, Great Ravine); needle with drainage. **Damp-heat:** Prolapse of the rectum due to damp-heat brewing and amassing is characterized by redness, swelling and pain of the prolapsed part. There may be thirst and dry stool. The facial complexion and lips are red. The tongue body is red with a yellow fur. The pulse is stringlike and rapid. [MED] Treat by clearing heat and disinhibiting dampness assisted by raising the fall using Four Agents Decoction (*sì wù tāng*) plus scutellaria (*huáng qín*), coptis (*huáng lián*), sophora flower (*huái huā*), cimicifuga (*shēng má*), and bupleurum (*chái hú*). Sumac gallnut (*wǔ bèi zǐ*) and alum (*bái fán*) can be decocted to make a wash. Pay attention to physical exercise to improve the constitution. [ACU] Base treatment mainly on back transport points, GV, BL, SP, and LI. Needle with even supplementation and drainage at GV-20 (*bǎi huì*, Hundred Convergences), BL-25 (*dà cháng shū*, Large Intestine Transport), GV-1 (*cháng qiáng*, Long Strong), and BL-57 (*chéng shān*, Mountain Support), and with drainage at LI-4 (*hé gǔ*, Union Valley), LI-11 (*qū chí*, Pool at the Bend), and SP-9 (*yīn líng quán*, Yin Mound Spring). ◇ Chin The Chinese term literally means shedding or desertion of the anus, hence "anal desertion" has been included as a synonym. [26: 646] [50: 1408] [92: No. 389] [46: 596, 672] [37: 462] [113: 106]

prolapse of the uterus 子宫脱垂 *zǐ gōng tuō chuí*, 子宫下垂 *zǐ gōng xià chuí*, 子肠不收 *zǐ cháng bù shōu*: Downward displacement of the uterus, in severe cases beyond the mouth of the vagina. Prolapse of the uterus is attributed to qi vacuity fall, loss of retention power of the girdling (*dài*) vessel and damage to the thoroughfare (*chōng*) and controlling (*rèn*) vessels, or to excessive childbirth, difficult childbirth or excessive straining during childbirth. **Qi vacuity** patterns are characterized by shortage of qi and laziness to speak, bright white facial complexion, and empty sagging in the smaller abdomen. [MED] Supplement qi and upbear yang using formulas such as Center-Supplementing Qi-Boosting Decoction (*bǔ zhōng yì qì tāng*). [ACU] Base treatment on CV and GV. Main points: CV-4 (*guān yuán*, Pass Head), CV-6 (*qì hǎi*, Sea of Qi), GV-20 (*bǎi huì*, Hundred Convergences), and Infant's Palace (*zǐ gōng*). For qi vacuity fall, add ST-36 (*zú sān lǐ*, Leg Three Li) and SP-6 (*sān yīn jiāo*, Three Yin Intersection); needle with supplementation and add moxa. **Kidney vacuity** patterns are characterized by dizziness, tinnitus, and limp aching lumbus and knees. [MED] Supplement the kidney and boost qi using formulas such as Major Origin-Supplementing Brew (*dà bǔ yuán jiān*) plus deerhorn glue (*lù jiǎo jiāo*), cimicifuga (*shēng má*), and bitter orange (*zhǐ ké*). [ACU] Use the main points given above, and add KI-12 (*dà hè*, Great Manifestation), and KI-6 (*zhào hǎi*, Shining Sea), needling with supplementation and adding moxa. Compare YIN PROTRUSION. [27: 484] [97: 522] [46: 694] [37: 436]

prolonged menstruation 经期延长 *jīng qī yán cháng*: Menstrual periods of more than seven days. [67: 99]

prominence 瘑 *tuí*: BULGING.

prominent green-blue abdominal veins 腹露青筋 *fù lù qīng jīn*: The appearance of veins on the surface of the abdomen, accompanying severe cases of drum distention. Prominent green-blue abdominal vessels are observed in qi stagnation and damp obstruction, liver-spleen static blood, spleen-kidney yang vacuity, and liver-kidney yin vacuity. [WMC] caput medusae. **Qi stagnation and damp obstruction** gives rise to abdominal enlargement, distention, and fullness with prominent green-blue veins, accompanied by distending pain in the rib-sides, poor appetite with abdominal distention worsening after eating, fatigued cumbersome limbs, short voidings of scant urine, sloppy diarrhea, slimy white tongue fur, and a stringlike pulse. It arises in liver depression and qi stagnation when liver qi runs cross counterflow to invade the spleen and nonmovement of spleen qi gives rise to internal collection of water-damp and phlegm turbidity congestion. [MED] Course the liver and fortify the spleen; disinhibit dampness and eliminate fullness. Use Bupleurum Liver-Coursing Powder (*chái hú shū gān sàn*) combined with Stomach-Calming Poria (Hoelen) Five Decoction (*wèi líng* *tāng*). **Liver-spleen blood stasis** gives rise to abdominal enlargement, distention, and fullness with prominent green-blue veins, accompanied by a lump under the rib-side with stabbing pain, a dry mouth with the desire only wash the mouth with fluid rather than swallowing it, black stool, dark black face, filiform blood moles on the head, neck, chest, and arms, dark purple lips, a dark purple tongue with stasis macules, and a fine rough pulse. MED Quicken the blood and transform stasis; disinhibit water and disperse swelling. Use variations of Construction-Regulating Beverage (*tiáo yíng yǐn*). **Spleen-kidney yang vacuity** causes abdominal enlargement, distention, and fullness with prominent green-blue veins, accompanied by fear of cold and coldlimbs, oppression in the stomach duct, torpid intake, limp aching lumbus and knees, inhibited urination, sloppy stool, puffy swelling of the lower limbs, somber yellow facial complexion, an enlarged purplish pale tongue, a glossy white tongue fur and a fine sunken pulse. MED Supplement the spleen and kidney; move qi and disinhibit water. Use variations of Spleen-Firming Beverage (*shí pí yǐn*). **Liver-kidney yin vacuity** causes abdominal enlargement, distention, and fullness with prominent green-blue veins, associated with dizzy head and vision, heart palpitations and insomnia, dry mouth and throat, spontaneous bleeding from the nose and gums, short voidings of scant urine, dark dull facial complexion, a red tongue with little liquid, and a fine rapid stringlike pulse. MED Enrich and nourish the liver and kidney; disinhibit water and disperse distention. Use All-the-Way-Through Brew (*yī guàn jiān*) combined with Polyporus Decoction (*zhū líng tāng*). See DRUM DISTENTION. [92: No. 205]

prominent mounting 癀疝 *tuí shàn*: A MOUNTING (*shàn*) pattern characterized by hypertonicity and pain of the lesser abdomen stretching into the testicles, or a lump in the abdomen with pus and blood; attributed to cold evil invading the liver and stomach channels. MED Dissipate cold, move qi, and transform stasis. Use Life Saver Tangerine Pip Pill (*jì shēng jú hé wán*) plus flying squirrel's droppings (*wǔ líng zhī*), red peony (*chì sháo yào*), cyathula (*chuān niú xī*), and tangkuei (*dāng guī*). Compare YIN MOUNTING. See MOUNTING. [26: 930] [48: 441]

promoting absorption of qi by the kidney 摄纳肾气 *shè nà shèn qì*: To treat failure of the kidney to ensure the absorption of qi through the lung, a condition known as the *kidney failing to absorb qi* and characterized by short rapid breathing, panting at the slightest exertion, vacuity sweating, cold limbs, a bright white or dark green-blue complexion, or upbearing fire flush, and a fine sunken pulse. MED Kidney-supplementing medicinals such as aconite (*fù zǐ*), cinnamon bark (*ròu*

guì), cooked rehmannia (*shú dì huáng*), cornus (*shān zhū yú*), walnut (*hú táo rén*), amethyst/fluorite (*zǐ shí yīng*), stalactite (*zhōng rǔ shí*), and galenite (*qiān*) are used. ACU Base treatment mainly on KI, CV, GV, and BL. Select CV-4 (*guān yuán*, Pass Head), BL-23 (*shèn shū*, Kidney Transport), BL-13 (*fèi shū*, Lung Transport), BL-43 (*gāo huāng shū*, Gao-Huang Transport), KI-3 (*tài xī*, Great Ravine), LU-5 (*chǐ zé*, Cubit Marsh), LU-9 (*tài yuān*, Great Abyss), and CV-6 (*qì hǎi*, Sea of Qi); needle with supplementation and add moxa. [46: 574] [6: 270]

promoting heart-kidney interaction 交通心肾 *jiāo tōng xīn shèn*: Synonym: *promote interaction of the heart and kidney*. To treat NONINTERACTION OF THE HEART AND KIDNEY characterized by heart palpitations, headache, insomnia, forgetfulness, seminal emission, tinnitus, deafness, aching lumbus and limp legs, short voidings of reddish urine, red tongue, and fine rapid pulse. MED Medicinals that promote heart-kidney interaction include dried/fresh rehmannia (*shēng dì huáng*), ophiopogon (*mài mén dōng*), lily bulb (*bǎi hé*), lycium berry (*gǒu qǐ zǐ*), ligustrum (*nǚ zhēn zǐ*), eclipta (*mò hàn lián*), and flowery knotweed (*hé shǒu wū*). Commonly used formulas include Peaceful Interaction Pill (*jiāo tài wán*) and Coptis, Ass Hide Glue, and Egg Yolk Decoction (*huáng lián ē jiāo jī zǐ huáng tāng*). ACU Base treatment mainly on back transport points, HT, and KI. Select BL-15 (*xīn shū*, Heart Transport), BL-23 (*shèn shū*, Kidney Transport), KI-3 (*tài xī*, Great Ravine), KI-1 (*yǒng quán*, Gushing Spring), HT-7 (*shén mén*, Spirit Gate), PC-8 (*láo gōng*, Palace of Toil), PC-7 (*dà líng*, Great Mound), and SP-6 (*sān yīn jiāo*, Three Yin Intersection); needle with even supplementation and drainage, or supplement the kidney and drain the heart. See NONINTERACTION OF THE HEART AND KIDNEY. [26: 236] [27: 287] [46: 678] [37: 348] [113: 145]

promoting interaction of the heart and kidney 交通心肾 *jiāo tōng xīn shèn*: PROMOTING HEART-KIDNEY INTERACTION.

promoting lactation 催乳 *cuī rǔ*, 下乳 *xià rǔ*: FREEING MILK.

promoting menstruation 通经 *tōng jīng*: FREEING MENSTRUATION.

promoting qi transformation and disinhibiting water 化气利湿 *huà qì lì shī*: WARMING YANG AND DISINHIBITING DAMPNESS.

promoting sweat 发汗 *fā hàn*: SWEATING[2]

propping 支 *zhī*: See following entries. ◇ Chin 支 *zhī*, prop, support, describing in this context the way in which the discomfort keeps the patient "propped up." [6: 220] [26: 109]

propping bind below the heart 心下支结 *xīn xià zhī jié*: Compare PROPPING FULLNESS. [26: 89]

propping fullness 支满 *zhī mǎn*: A feeling of fullness under the arch of the ribs. [26: 89]

propping fullness in the chest and rib-side 胸胁支满 *xiōng xié mǎ*: See CHEST AND RIB-SIDE FULLNESS. [26: 549]

propping rheum 支饮 *zhī yǐn*: One of the FOUR RHEUMS; water below the heart, causing signs such as cough, copious phlegm, rapid breathing, inability to lie flat, facial swelling, soot black complexion, and dizziness. [MED] Warm the lung, transform rheum, and calm panting with formulas such as Minor Green-Blue Dragon Decoction (*xiǎo qīng lóng tāng*) or Tingli and Jujube Lung-Draining Decoction (*tíng lì dà zǎo xiè fèi tāng*). For vacuity-repletion cold-heat complexes, use variations of Woody Fangji Decoction (*mù fáng jǐ tāng*). See PHLEGM-RHEUM. Compare PROPPING FULLNESS.

protracted tongue 舌纵 *shé zòng*: See EXTENDED TONGUE. [26: 337]

protrusion and worrying of the tongue 吐弄舌 *tǔ nòng shé*: Protrusion of the tongue is a state in which the tongue is loosely stretched and hangs out of the mouth. Worrying is when the tongue moves in a circular motion whereby the tip is extended from and retracted back into the mouth, or licks the upper and lower lips or the corners of the mouth. The combined sign is usually observed in infants and children, and is attributed to exuberant heart-spleen heat. Compare EXTENDED TONGUE. [26: 258] [27: 188] [97: 186] [6: 122]

protrusion of the umbilicus 脐突 *qí tú*: Enlargement and projection of the umbilicus in the newly born. Protrusion of the umbilicus is attributed to failure to tie the umbilical cord tightly allowing bathing water to enter. It usually requires no treatment and disappears with time. [26: 966] [27: 429] [97: 468]

protuberant bone 兑骨 *duì gǔ*, 锐骨 *ruì gǔ*: The protruding bone on the back of the wrist on the side of the little·finger. [WMC] styloid process of the ulna (processus styloideus ulnae). [27: 70] [97: 567]

proximal bleeding 近血 *jìn xuè*: Internal bleeding from a point close to the anus (i.e., in the rectum) or from the anus itself, manifesting in bright red blood in the stool or blood followed by stool. Proximal bleeding is observed in INTESTINAL WIND, HEMORRHOIDS, ANAL FISTULA, and VISCERAL TOXIN.[3] [26: 389]

pubic louse sore 阴虱疮 *yīn shī chuāng*: A papular eruption occurring in the pubic region, caused by pubic lice (identified in Western medicine as *Phthirus pubis*). The eruption consists of red or pink small itchy pimples that turn into sores when

scratched. [MED] Treat by applying Mercury and Apricot Kernel Carefree Powder (*yín xìng wú yōu sǎn*) topically. [26: 618] [27: 68] [61: 404]

pudendal itch 阴痒 *yīn yǎng*: Itching of the female external genitals or vagina; attributed either to damp-heat pouring downward or liver-kidney yin vacuity. **Damp-heat pouring downward** causes pudendal itch characterized by itching that is often severe and accompanied by a yellow pus-like vaginal discharge with a fishy smell, heart vexation, difficulty sleeping, bitter taste and slimy sensation in the mouth, bitter oppression in the chest and rib-side, frequent short voidings of urine, yellow slimy tongue fur, and a slippery stringlike pulse. In some cases, poor hygiene combines with damp-heat to nurture "invisible worms" that cause ulceration (see GENITAL EROSION). [MED] Damp-heat patterns are treated by clearing heat and disinhibiting dampness with Gentian Liver-Draining Decoction (*lóng dǎn xiè gān tāng*) plus dictamnus (*bái xiǎn pí*) and carpesium seed (*hè shī*) or with Fish Poison Yam Dampness-Percolating Decoction (*bì xiè shèn shī tāng*). Itching can be relieved by an external steam-wash of decocted Cnidium Seed Powder (*shé chuáng zǐ sǎn*), which contains cnidium seed (*shé chuáng zǐ*), zanthoxylum (*huā jiāo*), calcined alum (*kū fán*), flavescent sophora (*kǔ shēn*), and stemona (*bǎi bù*), and to which mugwort (*ài yè*) may also be added. [ACU] Base treatment on CV, SP, and LR. Main points for both patterns: CV-3 (*zhōng jí*, Central Pole), BL-34 (*xià liáo*, Lower Bone-Hole), and SP-6 (*sān yīn jiāo*, Three Yin Intersection). For damp-heat pouring downward, add SP-10 (*xuè hǎi*, Sea of Blood), SP-9 (*yīn líng quán*, Yin Mound Spring), and LR-5 (*lǐ gōu*, Woodworm Canal); needle with drainage. **Yin vacuity and blood dryness** patterns, observed in enduring disease or old age (after menopause), are characterized by itching with dryness and burning sensation that worsens at night. These patterns are associated with scant yellow or bloody vaginal discharge, tinnitus, dizziness, lumbar and leg pain, sometimes baking heat [effusion] with sweating, a red tongue with scant fur, and a fine stringlike or forceless rapid fine pulse. [WMC] This condition may occur in trichomonas vaginitis, colpomycosis, or senile vaginitis. [MED] Supplement the blood and eliminating wind. Use Tangkuei Beverage (*dāng guī yǐn*). The topical treatment given above can also be given (although it is more effective for damp-heat). [ACU] To the main points given above add KI-6 (*zhào hǎi*, Shining Sea), LR-8 (*qū quán*, Spring at the Bend), GB-20 (*fēng chí*, Wind Pool), and LR-3 (*tài chōng*, Supreme Surge), needling with supplementation. ◇ Chin 阴 *yīn*, yin (the complement of yang); 痒 *yǎng*, itch. [26: 625] [27: 454] [97: 232] [92: No. 320] [46: 596, 696] [37: 436]

puffy face 面浮 *miàn fú*: Synonym: *puffy swelling of the face and eyes*. A face affected by vacuity swelling that springs back up with the hand after being pressed. Puffy face is qi swelling caused by qi vacuity. It differs from the puffy swelling of the head and face with SLEEPING SILKWORMS BENEATH THE EYES that pit under pressure, which is a sign of water swelling due to water evil. Puffy face is attributable to lung qi vacuity or insufficiency of spleen yang. **Lung qi vacuity** gives rise to puffy face with bright white facial complexion, panting and shortness of breath, laziness to speak, rapid breathing on exertion, physical cold and fear of wind, spontaneous sweating, persistent cough, a pale tongue with thin white fur, and a vacuous pulse. [MED] Supplement the lung and boost qi. Use Ass Hide Glue Decoction (*bǔ fèi ē jiāo tāng*). **Insufficiency of spleen yang** causes a puffy face with a feeling of distention, withered-yellow facial complexion, lack of warmth in the limbs, fatigue and lack of strength, small intake of food, thin sloppy stool, emaciated flesh, pale soft tongue with dental impressions, a thin white tongue fur, and a weak vacuous pulse. [MED] Fortify the spleen, boost qi, and upbear yang. Use Center-Supplementing Qi-Boosting Decoction (*bǔ zhōng yì qì tāng*) plus aconite (*fù zǐ*) and dried ginger (*gān jiāng*). [92: No. 76]

puffy swelling 浮肿 *fú zhǒng*: Elementary Questions (*sù wèn, qì jiāo biàn dà lùn*). WATER SWELLING or vacuity puffiness. A distinction is sometimes made between swelling and puffiness, swelling being repletion and puffiness being vacuity. Puffy swelling is caused by debilitation of the visceral qi of the lung, spleen, and kidney. Lung vacuity deprives water of transformation; spleen vacuity means that water is not dammed; kidney vacuity means that water is not governed. When the spleen is affected, there is puffy swelling of the flesh; when the lung is affected, there is rapid panting. See WATER SWELLING. Consult *Jing-Yue's Complete Compendium* (*jǐng yuè quán shū*). See WATER SWELLING. Compare also VACUOUS PUFFINESS. [26: 483] [25: 264] [44: 1105] [50: 1312]

puffy swelling of the face and eyes 面目浮种 *miàn mù fú zhǒng*: PUFFY FACE.

pulling heart 心掣 *xīn chè*: HEART PALPITATIONS characterized by a pulling or contracting sensation and even pain, accompanied by shortness of breath and diarrhea. Pulling heart is usually caused by heart qi vacuity cold. [26: 94] [97: 118]

pulling pain 掣痛 *chè tòng*: Pain that is associated with a pulling sensation or pain that stretches to another location. See PAIN. [29: 190]

pulmonary 肺 *fèi*: Of, pertaining to, connected with, or affecting the lung.

pulmonary consumption 肺痨 *fèi láo*: CONSUMPTION.

pulmonary dispersion 肺消 *fèi xiāo*: LUNG DISPERSION.

pulmonary distention 肺胀 *fèi zhàng*: Synonym: *distention of the lung*. From *The Magic Pivot* (*líng shū, zhàng lùn*). Fullness in the chest due to evils settling in the lung. Pulmonary distention is accompanied by cough and panting, and pain in the supraclavicular fossa. [MED] Diffuse the lung and dispel the evil using Spleen-Effusing Decoction Plus Pinellia (*yuè bì jiā bàn xià tāng*) or Minor Green-Blue Dragon Decoction Plus Gypsum (*xiǎo qīng lóng jiā shí gāo tāng*). When there is a tendency to heat, use Supplemented White-Draining Powder (*jiā wèi xiè bái sǎn*). Where right is left vacuous after the evil has abated, use Pulse-Engendering Powder (*shēng mài sǎn*). [26: 449] [80: 121] [97: 350]

pulmonary epilepsy 肺痫 *fèi xián*: EPILEPSY in which episodes are marked by a gray-white complexion, upward staring eyes, convulsions, arched rigidity of the neck, loose open hands, open mouth and protrusion of the tongue, and utterance of a sheep-like cry; attributed to lung vacuity and damage to the liver and kidney. [27: 394]

pulmonary gan 肺疳 *fèi gān*: gan of the lung.

pulmonary impediment 肺痹 *fèi bì*: See LUNG IMPEDIMENT.

pulmonary liquid 肺津 *fèi jīn*: LUNG YIN.

pulmonary mounting 肺疝 *fèi shàn*: LUNG MOUNTING.

pulmonary welling-abscess 肺痈 *fèi yōng*: From *Essential Prescriptions of the Golden Coffer* (*jīn guì yào lüè*). A WELLING-ABSCESS (*yōng*) in the lung; arising when externally contracted wind evil and heat toxin brew and obstruct the lung, and when the heat causes congestion and blood stasis, which binds to form a welling-abscess (*yōng*) that in time starts to suppurate. The classic signs are coughing up of pus and blood. Pulmonary welling-abscess (*yōng*) is associated with heat effusion and shivering, cough, chest pain, rapid respiration, expectoration of sticky fishy-smelling purulent phlegm in severe cases producing phlegm and blood. [WMC] pulmonary abscess, bronchiectasis. [MED] Clear the lung and transform phlegm; resolve toxin and expel pus. Use Lonicera and Forsythia Powder (*yín qiào sǎn*), Tingli and Jujube Lung-Draining Decoction (*tíng lì dà zǎo xiè fèi tāng*), or Platycodon Decoction (*jié gěng tāng*) with judicious addition of houttuynia (*yú xīng cǎo*) and wild buckwheat root (*tiān qiáo mài gēn*). [26: 450] [61: 175]

pulmonary wilting 肺痿 *fèi wěi*: See LUNG WILTING.

pulse 脉 *mài*, 脉搏 *mài bó*, 脉象 *mài xiàng*: The throbbing of a blood vessel, especially one, such as at the wrist, palpated to determine the state of health of the body. Up to the Han Dynasty, the pulse was commonly taken at three positions: "Man's Prognosis" (*rén yíng*), i.e., the common carotid artery of the neck; "inch opening" (*cùn kǒu*), the radial styloid pulse on the wrist, and the "instep yang" pulse (*fū yáng*), dorsalis pedis artery. Nowadays, the first and third positions are rarely used, and the pulse palpated is that of the wrist. The wrist pulse is felt on the inner (palmar) face of the wrist, at the location described in modern anatomy as the styloid process of the radius. Anomalies of the pulse include OBLIQUE-RUNNING PULSE and PULSE ON THE BACK OF THE WRIST. The pulse is divided into three sections: inch (*cùn*), bar (*guān*), and cubit (*chǐ*), which in standard procedure are felt with the index, middle, and third fingers respectively. It is generally agreed that, on the left wrist, the inch pulse reflects the heart, the bar reflects the liver, and the cubit reflects the kidney, whereas on the right wrist, the inch reflects the lung, the bar the spleen and stomach, and the cubit the life gate. See Tables 10, 11; PULSE EXAMINATION; PULSE CONDITION. [26: 550] [27: 188]

10.	The Three Positions of the Pulse	
Position		Bowels and Viscera
Left	Inch	Heart (and pericardium), small intestine
	Bar	Liver and gallbladder
	Cubit	Kidney and bladder
Right	Inch	Lung (chest), large intestine
	Bar	Spleen and stomach
	Cubit	Kidney and life gate

11.	Correspondences of Pulse Positions to Organs in the Classics				
Position		*Nàn jīng*	*Mài jīng*	*Jīng yuè quán shū*	*Yī zōng jīn jiàn*
Inch (*cùn*)	Left	HT, SI	HT, SI	HT, PC	HT, Chest Center[1]
	Right	LU, LI	LU, LI	LU, Chest Center	LU, interior of the chest[2]
Bar (*guān*)	Left	LI, GB	LI, GB	LI, GB	LI, Diaphragm, GB
	Right	SP, ST	SP, ST	SP, ST	SP, ST
Cubit (*chǐ*)	Left	KI, BL	KI, BL	KI, BL, LI	KI, BL, SI
	Right	KI, life gate	KI, TB	KI, TB, life gate, SI	KI, LI

(1) Chest center (*dàn zhōng*): The part of the anterior chest between the nipples. (2) Interior of the chest (*xiōng zhōng*): The thoracic cavity.

pulse bereft of stomach qi 脉无胃气 *mài wú wèi qì*: A pulse lacking the regular and relaxed qualities that indicate the presence of stomach qi. A pulse that is excessively tight and hard, and that beats against the finger, a forceless vacuous, floating pulse, or a chaotic irregular pulse is a sign that the stomach qi is about to expire, and that the true qi of the wasted viscera is being exposed. If the true qi of the liver is exposed, the pulse is so tight that it feels as sharp as a knife blade. This is called *stringlike only, without stomach*. If the spleen's true qi is exposed, there are intervals between the beats of the pulse as long as between the drips from a leaky roof. This is called *intermittent only, without stomach*. See STOMACH, SPIRIT, AND ROOT, the three aspects of a healthy pulse; TRUE VISCERAL PULSE. [47: 92] [50: 1129]

pulse condition 脉象 *mài xiàng*: The form and pace of the pulsation of the vessels, especially at the wrist, as detected by palpation. **Normal pulse** (正常脉 *zhèng cháng mài*): A steady, even pulse with approximately four beats per respiration. Its significance is threefold. Its smoothness and forceful indicate the presence of spirit. It is neither sunken nor floating, and the beat arrives and departs evenly and effortlessly, indicating the presence of stomach qi. Forcefulness at the deep level indicates the presence of root. The pulse may be affected by such factors as age, sex, build, and constitution. The pulse of a child tends to be soft and rapid; that of a woman is softer and slightly faster than a man's. Obese people tend to have fine and sunken pulses, whereas thin people have large pulses; athletes have moderate pulses, and pregnant women usually have slippery, slightly rapid pulses. These variations are all within the bounds of normal health. Some people display congenital irregularities, such as a particularly narrow artery, which makes the pulse comparatively fine, or a PULSE ON THE BACK OF THE WRIST, in which the artery runs around the posterior face of the styloid process of the radius, or OBLIQUE-RUNNING PULSE, in which the pulse runs from the cubit position over the posterior face of the styloid process of the radius toward LI-4 (hé gǔ, Union Valley). These irregularities have no significance in pattern identification. **Floating pulse** (浮脉 fú mài): A pulse pronounced at the superficial level, but vacuous at the deep level, described as being "like wood floating on water." A floating pulse is felt as soon as the fingers touch the skin, but becomes markedly less perceptible when further pressure is applied. Although classically associated with exterior patterns, the floating pulse may be indistinct in patients of heavy build, with weak constitutions, or suffering from severe water swelling, even when an exterior pattern is present. A floating pulse may also occur in enduring illnesses or after a major loss of blood, indicating a severe insufficiency of right qi rather than an exterior pattern. It is said, "A floating pulse seen in enduring illness is cause for great concern." A floating pulse in these cases differs slightly from the floating pulse occurring in external disease in that it is somewhat less pronounced at the superficial level, and markedly less pronounced at the deep level, for which reason it is sometimes referred to as a vacuous floating pulse. A *dissipated pulse* (散脉 sàn mài) is a large floating pulse without root, i.e., one that is large at the superficial level but ceases to be felt as soon as the slightest pressure is applied; it is attended by other critical signs, and indicates the dissipation of qi and blood and the impending expiration of the essential qi of the organs. A *scallion-stalk pulse* (芤脉 kōu mài) is a large floating pulse that when pressure is applied feels empty in the middle; it is a sign of heavy blood loss and usually occurs in cases of major hemorrhage. **Sunken pulse** (沉脉 chén mài): A pulse that is distinct only at the deep level. A sunken pulse is associated essentially with interior patterns, although the exterior patterns of external diseases may temporarily present with a tight sunken pulse when the body's yang qi is obstructed. The *hidden pulse* (伏脉 fú mài) is even deeper than the sunken pulse and considerable pressure has to be applied in order to feel it. *The Bin-Hu Sphygmology* (bīn hú mài xué) states, "The hidden pulse is found by pressing through the sinews right to the bone." It is associated with fulminant desertion of yang qi and deep-lying cold, and generally appears in conjunction with severe vomiting, diarrhea, and pain. The *weak pulse*

(弱脉 ruò mài) is sunken and without force, and is associated with vacuity of qi and blood. The *firm pulse* (牢脉 láo mài) is sunken and forceful, and firm and unmoving, hence its name. It is associated with cold pain. In clinical practice, this term is no longer in popular use. The pulse is described as a stringlike sunken pulse or a sunken replete pulse. **Slow pulse** (迟脉 chí mài): A pulse that has three or less beats per respiration. The slow pulse is principally associated with cold and with yang vacuity. It may occur in any disease involving insufficiency of yang qi or obstruction of qi dynamic, such as cold, phlegm turbidity, and static blood. Occurring during pregnancy, this pulse signifies uterine vacuity cold or insecurity of fetal qi. The *moderate pulse* (缓脉 huǎn mài), like the slow pulse, is also slower than the standard pulse, although usually it has more than three beats per respiration, and is not an indication of morbidity. **Rapid pulse** (数脉 shuò mài): A pulse that has six beats per respiration is a rapid pulse; one having between five and six beats is termed a slightly rapid pulse. The rapid pulse is usually quite smooth-flowing, so it is often confused with a slippery pulse. However, the term "rapid" refers exclusively to the pace, whereas "slippery" denotes a quality. *The Bin-Hu Sphygmology* (bīn hú mài xué) clearly points out, "Rapid and slippery should not be considered as being the same; rapid refers to the pace only." The rapid pulse is associated with heat, but may sometimes be an indication of vacuity. A forceful rapid pulse indicates repletion heat and is most commonly seen in externally contracted heat (febrile) disease. A forceless fine rapid pulse indicates yin vacuity fire effulgence and is generally seen in depletion patterns, such as are described in Western medicine as pulmonary tuberculosis. A forceless large rapid pulse generally indicates qi vacuity. Most healthy infants have rapid pulses, and a slippery rapid pulse is a normal sign in pregnancy. A pulse with seven or more beats per respiration is known as a *racing pulse* (疾脉 jí mài). Its significance is basically the same as that of the rapid pulse, although the possibility of vacuity is greater. **Slippery pulse** (滑脉 huá mài): A smooth-flowing pulse classically described as "pearls rolling in a dish" or "small fish swimming." A slippery pulse is commonly seen in pregnancy, particularly in the early stages where extra blood is needed to nourish the fetus. It is also sometimes seen in healthy people, indicating an abundance of qi and blood. Phlegm-rheum patterns and food accumulation may also be characterized by a slippery pulse. The *stirred pulse* (动脉 dòng mài) is a forceful rapid slippery pulse, like a bean that is bobbing. It is seen in pain, fright, high fevers associated with external diseases, and in pregnancy. **Rough pulse** (涩脉 sè mài): A pulse opposite to the slippery pulse, i.e., one that does not flow smoothly and that is classically described as "a knife scraping bamboo." The rough pulse is sometimes termed a choppy or dry pulse in English. It tends to be somewhat fine, is generally slightly slower than the normal pulse, and has been described as being "fine, slow, short, dry, and beating with difficulty." The rough pulse is often seen in blood stasis patterns and dual vacuity of blood and qi. **Stringlike pulse** (弦脉 *xián mài*): A long taut pulse that feels like a the string of a musical instrument. It is sometimes called a wiry or bowstring pulse in English. The stringlike pulse is associated with diseases of the liver and gallbladder, and in particular with ascendant hyperactivity of liver yang. It is also associated with pain and with phlegm-rheum patterns. It may be commonly seen in diseases classified by Western medicine as hypertension, arteriosclerosis, chronic bronchitis, and in diseases characterized by severe pain. The stringlike pulse is generally strong; if forceless, it is termed a vacuous stringlike pulse, indicating vacuity of yin and hyperactivity of yang. A *tight pulse* (紧脉 *jǐn mài*) is a stringlike pulse that has marked forcefulness. "Stringlike" denotes a quality, whereas "tight" denotes a quality and forcefulness. A tight pulse is always stringlike, but a stringlike pulse is not necessarily tight. A tight pulse is associated with cold and pain. A *drumskin pulse* (革脉 *gé mài*) is stringlike and empty in the middle. Its significance is the same as that of the scallion-stalk pulse, the name by which it is more commonly denoted. **Soggy pulse** (濡脉 *rú mài*): A pulse that is fine, though less distinctly so than a fine pulse, and that tends to be floating. "Soggy" signifies softness and relative lack of force. The soggy pulse is associated with dual vacuity of blood and qi and with damp encumbrance. A *faint pulse* (微脉 *wēi mài*) is extremely fine and forceless, indistinct, and almost imperceptible; it indicates qi and blood vacuity desertion. The *vacuous pulse* (虚脉 *xū mài*), like the soggy pulse, is forceless, but differs as it is large rather than fine. The term is also generally used to connote forcelessness, particularly in combinations such as vacuous rapid pulse, vacuous stringlike pulse, etc. **Surging pulse** (洪脉 *hóng mài*): A broad and large pulse that is forceful at all levels, especially the superficial. The the coming of each beat is longer and more forceful than the going away, which accounts for the description, "Coming forcefully, going away feebly." It is thought of as "tempestuous billowing waves," "surging over the whole of the finger[tip]," with an initial strong swell followed by a sharp but calm ebbing away. A surging pulse indicates exuberant heat, and is usually a sign of repletion. Observed in enduring diseases (such as tuberculosis) or in vacuity patterns due to massive bleeding, it

indicates that right qi is extremely weak and that the condition is deteriorating. A *replete pulse* (实脉 *shí mài*) is similar to a surging pulse, but is as forceful when it departs as when it arrives. It indicates that the body is afflicted by an exuberant evil, but that right qi is still holding firm. A large pulse in clinical practice has roughly the same significance as the surging pulse. However, it should be noted that "large" refers only to the breadth of the blood vessel as it feels to the touch. It bears no connotations of forcefulness. **Fine pulse** (细脉 *xì mài*), sometimes call a small pulse: A pulse that feels like a well-defined thread under the fingers. The fine pulse indicates dual vacuity of qi and blood or of yin and yang, and in particular points to blood and yin vacuities. **Skipping, bound, and intermittent pulses:** The *skipping pulse*, or rapid irregularly interrupted pulse (促脉 *cù mài*), is also broken by irregular pauses, but is relatively fast. The *bound pulse*, or slow irregularly interrupted pulse (结脉 *jié mài*), is slow with pauses at irregular intervals. The *intermittent pulse*, or a regularly interrupted pulse (代脉 *dài mài*), is a pulse interspersed with more relatively regular pauses. These three are often loosely referred to by term interrupted (结代 *jié dài*) pulses. The interrupted pulses indicate debilitation of visceral qi, and in particular insufficiency of heart qi. They may also indicate blood stasis or phlegm turbidity obstructing yang qi in the chest, and can be seen in heart bi patterns. Interrupted pulses may also occur in healthy individuals and in patients suffering from emotional depression. **Long pulse** (长脉 *cháng mài*): A long pulse is one that can be felt beyond the inch and cubit positions. If runs straight from head to tail, a feels like long stick. A long pulse that is harmonious and moderate is a sign of effulgent center qi. A long, stringlike and hard pulse that feels like a rope pulled taut indicates a repletion pattern in which evil and right are both exuberant, and is seen in repletion heat binding internally or exuberant heat stirring wind. **Short pulse:** (短脉 *duǎn mài*): A pulse that is felt only at the bar point. The short pulse signifies dual vacuity of blood and qi, or impaired flow of blood and qi. See TWENTY-EIGHT PULSES; STOMACH, SPIRIT, AND ROOT; PULSE BEREFT OF STOMACH QI; SEVEN STRANGE PULSES; TEN STRANGE PULSES. [6: 137] [9: 336]

pulse examination 脉诊 *mài zhěn*: Examination of the pulsating vessel, especially that of the wrist, in order to determine the state of health. Pulse examination involves feeling with the fingertips the pulsation of the blood vessels, especially that felt on the inner face of the wrist (see PULSE). The procedure for examining the wrist pulse is as follows: **Time:** *Elementary Questions* (*sù wèn*) states, "The pulse should be taken in the CALM DAWN."

Calm dawn is the two-hour period between 3 and 5 a.m. This is the time when the body is least subject to external influences. Usually, however, it is sufficient to ensure that the patient is rested and relaxed so that external and emotional factors will distort the patient's pulse the least. The pulse should be felt for at least one or two minutes in order to ensure maximum accuracy. **Position of fingers:** The radial pulse is divided into three positions: the inch, the bar, and the cubit. The bar point is located on the anterior face of the radial styloid process. The inch point is located on its distal side, and the cubit point on its proximal side. Since the pulse is taken on both wrists, there are six positions in all, known as the six pulses. **Posture:** The patient should either be seated upright or be lying supine. The forearm should be in a horizontal position level with the heart. The palm of the hand should be facing upward, and the wrist, resting on a soft pad, is kept straight and relaxed. Incorrect posture may affect the flow of qi and blood, and thus falsify the pulse. **Normal breathing:** To ensure maximum accuracy when taking a patient's pulse, the pulse-taker's respiration should be natural and even. The mind should be fully collected and thus able to detect even the slightest changes. **Finger technique:** The physician places the index finger on the inch point. The middle and fourth fingers rest on the bar and cubit points respectively. When taking the pulse, the following considerations should be noted: (1) The spacing of the three fingers used in taking the pulse should depend on the height of the patient. For a tall patient, the fingers should be spaced apart, whereas with short patients, the fingers should be kept close together. For infants, the use of only one finger may be necessary. (2) To ensure the greatest accuracy in pulse reading, it is important to use only the very tips of the fingers, and to apply even pressure with all three fingers. (3) The practitioner should note the difference in the pulse at the various levels of pressure applied. There are three basic pressure levels: the superficial level is found by placing the fingertips lightly on the skin. The deep level is felt by pressing firmly. Between these two is the mid-level. The practitioner feels for the different levels by moving the fingers slightly across the skin and by applying different amounts of pressure. (4) Simultaneous palpation is the normal method of pulse-taking, involving the application of all three fingers at the same time. However, sometimes a clearer picture of the patient's condition can be gained by applying the fingers individually to the three positions. (5) The practitioner is said to have "found" the pulse when the pulsation is distinctly felt. The practitioner concentrates on the different aspects of the pulse. The rate is measured by counting the number of

beats to one complete respiration (one inhalation and one exhalation). The quality is judged by the thickness and length, the smoothness of the flow, and the regularity of the beat. Taking the pulse involves counting the number of beats, and identifying a form and pattern. It should be borne in mind that each of the types represents only one aspect of a given pulse. For example, floating and sunken describe the depth; slow and rapid describe the rate, whereas surging and fine describe the size of the pulse. In actual practice, these qualities occur in combinations. In most cases a patient's pulse is described with a composite term such as floating, slippery, and rapid, or sunken, stringlike, and thin. [26: 551]

pulse on the back of the wrist 反关脉 *fǎn guān mài*: A congenital anomaly in which the radial pulse is located on the posterior face of the medial styloid process. [27: 189] [27: 115] [97: 115]

pungency 辛 *xīn*: ACRIDITY.

pupil 瞳子 *tóng zǐ*, 瞳仁 *tóng rén*: The black spot in the center of the eye. Also called *water wheel.* ◇ Chin 瞳 *tóng*, composed of 目 *mù*, eye, with 童 *tóng*, child. 子 *zǐ*, noun suffix. Eng from L. *pupilla*, girl, doll, puppet. The origin of both Chinese and English names is apparently explained by the tiny image of oneself seen reflected in another's eye. [26: 940] [27: 17] [27: 65] [97: 652]

pupil spirit 瞳神 *tóng shén*: **1.** The black part of the center of the eye; the pupil. **2.** The pupil, the spirit water (aqueous humor), and spirit jelly (vitreous humor), and visual lining (retina), etc. ◇ Chin 瞳 *tóng*, pupil; 神 *shén*, spirit. [26: 941]

pure heat 瘅 *dān*: Exuberance of heat evil or heat qi. *Elementary Questions* (*sù wèn, jǔ tòng lùn*) states, "Pure heat turns into center dispersion." [26: 929] [48: 384]

pure-heat malaria 瘅疟 *dàn nüè*: **1.** MALARIA characterized by heat effusion without aversion to cold. See WARM MALARIA. **2.** MALARIA in the three yin channels. **3.** SUMMERHEAT MALARIA. [50: 1630] [26: 929] [27: 358] [97: 613]

purple and white patch wind 紫白癜风 *zǐ bái diàn fēng*: Synonym: *sweat macules.* A condition characterized by purple-brown or gray-white patches; attributed to stagnant qi and congealing blood traceable to accumulated heat in the organs and contraction of summerheat-damp (or wind-damp). Purple and white patch wind first appears as small speckles or patches, that gradually merge. The patches are clearly circumscribed and are characterized by smooth skin that bears a sheen, that may scale on scratching, and that may sometimes itch. The condition is milder in the winter than in the summer. WMC dermatomycosis microsporina (tinea versicolor, pityriasis versicolor). MED Apply Litharge Powder (*mì tuó* *sēng sǎn*) topically. [26: 723] [50: 1494] [96: 265] [27: 473] [97: 550] [61: 321]

purple menstrual flow 经来紫色 *jīng lái zǐ sè*: MENSTRUAL FLOW that is purple in color, i.e., much darker than the normal color. Purple menstrual flow is a repletion heat pattern arising when liver depression transforms into fire, which damages qi, causing qi heat that scorches the blood. MED Clear heat and regulate the menses with Four Agents Decoction (*sì wù tāng*) plus coptis (*huáng lián*) and cyperus (*xiāng fù zǐ*). [26: 815]

purple tongue 舌紫 *shé zǐ*: A purple coloration of the tongue indicates an impaired flow of blood and qi leading to congealing blood stasis. A purple tongue is observed in either heat or cold patterns. A generalized green-blue or purple coloration indicates severe blood stasis. Purple macules indicate less severe or localized blood stasis. A glossy green-blue or purple tongue characterizes cold patterns caused by failure of yang qi to warm and move the blood. A dry reddish purple tongue indicates binding blood stasis due to penetration of heat to the blood aspect. [6: 122]

pursed mouth 撮口 *cuō kǒu*: UMBILICAL WIND.

purulent ear 聤耳 *tíng ěr*: Synonym: *kidney gan*; *wind ear*. A condition characterized by the leaking of pus or pus-like yellow discharge from the ear. Purulent ear is attributed to taxation damage to qi and blood, and to evils following blood into the ear causing heat qi to gather and produce pus. WMC suppurative otitis media. A distinction is made between vacuity and repletion patterns. **Repletion** patterns are attributed to depressed liver-gallbladder fire and triple-burner damp-heat, and are characterized by pain in the ear, discharge of sticky yellow pus, green-blue facial complexion, oppression in the stomach duct and constipation, yellow tongue fur, and stringlike rapid. MED Treat with variations of Gentian Liver-Draining Decoction (*lóng dǎn xiè gān tāng*). ACU For repletion patterns, base treatment on the TB and GB. Select GB-20 (*fēng chí*, Wind Pool), TB-17 (*yì fēng*, Wind Screen), GB-2 (*tīng huì*, Auditory Convergence), TB-3 (*zhōng zhǔ*, Central Islet), GB-41 (*zú lín qì*, Foot Overlooking Tears), TB-21 (*ěr mén*, Ear Gate), TB-5 (*wài guān*, Outer Pass), and GV-14 (*dà zhuī*, Great Hammer); needle with drainage. **Vacuity** patterns are ascribed to kidney yin depletion and vacuity fire flaming upward, and are characterized by discharge of clear thin pus that continues for months. MED Enrich yin and downbear fire with formulas such as Anemarrhena, Phellodendron, and Rehmannia Pill (*zhī bǎi dì huáng wán*). In addition to oral medication, coptis (*huáng lián*) and aconite (*fù zǐ*) can be ground to a powder and insufflated into the ear after wiping the area clean of discharge. ACU For vacu-

ity patterns, base treatment on KI and TB. Select BL-23 (*shèn shū*, Kidney Transport), KI-3 (*tài xī*, Great Ravine), TB-17 (*yì fēng*, Wind Screen), and TB-3 (*zhōng zhǔ*, Central Islet); needle with supplementation. [26: 878] [46: 722]

push-cupping 推罐法 *tuī guàn fǎ*: Synonym: *slide-cupping*. A method of CUPPING whereby the cup is pushed back and forth over a wide area that has been lubricated with sesame oil, and now often petroleum jelly (Vaseline). **Method**: First, smear the area to be cupped with petroleum jelly or other lubricant, and then apply the cup in the same manner as for regular stationary cupping. Once the cup is firmly attached, hold it firmly in two hands, and move it around over the affected area. Remove the cup once the skin is evenly reddened to the desired degree. **Application**: This method is applied to large flat fleshy areas such as the back, lumbus, or thighs. It is used for IMPEDIMENT (*bì*) or other patterns of pain or numbness. See CUPPING. [26: 605] [27: 495] [97: 634]

putrefaction 腐烂 *fǔ làn*, 腐 *fǔ*: Rotting; the destruction of skin and flesh through disease that manifests in soreness and suppuration. Compare ULCERATION.

putrefying throat sand 烂喉痧 *làn hóu shā*: EPIDEMIC THROAT SAND.

putrefying throat wind 烂喉风 *làn hóu fēng*: THROAT WIND (sudden severe swelling and soreness of the throat) marked by putrefaction and ulceration. Putrefying throat wind attributed to lung-stomach heat toxin scorching the throat. The throat is swollen, sore, and ulcerated, with a gray-white or gray-yellow surface that is easily wiped off. The edge of the affected area is irregular. Other signs include foul breath, sore tongue, and alternating generalized heat [effusion] and aversion to cold. WMC Vincent's angina. MED Resolve toxin, drain heat, and disperse swelling. Use variations of Scourge-Clearing Toxin-Vanquishing Beverage (*qīng wēn bài dú yǐn*). See THROAT WIND. [26: 990]

putrid belching 嗳气腐臭 *ài qì fǔ chòu*: Synonym: *belching of putrid qi*. Belching with the expulsion of putrid sour-smelling qi (gas). Putrid belching is usually attributed to spleen-stomach vacuity or nontransformation of food due to dietary irregularities causing food to accumulate in the stomach and intestines. It is a principal sign of FOOD DAMAGE. ACU GB-40 (*qiū xū*, Hill Ruins) and GB-34 (*yáng líng quán*, Yang Mound Spring) are commonly used points. [26: 917] [27: 487] [97: 649] [46: 662] [113: 223]

putrid smell 腐臭 *fǔ chòu*: The odor characteristic of putrefaction.

putting forth oily sweat 汗出如油 *hàn chū rú yóu*: See OILY SWEAT.

Q

qi 气 *qì*: **1.** Air, gas, vapor, flatus (e.g., BELCH-ING OF PUTRID QI). **2.** Smell. **3.** Aura. **4.** Environmental forces (e.g., COLD; DAMPNESS; DRYNESS, etc.) **5.** Nature (e.g., the FOUR QI). **6.** Anything of a particular nature (e.g., YIN QI). **7.** Breath. (e.g., SHORTAGE OF QI and QI SHORTAGE). **8.** Any of various dynamic phenomena of the body (e.g., SOURCE QI; CONSTRUCTION QI; DEFENSE QI; BOWEL AND VISCERAL QI; CHANNEL QI) that are described in terms of the following functions: **8a.** Activity: Qi is highly active; human growth and development, as well as all physiological activity and metabolism, are manifestations of the activity of qi. **8b.** Warming: The temperature of the human body and the ability of the organs and tissues to perform their functional activities are dependent on the warming action of qi. **8c.** Defense: Qi is the outer defense of the body, and prevents evils from entering. **8d.** Transformation: Production of blood and fluids, the distribution of fluids, and the conversion of fluids into sweat and urine are all the result of qi transformation. Implicit in this notion is the movement, or bearing, of qi. Qi bears upward, downward, inward and outward, carrying blood and fluids with it. Combinations of these four movements explain all movement in the body. See QI TRANSFORMATION. **8e.** Containment: Under normal circumstances, spillage of blood from the vessels is prevented by the containing function of qi. Hence it is said, "Qi contains the blood." This function also prevents excessive loss of fluids through oversecretion of sweat and other fluids or excessive urination. **9.** Strength. **10.** Anger. **11.** Disease (e.g., LEG QI, MOUNTING QI), PLUM-PIT QI. **12.** An abbreviation for diseases of qi (qi vacuity, qi stagnation), as appearing in the terms QI BLOCK, QI CONSTIPATION, QI FETUS, QI TUMOR, QI COUGH, QI ACCUMULATION, QI VOMITING. ◇ Chin 气 *qì*, air, gas, vapor, smell, force; pronounced "chee" as in "cheese," transcribed in Wade-Giles as *ch'i*, and sometimes written as "ki" and pronounced as the English "key" in the Japanese tradition. [6: 37] [27: 78] [97: 89]

Qi 齐 *qí*: The name of a dynasty (A.D. 479–502).

qi absorption 纳气 *nà qì*: See KIDNEY GOVERNS QI ABSORPTION.

qi absorption failure 肾不纳气 *shèn bù nà qì*: KIDNEY FAILING TO ABSORB QI.

qi accumulation 气积 *qì jī*: An accumulation attributed to disharmony of qi dynamic stemming from anxiety, thought, depression, or anger. Qi accumulation is characterized by oppression in the chest, belching, and rib-side and abdominal distention. Sometimes there is the intermittent appearance of a lump and distending pain of unfixed location. ⟨MED⟩ Course the liver and rectify qi using Major Seven Qi Decoction (*dà qī qì tāng*) or Counterflow Cold Powder (*sì nì sǎn*) plus cyperus (*xiāng fù zǐ*), curcuma (*yù jīn*), unripe tangerine peel (*qīng pí*), and tangerine peel (*chén pí*). ⟨ACU⟩ Base treatment mainly on LR, PC, GB, CV, and back transport points. Select LR-3 (*tài chōng*, Supreme Surge), PC-6 (*nèi guān*, Inner Pass), GB-34 (*yáng líng quán*, Yang Mound Spring), CV-6 (*qì hǎi*, Sea of Qi), CV-17 (*shān zhōng*, Chest Center), BL-18 (*gān shū*, Liver Transport), BL-17 (*gé shū*, Diaphragm Transport), TB-6 (*zhī gōu*, Branch Ditch), and LI-4 (*hé gǔ*, Union Valley); needle with drainage. See ACCUMULATION. [26: 545] [46: 594]

qian 钱 *qián*: Synonym: *mace*. A unit of measure equal to the tenth part of a LIANG, and now roughly equal to 500 g. See tables 21 and 23, page 717.

qi and blood both ablaze 气血两燔 *qì xuè liǎng fán*: Synonym: *blazing of both qi and blood*. Pronounced heat in the construction and blood aspects occurring before heat has been eliminated from the qi aspect in warm heat disease. Signs of qi and blood both ablaze include vigorous heat effusion, thirst, vexation and agitation, delirious raving, maculopapular eruptions, crimson tongue with yellow fur, and a rapid fine pulse, and, in severe cases, blood ejection or spontaneous external bleeding. [26: 537]

qi and construction both ablaze 气营两燔 *qì yíng liǎng fán*: Synonyms: *blazing of both qi and construction*; *dual disease of qi and construction*. Exuberant heat in both the qi aspect and construction aspect in warm heat disease. Blazing of both qi and construction is characterized by vigorous heat [effusion], vexation and thirst, clouded spirit, and faintly visible macules or papules, and crimson tongue with dry yellow fur. [26: 546] [27: 134] [97: 97]

qi and flavor 气味 *qì wèi*: Qi is the hot, cold, warm, or cool nature of a medicinal; flavor is the taste a medicinal produces in the mouth. See FOUR QI; FIVE FLAVORS.

qi ascent 上气 *shàng qì*: Rapid breathing characterized by more exhalation than inhalation and attributed to inhibited lung qi. Distinction is made between vacuity and repletion. Repletion patterns are caused by phlegm-rheum obstructing the lung or external evils assailing the lung. Phlegm-rheum obstructing the lung is characterized by rapid breathing with coughing of copious thick white phlegm, phlegm rale in the throat, relief felt on exhalation, and inability to lie flat. Qi ascent caused by external evils assailing the lung is characterized by distressed rapid breathing, cough and panting with copious phlegm, aversion to cold and heat effusion, and, in severe cases, by puffy swelling of the face and eyes. Vacuity patterns are usually attributable to effulgent yin vacuity fire in which qi ascent is accompanied by cough without phlegm, scant phlegm that is not easily expectorated, short distressed breathing, generalized heat [effusion], night sweating, and vexing heat in the five hearts. [29: 165] [26: 59] [27: 384] [97: 28]

qi aspect 气分 *qì fèn*: DEFENSE, QI, CONSTRUCTION, AND BLOOD.

qi-aspect damp obstruction 湿阻气分 *shī zǔ qì fèn*: DAMPNESS OBSTRUCTING THE QI ASPECT.

qi-aspect pattern 气分证 *qì fèn zhèng*: Any warm disease pattern of heat effusion, aversion to heat rather than cold, thirst, bitter taste in the mouth, and yellow or reddish urine, a rapid pulse, and a yellow or yellow and white tongue fur. Qi-aspect disease is broad in scope, including a large variety of exuberant heat effusion stage externally contracted febrile diseases. These may be divided as follows: (1) INITIAL-STAGE QI-ASPECT HEAT characterized by generalized heat EFFUSION, thirst, heart vexation, burning sensation in the heart [region], and mixed yellow and white tongue fur. (2) EXUBERANT LUNG-STOMACH HEAT characterized by the classical signs of wind warmth: high fever, cough, rapid breathing, thirst, and yellow tongue fur. (3) GREAT HEAT IN THE QI ASPECT: Equivalent to yang brightness (*yáng míng*) channel disease. (4) GASTROINTESTINAL HEAT BIND: Equivalent to the yang brightness bowel pattern. (5) DAMP-HEAT LODGED IN THE TRIPLE BURNER characterized by the classical signs of damp warmth: persistent remittent heat effusion, oppression in the chest, thirst without great intake of fluids, upflow nausea, abdominal distention, short voidings of scant urine, a slimy tongue fur that is either white or slightly yellow in color, and soggy rapid pulse. Also observable at this stage is brewing damp-heat steaming the stomach and intestines, characterized either by oppression in the chest and hard stool or by foul-smelling diarrhea, a slimy yellow tongue fur, and a slippery rapid pulse. These five patterns show marked differences between WIND WARMTH and DAMP WARMTH in the qi aspect. Wind warmth may take the form of initial-stage qi-aspect heat, great heat in the qi aspect, gastrointestinal heat bind, or exuberant heat in the lung and stomach. This latter pattern is characterized by four main signs of exuberant heat: heat effusion, thirst, cough, and panting. Damp warmth presents differently. It is marked by unsurfaced heat and steaming of the stomach by brewing damp-heat. It develops slowly over a relatively long period of time. [6: 233]

qi bar 气关 *qì guān*: One of the THREE BARS OF THE FINGER. See INFANT'S FINGER EXAMINATION. [26: 546] [27: 177] [97: 90]

qi bind abdominal pain 气结腹痛 *qì jié fù tòng*: QI STAGNATION ABDOMINAL PAIN.

qi block 气闭 *qì bì*: **1.** DRIBBLING URINARY BLOCK due to qi vacuity or qi stagnation. **2.** Blockage and derangement of qi dynamic due to congestion of wind, phlegm, fire, or stasis evil and manifesting in signs such as coma, clenched jaw, clenched fists, and urinary and fecal stoppage. [57: 14] [116: 166] [72: 19] [50: 272]

qi block deafness 气闭耳聋 *qì bì ěr lóng*: DEAFNESS due to blockage of qi. Counterflow ascent of qi due to anger causing qi to congest in the upper body and block the ear orifices. Deafness due to contraction of external wind with headache is treated with Ledebouriella Sage-Inspired Powder (*fáng fēng tōng shèng sǎn*). Deafness due to stirring yin vacuity fire can be treated with Anemarrhena and Phellodendron Eight-Ingredient Pill (*zhī bǎi bā wèi wán*) plus polygala (*yuǎn zhì*), and acorus (*shí chāng pú*). Deafness due to great noise, shouting, or fright can be treated with Gallbladder-Clearing Decoction (*qīng dǎn tāng*) [57: 14] [116: 166]

qi-blood 气血 *qì xuè*: Qi and blood.

qi-blood pattern identification 气血辨证 *qì xuè biàn zhèng*: See QI, BLOOD, PHLEGM, AND FOOD PATTERN IDENTIFICATION. [26: 537]

qi, blood, phlegm, and food pattern identification 气血痰食辨证 *qì xuè tán shí biàn zhèng*: The process of identifying disease patterns of qi, blood, phlegm(-rheum) and food. Qi patterns include QI VACUITY, QI STAGNATION, QI COUNTERFLOW, and QI REVERSAL. Blood patterns include QI VACUITY, BLOOD STASIS, BLEEDING, and BLOOD REVERSAL. Phlegm (and rheum) patterns are patterns caused by phlegm (thick fluid) and rheum (thin fluid); see PHLEGM-RHEUM. Food patterns include FOOD DAMAGE, FOOD ACCUMULATION, LODGED FOOD, and FOOD REVERSAL. [26: 537] [6: 161] [27: 226] [97: 96]

qi-blood vacuity menstrual pain 气血虚弱痛经 *qì xuè xū ruò tòng jīng*: Continual unabating pain in the smaller abdomen when insufficiency of qi and blood has been exacerbated by menstruation. The pain likes warmth and pressure and the menstrual flow is scant, thin, and pale. MED Supplement qi and nourish the blood; support the spleen and relieve pain. Use Tangkuei Center-Fortifying Decoction (*dāng guī jiàn zhōng tāng*) or brown sugar steamed with fresh ginger. ACU Base treatment mainly on CV, back transport points, SP, and ST. Select CV-4 (*guān yuán*, Pass Head), CV-6 (*qì hǎi*, Sea of Qi), BL-23 (*shèn shū*, Kidney Transport), BL-20 (*pí shū*, Spleen Transport), ST-36 (*zú sān lǐ*, Leg Three Li), SP-6 (*sān yīn jiāo*, Three Yin Intersection), and LR-3 (*tài chōng*, Supreme Surge); needle with supplementation and add moxa. [26: 537] [27: 518] [97: 281] [113: 281]

Qi Bo and the Yellow Emperor 岐黄 *qí huáng*: The interlocutors of *The Yellow Emperor's Inner Canon* (*huáng dì nèi jīng*).

qi constipation 气秘 *qì bì*: Constipation attributed to either qi stagnation or qi vacuity. **Qi stagnation:** Qi stagnation constipation is constipation arising as a result of binding depression of the seven affects and is characterized by fullness in the stomach duct and abdomen, stabbing pain in the chest and rib-side, belching, and the desire but inability to defecate. MED Normalize qi and moisten the intestines using Four Milled Ingredients Decoction (*sì mò tāng*) or, in the elderly, with Tangerine Peel and Apricot Kernel Pill (*jú xìng wán*). Constipation attributed to impaired downbearing of lung qi is treated with Perilla Seed Qi-Downbearing Decoction (*sū zǐ jiàng qì tāng*) plus bitter orange (*zhǐ ké*). ACU Base treatment mainly on alarm, back transport, and lower uniting points of LI, and on CV and LR. Main points: BL-25 (*dà cháng shū*, Large Intestine Transport), ST-25 (*tiān shū*, Celestial Pivot), and ST-37 (*shàng jù xū*, Upper Great Hollow). For qi stagnation, add TB-6 (*zhī gōu*, Branch Ditch), CV-12 (*zhōng wǎn*, Center Stomach Duct), CV-6 (*qì hǎi*, Sea of Qi), PC-6 (*nèi guān*, Inner Pass), LR-3 (*tài chōng*, Supreme Surge), LR-2 (*xíng jiān*, Moving Between), and needle with even supplementation and drainage. For impaired downbearing of lung qi, add BL-13 (*fèi shū*, Lung Transport), LU-9 (*tài yuān*, Great Abyss), SP-3 (*tài bái*, Supreme White), and LI-4 (*hé gǔ*, Union Valley); needle with drainage. **Qi vacuity:** Constipation due to qi vacuity is attended by lassitude of spirit, laziness to speak, pale tongue, and a weak pulse. MED Boost qi and moisten the intestines with Astragalus Decoction (*huáng qí tāng*) or Clematis Pill (*wēi líng xiān wán*). ACU To the main points given above add CV-12 (*zhōng wǎn*, Center Stomach Duct), BL-21 (*wèi shū*, Stomach Trans-

port), BL-20 (*pí shū*, Spleen Transport), CV-4 (*guān yuán*, Pass Head), TB-6 (*zhī gōu*, Branch Ditch), and CV-17 (*shān zhōng*, Chest Center); needle with supplementation. [26: 539] [97: 92] [113: 102] [37: 327] [46: 670]

qi cough 气嗽 *qì sòu*: **1.** Cough with inhibited qi dynamic and fullness and oppression in the chest and diaphragm, attributed to lung vacuity and congestion of evil qi. MED Diffuse the lung and transform phlegm; support right and dispel the evil. Use formulas such as Schisandra Powder (*wǔ wèi zǐ sǎn*). ACU Base treatment mainly on LU, CV, PC, LI, and ST. Supplement BL-13 (*fèi shū*, Lung Transport), LU-7 (*liè quē*, Broken Sequence), LU-9 (*tài yuān*, Great Abyss), and SP-3 (*tài bái*, Supreme White); drain CV-22 (*tiān tú*, Celestial Chimney), CV-17 (*shān zhōng*, Chest Center), PC-6 (*nèi guān*, Inner Pass), LI-4 (*hé gǔ*, Union Valley), ST-40 (*fēng lóng*, Bountiful Bulge), and ST-36 (*zú sān lǐ*, Leg Three Li). **2.** Cough attributed to internal damage by the seven affects, characterized by cough and rapid breathing, thick sticky phlegm that may be like rotten threads, a feeling of something stuck in the throat that can be neither brought up nor swallowed, and a rapid slippery surging floating pulse. MED Transform phlegm and resolve depression with formulas such as Perilla Fruit Qi-Downbearing Decoction (*sū zǐ jiàng qì tāng*). ACU Base treatment mainly on LU, CV, PC, LR, SP, and ST. Select BL-13 (*fèi shū*, Lung Transport), LU-7 (*liè quē*, Broken Sequence), CV-22 (*tiān tú*, Celestial Chimney), PC-6 (*nèi guān*, Inner Pass), LR-3 (*tài chōng*, Supreme Surge), SP-6 (*sān yīn jiāo*, Three Yin Intersection), LI-4 (*hé gǔ*, Union Valley), ST-40 (*fēng lóng*, Bountiful Bulge), and BL-18 (*gān shū*, Liver Transport); needle with drainage. [26: 545]

qi counterflow 气逆 *qì nì*: A REVERSAL of the normal bearing of qi. The qi of the lung and stomach normally flows downward. When lung qi runs counterflow, there is hasty breathing and cough; when stomach qi flows counterflow, there is vomiting and hiccough, etc. Liver qi normally bears upward and effuses. However, when depressed anger damages the liver, then upbearing and effusion become excessive or liver fire ascends counterflow, causing headache, dizziness, clouding collapse, or blood ejection. See COUNTERFLOW; LIVER QI ASCENDING COUNTERFLOW; STOMACH QI ASCENDING COUNTERFLOW. [26: 539] [27: 143] [97: 92]

qi cultivation 气功 *qì gōng*: Synonym: *qi-gong*. Exercises consisting in controlling respiration and calming the mind and having the ultimate goal of improving physical health, mental alertness, and preventing and treating disease. Nowadays, a broad distinction is made between quiescent qi cultivation 静功 *jìng gōng*) and active qi cultivation

(动功 *dòng gōng*). Quiescent qi cultivation consists in breathing exercises in lying, sitting, or standing posture aimed at regulating and containing true qi. Active qi cultivation consists in gentle rhythmical movements and self massage. [26: 536]

qi depression 气郁 *qì yù*: One of the SIX DEPRESSIONS. Qi stagnation arising when affect-mind binding depression causes binding depression of liver qi. See BINDING DEPRESSION OF LIVER QI. [26: 546]

qi depression dizziness 气郁眩晕 *qì yù xuàn yūn*: DIZZINESS due to qi depression. Qi depression dizziness arises when binding depression of the seven affects causes qi depression which in turn engenders phlegm. Accompanying signs include mental depression, heart palpitations or fearful throbbing, periodic heat effusion, and eyebrow pain. [MED] Quiet the spirit and transform phlegm using formulas like Jade Flask Pill (*yù hú wán*). [ACU] Base treatment mainly on LR, PC, SP, GB, and ST. Select GB-20 (*fēng chí*, Wind Pool), Greater Yang (*tài yáng*), GV-23 (*shàng xīng*, Upper Star), LR-3 (*tài chōng*, Supreme Surge), PC-6 (*nèi guān*, Inner Pass), SP-6 (*sān yīn jiāo*, Three Yin Intersection), TB-6 (*zhī gōu*, Branch Ditch), ST-40 (*fēng lóng*, Bountiful Bulge), and HT-7 (*shén mén*, Spirit Gate), and needle with drainage. See DIZZINESS. [26: 546] [113: 19, 166] [46: 688]

qi depression flooding 气郁血崩 *qì yù xuè bēng*: FLOODING (profuse abnormal discharge of blood via the vagina) attributable to qi depression, occurring when sudden anger damages the liver and upsets its function of storing the blood, causing blood to move chaotically and the thoroughfare and controlling vessels to fall into imbalance. Qi depression flooding is characterized by sudden copious discharge of purple clotted blood, by vexation, agitation, and irascibility, and by rib-side discomfort. [MED] Treat the tip by stanching bleeding with Thoroughfare-Securing Decoction (*gù chōng tāng*). When bleeding has been reduced, Free Wanderer Powder (*xiāo yáo sǎn*) plus stir-fried cyperus (*xiāng fù zǐ*) and unripe tangerine peel (*qīng pí*) can be prescribed to course the liver and resolve depression. Alternatively, stir-fried cyperus (*xiāng fù zǐ*) ground to a powder can be taken in doses of 10 g at a time with water in which rice has been cooked. [ACU] Base treatment mainly on CV, SP, LR, and PC. Select CV-6 (*qì hǎi*, Sea of Qi), SP-6 (*sān yīn jiāo*, Three Yin Intersection), SP-1 (*yǐn bái*, Hidden White), LR-3 (*tài chōng*, Supreme Surge), PC-6 (*nèi guān*, Inner Pass), TB-6 (*zhī gōu*, Branch Ditch), and LR-1 (*dà dūn*, Large Pile). Needle with drainage. [26: 546] [46: 688] [37: 426]

qi depression rib-side pain 气郁胁痛 *qì yù xié tòng*: Pain in the rib-side due to binding depres-

sion of liver qi. See BINDING DEPRESSION OF LIVER QI. [26: 546]

qi depression stomach duct pain 气郁脘痛 *qì yù wǎn tòng*: Synonym: *liver-stomach qi pain*. Stomach pain resulting from affect-mind binding depression (mental or emotional imbalance) and liver qi invading the stomach. The pain is not confined to a fixed location, is relieved by pressure, and is often accompanied by pain in both rib-sides. Other signs include frequent belching, clamoring stomach, or vomiting of sour fluid. [MED] Course the liver and rectify qi. Use Bupleurum Liver-Coursing Powder (*chái hú shū gān sǎn*), Aquilaria Qi-Downbearing Decoction (*chén xiāng jiàng qì tāng*), or Toosendan Powder (*jīn líng zǐ sǎn*). For vomiting of acid fluid, Left-Running Metal Pill (*zuǒ jīn wán*), ark shell (*wǎ léng zǐ*), and cuttlefish bone (*hǎi piāo xiāo*) can be added. [ACU] Base treatment mainly on alarm and uniting points of ST, PC, LR, and SP. Select CV-12 (*zhōng wǎn*, Center Stomach Duct), ST-36 (*zú sān lǐ*, Leg Three Li), PC-6 (*nèi guān*, Inner Pass), SP-4 (*gōng sūn*, Yellow Emperor), LR-3 (*tài chōng*, Supreme Surge), BL-18 (*gān shū*, Liver Transport) LR-14 (*qī mén*, Cycle Gate), GB-34 (*yáng líng quán*, Yang Mound Spring), and SP-6 (*sān yīn jiāo*, Three Yin Intersection); needle with drainage. For pronounced qi stagnation, add CV-17 (*shān zhōng*, Chest Center). See LIVER-STOMACH QI PAIN. Compare STOMACH QI PAIN. [26: 547] [50: 280] [46: 660] [113: 216]

qi deserting with the blood 气随血脱 *qì suí xuè tuō*: Synonym: *blood desertion with qi desertion*. QI DESERTION developing as a result of heavy blood loss. Blood is the mother of qi, i.e., original qi requires the nourishing action of the blood in order to perform its functions. When heavy blood loss (BLOOD DESERTION) in severe cases deprives original qi of its support, qi also deserts. This condition may be characterized by a bright white or somber white complexion, a rapid pulse that is feeble at the deep level, or a great dripping sweat, and a faint pulse on the verge of expiration. [WMC] hemorrhagic shock. [MED] Treat by boosting qi to stem desertion, which is based on the principle that the first priority in blood desertion is to boost qi. Use formulas such as Pure Ginseng Decoction (*dú shēn tāng*), which both checks vacuity desertion and, by containing the bleed, helps to stanch bleeding. [ACU] Base treatment on GV and CV. For emergency treatment to revive the patient, needle GV-26 (*shuǐ gōu*, Water Trough), GV-20 (*bǎi huì*, Hundred Convergences), CV-4 (*guān yuán*, Pass Head), GV-25 (*sù liáo*, White Bone-Hole), and KI-1 (*yǒng quán*, Gushing Spring), needling with supplementation and moxa. Then needle SP-1 (*yǐn bái*, Hidden White), CV-6 (*qì hǎi*, Sea of Qi), ST-36 (*zú sān lǐ*, Leg Three

Li), CV-4 (*guān yuán*, Pass Head), GV-20 (*bǎi huì*, Hundred Convergences), and SP-6 (*sān yīn jiāo*, Three Yin Intersection), applying moxibustion to supplement qi and contain the blood. See BLOOD DESERTION. [26: 282] [27: 144]

qi desertion 气脱 *qì tuō*: Damage to and loss of. Excessive sweating, excessive precipitation, loss of semen, and blood collapse can deprive qi of support and containment so that qi deserts outward. *The Magic Pivot* (*líng shū*) states, "In the case of qi desertion, the eyes are not clear." In addition to unclear vision arising when the eyes are deprived of nourishment, other signs include low faint breathing, bright white facial complexion, weak faint pulse, dripping cold sweat, and clouding with failure to recognize people. [50: 276]

qi diarrhea 气泻 *qì xiè*, 气泄 *qì xiè*: Diarrhea attributed to qi depression, usually arising when depression and anger cause depressed liver qi to invade the spleen. Qi diarrhea is attended by glomus and oppression in the chest and diaphragm, rumbling intestines, and abdominal pain relieved temporarily by defecation and exacerbated by annoyance and anger. MED Course the liver and rectify qi; harmonize the liver and spleen. Use Major Seven Qi Decoction (*dà qī qì tāng*) or Pain and Diarrhea Formula (*tòng xiè yào fāng*). ACU Base treatment on PC, LR, CV, ST, and SP. Select PC-6 (*nèi guān*, Inner Pass), LR-3 (*tài chōng*, Supreme Surge), SP-6 (*sān yīn jiāo*, Three Yin Intersection), BL-18 (*gān shū*, Liver Transport), LR-14 (*qī mén*, Cycle Gate), CV-12 (*zhōng wǎn*, Center Stomach Duct), LR-13 (*zhāng mén*, Camphorwood Gate), ST-25 (*tiān shū*, Celestial Pivot), and ST-36 (*zú sān lǐ*, Leg Three Li); needle with even supplementation and drainage. [26: 546]

qi disease pattern 气病证候 *qì bìng zhèng hòu*: Any disease of qi, i.e., QI VACUITY, QI FALL, QI STAGNATION, QI COUNTERFLOW, or QI BLOCK. MED Qi vacuity and qi fall are treated by supplementing (sometimes called boosting) qi; qi stagnation and qi counterflow are treated by rectifying qi. [36: 266]

Qi Disease Patterns

QI VACUITY (*qì xū*)

QI FALL (*qì xiàn*)

QI STAGNATION (*qì zhì*)

QI COUNTERFLOW (*qì nì*)

QI BLOCK (*qì bì*)

qi distention 气胀 *qì zhàng*: **1.** Distention arising from congestion of the pathways of qi as a result of affect-mind binding depression and characterized by abdominal fullness and distention, emaciated limbs, and reduced food intake. MED Course the

liver and rectify qi. Use Bupleurum Liver-Coursing Powder (*chái hú shū gān sǎn*) plus barley sprout (*mài yá*). ACU Base treatment mainly on ST, SP, LR, and back transport points. Select ST-25 (*tiān shū*, Celestial Pivot), CV-6 (*qì hǎi*, Sea of Qi), PC-6 (*nèi guān*, Inner Pass), ST-36 (*zú sān lǐ*, Leg Three Li), BL-18 (*gān shū*, Liver Transport), LR-3 (*tài chōng*, Supreme Surge), SP-6 (*sān yīn jiāo*, Three Yin Intersection), and KI-13 (*qì xué*, Qi Point); needle with drainage. **2.** *Synonym: drum distention*. Abdominal distention and fullness that is empty. [26: 543] [27: 414] [97: 91] [46: 602, 646]

qi drum 气鼓 *qì gǔ*: *Synonym: qi drum distention*. DRUM DISTENTION (pronounced abdominal distention) caused by qi stagnation. The abdomen is distended and its skin is taught. Tapping produces an empty sound. In severe cases, the abdomen is greatly enlarged with prominent green-blue veins (caput medusae), generalized swelling, and somber yellow skin. MED Fortify the spleen and move qi. ACU Two groups of points can be used: (1) CV-12 (*zhōng wǎn*, Center Stomach Duct), ST-25 (*tiān shū*, Celestial Pivot), ST-36 (*zú sān lǐ*, Leg Three Li), BL-18 (*gān shū*, Liver Transport), LR-13 (*zhāng mén*, Camphorwood Gate), and LR-14 (*qī mén*, Cycle Gate). (2) SP-15 (*dà hèng*, Great Horizontal), CV-6 (*qì hǎi*, Sea of Qi), SP-6 (*sān yīn jiāo*, Three Yin Intersection), BL-18 (*gān shū*, Liver Transport), LR-13 (*zhāng mén*, Camphorwood Gate), and LR-14 (*qī mén*, Cycle Gate). Needle with drainage in treatments every 3–5 days. Alternate the groups, and moxa CV-12 (*zhōng wǎn*, Center Stomach Duct), CV-4 (*guān yuán*, Pass Head), and bilateral SP-15 (*dà hèng*, Great Horizontal) for 30–60 minutes each time after needling. [26: 543] [27: 413] [97: 94]

qi drum distention 气臌 *qì gǔ*: QI DRUM.

qi dynamic 气机 *qì jī*: The activity, particularly the movement, of qi. See QI. [26: 545] [27: 81] [97: 93]

qi dysentery 气痢 *qì lì*: **1.** Dysentery attributed to qi vacuity and characterized by efflux desertion and discharge of stool with flatus. MED Stem desertion with warm astringent medicinals. Use Chebule Powder (*hē lí lè sǎn*). **2.** Dysentery attributed to qi stagnation. MED Six Milled Ingredients Decoction (*liù mò tāng*). [26: 542]

qi failing to contain the blood 气不摄血 *qì bù shè xuè*: Qi failing to ensure that blood flows within the vessels, giving rise to blood loss. Qi failing to contain the blood is usually related to enduring illness damaging the spleen and giving rise to insufficiency of center qi. When there is qi vacuity fall, blood flows down with the qi (this is often called BLOOD FALLING WITH QI), giving rise to BLOODY STOOL, BLOODY URINE, or FLOODING AND SPOTTING. In addition, vacuous qi failing to control the blood can allow blood to leave its regular channels, spill out of the vessels, and seep out through the interstices, giving rise to subcutaneous hemorrhage or purple macules. [36: 270]

qi fall 气陷 *qì xiàn*: CENTER QI FALL.

qi fall diarrhea 气陷泄泻 *qì xiàn xiè xiè*: Diarrhea due to qi vacuity fall. Qi fall diarrhea is characterized by diarrhea immediately after eating with non-transformation of food, decreased food intake, emaciation, fatigue, prolapse of the rectum, and spontaneous sweating. MED Use Sweet Relief Decoction (*gān huǎn tāng*). If great diarrhea leads to qi desertion and loss of consciousness, use large amounts of of ginseng (*rén shēn*) and aconite (*fù zǐ*) to warm and supplement. See VACUITY DIARRHEA; SPLEEN VACUITY DIARRHEA. [50: 281]

qi fetus 气胎 *qì tāi*: Phantom pregnancy characterized by absence of the menses and enlargement of the abdomen arising when agitation and anger cause binding depression of liver qi, and consequent stagnation of the controlling (*rèn*), thoroughfare (*chōng*), and uterine vessels. MED Use Free Wanderer Powder (*xiāo yáo sǎn*) with the addition of saussurea (*mù xiāng*), cyperus (*xiāng fù zǐ*), and ligusticum (*chuān xiōng*). [26: 538]

qi gan 气疳 *qì gān*: GAN OF THE LUNG. [26: 539]

qi gate 气门 *qì mén*: The pores of the skin through which sweat flows and through which yang qi is discharged. See LUNG GOVERNS THE SKIN AND [BODY] HAIR. [97: 90]

qi glomus 气痞 *qì pǐ*: GLOMUS attributed to qi stagnation. [26: 542] [97: 93]

qi goiter 气瘿 *qì yǐng*: A goiter that is soft to the touch and of normal skin color and that swells and shrinks with the patient's moods. Qi goiter is attributed to emotional depression or environmental factors. WMC endemic goiter. MED Rectify qi and resolve depression; transform phlegm and soften hardness; fortify the spleen and eliminate dampness. Use Four Seas Depression-Soothing Pill (*sì hǎi shū yù wán*) or Sargassum Jade Flask Decoction (*hǎi zǎo yù hú tāng*). ACU Base treatment mainly on TB, ST, LI, GB, and empirical points. Select TB-13 (*nào huì*, Upper Arm Convergence), LI-4 (*hé gǔ*, Union Valley), ST-36 (*zú sān lǐ*, Leg Three Li), GB-34 (*yáng líng quán*, Yang Mound Spring), CV-22 (*tiān tú*, Celestial Chimney), LI-17 (*tiān dǐng*, Celestial Tripod), and SI-17 (*tiān róng*, Celestial Countenance); needle with even supplementation and drainage. For thyroid enlargement, add Qi Goiter (*qì yǐng*) and the paravertebrals of the neck (3-5). [26: 546] [27: 134] [97: 97] [113: 387] [37: 466]

qi-gong 气功 *qì gōng*: QI CULTIVATION.

qi hemorrhoids 气痔 *qì zhì*: HEMORRHOIDS attributed to qi stagnation in the triple burner stemming from wind-cold and anxiety, thought, depres-

sion, and anger. Qi hemorrhoid patterns occur in episodes associated with emotional difficulties and are characterized by abdominal and rib-side fullness and distention, painful swollen anus, difficult defecation, bloody stool, and in some cases prolapse of the rectum. MED Resolve depression and dissipate the evil using Cyperus and Perilla Powder (*xiāng sū sǎn*). ACU Base treatment mainly on BL, PC, TB, LR, and SP. Select BL-32 (*cì liáo*, Second Bone-Hole), GV-1 (*cháng qiáng*, Long Strong), BL-57 (*chéng shān*, Mountain Support), TB-6 (*zhī gōu*, Branch Ditch), TB-5 (*wài guān*, Outer Pass), LR-3 (*tài chōng*, Supreme Surge), PC-6 (*nèi guān*, Inner Pass), and SP-6 (*sān yīn jiāo*, Three Yin Intersection); needle with drainage or with even supplementation and drainage. Selection of points according to signs: For abdominal fullness and distention, add ST-25 (*tiān shū*, Celestial Pivot), CV-6 (*qì hǎi*, Sea of Qi), and ST-36 (*zú sān lǐ*, Leg Three Li). For rib-side fullness and distention, add LR-14 (*qī mén*, Cycle Gate), GB-34 (*yáng líng quán*, Yang Mound Spring), and GB-24 (*rì yuè*, Sun and Moon). For painful swollen anus, add BL-54 (*zhì biān*, Sequential Limit), and BL-58 (*fēi yáng*, Taking Flight). For difficult defecation, add CV-12 (*zhōng wǎn*, Center Stomach Duct), CV-6 (*qì hǎi*, Sea of Qi), and LR-2 (*xíng jiān*, Moving Between). For prolapse of the rectum, add GV-20 (*bǎi huì*, Hundred Convergences), and BL-25 (*dà cháng shū*, Large Intestine Transport). [26: 539] [46: 670, 714] [37: 324, 458]

qi hiccough 气呃 *qì è*: Hiccough attributed to depressed qi dynamic or qi vacuity. **Center qi vacuity:** See VACUITY HICCOUGH. **Yang qi verging on expiration:** See VACUITY HICCOUGH. **Qi stagnation:** Hiccough due to qi stagnation is characterized by continuous hiccough. It is associated with distention and oppression in the chest and rib-side, depression and anger, a thin tongue fur, and a stringlike pulse. MED Regulate qi and resolve depression. Use Saussurea Qi-Regulating Powder (*mù xiāng tiáo qì sǎn*) or Qi Depression Decoction (*qì yù tāng*). ACU Base treatment mainly on ST, LR, and PC. Main points: Select BL-17 (*gé shū*, Diaphragm Transport), CV-17 (*shān zhōng*, Chest Center), PC-6 (*nèi guān*, Inner Pass), ST-36 (*zú sān lǐ*, Leg Three Li), and LR-3 (*tài chōng*, Supreme Surge). For qi stagnation, add LR-14 (*qī mén*, Cycle Gate), GB-34 (*yáng líng quán*, Yang Mound Spring), and SP-6 (*sān yīn jiāo*, Three Yin Intersection). Drain all points. **Impeded lung qi:** Hiccough attributed to impeded lung qi is characterized frequent hiccough, attended by inhibited throat and cold face. MED Diffuse lung qi with medicinals such as loquat leaf (*pí pá yè*), Sichuan fritillaria (*chuān bèi mǔ*), curcuma (*yù jīn*), belamcanda (*shè gān*), rice-paper plant pith (*tōng cǎo*), and fermented soybean (*dàn dòu chǐ*). ACU To the main points given above add BL-13 (*fèi shū*, Lung Transport) and LU-7 (*liè quē*, Broken Sequence). Drain all points. See HICCOUGH. [50: 273] [26: 538] [113: 76] [46: 584, 646, 652]

qi impediment 气痹 *qì bì*: An IMPEDIMENT (*bì*) pattern brought on by emotional stimulus. [26: 543]

qi is the commander of the blood 气为血之帅 *qì wéi xuè zhī shuài*: Qi produces and moves the blood. Blood is produced by construction qi, which carries the essence assimilated from food by the stomach and spleen upward into the lung, combining it with lung qi. Once formed, it then flows with qi through the vessels. The heart's function of governing the blood, the liver's function of storing the blood, and the spleen's function of keeping the blood in the vessels are all ascribed to the qi of these organs. From this it can be seen that qi is indispensable for both the production and the circulation of blood. Qi engenders, moves, and contains the blood. This is why it is said that "qi is the commander of the blood." [26: 538]

qi lump 气块 *qì kuài*: Any lump caused by stagnation of qi.

qi mounting 气疝 *qì shàn*: **1.** A MOUNTING (*shàn*) pattern characterized by abdominal pain of varying intensity arising from blockage of qi dynamic from irregularities of diet or from excessive warmth or cold. MED Rectify qi using Litchee Pit and Fennel Powder (*lì xiāng sǎn*). ACU Base treatment mainly on points of the CV and LR. Select CV-6 (*qì hǎi*, Sea of Qi), LR-2 (*xíng jiān*, Moving Between), LR-5 (*lǐ gōu*, Woodworm Canal), LR-6 (*zhōng dū*, Central Metropolis), LR-3 (*tài chōng*, Supreme Surge), and SP-6 (*sān yīn jiāo*, Three Yin Intersection); needle with drainage. **2.** Painful sagging of the scrotum attributed to qi depression. MED Course the liver and rectify qi with formulas such as Qi-Abducting Decoction (*dǎo qì tāng*). See FOXY MOUNTING. [26: 538] [37: 455] [46: 680] [113: 196]

qi-moving technique 行气法 *xíng qì fǎ*: Any of several techniques applied in acupuncture after needles have been inserted and qi has been obtained to help the movement of qi to and from the disease locus. Qi-moving techniques include the following three. **Needle-driving method:** Pressure is applied at the location of the tip of the needle where qi is obtained; the needle is made to point in the direction of the desired flow of qi. The practitioner then concentrates his qi at the needle to force the qi to move. To drain, the action is performed while the patient breathes out, whereas to supplement, it is performed while the patient breathes in. **Qi-pushing method:** The flesh is lifted between the thumb and index finger

at the point of insertion, and the needle is angled in the desired direction of qi flow, thrust forcefully while being rotated up to the crease on the inside of the thumb, and then retracted. The action is performed several times. **Damming method:** After obtaining qi, lifting and thrusting and rotation are performed with the right hand, while left presses one side of the insertion point. If the qi is required to flow down the channel, the pressure is applied just above the insertion point; if it needs to move up the channel, pressure is applied just below it. [46: 466]

Qin 秦 *qín*: The name of a dynasty (221–207 B.C.).

Qing 清 *qīng*: The name of a dynasty (A.D. 1644–1911) under which China was controlled by the Manchus.

qi not homing to its root 气不归根 *qì bù guī gēn*: The KIDNEY IS THE ROOT OF QI, and qi (air) drawn in by the lungs is absorbed by the kidney. When qi fails to reach the kidney, this is called "qi not homing to its root." See KIDNEY FAILING TO ABSORB QI. ◇ Chin 归 *guī*, to return or go to its proper place.

qi occlusion 气膈 *qì gé*: Blockage of the throat accompanied by counterflow fullness in the chest and rib-side, and putrid belching. See DYSPHAGIA-OCCLUSION (*yē gé*). [26: 545] [97: 94]

qi opening 气口 *qì kǒu*: The *wrist pulse*, so called because it is, as it were, an "opening" in the body where the qi can be felt. Also called *vessel opening* for the same reason. [27: 188] [97: 90]

qi pain 气痛 *qì tòng*: Pain attributed to qi stagnation arising from binding depression of the seven affects, from stagnation of phlegm-heat, from damage by dietary irregularities, or from taxation fatigue. It may affect the chest, rib-side, abdomen, or lumbus. **Upper burner:** Qi stagnating in the upper burner with glomus and pain in the chest and heart [region]. MED Use Bitter Orange and Tangerine Peel Decoction (*zhǐ jú tāng*). **Center burner:** Qi stagnating in center burner is marked by stabbing pain in the abdomen and rib-side. MED Use Saussurea Qi-Breaking Powder (*mù xiāng pò qì sǎn*). **Lower burner:** Qi stagnating in the lower burner is marked by MOUNTING-CONGLOMERATION (*shàn jiǎ*) or lumbar pain and can be treated Four Milled Ingredients Beverage (*sì mò yǐn*) or Saussurea and Areca Pill (*mù xiāng bīng láng wán*). **External body:** Qi stagnating in the external body with generalized stabbing pain can be treated with Qi Flow Drink (*liú qì yǐn zi*) or Saussurea Qi Flow Beverage (*mù xiāng liú qì yǐn*). Wherever there are signs of qi stagnation causing blood stasis, blood-quickening stasis-transforming medicinals can be included. ACU Main points: CV-6 (*qì hǎi*, Sea of Qi), PC-6 (*nèi guān*, Inner Pass), and LR-3 (*tài chōng*, Supreme Surge); needle with drainage. Selection of points according to location of qi stagnation: For qi stagnation in the upper burner, add CV-17 (*shān zhōng,* Chest Center), CV-15 (*jiū wěi,* Turtledove Tail), and PC-5 (*jiān shǐ,* Intermediary Courier). For qi stagnation in the center burner, add CV-12 (*zhōng wǎn,* Center Stomach Duct), ST-25 (*tiān shū,* Celestial Pivot), ST-36 (*zú sān lǐ,* Leg Three Li), TB-6 (*zhī gōu,* Branch Ditch), and GB-34 (*yáng líng quán,* Yang Mound Spring). For qi stagnation in the lower burner, add BL-23 (*shèn shū,* Kidney Transport) and ST-36 (*zú sān lǐ,* Leg Three Li), and moxa CV-4 (*guān yuán,* Pass Head). For qi stagnation in the outer body, add LI-4 (*hé gǔ,* Union Valley), TB-5 (*wài guān,* Outer Pass), and GV-20 (*bǎi huì,* Hundred Convergences). For qi stagnation causing blood stasis, add BL-17 (*gé shū,* Diaphragm Transport), SP-10 (*xuè hǎi,* Sea of Blood), LI-4 (*hé gǔ,* Union Valley), and SP-6 (*sān yīn jiāo,* Three Yin Intersection), needling with drainage. [26: 543] [97: 93]

qi phlegm 气痰 *qì tán:* **1.** DRYNESS PHLEGM. **2.** PLUM-PIT QI. [26: 543]

qi-pushing method 推气法 *tuī qì fǎ:* QI-MOVING TECHNIQUE.

qi reversal 气厥 *qì jué:* Reversal attributed to qi vacuity or qi repletion. **Qi vacuity** reversal is characterized by dizziness and clouding collapse, bright white facial complexion, sweating, cold limbs, and faint weak pulse. ⃞MED⃞ Supplement qi and the blood using formulas such as Major Origin-Supplementing Brew (*dà bǔ yuán jiān*) or Pure Ginseng Decoction (*dú shēn tāng*). **Qi repletion** reversal is characterized by sudden CLOUDING REVERSAL, panting and fullness in the chest and diaphragm, and a slippery stringlike pulse. ⃞MED⃞ Normalize qi and resolve depression using formulas such as Four Milled Ingredients Beverage (*sì mò yǐn*). ⃞ACU⃞ Base treatment mainly on LR, TB, and PC. Select LR-3 (*tài chōng,* Supreme Surge), LR-2 (*xíng jiān,* Moving Between), LR-14 (*qī mén,* Cycle Gate), LR-13 (*zhāng mén,* Camphorwood Gate), TB-6 (*zhī gōu,* Branch Ditch), PC-6 (*nèi guān,* Inner Pass), GV-26 (*shuǐ gōu,* Water Trough), and CV-17 (*shān zhōng,* Chest Center). Needle with drainage. See REVERSAL. [26: 542] [37: 401] [27: 400] [97: 93]

qi screen 气翳 *qì yì:* MURKY EYE OBSTRUCTION. [26: 546]

qi scrofula 气疬 *qì lì:* From *The Golden Mirror of Medicine* (*yī zōng jīn jiàn*). Soft round scrofulous lumps on either side of the neck that move when pushed and that swell up in response to anger. ⃞MED⃞ Course the liver and resolve depression. Use variations of Free Wanderer Powder (*xiāo yáo sǎn*). [26: 546] [50: 274]

qi shortage 气少 *qì shǎo:* **1.** Shortage of breath, i.e., shallow rapid breathing with a feeling of being unable to catch one's breath; a sign of qi vacuity. **2.** Qi vacuity. Compare SHORTNESS OF BREATH and SHORTAGE OF QI. [26: 536] [27: 142] [97: 90]

qi stagnation 气滞 *qì zhì:* Decrease in the normal activity of qi that is attributed to the obstructive effect of mental and emotional problems, external injury, evil qi (cold, dampness), static blood, or qi vacuity, and that is capable of causing static blood, water-damp, or phlegm-rheum. Qi stagnation is characterized by distention, fullness, and oppression in the affected area. "Where there is stoppage, there is pain." The pain associated with qi stagnation is of unfixed location or "scurrying," as distinct from pain of fixed location associated with blood stasis. Often, discomfort associated with qi stagnation is temporarily relieved by belching or the passing of flatus. **Affect damage:** Mental and emotional problems, traditionally understood as excesses among the seven affects, can affect health in a number of ways. This is known as *affect damage.* The most important way in which the seven affects can damage health is when affect-mind depression impairs the liver's free coursing action causing "binding depression of liver qi." This mechanism is often referred to as "binding depression of affect-mind," and the condition that results from it, which is one of the main forms of qi stagnation, is called *qi depression.* Qi depression manifests as sighing, pain and distention in the chest and rib-side (pain of unfixed location), oppression in the stomach duct, torpid intake, and in some cases vomiting. These signs are accompanied by mental or emotional problems that are the root cause, and intensify in periods of depression. Qi depression can also manifest in the form of abdominal pain, stomach pain, and even lumbar pain. Depressed qi sometimes produces abdominal glomus lump that is soft to the touch and that disperses and reforms periodically. In women, qi depression often manifests in swelling of the breasts and menstrual irregularities. It can combine with phlegm to cause plum-pit qi. Whatever form it takes, qi depression easily turns into fire causing rashness, impatience, irascibility, oppression in the chest and rib-side distention, clamoring stomach, dry mouth with bitter taste, constipation, red tongue with yellow fur and stringlike rapid pulse, and in some cases with headache, red eyes, or tinnitus. **External injury:** Qi stagnation can also arise as a result of internal injury when blows to the chest or abdomen cause pain in the rib-side, cough, panting, and pain and distention in the abdomen and stomach duct. **Evil qi:** Qi stagnation can be the result of the obstructive effect of evils, especially cold and dampness. For example, in *cold stagnating in the liver vessel,* abdominal pain and distention is attributed to qi stagnation caused by cold evil. See also COLD; COLD-DAMP. Dampness can cause qi stagnation, as when dampness obstructing the center burner causes abdominal distention. See DAMPNESS; DAMP DEPRESSION. Damp-heat can also cause qi stagnation as seen in DAMP-HEAT DYSENTERY (manifesting in the form of tenesmus) and DAMP-HEAT RIB-SIDE PAIN. Qi stagnation can cause, or be caused by, blood stasis. This dual pathology is observed in MENSTRUAL BLOCK, LIVER FIXITY, DYSPHAGIA-OCCLUSION (*yē gé*), and CONCRETIONS, CONGLOMERATIONS, ACCUMULATIONS, AND GATHERINGS (including strings and aggregations, deep-lying beam etc.), WELLING-ABSCESS and FLAT-ABSCESS (*jū*) (intestinal welling-abscess (*yōng*), effusions of the back (*fā bèi*), sloughing flat-abscess (*tuō jū*), etc.), and INTERNAL OBSTRUCTION. **Qi vacuity:** Qi vacuity can cause qi stagnation, e.g., spleen vacuity causing qi stagnation abdominal distention in GREATER YIN DISEASE. WMC Qi stagnation is seen in gastrointestinal neurosis, chronic gastritis, chronic enteritis, ulcers, diseases of the biliary tract, and chronic hepatitis. MED Qi stagnation is treated by the methods of rectifying and moving qi. Agents such as cyperus (*xiāng fù zǐ*), saussurea (*mù xiāng*), bitter orange (*zhǐ ké*), and tangerine peel (*chén pí*) are especially suitable for gastrointestinal qi stagnation. Unripe tangerine peel (*qīng pí*), curcuma (*yù jīn*), and toosendan (*chuān liàn zǐ*) are appropriate for binding depression of liver qi or for liver channel qi stagnation. Since most cases of qi stagnation are related to impaired liver free coursing, formulas designed for liver qi stagnation contain liver-coursing qi-rectifying medicinals such as bupleurum (*chái hú*). Liver-coursing qi-rectifying formulas include Counterflow Cold Powder (*sì nì sǎn*) and Bupleurum Liver-Coursing Powder (*chái hú shū gān sǎn*). ACU To rectify qi and move qi, select as main points CV-6 (*qì hǎi*, Sea of Qi), CV-17 (*shān zhōng*, Chest Center), PC-6 (*nèi guān*, Inner Pass), LI-4 (*hé gǔ*, Union Valley), LR-3 (*tài chōng*, Supreme Surge), TB-6 (*zhī gōu*, Branch Ditch), and GB-34 (*yáng líng quán*, Yang Mound Spring). To these add further points chosen according to cause. Needle stimulus depends on cause. See DEPRESSION PATTERN; DISHARMONY OF QI AND BLOOD. [6: 164] [27: 339] [36: 267] [46: 594]

qi stagnation abdominal pain 气滞腹痛 *qì zhì fù tòng:* Synonym: *qi bind abdominal pain.* ABDOMINAL PAIN attributed to qi stagnation arising when constrained affect-mind or careless living depress qi dynamic. Qi stagnation abdominal pain is distending pain or attacks of pain of unfixed location, with oppression in the chest, and rib-side pain. Pain may be relieved by belching or passing of flatus, and exacerbated by emotional imbalance.

MED Course the liver and resolve depression; rectify qi and relieve pain. If depressed qi transforms into fire, it is also necessary to clear fire. Formulas include Saussurea Qi-Normalizing Decoction (*mù xiāng shùn qì tāng*) or Counterflow Cold Powder (*sì nì sǎn*) and Bupleurum Liver-Clearing Beverage (*chái hú qīng gān yǐn*). ACU Base treatment mainly on LR, PC, and SP. Select CV-17 (*shān zhōng*, Chest Center), PC-6 (*nèi guān*, Inner Pass), CV-6 (*qì hǎi*, Sea of Qi), ST-36 (*zú sān lǐ*, Leg Three Li), LR-3 (*tài chōng*, Supreme Surge), SP-3 (*tài bái*, Supreme White), LR-14 (*qī mén*, Cycle Gate), and ST-25 (*tiān shū*, Celestial Pivot); needle with drainage. Selection of points according to signs: For depressed qi transforming into fire, add PC-8 (*láo gōng*, Palace of Toil), GB-34 (*yáng líng quán*, Yang Mound Spring), and LR-2 (*xíng jiān*, Moving Between), needling with drainage. See ABDOMINAL PAIN. [26: 544] [46: 662] [37: 318]

qi stagnation and blood stasis 气滞血瘀 *qì zhì xuè yū:* The simultaneous occurrence of qi stagnation and blood stasis, characterized by signs such as menstrual block, stasis clots in the menstrual discharge, abdominal pain at the onset of menstruation, or painful distention of the breasts. Qi stagnation and blood stasis may also arise together as a result of external injury. When qi fails to move the blood, qi stagnation may cause—and be further exacerbated by—blood stasis. This frequently occurs in conditions described by Western medicine as chronic nephritis and ulcerative diseases. MED Dual patterns of qi stagnation and blood stasis are treated with blood-quickening and qi-rectifying medicinals. Toosendan Powder (*jīn líng zǐ sǎn*), commonly used to relieve pain, is a representative formula. ACU Base treatment mainly on back transport points, SP, LR, CV, PC, and GB. BL-17 (*gé shū*, Diaphragm Transport), SP-10 (*xuè hǎi*, Sea of Blood), LR-3 (*tài chōng*, Supreme Surge), SP-6 (*sān yīn jiāo*, Three Yin Intersection), CV-6 (*qì hǎi*, Sea of Qi), PC-6 (*nèi guān*, Inner Pass), LI-4 (*hé gǔ*, Union Valley), TB-6 (*zhī gōu*, Branch Ditch), and GB-34 (*yáng líng quán*, Yang Mound Spring) can be selected as main points; and needle with even supplementation and drainage or bleed with a three-edged needle to rectify qi and dissipate stasis. Selection of points according to signs: For menstrual block, add CV-3 (*zhōng jí*, Central Pole) and SP-8 (*dì jī*, Earth's Crux). For menstrual pain, add CV-3 (*zhōng jí*, Central Pole), and ST-29 (*guī lái*, Return). For painful distention of the breasts, add CV-17 (*shān zhōng*, Chest Center), ST-18 (*rǔ gēn*, Breast Root), and LR-14 (*qī mén*, Cycle Gate). For external injury, add local points. [6: 168] [46: 594, 686, 694] [37: 421]

qi stagnation blood stasis heart palpitations 气滞血瘀心悸 *qì zhì xuè yū xīn jì:* HEART PAL-

PITATIONS attributed to qi stagnation and blood stasis and associated with shortness of breath and panting, oppression or pain in the chest, dark purple tongue, and a rough pulse. [MED] Quicken the blood and transform stasis with House of Blood Stasis-Expelling Decoction (xuè fǔ zhú yū tāng) and Peach Kernel and Carthamus Brew (táo rén hóng huā jiān). Salvia Beverage (dān shēn yǐn). Nowadays, Coronary No.2 (guàn xīn èr hào) is used for coronary heart disease and angina pectoris, and is suitable for heart palpitations from these conditions. [ACU] Base treatment mainly on back transport points, CV, HT, PC, LR, and SP. Select BL-15 (xīn shū, Heart Transport), HT-7 (shén mén, Spirit Gate), PC-6 (nèi guān, Inner Pass), CV-17 (shān zhōng, Chest Center), BL-17 (gé shū, Diaphragm Transport), SP-10 (xuè hǎi, Sea of Blood), LI-4 (hé gǔ, Union Valley), and LR-3 (tài chōng, Supreme Surge); needle with even supplementation and drainage. See HEART PALPITATIONS. [26: 544]

qi stagnation blood stasis menstrual block 气滞血瘀经闭 qì zhì xuè yū jīng bì: Absence of menses attributed to qi and blood stagnation causing stagnation in the thoroughfare (chōng) and controlling (rèn) vessels and traceable either to affect damage affecting liver, heart, or spleen qi or to the cold evil. [MED] Rectify qi and quicken the blood; dispel stasis and free menstruation. Use House of Blood Stasis-Expelling Decoction (xuè fǔ zhú yū tāng) or Free Wanderer Powder (xiāo yáo sǎn) combined with Four Agents Decoction (sì wù tāng) plus millettia (jī xuè téng) and leonurus fruit (chōng wèi zǐ). [ACU] Base treatment mainly on CV, SP, and LR. Main points: CV-3 (zhōng jí, Central Pole), LI-4 (hé gǔ, Union Valley), SP-6 (sān yīn jiāo, Three Yin Intersection), SP-10 (xuè hǎi, Sea of Blood), LR-3 (tài chōng, Supreme Surge), and ST-29 (guī lái, Return). If qi stagnation is prominent, add CV-6 (qì hǎi, Sea of Qi) and LR-2 (xíng jiān, Moving Between), needling with drainage; if blood stasis is prominent, add BL-17 (gé shū, Diaphragm Transport), SP-8 (dì jī, Earth's Crux), LR-8 (qū quán, Spring at the Bend), and ST-30 (qì chōng, Qi Thoroughfare), needling with even supplementation and drainage or bleeding with three-edged needle. See MENSTRUAL BLOCK. [26: 544] [67: 121]

qi stagnation delayed menstruation 气滞经行后期 qì zhì jīng xíng hòu qī: DELAYED MENSTRUATION (lengthening of menstrual cycle) attributed to qi stagnation arising when depression and anger damage the liver, inhibiting qi dynamic and hampering the flow of blood in the thoroughfare (chōng) and controlling (rèn) vessels. Qi stagnation delayed menstruation is often associated with pain and distention in the smaller abdomen and breasts that refuses pressure. Menstrual flow

is scant and disfluent. [MED] Move qi and resolve depression using Supplemented Lindera Decoction (jiā wèi wū yào tāng) or Sevenfold Processed Cyperus Pill (qī zhì xiāng fù wán). [ACU] Base treatment mainly on CV and the three yin channels of the foot. Select CV-6 (qì hǎi, Sea of Qi), KI-13 (qì xué, Qi Point), SP-6 (sān yīn jiāo, Three Yin Intersection), LR-3 (tài chōng, Supreme Surge), and LR-5 (lí gōu, Woodworm Canal); needle with drainage. See DELAYED MENSTRUATION. [26: 545] [46: 683]

qi stagnation lumbar pain 气滞腰痛 qì zhì yāo tòng: Lumbar pain arising when either anger, depression, thought or anxiety, or sprains and falls cause qi stagnation in the sinews. Qi stagnation lumbar pain is characterized by pain that stretches into the abdomen and rib-side that seems to wander, and is intermittent. [MED] Move qi and course stagnation with formulas such as Aquilaria Qi-Downbearing Decoction (chén xiāng jiàng qì tāng). [ACU] Base treatment mainly on back transport points, BL, CV, LR, and PC. Select BL-23 (shèn shū, Kidney Transport), BL-40 (wěi zhōng, Bend Center), ouch points (ā shì xué), CV-6 (qì hǎi, Sea of Qi), PC-6 (nèi guān, Inner Pass), LR-3 (tài chōng, Supreme Surge), and GB-34 (yáng líng quán, Yang Mound Spring); needle with drainage. For enduring conditions, add ST-36 (zú sān lǐ, Leg Three Li), BL-20 (pí shū, Spleen Transport), and BL-17 (gé shū, Diaphragm Transport); needle with supplementation. See LUMBAR PAIN. [26: 544] [46: 622] [37: 388] [113: 229]

qi stagnation menstrual pain 气滞痛经 qì zhì tòng jīng: Lower abdominal distention and pain before or during menstruation, arising when emotional depression causes qi stagnation, which in turn obstructs the movement of blood in the thoroughfare (chōng) and controlling (rèn) vessels. Qi stagnation menstrual pain is often accompanied by oppression in the chest and distention of the breasts and by disfluent menstrual flow. [MED] Use formulas such as Supplemented Lindera Decoction (jiā wèi wū yào tāng) or Sevenfold Processed Cyperus Pill (qī zhì xiāng fù wán). [ACU] Base treatment mainly on CV, LR, PC, and SP. Select CV-6 (qì hǎi, Sea of Qi), LR-3 (tài chōng, Supreme Surge), PC-6 (nèi guān, Inner Pass), LR-2 (xíng jiān, Moving Between), and SP-6 (sān yīn jiāo, Three Yin Intersection); needle with drainage. Selection of points according to signs: For lower abdominal distention, add ST-25 (tiān shū, Celestial Pivot), KI-13 (qì xué, Qi Point), and SP-8 (dì jī, Earth's Crux). For oppression in the chest and distention of the breasts, add CV-17 (shān zhōng, Chest Center) and PC-6 (nèi guān, Inner Pass). See MENSTRUAL PAIN. [26: 544] [46: 685]

qi strangury 气淋 qì lín: STRANGURY (painful dribbling urination) attributed either to qi vacuity or to qi stagnation, and characterized in either case by pronounced smaller-abdominal distention and fullness. **Qi vacuity** patterns are attributed to insufficiency of center qi and are characterized by sagging distention in the lesser abdomen (attributed to center qi fall), forceless discharge of urine, dribble after voiding, bright white facial complexion, pale tongue, and forceless vacuous weak pulse. **Qi stagnation** (repletion) patterns are attributed to binding depression of liver qi and are characterized by a tongue with a green-blue tinge, and a stringlike sunken pulse. MED Treat qi vacuity patterns with Center-Supplementing Qi-Boosting Decoction (*bǔ zhōng yì qì tāng*) or Eight-Gem Decoction (*bā zhēn tāng*) plus eucommia (*dù zhòng*) and achyranthes (*niú xī*). Treat qi stagnation patterns with Aquilaria Powder (*chén xiāng sǎn*). ACU Base treatment mainly on the three yin channels of the foot and alarm and back transport points of BL (CV-3 and BL-28). Main points: CV-3 (*zhōng jí*, Central Pole), BL-28 (*páng guāng shū*, Bladder Transport), SP-9 (*yīn líng quán*, Yin Mound Spring), LR-2 (*xíng jiān*, Moving Between), and KI-3 (*tài xī*, Great Ravine). For vacuity patterns of insufficiency of center qi, add BL-20 (*pí shū*, Spleen Transport), CV-6 (*qì hǎi*, Sea of Qi), and ST-36 (*zú sān lǐ*, Leg Three Li), and needle with supplementation. For repletion patterns of qi stagnation, add PC-6 (*nèi guān*, Inner Pass), LR-3 (*tài chōng*, Supreme Surge), and GB-34 (*yáng líng quán*, Yang Mound Spring), and needle with drainage. See STRANGURY. [26: 539] [46: 674] [27: 425] [97: 93]

qi street 气街 *qì jiē*: **1.** A pathway along which qi flows. There are four qi streets in the body. *The Magic Pivot* (*líng shū*), "The chest has a qi street; the abdomen has a qi street; the head has a qi street; the lower leg has a qi street." **2.** The area of the pulsating vessel in the groin. It is said, for example, that the yang brightness (*yáng míng*) stomach channel descends from the supraclavicular, down the inner face of the breast, and past the umbilicus to enter the qi street. [26: 543] [27: 68] [97: 93]

qi surging up into the heart 气上冲心 *qì shàng chōng xīn*: A subjective feeling of an upward rush into the region of the heart. Qi surging up into the heart is observed in RUNNING PIGLET where the qi rises from the lesser abdomen, and in reverting yin (*jué yīn*) disease, where it is a manifestation of cross counterflow of liver qi. [6: 229] [51: 124, 497]

qi stroke 气中 *qì zhòng*: A form of WIND-LIKE STROKE arising when seven-affect qi bind or anger stirring liver qi causes qi to ascend counterflow. Signs include sudden collapse, loss of consciousness, clenched jaw, and hypertonicity of the limbs. It is very similar to wind stroke, but the body is

cool, and although there may be a small amount of phlegm-drool, there is no sound of drool in the mouth; hence the condition is different. MED Rectify qi, dissipate binds, and downbear counterflow. Use formulas such as Seven Qi Decoction (*qī qì tāng*). In severe cases, pour liquid storax (*sū hé xiāng*) mixed with ginger juice into the mouth. ACU Base treatment mainly on GV, LI, and hand and foot reverting yin (*jué yīn*) PC/LR. Select GV-26 (*shuǐ gōu*, Water Trough), GV-20 (*bǎi huì*, Hundred Convergences), PC-9 (*zhōng chōng*, Central Hub), LI-4 (*hé gǔ*, Union Valley), PC-6 (*nèi guān*, Inner Pass), LR-3 (*tài chōng*, Supreme Surge), LR-2 (*xíng jiān*, Moving Between), ST-36 (*zú sān lǐ*, Leg Three Li), ST-6 (*jiá chē*, Cheek Carriage), and ST-7 (*xià guān*, Below the Joint); needle with drainage. [26: 535] [113: 34]

qi swelling 气肿 *qì zhǒng*: **1.** WATER SWELLING with signs of qi depression. Qi swelling is caused by qi stagnation and damp depression. Accompanying signs include somber skin complexion, emaciation, and fullness and distention in the abdomen and rib-side, sometimes with abdominal pain stretching into the rib-side. The swelling may occur suddenly, and may spread from the upper body downward. The skin feels thick to the touch, and the swelling rebounds after pressure is relieved. MED Rectify qi and transform dampness; disperse swelling and eliminate fullness. Use Tangerine Peel Decocted Pill (*jú pí jiān wán*). ACU Base treatment mainly on CV, back transport points, ST, PC, LR, and SP. Select CV-9 (*shuǐ fēn*, Water Divide), CV-6 (*qì hǎi*, Sea of Qi), BL-20 (*pí shū*, Spleen Transport), BL-22 (*sān jiāo shū*, Triple Burner Transport), ST-25 (*tiān shū*, Celestial Pivot), PC-6 (*nèi guān*, Inner Pass), LR-3 (*tài chōng*, Supreme Surge), ST-36 (*zú sān lǐ*, Leg Three Li), TB-6 (*zhī gōu*, Branch Ditch), SP-6 (*sān yīn jiāo*, Three Yin Intersection), and SP-9 (*yīn líng quán*, Yin Mound Spring); needle with drainage and add moxa. See WATER SWELLING. **2.** Local painful swelling of the skin. *The Origin and Indicators of Disease* (*zhū bìng yuán hòu lùn, qì zhǒng hòu*). states, "Qi swelling is like a welling-abscess without a head, marked by vacuity swelling, no change in skin color, and painful taughtness in the skin that hurts whenever it is pressed. This is caused by wind evil binding contending with qi." **3.** VACUOUS PUFFINESS. [50: 273] [26: 544] [46: 676, 602, 595] [97: 92] [25: 59] [92: No. 76] [29: 261]

qi timidity 气怯 *qì qiè*: Qi vacuity as manifest in the form of shortage of breath with fear, lack of courage, and susceptibility to fright. Qi timidity arises when insufficiency of spleen qi engenders phlegm, which singly or in combination with heat obstructs the liver's free coursing action and disturbs bile flow. See GALLBLADDER VACUITY AND QI TIMIDITY. [26: 538] [27: 143] [97: 92]

qi transformation 气化 *qì huà*: The movement, mutation, and conversion of qi. In ancient Chinese thought, qi is considered to be a material entity having yin and yang aspects which are interdependent and opposing. Yang qi is formless and intangible, yet can evolve to assume tangible forms, which are yin qi. Yin qi and yang qi form a unity of opposites and undergo constant mutation from which the material world springs. This constant mutation is called "qi transformation." In the human body, qi in a wider sense denotes essence, qi (yang qi), liquid, humor, and blood (see SIX QI). Qi transformation refers to the processes by which these qi produce each other and convert from one to another. Qi transformation is therefore life activity. The five viscera and six bowels, the limbs and bones, etc., are all involved in the process of qi transformation. The movement of blood and essential qi, the distribution of fluids, the digestion and assimilation of food, the discharge of waste, the moistening of the sinew and bones, the warming of the skin, the maintenance of the sheen of the hair of the head and body, and the regulation of the organs all rely upon qi transformation. For this reason, some writers have said that qi transformation is roughly equivalent to metabolism. Growth and development of the body, and defense against external evils, are similarly dependent upon qi transformation. Cessation of qi transformation is the cessation of life. This is the broadest meaning of "qi transformation." In a narrower meaning, the term denotes the qi transformation of the triple burner, especially in the context of fluid metabolism. See QI; WATER FAILING TO TRANSFORM INTO QI. [45: 48–64] [26: 536] [27: 80] [97: 90] [36: 147–148]

qi tumor 气瘤 *qì liú*: A TUMOR (a growth on the outside of the body) caused by taxation damaging lung qi and by invasion of external evil is soft, with normal skin color, unassociated with cold or heat, and becomes larger or smaller with changing moods. MED Boost the lung and regulate qi; transform phlegm and dissipate binds. An appropriate formula is Qi-Freeing Hardness-Dissipating Pill (*tōng qì sàn jiān wán*). [26: 545]

qi vacuity 气虚 *qì xū*: **1.** *Synonym: original qi vacuity.* Weakness of qi; the manifestation of insufficiency of original qi. Qi vacuity is associated with poor organ function, general weakening through illness or overwork, dietary imbalance, or damage to yin-blood. General signs include fatigue, lack of strength, spontaneous sweating at the slightest movement, bright white facial complexion, dizziness, faint voice, shortness of breath, and a weak fine soft pulse. If qi's securing function breaks down, there may be flooding and spotting

or bloody stool, prolapse of the rectum or prolapse of the uterus, and reduced resistance to evils. A focus among the organs is usually detectable, and is identified by weak organ function. Since qi is yang in nature, qi vacuity and yang vacuity present with similar signs. Yang vacuity is characterized by qi vacuity signs as well as cold signs such as cold limbs, aversion to cold, cold sweating, and slow pulse. MED Qi vacuity is treated according to the principle that vacuity is treated by supplementation. Qi-supplementing medicinals include codonopsis (*dǎng shēn*), astragalus (*huáng qí*), and licorice (*gān cǎo*). Since the spleen and stomach are the root of later heaven (the acquired constitution), qi-supplementing medicinals are complemented by spleen-strengthening medicinals such as ovate atractylodes (*bái zhú*) and poria (*fú líng*). A formula that treats any form of qi vacuity is Four Gentlemen Decoction (*sì jūn zǐ tāng*). ACU Select CV-6 (*qì hǎi*, Sea of Qi), BL-43 (*gāo huāng shū*, Gao-Huang Transport), ST-36 (*zú sān lǐ*, Leg Three Li), BL-20 (*pí shū*, Spleen Transport), BL-21 (*wèi shū*, Stomach Transport), SP-3 (*tài bái*, Supreme White), LU-9 (*tài yuān*, Great Abyss), and GV-20 (*bǎi huì*, Hundred Convergences) as the main points; needle with supplementation and add moxa. To these add further points according to accompanying signs. **2.** Lung vacuity. *Elementary Questions* (*sù wèn, tōng píng xū shí lùn*) states, "Qi vacuity is lung vacuity." The lung governs qi, and lung qi is engendered by spleen-earth; hence qi vacuity principally denotes spleen-lung qi vacuity. MED Bank up earth to engender metal. Use Six Gentlemen Decoction (*liù jūn zǐ tāng*) or variations of Ginseng, Poria (Hoelen), and Ovate Atractylodes Powder (*shēn líng bái zhú sǎn*). ACU Base treatment mainly on back transport points, LU, and SP. Select BL-13 (*fèi shū*, Lung Transport), BL-20 (*pí shū*, Spleen Transport), BL-43 (*gāo huāng shū*, Gao-Huang Transport), BL-21 (*wèi shū*, Stomach Transport), SP-3 (*tài bái*, Supreme White), LU-9 (*tài yuān*, Great Abyss), and ST-36 (*zú sān lǐ*, Leg Three Li); needle with supplementation and add moxa. [26: 410] [27: 142] [97: 91] [6: 162]

qi vacuity abdominal pain 气虚腹痛 *qì xū fù tòng*: ABDOMINAL PAIN attributed to qi vacuity that occurs when enduring illness, dietary irregularities, or taxation fatigue (overwork, stress) damages center qi. Qi vacuity abdominal pain is a continual pain exacerbated by fatigue and relieved by pressure and eating. It is accompanied by a withered-yellow facial complexion, low faint voice, and shortness of breath. The pulse is fine and rough or large and vacuous, and in cases of original qi vacuity, it may be urgent or racing. MED Supplement qi and fortify the center using formulas such as Saussurea and Amomum Six Gentlemen

Decoction (*xiāng shā liù jūn zǐ tāng*), Center-Supplementing Qi-Boosting Decoction (*bǔ zhōng yì qì tāng*) or Minor Center-Fortifying Decoction (*xiǎo jiàn zhōng tāng*). ACU Base treatment mainly on back transport points and CV. Select BL-20 (*pí shū*, Spleen Transport), BL-21 (*wèi shū*, Stomach Transport), CV-12 (*zhōng wǎn*, Center Stomach Duct), LR-13 (*zhāng mén*, Camphorwood Gate), CV-6 (*qì hǎi*, Sea of Qi), and ST-36 (*zú sān lǐ*, Leg Three Li); needle with supplementation and add moxa. [26: 541] [37: 318]

qi vacuity advanced menstruation 气虚经行先期 *qì xū jīng xíng xiān qī*: ADVANCED MENSTRUATION (i.e., premature arrival of periods) due to qi vacuity. Qi vacuity advanced menstruation occurs when constitutional vacuity, damage to the spleen by anxiety and thought, or dietary irregularities lead to center qi vacuity. It is marked by continual unabating abdominal pain that is exacerbated by taxation fatigue and relieved by pressure. There is reduced food intake, withered-yellow facial complexion, low faint voice, shortness of breath, and a rough fine or large vacuous pulse. In severe original qi vacuity, there may be a racing pulse. MED Supplement qi and contain the blood; fortify the spleen and secure the thoroughfare (*chōng*) vessel. Use Center-Supplementing Qi-Boosting Decoction (*bǔ zhōng yì qì tāng*) or Major Origin-Supplementing Brew (*dà bǔ yuán jiān*). ACU Base treatment mainly on the CV and three yin channels of the foot. Select CV-4 (*guān yuán*, Pass Head), SP-10 (*xuè hǎi*, Sea of Blood), ST-36 (*zú sān lǐ*, Leg Three Li), CV-6 (*qì hǎi*, Sea of Qi), BL-20 (*pí shū*, Spleen Transport), SP-2 (*dà dū*, Great Metropolis), and LR-8 (*qū quán*, Spring at the Bend); needle with supplementation and add moxa. [26: 541] [46: 682]

qi vacuity center fullness 气虚中满 *qì xū zhōng mǎn*: Abdominal fullness attributed to spleen vacuity. The spleen and stomach are located in the center burner and are responsible for movement and transformation. Spleen-stomach qi vacuity manifests as impaired movement and transformation, which is characterized by poor appetite and abdominal glomus, fullness, and distention sometimes accompanied by sloppy diarrhea. MED Use Saussurea and Amomum Six Gentlemen Decoction (*xiāng shā liù jūn zǐ tāng*). ACU Base treatment mainly on back transport points, CV, ST, and SP. Select BL-20 (*pí shū*, Spleen Transport), BL-21 (*wèi shū*, Stomach Transport), CV-6 (*qì hǎi*, Sea of Qi), CV-12 (*zhōng wǎn*, Center Stomach Duct), ST-36 (*zú sān lǐ*, Leg Three Li), ST-25 (*tiān shū*, Celestial Pivot), SP-4 (*gōng sūn*, Yellow Emperor), and PC-6 (*nèi guān*, Inner Pass); needle with supplementation and moxa. [26: 540]

qi vacuity deafness 气虚耳聋 *qì xū ěr lóng*: DEAFNESS attributed to qi vacuity, occurring most

commonly in advancing years or after illness. Qi vacuity deafness is often associated with tinnitus and is accompanied by shortage of qi, fatigue, heart palpitations, bland taste in the mouth, torpid intake, and forceless weak pulse. MED Supplement the center and boost qi using variations of Center-Supplementing Qi-Boosting Decoction (*bǔ zhōng yì qì tāng*). See DEAFNESS. ACU See DEAFNESS. [26: 540]

qi vacuity dizziness 气虚眩晕 *qì xū xuàn yūn*: DIZZINESS attributed to qi vacuity and yang debilitation preventing normal upbearing of clear yang. Qi vacuity dizziness also includes yang vacuity dizziness. When caused by spleen qi vacuity, dizziness and flowery vision brought on by taxation are associated with lassitude of spirit and lack of strength, reduced food intake and sloppy stool, and a vacuous pulse. MED Boost qi and fortify the spleen using Four Gentlemen Panting Decoction (*chuǎn sì jūn zǐ tāng*) or Center-Supplementing Qi-Boosting Decoction (*bǔ zhōng yì qì tāng*). ACU Base treatment mainly on GV, CV, ST, and back transport points. Select GV-20 (*bǎi huì*, Hundred Convergences), ST-36 (*zú sān lǐ*, Leg Three Li), CV-12 (*zhōng wǎn*, Center Stomach Duct), CV-6 (*qì hǎi*, Sea of Qi), BL-20 (*pí shū*, Spleen Transport), BL-21 (*wèi shū*, Stomach Transport), and ST-8 (*tóu wéi*, Head Corner); needle with supplementation and add moxa. For yang vacuity patterns, see YANG VACUITY DIZZINESS. See also DIZZINESS. [26: 540] [46: 619 575]

qi vacuity fall 气虚下陷 *qì xū xià xiàn*: CENTER QI FALL. [26: 540]

qi vacuity flooding and spotting 气虚崩漏 *qì xū bēng lòu*: FLOODING AND SPOTTING (abnormal discharge of blood via the vagina) attributed to qi vacuity. Qi vacuity flooding and spotting occurs when constitutional vacuity, damage to the spleen by anxiety or thought, or dietary irregularities cause center qi fall and insecurity of the thoroughfare (*chōng*) vessel. It is characterized by copious or dribbling discharge of pale thin blood, accompanied by lassitude of spirit, shortness of breath and laziness to speak, no thought of food and drink, and in some cases by a bright white facial complexion, heart palpitations, and empty sagging in the smaller abdomen. MED Supplement qi to contain the blood; fortify the spleen and secure the thoroughfare (*chōng*) vessel. Use formulas like Center-Supplementing Qi-Boosting Decoction (*bǔ zhōng yì qì tāng*) or Origin-Lifting Brew (*jǔ yuán jiān*). ACU Base treatment mainly on CV and SP. Select GV-20 (*bǎi huì*, Hundred Convergences), CV-12 (*zhōng wǎn*, Center Stomach Duct), CV-6 (*qì hǎi*, Sea of Qi), BL-20 (*pí shū*, Spleen Transport), CV-4 (*guān yuán*, Pass Head), ST-36 (*zú sān lǐ*, Leg Three Li), and SP-6 (*sān yīn* *jiāo*, Three Yin Intersection), needling with supplementation and adding moxa. [26: 541] [46: 689, 575, 595]

qi vacuity generalized heat [effusion] 气虚身热 *qì xū shēn rè*: HEAT EFFUSIONheat effusion (fever) due to damage by summerheat-damp in patients suffering from vacuity of original qi. *Elementary Questions* (*sù wèn, cì zhì lùn*) states, "Qi vacuity generalized heat-[effusion] comes from damage by summerheat." This can be treated with Li's Summerheat-Clearing Qi-Boosting Decoction (*lǐ shì qīng shǔ yì qì tāng*) or Wang's Summerheat-Clearing Qi-Boosting Decoction (*wáng shì qīng shǔ yì qì tāng*). Qi vacuity generalized heat [effusion] may also be the result of damage to the spleen and stomach as a result of diet or taxation fatigue. This is treated by eliminating heat with warmth and sweetness. See QI VACUITY HEAT. [50: 282]

qi vacuity habitual miscarriage 气虚滑胎 *qì xū huá tāi*: Habitual miscarriage attributed to qi vacuity. Qi vacuity habitual miscarriage arises when spleen-stomach vacuity develops in pregnancy and causes insecurity of the thoroughfare (*chōng*) and controlling (*rèn*) vessels that deprives the fetus of its bearing. Accompanying signs include aching lumbus, abdominal distention, stirring fetus sometimes with bleeding, shortness of breath and lack of strength. MED Boost qi and quiet the fetus. A basic formula is Origin-Lifting Brew (*jǔ yuán jiān*), to which eucommia (*dù zhòng*) and mistletoe (*sāng jì shēng*) may be added for aching lumbus and sagging pain in the abdomen. Ass hide glue (*ē jiāo*) and charred mugwort (*ài yè tàn*) may be added if there is bleeding. See HABITUAL MISCARRIAGE. [26: 541]

qi vacuity headache 气虚头痛 *qì xū tóu tòng*: HEADACHE attributed to insufficiency of the stomach and spleen and to qi vacuity preventing the upbearing of clear yang. Qi vacuity headache is exacerbated by taxation and is accompanied by tinnitus, inhibition of the nine orifices, lassitude of spirit, inability to taste food, and a pulse that is either weak or large and forceless. MED Fortify the spleen and boost qi using formulas such as Center-Supplementing Qi-Boosting Decoction (*bǔ zhōng yì qì tāng*), or Four Gentlemen Decoction (*sì jūn zǐ tāng*) plus astragalus (*huáng qí*) and vitex (*màn jīng zǐ*). ACU Base treatment mainly on CV and ST. Select GV-20 (*bǎi huì*, Hundred Convergences), CV-12 (*zhōng wǎn*, Center Stomach Duct), CV-6 (*qì hǎi*, Sea of Qi), CV-4 (*guān yuán*, Pass Head), ST-36 (*zú sān lǐ*, Leg Three Li), and SP-3 (*tài bái*, Supreme White), and needle with supplementation and add moxa. For selection of points according to affected area, see HEADACHE. For tinnitus, add TB-21 (*ěr mén*, Ear Gate). [26: 452] [37: 362] [46: 575]

qi vacuity heart palpitations 气虚心悸 *qì xū xīn jì*: HEART PALPITATIONS attributed to yang qi vacuity and attended by emptiness below the heart, with palpitations usually preceded by vexation. The pulse is large and forceless. MED Warm yang and boost qi with Minor Center-Fortifying Decoction (*xiǎo jiàn zhōng tāng*), True Warrior Decoction (*zhēn wǔ tāng*), or Counterflow Cold Decoction (*sì nì tāng*) plus cinnamon bark (*ròu guì*). ACU Base treatment mainly on back transport points, CV, HT, and PC. Select BL-15 (*xīn shū*, Heart Transport), CV-14 (*jù què*, Great Tower Gate), HT-7 (*shén mén*, Spirit Gate), PC-6 (*nèi guān*, Inner Pass), CV-6 (*qì hǎi*, Sea of Qi), CV-4 (*guān yuán*, Pass Head), ST-36 (*zú sān lǐ*, Leg Three Li), and GV-4 (*mìng mén*, Life Gate); needle with even supplementation and drainage. See HEART PALPITATIONS. [26: 540]

qi vacuity heat 气虚热 *qì xū rè*: **1.** A heat pattern due to qi vacuity. Qi vacuity heat usually stems from spleen-stomach qi vacuity or spleen-lung qi vacuity and arising when dietary irregularities or taxation fatigue causes damage to the spleen and stomach. It is characterized by generalized heat [effusion], heart vexation, spontaneous sweating and aversion to cold, headache, fatigue, and laziness to speak, panting and lack of strength at the slightest exertion, and a large vacuous surging pulse. MED Eliminate heat with warmth and sweetness. Use Center-Supplementing Qi-Boosting Decoction (*bǔ zhōng yì qì tāng*) or variations of Eight-Gem Decoction (*bā zhēn tāng*). **2.** HEAT EFFUSION due to summerheat-damp damaging qi, and associated with fatigued cumbersome limbs, fatigued essence-spirit, heart vexation, hasty breathing, thirst, spontaneous sweating, yellow urine, and a vacuous pulse. If summerheat-heat evil wears qi and damages fluid, there is generalized fever and vacuity pulse, spontaneous sweating, and more pronounced vexation and thirst. MED Clear summerheat-heat; boost qi and engender liquid. Use Wang's Summerheat-Clearing Qi-Boosting Decoction (*wáng shì qīng shǔ yì qì tāng*). [26: 541]

qi vacuity heat effusion 气虚发热 *qì xū fā rè*: Heat effusion due to qi vacuity. Qi vacuity heat effusion is a low intermittent heat effusion associated with fatigue and lack of strength. See QI VACUITY HEAT. [6: 131]

qi vacuity impediment 气虚痹 *qì xū bì*: An IMPEDIMENT (*bì*) pattern arising when vacuity of yang qi allows internal cold-damp to become exuberant. Qi vacuity impediment is characterized by inhibited movement of the joints, lack of bodily warmth, and in some case numbness of the limbs. MED Boost qi and warm yang with Four Gentlemen Decoction (*sì jūn zǐ tāng*) plus cinnamon bark (*róu guì*) and aconite (*fù zǐ*). If there is numbness, use Wondrous Effect Astragalus Decoction (*shén xiào huáng qí tāng*). ACU Base treatment mainly on back transport points, GV, CV, ST, and SP. Needle with supplementation and moxa at BL-23 (*shèn shū*, Kidney Transport), BL-20 (*pí shū*, Spleen Transport), GV-4 (*mìng mén*, Life Gate), CV-4 (*guān yuán*, Pass Head), CV-6 (*qì hǎi*, Sea of Qi), and needle with drainage and moxa at ST-36 (*zú sān lǐ*, Leg Three Li), SP-9 (*yīn líng quán*, Yin Mound Spring), and SP-5 (*shāng qiū*, Shang Hill). Apply moxa on salt or ginger at CV-8 (*shén què*, Spirit Gate Tower). See IMPEDIMENT for selection of points according to affected area. [26: 541]

qi vacuity panting 气虚喘 *qì xū chuǎn*: PANTING (labored breathing) attributed to insufficiency of original qi or spleen-lung qi vacuity. Qi vacuity panting is characterized by hasty breathing and discontinuity between breaths, fatigue and lack of strength, low faint voice, and sweating and exacerbation of panting at the slightest exertion. MED Supplement qi and calm panting with Four Gentlemen Panting Decoction (*chuǎn sì jūn zǐ tāng*). For qi vacuity with cold, use Clove and Evodia Center-Rectifying Decoction (*dīng yú lǐ zhōng tāng*) or Center-Rectifying Decoction (*lǐ zhōng tāng*). For severe vacuity, use Pure Ginseng Decoction (*dú shēn tāng*). ACU Base treatment mainly on back transport points, LU, CV and SP. Select BL-13 (*fèi shū*, Lung Transport), Panting Stabilizer (*dìng chuǎn*), BL-43 (*gāo huāng shū*, Gao-Huang Transport), LU-9 (*tài yuān*, Great Abyss), and ST-36 (*zú sān lǐ*, Leg Three Li), BL-20 (*pí shū*, Spleen Transport), BL-21 (*wèi shū*, Stomach Transport), CV-6 (*qì hǎi*, Sea of Qi), and SP-3 (*tài bái*, Supreme White); needle with supplementation and add moxa. See VACUITY PANTING. [26: 541] [46: 655]

qi vacuity profuse menstruation 气虚月经过多 *qì xū yuè jīng guò duō*: Excessively copious or prolonged menstrual flow attributed to qi vacuity. Qi vacuity profuse menstruation arises when constitutional qi vacuity or center qi vacuity or damage to the spleen due to excessive anxiety and thought leads to insecurity of the thoroughfare (*chōng*) and controlling (*rèn*) vessels. This pattern is characterized by pale menstrual flow, bright white facial complexion, lassitude of spirit, shortness of breath and laziness to speak, no thought of food or drink, and empty sagging in the smaller abdomen. MED Supplement qi and contain the blood; fortify the spleen and secure the thoroughfare (*chōng*) vessel. Use Center-Supplementing Qi-Boosting Decoction (*bǔ zhōng yì qì tāng*), Origin-Lifting Brew (*jǔ yuán jiān*), or Spleen-Returning Decoction (*guī pí tāng*). ACU Base treatment mainly on CV, SP, and ST. Select CV-6 (*qì hǎi*,

Sea of Qi), CV-4 (*guān yuán*, Pass Head), SP-10 (*xuè hǎi*, Sea of Blood), ST-36 (*zú sān lǐ*, Leg Three Li), BL-20 (*pí shū*, Spleen Transport), SP-6 (*sān yīn jiāo*, Three Yin Intersection), SP-2 (*dà dū*, Great Metropolis), and LR-8 (*qū quán*, Spring at the Bend); needle with supplementation and add moxa. [26: 540] [37: 439] [59: 10]

qi vacuity spontaneous sweating 气虚自汗 *qì xū zì hàn*: Spontaneous sweating attributed to qi vacuity and insecurity of the defensive exterior. Qi vacuity spontaneous sweating is associated with aversion to cold, fatigue and lack of strength, faint moderate pulse or large vacuous pulse. MED Boost qi and secure the exterior using Jade Wind-Barrier Powder (*yù píng fēng sǎn*) or Center-Supplementing Qi-Boosting Decoction (*bǔ zhōng yì qì tāng*). ACU Base treatment mainly on CV, back transport points, ST, LI, HT, and SI. Select LI-4 (*hé gǔ*, Union Valley), HT-6 (*yīn xī*, Yin Cleft), SI-3 (*hòu xī*, Back Ravine), CV-6 (*qì hǎi*, Sea of Qi), ST-36 (*zú sān lǐ*, Leg Three Li), BL-13 (*fèi shū*, Lung Transport), and BL-20 (*pí shū*, Spleen Transport); needle with supplementation and, if appropriate, moxa. See SPONTANEOUS SWEATING. [26: 540] [42: 186] [14: 174]

qi vacuity tinnitus 气虚耳鸣 *qì xū ěr míng*: Tinnitus attributed to qi vacuity. It is accompanied by fatigue and lack of strength and bright white facial complexion. The inch and bar pulses of the right wrist are larger than those of the left. MED Use formulas such as Four Gentlemen Panting Decoction (*chuǎn sì jūn zǐ tāng*) and Center-Supplementing Qi-Boosting Decoction (*bǔ zhōng yì qì tāng*). ACU See TINNITUS. [26: 540]

qi vacuity wilting 气虚痿 *qì xū wěi*: Wilting attributed to qi vacuity, arising when taxation fatigue or dietary irregularities cause damage to spleen-stomach qi, depriving the limbs of adequate nourishment. Qi vacuity wilting is characterized by weak wilting extremities and lack of strength to lift them. MED Supplement the spleen and boost qi using Four Gentlemen Panting Decoction (*chuǎn sì jūn zǐ tāng*) combined with Mysterious Two Powder (*èr miào sǎn*), or with variations of Center-Supplementing Qi-Boosting Decoction (*bǔ zhōng yì qì tāng*) or Six Gentlemen Decoction (*liù jūn zǐ tāng*). ACU Use the general points listed under WILTING and add qi-supplementing points such as CV-4 (*guān yuán*, Pass Head), CV-6 (*qì hǎi*, Sea of Qi), BL-43 (*gāo huāng shū*, Gao-Huang Transport), SP-3 (*tài bái*, Supreme White), and LU-9 (*tài yuān*, Great Abyss), needling with supplementation and adding moxa. [27: 541]

qi vomiting 气呕 *qì ǒu*: VOMITING that arises when anger or anxiety and general emotional imbalance cause binding depression of spleen qi. Signs include distention and fullness in the chest and diaphragm, a feeling of satiety without eating, and vomiting of ingested food. In some cases, the patient may eat normally and vomit during the night. [MED] Move qi and harmonize the spleen with formulas such as Clove and Aquilaria Diaphragm-Freeing Decoction (*dīng chén tòu gé tāng*). [ACU] Base treatment on alarm and lower uniting points of ST, and on PC, CV, back transport points and SP. Select CV-12 (*zhōng wǎn*, Center Stomach Duct), ST-36 (*zú sān lǐ*, Leg Three Li), PC-6 (*nèi guān*, Inner Pass), CV-6 (*qì hǎi*, Sea of Qi), BL-20 (*pí shū*, Spleen Transport), LR-3 (*tài chōng*, Supreme Surge), SP-6 (*sān yīn jiāo*, Three Yin Intersection), and SP-4 (*gōng sūn*, Yellow Emperor); needle with even supplementation and drainage. [26: 545] [46: 595, 658]

qi wheel 气轮 *qì lún*: One of the FIVE WHEELS. The white of the eye, i.e., the sclera. [26: 545] [27: 500] [97: 65]

quartan malaria 三日疟 *sān rì nüè*: See TRIPLE-YIN MALARIA. [WMC] quartan malaria ◇ Chin 三 *sān*, three; 日 *rì*, day; 疟 *nüè*, malaria. Malaria occurring at three days intervals. **Eng** *quartan*, occurring every fourth day. [26: 28]

quelling the liver 伐肝 *fā gān*: Synonym: *repress the liver*. A method of treatment used to control excessively exuberant liver qi invading the spleen. [MED] Liver-quelling medicinals include bupleurum (*chái hú*), unripe tangerine peel (*qīng pí*), costusroot (*guǎng mù xiāng*), and Buddha's hand (*fó shǒu gān*). Quelling the liver is similar to COURSING THE LIVER. [27: 264]

quick and slow supplementation and drainage 徐疾补泻 *xú jí bǔ xiè*, 疾徐补泻 *jí xú bǔ xiè*: A method of achieving supplementation and drainage that involves varying the relative speed of insertion and extraction of the needle. A slow insertion followed by a quick extraction supplements, whereas a quick insertion followed by a slow extraction drains. See NEEDLE MANIPULATION. [26: 560] [27: 341] [97: 490]

quicken 活 *huó*: To increase activity, to enliven. ◇ Chin 活 *huó*, move, be alive; move, enliven. **Eng** quicken, from *quick*, alive, moving, rapid, akin to from L. *vivus*.

quickening the blood 活血 *huó xuè*: A method of treatment used to stimulate blood flow and eliminate blood stasis. See DISPELLING STASIS AND QUICKENING THE BLOOD.

quickening the blood and engendering the new 活血生新 *huó xuè shēng xīn*: See DISPELLING STASIS AND QUICKENING THE BLOOD.

quickening the blood and dispelling stasis 活血祛瘀 *huó xuè qū yū*: See DISPELLING STASIS AND QUICKENING THE BLOOD.

quickening the blood and transforming stasis 活血化瘀 *huó xuè huà yū*: See DISPELLING STASIS AND QUICKENING THE BLOOD. [41: 246]

quickening the network vessels 活络 *huó luò*: Stimulating blood flow in the network vessels.

quiet 安 *ān*: To reduce movement or activity; to calm. ◇ Chin The ideogram 安 is a pictorial representation of a woman covered by a roof (a woman at home). It connotes security, peace, calm, and quiet.

quieting the center 安中 *ān zhōng*: Harmonizing the stomach or liver and stomach.

quieting the fetus 安胎 *ān tāi*: Treating *stirring fetus*, or safeguarding the fetus in women suffering from habitual miscarriage, or other otherwise prevent miscarriage. [26: 235]

quieting the heart 安心 *ān xīn*: See QUIETING THE SPIRIT.

quieting the spirit 安神 *ān shén*: A method of treatment used to address disquieted spirit (heart palpitations, insomnia, agitation, mania). See NOURISHING THE HEART AND QUIETING THE SPIRIT; QUIETING THE SPIRIT WITH HEAVY SETTLERS. [26: 235] [27: 284] [97: 222] [60: 286] [126: 681]

Spirit-Quieting Medicinals

Heavy settling spirit-quieting medicinals
朱砂 (*zhū shā*) cinnabar (Cinnabaris)
磁石 (*cí shí*) loadstone (Magnetitum)
龙骨 (*lóng gǔ*) dragon bone (Mastodi Ossis Fossilia)
龙齿 (*lóng chǐ*) dragon tooth (Mastodi Dentis Fossilia)
牡蛎 (*mǔ lì*) oyster shell (Ostreae Concha)
琥珀 (*hǔ pò*) amber (Succinum)
珍珠母 (*zhēn zhū mǔ*) mother-of-pearl (Concha Margaritifera)
珍珠 (*zhēn zhū*) pearl (Margarita)
紫石英 (*zǐ shí yīng*) amethyst/fluorite (Amethystum seu Fluoritum)

Heart-nourishing spirit-quieting medicinals
酸枣仁 (*suān zǎo rén*) spiny jujube (Ziziphi Spinosi Semen)
柏子仁 (*bǎi zǐ rén*) biota seed (Biotae Semen)
远志 (*yuǎn zhì*) polygala (Polygalae Radix)
茯神 (*fú shén*) root poria (Poria cum Pini Radice)
夜交藤 (*yè jiāo téng*) flowery knotweed stem (Polygoni Multiflori Caulis)
龙眼肉 (*lóng yǎn ròu*) longan flesh (Longanae Arillus)
莲子 (*lián zǐ*) lotus fruit/seed (Nelumbinis Fructus seu Semen)
五味子 (*wǔ wèi zǐ*) schisandra (Schisandrae Fructus)

合欢皮 (*hé huān pí*) silk tree bark (Albizziae Cortex)

夜合花 (*yè hé huā*) dwarf magnolia (Magnoliae Coco Flos)

灵芝 (*líng zhī*) ganoderma (Ganoderma)

quieting the spirit with heavy settlers 重镇安神 *zhòng zhèn ān shén*: A method of treatment used to address disquieted heart spirit (heart palpitations, fearful throbbing, insomnia, fright mania) using heavy mineral and shell medicinals. Heavy settling spirit-quieting formulas include Spirit-Quieting Pill (*ān shén wán*). [26: 442] [27: 285] [97: 419]

R

racing pulse 疾脉 *jí mài*: A pulse having seven or more beats per respiration, i.e., at least one beat or more per respiration than the rapid pulse. It is a sign of in exhaustion of yin and yang and original qi about to desert, and is observed in acute febrile disease and vacuity traxation. It is usually a critical sign. A racing pulse in a healthy pregnant women is a sign of imminent birth. [50: 1290] [27: 196] [97: 490]

raised chest 胸高 *xiōng gāo*: Abnormal elevation of the anterior chest; observed in PULMONARY DISTENTION. [29: 264]

raised-shoulder breathing 肩息 *jiān xī*: Raising of the shoulders to assist breathing in severe panting patterns. See GAPING MOUTH AND RAISED SHOULDERS. [26: 350]

raising pus and dispelling putridity 提脓祛腐 *tí nóng qū fǔ*: Treating welling-abscess *yōng* and other sores to draw out pus and reduce ulceration. Representative formulas include Five-to-Five Elixir (*wǔ wǔ dān*) or Nine-to-One Elixir (*jiǔ yī dān*).

raising the pot and removing the lid 提壶揭盖法 *tí hú jiē gài fǎ*: To free urine by diffusing the lung or by upraising. The lung together with the spleen, kidney, triple burner, and bladder are responsible for water metabolism and keep the waterways free and regulated. The lung governs qi, and is the upper source of the waterways. When lung qi is blocked, and depurative downbearing fails, this can cause qi transformation failure in other organs, causing hasty panting, fullness in the chest, inhibited urination, and puffy swelling. This is treated by the method of diffusing the lung and downbearing qi, which is referred to by the metaphor of raising the pot and removing the lid, the pot apparently having a hole in its bottom from which water drains only when the lid is removed. [25: 292] [50: 1486]

raking the firewood from beneath the cauldron 釜底抽薪 *fǔ dǐ chōu xīn*: A method of eliminating repletion heat by freeing the stool with cold-natured draining precipitants. See COLD PRECIPITATION; EMERGENCY PRECIPITATION TO PRESERVE YIN. [50: 1269]

rapid hungering 善饥 *shàn jī*, 易饥 *yì jī*: Tendency to become hungry soon after eating. See INCREASED EATING WITH RAPID HUNGERING.

rapid pulse 数脉 *shuò mài*: A rapid pulse has six beats per respiration. The rapid pulse is usually associated with heat, but may also be an indication of vacuity. A forceful rapid pulse indicates repletion heat and is most commonly seen in external heat (febrile) disease. A fine weak rapid pulse indicates effulgent yin vacuity fire. A large weak rapid pulse generally indicates qi vacuity. A rapid pulse is normal in infants, and a slippery rapid pulse is normal in pregnancy. **Similar pulses**: The rapid pulse is usually quite smooth-flowing, so it is often confused with a *slippery pulse*. However, the term "rapid" refers exclusively to the pace, whereas "slippery" denotes a quality. *The Bin-Hu Sphygmology* (*bīn hú mài xué*) (1564) clearly points out, "Rapid and slippery should not be considered as being the same; rapid refers to the pace only." A pulse having seven or more beats per respiration is known as a *racing pulse*. Its significance is basically the same as that of the rapid pulse, though the possibility of vacuity is higher. [6: 140] [27: 385] [97: 364]

rashness, impatience, and irascibility 急燥易怒 *jí zào yì nù*: A sign of binding depression of liver qi.

raw 生 *shēng*: *Synonym: crude*. Uncooked or unprocessed.

reachable sore 搭手 *dā shǒu*: An effusion of the back, so called because the patient can reach it with his or her own hand. See EFFUSION OF THE BACK. [27: 463] [97: 547]

rebellion 相侮 *xiāng wǔ*: In the doctrine of the five phases, a reversal of the restraining relationship, where one of the five phases is disproportionately strong and rebels against the phase that should normally restrain it. For example, wood is normally restrained by metal, but if it becomes too strong it will rebel against metal. Powerless to withstand the attack, metal will succumb. In terms of the bowels and viscera, this means that when the liver, normally restrained by the lung, becomes too strong, it will rebel against the lung and overcome it. [6: 30]

rebounding 引手 *yǐn shǒu*, 应指 *yìng zhǐ*: Springing back against the hand as pressure is released. Rebounding is a test used in external medicine to determines whether or not pus has formed. If a sore springs back after the pressure applied to it is released, there is pus. If the sore does not spring back immediately, there is no pus. [26: 133]

rectal prolapse hemorrhoids 脱肛痔 *tuō gāng zhì*: HEMORRHOIDS with prolapse of the rectum.

Prolapse of the rectum may occur in patients who have suffered from hemorrhoids for a long time, when repeated contractions of damp-heat evil leads to qi vacuity and loss of containing power. The condition is characterized by prolapse when straining during defecation with pain and bleeding, and in some cases with exudation of yellow watery fluid. MED Clear heat and transform dampness; boost qi and raise the fall. Use Rectum-Lifting Powder (*tí gāng sǎn*). ACU Base treatment mainly on back transport points GV, BL, ST, and LI. Select GV-20 (*bǎi huì*, Hundred Convergences), BL-25 (*dà cháng shū*, Large Intestine Transport), GV-1 (*cháng qiáng*, Long Strong), BL-35 (*huì yáng*, Meeting of Yang), BL-57 (*chéng shān*, Mountain Support), LI-4 (*hé gǔ*, Union Valley), LI-11 (*qū chí*, Pool at the Bend), and SP-9 (*yīn líng quán*, Yin Mound Spring); needle with drainage. [26: 646]

rectify 理 *lǐ*: To correct (counterflow, stagnant qi, or static blood). See RECTIFYING QI; RECTIFYING THE BLOOD.

rectifying qi 理气 *lǐ qì*: Correction of any morbidity of qi (qi stagnation, qi counterflow, qi vacuity, qi fall), and especially to treat qi stagnation or qi counterflow. See MOVING QI (which includes COURSING DEPRESSION AND RECTIFYING QI and HARMONIZING THE STOMACH AND RECTIFYING QI); DOWNBEARING COUNTERFLOW AND PRECIPITATING QI (which includes DOWNBEARING COUNTERFLOW AND CHECKING VOMITING and DOWNBEARING QI AND CALMING PANTING). [26: 594] [27: 270] [97: 506]

Qi-Rectifying Medicinals

陈皮 (*chén pí*) tangerine peel (Citri Exocarpium)

橘白 (*jú bái*) white tangerine peel (Citri Exocarpium Album)

橘红 (*jú hóng*) red tangerine peel (Citri Exocarpium Rubrum)

橘核 (*jú hé*) tangerine pip (Citri Semen)

橘络 (*jú luò*) tangerine pith (Citri Fructus Fasciculus Vascularis)

橘叶 (*jú yè*) tangerine leaf (Citri Folium)

化橘红 (*huà jú hóng*) Huazhou pomelo rind (Citri Grandis Exocarpium Rubrum)

青皮 (*qīng pí*) unripe tangerine peel (Citri Exocarpium Immaturum)

枳壳 (*zhǐ ké*) bitter orange (Aurantii Fructus)

枳实 (*zhǐ shí*) unripe bitter orange (Aurantii Fructus Immaturus)

川楝子 (*chuān liàn zǐ*) toosendan (Toosendan Fructus)

荔枝核 (*lì zhī hé*) litchee pit (Litchi Semen)

香附子 (*xiāng fù zǐ*) cyperus (Cyperi Rhizoma)

木香 (*mù xiāng*) saussurea (Saussureae (seu Vladimiriae) Radix), including the next three items

川木香 (*chuān mù xiāng*) Sichuan saussurea (Vladimiriae Souliei Radix)

广木香 (*guǎng mù xiāng*) costusroot (Saussureae Radix)

青木香 (*qīng mù xiāng*) vladimiria (Vladimiriae Radix)

乌药 (*wū yào*) lindera (Linderae Radix)

薤白 (*xiè bái*) Chinese chive (Allii Bulbus)

檀香 (*tán xiāng*) sandalwood (Santali Lignum)

沉香 (*chén xiāng*) aquilaria (Aquilariae Lignum)

柿蒂 (*shì dì*) persimmon calyx (Kaki Calyx)

甘松 (*gān sōng*) nardostachys (Nardostachydis Rhizoma et Radix)

佛手柑 (*fó shǒu gān*) Buddha's hand (Citri Sarcodactylidis Fructus)

佛手花 (*fó shǒu huā*) Buddha's hand flower (Citri Sarcodactylidis Flos)

刀豆 (*dāo dòu*) sword bean (Canavaliae Semen)

娑罗子 (*suō luó zǐ*) horse chestnut (Aesculi Fructus)

八月札 (*bā yuè zhá*) akebia (Akebiae Fructus)

玫瑰花 (*méi guī huā*) rose (Rosae Flos)

梅花 (*méi huā*) mume flower (Mume Flos)

九香虫 (*jiǔ xiāng chóng*) stinkbug (Aspongopus)

---

rectifying qi and harmonizing construction 理气和营 *lǐ qì hé yíng*: A method of treatment used to address binding depression of liver qi and construction-blood disharmony in the treatment of pathoconditions characterized by emotional depression, vexation and agitation, rib-side pain, qi stagnation in the chest, and in some cases distention of the breasts, menstrual irregularities, and menstrual pain. MED medicinals used include liver-coursing and qi rectifying medicinals such as bupleurum (*chái hú*), unripe tangerine peel (*qīng pí*), cyperus (*xiāng fù zǐ*), and toosendan (*chuān liàn zǐ*), combined with blood-nourishing, construction-harmonizing medicinals like tangkuei (*dāng guī*), peony (*sháo yào*), and salvia (*dān shēn*). Blood-quickening stasis-transforming medicinals such as corydalis (*yán hú suǒ*), carthamus (*hóng huā*), madder (*qiàn cǎo gēn*), and curcuma (*yù jīn*) may be added where pain is particularly pronounced or static blood signs are present. Conditions involving liver fire may call for the admixture of medicinals such as gardenia (*shān zhī zǐ*) and moutan (*mǔ dān pí*). A representative formula is Free Wanderer Powder (*xiāo yáo sǎn*). ACU Base treatment on PC, LR, and SP. Select PC-6 (*nèi guān*, Inner Pass), LR-3 (*tài chōng*, Supreme Surge), SP-6 (*sān yīn jiāo*, Three Yin Intersection), BL-18 (*gān shū*, Liver Transport), BL-17 (*gé shū*, Diaphragm Transport), BL-20 (*pí shū*, Spleen Transport), LR-14 (*qī mén*, Cycle Gate), and ST-36 (*zú sān lǐ*, Leg Three Li); needle with even supplementation and drainage. [6: 255]

rectifying qi and harmonizing the stomach 理气和胃 *lǐ qì hé wèi*: HARMONIZING THE STOMACH AND RECTIFYING QI.

rectifying the blood 理血 *lǐ xuè*: Correction of any blood-aspect pathologies; includes SUPPLE-MENTING THE BLOOD; COOLING THE BLOOD; DISPELLING STASIS AND QUICKENING THE BLOOD; WARMING THE BLOOD; STANCHING BLEEDING. [27: 274] [97: 506]

rectifying the center 理中 *lǐ zhōng*: A method of treatment used to regulate the stomach and spleen, especially WARMING THE CENTER AND DISSIPATING COLD.

red 赤 *chì*, 红 *hóng*: The color of pale cinnabar; the color of fire. Red is associated with fire in the five phases. Diagnostically, it is associated with fire or heat. Generally speaking, the darker the red, the more severe the heat, and in externally contracted disease, the deeper the level of penetration into the body. See also CRIMSON. ◇ Chin 赤 *chì*, red; according to *Explanation of Characters* (说文解字 *shuō wén jiě zì*), originally composed of 大 *dà*, great, above 火 *huǒ*, fire; *hóng*, red (sometimes denoting a color paler than *chì*) in premodern texts. [19: 13914] [48: 108]

red and white dysentery 赤白痢 *chì bái lì*: Dysentery with sticky stool that contains red blood and white pus. See DYSENTERY. [26: 302]

red and white turbidity 赤白浊 *chì bái zhuó*: *Synonym: two turbidities.* The generic term for RED TURBIDITY and WHITE TURBIDITY, in both of which a distinction is made between URINARY TURBIDITY and ESSENCE TURBIDITY. [26: 302] [27: 361] [97: 246]

red and white vaginal discharge 赤白带下 *chì bái dài xià*: Mixed red and white vaginal discharge, i.e., a discharge part white and part tinged with red, that flows continuously from the vagina. Red and white vaginal discharge is attributable to liver qi invading the stomach and damp-heat pouring into the thoroughfare (*chōng*), controlling (*rèn*), and girdling (*dài*) vessels. In modern practice, red and white vaginal discharge usually prompts tests for cancer. See LIVER CHANNEL DAMP-HEAT VAGINAL DISCHARGE; DAMP TOXIN VAGINAL DISCHARGE. [26: 302]

red and white wandering wind 赤白游风 *chì bái yóu fēng*: *Synonym: wandering wind.* A disease characterized by the sudden appearance, usually on the lips, eyelids, and earlobes, or the chest and abdomen or shoulder and back, of red or white cloud-shaped patches of smooth, puffy skin that feel hard to the touch, associated with burning sensation, numbness, and mild itching. Red and white wandering wind is attributed to spleen-lung dryness-heat or insecurity of exterior qi allowing wind evil to invade the interstices, cause conges-

tion, and disturb construction and defense. When the evil is stagnating in the blood aspect, the patches are red in color (RED WANDERING WIND); when stagnating in the qi aspect, the patches are white (WHITE WANDERING WIND). Usually there are no generalized signs, but abdominal pain, diarrhea, and vomiting may be observed. ⬚WMC⬚ angioneurotic edema (called also Quincke's edema, Milton's edema, wandering edema, angioedema, and giant urticaria). ⬚MED⬚ Treat by dissipating wind, clearing heat, and disinhibiting dampness, assisted by regulating construction and defense. Oral: Wind-Dispersing Powder (*xiāo fēng sǎn*). Topical: apply Jade Dew Powder (*yù lù sǎn*) or Golden Yellow Powder (*jīn huáng sǎn*). See also KIDNEY QI WANDERING WIND. [50: 693] [26: 662] [27: 471] [97: 586] [96: 110]

red areola surrounding the dark of the eye 乌轮赤晕 *wū lún chì yūn*, 抱轮红 *bào lún hong*, 赤带抱轮 *chì dài bào lún*: A condition characterized by reddening of the white of the eye in the area surrounding the dark of the eye in which "red blood threads" (i.e., blood vessels) are dimly distinguishable and do not disappear if pressure is applied. Red areola surrounding the dark of the eye it observed in a number of eye diseases including GREEN WIND INTERNAL OBSTRUCTION (glaucoma). ⬚WMC⬚ ciliary congestion. [26: 364]

red bayberry sore 杨梅疮 *yáng méi chuāng*: Sores that occur after LOWER BODY GAN and BUBO SORE, that are heralded by generalized heat [effusion], headache, and joint pain, that start with faint red areolas, and then develop into red bayberry patches, red bayberry pox, red bayberry papules, and everted-flower red bayberry. In the advanced stage, the toxin invades the bones, joints, and internal organs in what is called "red bayberry toxin bind." Red bayberry sores were first recorded in the Jin-Yuan period. By the Qing Dynasty, the disease was understood to be transmitted directly through sexual intercourse (by "essence transformation"), indirectly (by "qi transformation"), and from mother to fetus. ⬚WMC⬚ syphilis. ⬚MED⬚ Clear the blood and resolve toxin. Oral: One-Packet Red Bayberry Powder (*yáng méi yī jì sǎn*) or Smooth Greenbrier Mixture (*tǔ fú líng hé jì*). Topical: Gosling Yellow Powder (*é huáng sǎn*). [26: 776] [27: 487] [61: 279] [50: 715] [56: 330] [54: 406]

red blood threads 红赤血丝 *hóng chì xuè sī*: Red filiform markings in the white of the eye observed in blood-shot eyes (ciliary congestion). Compare RED AREOLA SURROUNDING THE DARK OF THE EYE.

reddening of the cheeks 颧红 *quán hóng*, 颧赤 *quán chì*, 两颧发赤 *liǎng quán fā chì*: Diffuse flushing of cheeks that usually occurs in liver-kidney yin depletion with vacuity fire flaming upward. Reddening of the cheeks is often seen in enduring illness and consumption. It usually recurs in the afternoon (hence also the term *tidal reddening of the face*) and is associated with tidal heat [effusion], vexing heat in the five hearts, red tongue with little liquid, and a forceless rapid fine pulse. NB: The term *reddening of the cheeks* is not conventionally used to denote rosy cheeks of healthy individuals. ⟨MED⟩ Enrich yin and subdue yang. Anemarrhena, Phellodendron, and Rehmannia Pill (*zhī bǎi dì huáng wán*) plus abalone shell (*shí jué míng*) and oyster shell (*mǔ lì*). ⟨ACU⟩ Base treatment mainly on KI and LR. Needle with supplementation at BL-23 (*shèn shū*, Kidney Transport), KI-3 (*tài xī*, Great Ravine), LR-3 (*tài chōng*, Supreme Surge), KI-6 (*zhào hǎi*, Shining Sea), and SP-6 (*sān yīn jiāo*, Three Yin Intersection), and with drainage at KI-1 (*yǒng quán*, Gushing Spring), HT-8 (*shào fǔ*, Lesser Mansion), LR-3 (*tài chōng*, Supreme Surge), and LR-2 (*xíng jiān*, Moving Between). See RED FACIAL COMPLEXION. [26: 1009] [25: 349] [46: 595, 622]

reddening of the eyes 目赤 *mù chì*: See RED EYES.

reddish urine 尿赤 *niào chì*: Synonym: *dark-colored urine*. Urine that is considerably darker than normal color; a sign of heat. Not to be confused with bloody urine. See URINE. ◇ Chin 尿 *niào*, urine; 赤 *chì*, red.

red dysentery 赤痢 *chì lì*: Dysentery with bloody stool, i.e., BLOOD DYSENTERY. See DYSENTERY. [27: 361] [97: 246]

red ears 耳赤 *ěr chì*: Pronounced flushing of the ears. Red face and ears indicate yang heat, and are observed in patterns such as LARGE INTESTINAL HEAT BIND.

red eyes 目赤 *mù chì*: From *Elementary Questions* (*sù wèn, wǔ cháng zhèng dà lùn*). Red whites of the eye of either or both eyes. *Zhāng's Clear View of Medicine* (*zhāng shì yī tōng*) states, "There are three [kinds of] red eyes: the first is wind assisting fire to become depressed in the upper body; the second is exuberant fire; the third is dryness damaging the liver." Sudden reddening of the eyes is observed in externally contracted wind-fire (wind-heat) and in HEAVEN-CURRENT RED EYE. In wind-fire patterns, the eyes are swollen and painful with hot tears and aversion to light. Accompanying signs include aversion to cold and heat effusion, headache and nasal congestion, a thin white tongue fur, and a rapid floating pulse. Heaven-current red eye, also associated with discharge, is marked by being contagious. Reddening of the eyes of gradual onset is observed in internal damage patterns such as a) liver heat attacking the upper body (liver fire flaming upward) marked by red whites

of eyes or RED AREOLA SURROUNDING THE DARK OF THE EYE; and b) liver-kidney yin vacuity or liver-lung yin vacuity, characterized by pale red whites of the eyes with mild intermittent pain and clouded vision. In alcoholics, red or yellow-red eyes are attributable to internally brewing liquor toxin. ⟨MED⟩ For wind-fire eye or heaven-curent red eye, course wind, discharge heat, and resolve toxin, use Wind-Expelling Heat-Dissipating Drink (*qū fēng sàn rè yǐn zi*). For liver heat attacking upward, clear the liver and drain fire, using Gentian Liver-Draining Decoction (*lóng dǎn xiè gān tāng*). For liver-kidney yin vacuity or liver-lung yin vacuity, enrich yin and nourish the blood, and clear the liver and downbear fire. Use Ten-Gem Decoction (*shí zhēn tāng*) which contains dried/ fresh rehmannia (*shēng dì huáng*), tangkuei (*dāng guī*), white peony (*bái sháo yào*), lycium root bark (*dì gǔ pí*), anemarrhena (*zhī mǔ*), moutan (*mǔ dān pí*), asparagus (*tiān mén dōng*), ophiopogon (*mài mén dōng*), ginseng (*rén shēn*), and licorice (*gān cǎo*). For internally brewing liquor toxin in alcoholics, clear heat and disinhibit dampness, using Capillaris and Poria (Hoelen) Five Powder (*yīn chén wǔ líng sǎn*). ⟨ACU⟩ Points in the region of the eye should only be given mild stimulation. For wind-fire eye or heaven-curent red eye, base treatment mainly on BL, GB, LI, and LR. Draim BL-1 (*jīng míng*, Bright Eyes), GB-20 (*fēng chí*, Wind Pool), and LI-4 (*hé gǔ*, Union Valley); prick Greater Yang (*tài yáng*), GV-23 (*shàng xīng*, Upper Star), and LU-11 (*shào shāng*, Lesser Shang) to bleed. For liver heat attacking upward, base treatment mainly on GB and LR. Select BL-18 (*gān shū*, Liver Transport), LR-2 (*xíng jiān*, Moving Between), GB-43 (*xiá xī*, Pinched Ravine), LR-3 (*tài chōng*, Supreme Surge), GB-1 (*tóng zǐ liáo*, Pupil Bone-Hole), GB-15 (*tóu lín qì*, (Head) Overlooking Tears), and Greater Yang (*tài yáng*); needle with drainage. For liver-kidney yin vacuity or liver-lung yin vacuity, base treatment mainly on KI, LR, BL, and GB. Select BL-1 (*jīng míng*, Bright Eyes), GB-37 (*guāng míng*, Bright Light), ST-1 (*chéng qì*, Tear Container), LI-4 (*hé gǔ*, Union Valley), SP-6 (*sān yīn jiāo*, Three Yin Intersection), KI-3 (*tài xī*, Great Ravine), KI-6 (*zhào hǎi*, Shining Sea), LR-3 (*tài chōng*, Supreme Surge), BL-18 (*gān shū*, Liver Transport), and BL-23 (*shèn shū*, Kidney Transport); needle with supplementation. See also TANGLED RED-THREAD VESSELS; RED AREOLA SURROUNDING THE DARK OF THE EYE; RED VESSELS INVADING THE EYE. [6: 125] [92: No. 468] [50: 402] [46: 596] [4: 140] [37: 465] [113: 468]

red face 面赤 *miàn chì*, 面红 *miàn hóng*: RED FACIAL COMPLEXION.

red face wind 赤面风 *chì miàn fēng*: A condition that begins with reddening and itching of the face, subsequently giving way to swelling and scorching heat. WMC allergic dermatitis (including drug-induced dermatitis). [26: 303]

red facial complexion 面色红 *miàn sè hóng*: Synonym: *red face*. A complexion redder than normal; a sign of heat. External wind-heat exterior patterns are characterized by a red face with pronounced heat effusion and mild aversion to cold, thirst, sweating, red sore swollen throat, a red tongue tip and margins, a thin yellow tongue fur, and a rapid floating pulse. Yang brightness (*yáng míng*) channel heat is marked by a *continuous full red facial complexion* (面色缘缘正赤 *miàn sè yuán yuán zhèng chì*) with high fever, sweating, aversion to heat rather than to cold, thirst with intake of fluids, a dry yellow tongue fur, and a large surging pulse. Heat entering construction-blood is characterized by *redness of the whole face* (满面通红 *mǎn miàn tōng hóng*) with a generalized heat [effusion] that is most pronounced at night, dry mouth with little intake of fluid, heart vexation and sleepless, periodic delirious speech, maculopapular eruptions, ejection of blood and spontaneous external bleeding, bloody stool, bloody urine, a red or crimson tongue body, and a fine rapid pulse. Yin vacuity internal heat is characterized by a somber white facial complexion with *postmeridian reddening of the cheeks*; (午后 @ 两颧发赤 *wǔ hòu liǎng quán fā chì*) this is associated with emaciation, dry mouth and throat dizziness, insomnia, tidal heat [effusion], night sweating, vexing heat in the five hearts, red tongue with scant fur, and fine rapid pulse. Vacuous yang floating astray (also called UPCAST YANG) is marked by *cheeks that are a floating red as if dabbed with rouge* (两颧泛红如妆 *liǎng quán fàn hóng rú zhuāng*) ("floating" describes how the patches constantly change location); this is observed in severe illnesses and is accompanied by generalized heat [effusion] despite a desire to keep well wrapped, thirst with liking for warm drinks, short hasty breathing, cold sweating, reversal cold of the limbs, clear urine and sloppy stool, pale lips and tongue, white or gray-black moist tongue fur, and a faint pulse on the verge of expiration. [6: 117] [92: No. 69] [29: 44]

red flaming sore 赤炎疮 *chì yán chuāng*: A disease characterized by the intermittent appearance over the whole body of small red speckles. Red flaming sore is attributable to wind-heat that invades the lung and becomes depressed in the skin or to heart fire invading the lung. MED Course wind, clear heat, and cool the blood. Take Ledebouriella Sage-Inspired Powder (*fáng fēng tōng shèng sǎn*) orally. [26: 303] [27: 74]

red flesh 赤肉 *chì ròu*: **1.** The dorsal aspect of the hands and feet that is dark in color, in contradistinction to WHITE FLESH, i.e., the paler flesh of the

palmar or plantar aspect. **2.** The deeper layer of flesh that is red in color (muscle). [25: 149]

red-hot needling 焠刺 *cuì cì*: FIRE NEEDLING. [27: 335]

red nose 鼻赤 *bí chì*, 赤鼻 *chì bí*: DRINKER'S NOSE. [27: 495] [97: 622]

red sore swollen eyes 眼睛红肿痛 *yǎn jīng hóng zhǒng tòng*: Observed, for example, in CINNABAR EYE.

red-thread clove sore 红丝疗 *hóng sī dīng*: A CLOVE SORE (*dīng chuāng*) with a red threadlike line running from it toward the trunk. If the thread is fine, recovery can be rapid. A thick long thread is an unfavorable sign, especially if there are signs of traveling. ACU Apply the treatment given under (*clove sore*) and prick the red thread from the tail upward with a three-edged needle to drain the malign blood. See CLOVE SORE; RUNNING YELLOW. [26: 475] [27: 469] [97: 242]

red thread mark 红缕赤痕 *hóng lǚ chì hén*: Small red markings on the surface of the skin composed of red thread-like lines up to a few millimeters long radiating from a central point. WMC spider nevi. Red threat marks are a sign of blood amassment creating distention. [6: 119]

red tongue 舌红 *shé hóng*: A tongue redder than normal. A red tongue indicates either vacuity heat or repletion heat. Crimson (deep red or maroon), is also associated with heat, but the added depth of color indicates that the heat is located in the construction or blood aspect. [6: 122] [27: 178] [97: 194]

red turbidity 赤浊 *chì zhuó*: **1.** Murky urine that is red in color. See BLOODY URINE. **2.** The discharge of a turbid substance containing blood from the urethra associated with burning or stabbing pain on urination, but no blood in the urine. This is one form of ESSENCE TURBIDITY. [26: 304]

reduced food intake 纳少 *nà shǎo*, 少食 *shǎo shí*, 胃纳减少 *wèi nà jiǎn shǎo*, 纳谷减退 *nà gǔ jiǎn tuì*: See POOR APPETITE.

reducing urine 缩尿 *suō niào*: A method of treatment used to address enuresis and frequent long voidings of clear urine. MED The most commonly used urine-reducing medicinals include mantis egg-case (*sāng piāo xiāo*), dioscorea (*shān yào*), rubus (*fù pén zǐ*), and alpinia (*yì zhì rén*). Certain essence-securing medicinals such as Cherokee rose fruit (*jīn yīng zǐ*), euryale (*qiàn shí*), and lotus stamen (*lián xū*) may also be used to reduce urine. Among formulas, Mantis Egg-Case Powder (*sāng piāo xiāo sǎn*) has the added action of promoting interaction between the heart and kidney, and is most used for enuresis in children. Stream-Reducing Pill (*suō quán wán*), which warms and supplements kidney qi, is used to treat copious urine in vacuity patterns in elderly patients. ACU Base treatment mainly on CV, SP, and back transport points. Select BL-23 (*shèn shū,* Kidney Transport), CV-4 (*guān yuán,* Pass Head), CV-3 (*zhōng jí,* Central Pole), SP-6 (*sān yīn jiāo,* Three Yin Intersection), and CV-2 (*qū gŭ,* Curved Bone)ⓜ; needle with supplementation and moxa. [6: 268] [4: 116]

red vaginal discharge 赤带 *chì dài:* The continuous dribbling discharge of a sticky mucus from the vagina that is red like blood, but not completely composed of blood. Red vaginal discharge arises when anxiety and thought damage the spleen, disturbing movement and transformation. It also arises when depression and anger damage the liver and liver depression transforms into fire, and blood thus fails to be stored and flows with damp-heat down to the girdling (*dài*) vessel. In modern clinical practice, red vaginal discharge is taken as a prompt for cancer tests. MED Clear the liver and support the spleen. Use variations of Free Wanderer Powder (*xiāo yáo săn*) combined with Gentian Liver-Draining Decoction (*lóng dăn xiè gān tāng*). ACU Base treatment on CV, GIV, SP, and LR. Select GB-26 (*dài mài,* Girdling Vessel), BL-30 (*bái huán shū,* White Ring Transport), CV-6 (*qì hăi,* Sea of Qi), SP-6 (*sān yīn jiāo,* Three Yin Intersection), BL-20 (*pí shū,* Spleen Transport), BL-18 (*gān shū,* Liver Transport), CV-3 (*zhōng jí,* Central Pole), SP-10 (*xuè hăi,* Sea of Blood), LR-2 (*xíng jiān,* Moving Between), and PC-5 (*jiān shĭ,* Intermediary Courier); needle with drainage. See LIVER CHANNEL DAMP-HEAT VAGINAL DISCHARGE; DAMP TOXIN VAGINAL DISCHARGE. [26: 303] [46: 690] [113: 298]

red vessels invading the eye 赤脉侵睛 *chì mài qīn jīng:* RED VESSELS SPREADING ACROSS THE EYE.

red vessels spreading across the eye 赤脉传睛 *chì mài chuán jīng: Synonym: red vessels invading the eye.* A pathocondition characterized by visible red vessels ramifying outward from the inner or outer canthus, sometimes stretching into the dark of the eye, and associated with dry itchy eyes, in some cases tearing and discharge. Red vessels invading the eye are attributable to ascendant hyperactivity of heart fire, kidney water vacuity, or triple burner accumulated heat. WMC ciliary hyperemia. **Repletion fire** is characterized by large thick red vessels, itching, dryness, a stabbing pain, and dry discharge and hot tears. MED Clear heat and drain fire. Use Three Yellows Heart-Draining Decoction (*sān huáng xiè xīn tāng*) plus forsythia (*lián qiào*), schizonepeta (*jīng jiè*), red peony (*chì sháo yào*), plantago seed (*chē qián zĭ*), mint (*bò hé*), and chrysanthemum (*jú huā*). **Vacuity fire** is characterized by pale red vessels, and only slight itching and pain. MED Enrich yin and downbear

fire. Use Heart-Supplementing Decoction (*bŭ xīn tāng*) or variations of Six-Ingredient Rehmannia Pill (*liù wèi dì huáng wán*). Compare TANGLED RED-THREAD VESSELS. [26: 303] [50: 695]

red wandering cinnabar 赤游丹 *chì yóu dān: Synonym: red wandering cinnabar toxin.* A type of INFANTILE CINNABAR TOXIN, attributed to contraction of heat in the uterus, heralded by generalized heat [effusion], crying, fright, and spasm, and characterized by the appearance of red swollen areolas the color of cinnabar that gradually spread and wander with no fixed location. Spreading from abdomen and back to the limbs is favorable; starting at the limbs and moving into the chest and abdomen is unfavorable. MED Clear heat and resolve toxin. Oral: In the initial stage, use Forsythia Drink (*lián qiào yĭn zi*) followed by Toxin-Dispersing Rhinoceros Beverage (*xiāo dú xī jiăo yĭn*). Topical: Remove malign blood with alum (*bái fán*), and then place thin slices of beef or goat's meat on the patches, and allow them to dry slightly before changing them. If the meat slices do not dry, use Agreeable Golden Yellow Powder (*rú yì jīn huáng săn*) mixed with the juice of indigo residue (*lán diàn*). See CINNABAR TOXIN. [50: 693] [26: 304] [27: 471] [97: 247]

red wandering wind 赤游风 *chì yóu fēng:* **1.** The red form of RED AND WHITE WANDERING WIND. **2.** FETAL HEAT CINNABAR TOXIN. [50: 693] [26: 662]

red wandering cinnabar toxin 赤游丹毒 *chì yóu dān dú:* RED WANDERING CINNABAR.

redworm 赤虫 *chì chóng:* See REDWORM DISEASE.

redworm disease 赤虫病 *chì chóng bìng:* From *The Origin and Indicators of Disease* (*zhū bìng yuán hòu lùn*). One of the NINE WORM DISEASES. A worm disease characterized by rumbling intestines, diarrhea, and sometimes stool containing pus and blood. [26: 305]

refloating the grounded ship 增水行舟 *zēng shuĭ xíng zhōu:* INCREASING WATER TO MOVE THE SHIP.

refuse pressure 拒按 *jù àn:* (Of pain or discomfort, especially in the chest or abdomen) to be exacerbated by pressure; as sign of interior repletion. [50: 728]

[region] below the heart 心下 *xīn xià:* The area below the heart, i.e., the stomach duct. See also HEART. [29: 266]

[region] below the lower extreme 下极之下 *xià jí zhī xià: Synonyms: nose pillar; nose beam.* The stem of the nose. [27: 66]

regular channel 正经 *zhèng jīng:* Any one of the TWELVE CHANNELS. [27: 84] [97: 141]

regularly interrupted pulse 代脉 *dài mài:* INTERMITTENT PULSE.

regular water 正水 *zhèng shuǐ*: From *Essential Prescriptions of the Golden Coffer* (*jīn guì yào lüè, shuǐ qì bìng mài zhèng bìng zhì*). WATER SWELLING arising when spleen-kidney yang vacuity allow water to collect in the interior and ascend to distress the lung. Regular water is marked by general water swelling, abdominal fullness, rapid panting, and a slow sunken pulse. The lung is the tip, whereas the spleen and kidney are the root. It is treated by fortifying the spleen, warming the kidney, and promoting qi absorption. See WATER SWELLING. [26: 181] [27: 419] [97: 140]

regulate 调 *tiáo*: To restore normal regular activity.

regulating menstruation 调经 *tiáo jīng*: A method of treatment used to eliminate menstrual irregularities such as ADVANCED MENSTRUATION, DELAYED MENSTRUATION, MENSTRUATION AT IRREGULAR INTERVALS, and PROFUSE MENSTRUATION or SCANT MENSTRUATION. [27: 287] [97: 494]

regulating qi 调气 *tiáo qì*: **1.** A method of treatment used to eliminate qi stagnation or qi counterflow, thus restoring the normal smooth flow of qi; to move or downbear qi. **2.** In acupuncture, the use of supplementation and drainage to balance yin and yang in the body and improve physiological functioning. [27: 271, 339] [97: 494]

reinforcing yang 助阳 *zhù yáng*: SUPPLEMENTING YANG.

relaxing tension 缓急 *huǎn jí*: See RELAXING TENSION AND RELIEVING PAIN.

relaxing tension and relieving pain 缓急止痛 *huǎn jí zhǐ tòng*: A method of treatment used to alleviate hypertonicity and pain with agents such as licorice (*gān cǎo*). For this purpose, licorice is often combined with white peony (*bái sháo yào*), which nourishes the blood and constrains yin, and emolliates the liver and relieves pain. [126: 833, 760]

repelled yang 格阳 *gé yáng*: See EXUBERANT YIN REPELLING YANG.

repelling foulness 辟秽 *bì huì*: A method of treatment used to eliminate foul turbidity.

replete metal failing to sound 金实不鸣 *jīn shí bù míng*: SUDDEN LOSS OF VOICE. [27: 162] [97: 347]

replete pulse 实脉 *shí mài*: A large pulse that is forceful at all levels; its beats are equally forceful when coming as when going away. Compare SURGING PULSE. [26: 820] [6: 142] [27: 193] [97: 368]

repletion 实 *shí*: The opposite of vacuity. See VACUITY AND REPLETION; REPLETION PATTERN.

repletion cold 寒实 *hán shí*: COLD REPLETION.

repletion constipation 实秘 *shí bì*: CONSTIPATION occurring in repletion patterns such as HEAT CONSTIPATION, PHLEGM CONSTIPATION, QI CONSTIPATION, etc. [26: 820] [27: 408] [97: 416]

repletion distention 实胀 *shí zhàng*: DISTENTION occurring in repletion patterns of qi stagnation and damp obstruction, brewing damp-heat, depressed heat and static blood, or food accumulation; characterized by a firm tender abdomen, constipation, yellow or reddish urine, and a forceful slippery rapid pulse. ⌷MED⌷ Treatment focuses on dispelling the evil. See HEAT DISTENTION; QI DISTENTION; BLOOD DRUM; FOOD DISTENTION. [26: 820] [27: 108] [97: 386]

repletion evil 实邪 *shí xié*: **1.** An evil giving rise to a repletion pattern; exuberant evil qi. *Elementary Questions* (*sù wèn, tōng píng xū shí lùn*) states, "When evil qi is exuberant, there is repletion. **2.** One of the FIVE EVILS. Evil qi transmitted from the child viscus in disease arising when the child steals the mother's qi. [26: 820]

repletion fire 实火 *shí huǒ*: Repletion heat patterns caused by exuberant evil heat. The most common repletion fire patterns are gastrointestinal repletion fire or liver-gallbladder repletion fire. They are characterized by high fever, headache, red eyes, bitter taste in the mouth, dry mouth, thirst with desire for cold drinks, vexation and agitation, rib-side pain, abdominal pain that refuses pressure, constipation, red tongue with dry yellow and sometimes prickly fur, and a rapid replete pulse. In severe cases, there is blood ejection or spontaneous external bleeding, or maculopapular eruptions. [26: 819] [27: 216] [97: 386]

repletion glomus 实痞 *shí pǐ*: Fullness, oppression, and sensation of blockage in the stomach duct attributed to stagnating evils. Repletion glomus can arise in damp turbidity obstruction, cold stagnating in the spleen and stomach, and binding of phlegm-food. It may also occur in patterns of liver qi depression or external evils lodged in the inner body. In severe cases, there may be pain, vomiting, constipation, or inability to eat. ⌷MED⌷ Regulate qi dynamic, dispel damp-phlegm, and free bowel qi. Use formulas such as Stomach-Calming Powder (*píng wèi sǎn*) or Unripe Bitter Orange and Glomus-Dispersing Pill (*zhǐ shí xiāo pǐ wán*). ⌷ACU⌷ Base treatment mainly on CV, ST, and SP. Main points: PC-6 (*nèi guān*, Inner Pass), ST-25 (*tiān shū*, Celestial Pivot), CV-12 (*zhōng wǎn*, Center Stomach Duct), CV-6 (*qì hǎi*, Sea of Qi), and ST-36 (*zú sān lǐ*, Leg Three Li). Selection of points according to pattern: For internal damp turbidity obstruction, add SP-9 (*yīn líng quán*, Yin Mound Spring), LR-13 (*zhāng mén*, Camphorwood Gate), and BL-20 (*pí shū*, Spleen Transport), needle with even supplementation and drainage and add moxa. For cold stagnating in the spleen and stomach, add BL-20 (*pí shū*, Spleen Transport), BL-21 (*wèi shū*, Stomach Transport), and CV-4 (*guān yuán*, Pass Head), needling with drainage and adding moxa. For phlegm and food binding internally, add ST-40 (*fēng lóng*, Bountiful Bulge), LI-4 (*hé gǔ*, Union Valley), and SP-4 (*gōng sūn*, Yellow Emperor), needling with drainage and adding moxa. For liver qi depression, add LR-3 (*tài chōng*, Supreme Surge), SP-6 (*sān yīn jiāo*, Three Yin Intersection), BL-18 (*gān shū*, Liver Transport), BL-17 (*gé shū*, Diaphragm Transport), BL-20 (*pí shū*, Spleen Transport), and LR-13 (*zhāng mén*, Camphorwood Gate), needling with drainage. For lodged external evils, add GB-20 (*fēng chí*, Wind Pool), TB-5 (*wài guān*, Outer Pass), and LI-4 (*hé gǔ*, Union Valley), needling with drainage and, for cold evil, moxa. [26: 820] [14: 155] [46: 594, 597, 602]

repletion heat 实热 *shí rè*: Signs include high fever, vexation and thirst with intake of fluid, constipation sometimes with abdominal pain that refuses pressure, yellow or reddish urine, dry yellow tongue fur, and a surging rapid pulse. [26: 821] [27: 216] [97: 369]

repletion hiccough 实呃 *shí è*: Powerful sonorous HICCOUGH associated with a large slippery pulse. Repletion hiccough is usually attributable to stomach repletion with fire, or phlegm-damp obstruction. The root cause may be damage to the stomach by voracious eating causing food to stagnate in the stomach duct. WMC observed in gastric neurosis and acute gastritis. MED Treat by harmonizing the stomach and downbearing qi, and by clearing stomach fire or transforming phlegm-damp. For stomach fire, use variations of Bamboo Leaf and Gypsum Decoction (*zhú yè shí gāo tāng*) or Minor Qi-Coordinating Decoction (*xiǎo chéng qì tāng*), adding persimmon calyx (*shì dì*) to downbear qi. For phlegm-damp, use Inula and Hematite Decoction (*xuán fù huā dài zhě shí tāng*) minus ginseng (*rén shēn*), raw licorice (*shēng gān cǎo*), and jujube (*dà zǎo*), plus poria (*fú líng*) and tangerine peel (*chén pí*). If the root cause is food damage, add stir-fried barley sprout (*mài yá*), stir-fried rice sprout (*gǔ yá*), crataegus (*shān zhā*), and medicated leaven (*shén qū*) to rectify qi and disperse food. ACU Base treatment mainly on ST, LR, and PC. Main points: BL-17 (*gé shū*, Diaphragm Transport), PC-6 (*nèi guān*, Inner Pass), CV-17 (*shān zhōng*, Chest Center), ST-36 (*zú sān lǐ*, Leg Three Li), CV-14 (*jù què*, Great Tower Gate), ST-25 (*tiān shū*, Celestial Pivot), and LR-3 (*tài chōng*, Supreme Surge). Selection of points according to cause: For stomach fire, add LI-4 (*hé gǔ*, Union Valley) and ST-44 (*nèi tíng*, Inner Court). For phlegm-damp, add ST-40 (*fēng lóng*, Bountiful Bulge) and SP-9 (*yīn líng quán*, Yin Mound Spring). For food damage, add CV-10 (*xià wǎn*,

Lower Stomach Duct), Li Inner Court (*lǐ nèi tíng*), and CV-21 (*xuán jī*, Jade Swivel); Drain all points. [26: 820] [50: 995] [37: 308] [113: 76] [80: 302] [46: 662]

repletion is treated by draining 实则泻之 *shí zé xiè zhī*: From *Elementary Questions* (*sù wèn, sān bù jiǔ hóu lùn*). Disease patterns that arise when evil qi is exuberant and right qi is not debilitated (e.g., external contractions, phlegm-rheum, static blood, food stagnation, and cold accumulation patterns) are treated by methods that remove the evil qi such as resolving the exterior, dispelling phlegm, quickening the blood and transforming stasis, softening hardness, draining precipitation, and abductive stagnation. [27: 238] [97: 369]

repletion is treated by draining the child 实则泻其子 *shí zé xiè qí zǐ*: Use of the mother-child, i.e., the engendering, relationship of the five phases involving the draining of the viscus that is the child of a viscus affected by repletion. For example, since liver-wood engenders heart-fire, the liver is the mother and the heart is the child. Hence, liver repletion can be treated not only by draining the liver, but also by draining heart-fire. Thus, for example, the method of draining heart fire can be combined with that of calming and draining the liver to treat repletion fire signs such as headache, dizziness, tinnitus, rashness, impatience and irascibility, red face and red ears, scorching pain in the chest and rib-side, yellow or reddish urine, bitter taste in the mouth, constipation, yellow tongue fur, and a rapid stringlike pulse. [26: 820] [97: 369]

repletion panting 实喘 *shí chuǎn*: PANTING due to exuberant evil qi repletion. Repletion panting is attributable to congestion of lung qi and impairment of depurative downbearing by six excesses invading the body, depressed phlegm-fire, or water rheum intimidating the heart. It is of rapid onset and short duration, and characterized by forceful, rough, hasty rapid breathing. See WIND-COLD RAPID PANTING; COLD PANTING; HEAT PANTING; PHLEGM PANTING; WATER PANTING; FIRE DEPRESSION PANTING. [26: 820] [6: 157] [27: 214] [97: 369]

repletion pattern 实证 *shí zhèng*: Any condition in which the presence of an evil is resisted by the body; the opposite of VACUITY PATTERN. Repletion patterns are attributed to external evils, water-damp, phlegm-rheum, static blood, worm accumulations, or food accumulations. They reflect the nature of the evil (e.g., cold being characterized by pale or green-blue complexion, clear thin cold fluids), and the location (e.g., stomach disease being marked by vomiting, belching etc., or exterior disease being characterized by heat effusion, aversion to cold, and sweating). Most importantly, however, there are signs of right qi fighting the evil such as pulses that are forceful at the deep level (e.g., rapid surging pulses, slippery stringlike pulses, and large replete pulses), pain or discomfort that refuses pressure, and sudden onset of disease. [26: 821]

repletion swelling 实肿 *shí zhǒng*: See WATER SWELLING.

repletion with vacuity complication 实中夹虚 *shí zhōng jiā xū*: Disease patterns characterized by evil exuberance and vacuity of right, i.e., disease patterns caused by repletion evils, but in which there are also signs of vacuity. For example, drum distention characterized by abdominal distention, inhibited stool and urine, emaciation, withered-yellow facial complexion, reduced food intake, shortness of breath and lack of strength, and a fine stringlike pulse, repletion pattern of binding depression of qi and blood complicated by insufficiency of the spleen and kidney. [26: 820] [97: 369]

repress the liver 抑肝 *yì gān*: See QUELLING THE LIVER.

residual heat 余热 *yú rè*: The continuing presence of heat, as manifest if heat and dryness signs, after its abatement in heat (febrile) disease.

residual screen 宿翳 *sù yì*: A screen scar left when any disease of the dark of the eye manifesting in redness, soreness, and aversion to light has abated. [MED] Supplement vacuity and drain repletion; brighten the eyes and abate screens. Use Abalone Shell Powder (*shí jué míng sǎn*) as oral medication; apply Seven-Jewel Powder (*qī bǎo sǎn*) topically. [ACU] Main points: TB-23 (*sī zhú kōng*, Silk Bamboo Hole), BL-2 (*zǎn zhú*, Bamboo Gathering), Thumb Bone Hollow (*dà gǔ kōng*), and Little Finger Bone Hollow (*xiǎo gǔ kōng*). For repletion, add TB-20 (*jiǎo sūn*, Angle Vertex), BL-1 (*jīng míng*, Bright Eyes), and GB-41 (*zú lín qì*, Foot Overlooking Tears), needling with drainage and retaining the needles for 20–30 minutes. For vacuity, add BL-18 (*gān shū*, Liver Transport), BL-23 (*shèn shū*, Kidney Transport), and KI-3 (*tài xī*, Great Ravine), needling with supplementation (needles can be retained for 10 minutes). [26: 563] [37: 468]

resolve 解 *jiě*: To terminate (disease patterns), eliminate (evils), or free (parts of the body from evils). "Resolve" appears in the following terms: resolve the exterior (liberate it from an evil): resolve the flesh (liberate them from an evil); resolve toxin (dispel); resolve depression (relieve, dispel). ◊ Chin 解 *jiě* consists of a horn 角 *jiǎo*, a knife 刀 *dāo*, and a bull 牛 *niú*. Its original meaning may have been a knife that was made from bovine horn, or the act of separating the horn from the bull. Its meaning in everyday Chinese is that of to separate, untie, liberate, relieve, and dispel.

resolving both exterior and interior 表里双解 *biǎo lǐ shuāng jiě*: A method of treatment used to address interior and exterior patterns at the same time. There are two main forms: (1) Treating exterior evils in the outer body with repletion accumulation in the interior marked by aversion to cold, heat effusion, abdominal distention and pain, nausea and constipation, and a slippery floating pulse. A representative formula is Magnolia Bark Seven Agents Decoction (*hòu pò qī wù tāng*), which contains Cinnamon Twig Decoction (*guì zhī tāng*) minus peony (*sháo yào*) to resolve the exterior, and Magnolia Bark Three Agents Decoction (*hòu pò sān wù tāng*) to treat the interior. (2) Treating exuberant interior heat with a concurrent exterior pattern, marked by high fever without sweating, red face and eyes, generalized hypertonicity, dry nose, thirst, bitter taste in the mouth, vexation and agitation, delirious speech, dry tongue, and a rapid surging pulse. A representative formula is Three Yellows and Gypsum Decoction (*sān huáng shí gāo tāng*) in which ephedra (*má huáng*) and litsea (*dòu chǐ jiāng*) resolve the exterior, while gypsum (*shí gāo*), scutellaria (*huáng qín*), coptis (*huáng lián*), and gardenia (*shān zhī zǐ*) clear the interior. See RESOLVING THE EXTERIOR. [50: 871]

resolving depression 解郁 *jiě yù*: COURSING DEPRESSION AND RECTIFYING QI.

resolving tetany 解痉 *jiě jìng*: A method of treatment used to address TETANIC DISEASE characterized by signs such as tremor, convulsions, or arched-back rigidity with liver-calming, settling and subduing, and wind-dispelling agents. See EXTINGUISHING WIND; TETANY. [26: 802] [27: 268] [97: 605]

resolving the exterior 解表 *jiě biǎo*: A method of treatment used to eliminate evil from the FLESHY EXTERIOR by effusing sweat (see SWEATING[2]). Exterior-resolving medicinals include schizonepeta (*jīng jiè*), ledebouriella (*fáng fēng*), notopterygium (*qiāng huó*), perilla leaf (*zǐ sū yè*), fresh ginger (*shēng jiāng*), scallion white (*cōng bái*), ephedra (*má huáng*), and cinnamon twig (*guì zhī*). The method of resolving the exterior takes various forms depending on the evil. See the entries listed below.

Resolving the Exterior

RESOLVING THE EXTERIOR WITH COOLNESS AND ACRIDITY (*xīn liáng jiě biǎo*)

RESOLVING THE EXTERIOR WITH WARMTH AND ACRIDITY (*xīn wēn jiě biǎo*)

ENRICH YIN AND RESOLVE THE EXTERIOR (*zī yīn jiě biǎo*)

BOOSTING QI AND RESOLVING THE EXTERIOR (*bǔ qì jiě biǎo*)

ASSISTING YANG AND RESOLVING THE EXTERIOR
(zhù yáng jiě biǎo)
RESOLVING THE FLESH (jiě jī)
OUTTHRUSTING PAPULES (tòu zhěn)
COURSING THE EXTERIOR (shū biǎo)

ACU Base treatment mainly on LU, LI, GB, and TB. Main points: GV-20 (bǎi huì, Hundred Convergences), GB-20 (fēng chí, Wind Pool), and TB-5 (wài guān, Outer Pass). Point selection according to pattern: For wind-cold, add BL-11 (dà zhù, Great Shuttle), GV-16 (fēng fǔ, Wind Mansion), BL-12 (fēng mén, Wind Gate), LI-4 (hé gǔ, Union Valley), and LU-7 (liè quē, Broken Sequence); needle with drainage and moxa. For wind-heat, add GV-14 (dà zhuī, Great Hammer), LI-4 (hé gǔ, Union Valley), LI-11 (qū chí, Pool at the Bend), LU-5 (chǐ zé, Cubit Marsh), and LU-10 (yú jì, Fish Border); needle with drainage and prick LU-11 (shào shāng, Lesser Shang) to bleed with a three-edged needle. [26: 801]

resolving the exterior with coolness and acridity 辛涼解表 xīn liáng jiě biǎo: A method of treatment used to address exterior heat patterns with mild aversion to cold and pronounced heat signs, thirst, red sore pharynx, red tongue with dry thin white fur, and rapid floating pulse. The main medicinals are mint (bò hé), mulberry leaf (sāng yè), fermented soybean (dàn dòu chǐ), arctium (niú bàng zǐ), pueraria (gé gēn), and tamarisk (chēng liǔ),

---

Cool Acrid Exterior-Resolving Agents

薄荷 (bò hé) mint (Menthae Herba)
桑叶 (sāng yè) mulberry leaf (Mori Folium)
淡豆豉 (dàn dòu chǐ) fermented soybean (Glycines Semen Fermentatum Insulsum)
牛蒡子 (niú bàng zǐ) arctium (Arctii Fructus)
葛根 (gé gēn) pueraria (Puerariae Radix)
柽柳 (chēng liǔ) tamarisk (Tamaricis Ramulus et Folium)

Of these, mint (bò hé), mulberry leaf (sāng yè), fermented soybean (dàn dòu chǐ), and arctium (niú bàng zǐ) are the most commonly used. Mint has the strongest sweat-effusing and heat-abating effect of all cool exterior-resolving medicinals. Also, mulberry leaf can clear lung and liver heat and is thus particularly suitable for patterns involving headache, red eyes and cough. Fermented soybean is effective in outthrusting evils and abating heat effusion. Arctium has the additional effect of clearing the throat, promoting lung qi diffusion, and clearing phlegm-heat. Pueraria is suitable for patterns also involving diarrhea and stiffness in the

neck and back. Tamarisk may be used to outthrust papules in measles and can also dispel wind-damp. In cool acrid exterior resolution, the emphasis is on cool rather than acrid. For intense heat patterns, medicinals that clear heat and resolve toxin such as scutellaria (huáng qín), gardenia (shān zhī zǐ), lonicera (jīn yín huā), forsythia (lián qiào), isatis root (bǎn lán gēn), and dandelion (pú gōng yīng) may also be used. The use of certain warm exterior-resolving medicinals such as schizonepeta (jīng jiè), ledebouriella (fáng fēng), notopterygium (qiāng huó), and ephedra (má huáng) is not excluded in the treatment of exterior heat patterns when used with large quantities of heat-clearing medicinals. For example, Lonicera and Forsythia Powder (yín qiào sǎn) includes schizonepeta, and Notopterygium, Arctium, Dandelion, and Mint Decoction (qiāng bàng pú bò tāng) includes notopterygium although both are cool acrid exterior-resolving formulas. Cool acrid exterior-resolving formulas include Lonicera and Forsythia Powder (yín qiào sǎn), Mulberry Leaf and Chrysanthemum Beverage (sāng jú yǐn), and Notopterygium, Arctium, Dandelion, and Mint Decoction (qiāng bàng pú bò tāng). The most commonly used is Lonicera and Forsythia Powder. Notopterygium, Arctium, Dandelion, and Mint Decoction, a formula tested in modern clinical practice, contains cool and warm acrid medicinals, with the addition of heat-clearing toxin-resolving medicinals. For treatment of measles, see OUTTHRUSTING PAPULES. See also RESOLVING THE EXTERIOR; WIND-HEAT. [26: 296] [6: 247]

resolving the exterior with warmth and acridity 辛温解表 xīn wēn jiě biǎo: To treat exterior cold patterns marked by marked aversion to cold, pronounced headache and aching bones, high or low fever moist white tongue fur, tight floating pulse, and absence of any heat signs such as red tongue, dry mouth, or red sore swollen tongue. MED The main warm acrid exterior-resolving medicinals are listed below.

Warm Acrid Exterior-Resolving Agents

麻黄 (má huáng) ephedra (Ephedrae Herba)
桂枝 (guì zhī) cinnamon twig (Cinnamomi Ramulus)
紫苏叶 (zǐ sū yè) perilla leaf (Perillae Folium)
荆芥 (jīng jiè) schizonepeta (Schizonepetae Herba et Flos)
生姜 (shēng jiāng) fresh ginger (Zingiberis Rhizoma Recens)
防风 (fáng fēng) ledebouriella (Ledebouriellae Radix)
羌活 (qiāng huó) notopterygium (Notopterygii Rhizoma)

连须葱白 (*lián xū cōng bái*) scallion white with root (Allii Fistulosi Bulbus cum Radice)

Of these, schizonepeta (*jīng jiè*) and ledebouriella (*fáng fēng*) are the most commonly used. Notopterygium (*qiāng huó*) possesses a much stronger sweat-effusing heat-abating and pain-relieving effect than either of these, and is mainly prescribed for severe joint pain. Fresh ginger (*shēng jiāng*) and scallion white (*cōng bái*) are often used in combination with other warm acrid exterior-resolving medicinals, but may also be used alone. Perilla (*zǐ sū yè*) warms and dissipates, and can also harmonize the center; it is mainly used in exterior cold patterns where gastrointestinal signs are also present. Ephedra (*má huáng*) is mainly used in exterior cold patterns where cough, panting, or water swelling are also present. Cinnamon twig (*guì zhī*) and white peony (*bái sháo yào*) are used in exterior cold patterns involving construction-defense disharmony. The main formulas are Ephedra Decoction (*má huáng tāng*), Cinnamon Twig Decoction (*guì zhī tāng*), and Schizonepeta and Ledebouriella Toxin-Vanquishing Powder (*jīng fáng bài dú sǎn*). Ephedra Decoction is for repletion patterns with cough and panting. Cinnamon Twig Decoction is for patterns of construction-defense disharmony, exterior vacuity and heat effusion unabated by sweating. Schizonepeta and Ledebouriella Toxin-Vanquishing Powder is used for general colds and influenza caused attributable to wind-cold. See also RESOLVING THE EXTERIOR; WIND-COLD. [6: 246] [26: 296]

resolving the flesh 解肌 *jiě jī*: A method of treatment used to address exterior patterns marked by sweating. Warm acrid flesh-resolving formulas such as Cinnamon Twig Decoction (*guì zhī tāng*) are used when there is headache, heat effusion, sweating, aversion to cold, noisy nose, dry retching, weak floating pulse, white glossy tongue fur, and no thirst and drinking. Cool acrid flesh-resolving formulas such as Bupleurum and Pueraria Flesh-Resolving Decoction (*chái gé jiě jī tāng*) are used for pronounced generalized heat [effusion], slight aversion to cold, slight sweating, thirst, thin yellow tongue fur, and a rapid floating pulse. Flesh-resolving formulas help, without additional clothing or bedclothes, to encourage a mild generalized sweat that brings about resolution. See RESOLVING THE EXTERIOR. [27: 248] [26: 801] [44: 278]

respiration 呼吸 *hū xī*: BREATHING.

respiratory supplementation and drainage 呼吸补泻 *hū xī bǔ xiè*: A method of achieving supplementation and drainage that involves asking the patient to breath in or out on insertion and extraction of the acupuncture needle. Insertion on exhalation and extraction on inhalation supplement, whereas insertion on inhalation and extraction on exhalation drain. See NEEDLE MANIPULATION.

restore flow 通 *tōng*: See FREE.

restraining 相克 *xiāng kè*: The sequence in which the five phases keep each other in check, i.e., wood (liver) → earth (spleen) → water (kidney) → fire (heart) → metal (lung) → wood (liver). When the restraining cycle breaks down, the resulting disharmony can be explained in terms of the REBELLION or OVERWHELMING. [6: 29]

retained cupping 留罐法 *liú guàn fǎ*: STATIONARY CUPPING.

retainer 约束 *yuē shù*: EYELID.

retarded closure of the fontanel gate 囟门迟闭 *xìn mén chí bì*: See UNUNITED SKULL.

retching 呕 *ǒu*: See VOMITING.

retching of blood 呕血 *ǒu xuè*: The bringing up of blood with relatively little food from the stomach. Retching of blood is attributed to anger damaging the liver, excessive liquor consumption, dietary irregularities and taxation fatigue damaging the spleen and stomach, or sexual taxation damaging the kidney causing lower body vacuity and upper body exuberance. MED For anger damaging the liver, treat by coursing the liver and draining fire. Use Bupleurum Liver-Coursing Powder (*chái hú shū gān sǎn*) plus wine-processed rhubarb (*dà huáng*) or Moutan and Gardenia Free Wanderer Powder (*dān zhī xiāo yáo sǎn*). For excessive liquor consumption with accumulated heat stirring the blood, treat by draining fire and stanching bleeding, using Coptis and Pueraria Flower Pill (*gé huáng wán*). For dietary irregularities or taxation fatigue damaging the spleen, fortify the spleen and contain the blood with Spleen-Returning Decoction (*guī pí tāng*) with judicious addition of agrimony (*xiān hè cǎo*), bletilla (*bái jí*), and cuttlefish bone (*hǎi piāo xiāo*). For sexual taxation damaging the kidney with lower body vacuity and upper body exuberance, with signs such as vexation, agitation, and thirst, red face and cold lower extremities, base treatment mainly on supplementing the kidney. Use Six-Ingredient Rehmannia Pill (*liù wèi dì huáng wán*) plus cinnamon bark (*ròu guì*) and schisandra (*wǔ wèi zǐ*) combined with Pulse-Engendering Powder (*shēng mài sǎn*). See VOMITING; BLOOD EJECTION. [26: 846] [27: 420] [97: 276]

retention of dead fetus 胎死不下 *tāi sǐ bù xià*, 死胎不下 *sǐ tāi bù xià*: Failure to expel a fetus that has died in the uterus. This may happen at any time during pregnancy or during labor. Retention of dead fetus is attributable either to qi-blood vacuity or to uterine stasis obstruction. **Qi-blood vacuity** retention of a dead fetus is characterized by discontinuation of growth and slight shrinkage of the abdomen, pale red discharge, fatigued essence-spirit, somber complexion, and poor appetite with bad breath. MED Treat by supplementing qi and boosting the blood, assisted by precipitating the fetus, using formulas such as Child-Curing Powder (*liáo ér sǎn*), which contains ginseng (*rén shēn*), tangkuei (*dāng guī*), achyranthes (*niú xī*), frankincense (*rǔ xiāng*), myrrh (*mò yào*), and common dysosma (*guǐ jiù*). **Static blood obstruction** retention of dead fetus is characterized by cessation of movement of the fetus and a discharge of purple-black blood from the vagina. When the fetus dies shortly before birth, lumbar pain, and fullness and oppression in the chest with panting, and a dark green-blue complexion are observed. MED Move the blood and dispel stasis with formulas such as Falling Flower Brew (*tuō huā jiān*), which contains tangkuei (*dāng guī*), ligusticum (*chuān xiōng*), cinnamon bark (*ròu guì*), achyranthes (*niú xī*), plantago (*chē qián*), and carthamus (*hóng huā*). ACU Base treatment mainly on LI, CV, and SP. Select LR-3 (*tài chōng*, Supreme Surge), LI-4 (*hé gǔ*, Union Valley), SP-6 (*sān yīn jiāo*, Three Yin Intersection), CV-12 (*zhōng wǎn*, Center Stomach Duct), and CV-6 (*qì hǎi*, Sea of Qi) to move qi, quicken blood, and expel the fetus. Use filiform needles, and needle more than moxa. Selection of points according to pattern: For qi-blood vacuity, add ST-36 (*zú sān lǐ*, Leg Three Li), CV-4 (*guān yuán*, Pass Head), BL-20 (*pí shū*, Spleen Transport), and BL-21 (*wèi shū*, Stomach Transport); needle with supplementation. For static blood obstruction, add SP-8 (*dì jī*, Earth's Crux) and SP-10 (*xuè hǎi*, Sea of Blood); needle with even supplementation and drainage or with drainage. [26: 253] [27: 450] [97: 179] [37: 414] [46: 594–5]

retention of the lochia 恶露不下 *è lù bù xià*: *Synonym: postpartum retention of the lochia.* Absence of normal postpartum discharge. Retention of the lochia is when cold evil exploits the sudden vacuity of qi and blood created by childbirth, and invades the uterine vessels, where it congeals and causes blood stasis. It may also arise in patients with constitutional vacuity when damage to qi and blood through childbirth causes sluggish movement of the blood. **Cold qi invading the uterus** is marked by smaller-abdominal fullness with stabbing pain at irregular intervals. WMC lochioschesis, lochiostasis. MED Dissipate cold, quicken the blood, and transform stasis. Use variations of Engendering Transformation Decoction (*shēng huà tāng*). ACU Base treatment mainly on CV and SP. Select CV-3 (*zhōng jí*, Central Pole), ST-30 (*qì chōng*, Qi Thoroughfare), SP-8 (*dì jī*, Earth's Crux), CV-4 (*guān yuán*, Pass Head), and SP-6 (*sān yīn jiāo*, Three Yin Intersection); needle with supplementation and add moxa. **Vacuity** is characterized by intermittent or continual unabating mild smaller-abdominal distention without

pain. MED Supplement qi and blood with formulas such as Eight-Gem Decoction (*bā zhēn tāng*) plus blast-fried ginger (*páo jiāng*) and cinnamon bark (*ròu guì*). ACU Base treatment mainly on CV, SP, ST, and back transport points. Select CV-6 (*qì hǎi*, Sea of Qi), BL-20 (*pí shū*, Spleen Transport), BL-17 (*gé shū*, Diaphragm Transport), ST-36 (*zú sān lǐ*, Leg Three Li), SP-6 (*sān yīn jiāo*, Three Yin Intersection), CV-3 (*zhōng jí*, Central Pole), SP-10 (*xuè hǎi*, Sea of Blood), and SP-8 (*dì jī*, Earth's Crux); needle with supplementation and add moxa. See POSTPARTUM BLOOD DIZZINESS; POSTPARTUM PANTING; POSTPARTUM VACUITY SWELLING OF THE LIMBS; POSTPARTUM FEARFUL THROBBING; THREE POSTPARTUM SURGES; POSTPARTUM RAVING AND HALLUCINATION. [26: 579] [50: 618] [97: 462] [27: 452] [59: 179]

retention of the afterbirth 胞衣不下 *bāo yī bù xià*, 胎衣不下 *tāi yī bù xià*: Failure of the afterbirth to be discharged within half an hour after birth; attributable to major qi vacuity. This was traditionally treated by introducing the hand into the womb and following the umbilical cord to its end to locate the placenta, which was then detached from the uterus. This was followed by medicinal therapy and/or acupuncture. WMC retained placenta; incarcerated placenta. MED Use Perfect Major Supplementation Decoction (*shí quán dà bǔ tāng*). ACU Base treatment mainly on CV, GB, LI, SP, BL, and empirical points. Select CV-3 (*zhōng jí*, Central Pole), GB-21 (*jiān jǐng*, Shoulder Well), LI-4 (*hé gǔ*, Union Valley), SP-6 (*sān yīn jiāo*, Three Yin Intersection), BL-60 (*kūn lún*, Kunlun Mountains); needle with even supplementation and drainage or with drainage. Moxa Solitary Yin (*dú yīn*). For pronounced vacuity cold, pole CV-6 (*qì hǎi*, Sea of Qi) and CV-4 (*guān yuán*, Pass Head). [26: 451, 453] [97: 411] [59: 169]

retracted external kidney 外肾缩入 *wài shèn suō rù*: Retraction of the male genitals. See RETRACTED GENITALS.

retracted genitals 阴缩 *yīn suō*, 阳缩 *yáng suō*, 缩阴 *suō yīn*, 缩阳 *suō yáng*: The drawing into the body of the anterior yin (i.e., the genitals) in either males or females. It may be the result of cold entering the reverting yin (*jué yīn*), yang brightness (*yáng míng*) heat entering the reverting yin, or vacuity fall of original qi due to great vomiting and diarrhea. **Cold entering the reverting yin** is associated with cold pain and tension in the lesser abdomen. Other signs include fear of cold and cold limbs, and, in severe cases, green-blue lips and curled tongue, heavy body and body pains, long clear voidings of urine or possibly incontinence, and clear-food diarrhea.

MED Warm and dissipate the evil with Tangkuei Counterflow Cold Decoction (*dāng guī sì nì tāng*). ACU Base treatment mainly on CV and LR. Select LR-12 (*jí mài*, Urgent Pulse), CV-6 (*qì hǎi*, Sea of Qi), CV-4 (*guān yuán*, Pass Head), and LR-1 (*dà dūn*, Large Pile); needle with supplementation and add moxa. **Yang brightness heat evil entering the reverting yin** is characterized by yang brightness heat signs including constipation. MED Treat by swift precipitation with Major Qi-Coordinating Decoction (*dà chéng qì tāng*). ACU Base treatment mainly on ST, LR, and GB. Select ST-44 (*nèi tíng*, Inner Court), ST-36 (*zú sān lǐ*, Leg Three Li), LI-4 (*hé gǔ*, Union Valley), LR-3 (*tài chōng*, Supreme Surge), LR-2 (*xíng jiān*, Moving Between), and GB-34 (*yáng líng quán*, Yang Mound Spring); needle with drainage. **Vacuity fall of original qi** patterns are characterized by counterflow cold of the limbs, black facial complexion, panting, cold sweating, and, in severe cases, loss of consciousness. MED Immediate treatment should be given to return yang and stem desertion using Counterflow Cold Decoction (*sì nì tāng*) plus ginseng (*rén shēn*) and cinnamon bark (*ròu guì*). ACU Base treatment mainly on CV and GV. Select GV-26 (*shuǐ gōu*, Water Trough), GV-25 (*sù liáo*, White Bone-Hole), PC-6 (*nèi guān*, Inner Pass), GV-20 (*bǎi huì*, Hundred Convergences), CV-4 (*guān yuán*, Pass Head), and KI-1 (*yǒng quán*, Gushing Spring); needle with supplementation or direct moxa. Apply moxa on salt or ginger at CV-8 (*shén què*, Spirit Gate Tower). Compare RETRACTED SCROTUM. [56: 68] [26: 624] [97: 232]

retracted scrotum 囊缩 *náng suō*: Synonym: *retracted testicles*. The drawing of the scrotum into the body. Retracted scrotum is usually a severe condition and is observed in both heat and cold patterns. Yang brightness (*yáng míng*) exuberant heat passing to reverting yin (*jué yīn*) is treated by emergency precipitation to preserve yin with formulas such as Major Qi-Coordinating Decoction (*dà chéng qì tāng*), whereas cold evil directly striking the lesser yin (*shào yīn*) is treated with Counterflow Cold Decoction (*sì nì tāng*) or Tangkuei Counterflow Cold Decoction (*dāng guī sì nì tāng*). Compare RETRACTED GENITALS. [50: 1747] [26: 995]

retracted testicles 卵缩 *luǎn suō*: Testicles drawn upward and into the body. Retracted testicles are usually attributed to disease of the foot reverting yin (*jué yīn*) liver channel. *The Magic Pivot* (*líng shū, jīng mài*) states, "When reverting yin (*jué yīn*) qi expires, the sinew expires. The reverting yin (*jué yīn*) is the liver vessel. The liver is the union of the sinews. The sinew gather at the yin organs (genitals) and net the root of the tongue. When the vessel loses its luxuriance, the sinews become tense. When the sinews become

tense, they pull the tongue and testicles. Hence, green-blue lips, curled tongue, and retracted testicle mean the death of the sinews." This falls within the scope of RETRACTED GENITALS and RETRACTED SCROTUM. [50: 798]

return 回 *huí*, 归 *guī*: See following entries.

returning fire to its source 引火归原 *yǐn huǒ guī yuán*: A method of treatment used to address upbearing kidney fire using medicinals that enrich kidney yin and conduct fire downward. Upbearing kidney fire is a pattern of upper body heat and lower body cold characterized by floating red complexion, dizziness, tinnitus, ulceration of the mouth and tongue, loose teeth, aching lumbus and weak legs, cold in the lower extremities, tender-red tongue, and a vacuous pulse. MED Combine kidney-enriching medicinals such as cooked rehmannia (*shú dì huáng*), dioscorea (*shān yào*), cornus (*shān zhū yú*), schisandra (*wǔ wèi zǐ*), and ligustrum (*nǚ zhēn zǐ*), with aconite (*fù zǐ*) and cinnamon bark (*ròu guì*), which supplement true yang and conduct fire downward. [26: 133] [27: 287] [70: 352]

returning yang and stemming counterflow 回阳救逆 *huí yáng jiù nì*: A method of treatment used to address great yang collapse vacuity desertion, characterized by aversion to cold, curled-up lying posture, counterflow cold of the limbs, drop in both body temperature and blood pressure, cold sweats, a somber white complexion, and a faint, fine pulse or vacuous rapid pulse. MED Base treatment on yang-warming medicinals such as aconite (*fù zǐ*), dried ginger (*gān jiāng*), and cinnamon bark (*ròu guì*), combined with qi-boosting medicinals such as licorice (*gān cǎo*) and codonopsis (*dǎng shēn*). In severe cases, add ginseng (*rén shēn*). If copious sweat indicates a desertion trend, include medicinals such as dragon bone (*lóng gǔ*) and oyster shell (*mǔ lì*) to constrain sweat and stem desertion. For yin humor depletion, use yin-constraining and humor-nourishing medicinals such as schisandra (*wǔ wèi zǐ*) and cooked rehmannia (*shú dì huáng*). A commonly used formula is Counterflow Cold Decoction (*sì nì tāng*). ACU See YANG COLLAPSE. [6: 257] [26: 260] [27: 277]

reversal 厥 *jué*: The term *jué* is explained as meaning (1) sudden CLOUDING REVERSAL, i.e., fainting or syncope. (2) counterflow cold spreading upward from the extremity of the limbs. Thus, *jué* means disruption (in the flow of qi, blood) and recession of the outward spread (of yang qi). The term "reversal" is closely related in meaning to "counterflow." Reversal cold of the limbs and counterflow cold of the limbs are identical in meaning. "Counterflow," unlike "reversal," is commonly used to denote disruption of the qi dynamic of organs such as the liver, stomach and lung and does not appear in terms denoting loss of consciousness. See REVERSAL PATTERN; REVERSE-FLOW. ◇ Chin 厥 *jué*, reverse, adverse; ebb; disrupt. [26: 706] [27: 399] [97: 545] [19: 2164] [48: 349]

reversal cold of the extremities 手足厥冷 *shǒu zú jué lěng*: Synonyms: *counterflow cold of the extremities*; *counterflow cold of the limbs*; *reversal cold of the limbs*; *limb reversal*. Pronounced cold in the extremities up to the knees and elbows or beyond, as occurs in yang collapse or internal heat evil block. Reversal cold of the extremities is similar to lack of warmth in the extremities. However, the latter differs in that it is less pronounced, does not reach as far as the knees and elbows, and is observed in general yang vacuity patterns. Reversal cold of the extremities is called *reversal* because yang qi recedes away from the extremities. Distinction is made between cold and heat. **Cold** patterns are attributed to debilitation of yang qi and exuberant internal yin cold, and are associated with fear of cold, clear-food diarrhea, and a faint sunken pulse. ⌊MED⌋ Return yang and stem counterflow with Counterflow Cold Decoction (*sì nì tāng*) or Aconite Main Tuber Brew (*wū tóu jiān*). **Heat** patterns are attributed to depressed heat evil preventing yang qi from reaching the four limbs, and are associated with heat vexation in the chest and abdomen and with thirst. ⌊MED⌋ Diffuse depressed heat with Counterflow Cold Powder (*sì nì sǎn*), White Tiger Decoction (*bái hǔ tāng*), or one of the Qi-Coordinating Decoctions (*chéng qì tāng*). Reversal cold of the extremities is observed in COLD DAMAGE, REVERSAL PATTERNS, and in MOUNTING (*shàn*). See REVERSAL. [26: 161]

reversal cold of the limbs 四肢厥冷 *sì zhī jué lěng*: REVERSAL COLD OF THE EXTREMITIES.

reversal desertion 厥脱 *jué tuō*: A desertion pattern characterized by reversal cold of the limbs. [26: 209]

reversal headache 厥头痛 *jué tóu tòng*: LIVER REVERSAL HEADACHE.

reversal heart pain 厥心痛 *jué xīn tòng*: Heart pain stretching to the back. See COLD REVERSAL HEART PAIN; HEAT REVERSAL HEART PAIN. [26: 706]

reversal mounting 厥疝 *jué shàn*: See YIN MOUNTING (*shàn*)[2].

reversal pattern 厥证 *jué zhèng*: Any condition a) clouding collapse (fainting) and loss of consciousness and/or b) reversal cold of the limbs (marked cold in the extremities). Reversal patterns occur in the follow circumstances. (1) They occur in patients usually suffering from effulgent liver yang or dietary irregularities when mental stimulus or acute pain causes counterflow and derangement of qi dynamic. The blood moves counterflow with the qi or phlegm rises with the qi,

causing clouding of the heart spirit. (2) They occur in patients suffering from weak original qi, damage to qi and liquid after enduring illness, or loss of blood, when the supply of qi and blood fails. In reversal patterns, loss of consciousness comes suddenly and is usually temporary. The patient in most cases gradually recovers. Reversal patterns can be divided into ones characterized by loss of consciousness and ones characterized by reversal cold of the extremities. See the entries listed below. Note that all the reversal patterns listed were mentioned in *The Inner Canon* (*nèi jīng, lùn jué zhèng*) except for LIVER REVERSAL. See REVERSAL. [26: 707] [27: 399] [97: 545]

Reversal Patterns

Patterns marked by loss of consciousness
PHLEGM REVERSAL (*tán jué*)
FOOD REVERSAL (*shí jué*)
QI REVERSAL (*qì jué*)
BLOOD REVERSAL (*xuè jué*)
LIVER REVERSAL (*gān jué*)
SUDDEN REVERSAL (*bó jué*)
FULMINANT REVERSAL (*bào jué*)
DEATHLIKE REVERSAL (*shī jué*)
BOILING REVERSAL (*jiān jué*)

Patterns marked by cold limbs
COLD REVERSAL (*hán jué*)
HEAT REVERSAL (*rè jué*)
ROUNDWORM REVERSAL (*huí jué*)

---

reverse-flow 厥逆 *jué nì*: **1.** REVERSAL COLD OF THE EXTREMITIES. *On Cold Damage* (*shāng hán lùn, biàn shào yīn bìng mài zhèng bìng zhì*) states, "Lesser yin (*shào yīn*) disease with clear-food diarrhea, interior cold and external heat, reverse-flow of the extremities, faint pulse on the verge of expiration... is treated with Vessel-Freeing Counterflow Cold Decoction (*tōng mài sì nì tāng*). **2.** From *The Magic Pivot* (*líng shū, diān kuáng*). Acute pain in the chest with sudden cold of the lower extremities, heart vexation, inability to eat, and a rough pulse. **3.** From *Elementary Questions* (*sù wèn, qī bìng piàn*). A kind of enduring headache. *Elementary Questions* (*sù wèn, qí bìng lùn*) states, "When a person is ill, with a headache that has lasted incessantly for years... he must have been invaded by great cold that has reached the bone and marrow. The marrow is mainly the brain. Counterflow to the brain causes headache with pain in the teeth too. This disease is called reverse-flow. See REVERSAL PATTERN. [26: 706] [27: 546] [25: 291]

reverse-flow headache 厥逆头痛 *jué nì tóu tòng*: HEADACHE characterized by pain in the head stretching into the teeth and attributed to cold evil invading the brain. MED Warm and dissipate cold evil using formulas such as Notopterygium and Aconite Decoction (*qiāng huó fù zǐ tāng*). ACU Base treatment mainly on GV. Select GV-20 (*bǎi huì*, Hundred Convergences), SI-3 (*hòu xī*, Back Ravine), Greater Yang (*tài yáng*), GB-8 (*shuài gǔ*, Valley Lead), LI-4 (*hé gǔ*, Union Valley), GV-16 (*fēng fǔ*, Wind Mansion), and GV-4 (*mìng mén*, Life Gate); needle with drainage and moxa. See HEADACHE. Compare REVERSAL HEADACHE. [26: 707] [113: 208] [37: 400]

reverse-flow of the extremities 手足厥逆 *shǒu zú jué nì*: See REVERSE-FLOW.

reverse-flow of the limbs 四肢厥逆 *sì zhī jué nì*: See REVERSE-FLOW.

reverting yin 厥阴 *jué yīn*: The hand reverting yin pericardium and foot reverting yin liver channels. The name reverting yin indicates yin qi developing to its final stage and then reverting toward yang. The reverting yin is located within the greater yin (*tài yīn*) and lesser yin (*shào yīn*), and hence it is said that "reverting yin is the closedness." [27: 91] [97: 545]

reverting yin channel 厥阴经 *jué yīn jīng*: See REVERTING YIN.

reverting yin disease 厥阴病 *jué yīn bìng*: In the classical sequence, the reverting yin is the last of the three yin channels. Hence, it should theoretically be associated with the most severe diseases. *Elementary Questions* (*sù wèn*), states, "The reverting yin channel skirts round the genitals and connects with the liver, so that diseases include vexation and fullness, and retracted scrotum." The same chapter also mentions, among the signs of reverting yin disease, "deafness, retraction of the scrotum, inability to ingest [even] liquid foods, and unconsciousness." *Elementary Questions* (*sù wèn*) enumerates symptoms but prescribes no formulas. Because the reverting yin patterns described in *On Cold Damage* (*shāng hán lùn*) are less severe, the real nature of reverting yin disease is still in question. Further research is required to clarify the matter fully. Reverting yin disease as described in *On Cold Damage* (*shāng hán lùn*) is characterized by upper body heat and lower body cold, and may take the form of dispersion-thirst, qi surging up into the heart [region], pain and heat in the heart [region], hunger with no desire to eat, or vomiting of roundworm. Reversal cold of the limbs is also observed in some cases. Pathomechanically, upper body heat and lower body cold is explained as a cold-heat complex resulting from interior vacuity. Dispersion-thirst, qi surging up into the heart [region], pain and heat in the heart [region], and clamoring stomach discomfort are the manifestations of upper body heat (heat in the area just above the diaphragm). No desire for food and vom-

iting of roundworm reflect lower body cold (in the intestines). This impairs movement and transformation of the food, which disquiets the roundworm and causes it to rise counterflow. The reversal cold of the limbs indicates failure of yang qi to reach the periphery of the body, arising when a cold-heat complex disrupts qi dynamic. [6: 229] [27: 220] [97: 546]

reverting yin headache 厥阴头痛 *jué yīn tóu tòng*: **1.** HEADACHE due to reverting yin (*jué yīn*) disease in cold damage, characterized by headache and neck pain, dry retching, ejection of foaming drool, and reversal cold of the limbs. MED Treat with Evodia Decoction (*wú zhū yú tāng*). ACU Select GV-20 (*bǎi huì*, Hundred Convergences), CV-12 (*zhōng wǎn*, Center Stomach Duct), and ST-36 (*zú sān lǐ*, Leg Three Li); needle with drainage and add moxa. Apply moxa at LR-1 (*dà dūn*, Large Pile). **2.** HEADACHE located on the reverting yin (*jué yīn*) channel (i.e., the vertex), for which evodia (*wú zhū yú*) can be used as a channel conductor. ACU Select GV-20 (*bǎi huì*, Hundred Convergences), Alert Spirit Quartet (*sì shén cōng*), LR-8 (*qū quán*, Spring at the Bend), LR-3 (*tài chōng*, Supreme Surge), CV-12 (*zhōng wǎn*, Center Stomach Duct), ST-36 (*zú sān lǐ*, Leg Three Li), and KI-1 (*yǒng quán*, Gushing Spring). See HEADACHE. [113: 9] [27: 392] [97: 546] [75: 275] [113: 9]

reverting yin transforming into wind 厥阴化风 *jué yīn huà fēng*: LIVER YANG TRANSFORMING INTO WIND. See LIVER WIND STIRRING INTERNALLY.

rheum 饮 *yǐn*: See PHLEGM-RHEUM. [26: 738]

rheum aggregation 饮癖 *yǐn pì*: A condition characterized by a stringlike tautness under the ribs, with periodic sound of water, pain brought on by exposure to cold, and periodic vomiting of foamy drool, and attributed to devitalization of center yang and gathering of water rheum. MED Treat with Drool-Controlling Elixir (*kòng xián dān*). [26: 738] [97: 295]

rheumatism 风湿 *fēng shī*: See WIND-DAMP.[1]

rheum evil congesting the lung 饮邪壅肺 *yǐn xié yōng fèi*: A form of PROPPING RHEUM characterized by panting and fullness in the chest, thin clear phlegm, and, in severe cases, scant urine, white slimy tongue fur, and a stringlike sunken pulse. MED Drain the lung and expel rheum with Tingli and Jujube Lung-Draining Decoction (*tíng lì dà zǎo xiè fèi tāng*). ACU Base treatment mainly on LU, LI, SP, and ST. Select BL-13 (*fèi shū*, Lung Transport), LU-5 (*chǐ zé*, Cubit Marsh), CV-22 (*tiān tú*, Celestial Chimney), LI-4 (*hé gǔ*, Union Valley), CV-17 (*shān zhōng*, Chest Center), SP-9 (*yīn líng quán*, Yin Mound Spring), and ST-40 (*fēng lóng,* Bountiful Bulge); needle with drainage. [80: 151] [46: 597, 653]

rib-side 胁 *xié*: The area from the armpit down to bottom of the ribs. (i.e., to lowest of the 12 ribs).
WMC The rib-side includes the hypochondrium. See CHEST AND RIB-SIDE. [123: 289] [26: 511]

rib-side pain 胁痛 *xié tòng,* 胁肋疼痛 *xié lè téng tòng*: Pain in the area between the armpits and the lowest rib. The rib-side is traversed by the foot reverting yin (*jué yīn*) liver and foot lesser yang (*shào yáng*) gallbladder channels; hence pain in this area is associated with disease of the liver and gallbladder. In addition, heart, lung, spleen, and kidney disease can also affect the chest and rib-side or rib-side and abdomen. Rib-side pain is observed in both external contractions and internal damage patterns. External contraction patterns include wind-damp, summerheat-heat, and epidemic scourges. Internal damage includes qi depression, phlegm-rheum, static blood, and food accumulations. See entries listed below.

Rib-Side Pain

WIND-COLD RIB-SIDE PAIN (*fēng hán xié tòng*)

SUMMERHEAT-HEAT RIB-SIDE PAIN (*shǔ rè xié tòng*)

LUNG EVIL RIB-SIDE PAIN (*fèi xié xié tòng*)

MOVING QI RIB-SIDE PAIN (*yùn qì xié tòng*)

LIVER DEPRESSION RIB-SIDE PAIN (*gān yù xié tòng*)

LIVER QI RIB-SIDE PAIN (*gān qì xié tòng*)

DEAD BLOOD RIB-SIDE PAIN (*sǐ xuè xié tòng*)

COLLECTING RHEUM RIB-SIDE PAIN (*tíng yǐn xié tòng*)

DAMP-HEAT RIB-SIDE PAIN (*shī rè xié tòng*)

FOOD ACCUMULATION RIB-SIDE PAIN (*shí jī xié tòng*)

DRY RIB-SIDE PAIN (*gān xié tòng*)

FREE-RIB PAIN (*jì xié tòng*)

Rib-side pain may also occur in disharmony of liver qi, liver blood vacuity, liver yin vacuity, liver-kidney yin vacuity, depletion of liver-spleen qi and blood, and depressed liver-gallbladder heat. It may be observed in jaundice. From the modern clinical viewpoint, rib-side pain is also noted in hepatomegaly or splenomegaly. [26: 516]

rib-side pain and distention 胁肋胀痛 *xié lè zhàng tòng*: Pain and subjective feeling of distention in the rib-side region. Rib-side pain and distention is variously attributed to qi depression, congealing phlegm, and stagnation in the vessels. See RIB-SIDE PAIN. [97: 356]

rich paste 膏滋 *gāo zī*: A paste preparation to be taken orally. **Preparation**: The ingredients are usually boiled 2–3 times, for 2–3 hours each time, until the smell is only faint. After each boiling, the decoction should be strained off, and fresh water added to the pot for the next boiling. Then, all the decoctions are slow-boiled together until they are reduced to a thick, viscous paste. The correct consistency is reached as soon as no water separates out from a globule of the paste when dropped on paper. If the paste becomes too thick, it is likely to stick to the pot and burn. If too thin, it is difficult to store. Then, a quantity of honey or sugar, equal to a specified proportion of the original materials (usually an equal proportion) is added before a final boiling. The paste is then put in earthenware or glass jars. Pastes keep for long periods, and are usually used for chronic diseases. See PASTE. ◇ Chin 膏 *gāo*, paste; 滋 *zī*, rich, wholesome, moisten, enrich. [97: 629]

right 正 *zhèng*: Synonym: *correct (obs)*. **1.** *adj.* Normal or rendering normal. RIGHT COMPLEXION refers to the normal complexion of the healthy individual. RIGHT QI denotes the forces that maintain normal bodily functions and that seek to reestablish them when evil qi is present. **2.** *n.* (usually 'the right') RIGHT QI. Compare EVIL.

right complexion 正色 *zhèng sè*: A normal complexion. The healthy complexion of the Chinese is traditionally described as a "bright, lustrous, contained complexion with a faint red and yellow hue." A bright, lustrous complexion indicates the presence of spirit. A "contained" complexion, i.e., one in which color is held within the skin and is not exposed (see TRUE VISCERAL COMPLEXION), indicates the presence of stomach. A right complexion indicates harmony of qi and blood and internal fullness of essential qi. A distinction is made between the *governing complexion* and the *visiting complexion*. The governing complexion is each person's basic complexion; the visiting complexion is any deviation from governing complexion brought about by changes in the weather and environment or in physiological state. Neither the governing nor the visiting complexion is pathological. [50: 365] [29: 35]

righting qi 正气 *zhèng qì*: RECTIFYING QI. [26: 182] [27: 78, 107]

right qi 正气 *zhèng qì*: **1.** True qi, especially in opposition to disease. Right qi is the active aspect of all components including the organs, blood, fluids, and essence and the above-mentioned forms of qi in maintaining health and resisting disease. Right qi stands in opposition to evil qi, which is any entity in its active aspect of harming the body. **2.** The normal qi of the seasons, warmth in spring, heat in summer, coolness in autumn, and cold in winter.

right vacuity and evil repletion 正虚邪实 *zhèng xū xié shí*: Simultaneous existence in one patient of vacuity and repletion. Rich vacuity and evil repletion occurs when a disease is not treated properly or evil qi is excessively exuberant, or when vacuity of right develops while evil repletion is still present. It may also occur when patients suffering from constitutional vacuity contract an evil and display signs of both vacuity and repletion. *Elementary Questions* (*sù wèn, tōng píng xū shí lùn*) states, "When evil qi is exuberant, there is repletion; when essential qi is despoiled, there is vacuity." In most cases, the right vacuity is the root, whereas the evil repletion is the tip. [26: 182]

rigid 强直 *qiáng zhí*: Severe stiffness, such as of the neck or back.

rigid center 强中 *qiáng zhōng*: **1.** *Synonym: yin protrusion*[1]. Lasting stiff erections with spontaneous discharge of semen or inability to ejaculate. Rigid center has been attributed to excessive consumption of "elixirs" containing metals, exuberant internal fire toxin, and to excessive libido causing liver-kidney yin depletion and yang hyperactivity. ⟨MED⟩ Enrich yin and drain fire. Use Gypsum and Apricot-Leaved Adenophora Decoction (*shí zǐ jì ní tāng*) or Coptis and Pig's Stomach Pill (*huáng lián zhū dǔ wán*). For exuberant fire and yin vacuity, add scrophularia (*xuán shēn*), ophiopogon (*mài mén dōng*), and dried/fresh rehmannia (*shēng dì huáng*). For debilitation of kidney qi and frenetic stirring of vacuity fire, warm and supplement the kidney origin using Cistanche Pill (*cōng róng wán*) from *A Unified Treatise on Diseases, Patterns, and Remedies According to the Three Causes* (*sān yīn jí yī bìng zhèng fāng lùn*) or Velvet Deerhorn Pill (*lù róng wán*) from *The Great Peace Sagacious Benevolence Formulary* (*tài píng shèng huì fāng*). See YANG RIGIDITY. **2.** A type of dispersion-thirst pattern. [112: 164] [50: 1584] [26: 611] [27: 428] [97: 592]

rigidity of the neck 项强 *xiàng qiáng*: From *Elementary Questions* (*sù wèn, zhì zhēn yào dà lùn*). Tension in the muscles of the neck; attributed a) to contraction of wind, cold, or damp evil in the greater yang (*tài yáng*) channel, b) to invasion of disease evil through wounds of the skin and flesh, or c) to damage to yin through loss of blood, great sweating, or great heat [effusion] with insufficiency of liquid and blood depriving the sinews of nourishment. Rigidity of the neck is observed in COLD DAMAGE, WIND STROKE, TETANY, and CRICK IN THE NECK. ⟨ACU⟩ Base treatment mainly on GV, GB, and SI. Main points: GB-20 (*fēng chí*, Wind Pool), GV-14 (*dà zhuī*, Great Hammer), GB-39 (*jué gǔ*, Severed Bone), and SI-3 (*hòu xī*, Back Ravine); add points and select appropriate stimulus according to the cause. [26: 686] [44: 330] [37: 440] [46: 718]

rigidity of the penis 茎强 *jīng qiáng*: YANG RIGIDITY.

river point 经穴 *jīng xué*: CHANNEL POINT[2].

roasting 煨 *wēi*: A method of drawing out unwanted oils or irritants from medicinal materials and reducing their toxicity by exposure to heat. Method: Materials are usually wrapped in wet paper or coated in flour and water paste, and then placed in hot embers until the wrapping becomes burnt and black. They may also be put at the side of the fire, in an oven, or tossed in a wok. Nutmeg (*ròu dòu kòu*) and kansui (*gān suì*) may be treated in this way. [27: 342] [97: 617]

rock 岩 *yán*: A hard uneven swelling on the surface of the body, of fixed location, and unassociated with change in skin color. After it has ruptured, it appears like a pomegranate with the skin peeling away, purple in color, giving off a malign odor, acutely painful, and healing readily. See TONGUE MUSHROOM; COCOON LIP; LOSS-OF-LUXURIANCE; MAMMARY ROCK; KIDNEY ROCK. [27: 481] [97: 344] [96: 205]

root and tip 标本 *biāo běn*: Primary and secondary aspects of disease. The word "root" is used in opposition to "tip," the two terms being of varying significance according to context. Root refers to (1) the essential nature of the disease, when tip is the signs; (2) the cause of disease, when the tip is clinically observable changes in the body; (3) right qi, when the tip is the evil; or (4) the primary condition, when tip are the resulting secondary condition. ◇ Chin 标 *biāo*, tip, topmost branch, a mark, beacon, signal, streamer; 本 *běn* root, source, stem. [26: 879]

root of earlier heaven 先天之本 *xiān tiān zhī běn*: The kidney as the seat of that which is inherited at conception in the FETAL ORIGIN and which provides the basis for growth, development, reproductive ability, and resistance to disease. The root of earlier heaven stands in complementary opposition to the ROOT OF LATER HEAVEN, which is the stomach and spleen as the source of engendering transformation, i.e., producing from food what is required for the growth, development, and life activity. See EARLIER HEAVEN; KIDNEY IS THE ROOT OF EARLIER HEAVEN. [44: 749]

root of later heaven 后天之本 *hòu tiān zhī běn*: The spleen and stomach as the source of engendering transformation, i.e., producing from food what is required for the growth, development, and life activity. See SPLEEN IS THE ROOT OF LATER HEAVEN. [44: 341]

root-severing therapy 截根疗法 *jié gēn liáo fǎ*: PICKING THERAPY.

rot 烂 *làn*: **1.** The state of rotting. See PUTREFACTION. **2.** A disease characterized by rotting, e.g., FOOT ROT.

rotating supplementation and drainage 捻转补泻 *niǎn zhuǎn bǔ xiè*: TWIRLING SUPPLEMENTATION AND DRAINAGE.

rough breathing 气粗 *qì cū*: Breathing characterized by a rough sound in the nose. Rough breathing generally occurs in repletion patterns and arises when contraction of external evils or exuberant internal phlegm turbidity inhibits qi dynamic. Vacuity patterns are characterized by faint weak breathing and are attributed to lung-kidney qi vacuity. See BREATHING. [29: 165]

rough pulse 涩脉 *sè mài*: The opposite of a slippery pulse. A pulse that does not flow smoothly, felt to be like a knife lightly scratching bamboo. The rough tends to be somewhat fine, is generally slightly slower than the normal pulse. *The Bin-Hu Sphygmology* (*bīn hú mài xué*) states, "The rough pulse is fine and slow, comes with difficulty, is short and scattered, or stops and then returns, at threes and fives, like a knife lightly scratching bamboo, like rain wetting sand, or like sick silkworms eating leaves." (NB: "at threes and fives," 三五不调 *sān wǔ bù tiáo*, means irregular; "like rain wetting sand," 如雨沾沙 *rú yǔ zhān shā*, refers to splodgy patterns created by raindrops on a smooth sandy surface; "sick silkworms eating leaves" 病蚕食叶 *bìng cán shí yè*, refers to the fact that sick silkworms leave irregular edges on leaves after gnawing at them, as opposed to the smooth edges left by healthy silkworms.) The rough pulse is often seen in blood stasis patterns and dual vacuity of blood and qi. A forceful rough pulse indicates repletion, whereas a forceless rough pulse indicates vacuity. [27: 193] [6: 141]

rough tongue fur 糙苔 *cāo tāi*: A dry tongue fur that is rough to the touch. See DRY TONGUE FUR. [26: 123]

rough voidings of reddish urine 小便赤涩 *xiǎo biàn chì sè*: Scant dark-colored urine passed in short inhibited (disfluent) voidings. Rough voidings of reddish urine are observed in repletion patterns of heat or damp-heat pouring downward. ◇ Chin 赤 *chì*, red, here refers to a deep color of the urine and is rendered as 'reddish' to avoid suggesting that 'bloody urine' is meant.

roundworm 蛔虫 *huí chóng*: Synonyms: *heart worm disease*; *long worm*. One of the NINE WORM DISEASES. See ROUNDWORM DISEASE. [26: 359]

roundworm disease 蛔虫病 *huí chóng bìng*, 蚘 虫病 *huí chóng bìng*: Synonyms: *heart worm disease*; *long worm disease*. One of the NINE WORM DISEASES. A disease caused by the presence of roundworm in the body; attributed to spleen-stomach vacuity, indiscriminate eating of cold, raw, sweet, and fatty foods, or of unclear gourds, fruits, and vegetables. Roundworm disease is characterized by intermittent abdominal pain. A lump may form at the painful spot, which wriggles up and down. Pain abates when the movement ceases. The face is bright white or mixed yellow and white,

sometimes with whitish patches called *worm macules*. Other signs include emaciation and vomiting of clear water sometimes containing roundworm. MED Treat principally by expelling worms. If there is spleen-stomach vacuity or accumulation and stagnation, the methods of fortifying the spleen and abductive dispersion may also be applied. Medicinals used to expel roundworm include. quisqualis (*shǐ jūn zǐ*), chinaberry root bark (*kǔ liàn gēn pí*), toosendan (*chuān liàn zǐ*), Levant wormseed flower and leaf (*shān dào nián hāo*), and torreya (*fěi zǐ*). Formulas include Mume Pill (*wū méi wán*), Worm-Transforming Pill (*huà chóng wán*), and Myriad Applications Pill (*wàn yìng wán*). ACU Base treatment mainly on SP, ST, LI, and points for expelling worms. Select Hundred Worm Nest (*bǎi chóng wō*), SP-15 (*dà héng*, Great Horizontal), LI-4 (*hé gǔ*, Union Valley), ST-36 (*zú sān lǐ*, Leg Three Li), and ST-4 (*dì cāng*, Earth Granary); needle with drainage. [26: 737] [37: 320]

roundworm gan 蛔疳 *huí gān*: Gan disease due to persistent worm accumulation. Roundworm gan is characterized by emaciation, disquieted spirit, abdominal pain, knitting of the eyebrows, crying, vomiting of clear fluid, grinding of teeth at night, rapid hungering, and perverted appetite. MED Expel worms and supplement the spleen, taking care to avoid indiscriminate use of attack (offensive treatment). Initial medication can take the form of Center-Rectifying Roundworm-Quieting Decoction (*lǐ zhōng ān huí tāng*), which can be followed by Worm-Transforming Pill (*huà chóng wán*) or Chubby Child Pill (*féi ér wán*). For worms coming out of the mouth or nose, use Mume Pill (*wū méi wán*). [26: 736] [97: 556]

roundworm reversal 蛔厥 *huí jué*: From *On Cold Damage* (*shāng hán lùn, biàn jué yīn bìng mài zhèng bìng zhì*). Episodic abdominal pain, vexation and agitation, and reversal cold of the limbs due to roundworm. WMC biliary ascariasis, ascaris intestinal obstruction. MED Quiet and kill roundworm using formula such as Mume Pill (*wū méi wán*). See REVERSAL. ACU Base treatment mainly on CV, LR, and ST. Select CV-12 (*zhōng wǎn*, Center Stomach Duct), LR-13 (*zhāng mén*, Camphorwood Gate), ST-36 (*zú sān lǐ*, Leg Three Li), Hundred Worm Nest (*bǎi chóng wō*), BL-25 (*dà cháng shū*, Large Intestine Transport), BL-27 (*xiǎo cháng shū*, Small Intestine Transport), and ST-25 (*tiān shū*, Celestial Pivot). Needle with supplementation and add moxa. [26: 528] [27: 401] [97: 556] [37: 402]

roundworm stomach duct pain 蚘动胃脘痛 *huí dòng wèi wǎn (guǎn) tòng*: Stomach pain due to roundworm, characterized by episodes of acute pain associated with somber white complexion, reversal cold of the limbs, and in some cases vomiting of roundworm. Between episodes the complexion is yellow, sometimes with white patches, and despite normal appetite the body is emaciated. ‖MED‖ The condition can be treated with a decoction of mume (*wū méi*), areca (*bīng láng*), and chinaberry root bark (*kǔ liàn gēn pí*). ‖ACU‖ Base treatment mainly on alarm and uniting points of ST, PC, SP, and empirical points. Select CV-12 (*zhōng wǎn*, Center Stomach Duct), ST-36 (*zú sān lǐ*, Leg Three Li), PC-6 (*nèi guān*, Inner Pass), ST-25 (*tiān shū*, Celestial Pivot), SP-4 (*gōng sūn*, Yellow Emperor), and Hundred Worm Nest (*bǎi chóng wō*); needle with drainage. [26: 528]

roundworm vomiting 吐蚘 *tù huí*: Expulsion of vomitus containing roundworm. Vomiting of roundworm is mentioned in the *On Cold Damage* (*shāng hán lùn, biàn jué yīn bìng mài zhèng bìng zhì*). The *Zhang's Clear View of Medicine* (*zhāng shì yī tōng*) states, "When there is roundworm in the stomach and intestines, if there is cold, or heat, or a cold-heat complex in the stomach and spleen, this can disquiet roundworm, which ascend counterflow to be vomited out. If there is cold, there is reversal cold of the extremities, and the vomited roundworm are pale white in color; for this, use Center-Rectifying Decoction (*lǐ zhōng tāng*) plus mume (*wū méi*), coptis (*huáng lián*), and dichroa leaf (*shǔ qī*). If there is heat, the vomited roundworm are red and lively; for this, use Roundworm-Quieting Powder (*ān huí sǎn*). For a cold-heat complex with periodic heart heart vexation, and vomiting after eating, use Mume Pill (*wū méi wán*). [26: 259]

rumbling intestines 肠鸣 *cháng míng*: Synonym: *borborygmus*. Any sound made by food in the intestines. See also GURGLING INTESTINES. [97: 289]

running piglet 奔豚 *bēn tún*: One of the FIVE ACCUMULATIONS (kidney accumulation). A sen-

sation of upsurge from the lower abdomen to the chest and throat, accompanied by gripping abdominal pain, oppression in the chest, rapid breathing, dizziness, heart palpitations, and heart vexation. This pattern is considered to be one of the five accumulations, and is a result of an upsurging of yin cold qi of the kidney or liver channel qi fire ascending counterflow. ‖MED‖ For an upsurging of yin cold qi of the kidney, use Cinnamon Twig Decoction Plus Extra Cinnamon (*guì zhī jiā guì tāng*) or Poria (Hoelen), Cinnamon Twig, Licorice, and Jujube Decoction (*fú líng guì zhī gān cǎo dà zào tāng*) to warm and dissipate cold evil. For liver channel qi fire ascending counterflow, use Running Piglet Decoction (*bēn tún tāng*) to clear the liver and downbear counterflow. [26: 367] [50: 891]

running yellow 走黄 *zǒu huáng*: CLOVE SORE RUNNING YELLOW.

runny nose 流鼻涕 *liú bí tì*: Profuse production of snivel (nasal mucus).

rushing gate 贲门 *bēn mén*: The upper orifice of the stomach, i.e., the cardia. One of the SEVEN GATES. [26: 30]

rushing respiration 息贲 *xī bēn*: Hasty rapid breathing with qi rushing counterflow upward; the LUNG ACCUMULATION among the FIVE ACCUMULATIONS. Rushing respiration is marked by upward rush of qi, a lump under the left rib-side like an upturned cup, heat effusion and aversion to cold, oppression in the chest, counterflow retching, and coughing up of blood and pus. In enduring cases, it can develop into a PULMONARY WELLING-ABSCESS (*yōng*). ‖MED‖ Clear and downbear lung qi; flush phlegm and discharge heat. Use Rushing Respiration Decoction (*xī bēn tāng*). ◇ Chin 息 *xī*, breath, respiration; 贲 *bēn*, rush, hasty, distressed. [26: 533]

S

S1-wood 甲木 *jiǎ mù*: The gallbladder.

S2-wood 乙木 *yǐ mù*: The liver.

S3-fire 丙火 *bǐng huǒ*: The small intestine.

S4-fire 丁火 *dīng huǒ*: The heart.

S5-earth 戊土 *wù tǔ*: The stomach.

S6-earth 己土 *jǐ tǔ*: The spleen.

S7-metal 庚金 *gēng jīn*: The large intestine.

S8-metal 辛金 *xīn jīn*: The lung.

S9-water 壬水 *rén shuǐ*: The bladder.

S10-water 癸水 *guǐ shuǐ*: The kidney.

saber and pearl-string lumps 马刀侠瘿 *mǎ dāo xiá yǐng*: Scrofula. Saber lumps are scrofula occurring in a configuration that looks like the shape of a saber; pearl-string lumps occur on the neck giving the appearance of a pearl necklace. ◇ Chin *mǎ dāo*, horse knife, i.e., saber; 侠 *xiá* kungfu fighter, probably a substitute for 夹 *jiá*, to clasp, border; 瘿 *yǐng* knobble, goiter, is explained as 缨络 *yīng luò*, a string of gems. [27: 478] [97: 37]

sagging distention in the stomach duct and abdomen 脘腹坠胀 *wǎn fù zhuì zhàng*: Fullness and distention with a heavy downbearing sensation in the stomach duct and abdomen; a sign of center qi fall.

sagging of one testicle 偏坠 *piān zhuì*: Synonym: *hemilateral sagging*. Painful swelling and sagging of one testicle attributable to phlegm-damp, static blood, or liver channel fire-heat. Sagging of the left testicle is usually due to static blood or liver fire; sagging of the right testicle is usually due to phlegm-damp or food accumulation. ⎣MED⎦ Phlegm-damp or static blood patterns can be treated with Tangerine Pip Pill (*jú hé wán*), whereas liver channel fire-heat can be treated with Gentian Liver-Draining Decoction (*lóng dǎn xiè gān tāng*). ⎣ACU⎦ Base treatment mainly on CV, LR, SP, and ST. Main points: LR-1 (*dà dūn*, Large Pile), LR-4 (*zhōng fēng*, Mound Center), LR-3 (*tài chōng*, Supreme Surge), SP-6 (*sān yīn jiāo*, Three Yin Intersection), and CV-4 (*guān yuán*, Pass Head). Selection of points according to pattern: For phlegm-damp and static blood, add ST-40 (*fēng lóng*, Bountiful Bulge), ST-36 (*zú sān lǐ*, Leg Three Li), SP-9 (*yīn líng quán*, Yin Mound Spring), BL-17 (*gé shū*, Diaphragm Transport), SP-10 (*xuè hǎi*, Sea of Blood), and LI-4 (*hé gǔ*, Union Valley); needle with drainage, or prick to bleed with a three-edged needle. For liver channel fire-heat, add BL-18 (*gān shū*, Liver Transport),

BL-17 (*gé shū*, Diaphragm Transport), LR-2 (*xíng jiān*, Moving Between), GB-43 (*xiá xī*, Pinched Ravine), SP-9 (*yīn líng quán*, Yin Mound Spring), GB-34 (*yáng líng quán*, Yang Mound Spring), and KI-1 (*yǒng quán*, Gushing Spring); needle with drainage. ◇ Chin 偏 *piān*, biased, to one side; 坠 *zhuì*, sag. Hemilateral sagging. [26: 651] [4: 150] [46: 596–7]

saltiness 咸 *xián*: One of the FIVE FLAVORS. Saltiness enters the kidney; it can soften hardness and induce moist precipitation. See FIVE FLAVORS; FIVE FLAVOR ENTRIES. [27: 62]

saltiness enters the kidney 咸入肾 *xián rù shèn*: Salty medicinals tend to act upon the kidney. Salty medicinals that enter the kidney notably include products from the sea such as abalone shell (*shí jué míng*), clamshell (*hǎi gé ké*), oyster shell (*mǔ lì*), pumice (*hǎi fú shí*), sargassum (*hǎi zǎo*), and seal's genitals (*hǎi gǒu shèn*). Other animal products include gecko (*gé jiè*), mantis egg-case (*sāng piāo xiāo*), placenta (*zǐ hé chē*), tortoise plastron (*guī bǎn*), and velvet deerhorn (*lù róng*). Other vegetable products include baiwei (*bái wēi*), cistanche (*ròu cōng róng*), cuttlefish bone (*hǎi piāo xiāo*), dendrobium (*shí hú*), and scrophularia (*xuán shēn*). Minerals include actinolite (*yáng qǐ shí*) and loadstone (*cí shí*). [27: 62]

salt wheezing 盐哮 *yán xiāo*: Wheezing exacerbated by excessive consumption of salty or sour foods in enduring vacuity. Saltiness and sourness seep into the bronchioles allowing phlegm to enter and gather, causing phlegm-damp to gather in the bronchioles. In such conditions, exposure to wind-cold causes qi to become depressed and phlegm to congest. Salt wheezing is essentially a vacuity pattern, and may present as heat or cold. ⎣MED⎦ Salt wheezing requires medicinals to disinhibit the lung, regulate qi, and sweep phlegm in addition to a basic formula for heat or cold wheezing. Malt sugar (*yí táng*) or granulated sugar (*shā táng*) can be added to the formula. If necessary, decoct ginseng top (*rén shēn lú*) and apply mechanical ejection. See WHEEZING. [26: 1007]

salty 咸 *xián*: See SALTINESS.

salty taste in the mouth 口咸 *kǒu xián*: A subjective sensation of saltiness in the mouth, which may be associated with periodic ejection of salty drool. A salty taste in the mouth is a sign of kidney vacuity. **Kidney yin vacuity** causes a salty taste in the mouth with ejection of small amounts of salty drool. Accompanying signs include dry throat and mouth, dizzy head, tinnitus, limb aching lumbus and knees, vexing heat in the five hearts, unquiet sleep, red tongue with thin fur, and a sunken fine rapid pulse that is forceless at the cubit. [MED] Enrich the kidney and downbear fire; invigorate the governor of water. Use Major Yin Supplementation Pill (*dà bǔ yīn wán*) or Anemarrhena, Phellodendron, and Rehmannia Pill (*zhī bǎi dì huáng wán*). **Kidney yang vacuity** causes a salty taste in the mouth with generalized fatigue, shortness of breath and lack of strength, fear of cold and cold limbs, limp wilting lumbus and legs, frequent nocturnal urination, a pale enlarged tongue with dental impressions, and a forceless fine sunken pulse. [MED] Warm and supplement kidney yang with Kidney Qi Pill (*shèn qì wán*) plus schisandra (*wǔ wèi zǐ*). See TASTE IN THE MOUTH. [92: No. 83]

same-name channel 同名经 *tóng míng jīng*: Channels of the hand and foot that otherwise share the same name. For example, the foot greater yang (*tài yáng*) channel and hand greater yang (*tài yáng*) channel are same-name channels. See SELECTION OF SAME-NAME CHANNEL POINTS; COMBINING SAME-NAME CHANNEL POINTS.

sand 痧 *shā*: Synonym: *sand qi*. Any of various externally contracted heat (febrile) disease patterns characterized by distention or papules. (1) Disease characterized by pain, distention, and oppression in the chest attributable to wind-cold, summerheat, and epidemic qi blocking the stomach and intestines is called *sand distention*. (2) Sand in the skin and qi aspect manifests as faint red papules the size of millet seeds; when it brews in the blood aspect, the whole body is painfully swollen, and there are blackish patches ("black sand"). (3) Papules. *A Clinical Guide with Case Histories* (*lín zhèng zhǐ nán yī àn*) states, "Sand is a general word for papules." See also GUA-SHA and MACULOPAPULAR ERUPTION. ◇ Chin 痧 *shā* is composed of the illness signifier 疒 with 沙 *shā*, sand, the latter element being descriptive of the papules. The precise etiological connection between a granular eruption and disease characterized by abdominal signs is not clear. [27: 370] [26: 670] [97: 587] [48: 338]

sand distention 痧胀 *shā zhàng*: See SAND.

sand-heap perverse crop 堆沙鬎鬁 *duī shā là lì*: FAT SORE. See also PERVERSE CROP.

sand lump 痧块 *shā kuài*: A lump in the rib-side, chest, or abdomen, observed in sand patterns and that forms when release of sand by gua-sha leaves residual toxin that gathers and binds. [MED] Clear and separate the toxin bind using a) medicinals that course the qi aspect such as aquilaria (*chén xiāng*) and amomum (*shā rén*), b) medicinals that

address toxin bind in the blood aspect such as peach kernel (*táo rén*), carthamus (*hóng huā*), madder (*qiàn cǎo gēn*), sparganium (*sān léng*), and dalbergia (*jiàng zhēn xiāng*), and c) abductive dispersers that address toxin binding with stagnant food such as radish seed (*lái fú zǐ*) and areca (*bīng láng*). [26: 670]

sand qi 痧气 *shā qì*: See SAND.

sand scraping 刮痧 *guā shā*: See GUA-SHA.

sand strangury 砂淋 *shā lín*, 砂石淋 *shā shí lín*: Stone strangury, especially when the stones passed in the urine are small. See STONE STRANGURY. ◇ Chin 砂 *shā*, sand, grit; *lín*, dribble, drip. [27: 425]

sand toxin 痧毒 *shā dú*: The toxin to which sand is attributed. See SAND.

sand veins 痧筋 *shā jīn*: The appearance of dark green-blue, purple, or red veins above and below the knees and elbows in sand patterns. Sand veins are attributable to sand toxin. Clearly visible sand veins are a sign of the toxin in the blood aspect. Veins that are sometimes visible and sometimes not are an indication of toxin entering the qi aspect. If they are slightly visible, this is usually a sign that the toxin is obstructing the qi aspect. Sand veins can be treated by pricking with a three-edged needle to discharge the toxin. [26: 670]

sapping of kidney yin 下汲肾阴 *xià jí shèn yīn*: Exuberant heart fire causing the life gate fire to stir and wear kidney yin, and causing such signs as seminal emission, premature ejaculation, and vacuity vexation and insomnia. Such conditions are sometimes described as "sapping of kidney yin" because the kidney yin and kidney yang are the root of all the viscera, and disease among them naturally take their toll on the kidney. ◇ Chin 汲 *jí*, to draw water, as from a well. [6: 96] [27: 148] [97: 26]

sauce receptacle 承浆 *chéng jiāng*: The depression below the lip and above the chin. [WMC] mentolabial groove. [27: 66]

sauce receptacle clove sore 承浆疔 *chéng jiāng dīng*: A clove sore in the source receptacle (infralabial fossa). See HUMAN CENTER CLOVE SORE.

¹**scab** 痂 *jiā*: The crust that forms over a wound and protects it until the flesh has grown back. [48: 355]

²**scab** 疥 *jiè*, 疥疮 *jiè chuāng*: A disease characterized by small papules the size of a pinhead that are associated with insufferable penetrating itching and that, when scratched, may suppurate or crust without producing any exudate. Scab commonly occurs between the fingers and may also be observed on the inside of the elbow, in the armpits, on the lower abdomen, in the groin, and on the buttocks and thighs, and, in severe cases, over the

whole body. It is attributed to damp-heat depressed in the skin, and is transmitted by contact. In *The Origin and Indicators of Disease* (*zhū bìng yuán hòu lùn*) of the Sui Dynasty, the author, Chao Yuan-fang, attributed it to "worms," which he said were "small and very difficult to see." WMC Scabies. NB: Scabies is caused by the common itch mite, *Sarcoptes scabiei*, which is 0.3–0.5 mm long and 0.2–0.4 mm wide. MED Wash with a decoction of 9 g of zanthoxylum (*huā jiāo*) and 30 g of kochia (*dì fū zǐ*); then apply Cnidium Seed Powder (*shé chuáng zǐ sǎn*). This disease is less commonly seen nowadays because of improved hygiene. See SORE. ◇ Chin The character 疥 is composed of 介 *jiè*, a shell or crust with the illness signifier 疒. Eng *scab* akin to Old Swed. *skabbr* and L. *scabies* mange, *scabere* to scratch. The meaning of crust (a protective coating that forms over a wound) developed from scab as a disease name. Thus *scab* and 疥 are almost identical in their linguistic meaning. [26: 403] [27: 474] [97: 430] [61: 349]

scald 烫伤 *tàng shān*: See BURNS AND SCALDS.

scalding 燀 *shǎn*: Soaking in hot water to facilitate removal of skin and tips. Peach kernel (*táo rén*) and apricot kernel (*xìng rén*) are treated in this way. [27: 323]

scallion-stalk pulse 芤脉 *kōu mài*: A large floating pulse that when pressure is applied is empty in the middle, like a scallion or green onion stalk. Li Zhong-Zi states that "It is as if the finger is feeling a scallion. At the superficial level, the skin of the scallion is felt. At the mid-level, the empty middle of the scallion is felt. At the deep level, the finger touches the under side of the scallion." This is why this pulse is likened to a scallion stalk. The scallion-stalk pulse is a sign of heavy blood loss, and usually occurs in major bleeding. [27: 194] [97: 259] [93: 274]

scalp acupuncture 头针疗法 *tóu zhēn liáo fǎ*, 头皮针 *tóu pí zhēn*: Acupuncture involving the needling of points on the scalp in accordance with a system that purportedly combines traditional Chinese medical understanding with modern theories of cerebral cortical function. [26: 906]

scant breast milk 缺乳 *quē rǔ*, 乳汁少 *rǔ zhī shǎo*, 乳少 *rǔ shǎo*: Synonym: *breast milk stoppage*. Insufficient milk to suckle the infant. Scant breast milk is due to postpartum depletion of qi and blood or to liver qi depression. The latter is easily distinguishable by the presence of distention and fullness of the breasts. **Qi-blood vacuity** causes scant breast milk by causing insufficiency of the source of milk transformation (i.e., reduced milk production). The chief characteristic is absence of pain and distention in the breast. Other signs include white lips, low food intake, and fatigue. MED Treat by the method of supplement-

ing qi and nourishing the blood, assisted by freeing breast milk. Use Lactation Elixir (*tōng rǔ dān*). ACU Base treatment mainly on ST and LR. Main points: CV-17 (*shān zhōng*, Chest Center), ST-18 (*rǔ gēn*, Breast Root), and SI-1 (*shào zé*, Lesser Marsh). For qi-blood vacuity, add BL-20 (*pí shū*, Spleen Transport) and ST-36 (*zú sān lǐ*, Leg Three Li), needling with supplementation. **Liver depression and qi stagnation** is characterized by fullness, distention, and pain in the breast, sometimes associated with generalized heat [effusion] and oppression in the chest. MED Course the liver, resolve depression, and free milk. Use Free Wanderer Powder (*xiāo yáo sǎn*) plus pangolin scales (*chuān shān jiǎ*) and vaccaria (*wáng bù liú xíng*). ACU Use the main points listed above, and add PC-6 (*nèi guān*, Inner Pass) and LR-3 (*tài chōng*, Supreme Surge), needling with even supplementation and drainage. [26: 547] [27: 453] [97: 480] [46: 693] [67: 326]

scant inhibited menstruation 月经涩少 *yuè jīng sè shǎo*: See SCANT MENSTRUATION.

scant menstruation 月经过少 *yuè jīng guò shǎo*: A smaller menstrual flow or shorter menstrual period than normal (in some cases reduced to spotting). Because the flow is disfluent, scant menstruation it often called UNGRATIFYING MENSTRUATION or INHIBITED MENSTRUATION, and SCANT INHIBITED MENSTRUATION. It is attributed to blood vacuity, blood cold and blood stasis, phlegm-damp, or kidney vacuity. Compare PROFUSE MENSTRUATION. See entries listed below. [26: 168] [27: 441] [97: 110]

Scant Menstruation

BLOOD VACUITY SCANT MENSTRUATION (*xuè xū yuè jīng guò shǎo*)

BLOOD COLD SCANT MENSTRUATION (*xuè hán yuè jīng guò shǎo*)

BLOOD STASIS SCANT MENSTRUATION (*xuè yū yuè jīng guò shǎo*)

KIDNEY VACUITY SCANT MENSTRUATION (*shèn xū yuè jīng guò shǎo*)

---

scant semen 精少 *jīng shǎo*: Scant ejaculate, sometimes of only two or three drops, affecting the ability to produce children. Scant semen is attributable to congenital insufficiency, sexual intemperance, or excessive mental taxation wearing essential qi. MED Supplement essence and replenish the marrow with Marrow-Engendering Unicorn-Fostering Elixir (*shēng suǐ yù lín dān*). Compare SEMINAL COLD. ACU Base treatment mainly on CV, back transport points, KI, and SP. Select CV-4 (*guān yuán*, Pass Head), BL-23 (*shèn shū*, Kidney Transport), BL-52 (*zhì shì*, Will Chamber), KI-3 (*tài xī*, Great Ravine), BL-20 (*pí* *shū*, Spleen Transport), SP-6 (*sān yīn jiāo*, Three Yin Intersection), and BL-52 (*jīng gōng*, Palace of Essence); needle with supplementation. If there is a tendency to yang vacuity, add GV-4 (*mìng mén*, Life Gate) and KI-7 (*fù liū*, Recover Flow), and add moxa. For excessive mental taxation, add BL-15 (*xīn shū*, Heart Transport) and HT-7 (*shén mén*, Spirit Gate). [26: 831] [37: 41] [46: 678]

scant urine 尿少 *niào shǎo*: Less urine than normal. See URINE.

scapula 胛 *jiǎ*: SHOULDER BLADE. [27: 70]

scarring moxibustion 瘢痕灸 *bān hén jiǔ*: The method of treatment whereby moxa is burned on the body and leaves a scar. Scarring moxibustion employs a small cone of moxa wool (some less than 1 cm in diameter) that is placed directly on the skin and completely burned. The area is then wiped clean with a cloth and the process is repeated until the prescribed number of cones has been burned. When this has been done, the area should be carefully cleaned and dressed. After one to three days, the patient will develop a blister that will eventually leave a small scar. The blister generally takes about a month to heal. During this time, the patient must keep the area clean and frequently change the dressing to prevent infection. The scarring method is the most drastic form of moxibustion. The formation of a blister was traditionally considered important in the healing process and thus it is said that if moxibustion does not form a blister, the disease will not be cured. This method is currently used in China to treat severe vacuity cold or cold-damp diseases. When performing scarring moxibustion, note the following: (1) The pre-burning of a cone or two not quite down to the skin is a way to accustom the patient gradually to the burning pain. These pre-burned cones, however, should not be counted toward the prescribed number. (2) When the moxa is burning, the practitioner should scratch or tap the area around the point to reduce the burning pain. (3) The number of recommended cones should be adjusted to the patient's condition. Strong young patients can withstand more burnings and larger cones than weak elderly patients. (4) The patient should be given a full explanation about the procedure and be forewarned of the formation of a scar. (5) Garlic juice or some other liquid is usually placed on the point being treated in order to secure the moxa cone. [27: 242] [97: 639]

scattered pulse 散脉 *sàn mài*: DISSIPATED PULSE.

scorch 灼 *zhuó*: Describes the drastic damaging effect of heat on the blood and fluids. See HEAT.

scorch-frying 炒焦 *chǎo jiāo*: Stir-frying materials in a wok over a high flame until they become burnt on the outside and emit a burnt smell. Ab-

ductive dispersing medicinals such as medicated leaven (*shén qū*) and crataegus (*shān zhā*) are scorch-fried to strengthen their spleen-fortifying food-dispersing action. [27: 324]

scorching heat 灼热 *zhuó rè*: Intense heat of which the patient is subjectively aware and very often can also be felt with the hands. Scorching heat may be experienced subjectively in the stomach or anus. Heat toxin sores characterized by redness and swelling are often scorching hot to the touch.

scorching pain 灼痛 *zhuó tòng*: Pain associated with a heat sensation, and when located at the surface of the body, with palpable heat. Scorching pain is observed in both repletion and vacuity heat patterns, and notably sore patterns and stomach yin vacuity. See PAIN. [29: 190]

scourge 瘟 *wēn*: SCOURGE EPIDEMIC. [26: 828]

scourge epidemic 瘟疫 *wēn yì*: Synonym: *scourge; warm epidemic*. From *Elementary Questions* (*sù wèn, běn bìng lùn*). Any contagious disease attributed to the contraction of EPIDEMIC PESTILENTIAL QI. The two most commonly observed kinds are pestilential qi epidemic toxin hidden in the membrane source and summerheat-heat epidemic toxin hidden the stomach. **Pestilential qi epidemic toxin hidden in the membrane source** (*mò yuán*) starts with abhorrence of cold and vigorous heat [effusion], quickly shifting to a pattern of heat without headache and generalized pain, red or crimson tongue with a chalky white tongue fur, and a rapid pulse. MED Course, disinhibit, and outthrust using Membrane-Source–Opening Beverage (*dá yuán yǐn*) or Three Dispersers Beverage (*sān xiāo yǐn*). **Summerheat-heat epidemic toxin hidden in the stomach** is marked by vigorous heat [effusion], vexation and agitation, splitting headache, abdominal pain, diarrhea, crimson tongue with parched fur, and in some cases by spontaneous external bleeding, macules, and clouded spirit or coma. MED Clear the scourge and resolve toxin with Scourge-Clearing Toxin-Vanquishing Beverage (*qīng wēn bài dú yǐn*). [26: 828] [27: 353] [97: 630]

scourge jaundice 瘟黄 *wēn huáng*: **1.** Any severe contagious jaundice. Scourge jaundice is attributed to heaven-current epidemic pestilence or damp-heat seasonal toxin scorching construction blood. Scourge jaundice is characterized by body and eyes that are deep yellow in color, high fever, clouded spirit, urine the color of phellodendron (*huáng bǎi*) juice, abdominal distention with water, rib-side pain, and blood ejection and bloody stool. In some cases, there are maculopapular eruptions. The tongue is red or crimson; the pulse is surging and rapid. MED Clear construction, cool the blood, and open the orifices. See ACUTE JAUNDICE. **2.** ACUTE JAUNDICE. [26: 828]

scourge sand 瘟痧 *wēn shā*: A disease caused by depressed deep-lying cold qi that emerges in the spring, or stagnant summerheat-heat that emerges in the autumn, the latter form being by far the more common and more highly contagious. Scourge sand is characterized by heat effusion and aversion to cold that makes it seem similar to but not the same as malaria. Other signs include swelling of the head and face, and in some cases signs such as rapid breathing with fullness and oppression, bloating in the chest and diaphragm, abdominal pain, or dysentery with stool containing pus and blood. [TRT] Treat by letting blood to discharge the sand toxin. Use Aquilaria and Asafetida Pill (*chén xiāng ē wèi wán*). [26: 828]

screen gate 阑门 *lán mén*: One of the SEVEN GATES. [WMC] ileocecal valve. [97: 589]

scrofula 瘰疬 *luǒ lì*: *Synonym: mouse sores.* From *Elementary Questions* (*sù wèn*). Lumps beneath the skin down the side of the neck and under the armpits. These are often referred to in older books as SABER AND PEARL-STRING LUMPS because of the saberlike formation they can make below the armpit, and the necklace-like formation they make on the neck. Scrofula occurs when phlegm gathers in the neck, armpits or groin. The phlegm is produced by the scorching of fluids by vacuity fire arising in lung-kidney vacuity. In some cases, wind-fire evil toxin is also a factor. Scrofula starts as bean-like lumps, associated with neither pain nor heat. Subsequently the lumps expand and assume a stringlike formation, merge, and even bunch up into heaps. They are hard and do not move under pressure. In the latter stages they may become slightly painful. They can rupture to exude a thin pus and sometimes contain matter that resembles bean curd dregs (residue of ground soybeans in the production of soybean milk and tofu). They can take a long time to heal, old ones healing while new ones arise. In some cases, fistulas may form. [WMC] tuberculosis of lymph node; lymphadenitis. [MED] Course the liver and resolve depression; soften hardness and transform phlegm. Use Free Wanderer Powder (*xiāo yáo sǎn*) combined with Two Matured Ingredients Decoction (*èr chén tāng*). In advanced stages, base treatment on enriching the lung and supplementing the kidney, using Six-Ingredient Rehmannia Pill (*liù wèi dì huáng wán*) plus adenophora/glehnia (*shā shēn*) and ophiopogon (*mài mén dōng*). [ACU] Use principally local points and points selected according to the affected channel. Main points: Ouch points (*ā shì xué*) (i.e., the nodes themselves), Hundred Taxations (*bǎi láo*) and Tip of the Elbow (*zhǒu jiān*). Apply treatment in the following way: Prior

to rupture, fire-needle the center of each node once every 2–3 days. After rupture, for wounds that fail to heal, pole the affected areas or apply 3–5 cones of moxa on garlic or aconite cake every 3–5 days; complement acupuncture treatment with medicinal therapy and dressings. At Hundred Taxations (*bǎi láo*) and Tip of the Elbow (*zhǒu jiān*), apply moxa pole or 5–7 cones directly or on ginger, repeating the treatment every other day. These points may also be needled with supplementation, retaining the needles for 15–30 minutes. Selection of points according to affected area: For scrofula on the nape, add TB-17 (*yì fēng*, Wind Screen), TB-6 (*zhī gōu*, Branch Ditch), and TB-10 (*tiān jǐng*, Celestial Well), and moxa GB-41 (*zú lín qì*, Foot Overlooking Tears). For the neck, add LI-14 (*bì nào*, Upper Arm) and ST-5 (*dà yíng*, Great Reception), and moxa LI-10 (*shǒu sān lǐ*, Arm Three Li). For the armpit, add GB-21 (*jiān jǐng*, Shoulder Well), HT-3 (*shào hǎi*, Lesser Sea), and GB-38 (*yáng fǔ*, Yang Assistance). Needle with drainage. Selection of points according to progression of the disease: For initial-stage scrofula, needle with drainage at BL-18 (*gān shū*, Liver Transport), LR-3 (*tài chōng*, Supreme Surge), ST-36 (*zú sān lǐ*, Leg Three Li), and ST-40 (*fēng lóng*, Bountiful Bulge) to course the liver and resolve depression, soften hardness and transform phlegm. For pronounced phlegm-fire, further add LI-4 (*hé gǔ*, Union Valley), ST-44 (*nèi tíng*, Inner Court), and SP-6 (*sān yīn jiāo*, Three Yin Intersection). For advanced stages, needle with supplementation at BL-23 (*shèn shū*, Kidney Transport), BL-13 (*fèi shū*, Lung Transport), BL-43 (*gāo huāng shū*, Gao-Huang Transport), LU-9 (*tài yuān*, Great Abyss), KI-3 (*tài xī*, Great Ravine), and ST-36 (*zú sān lǐ*, Leg Three Li) to enrich the lung and supplement the kidney. For binding wind-heat toxin, needle with drainage at GV-20 (*bǎi huì*, Hundred Convergences), GB-20 (*fēng chí*, Wind Pool), TB-5 (*wài guān*, Outer Pass), GV-14 (*dà zhuī*, Great Hammer), LI-4 (*hé gǔ*, Union Valley), and ST-40 (*fēng lóng*, Bountiful Bulge), and prick LU-11 (*shào shāng*, Lesser Shang) to bleed. **Caution:** Modern medicine observes that malign tumors of the nose, mouth, throat, and breast can spread to the lymph nodes of the neck and armpits. It is important to be able to differentiate these forms of metastasis from scrofula. ◇ **Eng** from L. little sows. [26: 902] [27: 477] [37: 446] [113: 383] [61: 118]

scrotal itch 阴囊瘙痒 *yīn náng sāo yǎng*: *Synonym: yin sac itch.* Itching of the scrotum, in severe cases with thickening of the skin, and rupture by scratching causing exudation of yellow water and subsequent scabbing. Scrotal itch is caused by brewing damp-heat, yin vacuity and blood dryness, or by lower burner cold-damp. **Brewing damp-heat** scrotal itch starts with severe itching relieved by bathing in hot water, and with pimples like millet grains. Scratching produces a watery exudate and burning soreness. The tongue is yellow and slimy, and the pulse is stringlike, slippery, and rapid. MED Clear and drain liver-gallbladder heat with Gentian Liver-Draining Decoction (*lóng dăn xiè gān tāng*). Bathe with a decoction of purslane (*mă chĭ xiàn*). ACU Base treatment mainly on SP, ST, LR, and LI. Select GV-14 (*dà zhuī*, Great Hammer), LI-11 (*qū chí*, Pool at the Bend), SP-10 (*xuè hăi*, Sea of Blood), SP-6 (*sān yīn jiāo*, Three Yin Intersection), SP-9 (*yīn líng quán*, Yin Mound Spring), ST-36 (*zú sān lĭ*, Leg Three Li), LR-3 (*tài chōng*, Supreme Surge), and GB-34 (*yáng líng quán*, Yang Mound Spring); needle with drainage. **Yin vacuity and blood dryness** patterns are characterized by severe itching with roughening and thickening of the skin. Scratching produces blood (no watery exudate), which dries to form a regular blood scab. It is associated with thirst, heart vexation, red tongue, and fine rapid pulse. MED Use medicinals such as dried/fresh rehmannia (*shēng dì huáng*), tangkuei (*dāng guī*), white peony (*bái sháo yào*), salvia (*dān shēn*), millettia (*jī xuè téng*), earthworm (*dì lóng*), kochia (*dì fū zĭ*), fish poison yam (*bì xiè*), cnidium seed (*shé chuáng zĭ*), raw licorice (*shēng gān căo*), and cyathula (*chuān niú xī*), ACU Base treatment mainly on back transport points, SP, LR, KI, and ST. Select BL-17 (*gé shū*, Diaphragm Transport), BL-20 (*pí shū*, Spleen Transport), BL-23 (*shèn shū*, Kidney Transport), SP-10 (*xuè hăi*, Sea of Blood), SP-6 (*sān yīn jiāo*, Three Yin Intersection), LR-8 (*qū quán*, Spring at the Bend), LR-3 (*tài chōng*, Supreme Surge), KI-6 (*zhào hăi*, Shining Sea), and ST-36 (*zú sān lĭ*, Leg Three Li); needle with even supplementation and drainage. For pronounced itching, add HT-8 (*shào fŭ*, Lesser Mansion), and Itch Reliever (*zhĭ yăng*). **Lower burner cold-damp** patterns are characterized by damp scrotum, mild itching, limp aching lumbus and knees, sagging distention in the smaller abdomen, inhibited urination, heavy swollen lower limbs, moist white tongue fur and a forceless sunken moderate pulse. MED Warm the channels and dissipate cold; eliminate dampness and relieve itch. An effective formula is Five Accumulations Powder (*wŭ jī săn*). ACU Base treatment mainly on CV, SP, and ST. Select CV-4 (*guān yuán*, Pass Head), CV-3 (*zhōng jí*, Central Pole), ST-36 (*zú sān lĭ*, Leg Three Li), SP-9 (*yīn líng quán*, Yin Mound Spring), and SP-10 (*xuè hăi*, Sea of Blood); needle with drainage and moxa. See SCROTAL WIND. [92: No. 244] [61: 348] [96: 380] [4: 116] [113: 434, 435] [46: 594, 597]

scrotal welling-abscess 肾囊痈 *shèn náng yōng*, 囊痈 *náng yōng*: Synonym: *kidney sac welling-abscess*. A large suppurative swelling of the scrotum. A scrotal welling-abscess starts with painful swelling of the scrotum with heat and redness. In severe cases, the skin is fully stretched so that it becomes smooth and shiny, and the scrotum becomes heavy and sags. With time, it begins to suppurate. A scrotal welling-abscess is accompanied by heat effusion and aversion to cold, dry mouth with desire for cold fluids, and rough voidings of reddish urine. It is attributed to liver and kidney channel damp-heat pouring downward or to invasion of external dampness. MED Clear heat and disinhibit dampness with Gentian Liver-Draining Decoction (*lóng dăn xiè gān tāng*). When pus forms, the same formula can be used with the addition of pangolin scales (*chuān shān jiă*) and gleditsia thorn (*zào jiăo cì*), although lancing may be necessary. The condition is distinguished from *welling-abscess of the testicle* by absence of swelling of the testicles. [26: 693, 995] [61: 264]

scrotal wind 肾囊风 *shèn náng fēng*: Synonyms: *kidney sac wind*; *bobble wind*. A condition of dryness and itchiness of the scrotum relieved by bathing in hot water, and, in severe cases, with red pimples the size of millet seed, that exude fluid when scratched and are sometimes associated with scorching heat pain. Scrotal wind is caused by liver channel damp-heat pouring downward and invasion of external wind evil. It is usually difficult to cure. WMC scrotal eczema; neurodermatitis; riboflavin deficiency. MED Oral: Clear heat, dispel wind, and eliminate dampness with Gentian Liver-Draining Decoction (*lóng dăn xiè gān tāng*). Topical: Dab on Indigo Powder (*qīng dài săn*) plus Three Stones Powder (*sān shí săn*) after bathing the affected area with decocted Cnidium Seed Powder (*shé chuáng zĭ săn*). In persistent cases, use Chinese Wolfsbane Paste (*láng dú gāo*). ACU Base treatment mainly on GV, ST, LI, SP, LR, and GB. Main points: GV-14 (*dà zhuī*, Great Hammer), LI-11 (*qū chí*, Pool at the Bend), SP-10 (*xuè hăi*, Sea of Blood), ST-36 (*zú sān lĭ*, Leg Three Li), and SP-6 (*sān yīn jiāo*, Three Yin Intersection); needle with drainage. Selection of points according to pattern: For liver channel damp-heat, add LR-3 (*tài chōng*, Supreme Surge), GB-34 (*yáng líng quán*, Yang Mound Spring), and SP-9 (*yīn líng quán*, Yin Mound Spring). For wind evil, add GB-20 (*fēng chí*, Wind Pool), TB-5 (*wài guān*, Outer Pass), and GV-20 (*băi huì*, Hundred Convergences). See also SCROTAL ITCH. [26: 694]

scrotum 肾囊 *shèn náng*, 阴囊 *yīn náng*: Synonyms: *kidney sac*; *yin sac*. The sac that contains the testicles. See SCROTAL WIND; COLD MOUNTING; FOXY MOUNTING; SAGGING OF ONE TESTICLE; SCROTAL WELLING-ABSCESS. ◇ Chin 肾 *shèn*, kidney; 囊 *náng*, bag, pouch, sack, sac.

scurrying pain 窜痛 *cuàn tòng*: Pain that repeatedly changes location; attributable to qi stagnation or wind evil. Pain that moves from one location to another. Scurrying pain is a sign of wind evil in the channels obstructing qi dynamic. Wind is swift and changeable; the pain that it causes changes from one position to another. It is observed in wind-damp impediment (*bì*) patterns with a prevalence of wind evil. WMC wandering pain. See PAIN. [29: 190] [27: 24, 38] [97: 188]

sea of blood 血海 *xuè hǎi*: 1. *Synonym: sea of the twelve channels.* One of the FOUR SEAS. The thoroughfare (*chōng*) vessel. 2. The liver. 3. SP-10 (*xuè hǎi*, Sea of Blood). [26: 279] [50: 582]

sea of grain and water 水谷之海 *shuǐ gǔ zhī hǎi*: One of the FOUR SEAS. The stomach. [26: 154] [27: 21] [97: 132]

sea of marrow 髓海 *suǐ hǎi*: One of the FOUR SEAS. The brain. [27: 25] [97: 660]

sea of qi 气海 *qì hǎi*: One of the FOUR SEAS. Chest center. 1. Cinnabar field. 2. CV-6 (*qì hǎi*, Sea of Qi). [27: 34] [97: 92]

sea of the channels 经脉之海 *jīng mài zhī hǎi*: The thoroughfare (*chōng*) vessel. [27: 93] [97: 379]

sea of the twelve channels 十二经之海 *shí èr jīng zhī hǎi*: Synonym: *sea of blood.* The thoroughfare (*chōng*) vessel. [27: 93]

sea of the yang vessels 阳脉之海 *yáng mài zhī hǎi*: The governing (*dū*) vessel. [27: 93]

sea of the yin vessels 阴脉之海 *yīn mài zhī hǎi*: The controlling (*rèn*) vessel. [27: 93]

seasonal cold epidemic 时行寒疫 *shí xíng hán yì*: A contagious disease caused by fulminant cold in spring or summer, characterized by headache and generalized pain, cold and heat without sweating, or retching counterflow, white fur, absence of thirst, a pulse that is tight and floating. Seasonal cold epidemic is similar to the cold damage greater yang pattern. MED Resolve the exterior with warmth and acridity. [26: 527]

seasonal cough 时行嗽 *shí xíng sòu*: *Synonyms: fulminant seasonal cough; heaven-current cough.* Cough due to a seasonal qi that is contagious. A seasonal cough is characterized by bouts of continuous coughing with heat effusion, aversion to cold, headache, and nasal congestion. MED Diffuse the lung and resolve the exterior. Use Ginseng and Perilla Beverage (*shēn sū yǐn*), Toxin-Vanquishing Powder (*bài dú sǎn*), and variations. ACU Base treatment mainly on LU, LI, and BL. Select BL-13 (*fèi shū*, Lung Transport), LU-7 (*liè quē*, Broken Sequence), LI-4 (*hé gǔ*, Union Valley), GB-20 (*fēng chí*, Wind Pool), BL-12 (*fēng mén*, Wind Gate), and BL-11 (*dà zhù*, Great Shuttle); needle with drainage. [26: 526] [113: 51] [46: 652]

seasonal current 时行 *shí xíng*: SEASONAL QI. [26: 527] [27: 347] [97: 273]

seasonal epidemic 时疫 *shí yì*: SEASONAL QI. [26: 527]

seasonal epidemic dysentery 时疫痢 *shí yì lì*: EPIDEMIC DYSENTERY. [26: 527]

seasonal evil 时邪 *shí xié*: Any evil whose occurrence is seasonally related. [26: 527]

seasonal qi 时气 *shí qì*: 1. Any contagious epidemic qi, whose occurrence is associated with a given season. 2. *Synonym: epidemic scourge; heaven current; seasonal current; seasonal epidemic.* Epidemic disease. [27: 108] [97: 278]

seasonal toxin 时毒 *shí dú*: Any seasonally related contagious epidemic disease evil or disease caused by it. See WARM TOXIN. [26: 527] [27: 108] [97: 278] [61: 157]

seat board bone 坐板骨 *zuò bǎn gǔ*: *bolt bone.* The bone on which the body rests when sitting. In women, the seat bone is sometimes called the *interlocking bones.* See FAILURE OF THE INTERLOCKING BONES TO OPEN. WMC ischium. [27: 70] [27: 71]

seat sores 坐板疮 *zuò bǎn chuāng*: Pock pimples of the buttocks. See POCK PIMPLES. [97: 298, 588] [26: 326, 673]

second yang channel 二阳 *èr yáng*: Yang brightness (*yáng míng*) channel. [27: 91]

second yin channel 二阴 *èr yīn*: Lesser yin (*shào yīn*) channel. [27: 90]

secret formula 秘方 *mì fāng*: A formula kept secret by its inventor or anyone to whom he passes it on. [26: 457]

secure 固 *gù*: To prevent or arrest the loss of qi, blood, fluids, or essence, and the invasion of evil, as through the exterior. Examples: *secure essence* (also called *astringe essence),* to arrest seminal loss; *secure the exterior,* to treat insecurity of exterior qi, characterized by spontaneous or night sweating. See also INSECURITY.

securing and astriction 固涩法 *gù sè fǎ*: The method of treating efflux desertion patterns (i.e., enduring or critical discharge or loss of sweat, blood, semen etc.). Securing and astriction involves the use of supplementing and astringent medicinals to **constrain sweat** in the treatment of spontaneous or night sweating; **constrain the lung** in the treatment of persistent cough; **astringe the intestines** in the treatment of persistent diarrhea culminating in prolapse of the anus (called *enduring diarrhea efflux desertion*); **secure essence** in the treatment of seminal emission or seminal efflux; **reduce urine** in the treatment of copious urine or enuresis; **stanch bleeding** to treat severe bleeding; **secure the menses** to treat flooding and spotting; or **check vaginal discharge** to treat persistent vaginal discharge.

Securing and Astriction

CONSTRAINING SWEAT AND SECURING THE EXTERIOR (*liǎn hàn gù biǎo*)

CONSTRAINING THE LUNG AND SUPPRESSING COUGH (*liǎn fèi zhǐ ké*)

ASTRINGING THE INTESTINES AND STEMMING DESERTION (*sè cháng gù tuō*)

ASTRINGING ESSENCE AND CHECKING SEMINAL EMISSION AND ENURESIS (*sè jīng zhǐ yí*)

SECURING THE KIDNEY AND ASTRINGING ESSENCE (*gù shèn sè jīng*)

SECURING ESSENCE (*gù jīng*)

REDUCING URINE (*suō niào*)

STEMMING FLOODING AND VAGINAL BLEEDING (*gù bēng zhǐ dài*)

STANCHING BLEEDING (*zhǐ xuè*)

Efflux desertion patterns are all at root vacuity patterns, the loss of sweat, blood, or semen etc., being the tip. For this reason securing astriction formulas usually comprise supplementing medicinals combined with astringent medicinals, the former usually being used in large number or quantity than the latter. Rarely, securing medicinals are used alone. In general, securing astriction is a method of treatment that is not used too early in the development of a condition. See the entries listed above.

Astringent Medicinals

五味子 (*wǔ wèi zǐ*) schisandra (Schisandrae Fructus)

乌梅 (*wū méi*) mume (Mume Fructus)

五倍子 (*wǔ bèi zǐ*) sumac gallnut (Rhois Galla)

浮小麦 (*fú xiǎo mài*) light wheat (Tritici Semen Leve)

麻黄根 (*má huáng gēn*) ephedra root (Ephedrae Radix)

糯稻根须 (*nuò dào gēn xū*) glutinous rice root (Oryzae Glutinosae Rhizoma et Radix)

石榴皮 (*shí liú pí*) pomegranate rind (Granati Pericarpium)

诃子 (*hē zǐ*) chebule (Chebulae Fructus)

肉豆蔻 (*ròu dòu kòu*) nutmeg (Myristicae Semen)

赤石脂 (*chì shí zhī*) halloysite (Halloysitum Rubrum)

禹余粮 (*yǔ yú liáng*) limonite (Limonitum)

罂粟壳 (*yīng sù ké*) poppy husk (Papaveris Pericarpium)

莲肉 (*lián ròu*) lotus seed (Nelumbinis Semen)

莲子 (*lián zǐ*) lotus fruit/seed (Nelumbinis Fructus seu Semen)

莲房 (*lián fáng*) lotus receptacle (Nelumbinis Receptaculum)

莲须 (*lián xū*) lotus stamen (Nelumbinis Stamen)

芡实 (*qiàn shí*) euryale (Euryales Semen)

山茱萸 (*shān zhū yú*) cornus (Corni Fructus)

金樱子 (*jīn yīng zǐ*) Cherokee rose fruit (Rosae Laevigatae Fructus)

桑螵蛸 (*sāng piāo xiāo*) mantis egg-case (Mantidis Oötheca)

覆盆子 (*fù pén zǐ*) rubus (Rubi Fructus)

海螵蛸 (*hǎi piāo xiāo*) cuttlefish bone (Sepiae seu Sepiellae Os)

刺猬皮 (*cì wèi pí*) hedgehog's pelt (Erinacei Pellis)

securing essence 固精 *gù jīng*: Synonym: *astringing essence*. A method of treatment used to address SEMINAL EMISSION and SEMINAL EFFLUX in vacuity patterns, using essence-securing medicinals such as dragon bone (*lóng gǔ*), oyster shell (*mǔ lì*), Cherokee rose fruit (*jīn yīng zǐ*), euryale (*qiàn shí*), and lotus stamen (*lián xū*), combined with kidney-supplementing medicinals like cuscuta (*tù sī zǐ*), tribulus (*cì jí lí*), and cornus (*shān zhū yú*). A representative essence-securing formula is Golden Lock Essence-Securing Pill (*jīn suǒ gù jīng wán*). ☐ACU☐ Base treatment mainly on back transport points, CV, and KI. Select CV-4 (*guān yuán*, Pass Head), BL-23 (*shèn shū*, Kidney Transport), BL-15 (*xīn shū*, Heart Transport), BL-52 (*zhì shì*, Will Chamber), KI-3 (*tài xī*, Great Ravine), KI-12 (*dà hè*, Great Manifestation), CV-3 (*zhōng jí*, Central Pole), and SP-6 (*sān yīn jiāo*, Three Yin Intersection); needle with supplementation. [6: 267] [27: 286] [97: 343] [46: 678] [14: 177] [37: 384]

securing the kidney and astringing essence 固肾涩精 *gù shèn sè jīng*: A method of treatment used to address SEMINAL EMISSION or FREQUENT URINATION due to INSECURITY OF KIDNEY QI. Securing the kidney and astringing essence includes treating seminal emission or unconscious loss of semen, night sweating, lumbar pain, tinnitus, and lack of strength in the limbs with Golden Lock Essence-Securing Pill (*jīn suǒ gù jīng wán*) or treating frequent voidings of clear scant urine with Mantis Egg-Case Powder (*sāng piāo xiāo sǎn*). ☐ACU☐ Base treatment mainly on KI, CV, and BL. Select BL-23 (*shèn shū*, Kidney Transport), CV-4 (*guān yuán*, Pass Head), BL-52 (*zhì shì*, Will Chamber), KI-3 (*tài xī*, Great Ravine), KI-12 (*dà hè*, Great Manifestation), and BL-52 (*jīng gōng*, Palace of Essence); needle with supplementation. For tendency to yang vacuity, add GV-4 (*mìng mén*, Life Gate) and KI-7 (*fù liū*, Recover Flow) and use moxa. [26: 376] [27: 286] [97: 343]

securing the kidney to promote qi absorption 固肾纳气 *gù shèn nà qì*: See PROMOTING ABSORPTION OF QI BY THE KIDNEY.

securing the menses 固经 *gù jīng*: To stanch persistent FLOODING AND SPOTTING. Securing the menses treats the tip rather than the root of flooding and spotting. [MED] Among medicinals used are general blood-stanching medicinals like ass hide glue (*ē jiāo*), dried/fresh rehmannia (*shēng dì huáng*), and agrimony (*xiān hè cǎo*), and securing astringents like ox horn bone (*niú jiǎo sāi*), limonite (*yǔ yú liáng*), halloysite (*chì shí zhī*), and amethyst/fluorite (*zǐ shí yīng*). A representative menses-securing formula is Rousing Spirit Elixir (*zhèn líng dān*). [6: 268]

seeing one as two 视一为二 *shì yī wéi èr*: Seeing one object as two, usually overlapping images. [WMC] double vision. Seeing one as two is observed in SQUINT.

seeing red as white 视赤如白 *shì chì rú bái*: Synonym: *seeing things in changed colors*. Improper perception of colors. Seeing red as white is attributed to poor congenital constitution or to obstruction of the vessels in the eye. [WMC] color blindness. [MED] Enrich yin and nourish essence; regulate qi and blood. Use variations of Light-Restoring Powder (*fù míng sǎn*) and acupuncture, but expect no marked results.

seeing things in changed colors 视物易色 *shì wù yì sè*: SEEING RED AS WHITE.

seeking the cause from patterns identified 辨证求因 *biàn zhèng qiú yīn*: IDENTIFYING PATTERNS AND SEEKING THE CAUSE. [6: 266] [27: 255] [97: 343] [26: 899]

seething cauldron pulse 釜沸脉 *fǔ fèi mài*: See SEVEN STRANGE PULSES. [27: 199]

selection of adjacent points 邻近部位选穴 *lín jìn bù wèi xuǎn xué*: See SELECTION OF LOCAL POINTS.

selection of contralateral points 交叉取穴 *jiāo chā qǔ xué*: Selection of points lying on the opposite side of the body to that of the disease site. Selection of contralateral points includes GREAT NEEDLING and CROSS NEEDLING. See SELECTION OF DISTANT POINTS.

selection of distant points 远部选穴 *yuǎn bù xuǎn xué*, 远道取穴 *yuǎn dào qǔ xué*, 远道选穴 *yuǎn dào xuǎn xué*: Selecting points far from the disease site. Distant points are usually connected with the disease site directly or indirectly through the channel system. Methods of selecting distant points include: selection of same-channel points; selection of opposite-channel points; selection of same-name channel points; selection of contralateral points; selection of same-channel points of corresponding location. **Selection of same-channel points:** After determining the channel

on which the disease site is located, points can be selected on that channel for treatment. For instance, if a headache is identified as a yang brightness (*yáng míng*) channel headache in the forehead, ST-8 (*tóu wéi*, Head Corner), LI-4 (*hé gǔ*, Union Valley), and ST-41 (*jiě xī*, Ravine Divide) may be chosen. For a lesser yang (*shào yáng*) headache on the sides of the head, GB-8 (*shuài gǔ*, Valley Lead), GB-32 (*zhōng dú*, Central River), and GB-43 (*xiá xī*, Pinched Ravine) may be selected. **Selection of opposite-channel points:** In some cases, a disease located on one channel may be treated by needling points located on the channel with which it stands in interior-exterior relationship, often in combination with same-channel points. For example, the nose lies on the hand yang brightness (*yáng míng*) channel, so that disorders of the nose can be treated by combining the opposite-channel point LU-7 (*liè quē*, Broken Sequence) with the same-channel point LI-4 (*hé gǔ*, Union Valley). The throat is considered to belong to the hand greater yin (*tài yīn*) lung channel, and hence it can be treated by combining the same-channel point LU-11 (*shào shāng*, Lesser Shang) with the opposite-channel point LI-4 (*hé gǔ*, Union Valley). The stomach belongs to the foot yang brightness (*yáng míng*) stomach channel, and stomach disorders are often treated by combining ST-36 (*zú sān lǐ*, Leg Three Li) with SP-4 (*gōng sūn*, Yellow Emperor). Abdominal distention is considered to be a foot greater yin (*tài yīn*) disease, and is often treated by combining SP-3 (*tài bái*, Supreme White) and SP-4 (*gōng sūn*, Yellow Emperor) with ST-36 (*zú sān lǐ*, Leg Three Li). **Selection of same-name channel points:** Disorders can also be treated by needling points on the channel that bears the same yin-yang name as the affected channel. For example headache and pain in the nape and back can be treated by combining the foot greater yang (*tài yáng*) channel points BL-60 (*kūn lún*, Kunlun Mountains) and BL-62 (*shēn mài*, Extending Vessel) with the hand greater yang (*tài yáng*) channel point SI-3 (*hòu xī*, Back Ravine). Frontal headache and red sore swollen eyes can be treated by combining the foot yang brightness (*yáng míng*) channel points ST-44 (*nèi tíng*, Inner Court) and ST-41 (*jiě xī*, Ravine Divide) with the hand yang brightness (*yáng míng*) channel point LI-4 (*hé gǔ*, Union Valley). Stomach pain or distention and fullness in the stomach duct can be treated by combining ST-36 (*zú sān lǐ*, Leg Three Li) with LI-4 (*hé gǔ*, Union Valley). Rib-side pain can be treated by combining the foot lesser yang (*shào yáng*) point GB-34 (*yáng líng quán*, Yang Mound Spring) with the hand lesser yang (*shào yáng*) point TB-6 (*zhī gōu*, Branch Ditch). **Selection of contralateral points:** Points on one side of the body may be selected to treat disorders of the other. Contralateral points may be selected according to channel or according to corresponding location of the disorders. For example, toothache on the left can be treated by needling the LI-4 (*hé gǔ*, Union Valley) of the right hand. Paralysis of the left side of the face can be treated by needling the LI-4 (*hé gǔ*, Union Valley) and TB-5 (*wài guān*, Outer Pass) of the right extremity. Left-sided hemilateral headache can be treated by needling the TB-9 (*sì dú*, Four Rivers) of the right arm. The left shoulder can be treated by needling the LU-5 (*chǐ zé*, Cubit Marsh), LI-4 (*hé gǔ*, Union Valley), TB-5 (*wài guān*, Outer Pass), and SI-3 (*hòu xī*, Back Ravine) of right. Finally, left hip pain can be treated by needling GB-34 (*yáng líng quán*, Yang Mound Spring) of the right side. An example of treating disorders by the contralateral point corresponding to the location of the disorder is to treat pain on the left by needling LI-15 on right. Selection of contralateral points includes the method described in *The Inner Canon* (*nèi jīng*), GREAT NEEDLING, sometimes referred to by its French name *grande piqûre*, and CROSS NEEDLING. **Selection of same-name channel points of corresponding location:** The twelve regular channels comprise six pairs of channels, each pair of which shares the same yin-yang denomination. One channel of each pair is a foot channel, whereas the other is a hand channel. The arms and legs have corresponding locations, e.g., the fingers and toes, wrists and ankles, elbows and knees, etc. Selecting the same-name channel point of corresponding locations means that a disease affecting the channel at a point on the arm can be treated by needling a point on the same-name channel of the foot at the corresponding location on the opposite side of the body. Thus a disorder at LU-11 (*shào shāng*, Lesser Shang) on the hand greater yin (*tài yīn*) channel can be treated by needling the corresponding point on the foot greater yin channel, which is SP-1 (*yīn bái*, Hidden White). See more examples in the list below. [46: 599]

Selection of Same-Name Channel points of corresponding location

Pairs on the greater yin (tài yīn)

LU-11 (*shào shāng*, Lesser Shang) and SP-1 (*yīn bái*, Hidden White)

LU-10 (*yú jì*, Fish Border) and SP-3 (*tài bái*, Supreme White)

LU-9 (*tài yuān*, Great Abyss) and SP-5 (*shāng qiū*, Shang Hill)

LU-7 (*liè quē*, Broken Sequence) and SP-6 (*sān yīn jiāo*, Three Yin Intersection)

LU-6 (*kǒng zuì*, Collection Hole) and SP-8 (*dì jī*, Earth's Crux)

LU-5 (*chǐ zé*, Cubit Marsh) and SP-9 (*yīn líng quán*, Yin Mound Spring)

LU-4 (*xiá bái*, Guarding White) and SP-11 (*jī mén*, Winnower Gate)

Pairs on the yang brightness (yáng míng)

LI-1 (*shāng yáng*, Shang Yang) and ST-45 (*lì duì*, Severe Mouth)

LI-2 (*èr jiān*, Second Space) and ST-44 (*nèi tíng*, Inner Court)

LI-4 (*hé gǔ*, Union Valley) and ST-43 (*xiàn gǔ*, Sunken Valley)

LI-5 (*yáng xī*, Yang Ravine) and ST-41 (*jiě xī*, Ravine Divide)

LI-10 (*shǒu sān lǐ*, Arm Three Li) and ST-36 (*zú sān lǐ*, Leg Three Li)

LI-11 (*qū chí*, Pool at the Bend) and ST-35 (*dú bí*, Calf's Nose)

LI-12 (*zhǒu liáo*, Elbow Bone-Hole) and ST-34 (*liáng qiū*, Beam Hill)

LI-14 (*bì nào*, Upper Arm) and ST-32 (*fú tù*, Crouching Rabbit)

---

selection of interior-exterior–related channel points 表里经选穴 *biǎo lǐ jīng xuǎn xué*: SELECTION OF OPPOSITE-CHANNEL POINTS.

selection of local points 近部选穴 *jìn bù xuǎn xué*, 局部取穴 *jú bù qǔ xué*: Local points are acupuncture points located at the site of the sign or bowels or viscus being treated. Any point can be employed as a local point. Local points are most effective for chronic local diseases, but are occasionally used to treat acute local diseases too. Local points also include adjacent points—those situated near the disease site. These can replace local points in the treatment of acute conditions, and can strengthen the effects of local (and distant) points. Although any point can function as an adjacent point, those that have a salient location are usually chosen. A number of commonly used local points are conventionally used for certain local diseases. [46: 598] [46: 629]

Selection of Local Points

Vertex

GV-20 (*bǎi huì*, Hundred Convergences)

Alert Spirit Quartet (*sì shén cōng*)

BL-7 (*tōng tiān*, Celestial Connection)

Forehead

GB-14 (*yáng bái*, Yang White)

Greater Yang (*tài yáng*)

GB-15 (*tóu lín qì*, (Head) Overlooking Tears)

BL-5 (*wǔ chù*, Fifth Place)

Eyes

BL-1 (*jīng míng*, Bright Eyes)

GB-1 (*tóng zǐ liáo*, Pupil Bone-Hole)

Back of the Ball (*qiú hòu*)
BL-2 (*zǎn zhú*, Bamboo Gathering)

Nose
LI-20 (*yíng xiāng*, Welcome Fragrance)
ST-3 (*jù liáo*, Great Bone-Hole)
GV-23 (*shàng xīng*, Upper Star)

Ear diseases
TB-21 (*ěr mén*, Ear Gate)
TB-17 (*yì fēng*, Wind Screen)
GB-20 (*fēng chí*, Wind Pool)
GB-2 (*tīng huì*, Auditory Convergence)
SI-19 (*tīng gōng*, Auditory Palace)

Mouth and teeth
ST-5 (*dà yíng*, Great Reception)
CV-24 (*chéng jiāng*, Sauce Receptacle)
ST-6 (*jiá chē*, Cheek Carriage)
ST-7 (*xià guān*, Below the Joint)

Throat
CV-23 (*lián quán*, Ridge Spring)
CV-22 (*tiān tú*, Celestial Chimney)
SI-17 (*tiān róng*, Celestial Countenance)

Shoulder
LI-15 (*jiān yú*, Shoulder Bone)
TB-14 (*jiān liáo*, Shoulder Bone-Hole)
SI-10 (*nào shū*, Upper Arm Transport)
SI-11 (*tiān zōng*, Celestial Gathering)

Elbows
LI-11 (*qū chí*, Pool at the Bend)
LU-5 (*chǐ zé*, Cubit Marsh)
TB-10 (*tiān jǐng*, Celestial Well)

Wrists
TB-4 (*yáng chí*, Yang Pool)
LI-5 (*yáng xī*, Yang Ravine)
SI-4 (*wàn gǔ*, Wrist Bone)

Stomach
CV-12 (*zhōng wǎn*, Center Stomach Duct)
ST-21 (*liáng mén*, Beam Gate)
LR-13 (*zhāng mén*, Camphorwood Gate)

Kidney
BL-23 (*shèn shū*, Kidney Transport)
BL-52 (*zhì shì*, Will Chamber)

Lumbus
BL-23 (*shèn shū*, Kidney Transport)
GV-4 (*mìng mén*, Life Gate)
GV-25 (*sù liáo*, White Bone-Hole)
GV-3 (*yāo yáng guān*, Lumbar Yang Pass)

Knees
ST-34 (*liáng qiū*, Beam Hill)
GB-33 (*xī yáng guān*, Knee Yang Joint)
GB-34 (*yáng líng quán*, Yang Mound Spring)
Crane Top (*hè dǐng*)
Eye of the Knee (*xī yǎn*)

Ankles
GB-40 (*qiū xū*, Hill Ruins)
KI-3 (*tài xī*, Great Ravine)

BL-60 (*kūn lún*, Kunlun Mountains)
KI-6 (*zhào hǎi*, Shining Sea)

selection of opposite-channel points 异经选穴
yì jīng xuǎn xué: Synonym: *selection of exterior-interior related points*. Selection of points that lie on the channel that stands in exterior-interior relationship to the channel on which the disease is located. See SELECTION OF DISTANT POINTS.

selection of pathocondition points 对症选穴
duì zhèng xuǎn xué: Some points are traditionally noted for their effectiveness in treating specific signs, helping to relieve the tip of an illness. See list below. [46: 602]

Selection of Pathocondition Points

Heat effusion
GV-14 (*dà zhuī*, Great Hammer)
LI-11 (*qū chí*, Pool at the Bend)
LI-4 (*hé gǔ*, Union Valley)

Coma
GV-26 (*shuǐ gōu*, Water Trough)
Ten Diffusing Points (*shí xuān*)

Vacuity desertion
CV-4 (*guān yuán*, Pass Head)ⓜ
CV-8 (*shén què*, Spirit Gate Tower)ⓜ
ST-36 (*zú sān lǐ*, Leg Three Li)

Profuse sweating
LI-4 (*hé gǔ*, Union Valley)
KI-7 (*fù liū*, Recover Flow)

Night sweating
SI-3 (*hòu xī*, Back Ravine)
HT-6 (*yīn xī*, Yin Cleft)

Insomnia
HT-7 (*shén mén*, Spirit Gate)
SP-6 (*sān yīn jiāo*, Three Yin Intersection)

Profuse dreaming
BL-15 (*xīn shū*, Heart Transport)
HT-7 (*shén mén*, Spirit Gate)
GB-44 (*zú qiào yīn*, Foot Orifice Yin)

Loss of voice
LI-18 (*fú tú*, Protuberance Assistant)
LI-4 (*hé gǔ*, Union Valley)
PC-5 (*jiān shǐ*, Intermediary Courier)

Clenched jaw
ST-7 (*xià guān*, Below the Joint)
ST-6 (*jiá chē*, Cheek Carriage)
LI-4 (*hé gǔ*, Union Valley)

Stiff tongue
LI-4 (*hé gǔ*, Union Valley)
CV-23 (*lián quán*, Ridge Spring)
HT-5 (*tōng lǐ*, Connecting Li)

Sore throat impediment (hóu bì)
LI-4 (*hé gǔ*, Union Valley)

LU-11 (*shào shāng*, Lesser Shang)

Drooling
GV-26 (*shuǐ gōu*, Water Trough)
ST-6 (*jiá chē*, Cheek Carriage)
LI-4 (*hé gǔ*, Union Valley)

Heart palpitations
PC-6 (*nèi guān*, Inner Pass)
PC-4 (*xī mén*, Cleft Gate)

Cough
CV-22 (*tiān tú*, Celestial Chimney)
LU-7 (*liè quē*, Broken Sequence)

Gan accumulation
Four Seams (*sì fèng*)

Insufficient breast milk
SI-1 (*shào zé*, Lesser Marsh)

Flooding and spotting
CV-6 (*qì hǎi*, Sea of Qi)
SP-6 (*sān yīn jiāo*, Three Yin Intersection)
SP-1 (*yǐn bái*, Hidden White)

Pudendal itch
LR-5 (*lǐ gōu*, Woodworm Canal)

Dysphagia-occlusion (yē gé)
CV-22 (*tiān tú*, Celestial Chimney)
PC-6 (*nèi guān*, Inner Pass)

Oppression in the chest
CV-12 (*zhōng wǎn*, Center Stomach Duct)
PC-6 (*nèi guān*, Inner Pass)

Chest pain
CV-17 (*shān zhōng*, Chest Center)
PC-6 (*nèi guān*, Inner Pass)

Nausea and vomiting
PC-6 (*nèi guān*, Inner Pass)
ST-36 (*zú sān lǐ*, Leg Three Li)

Hiccough
BL-17 (*gé shū*, Diaphragm Transport)
PC-6 (*nèi guān*, Inner Pass)
PC-8 (*láo gōng*, Palace of Toil)

Abdominal distention
ST-25 (*tiān shū*, Celestial Pivot)
CV-6 (*qì hǎi*, Sea of Qi)
PC-6 (*nèi guān*, Inner Pass)
ST-36 (*zú sān lǐ*, Leg Three Li)

Rib-side pain
TB-6 (*zhī gōu*, Branch Ditch)
GB-34 (*yáng líng quán*, Yang Mound Spring)

Indigestion
ST-36 (*zú sān lǐ*, Leg Three Li)
SP-4 (*gōng sūn*, Yellow Emperor)

Urinary stoppage
SP-6 (*sān yīn jiāo*, Three Yin Intersection)
SP-9 (*yīn líng quán*, Yin Mound Spring)

Seminal emission, impotence, and premature ejaculation
CV-4 (*guān yuán*, Pass Head)

SP-6 (*sān yīn jiāo*, Three Yin Intersection)

Frequent urination
CV-3 (*zhōng jí*, Central Pole)
KI-3 (*tài xī*, Great Ravine)
KI-7 (*fù liū*, Recover Flow)

Urinary incontinence
CV-2 (*qū gǔ*, Curved Bone)
SP-6 (*sān yīn jiāo*, Three Yin Intersection)

Vaginal discharge
GB-26 (*dài mài*, Girdling Vessel)
BL-30 (*bái huán shū*, White Ring Transport)
CV-6 (*qì hǎi*, Sea of Qi)
SP-6 (*sān yīn jiāo*, Three Yin Intersection)

Constipation
ST-25 (*tiān shū*, Celestial Pivot)
TB-6 (*zhī gōu*, Branch Ditch)

Prolapse of the rectum
GV-1 (*cháng qiáng*, Long Strong)
BL-57 (*chéng shān*, Mountain Support)

Itchy skin
LI-11 (*qū chí*, Pool at the Bend)
SP-10 (*xuè hǎi*, Sea of Blood)
SP-6 (*sān yīn jiāo*, Three Yin Intersection)
Itch Reliever (*zhǐ yǎng*)

Vacuity
CV-4 (*guān yuán*, Pass Head)
ST-36 (*zú sān lǐ*, Leg Three Li)

Worm accumulation
Hundred Worm Nest (*bǎi chóng wō*)

---

selection of points on the affected channel 循经取穴 *xún jīng qǔ xué: Synonym: selection of same-channel points.* Selection of points on the same channel as the disease site. Points are selected at either local or distant locations. Disease sites in the head, face or trunk are often treated by distant points below the elbows and knees on the affected channel. For example, yang brightness (*yáng míng*) headache can be treated by needling LI-4 (*hé gǔ*, Union Valley), and stomach pain can be treated by needling ST-36 (*zú sān lǐ*, Leg Three Li). In some cases, points close to the affected area are chosen, e.g., LR-13 (*zhāng mén*, Camphorwood Gate) for liver vomiting and pain or LI-20 (*yíng xiāng*, Welcome Fragrance) for nasal congestion and loss of sense of smell. See Table 12. POINT SELECTION. [26: 753]

12.	Selecting Points on the Affected Channel	
Affected area	Local and Adjacent Points	Distant Points
Forehead	Hall of Impression (*yìn táng*) GB-14 (*yáng bái*) GV-23 (*shàng xīng*) ST-8 (*tóu wéi*)	LI-4 (*hé gǔ*) ST-44 (*nèi tíng*)
Temples	Greater Yang (*tài yáng*) GB-4 (*hàn yàn*) GB-8 (*shuài gǔ*) GB-20 (*fēng chí*)	TB-5 (*wài guān*) GB-41 (*zú lín qì*)
Back of head	BL-9 (*yù zhěn*) GV-19 (*hòu dǐng*) GB-20 (*fēng chí*)	SI-6 (*yǎng lǎo*) BL-63 (*jīn mén*) BL-67 (*zhì yīn*)
Nose	LI-20 (*yíng xiāng*) Hall of Impression (*yìn táng*) GV-23 (*shàng xīng*)	LI-4 (*hé gǔ*) LU-7 (*liè quē*)
Teeth	ST-7 (*xià guān*) ST-6 (*jiá chē*) Greater Yang (*tài yáng*)	LI-4 (*hé gǔ*) ST-44 (*nèi tíng*)
Ear	TB-21 (*ěr mén*) SI-19 (*tīng gōng*) GB-2 (*tīng huì*) TB-17 (*yì fēng*)	GB-32 (*zhōng dú*) GB-41 (*zú lín qì*) KI-3 (*tài xī*)
Tongue	CV-23 (*lián quán*) GV-15 (*yǎ mén*)	HT-5 (*tōng lǐ*) PC-7 (*dà líng*) KI-6 (*zhào hǎi*) SP-5 (*shāng qiū*)
Throat	SI-17 (*tiān róng*)	LU-7 (*liè quē*) KI-6 (*zhào hǎi*) ST-44 (*nèi tíng*)
Chest	CV-17 (*dàn zhōng*) BL-13 (*fèi shū*) LU-1 (*zhōng fǔ*)	LU-5 (*chǐ zé*) PC-6 (*nèi guān*)
Upper abdomen	CV-12 (*zhōng wǎn*) ST-21 (*liáng mén*) BL-21 (*wèi shū*)	ST-36 (*zú sān lǐ*) SP-4 (*gōng sūn*)
Umbilical region	ST-25 (*tiān shū*) CV-6 (*qì hǎi*) BL-25 (*dà cháng shū*)	ST-37 (*shàng jù xū*) ST-36 (*zú sān lǐ*)
Lower abdomen	CV-4 (*guān yuán*) CV-3 (*zhōng jí*) CV-6 (*qì hǎi*)	SP-6 (*sān yīn jiāo*)
Rib-side	LR-14 (*qí mén*) GB-24 (*rì yuè*) BL-18 (*gān shū*)	TB-6 (*zhī gōu*) PC-6 (*nèi guān*) GB-34 (*yáng líng quán*) LR-3 (*tài chōng*)
Anterior Yin	CV-3 (*zhōng jí*) CV-4 (*guān yuán*)	LR-1 (*dà dūn*) LR-3 (*tài chōng*) KI-3 (*tài xī*)
Anus	GV-1 (*cháng qiáng*) BL-30 (*bái huán shū*)	BL-57 (*chéng shān*) BL-65 (*shù gǔ*) GV-20 (*bǎi huì*)

selection of same-channel points 本经选穴 *běn jīng xuǎn xué*: Selection of points on the same channel as the disease. See SELECTION OF DISTANT POINTS.

selection of same-name channel points 同名经选穴 *tóng míng jīng xuǎn xué*: See SELECTION OF DISTANT POINTS.

selection of special group points 特定穴组选穴 *tè dìng xué zǔ xuǎn xué*: Selection of points belonging to groups such as the SOURCE POINT; NETWORK POINT; CLEFT POINT; MEETING POINTS; LOWER UNITING POINT; FOUR COMMAND POINTS; ALARM POINT; BACK TRANSPORT POINT; TRANSPORT POINT; INTERSECTION POINT. See these entries. [46: 603]

selection of same-name channel points of corresponding location 同经相应取穴法 *tóng jīng xiāng yìng qǔ xué fǎ*: Selection of points on the channel of the same yin-yang denomination at anatomically corresponding positions on the channel of the same yin-yang denomination on the opposite side of the body. See SELECTION OF DISTANT POINTS.

semen 精 *jīng*: The viscid white fluid released during ejaculation, a tangible form of essence. Diseases of or relating to semen include SCANT SEMEN, SEMINAL COLD, and SEMINAL LOSS. See ESSENCE; ESSENCE GATE; ESSENCE CHAMBER. ◇ Chin 精 *jīng*, essence, semen. There is no distinction in Chinese between essence and semen—both are called *jīng*.

seminal cold 精冷 *jīng lěng*, 精寒 *jīng hán*: A condition characterized by cold, thin, scant semen; a major cause of male sterility. Seminal cold is attributed to insufficiency of kidney qi or to kidney yang vacuity. **Insufficiency of kidney qi:** Seminal cold due to insufficiency of kidney qi is accompanied by weak constitution, marked emaciation, lusterless facial complexion, lack of strength and shortness of breath, aching lumbus and limp knees, hair loss, loosening of the teeth, frequent urination or profuse urination at night, a pale tongue and a fine pulse weak at the cubit. MED Treat by neutral supplementation of kidney. Use variations of Five-Seed Progeny Pill (*wǔ zǐ yǎn zōng wán*). ACU Base treatment mainly on KI, CV, and back transport points. BL-23 (*shèn shū*, Kidney Transport), CV-6 (*qì hǎi*, Sea of Qi), CV-4 (*guān yuán*, Pass Head), ST-36 (*zú sān lǐ*, Leg Three Li), and KI-3 (*tài xī*, Great Ravine); needle with supplementation. **Kidney yang vacuity:** Seminal cold due to kidney yang vacuity is accompanied by physical cold and coldlimbs, a bright white facial complexion, and impotence. Other signs include aching lumbus and limp knees, dizziness, tinnitus, devitalized essence-spirit, long voidings of clear urine or profuse urination at night, pale enlarged tongue with thin white fur, and forceless fine sunken pulse. MED Warm the kidney and invigorate yang. Use formulas such as Cuscuta Seed Pill (*tù sī zǐ wán*), Golden Coffer Kidney Qi Pill (*jīn guì shèn qì wán*), Right-Restoring [Life Gate] Pill (*yòu guī wán*), and Striped Dragon Pill (*bān lóng wán*). ACU Base treatment mainly on CV, KI, and GV.

Select BL-23 (*shèn shū*, Kidney Transport), KI-3 (*tài xī*, Great Ravine), BL-52 (*zhì shì*, Will Chamber), GV-4 (*mìng mén*, Life Gate), CV-4 (*guān yuán*, Pass Head), ST-29 (*guī lái*, Return), and KI-7 (*fù liū*, Recover Flow); needle with supplementation and add moxa. [92: No. 234] [56: 122] [46: 587, 677] [37: 383, 415]

seminal efflux 滑精 *huá jīng*: Involuntary loss of semen (essence) occurring in sleep without dreaming or when awake, in severe cases several times a day. Mentioned *Jing-Yue's Complete Compendium* (*jǐng yuè quán shū*). states, "Emission of semen not due to dreaming is called seminal efflux." Seminal efflux sexual performance incommensurate with libido, sexual intemperance, or excessive masturbation, causing depletion of the kidney origin and insecurity of the essence gate. MED Treat with formulas such as Golden Lock Essence-Securing Pill (*jīn suǒ gù jīng wán*), Left-Restoring [Kidney Yin] Pill (*zuǒ guī wán*), or Right-Restoring [Life Gate] Pill (*yòu guī wán*). In some cases it may be attributable to damp-heat or phlegm congestion. ACU Base treatment mainly on CV, KI, and back transport points. Select BL-23 (*shèn shū*, Kidney Transport), BL-20 (*pí shū*, Spleen Transport), CV-6 (*qì hǎi*, Sea of Qi), CV-4 (*guān yuán*, Pass Head), KI-3 (*tài xī*, Great Ravine), KI-12 (*dà hè*, Great Manifestation), BL-52 (*jīng gōng*, Palace of Essence), and ST-36 (*zú sān lǐ*, Leg Three Li). Needle with supplementation and add moxa. For seminal efflux due to damp-heat or phlegm congestion, see DAMP-HEAT SEMINAL EMISSION and PHLEGM CONGESTION SEMINAL EMISSION. See also SEMINAL LOSS. [26: 760] [27: 427] [50: 1556] [97: 585] [113: 131] [80: 591]

seminal emission 遺精 *yí jīng*: **1.** *Synonym: seminal loss.* Involuntary loss of semen (essence). In a broad sense, *seminal emission* refers to any involuntary loss of semen (seminal loss); in a narrower sense, it refers to loss of semen during sleep, the most common form. Seminal emission is mildest when it occurs while dreaming (DREAM EMISSION). It is more severe if it occurs without dreaming (SEMINAL EMISSION WITHOUT DREAMING), or while awake in the daytime (SEMINAL EFFLUX and when profuse GREAT SEMINAL DISCHARGE). It is said that "essence [i.e., semen] is moved by the spirit in response to the heart." In dream emission, the disease is mostly in the heart, whereas in seminal emission without dreaming, the disease is usually in the kidney. If evil is involved, the patterns are repletion and heat; if no evil is involved, the patterns are vacuity and cold. Seminal emission at the onset of illness is usually caused by evil fire stirring the essence chamber. In enduring illness it is usually due to internal damage by the seven affects and dishar-

mony of the organs. The main causes are effulgent sovereign and ministerial fire, heart vacuity and liver depression, insecurity of kidney qi, noninteraction of the heart and kidney, and spleen vacuity qi fall. **Effulgent sovereign and ministerial fire** causes dream emission and frequent erections. Other signs include a) heart palpitations or fearful throbbing, vexation, red face, b) dizzy head and flowery vision, c) aching lumbus and tinnitus, and d) tidal heat [effusion], night sweating, and emaciation. The tongue is red with little fur, the pulse fine stringlike and rapid, large and vacuous, or stringlike and vacuous at the cubit. MED Treat by enriching yin and downbearing fire, assisted by subduing and settling. Use Heaven, Human, and Earth Marrow-Retaining Elixir (*sān cái fēng suǐ dān*) plus dragon bone (*lóng gǔ*), oyster shell (*mǔ lì*), tortoise plastron (*guī bǎn*), gardenia (*zhī zǐ*), and coptis (*huáng lián*). ACU Base treatment mainly on back transport points, HT, KI, and LR. Drain BL-15 (*xīn shū*, Heart Transport), HT-7 (*shén mén*, Spirit Gate), HT-8 (*shào fǔ*, Lesser Mansion), and LR-3 (*tài chōng*, Supreme Surge); supplement BL-23 (*shèn shū*, Kidney Transport), KI-6 (*zhào hǎi*, Shining Sea), BL-52 (*zhì shì*, Will Chamber), and SP-6 (*sān yīn jiāo*, Three Yin Intersection). **Heart vacuity and liver depression** causes frequent alternating dream emission and seminal emission. Accompanying signs include: a) distention and fullness in the rib-side, sighing; b) heart palpitations, insomnia, dizziness, and lassitude of spirit, c) heart vexation, susceptibility to fright, reduced sleep, and mental depression; d) intermittent alternating heat [effusion] and [aversion to] cold, bitter taste in the mouth, and reduced food intake. The tongue is red at the tip with a white fur, while the pulse is large, stringlike, vacuous and rapid. MED Course the liver and eliminate depression; nourish the heart and quiet the spirit. Use Free Wanderer Powder (*xiāo yáo sǎn*) plus cinnabar (*zhū shā*), or use Biota Seed Heart-Nourishing Pill (*bǎi zǐ yǎng xīn wán*) combined with Free Wanderer Powder (*xiāo yáo sǎn*). ACU Base treatment mainly on PC, LR, SP, HT, and back transport points. Supplement HT-7 (*shén mén*, Spirit Gate), BL-15 (*xīn shū*, Heart Transport), and BL-43 (*gāo huāng shū*, Gao-Huang Transport) to nourish the heart and quiet the spirit. Drain PC-6 (*nèi guān*, Inner Pass), LR-3 (*tài chōng*, Supreme Surge), and SP-6 (*sān yīn jiāo*, Three Yin Intersection) to soothe the liver and eliminate depression. A combination of supplementing and draining nourishes the heart and regulates the liver, quiets the spirit and secures essence. **Insecurity of kidney qi** causes seminal emission unassociated with dreaming or frequent seminal emission. Accompanying signs are: a) limp aching lumbus and knees and listlessness of essence-spirit; b) clouded head and tinnitus, panting on physical exertion, bright white facial complexion and emaciation; c) increased urination at night or frequent urination. The tongue is pale with white fur, and the pulse is sunken and weak. MED Supplement the kidney and astringe essence. Use Essence-Containing Pill (*mì jīng wán*). ACU Base treatment mainly on back transport points, CV, and KI. Select CV-4 (*guān yuán*, Pass Head), KI-12 (*dà hè*, Great Manifestation), BL-52 (*zhì shì*, Will Chamber), BL-23 (*shèn shū*, Kidney Transport), and ST-36 (*zú sān lǐ*, Leg Three Li): needle with supplementation and add moxa. **Noninteraction of the heart and kidney** causes dream emission accompanied a) vexation and insomnia and limp aching lumbus and knees; and b) dizziness and tinnitus, dry mouth and pharynx, and in some cases tidal heat [effusion] and night sweating. The tongue is red with scant fur, and the pulse is rapid at the inch and sunken at the cubit, or large, vacuous and rapid. MED Promote heart-kidney interaction; enrich water and quiet the spirit. Use Cinnabar Spirit-Quieting Pill (*zhū shā ān shén wán*) combined either with Celestial Emperor Heart-Supplementing Elixir (*tiān wáng bǔ xīn dān*) or with Coptis and Ass Hide Glue Decoction (*huáng lián ē jiāo tāng*). ACU Base treatment mainly on back transport points, HT, and KI. Drain BL-15 (*xīn shū*, Heart Transport), HT-7 (*shén mén*, Spirit Gate), and PC-7 (*dà líng*, Great Mound); supplement BL-23 (*shèn shū*, Kidney Transport), KI-3 (*tài xī*, Great Ravine), KI-6 (*zhào hǎi*, Shining Sea), and SP-6 (*sān yīn jiāo*, Three Yin Intersection). **Spleen vacuity qi fall** causes seminal efflux with a) shortness of breath and laziness to speak, fatigued limbs and lack of strength, and withered-yellow facial complexion; b) torpid intake, bland taste in the mouth, diarrhea with sloppy stool, distention and sagging in the stomach duct and abdomen after eating, and lack of warmth in the limbs. The tongue is pale with white fur, while the pulse is sunken and weak or sunken and fine. MED Supplement the center and boost qi; fortify the spleen and secure essence. Use Center-Supplementing Qi-Boosting Decoction (*bǔ zhōng yì qì tāng*) plus lotus fruit/seed (*lián zǐ*), dragon bone (*lóng gǔ*), and oyster shell (*mǔ lì*) to fortify the spleen and upbear qi and to secure essence. Alternatively, use Mysterious Fragrance Powder (*miào xiāng sǎn*) or Origin-Securing Brew (*mì yuán jiān*). ACU Base treatment mainly on back transport points, CV, SP, and ST. Select BL-23 (*shèn shū*, Kidney Transport), BL-20 (*pí shū*, Spleen Transport), KI-3 (*tài xī*, Great Ravine), SP-6 (*sān yīn jiāo*, Three Yin Intersection), CV-6 (*qì hǎi*, Sea of Qi), ST-36 (*zú sān lǐ*, Leg Three Li), and SP-9 (*yīn líng quán*, Yin Mound Spring); needle with supplementation

and add moxa. For other patterns, see DAMP-HEAT SEMINAL EMISSION; DEPRESSED HEAT SEMINAL EMISSION; PHLEGM CONGESTION SEMINAL EMISSION. See also WHITE OOZE. **2.** Specifically, involuntary loss of semen during sleep. [26: 918] [50: 1556] [56: 47] [46: 596, 646, 678] [37: 384] [113: 130] [80: 591]

seminal emission without dreaming 不梦而遗 *bù mèng ér yí*, 无梦而遗 *wú mèng ér yí*: See SEMINAL EMISSION.

seminal loss 失精 *shī jīng*: SEMINAL EMISSION.[1]

sensation of pressure in the head 头胀 *tóu zhàng*: See DISTENTION IN THE HEAD.

separate decoction 另煎 *lìng jiān*: Decocting certain medicinals separately from others used in the same formula. Some costly materials such as ginseng (*rén shēn*) and rhinoceros horn (*xī jiǎo*) are boiled separately to ensure maximum extraction of their active constituents and prevent loss. The fluid is strained off and the dregs are then boiled with the other ingredients. The two decoctions are blended before taking.

separating the clear and the turbid 分清别浊 *fēn qīng bié zhuó*, 分别清浊 *fēn bié qīng zhuó*: To promote the separation of the clear and the turbid.

separation of the clear and the turbid 泌别清浊 *mì bié qīng zhuó*: The absorption in the small intestine of the essence of grain and water (the clear) by the action of the spleen, and the transference of solid waste to the large intestine and fluid waste to the bladder (the turbid). [27: 38]

separation of yin and yang 阴阳离决 *yīn yáng lí jué*: The parting of two interdependent paired yin-yang phenomena that inherently brings the destruction of both. In the body, when the yin or yang aspect of the body has been worn away excessively, the opposite pole is deprived of its basis for survival. *Elementary Questions* (*sù wèn*, *shēng qì tōng tiān lùn*) states, "When yin and yang separate, essential qi expires." See YIN COLLAPSE; YANG COLLAPSE. [27: 5] [27: 5]

settle 镇 *zhèn*: To calm; (in medicinal therapy) to calm (the spirit) with heavy settling medicinals.

settling and absorption 镇纳 *zhèn nà*: Any method of treatment involving the use of minerals and animal shells, and other medicinals to settle fright and calm the spirit, to subdue yang and extinguish wind, and to secure the kidney and promote qi absorption. **Settling fright and quieting the spirit** is used to treat heart palpitations, fearful throbbing, insomnia, or mania and withdrawal. This method makes use of heavy settlers, i.e., medicinals that are heavy in substance and have a settling effect on bodily functions, such as loadstone (*cí shí*), dragon bone (*lóng gǔ*), dragon tooth (*lóng chǐ*), oyster shell (*mǔ lì*), mother-of-pearl (*zhēn zhū mǔ*), cinnabar (*zhū shā*), and iron flakes (*tiě luò*). Heavy settlers may be combined with yang-freeing medicinals such as cinnamon twig (*guì zhī*) and acorus (*shí chāng pú*), with heart-qi–supplementing medicinals such as codonopsis (*dǎng shēn*) and licorice (*gān cǎo*), with heart-blood-nourishing medicinals such as salvia (*dān shēn*), dried rehmannia (*gān dì huáng*), tangkuei (*dāng guī*), and ass hide glue (*ē jiāo*), with heart-spirit–quieting medicinals such as spiny jujube (*suān zǎo rén*) and biota seed (*bǎi zǐ rén*), and with heat-clearing phlegm-transforming medicinals such as coptis (*huáng lián*) and bamboo shavings (*zhú rú*) according to need. A commonly used formula is Loadstone and Cinnabar Pill (*cí zhū wán*). **Subduing yang and extinguishing wind** is used to treat a) ascendant liver yang or liver wind characterized by headache, dizziness, agitation, twitching muscles, and trembling hands, b) extreme heat engendering wind on externally contracted disease, characterized by high fever, clouded spirit, TETANIC REVERSAL, and convulsions of the limbs, or c) yin vacuity stirring external wind in final-stage externally contracted heat (febrile) diseases, characterized by heat in the palms of the hands and soles of the feet, trembling limbs, or tetanic reversal. MED Yang-subduing wind-extinguishing medicinals such as oyster shell (*mǔ lì*), mother-of-pearl (*zhēn zhū mǔ*), dragon tooth (*lóng chǐ*), and loadstone (*cí shí*) combined with liver-clearing medicinals such as uncaria (*gōu téng*), chrysanthemum (*jú huā*), mulberry leaf (*sāng yè*), prunella (*xià kū cǎo*), moutan (*mǔ dān pí*), and gardenia (*shān zhī zǐ*) or with yin-enriching medicinals such as dried rehmannia (*gān dì huáng*), scrophularia (*xuán shēn*), ophiopogon (*mài mén dōng*), ligustrum (*nǔ zhēn zǐ*), tortoise plastron (*guī bǎn*), and ass hide glue (*ē jiāo*). If necessary, wind-extinguishing tetany-settling medicinals such as scorpion (*quán xiē*), silkworm (*bái jiāng cán*), earthworm (*dì lóng*), and antelope horn (*líng yáng jiǎo*) may be employed. Gastrodia and Uncaria Beverage (*tiān má gōu téng yǐn*) is used to treat liver yang transforming into wind. Triple-Armored Pulse-Restorative Decoction (*sān jiǎ fù mài tāng*) is used to treat yin vacuity stirring wind. **Securing the kidney and promoting qi absorption** is used to treat failure of the kidney to absorb qi, marked by short rapid breathing, panting at the slightest exertion, vacuity sweating, cold limbs, a bright white or dark green-blue complexion or upbearing fire flush (red complexion due fire in bowels and viscera), and a fine sunken pulse. Treatment employs kidney-supplementing medicinals such as aconite (*fù zǐ*), cinnamon bark (*ròu guì*), cooked rehmannia (*shú dì huáng*), cornus (*shān zhū yú*), walnut (*hú táo rén*), and gecko (*gé jiè*). To these should added

heavy settlers such as loadstone (*cí shí*), amethyst/fluorite (*zǐ shí yīng*), stalactite (*zhōng rǔ shí*), and galenite (*qiān*) to promote the kidney's action of absorbing qi. A commonly used formula is Galenite Elixir (*hēi xí dān*) [6: 269]

settling and subduing 镇潜 *zhèn qián*: SUBDUING AND SETTLING.

settling fright and quieting the spirit 镇惊安神 *zhèn jīng ān shén*: A method of treatment used to address heart palpitations or fearful throbbing, insomnia, and mania and withdrawal (mental disturbances). MED Fright-settling spirit-quieting medicinals include loadstone (*cí shí*), dragon bone (*lóng gǔ*), oyster shell (*mǔ lì*), mother-of-pearl (*zhēn zhū mǔ*), cinnabar (*zhū shā*), and iron flakes (*tiě luò*). These may be combined with heart yang freeing medicinals such as cinnamon twig (*guì zhī*) and acorus (*shí chāng pú*). They also include medicinals that boost heart qi such as codonopsis (*dǎng shēn*), dried/fresh rehmannia (*shēng dì huáng*), tangkuei (*dāng guī*), and ass hide glue (*ē jiāo*), as well as spirit-quieting medicinals like spiny jujube (*suān zǎo rén*) and biota seed (*bǎi zǐ rén*). Representative formula: Loadstone and Cinnabar Pill (*cí zhū wán*). ACU BL-15 (*xīn shū*, Heart Transport), HT-7 (*shén mén*, Spirit Gate), PC-6 (*nèi guān*, Inner Pass), and SP-6 (*sān yīn jiāo*, Three Yin Intersection) can be selected as the main points, adding other points for particular patterns and signs. See HEART PALPITATIONS; FRIGHT PALPITATIONS; SLEEPLESSNESS; FORGETFULNESS; MANIA; WITHDRAWAL. [6: 269] [46: 602, 644] [?: 66–70]

settling tetany 镇痉 *zhèn jìng*: RESOLVING TETANY.

settling the liver and extinguishing wind 镇肝熄风 *zhèn gān xī fēng*: CALMING THE LIVER AND EXTINGUISHING WIND.

seven affects 七情 *qī qíng*: Joy, anger, anxiety, thought, sorrow, fear, and fright. The seven affects in excess can be a cause of disease. See INTERNAL DAMAGE BY THE SEVEN AFFECTS; AFFECT. Compare FIVE MINDS. NB: The Chinese term for seven affects is identical with the term rendered as SEVEN RELATIONS. [27: 117]

seven damages 七伤 *qī shāng*: **1.** From *Essential Prescriptions of the Golden Coffer* (*jīn guì yào lüè, xuè bì xū láo bìng mài zhèng bìng zhì*). Food damage, anxiety damage, drink damage, sexual intemperance damage, hunger damage, taxation damage, and channel-network and construction-defense damage. **2.** From *The Origin and Indicators of Disease* (*zhū bìng yuán hòu lùn*). Great overeating damages the spleen; great anger and qi counterflow damages the liver; exertion or lifting heavy weights and long sitting on wet ground damages the kidney; cold in the body and cold drinks damage the lung; anxiety, worry, and thought and cogitation damage the heart; wind, rain, cold, and summerheat damage the body; great fear damages the mind. [26: 13] [27: 118]

seven gates 七冲门 *qī chōng mén*: Seven points between the mouth and anus: (1) *flying gates* (lips); (2) *door gates* (teeth); (3) *respiration gate* (epiglottis); (4) *rushing gate* (cardia, the upper mouth of the stomach); (5) *dark gate* (pylorus, lower mouth of the stomach); (6) *screen gate* (ileocecal valve); (7) *corporeal soul gate* (anus). [27: 30] [26: 14]

seven orifices 七窍 *qī qiào*: The two eyes, two ears, two nostrils, and the mouth. Compare NINE ORIFICES. [27: 27]

seven relations 七情 *qī qíng*: Seven relationships or interactions of medicinals, namely: going alone; mutual need; empowering; fear; aversion; killing; clashing. **Going alone** (单行 *dān xíng*): The ability of a medicinal to be used alone, as in Licorice Decoction (*gān cǎo tāng*) and Pure Ginseng Decoction (*dú shēn tāng*). **Mutual need** (相须 *xiāng xū*): The combined use of two medicinals of similar action used together to enhance each other's action. The implication is that the combined use of the two medicinals is greater than the sum of their individual action. Mutual need medicinals include anemarrhena (*zhī mǔ*) and phellodendron (*huáng bǎi*). **Empowering** (相使 *xiāng shǐ*): The use of one or more agents to enhance the action of a main agent. For example, apricot kernel (*xìng rén*) empowers tussilago (*kuǎn dōng huā*) to moisten the lung and downbear qi, and to suppress cough and transform phlegm. **Fear** (相畏 *xiāng wèi*): Toxicity of a medicinal being counteracted by another. For example, pinellia (*bàn xià*) fears fresh ginger (*shēng jiāng*) because its toxicity is reduced by it. Astragalus (*huáng qí*) was traditionally said to fear ledebouriella (*fáng fēng*), although in Jade Wind-Barrier Powder (*yù píng fēng sǎn*) astragalus (*huáng qí*) is said to be empowered by ledebouriella (*fáng fēng*). NB: The Chinese 畏 *wèi* means fear, but in this context the term implies the fear of a benevolent power as the English word awe. **Aversion** (相恶 *xiāng wù*): The weakening of a medicinal action by another. For example scutellaria (*huáng qín*) is averse to fresh ginger (*shēng jiāng*) because its action is weakened by it; ginseng (*rén shēn*) is averse to radish (*lái fú*), since its supplementing action is reduced by it. NB: The Chinese 恶 (*wù*) implies dislike, sickening, ailing, hence weakening; see NAUSEA. **Killing** (相杀 *xiāng shā*): The elimination of side-effects of a medicinal. For example, mung bean (*lǜ dòu*) kills croton (*bā dòu*), i.e., it eliminates the croton's noxious effects. NB: The Chinese 杀 *shā* has connotations of purification as well as slaughter.

Clashing (相反 *xiāng fǎn*:) The creation of noxious effects when two medicinals are used together. For example, aconite main tuber (*chuān wū tóu*) clashes with pinellia (*bàn xià*), so the two should not be used together. ◇ Chin 七 *qī*, seven; 情 *qíng*, affinity, affection, emotion; fact. The Chinese term *qī qíng* is identical with the term rendered in other contexts as SEVEN AFFECTS. The Chinese names of six of the seven relations contain the character 相 *xiāng*, usually rendered as mutual or reciprocal; however only in two of the terms, 相须 *xiāng xū*, mutual need, and 相反 *xiāng fǎn*, clashing, is any reciprocity implied. The technical meaning of the terms denoting the seven relations is poorly reflected in social metaphor used to describe it. [126: 48] [26: 12] [27: 307]

seven-star needle 七星针 *qī xīng zhēn*: A cutaneous needle, traditionally made by binding sewing needles to a bamboo stick, and used to provide a therapeutic stimulus when tapped lightly on the skin. See CUTANEOUS NEEDLE. [27: 330]

seven strange pulses 七怪脉 *qī guài mài*: Seven pulses signifying critical conditions: **Pecking sparrow pulse** 雀啄脉 (*què zhuó mài*): An urgent rapid pulse of irregular rhythm that stops and starts, like a sparrow pecking for food. **Leaking roof pulse** 屋漏脉 (*wū lòu mài*): A pulse that comes at long and irregular intervals, like water dripping from a leaky roof. **Flicking stone pulse** 弹石脉 (*tán shí mài*): A sunken replete pulse that feels like flicking a stone with a finger. **Untwining rope pulse** 解索脉 (*jiě suǒ mài*): A pulse described as being now loose, now tight, with an irregular rhythm like an untwining rope. Damage to a hemp rope made of tightly twined strands can cause a local slackening of the twine, so that it is tight in some places and loose in others; hence the image used to describe this pulse. **Waving fish pulse** 鱼翔脉 (*yú xiáng mài*): A pulse that seems to be yet seems not to be present, like a fish waving in the water. **Darting shrimp pulse** 虾游脉 (*xiā yóu mài*): A pulse that arrives almost imperceptibly and vanishes with flick, like a darting shrimp. **Seething cauldron pulse** 釜沸脉 (*fǔ fèi mài*): an extremely rapid floating pulse that is all outward movement with no inward movement, like water seething in a cauldron. See also TEN STRANGE PULSES. [26: 12] [27: 199]

severe conditions are treated by coaction 甚者从之 *shèn zhě cóng zhī*: From *Elementary Questions* (*sù wèn, zhì zhēn yào dà lùn*). Critical conditions of extreme heat resembling cold (true heat and false cold) and extreme cold resembling heat (true cold and false heat) are handled by the paradoxical method of treatment whereby the nature of the treatment coincides with that of the false signs. [27: 241]

severe heat and severe reversal 热深厥深 *rè shēn jué shēn*: The deeper heat evil lies in the body, the more pronounced REVERSAL COLD OF THE EXTREMITIES. Severe heat and severe reversal occurs in warm heat disease when deep-lying heat damages right qi and prevents yang qi from reaching the extremities of the body. Although there is high fever and clouded spirit, the extremities are cold. The more severe the heat, the more pronounced the cold signs. [26: 873] [27: 135] [97: 455]

sexual taxation 房室劳伤 *fáng shì láo shāng*: Excessive in sexual activity (sex, childbirth), which wears kidney essence, thereby weakening the health and increasing vulnerability to disease. Commonly observed signs include lumbar pain, seminal emission, fatigued spirit, lack of strength, and dizziness. Excessive childbirth may cause damage to the thoroughfare (*chōng*) and controlling (*rèn*) vessels, characterized by menstrual irregularities, menstrual block, and vaginal discharge. [27: 119] [97: 364]

shaking 掉 *diào*: Any shaking or tremulous movement of the head or limbs. "Shaking" occurs in the phrase: "All wind with shaking and [visual] dizziness is ascribed to the liver." ◇ Chin 掉 *diào*, move, shake (among other meanings).

shaking of the head 头摇 *tóu yáo*: Tremor or wobbling of the head that the patient cannot control. There are repletion and vacuity patterns. **Repletion** patterns usually take the form of mutual exacerbation of wind and fire or liver wind stemming from yang brightness (*yáng míng*) repletion heat; signs include sudden shaking of the head, dizziness, deafness, stiff painful neck, and in some cases high fever, vexation and agitation, and abdominal pain and constipation. MED Calm the liver and extinguish wind; drain fire and clear heat. **Vacuity** patterns mostly arise when insufficiency of the liver and kidney in old age or to vacuity weakness after enduring disease stirs internal vacuity wind. They are characterized by enduring tremor of the head with other vacuity signs. MED Supplement the liver and kidney; boost qi and blood; support the right and extinguish wind. [26: 910]

shaman healer 巫医 *wū yī*: A person who professes to heal by incantations or magic figures. Shaman healers were popular in the Shang (21st to 16th century B.C.) and Zhou (16th to 11th century B.C.). By the period of the Warring States, folk doctors were more common than before, and (the legendary) Bian Que (Qin Yue Ren) advocated that doctors should not treat patients who believed in shamans rather than healers. Despite this, shamanism has continued to the present. [27: 516] [129] [130: 17–50, 251]

shan 疝 *shàn*: MOUNTING.

Shang 商 *shāng*: The name of a dynastic period (approx. 16th cent. B.C.–11th cent. B.C.).

shank sore 臁疮 *lián chuāng*: *Synonyms: trouser-bottom sore; trouser-bottom toxin sore; skirt-hem sore.* A sore on the shin, characterized by redness, swelling, and itching. The local skin and flesh turns gray and dark. When scratched open, it suppurates. Shank sores can persist for a long time without healing. It arises mostly when damp-heat pours downward and causes blood stasis and qi stagnation. Accordingly, it is accompanied by a thin slimy yellow tongue fur, and a slippery rapid pulse. If the sore persists without healing, it becomes grayish white in color, and exudes thin dirty gray or green pus, and tends to swell in the evening. Such conditions indicate center qi fall, which often attended by bright white facial complexion, thin sloppy stool, pale tongue with thin fur, and a fine pulse. WMC ulceration of the lower leg. MED Oral: Clear heat and disinhibit dampness; harmonize construction and resolve toxin. Take Fish Poison Yam Toxin-Transforming Decoction (*bì xiè huà dú tāng*) or Mysterious Three Pill (*sān miào wán*) combined with Fish Poison Yam Dampness-Percolating Decoction (*bì xiè shèn shī tāng*). Apply Golden Yellow Paste (*jīn huáng gāo*) with Nine-to-One Elixir (*jiǔ yī dān*). For those who are allergic to Nine-to-One Elixir, use Black Tiger Elixir (*hēi hǔ dān*) topically. Center qi fall is treated by nourishing the blood and harmonizing construction, and by freeing the network vessels and relieving pain. Use variations of Cinnamon Twig Decoction Plus Tangkuei (*guì zhī jiā dāng guī tāng*). For liver-kidney yin vacuity, use Six-Ingredient Rehmannia Pill (*liù wèi dì huáng wán*), Left-Restoring [Kidney Yin] Pill (*zuǒ guī wán*), or Double Supreme Pill (*èr zhì wán*). For spleen-kidney vacuity cold with a sore that is black and painless, add Perfect Major Supplementation Decoction (*shí quán dà bǔ tāng*). Topical: Dab on Flesh-Engendering Powder (*shēng jī sǎn*) and cover with White Jade Plaster (*bái yù gāo*). NB: Some older literature makes a distinction between inner shank sores (on the medial face of the shin) and outer shank sore (on the lateral face). It attributes inner shank sores to dampness in the three yin channels of the foot, with vacuity heat in the blood aspect, and attributes outer shank sores to damp-heat gathering in the three yang channels of the foot. *The Great Compendium of External Medicine* (*wài kē dà chéng*) states inner shank sores are hard to cure, whereas outer shank sores are easy to cure. [26: 943] [96: 439] [61: 352]

shedding of flesh and loss of bulk 脱肉破䐃 *tuō ròu pò jiǒng (jùn)*: *Synonym: loss of bulk and shedding of flesh.* From *Elementary Questions* (*sù* *wènyù jī zhēn zàng lùn*). Severe emaciation, a sign of debilitation of spleen qi. It is seen in enduring illness and cachexia. See EMACIATION. ◇ Chin 脱 *tuō*, shed, desert; 肉 *ròu*, flesh; 破 *pò*, break (down); 䐃 *jùn*, also read as *jiŏng*, protuberant flesh (rendered here as bulk). [81: 443] [50: 1231]

shell-bursting mammary welling-abscess 脱壳乳痈 *tuō ké rŭ yōng*: EFFUSION OF THE BREAST.

shell-bursting scrotal welling-abscess 脱壳囊痈 *tuō ké náng yōng*: SCROTAL WELLING-ABSCESS.

shelter 蔽 *bì*: The tonguelike protuberance in front of the ear, i.e., the tragus. Also called *ear gate*, *fleshy protuberance in front of the ear*, and *pearl of the ear*. [27: 67]

sheng 升 *shēng*: A unit of volume that in the Ming and Qing Dynasty was slightly greater than 1 liter (1,073.7 and 1,035.5 ml respectively), and that in previous dynasties was considerably less, e.g., 594.4 ml in the Tang. See Table 22, page 717. [27: 578]

shiatsu 指压 *zhĭ ya*: ACUPRESSURE. ◇ Chin 指 *zhĭ*, finger; 压 *yā*, pressure. Eng from J. pronunciation of *zhĭ yā*.

shift 传变 *chuán biàn*: PASSAGE AND TRANSMUTATION. Any passage from one channel to another or change in the manifestation of disease, i.e., all regular and irregular developments in cold-damage diseases. Shift includes the normal passage of disease through the channels, such as from greater yang (*tài yáng*) to yang brightness (*yáng míng*) or lesser yang (*shào yáng*), and major or irregular changes such as of yang patterns into yin patterns or cold-heat complexes. [27: 222]

shifted bladder 转胞 *zhuăn bāo*: Urinary stoppage or frequent voiding of small amounts of urine occurring in the seventh or eighth month of pregnancy; attributable to qi vacuity or kidney vacuity. **Qi vacuity** shifted bladder is marked by urinary stoppage or frequent voidings of small amounts of urine, pain and distention in the smaller abdomen, and fidgetiness. General signs include bright white facial complexion, lassitude of essence-spirit, heavy-headedness and dizziness, shortness of breath, laziness to speak, ungratifying defecation, pale tongue with thick white fur, and a moderate vacuous slippery pulse. [MED] Supplement qi, upbear the fall, and raise the fetus. Use Qi-Boosting Urine-Abducting Decoction (*yì qì dăo niào tāng*). **Kidney vacuity** shifted bladder is characterized by frequent inhibited urination that may gradually turn into urinary stoppage. There is distention, fullness, and pain in the abdomen, and fidgetiness. General signs include fear of cold and cold limbs, limp aching lumbus and legs, pale tongue with thin moist tongue fur, and a forceless slippery sunken pulse. [MED] Warm the kidney and support yang; transform qi (promote qi transfor-

mation) and move water. Use Golden Coffer Kidney Qi Pill (*jīn guì shèn qì wán*) minus aconite (*fù zĭ*) and moutan (*mŭ dān pí*), and plus morinda (*bā jĭ tiān*) and cuscuta (*tù sī zĭ*). [ACU] Base treatment on back transport points and CV. Main points: Needle CV-6 (*qì hăi*, Sea of Qi), bilateral BL-28 (*páng guāng shū*, Bladder Transport), bilateral SP-9 (*yīn líng quán*, Yin Mound Spring); moxa CV-4 (*guān yuán*, Pass Head). Supporting points: GV-14 (*dà zhuī*, Great Hammer) and bilateral ST-36 (*zú sān lĭ*, Leg Three Li). Apply a strong stimulus and retain needles for 15–20 minutes, rotating every 1–2 minutes. Moxa after needling. For qi vacuity, add BL-20 (*pí shū*, Spleen Transport). For kidney vacuity, add BL-23 (*shèn shū*, Kidney Transport) and KI-3 (*tài xī*, Great Ravine). ◇ Chin 转 *zhuăn*, turn, rotate, pass on; 胞 *bāo*, bladder, uterus. *Essential Prescriptions of the Golden Coffer* (*jīn guì yào lüè*) describes this condition as being caused by "twisting of the bladder tie," where 'tie', 系 *xì*, is believed to refer to the urethra. *Essential Rhymes for Patterns and Treatment* (*zhèng zhì yào jué*) says that the condition is so named because "as the fetus grows it forces downward close to the bladder and the bladder is forced to the side." [67: 251] [26: 951] [27: 447] [50: 897] [5: 1154]

shivering 战栗 *zhàn lì*, 振栗 *zhèn lì*, 战寒 *zhàn hán*, 寒战 *hán zhàn*: Trembling with a subjective sensation of cold. Occurring in malaria, it comes at regular intervals and is followed by high fever. In other febrile diseases, it is a sign of exuberant interior heat preventing yang qi from effusing to the exterior and is treated by clearing heat or outthrusting evil. Shivering may also occur in yang qi vacuity patterns without heat effusion and with a fine vacuous pulse. In such cases, it is treated by supporting yang using formulas such as Astragalus Center-Fortifying Decoction (*huáng qí jiàn zhōng tāng*) or Cinnamon Twig Decoction Plus Aconite (*guì zhī jiā fù zĭ tāng*). [27: 389] [97: 405]

shiver sweating 战汗 *zhàn hàn*: Perspiration accompanied by pronounced shivering is a sign of the struggle between the evil and right in externally contracted heat (febrile) diseases. Shiver sweating is a favorable sign when the disease resolves after it. If the disease does not resolve, right qi, severely debilitated by the struggle, may desert outward leaving the patient in a critical state. Shivering without sweating is a sign of insufficiency of right qi, and heralds the inward fall of the evil. [6: 131]

shoot 射 *shè*: To thrust or surge, as in the term *water-cold shooting into the lung*.

shortage of qi 少气 *shăo qì*: Weak, short, hasty breathing, a weak voice, and a tendency to take deep breaths in order to continue speaking; mainly attributable to visceral qi vacuity, especially of center and lung-kidney qi, but also observed in phlegm turbidity, water-rheum, food stagnation, and qi stagnation. See BREATHING. Compare QI SHORTAGE. [26: 148] [29: 165] [27: 384] [97: 86]

shortness of breath 气短 *qì duǎn*, 短气 *duǎn qì*: Breathing characterized by short rapid shallow breaths. Shortness of breath is observed in many different diseases and in both vacuity and repletion patterns. In repletion patterns, it is characterized by a rough sound usually associated with distention and fullness in the chest and abdomen, and is attributable to phlegm or stagnant food affecting the normal bearing of qi. In vacuity patterns, it is generally a sign of major vacuity of original qi in enduring disease, and is characterized by weak faint breathing and associated with physical fatigue and lassitude of spirit. Comparison: Shortness of breath is similar to PANTING in that there is discontinuity between breaths (inability to catch one's breath), but differs from panting by the absence of raising of the shoulders, of flaring nostrils, or of inability to lie flat. SHORTAGE OF QI is weak breathing and a faint voice. Patients suffering from repletion shortness of breath may tend to suffer from cough and panting. Those with vacuity shortness of breath tend also to have shortage of qi. Thus the dividing lines are not clear-cut. See also BREATHING. [27: 384] [29: 165] [26: 543] [97: 569]

short pulse 短脉 *duǎn mài*: A short pulse is one that is felt only at the bar point. The short pulse signifies dual vacuity of blood and qi, or impaired flow of blood and qi. [26: 742] [27: 194] [6: 143]

short voidings of reddish urine 小便短赤 *xiǎo biàn duǎn chì*: Scant urine that is darker in color than normal. Short voidings of reddish urine normally signify repletion heat unless the patient has been given sweating, ejection, or precipitation treatment. The presence of water swelling with short voidings indicates disease among the lung, spleen, and kidney. See URINE. [92: 220]

short voidings of scant urine 小便短少 *xiǎo biàn duǎn shǎo*: Scant urine (oliguria) characterized by short voidings. See URINE.

shoulder 肩 *jiān*, 肩膀 *jiān bǎng*: The joint between the arm and the trunk and the surrounding area. [97: 364]

shoulder and back pain 肩背痛 *jiān bèi tòng*: Pain in the shoulder and back. The shoulder and back are traversed by the foot greater yang (*tài yáng*) and are associated with the lung. Pain in this area may be due to wind-cold or wind-heat invasion, or else to injury or taxation. See BACK PAIN; SHOULDER PAIN. [26: 350]

shoulder blade 胛 *jiǎ*: Either of two flat triangular bones each forming the back part of the shoulder. WMC scapula. [27: 70]

shoulder pain 肩痛 *jiān tòng*, 肩膀痛 *jiān bǎng tòng*: Any pain in the shoulder. The shoulder is a convergence point of the three yang channels of the hand and is close to the lung. Shoulder pain if not due to injury or taxation (best treated by manipulation and acupuncture), is usually caused by wind-damp. Distinction is made between pain on the anterior and posterior aspects. Pain in the anterior aspect is usually caused by wind-heat in the lung, whereas pain in the posterior aspect, which is often associated with back pain (see SHOULDER AND BACK PAIN), is usually caused by wind-damp. MED For wind-heat in the lung causing pain in the anterior aspect, dispel wind and clear heat with Major Ledebouriella Decoction (*dà fáng fēng tāng*) and variations. For pain in the posterior aspect due to wind-damp, dispel wind and transform dampness using Notopterygium Dampness-Overcoming Decoction (*qiāng huó shèng shī tāng*). ACU Base treatment mainly on LI, TB, and SI. Main points: LI-15 (*jiān yú*, Shoulder Bone), TB-14 (*jiān liáo*, Shoulder Bone-Hole), Shoulder Front (*jiān qián*), SI-11 (*tiān zōng*, Celestial Gathering), LI-16 (*jù gǔ*, Great Bone), GB-20 (*fēng chí*, Wind Pool), TB-5 (*wài guān*, Outer Pass), and LU-9 (*tài yuān*, Great Abyss). Needle with drainage. Selection of points according to pattern: For wind-heat, add LU-7 (*liè quē*, Broken Sequence), LI-4 (*hé gǔ*, Union Valley), and LI-11 (*qū chí*, Pool at the Bend). For wind-damp, add LU-5 (*chǐ zé*, Cubit Marsh), TB-4 (*yáng chí*, Yang Pool), SP-9 (*yīn líng quán*, Yin Mound Spring), and ST-36 (*zú sān lǐ*, Leg Three Li). If necessary add moxa. Selection of points according to affected channel: For pain on the yang brightness (*yáng míng*) or lesser yang (*shào yáng*) channels, add ST-36 (*zú sān lǐ*, Leg Three Li) and GB-34 (*yáng líng quán*, Yang Mound Spring). For pain on the greater yang (*tài yáng*) channel, add SI-3 (*hòu xī*, Back Ravine) and ST-38 (*tiáo kǒu*, Ribbon Opening) joined to BL-57 (*chéng shān*, Mountain Support). Selection of points according to signs: For pain in the shoulder and arm, add LI-11 (*qū chí*, Pool at the Bend) and GB-21 (*jiān jǐng*, Shoulder Well). For inability to lift the shoulder, add ST-38 (*tiáo kǒu*, Ribbon Opening) joined to BL-57 (*chéng shān*, Mountain Support). For inability to adduct the arm, add SI-10 (*nào shū*, Upper Arm Transport) and SI-9 (*jiān zhēn*, True Shoulder). For inability to rotate the shoulder and stretch out the arm, add SI-3 (*hòu xī*, Back Ravine) and SI-6 (*yǎng lǎo*, Nursing the Aged). See also LEAKY SHOULDER WIND. [26: 350]

shrunken tongue 舌瘦瘪 *shé shòu biě*: A thin, shrunken tongue indicates insufficiency of yin liquid or a dual vacuity of yin and qi. A shrunken tongue resulting from damage to yin humor by exuberant heat is crimson in color and dry. In dual yin and qi vacuity, the tongue is pale in color. Modern clinical observation shows that shrinkage generally occurs in the latter stages of external heat (febrile) diseases, and in conditions described in Western medicine as pulmonary tuberculosis, and also in advanced-stage carcinoma. It is explained as the atrophy of the lingual muscle and epithelium due to malnutrition. [6: 120]

Shu Han 蜀汉 *shǔ hàn*: The name of a dynasty (A.D. 221–263).

shuttle bone 杼骨 *zhù gǔ*: SPINE BONE.

SI 小肠 *xiǎo cháng*, 手太阳小肠经 *shǒu tài yáng xiǎo cháng jīng*: Abbreviation for the hand greater yang (*tài yáng*) small intestine channel.

side head wind 边头风 *biān tóu fēng*: HEMILATERAL WIND.

side-lock bone 鬓骨 *bìn gǔ*: TEMPLE. ◇ Chin *bìn*, the side locks, the hair at the side of the face; 骨 *gǔ*, bone. [26: 1007] [27: 64]

sighing 叹息 *tàn xī*: A long deep audible exhalation, commonly observed in depression of liver qi, but may also be observed in qi vacuity patterns. Compare GREAT RESPIRATION. [50: 214] [92: 54] [81: 148]

sign 证 *zhèng*, 证候 *zhèng hòu*, 象 *xiàng*: **1.** Any indication of disease, e.g., pain or other localized discomfort, heat effusion, poor appetite, abnormalities of stool, urine, menses, etc. In most cases, a sign is insufficient to determine the nature of the disease. A group of signs of diagnostic significance is called a *pattern*. The most important signs are listed below. **2.** Any disease sign other than the pulse. See PRECEDENCE OF SIGNS OVER THE PULSE; PRECEDENCE OF PULSE OVER SIGNS. [27: 347]

Signs

AVERSION TO COLD (*wù hán*)
  COLD BACK (*bèi hán*)
HEAT EFFUSION (*fā rè*)
  BAKING HEAT [EFFUSION] (*hōng rè*)
  VIGOROUS HEAT [EFFUSION] (*zhuàng rè*)
  TIDAL HEAT [EFFUSION] (*cháo rè*)
  UNSURFACED HEAT (*shēn rè bú wài yáng*)
  VEXING HEAT IN THE FIVE HEARTS (*wǔ xīn fán rè*)
  HOT BACK (*bèi rè*)
  HOT HEAD (*tóu rè*)
ALTERNATING HEAT [EFFUSION] AND [AVERSION TO] COLD (*hán rè wǎng lái*)
SWEATING (*hàn chū*)
  SPONTANEOUS SWEATING (*zì hàn*)
  NIGHT SWEATING (*dào hàn*)
RUNNY NOSE (*liú bí tì*)
TEARING (*liú lèi*)
  TEARING ON EXPOSURE TO WIND (*yíng fēng liú lèi*)
DELIRIOUS SPEECH (*zhān yǔ*)
MUSSITATION (*zhèng shēng*)

SOLILOQUY (*dú yǔ*)
CLOUDED SPIRIT (*shén hūn*)
TUGGING AND SLACKENING (*jì zòng*) (convulsions)
HEMIPLEGIA (*bàn shēn bú suì*)
ARCHED-BACK RIGIDITY (*jiǎo gōng fǎn zhāng*)
HEAVY BODY (*shēn zhòng*)
SPONTANEOUS EXTERNAL BLEEDING (*nǜ xuè*)
HEADACHE (*tóu tòng*)
DIZZINESS (*xuàn yūn*)
HEAVY-HEADEDNESS (*tóu zhòng*)
DISTENTION IN THE HEAD (*tóu zhàng*)
FLOWERY VISION (*mù huā*)
DRY EYES (*mù gān sè*)
RED EYES (*mù chì*)
DEVIATED EYES AND MOUTH (*kǒu yǎn wāi (kuāi) xié*)
CLENCHED JAW (*kǒu jìn*)
LUSTERLESS NAILS (*jiǎ zhuǎ bù róng*)
THIRST (*kǒu kě*)
SORE THROAT (*yān hóu tòng*)
DRY THROAT (*hóu yān gān zào*)
BITTER TASTE IN THE MOUTH (*kǒu kǔ*)
COUGH (*ké sòu*)
COUGHING OF BLOOD (*ké xuè*)
PANTING (*chuǎn*)
FROG RALE IN THE THROAT (*hóu zhōng yǒu shuǐ jī shēng*)
SHORTNESS OF BREATH (*duǎn qì*)
QI ASCENT (*shàng qì*)
SHORTAGE OF QI (*shǎo qì*)
HEART PALPITATIONS (*xīn jì*)
FORGETFULNESS (*jiàn wàng*)
VEXATION (*xīn fán*)
SUSCEPTIBILITY TO FRIGHT (*yì jīng*)
IRASCIBILITY (*yì nù*)
PROFUSE DREAMING (*duō mèng*)
SLEEPLESSNESS (*bù mèi*)
SOMNOLENCE (*shì shuì*)
CLOUDING SLEEP (*hūn shuì*)
POOR APPETITE (*shí yù bù zhèn*)
TORPID INTAKE (*nà dāi*)
PREDILECTION FOR STRANGE FOODS (*shì shí yì wù*)
ACID UPFLOW (*fàn suān*)
SWALLOWING OF UPFLOWING ACID (*tūn suān*)
ACID VOMITING (*tù suān*)
VOMITING (*ǒu tù*)
BELCHING (*ài qì*)
VOMITING OF BLOOD (*tù xuè*)
CHEST PAIN (*xiōng tòng*)
OPPRESSION IN THE CHEST (*xiōng mèn*)
RIB-SIDE PAIN (*xié tòng*)
STOMACH DUCT PAIN (*wèi wǎn (guǎn) téng tòng*)
ABDOMINAL PAIN (*fù tòng*)
ABDOMINAL FULLNESS (*fù mǎn*)
ABDOMINAL DISTENTION (*fù zhàng*)
PUFFY SWELLING (*fú zhǒng*)

DIARRHEA (*xiè xiè*)

TENESMUS (*lǐ jí hòu zhòng*)

BLOODY STOOL (*biàn xuè*)

PUS AND BLOOD IN THE STOOL (*dà biàn nóng xuè*)

NONTRANSFORMATION OF FOOD (*wán gǔ bù huà*)

CONSTIPATION (*biàn bì*)

BLOODY STOOL (*biàn xuè*)

PROFUSE URINATION AT NIGHT (*yè jiān duō niào*)

SHORT VOIDINGS OF REDDISH URINE (*xiǎo biàn duǎn chì*)

LONG VOIDINGS OF CLEAR URINE (*xiǎo biàn qīng cháng*)

INHIBITED URINATION (*xiǎo biàn bù lì*)

PAINFUL URINATION (*niào tòng*)

BLOODY URINE (*niào xuè*)

FREQUENT URINATION (*xiǎo biàn pín shuò*)

DRIBBLING URINATION (*xiǎo biàn lín lì*)

LUMBAR PAIN (*yāo tòng*)

TINNITUS (*ěr míng*)

DEAFNESS (*ěr lóng*)

YELLOWING (*fā huáng*)

NUMBNESS (*má mù*)

EMACIATION (*xíng tǐ xiāo shòu*)

HYPERTONICITY (*jū jí*)

LASSITUDE OF SPIRIT AND LACK OF STRENGTH (*shén pí fá lì*)

HEMIPLEGIA (*bàn shēn bù suì*)

MENSTRUAL IRREGULARITIES (*yuè jīng bù tiáo*)

VAGINAL DISCHARGE (*dài xià*)

IMPOTENCE (*yáng wěi*)

SEMINAL EMISSION (*yí jīng*)

---

silvery internal obstruction 如银内障 *rú yín nèi zhàng*: COIN SCREEN. ◇ Chin 如 *rú*, as, like; 银 *yín*, silver, silver coin; 内 *nèi*, internal; 障 *zhàng*, obstruction.

simple abdominal distention 单腹胀 *dān fù zhàng*, 单腹胀大 *dān fù zhàng dà*: Synonyms: *simple abdominal drum*; *simple drum*. Pronounced abdominal distention without generalized water swelling. See DRUM DISTENTION; STONE WATER.[2] [26: 730]

simple abdominal drum 单腹鼓 *dān fù gǔ*: See SIMPLE ABDOMINAL DISTENTION.

simple drum 单鼓 *dān gǔ*: See SIMPLE ABDOMINAL DISTENTION.

simple supplementation and drainage manipulation 单式补泻手法 *dān shì bǔ xiè shǒu fǎ*: A method of achieving supplementation or drainage in acupuncture by manipulating the needles. Simple supplementation and drainage techniques are listed below. See NEEDLE MANIPULATION. [27: 340]

Simple Supplementation and Drainage Manipulation

DIRECTIONAL SUPPLEMENTATION AND DRAINAGE (*yíng suí bǔ xiè*)

ROTATING SUPPLEMENTATION AND DRAINAGE (*niǎn zhuǎn bǔ xiè*)

QUICK AND SLOW SUPPLEMENTATION AND DRAINAGE (*jí xú bǔ xiè*)

LIFTING AND THRUSTING SUPPLEMENTATION AND DRAINAGE (*tí chā bǔ xiè*)

RESPIRATORY SUPPLEMENTATION AND DRAINAGE (*hū xī bǔ xiè*)

OPEN AND CLOSED SUPPLEMENTATION AND DRAINAGE (*kāi hé bǔ xiè*)

NINE AND SIX SUPPLEMENTATION AND DRAINAGE (*jiǔ liù bǔ xiè*)

---

simultaneous supplementation and attack 攻补兼施 *gōng bǔ jiān shī*: The principle of simultaneously supporting right and dispelling an evil. Simultaneous supplementation and attack applies in two cases: (1) where the evil is strong but right is not too severely weakened, or (2) where evil qi is strong and the first consideration is to expel it, whereas right qi is weak and cannot withstand attack (offensive treatment). An example of the first case is were there is cold diarrhea due to mild interior vacuity (not persistent clear-food diarrhea which would be more severe). Such conditions may be treated by simultaneously resolving the exterior and warming the interior, using a formula such as Cinnamon Twig and Ginseng Decoction (*guì zhī rén shēn tāng*) as prescribed in *On Cold Damage* (*shāng hán lùn*) for dual resolution of interior and exterior. An example of the second case is a condition requiring swift precipitation to preserve yin, for which the normally prescribed Major Qi-Coordinating Decoction (*dà chéng qì tāng*) is contraindicated because of the presence of a forceless soft pulse. Instead, Yellow Dragon Decoction (*huáng lóng tāng*) or Humor-Increasing Qi-Coordinating Decoction (*zēng yè chéng qì tāng*) is used, to prevent sudden desertion following precipitation. [6: 244] [27: 257]

sinew 筋 *jīn*, 筋脉 *jīn mài*: Tough, stringy, elastic parts of the body. (1) A tendon. See SINEW MEMBRANE. (2) A palpable muscle. (3) The *sinew gathering*, i.e., the penis. See SINEW WILTING for an example of this usage. (4) A vain visible at the surface of the body, especially one that is abnormal in size or form. ◇ Chin 筋 *jīn*, tendon, sinew, or anything similar such as veins or stringy parts of plants. Modern Chinese dictionaries tend to equate the term with 'tendon' as used in modern medicine. However, both old and new literature applies the term in a wider meaning: a) 'sinews' referred to in descriptions of acupuncture point locations are often muscles rather than tendons, e.g., GB-31 (*fēng shì*, Wind Market); b) the *sinew channels* cover areas beyond tendons; c) in explanations of *wilting wěi* and *tetany* in terms of the liver's governing of the sinews, 'sinew' refers to what are called muscles in modern anatomy, and it is unlikely that the Chinese thought of it exclusively as the tough white substance attached to the bone. Anatomically, therefore, the Chinese concept of 筋 *jīn* cannot be equated with the meaning of the English *tendon*. It should, rather, be understood to overlap with that of the flesh, which anatomically includes the muscle and fat. The sinew in its relationship to the liver explains the etiology and treatment of diseases affecting the muscles such as WILTING *wěi* and TETANY, whereas 'flesh' in its relationship to the spleen explains the etiology and treatment of other diseases affecting the muscles such as emaciation and general lack of strength. *The Magic Pivot* (*líng shū*) says, "Sinew is toughness." *Explanation of Characters* (说文解字 *shuō wén*) states, "筋 is the strength of the flesh; [the character] is derived from [the meaning of its components] 肉 *ròu*, flesh, and 力 *lì*, strength, and 竹 *zhú*, bamboo, a thing that is very sinewy." The sinew must be understood in its relationship to the liver and the five-phase concept of wood. Wood is the "bending and stretching." It corresponds to "woody" or "sinewy" parts of the body that have the power to bend and stretch. These include include tendons and functional aspect of the muscles. Note also that the liver is described as the "unyielding viscus" and a "(military) general," which also reflect the notion of strength associated with liver-wood. See LIVER. Finally, it should also be pointed out that the 筋 also refers to visible blood vessels, especially in the compound 青筋 *qīng jīn*, "blue-green *jin*." Both sinew goiter (see GOITER) and SINEW TUMOR are characterized by and so named because of knotted veins (varicosity) appearing on their surface. Note that the term 筋脉 *jīn mài* nowadays usually means simply 'sinew', but in earlier texts, it may be interpreted as 'sinews and vessels'. [26: 740] [81: 394]

sinew and bone pain 筋骨疼痛 *jīn gǔ téng tòng*: Pain experienced as coming from the sinew and bone.

sinew gan 筋疳 *jīn gān*: See GAN OF THE LIVER. [26: 741]

sinew goiter 筋瘿 *jīn yǐng*: Goiter on whose surface green-blue veins like earthworms are clearly visible. Sinew goiter is attributed to anger damaging the liver, effulgent fire, and blood dryness. MED Clear the liver and resolve depression; nourish the blood and soothe the sinews. An appropriate formula is Liver-Clearing Aloe Pill (*qīng gān lú huì wán*). [26: 741]

sinew impediment 筋痹 *jīn bì*: An IMPEDIMENT (*bì*) pattern characterized by hypertonicity of sinews and joint pain preventing normal move-

ment. Sinew impediment is caused by wind-cold-damp invading the sinews. Long-standing sinew impediment can develop in *liver impediment*. [26: 741] [27: 404]

sinew membrane 筋膜 *jīn mó*: The thin coating of the muscle, as distinct from the thick sinews (tendons) that are attached to the bone. The sinew membrane, like the sinew itself, is governed by the liver. See SINEW. [27: 30] [97: 565]

sinew mounting 筋疝 *jīn shàn*: Pain and shrinkage of the penis, sometimes associated with itching, swelling, suppuration, impotence, and discharge of white mucus with the urine. Sinew mounting is attributed to liver channel damp-heat and damage to the kidney through sexual intemperance. MED Treat by clearing damp-heat, using formulas such as Gentian Liver-Draining Decoction (*lóng dǎn xiè gān tāng*) or Coptis Toxin-Resolving Decoction (*huáng lián jiě dú tāng*). If there is swelling and rupture, Coptis Paste (*huáng lián gāo*) may be applied topically. When the tip has been treated, treatment can be given to boost the kidney. ACU Base treatment mainly on LR, SP, and CV. Select LR-2 (*xíng jiān*, Moving Between), LR-3 (*tài chōng*, Supreme Surge), SP-9 (*yīn líng quán*, Yin Mound Spring), SP-6 (*sān yīn jiāo*, Three Yin Intersection), CV-3 (*zhōng jí*, Central Pole); and BL-28 (*páng guāng shū*, Bladder Transport); needle with drainage. ◇ Chin 筋 *jīn*, sinew; 疝 *shàn*, an accumulation. See MOUNTING. The term probably derives from the euphemistic attribute of the penis as the "gathering place of the sinews." [26: 740] [27: 430] [97: 565] [56: 67] [37: 454]

sinew network vessel 筋络 *jīn luò*: See SINEW VESSEL.

sinew pain 筋痛 *jīn tòng*: Pain in the sinews. Sinew pain is attributed to blood vacuity, obstruction of qi and blood, or vacuity of the fluids depriving the sinews of nourishment. [26: 741]

sinew scrofula 筋疬 *jīn lì*: Hard scrofula of varying size on the side of the neck, associated with heat effusion and aversion to cold, and exacerbated by taxation and anger. MED Clear the liver and resolve depression with Bupleurum Liver-Clearing Decoction (*chái hú qīng gān tāng*). ACU Use appropriate points given under SCROFULA, and select BL-18 (*gān shū*, Liver Transport), BL-17 (*gé shū*, Diaphragm Transport), PC-6 (*nèi guān*, Inner Pass), LR-3 (*tài chōng*, Supreme Surge), SP-6 (*sān yīn jiāo*, Three Yin Intersection), and ST-36 (*zú sān lǐ*, Leg Three Li) as main points; needle with even supplementation and drainage to clear the liver and resolve depression. See SCROFULA. [26: 741] [27: 478]

sinew tumor 筋瘤 *jīn liú*: A TUMOR (a growth on the outside of the body) characterized by purple coloration, with green-blue veins entwined over it and some protruding like worms. [WMC] phlebangioma; varicosity. A sinew tumor is attributable to anger stirring liver fire, blood dryness, and sinew hypertonicity. [MED] Clear the liver, nourish the blood, and soothe the sinews. Use Liver-Clearing Aloe Pill (*qīng gān lú huì wán*). ◇ Chin 筋 *jīn*, sinew, visible vein; 瘤 *liú*, tumor. [26: 741]

sinew vessel 筋脉 *jīn mài*: Synonym: *sinew network vessel*. Any of the vessels that bring nourishment to the sinews. See SINEW. [81: 394] [46: 13]

sinew wilting 筋痿 *jīn wěi*: From *Elementary Questions* (*sù wèn, wěi lùn*). **1.** Synonym: *liver wilting*. A WILTING (*wěi*) pattern attributable to liver heat causing insufficiency of liver yin, in turn causing desiccation of the sinews and membranes. Sinew wilting is characterized by hypertonicity of the sinews gradually giving way to wilting that prevents normal movement. It is accompanied by bitter taste in the mouth and dry nails. [MED] Clear heat, supplement the blood, and nourish the liver. Use formulas such as Blood-Supplementing Sinew-Enhancing Pill (*bǔ xuè róng jīn wán*). [ACU] Base treatment mainly on back transport points, LR, GB, and KI. Needle with supplementation at BL-18 (*gān shū*, Liver Transport), BL-23 (*shèn shū*, Kidney Transport), BL-20 (*pí shū*, Spleen Transport), BL-17 (*gé shū*, Diaphragm Transport), and LR-3 (*tài chōng*, Supreme Surge), and with drainage at GB-34 (*yáng líng quán*, Yang Mound Spring), LR-2 (*xíng jiān*, Moving Between), and KI-1 (*yǒng quán*, Gushing Spring). See WILTING. **2.** SLACKNESS OF THE ANCESTRAL SINEW, i.e., impotence; attributed to stirring of wild desires and excessive sexual taxation. See IMPOTENCE. [26: 741] [27: 402] [97: 565] [113: 242] [46: 638]

single-handed needle insertion 单手进针法 *dān shǒu jìn zhēn fǎ*: A needle insertion technique using one hand only. **Method:** (1) The needle is held between the thumb and index finger, and the middle finger is placed next to the insertion site. The tip and lower part of the needle rest against the middle finger. (2) The needle is thrust sharply into the body, the middle finger bending in the action. **Application:** This method is used in the insertion of short filiform needles. The technique of the single-handed insertion can also be applied with the techniques of SKIN-SPREADING NEEDLE INSERTION, SKIN-PINCHING NEEDLE INSERTION, and the NAIL PRESS NEEDLE INSERTION. See NEEDLE INSERTION; NEEDLE MANIPULATION. [46: 461]

six bowels 六腑 *liù fǔ*: The gallbladder, stomach, large intestine, small intestine, triple burner, and bladder. See BOWELS AND VISCERA. [26: 87]

six-channel pattern identification 六经辨证 *liù jīng biàn zhèng*: Six-channel pattern identification was first mentioned in *The Inner Canon* (*nèi jīng*) and subsequently refined in *On Cold Damage* (*shāng hán lùn*). The latter represents a systematic synthesis of pre-Han experience and theory concerning external heat (febrile) diseases, and elaborated on the six-channel patterns discussed in *Elementary Questions* (*sù wèn*), in which observable signs and disease shifts are explained in terms of greater yang (*tài yáng*), yang brightness (*yáng míng*), and lesser yang (*shào yáng*) diseases (collectively known as the three yang channel diseases), and greater yin (*tài yīn*), lesser yin (*shào yīn*), and reverting yin (*jué yīn*) diseases (collectively known as the three yin channel diseases). It describes the principal patterns, the methods, and formulas used to treat them, as well as combined and transmuted patterns and sequences of channel passage. *On Cold Damage* (*shāng hán lùn*) is considered the basis of identification and treatment of external heat (febrile) disease patterns; the pathology, methods of treatment, formulas, and medicinals it discusses are used as a guide for internal damage miscellaneous disease as well. [6: 224] [27: 218] [97: 128]

six-channel patterns 六经形证 *liù jīng xíng zhèng*: From *Elementary Questions* (*sù wèn*). "On the first day of cold damage, greater yang (*tài yáng*) is affected, and signs include headache and pain in the neck, and stiffness in the lower back. On the second day, yang brightness (*yáng míng*) is affected. Since the yang brightness (*yáng míng*) governs the flesh, and its channel passes up the side of the nose to connect with the eyes, there is generalized heat [effusion], eye pain and dry nose. On the third day, the lesser yang (*shào yáng*) is affected. Since the lesser yang (*shào yáng*) governs the gallbladder, and its channel passes through the rib-side and connects with the ears, signs include pain in the chest and rib-side and tinnitus. On the fourth day, the greater yin (*tài yīn*) is affected. Since the greater yin (*tài yīn*) channel passes through the stomach and connects with the throat, signs include fullness in the stomach and dry throat. On the fifth day, the lesser yin (*shào yīn*) is affected. Since the lesser yin (*shào yīn*) channel passes through the kidney, connects with the lung, and penetrates through to the root of the tongue, signs include dry mouth and tongue, and thirst. On the sixth day, the reverting yin (*jué yīn*) is affected. Since the reverting yin (*jué yīn*) channel passes through the genitals and connects with the liver, signs include agitation and retracted scrotum." This passage is considered to be the basis of six-channel pattern identification and treatment on which *On Cold Damage* (*shāng hán lùn*) is founded. [6: 224]

six depressions 六郁 *liù yù*: Stagnation of qi, blood, damp, fire, phlegm, and food. Each is readily identifiable: QI DEPRESSION, by pain in the chest and rib-side, and a rough sunken pulse; DAMP DEPRESSION, by general heaviness and pain, or pain in the joints, usually associated with damp weather, and a fine sunken pulse; FIRE DEPRESSION (or heat depression), by visual distortion, oppression and vexation, reddish urine, and a rapid sunken pulse; PHLEGM DEPRESSION, by panting associated with physical exertion, and a slippery sunken pulse; BLOOD DEPRESSION, by loss of power in the lower limbs, bloody stool, and a sunken, scallion-stalk pulse; and FOOD DEPRESSION, which denotes lodged food, by belching of sour gas, abdominal distention, and no thought of food and drink. Of these six, qi depression is the most important, as it underlies all the others; when qi depression is eliminated, the other forms naturally disappear. See also DEPRESSION. [26: 88]

six excesses 六淫 *liù yín*: Excess or untimeliness of the six qi (wind, cold, summerheat, damp, dryness, and fire) that invade the body through the exterior to cause disease. Wind diseases are most common in spring, summerheat in summer, damp disease in long summer, dryness diseases in autumn, and cold diseases in winter. *The Inner Canon* (*nèi jīng*) referred to the six excesses as the "six qi" (the six kinds of weather), but recognized them as causes of diseases. *Elementary Questions* (*sù wèn*) states, "The hundred diseases are all engendered by wind, cold, summerheat, dampness, and fire." The name *liù yín* is a later coining, thought to have been based on a passage in *Elementary Questions* (*sù wèn, zhì zhēn yào dà lùn*) which states, "when wind is excessive (淫) in the inner body...", "when dampness is excessive in the inner body..." The term was first recorded in SP-6 (*sān yīn jiāo*, Three Yin Intersection), published in A.D. 1174, in which they are referred to as cold, summerheat, dryness, dampness, wind, and heat (not fire). Each of the six excesses is associated with a season. Fire and summerheat are both forms of heat. Heat in the summer (from the Summer Solstice to Beginning of Autumn) is generally called summerheat, whereas heat that occurs untimely in other seasons is called fire (or heat). Fire is other contexts denotes an intense form of heat and is contrasted with a milder form, warmth. ◇ Chin 淫 *yín*, dissolute, licentious; excess; evil. [26: 87] [36: 204–210] [97: 125] [81: 329]

six extremes 六极 *liù jí*: From *Essential Prescriptions of the Golden Coffer* (*jīn guì yào lüè, zàng fǔ jīng luò xī hòu bìng mài*). Six extreme forms of VACUITY DETRIMENT affecting the blood, sinews, flesh, qi, bone, and essence. Each is identifiable by signs: **extreme of the blood** by hair loss and forgetfulness; **extreme of the sinew** by hypertonic-ity; **extreme of the flesh** by wasting of the flesh and withered-yellow facial complexion; **extreme of qi** by shortness of breath and rapid panting; **extreme of the bone** by loose teeth and wilting legs; **extreme of essence** by dark vision and tinnitus. [26: 88] [27: 387]

six qi 六气 *liù qì*: **1.** From *Elementary Questions* (*sù wèn, tiān yuán jì dà lùn*). Six environmental phenomena, wind, cold, summerheat, dampness, dryness, and fire, which in excess are believed to cause disease and as such are known as the *six excesses*. **2.** Essence, qi, liquid, humor, blood, and vessels (or pulse). [26: 87] [27: 107] [97: 124]

skin 皮 *pí*, 皮肤 *pí fū*: The outer integument of the body; governed by the lung. See LUNG GOVERNS THE SKIN AND [BODY] HAIR. *adj. cutaneous.* [26: 197]

skin and [body] hair 皮毛 *pí máo*: The outer covering of the body and the hair that grows from it. The skin and [body] hair are closely associated with defense qi, which repels invading evils. See LUNG GOVERNS SKIN AND [BODY] HAIR.

skin and [body] hair wilting 皮毛痿 *pí máo wěi*: LUNG WILTING (*fèi wěi*) that affects the skin and [body] hair. Skin and [body] hair wilting is attributed to lung heat scorching the lobes. The skin is desiccated and withered and is possibly associated with cough and rapid breathing. If it does not go away, the sinews, vessels, bones, and flesh may be deprived of nourishment, giving rise to crippling wilt. ⎡MED⎤ Clear heat and engender liquid; nourish yin and moisten the lung. Use formulas such as Lung-Clearing Decoction (*qīng fèi tāng*). ⎡ACU⎤ Use the general points listed under WILTING (*wěi*) and add points such as BL-13 (*fèi shū*, Lung Transport), LU-5 (*chǐ zé*, Cubit Marsh), KI-6 (*zhào hǎi*, Shining Sea), KI-2 (*rán gǔ*, Blazing Valley), and SP-6 (*sān yīn jiāo*, Three Yin Intersection), needling with supplementation to clear heat, nourish yin, and moisten the lung. See LUNG WILTING. [26: 197]

skin impediment 皮痹 *pí bì*: Synonym: *cold impediment*. An IMPEDIMENT (*bì*) pattern described in *Zhang's Clear View of Medicine* (*zhāng shì yī tōng*) in the following ways: "Skin impediment is cold impediment. The evil is in the skin and [body] hair, causing dormant papules and wind sores that are not made sore by scratching, and in the initial stages, produces a sensation of "bugs creeping in the skin." ⎡MED⎤ Course wind and nourish the blood using Large Gentian and Rehmannia Decoction (*qín jiāo dì huáng tāng*). [26: 198] [27: 404]

skin-pinching needle insertion 夹持进针法 *jiā chí jìn zhēn fǎ*: PINCH-AND-LIFT NEEDLE INSERTION.

skin-spreading needle insertion 舒张进针法 *shū zhāng jìn zhēn fǎ*: A two-hand needle insertion technique whereby the skin is stretched to facilitate needle insertion. **Method:** (1) While holding the handle of the needle between the thumb and forefinger of the right hand, bring the needle tip to rest lightly on the skin surface above the point. (2) Stretch the skin on either side of the point with the thumb and forefinger of the left hand. (3) Insert the needle using a quick, firm downward movement with the right hand while keeping the skin spread taught with the left hand. **Application:** By increasing the surface tension of the skin, areas of loose or folded skin (such as on the abdomen and on elderly patients) are more easily penetrated. See NEEDLE INSERTION. [46: 461]

skin water 皮水 *pí shuǐ*: From *Essential Prescriptions of the Golden Coffer* (*jīn guì yào lüè, shuǐ qì bìng mài zhèng bìng zhì*). WATER SWELLING of gradual onset that engulfs the fingers, associated with drum-like enlargement of the abdomen, with absence of both sweating and thirst, and with a floating pulse. Skin water is attributed to spleen vacuity with severe dampness causing water to spill into the skin. [MED] Free yang, fortify the spleen, and disinhibit water using formulas like Fangji and Poria (Hoelen) Decoction (*fáng jǐ fú líng tāng*). [ACU] See WATER SWELLING. [26: 197] [27: 419] [97: 170]

skipping channels 越经传 *yuè jīng chuán*: In six-channel pattern identification, the missing of a channel in the normal sequence of passage, e.g., when greater yang (*tài yáng*) disease passes directly to lesser yang (*shào yáng*) without first affecting yang brightness (*yáng míng*). [27: 223] [97: 543]

skipping pulse 促脉 *cù mài*: Synonym: *rapid irregularly interrupted pulse*. A pulse that is urgent and forceful and that pauses at irregular intervals. It indicates: a) exuberant heat repletion; b) blood, qi, phlegm, or food stagnation; or c) painful swelling. See PULSE CONDITION. [50: 1105] [6: 142]

skirt-hem sore 裙边疮 *quán biān chuāng*: SHANK SORE.

slackness of the ancestral sinew 宗筋弛纵 *zōng jīn chí zòng*: **1.** An etiological factor of *crippling wilt*. *Elementary Questions* (*sù wèn, wěi lùn*) states, "When yang brightness (*yáng míng*) is vacuous, then the ancestral sinews are slack, the girdling (*dài*) vessel fails to conduct; hence the legs become wilted and useless." **2.** IMPOTENCE. *Elementary Questions* (*sù wèn, wěi lùn*) states, "When the ancestral sinew is slack, sinew wilting develops." [97: 370] [25: 205]

slack sinews 筋缓 *jīn huǎn*: Limpness or lack of contractile strength of the sinews hampering normal voluntary movements. Slack sinews are the result of liver-kidney depletion, excessive consump-

tion of sour food, or damage by damp-heat. It occurs in WILTING, IMPEDIMENT, and VACUITY TAXATION patterns. [26: 741]

slanted insertion 斜刺 *xié cì*: OBLIQUE INSERTION. See also NEEDLE INSERTION.

sleep 睡眠 *shuì mián*: The naturally recurring (especially nightly) condition of repose and inactivity in which consciousness and response to external stimuli are largely suspended. Sleep is understood in terms of the heart, kidney, and construction and defense. A healthy person under normal circumstances is alert in the daytime and has undisturbed sleep at night. In the daytime, defense qi moves in the yang channels, the heart and kidney work together, and essence-spirit is vigorous. At night, defense qi enters the yin channels, the heart spirit returns to its abode and the kidney mind (see MIND) becomes calm. See ETHEREAL SOUL. Disturbances of sleep primarily include INSOMNIA, reduced sleeping time, SOMNOLENCE, which is the ability to sleep night and day and to fall asleep quickly and return to sleep after waking, and DROWSINESS AFTER EATING, which is the tendency to sleep after meals. Excessive or confused dreaming, called PROFUSE DREAMING attends some forms of insomnia. Somnolence with clouded spirit is called CLOUDING SLEEP, observed in heat entering the pericardium. Other sleep-related conditions include PROFUSE URINATION AT NIGHT, ENURESIS, SEMINAL EMISSION, DREAM EMISSION, and GRINDING OF THE TEETH. Sleeping with the head in poor posture may cause CRICK IN THE NECK. Excessive snoring may indicate NASAL POLYP. [29: 206] [66: 257]

sleeping silkworms beneath the eyes 目下有卧蚕 *mù xià yǒu wò cán*: From *Essential Prescriptions of the Golden Coffer* (*jīn guì yào lüè, shuǐ qì bìng mài zhèng bìng zhì*). Swelling of the lower lids. A sign of water qi in the abdomen. [97: 151] [27: 172] [44: 1179]

sleeplessness 不寐 *bù mèi*, 不得眠 *bù dé mián*, 不得卧 *bù dé wò*: Synonym: *insomnia*. Total or partial reduction in sleeping time. Sleeplessness may take the form of difficulty getting to sleep (initial insomnia), tendency to awake and difficulty getting back to sleep, or tendency to sleep on and off through the night (failure to sleep soundly). In severe cases, there may be nightlong sleeplessness. Sleeplessness arises through a variety of pathomechanisms most of which involve insufficiency of heart blood, heart-spleen vacuity, qi vacuity and blood depletion, water qi intimidating the heart, noninteraction of the heart and kidney, heart-gallbladder qi vacuity, effulgent yin vacuity fire, intense heart fire, liver depression transforming into fire, gallbladder fire, and phlegm-heat harassing the inner body. **Insufficiency of heart**

blood sleeplessness arises when insufficiency of yin-blood deprives the heart of nourishment. It is associated with signs of yin-blood insufficiency and vacuity fire such as vexing heat in the five hearts, profuse sweating, dry mouth and red tongue, and a fine rapid pulse. There may be kidney yin vacuity signs such as lumbar pain, dizziness, and tinnitus, or signs of noninteraction of the heart and kidney, such as dream emission. [MED] Enrich yin and boost the kidney; drain fire and quiet the spirit. Use Coptis and Ass Hide Glue Decoction (*huáng lián ē jiāo tāng*), Heart-Supplementing Elixir (*bǔ xīn dān*), Cinnabar Spirit-Quieting Pill (*zhū shā ān shén wán*), and Celestial Emperor Heart-Supplementing Elixir (*tiān wáng bǔ xīn dān*). [ACU] Base treatment for sleeplessness mainly on HT and the three yin channels of the foot. Main points: Alert Spirit Quartet (*sì shén cōng*), HT-7 (*shén mén*, Spirit Gate), and SP-6 (*sān yīn jiāo*, Three Yin Intersection). For yin-blood depletion, add BL-15 (*xīn shū*, Heart Transport), BL-20 (*pí shū*, Spleen Transport), BL-17 (*gé shū*, Diaphragm Transport), CV-14 (*jù què*, Great Tower Gate), and CV-6 (*qì hǎi*, Sea of Qi); needle with supplementation. Acupuncture treatment for sleeplessness is most effective when applied in the afternoon or in the evening before bed. If yin-blood depletion is accompanied by hyperactive vacuity fire, add BL-23 (*shèn shū*, Kidney Transport), KI-1 (*yǒng quán*, Gushing Spring), KI-6 (*zhào hǎi*, Shining Sea), and PC-8 (*láo gōng*, Palace of Toil). **Center qi vacuity** sleeplessness is insomnia accompanied by lassitude and lack of strength and reduced appetite. If there is copious phlegm, signs include nausea and vomiting, oppression in the chest, a slimy tongue fur, and slippery pulse. [MED] Supplement qi with Six Gentlemen Decoction (*liù jūn zǐ tāng*). For copious phlegm, base treatment on transforming phlegm using Gallbladder-Warming Decoction (*wēn dǎn tāng*) or Center-Supplementing Qi-Boosting Decoction (*bǔ zhōng yì qì tāng*). [ACU] Use the main points for insomnia given above, and add BL-15 (*xīn shū*, Heart Transport), BL-20 (*pí shū*, Spleen Transport), CV-6 (*qì hǎi*, Sea of Qi), and ST-36 (*zú sān lǐ*, Leg Three Li), needling with supplementation and adding moxa. For copious phlegm, use the main points for insomnia combined with ST-40 (*fēng lóng*, Bountiful Bulge), CV-12 (*zhōng wǎn*, Center Stomach Duct), ST-36 (*zú sān lǐ*, Leg Three Li), and PC-6 (*nèi guān*, Inner Pass), needling with drainage. **Heart-spleen vacuity** causes sleeplessness characterized by failure to sleep soundly, sleeping on and off, profuse dreaming, heart palpitations, forgetfulness, dizziness, fatigued limbs and lassitude of the spirit, tastelessness of food, lusterless complexion, pale tongue with thin fur, and a fine weak pulse. The heart governs the blood, and the spleen is the source of blood production. Vacuity of the heart and spleen creates blood vacuity that deprives the heart of nourishment, so the spirit does not keep to its abode. Excessive thought can damage both the spleen and heart, and tends to prevent the heart spirit from "returning to its abode," hence the tendency to profuse dreaming. Sleeplessness due to dual vacuity of the heart and spleen is treated by boosting qi and fortifying the spleen and by nourishing the heart and quieting the spirit. [MED] Supplement the heart and spleen with Spleen-Returning Decoction (*guī pí tāng*). For pronounced insufficiency of heart blood, cooked rehmannia (*shú dì huáng*), white peony (*bái sháo yào*), and ass hide glue (*ē jiāo*) may be added. For pronounced sleeplessness, heart-nourishing spirit-quieting medicinals such as schisandra (*wǔ wèi zǐ*) and biota seed (*bǎi zǐ rén*), spirit-quieting medicinals such as silk tree bark (*hé huān pí*) and flowery knotweed stem (*yè jiāo téng*), or heavy settlers such as dragon bone (*lóng gǔ*) and oyster shell (*mǔ lì*) can be added. Another formula used to treat sleeplessness due to heart-spleen vacuity is Spleen Longevity Brew (*shòu pí jiān*). [ACU] To the main points for sleeplessness add BL-15 (*xīn shū*, Heart Transport), BL-20 (*pí shū*, Spleen Transport), LR-13 (*zhāng mén*, Camphorwood Gate), CV-6 (*qì hǎi*, Sea of Qi), needling with supplementation and adding moxa. **Qi vacuity and blood depletion** is a common cause of sleeplessness in the elderly. [MED] Supplement qi or the blood. Use the formulas for qi vacuity given above for insufficiency of yin-blood and center qi vacuity. [ACU] To the main points for sleeplessness add CV-6 (*qì hǎi*, Sea of Qi), ST-36 (*zú sān lǐ*, Leg Three Li), LR-3 (*tài chōng*, Supreme Surge), BL-20 (*pí shū*, Spleen Transport), BL-21 (*wèi shū*, Stomach Transport), and BL-17 (*gé shū*, Diaphragm Transport). Supplement and add moxa. **Water qi intimidating the heart** causes sleeplessness accompanied by stirring palpitations below the heart. [MED] Free yang and disinhibit water with Poria (Hoelen), Cinnamon Twig, Ovate Atractylodes, and Licorice Decoction (*líng guì zhú gān tāng*) or variations. [ACU] To the main points for sleeplessness add BL-15 (*xīn shū*, Heart Transport), BL-21 (*wèi shū*, Stomach Transport), BL-23 (*shèn shū*, Kidney Transport), BL-22 (*sān jiāo shū*, Triple Burner Transport), PC-6 (*nèi guān*, Inner Pass), CV-17 (*shān zhōng*, Chest Center), CV-9 (*shuǐ fēn*, Water Divide), CV-6 (*qì hǎi*, Sea of Qi), and ST-36 (*zú sān lǐ*, Leg Three Li); needle with drainage and add moxa. See also LIVER FIRE SLEEPLESSNESS. **Noninteraction of the heart and kidney** is characterized by difficulty getting to sleep or, in severe cases, nightlong sleeplessness, associated with dizziness, tinnitus, tidal heat [effusion], night sweating, vexing heat in the five hearts, forgetfulness, limp aching lumbus and limbs, seminal emission, red tongue with scant fur, and rapid fine pulse. ⟦MED⟧ Enrich kidney water, downbear heart fire, and promote heart-kidney interaction. Use Coptis and Ass Hide Glue Decoction (*huáng lián ē jiāo tāng*) combined with Peaceful Interaction Pill (*jiāo tài wán*). *Medical Discussions of the Cold Shack* (*lěng lú yī huà*) recommends using pinellia (*bàn xià*) and prunella (*xià kū cǎo*) to promote heart-kidney interaction. These medicinals can be combined with the formulas suggested. ⟦ACU⟧ To the main points for sleeplessness add BL-15 (*xīn shū*, Heart Transport), BL-23 (*shèn shū*, Kidney Transport), and PC-7 (*dà líng*, Great Mound), needling with even supplementation and drainage. For pronounced yin vacuity, add KI-6 (*zhào hǎi*, Shining Sea). For profuse dreaming, add GB-44 (*zú qiào yīn*, Foot Orifice Yin) and ST-45 (*lì duì*, Severe Mouth). **Heart-gallbladder qi vacuity** causes sleeplessness with profuse dreaming and a tendency to awake with fright. Signs of gallbladder vacuity include susceptibility to fright and fear, lack of decisiveness, and a tendency to get nervous about small matters. Signs of qi vacuity include shortness of breath, fatigue, and long voidings of clear urine. Qi-blood vacuity and gallbladder involvement are reflected in a pale tongue and a fine stringlike pulse. ⟦MED⟧ Boost qi and settle fright; quiet the spirit. Use formulas such as Spirit-Quieting Mind-Stabilizing Pill (*ān shén dìng zhì wán*). ⟦ACU⟧ To the main points add BL-15 (*xīn shū*, Heart Transport), BL-19 (*dǎn shū*, Gallbladder Transport), GB-34 (*yáng líng quán*, Yang Mound Spring), and GB-40 (*qiū xū*, Hill Ruins), needling with supplementation. **Effulgent yin vacuity fire** patterns are marked by heart palpitations, dizziness, tinnitus, forgetfulness, lumbar pain, dry mouth with little liquid, vexing heat in the five hearts, red tongue, and a fine rapid pulse. ⟦MED⟧ Enrich yin and downbear fire; clear the heart and quiet the spirit. Use Six-Ingredient Rehmannia Pill (*liù wèi dì huáng wán*) combined with Coptis, Ass Hide Glue, and Egg Yolk Decoction (*huáng lián ē jiāo jī zǐ huáng tāng*). ⟦ACU⟧ To the main points add BL-15 (*xīn shū*, Heart Transport), BL-23 (*shèn shū*, Kidney Transport), and KI-6 (*zhào hǎi*, Shining Sea), needling with even supplementation and drainage. **Intense heart fire** is characterized by agitation, dry mouth and tongue, possibly with sores, short voidings of reddish urine, red-tipped tongue, and thin yellow tongue fur. ⟦MED⟧ Clear heat and drain fire; quiet the heart and spirit. Use Cinnabar Spirit-Quieting Pill (*zhū shā ān shén wán*) plus scutellaria (*huáng qín*), and gardenia (*shān zhī zǐ*). ⟦ACU⟧ To the main points add PC-8 (*láo gōng*, Palace of Toil), CV-14 (*jù què*, Great Tower Gate), PC-4 (*xī mén*, Cleft Gate), and HT-5 (*tōng lǐ*, Connecting Li), needling with drainage. Prick HT-9 (*shào chōng*, Lesser Surge)

to bleed. **Liver depression transforming into fire** causes sleeplessness with rashness, impatience, and irascibility, the classic signs of liver depression. Fire harassing the upper body can cause red eyes. When liver qi invades the stomach, there is no thought of food and drink. Thirst with desire for fluids, reddish urine, constipation, bitter taste in the mouth, red tongue with yellow fur, and a rapid slippery stringlike pulse indicate heat. ⟦MED⟧ Treat by clearing the liver and draining fire, supported by quieting the spirit. Use variations of Gentian Liver-Draining Decoction (*lóng dǎn xiè gān tāng*). For oppression in the chest and sighing, add cyperus (*xiāng fù zǐ*), curcuma (*yù jīn*), and bitter orange (*zhǐ ké*). If the formula fails to deal with the sleeplessness, add abalone shell (*shí jué míng*), mother-of-pearl (*zhēn zhū mǔ*), loadstone (*cí shí*), and dragon tooth (*lóng chǐ*). ⟦ACU⟧ To the main points add BL-18 (*gān shū*, Liver Transport), LR-3 (*tài chōng*, Supreme Surge), PC-6 (*nèi guān*, Inner Pass), LR-2 (*xíng jiān*, Moving Between), GB-34 (*yáng líng quán*, Yang Mound Spring), and PC-7 (*dà líng*, Great Mound), needling with drainage. **Gallbladder fire** sleeplessness results from depressed gallbladder qi transforming into fire, usually stemming from emotional depression or anger or dietary irregularities causing phlegm and heat to gather in the gallbladder. The sleeplessness is accompanied by rib-side distention and fullness, heart vexation, yellow or red eyes, and stringlike pulse. ⟦MED⟧ Clear and drain the liver and gallbladder with Gentian Liver-Draining Decoction (*lóng dǎn xiè gān tāng*), Sweet Wormwood and Scutellaria Gallbladder-Clearing Decoction (*hāo qín qīng dǎn tāng*), or Bovine Bezoar Heart-Clearing Pill (*niú huáng qīng xīn wán*). ⟦ACU⟧ To the main points add BL-19 (*dǎn shū*, Gallbladder Transport), GB-43 (*xiá xī*, Pinched Ravine), and GB-34 (*yáng líng quán*, Yang Mound Spring), needling with drainage. **Phlegm-heat harassing the inner body** causes sleeplessness with dizziness and heavy-headedness. This is a phlegm-food pattern that develops when lodged food engenders phlegm, which in turn engenders heat. Lodged food and phlegm manifest as oppression in the chest. Phlegm-heat causes sleepless and vexation, dizziness, heavy-headedness, and canthus discharge. Phlegm heat also accounts for a slimy yellow tongue fur and a slippery rapid pulse. Phlegm-food stagnating in the center burner causes stomach qi to ascend counterflow, manifesting in signs such as aversion to food, belching, nausea, and vomiting. For this reason, this pattern falls into the category of "unquiet sleep due to stomach disharmony." Phlegm-heat sleeplessness is treated by transforming phlegm and clearing heat, and by harmonizing the stomach and quieting the spirit. An appropriate formula is Gallbladder-Warming

Decoction (*wēn dǎn tāng*) plus coptis (*huáng lián*) and gardenia (*shān zhī zǐ*). For heart palpitations and susceptibility to fright, add dragon tooth (*lóng chǐ*), mother-of-pearl (*zhēn zhū mǔ*), loadstone (*cí shí*), and lily bulb (*bǎi hé*). For severe phlegm-damp, Chlorite/Mica Phlegm-Rolling Pill (*méng shí gǔn tán wán*) can be considered. ACU To the main points add ST-40 (*fēng lóng*, Bountiful Bulge), CV-12 (*zhōng wǎn*, Center Stomach Duct), ST-36 (*zú sān lǐ*, Leg Three Li), LI-4 (*hé gǔ*, Union Valley), PC-6 (*nèi guān*, Inner Pass), sCV-17 (*shān zhōng*, Chest Center), and ST-8 (*tóu wéi*, Head Corner), needling with drainage. See also INTERNAL DAMAGE SLEEPLESSNESS and EXTERNAL CONTRACTION SLEEPLESSNESS. ◇ Chin 不寐 *bù mèi* means literally "not sleep"; 不得眠 *bù dé mián*, "cannot sleep"; 不得卧 *bù dé wò*, "cannot lie/sleep". The last of these terms is ambiguous, and in some contexts it denotes inability to lie flat. 失眠 *shī mián* is the equivalent of 'insomnia' in Western medicine, and is now the term most commonly used in modern Chinese medical literature literature. [26: 128] [27: 395] [92: No. 53] [80: 216] [37: 346]

sleep talking 梦呓 *mèng yì*: Talking during sleep; a sign of the ethereal soul failing to be stored. See ETHEREAL SOUL.

sleep walking 梦游 *mèng yóu*: Walking during sleep; a sign of the ethereal soul failing to be stored. See ETHEREAL SOUL.

slide-cupping 走罐 *zǒu guàn*: PUSH-CUPPING.

slight swelling of the eye nest 目窠上微肿 *mù kē shàng wēi zhǒng*: Mild swelling of the upper and lower eyelids. Slight swelling of the eye nest is attributable to the spleen failing to control water and kidney failing to perform qi transformation, or to externally contracted wind evil contending with water. See EYE NEST. [26: 201]

sliminess in the mouth 口腻 *kǒu nì*: A slimy or sticky feeling in the mouth. Sliminess in the mouth is often associated with bitter taste in the mouth, sweet taste in the mouth, or especially bland taste in the mouth. It is attributed to cold-damp encumbering the spleen, damp-heat obstructing the center, or phlegm-heat obstruction. **Cold-damp encumbering the spleen** causes a sticky slimy sensation in the mouth, bland taste in the mouth, absence of thirst, no thought of food and drink, fullness and oppression in the stomach duct, fatigue and lack of strength, thin sloppy stool, inhibited urination, pale enlarged tongue, and a white slimy watery glossy tongue fur, and a moderate soggy pulse. MED Transform turbidity with aroma; fortify the spleen and dry dampness. Use Agastache/Patchouli Qi-Righting Powder (*huò xiāng zhèng qì sǎn*) or Stomach-Calming Powder (*píng wèi sǎn*). **Damp-heat obstructing the center** causes a

sticky slimy dry sensation in the mouth, foul turbid breath, inability to taste ingested food, dry mouth with no desire to drink, fullness and distention in the stomach duct and abdomen, grimy sloppy stool, reddish or yellow urine, red tongue with slimy yellow tongue fur, and a soggy rapid or stringlike rapid pulse. A sweet taste in the mouth indicates that the damp-heat is mostly in the spleen and stomach, whereas bitter taste in the mouth with rib-side pain indicates damp-heat affecting the liver and gallbladder. MED Clear heat and transform dampness. Use Three Kernels Decoction (*sān rén tāng*) or Agastache/Patchouli, Pinellia, and Poria (Hoelen) Decoction (*huò pò xià líng tāng*). If there is a sweet taste in the mouth, apply the method of repelling foulness with aroma and arousing the spleen; use Sweet Dew Toxin-Dispersing Elixir (*gān lù xiāo dú dān*) or Basil Drink (*lán xiāng yǐn zi*). If there is a bitter taste in the mouth with rib-side pain, use Gentian Liver-Draining Decoction (*lóng dǎn xiè gān tāng*) or variations of Coptis and Magnolia Bark Beverage (*lián pò yǐn*). **Phlegm-heat obstruction** causes a sticky slimy sensation in the mouth with thirst but no desire to drink, fullness and oppression in the chest and diaphragm, heart vexation, yellow sticky phlegm that is difficult to expectorate, torpid intake and reduced eating, red tongue with dry slimy yellow tongue, and a slippery rapid pulse. MED Clear heat and transform phlegm. Use Coptis Gallbladder-Warming Decoction (*huáng lián wēn dǎn tāng*). [92: 116]

slimy tongue fur 腻苔 *nì tāi*: A tongue with a turbid slimy coating that is not easily removed and that does not have the grainy appearance of a healthy tongue fur. A slimy tongue fur is a sign of damp turbidity, phlegm-rheum, or food accumulation, the evil being judged as strong when the slimy coating is generalized. A slimy fur that covers only the center or the root of the tongue indicates a chronic condition, and disappears easily. [6: 123]

slippery pulse 滑脉 *huá mài*: The slippery pulse is very smooth-flowing, and is classically described as "pearls rolling in a dish" or "small fish swimming." A slippery pulse is commonly seen in: (1) pregnancy, particularly in the early stages where extra blood is needed to nourish the fetus; (2) some healthy people, indicating an abundance of qi and blood; (3) phlegm-rheum patterns and food stagnation. **Similar pulse:** The *stirred pulse* is a combination of the rapid, short, and slippery pulses, and is smooth-flowing. It differs from the slippery pulse mainly in bobbing like a bean. It is a sign of pain or fright, and may be seen in sweating, heat effusion, diarrhea, seminal collapse, and flooding and spotting. It is also observed in pregnancy. [29: 228, 251] [6: 141]

sloppy diarrhea 溏泄 *táng xiè*: Mild diarrhea characterized by sloppy stool. [27: 364] [97: 615]

sloppy stool 便溏 *biàn táng*: Semiliquid stool. See also DUCK'S SLOP.

sloughing flat-abscess 脱疽 *tuō jū*: A sore of gradual onset appearing on the hands and feet, and more frequently on the toes. It starts as a yellow blister the size of a millet seed. The skin is maroon like the color of boiled jujubes. It gradually putrefies and ulcerates, spreads outward, and penetrates inward to the flesh, sinew, and bone. It gives off a malign smell. On the toes, it can spread up onto the feet, or to other toes. The sore is associated with a burning pain that is usually intermittent and that usually occurs suddenly when walking or at night. It arises when as a result of rich food, lack of exercise, or excessive consumption of hot kidney-supplementing medicinals, depressed fire toxic evil brews in the bowels and viscera and disperses yin humor. It may also arise when cold-damp evil toxin causes disharmony of construction and defense and stagnation of qi and blood. A sloughing flat-abscess is difficult to cure, especially if treatment is not administered early in its development. ⌷WMC⌷ thromboangiitis (thrombotic angiitis). ⌷MED⌷ Depending on the cause, Mysterious Four Resting Hero Decoction (*sì miào yǒng ān tāng*), Harmonious Yang Decoction (*yáng hé tāng*), or Peach Kernel and Carthamus Four Agents Decoction (*táo hóng sì wù tāng*) can be selected as the basic formula to treat fire toxin, cold-damp evil toxin, and blood stasis respectively. Add wingless cockroach (*zhè chóng*), notoginseng (*sān qī*), frankincense (*rǔ xiāng*), myrrh (*mò yào*), salvia (*dān shēn*), moutan (*mǔ dān pí*), lonicera stem and leaf (*rěn dōng téng*) smooth greenbrier root (*tǔ fú líng*), and bushy knotweed (*hǔ zhàng*) to quicken the blood and dissipate stasis and to clear heat and relieve pain. For qi and blood vacuity, use Perfect Major Supplementation Decoction (*shí quán dà bǔ tāng*) or Ginseng Construction-Nourishing Decoction (Pill) (*rén shēn yǎng róng tāng (wán)*). ⌷ACU⌷ Base treatment mainly on LI and GB. Selection of points according to affected area: On the upper limbs, select LI-4 (*hé gǔ*, Union Valley) joined to SI-3 (*hòu xī*, Back Ravine), LI-11 (*qū chí*, Pool at the Bend) joined to HT-3 (*shào hǎi*, Lesser Sea), and HT-2 (*qīng líng*, Green-Blue Spirit); add LI-10 (*shǒu sān lǐ*, Arm Three Li) for the thumb, PC-6 (*nèi guān*, Inner Pass) for the middle finger, TB-5 (*wài guān*, Outer Pass) for the fourth finger (ring finger), and HT-5 (*tōng lǐ*, Connecting Li) for the little finger. On the lower limbs, select GB-34 (*yáng líng quán*, Yang Mound Spring) joined to SP-9 (*yīn líng quán*, Yin Mound Spring), GB-39 (*xuán zhōng*, Suspended Bell) joined to SP-6 (*sān yīn jiāo*, Three Yin Intersection), and Vessel's Root (*mài gēn*); add ST-36

(*zú sān lǐ*, Leg Three Li), and ST-40 (*fēng lóng*, Bountiful Bulge) for the back of the foot and the second and third toes; add SP-8 (*dì jī*, Earth's Crux); for the great toe. Needle with drainage and add moxa. Selection of points according to cause: For depressed fire toxin, add PC-3 (*qū zé*, Marsh at the Bend), BL-40 (*wěi zhōng*, Bend Center), Eight Evils (*bā xié*), and Eight Winds (*bā fēng*), needling with drainage. For cold-damp evil toxin, add CV-12 (*zhōng wǎn*, Center Stomach Duct), ST-25 (*tiān shū*, Celestial Pivot), LI-4 (*hé gǔ*, Union Valley), SP-9 (*yīn líng quán*, Yin Mound Spring); and ST-36 (*zú sān lǐ*, Leg Three Li), needling with drainage and adding moxa. For blood stasis, add BL-17 (*gé shū*, Diaphragm Transport), SP-10 (*xuè hǎi*, Sea of Blood), and LR-3 (*tài chōng*, Supreme Surge), needling with even supplementation and drainage or with drainage. ◇ Chin 脱 *tuō*, shed, cast off. [97: 522] [26: 646] [61: 109] [113: 403] [73: 525] [96: 449]

sloughing scrotum 脱囊 *tuō náng*, 囊脱 *náng tuō*: Redness and swelling of the scrotum causing ulceration that, in severe cases, leaves the testicles exposed. Sloughing scrotum is attributed to damp-heat fire toxin pour down into the liver channel. ⌷MED⌷ Drain liver fire; disinhibit damp-heat. In the initial stages, use Gentian Liver-Draining Decoction (*lóng dǎn xiè gān tāng*). Before ulceration, apply Jade Dew Powder (*yù lù sǎn*) or Golden Yellow Powder (*jīn huáng sǎn*). After ulceration, first wash with brine or a decoction of perilla stem (*zǐ sū gěng*), and then apply Flesh-Engendering Powder (*shēng jī sǎn*) or Flesh-Engendering Jade and Red Paste (*shēng jī yù hóng gāo*) and dress with gauze. Change the dressing each day. [50: 1409] [26: 647] [56: 155]

slowness to grow hair 发迟 *fà chí*: One of the FIVE SLOWNESSES. Delayed hair growth or sparse hair growth in infants. Slowness to grow hair is attributed to constitutional insufficiency with qi and blood vacuity depriving the hair of proper nourishment. ⌷TRT⌷ Supplement the blood. Improve diet. [26: 869]

slowness to speak 语迟 *yǔ chí*: One of the FIVE SLOWNESSES. Slowness of children in learning to speak. Children normally begin speaking between the age of two or three. Failure to begin speaking by the age of four or five is called slowness to speak. **Earlier heaven kidney vacuity and disharmony of heart qi,** two major causes of slowness to speak, are explained by the heart's being the sprout of the tongue and the kidney vessel's connection with the root of the tongue. ⌷MED⌷ When due to insufficiency of kidney qi, treat with Six-Ingredient Rehmannia Pill (*liù wèi dì huáng wán*) plus acorus (*shí chāng pú*) and polygala (*yuǎn zhì*). When due to insufficiency of heart qi, treat with Heart-Supplementing Elixir (*bǔ xīn dān*). **Spleen-stomach depletion** preventing liquid qi from nourishing the tongue may also be a cause. MED Treat with Center-Supplementing Qi-Boosting Decoction (*bǔ zhōng yì qì tāng*). In addition, proper attention to speech training should be given, and if there are signs of poor hearing, tests should be performed to identify possible congenital deaf-mutism. [26: 825]

slowness to stand 立迟 *lì chí*: One of the FIVE SLOWNESSES. Slowness of infants in learning to stand erect. Infants normally learn to stand within their first year. Failure to be able to stand erect after this time is called slowness to stand. It may be due to such factors as liver-kidney vacuity or poor feeding affecting the development of the sinew and bone and causing limpness of the knee and lower leg. MED Ensure correct diet; supplement the liver and kidney with formulas such as Six-Ingredient Rehmannia Pill (*liù wèi dì huáng wán*) plus lycium berry (*gǒu qǐ zǐ*) and deerhorn glue (*lù jiǎo jiāo*). [26: 173]

slowness to teethe 齿迟 *chǐ chí*: One of the FIVE SLOWNESSES. Slowness of infants to grow teeth. Teeth usually start to erupt at the age of 6–7 months. Any delay in this process is known as slowness to teethe. Since the teeth are the surplus of the bone and the kidney governs the bone, slowness to teeth is attributed to congenital kidney vacuity. MED Use formulas such as Six-Ingredient Rehmannia Pill (*liù wèi dì huáng wán*) prepared as a decoction. [26: 886] [97: 213]

slowness to walk 行迟 *xíng chí*: One of the FIVE SLOWNESSES. Slowness of children in learning to walk. Children normally learn to walk soon after they have learned to stand. A child that has not learned to walk by the age of two to three is said to suffer from slowness to walk. Slowness to walk is attributable to the same causes and treated in the same way as slowness to stand. In modern clinical practice, slowness to walk is a prompt for tests to identify possible infantile paralysis, myodystrophy, or bone damage from external injury. [26: 289]

slow pulse 迟脉 *chí mài*: A slow pulse is one that has three or less beats per respiration. The slow pulse is principally associated with cold and with yang vacuity. It may occur in any disease involving insufficiency of yang qi or obstruction of qi dynamic, such as cold, phlegm turbidity, and static blood. Occurring during pregnancy, this pulse signifies uterine vacuity cold or insecurity of fetal qi. Similar pulse: The *moderate pulse* is also slower than the standard pulse, though with more than three beats per respiration, and is not an indication of morbidity. [6: 140] [27: 193] [97: 324]

sluggish speech 言语謇（謇）涩 *yán yǔ jiǎn (jiǎn) sè*: Inhibited movement of the tongue that makes speech unclear. Sluggish speech is observed in wind stroke. See SLUGGISH TONGUE.

sluggish tongue 舌謇（謇）*shé jiǎn (jiǎn)*: Synonym: *difficult speech*. A condition in which the tongue is curled and shrunken, cannot move freely, and makes speech indistinct. A sluggish tongue is attributed to spleen-stomach accumulated heat scorching the fluids or to phlegm obstructing the orifices of the heart in wind stroke or summerheat tetany. MED Treat spleen-stomach accumulated heat by clearing heat and engendering liquid, using Red-Abducting Powder (*dǎo chì sǎn*) plus coptis (*huáng lián*), ophiopogon (*mài mén dōng*), and scrophularia (*xuán shēn*). Treat phlegm obstructing the orifices of the heart by sweeping phlegm and opening the orifices using Gallbladder-Warming Decoction (*wēn dǎn tāng*) plus acorus (*shí chāng pú*), bile arisaema (*dǎn xīng*), scorpion (*quán xiē*), and bamboo sugar (*tiān zhú huáng*). [26: 269] [25: 114]

smaller abdomen 小腹 *xiǎo fù*: Lower abdomen, i.e., the part of the abdomen below the umbilicus is referred to as the smaller abdomen. Compare LESSER ABDOMEN. *adj.* smaller-abdominal. [27: 68]

smaller-abdominal fullness 小腹满 *xiǎo fù mǎn*: A subjective feeling of fullness in the smaller abdomen. Smaller-abdominal fullness that is painful when pressure is applied and that is accompanied by reversal cold of the extremities is a sign of cold binding in the bladder. MED Treat with True Warrior Decoction (*zhēn wǔ tāng*). Smaller-abdominal fullness also occurs in DRIBBLING URINARY BLOCK and COLD DAMAGE BLOOD AMASSMENT PATTERN. ACU Base treatment mainly on CV and BL-28 (*páng guāng shū*, Bladder Transport), and alarm points. Select CV-4 (*guān yuán*, Pass Head), CV-6 (*qì hǎi*, Sea of Qi), CV-3 (*zhōng jí*, Central Pole), and BL-28 (*páng guāng shū*, Bladder Transport); needle with even supplemenation and drainage or with drainage, and add moxa. [26: 79] [46: 588]

smaller-abdominal pain 小腹痛 *xiǎo fù tòng*: Pain in the SMALLER ABDOMEN due to various factors including damp-heat, static blood, bowel qi stoppage, or kidney vacuity. When due to bladder damp-heat, abdominal pain and distention is accompanied by inhibited urination and sometimes thirst with desire for fluids, and a rapid pulse, and is treated by clearing and disinhibiting damp-heat with formulas like Polyporus Decoction (*zhū líng tāng*), and Poria (Hoelen) Five Powder (*wǔ líng sǎn*) and their variations. When due to blood binding in the bladder, abdominal pain and distention is accompanied by disinhibited urination and urinary urgency, and is treated by quickening the blood and expelling stasis with formulas such as

Substitute Dead-On Pill (*dài dǐ dàng wán*). Pain in the smaller abdomen and around the umbilicus accompanied by dry bound stool calls for moistening the intestines or precipitation with Honey Enema (*mì jiān dǎo fǎ*), Hemp Seed Pill (*má rén wán*), or Major Qi-Coordinating Decoction (*dà chéng qì tāng*). Lower abdominal pain and distention due to excessive drinking and sexual activity is accompanied by frequent inhibited urination, and is treated by supplementing the kidney with Life Saver Kidney Qi Pill (*jì shēng shèn qì wán*). Smaller-abdominal pain is also seen in MOUNTING QI, MENSTRUAL PAIN, VAGINAL DISCHARGE, INTESTINAL WELLING-ABSCESS, POSTPARTUM ABDOMINAL PAIN, and STRANGURY. [ACU] Base treatment mainly on CV, LR, and LI. Use CV-4 (*guān yuán*, Pass Head), LR-1 (*dà dūn*, Large Pile), LR-4 (*zhōng fēng*, Mound Center), and LI-8 (*xià lián*, Lower Ridge) as the main points. Secondary points and needle stimulus should be chosen in accordance with the cause. For unbearable acute abdominal pain, burn five cones of moxa Solitary Yin (*dú yīn*) at the crease below the middle joint of the second toe. Compare also LESSER-ABDOMINAL PAIN. [26: 78] [113: 6] [4: 146]

small intestinal cough 小肠咳 *xiǎo cháng ké*: A COUGH occurring in bouts that stimulate that passing of flatus. [27: 380]

small intestinal disease 小肠病 *xiǎo cháng bìng*: Any disease of the small intestine. Disease of the small intestine can arise when damage to the stomach and spleen from dietary irregularities passes to the intestine, or when heart fire spreads to the small intestine. Distinction is made between vacuity cold and repletion heat patterns. Vacuity cold patterns are characterized by dull abdominal pain, rumbling intestines, sloppy stool, and ungratifying frequent urination. Repletion heat patterns are characterized by vexation and mouth sores, reddish disfluent urine, and distention in abdomen and umbilical region. Vacuity cold is treated by warming and supplementing; repletion heat is treated by clearing and disinhibiting. [26: 78]

small intestinal mounting 小肠疝 *xiǎo cháng shàn*: A MOUNTING disease characterized by cold pain in the smaller abdomen stretching into the testicles and the lumbus and back. Small intestinal mounting is attributed to small intestinal vacuity and the invasion of wind-cold. [MED] Warm, promote qi transformation, and move qi with medicinals such as fennel (*huí xiāng*), toosendan (*chuān liàn zǐ*), evodia (*wú zhū yú*), tangerine peel (*chén pí*), kalimeris (*mǎ lán*), and coriander (*hú suī*). [ACU] Base treatment mainly on SI, LR, and CV. Select CV-4 (*guān yuán*, Pass Head), CV-6 (*qì hǎi*, Sea of Qi), SI-3 (*hòu xī*, Back Ravine), SI-1 (*shào zé*, Lesser Marsh), LR-1 (*dà dūn*, Large Pile), LR-2

(*xíng jiān*, Moving Between), and SP-6 (*sān yīn jiāo*, Three Yin Intersection); needle with drainage and moxa. [26: 79] [113: 12, 190] [37: 454]

small intestinal qi 小肠气 *xiǎo cháng qì*: Mentioned in *A Unified Treatise on Diseases, Patterns, and Remedies According to the Three Causes* (*sān yīn jí yī bìng zhèng fāng lùn*). See MOUNTING QI. [26: 78]

small intestinal qi pain 小肠气痛 *xiǎo cháng qì tòng*: MOUNTING QI PAIN. [27: 428]

small intestinal repletion heat 小肠实热 *xiǎo cháng shí rè*: Heat brewing in the small intestine, with signs such as heart vexation, tinnitus, sore throat, mouth sores, rough painful voidings of reddish urine, abdominal pain, yellow tongue fur, and a slippery rapid pulse. In modern clinical practice, this is most commonly seen in urinary tract infections and in stomatatis. [MED] Use Red-Abducting Powder (*dǎo chì sǎn*). [ACU] Base treatment mainly on SI, HT and CV. Select SI-3 (*hòu xī*, Back Ravine), CV-3 (*zhōng jí*, Central Pole), HT-8 (*shào fǔ*, Lesser Mansion), CV-4 (*guān yuán*, Pass Head), SI-2 (*qián gǔ*, Front Valley), and SP-9 (*yīn líng quán*, Yin Mound Spring); needle with drainage or prick to bleed. [27: 150] [97: 35] [113: 12, 124] [46: 591, 596]

small intestinal vacuity cold 小肠虚寒 *xiǎo cháng xū hán*: Damage to the small intestine by cold evil affecting the separation of the clear and turbid. Small intestinal vacuity cold is usually seen in spleen vacuity, and is characterized by dull pain in the smaller abdomen that likes pressure, rumbling intestines, frequent inhibited urination, pale tongue with white fur, and a weak moderate pulse. [ACU] Base treatment mainly on back transport points, SI, and CV. Select BL-27 (*xiǎo cháng shū*, Small Intestine Transport), BL-28 (*páng guāng shū*, Bladder Transport), BL-23 (*shèn shū*, Kidney Transport), SI-3 (*hòu xī*, Back Ravine), CV-4 (*guān yuán*, Pass Head), and CV-6 (*qì hǎi*, Sea of Qi); needle with supplementation and moxa. **Comparison**: Small intestinal vacuity cold is closely related to spleen yang vacuity. Both may manifest in white face and lassitude of the spirit, fear of cold and cold limbs, abdominal pain and sloppy stool, a pale tongue, and sunken slow fine weak pulse. However, small intestinal vacuity cold centers around failure to separate the clear and turbid, so that the main clinical signs are rumbling intestines, diarrhea, frequent ungratifying urination, accompanied by continuous smaller-abdominal pain that likes warmth and pressure. Spleen yang vacuity is characterized by a wider range of signs, Apart from the signs common to both patterns (white face and lassitude of the spirit, fear of cold and cold limbs, etc.), there may also be reduced eating and abdominal distention especially after eating, and signs of exuberant internal cold-damp such as heavy cumbersome limbs, puffy swelling, reduced urination, and in women copious thin white vaginal discharge. Furthermore, abdominal pain tends to be in the larger abdomen (above the umbilicus) rather than smaller abdomen (below the umbilicus). [27: 150] [97: 35] [113: 12]

small intestinal welling-abscess 小肠痈 *xiǎo cháng yōng*: A WELLING-ABSCESS (*yōng*) of the small intestine; an INTESTINAL WELLING-ABSCESS characterized by pain at CV-4 (*guān yuán*, Pass Head). [27: 461] [44: 574]

small intestine 小肠 *xiǎo cháng*: One of the SIX BOWELS, joined to stomach at its upper extremity, and the large intestine at the lower extremity. The SMALL INTESTINE HOLDS THE OFFICE OF RECEPTION, i.e., it receives grain and water that has been decomposed in the stomach. It transforms this food further, extracting nutrients for the body. It governs the transformation of matter and the separation of the clear turbid. It passes the waste on to the large intestine and the water humor to the bladder; hence it is said that the SMALL INTESTINE GOVERNS SEPARATION OF THE CLEAR AND THE TURBID. The small intestine stands in interior-exterior relationship with the lung, and belongs to metal among the five phases. Its channel is the hand greater yang (*tài yáng*) channel. Diseases of the small intestine are attributable to failure to separate the clear and the turbid, manifesting as stool and urinary disturbances. Common signs are abdominal pain, diarrhea, and scant urine. See SMALL INTESTINAL DISEASE. [26: 78] [27: 21] [97: 33]

small intestine channel 小肠经 *xiǎo cháng jīng*: HAND GREATER YANG SMALL INTESTINE CHANNEL. [26: 78]

small intestine governs humor 小肠主液 *xiǎo cháng zhǔ yè*: See SMALL INTESTINE GOVERNS SEPARATION OF THE CLEAR AND THE TURBID.

small intestine governs reception 小肠主受盛 *xiǎo cháng zhǔ shòu chéng*: The small intestine receives food from the stomach. [27: 38]

small intestine governs separation of the clear and the turbid 小肠主分别清浊 *xiǎo cháng zhǔ fēn bié qīng zhuó*: The small intestine's function of further transforming food already decomposed by the stomach. The clear refers to what is useful to the body, while the turbid denotes waste. In the small intestine, the essence of grain and water is assimilated into the body by the action of the spleen. Waste water is absorbed and, by kidney qi transformation, is conveyed to the bladder. Hence, "The small intestine governs humor." [6: 87]

small intestine holds the office of reception, whence the transformation of things emanates 小肠者，受盛之官也，化物出焉 *xiǎo cháng zhě, shòu chéng zhī guān yě, huà wù chū yān*: The small intestine receives food from the stomach, and transforms it further. [27: 38]

smallpox 天花 *tiān huā*: Synonym: *pox*. A disease characterized by heat effusion, cough, sneezing, yawning, red face, fright palpitations, cold extremities and ears, and eruption of pox. This disease is prevented by modern medical inoculation. It is noteworthy that there are records suggesting that inoculation against smallpox was practiced as early as the Northern Song under the reign of Emperor Zhengzong (998-1022), and that nasal inoculation was discovered in the Ming dynasty between 1567 and 1572. See NASAL INOCULATION. ◇ Chin 天 *tiān*, heaven; 花 *huā*, flower. [26: 104]

small pulse 小脉 *xiǎo mài*: FINE PULSE.

snake body 蛇身 *shé shēn*, 蛇体 *shé tǐ*: ENCRUSTED SKIN.

snake lice 蛇虱 *shé shī*: WHITE CRUST.

snake scales 蛇鳞 *shé lín*: ENCRUSTED SKIN.

snake tongue 蛇舌 *shé shé*: WORRYING TONGUE.

snivel 涕 *tì*: Synonym: *nasal mucus*. Snivel is the humor of the lung. Abnormalities of nasal mucus indicate either nondiffusion of lung qi due to the presence of evil or lung vacuity. Nasal congestion with turbid snivel is observed in external contraction of wind-heat, whereas nasal congestion and runny nose with clear snivel indicates wind-cold invading the lung (common cold). In the latter case, it thickens and turns yellow on recovery. Thin clear snivel and pronounced sneezing indicates SNIVELING NOSE, which would appear to correspond to allergic rhinitis in Western medicine. Foul-smelling turbid yellow snivel accompanied by recurrent headaches indicates DEEP-SOURCE NASAL CONGESTION, which corresponds to paranasal sinusitis. [26: 479] [97: 481]

sniveling 鼽 *qiú*: SNIVELING NOSE.

sniveling nose 鼻鼽 *bí qiú*, 鼽鼻 *qiú bí*: Synonyms: *sniveling*; *watery sniveling*. A condition characterized by runny nose with clear snivel (nasal mucus), nasal congestion, and sneezing, and attributed to lung qi depletion, insecurity of defense qi, and external contraction of wind-cold. This disease was described in *Elementary Questions* (*sù wèn, xuán jī yuán bìng shì*) as follows, "Sniveling is the running of clear snivel from the nose." MED Course wind and diffuse the lung with variations of Magnolia Flower Powder (*xīn yí sǎn*). ACU Base treatment mainly on LU and LI points that course wind and resolve the exterior and free the nasal orifices. Select LI-20 (*yíng xiāng*, Welcome Fragrance), Hall of Impression (*yìn táng*), LI-4 (*hé gǔ*, Union Valley), and Clear Nose (*bí* *tōng*); needle with drainage. For nasal congestion, add GB-20 (*fēng chí,* Wind Pool) and GV-23 (*shàng xīng,* Upper Star). For pronounced externally contracted wind-cold, add GB-20 (*fēng chí,* Wind Pool), GV-20 (*bǎi huì,* Hundred Convergences), TB-5 (*wài guān,* Outer Pass), and LU-7 (*liè quē,* Broken Sequence), needling with drainage and adding moxa. [26: 921] [27: 415] [97: 623] [113: 495]

snivel is the humor of the lung 涕为肺液 *tì wéi fèi yè*: The lung opens at the nose; hence the snivel (nasal mucus) is the humor of the lung. [27: 499] [97: 510]

snow mouth 雪口 *xuě kǒu*: GOOSE-MOUTH SORE.

soaking 浸泡 *jìn pào*: STEEPING.

softening hardness 软坚 *ruǎn jiān*: To treat any morbid induration in the body, notably a) scrofula, phlegm nodes, and goiter (including what Western medicine calls lymphadenhypertrophy and thyrocele), b) urinary calculi and gallstones, and c) abdominal concretions (including hepatomegaly, splenomegaly, and abdominal masses). MED Sargassum (*hǎi zǎo*), kelp (*kūn bù*), prunella (*xià kū cǎo*), fritillaria (*bèi mǔ*), oyster shell (*mǔ lì*), shancigu (*shān cí gū*), dried taro (*qīng yù nǎi gān*), and air potato (*huáng yào zǐ*) are hardness-softening medicinals commonly used for scrofula, phlegm nodes, and goiter. They are often combined with blood-quickening stasis-transforming medicinals and heat-clearing toxin-resolving medicinals. Moneywort (*jīn qián cǎo*), gizzard lining (*jī nèi jīn*), and niter (*xiāo shí*) are hardness-softening agents used to disperse stones. To treat urinary calculi, these agents are frequently combined with water-disinhibiting strangury-freeing agents; to treat biliary tract calculi, they may be combined with liver-coursing qi-rectifying medicinals, and in some cases with draining precipitants such as rhubarb (*dà huáng*), unripe bitter orange (*zhǐ shí*), and mirabilite (*máng xiāo*). For agents that disperse concretions, see DISPELLING STASIS AND QUICKENING THE BLOOD. Among formulas used, Sargassum Jade Flask Decoction (*hǎi zǎo yù hú tāng*) is used for dispersing goiter. Scrofula Internal Dispersion Pill (*nèi xiāo luǒ lì wán*) disperses scrofula. Biliary Calculus Decoction (*dǎn dào pái shí tāng*), expels gallstones. Pyrrosia Powder (*shí wéi sǎn*) disperses urinary tract calculi. All these are specific-use formulas. [6: 262]

softening hardness and dissipating binds 软坚散结 *ruǎn jiān sàn jié*: To treat turbid phlegm or static blood gathering to form lumps. Softening hardness and dissipating binds is used to treat SCROFULA, GOITER, MOTHER OF MALARIA, and dry stool. **Scrofula or goiter** due to turbid phlegm congealing and gathering. MED Dis-

perse phlegm, soften hardness, and dissipate binds with agents such as Zhejiang fritillaria (*zhè bèi mǔ*), sargassum (*hǎi zǎo*), kelp (*kūn bù*), and oyster shell (*mǔ lì*), ACU Select Hundred Taxations (*bǎi láo*)ⓜ, and Tip of the Elbow (*zhǒu jiān*), ST-36 (*zú sān lǐ,* Leg Three Li), ST-40 (*fēng lóng,* Bountiful Bulge), LI-4 (*hé gǔ,* Union Valley), and CV-22 (*tiān tú,* Celestial Chimney); needle with even supplemenation and drainage or with supplementation, and add moxa. **Mother of malaria** (recognized in modern medicine as splenomegaly) due to enduring malaria. MED Soften hardness and break binds with turtle shell (*biē jiǎ*), sparganium (*sān léng*), and zedoary (*é zhú*). ACU Select GV-14 (*dà zhuī,* Great Hammer), PC-5 (*jiān shǐ,* Intermediary Courier), SI-3 (*hòu xī,* Back Ravine), LR-13 (*zhāng mén,* Camphorwood Gate), and Glomus Root (*pǐ gēn*); needle with drainage. **Dry stool** due to heat binding in the stomach and large intestines. MED This is treated by draining precipitation. However, the use of cold salty mirabilite (*máng xiāo*) in precipitant formulas can also said to be a form of softening hardness and dissipating binds. ACU Select SP-14 (*fù jié,* Abdominal Bind), LI-4 (*hé gǔ,* Union Valley), LI-11 (*qū chí,* Pool at the Bend), and ST-37 (*shàng jù xū,* Upper Great Hollow); needle with drainage. [26: 596] [27: 273] [46: 597, 649, 670] [113: 169]

soft ribs 软肋 *ruǎn lè*: FREE RIBS. [27: 69]

soft tetany 柔痉 *róu cì (jìng)*: A TETANY (*jìng*) pattern characterized by generalized heat [effusion], sweating, rigidity of the neck, shaking of the heat, clenched jaw, hypertonicity of the extremities, arched-back rigidity, and a slow sunken pulse. MED Soft tetany can be treated with variations of Trichosanthes and Cinnamon Twig Decoction (*guā lóu guì zhī tāng*). Compare HARD TETANY; YIN TETANY. [26: 428] [27: 373] [97: 446]

soggy diarrhea 濡泻 *rú xiè*: See DAMP DIARRHEA. [26: 923] [50: 1728] [27: 363] [97: 655]

soggy pulse 濡脉 *rú mài*: A soft pulse lacking in force. A soggy pulse tends to float, and is thin, though less distinctly so than a thin pulse. The soggy pulse is associated with dual vacuity of blood and qi and with damp encumbrance. Similar pulses: A *faint pulse* is extremely fine and weak, indistinct, and almost imperceptible. It indicates qi and blood vacuity desertion. The *vacuous pulse,* like the soggy pulse, is weak, but differs in that it is large rather than thin. The term *vacuous* is also generally used to connote weakness, particularly in combinations such as vacuous rapid pulse, vacuous stringlike pulse, etc. [27: 195] [97: 655]

soliloquy 独语 *dú yǔ*: Talking to oneself, but ceasing when another approaches. Soliloquy is a sign of a deranged heart-spirit (insanity). See WITHDRAWAL; SPIRIT. [27: 186] [97: 423]

solitary yang straying upward 孤阳上越 *gū yáng shàng yuè*: VACUOUS YANG FLOATING UPWARD.

soluble granules 冲剂 *chōng jì*: A newly developed preparation made by combining an extract of the materials with glucose and lactose and shaping them into granules, which can be dissolved in water and swallowed. Soluble granules are a pure medicinal form, and are easy to use. [26: 294]

somber white facial complexion 面色苍白 *miàn sè cāng bái*: A white complexion with a hint of dull blue or gray, often seen, for example, in desertion patterns. Compare BRIGHT WHITE FACIAL COMPLEXION and PALE WHITE FACIAL COMPLEXION. More at WHITE FACIAL COMPLEXION. ◇ Chin 苍 *cāng*, blue, black; 白 *bái*, white. [6: 116] [48: 113]

somber yellow skin 皮色苍黄 *pí sè cāng huáng*: The dull yellow coloring of the skin seen in *drum distention*.

somnolence 嗜睡 *shì shuì*: Synonym: *tendency to sleep*. Pronounced drowsiness and tendency to sleep for long periods. If accompanied by heavy-headedness and heavy body, it is a sign that the spleen is encumbered by phlegm-damp, which may either stem from external contraction of summerheat-damp or from phlegm-damp arising from within. When accompanied by dizziness, headache, and hypertonicity of the shoulder and back, it is a sign of wind-phlegm. With cold limbs and faint pulse, and pronounced general weakness, it is a sign of heart-kidney yang vacuity, and is referred to in *On Cold Damage* (*shāng hán lùn*), where it states, "When the lesser yin (*shào yīn*) is affected by disease..., there is desire only for sleep." DROWSINESS AFTER EATING with poor appetite, shortage of qi, and lack of strength is a sign of spleen qi vacuity. ◇ Chin 嗜 *shì*, like to; 睡 *shuì*, sleep. [97: 600]

Song 宋 *sòng*: The name of two dynasties, one running from A.D. 420–479, and the other (better known), running from A.D. 960–1279.

soot black 黧黑 *lí hēi*: A blackish color with a yellow or brown hue. [19: 17085] [48: 486]

soothe 舒 *shū*: To relax. Soothing the sinews is a general term that means relax the sinews when they are tensed and heal them when they are damaged. Soothing the liver is synonymous with coursing the liver. See COURSE.

soothe the liver 舒肝 *shū gān*: COURSING THE LIVER AND RECTIFYING QI. [27: 264]

¹**sore** 酸（痠） *suān*, 酸痛 *suān tòng*: adj. See SORENESS.

²**sore** 痛 *tòng*: adj. See SORENESS.

³**sore** 疮 *chuāng*, 疮疡 *chuāng yáng*: n. **1.** A generic term for diseases of EXTERNAL MEDICINE, such as WELLING-ABSCESS (*yōng*), FLAT-ABSCESS (*jū*), CLOVE SORE (*dīng chuāng*), BOIL (*jié*), STREAMING SORE (*liú zhù*), FLOWING PHLEGM (*liú tán*), and SCROFULA (*luǒ lì*), generally caused by toxic evils invading the body, evil heat scorching the blood, and congestion of qi and blood. Sores are treated differently according to the whether they are yin or yang, according to their stage of development, and according to the channel affected. **Yin-yang:** Most common are yang sores, which appear suddenly and develop swiftly, and are characterized by clearly circumscribed elevated swelling, redness, heat, pain, and glossy skin. Usually, yang sores that fail to disperse within a week will suppurate and burst, but heal quickly. Even though there may be general signs such as physical cold, heat effusion, thirst, constipation, reddish urine, and a forceful surging rapid pulse, essence-spirit and appetite are not endangered. Yin sores, by contrast, develop more slowly, are flat or sunken and diffuse, and are associated with dull or pulling if any pain, purple or black if any discoloration, and mild if any heat. Since they disperse, burst, and heal with difficulty, they are of long duration. They produce pus that is often watery and clear. They are associated with general signs such as lack of strength, bright white facial complexion, spontaneous or night sweating, torpid intake, and a forceless fine sunken pulse, which indicate dual vacuity of qi and blood. Half-yin half-yang sores are without pronounced yin or yang signs such as heat or cold and elevated swelling or sunkenness. They resemble yang sores though redness, pain, and swelling are mild; they resemble yin sores though they are not hard or sunken. They are associated with swelling of a vacuity rather than a repletion type and that do not easily disperse. They are painful, but do not easily suppurate and burst. Pain continues after bursting, and they heal slowly. Prognosis improves if the yang signs come into greater evidence, and poor if the yin signs increase. Successful treatment of half-yin half yang sores lies in mastering yin-yang conversion. **Stage of development:** Sores are treated differently at different stages of their development. Before suppuration the method of INTERNAL DISPERSION is used to prevent the sore from developing. When suppuration begins, INTERNAL EXPRESSION is used to hasten the sore through its development. After a sore has burst, SUPPLEMENTATION is applied to speed the healing. The stage of development is judged in the following way. A sore associated with mild local heat, hardness and tenderness accompanied by a tight pulse whether rapid or slow indicates that pus has not formed. If the sore is hot and tender, fails to rebound after pressure is released, and is accompanied by a rapid pulse, pus has already formed. If the swelling is markedly elevated

with thin skin, is soft and depressed in the middle, has thick skin, is hot, red, and shiny, is painful at the slightest pressure, and rebounds after pressure is released, there is pus close to the surface. If the swelling is diffuse and hard with sheenless skin, pits slightly when pressed, is slightly hot, and is only painful when heavy pressure is applied, the pus is deep in the body. A sore that bursts to discharge thick clean-looking, slightly fishy smelling pus that is yellow-white or the color of peach blossom indicates favorable development. Discharge of thin turbid dull dark pus with a foul smell indicates an unfavorable development. **Channel:** Sores may develop differently and may be treated differently depending on their location on or proximity to channels. The yang brightness (*yáng míng*) channel has copious qi and copious blood, hence sores of the extremities on this channel tend to heal quickly. The greater yang (*tài yáng*) and reverting yin (*jué yīn*) channels have copious blood and scant qi, hence sores on these channels have a tendency to inward fall, so that in treatment attention must be paid to timely and effective INTERNAL EXPRESSION. The lesser yang (*shào yáng*), lesser yin (*shào yīn*), and greater yin (*tài yīn*) channels have copious qi and scant blood; hence sores of the extremities located on these channels do not heal easily, so that it becomes important to supplement yin and nourish the blood. Sores on different channels are treated with formulas that include appropriate channel conductors, as the table below shows.

Channel Conductors Used to Treat Sores

Greater Yang
notopterygium (*qiāng huó*) for the upper body
charred phellodendron (*huáng bǎi tàn*) for the lower body

Yang Brightness
angelica (*bái zhǐ*) and cimicifuga (*shēng má*) for the upper body
gypsum (*shí gāo*) for the lower body

Lesser Yang
bupleurum (*chái hú*) for the upper body
unripe tangerine peel (*qīng pí*) for the lower body

Greater Yin
platycodon (*jié gěng*) for the upper body
white peony (*bái sháo yào*) for the lower body

Reverting Yin
bupleurum (*chái hú*) for the upper body
unripe tangerine peel (*qīng pí*) for the lower body
(as for lesser yang)

Lesser Yin
duhuo (*dú huó*) for the upper body
anemarrhena (*zhī mǔ*) for the lower body

2. In a wider sense, the term sore includes shallow skin diseases such as scab (*jiè*), lichen (*xiǎn*), and cinnabar toxin (*dān dú*). ◇ Chin 疮 *chuāng*, sore; 疡 *yáng*, open sore, ulceration. [26: 863-866] [27: 456] [97: 427] [61: 31]

sore dry throat 咽喉燥痛 *yān hóu zào tòng*: See SORE THROAT; DRY THROAT.

[1]**soreness** 酸 *suān*, 酸痛 *suān tòng*: Tenderness of the limbs produced by prolonged physical exertion. See PAIN. [29: 190]

[2]**soreness** 痛 *tòng*: Tenderness associated with a smarting wound, red swollen throat, or red swollen eyes. See PAIN. [29: 190]

sore of the head or face 头面疮 *tóu miàn chuāng*: A sore located on the head or face, usually attributable to contention between dampness and heat in patients suffering from accumulated heat in the bowels and viscera who contract wind-dampness, and are most commonly seen in children. A sore of the head and face begins with tidal heat [effusion] of the head and face, itching, and the development of a papule that releases pus when it bursts. It may be recurrent, and, in severe cases, can spread to other parts of the body. It is treated by clearing heat, coursing wind, and disinhibiting dampness. Variants of Ledebouriella Sage-Inspired Powder (*fáng fēng tōng shèng sǎn*) can be taken orally, and Indigo Powder (*qīng dài sǎn*) can be applied topically. ACU Select GV-14 (*dà zhuī*, Great Hammer), LI-11 (*qū chí*, Pool at the Bend), LI-4 (*hé gǔ*, Union Valley), SP-6 (*sān yīn jiāo*, Three Yin Intersection), SP-9 (*yīn líng quán*, Yin Mound Spring), and GB-20 (*fēng chí*, Wind Pool); needle with drainage. Selection of points according to the affected channel: For the yang brightness (*yáng míng*) channel, add ST-44 (*nèi tíng*, Inner Court), and prick LI-1 (*shāng yáng*, Shang Yang) to bleed. For the lesser yang (*shào yáng*) channel, add GB-34 (*yáng líng quán*, Yang Mound Spring), and GB-44 (*zú qiào yīn*, Foot Orifice Yin), For the greater yang (*tài yáng*) channel, add BL-40 (*wěi zhōng*, Bend Center). [26: 906] [46: 595, 709]

sore of the mouth or tongue 口舌生疮 *kǒu shé shēng chuāng*, 口舌疮 *kǒu shé chuāng*: MOUTH SORE.

sore-opening 疮口 *chuāng kǒu*: The opening of a sore through which pus and blood may be discharged.

sores in pregnancy 妊娠疮疡 *rèn shēn chuāng yáng*: WELLING-ABSCESS (*yōng*), FLAT-ABSCESS (*jū*), CLOVE SORES (*dīng chuāng*), and toxin sores during pregnancy. In general, they are treated by regulating qi and quieting the fetus, and by internal expression and toxin resolving. Attention should be paid to contraindications of medicinals in pregnancy. Indiscriminate use of interior-freeing draining precipitant agents should be avoided. [26: 341]

sore swollen throat 咽喉肿痛 *yān hóu zhǒng tòng*: A sore throat with swelling, usually attributable to the presence of an external evil. Compare SORE THROAT.

sore throat 咽喉痛 *yān hóu tòng*, 咽喉疼痛 *yān hóu téng tòng*, 喉咙痛 *hóu lóng tòng*, 咽嗌痛 *yān yì tòng*: Painful pharynx or larynx. Sore throat may be a repletion or vacuity sign. **Wind-cold sore throat** is characterized by usually only mild pain, by redness and swelling in the throat, and is often attended by nasal congestion, sneezing, clear snivel (nasal mucus), cough with thin phlegm, headache and generalized pain, heat effusion without sweating, thin tongue fur, and a tight floating pulse. [MED] Course wind and dissipate cold with Six-Ingredient Decoction (*liù wèi tāng*) plus perilla leaf (*zǐ sū yè*) and fresh ginger (*shēng jiāng*). [ACU] Base treatment mainly on LI, LU, and BL. Select GB-20 (*fēng chí*, Wind Pool), BL-12 (*fēng mén*, Wind Gate), LI-4 (*hé gǔ*, Union Valley), LU-7 (*liè quē*, Broken Sequence), and CV-22 (*tiān tú*, Celestial Chimney); needle with drainage and add moxa, if appropriate, and prick LU-11 (*shào shāng*, Lesser Shang) to bleed. **Wind-heat sore throat** is characterized by more pronounced pain felt particularly when swallowing, with redness and swelling. It is accompanied by heat effusion, aversion to cold, sweating, and headache, by a red tongue with thin yellow fur, and by a rapid floating pulse. [MED] Course wind and dissipate heat with Lonicera and Forsythia Powder (*yín qiào sǎn*). [ACU] Base treatment mainly on LU and LI. Select LI-11 (*qū chí*, Pool at the Bend), LI-4 (*hé gǔ*, Union Valley), LU-5 (*chǐ zé*, Cubit Marsh), GV-14 (*dà zhuī*, Great Hammer), TB-5 (*wài guān*, Outer Pass), and GB-20 (*fēng chí*, Wind Pool); needle with drainage, and prick LU-11 (*shào shāng*, Lesser Shang) to bleed. **Damp-heat sore throat** is characterized by acute pain, swelling and redness, and small vesicles that give way to ulceration after bursting. There is usually heat effusion, cough, ejection of yellow phlegm, inhibited feeling in the chest and diaphragm, red tongue with slimy yellow tongue fur, and a rapid pulse. [MED] Clear heat and resolve toxin and disinhibit dampness, using Sweet Dew Beverage (*gān lù yǐn*) plus isatis leaf (*dà qīng yè*). [ACU] Base treatment mainly on LI, ST, and SP. Select LI-11 (*qū chí*, Pool at the Bend), LI-4 (*hé gǔ*, Union Valley), SP-9 (*yīn líng quán*, Yin Mound Spring), ST-44 (*nèi tíng*, Inner Court), CV-22 (*tiān tú*, Celestial Chimney), ST-43 (*xiàn gǔ*, Sunken Valley), and TB-1 (*guān chōng*, Passage Hub); needle with drainage, and prick LI-1 (*shāng yáng*, Shang Yang) to bleed. **Depressed fire sore throat** is characterized by rapid development into a severe

condition with difficulty in swallowing even small amounts of fluids. The throat is hot and red, and, characteristically, the uvula is swollen, constituting what is called "THROAT IMPEDIMENT." Other signs include hasty rapid breathing, red tongue with scant fur or thin yellow fur, and a large floating rapid pulse. [MED] Downbear fire and dissipate binds with Impediment-Diffusing Decoction (*xuān bì tāng*) plus moutan (*mǔ dān pí*) and gardenia (*shān zhī zǐ*). [ACU] Base treatment mainly on LU, LI, KI, LR, and back transport points. Select LU-10 (*yú jì*, Fish Border), LU-5 (*chǐ zé*, Cubit Marsh), LI-4 (*hé gǔ*, Union Valley), LI-2 (*èr jiān*, Second Space), TB-1 (*guān chōng*, Passage Hub), KI-1 (*yǒng quán*, Gushing Spring), LR-2 (*xíng jiān*, Moving Between), BL-13 (*fèi shū*, Lung Transport), and BL-18 (*gān shū*, Liver Transport); needle with drainage, and prick Ten Diffusing Points (*shí xuān*), LU-11 (*shào shāng*, Lesser Shang), and HT-9 (*shào chōng*, Lesser Surge) to bleed. **Yin vacuity sore throat** is a dry sore throat accompanied by dry mouth and desire for fluids, and a sensation that the throat is blocked by phlegm that is not easily expectorated. The pain is worse after midday. Other signs include postmeridian tidal heat [effusion], heat in the hearts of the soles and palms, night sweating, dry stool, yellow urine, red tongue with scant fur, and a rapid fine pulse. [MED] Supplement the lung and kidney and clear vacuity heat. Use formulas such as Anemarrhena, Phellodendron, and Rehmannia Pill (*zhī bǎi dì huáng wán*). [ACU] Base treatment mainly on KI and LU. Select KI-3 (*tài xī*, Great Ravine), KI-6 (*zhào hǎi*, Shining Sea), KI-7 (*fù liū*, Recover Flow), LU-10 (*yú jì*, Fish Border), LI-4 (*hé gǔ*, Union Valley), and TB-2 (*yè mén*, Humor Gate); needle with even supplementation and drainage and prick LU-11 (*shào shāng*, Lesser Shang) to bleed. **Dual vacuity of qi and yin sore throat** is usually characterized by dryness and soreness, is exacerbated by taxation, and is accompanied by shortness of breath, lack of strength, tidal heat [effusion], dry stool, pale tongue with thin fur, and a forceless fine pulse. [MED] Boost qi and nourish yin with Lily Bulb Metal-Securing Decoction (*bǎi hé gù jīn tāng*) with the addition of qi-boosting agents. [ACU] Base treatment mainly on KI, LU, CV, and back transport points. Select KI-3 (*tài xī*, Great Ravine), KI-6 (*zhào hǎi*, Shining Sea), KI-7 (*fù liū*, Recover Flow), LU-5 (*chǐ zé*, Cubit Marsh), TB-2 (*yè mén*, Humor Gate), ST-36 (*zú sān lǐ*, Leg Three Li), CV-6 (*qì hǎi*, Sea of Qi), BL-23 (*shèn shū*, Kidney Transport), BL-20 (*pí shū*, Spleen Transport), and BL-13 (*fèi shū*, Lung Transport); needle with supplementation. [92: No. 449] [46: 726] [113: 505] [37: 470]

sore throat in measles 麻疹喉痛 *má zhěn hóu tòng*: Sore throat due to measles toxin attacking the throat. Sore throat in measles usually arises when the exterior evil is depressed so that the measles toxin cannot effuse smoothly, or when there is intense heat in the interior. Mild cases are marked by sore swollen throat; severe cases by difficulty in swallowing even soup or water. MED For exterior depression, clear, resolve, and outthrust the evil with Scrophularia and Cimicifuga Decoction (*xuán shēn shēng má tāng*). For intense interior heat, clear the interior and resolve toxin with schizonepeta (*jīng jiè*), ledebouriella (*fáng fēng*), forsythia (*lián qiào*), mint (*bò hé*), scutellaria (*huáng qín*), gardenia (*shān zhī zǐ*), licorice (*gān cǎo*), mirabilite (*máng xiāo*), rhubarb (*dà huáng*), and arctium (*niú bàng zǐ*). [26: 588]

sore-toxin 疮毒 *chuāng dú*: The toxin that causes sores and pox. [50: 1146] [111: 3972]

sorrow 悲 *bēi*: One of the SEVEN AFFECTS. Sorrow is the affect of the lung, and in excess it can damage the lung. Wailing is the voice of the lung, and is associated with sorrow. Damage to the lung by sorrow is characterized by crying, heat vexation and agitation, pale white complexion, insufficiency of spirit qi (lack of vigor), and a tight or bound pulse.

sorrow causes qi to disperse 悲则气消 *bēi zé qì xiāo*: Excessive sorrow and grief can cause depression in the upper burner that transforms into heat, which disperses and wears lung qi. [27: 145] [97: 559]

sound like the rasping of a saw 声如拽锯 *shēng rú zhuài jù*: Labored breathing that produces a rasping sound like a wood saw. It occurs in sudden collapse and certain conditions involving blockage of the throat. [26: 933] [27: 185]

sound of cicadas in the ear 耳作蝉鸣 *ěr zuò chán míng*: See TINNITUS.

sour 酸 *suān*: See SOURNESS.

source of engendering transformation 脾为生化之源 *shēng huà zhī yuán*: See SPLEEN IS THE SOURCE OF ENGENDERING TRANSFORMATION.

source point 原穴 *yuán xué*: From *The Magic Pivot* (*líng shū*). Any of the points that lie on one of the twelve channels at which the source qi of the bowels or viscus related to that channel collects. The source points of the six yin channels are the same as the STREAM POINTS of the six yin channels, and are located one point proximal to the stream points on the six yang channels. Source points can be palpated to identify repletion or vacuity of source qi in the channel's associated bowel or viscus (repletion being characterized by swelling or distention, and vacuity by a depression at the point). These points are primarily used for the treatment of diseases affecting the bowels and viscera. They can be drained or supplemented to treat vacuity or repletion in the channel or its associated organ.

Source Points

LU-9 (*tài yuān*, Great Abyss)
HT-7 (*shén mén*, Spirit Gate)
PC-7 (*dà líng*, Great Mound)
SP-3 (*tài bái*, Supreme White)
KI-3 (*tài xī*, Great Ravine)
LR-3 (*tài chōng*, Supreme Surge)
LI-4 (*hé gǔ*, Union Valley)
SI-4 (*wàn gǔ*, Wrist Bone)
TB-4 (*yáng chí*, Yang Pool)
ST-42 (*chōng yáng*, Surging Yang)
BL-64 (*jīng gǔ*, Capital Bone)
GB-40 (*qiū xū*, Hill Ruins)

Combinations: Source points can be combined with network points. See COMBINING SOURCE AND NETWORK POINTS. [27: 101] [97: 463] [46: 154] [50: 1230]

source qi 原气 *yuán qì*: The basic form of qi in the body, which is made up of a combination of three other forms: the essential qi of the kidney; qi of grain and water, derived through the transformative function of the spleen; and air (great qi) drawn in through the lung. Source qi springs from the kidney (or life gate), and is stored in the cinnabar field (*dān tián*), the area three body-inches below the umbilicus); it reaches all parts of the body through the pathways of the triple burner, activating all the organs. It is the basis of all physiological activity. All other forms of qi inherent in the body are considered to be manifestations or derivatives of source qi. Source qi can be stimulated through the source points of each channel. Compare ORIGINAL QI. [27: 79] [97: 463]

sourness 酸 *suān*: One of the FIVE FLAVORS. Sourness enters the liver; it can contract and astringe. See FIVE FLAVORS and FIVE-FLAVOR ENTRIES.

sourness enters the liver 酸入肝 *suān rù gān*: Sour medicinals tend to act on the liver. Sour medicinals that enter the liver include achyranthes (*niú xī*), chaenomeles (*mù guā*), cornus (*shān zhū yú*), crataegus (*shān zhā*), eclipta (*mò hàn lián*), litchee (*lì zhī*), mume (*wū méi*), ophicalcite (*huā ruǐ shí*), red peony (*chì sháo yào*), rhinoceros horn (*xī jiǎo*), rubus (*fù pén zǐ*), sanguisorba (*dì yú*), and white peony (*bái sháo yào*). [27: 63]

sour-sore nose 鼻痠 *bí suān*: An aching or sore nose described as feeling "sour." *The Complete Compendium of Medical Works, Ancient and Modern* (*gǔ jīn yī tǒng dà quán*) states, "Sour-sore nose is caused by phlegm-fire, and is treated with Diaphragm-Cooling Powder (*liáng gé sǎn*) with the addition of schizonepeta spike (*jīng jiè suì*) and platycodon (*jié gěng*). [50: 1661]

sour taste in the mouth 口酸 *kǒu suān*: A subjective feeling of sourness in the mouth that in severe cases may be accompanied by a sour smell on the breath, and that differs from *swallowing of upflowing acid*, which refers to the upflow of acid fluid that is then quickly swallowed before it can be spat out. Sour taste in the mouth is attributed to liver heat, to spleen vacuity being exploited by wood, or to food stagnation. **Liver heat** gives rise to a sour-bitter taste in the mouth with fullness and pain in the chest and rib-side, rashness, impatience, and irascibility. There may be red eyes and dizziness, and anguish in the heart, dry stool, and yellow urine. The tongue tends to be red with a thin yellow tongue fur; the pulse is stringlike and slightly rapid. MED Course the liver and clear heat. Use Bupleurum Liver-Clearing Decoction (*chái hú qīng gān tāng*) or Tangkuei, Gentian, and Aloe Pill (*dāng guī lóng huì wán*). **Spleen vacuity being exploited by wood** gives rise to a sour taste in the mouth that may be accompanied by swallowing of upflowing acid and retching of bitter fluid. Other signs include belching, sighing, no enjoyment in food, stomach duct glomus and abdominal distention after eating, fatigue and lack of strength, and thin sloppy stool. The tongue fur is white, and the pulse is fine and stringlike or moderate and stringlike. MED Use fortifying the spleen and harmonizing the stomach as the main method, complemented by calming the liver. Use Six Gentlemen Decoction (*liù jūn zǐ tāng*) combined with Left-Running Metal Pill (*zuǒ jīn wán*). **Food stagnation** gives rise to a sour taste in the mouth with sour and putrid belching, torpid intake and aversion to food, glomus, oppression, distention, and fullness in the stomach duct and abdomen, and foul putrid stool that is either bound or sloppy, and possibly associated with ungratified defecation. The tongue fur is thick and slimy, and sometimes yellow. The pulse is slippery and forceful. MED Disperse food and abduct dispersion; harmonize the stomach and downbear qi. Use Harmony-Preserving Pill (*bǎo hé wán*) or Saussurea and Areca Pill (*mù xiāng bīng láng wán*). See TASTE IN THE MOUTH. [92: No. 84]

Southern Dynasties 南朝 *nán cháo*: The name of a dynastic period (A.D. 420–589).

Southern Song 南宋 *nán sòng*: The name of a dynasty (A.D. 1127–1279).

sovereign 君 *jūn*: See SOVEREIGN, MINISTER, ASSISTANT, AND COURIER.

sovereign fire 君火 *jūn huǒ*: The heart fire. The name sovereign fire derives from the statement contained in the *The Inner Canon* (*nèi jīng*) that the "heart holds the office of sovereign." The sovereign

fire stands in complementary opposition to the *ministerial fire*. See HEART FIRE. [27: 59] [97: 323]

sovereign, minister, assistant, and courier 君臣佐使 *jūn chén zuǒ shǐ*: Synonym: *medicinal roles*. The four roles performed by medicinals within a formula. The *sovereign* performs the principal action of the formula, addressing the principal sign pattern. The sovereign may be one or more medicinals. The *minister* provides direct assistance to the sovereign. The *assistant* addresses secondary patterns or reduces the toxicity or harshness of the sovereign. The *courier* makes other medicinals act on the desired part of the body or harmonizes the other medicinals. NB: Socialist fervor in China led to efforts to rename the four medicinal roles have been as *chief, support, assistant, and conductor,* to avoid the feudal connotations of the traditional terms. With the liberalization over the past few years, the new terms have slipped into oblivion. [27: 300]

SP 脾 *pí*, 足太阴脾经 *zú tài yīn pí jīng*: The spleen or leg greater yin (*tài yīn*) spleen channel.

sparrow blindness 雀盲 *què máng*: SPARROW VISION.

sparrow vision 雀目 *què mù*: Synonyms: *sparrow blindness; night blindness*. Reduced visual acuity in poor lighting. Distinction is made between the earlier heaven type, called HIGH-ALTITUDE WIND SPARROW-VISION INTERNAL OBSTRUCTION, and a later heaven type, called *liver vacuity sparrow-vision internal obstruction*, which is due to splenic movement and transformation failure and gan disease ascending to the eyes. WMC vitamin A deficiency; pigmentary degeneration of retina. MED For the earlier heaven type, warm and supplement kidney yang using Right-Restoring [Life Gate] Pill (*yòu guī wán*). For the later heaven type, kill worms and disperse gan; fortify the spleen and boost qi. Use variations of Chubby Child Pill (*féi ér wán*). Include pig's liver in medication or diet. ACU Base treatment mainly on back transport points, LR, SI, and BL. Main points: BL-18 (*gān shū*, Liver Transport), BL-23 (*shèn shū*, Kidney Transport), LR-2 (*xíng jiān*, Moving Between), BL-1 (*jīng míng*, Bright Eyes), GB-37 (*guāng míng*, Bright Light), and SI-6 (*yǎng lǎo*, Nursing the Aged); needle with supplementation and add moxa. Selection of points according to pattern: For the earlier heaven typen, add GV-4 (*mìng mén*, Life Gate), CV-4 (*guān yuán*, Pass Head), and KI-3 (*tài xī*, Great Ravine), to warm and supplement kidney yang. For the later heaven type, add BL-20 (*pí shū*, Spleen Transport), CV-12 (*zhōng wǎn*, Center Stomach Duct), and ST-36 (*zú sān lǐ*, Leg Three Li) to fortify the spleen and boost qi, and Hundred Worm Nest (*bǎi chóng wō*) to kill worms. ◇ Chin 雀 *què,* sparrow; 目 *mù,* eye, vision. [27: 505] [50: 1379] [37: 466]

spasm 痉挛 *jìng luán:* Western medical term now widely used in Chinese medicine. Spasm is traditionally discussed in variety of terms: Any stiffness or tension in the limbs is referred to as HYPERTONICITY. A painful pulling of the sinews that can be felt as a bulging and knotting is called CRAMP. Spasm preventing the mouth from opening is called CLENCHED JAW, and stiffness of the back that pulls the back in an arch is called ARCHED-BACK RIGIDITY. These two signs are signs of TETANY, which may be observed in FRIGHT WIND or LOCKJAW. Alternating contraction and relaxation of the muscles is traditionally called TUGGING AND SLACKENING, CONVULSIONS, or TUGGING WIND and is observed in EPILEPSY and lockjaw. Mild contraction and relaxation due to insufficiency of blood or fluids, cold-damp, or yang vacuity patterns is called JERKING SINEWS AND TWITCHING FLESH.

spider drum 蜘蛛鼓 *zhī zhū gǔ:* From *The Gateway to Medicine (yī xué rù mén).*
Simple abdominal distention. Spider drum is so called because of the large abdomen and thin legs. See DRUM DISTENTION. [26: 846]

spillage rheum 溢饮 *yì yǐn:* One of the FOUR RHEUMS. Water in the limbs, characterized by heavy painful and sometimes swollen limbs and sometimes accompanied by panting and cough; so called because rheum spills outward to the body surface. Spillage rheum is at root attributable to spleen vacuity. ⎡MED⎤ Warm the lung and effuse sweat with Major Green-Blue Dragon Decoction (*dà qīng lóng tāng*) or Minor Green-Blue Dragon Decoction (*xiǎo qīng lóng tāng*). ⎡ACU⎤ Base treatment mainly on CV, ST, SP, LU, and LI. Select CV-12 (*zhōng wǎn,* Center Stomach Duct), ST-36 (*zú sān lǐ,* Leg Three Li), ST-40 (*fēng lóng,* Bountiful Bulge), SP-9 (*yīn líng quán,* Yin Mound Spring), BL-20 (*pí shū,* Spleen Transport), BL-13 (*fèi shū,* Lung Transport), LI-4 (*hé gǔ,* Union Valley), and KI-7 (*fù liū,* Recover Flow); needle with drainage and add moxa. For panting and cough, add Panting Stabilizer (*dìng chuǎn*), and LU-9 (*tài yuān,* Great Abyss). See PHLEGM-RHEUM. [26: 757] [6: 221] [27: 382] [97: 615] [46: 595, 653]

spinal column 脊骨 *lǚ gǔ:* The back bone. [27: 69] [97: 631]

spine bone 脊骨 *lǚ gǔ:* Synonym: *shuttle bone.* The protruding bone of the spine at the level of the shoulder; just below GV-14 (*dà zhuī,* Great Hammer) and just above GV-13 (*táo dào,* Kiln Path). ; i.e., the spinous process of the first thoracic vertebra (T$_1$) of modern medicine. [27: 69]

spine pinching 捏脊 *nēi jǐ:* A tui-na method of spine manipulation used in the treatment of gan accumulation in infants. **Method:** The manipu-

lator places the child is placed prone posture in front of him. He places both index fingers on the ridge of the spine, and pinches the flesh on either side of the spine between the thumb and second joint of the middle finger of each hand. The action is performed running up the spine from GV-1 (*cháng qiáng,* Long Strong) to GV-14 (*dà zhuī,* Great Hammer), alternating left and right hand pinches. This sequence is performed 3–6 times in each session. This method can also be used treat enuresis and insomnia. [50: 1234]

spinning bean pulse 转豆脉 *zhuǎn dòu mài:* See TEN STRANGE PULSES. [27: 199]

spinning pill pulse 转丸脉 *zhuǎn wán mài:* SPINNING BEAN PULSE. See TEN STRANGE PULSES. [27: 199]

spirit 神 *shén:* Synonyms: *spirit light; heart spirit; spirit-mind.* **1.** (In the narrow sense) that which is said to be stored by the heart, to return to the abode of the heart during sleep, to be disquieted in conditions of heart palpitations, susceptibility to fright, heart vexation, and insomnia, and to be clouded in wind stroke or when evils enter the pericardium. The Chinese concept of spirit is what normally makes us conscious and alert during the day, what becomes inactive during sleep, and thus corresponds to the concept of the English word 'mind' in the sense of the mental capacity to think, feel, and respond. See the entries listed below.

Conditions of or Affecting the "Spirit"

DISQUIETED HEART SPIRIT (*xīn shén bù ān*)

INSOMNIA (*shī mián*)

CLOUDED SPIRIT (*shén hūn*)

CLOUDING SLEEP (*hūn shuì*)

DELIRIOUS SPEECH (*zhān yǔ*)

LOSS OF CONSCIOUSNESS (*bù xǐng rén shì*)

SOLILOQUY (*dú yǔ*)

MUSSITATION (*zhèng shēng*)

SPIRIT FAILING TO KEEP TO ITS ABODE (*shén bù shǒu shè*)

PERICARDIAC PATTERN (*xīn bāo zhèng*)

HEAT ENTERING THE PERICARDIUM (*rè rù xīn bāo*)

PHLEGM CONFOUNDING THE ORIFICES OF THE HEART (*tán mí xīn qiào*)

EPILEPSY (*xián*)

MANIA AND WITHDRAWAL (*diān kuáng*)

See also ESSENCE-SPIRIT; MIND; AFFECT. **2.** (In a wider sense) that which is said to present in individuals with healthy complexion, bright eyes, erect bearing, physical agility, and clear coherent speech. It is said, "If the patient is spirited, he is fundamentally healthy; if he is spiritless, he is doomed."

Thus, the spirit sheds useful light on the severity of a given complaint. Conditions of the spirit may be arranged in three fundamental categories: spiritedness, spiritlessness, and false spiritedness. **Spiritedness:** If the patient has bright eyes, normal bearing, clear speech, and responds coherently to inquiry, the condition is said to be spirited, indicating that right qi is undamaged and the complaint is relatively minor. Although certain aspects of the patient's health may be seriously affected, swift improvement may be expected. **Spiritlessness:** Essence-spirit debilitation (lack of mental energy), apathy, abnormal bearing, torpid expression, dark complexion and dull eyes, low voice, slow, halting speech, and incoherent response to inquiry are signs of a spiritless condition. They indicate a relatively serious condition in which right qi has suffered damage. Although no critical signs may be present, extreme care is necessary. Where a spiritless condition is particularly marked, there may be signs of deranged speech, stupor of the spirit-mind, carphology (involuntary picking at bedclothes), and a general feeling of heaviness preventing the patient from turning over in bed. **False spiritedness:** False spiritedness generally occurs in enduring or severe illness and extremely severe cases of debilitation of essence-spirit. If, suddenly, during a disease characterized by taciturnity, a low voice, halting speech, and an extremely dark complexion, the patient becomes strangely garrulous and his cheeks are flushed and unusually rosy, this new condition is said to be one of false spiritedness. Such conditions are extremely serious and should not be mistaken for improvement. False spiritedness implies a superficial improvement in certain aspects of the patient's mental state, which does not fit in with other aspects of the condition. It is a sign that the patient's condition will soon deteriorate dramatically, and therefore demands special attention. See also STOMACH, SPIRIT, AND ROOT. Note also that the word spirit occurs in several terms pertaining to the eye. See SPIRIT WATER; SPIRIT JELLY; SPIRIT BALL; PUPIL SPIRIT. [26: 405] [27: 82] [97: 424]

spirit-affect 神情 *shén qíng*: The spirit and the outwardly manifest emotions, as seen in the facial expression.

spirit ball 神珠 *shén zhū*: Eyeball. [97: 424]

spiritedness 得神 *dé shén*: The presence of general signs of vitality such as bright eyes, normal bearing, clear speech, and coherent response to inquiry indicating that right qi is undamaged and the complaint is relatively minor. Although certain aspects of the patient's health may be seriously affected, swift improvement may be expected. [6: 115]

spirit failing to keep to its abode 神不守舍 *shén bù shǒu shè*: Mental derangement. *The Magic Pivot* (*líng shū, zhì zhēn yào dà lùn*) states "The heart... is the abode of essence-spirit." The spirit failing to keep to its abode reflects the conception that under normal circumstances the spirit resides in the heart, and that when it is made to leave the heart (by disease evil invading the heart or by mental stimulus), normal clarity of mind and composure is lost. [27: 371] [27: 371] [97: 424]

spirit jelly 神膏 *shén gāo*: The jelly-like substance in the eye. WMC vitreous humor. [26: 405]

spiritlessness 失神 *shī shén*: Presence of signs of lack of general vitality such as mental debilitation, apathy, abnormal bearing, torpid expression, dark complexion and dull eyes, low voice, slow, halting speech, and incoherent response to inquiry, indicating a relatively serious condition in which right qi has suffered damage. Although no critical signs may be present, extreme care is necessary in devising treatment. [6: 115]

spirit light 神明 *shén míng*: Spirit or essence-spirit. [27: 82]

spirit-mind 神志 *shén zhì*: The spirit. See SPIRIT and MIND. [27: 82] [97: 424]

spirit qi 神气 *shén qì*: **1.** Spirit, vigor. **2.** In *The Inner Canon* (*nèi jīng*), 'spirit qi' refers to the spirit, channel qi, right qi, the blood, and the yang qi of the bowels and viscera. [81: 382]

spirit water 神水 *shén shuǐ*: **1.** Watery substance in the eye. WMC aqueous humor. **2.** Tears. [26: 405] [97: 424]

spitting of blood 唾血 *tuò xuè*: **1.** Coughing of phlegm-blood. *Elementary Questions* (*sù wèn, ké lùn*) states, "The signs of lung cough are cough with noisy panting, and in severe cases spitting of blood." **2.** Expulsion of blood with saliva; attributed to the spleen failing to manage the blood, effulgent yin vacuity fire, or the liver failing to store the blood. **Spleen failing to manage the blood** causes spitting of blood accompanied by heart palpitations or fearful throbbing, vexation, and insomnia, reduced eating and lassitude of spirit. MED Use Spleen-Returning Decoction (*guī pí tāng*). ACU Base treatment mainly on SP, ST, HT, CV, and back transport points. Select BL-20 (*pí shū*, Spleen Transport), BL-15 (*xīn shū*, Heart Transport), CV-12 (*zhōng wǎn*, Center Stomach Duct), ST-36 (*zú sān lǐ*, Leg Three Li), SP-4 (*gōng sūn*, Yellow Emperor), SP-1 (*yǐn bái*, Hidden White), PC-6 (*nèi guān*, Inner Pass), and HT-7 (*shén mén*, Spirit Gate); needle with supplementation and moxa. **Effulgent yin vacuity fire** spitting of blood is accompanied by fine rapid pulse. MED Use Yin-Enriching Fire-Downbearing Decoction (*zī yīn jiàng huǒ tāng*). ACU Base treatment mainly on KI, SP, and PC.

Select KI-3 (*tài xī*, Great Ravine), KI-6 (*zhào hǎi*, Shining Sea), KI-2 (*rán gǔ*, Blazing Valley), SP-6 (*sān yīn jiāo*, Three Yin Intersection), BL-17 (*gé shū*, Diaphragm Transport), PC-6 (*nèi guān*, Inner Pass), and PC-7 (*dà líng*, Great Mound); needle with drainage or with even supplementation and drainage. **Liver failing to store the blood** can cause spitting of blood attended by headache, thirst, and constipation. MED Use Tangkuei, Gentian, and Aloe Pill (*dāng guī lóng huì wán*) or Heart-Draining Decoction (*xiè xīn tāng*). ACU Base treatment mainly on LR and CV. Select LR-3 (*tài chōng*, Supreme Surge), LR-2 (*xíng jiān*, Moving Between), PC-8 (*láo gōng*, Palace of Toil), PC-7 (*dà líng*, Great Mound), PC-6 (*nèi guān*, Inner Pass), BL-18 (*gān shū*, Liver Transport), and BL-17 (*gé shū*, Diaphragm Transport); needle with drainage. [26: 633] [97: 521] [46: 738] [37: 310]

spittle 唾 *tuò*: One of the FIVE HUMORS. Spittle is one of the fluids of the mouth, the other being DROOL. These two together are known as drool-spittle or spittle humor (saliva). The kidney clasps the root of the tongue connecting with CV-23 (*lián quán*, Ridge Spring) under the tongue. Kidney vacuity water flood is characterized by clear cold spittle humor. Kidney yin vacuity with vacuity fire flaming upward can cause scant spittle and dry throat accompanied by a strange fishy, salty taste in the mouth. [27: 521] [29: 116]

spittle humor 唾液 *tuò yè*: See SPITTLE.

spittle is the humor of the kidney 唾为肾液 *tuò wéi shèn yè*: The kidney channel rises to the root of the tongue, to communicate with Ridge Spring (CV-23) and Jade's Beauty (CV-18), from where spittle springs. Spittle is therefore the humor of the kidney. [26: 121]

spleen 脾 *pí*: The organ that lies against the lower face of the stomach. The spleen is ascribed the function of assimilating nutrients from food in the stomach to make qi, blood, and fluids. It is associated in the five phases with earth. The SPLEEN GOVERNS MOVEMENT AND TRANSFORMATION of grain and water and distribution of its essence. This is the spleen's main function. It plays an important role in the formation of qi and blood. For this reason it is said that the spleen is the source of qi and blood formation. The stomach is responsible for initial decomposition of "grain and water" (i.e., food). The spleen then extracts the essence of grain and water (nutrients) and dispatches it to the other organs, so that it reaches all parts of the body. *Elementary Questions* (*sù wèn, tài yīn yáng míng lùn*) states that the spleen "moves the fluids of the stomach." *Elementary Questions* (*sù wèn, jīng mài bié lùn*) further states, "Drink (饮 *yǐn*, imbibed fluid) enters the stomach, where it

is churned and its its essential qi is strained off. This is then carried to the spleen and further distributed by spleen qi. It passes up to the lung, which regulates the waterways down to the bladder. Thus water essence is distributed to the four parts, passing through the five channels." These statements explain the spleen's function of moving and transforming grain and water and distributing their essence. In actual fact, these functions include digestion, assimilation, and distribution of nutrients spoken of in Western medicine. Failure of splenic movement and transformation can lead to a variety of pathologies. If, for any reason, digestion and assimilation are upset, this can cause abdominal distention, diarrhea, or nutritional disorders. If the distributive function is impaired, improper movement of fluids may give rise to INTERNAL DAMPNESS, PHLEGM, RHEUM, or WATER SWELLING; hence it is said that the spleen ails by dampness and is "the source of phlegm formation." Diseases resulting from impaired movement and transformation are commonly denoted by the term spleen vacuity (spleen vacuity dampness, spleen vacuity phlegm, spleen vacuity diarrhea, and spleen vacuity water swelling). These pathologies are neatly summed up by the statement in *Elementary Questions* (*sù wèn, zhì zhēn yào dà lùn*) "All dampness with swelling and fullness is ascribed to the spleen." The SPLEEN MANAGES THE BLOOD; it plays an important role in blood formation and also prevents extravasation of blood. The spleen is the source of blood and qi formation, and when healthy it ensures plentiful supplies of qi and blood in the body, and since qi contains the blood, the spleen both engenders the blood and contains it. Thus the notion of the spleen managing the blood includes the notion of qi containing the blood. In pathology, bleeding that occurs in qi and blood vacuity patterns stemming from impairment of splenic movement and transformation is explained as the spleen failing to manage the blood. Considered strictly from the point of view of bleeding, such conditions could also be described as failure of qi to contain the blood. However, FLOODING AND SPOTTING due to heart-spleen vacuity and blood in the stool due to qi vacuity are conventionally attributed to the spleen failing to manage the blood. The SPLEEN GOVERNS THE FLESH AND LIMBS: Because the spleen is the source of blood and qi formation, the flesh of the whole body relies for its nourishment on the capacity of the stomach and spleen to move and transform the essence of grain and water. Only when the stomach and spleen are functioning properly is the flesh full and firm and the limbs powerful. Impairment of splenic function may therefore lead to emaciation, lack of strength, and, in severe cases, wilting weakness of the limbs with loss of their use. "The SPLEEN OPENS AT THE MOUTH" refers to the relationship of splenic movement and transformation to appetite and taste in the mouth. If the stomach and the spleen are functioning normally, the individual has a good appetite and normal taste in the mouth. *The Magic Pivot* (*líng shū*) states, "Spleen qi flows through to the mouth; if the spleen is in harmony, then the mouth can taste the five flavors." Diseases of the spleen and stomach are often reflected in changes in appetite and changes in taste in the mouth (blandness, sweetness, sliminess). The spleen's relationships to other bowels and viscera are as follows: **Spleen and stomach:** The spleen and stomach stand in interior-exterior relationship: The spleen and stomach are interlinked by the "homing and "netting" connections between their channels, and stand in interior-exterior relationship with each other. Physiologically, the spleen governs movement and transformation, whereas the stomach governs intake. The spleen governs upbearing, whereas the stomach governs downbearing. The stomach and the spleen thus complement and counterbalance each other. Together the spleen and stomach perform the main part of digestion and assimilation. The stomach governs intake and decomposition, thus preparing for movement and transformation. The spleen "moves the fluids of the stomach," adapting to the stomach's continual need for food intake. Both organs function in close cooperation in performing digestive activity. A poor appetite (poor stomach intake) leaves the spleen with fewer raw materials from which to form qi and blood. Yet a good appetite with indigestion is an equally pathological state. *Medical Remedies Researched* (*yī fāng kǎo*) states, "The stomach governs intake, and the spleen governs the grinding down. So if the patient can take in food but cannot transform it, spleen vacuity is to blame." A clear distinction is made between the stomach's governing of intake and the spleen's governing of movement and transformation. In clinical practice, poor appetite or CLAMORING STOMACH with rapid hungering is attributed to the stomach, while indigestion, bloating after eating, and sloppy stool, are attributed to the spleen. In the first instance, treatment must be directed to increasing the appetite and harmonizing the stomach; in the second case, it must aim to fortify the spleen and assist movement. The spleen's governing of upbearing and the stomach's governing of downbearing again show the antagonism and complementarity of the two organs. The spleen not only moves and transforms the essence of grain and water, but also carries it up to the heart and lung. This is why it is said, "The spleen governs upbearing." Failure of spleen qi to bear upward leads to center qi fall, characterized by

sagging distention in the stomach duct and abdomen, diarrhea, and prolapse of the rectum. The stomach's governing of downbearing refers to conveyance of the food to the small intestine and, in a broader sense, to downward flow throughout the whole of the digestive tract. "Stomach qi is normal when there is free downbearing" highlights the advantage to the stomach of unimpaired downbearing. However, should stomach qi bear upward instead of downward, such signs as nausea, vomiting, belching, and hiccough are observed. Ye Tian-Shi (A.D. 1667–1746, Qing) wrote: "Intake of food is governed by the stomach, while movement and transformation are governed by the spleen; the spleen is healthy when it bears upward, whereas the stomach is in harmony when it bears downward." Upbearing and downbearing are mutually serving. The spleen upbears clear qi (the essential qi extracted from the grain and water), whereas the stomach downbears turbid qi (the remains). Failure of the clear qi to bear upward may impair the downbearing of turbid qi. Similarly, failure of the turbid qi to bear downward may affect the bearing upward of the clear qi. For this reason, signs such as poor appetite, bloating of the stomach duct and abdomen, nausea, belching, indigestion, diarrhea, and thick slimy tongue fur often occur simultaneously. *Elementary Questions* (*sù wèn, yīn yáng yìng xiàng dà lùn*) says, "When clear qi is below, there is swill diarrhea; where turbid qi is above, there is distention." In clinical practice, such conditions are treated by fortifying the spleen (upbearing the clear) and harmonizing the stomach (downbearing the turbid). Furthermore, the spleen "likes dryness" and "is averse to dampness" while the stomach "likes dampness" and "is averse to dryness." There is a difference in nature between diseases of the spleen and those of the stomach. The spleen is particularly susceptible to invasion by dampness evil, which affects movement and transformation; impairment of movement and transformation due to other causes may easily give rise to dampness. When dampness affects movement and transformation, the spleen is said to be "encumbered by dampness." This condition is treated with warm bitter medicinals that dry dampness and fortify the spleen. The stomach, by contrast, is vulnerable to heat evil that "scorch" the stomach juices. The stomach juices are easily damaged in exuberant lung and stomach heat patterns, which are characterized by heat effusion, dry mouth, dry pharynx, constipation, red tongue with scant fur, and a rapid fine pulse. Frequent vomiting due to counterflow ascent causes detriment to the stomach juices characterized by signs of dryness. Such patterns are treated by moistening dryness and nourishing the stomach. Physiologically, the stomach and the spleen are closely related; the antagonistic and complementary nature of spleen upbearing and stomach downbearing constitute the dynamics of the digestive process. Destruction of this balance constitutes the main cause of digestive disturbances, while the treatment of spleen and stomach disease mostly rests on the principle of restoring normal spleen upbearing and stomach downbearing. **Spleen and liver:** The normal functioning of the stomach and spleen is related to the liver's governing of free coursing. When the liver's free coursing action is impaired, the resulting depression of liver qi affects digestive function, causing distention and pain in the stomach duct and abdomen, torpid intake, belching, nausea, vomiting, and diarrhea. *The Magic Pivot* (*líng shū*) states, "Diseases to which the liver gives rise include fullness in the chest, belching, and swill diarrhea." Such conditions are termed "liver qi invading the stomach" and "liver-spleen disharmony." **Spleen and kidney:** Kidney yang, also known as "life gate fire," is a motor force in the digestive process. Insufficiency of kidney yang (debilitation of the life gate fire) leads to impairment of the digestive function. This pathology is called "spleen-kidney yang vacuity" and is characterized by cold pain in the abdomen, persistent diarrhea, fifth-watch diarrhea, nontransformation food, and water swelling. ◇ Chin 脾 *pí* is composed of the flesh signifier 月, an abbreviated form of 肉 *ròu* combined with 卑 *bēi*, which gives the character its sound, and by its meaning of low or below, may contribute to meaning by indicating that the spleen is the organ located below the stomach. [26: 746]

spleen accumulation 脾积 *pí jī*: From *The Pulse Canon* (*mài jīng, píng wǔ zàng jī jù mài zhèng*). See GLOMUS QI. [26: 750]

spleen and stomach hold the office of the granaries, whence the five flavors emanate 脾胃者，仓廪之官，五味出焉 *pí wèi zhě, cāng lǐn zhī gān, wǔ wèi chū yān*: This phrase comes from *Elementary Questions* (*sù wèn, líng lán mì diǎn lùn*). The spleen and stomach are like an official responsible for the national grain stores; they provide nourishment for the whole body. Since traditionally the effect not only of medicinals but also foodstuffs was understood in terms of qi and flavor, the term "five flavors" denotes five different nutritive properties of food. [27: 47]

spleen and stomach stand in interior-exterior relationship 脾与胃相表里 *pí yǔ wèi xiāng biǎo lǐ*: See SPLEEN IS CONNECTED WITH THE STOMACH. [27: 147]

spleen channel 脾经 *pí jīng*: FOOT GREATER YIN SPLEEN CHANNEL. [27: 750]

spleen channel cough 脾经咳嗽 *pí jīng ké sòu*: SPLEEN COUGH.

spleen cough 脾咳 *pí ké*: *Synonym: spleen channel cough*. COUGH occurring in bouts and causing pain in right rib-side, stretching into the shoulder and back. In severe cases, the patient can barely move, and any movement exacerbates the cough. See FIVE BOWELS AND SIX VISCERA COUGH. [26: 747] [27: 370] [97: 560]

spleen dampness and liver depression 脾湿肝郁 *pí shī gān yù*: A disease pattern arising when persistent dampness encumbering the spleen and stomach affects the liver's free coursing function. The main signs are distention and pain in the chest, rib-side, stomach duct, and abdomen, and torpid intake with sloppy stool. Other signs include constrained affect-mind, vexation, agitation, and irascibility, rib-side pain and distention, nausea, lassitude of spirit and lack of strength, fatigued cumbersome limbs, withered-yellow facial complexion, short voidings of scant urine, in severe cases with puffy swelling, and yellowing of the eyes and skin. The tongue fur is yellow and slimy or thick and slimy. The pulse is soggy and moderate or fine and stringlike. ⟨MED⟩ Use Saussurea and Amomum Six Gentlemen Decoction (*xiāng shā liù jūn zǐ tāng*) combined with Bupleurum Liver-Coursing Powder (*chái hú shū gān sǎn*). ⟨ACU⟩ Base treatment mainly on CV, back transport points, ST, SP, and LR. Select CV-12 (*zhōng wǎn*, Center Stomach Duct), LR-13 (*zhāng mén*, Camphorwood Gate), ST-25 (*tiān shū*, Celestial Pivot), ST-36 (*zú sān lǐ*, Leg Three Li), SP-9 (*yīn líng quán*, Yin Mound Spring), BL-20 (*pí shū*, Spleen Transport), BL-18 (*gān shū*, Liver Transport), GB-34 (*yáng líng quán*, Yang Mound Spring), PC-6 (*nèi guān*, Inner Pass), LR-3 (*tài chōng*, Supreme Surge), and SP-6 (*sān yīn jiāo*, Three Yin Intersection); needle with drainage or with even supplementation and drainage, and, if appropriate, add moxa. **Analysis:** When dampness evil causes internal obstruction, qi dynamic is inhibited, hence the distention and pain in the chest, rib-side, stomach duct, and abdomen. When the spleen's movement and the stomach's harmonious downbearing are impaired, there is torpid intake, sloppy stool, and nausea. When dampness obstructs qi dynamic, and the movement of qi and blood is inhibited, there is lassitude of spirit, fatigued cumbersome limbs, and withered-yellow facial complexion. When dampness obstructs the liver and gallbladder, bile does not keep to its normal path, but spills out, hence the yellow skin and eyes. When exuberant internal dampness affects bladder qi transformation, there are short voidings of scant urine. When dampness floods the skin and flesh, there is puffy swelling of the limbs. When the liver's free coursing action is impaired, constrained affect mind, or vexation, agitation, and irascibility are observed. The slimy tongue fur reflects the spleen dampness. The pulse is soggy and moderate when spleen dampness is dominant, and is fine and stringlike when liver depression is dominant. [116: 148] [46: 585, 646, 662]

spleen diarrhea 脾泻 *pí xiè*, 脾泄 *pí xiè*: Synonym: *throughflux diarrhea*. DIARRHEA due to spleen disease; associated with distention and fullness or abdominal discomfort, vomiting, heavy limbs, and vacuity yellow facial complexion. MED Fortify the spleen and regulate the center with the Center-Fortifying Decoctions (*jiàn zhōng tāng*) or variations of Center-Rectifying Decoction (*lǐ zhōng tāng*). ACU Base treatment mainly on back transport points, CV, PC, and ST. Select BL-20 (*pí shū*, Spleen Transport), CV-6 (*qì hǎi*, Sea of Qi), PC-6 (*nèi guān*, Inner Pass), CV-12 (*zhōng wǎn*, Center Stomach Duct), LR-13 (*zhāng mén*, Camphorwood Gate), ST-25 (*tiān shū*, Celestial Pivot), and ST-36 (*zú sān lǐ*, Leg Three Li); needle with supplementation and add moxa. If caused by summerheat-damp, see SUMMERHEAT DIARRHEA. [26: 747] [97: 585]

spleen disease 脾病 *pí bìng*: Any disease of the spleen. The spleen governs movement and transformation of grain and water (i.e., food), and is the source qi and blood formation; hence spleen disease, whatever form it takes, is a failure of these functions. Spleen disease is attributable to damage by dietary irregularities, affect damage, and dampness. Spleen disease patterns include the following:

Spleen Disease Patterns

Simple patterns

SPLEEN QI VACUITY (*pí qì xū*)

SPLEEN YANG VACUITY (*pí yáng xū*)

SPLEEN YIN VACUITY (*pí yīn xū*)

CENTER QI FALL (*zhōng qì xià xiàn*)

SPLEEN VACUITY WITH FOOD DAMAGE (*pí xū jiā shí*)

SPLEEN VACUITY WITH DAMP ENCUMBRANCE (*pí xū shī kùn*)

COLD-DAMP ENCUMBERING THE SPLEEN (*hán shī kùn pí*)

SPLEEN FAILING TO MANAGE THE BLOOD (*pí bù tǒng xuè*)

DAMP-HEAT BREWING IN THE SPLEEN (*shī rè yùn pí*)

Combined patterns

SPLEEN-STOMACH VACUITY (*pí wèi xū ruò*)

SPLEEN-STOMACH YANG VACUITY (*pí wèi yáng xū*)

STRONG STOMACH AND WEAK SPLEEN (*wèi qiáng pí ruò*)

SPLEEN-KIDNEY YANG VACUITY (*pí shèn yáng xū*)

DUAL VACUITY OF THE SPLEEN AND LUNG (*pí fèi liǎng xū*)

YANG VACUITY WATER FLOOD (*yáng xū shuǐ fàn*)

DUAL VACUITY OF THE HEART AND SPLEEN (*xīn pí liǎng xū*)

LIVER-SPLEEN DISHARMONY (*gān pí bù hé*)

SPLEEN DAMPNESS AND LIVER DEPRESSION (*pí shī gān yù*)

Of these, the most main basic patterns are spleen qi vacuity, spleen yang vacuity, spleen yin vacuity, center qi fall, spleen failing to manage the blood, cold-damp encumbering the spleen, spleen vacuity with food damage, and damp-heat brewing in the spleen. **Spleen qi vacuity** is a pattern of insufficiency of spleen qi impairing movement and transformation. It is caused by dietary irregularities or overwork, or it may be a consequence of other diseases. It is characterized by reduced food intake, abdominal distention exacerbated by eating, sloppy stool, fatigued limbs, shortage of qi and laziness to speak, and withered-yellow or bright white facial complexion, a pale tongue with white fur, and a weak moderate pulse. In some cases there may be water swelling or emaciation. **Spleen yang vacuity** is the result of debilitation of spleen yang and the consequent development of exuberant internal yin cold. It may develop from spleen qi vacuity, arise from excessive consumption of raw or cold foods, or may stem from spleen yang vacuity with fire (kidney yang) failing to engender earth. It is characterized by abdominal distention, abdominal pain that likes warmth and pressure, clear sloppy stool, reduced food intake, lack of warmth in the extremities, a pale enlarged tongue with glossy white fur, and a forceless slow sunken pulse. In some cases, signs may also include heavy cumbersome limbs, generalized swelling and inhibited urination, or copious white vaginal discharge. **Spleen yin vacuity** is failure of the spleen to distribute essence, characterized by emaciation, and most often resulting from enduring illness or from wear on the yin humor of the stomach and spleen in febrile disease. Spleen yin vacuity is actually dual vacuity of spleen qi and yin. **Center qi fall** is impairment of the upbearing power of the spleen. It may develop from spleen qi vacuity, or may result from enduring diarrhea or dysentery, or from overwork. It is characterized by abdominal distention with a heavy sagging sensation that is exacerbated by eating. There may be a frequent desire to defecate with a heavy sagging sensation in the anus, or enduring diarrhea or dysentery that can culminate in prolapse of the rectum. Alternatively their may be prolapse of the uterus. Yet another pattern is murky urine like rice water (see URINARY TURBIDITY). Attendant signs include qi shortage and lack of strength, fatigued limbs, low voice and laziness to speak, dizziness, pale tongue with white fur, and a weak pulse. The **spleen failing to manage the blood** is depletion of spleen qi manifesting in failure to contain blood. It is characterized by profuse menstruation or flooding and spotting, or in bloody stool, blood in the urine, spontaneous bleeding of the flesh, or spontaneous bleeding of the gums. It is often accompanied by reduced food intake, sloppy stool, lassitude of spirit, shortage of qi and laziness to speak, lusterless complexion, pale tongue with white fur, and a weak fine pulse. **Spleen vacuity with damp encumbrance** in which splenic movement and transformation causes water-damp water-damp gathers and stagnates. Signs include reduced food intake, fullness and oppression in the stomach duct, sloppy diarrhea, cumbersome fatigued limbs that may be swollen, a thick slimy tongue fur, and a moderate pulse. **Cold-damp encumbering the spleen** is a pattern of exuberant cold-damp hampering spleen yang. It is similar to spleen vacuity with damp encumbrance, but cold and dampness resulting from excessive consumption of cold food and drinks are prominent. It is attributed to dietary irregularities, excessive consumption of raw or cold foods, getting soaked in the rain, wading through water, or living in damp places. It is marked by glomus, oppression, distention and pain in the stomach duct and abdomen, reduced food intake, sloppy stool, nausea and vomiting, bland taste in the mouth, lack of thirst, heavy cumbersome head and body, somber yellow facial complexion, short scant voidings of urine, pale enlarged tongue with slimy white tongue fur, and a moderate soggy pulse. Cold-damp encumbering the spleen is a pattern of cold and dampness due to excessive consumption of raw or cold foods or due exposure to dampness in the environment; spleen vacuity with damp encumbrance, by contrast, is spleen vacuity giving rise to internal dampness. The two patterns differ in the importance of vacuity and the presence of cold. **Spleen vacuity with food damage** is nontransformation of ingested food attributable to spleen-stomach vacuity, marked by bloating after eating and by sloppy stool containing untransformed food. **Damp-heat brewing in the spleen** is caused by contraction of external damp-heat or by damp-heat arising internally as a result of excessive consumption of alcohol or sweet fatty foods. It is characterized by glomus and oppression in the abdomen, torpid intake, nausea and vomiting, sloppy stool, yellow urine, and heavy cumbersome limbs, a red tongue with slimy yellow fur and a rapid soggy pulse. In some cases, there is yellowing of the skin and eyes marked by the color of tangerines (see JAUNDICE). There may also be itchy skin, or remittent generalized heat effusion unresolved by sweating. Combined patterns of the spleen such as SPLEEN-STOMACH VACUITY and SPLEEN-KIDNEY YANG VACUITY are given in

the list of spleen disease pattern above. [26: 748] [29: 415] [6: 178]

spleen dispersion 脾消 *pí xiāo*: CENTER DISPERSION. [27: 424]

spleen distention 脾胀 *pí zhàng*: **1.** A condition described in *The Magic Pivot* (*líng shū*) as follows: "In the case of [distention of] the spleen, there is hiccough, vexation in the limbs, heavy body that makes dressing difficult, and unquiet sleep." Spleen distention is usually caused by cold qi exploiting the spleen. [MED] Use formulas such as Stomach-Calming Poria (Hoelen) Five Decoction (*wèi líng tāng*). **2.** The same signs occurring in distention disease. [26: 749]

spleen-earth 脾土 *pí tǔ*: The spleen viewed as corresponding to earth in the five phases. [97: 559]

spleen failing to manage the blood 脾不统血 *pí bù tǒng xuè*: Synonym: *blood management failure*. Impairment of the spleen's function of managing the blood, resulting in bleeding. Since the spleen is the source of blood and qi formation, the pathomechanism of this disease may be explained as failure of qi to contain the blood. Although blood management failure and containment failure are technically considered to be interchangeable terms, bloody stool and FLOODING AND SPOTTING are conventionally attributed to the spleen failing to manage the blood. Bleeding that results from blood management failure includes blood in the stool or flooding and spotting with a somber white or withered-yellow complexion, weakness and fatigued spirit, dizziness, heart palpitations, and shortness of breath. The tongue is generally pale and the pulse is fine and soggy. Such signs indicate vacuity of the stomach and spleen and insufficiency of blood and qi. Spleen yang vacuity signs may also be observed. [MED] Treat by boosting qi to contain blood. This can be combined with spleen warming where signs of spleen yang vacuity are present. Commonly used medicinals that boost qi and contain the blood include codonopsis (*dǎng shēn*), astragalus (*huáng qí*), and licorice (*gān cǎo*). Concurrent spleen yang vacuity calls for addition of spleen-warming medicinals such as oven earth (*fú lóng gān*), blast-fried ginger (*páo jiāng*), and aconite (*fù zǐ*). Yellow Earth Decoction (*huáng tǔ tāng*) warms the spleen and enhances blood management, and is used where spleen vacuity blood in the stool is accompanied by cold signs. Spleen-Returning Decoction (*guī pí tāng*), which not only nourishes the heart and spleen but also boosts qi and contains the blood, is more suitable for flooding and spotting. Since blood management failure is pathomechanically the same as failure of qi to contain the blood, boosting qi represents the basis of treatment. However, given the danger that bleeding may lead to blood vacuity, addition of blood-nourishing medicinals such as dried rehmannia (*gān dì huáng*) and ass hide glue (*ē jiāo*) is advisable. If bleeding gives rise to signs of disquieted heart spirit such as heart palpitations and insomnia, blood-nourishing spirit-quieting medicinals such as spiny jujube (*suān zǎo rén*) and polygala (*yuǎn zhì*) can be added. Addition of blood-quickening medicinals may be indicated where blood stasis occurs in the course of enduring bleeding. [ACU] Base treatment mainly on SP, ST, CV, and back transport points. Main points: BL-20 (*pí shū*, Spleen Transport), BL-21 (*wèi shū*, Stomach Transport), CV-12 (*zhōng wǎn*, Center Stomach Duct), ST-36 (*zú sān lǐ*, Leg Three Li), SP-3 (*tài bái*, Supreme White), and SP-1 (*yǐn bái*, Hidden White); needle with supplementation and add moxa. For blood in the stool, add CV-4 (*guān yuán*, Pass Head), and BL-35 (*huì yáng*, Meeting of Yang). For flooding and spotting, add CV-4 (*guān yuán*, Pass Head), CV-6 (*qì hǎi*, Sea of Qi), and SP-6 (*sān yīn jiāo*, Three Yin Intersection). For spleen yang vacuity, add large amounts of moxa. [46: 688, 738] [27: 156] [97: 562]

spleen failing to move and transform 脾失健运 *pí shī jiàn yùn*: SPLENIC MOVEMENT AND TRANSFORMATION FAILURE.

spleen forms drool 脾为涎 *pí wéi xián*: From *Elementary Questions* (*sù wèn, xuān míng wǔ qì piān*). The spleen opens at the mouth. Drool is produced in the mouth. Same in meaning as *drool is the humor of the spleen*. [27: 161]

spleen gan 脾疳 *pí gān*: Synonym: *gan accumulation*; *food gan*; *fat gan*. A GAN pattern infants and children arising when improper feeding or diet leads to spleen-stomach vacuity and accumulation and stagnation of food. Spleen gan is characterized by yellow face and emaciated flesh, ability to eat with rapid hungering, stool that is sometimes dry and sometimes thin, unquiet sleep, profuse sweating, grinding of the teeth, and tendency to lie prone. *The Level-Line of Pattern Identification and Treatment* (*zhèng zhì zhǔn shéng*) states, "Accumulation is the mother of gan; hence accumulations that are not treated result in gan." [MED] To treat accumulation, regulate the spleen and stomach with Harmony-Preserving Pill (*bǎo hé wán*) with additions. If the accumulation persists and signs appear such as marked emaciation, withered-yellow facial complexion, congestion and oppression in the chest and diaphragm, distention and enlargement of the abdomen, taking of little milk, frequent diarrhea with sour-smelling stool, lassitude of spirit and physical fatigue, and laziness to speak and move, gan accumulation has set in. This is treated by dispersing gan and fortifying the spleen with variations of Chubby Child Pill (*féi ér wán*) and Ginseng, Poria (Hoelen), and Ovate Atracty-

lodes Powder (*shēn líng bái zhú sǎn*). [ACU] Base treatment mainly on SP and ST. Select BL-20 (*pí shū*, Spleen Transport), BL-21 (*wèi shū*, Stomach Transport), CV-10 (*xià wǎn*, Lower Stomach Duct), CV-12 (*zhōng wǎn*, Center Stomach Duct), LR-13 (*zhāng mén*, Camphorwood Gate), ST-36 (*zú sān lǐ*, Leg Three Li), SP-4 (*gōng sūn*, Yellow Emperor), SP-5 (*shāng qiū*, Shang Hill), and Four Seams (*sì fèng*); needle with supplementation. [26: 748] [46: 702] [37: 410]

spleen governs center-earth 脾主中土 *pí zhǔ zhōng tǔ*: The spleen is located in the middle of the body, in the center burner, and among the five phases is associated with earth, to which the center position is also associated. Earth is the mother of the myriad things, bringing forth the crops that sustain humanity. The spleen holds a corresponding function in the body: producing the nutrients for the body from ingested foods. [27: 45]

spleen governs later heaven 脾主后天 *pí zhǔ hòu tiān*: The spleen moves and transforms ingested food to produce the body's day-to-day requirements in nutrients. 'Later heaven' means the constitution of the body determined by factors prevailing after birth, i.e., it is the acquired constitution. The spleen is the basis of later heaven (acquired constitution), its health being a prerequisite for the assimilation on which all the other organs depend. [27: 45]

spleen governs movement and transformation 脾主运化 *pí zhǔ yùn huà*: The spleen is in charge of digestion. Food enters the stomach where it is decomposed. The spleen "moves the fluids of the stomach," extracts the essence of grain and water (nutrients in food), and dispatches it to the other organs, so that the essence is ultimately carried to all parts of the body. Modern writers explain this function as comprising digestion, assimilation, and distribution of nutrients. *Elementary Questions* (*sù wèn*) explains it in the following terms: "Drink (饮 *yǐn*, imbibed fluid) enter the stomach, where it is churned and its essential qi is strained off. The essential qi is then carried to the spleen and further distributed by spleen qi. It passes up to the lung, which ensures regular flow through the waterways down to the bladder. In this way, water essence is distributed throughout the five channels and the four parts of the body." Because of its importance in providing nutrients for the production of blood and qi that maintain the life and health of the organism, the spleen is described as the SOURCE OF ENGENDERING TRANSFORMATION (i.e., the basis of qi and blood production), and the ROOT OF LATER HEAVEN (i.e., the chief factor in the acquired constitution). This productive aspect of the spleen explains the five-phase association with earth. Abnormality of the spleen's government of movement and transformation is called SPLENIC MOVEMENT AND TRANSFORMATION FAILURE. [6: 85] [27: 562]

spleen governs movement of stomach liquid 脾主为胃行其津液 *pí zhǔ wèi wèi xíng qí jīn yè*: The spleen moves the liquid in the stomach, i.e., it is by the action of the spleen that liquid (nutrients) are removed from the stomach. Compare SPLEEN GOVERNS MOVEMENT AND TRANSFORMATION. [6: 86]

spleen governs the central region 脾主中州 *pí zhǔ zhōng zhōu*: See SPLEEN GOVERNS CENTER-EARTH. [27: 45] [97: 562]

spleen governs the flesh 脾主肌肉 *pí zhǔ jī ròu*: The fullness of the flesh is dependent upon the spleen's movement and transformation function. [6: 86] [27: 45] [97: 560]

spleen governs the flesh and limbs 脾主肌肉、四肢 *pí zhǔ jī ròu, sì zhī*: The fullness of the flesh and the strength of the limbs are dependent upon the spleen's movement and transformation function. Because the spleen is the source of blood and qi formation, all the muscles of the body rely for their nourishment on the capacity of the stomach and spleen to move and transform the essence of grain and water. Only when the stomach and spleen are functioning properly are the muscles full and sound and the limbs powerful. Impairment of spleen function may therefore lead to wasting of the flesh, loss of limb power, and, in severe cases, wilting of the flesh and paralysis. [6: 86]

spleen governs the four limbs 脾主四肢 *pí zhǔ sì zhī*: The fullness and strength of the limbs is dependent upon splenic movement and transformation. In addition, the activity of the limbs is dependent upon yang qi produced by the spleen. [6: 86]

spleen governs the mouth 脾主口 *pí zhǔ kǒu*: From *Elementary Questions* (*sù wèn, yīn yáng yìng xiàng dà lùn*). See SPLEEN OPENS AT THE MOUTH. [26: 746]

spleen governs upbearing of the clear 脾主升清 *pí zhǔ shēng qīng*: Upbearing of the clear refers to the spleen's governing of movement and transformation. The clear refers to essence of grain and water (nutrients absorbed from food), which by the action of spleen qi is carried upward and outward around the whole body. Compare SPLEEN QI GOVERNS UPBEARING. [6: f88] [27: 46] [97: 562]

spleen heat 脾热 *pí rè*: A heat pattern arising from contraction of heat evil or excessive consumption of hot dry foods or liquor; characterized by red lips, dry throat, heart vexation, abdominal fullness or abdominal pain, constipation, and short voidings of yellow urine. [27: 155] [97: 560] [50: 1532]

spleen heat copious drool 脾热多涎 *pí rè duō xián*: Copious drool in infants arising when con-

gesting wind-heat causes phlegm to gather in the spleen. The drool is thick and foamy and is accompanied by inability to swallow milk and by vigorous heat [effusion]. ⟮MED⟯ Clear the spleen and drain heat using Yellow-Draining Powder (*xiè huáng sǎn*) or Bamboo Leaf and Gypsum Decoction (*zhú yè shí gāo tāng*). [26: 749]

spleen impediment 脾痹 *pí bì*: An IMPEDIMENT (*bì*) pattern developing from long-standing flesh impediment when further contraction of evils or dietary irregularities cause damage to the spleen. Spleen impediment is characterized by slothfulness of the limbs, vomiting of clear fluid, oppression in the chest and qi stagnation, abdominal distention, no desire for food and drink, and cough. ⟮MED⟯ Boost qi and warm the center; fortify the spleen and disperse food. Appropriate formulas include Unripe Bitter Orange and Glomus-Dispersing Pill (*zhǐ shí xiāo pǐ wán*) and Ginseng, Poria (Hoelen), and Ovate Atractylodes Powder (*shēn líng bái zhú sǎn*). ⟮ACU⟯ Base treatment mainly on CV, SP, and ST. Select BL-20 (*pí shū*, Spleen Transport), CV-12 (*zhōng wǎn*, Center Stomach Duct), LR-13 (*zhāng mén*, Camphorwood Gate), ST-25 (*tiān shū*, Celestial Pivot), ST-36 (*zú sān lǐ*, Leg Three Li), SP-4 (*gōng sūn*, Yellow Emperor), CV-6 (*qì hǎi*, Sea of Qi); and Li Inner Court (*lǐ nèi tíng*); needle with supplementation and add moxa. [26: 750] [27: 405] [97: 56] [46: 594, 662, 666]

spleen is averse to dampness 脾恶湿 *pí wù shī*: The activity of the spleen is easily affected by dampness invading the body from outside. And when spleen qi is weak, so that splenic movement and transformation is affected, fluids can accumulate as dampness in the body. Dampness is identified by the presence of sloppy stool diarrhea, heavy-headedness, generalized feeling of heaviness, cumbersome fatigued limbs, and fullness in the stomach duct and abdomen, and by a white slimy tongue fur. This condition is often described by *damp encumbering spleen-earth*. [26: 749] [27: 47] [97: 561]

spleen is connected with the stomach 脾合胃 *pí hé wèi*: The spleen is in the interior, and its corresponding bowel in the exterior is the stomach, to which it is connected by channel. The spleen and stomach are complementary in their functions: the spleen governs movement and transformation, while the stomach governs intake; the spleen governs upbearing of the clear, while the stomach governs downbearing of the turbid; the spleen is averse to dampness, while the stomach likes moisture. Furthermore, the stomach's governing decomposition of grain and water is to some extent attributable to the spleen since, the spleen "moves of stomach fluids of the stomach." [27: 47] [97: 561]

spleen is the root of later heaven 脾为后天之本 *pí wéi hòu tiān zhī běn*: SPLEEN GOVERNS LATER HEAVEN.

spleen is the source of engendering transformation 脾为生化之源 *pí wéi shēng huà zhī yuán*: In the five phases, the spleen belongs to earth, which is the "mother of the myriad things." The production of qi and blood, which nourish the whole body, is dependent up splenic movement and transformation. ◇ Chin 生 *shēng*, engender; 化 *huà*, transform. Engendering transformation means productive change, production. [27: 45]

spleen is the source of phlegm formation 脾为生痰之源 *pí wéi shēng tán zhī yuán*: Phlegm most commonly arises as dampness accumulates and congeals; dampness is closely related to disease of the spleen. More at SPLENIC MOVEMENT AND TRANSFORMATION FAILURE and SPLEEN IS AVERSE TO DAMPNESS. [6: 84]

spleen is the source of qi and blood formation 脾为生化气血之源 *pí wéi shēng huà qì xuè zhī yuán*: See SPLEEN IS THE SOURCE OF ENGENDERING TRANSFORMATION. [27: 45]

spleen, its bloom is in the four whites of the lips 脾，其华在唇四白 *pí, qí huá zài chún sì bái*: The health of the spleen is reflected in the lips and surrounding area, which is generally slightly paler than other parts of the face. Strong movement of spleen qi is also reflected in red, moist, and lustrous lips. The "four whites of the lips" (*chún sì bái*) is understood to mean the pale flesh above, below, and either side of the mouth. [27: 46]

spleen-kidney yang vacuity 脾肾阳虚 *pí shèn yáng xū*: A disease pattern characterized by signs of both SPLEEN YANG VACUITY and KIDNEY YANG VACUITY. Spleen yang vacuity and kidney yang vacuity are mutually conducive, and often develop when enduring illness damages yang. In most cases, the spleen yang vacuity is the root, and hence in the language of the five phases can be expressed as fire (kidney yang) failing to engender earth, and earth failing to dam water. The chief signs are cold pain in the lumbus and knees, enduring diarrhea, and puffy face and swollen limbs. Other signs include bright white facial complexion, physical cold and cold limbs, and lower abdominal cold pain. In some cases, there is fifth watch diarrhea, clear-food diarrhea, inhibited urination, or drumlike abdominal distention. The tongue is pale and enlarged with a white glossy fur. The pulse is sunken, fine, slow and weak or fine and faint. Analysis: When kidney yang fails to warm the lumbus and knees, there is cold pain in the lumbus and knees. When spleen yang fails to move and transform the essence of grain and water, there is enduring diarrhea. When spleen yang is vacuous, it cannot warm the body, hence the physical cold and cold limbs, bright white facial complexion, pale enlarged tongue with glossy white fur, and a sunken fine slow weak or faint fine pulse. When spleen and kidney yang are vacuous, exuberant internal yin cold causes stagnation of qi dynamic, hence the lower abdominal cold pain. When spleen and kidney yang fail to warm and transform water-damp, dampness percolates into the intestines, hence the fifth-watch diarrhea or clear-food diarrhea. Yang vacuity water-damp collecting internally causes bladder qi transformation failure, hence the inhibited urination. Water-damp flooding the flesh and skin gives rise to puffy face and swollen limbs. When water fails to dam water, water percolates into the abdomen, there is drumlike abdominal distention (drum distention). MED Warm and supplement the spleen and kidney. Use Aconite Center-Rectifying Decoction (*fù zǐ lǐ zhōng tāng*), or Spleen-Firming Beverage (*shí pí yǐn*). ACU Base treatment mainly on back transport points, CV, SP, ST, and KI. Select BL-20 (*pí shū*, Spleen Transport), BL-23 (*shèn shū*, Kidney Transport), GV-4 (*mìng mén*, Life Gate), CV-4 (*guān yuán*, Pass Head), CV-12 (*zhōng wǎn*, Center Stomach Duct), SP-4 (*gōng sūn*, Yellow Emperor), ST-36 (*zú sān lǐ*, Leg Three Li), KI-3 (*tài xī*, Great Ravine), and KI-7 (*fù liū*, Recover Flow); needle with supplementation and large amounts of moxa. Selection of points according to signs: For cold pain in the lumbus and knees, add GV-3 (*yāo yáng guān*, Lumbar Yang Pass), BL-40 (*wěi zhōng*, Bend Center), and SP-9 (*yīn líng quán*, Yin Mound Spring). For enduring diarrhea, add ST-25 (*tiān shū*, Celestial Pivot), and GV-20 (*bǎi huì*, Hundred Convergences). For puffy face and swollen limbs, add CV-9 (*shuǐ fēn*, Water Divide), CV-6 (*qì hǎi*, Sea of Qi), and BL-22 (*sān jiāo shū*, Triple Burner Transport). [116: 149] [97: 563] [46: 586, 587, 666]

spleen-lung vacuity 脾虚肺弱 *pí xū fèi ruò*: DUAL VACUITY OF THE SPLEEN AND LUNG.

spleen manages the blood 脾统血 *pí tǒng xuè*: The spleen produces blood and prevents it from spilling out of the vessels. The spleen is the source of blood and qi formation, and when healthy, it ensures plentiful supplies of blood, and of qi, which moves the blood and keeps it within the vessels. Thus, the spleen engenders the blood and indirectly keeps it from spilling out of the vessels. The two phrases "the spleen manages the blood" and "qi contains the blood" are therefore essentially synonymous. Flooding and spotting and bloody stool, considered strictly from the point of view of bleeding, could also be described as failure of qi to contain the blood. By convention, however, these patterns are ascribed to blood management failure. ◇ Chin 统 *tǒng*, to rule, dominate, hold together. [26: 750] [27: 44] [97: 561]

spleen opens at the mouth 脾开窍于口 *pí kāi qiào yú kǒu*: Synonym: *spleen governs the mouth*. The mouth is the outer orifice of the spleen. This phrase refers to the relationship of the splenic movement and transformation to appetite and taste in the mouth. If the stomach and the spleen are functioning normally, the individual has a good appetite and normal taste in the mouth. *The Magic Pivot* (*líng shū*) states, "Spleen qi passes through to the mouth; if the spleen is in harmony, then the mouth can taste the five flavors." Diseases of the spleen and stomach are often reflected in changes in appetite and changes in taste in the mouth (a bland or sweet taste or slimy sensation). See also STOMACH GOVERNS INTAKE. [27: 46] [97: 563]

spleen pulse is moderate 脾脉缓 *pí mài huǎn*: A moderate pulse, a pulse of four beats per respiration; it is neither floating nor sunken, neither large nor small, neither slow nor racing, neither faint nor weak, and is harmonious and forceful. *The Inner Canon* (*nèi jīng, xuān míng wǔ qì piān*) states, "The spleen pulse is changing." The word "changing" (代 *dài*) is interpreted to mean harmonious and soft, but changing with the seasons (stringlike in spring, surging in summer, floating in autumn, and sunken and hard in winter). This notion also also thought to be implied by term Thus the spleen pulse is often described as moderate. [93: 440] [9: 336]

spleen qi 脾气 *pí qì*: What is active in the spleen. [26: 748] [27: 44] [97: 559]

spleen qi fall 脾气下陷 *pí qì xià xiàn*: CENTER QI FALL.

spleen qi flows to the mouth 脾气通于口 *pí qì tōng yú kǒu*: The spleen is paired with the stomach, whose upper opening is the mouth. The spleen governs movement and transformation of food, which enters the body through the mouth. Ability to taste and enjoy food is dependent on the spleen and stomach. *The Magic Pivot* (*líng shū, mài dù piān*) says, "Spleen qi flows to the mouth; when the spleen is in harmony, one can taste the five grains." This means that the ability to distinguish flavors is dependent upon the spleen. In spleen vacuity, there is a bland taste in the mouth. When there is damp-heat in the spleen, there is a sweet flavor in the mouth. [27: 46]

spleen qi governs upbearing 脾气主升 *pí qì zhǔ shēng*: The spleen, by its movement and transformation function, bears the essence of grain and water (food extracted from nutrients) upward. This upward movement is complementary and opposite to the downbearing of stomach qi, which carries food down from the stomach into the intestines. [27: 46]

spleen-lung qi vacuity 脾肺气虚 *pí fèi qì xū*: DUAL VACUITY OF THE SPLEEN AND LUNG.

spleen qi vacuity 脾气虚 *pí qì xū*, 脾气虚弱 *pí qì xū ruò*: Synonym: *spleen-stomach vacuity*; *insufficiency of spleen qi*. From *Elementary Questions* (*sù wèn, fāng shèng shuāi lùn*). A condition arising when irregular eating or anxiety, thought, and taxation fatigue damage the spleen and stomach. It may take different forms depending on the aspect of spleen function affected: SPLENIC MOVEMENT AND TRANSFORMATION FAILURE is a disturbance of the spleen's governing movement and transformation and the upbearing of the clear; characterized by abdominal distention, torpid intake, rumbling intestines, diarrhea, and other signs of poor digestion. INSUFFICIENCY OF CENTER QI is a general disturbance of the spleen and stomach function characterized by yellow face with little luster, pale or dark lips, poor appetite, abdominal distention after eating, dizziness, low voice, shortness of breath, fatigue and lack of strength, sloppy stool, tender-soft tongue with thick tongue fur and a vacuous pulse. If there stomach pain, it is relieved by pressure. *The Magic Pivot* (*líng shū, kǒu wèn*) states, "When center qi is insufficient, there are changes in stool and urine, and the intestines rumble." CENTER QI FALL is failure of the spleens governing of upbearing, which manifests in sinking effects such as prolapse of the anus, enduring diarrhea, prolapse of the uterus, or, in infants, depressed fontanel. SPLEEN FAILING TO MANAGE THE BLOOD is a disturbance of the spleen's function of function of managing the blood, resulting in bleeding. [50: 1533] [27: 154] [26: 749] [97: 560] [6: 179] [46: 586, 595]

spleen-stomach damp-heat 脾胃湿热 *pí wèi shī rè*: Synonyms: *damp-heat obstructing the spleen and stomach*; *damp-heat brewing in the spleen*; *center burner damp-heat*. A disease pattern that results when damp-heat arises in the center burner or is externally contracted, and brews in the spleen, disturbing normal movement and transformation. Spleen-stomach damp-heat is characterized by glomus and oppression in the stomach duct, torpid intake, nausea, sloppy stool, and yellow urine, and heavy cumbersome limbs. Other possible signs include: yellowing of the skin (the color of tangerines); fluctuating heat effusion unabated by sweating. The tongue is red with yellow slimy fur, and the pulse is soggy. ACU Base treatment mainly on ST, LI, and SP. Select SP-9 (*yīn líng quán*, Yin Mound Spring), SP-6 (*sān yīn jiāo*, Three Yin Intersection), LI-11 (*qū chí*, Pool at the Bend), LI-4 (*hé gǔ*, Union Valley), ST-44 (*nèi tíng*, Inner Court), ST-36 (*zú sān lǐ*, Leg Three Li), ST-43 (*xiàn gǔ*, Sunken Valley), and ST-25 (*tiān shū*, Celestial Pivot); needle with drainage. Do not use moxa. For yellowing of the body and eyes, drain LR-3 (*tài chōng*, Supreme Surge) and GB-34 (*yáng líng quán*, Yang Mound Spring). For itchy skin, add Itch Reliever (*zhǐ yǎng*) and SP-10 (*xuè hǎi*, Sea of Blood). For pronounced heat, drain GV-14 (*dà zhuī*, Great Hammer), or prick LI-1 (*shāng yáng*, Shang Yang) to bleed. Compare DAMP-HEAT BREWING INTERNALLY. [29: 412] [116: 83] [57: 106] [46: 597, 665] [27: 156] [97: 563]

spleen-stomach disharmony 脾胃不和 *pí wèi bù hé*: A pathology of the spleen and stomach characterized by glomus, oppression, and continuous pain in the stomach duct exacerbated by hunger, abdominal distention and poor transformation of food, belching, hiccough, and, in severe cases, vomiting, a liking for pressure and warmth, a pale tongue with dental impressions on the margins and a thin white fur, and a forceless sunken fine or sunken moderate pulse. MED Fortify the spleen and nourish the stomach. Use Saussurea and Amomum Six Gentlemen Decoction (*xiāng shā liù jūn zǐ tāng*) or Spleen-Returning Decoction (*guī pí tāng*) plus amomum (*shā rén*), corydalis (*yán hú suǒ*), and evodia (*wú zhū yú*). ACU Base treatment mainly on back transport points, CV, SP, and ST. Select BL-20 (*pí shū*, Spleen Transport), BL-21 (*wèi shū*, Stomach Transport), CV-12 (*zhōng wǎn*, Center Stomach Duct), ST-36 (*zú sān lǐ*, Leg Three Li), ST-25 (*tiān shū*, Celestial Pivot), CV-6 (*qì hǎi*, Sea of Qi), PC-6 (*nèi guān*, Inner Pass), and SP-6 (*sān yīn jiāo*, Three Yin Intersection); needle with supplementation and add moxa. [36: 135] [90: 173] [46: 602]

spleen-stomach harmonization 调和脾胃 *tiáo hé pí wèi*: HARMONIZING THE SPLEEN AND STOMACH.

spleen-stomach qi vacuity 脾胃气虚 *pí wèi qì xū*: INSUFFICIENCY OF CENTER QI.

spleen-stomach vacuity 脾胃虚弱 *pí wèi xū ruò*: SPLEEN QI VACUITY.

spleen-stomach vacuity cold 脾胃虚寒 *pí wèi xū hán*: SPLEEN-STOMACH YANG VACUITY. [25: 303]

spleen-stomach vacuity cold stomach duct pain 脾胃虚寒胃脘痛 *pí wèi xū hán wèi wǎn* (*guǎn*) *tòng*: See INTERNAL DAMAGE STOMACH DUCT PAIN.

spleen-stomach yang vacuity 脾胃阳虚 *pí wèi yáng xū*: Synonyms: *devitalized center yang*; *insufficiency of center yang*. Vacuity of spleen-stomach yang qi of the center burner with poor digestion. Signs include reduced food intake, vomiting, diarrhea, cold limbs, fatigue, withered-yellow facial complexion, dizziness, pale tongue, soft enlarged tongue, thick turbid tongue fur, and a large vacuous pulse. **Comparison:** Spleen-stomach yang

vacuity differs from stomach vacuity cold by the presence of diarrhea, which is a spleen sign. It differs from spleen yang vacuity by the presence of vomiting, which is a stomach sign. MED Treat by warming and moving center yang. Use Center-Rectifying Decoction (*lǐ zhōng tāng*) or Magnolia Bark Center-Warming Decoction (*hòu pò wēn zhōng tāng*). ACU Base treatment mainly on SP, ST, CV, and back transport points. Select BL-20 (*pí shū*, Spleen Transport), BL-21 (*wèi shū*, Stomach Transport), CV-12 (*zhōng wǎn*, Center Stomach Duct), LR-13 (*zhāng mén*, Camphorwood Gate), CV-6 (*qì hǎi*, Sea of Qi), ST-36 (*zú sān lǐ*, Leg Three Li), and PC-6 (*nèi guān*, Inner Pass); needle with supplementation and add moxa. CROSS MOXA and the five pillar points can also be used. [26: 139] [25: 50] [46: 660, 662] [57: 107]

spleen-stomach yin vacuity 脾胃阴虚 *pí wèi yīn xū*: The combined manifestation of spleen and stomach yin vacuity. The spleen and stomach stand in exterior-interior relationship. Together they are responsible for later heaven management of grain and water. Stomach yin vacuity often causes spleen yin vacuity; hence the two often occur together. See SPLEEN YIN VACUITY; STOMACH YIN VACUITY. [26: 747] [27: 154] [97: 563]

spleen stores construction 脾藏营 *pí cáng yíng*: From *The Magic Pivot* (*líng shū, běn shén*). Construction is the essential qi that flows in the vessels; it is generated from grain and water (food), has its source in the spleen and stomach, and has the function of engendering blood; hence construction and blood are often referred to together. *The Classic of Difficult Issues* (*nàn jīng, 42*) states "The spleen... governs the containment of blood." This means that the spleen has the function of storing and containing the blood. [25: 301]

spleen stores reflection 脾藏意 *pí cáng yì*: From *Elementary Questions* (*sù wèn, xuān míng wǔ qì piān*). Thinking capacity is dependent upon a healthy spleen. Excessive thought can damage the spleen, affecting movement and transformation, and causing poor appetite, glomus and fullness in the chest and abdomen, etc. [25: 301]

spleen taxation 脾劳 *pí láo*: See FIVE TAXATIONS. [27: 118] [27: 368] [97: 560]

spleen vacuity 脾虚 *pí xū*: From *Elementary Questions* (*sù wèn, zàng qì fǎ shí lùn*). **1.** Any disease pattern of spleen yin or spleen yang vacuity or of qi-blood insufficiency, usually arising from dietary imbalance, inappropriate temperatures, anxiety and thought, taxation fatigue (overwork etc.), or damage to the spleen through enduring sickness. Signs include emaciation with yellow face, lack of strength in the limbs, reduced food intake, nontransformation of food, abdominal pain, rumbling intestines, sloppy stool or diarrhea, puffy swelling, bloody stool, or flooding and spotting. MED The principal method of treatment is that of fortifying the spleen. Use formulas like Ginseng, Poria (Hoelen), and Ovate Atractylodes Powder (*shēn líng bái zhú sǎn*). ACU Base treatment mainly on the back transport points, CV, SP, and ST. Main points: BL-20 (*pí shū*, Spleen Transport), BL-21 (*wèi shū*, Stomach Transport), CV-12 (*zhōng wǎn*, Center Stomach Duct), SP-3 (*tài bái*, Supreme White), and ST-36 (*zú sān lǐ*, Leg Three Li); needle with supplementation and add moxa. For selection of points according to signs, see the following entries. **2.** SPLEEN QI VACUITY. [26: 749] [27: 154] [97: 560] [46: 585]

spleen vacuity abdominal distention 脾虚腹胀 *pí xū fù zhàng*: Abdominal distention arising when, owing to habitual spleen qi vacuity, and splenic movement and transformation failure, food and drink have difficulty in transforming and accumulate in the stomach and intestines. MED Base treatment primarily on fortifying the spleen and dispersing food. If spleen qi is unreplete, use Ginseng, Poria (Hoelen), and Ovate Atractylodes Powder (*shēn líng bái zhú sǎn*); if speech is faint, use Four Gentlemen Decoction (*sì jūn zǐ tāng*); if there is periodic fullness in the region of the heart and abdomen and difficulty in digesting food and drink, use Unripe Bitter Orange and Ovate Atractylodes Variant Decoction (*jiā jiǎn zhǐ zhú tāng*). ACU Base treatment mainly on the back transport points, CV, SP, ST, and PC. Select BL-20 (*pí shū*, Spleen Transport), ST-25 (*tiān shū*, Celestial Pivot), CV-6 (*qì hǎi*, Sea of Qi), LR-13 (*zhāng mén*, Camphorwood Gate), PC-6 (*nèi guān*, Inner Pass), and ST-36 (*zú sān lǐ*, Leg Three Li); needle with supplementation and add moxa. Five Pillar Points (*wǔ zhù xué*), can be moxaed. See ABDOMINAL DISTENTION. [50: 1537] [46: 585, 602]

spleen vacuity cold 脾虚寒 *pí xū hán*: SPLEEN YANG VACUITY.

spleen vacuity copious drool 脾虚多涎 *pí xū duō xián*: Copious thin clear drool in infants arising when insufficiency of spleen qi prevents normal distribution of fluids. Spleen vacuity copious drool is associated with lassitude of spirit and withered-yellow facial complexion. MED Supplement the spleen and stomach, and nourish qi and the blood. Use variations of Center-Supplementing Qi-Boosting Decoction (*bǔ zhōng yì qì tāng*). [26: 749] [50: 1537]

spleen vacuity diarrhea 脾虚泄泻 *pí xū xiè xiè*: DIARRHEA due to habitual spleen qi vacuity or to damage to the spleen and stomach by excessive consumption of cold things after illness or by dietary irregularities. Thin diarrhea is a associated with weak health, fear of cold, withered-yellow facial complexion, cold extremities, fatigued

limbs, no thought of food and drink, faint weak or slow to moderate pulse. MED Fortify and warm splenic movement. Center-Rectifying Decoction (*lǐ zhōng tāng*), Four Gentlemen Decoction (*sì jūn zǐ tāng*), and Ginseng, Poria (Hoelen), and Ovate Atractylodes Powder (*shēn líng bái zhú sǎn*) ACU Base treatment mainly on the back transport and alarm points of the SP and ST. Select BL-20 (*pí shū*, Spleen Transport), BL-21 (*wèi shū*, Stomach Transport), CV-12 (*zhōng wǎn*, Center Stomach Duct), LR-13 (*zhāng mén*, Camphorwood Gate), ST-25 (*tiān shū*, Celestial Pivot), SP-4 (*gōng sūn*, Yellow Emperor), and ST-36 (*zú sān lǐ*, Leg Three Li); needle with supplementation and add moxa. Five Pillar Points (*wǔ zhù xué*), can also be moxaed. See SPLEEN DIARRHEA; QI FALL DIARRHEA. [50: 1537] [46: 666] [37: 323]

spleen vacuity enduring cough 脾虚久嗽 *pí xū jiǔ sòu*: A long-standing COUGH due to spleen qi vacuity. In children, the spleen is often insufficient and is susceptible to milk feeding damage, which in turn causes movement and transformation failure and makes dampness transform into phlegm. Phlegm and dampness obstructing each other disturb lung qi diffusion, giving rise to cough. Spleen vacuity enduring cough is a persistent cough with copious phlegm, accompanied by poor food intake, abdominal distention, sloppy stool, yellow face, and emaciation. MED Fortify the spleen and disinhibit qi; suppress cough and transform phlegm. Use variations of Six Gentlemen Decoction (*liù jūn zǐ tāng*). ACU Base treatment mainly on the back transport points, CV, LU, SP, and ST. Select BL-20 (*pí shū*, Spleen Transport), BL-13 (*fèi shū*, Lung Transport), LU-9 (*tài yuān*, Great Abyss), SP-3 (*tài bái*, Supreme White), ST-40 (*fēng lóng*, Bountiful Bulge), LI-4 (*hé gǔ*, Union Valley), and ST-36 (*zú sān lǐ*, Leg Three Li); needle with supplementation and add moxa. [50: 1537] [46: 653] [37: 274]

spleen vacuity engendering wind 脾虚生风 *pí xū shēng fēng*: INTERNAL WIND due to spleen vacuity. Spleen vacuity engendering wind is mostly the result of damage to the spleen by vomiting and diarrhea or medication. It is characterized by mild convulsions of the extremities accompanied by counterflow cold of the limbs, faint nose and mouth breath, and clouding sleep with exposed eyeballs. MED Warm and supplement the spleen and stomach. Use Spleen-Returning Decoction (*guī pí tāng*) plus uncaria (*gōu téng*) and notopterygium (*qiāng huó*), or use Six Gentlemen Decoction (*liù jūn zǐ tāng*) plus blast-fried ginger (*páo jiāng*), cinnamon bark (*ròu guì*), and scorpion tail (*xiē shāo*). [50: 1537]

spleen vacuity menstrual block 脾虚经闭 *pí xū jīng bì*: MENSTRUAL BLOCK arising when damage to the spleen and stomach and reduced appetite causes insufficiency of the source and qi and blood formation so that there is no blood to reach the thoroughfare and controlling vessels. Spleen vacuity menstrual block is often associated with poor appetite, glomus and fullness, and unsolid stool. MED Supplement the spleen and stomach; nourish qi and blood. Use Center-Supplementing Qi-Boosting Decoction (*bǔ zhōng yì qì tāng*) or Ginseng, Poria (Hoelen), and Ovate Atractylodes Powder (*shēn líng bái zhú sǎn*). ACU Base treatment mainly on the back transport points, CV, SP, and ST. Select BL-20 (*pí shū*, Spleen Transport), BL-23 (*shèn shū*, Kidney Transport), BL-17 (*gé shū*, Diaphragm Transport), CV-12 (*zhōng wǎn*, Center Stomach Duct), SP-6 (*sān yīn jiāo*, Three Yin Intersection), SP-10 (*xuè hǎi*, Sea of Blood), CV-4 (*guān yuán*, Pass Head), and ST-36 (*zú sān lǐ*, Leg Three Li); needle with supplementation and add moxa. [50: 1538] [37: 422] [46: 686] [59: 43]

spleen vacuity qi stagnation 脾虚气滞 *pí xū qì zhì*: Spleen vacuity causing qi stagnation manifesting as abdominal distention. See, for example, GREATER YIN DISEASE.

spleen vacuity spontaneous sweating 脾虚自汗 *pí xū zì hàn*: SPONTANEOUS SWEATING due to spleen vacuity, accompanied by fatigue and reduced eating. MED Use Center-Supplementing Qi-Boosting Decoction (*bǔ zhōng yì qì tāng*) or Four Gentlemen Decoction (*sì jūn zǐ tāng*). ACU Base treatment mainly on back transport points, ST, and SP. Select BL-20 (*pí shū*, Spleen Transport), BL-21 (*wèi shū*, Stomach Transport), CV-12 (*zhōng wǎn*, Center Stomach Duct), ST-36 (*zú sān lǐ*, Leg Three Li), LI-4 (*hé gǔ*, Union Valley), and KI-7 (*fù liū*, Recover Flow); needle with supplementation and add moxa. [50: 1537] [46: 585, 602] [14: 174]

spleen vacuity vaginal discharge 脾虚带下 *pí xū dài xià*: VAGINAL DISCHARGE arising from splenic movement and transformation failure due to spleen vacuity (or liver depression and spleen vacuity), causing dampness to gather and pour downward and damage the controlling and girdling vessels. Spleen vacuity vaginal discharge is a copious, white or pale yellow discharge that is like spittle or snivel (nasal mucus) in consistency, and that flows continuously. It is attended by a pale yellow facial complexion, lassitude of spirit, no thought of food or drink, aching lumbus with sagging sensation in the abdomen, unsolid stool, and in some cases swelling of the lower limbs. MED Fortify the spleen and boost qi; upbear yang and eliminate dampness. An appropriate formula is Discharge-Ceasing Decoction (*wán dài tāng*). ACU Base treatment mainly on CV, GIV, SP, and ST. Select GB-26 (*dài mài*, Girdling Vessel), BL-30 (*bái

huán shū*, White Ring Transport), BL-20 (*pí shū*, Spleen Transport), CV-6 (*qì hǎi*, Sea of Qi), SP-6 (*sān yīn jiāo*, Three Yin Intersection), ST-36 (*zú sān lǐ*, Leg Three Li), and SP-9 (*yīn líng quán*, Yin Mound Spring); needle with supplementation and add moxa. [26: 749] [50: 1537] [46: 646, 690]

spleen vacuity vomiting 脾虚呕吐 *pí xū ǒu tù*: VOMITING due to spleen vacuity and exuberant dampness. MED Rectify the spleen and harmonize the stomach. Use variations of Six Gentlemen Decoction (*liù jūn zǐ tāng*). [50: 1537]

spleen vacuity with damp encumbrance 脾虚湿困 *pí xū shī kùn*: Spleen vacuity giving rise to damp obstruction. The spleen governs movement and transformation of water-damp, and moves the fluid of the stomach. In spleen vacuity, movement and transformation breaks down, and as a result, water-damp gathers and stagnates, further weakening movement and transformation. Signs include reduced food intake, fullness and oppression in the stomach duct, sloppy diarrhea, cumbersome fatigued limbs that may be swollen, thick slimy tongue fur, and a moderate pulse. There may be a sticky sensation in the mouth and absence of thirst or thirst with desire for warm drinks. In severe cases, there may also be nausea and vomiting. MED Fortify the spleen and disinhibit dampness. Use Stomach-Calming Powder (*píng wèi sǎn*) or Stomach-Calming Poria (Hoelen) Five Decoction (*wèi líng tāng*). ACU Base treatment mainly on SP, ST, and CV. Select BL-20 (*pí shū*, Spleen Transport), CV-12 (*zhōng wǎn*, Center Stomach Duct), LR-13 (*zhāng mén*, Camphorwood Gate), ST-36 (*zú sān lǐ*, Leg Three Li), and SP-9 (*yīn líng quán*, Yin Mound Spring); needle with even supplementation and drainage and moxa. [26: 749] [50: 1538] [27: 155] [46: 597]

spleen vacuity with food damage 脾虚夹食 *pí xū jiā shí*: Nontransformation of ingested food attributable to spleen-stomach vacuity. It is characterized by bloating after eating and by sloppy stool containing untransformed food. In general, there is no abdominal pain and the tongue fur may be completely normal. Signs such as no thought of food and drink and no pleasure in eating indicate prominence of stomach vacuity, while nontransformation of ingested food indicates prominence of spleen vacuity. Yellow face, emaciation, and rapacious appetite with nonmovement of ingested food indicate a strong stomach and weak spleen. MED Open the stomach and fortify the spleen; or disperse and supplement simultaneously. Use medicinals such as codonopsis (*dǎng shēn*), ovate atractylodes (*bái zhú*), poria (*fú líng*), lablab (*biǎn dòu*), and dioscorea (*shān yào*) to supplement the spleen and stomach, combined with tangerine peel (*chén pí*), rice sprout (*gǔ yá*), barley sprout (*mài yá*), unripe bitter orange (*zhǐ shí*), and amomum (*shā rén*) to open the stomach and disperse food. Formulas such as Ginseng, Poria (Hoelen), and Ovate Atractylodes Powder (*shēn líng bái zhú sǎn*) are used to supplement spleen-stomach vacuity in patients with little thought of food and drink or thin sloppy stool due to non-transformation of ingested food. Great Tranquility Pill (*dà ān wán*) can be used for spleen-stomach vacuity with food stagnation. ACU Base treatment mainly on CV, back transport points, and ST. Select BL-20 (*pí shū*, Spleen Transport), BL-21 (*wèi shū*, Stomach Transport), CV-12 (*zhōng wǎn*, Center Stomach Duct), CV-10 (*xià wǎn*, Lower Stomach Duct), ST-25 (*tiān shū*, Celestial Pivot), CV-6 (*qì hǎi*, Sea of Qi), ST-36 (*zú sān lǐ*, Leg Three Li), Li Inner Court (*lǐ nèi tíng*), and CV-21 (*xuán jī*, Jade Swivel); needle with supplementation and add moxa. [6: 215] [46: 662] [113: 18]

spleen vacuity yellowing 脾虚发黄 *pí xū fā huáng*: JAUNDICE arising when spleen qi vacuity causes damp-heat to become depressed and stagnant. MED Disinhibit damp-heat using Capillaris and Poria (Hoelen) Five Powder (*yīn chén wǔ líng sǎn*). After jaundice abates, fortify the spleen. For yellow face and eyes with vacuity swelling, supplement the spleen and fortify the stomach using variations of Six Gentlemen Decoction (*liù jūn zǐ tāng*). ACU To abate jaundice, base treatment mainly on GB, SP, LR, and ST. Select BL-19 (*dǎn shū*, Gallbladder Transport), GB-34 (*yáng líng quán*, Yang Mound Spring), LR-3 (*tài chōng*, Supreme Surge), SP-9 (*yīn líng quán*, Yin Mound Spring), GV-9 (*zhì yáng*, Extremity of Yang), ST-44 (*nèi tíng*, Inner Court), and SP-6 (*sān yīn jiāo*, Three Yin Intersection); needle with drainage. To fortify the spleen after jaundice abates, select BL-20 (*pí shū*, Spleen Transport), BL-21 (*wèi shū*, Stomach Transport), CV-12 (*zhōng wǎn*, Center Stomach Duct), LR-13 (*zhāng mén*, Camphorwood Gate), and ST-36 (*zú sān lǐ*, Leg Three Li); needle with supplementation and add moxa. [50: 1537] [46: 664] [37: 398] [43: 162]

spleen vacuous as a ball 脾虚如球 *pí xū rú qiú*: Synonyms: *eyelid vacuous as a ball*; *suspended ball*. Puffy swelling of the eyelids making them appear as balls, without redness or pain. It is mostly caused by spleen vacuity complicated by dampness or insufficiency of qi and blood, and vacuity fire congesting the qi aspect. MED Treat by supplementing the spleen and boosting qi, assisted by dispelling evil. Use Wondrous Effect Astragalus Decoction (*shén xiào huáng qí tāng*) or Center-Supplementing Qi-Boosting Decoction (*bǔ zhōng yì qì tāng*). [50: 1537]

spleen water 脾水 *pí shuǐ*: One of the FIVE WATERS spoken of in *Essential Prescriptions of the Golden Coffer* (*jīn guì yào lüè*). WATER SWELLING in spleen disease characterized by abdominal distention with difficult urination, shortage of qi, and cumbersome heavy limbs. [27: 44] [97: 559]

spleen wilting 脾痿 *pí wěi*: FLESH WILTING. [26: 750]

spleen worm disease 脾虫病 *pí chóng bìng*: INCH WHITEWORM. [26: 750]

spleen yang 脾阳 *pí yáng*: Splenic movement and transformation, and the warming effect it produces. When spleen yang is vacuous splenic transformation breaks down, and signs such as non-transformation of food, abdominal fullness, diarrhea, and lack of warmth in extremities are observed. In some cases, phlegm-rheum may develop or water-damp may cause swelling of the extremities. Spleen yang requires the warmth of the life gate fire; hence insufficiency of the life gate fire can cause spleen yang vacuity. [26: 749] [27: 44] [97: 559]

spleen yang vacuity 脾阳虚 *pí yáng xū*: Synonyms: *devitalized spleen yang*; *spleen vacuity cold*. A further development of spleen qi vacuity. Spleen yang vacuity presents with pronounced cold signs in addition to spleen vacuity signs. It may thus be differentiated from spleen qi vacuity by the presence of a bright white facial complexion, fatigued spirit, physical cold, abdominal pain relieved by warmth and pressure, and diarrhea containing untransformed food. The pulse is sunken and weak, while the tongue is pale with white fur. It is often accompanied by signs of kidney yang debilitation. MED Warm yang and enhance movement. Use spleen-fortifying medicinals such as ovate atractylodes (*bái zhú*), dioscorea (*shān yào*), and lablab (*biǎn dòu*), combined with yang-warming medicinals blast-fried ginger (*páo jiāng*), cinnamon bark (*ròu guì*), and aconite (*fù zǐ*). Formulas for treating spleen yang vacuity include Center-Rectifying Pill (*lǐ zhōng wán*), Aconite Center-Rectifying Decoction (*fù zǐ lǐ zhōng tāng*) and variations. ACU Base treatment mainly on CV, SP, and ST. Select BL-20 (*pí shū*, Spleen Transport), CV-12 (*zhōng wǎn*, Center Stomach Duct), ST-36 (*zú sān lǐ*, Leg Three Li), SP-4 (*gōng sūn*, Yellow Emperor), CV-4 (*guān yuán*, Pass Head), CV-6 (*qì hǎi*, Sea of Qi), and GV-4 (*mìng mén*, Life Gate); needle with supplementation and large amounts of moxa. [6: 179]

spleen yin 脾阴 *pí yīn*: 1. The yin essence of the spleen. 2. The spleen as a yin viscus in relation to the stomach which is yang. [26: 748]

spleen yin vacuity 脾阴虚 *pí yīn xū*: Synonym: *spleen-stomach yin vacuity*. The manifestation of the spleen failing to distribute essence. The spleen and stomach are the root of later heaven. The whole of the body relies on the spleen's function of distributing essence. Since essence is distributed by splenic movement and transformation, spleen yin vacuity is actually dual vacuity of spleen qi and yin. It most often results from enduring illness or from wear on the yin humor of the stomach and spleen in febrile disease. The nondistribution of essence is reflected in emaciation. Spleen qi vacuity due to splenic movement and transformation failure may be reflected on the one hand in fatigue and lack of strength, and on the other in abdominal distention and sloppy stool. Insufficiency of stomach yin, which may be a cause or result of spleen yin vacuity, leads to failure of harmony and downbearing and, in severe cases, to counterflow ascent; hence there is hunger with no desire for food and drink, torpid intake, or dry retching and hiccough. In spleen yin vacuity, yin may fail to restrain yang, causing vacuity heat signs such as dry mouth and tongue, and red tongue with scant fur. MED Supplement qi and fortify the spleen; boost the stomach and nourish yin. Use Ginseng, Poria (Hoelen), and Ovate Atractylodes Powder (*shēn líng bái zhú sǎn*) plus dendrobium (*shí hú*), ophiopogon (*mài mén dōng*), and adenophora/glehnia (*shā shēn*). ACU Base treatment mainly on back transport points, CV, SP, and ST. Select BL-20 (*pí shū*, Spleen Transport), BL-21 (*wèi shū*, Stomach Transport), CV-12 (*zhōng wǎn*, Center Stomach Duct), LR-13 (*zhāng mén*, Camphorwood Gate), ST-36 (*zú sān lǐ*, Leg Three Li), SP-6 (*sān yīn jiāo*, Three Yin Intersection), and KI-6 (*zhào hǎi*, Shining Sea); needle with supplementation. [26: 748] [50: 1534] [85: 50][36: 294] [27: 154] [97: 561] [46: 584, 660]

splenic 脾 *pí*: Of, pertaining to, connected with, or affecting the spleen.

splenic blood management failure 脾不统血 *pí bù tǒng xuè*: SPLEEN FAILING TO MANAGE BLOOD.

splenic dispersion 脾消 *pí xiāo*: See SPLEEN DISPERSION.

splenic fortification 健脾 *jiàn pí*: FORTIFYING THE SPLEEN.

splenic movement and transformation failure 脾失健运 *pí shī jiàn yùn*: Synonym: *spleen failing to move and transform*. The pathomechanism in which the spleen ceases to perform its movement and transformation function normally. The spleen governs movement and translation. and when spleen yang is vacuous, the spleen fails to move and transform, and cannot upbear the clear. In mild cases, abdominal distention, torpid intake, rumbling intestines, diarrhea and other signs of poor digestion are observed. In enduring conditions, the face becomes yellow, the flesh becomes emaciation, and limbs lack in strength. If the spleen fails to move and transform water-damp, either there is either puffy swelling of the limbs

or phlegm or rheum develops. MED Fortify the spleen and boost qi. Use variations of Saussurea and Amomum Six Gentlemen Decoction (*xiāng shā liù jūn zǐ tāng*) or Ginseng, Poria (Hoelen), and Ovate Atractylodes Powder (*shēn líng bái zhú sǎn*). ACU Base treatment mainly on back transport points, CV, SP, and ST. Select BL-20 (*pí shū*, Spleen Transport), BL-21 (*wèi shū*, Stomach Transport), CV-12 (*zhōng wǎn*, Center Stomach Duct), ST-36 (*zú sān lǐ*, Leg Three Li), SP-4 (*gōng sūn*, Yellow Emperor), and LR-13 (*zhāng mén*, Camphorwood Gate); needle with supplementation and add moxa. Selection of points according to signs: For diarrhea, add ST-25 (*tiān shū*, Celestial Pivot). For abdominal distention, PC-6 (*nèi guān*, Inner Pass), and CV-6 (*qì hǎi*, Sea of Qi). For the spleen fails to move and transform water-damp, add SP-9 (*yīn líng quán*, Yin Mound Spring), ST-40 (*fēng lóng*, Bountiful Bulge), and LI-4 (*hé gǔ*, Union Valley). See SPLEEN DISEASE. [50: 1536] [6: 179] [46: 594, 597, 666] [43: 162]

splenic pure heat 脾瘅 *pí dān*: Heat in the spleen from eating sweet and fatty foods, causing upflow of hot turbid qi. Splenic pure heat is characterized by sweet taste in the mouth with a slimy sensation. MED Repel turbidity with aroma. Use Basil Drink (*lán xiāng yǐn zi*). A slippery stringlike pulse with clamoring stomach and sweet taste in the mouth is a sign of phlegm-damp, which is treated with Phlegm-Rolling Pill (*gǔn tán wán*). Sweet taste in the mouth due to spleen-stomach vacuity heat preventing retention of fluids is treated by supplementing spleen qi with Center-Supplementing Qi-Boosting Decoction (*bǔ zhōng yì qì tāng*). [26: 750]

splitting of the anus 肛裂 *gāng liè*: Splitting and bleeding of the anus due to blood heat intestinal dryness, dry bound stool, and straining in defecation. Splitting of the anus is associated with constipation, burning pain on defecation, and minor bleeding after the passage of stool. MED Oral: Intestine-Moistening Decoction (*rùn cháng tāng*). Topical: For new splitting with a clean wound, apply Flesh-Engendering Powder (*shēng jī sǎn*) or Flesh-Engendering Jade and Red Paste (*shēng jī yù hóng gāo*). For old wounds, use Alum Hemorrhoid-Desiccating Powder (*kū zhì sǎn*) to erode the wound, followed by Flesh-Engendering Powder (*shēng jī sǎn*) to close it. [26: 334] [97: 291]

spontaneous bleeding of the ear 耳衄 *ěr nǜ*: Bleeding from the ear not attributable to injury. There are two patterns, lesser yin (*shào yīn*) vacuity fire and reverting yin (*jué yīn*) liver fire. **Lesser yin vacuity fire** patterns are characterized by pale red blood, absence of pain or swelling, and forceless fine rapid pulse that is especially weak at the two cubit positions. MED Nourish yin, clear heat, and stanch bleeding with Six-Ingredient Rehmannia Pill (*liù wèi dì huáng wán*) plus schisandra (*wǔ wèi zǐ*) and white peony (*bái sháo yào*). ACU Base treatment mainly on TB, GB, and KI. Select SI-19 (*tīng gōng*, Auditory Palace), TB-17 (*yì fēng*, Wind Screen), TB-3 (*zhōng zhǔ*, Central Islet), KI-3 (*tài xī*, Great Ravine), KI-2 (*rán gǔ*, Blazing Valley), KI-1 (*yǒng quán*, Gushing Spring), SP-6 (*sān yīn jiāo*, Three Yin Intersection), BL-40 (*wěi zhōng*, Bend Center), and LR-3 (*tài chōng*, Supreme Surge); needle with drainage or with even supplementation and drainage. **Reverting yin liver fire** is marked by sudden flow of bright red blood from within the ear, swelling and pain, and a forceful stringlike pulse. MED Cool the liver and drain fire with variations of Gentian Liver-Draining Decoction (*lóng dǎn xiè gān tāng*). Calcined dragon bone (*duàn lóng gǔ*) can be dabbed on. ACU Base treatment mainly on TB, GB, LR, and PC. Select GB-2 (*tīng huì*, Auditory Convergence), TB-3 (*zhōng zhǔ*, Central Islet), TB-17 (*yì fēng*, Wind Screen), LR-3 (*tài chōng*, Supreme Surge), LR-2 (*xíng jiān*, Moving Between), LR-8 (*qū quán*, Spring at the Bend), PC-8 (*láo gōng*, Palace of Toil), BL-18 (*gān shū*, Liver Transport), and BL-17 (*gé shū*, Diaphragm Transport); needle with drainage. [26: 248] [46: 595, 738]

spontaneous bleeding of the flesh 肌衄 *jī nǜ*: *Synonym: sweating of blood.* Bleeding through the pores of the skin unassociated with injury. It is attributed to qi-blood vacuity, effulgent yin vacuity fire, or intense liver-stomach fire. MED When attributable to qi-blood vacuity with blood dissipating with qi, it is treated by supplementing qi and boosting the blood using formulas such as Tangkuei Blood-Supplementing Decoction (*dāng guī bǔ xuè tāng*), Origin-Preserving Decoction (*bǎo yuán tāng*), and Astragalus Center-Fortifying Decoction (*huáng qí jiàn zhōng tāng*). When attributable to effulgent yin vacuity fire, it is treated by nourishing yin and clearing heat, using Blood-Cooling Rehmannia Decoction (*liáng xuè dì huáng tāng*). When attributable to intense liver-stomach fire, it can be treated with Tangkuei, Gentian, and Aloe Pill (*dāng guī lóng huì wán*). See SPONTANEOUS EXTERNAL BLEEDING. Compare BLOOD ARROW. [26: 272] [97: 214]

spontaneous bleeding of the gums 齿衄 *chǐ nǜ*: *Synonym: bleeding gums.* Bleeding of the gums unattributable to injury. Spontaneous bleeding of the gums is due to accumulated heat in the stomach from excessive consumption of acrid spicy and rich foods, and less commonly due to insufficiency of stomach yin with vacuity fire flaming upward or spleen vacuity with blood management failure. **Stomach heat** spontaneous bleeding of the gums is accompanied by bad breath, consti-

pation, slimy yellow tongue fur, and copious oozing of blood. MED Clear the stomach and drain fire. Use formulas such as Stomach-Clearing Powder (*qīng wèi sǎn*) or Jade Lady Brew (*yù nǚ jiān*). ACU Base treatment mainly on ST and SP. Select ST-44 (*nèi tíng*, Inner Court), ST-36 (*zú sān lǐ*, Leg Three Li), LI-4 (*hé gǔ*, Union Valley), SP-1 (*yǐn bái*, Hidden White), and PC-4 (*xī mén*, Cleft Gate); needle with drainage. **Kidney yin vacuity** causes mild redness and swelling of the gums, loosening of the teeth with mild pain, and scant oozing of blood. MED Enrich yin and downbear fire. Use formulas such as variations of Anemarrhena, Phellodendron, and Rehmannia Pill (*zhī bǎi dì huáng wán*). ACU Base treatment mainly on KI and LI. Select KI-3 (*tài xī*, Great Ravine), KI-6 (*zhào hǎi*, Shining Sea), KI-2 (*rán gǔ*, Blazing Valley), KI-1 (*yǒng quán*, Gushing Spring), LI-4 (*hé gǔ*, Union Valley), SP-6 (*sān yīn jiāo*, Three Yin Intersection), and LR-2 (*xíng jiān*, Moving Between); needle with even supplementation and drainage. **Spleen vacuity with blood containment failure** can give rise to spontaneous bleeding of the gums marked by continuous scant bleeding. MED Supplement the spleen, boost qi, and contain the blood. Use Center-Supplementing Qi-Boosting Decoction (*bǔ zhōng yì qì tāng*). ACU Base treatment mainly on SP, ST, and CV. Select CV-12 (*zhōng wǎn*, Center Stomach Duct), ST-36 (*zú sān lǐ*, Leg Three Li), BL-20 (*pí shū*, Spleen Transport), SP-1 (*yǐn bái*, Hidden White), and SP-6 (*sān yīn jiāo*, Three Yin Intersection); needle with supplementation and add moxa. [46: 595, 596, 737] [26: 887] [27: 442] [97: 342]

spontaneous bleeding of the nipple 乳衄 *rǔ nǜ*: Bleeding from the nipple unattributable to external injury. Spontaneous bleeding of the nipples is bleeding of the nipples without any hardness, swelling, or nodes. It is attributed to excessive anxiety and thought causing damage to the liver and spleen and preventing the blood from being contained. WMC intracanalicular papilloma. MED Calm the liver and support the spleen; nourish the blood and stanch bleeding. An appropriate formula is Black Free Wanderer Powder (*hēi xiāo yáo sǎn*). [26: 377] [97: 357]

spontaneous bleeding of the tongue 舌衄 *shé nǜ*: Bleeding from the tongue not due to injury. It is attributed to heat brewing in the heart channel or spleen and kidney channel vacuity fire flaming upward. **Heat brewing in the heart channel** can cause spontaneous bleeding of the tongue marked by blood gushing from the top of the tongue and a tongue that is swollen and hard as wood. MED Clear heat and cool the blood with Coptis Toxin-Resolving Decoction (*huáng lián jiě dú tāng*) plus imperata (*bái máo gēn*) and sophora flower (*huái huā*) for mild cases and Rhinoceros

Horn and Rehmannia Decoction (*xī jiǎo dì huáng tāng*) plus child's urine (*tóng biàn*) for severe cases. ACU Select PC-8 (*láo gōng*, Palace of Toil), HT-8 (*shào fǔ*, Lesser Mansion), PC-9 (*zhōng chōng*, Central Hub), PC-4 (*xī mén*, Cleft Gate), GV-26 (*shuǐ gōu*, Water Trough); and KI-3 (*tài xī*, Great Ravine), needle with drainage, or prick to bleed with a three-edged needle. **Spleen and kidney channel vacuity fire flaming upward** causes spontaneous bleeding of the tongue characterized by oozing of blood from the upper surface of the tongue often accompanied by tidal heat [effusion] and night sweating. MED Oral: Enrich yin and cool the blood with Six-Ingredient Rehmannia Pill (*liù wèi dì huáng wán*) plus white peony (*bái sháo yào*) and licorice (*gān cǎo*). Topical: Apply a concentrated decoction of sumac gallnut (*wǔ bèi zǐ*) on a ball of gauze, or apply sophora flower (*huái huā*), stir-fried typha pollen (*pú huáng*), and charred hair (*xuè yú tàn*) in powder form. Persistent bleeding may call for cauterization. ACU Base treatment mainly the three yin channels of the foot. Select KI-3 (*tài xī*, Great Ravine), KI-6 (*zhào hǎi*, Shining Sea), KI-2 (*rán gǔ*, Blazing Valley), KI-1 (*yǒng quán*, Gushing Spring), SP-6 (*sān yīn jiāo*, Three Yin Intersection), SP-10 (*xuè hǎi*, Sea of Blood), LR-3 (*tài chōng*, Supreme Surge), LR-2 (*xíng jiān*, Moving Between), and ST-44 (*nèi tíng*, Inner Court); needle with even supplementation and drainage. [26: 267] [27: 422] [97: 195] [46: 595, 737]

spontaneous diarrhea 自下利 *zì xià lì*: Diarrhea not attributable to precipitation. [118: 85]

spontaneous external bleeding 衄血 *nǜ xuè*: Bleeding not attributable to external injury, especially nosebleed. See NOSEBLEED; SPONTANEOUS BLEEDING OF THE NIPPLE; SPONTANEOUS BLEEDING OF THE EAR; SPONTANEOUS BLEEDING OF THE FLESH; SPONTANEOUS BLEEDING OF THE GUMS; SPONTANEOUS BLEEDING OF THE TONGUE. [26: 559]

spontaneous sweating 自汗 *zì hàn*: **1.** Sweating that occurs with heat effusion. The term is used in this sense in *On Cold Damage* (*shāng hán lùn*). **2.** Excessive sweating during the daytime or sweating at the slightest physical exertion. It occurs in patients suffering from qi or yang vacuity and is an indication of vacuous defense qi and a slackening of the interstices. It also occurs in blood vacuity, phlegm obstruction, and dampness damage. See QI VACUITY SPONTANEOUS SWEATING; YANG VACUITY SPONTANEOUS SWEATING; BLOOD VACUITY SPONTANEOUS SWEATING; PHLEGM-PATTERN SPONTANEOUS SWEATING; DAMPNESS DAMAGE SPONTANEOUS SWEATING. It may also occur in WIND DAMAGE, SUMMERHEAT STROKE, WARM

DISEASE, SOFT TETANY, and CHOLERA. [26: 276] [27: 389] [97: 215] [50: 591]

spotting 漏下 *lòu xià*: Scant nonmenstrual bleeding from the uterus. See FLOODING AND SPOTTING. [27: 443]

sprain 扭伤 *niǔ shāng*: Damage to the sinew and flesh, and blood vessels around the joints such as the shoulder, elbow, wrist, lumbus, hip, knee, and ankle joints, due to twisting, pulling, or knocks and falls. They are characterized by pain, by swelling, and by discoloration of the skin due to stasis and blockage. Red indicates damage to the skin and flesh; blue-green indicates damage to the sinews; purple indicates blood stasis. Slight local swelling and tenderness indicate mild injury. Pronounced swelling and difficulty in flexing the joint are signs of a severe sprain. MED Quicken the blood and transform stasis; soothe the sinews and free the network vessels. Use Sinew-Strengthening Blood-Nourishing Decoction (*zhuàng jīn yǎng xuè tāng*). ACU Base treatment mainly on points in the affected area and at distant points on affected channels. Shoulder: LI-15 (*jiān yú*, Shoulder Bone) and TB-14 (*jiān liáo*, Shoulder Bone-Hole), and SI-9 (*jiān zhēn*, True Shoulder). Elbow: LI-11 (*qū chí*, Pool at the Bend), SI-8 (*xiǎo hǎi*, Small Sea), and TB-10 (*tiān jǐng*, Celestial Well). Wrist: TB-4 (*yáng chí*, Yang Pool), LI-5 (*yáng xī*, Yang Ravine), and SI-5 (*yáng gǔ*, Yang Valley). Lumbus: BL-23 (*shèn shū*, Kidney Transport), GV-3 (*yāo yáng guān*, Lumbar Yang Pass), and BL-40 (*wěi zhōng*, Bend Center). Thigh and buttock: GB-30 (*huán tiào*, Jumping Round), BL-54 (*zhì biān*, Sequential Limit), and BL-36 (*chéng fú*, Support). Knee: Eye of the Knee (*xī yǎn*) ST-34 (*liáng qiū*, Beam Hill), and GB-33 (*xī yáng guān*, Knee Yang Joint). Ankle: ST-41 (*jiě xī*, Ravine Divide), BL-60 (*kūn lún*, Kunlun Mountains), and GB-40 (*qiū xū*, Hill Ruins). Needle with drainage or prick to bleed with a three-edged needle. Selection of points according to signs: (1) Select contralateral points of corresponding location, i.e., for pain at TB-4 (*yáng chí*, Yang Pool) on the left wrist, needle TB-4 on the right wrist; for pain at BL-62 (*shēn mài*, Extending Vessel) on the left ankle, treat BL-62 on the right ankle. If pain is not located on a channel, use corresponding ouch points (*ā shì xué*) on the opposite side. (2) Select same-name channel points of corresponding location e.g., for pain at a point on the left wrist, apply treatment at the corresponding point of the left ankle. See SELECTION OF DISTANT POINTS. [26: 310] [46: 716] [27: 488] [97: 265]

Spring and Autumn 春秋 *chūn qiū*: Name of a dynastic period (770–476 B.C.).

spring point 荥穴 *yíng xué*: See TRANSPORT POINTS.

spring warmth 春温 *chūn wēn*: **1.** A latent qi warm disease arising when cold evil is contracted in winter and remains latent until the spring when it erupts as an acute febrile disease. See LATENT QI WARM DISEASE. **2.** A new contraction warm disease. An acute febrile disease due to contraction of wind-heat in spring. See NEW CONTRACTION WARM DISEASE. [26: 409]

squint 斜视 *xié shì*, 目偏视 *mù piān shì*, 目珠偏斜 *mù zhū piān xié*: A disease of vision marked by a deviation from the normal direction of one or both eyeballs that prevents the eyes from being directed at one object at the same time. One or both eyes may point toward the inner or outer canthus and are restricted in movement. The patient experiences what was traditionally called *seeing one as two*, i.e., double vision. *The Level-Line of Pattern Identification and Treatment* (*zhèng zhì zhǔn shéng*) refers to squint as *backward turning spirit ball* (神珠将反 *shén zhū jiāng fǎn*) and severe squint with the pupil disappearing into the socket as *backward turned pupil spirit* (瞳神反背 *tóng shén fǎn bèi*). The term *wind-induced squint* (风牵偏视 *fēng qiān piān shì*) highlights the underlying cause of nearly all squints. The terms *converging eyes* (双目通睛 *shuāng mù tōng jīng*), *dropped eye* (坠睛 *zhuì jīng*), *heaven-turned [eye]* (天旋 *tiān xuán*), and *upward-looking eye* (目仰视 *mù yǎng shì*) refer to various kinds of squint. ⎡WMC⎤ strabism. Squint patterns include wind evil striking the network vessels either due to insecurity of exterior defense, or due to insufficiency of liver blood, wind-phlegm obstructing the network vessels, liver yang transforming into wind, static blood, and wind-heat attacking upward. **Wind evil striking the network vessels** owing to insecurity of external defense causes a sudden squint and restricted movement of the eyeballs. It is associated at onset with aversion to cold and heat effusion, headache, a thin white tongue fur, and a floating pulse. Wind striking the network vessels due to insufficiency of liver blood causes a squint with exterior signs such as aversion to cold and heat effusion. It differs from the first pattern by the fact that it is observed in patients with lusterless complexion, dizziness, tinnitus, a pale tongue, and a fine pulse. ⎡MED⎤ For insecurity of external defense, course wind and free the network vessels; support right and dispel evil. Use Minor Life-Prolonging Decoction (*xiǎo xù mìng tāng*). For insufficiency of liver blood, nourish the blood and dispel wind. Use Blood-Nourishing Tangkuei and Rehmannia Decoction (*yǎng xuè dāng guī dì huáng tāng*). ⎡ACU⎤ Base treatment on BL, GB, and ST. The main points for squint are: For an inward squint, select Back of the Ball (*qiú hòu*), Greater Yang (*tài yáng*), and GB-1 (*tóng zǐ liáo*, Pupil Bone-Hole). For an outward squint, select BL-1

(*jīng míng*, Bright Eyes), BL-2 (*zǎn zhú*, Bamboo Gathering), and ST-2 (*sì bái*, Four Whites). Use a mild stimulus at points in the region of the eye. Selection of points according to pattern: For wind evil striking the network vessels due to insecurity of external defense, add GB-20 (*fēng chí*, Wind Pool), LI-4 (*hé gǔ*, Union Valley), and TB-5 (*wài guān*, Outer Pass); needle with drainage. For wind striking the network vessels due to insufficiency of liver blood, add GB-20 (*fēng chí*, Wind Pool), LR-3 (*tài chōng*, Supreme Surge), SP-6 (*sān yīn jiāo*, Three Yin Intersection), LR-8 (*qū quán*, Spring at the Bend), and KI-1 (*yǒng quán*, Gushing Spring); needle with even supplementation and drainage. **Wind-phlegm obstructing the network vessels** causes a squint when externally contracted wind evil carries phlegm upward to obstruct the network vessels. It occurs in patients with small food intake, torpid intake, ejection of phlegm-drool, thick slimy tongue fur, and a slippery stringlike pulse. ⎡MED⎤ Fortify the spleen and transform phlegm; dispel wind and free the network vessels. Use Bupleurum and Peony Six Gentlemen Decoction (*chái sháo liù jūn zǐ tāng*) combined with Face-Righting Decoction (*zhèng róng tāng*). ⎡ACU⎤ To the main points given above add GB-20 (*fēng chí*, Wind Pool), LI-4 (*hé gǔ*, Union Valley), LR-3 (*tài chōng*, Supreme Surge), ST-40 (*fēng lóng*, Bountiful Bulge), and ST-36 (*zú sān lǐ*, Leg Three Li); needle with drainage. **Liver yang transforming into wind** and carrying phlegm upward to harass the upper body causes a squint in patients suffering from dizziness, tinnitus, profuse dreaming, limp aching lumbus and knees, red tongue with yellow fur, and a fine stringlike or slippery stringlike pulse. ⎡MED⎤ Calm the liver and subdue yang; transform phlegm and extinguish wind. Use Gastrodia and Uncaria Beverage (*tiān má gōu téng yǐn*). ⎡ACU⎤ To the main points given above add BL-18 (*gān shū*, Liver Transport), GB-20 (*fēng chí*, Wind Pool), LR-3 (*tài chōng*, Supreme Surge), GB-43 (*xiá xī*, Pinched Ravine), BL-23 (*shèn shū*, Kidney Transport), KI-6 (*zhào hǎi*, Shining Sea), SP-6 (*sān yīn jiāo*, Three Yin Intersection), and ST-40 (*fēng lóng*, Bountiful Bulge); needle with drainage or with even supplementation and drainage. **Static blood** due to qi vacuity and blood stagnation can cause a squint in wind stroke patients. It may be accompanied by hemiplegia or numbness of the limbs. ⎡MED⎤ Boost qi and quicken the blood; transform stasis and free the network vessels. Use Yang-Supplementing Five-Returning Decoction (*bǔ yáng huán wǔ tāng*). ⎡ACU⎤ To the main points given above add BL-17 (*gé shū*, Diaphragm Transport), SP-10 (*xuè hǎi*, Sea of Blood), LI-4 (*hé gǔ*, Union Valley), LR-3 (*tài chōng*, Supreme Surge), and SP-6 (*sān yīn jiāo*, Three Yin Intersection); needle with even supplementation and drainage. **Wind-heat attacking upward** causes a squint in child fright wind with high fever and clouded spirit. MED Dispel wind and clear heat; soothe the channels and quicken the network vessels. Use Bovine Bezoar Dragon-Embracing Pill (*niú huáng bào lóng wán*) or Face-Righting Decoction (*zhèng róng tāng*) with the addition of scutellaria (*huáng qín*), ground pine (*shēn jīn cǎo*), limestone (*shí huī*), and ophiopogon (*mài mén dōng*). ACU To the main points given above add GB-20 (*fēng chí*, Wind Pool), LI-4 (*hé gǔ*, Union Valley), LI-11 (*qū chí*, Pool at the Bend), GV-14 (*dà zhuī*, Great Hammer), and PC-6 (*nèi guān*, Inner Pass), and prick LU-11 (*shào shāng*, Lesser Shang) to bleed; needle with drainage. **Poor constitution:** Squint may occur congenitally and is usually associated with slowness to teethe and walk, low I.Q., and weak health. MED Supplement the liver and boost the kidney; soothe the sinews and quicken the network vessels. If yang vacuity is prominent, use Golden Coffer Kidney Qi Pill (*jīn guì shèn qì wán*); if yin vacuity is prominent, use Six-Ingredient Rehmannia Pill (*liù wèi dì huáng wán*). In either case, add loofah (*sī guā luò*), ground pine (*shēn jīn cǎo*), and earthworm (*dì lóng*). ACU To the main points given above add BL-18 (*gān shū*, Liver Transport), BL-23 (*shèn shū*, Kidney Transport), LR-3 (*tài chōng*, Supreme Surge), KI-3 (*tài xī*, Great Ravine), KI-7 (*fù liū*, Recover Flow), and GV-4 (*mìng mén*, Life Gate); for yang vacuity needle with supplementation and moxa; add BL-18 (*gān shū*, Liver Transport), BL-23 (*shèn shū*, Kidney Transport), LR-3 (*tài chōng*, Supreme Surge), KI-3 (*tài xī*, Great Ravine), KI-6 (*zhào hǎi*, Shining Sea), and BL-52 (*zhì shì*, Will Chamber); for yin vacuity, needle with supplementation. [125: 313] [97: 528] [92: No. 489] [113: 476] [42: 210]

ST 胃 *wèi*, 足阳明胃经 *zú yáng míng wèi jīng*: The stomach or foot yang brightness (*yáng míng*) stomach channel.

stabbing pain 刺痛 *cì tòng*: A pain of fixed location that feels like the stabbing of a knife. Stabbing pain is attributed to static blood. See PAIN. [29: 190]

stabilizing panting 定喘 *dìng chuǎn*: CALMING PANTING.

stabilizing the mind 定志 *dìng zhì*: To treat disquieted essence-spirit. See QUIETING THE SPIRIT. [44: 879]

stabilizing wind 定风 *dìng fēng*: Treating the stirring of internal vacuity wind due to damage to yin by exuberant heat in the final stages of warm heat disease; effectively the same as ENRICHING YIN AND EXTINGUISHING WIND. MED Major Wind-Stabilizing Pill (*dà dìng fēng zhū*) is a commonly used wind-stabilizing formula. [97: 369]

stagnant 滞 *zhì*: **1.** Affected by stagnation. **2.** Presenting a stagnant appearance, i.e., dull and blotchy. A stagnant complexion may be observed in qi stagnation and blood stasis, especially when stemming from severe heart yang vacuity.

stagnant diarrhea 滞下 *zhì xià*: An old name for dysentery. "Stagnant diarrhea" describes the stagnation of the intestines and difficulty in defecation associated with the disease. See DYSENTERY.

stagnation 滞 *zhì*: Sluggishness of movement, particularly of qi and the food. See STOPPAGE.

stained fur 染苔 *rǎn tāi*: A tongue fur stained by foodstuffs or medicines. Milk and soybean milk stain the tongue fur white; coffee, tea, and tobacco leave brown stains; egg yolk, oranges, coptis (*huáng lián*), and ass hide glue (*ē jiāo*) leave yellow stains. Blackberries and similar fruits leave purple stains. Staining normally affects only the surface of the tongue fur, and is washed away by saliva. When examining the tongue, it is important that these factors are ruled out before the color of the tongue fur is taken as a diagnostic datum. [6: 120] [27: 183] [97: 438]

stanching bleeding 止血 *zhǐ xuè*: *Synonym: containing bleeding.* Any of various methods of treatment used to address bleeding. Different medicinals are used depending on whether it occurs in cold or heat patterns. MED Cool blood-stanching medicinals, which are used for bleeding in heat patterns, include eclipta (*mò hàn lián*), biota leaf (*cè bǎi yè*), imperata (*bái máo gēn*), trachycarpus (*zōng lǘ pí*), lotus leaf (*hé yè*), cephalanoplos (*xiǎo jì*), sophora flower (*huái huā*), and Madaio dock root (*tǔ dà huáng*). Warm blood-stanching medicinals, which are used for bleeding in cold patterns, include mugwort (*ài yè*), agrimony (*xiān hè cǎo*), notoginseng (*sān qī*), blast-fried ginger (*páo jiāng*), and oven earth (*fú lóng gān*). Agents are also chosen according to the location of the bleeding. Mugwort (*ài yè*) and ox horn bone (*niú jiǎo sāi*) are used for flooding and spotting. Typha pollen (*pú huáng*), cirsium (*dà jì*), and cephalanoplos (*xiǎo jì*) are used for bloody urine. Bletilla (*bái jí*) and imperata (*bái máo gēn*) are used for blood ejection (vomiting or expectoration of blood). Sanguisorba (*dì yú*), sophora flower (*huái huā*), and oven earth (*fú lóng gān*) are used for bloody stool. Blood-stanching medicinals with a pronounced securing effect include biota leaf (*cè bǎi yè*), trachycarpus (*zōng lǘ pí*), lotus leaf (*hé yè*), bletilla (*bái jí*), and oven earth (*fú lóng gān*). Charring (char-frying, or blast-frying) is frequently used to increase the astringent and blood-stanching effect of other medicinals. A representative blood-stanching formula is Ten Cinders Pill (*shí huī wán*). ACU For frenetic movement of hot blood, cool the blood and stanch bleeding with points such as PC-7 (*dà* *líng*, Great Mound), PC-4 (*xī mén*, Cleft Gate), LU-6 (*kǒng zuì*, Collection Hole), LU-9 (*tài yuān*, Great Abyss), KI-3 (*tài xī*, Great Ravine), LR-3 (*tài chōng*, Supreme Surge), SP-6 (*sān yīn jiāo*, Three Yin Intersection), and ST-44 (*nèi tíng*, Inner Court); needle with drainage. For qi failing to contain the blood, supplement qi to contain the blood using points such as SP-1 (*yǐn bái*, Hidden White), ST-36 (*zú sān lǐ*, Leg Three Li), CV-4 (*guān yuán*, Pass Head), CV-6 (*qì hǎi*, Sea of Qi), GV-14 (*dà zhuī*, Great Hammer), and GV-20 (*bǎi huì*, Hundred Convergences); needle with supplementation and moxa. See CLEARING HEAT AND STANCHING BLEEDING; SUPPLEMENTING QI AND STANCHING BLEEDING; DISPELLING STASIS AND STANCHING BLEEDING; FLOODING AND SPOTTING; BLOODY URINE; BLOOD EJECTION. [6: 268] [46: 595]

stasis 瘀 *yū*: **1.** Sluggishness or cessation of movement (of the blood), specifically of the blood. **2.** Static blood. See BLOOD STASIS.

stasis clot 瘀块 *yū kuài*: Blood clot due to blood stasis. Clotting of menstrual flow indicates the presence of static blood.

stasis heat 瘀热 *yū rè*: **1.** Depressed accumulated heat in the inner body. Stasis heat is observed, for example, when heat binds with dampness internally, and after stagnating for a long time, eventually causes jaundice, which can be treated with Capillaris Decoction (*yīn chén hāo tāng*). **2.** Blood stasis transforming into heat. [26: 762] [27: 136] [97: 611]

stasis heat in the interior 瘀热在里 *yū rè zài lǐ*: **1.** Yang brightness (*yáng míng*) heat patterns with sweating and with inhibited urination and water-damp collecting internally, eventually causing jaundice. **2.** Static blood lodged in the interior giving rise, in certain circumstances, to heat effusion. See STASIS HEAT. [26: 762]

stasis hiccough 瘀呃 *yū è*: HICCOUGH due to static blood causing obstruction in the chest and diaphragm. Stasis hiccough is characterized by hiccough immediately after drinking and is accompanied by stabbing pain in the heart [region] and chest, mild yellow of the eyes, mild cold of the limbs, and thin black stool. MED Quicken the blood and transform stasis with Peach Kernel Qi-Coordinating Decoction (*táo hé chéng qì tāng*) or House of Blood Stasis-Expelling Decoction (*xuè fǔ zhú yū tāng*). ACU Base treatment mainly on ST, LR, PC, and SP. Select BL-17 (*gé shū*, Diaphragm Transport), PC-6 (*nèi guān*, Inner Pass), CV-17 (*shān zhōng*, Chest Center), ST-36 (*zú sān lǐ*, Leg Three Li), LR-3 (*tài chōng*, Supreme Surge), SP-10 (*xuè hǎi*, Sea of Blood), and SP-6 (*sān yīn jiāo*, Three Yin Intersection); needle with drainage or

prick to bleed with a three-edged needle. See HICCOUGH. [26: 763] [46: 594] [37: 307]

stasis macule 瘀斑 *yū bān*: A small purple patch on the skin due to and indicating the presence of blood stasis. Compare STASIS SPECKLE.

stasis pain 瘀痛 *yū tòng*: The pain caused with static blood. Stasis pain is a pain of fixed location. See BLOOD STASIS.

stasis speckle 瘀点 *yū diǎn*: Green-blue or purple speckles on the tongue indicating the presence of static blood. Compare STASIS MACULE.

stasis swelling 瘀肿 *yū zhǒng*: Swelling due static blood resulting from knocks and falls; bruise.

static 守而不走 *shǒu ér bù zǒu*: Tending to remain still. Yin-supplementing medicinals, especially when heavy in substance, are described as static. Cooked rehmannia (*shú dì huáng*) and deerhorn (*lù jiǎo*) are examples of static medicinals.

static blood 瘀血 *yū xuè*: Blood affected by stasis, i.e., blood that does not move freely, stagnates in the vessels, or accumulates outside the vessels. Static blood and the morbid changes to which it gives rise are identified by localized pain, stasis macules, and masses; these changes indicate the presence of concretions and gatherings. When blood vessels are blocked by static blood and can no longer withstand the pressure, bleeding may occur. This is most commonly seen in gynecological diseases. Generalized signs of blood stasis include a dull complexion, blue-green or purple lips and tongue, and stasis macules on the edge of the tongue. The pulse is fine or rough. See BLOOD STASIS. [26: 762] [27: 119] [97: 611]

static blood abdominal pain 瘀血腹痛 *yū xuè fù tòng*: Synonym: *blood stagnation abdominal pain*. ABDOMINAL PAIN due to static blood that arises when persistent qi stagnation affects the network vessels. Static blood abdominal pain is a pain of fixed location that refuses pressure. The tongue is purple and dark, and the pulse is rough. MED Treat by quickening the blood and eliminating stasis with formulas such as Stasis-Dispersing Beverage (*xiāo yū yǐn*), Blood-Quickening Decoction (*huó xuè tāng*), or Infradiaphragmatic Stasis-Expelling Decoction (*gé xià zhú yū tāng*). ACU Base treatment on SP and LR. Select SP-10 (*xuè hǎi*, Sea of Blood), SP-6 (*sān yīn jiāo*, Three Yin Intersection), LR-3 (*tài chōng*, Supreme Surge), LR-2 (*xíng jiān*, Moving Between), BL-25 (*dà cháng shū*, Large Intestine Transport), and ST-25 (*tiān shū*, Celestial Pivot); needle with drainage. [26: 763] [37: 319]

static blood cough 瘀血咳 *yū xuè ké*: Cough attributable to static blood obstructing the network vessels of the lung. Static blood cough is characterized by cough with a fishy smell in the throat, and ejection of purple black blood. In some cases, there is only one side on which the patient can lie without experience cough and rapid breathing. [MED] Quicken the blood and harmonize the network vessels. Use House of Blood Stasis-Expelling Decoction (*xuè fǔ zhú yū tāng*) plus apricot kernel (*xìng rén*) or schisandra (*wǔ wèi zǐ*). Alternatively, use Tangkuei Powder (*dāng guī sǎn*). [ACU] Base treatment mainly on LU, back transport points, and SP. Select BL-13 (*fèi shū*, Lung Transport), LU-5 (*chǐ zé*, Cubit Marsh), LU-9 (*tài yuān*, Great Abyss), BL-17 (*gé shū*, Diaphragm Transport), CV-17 (*shān zhōng*, Chest Center), SP-10 (*xuè hǎi*, Sea of Blood), and SP-6 (*sān yīn jiāo*, Three Yin Intersection); needle with drainage. [26: 762]

static blood headache 瘀血头痛 *yū xuè tóu tòng*: HEADACHE attributed to static blood resulting from external injury or from stagnation in the vessels in enduring sickness. Static blood headache is a continually intermittent pain of fixed location, like the piercing of an awl. Accompanying signs include stagnant complexion, stasis speckles on the tongue, and a rough pulse. [MED] Quicken the blood and transform stasis. Use formulas such as Orifice-Freeing Blood-Quickening Decoction (*tōng qiào huó xuè tāng*) or House of Blood Stasis-Expelling Decoction (*xuè fǔ zhú yū tāng*) or variations. [ACU] Base treatment mainly on LI, SP, and ouch points (*ā shì xué*). Drain ouch points (*ā shì xué*) on the head, and prick them to bleed in order to drain stasis and free the network vessels. Drain BL-17 (*gé shū*, Diaphragm Transport), SP-10 (*xuè hǎi*, Sea of Blood), LI-4 (*hé gǔ*, Union Valley), and SP-6 (*sān yīn jiāo*, Three Yin Intersection) to quicken the blood, and supplement LI-4 (*hé gǔ*, Union Valley) to move qi. See also HEADACHE. [26: 763] [27: 392] [97: 611] [46: 623]

static blood lumbar pain 瘀血腰痛 *yū xuè yāo tòng*: Synonym: *blood stasis lumbar pain*. LUMBAR PAIN due to blood stasis that congeals and accumulates either as a result of knocks and falls or wrenching, or as a result of enduring lumbar pain due to other causes. Static blood lumbar pain is characterized by pain of fixed location, like the piercing of an awl, mild in the day and more severe at night, and accompanied by a rough pulse. In some cases the stool may be black and the urine yellow, reddish, or blackish. [MED] Quicken the blood and transform stasis using Major Yin Supplementation Pill (*dà bǔ yīn wán*) plus peach kernel (*táo rén*) and carthamus (*hóng huā*), or using Peach Kernel Qi-Coordinating Decoction (*táo hé chéng qì tāng*). [ACU] Base treatment on back transport points and BL. Select BL-23 (*shèn shū*, Kidney Transport), GV-3 (*yāo yáng guān*, Lumbar Yang Pass), BL-17 (*gé shū*, Diaphragm Transport), and BL-32 (*cì liáo*, Second Bone-Hole); need with even supplementation and drainage. BL-40 (*wěi zhōng*, Bend Center) can be bled with a three-

edged needle or needled. Ouch points (*ā shì xué*) may also be needled. For long-standing pain, tap ouch points with a plum-blossom needle and firecup. [26: 763] [46: 633] [37: 391]

static blood stomach duct pain 瘀血胃脘痛 *yū xuè wèi wǎn (guǎn) tòng*: Pain in the stomach duct due to qi stagnation and congealing blood. Pain like the stabbing of knife, of fixed location, that refuses pressure and cold may be accompanied by the ejection of dark purple blood, black stool, or hiccough after drinking. The tongue fur is dark purple and the pulse is fine and rough. [MED] Treatment takes the approach of transforming stasis and freeing the network vessels and uses formulas like Instant Relief Powder (*shǒu niān sǎn*) or Sudden Smile Powder (*shī xiào sǎn*). [ACU] Base treatment mainly on ST, PC, LR, and SP. Select CV-12 (*zhōng wǎn*, Center Stomach Duct), ST-36 (*zú sān lǐ*, Leg Three Li), PC-6 (*nèi guān*, Inner Pass), SP-4 (*gōng sūn*, Yellow Emperor), BL-17 (*gé shū*, Diaphragm Transport), BL-18 (*gān shū*, Liver Transport), LR-14 (*qī mén*, Cycle Gate), and SP-6 (*sān yīn jiāo*, Three Yin Intersection). Needle with drainage. [26: 762] [46: 660]

static blood streaming sore 瘀血流注 *yū xuè liú zhù*: A STREAMING SORE that arises after knocks or falls or incomplete elimination of the LOCHIA have caused stasis in the network vessels and damp-heat exploits vacuity to enter the body and combine with the stasis. A static blood streaming sore in the initial stage is characterized by local swelling that is hard and painful to the touch. The affected area is marked by slightly red or green-blue to purple skin that subsequently becomes red and scorching hot. The affected area spreads outward, and signs such as aversion to cold, heat effusion, and joint pain develop. If the process through suppuration to rupture is smooth, prognosis is good. [MED] Move qi, quicken the blood, and resolve toxin. Use Stasis-Dissipating Pueraria Decoction (*sàn yū gé gēn tāng*). If caused by postpartum static blood, use variations Channel-Freeing Stagnation-Abducting Decoction (*tōng jīng dǎo zhì tāng*). When pus has formed, open and drain. Otherwise treat as for welling-abscesses (*yōng*) and flat-abscesses (*jū*) that have ruptured. [26: 762] [27: 470] [97: 612]

static blood yellowing 瘀血发黄 *yū xuè fā huáng*: See BLOOD AMASSMENT YELLOWING. [26: 763]

stationary cupping 坐罐法 *zuò guàn fǎ*: Synonym: *retained cupping*. A method of cupping whereby the cups are left in place for about ten minutes after they have been applied. [37: 237]

steam 蒸 *zhēng*: (Of heat in the body) to rise from a locus and affect other higher or peripheral areas. For, example heat sores on the mouth are explained as the product of "upward steaming of lung-stomach heat," and a normal tongue fur as the "upward steam of stomach qi." "Steaming bone" tidal heat [effusion] describes how heat seems to emanate from the depths of the body as a steam rising from the bones. See HEAT.

steaming 蒸 *zhēng*: A method of processing medicinals whereby medicinal materials are placed in pots or baskets, with or without adjuvants, over boiling water. The aim is to change the nature of the medicinal, improve its effectiveness, and facilitate slicing and storage. See PROCESSING OF MEDICINALS. [74: 10] [11: 20] [27: 235] [97: 596]

steaming bone 骨蒸 *gǔ zhēng*: A STEAMING DISEASE that is characterized by tidal heat [effusion], night sweating, forceless panting, heart vexation and reduced sleep, heat in the palms, and yellow or reddish urine. Steaming bone is so called because the heat appears to emanate from the bone or marrow. [MED] Nourish yin and clear heat using formulas such as Large Gentian and Turtle Shell Powder (*qín jiāo biē jiǎ sǎn*) or Bone-Clearing Powder (*qīng gǔ sǎn*). [ACU] Base treatment mainly on KI, HT, and GV. Select KI-6 (*zhào hǎi*, Shining Sea), KI-2 (*rán gǔ*, Blazing Valley), KI-1 (*yǒng quán*, Gushing Spring), HT-8 (*shào fǔ*, Lesser Mansion), and HT-7 (*shén mén*, Spirit Gate); needle with even supplementation and drainage. Selection of points according to signs: For tidal heat [effusion], add GV-14 (*dà zhuī*, Great Hammer), LU-10 (*yú jì*, Fish Border), and PC-5 (*jiān shǐ*, Intermediary Courier). For night sweating, add HT-6 (*yīn xī*, Yin Cleft), SI-3 (*hòu xī*, Back Ravine), and LI-4 (*hé gǔ*, Union Valley). For panting, add BL-13 (*fèi shū*, Lung Transport), LU-5 (*chǐ zé*, Cubit Marsh), and BL-43 (*gāo huāng shū*, Gao-Huang Transport). For heart vexation and reduced sleep, add BL-15 (*xīn shū*, Heart Transport), PC-6 (*nèi guān*, Inner Pass), SP-6 (*sān yīn jiāo*, Three Yin Intersection), and HT-5 (*tōng lǐ*, Connecting Li). A moxibustion formula suggested by Liu Wan-Su (1120–1200 A.D.) of the Jin Dynasty is to first moxa GV-20 (*bǎi huì*, Hundred Convergences), and then moxa GV-14 (*dà zhuī*, Great Hammer), burning 5–7 cones at each point. See also CONSUMPTION. [27: 387] [97: 400] [46: 596] [14: 49]

steaming bone tidal heat [effusion] 骨蒸潮热 *gǔ zhēng cháo rè*: Yin vacuity tidal heat [effusion] characteristic of steaming bone. See HEAT EFFUSION. [26: 530]

steaming disease 蒸病 *zhēng bìng*: Synonym: *taxation steaming*. From *The Origin and Indicators of Disease* (*zhū bìng yuán hòu lùn*). Various diseases characterized by tidal heat [effusion] that appears to emanate from within the body, "steaming" up to the surface; the most notable example is steaming bones. Steaming diseases include the

five steamings—steaming bone, steaming vessels, steaming skin, steaming flesh, and internal steaming. Of these, only STEAMING BONE is mentioned frequently in modern literature. [26: 843] [27: 387] [97: 50, 597]

steam-wash 熏洗 *xūn xǐ*: **1.** *vb.* To steam and/or bathe parts of the body, usually with a medicinal decoction. Steam-washing usually involves steaming followed by washing. The warmth of the steam and fluids helps to move qi and blood. The medicinals used also help the healing action. Steam-washing is commonly used in the treatment of eye diseases such as red swollen eyelids, red whites of the eye, and sore dry eyes averse to light. **2.** *n.* An act of steam-washing. **3.** *n.* A preparation used as in steam-washing. [125: 92]

steeping 浸泡 *jìn pào*: Synonym: *soaking*. Allow medicinal materials to stand in clear water or other fluid for a certain time. Steeping facilitates slicing, as in the case of areca (*bīng láng*) and lindera (*wū yào*). It can also reduce toxicity, as in the case of arisaema (*tiān nán xīng*) and pinellia (*bàn xià*). See PROCESSING OF MEDICINALS. [74: 5] [27: 323]

¹**stem** 固 *gù*: To stop or contain (a flow), e.g., to stem flooding and check vaginal discharge.

²**stem** 救 *jiù*: To curtail or relieve. See RETURNING YANG AND STEMMING COUNTERFLOW.

³**stem** 干 *gān*: See HEAVENLY STEMS AND EARTHLY BRANCHES.

stem and branch point selection 子午流注 *zǐ wǔ liú zhù*: MIDDAY-MIDNIGHT POINT SELECTION.

stemming flooding and checking (vaginal) discharge 固崩止带 *gù bēng zhǐ dài*: A method of treatment used to address uterine blooding, incessant menses, and vaginal discharge using astringent agents such as calcined dragon bone (*lóng gǔ*), calcined oyster shell (*mǔ lì*), ailanthus root bark (*shū gēn bái pí*), cuttlefish bone (*hǎi piāo xiāo*), madder (*qiàn cǎo gēn*), and sumac gallnut (*wǔ bèi zǐ*), combined with spleen-fortifying kidney-supplementing medicinals such as astragalus (*huáng qí*), ginseng (*rén shēn*), dioscorea (*shān yào*), cuscuta (*tù sī zǐ*), charred eucommia (*dù zhòng tàn*), and deer-horn glue (*lù jiǎo jiāo*), For flooding and spotting or incessant menses due to yin vacuity and blood heat, use Menses-Securing Pill (*gù jīng wán*). For dribbling vaginal discharge forming a damp-heat pattern, use Ailanthus Root Bark Pill (*shū shù pí wán*). [26: 376] [16: 359]

stewing 炖 *dù*: Slow cooking. See DOUBLE-BOILING.

sticky sweat 黏汗 *nián hàn*: OILY SWEAT.

stiff tongue 舌强 *shé qiáng*: A tongue that is stiff, moves sluggishly, and inhibits speech. A stiff tongue occurs in a number of serious diseases, such as heat entering the pericardium, phlegm confounding the orifices of the heart, phlegm obstructing the network vessels, and liver wind stirring internally. Other signs are therefore decisive in determining the nature of the disease. In Western medicine, a stiff tongue generally indicates diseases of the central nervous system. ACU Base treatment mainly on GV, CV, and HT. Select GV-15 (*yǎ mén*, Mute's Gate), CV-23 (*lián quán*, Ridge Spring), HT-5 (*tōng lǐ*, Connecting Li), and GV-16 (*fēng fǔ*, Wind Mansion); needle with drainage. Prick Gold Liquid and Jade Humor (*jīn jīn yù yè*) to bleed with a three-edged needle. Add other points according to cause. [6: 121] [26: 267] [27: 179] [46: 602] [14: 57]

stifling oppression in the heart and chest 心胸憋闷 *xīn xiōng biē mèn*: Pronounced OPPRESSION IN THE CHEST.

stinging pain 刺痛 *cì tòng*: An acute localized pain on the surface of the body, as in the urethra on urination. NB: The Chinese term 刺痛 *cì tòng* also denotes STABBING PAIN within the body. See PAIN. [29: 190]

stir-frying 炒 *chǎo*: Tossing (medicinal materials) in a heated wok. Stir-frying is the most commonly used method of heat processing. It is dry frying: oil should never be used unless specifically stated. The aims of stir-frying are threefold: (1) To eliminate unwanted constituents, change the nature of medicinals, and reduce irritation or other side-effects, and reduce extreme cold or dryness. For example, the fierce draining precipitant action of rhubarb (*dà huáng*) in its raw form is moderated by stir-frying, and even more markedly reduced by char-frying. (2) To increase the aromatic and spleen-fortifying qualities. For example, ovate atractylodes (*bái zhú*) and barley sprout (*mài yá*) are stir-fried until yellow, whereas crataegus (*shān zhā*) and medicated leaven (*shén qū*) are scorch-fried. (3) To facilitate crushing, storage, and extraction of active constituents through decoction. For example, some seeds when lightly fried, crispen and crack open facilitating decoction. Some materials become looser after stir-frying, so that they are not only more easily crushed, but also their active constituents are more easily extracted. Also stir-frying reduces moisture content and destroys ferments, thus preventing the breakdown of active constituents during storage. Stir-frying includes plain stir-frying (light-stir-frying, scorch-frying, char-frying etc), and stir-frying with adjuvants such as bran, earth, oven earth (*fú lóng gān*), or rice. Stir-frying with liquid adjuvants, especially honey, is usually referred to as mix-frying.

Stir-Frying

Plain stir-frying

   LIGHT STIR-FRYING (*wéi chǎo*)

   SCORCH-FRYING (*chǎo jiāo*)
   BLAST-FRYING (*páo*)
   CHAR-FRYING (*chǎo tàn*)
   EARTH-FRYING (*tǔ chǎo*)

Stir-frying with adjuvants

   STIR-FRYING WITH CLAMSHELL POWDER (*gé fěn chǎo*)
   STIR-FRYING WITH EARTH (*tǔ chǎo*)
   STIR-FRYING WITH BRAN (*fū chǎo*)
   STIR-FRYING WITH RICE (*mǐ chǎo*)

Mix-frying

   MIX-FRYING WITH BRINE (*yán zhì*)
   MIX-FRYING WITH GINGER (*jiāng zhì*)
   MIX-FRYING WITH HONEY (*mì zhì*)
   MIX-FRYING WITH VINEGAR (*cù zhì*)
   MIX-FRYING WITH WINE (*jiǔ zhì*)

---

stir-frying with adjuvants 副料炒 *fù liào chǎo*: Tossing (medicinal materials) with in a wok over a flame, with a secondary solid material that is sifted off when frying is completed. The aim of stir-frying with adjuvants is to enhance the physical or medicinal properties of medicinals. Stir-frying with adjuvants includes STIR-FRYING WITH CLAMSHELL POWDER, STIR-FRYING WITH EARTH, STIR-FRYING WITH BRAN, and STIR-FRYING WITH RICE. Compare PLAIN STIR-FRYING.

stir-frying with bran 麸炒 *fū chǎo*: Stir-frying (medicinal materials) in a wok with bran over a flame until a thick yellow-black smoke is given off. This process increases a medicinal's capacity to fortify the spleen and stomach and causes oils that would otherwise cause side effects and unpleasant smells to be absorbed by the bran. Ovate atractylodes (*bái zhú*) and bitter orange (*zhǐ ké*) may be processed in this way.

stir-frying with clamshell powder 蛤粉炒 *gé fěn chǎo*: Tossing (medicinal materials) with clamshell powder (*hǎi gé fěn*), in a wok over a flame. Clam shell powder is fine, and conducts heat slowly, and hence poses little danger of burning. For this reason, it is often used to treat gelatinous animal products, which are allowed to turn yellow or bubble up at the surface before removal. Ass hide glue pellets (*ē jiāo zhū*) are made in this way. Talcum (*huá shí*) is used in exactly the same way as clamshell.

stir-frying with earth 土炒 *tǔ chǎo*: Tossing (medicinal materials) with oven earth (*fú lóng gān*) in a wok over a flame. Stir-frying with earth makes use of the acridity and warmth of oven earth to warm the center and check both bleeding and vomiting. Materials fried with it have stronger capacity to supplement the spleen, harmonize the stomach, and check vomiting and diarrhea. Modern biomedical research shows that oven earth, due to its long exposure to high temperatures, contains zinc oxide and little water or organic matter, and being slightly alkaline it reduces stomach acidity. Ovate atractylodes (*bái zhú*) and dioscorea (*shān yào*) may be treated in this way.

stir-frying with ginger juice 姜汁炒 *jiāng zhī chǎo*: Stir-frying medicinal materials that have been soaked in a decoction of fresh ginger (*shēng jiāng*). Bamboo shavings (*zhú rú*), gardenia (*shān zhī zǐ*), tsaoko (*cǎo guǒ*), and coptis (*huáng lián*) may be stir-fried with ginger juice. Method: Boil 1 kg of crushed or finely sliced fresh ginger in 3 l of water in an earthenware pot (*shā guō*) for thirty minutes. Strain and reduce the liquid to 1 l. Stir in the materials thoroughly so that all the liquid is absorbed, and then stir-fry in the earthenware pot until dry. Do not use a steel wok. Stir-fry in small quantities, because the earthenware pots easily break. [82: 41]

stir-frying with rice 米炒 *mǐ chǎo*: Tossing (medicinal materials) with rice in a wok over a flame. Stir-frying with rice reduces the dryness of medicinals and increases their capacity to supplement the center and boost qi. Stir-frying with rice can also reduce the toxicity of a small number of medicinals. Codonopsis (*dǎng shēn*) and mylabris (*bān máo*) can be treated this way.

stir-frying with vinegar 醋炒 *cù chǎo*: Tossing medicinal materials with a certain amount of vinegar in a heated wok. Vinegar is sour, bitter, and slightly warm. It enters the liver channel and the blood aspect, and has the action of promoting astriction, resolving toxin, and dissipating stasis and relieving pain. Stir-frying with vinegar is therefore applied to medicinals used to course the liver and resolve depression, dissipate stasis and relieve pain, and expel water. It is applied, for example, to frankincense (*rǔ xiāng*), myrrh (*mò yào*), sparganium (*sān léng*), and zedoary (*é zhú*) in order to conduct them into the liver and increase their blood-quickening pain-relieving action; to bupleurum (*chái hú*), cyperus (*xiāng fù zǐ*), unripe tangerine peel (*qīng pí*), and corydalis (*yán hú suǒ*) to increase their liver-coursing and pain-relieving properties; to euphorbia/knoxia (*dà jǐ*), kansui (*gān suì*), genkwa (*yuán huā*), and phytolacca (*shāng lù*), to reduce their toxicity and moderate their drastic precipitating action; and to flying squirrel's droppings (*wǔ líng zhī*), frankincense (*rǔ xiāng*), and myrrh (*mò yào*) to remove unpleasant smells as well as to increase their blood-quickening stasis-dispelling action. [100: 93]

stirred pulse 动脉 *dòng mài*: A pulse that is forceful, rapid and slippery, like a bean that is bobbing. According to some sources, the stirred pulse is only felt at the bar (not generally recognized nowadays). The stirred pulse is a sign of pain or

fright, and may be seen in sweating, heat effusion, diarrhea, seminal collapse, and flooding and spotting. A stirred pulse is also observed in pregnancy. [97: 177] [29: 228, 251] [93: 284]

stirring 动 *dòng*: Provocation or development (of wind); agitation (of blood).

stirring fetus 胎动不安 *tāi dòng bù ān*, 胎动 *tāi dòng*: A disease pattern characterized by movement of the fetus, pain and sagging sensation in the abdomen, and, in severe cases, discharge of blood from the vagina; a sign of possible or impending miscarriage; can be caused by knocks and falls, qi vacuity, blood vacuity, kidney vacuity, or blood heat causing thoroughfare (*chōng*) and controlling (*rèn*) vessels. **Knocks and falls** causes sudden stirring fetus with aching lumbus and smaller-abdominal pain. ⌐MED⌐ Supplement qi, nourish the blood, and quiet the fetus with Ass Hide Glue and Mugwort Four Agents Decoction (*jiāo ài sì wù tāng*). **Qi vacuity** stirring fetus is accompanied by listlessness of essence-spirit, shortage of qi, and laziness to speak. ⌐MED⌐ Supplement qi and quiet the spirit with Origin-Lifting Brew (*jǔ yuán jiān*) plus ass hide glue (*ē jiāo*). **Blood vacuity** causes stirring fetus with pale yellow facial complexion, lassitude of spirit, and lack of strength. ⌐MED⌐ Supplement the blood and quiet the fetus with Fetal Origin Beverage (*tāi yuán yǐn*). **Kidney vacuity** stirring fetus is accompanied by dizzy head, tinnitus, limp legs, and frequent urination. ⌐MED⌐ Secure the kidney and quiet the fetus with Fetal Longevity Pill (*shòu tāi wán*). **Blood heat** stirring fetus is associated with dry mouth and throat and with heart vexation. ⌐MED⌐ Clear heat, cool the blood, and quiet the fetus with Yin-Safeguarding Brew (*bǎo yīn jiān*). [26: 455]

stirring heart palpitations 心动悸 *xīn dòng jì*: HEART PALPITATIONS that are not only subjective, but also palpable or even visible. [26: 93] [27: 388] [97: 119]

stirring of the ministerial fire 相火妄动 *xiàng huǒ wàng dòng*: Insufficiency of liver-kidney yin with vacuity fire flaming upward. It is characterized by dizziness, headache, unclear vision, tinnitus, deafness, irascibility, profuse dreaming, vexing heat in the palms, excessive libido, seminal emission, and premature ejaculation. If hyperactive liver yang is prominent, it is treated by fostering yin and subduing yang, using Gastrodia and Uncaria Beverage (*tiān má gōu téng yǐn*); if effulgent kidney fire is prominent, it is treated by enriching yin and downbearing fire, using Anemarrhena, Phellodendron, and Rehmannia Pill (*zhī bǎi dì huáng wán*). [26: 415] [27: 56] [97: 340]

stirring qi in the kidney region 肾间动气 *shèn jiān dòng qì*: True qi stored in the region of the kidneys, i.e., a manifestation of the life gate fire.

The qi of the organs and channels and qi transformation in the triple burner is dependent upon the stirring qi in the kidney region. [26: 692] [27: 56] [97: 340]

stomach 胃 *wèi*: **1.** The bowel standing in exterior-interior relationship with the spleen. The stomach is the place where food first collects after it enters the body before it passes to the intestines, and where it is broken down to enable its "essence" (nutrients) to be absorbed into the body. Traditionally, the stomach's function of controlling appetite and receiving food is referred to as the STOMACH GOVERNS INTAKE and its function of breaking down food is called the STOMACH GOVERNS DECOMPOSITION. Since food, after being decomposed in the stomach, passes on to the intestines, it is said that the STOMACH GOVERNS DOWNBEARING OF THE TURBID. The downward action of stomach qi that carries food down to the intestines stands in complementary opposition to the spleen's function extracting the "essence" (see SPLEEN GOVERNS UPBEARING OF THE CLEAR). The stomach is related to other organs largely through the its channel, the FOOT YANG BRIGHTNESS STOMACH CHANNEL. By an internal pathway, the stomach channel homes to the stomach and connects with the spleen. The external pathway starts at the side of the nose, crosses the side of the head, face and neck, runs down the chest, through the nipples, over the abdomen, and down the outer anterolateral surface of the leg, to end at the tip of the second toe. The channel's passage through the mandible partly explains how stomach heat can affect the mouth. The tongue fur is closely related to the stomach since it is considered to be a result of the upward steaming of stomach qi. **2.** An abbreviation for *stomach qi*. See also STOMACH DUCT. [26: 438] [6: 85]

stomach channel 胃经 *wèi jīng*: See FOOT YANG BRIGHTNESS STOMACH CHANNEL. [26: 440]

stomach cold 胃寒 *wèi hán*: See STOMACH VACUITY COLD; STOMACH REPLETION COLD. [26: 440]

stomach cold and intestinal heat 胃寒肠热 *wèi hán cháng rè*: Stomach cold preventing the normal decomposition of food, with intestinal heat characterized by dry stool or diarrhea. It occurs in the beginning of gastrointestinal disease and is marked by indigestion, abdominal distention, and dry stool giving way to diarrhea. [97: 399]

stomach cold hiccough 胃寒呃逆 *wèi hán è nì*: See COLD HICCOUGH. [27: 410]

stomach cold malign obstruction 胃寒恶阻 *wei hán è zǔ*: MALIGN OBSTRUCTION (vomiting in pregnancy) due to stomach vacuity cold and upsurge of cold rheum. Stomach cold malign obstruction is characterized by vomiting of clear fluid, fatigue, fear of cold, and a desire for warm drinks.

MED Treat by warming the stomach and checking vomiting with Saussurea and Amomum Six Gentlemen Decoction (*xiāng shā liù jūn zǐ tāng*).

ACU Base treatment mainly on CV and ST. Select CV-12 (*zhōng wǎn*, Center Stomach Duct), PC-6 (*nèi guān*, Inner Pass), ST-36 (*zú sān lǐ*, Leg Three Li), SP-4 (*gōng sūn*, Yellow Emperor), BL-20 (*pí shū*, Spleen Transport), and BL-21 (*wèi shū*, Stomach Transport). Needle with supplementation and add moxa. [26: 440]

stomach cough 胃咳 *wèi ké*: COUGH in bouts accompanied by retching and, in severe cases, by vomiting of roundworm. [27: 380] [97: 396]

stomach disease 胃病 *wèi bìng*: Any morbid condition of the stomach. Stomach disease is attributable to such factors as dietary irregularities (irregular eating habits, predilection for hot spicy or sweet fatty foods, excessive alcohol consumption, excessive consumption of raw or cold foods, voracious eating), cold or heat evils, or taxation fatigue, other illnesses etc.

Stomach Disease Patterns

Simple patterns

STOMACH VACUITY COLD (*wèi yáng xū*)

STOMACH REPLETION COLD (*wèi shí hán*)

FOOD STAGNATING IN THE STOMACH DUCT (*shí zhì wèi wǎn (guǎn)*)

STOMACH YIN VACUITY (*wèi yīn xū*)

STOMACH HEAT (*wèi rè*)

STOMACH QI ASCENDING COUNTERFLOW (*wèi qì shàng nì*)

Combined patterns

STRONG STOMACH AND WEAK SPLEEN (*wèi qiáng pí ruò*)

LIVER-STOMACH DISHARMONY (*gān wèi bù hé*)

EXUBERANT LUNG-STOMACH HEAT (*fèi wèi rè shèng*)

GASTROINTESTINAL ACCUMULATION (*wèi cháng jī*)

GASTROINTESTINAL HEAT BIND (*rè jié wèi cháng*)

EXUBERANT HEART-STOMACH FIRE (*xīn wèi huǒ shèng*)

LIVER-STOMACH DISHARMONY (*gān wèi bù hé*)

Stomach cold is the manifestation of yin cold congealing in the stomach which arises from catching cold in the abdomen, excessive consumption of raw or cold foods (vacuity), or from damage to the center by taxation fatigue and contraction of cold evil (vacuity, vacuity/repletion). It is characterized either by acute crampy pain or by continuous mild stomach duct pain. In either case exacerbated by exposure to cold and relieved by warmth. Other signs include bland taste in the mouth, absence of thirst, pale tongue with glossy white tongue fur, and a slow pulse that may be stringlike. In some cases there is lassitude of spirit and lack of strength, lack of warmth in the limbs; in others there may be gurgling of water in the stomach and upflow of clear fluid. See STOMACH REPLETION COLD; STOMACH VACUITY COLD. **Food stagnating in the stomach duct** arises when food is not decomposed in the stomach and is attributed to dietary irregularities such as voracious eating and drinking. Spleen-stomach vacuity with impaired movement and transformation is a predisposing factor. Signs include distention and oppression in the stomach duct with pain in severe cases, belching and swallowing of upflowing acid, vomiting of sour putrid matter, relief from distention and pain by vomiting, and a thick slimy tongue fur with a slippery pulse. In some cases, there is passing of flatus and thin stool that is putrid, sour, or foul-smelling. **Stomach yin vacuity** is the manifestation of stomach yin depletion that occurs in enduring illness or in advanced stages of febrile disease, or that arises from predilection for hot spicy foods, constrained emotions, or depressed qi transforming into heat. It is characterized by dull pain in the stomach duct, no desire to eat even when hungry, dry mouth and throat, dry bound stool, red tongue with little liquid, and a rapid fine pulse. In some cases, there may be glomus in the stomach duct or dry retching. **Stomach heat** is the manifestation of intense fire heat in the stomach attributable to a) a predilection for hot spicy or rich fatty foods that engender fire, b) constrained emotions giving rise to depressed qi, which then transforms into fire, or c) heat evil invading the inner body. It is characterized by scorching stomach duct pain, clamoring stomach with swallowing of upflowing acid, dry bound stool, short voidings of reddish urine, a red tongue with yellow fur, and a slippery rapid pulse. In some cases, there is immediate vomiting of ingested foods or thirst with desire for cold drinks with swift digestion with rapid hungering. When stomach fire flames upward, signs are observed such as sore swollen and even ulcerated gums, spontaneous bleeding of the gums, and bad breath. Combined stomach disease patterns include LIVER-STOMACH DISHARMONY, GASTROINTESTINAL ACCUMULATION, EXUBERANT LUNG-STOMACH HEAT, and GASTROINTESTINAL HEAT BIND. **Stomach qi ascending counterflow** is impaired harmonious downbearing of the stomach characterized by nausea, vomiting, belching, or hiccough. It results from a number of causes including cold, heat, phlegm, foul turbidity, food stagnation, and gastrointestinal qi stagnation, and can occur in any stomach disease. [26: 438]

stomach disharmony 胃不和 *wèi bù hé*: DISHARMONY OF STOMACH QI. [26: 437]

stomach disharmony sleeplessness 胃不和不得卧 *wèi bù hé bù dé wò*: From *A Unified Treatise on Diseases, Patterns, and Remedies According to the Three Causes (sān yīn jí yī bìng zhèng fāng lùn)*. See WHEN THE STOMACH IS IN DISHARMONY, THERE IS UNQUIET SLEEP. See SLEEPLESSNESS.

stomach dispersion 胃消 *wèi xiāo*: CENTER DISPERSION. [26: 438] [27: 424] [97: 396]

stomach domain 胃家 *wèi jiā*: The stomach, small intestine, and large intestine. *The Magic Pivot (líng shū, běn shū)* states, "The large intestine and small intestine both belong to the stomach, which is the foot yang brightness (*yáng míng*)." Commenting on *On Cold Damage (shāng hán lùn)*, Zhang Xu-Gu states, "Stomach domain means the interconnected system of the yang brightness and bowels." ◇ Chin 家 *jiā*, home, family. [44: 24] [51: 265]

stomach domain repletion 胃家实 *wèi jiā shí*: Yang brightness repletion. *On Cold Damage (shāng hán lùn, yáng míng bìng piān)* states, "Disease of the yang brightness is stomach domain repletion." See STOMACH DOMAIN. [51: 265]

stomach duct 胃脘 *wèi wǎn (guǎn)*, 脘 *wǎn (guǎn)*: Synonym: *venter (obs)*. The stomach cavity and adjoining sections of the small intestine and gullet. The stomach duct is divided into the upper, center, and lower stomach ducts. ◇ Chin 脘 pronounced as *wǎn* or *guǎn*, the stomach as a physical organ. In pre-modern literature, the character is sometimes written as 管 *guǎn*, tube pipe . [26: 439] [27: 22] [97: 396]

stomach duct pain 胃脘痛 *wèi wǎn (guǎn) tòng*, 胃脘疼痛 *wèi wǎn (guǎn) téng tòng*: Synonyms: *stomach pain; pain below the heart; heart pain*. Pain in the region of the STOMACH DUCT (epigastrium) and the [REGION] BELOW THE HEART (pit of the stomach). It arises a) when general vacuity, taxation fatigue, or enduring illness lead to spleen-stomach vacuity and insufficiency of center qi preventing normal movement and transformation, b) when disease evils invade the stomach (cold evil, raw or cold foods, rich fatty or hot spicy foods) and cause food to stagnate, and c) when anxiety and anger impair liver free coursing so that liver qi invades the stomach and obstructs normal qi dynamic. [WMC] epigastric pain. A broad distinction is made between EXTERNAL CONTRACTION STOMACH DUCT PAIN, which is caused by externally contracted evils, and INTERNAL DAMAGE STOMACH DUCT PAIN, which is a general term for stomach duct pain due other causes (vacuity, evils arising within the body, and dietary irregularities). [26: 439] [50: 1081]

stomach duct welling-abscess 胃脘痈 *wèi wǎn (guǎn) yōng*: WELLING-ABSCESS OF THE STOMACH DUCT.

stomach fire 胃火 *wèi huǒ*: **1.** The warming force of the stomach. **2.** A fire pattern of the stomach. **Comparison:** "Stomach heat" is a general term for morbid conditions of the stomach manifesting as patterns. "Stomach fire" refers specifically to such conditions causing marked upper body signs such as bleeding gums or toothache. See STOMACH HEAT.

stomach fire toothache 胃火牙痛 *wèi huǒ yá tòng*: Toothache attributable to stomach fire rising along the hand and foot yang brightness (*yáng míng*) channels, which pass through the lower and upper jaws respectively. See TOOTHACHE.

stomach governs decomposition 胃主腐熟 *wèi zhǔ fǔ shóu*: The stomach is responsible for breaking down food (grain and water) so that its essence can be extracted by the spleen. More at STOMACH GOVERNS INTAKE. [6: 87] [27: 48] [97: 398]

stomach governs downbearing of the turbid 胃主降浊 *wèi zhǔ jiàng zhuó*: The stomach sends food down to the small intestine. The spleen removes essence of grain and water, which is the "clear" part of the food. What remains is the "turbid" part, which after further transformation, is discharged from the anus. [6: 88] [27: 48] [97: 398]

stomach governs intake 胃主受纳 *wèi zhǔ shòu nà*: The function of the stomach is to receive ingested foods and perform the initial stage of digestion. Normal performance of this function is dependent on the "free downflow" of food to the small intestine. It is less important than the spleen, and to some extent dominated by it since "the spleen moves the fluids of the stomach." Impairment of stomach function may take the form of stomach qi disharmony, characterized by distention and fullness in the upper abdomen, torpid intake (sluggishness of the intake function manifesting in poor appetite and indigestion), stomach pain, or stomach qi ascending counterflow, presenting signs of nausea, vomiting, belching, or hiccough. [6: 88] [27: 48] [97: 398]

stomach heart pain 胃心痛 *wèi xīn tòng*: See STOMACH DUCT PAIN. [26: 437]

stomach heat 胃热 *wèi rè*: Any heat pattern of the stomach. It arises when evil heat enters the interior (see EXTERNALLY CONTRACTED HEAT (FEBRILE) DISEASE PATTERN IDENTIFICATION), when the stomach is damaged by excessive consumption of fried or otherwise rich fatty foods or hot spicy food, or when liver fire invades the stomach. Most cases of stomach heat are repletion heat. For stomach vacuity heat, see STOMACH YIN VACUITY. Stomach heat can take a number of forms: (1) Affecting the stomach's function of intake, it can manifest in swift digestion and rapid hungering. (2) Affecting the stomach downbearing, it manifests as pain or burning sensation in the stomach duct, vomiting, clamoring stomach, and hard stool. (3) Stomach heat can manifest in up-

per body signs such as bad breath, painful swollen gums, gaping gums, or bleeding gums. In such cases, it is referred to as *stomach fire* or *upbearing stomach fire*. Whatever form stomach heat takes, it is invariably attended by a bitter taste in the mouth, dry mouth, red tongue with yellow fur, and a rapid slippery pulse. MED Treatment involves clearing the stomach and draining fire. Commonly used medicinals include coptis (*huáng lián*), gypsum (*shí gāo*), phragmites (*lú gēn*), gardenia (*shān zhī zǐ*), scutellaria (*huáng qín*), and rhubarb (*dà huáng*). Representative formulas: Stomach-Clearing Powder (*qīng wèi sǎn*) and Jade Lady Brew (*yù nǚ jiān*). Intense (i.e., severe) invariably causes damage to yin fluids of the stomach, so that the judicious admixture of medicinals that nourish yin and engender liquid is indicated. These include dried/fresh rehmannia (*shēng dì huáng*), ophiopogon (*mài mén dōng*), and scrophularia (*xuán shēn*). ACU Base treatment mainly on ST points. Main points: ST-44 (*nèi tíng*, Inner Court), ST-36 (*zú sān lǐ*, Leg Three Li), and LI-4 (*hé gǔ*, Union Valley). For stomach repletion heat, add ST-45 (*lì duì*, Severe Mouth); needle with drainage. For vacuity heat, add BL-21 (*wèi shū*, Stomach Transport), KI-6 (*zhào hǎi*, Shining Sea), and SP-6 (*sān yīn jiāo*, Three Yin Intersection); needle with even supplementation and drainage. [27: 181] [6: 181] [116: 90]

stomach heat hiccough 胃热呃逆 *wèi rè è nì*: See HEAT HICCOUGH. [27: 410]

stomach heat malign obstruction 胃热恶阻 *wei rè è zǔ*: MALIGN OBSTRUCTION (vomiting in pregnancy) due to stomach heat. In pregnancy, thoroughfare (*chōng*) vessel qi is exuberant and easily causes nondownbearing of stomach qi when stomach heat is present. Stomach heat pregnancy vomiting is characterized by vomiting, heart vexation, tidal reddening of the face, thirst with a liking for cool drinks, and constipation. MED Clear stomach heat, downbear counterflow, and check vomiting. Use perilla leaf (*zǐ sū yè*), coptis (*huáng lián*), pinellia (*bàn xià*), bamboo shavings (*zhú rú*), and tangerine peel (*chén pí*). ACU Base treatment mainly on CV, PC, SP, ST, and LI. Select CV-12 (*zhōng wǎn*, Center Stomach Duct), PC-6 (*nèi guān*, Inner Pass), SP-4 (*gōng sūn*, Yellow Emperor), ST-44 (*nèi tíng*, Inner Court), LI-4 (*hé gǔ*, Union Valley), and ST-36 (*zú sān lǐ*, Leg Three Li). Needle with drainage. [26: 440] [59: 117] [46: 596]

stomach heat with rapid digestion 胃热杀谷 *wèi rè shā gǔ*: Stomach heat giving rise to accelerated decomposition of food and a tendency to get hungry quickly. See SWIFT DIGESTION AND RAPID HUNGERING. [27: 158]

stomach is the sea of grain and water 胃为水谷之海 *wèi wéi shuǐ gǔ zhī hǎi*: The stomach is the first collecting place of ingested food (grain and water). [26: 154] [27: 21] [97: 132]

stomach juices 胃汁 *wèi zhī*: STOMACH YIN.

stomach liquid 胃津 *wèi jīn*: STOMACH YIN.

stomach malaria 胃疟 *wèi nüè*: *Synonym: food malaria.* A kind of MALARIA described in *Elementary Questions* (*sù wèn, cì nüè piān*) as being characterized by rapid hungering and inability to eat, with propping fullness and enlarged abdomen after eating. [22: 245]

stomach pain 胃痛 *wèi tòng*: STOMACH DUCT PAIN.

stomach qi 胃气 *wèi qì*: **1.** The power manifest in stomach function. See STOMACH GOVERNS INTAKE; STOMACH GOVERNS DECOMPOSITION; STOMACH QI GOVERNS DOWNBEARING. Impairments of the stomach's governing of downbearing include DISHARMONY OF STOMACH QI and STOMACH QI ASCENDING COUNTERFLOW. **2.** Activity of the stomach and the spleen in general. **3.** Stomach (and spleen) function as reflected in the appetite. A healthy patient who has a good appetite is said to "have stomach qi," a patient with a poor appetite is said to have "weak stomach qi," whereas a patient who is severely ill and cannot eat is said to "have no stomach qi." Thus, it is often said, "The presence of stomach qi means life; the absence of stomach qi is death." See APPETITE. **4.** The strength of the spleen and stomach manifesting in the pulse. See STOMACH, SPIRIT, AND ROOT; PULSE BEREFT OF STOMACH QI. [26: 438] [27: 47] [97: 395]

stomach qi ascending counterflow 胃气上逆 *wèi qì shàng nì*: The chief manifestation of impaired harmonious downbearing of the stomach that causes nausea, vomiting, belching, or hiccough and that results from a number of causes including cold, heat, phlegm, foul turbidity, food stagnation, and gastrointestinal qi stagnation. Stomach qi ascending counterflow is a pattern that can occur in any stomach disease. Counterflow occurring in a cold pattern is usually characterized by a pale tongue, white face, vomiting of clear fluid, or vomiting in the evening of food ingested in the morning. Where heat is present, signs include red tongue with yellow fur, vomiting of sour or bitter fluid, and immediate vomiting of ingested food. If phlegm is the cause, a slimy tongue fur, repeated ejection of phlegm-drool, and occasionally dizziness are observed. Stomach qi ascending counterflow due to foul turbidity usually occurs in hot weather, is sudden in onset, and is characterized by abdominal pain, ungratified desire to vomit, and agonizing distention and oppression in the stomach duct. Where stomach qi ascending counterflow is a result of food stagnation, there is usually a history of food damage, and signs such as sour, putrid

vomitus, with improvement brought by vomiting. Finally, stomach qi ascending counterflow owing to gastrointestinal qi stagnation is characterized by glomus in the chest, abdominal pain, and belching. [MED] Harmonize the stomach and downbear counterflow. Frequently used medicinals include: pinellia (*bàn xià*), tangerine peel (*chén pí*), evodia (*wú zhū yú*), fresh ginger (*shēng jiāng*), coptis (*huáng lián*), bamboo shavings (*zhú rú*), inula flower (*xuán fù huā*), and hematite (*dài zhě shí*). Treatment should also be directed toward eliminating the relevant cause of disease, using methods such as warming the stomach, clearing heat, transforming phlegm, repelling turbidity, abductive dispersion, and rectifying qi. Stomach qi ascending counterflow due to stomach cold can be treated with Evodia Decoction (*wú zhū yú tāng*) or Clove and Persimmon Decoction (*dīng xiāng shì dì tāng*) (mainly used for hiccough). When the cause is stomach heat, Left-Running Metal Pill (*zuǒ jīn wán*) can be used. Minor Pinellia Decoction Plus Poria (Hoelen) (*xiǎo bàn xià jiā fú líng tāng*) or Gallbladder-Warming Decoction (*wēn dǎn tāng*) can be used to treat patterns caused by phlegm, and Gallbladder-Warming Decoction supplemented with coptis (*huáng lián*) can be used if an added heat complication is identified. Foul turbidity patterns are treated with Jade Pivot Elixir (*yù shū dān*). Harmony-Preserving Pill (*bǎo hé wán*) is appropriate for food stagnation. Inula and Hematite Decoction (*xuán fù huā dài zhě shí tāng*) and its variations can be used where qi stagnation is the cause. [ACU] Treatment varies according to the cause. The alarm and lower uniting points of ST, CV-12 (*zhōng wǎn*, Center Stomach Duct) and ST-36 (*zú sān lǐ*, Leg Three Li), and PC-6 (*nèi guān*, Inner Pass), can be selected as the main points to harmonize the stomach, downbear counterflow, and check vomiting. For cold patterns, add stomach-warming points BL-21 (*wèi shū*, Stomach Transport), CV-13 (*shàng wǎn*, Upper Stomach Duct), SP-4 (*gōng sūn*, Yellow Emperor), and CV-4 (*guān yuán*, Pass Head); needle with drainage and add moxa. For heat patterns, add stomach-heat-clearing points LI-4 (*hé gǔ*, Union Valley), LI-11 (*qū chí*, Pool at the Bend), and ST-44 (*nèi tíng*, Inner Court); needle with drainage. For phlegm, add phlegm-transforming counterflow-downbearing points ST-40 (*fēng lóng*, Bountiful Bulge), CV-17 (*shān zhōng*, Chest Center), SP-4 (*gōng sūn*, Yellow Emperor), and BL-20 (*pí shū*, Spleen Transport); needle with drainage or with even supplementation and drainage, and add moxa. For food complication, add food-dispersing stagnation-abducting points CV-10 (*xià wǎn*, Lower Stomach Duct), Li Inner Court (*lǐ nèi tíng*), and CV-21 (*xuán jī*, Jade Swivel); needle with drainage. For foul turbidity, add dampness-transforming turbidity-dispelling points LI-4 (*hé gǔ*, Union Valley), LI-11 (*qū chí*, Pool at the Bend), and SP-9 (*yīn líng quán*, Yin Mound Spring); needle with drainage. For qi stagnation, add qi-rectifying points CV-6 (*qì hǎi*, Sea of Qi), BL-20 (*pí shū*, Spleen Transport), LR-3 (*tài chōng*, Supreme Surge), and SP-4 (*gōng sūn*, Yellow Emperor); needle with even supplementation and drainage or with drainage. [6: 182] [27: 157] [97: 398] [46: 595–7, 602, 658] [14: 98] [113: 18, 71]

stomach qi governs downbearing 胃气主降 *wèi qì zhǔ jiàng*: The stomach decomposes food and bears it down to the intestines. The downward movement of stomach qi stands in complementary and opposite relationship to spleen qi, which governs upbearing (i.e., carries the essence of grain and water upward to be distributed around the body). [6: 88]

stomach qi pain 胃气痛 *wèi qì tòng*: STOMACH DUCT PAIN due to disturbance of qi dynamic in the stomach duct. See STOMACH DUCT PAIN. [50: 1080]

stomach qi stagnation 胃气滞 *wèi qì zhì*: See DISHARMONY OF STOMACH QI.

stomach qi vacuity 胃气虚 *wèi qì xū*: Impairment of the stomach's governing of food intake and decomposition. Stomach qi vacuity is attributed to persistent or repeated dietary irregularities, to splenic movement and transformation failure from insufficiency of spleen qi or to constitutional vacuity, or to damage to original qi through enduring illness. Disturbance of food intake and decomposition is characterized by torpid intake and reduced eating, tastelessness of food, and distention and fullness in the stomach duct. Stomach qi vacuity affects harmonious downbearing, and when stomach qi fails to bear downward and carry food with it, the qi ascends counterflow, causing distention and pain in the stomach duct or nausea and vomiting, or belching and hiccough. [36: 303] [27: 157] [97: 397]

stomach qi vacuity cold 胃气虚寒 *wèi qì xū hán*: STOMACH VACUITY COLD.

stomach reflux 反胃 *fǎn wèi*, 胃反 *wèi fǎn*, 翻胃 *fān wèi*: **1.** A disease pattern characterized by distention and fullness after eating, by vomiting in the evening of food ingested in the morning or by vomiting in the morning of food ingested in the evening (i.e., vomiting a long time after eating), untransformed food in the vomitus, lassitude of spirit, and lack of bodily strength. Its principal cause is spleen-stomach vacuity cold, but it may also be due to debilitation of the life gate fire or to dual vacuity of qi and yin. **Spleen-stomach vacuity cold:** The principal signs of stomach reflux, i.e., distention and fullness after eating, vomiting in the morning of food ingested in the evening

and vomiting in the evening of food ingested in the morning, untransformed food in the vomitus, and a feeling of comfort after vomiting indicate spleen-stomach vacuity cold preventing grain and water from being decomposed so that they remain in the stomach. Lassitude of spirit and lack of strength, as well as a lusterless complexion, indicate damage to qi by enduring vomiting and inability to produce essence from grain and water. A pale tongue with thin tongue fur and a forceless moderate fine pulse are further signs of spleen-stomach vacuity cold. MED Warm the center and fortify the spleen; downbear qi and harmonize the stomach. Use Clove and Aquilaria Diaphragm-Freeing Decoction (*dīng chén tòu gé tāng*). ACU Base treatment mainly on back transport points, CV, and ST. Select BL-20 (*pí shū*, Spleen Transport), BL-21 (*wèi shū*, Stomach Transport), CV-12 (*zhōng wǎn*, Center Stomach Duct), LR-13 (*zhāng mén*, Camphorwood Gate), CV-6 (*qì hǎi*, Sea of Qi), ST-36 (*zú sān lǐ*, Leg Three Li), and Central Eminence (*zhōng kuí*)ⓜ. The last point should only be moxaed, whereas the other points should be both needled to supplement and moxaed. **Debilitation of the life gate fire** patterns are marked by the addition of bright white facial complexion, aversion to cold, lack of warmth in the extremities, a pale enlarged tongue, and a fine sunken pulse. Other signs may include dizziness, tinnitus, limp lumbus and knees, impotence, seminal efflux, and profuse urination at night or inhibited urination. MED Warm and supplement the life gate using Cinnamon Bark and Aconite Eight-Ingredient Pill (*guì fù bā wèi wán*). ACU Base treatment mainly on back transport points, CV, and GV points. Select BL-23 (*shèn shū*, Kidney Transport), GV-4 (*mìng mén*, Life Gate), KI-3 (*tài xī*, Great Ravine), BL-20 (*pí shū*, Spleen Transport), CV-4 (*guān yuán*, Pass Head), ST-25 (*tiān shū*, Celestial Pivot), ST-36 (*zú sān lǐ*, Leg Three Li), and CV-12 (*zhōng wǎn*, Center Stomach Duct); needle with supplementation and add moxa. **Dual vacuity of qi and yin** from febrile disease, from vomiting for long periods or from inappropriate use of harsh warm, hot, or drying medicinals causes stomach reflux with poor appetite, dry bound stool, heart palpitations, spontaneous sweating, scorching heat in the hands and feet, shortness of breath, fatigue, dry mouth and lips, red tongue without fur or with peeling tongue fur, and a rapid vacuous fine pulse. MED Boost qi and nourish yin; downbear counterflow and check vomiting. Use Major Pinellia Decoction (*dà bàn xià tāng*). ACU Base treatment mainly on back transport points, ST, SP, PC, and KI. Select BL-20 (*pí shū*, Spleen Transport), BL-21 (*wèi shū*, Stomach Transport), PC-6 (*nèi guān*, Inner Pass), SP-6 (*sān yīn jiāo*, Three Yin Intersection), ST-36 (*zú sān lǐ*, Leg Three Li),

CV-12 (*zhōng wǎn*, Center Stomach Duct), CV-6 (*qì hǎi*, Sea of Qi), KI-6 (*zhào hǎi*, Shining Sea), and KI-3 (*tài xī*, Great Ravine); needle with supplementation. **2.** DYSPHAGIA-OCCLUSION (*yē gé*). [80: 296] [26: 170–1] [27: 411] [97: 115] [113: 82] [37: 290] [92: No. 197]

stomach repletion 胃实 *wèi shí*: A pattern characterized by distention and pain in the stomach duct, belching, constipation, heart vexation, and late afternoon tidal heat [effusion], and arising when accumulated gastrointestinal heat damages liquid and causes stagnation of stomach qi. [97: 397] [27: 365]

stomach repletion cold 胃实寒 *wèi shí hán*: A disease pattern caused by cold evil invading the stomach. This may be the result of excessive consumption of cold raw foods or external cold (EXTERNAL COLD INVADING THE STOMACH). The chief signs are acute cold pain in the stomach duct that is exacerbated by exposure to cold and relieved by warmth. Secondary signs include glomus and distention in the stomach duct, nausea with vomiting that relieves pain, as well as physical cold and cold limbs. Excessive consumption of raw and cold foods causes cold to accumulate in the center. Careless living such as eating in the wind and sleeping in the dew causes cold evil to invade the stomach and yin cold to congeal and stagnate. Cold causes contraction, hence the cold pain in the stomach duct. Exposure to cold exacerbates the congealing, whereas warmth causes the cold qi to dissipate. When cold congeals in the stomach, qi dynamic is obstructed, and the harmonious downbearing of the stomach is impaired, hence the glomus and distention in the stomach duct. Vomiting helps to get rid of the cold repletion evil and temporarily restores qi dynamic to normal, hence relief from pain after vomiting. When cold evil is in the stomach, it encumbers stomach yang and prevents it from warming the limbs and the FLESHY EXTERIOR, hence the physical cold and cold limbs. The white tongue fur and stringlike or tight sunken pulse are signs of disease due to cold evil. ⊡MED⊡ Warm the stomach and dissipate cold. Use Lesser Galangal and Cyperus Pill (*liáng fù wán*) or Agastache/Patchouli Qi-Righting Powder (*huò xiāng zhèng qì sǎn*). ⊡ACU⊡ Base treatment mainly on ST points. Select CV-12 (*zhōng wǎn*, Center Stomach Duct), ST-36 (*zú sān lǐ*, Leg Three Li), ST-44 (*nèi tíng*, Inner Court), ST-21 (*liáng mén*, Beam Gate), and PC-6 (*nèi guān*, Inner Pass). Needle with even supplementation and drainage or with drainage, and add large amounts of moxa. For external cold invading the stomach, add GB-20 (*fēng chí*, Wind Pool), TB-5 (*wài guān*, Outer Pass), LI-4 (*hé gǔ*, Union Valley), and BL-11 (*dà zhù*, Great Shuttle). [116: 95] [43: 280] [46: 595, 602, 658, 660]

stomach repletion hiccough 胃实呃逆 *wèi shí è nì*: See REPLETION HICCOUGH. [27: 410]

stomach, spirit, and root 胃、神、根 *wèi, shén, gēn*: Stomach function, general vitality, and fundamental constitution as reflected in the pulse. A healthy pulse is regular, smooth, and harmonious, indicating the presence of stomach qi. It is also supple and powerful, indicating the presence of spirit. It can also be felt at the deep level and at all three positions of the pulse (inch, bar, and cubit), which is a sign of the presence of root. In disease, these three factors help to determine the severity. When despite illness the pulse has stomach, spirit, and root, recovery is possible. [27: 198] [27: 198]

stomach stagnation 胃滞 *wèi zhì*: STOMACH QI STAGNATION. [27: 157] [97: 397]

stomach vacuity 胃虚 *wèi xū*: Any vacuity pattern of the stomach. See STOMACH YIN VACUITY and STOMACH QI VACUITY. [27: 156] [27: 157] [97: 397]

stomach vacuity cold 胃虚寒 *wèi xū hán*: Synonyms: *stomach qi vacuity cold*; *stomach yang vacuity*. A disease pattern characterized by stomach signs such as stomach pain and vomiting, and vacuity cold signs. It can be the result of damage to stomach qi by excessive consumption of raw and cold foods or other dietary irregularities. It may also occur when constrained emotions cause liver qi to invade the stomach and, in time, damages its qi. The stomach pain usually occurs on an empty stomach, and is relieved by eating or by pressure. Vomiting of clear cold sour fluid is sometimes observed. General signs include lusterless complexion, aversion to cold, lack of warmth in the extremities, and a pale enlarged tongue. The pulse is soggy, but may become stringlike or tight during pain attacks. Vacuity cold gives rise to signs of stomach qi disharmony such as belching and acid upflow. Stomach qi vacuity cold characterized by stomach duct pain that may be exacerbated by contraction of external cold. It differs, however, from fulminant strike by cold evil (from catching cold or from excessive consumption of raw or cold foods), as it is less sudden and violent in onset, of longer duration, and characterized by a prominence of vacuity signs. Fulminant strike by cold evil is associated with pronounced cold signs, less pronounced vacuity signs, and a more sudden onset. Compare STOMACH REPLETION COLD. ⊡WMC⊡ Stomach qi vacuity cold is often seen in diseases described by Western medicine as ulcers and gastric neurosis. ⊡MED⊡ Fortify the center and warm the stomach. Center-fortifying medicinals include malt sugar (*yí táng*), white peony (*bái sháo yào*), licorice (*gān cǎo*), and jujube (*dà zǎo*). Stomach-warming medicinals include cinnamon twig (*guì* *zhī*), fresh ginger (*shēng jiāng*), lesser galangal (*gāo liáng jiāng*), and evodia (*wú zhū yú*). A basic formula is Minor Center-Fortifying Decoction (*xiǎo jiàn zhōng tāng*), which fortifies the center and warms the stomach, as well harmonizing construction and relieving pain. For pronounced qi vacuity, astragalus (*huáng qí*) can be added to form Astragalus Center-Fortifying Decoction (*huáng qí jiàn zhōng tāng*). For pronounced qi stagnation and pain, add cyperus (*xiāng fù zǐ*), toosendan (*chuān liàn zǐ*), corydalis (*yán hú suǒ*), saussurea (*mù xiāng*), and tangerine peel (*chén pí*). For pronounced acid upflow, add cuttlefish bone (*hǎi piāo xiāo*) and ark shell (*wǎ léng zǐ*), which have an antacid effect. ACU Base treatment mainly on ST points. Select BL-20 (*pí shū*, Spleen Transport), BL-21 (*wèi shū*, Stomach Transport), CV-12 (*zhōng wǎn*, Center Stomach Duct), LR-13 (*zhāng mén*, Camphorwood Gate), ST-36 (*zú sān lǐ*, Leg Three Li), ST-44 (*nèi tíng*, Inner Court), ST-21 (*liáng mén*, Beam Gate), and ST-37 (*shàng jù xū*, Upper Great Hollow). Needle with supplementation and large amounts of moxa. Selection of points according to signs: For pronounced qi vacuity, add CV-6 (*qì hǎi*, Sea of Qi). For pronounced qi stagnation, add CV-17 (*shān zhōng*, Chest Center), PC-6 (*nèi guān*, Inner Pass), and LR-3 (*tài chōng*, Supreme Surge). See also SPLEEN-STOMACH VACUITY COLD. [6: 181] [116: 87] [46: 586, 660]

stomach vacuity hiccough 胃虚呃逆 *wèi xū è nì*: See VACUITY HICCOUGH. [27: 410]

stomach welling-abscess 胃痈 *wèi yōng*: WELLING-ABSCESS OF THE STOMACH DUCT. [26: 440] [50: 1081]

stomach wind 胃风 *wèi fēng*: **1.** An ancient disease name from *Elementary Questions* (*sù wèn*). A stomach disease that is caused by invasion of wind evil and characterized by sweating at the neck, aversion to wind, abdominal fullness, and diarrhea after taking cold food or drink. MED Dispel wind and dissipate cold; warm the center and rectify qi. Use formulas such as Tsaoko Pill (*dòu kòu wán*) or Stomach Wind Decoction (*wèi fēng tāng*). **2.** Accumulated heat in the stomach engendering wind and giving rise to vomiting. [26: 437] [27: 411] [50: 1078]

stomach yang 胃阳 *wèi yáng*: The activity or function of the stomach. [26: 440] [27: 47] [97: 396]

stomach yang vacuity 胃阳虚 *wèi yáng xū*: STOMACH VACUITY COLD.

stomach yin 胃阴 *wèi yīn*: Synonyms: *stomach juices*; *stomach liquid*. The fluids of the stomach; the opposite of stomach yang. Stomach yin is necessary for maintaining normal intake and transformation of food. Stomach yin is easily damaged by exuberant lung-stomach heat in warm heat dis-

ease, causing heat effusion, dry mouth, dry pharynx, constipation, red tongue with scant fur, and a rapid fine pulse. *On Warm Heat* (*wēn rè lùn*) "When the tongue is crimson and shiny, stomach yin is depleted. This requires urgent use of cool sweet moisturizing items." [26: 439] [27: 48] [97: 396]

stomach yin depletion 胃阴亏虚 *wèi yīn kuī xū*: Synonym: *insufficiency of stomach yin*. See STOMACH YIN VACUITY.

stomach yin vacuity 胃阴虚 *wèi yīn xū*: The manifestation of insufficiency of stomach yin (stomach yin depletion), i.e., insufficiency of the yin humor of the stomach; attributed to intense stomach heat, spleen-stomach damp-heat, or damage to liquid in externally contracted febrile (heat disease); characterized by dry lips and mouth, desire for fluids, reduced food intake, dry stool, short voidings of scant urine, and, in severe cases, dry retching or hiccough, a dry crimson area in the center of the tongue, and a rapid fine pulse. MED Treat by nourishing stomach yin, combined where necessary with clearing heat and harmonizing the stomach. Commonly used medicinals include ophiopogon (*mài mén dōng*), Solomon's seal (*yù zhú*), adenophora/glehnia (*shā shēn*), dendrobium (*shí hú*), dried/fresh rehmannia (*shēng dì huáng*), and trichosanthes root (*tiān huā fěn*). Formulas include Ophiopogon Decoction (*mài mén dōng tāng*) and Stomach-Nourishing Decoction (*yǎng wèi tāng*). The former clears qi and fire ascending counterflow, whereas the latter restores stomach yin with cool sweet moistening medicinals. ACU Base treatment mainly on ST, CV, KI, and back transport points. Select ST-36 (*zú sān lǐ*, Leg Three Li), CV-12 (*zhōng wǎn*, Center Stomach Duct), ST-25 (*tiān shū*, Celestial Pivot), BL-21 (*wèi shū*, Stomach Transport), BL-20 (*pí shū*, Spleen Transport), KI-6 (*zhào hǎi*, Shining Sea), SP-6 (*sān yīn jiāo*, Three Yin Intersection), and ST-44 (*nèi tíng*, Inner Court); needle with supplementation. [6: 182] [26: 439] [27: 157] [97: 397] [46: 586] [37: 296]

stone-baking 焙 *bèi*: Heating medicinal materials on a slab (or in a pan) without allowing them to change color. [27: 324] [97: 591]

stone moth 石蛾 *shí é*: A persistent nipple moth observed most commonly in children before qi and the physical body have reached their fullness, and attributed to weakness of the organs creating susceptibility to external evils and the lodging of (mild) evil toxin in the throat that congeals and binds to produce swelling. WMC chronic tonsillitis. MED Treat with Throat-Clearing Diaphragm-Disinhibiting Decoction (*qīng yān lì gé tāng*) used in pill form. Pay attention to diet and way of life, appropriate warmth and coolness, and preventing contraction of evils to allow right to gain strength and thereby all the disease to be eliminated in time. See NIPPLE MOTH. [26: 195]

stone strangury 石淋 *shí lín*: Synonym: *sand strangury*. STRANGURY (painful, dribbling urination) with the passing of stones. Patterns with the passing of fine stones are sometimes called *sand strangury*; however, this distinction probably has no clinical significance. The pain radiates into the lesser abdomen and is relieved by the passing of stones. The urine is normally yellow or reddish, and sometimes contains blood. It is attributed to lower burner accumulated heat. ⃞WMC urinary calculus, especially cystolith (vesical calculus). ⃞MED Clear heat and flush stones with Single Sage Powder (*dú shèng săn*) and medicinals such as moneywort (*jīn qián căo*), gizzard lining (*jī nèi jīn*), and mallow seed (*dōng kuí zĭ*). ⃞ACU Base treatment mainly on the three yin channels of the foot and on the alarm and back transport points of BL (CV-3 and BL-28). Select BL-28 (*páng guāng shū*, Bladder Transport), CV-3 (*zhōng jí*, Central Pole), SP-9 (*yīn líng quán*, Yin Mound Spring), LR-2 (*xíng jiān*, Moving Between), KI-3 (*tài xī*, Great Ravine), BL-39 (*wĕi yáng*, Bend Yang), KI-6 (*zhào hăi*, Shining Sea) KI-2 (*rán gŭ*, Blazing Valley), and KI-12 (*dà hè*, Great Manifestation); needle with drainage. [26: 194] [46: 674] [27: 425] [97: 135]

stone water 石水 *shí shuĭ*: From *Elementary Questions* (*sù wèn, yīn yáng bié lùn*). **1.** WATER SWELLING that arises when liver-kidney yin cold causes water qi to gather in the lower burner. Signs include enlarged swollen lesser abdomen that is a hard as stone, distention and pain under the rib-side, abdominal fullness without panting, and a sunken pulse. **2.** SIMPLE ABDOMINAL DISTENTION. *Axioms of Medicine* (*yī mén fă lù, zhàng bìng lùn*) states, "Wherever there is a concretion, a conglomeration, an accumulation lump or glomus lump, this is the root of distention disease. With the passage of days and months, the abdomen becomes as large as a winnowing basket or stone jar. This is called simple abdominal distention... What [Zhang] Jing-Yue called "stone water" is precisely this." **3.** MOUNTING-CONGLOMERATION (*shàn jiă*) type disease patterns. [26: 191] [27: 419] [97: 135]

stool 大便 *dà biàn*, 大溲 *dà sōu*, 屎 *shĭ*, 矢 *shĭ*: **1.** Waste discharged from the anus. Abnormalities of the stool are helpul in diagnosis. Malodorous sloppy yellow stool is associated with dampheat. Frequent evacuation of small amounts of sticky stool containing blood is a sign of DYSENTERY. Watery stool containing improperly digested food or DUCK'S SLOP may indicate colddamp. Stool with bright red blood indicates heavy

bleeding, usually in the anus or rectum is called PROXIMAL BLEEDING, i.e., bleeding in the digestive tract close to the anus, and is observed in INTESTINAL WIND, HEMORRHOIDS, ANAL FISTULA, and VISCERAL TOXIN.[3] INTESTINAL WIND BLEEDING. Blackish duck stool indicates DISTAL BLEEDING, i.e., bleeding in the digestive tract far from the anus, and is attributable to a variety of causes. Hard dry stool bearing the appearance of sheep droppings and accompanied by difficult defecation indicates dry intestines due to HEAT BIND and is generally associated with STOMACH REFLUX and DYSPHAGIA-OCCLUSION (*yē gé*). **2.** An act of defecation. [6: 127] [26: 46] [29: 202]

Stool

CONSTIPATION (*xiè xiè*)

DIARRHEA (*xiè xiè*)

    DUCK'S SLOP DIARRHEA (*táng xiè*)

    SIMULTANEOUS VOMITING AND DIARRHEA (*shàng tù xià xiè*)

    FECAL INCONTINENCE (*dà biàn shī jìn*)

DIFFICULT DEFECATION (*dà biàn nán*)

BLACK STOOL (*dà biàn hēi sè*)

BLOODY STOOL (*biàn xuē*)

STOOL CONTAINING PUS AND BLOOD (*dà biàn nóng xuè*)

STOOL IN THE URINE (*xiăo biàn chū fèn*)

TENESMUS (*lĭ jí hòu zhòng*)

---

stool containing pus and blood 大便脓血 *dà biàn nóng xuè*: Stool containing white sticky matter or red matter; a major sign of DYSENTERY. [92: No. 214]

stool in the urine 小便出粪 *xiăo biàn chū fèn*: The presence of particles of stool in the urine. A sign of COMMUNICATING BOWELS.

stoppage 不通 *bù tōng*: Synonym: *blockage*. Cessation of movement of body elements (qi, blood, fluids) and their derivatives phlegm and rheum, due either to intrinsic vacuity or to extrinsic obstruction. For example, qi may stop because it is vacuous, or may be stopped by static blood. Terms denoting specific forms of flow stoppage highlight the degree and nature of the stoppage. **Inhibition** (不利 *bù lì*) is a mild or partial stoppage or a difficult, halting flow, and is applied mainly to the movement of fluids (particularly urine) and the blood; it also describes motor impairment. See INHIBITED URINATION; INHIBITION OF LUNG QI. **Stagnation** (滞 *zhì*) describes the impaired movement of qi or of food. See QI STAGNATION; FOOD STAGNATION. **Stasis** (瘀 *yū*) most commonly denotes stagnation of blood, i.e., impairment or cessation of blood flow, and is attributable to heat, cold, qi stagnation, or injury; it sometimes describes cessation of movement resulting from exuberant heat. See BLOOD STASIS; BLOOD STASIS. **Depression** (郁 *yù*) describes stagnation of qi especially when due to affect damage (i.e., emotional causes); also describes stagnation of evils due either to qi stagnation or vacuity of right qi. See for example QI DEPRESSION; SIX DEPRESSIONS. **Bind** (*adj.* bound, 结 *jié*) describes the intensity of depression (particularly in the context of the emotions and liver qi), the concentration of evils and the hardening that results from either of these (e.g., phlegm nodes; hard bound stool). See BINDING DEPRESSION OF LIVER QI; CHEST BIND; DRY BOUND STOOL. **Accumulation** (积 *jī*) denotes the buildup of waste in the digestive tract. See FOOD ACCUMULATION. **Gathering** denotes the coming together in one place of evils. Both gathering and accumulation denote not only processes but specific abdominal masses. See CONCRETIONS, CONGLOMERATIONS, ACCUMULATIONS, AND GATHERINGS. **Collection** (停 *tíng*) usually denotes buildup of water in specific locations, particularly in the region of the stomach. See for example COLLECTING RHEUM RIB-SIDE PAIN. **Amassment** (蓄 *xù*) describes buildup of blood or water. See BLOOD AMASSMENT; COLD DAMAGE BLOOD AMASSMENT PATTERN. COLD DAMAGE WATER AMASSMENT PATTERN. **Congestion** (壅 *yōng*) denotes clogging by exuberant evils, especially in the lung. **Block** (闭 *bì*) denotes failure of body elements to escape through the exterior (e.g., fecal block, menstrual block, internal heat block); it is the opposite of insecurity insofar as the latter denotes failure to retain blood or fluids. **Obstruction** (阻、阻遏 *zǔ, zǔ è*) denotes the inhibitive effect of a substantial evil on pathways (e.g., the interstices) or bowels and viscera (e.g., the lung or spleen). **Impediment** (痹 *bì*) blockage (e.g., THROAT IMPEDIMENT), especially blockage and disturbance of channel flow, usually giving rise to signs such as numbness or pain. See IMPEDIMENT. ◇ Chin 不 *bù*, not; 通 *tōng*, get through, pervade, communicate.

straight treatment 正治 *zhèng zhì*: Synonym: *coacting treatment*. The principle of treatment whereby the nature and pathomechanism are addressed directly, as when a cold pattern is treated with hot medicinals and a heat pattern is treated with cold medicinals, or when vacuity patterns are treated by supplementing or repletion patterns are treated by attack. [50: 365]

straitened spleen 脾约 *pí yuē*: From *On Cold Damage* (*shāng hán lùn, biàn yáng míng bìng mài zhèng bìng zhì*). Constipation arising when splenic movement and transformation is impaired and the stool becomes dry. *The Annotated Cold Damage* (*zhù jiě shāng hán lùn*) states, "*Straitened* means tight of resources or constrained. A strong stomach and weak spleen constrains the fluids, preventing

their distribution in the four directions and allowing their transportation only to the bladder. This causes frequent urination and difficult defecation." [26: 748] [27: 413] [97: 559]

strangury 淋 *lín*: From *Elementary Questions* (*sù wèn, liù yuán zhèng jì dà lùn*). A disease pattern characterized by urinary urgency, frequent short painful rough voidings, and dribbling incontinence. Strangury is attributed to damp-heat gathering and pouring into the bladder. In persistent conditions or in elderly or weak patients, the cause may be center qi fall and kidney vacuity and impaired qi transformation. Distinction is made between STONE STRANGURY (which also includes sand strangury), QI STRANGURY, BLOOD STRANGURY, UNCTUOUS STRANGURY, and TAXATION STRANGURY, known collectively as the *five stranguries*. ⊠WMC urinary tract infections; tuberculosis of the urinary tract; urinary calculus; prostatitis; filariasis. ⊠MED For heat, use the method of clearing; for rough voidings of urine, disinhibit; for falls, apply upbearing, and for vacuity, supplement. ◇ Chin 淋 *lín*, dribble, drip. **Eng** from Gk. *stragx, stragg-*, a drop, *ouron*, urine. See also DRIBBLING URINARY BLOCK. [26: 572] [97: 532]

strangury of pregnancy 子淋 *zǐ lín*: From *The Origin and Indicators of Disease* (*zhū bìng yuán hòu lùn*). STRANGURY (painful, dribbling urination) during pregnancy. Strangury of pregnancy is due to yin vacuity, repletion heat, damp-heat, or qi vacuity disturbing bladder qi transformation. **Yin vacuity** causes strangury with tidal reddening of the cheeks and heart vexation. ⊠MED Clear heat, nourish yin, and free strangury. Use Anemarrhena and Phellodendron Eight-Ingredient Pill (*zhī bǎi bā wèi wán*). **Repletion heat** causes strangury with bitter taste in the mouth, thirst, and mouth and tongue sores. ⊠MED Clear heat, drain fire, and free strangury. Use Red-Abducting Powder (*dǎo chì sǎn*). **Damp-heat** causes strangury with heavy fatigued limbs and rough painful urination. ⊠MED Clear heat, disinhibit dampness, and free strangury. Use Five Stranguries Powder (*wǔ lín sǎn*). **Qi vacuity** preventing the retention of urine causes strangury marked by pain after urination. ⊠MED Boost qi and check strangury. Use formulas such as Qi-Boosting Strangury-Checking Decoction (*yì qì zhǐ lín tāng*). [26: 56]

strangury-turbidity 淋浊 *lín zhuó*: **1.** A generic name for strangury and turbidity. **2.** A venereal disease described in *Mysterious Pearl of Red Water* (*chì shuǐ xuán zhū, chì bái zhuó*) characterized by pain in the penis on urination, with semen dripping down like malodorous rotten pus and treated by resolving toxin and vanquishing turbidity with Eight Corrections Powder (*bā zhèng sǎn*) plus fish poison yam (*bì xiè*) and smooth greenbrier root (*tŭ fú líng*). See TURBIDITY³; STRANGURY. [26: 573]

straw-shoe wind 草鞋风 *căo xié fēng*: Itching, pain and sores that begin in the upper thigh and can spread down to the feet. This typically follows the kidney channel and results from damp-heat pouring down into the legs.

streaming sore 流注 *liú zhù*: A sore deep in the body, so called because of the tendency of its toxin to move from one place to another, as if flowing through the flesh. It begins with a lump or diffuse swelling of the flesh. Pus forms, and after rupture and thorough drainage, the sore can heal. See DAMP PHLEGM STREAMING SORE; STATIC BLOOD STREAMING SORE; SUMMERHEAT-DAMP STREAMING SORE; LEG-FLEXING STREAMING SORE. [26: 478] [27: 470] [97: 48] [61: 188]

streaming sweat 漐然汗出 *jí rán hán chū*: From *On Cold Damage* (*shāng hán lùn*). A continual, usually fluctuating discharging of sweat, usually associated with yang brightness (*yáng míng*) disease. [118: 274]

stream point 输穴 *shū xué*: See TRANSPORT POINTS. [27: 99] [97: 604]

strengthening yin 强阴 *qiáng yīn*: A method of treatment used to supplement yin essence. Yin-strengthening medicinals include cooked rehmannia (*shú dì huáng*), dried/fresh rehmannia (*shēng dì huáng*), lycium berry (*gŏu qǐ zǐ*), ligustrum (*nǚ zhēn zǐ*), and complanate astragalus seed (*shā yuàn zǐ*), which treat kidney yin vacuity with aching lumbus, seminal emission, and copious urine. ACU Yin-strengthening points include BL-23 (*shèn shū*, Kidney Transport), KI-3 (*tài xī*, Great Ravine), BL-52 (*zhì shì*, Will Chamber), and SP-6 (*sān yīn jiāo*, Three Yin Intersection); needle with supplementation. Compare SUPPLEMENTING YIN; CONSOLIDATING YIN. [27: 266] [46: 633, 677]

strength desertion yellowing 脱力黄 *tuō lì huáng*: YELLOW SWELLING.

strike 中 *zhòng*: Afflict, usually suddenly or severely, e.g., direct strike by an external evil on the viscera. See DIRECT STRIKE ON THE TRIPLE YIN. Compare STROKE.

strike-on-person 中人 *zhòng rén*: CHILD VISITING HOSTILITY.

stringlike only, without stomach 但弦无胃 *dàn xián wú wèi*: A pulse that has no sign of stomach (see STOMACH, SPIRIT, AND ROOT), and only has a stringlike quality. See PULSE BEREFT OF STOMACH QI. [27: 198]

stringlike pulse 弦脉 *xián mài*: Synonyms: *wiry pulse* (obs); *bowstring pulse*. A pulse that is long and taut and feels like a zither string to the touch. The stringlike pulse is associated with diseases of the liver and gallbladder, and in particular with as-

cendant liver yang. It is also associated with pain and with phlegm-rheum patterns. WMC observed in hypertension, arteriosclerosis, chronic bronchitis, and in diseases characterized by severe pain. The stringlike pulse is generally forceful; if forceless, it is termed a vacuous stringlike pulse, which indicates vacuity of yin and hyperactivity of yang. Similar pulses: A *tight pulse* is a stringlike pulse that has marked forcefulness. "Stringlike" denotes a quality, whereas "tight" denotes a quality and forcefulness. A tight pulse is always stringlike, whereas a stringlike pulse is not necessarily tight. A tight pulse is associated with cold and pain. A *drumskin pulse* is stringlike and empty in the middle. Its significance is the same as that of the scallion-stalk pulse, the name by which it is more commonly denoted. [6: 141] [97: 383]

strings and aggregations 痃癖 *xián pì*: Strings are elongated masses located at the side of the umbilicus; aggregations are masses located in the rib-side that occur intermittently with pain and at other times are not detectable by palpation. The two conditions belong to the category of concretions, conglomerations, accumulations, and gatherings, and are usually referred to together. Both are caused by dietary irregularities damaging the spleen and stomach, the gathering and binding of cold and phlegm, and congealing stagnation of qi and blood. Very often they are associated with emaciation, reduced food intake, and fatigue. Treatment takes the form of dispersing accumulations, dissipating cold, flushing phlegm, rectifying qi, harmonizing the blood, and dispersing stasis. See CONCRETIONS, CONGLOMERATIONS, ACCUMULATIONS, AND GATHERINGS. [26: 488] [27: 417]

stroke 中 *zhòng*: Affliction, usually sudden or severe, e.g., WIND STROKE. Compare STRIKE.

strong stomach and weak spleen 胃强脾弱 *wèi qiáng pí ruò*: A disease pattern of stomach heat scorching the fluids on the one hand and of spleen vacuity with little liquid and dryness of the intestinal humor on the other. It results from factors such as exuberant stomach yang, depressed fire due to affect-mind internal damage, and excessive consumption of hot spicy foods. The main signs are scorching pain in the stomach duct, thirst with a liking for fluids, frequent short voidings of urine, and hard stool that is difficult to pass. Other signs include swallowing of upflowing acid, immediate vomiting of ingested foods, and bad breath. In some cases, there may be sore swollen gums or bleeding gums. The tongue is red with yellow fur. The pulse is slippery and rapid. MED Drain heat, moisten the intestines, and free the stool. Use Hemp Seed Pill (*má zǐ rén wán*). ACU Base treatment mainly on the alarm, back transport, and lower uniting points of LI, and on ST and SP.

Drain BL-25 (*dà cháng shū*, Large Intestine Transport), ST-25 (*tiān shū*, Celestial Pivot), ST-37 (*shàng jù xū*, Upper Great Hollow), TB-6 (*zhī gōu*, Branch Ditch), LI-4 (*hé gǔ*, Union Valley), LI-11 (*qū chí*, Pool at the Bend), SP-14 (*fù jié*, Abdominal Bind), and ST-44 (*nèi tíng*, Inner Court); supplement KI-6 (*zhào hǎi*, Shining Sea), SP-6 (*sān yīn jiāo*, Three Yin Intersection), CV-12 (*zhōng wǎn*, Center Stomach Duct), and ST-36 (*zú sān lǐ*, Leg Three Li). [57: 110] [46: 670] [37: 296, 326] [43: 276]

stuck needle 滞针 *zhì zhēn*: A needle inserted in the body that resists turning, lifting, thrusting or performance of any other needle manipulation. Stuck needle occurs in spasm due to nervousness or to rotation in too wide an arc causing tissue to catch on the needle. **Method:** First allay any apprehension in the patient, and then massage the local area before trying to gently lift and thrust to free the needle. Sometimes insertion of another needle in the area helps to free the needle. [27: 339] [27: 338]

sty 针眼 *zhēn yǎn*: A small boil on the eyelid rim. A sty, when it first appears, is the size of wheat grain and is associated with mild pain and itching. Later it becomes hot, swollen, and tender. It is attributed to wind-heat or to spleen-stomach heat toxin. [MED] Dispel wind and clear heat; drain fire and resolve toxin; disperse swelling and relieve pain. Use Immortal Formula Life-Giving Beverage (*xiān fāng huó mìng yǐn*), which can be combined with topical application of Agreeable Golden Yellow Powder (*rú yì jīn huáng sǎn*). Severe cases require lancing. [ACU] For wind-heat, base treatment mainly on GB, BL, and LI. Select GB-20 (*fēng chí*, Wind Pool), BL-1 (*jīng míng*, Bright Eyes), and LI-4 (*hé gǔ*, Union Valley); needle with drainage and prick Tip of the Ear (*ěr jiān*) to bleed. For spleen-stomach heat toxin, base treatment mainly on LI, ST, SP, and HT. Select ST-1 (*chéng qì*, Tear Container), ST-36 (*zú sān lǐ*, Leg Three Li), ST-44 (*nèi tíng*, Inner Court), SP-6 (*sān yīn jiāo*, Three Yin Intersection), SP-9 (*yīn líng quán*, Yin Mound Spring), LI-4 (*hé gǔ*, Union Valley), and HT-9 (*shào chōng*, Lesser Surge); needle with drainage. Another method of acupuncture that can be applied regardless of the cause distinguishes between the initial stage marked by brewing heat toxin and the advanced stage marked by putrid flesh and formation of pus. Initial stage: People suffering from sties are usually found to have on their shoulder or back pink or flesh-colored papules that are each the size of a grain of rice and that do not change color under pressure. These should be picked open with a three-edged needle. Advanced stage: Use ouch points (*ā shì xué*) at the site of the sty. The hard lump is lifted and pricked once or twice with a red hot needle, which should be swiftly rotated

before removal. For heat effusion, add GV-14 (*dà zhuī*, Great Hammer) and LI-4 (*hé gǔ*, Union Valley). At GV-14, apply gentle lifting and thrusting and needle scraping. At LI-4, apply needle rotation every ten minutes for thirty minutes once a day. [26: 535] [46: 721] [42: 174]

subduing and settling 潜镇 *qián zhèn*: To settle fright and subdue yang, i.e., to treat fright palpitations due to straying of the heart spirit or headache and dizziness due to ascendant liver yang. Settling subduing medicinals are heavy minerals and shells such as loadstone (*cí shí*), cinnabar (*zhū shā*), iron flakes (*tiě luò*), dragon bone (*lóng gǔ*), oyster shell (*mǔ lì*), and mother-of-pearl (*zhēn zhū mǔ*). [27: 267]

subduing yang 潜阳 *qián yáng*: *Synonym: calming the liver and subduing yang.* A method of treatment used to address ascendant liver yang marked by headache and dizziness, tinnitus and deafness, and numbness or tremor of the limbs. Subduing yang uses heavy settling medicinals such as oyster shell (*mǔ lì*), crude dragon bone (*shēng lóng gǔ*), crude abalone shell (*shēng shí jué míng*), mother-of-pearl (*zhēn zhū mǔ*), loadstone (*cí shí*), and hematite (*dài zhě shí*). Since ascendant liver yang is at root a problem of yin vacuity, yang subduing medicinals are often combined with yin-enriching and liver-calming medicinals. [ACU] Base treatment mainly on GV, GB, LR, and KI. Drain GV-20 (*bǎi huì*, Hundred Convergences), GB-20 (*fēng chí*, Wind Pool), PC-6 (*nèi guān*, Inner Pass), LR-3 (*tài chōng*, Supreme Surge), and GB-43 (*xiá xī*, Pinched Ravine), and supplement KI-3 (*tài xī*, Great Ravine), and SP-6 (*sān yīn jiāo*, Three Yin Intersection). ◇ Chin 潜 *qián*, submerge, dive, latent; 阳 *yáng*, yang, the complement of yin. [27: 266] [26: 859] [46: 618, 622]

subduing yang and extinguishing wind 潜阳熄风 *qián yáng xī fēng*: CALMING THE LIVER AND EXTINGUISHING WIND.

submandibular region 颔 *hàn*: Region below the chin.

suckle 吮乳 *shǔn rǔ*: To take milk.

suckling lichen 奶癣 *nǎi xiǎn*, 乳癣 *rǔ xiǎn*: *Synonym: fetal lichen.* A papular skin disease in infants affecting the head and face, and capable of spreading to other parts of the body. Suckling lichen is attributed to wind-heat-damp brewing in the skin. Distinction is made between dry and damp forms. The dry form, attributed to predominance of wind-heat, is characterized by red millet-like papules of differing density that scale on scratching, a lichen-like appearance, and absence of watery discharge. The damp form, attributed to a predominance of damp-heat, is characterized by itchy papules that when scratched exude water and spread, sometimes to cover most of the body. ⬚WMC⬚ infantile eczema (lactigo). ⬚MED⬚ The dry form is treated by clearing heat and dispelling wind, whereas the damp form is treated by clearing heat and dispelling dampness. Wind-Dispersing Red-Abducting Decoction (*xiāo fēng dǎo chì tāng*) or Five-Jewel Powder (*wǔ bǎo sǎn*) can be used as oral medication for either. Apply Flesh-Moistening Paste (*rùn jī gāo*) to the dry form and Indigo Powder (*qīng dài sǎn*) to the damp form. ⬚ACU⬚ Base treatment mainly on GV, SP, ST, LI, and GB. Main points: GV-14 (*dà zhuī*, Great Hammer), SP-10 (*xuè hǎi*, Sea of Blood), ST-36 (*zú sān lǐ*, Leg Three Li), and SP-6 (*sān yīn jiāo*, Three Yin Intersection); needle with drainage. Selection of points according to pattern: For the dry form, add LI-11 (*qū chí*, Pool at the Bend) and GB-20 (*fēng chí*, Wind Pool). For the damp form, add SP-9 (*yīn líng quán*, Yin Mound Spring). [26: 232] [96: 282,232] [27: 476] [97: 173]

sudden blindness 暴盲 *bào máng*: Sudden loss of sight, attributable to liver qi ascending counterflow, qi stagnation and blood stasis, or major vacuity of original qi. ⬚WMC⬚ acute optic neuritis; thrombosis of the central artery of the retina; retinal hemorrhage; retinal detachment. ⬚MED⬚ For liver qi ascending counterflow, clear heat, calm the liver, and rectify qi with variations of Moutan and Gardenia Free Wanderer Powder (*dān zhī xiāo yáo sǎn*). If there is bleeding, treatment should take the form of cooling the blood and stanching bleeding assisted by dissipating stasis. Use a decoction of raw typha pollen (*shēng pú huáng*), eclipta (*mò hàn lián*), salvia (*dān shēn*), moutan (*mǔ dān pí*), charred schizonepeta (*jīng jiè tàn*), curcuma (*yù jīn*), dried/fresh rehmannia (*shēng dì huáng*), and ligusticum (*chuān xiōng*). For qi stagnation and blood stasis, dispel stasis and free the network vessels with House of Blood Stasis-Expelling Decoction (*xuè fǔ zhú yū tāng*). For major vacuity of original qi, use formulas such as Pure Ginseng Decoction (*dú shēn tāng*) or Pulse-Engendering Powder (*shēng mài sǎn*). ⬚ACU⬚ Select local eye points and points according to pattern. Any of the following sets of points can be used as main points: (1) BL-2 (*zǎn zhú*, Bamboo Gathering), Greater Yang (*tài yáng*), GV-21 (*qián dǐng*, Before the Vertex), GV-23 (*shàng xīng*, Upper Star), and Inner Welcome Fragrance (*nèi yíng xiāng*) and prick all of them to bleed (2) Drain BL-1 (*jīng míng*, Bright Eyes), GB-14 (*yáng bái*, Yang White), and Shielding Brightness (*yì míng*), and apply moxa on ginger at Thumb Bone Hollow (*dà gǔ kōng*) and Little Finger Bone Hollow (*xiǎo gǔ kōng*). (3) Drain Back of the Ball (*qiú hòu*), Greater Yang (*tài yáng*), GB-20 (*fēng chí*, Wind Pool), and GB-37 (*guāng míng*, Bright Light). (4) Drain ST-1 (*chéng qì*, Tear Container), TB-23 (*sī zhú kōng*, Silk Bamboo Hole), BL-17 (*gé shū*, Diaphragm Transport), and

LR-2 (*xíng jiān*, Moving Between). Selection of points according to pattern: For liver qi ascending counterflow, add ST-36 (*zú sān lǐ*, Leg Three Li), LR-3 (*tài chōng*, Supreme Surge), PC-6 (*nèi guān*, Inner Pass), SP-6 (*sān yīn jiāo*, Three Yin Intersection), and GB-34 (*yáng líng quán*, Yang Mound Spring), and needle with drainage. For qi stagnation and blood stasis, add BL-18 (*gān shū*, Liver Transport), BL-17 (*gé shū*, Diaphragm Transport), LR-3 (*tài chōng*, Supreme Surge), PC-6 (*nèi guān*, Inner Pass), SP-6 (*sān yīn jiāo*, Three Yin Intersection), SP-10 (*xuè hǎi*, Sea of Blood), and LI-4 (*hé gǔ*, Union Valley), needling with even supplementation and drainage. For major vacuity of original qi, add BL-20 (*pí shū*, Spleen Transport), BL-18 (*gān shū*, Liver Transport), BL-23 (*shèn shū*, Kidney Transport), CV-6 (*qì hǎi*, Sea of Qi), CV-4 (*guān yuán*, Pass Head), ST-36 (*zú sān lǐ*, Leg Three Li), and KI-3 (*tài xī*, Great Ravine), needling with supplementation and adding moxa. [26: 888] [27: 505] [97: 635]

sudden deafness 暴聾 *bào lóng*: DEAFNESS occurring suddenly. See DEAFNESS. [26: 889] [27: 493] [97: 635]

sudden loss of voice 暴瘖 *bào yīn*: Synonym: *replete metal failing to sound*. Loss of voice occurring suddenly, attributed to wind-heat or wind-cold invading the lung and obstructing the pathways of qi and congestion of the lung qi. ⬚WMC⬚ acute laryngitis; spastic aphonia. ⬚MED⬚ Wind-cold is treated by warm acrid effusion and dissipation with Nine-Ingredient Notopterygium Decoction (*jiǔ wèi qiāng huó tāng*). Wind-heat is treated by cool acrid coursing and dissipation with Lonicera and Forsythia Powder (*yín qiào sǎn*) or Throat-Clearing Diaphragm-Disinhibiting Decoction (*qīng yān lì gé tāng*). ⬚ACU⬚ Base treatment mainly on ST, LU, and LI. For wind-cold, select ST-9 (*rén yíng*, Man's Prognosis), LU-7 (*liè quē*, Broken Sequence), LI-4 (*hé gǔ*, Union Valley), BL-12 (*fēng mén*, Wind Gate), and GB-20 (*fēng chí*, Wind Pool). Needle with drainage; use moxa if appropriate. For wind-heat, select ST-9 (*rén yíng*, Man's Prognosis), LI-11 (*qū chí*, Pool at the Bend), LU-5 (*chǐ zé*, Cubit Marsh), ST-44 (*nèi tíng*, Inner Court), GV-14 (*dà zhuī*, Great Hammer), and TB-5 (*wài guān*, Outer Pass), needling with drainage. If there is high fever, prick the Ten Diffusing Points (*shí xuān*) to bleed. See LOSS OF VOICE. [26: 889] [27: 162] [97: 636] [42: 209] [46: 650]

sudden reversal 薄厥 *bó jué*: A REVERSAL PATTERN described in *Elementary Questions* (*sù wèn*, *shēng qì tōng tiān lùn*) marked by sudden reverse-flow, headache, and dizzy collapse. ⬚WMC⬚ cerebrovascular spasm, cerebral hemorrhage, subarachnoid hemorrhage. See REVERSAL PATTERN and

WIND STROKE. Compare FULMINANT REVERSAL. [26: 938]

sudden turmoil 霍乱 *huò luàn*: CHOLERA.

suffering of fullness in the chest and rib-side 胸胁苦满 *xiōng xié kǔ mǎn*: CHEST AND RIB-SIDE FULLNESS.

Sui 隋 *suí*: The name of a dynasty (A.D. 581–618).

summerheat 暑 *shǔ*: Hot summer weather as a cause of disease, or the disease caused by it. Distinction is made between summerheat-heat and summerheat-damp. Summerheat-heat is exposure to the heat of summer; this is called "summerheat stroke," and is what English speakers normally refer to as sunstroke or heatstroke. Summerheat-damp refers to certain externally-contracted diseases occurring in hot weather, that in China used to be loosely called "summerheat disease," and that include "summerheat warmth," which is equivalent to infectious encephalitis B. Summerheat-heat is associated with torrid summer weather, whereas summerheat-damp is associated with hot humid weather. This difference is reflected in signs: summerheat-heat is marked by high fever, thirst, heart vexation, absence of sweating, and a surging pulse. High fever can easily damage qi and fluids, causing lack of strength, short hasty breathing, and dry tongue fur. Summerheat-damp, by contrast, is marked by fluctuating generalized heat [effusion], fatigued limbs, poor appetite, oppression in the chest, nausea and vomiting, abnormal stool, short voidings of reddish urine, soggy pulse, and thick slimy tongue fur. Summerheat-heat patterns are essentially heat patterns, whereas summerheat-damp is heat with dampness complications. See SUMMERHEAT-HEAT; SUMMERHEAT-DAMP. [6: 105] [26: 734] [27: 112] [97: 554] [36: 207] [50: 235]

Summerheat Disease Patterns

SUMMERHEAT STROKE (*zhòng shǔ*)
SUMMERHEAT DAMAGE (*shāng shǔ*)
LATENT SUMMERHEAT (*fú shǔ*)
YANG SUMMERHEAT (*yáng shǔ*)
YIN SUMMERHEAT (*yīn shǔ*)
SUMMERHEAT WIND (*shǔ fēng*)
SUMMERHEAT REVERSAL (*shǔ jué*)
SUMMERHEAT EPILEPSY (*shǔ xián*)
SUMMER INFIXATION (*zhù xià*)

---

summerheat cholera 暑霍乱 *shǔ huò luàn*: DAMP CHOLERA.[2]

summerheat cough 暑咳 *shǔ ké*: COUGH due to damage to the lung by summerheat. Summerheat cough is characterized by cough without phlegm or with scant foamy phlegm, rapid breathing, generalized heat [effusion], red face, thirst, oppression

in the chest and rib-side pain, and a rapid slippery soggy pulse. MED Treat by clearing the lung and resolving summerheat. Use Gypsum and Anemarrhena Decoction (*shí gāo zhī mǔ tāng*) or White-Draining Origin-Boosting Powder (*xiè bái yì yuán sǎn*). ACU Base treatment mainly on LU, LI, ST, and PC. Select LU-5 (*chǐ zé*, Cubit Marsh), LI-4 (*hé gǔ*, Union Valley), LI-11 (*qū chí*, Pool at the Bend), PC-6 (*nèi guān*, Inner Pass), CV-17 (*shān zhōng*, Chest Center), ST-36 (*zú sān lǐ*, Leg Three Li), LU-1 (*zhōng fǔ*, Central Treasury), and PC-7 (*dà líng*, Great Mound); needle with drainage. For rib-side pain, add GB-34 (*yáng líng quán*, Yang Mound Spring). For thirst, add Gold Liquid and Jade Humor (*jīn jīn yù yè*), and KI-6 (*zhào hǎi*, Shining Sea). [26: 734] [113: 48] [37: 272] [27: 379] [97: 555]

summerheat damage 伤暑 *shāng shǔ*: **1.** Any disease resulting from summerheat stroke in the summer. *Elementary Questions* (*sù wèn, cì zhì lùn*) states, "When qi is exuberant and the body is cold, contraction will produce cold damage; when qi is vacuous and the body is hot, contraction produces summerheat damage." **2.** A mild summerheat pattern. *Medical Insights* (*yī xué xīn wù*) states, "Summerheat damage is a mild contraction... Summerheat stroke is a severe contraction." Distinction is made between YIN SUMMERHEAT and YANG SUMMERHEAT. [26: 809]

summerheat-damp 暑湿 *shǔ shī*: Disease occurring in hot, damp weather and caused by a combination of summerheat and dampness. Summerheat-damp is characterized by enduring low heat effusion, fatigued and cumbersome limbs, poor appetite, oppression in the chest, and nausea and vomiting. There is frequently sloppy diarrhea with ungratifying defecation, and short voidings of reddish urine. The pulse is soggy and the tongue fur thick and slimy. MED Clear summerheat and transform dampness using agastache/patchouli (*huò xiāng*), eupatorium (*pèi lán*), sweet wormwood (*qīng hāo*), Six-to-One Powder (*liù yī sǎn*), magnolia bark (*hòu pò*), atractylodes (*cāng zhú*), and poria (*fú líng*), which are often combined with coptis (*huáng lián*) and scutellaria (*huáng qín*). Pronounced exterior patterns can be treated with formulas containing elsholtzia (*xiāng rú*), which clears summerheat and resolves the exterior. General summerheat-damp patterns can be treated with Sweet Wormwood and Scutellaria Gallbladder-Clearing Decoction (*hāo qín qīng dǎn tāng*) and its variations. Summerheat-heat with pronounced exterior signs can be treated with Six-Ingredient Elsholtzia Beverage (*liù wèi xiāng rú yīn*). ACU Base treatment mainly on PC, ST, LI, and SP. Select PC-6 (*nèi guān*, Inner Pass), LI-11 (*qū chí*, Pool at the Bend), LI-4 (*hé gǔ*, Union Valley), CV-12 (*zhōng wǎn*, Center Stomach Duct),

ST-36 (*zú sān lǐ*, Leg Three Li), and SP-9 (*yīn líng quán*, Yin Mound Spring); needle with drainage. Selection of points according to signs: For enduring low fever, add GV-14 (*dà zhuī*, Great Hammer), and SI-3 (*hòu xī*, Back Ravine). For oppression in the chest, add CV-17 (*shān zhōng*, Chest Center). For nausea and vomiting, add ST-25 (*tiān shū*, Celestial Pivot), CV-17 (*shān zhōng*, Chest Center), and ST-40 (*fēng lóng*, Bountiful Bulge), [26: 736] [27: 116] [97: 555] [37: 304] [46: 597] [113: 48]

summerheat-damp dizziness 暑湿眩晕 *shǔ shī xuàn yūn*: DIZZINESS attributed to contraction of dampness in summer. Distinction is made between damp-heat dizziness and cold-damp dizziness. **Damp-heat** dizziness is characterized by clouded head and dizzy vision, generalized heat [effusion] and spontaneous sweating, grimy-looking face, and cold back, vexation and thirst with intake of fluid, and a vacuous rapid pulse. MED Clear heat and transform dampness with formulas such as White Tiger Decoction Plus Ginseng (*bái hǔ jiā rén shēn tāng*). ACU Base treatment mainly on ST, LI, and SP. Main points: ST-8 (*tóu wéi*, Head Corner), PC-6 (*nèi guān*, Inner Pass), LI-4 (*hé gǔ*, Union Valley), ST-36 (*zú sān lǐ*, Leg Three Li), CV-12 (*zhōng wǎn*, Center Stomach Duct), and SP-9 (*yīn líng quán*, Yin Mound Spring); needle with drainage. For damp-heat, add GV-14 (*dà zhuī*, Great Hammer), LI-11 (*qū chí*, Pool at the Bend), SI-3 (*hòu xī*, Back Ravine), and KI-6 (*zhào hǎi*, Shining Sea). **Cold-damp** dizziness is characterized by dizzy head with aversion to cold, generalized pain and heaviness, difficulty in turning sides, and vacuous moderate pulse. MED Transform dampness and dissipate cold. Notopterygium Dampness-Overcoming Decoction (*qiāng huó shèng shī tāng*) combined with Ovate Atractylodes and Aconite Decoction (*zhú fù tāng*). ACU Use the main points given under damp-heat, and use large mounts of moxa. [26: 736] [113: 48]

summerheat-damp streaming sore 暑湿流注 *shǔ shī liú zhù*: A STREAMING SORE arising when contraction of summerheat-damp is followed by contraction of cold evil that fetters construction and defense in the flesh and causes qi and blood to stagnate. A summerheat-damp streaming sore is marked by diffuse white local swelling and slight heat and pain, and is accompanied by general signs such as aversion to cold, heat effusion, oppression in the chest, reduced eating, and joint pain. MED Resolve toxin, clear summerheat, and transform dampness. Use Six-to-One Powder (*liù yī sǎn*) plus eupatorium (*pèi lán*), agastache/patchouli (*huò xiāng*), violet (*dì dīng*), scutellaria (*huáng qín*), gardenia (*shān zhī zǐ*), and peach kernel (*táo rén*). See also LEG-FLEXING STREAMING SORE. [26: 736] [27: 470] [97: 556]

summerheat diarrhea 暑泄 *shǔ xiè*: DIARRHEA occurring in a summerheat pattern. Contraction of summerheat-heat may cause diarrhea characterized by watery or thick slimy stool, accompanied by such signs as vexation and thirst, reddish urine, spontaneous sweating, dirty-looking complexion, and a soggy rapid pulse. Conventionally, the term also refers to diarrhea caused by heat stroke, excessive consumption of fluid, raw foods, or cold foods in summer. If heat is prominent, signs include vexation, thirst, reddish urine, spontaneous sweating, grimy face, and slimy yellow tongue fur. WMC bacillary food poisoning; acute enteritis. MED Transform dampness and resolve summerheat with Elsholtzia Beverage (*xiāng rú yǐn*). For pronounced heat, treat by clearing heat and transforming dampness with Coptis and Elsholtzia Powder (*huáng lián xiāng rú sǎn*), Saussurea and Coptis Pill (*xiāng lián wán*), or Six-to-One Powder (*liù yī sǎn*). ACU Base treatment mainly on PC, CV, ST, and SP. Main points: PC-6 (*nèi guān*, Inner Pass), LI-4 (*hé gǔ*, Union Valley), CV-12 (*zhōng wǎn*, Center Stomach Duct), ST-25 (*tiān shū*, Celestial Pivot), and ST-36 (*zú sān lǐ*, Leg Three Li); needle with drainage. If dampness is prominent, add LR-13 (*zhāng mén*, Camphorwood Gate) and SP-9 (*yīn líng quán*, Yin Mound Spring). If heat is prominent, add LI-11 (*qū chí*, Pool at the Bend), ST-44 (*nèi tíng*, Inner Court), and SP-6 (*sān yīn jiāo*, Three Yin Intersection). [26: 737] [27: 363] [97: 555]

summerheat disease 暑病 *shǔ bìng*: Various forms of febrile disease attributed to contraction of summerheat in the summer months, usually referring to summerheat warmth or summerheat stroke. See SUMMERHEAT and entries listed below. [26: 734] [27: 349] [97: 555]

summerheat dysentery 暑痢 *shǔ lì*: DYSENTERY that is attributed to summerheat and is associated with abdominal pain, generalized heat [effusion], and vacuous pulse. MED Use Elsholtzia Beverage (*xiāng rú yǐn*), Summerheat-Clearing Qi-Boosting Decoction (*qīng shǔ yì qì tāng*), Six-to-One Powder (*liù yī sǎn*), or Agastache/Patchouli Qi-Righting Tablet (*huò xiāng zhèng qì piàn*) plus saussurea (*mù xiāng*). If signs include spontaneous sweating, heat effusion, grimy face, vomiting, thirst with intake of fluid, attacks of abdominal pain, red and white dysentery, and inhibited urination, combine Coptis and Elsholtzia Powder (*huáng lián xiāng rú sǎn*) with Poria (Hoelen) Five Powder (*wǔ líng sǎn*). For contraction of summerheat-heat qi in the summer or autumn, with dysentery characterized by bloody stool and markedly frequent and incessant diarrhea, use white peony (*bái sháo yào*), tangkuei (*dāng guī*), bitter orange (*zhǐ ké*), areca (*bīng láng*), gypsum (*shí gāo*), saussurea (*mù xiāng*), and radish seed (*lái fú zǐ*). [ACU] Base treatment on ST, LI, and PC. Select LI-4 (*hé gǔ*, Union Valley), ST-25 (*tiān shū*, Celestial Pivot), ST-37 (*shàng jù xū*, Upper Great Hollow), PC-6 (*nèi guān*, Inner Pass), ST-36 (*zú sān lǐ*, Leg Three Li), ST-44 (*nèi tíng*, Inner Court), and LI-11 (*qū chí*, Pool at the Bend); needle with drainage. Selection of points according to signs: For generalized heat [effusion] and vacuous pulse, add GV-14 (*dà zhuī*, Great Hammer) and LU-9 (*tài yuān*, Great Abyss). For spontaneous sweating and heat effusion, add SI-3 (*hòu xī*, Back Ravine) and HT-6 (*yīn xī*, Yin Cleft). For thirst with desire to drink, add HT-5 (*tōng lǐ*, Connecting Li) and KI-6 (*zhào hǎi*, Shining Sea). For inhibited urination, add CV-3 (*zhōng jí*, Central Pole), KI-10 (*yīn gǔ*, Yin Valley), SP-9 (*yīn líng quán*, Yin Mound Spring), and CV-6 (*qì hǎi*, Sea of Qi). For dysentery with bloody stool, add SP-10 (*xuè hǎi*, Sea of Blood), and SP-9 (*yīn líng quán*, Yin Mound Spring). For incessant frequent diarrhea, add moxa at BL-20 (*pí shū*, Spleen Transport), CV-12 (*zhōng wǎn*, Center Stomach Duct), and BL-25 (*dà cháng shū*, Large Intestine Transport). [26: 735] [46: 667]

summerheat epilepsy 暑痫 *shǔ xián*: Synonym: *summerheat-wind*. CLOUDED SPIRIT and sudden TETANIC REVERSAL resulting from extreme heat after contraction of the summerheat evil. [MED] Clear heat and extinguish wind. Although this pattern is called "summerheat epilepsy," it cannot be treated as epilepsy. Appropriate formulas include Construction-Clearing Decoction (*qīng yíng tāng*) or Purple Snow Elixir (*zǐ xuě dān*). [ACU] Base treatment mainly on GV, HT, PC, LI, and GB. Select GV-20 (*bǎi huì*, Hundred Convergences), GV-26 (*shuǐ gōu*, Water Trough), HT-7 (*shén mén*, Spirit Gate), LI-4 (*hé gǔ*, Union Valley), PC-9 (*zhōng chōng*, Central Hub), PC-3 (*qū zé*, Marsh at the Bend), BL-40 (*wěi zhōng*, Bend Center), GB-34 (*yáng líng quán*, Yang Mound Spring), and BL-57 (*chéng shān*, Mountain Support). For high fever, add LI-11 (*qū chí*, Pool at the Bend), GV-14 (*dà zhuī*, Great Hammer), and PC-8 (*láo gōng*, Palace of Toil), needling with drainage. Prick Ten Diffusing Points (*shí xuān*) to bleed. See also SUMMERHEAT TETANY. [26: 736]

summerheat-heat 暑热 *shǔ rè*: A disease caused by summerheat, referred to as summerheat-heat by contradistinction to summerheat-damp. Summerheat-heat occurs mainly in the hot season, and is characterized by pronounced heat signs such as high fever, thirst, scant urine, and heart vexation. In severe cases, there may be clouding of the spirit and TETANIC REVERSAL. Other signs include either absence of sweating or great sweating, and a large rapid surging pulse. High fever poses the danger of damage to fluids and original qi, which is characterized by such signs as short-

age of qi, fatigue and lack of strength, dry tongue fur, and a thin and rapid or large and vacuous pulse. [MED] Clear summerheat-heat. Commonly used medicinals include gypsum (*shí gāo*), anemarrhena (*zhī mǔ*), licorice (*gān cǎo*), watermelon rind (*xī guā pí*), fresh bamboo leaf (lophatherum) (*xiān zhú yè*), Six-to-One Powder (*liù yī sǎn*), and coptis (*huáng lián*). Where qi and yin are damaged, adenophora/glehnia (*shā shēn*), ophiopogon (*mài mén dōng*), and dendrobium (*shí hú*) can be added to boost qi and engendering liquid. Where clouded spirit results from orifice block, orifice-opening medicinals can be used. Formulas such as White Tiger Decoction (*bái hǔ tāng*) mainly treat patterns involving high fever, copious sweating, thirst, and a large rapid surging pulse. Wang's Summerheat-Clearing Qi-Boosting Decoction (*wáng shì qīng shǔ yì qì tāng*) is mainly used for summerheat-heat with damage to qi and yin, characterized by copious perspiration, a dry red tongue, thirst, vexation and heat effusion, and a large vacuous pulse. Purple Snow Elixir (*zǐ xuě dān*) is mainly used for patterns including high fever, coma, and TETANIC REVERSAL. [ACU] Base treatment mainly on PC, ST, and LI. Select PC-6 (*nèi guān*, Inner Pass), LI-4 (*hé gǔ*, Union Valley), and ST-36 (*zú sān lǐ*, Leg Three Li); needle with drainage. Selection of points according to signs: For high fever, add GV-14 (*dà zhuī*, Great Hammer) and PC-8 (*láo gōng*, Palace of Toil), or prick Ten Diffusing Points (*shí xuān*) to bleed. For thirst, add HT-5 (*tōng lǐ*, Connecting Li), KI-6 (*zhào hǎi*, Shining Sea), and TB-2 (*yè mén*, Humor Gate). For heart vexation, add HT-7 (*shén mén*, Spirit Gate), and HT-5 (*tōng lǐ*, Connecting Li). In severe cases, select GV-20 (*bǎi huì*, Hundred Convergences), GV-26 (*shuǐ gōu*, Water Trough), and HT-7 (*shén mén*, Spirit Gate); needle with drainage, and prick PC-9 (*zhōng chōng*, Central Hub), PC-3 (*qū zé*, Marsh at the Bend), and BL-40 (*wěi zhōng*, Bend Center) to bleed to drain heat and open the block. For tetanic reversal, add SI-3 (*hòu xī*, Back Ravine), LI-11 (*qū chí*, Pool at the Bend), GB-34 (*yáng líng quán*, Yang Mound Spring), and BL-57 (*chéng shān*, Mountain Support). For absence of sweating, add LI-4 (*hé gǔ*, Union Valley), KI-7 (*fù liū*, Recover Flow), and BL-11 (*dà zhù*, Great Shuttle). For great sweating, add HT-6 (*yīn xī*, Yin Cleft), SI-3 (*hòu xī*, Back Ravine), and LI-4 (*hé gǔ*, Union Valley). [26: 735] [6: 105] [37: 304] [46: 597] [113: 18, 47]

summerheat-heat rib-side pain 暑热胁痛 *shǔ rè xié tòng*: A summerheat pattern with RIB-SIDE PAIN. [MED] Resolve summerheat; clear the liver and gallbladder. Use Six-to-One Powder (*liù yī sǎn*) plus watermelon rind (*xī guā pí*), loofah (*sī guā luò*), gardenia (*shān zhī zǐ*), capillaris (*yīn chén hāo*), and toosendan (*chuān liàn zǐ*).

ACU Base treatment on LI, ST, GB, and TB. Select PC-6 (*nèi guān*, Inner Pass), LI-4 (*hé gǔ*, Union Valley), ST-36 (*zú sān lǐ*, Leg Three Li), LR-14 (*qī mén*, Cycle Gate), GB-24 (*rì yuè*, Sun and Moon), TB-6 (*zhī gōu*, Branch Ditch), and GB-34 (*yáng líng quán*, Yang Mound Spring). Needle with drainage. [26: 735] [46: 636]

summerheat malaria 暑疟 *shǔ nüè*: **1.** MALARIA resulting from contraction of the summerheat evil, characterized by heat effusion without aversion to cold, emaciation, cold back, and grimy face. MED Clear summerheat with formulas such as Origin-Boosting Powder (*yì yuán sǎn*), Elsholtzia Beverage (*xiāng rú yǐn*), or Bupleurum White Tiger Decoction (*chái hú bái hǔ tāng*). ACU Base treatment mainly on GV, PC, SI, and LI. Select GV-14 (*dà zhuī*, Great Hammer), GV-13 (*táo dào*, Kiln Path), PC-5 (*jiān shǐ*, Intermediary Courier), SI-3 (*hòu xī*, Back Ravine), LI-4 (*hé gǔ*, Union Valley), LI-11 (*qū chí*, Pool at the Bend), LI-1 (*shāng yáng*, Shang Yang), and TB-1 (*guān chōng*, Passage Hub). Needle with drainage and, if appropriate, prick to bleed. For principles and methods of treatment, see MALARIA. **2.** See PURE-HEAT MALARIA. **3.** A form of damp malaria characterized by generalized pain and heaviness, pain in the joints, vomiting, distention and fullness, discomfort in the chest and diaphragm, and a pulse that is tight and floating, moderate and floating, or rapid and surging. MED Dry dampness and dissipate the evil. See MALARIA. [50: 1505] [26: 735] [113: 171] [27: 358] [97: 534]

summerheat reversal 暑厥 *shǔ jué*: An orifice block due to summerheat-heat and characterized by sudden oppression and collapse, inability to recognize people, generalized heat [effusion], slight sweating, REVERSAL COLD OF THE LIMBS, panting, loss of speech, slightly clenched jaws, and soggy surging or slippery rapid pulse. Summerheat reversal is similar to wind stroke except for the absence of deviated eyes and mouth. MED Open the orifices with aroma; drain heat and clear the heart. Take care to avoid excessive use of cold medicinals. Appropriate formulas include Liquid Storax Pill (*sū hé xiāng wán*) or Return Again Elixir (*lái fù dān*) poured into the mouth with garlic water. Garlic can also be stuffed into the nose. When the patient has regained consciousness, treatment can be given to eliminate summerheat and regulate the origin (support right). ACU Base treatment mainly on GV, HT, PC, and LI. GV-20 (*bǎi huì*, Hundred Convergences), GV-26 (*shuǐ gōu*, Water Trough), HT-7 (*shén mén*, Spirit Gate), LI-4 (*hé gǔ*, Union Valley), PC-9 (*zhōng chōng*, Central Hub), PC-3 (*qū zé*, Marsh at the Bend), and BL-40 (*wěi zhōng*, Bend Center). For high fever, add LI-11 (*qū chí*, Pool at the Bend), GV-14 (*dà zhuī*, Great Hammer), and PC-8 (*láo gōng*, Palace

of Toil), needling with drainage. Prick Ten Diffusing Points (*shí xuān*) to bleed. [26: 735] [113: 47] [27: 351] [97: 555]

summerheat sand 暑痧 *shǔ shā*: A condition attributed to contraction of the foul turbid SAND (*shā*) evil and characterized by nausea and vomiting, and diarrhea with foul-smelling stool, abdominal pain of fluctuating intensity, dizziness, sweating like rain, and a surging pulse. MED Clear summerheat and transform turbidity; harmonize the spleen and stomach. Use Bamboo Leaf and Gypsum Decoction (*zhú yè shí gāo tāng*) or Six-to-One Powder (*liù yī sǎn*). [26: 735]

summerheat stroke 中暑 *zhòng shǔ*: **1.** Contraction of summerheat evil in the torrid heat of summer. Summerheat stroke is characterized by sudden oppression and collapse, clouding and loss of consciousness, generalized heat [effusion], panting, loss of speech, mild clenching of the jaws, or open mouth and dry teeth, great sweating or absence of sweating, and a vacuous rapid pulse. In severe cases, there is coma with convulsions of the limbs. MED After moving the patient into a cool airy place, administer summerheat-clearing orifice-opening formulas such as Scourge-Averting Powder (*bì wēn sǎn*) or Jade Pivot Elixir (*yù shū dān*). ACU Base treatment mainly on GV, PC, LI, and BL. Select GV-20 (*bǎi huì*, Hundred Convergences), GV-26 (*shuǐ gōu*, Water Trough), HT-7 (*shén mén*, Spirit Gate), PC-9 (*zhōng chōng*, Central Hub), PC-3 (*qū zé*, Marsh at the Bend), and BL-40 (*wěi zhōng*, Bend Center); needle with drainage or prick to bleed. Selection of points according to signs: For high fever, add Ten Diffusing Points (*shí xuān*), LI-11 (*qū chí*, Pool at the Bend), LI-4 (*hé gǔ*, Union Valley), PC-6 (*nèi guān*, Inner Pass), GV-14 (*dà zhuī*, Great Hammer), and PC-8 (*láo gōng*, Palace of Toil). For sweating and expiring pulse, add LU-9 (*tài yuān*, Great Abyss), KI-7 (*fù liū*, Recover Flow), HT-6 (*yīn xī*, Yin Cleft), and CV-6 (*qì hǎi*, Sea of Qi)ⓜ.′ For convulsions of the limbs, add SI-3 (*hòu xī*, Back Ravine), LI-11 (*qū chí*, Pool at the Bend), GB-34 (*yáng líng quán*, Yang Mound Spring), and BL-57 (*chéng shān*, Mountain Support). Gua-sha is also effective for this condition, and is a commonly used home remedy. **2.** SUMMERHEAT-WIND. **3.** YIN SUMMERHEAT. **4.** Contraction of cold in the summer, with abdominal pain, vomiting, and diarrhea. [26: 140] [27: 350] [97: 79]

summerheat stroke dizziness 中暑眩晕 *zhòng shǔ xuàn yūn*: DIZZINESS attributed to summerheat stroke marked by sudden fainting collapse, generalized heat [effusion], thirst, vexation and agitation, vacuous pulse, and, in severe cases, clouding and inability to recognize people. MED Resolve summerheat and transform dampness using Summerheat-Clearing Qi-Boosting Decoction (*qīng shǔ yì qì tāng*). See SUMMERHEAT-DAMP DIZZINESS.

summerheat tetany 暑痉 *shǔ jìng*: FRIGHT WIND due to the contraction of summerheat characterized by generalized heat effusion, headache, rigidity of the neck, and absence of sweating. MED Use Newly Supplemented Elsholtzia Beverage (*xīn jiā xiāng rú yǐn*). If there is sweating, Lonicera and Forsythia Powder (*yín qiào sǎn*) with extra mulberry leaf (*sāng yè*) can be used. If there is generalized heaviness and scant sweating, Atractylodes White Tiger Decoction (*cāng zhú bái hǔ tāng*) is appropriate. If there is a scallion-stalk pulse, red facial complexion, garrulousness, panting, and thirst, indicating that the verge of desertion has been reached, Pulse-Engendering Variant Powder (*jiā jiǎn shēng mài sǎn*) can be used. If there is clouded spirit, Construction-Clearing Decoction (*qīng yíng tāng*) plus uncaria (*gōu téng*), moutan (*mǔ dān pí*), and antelope horn (*líng yáng jiǎo*) should be prescribed. ACU Base treatment mainly on PC, LI, ST, GV, GB, and BL. Select PC-6 (*nèi guān*, Inner Pass), LI-4 (*hé gǔ*, Union Valley), ST-36 (*zú sān lǐ*, Leg Three Li), GV-20 (*bǎi huì*, Hundred Convergences), HT-7 (*shén mén*, Spirit Gate), SI-3 (*hòu xī*, Back Ravine), LR-3 (*tài chōng*, Supreme Surge), GB-34 (*yáng líng quán*, Yang Mound Spring), GV-8 (*jīn suō*, Sinew Contraction), BL-57 (*chéng shān*, Mountain Support), and BL-60 (*kūn lún*, Kunlun Mountains); needle with drainage to clear summerheat and resolve tetany. For high fever, add GV-14 (*dà zhuī*, Great Hammer), and LI-11 (*qū chí*, Pool at the Bend). Prick Ten Diffusing Points (*shí xuān*) to bleed. [26: 735] [27: 351] [97: 555] [42: 187] [37: 486] [113: 48]

summerheat warmth 暑温 *shǔ wēn*: In warm heat diseases, a condition attributed to the contraction of summerheat-heat. Summerheat warmth is a highly varied condition whose basic traits are vigorous heat [effusion], spontaneous sweating, thirst, red facial complexion, shortage of qi, and a large left-wrist pulse. WMC epidemic encephalitis and similar diseases. MED Clear summerheat and discharge heat; boost qi and yin; constrain fluids. Appropriate formulas include White Tiger Decoction (*bái hǔ tāng*), White Tiger Decoction Plus Ginseng (*bái hǔ jiā rén shēn tāng*), Wang's Summerheat-Clearing Qi-Boosting Decoction (*wáng shì qīng shǔ yì qì tāng*), and Pulse-Engendering Variant Powder (*jiā jiǎn shēng mài sǎn*). If clouded spirit, convulsions, and arched-back rigidity are observed, the pattern is one of SUMMERHEAT EPILEPSY. ACU Base treatment mainly on PC, LI, ST, GV, KI, and SP. Select PC-6 (*nèi guān*, Inner Pass), LI-4 (*hé gǔ*, Union Valley), LI-11 (*qū chí*, Pool at the Bend), ST-36 (*zú sān lǐ*, Leg Three Li), GV-14 (*dà zhuī*, Great Hammer),

SI-3 (*hòu xī*, Back Ravine), KI-3 (*tài xī*, Great Ravine), KI-2 (*rán gǔ*, Blazing Valley), KI-6 (*zhào hǎi*, Shining Sea), and SP-6 (*sān yīn jiāo*, Three Yin Intersection); needle with drainage. For extreme heat causing coma and convulsions see SUMMERHEAT EPILEPSY. [26: 735] [27: 350] [97: 555] [113: 48] [37: 486]

summerheat-wind 暑风 *shǔ fēng*: **1.** Contraction of wind after damage by summerheat causing periodic convulsions of the extremities. MED Clear summerheat and dispel wind with Six-Ingredient Elsholtzia Beverage (*liù wèi xiāng rú yǐn*); if phlegm is copious, use variations of Six Harmonizations Decoction (*liù hé tāng*). ACU Base treatment mainly on PC, LI, ST, and GB. Select PC-6 (*nèi guān*, Inner Pass), LI-4 (*hé gǔ*, Union Valley), ST-36 (*zú sān lǐ*, Leg Three Li), GB-20 (*fēng chí*, Wind Pool), and TB-5 (*wài guān*, Outer Pass); needle with drainage. For convulsions of the limbs, add SI-3 (*hòu xī*, Back Ravine), LI-11 (*qū chí*, Pool at the Bend), GB-34 (*yáng líng quán*, Yang Mound Spring), and BL-57 (*chéng shān*, Mountain Support). For copious phlegm, add CV-12 (*zhōng wǎn*, Center Stomach Duct) and ST-40 (*fēng lóng*, Bountiful Bulge). **2.** See SUMMERHEAT EPILEPSY. **3.** Itching in the summertime like the pricking of needles and sometimes associated with redness and swelling. MED Dispel wind and clear the network vessels. Use formulas like Six Harmonizations Decoction (*liù hé tāng*) and Wind-Dispersing Powder (*xiāo fēng sǎn*). ACU Base treatment mainly on LI, SP, and ST. Select LI-4 (*hé gǔ*, Union Valley), PC-6 (*nèi guān*, Inner Pass), ST-36 (*zú sān lǐ*, Leg Three Li), LI-11 (*qū chí*, Pool at the Bend), SP-10 (*xuè hǎi*, Sea of Blood), SP-6 (*sān yīn jiāo*, Three Yin Intersection), and GB-31 (*fēng shì*, Wind Market); needle with drainage. Selection of points according to signs: For redness and swelling of the skin, add BL-17 (*gé shū*, Diaphragm Transport). For great heat [effusion], add GV-14 (*dà zhuī*, Great Hammer). For pronounced itching, add Itch Reliever (*zhǐ yǎng*). **4.** See SUMMERHEAT STROKE. [26: 734] [113: 48] [46: 597, 602]

summerheat-wind turning into fright 暑风成惊 *shǔ fēng chéng jīng*: Excessively exuberant summerheat-damp in infants and children causing great vomiting and diarrhea, heat effusion and sweating from the brow, REVERSAL COLD OF THE LIMBS, and CONVULSIONS. It arises when spleen-stomach vacuity and major damage to original qi conspire with the evil to cause FRIGHT WIND. MED Treat by boosting qi and fostering yin supported by clearing summerheat and extinguishing wind. Bovine Bezoar Dragon-Embracing Pill (*niú huáng bào lóng wán*) dissolved in Pulse-Engendering Variant Powder (*jiā jiǎn shēng mài sǎn*) prepared as a decoction is appropriate medication. [26: 734]

summer infixation 疰夏 *zhù xià*: Synonym: *summer influx*. Regular recurrence each summer of signs such as of poor appetite, fatigue and weakness, and low fever, with gradual recovery in the autumn. Summerheat infixation falls within the scope of damp obstruction. See INFIXATION; DAMP OBSTRUCTION. [27: 351] [97: 490]

summer influx 注夏 *zhù xià*: SUMMER INFIXATION. [27: 351] [97: 367]

sunken pulse 沉脉 *chén mài*: Synonym: *deep pulse (obs)*. A pulse that is distinct only at the deep level. The sunken pulse is usually associated with interior disease, although the exterior patterns of externally contracted diseases may temporarily present with a tight sunken pulse when the body's yang qi is obstructed. Similar pulses: The *hidden pulse* is even deeper than the sunken pulse and considerable pressure has to be applied in order to feel it. *The Bin-Hu Sphygmology (bīn hú mài xué)* states, "The hidden pulse is found by pressing through the sinews right to the bone." It is associated with fulminant desertion of yang qi and deep-lying cold, and generally appears in conjunction with severe vomiting, diarrhea, and pain. The *weak pulse* is sunken and forceless, and is associated with vacuity of qi and blood. The *firm pulse* is sunken and forceful and feels as though "tied to the bone," hence its name. It is associated with cold pain. In clinical practice, this pulse is described as a stringlike sunken pulse or a sunken replete pulse, the term "firm pulse" having fallen into disuse. [27: 193] [97: 306]

superabundance 有余 *yǒu yú*: Excess (of qi, blood, or fluids). Compare VACUITY AND REPLETION.

superabundance of qi gives rise to fire 气有于便是火 *qì yǒu yú biàn shì huǒ*: Exuberant yang qi gives rise to fire patterns. For example, exuberant yang qi due to insufficiency of yin humor can manifest in signs of vacuity fire flaming upward such as red eye, sore pharynx, and sore swollen gums. The five minds and seven affects can cause yang hyperactivity or depressed qi transforming into fire manifesting in various patterns such as liver fire, gallbladder fire, stomach fire, and heart fire. [26: 536] [27: 142]

superficial network vessel 浮络 *fú luò*: From *Elementary Questions (sù wèn, pí bù lùn)*. Network vessels in the surface of the body. The color and location of visible superficial network vessels are of value in diagnosis, and can be pricked to bleed in acupuncture therapy. [26: 483] [27: 96] [97: 483]

supplement 补 *bǔ*: To increase or strengthen. Yin, yang, qi and blood may all be supplemented; the organs that most commonly receive supplemen-

tation are the spleen and kidney. Because supplementation is often associated with qi, the term is frequently seen together with the word boost. Terms of similar meaning, but more specific usage include: **support** (扶 *fú*), to supplement right qi (see DISPELLING EVIL AND SUPPORTING RIGHT); **nourish** (养 *yǎng*) or **foster** (育 *yù*), to supplement (heart, stomach, kidney, and liver, in particular their yin aspect); **enrich** (滋 *zī*), to nourish and moisten (yin, especially kidney or liver yin); **increase** (增 *zēng*), to supplement (fluids to treat patterns including dry stool); **engender** (生 *shēng*), to supplement (fluids lost through disease); **moisten** (润 *rùn*), to eliminate dryness (especially of the lung or large intestine); **boost** (益 *yì*), to supplement (qi, spleen, and occasionally yin); **strengthen** (强 *qiáng*), to supplement (yin, especially kidney yin); **invigorate** (壮 *zhuàng*), to supplement (yang, especially kidney yang); **emolliate** (柔 *róu*), to supplement (liver blood); **return** (回 *huí*), to supplement (deserting yang); **fortify** (健 *jiàn*), to strengthen (spleen and stomach function); **upbear** (升 *shēng*) to restore normal upbearing or upward movement of qi; **raise, lift** (举 *jǔ*), to return a prolapsed or sagging organ back to its normal position. See SUPPLEMENTATION. ◇ Chin 补 *bǔ*, patch, repair, fill a gap; the cloth signifier 衣 suggests that 'to patch' was the original meaning of this character.

supplemental expression 补托 *bǔ tuō*: An INTERNAL EXPRESSION method involving the use of medicinals that supplement qi and blood, applied when right qi is weak. See INTERNAL EXPRESSION.

Supplementation

SUPPLEMENTING QI (*bǔ qì*)
SUPPLEMENTING THE BLOOD (*bǔ xuè*)
SUPPLEMENTING BOTH QI AND THE BLOOD (*qì xuè shuāng bǔ*)
SUPPLEMENTING YANG (*bǔ yáng*)
SUPPLEMENTING YIN (*bǔ yīn*)
ENRICHING YIN AND BOOSTING QI (*zī yīn yì qì*)

---

supplementation 补法 *bǔ fǎ*: One of the EIGHT METHODS. A method of treatment derived from the principles, "vacuity is treated by supplementation," and "detriment is treated by boosting." Supplementation is the method that supplies insufficiencies of yin and yang, blood and qi, and organ functions. When right qi is too weak to expel an evil, the method of supplementation can restore right qi to normal strength, helping it to eliminate the evil; hence the principle, "By supporting right, evils are dispelled." There are four fundamental objects of supplementation: qi, blood, yin, and yang. Supplementation methods are listed above, and supplementing medicinals are listed below. See also SUPPLEMENT.

Qi-Supplementing Medicinals

Qi-Supplementing Medicinals
人参 (*rén shēn*) ginseng (Ginseng Radix)

红参 (*hóng shēn*) red ginseng (Ginseng Radix Rubra)

高丽参 (*gāo lì shēn*) Korean ginseng (Ginseng Radix Coreensis)

西洋参 (*xī yáng shēn*) American ginseng (Panacis Quinquefolii Radix)

党参 (*dǎng shēn*) codonopsis (Codonopsitis Radix)

太子参 (*tài zǐ shēn*) pseudostellaria (Pseudostellariae Radix)

黄芪 (*huáng qí*) astragalus (Astragali (seu Hedysari) Radix)

白术 (*bái zhú*) ovate atractylodes (Atractylodis Ovatae Rhizoma)

山药 (*shān yào*) dioscorea (Dioscoreae Rhizoma)

扁豆 (*biǎn dòu*) lablab (Lablab Semen)

甘草 (*gān cǎo*) licorice (Glycyrrhizae Radix)

大枣 (*dà zǎo*) jujube (Ziziphi Fructus)

饴糖 (*yí táng*) malt sugar (Granorum Saccharon)

蜜 (*mì*) honey (Mel)

Yang-Supplementing Medicinals
鹿茸 (*lù róng*) velvet deerhorn (Cervi Cornu Parvum)

鹿角 (*lù jiǎo*) deerhorn (Cervi Cornu)

鹿角胶 (*lù jiǎo jiāo*) deerhorn glue (Cervi Gelatinum Cornu)

鹿角霜 (*lù jiǎo shuāng*) degelatinated deerhorn (Cervi Cornu Degelatinatum)

牡狗阴茎 (*mǔ gǒu yīn jīng*) dog's penis (Canis Penis)

紫河车 (*zǐ hé chē*) placenta (Hominis Placenta)

蛤蚧 (*gé jiè*) gecko (Gekko)

冬虫夏草 (*dōng chóng xià cǎo*) cordyceps (Cordyceps)

胡桃仁 (*hú táo rén*) walnut (Juglandis Semen)

肉苁蓉 (*ròu cōng róng*) cistanche (Cistanches Caulis)

锁阳 (*suǒ yáng*) cynomorium (Cynomorii Caulis)

巴戟天 (*bā jǐ tiān*) morinda (Morindae Radix)

淫羊藿 (*yín yáng huò*) epimedium (Epimedii Herba)

仙茅 (*xiān máo*) curculigo (Curculiginis Rhizoma)

杜仲 (*dù zhòng*) eucommia (Eucommiae Cortex)

续断 (*xù duàn*) dipsacus (Dipsaci Radix)

狗脊 (*gǒu jǐ*) cibotium (Cibotii Rhizoma)

骨碎补 (*gǔ suì bǔ*) drynaria (Drynariae Rhizoma)

补骨脂 (*bǔ gǔ zhī*) psoralea (Psoraleae Semen)

益智仁 (*yì zhì rén*) alpinia (Alpiniae Oxyphyllae Fructus)

沙苑子 (*shā yuàn zǐ*) complanate astragalus seed (Astragali Complanati Semen)

菟丝子 (*tù sī zǐ*) cuscuta (Cuscutae Semen)

韭菜 (*jiǔ cài*) Chinese leek (Allii Tuberosi Folium)

韭子 (*jiǔ zǐ*) Chinese leek seed (Allii Tuberosi Semen)

胡芦巴 (*hú lú bā*) fenugreek (Foeni-Graeci Semen)

阳起石 (*yáng qǐ shí*) actinolite (Actinolitum)

Blood-Supplementing Medicinals
当归 (*dāng guī*) tangkuei (Angelicae Sinensis Radix)

熟地黄 (*shú dì huáng*) cooked rehmannia (Rehmanniae Radix Conquita)

何首乌 (*hé shǒu wū*) flowery knotweed (Polygoni Multiflori Radix)

夜交藤 (*yè jiāo téng*) flowery knotweed stem (Polygoni Multiflori Caulis)

白芍药 (*bái sháo yào*) white peony (Paeoniae Radix Alba)

阿胶 (*ē jiāo*) ass hide glue (Asini Corii Gelatinum)

龙眼肉 (*lóng yǎn ròu*) longan flesh (Longanae Arillus)

鸡血藤 (*jī xuè téng*) millettia (Millettiae Radix et Caulis)

Yin-Supplementing Medicinals
北沙参 (*běi shā shēn*) glehnia (Glehniae Radix)

南沙参 (*nán shā shēn*) adenophora (Adenophorae Radix)

沙参 (*shā shēn*) adenophora/glehnia (Adenophorae seu Glehniae Radix)

麦门冬 (*mài mén dōng*) ophiopogon (Ophiopogonis Tuber)

天门冬 (*tiān mén dōng*) asparagus (Asparagi Tuber)

石斛 (*shí hú*) dendrobium (Dendrobii Caulis)

玉竹 (*yù zhú*) Solomon's seal (Polygonati Yuzhu Rhizoma)

黄精 (*huáng jīng*) polygonatum (Polygonati Huangjing Rhizoma)

百合 (*bǎi hé*) lily bulb (Lilii Bulbus)

枸杞子 (*gǒu qǐ zǐ*) lycium berry (Lycii Fructus)

桑椹 (*sāng shèn*) mulberry (Mori Fructus)

墨旱莲 (*mò hàn lián*) eclipta (Ecliptae Herba)

女贞子 (*nǚ zhēn zǐ*) ligustrum (Ligustri Fructus)

龟版 (*guī bǎn*) tortoise plastron (Testudinis Plastrum)

龟版胶 (*guī bǎn jiāo*) tortoise plastron glue (Testudinis Plastri Gelatinum)

鳖甲 (*biē jiǎ*) turtle shell (Amydae Carapax)

鳖甲胶 (*biē jiǎ jiāo*) turtle shell glue (Amydae Carapacis Gelatinum)

黑脂麻 (*hēi zhī má*) black sesame (Sesami Semen Atrum)

---

supplementation and drainage needling 针刺补泻法 *zhēn cì bǔ xiè fǎ*: The use of different needle manipulation techniques to supplement vacuity and drain repletion. See the entries listed below. [26: 534]

Supplementation and Drainage Needling

QUICK AND SLOW SUPPLEMENTATION AND DRAINAGE (*xú jí bǔ xiè*)

OPEN AND CLOSED SUPPLEMENTATION AND DRAINAGE (*kāi hé bǔ xiè*)

DIRECTIONAL SUPPLEMENTATION AND DRAINAGE (*yíng suí bǔ xiè*)

TWIRLING SUPPLEMENTATION AND DRAINAGE (*niǎn zhuǎn bǔ xiè*)

LIFTING AND THRUSTING SUPPLEMENTATION AND DRAINAGE (*tí chā bǔ xiè*)

---

supplementation followed by attack 先补后攻 *xiān bǔ hòu gōng*: The therapeutic principle of supplementing vacuity before eliminating an evil, applied where the evil is strong, and right is weak (with depletion of both yin and yang) and incapable of withstanding attack (offensive treatment). For example, a patient displaying an exterior pattern who is mistakenly given precipitation that damages the spleen and stomach may be left not only with the exterior pattern, but also an interior pattern of persistent clear-food diarrhea. Such a patient displays an interior pattern characterized by persistent clear-food diarrhea and an exterior pattern characterized by generalized pain. These signs mean that a strong evil is located in the exterior and a vacuity of right qi is in the interior. Persistent clear-food diarrhea indicates that right qi is severely weakened and is unable to expel the evil, and is also susceptible to yang-collapse vacuity desertion. Thus, the first concern is to support right qi. When the interior pattern has been treated and the bowels have returned to normal, further treatment may be directed toward resolving the exterior by expelling the evil before it passes into the interior, causing new complications. [6: 244] [27: 257]

supplementing both qi and blood 气血双补 *qì xuè shuāng bǔ*: A method of treatment used to address dual vacuity of qi and the blood characterized by somber white facial complexion, dizziness, heart palpitations, shortness of breath, lack of strength, a soft-red pale tongue, and a weak fine pulse. MED A formula that supplements both qi and the blood is Eight-Gem Decoction (*bā zhēn tāng*). ACU See DUAL VACUITY OF QI AND BLOOD. [26: 537]

supplementing fire to engender earth 补火生土 *bǔ huǒ shēng tǔ*: A method of treatment used to warm and supplement the life gate fire to restore spleen function. See WARMING AND SUPPLEMENTING THE LIFE GATE. [27: 263] [97: 301]

supplementing formula 补剂 *bǔ jì*: One of the TEN FORMULA TYPES. A formula that addresses vacuity. Supplementing can eliminate weakness. A commonly used supplementing formula is Four Gentlemen Decoction (*sì jūn zǐ tāng*), which contains ginseng (*rén shēn*), ovate atractylodes (*bái zhú*), poria (*fú líng*), and licorice (*gān cǎo*), fortifies the spleen and boosts qi in the treatment of spleen-stomach vacuity with poor appetite. [27: 305] [97: 301]

supplementing heart qi 补心气 *bǔ xīn qì*: A method used to treat HEART QI VACUITY characterized by heart palpitations, shortness of breath, fatigue, and lack of strength. MED Medicinals that supplement heart qi include mix-fried licorice (*gān cǎo*), astragalus (*huáng qí*), codonopsis (*dǎng shēn*), and ginseng (*rén shēn*). Appropriate formulas include Honey-Fried Licorice Decoction (*zhì gān cǎo tāng*) and Heart-Nourishing Decoction (*yǎng xīn tāng*). ACU Base treatment mainly on HT, back transport points and CV. Select BL-15 (*xīn shū*, Heart Transport), BL-20 (*pí shū*, Spleen Transport), CV-14 (*jù què*, Great Tower Gate), HT-7 (*shén mén*, Spirit Gate), CV-4 (*guān yuán*, Pass Head), CV-6 (*qì hǎi*, Sea of Qi), and ST-36 (*zú sān lǐ*, Leg Three Li); needle with supplementation and add moxa. [6: 171] [37: 282] [46: 594, 655]

supplementing kidney yang 补肾阳 *bǔ shèn yáng*: A method of treatment used to address KIDNEY YANG VACUITY. MED The principal formula for supplementing kidney yang is Right-Restoring [Life Gate] Beverage (*yòu guī yǐn*). ACU Base treatment mainly on KI, GV, and BL. Select BL-23 (*shèn shū*, Kidney Transport), GV-4 (*mìng mén*, Life Gate), KI-7 (*fù liū*, Recover Flow), KI-3 (*tài xī*, Great Ravine), and CV-4 (*guān yuán*, Pass Head); needle with supplementation and add moxa. See SUPPLEMENTING YANG. [26: 674] [46: 587, 679]

supplementing kidney yin 补肾阴 *bǔ shèn yīn*: A method of treatment used to address KIDNEY YIN VACUITY. MED Formulas that supplement kidney yin include Six-Ingredient Rehmannia Pill (*liù wèi dì huáng wán*) and Left-Restoring [Kidney Yin] Beverage (*zuǒ guī yǐn*). See SUPPLEMENTING YIN. ACU Base treatment mainly on KI and BL. Select BL-23 (*shèn shū*, Kidney Transport), KI-3 (*tài xī*, Great Ravine), BL-52 (*zhì shì*, Will Chamber), and SP-6 (*sān yīn jiāo*, Three Yin Intersection); needle with supplementation. [26: 674] [46: 587, 678]

supplementing qi 补气 *bǔ qì*: A method of treatment used to address qi vacuity presenting with general physical weakness, shortness of breath, fatigue, spontaneous sweating, soft weak soggy pulse, prolapse of the rectum or uterus, general physical debilitation following illness, and sequential desertion of blood and qi (qi following blood into desertion) in cases of massive bleeding. MED Use qi-supplementing medicinals such as astragalus (*huáng qí*), codonopsis (*dǎng shēn*), and licorice (*gān cǎo*), which are often combined with spleen-fortifying medicinals, and, if necessary, uplifting medicinals, blood-nourishing medicinals, dampness-transforming medicinals, and qi-moving medicinals. Among commonly used formulas, Four Gentlemen Decoction (*sì jūn zǐ tāng*) is a general qi-supplementing formula, Center-Supplementing Qi-Boosting Decoction (*bǔ zhōng yì qì tāng*) counters center qi fall, whereas Pure Ginseng Decoction (*dú shēn tāng*) treats massive bleeding where the primary concern is to secure original qi and contain the blood. ACU Base treatment mainly on back transport points and CV. Select points from the following: CV-6 (*qì hǎi*, Sea of Qi), BL-43 (*gāo huāng shū*, Gao-Huang Transport), ST-36 (*zú sān lǐ*, Leg Three Li), CV-4 (*guān yuán*, Pass Head), CV-12 (*zhōng wǎn*, Center Stomach Duct), BL-20 (*pí shū*, Spleen Transport), BL-21 (*wèi shū*, Stomach Transport), SP-3 (*tài bái*, Supreme White), LU-9 (*tài yuān*, Great Abyss), and GV-20 (*bǎi huì*, Hundred Convergences); needle with supplementation and add moxa. See SUPPLEMENTATION. [6: 258] [27: 282] [97: 299] [46: 594] [113: 18]

supplementing [medicinals] can eliminate weakness 补可去弱 *bǔ kě qù ruò*: Agents such as ginseng (*rén shēn*) and astragalus (*huáng qí*) can treat vacuity and weakness. Ginseng and astragalus may be boiled together to make a paste to supplement spleen and lung qi. See SUPPLEMENTING FORMULA.

supplementing qi and containing the blood 补气摄血 *bǔ qì shè xuè*: SUPPLEMENTING QI AND STANCHING BLEEDING.

supplementing qi and fortifying the spleen 补气健脾 *bǔ qì jiàn pí*: A method of treatment used to address spleen qi vacuity. See FORTIFYING THE SPLEEN; SUPPLEMENTING THE SPLEEN AND BOOSTING QI.

supplementing qi and resolving the exterior 补气解表 *bǔ qì jiě biǎo*: BOOSTING QI AND RESOLVING THE EXTERIOR.

supplementing qi and securing the exterior 补气固表 *bǔ qì gù biǎo*: A method of treatment used to address qi vacuity spontaneous sweating (insecurity of the exterior), which easily arises when there is heart qi or lung qi vacuity. MED Astragalus (*huáng qí*), and ovate atractylodes (*bái zhú*) are commonly used qi-supplementing exterior-securing medicinals. A representative qi-supplementing exterior-securing formula is Oyster Shell Powder (*mǔ lì sǎn*). ACU Base treatment on back transport points, CV, ST, LI, HT, and SI. Select LI-4 (*hé gǔ*, Union Valley), HT-6 (*yīn xī*, Yin Cleft), SI-3 (*hòu xī*, Back Ravine), CV-6 (*qì hǎi*, Sea of Qi), ST-36 (*zú sān lǐ*, Leg Three Li), BL-13 (*fèi shū*, Lung Transport), and

BL-20 (*pí shū*, Spleen Transport); needle with supplementation and, if appropriate, moxa. For heart qi vacuity, add BL-15 (*xīn shū*, Heart Transport) and CV-14 (*jù què*, Great Tower Gate). For lung qi vacuity add LU-9 (*tài yuān*, Great Abyss) and SP-3 (*tài bái*, Supreme White). [42: 186]

supplementing qi and stanching bleeding 补气止血 *bǔ qì zhǐ xuè*: Synonym: *supplementing qi and containing the blood*. A method of treatment used to address prolonged bleeding due to qi vacuity. This method is used, for example to treat FLOODING AND SPOTTING with thin pale blood. When such bleeding persists for a long time and signs such as somber white complexion, flusteredness and shortness of breath, cold limbs, pale tongue with white fur, and soft fine pulse appear, it can be treated with medicinals such as codonopsis (*dǎng shēn*), astragalus (*huáng qí*), ovate atractylodes (*bái zhú*), mix-fried licorice (*gān cǎo*), tangkuei (*dāng guī*), and cooked rehmannia (*shú dì huáng*). ACU Base treatment mainly on SP, ST, CV, and GV. Select SP-1 (*yǐn bái*, Hidden White), ST-36 (*zú sān lǐ*, Leg Three Li), CV-4 (*guān yuán*, Pass Head), CV-6 (*qì hǎi*, Sea of Qi), GV-14 (*dà zhuī*, Great Hammer), and GV-20 (*bǎi huì*, Hundred Convergences); needle with supplementation and add moxa. For qi vacuity flooding and spotting, add BL-43 (*gāo huāng shū*, Gao-Huang Transport), BL-23 (*shèn shū*, Kidney Transport), BL-20 (*pí shū*, Spleen Transport), and SP-6 (*sān yīn jiāo*, Three Yin Intersection). [27: 275] [97: 301]

supplementing the blood 补血 *bǔ xuè*: Synonym: *nourishing the blood*. A method of treatment used to address conditions of blood vacuity characterized by a drawn, withered-yellow or pale white complexion, dizzy head, tinnitus, heart palpitations, pale scant menstrual flow, fine pulse, and pale tongue. MED Blood-supplementing medicinals include dried/fresh rehmannia (*shēng dì huáng*), tangkuei (*dāng guī*), flowery knotweed (*hé shǒu wū*), lycium berry (*gǒu qǐ zǐ*), ass hide glue (*ē jiāo*), and longan flesh (*lóng yǎn ròu*). These can be combined with qi-supplementing medicinals and, depending on the condition of the patient, with blood-quickening, blood-stanching medicinals, and spirit-quieting medicinals. Among the formulas commonly used, Four Agents Decoction (*sì wù tāng*) is a basic formula for supplementing the blood, regulating menstruation and quickening the blood, Eight-Gem Decoction (*bā zhēn tāng*) treats dual vacuity of qi and blood, whereas Spleen-Returning Decoction (*guī pí tāng*) treats heart-spleen blood vacuity marked by heart palpitations, heart vexation, insomnia, and profuse dreaming. ACU Base treatment on back transport points, SP, LR, and ST. To boost qi and nourish blood, select from the following points:

LR-3 (*tài chōng,* Supreme Surge), ST-36 (*zú sān lǐ,* Leg Three Li), LR-13 (*zhāng mén,* Camphorwood Gate), SP-6 (*sān yīn jiāo,* Three Yin Intersection), BL-17 (*gé shū,* Diaphragm Transport), BL-20 (*pí shū,* Spleen Transport), and BL-21 (*wèi shū,* Stomach Transport); needling with supplementation. See SUPPLEMENTATION. [6: 258] [27: 284] [97: 299] [113: 18] [46: 594]

supplementing the center and boosting qi 补中益气 *bǔ zhōng yì qì:* SUPPLEMENTING THE SPLEEN AND BOOSTING QI.

supplementing the kidney 补肾 *bǔ shèn:* Any method of treatment used to address kidney yin or kidney yang vacuity. See SUPPLEMENTING KIDNEY YIN; SUPPLEMENTING KIDNEY YANG. [27: 287] [97: 300]

supplementing the kidney to promote qi absorption 补肾纳气 *bǔ shèn nà qì:* A method of treatment used to address panting due to kidney vacuity and nonabsorption of qi using medicinals such as codonopsis (*dǎng shēn*), walnut (*hú táo rén*), psoralea (*bǔ gǔ zhī*), cornus (*shān zhū yú*), schisandra (*wǔ wèi zǐ*), and cooked rehmannia (*shú dì huáng*). [ACU] Base treatment mainly on KI, CV, and back transport points. Select BL-23 (*shèn shū,* Kidney Transport), Panting Stabilizer (*dìng chuǎn*), CV-6 (*qì hǎi,* Sea of Qi), KI-3 (*tài xī,* Great Ravine), LU-9 (*tài yuān,* Great Abyss), and ST-36 (*zú sān lǐ,* Leg Three Li); needle with supplementation and, if appropriate, moxa. Compare PROMOTING ABSORPTION OF QI BY THE KIDNEY. [27: 287] [46: 655] [113: 64]

supplementing the lung and kidney and transforming phlegm 补益肺肾化痰 *bǔ yì fèi shèn huà tán:* A method of treatment used to address lung-kidney yin vacuity with exuberant internal damp phlegm marked by cough and nausea, counterflow panting, and copious phlegm with cough especially pronounced at night. [MED] This method uses a combination medicinals that dry dampness and transform phlegm and medicinals that supplement the lung and kidney. A representative lung-kidney-supplementing phlegm-transforming formula is Six Gentlemen Metal and Water Brew (*jīn shuǐ liù jūn jiān*). [ACU] Base treatment mainly on back transport points, LU, KI, and ST. Select BL-13 (*fèi shū,* Lung Transport), BL-23 (*shèn shū,* Kidney Transport), BL-43 (*gāo huāng shū,* Gao-Huang Transport), LU-5 (*chǐ zé,* Cubit Marsh), KI-3 (*tài xī,* Great Ravine), KI-6 (*zhào hǎi,* Shining Sea), LU-9 (*tài yuān,* Great Abyss), ST-36 (*zú sān lǐ,* Leg Three Li), and ST-40 (*fēng lóng,* Bountiful Bulge); needle with supplementation. [46: 597, 653]

supplementing the spleen 补脾 *bǔ pí:* See SUPPLEMENTING THE SPLEEN AND BOOSTING QI; FORTIFYING THE SPLEEN. [27: 262]

supplementing the spleen and boosting qi 补脾益气 *bǔ pí yì qì:* Synonym: *supplementing the center and boosting qi.* A method of treatment used to fortify the spleen to treat qi vacuity. Supplementing the spleen and boosting qi is the basic method for treating qi vacuity, since the spleen and stomach are the ROOT OF LATER HEAVEN (the acquired constitution) and are the source of qi and blood formation. [MED] Commonly used formulas include Four Gentlemen Decoction (*sì jūn zǐ tāng*) and Center-Supplementing Qi-Boosting Decoction (*bǔ zhōng yì qì tāng*). [ACU] Base treatment mainly on back transport points, CV, SP, and ST. Select BL-20 (*pí shū,* Spleen Transport), BL-21 (*wèi shū,* Stomach Transport), CV-12 (*zhōng wǎn,* Center Stomach Duct), LR-13 (*zhāng mén,* Camphorwood Gate), CV-6 (*qì hǎi,* Sea of Qi), SP-3 (*tài bái,* Supreme White), and ST-36 (*zú sān lǐ,* Leg Three Li); needle with supplementation and add moxa. Compare FORTIFYING THE SPLEEN AND BOOSTING QI. [26: 676] [46: 594]

supplementing the spleen to boost the lung 补脾益肺 *bǔ pí yì fèi:* Synonym: *banking up earth to engender metal.* A method of treatment used to supplement the spleen to treat lung depletion, as in enduring cough with copious clear phlegm, poor appetite, abdominal distention, sloppy stool, lack of strength, and, in severe cases, water swelling of the limbs, a pale tongue with white fur, and a fine soggy pulse. Agents such as codonopsis (*dǎng shēn*), poria (*fú líng*), ovate atractylodes (*bái zhú*), dioscorea (*shān yào*), saussurea (*mù xiāng*), tangerine peel (*chén pí*), and pinellia (*bàn xià*) are used. [27: 263]

supplementing yang 补阳 *bǔ yáng:* A method of treatment used to address yang vacuity, which is characterized by aversion to cold, cold extremities, aching and limpness of the lumbus and knees, impotence, seminal efflux, long voidings of copious clear urine, a pale tongue, and a sunken weak pulse. [MED] The medicinals used warm and supplement kidney yang such as: curculigo (*xiān máo*), epimedium (*yín yáng huò*), deerhorn (*lù jiāo*), and cistanche (*ròu cōng róng*). Fire-invigorating medicinals such as aconite (*fù zǐ*) and cinnamon bark (*ròu guì*) may be added where cold signs are especially pronounced, but if used over extended periods, must be complemented by medicinals that nourish kidney essence. Cinnamon Bark and Aconite Eight-Ingredient Pill (*guì fù bā wèi wán*) and Right-Restoring [Life Gate] Pill (*yòu guī wán*), both of which supplement yang and invigorate the body fire. With the addition of medicinals that nourish kidney essence, Right-Restoring [Life Gate] Pill (*yòu guī wán*) supplements yang while supporting yin. [ACU] Base treatment mainly on KI, GV, and BL. Select BL-23 (*shèn shū,* Kidney Transport), GV-4 (*mìng mén,* Life Gate),

KI-7 (*fù liū*, Recover Flow), KI-3 (*tài xī*, Great Ravine), and CV-4 (*guān yuán*, Pass Head); needle with supplementation and add moxa. Selection of points according to signs: For aching and limpness of the lumbus and knees, add GV-3 (*yāo yáng guān*, Lumbar Yang Pass), BL-40 (*wěi zhōng*, Bend Center), and GB-34 (*yáng líng quán*, Yang Mound Spring). For impotence, add SP-6 (*sān yīn jiāo*, Three Yin Intersection). For seminal efflux, add BL-52 (*zhì shì*, Will Chamber), and ST-36 (*zú sān lǐ*, Leg Three Li). For long voidings of copious clear urine, add BL-28 (*páng guāng shū*, Bladder Transport), and CV-3 (*zhōng jí*, Central Pole). See SUPPLEMENTATION. [6: 259] [27: 281] [97: 300] [46: 587, 678, 679]

supplementing yin 补阴 *bǔ yīn*: Synonym: *boosting yin*; *fostering yin*; *nourishing yin*; *enriching yin*. To treat yin vacuity, characterized by emaciation, vacuity heat, upbearing fire, night sweating, dry mouth, dry pharynx, expectoration of blood, insomnia, vexation, heat in the hearts of the palms and soles, red tongue with scant or peeling fur, and a fine rapid pulse. MED Agents commonly used to treat lung or stomach yin vacuity include glehnia (*běi shā shēn*), ophiopogon (*mài mén dōng*), dendrobium (*shí hú*), and Solomon's seal (*yù zhú*). The following medicinals clear heat as well as supplement yin, and treat yin vacuity in the recovery stage of externally contracted heat (febrile) disease: dried/fresh rehmannia (*shēng dì huáng*), dendrobium (*shí hú*), and scrophularia (*xuán shēn*). Some medicinals have a stronger enriching effect, and are generally used to treat liver-kidney yin vacuity: dried/fresh rehmannia (*shēng dì huáng*), ass hide glue (*ē jiāo*), asparagus (*tiān mén dōng*), tortoise plastron (*guī bǎn*), and turtle shell (*biē jiǎ*). Some medicinals used to treat liver-kidney yin vacuity have a lesser enriching effect, but have the advantage of supplementing without being glutinous: ligustrum (*nǔ zhēn zǐ*), eclipta (*mò hàn lián*), and mulberry (*sāng shèn*). Agents used to nourish heart, lung, and kidney yin include ophiopogon (*mài mén dōng*), lily bulb (*bǎi hé*), scrophularia (*xuán shēn*), and biota seed (*bǎi zǐ rén*). Representative formulas include: Anemarrhena, Phellodendron, and Rehmannia Pill (*zhī bǎi dì huáng wán*) and Major Yin Supplementation Pill (*dà bǔ yīn wán*), which treats yin vacuity with effulgent fire; Humor-Increasing Decoction (*zēng yè tāng*), which is mostly used in heat (febrile) diseases where heat evil is still present and yin humor is already showing signs of vacuity; and Stomach-Nourishing Decoction (*yǎng wèi tāng*), which engenders liquid and nourishes the stomach and is mostly used in the treatment of stomach yin vacuity after illness. ACU For lung yin vacuity, base treatment mainly on LU and KI. Select BL-13 (*fèi shū*, Lung Transport), BL-43 (*gāo huāng shū*, Gao-

Huang Transport), LU-5 (*chǐ zé*, Cubit Marsh), and KI-6 (*zhào hǎi*, Shining Sea); needle with supplementation. For stomach yin vacuity, base treatment mainly on ST, SP, and KI. Select BL-21 (*wèi shū*, Stomach Transport), KI-6 (*zhào hǎi*, Shining Sea), ST-36 (*zú sān lǐ*, Leg Three Li), and SP-6 (*sān yīn jiāo*, Three Yin Intersection); needle with supplementation. For liver-kidney yin vacuity, base treatment mainly on KI and LR. Select BL-23 (*shèn shū*, Kidney Transport), BL-18 (*gān shū*, Liver Transport), KI-3 (*tài xī*, Great Ravine), LR-3 (*tài chōng*, Supreme Surge), BL-52 (*zhì shì*, Will Chamber), KI-6 (*zhào hǎi*, Shining Sea), and SP-6 (*sān yīn jiāo*, Three Yin Intersection); needle with supplementation and add moxa. For heart yin vacuity, base treatment mainly on back transport points, HT, PC, and CV. Select BL-15 (*xīn shū*, Heart Transport), BL-20 (*pí shū*, Spleen Transport), BL-17 (*gé shū*, Diaphragm Transport), PC-6 (*nèi guān*, Inner Pass), HT-7 (*shén mén*, Spirit Gate), SP-6 (*sān yīn jiāo*, Three Yin Intersection), KI-3 (*tài xī*, Great Ravine), and KI-6 (*zhào hǎi*, Shining Sea); needle with supplementation. Selection of points according to signs: For vacuity heat, add KI-2 (*rán gǔ*, Blazing Valley), KI-1 (*yǒng quán*, Gushing Spring), and HT-8 (*shào fǔ*, Lesser Mansion). For night sweating, add HT-6 (*yīn xī*, Yin Cleft), LI-4 (*hé gǔ*, Union Valley), and SI-3 (*hòu xī*, Back Ravine). For insomnia or vexation, add HT-7 (*shén mén*, Spirit Gate), HT-5 (*tōng lǐ*, Connecting Li), and HT-8 (*shào fǔ*, Lesser Mansion), Compare CONSOLIDATING YIN; STRENGTHENING YIN. See SUPPLEMENTATION. [37: 296] [6: 259] [27: 281] [97: 299] [46: 596, 653, 660, 678]

¹**support** 扶 *fú*: To assist. See SUPPORTING RIGHT AND DISPELLING EVIL.

²**support** 辅 *fǔ*: n. See SOVEREIGN, MINISTER, ASSISTANT, AND COURIER.

supporting right and dispelling evil 扶正祛邪 *fú zhèng qū xié*: A method of treatment used to strengthen right qi so that it can eliminate the evil, and to dispel the evil so as to protect right qi. In practice, supporting right and dispelling evil is used in situations where right qi is vacuous and the evil has abated. The term implies an emphasis on supporting right. Compare DISPELLING EVIL AND SUPPORTING RIGHT. [27: 34]

supporting right and resolving the exterior 扶正解表 *fú zhèng jiě biǎo*: Any of several methods of treatment used to address constitutional vacuity with contraction of external evils. See ENRICHING YIN AND RESOLVING THE EXTERIOR; ASSISTING YANG AND RESOLVING THE EXTERIOR; BOOSTING QI AND RESOLVING THE EXTERIOR. [16: 80]

supreme physician 太医 *tài yī*: A physician of the supreme hospital, which served the emperor and his court. [27: 515]

surfeit 偏胜 *piān shèng*: In the doctrine of yin and yang, relative strengthening (of either yin or yang). Same as PREVALENCE.

surging pulse 洪脉 *hóng mài*: A pulse that is broad and large, and is forceful at all levels, especially the superficial. The arrival is longer and more forceful than the departure, which accounts for the description, "Coming forcefully, going away feebly," like "tempestuous billowing waves," "surging over the whole of the finger[tip]." It is characterized by a strong initial swell followed by a sharp, but calm, ebbing away. A surging pulse indicates exuberant heat, and is usually a sign of repletion. Observed in enduring diseases (such as tuberculosis) or in vacuity patterns due to massive bleeding, it indicates that right qi is extremely weak and that the condition is deteriorating. Similar pulses: A *replete pulse* is similar to a surging pulse, although it is as forceful when it falls as when it rises. It indicates that the body is afflicted by an exuberant evil, but that right qi is still holding firm. A *large pulse* in clinical practice has roughly the same significance as the surging pulse. However, it should be noted that "large" refers only to the breadth of the blood vessel as it feels to the touch. It bears no connotations of strength. [6: 142] [27: 194] [93: 249]

surreptitious menstruation 暗经 *àn jīng*: Complete lifelong absence of menstruation unassociated with infertility. Slight aching of the lumbus may occur at time when periods would otherwise normally occur, but there is no bleeding. [26: 788] [27: 442] [97: 601]

susceptibility to fright 易惊 *yì jīng*: Tendency to be easily frightened or get nervous. Susceptibility to fright is associated with liver and gallbladder disease and heart disease. See in particular GALL-BLADDER VACUITY AND QI TIMIDITY and DISQUI-ETED HEART SPIRIT.

suspended ball 悬球 *xuán qiú*: SPLEEN VACUOUS AS A BALL.

suspended rheum 悬饮 *xuán yǐn*: One of the FOUR RHEUMS. Water in the chest and rib-side causing local pain and cough with copious phlegm. [6: 220]

swallowing of upflowing acid 吞酸 *tūn suān*: The welling up of acid fluid that is swallowed before it can be spat out. Swallowing of upflowing acid occurs in liver qi invading the stomach, and is associated with either heat or cold signs: in heat patterns, accompanying signs include vexation, dry throat, bitter taste in the mouth, and yellow tongue fur; in cold patterns, signs include dull pain in the chest and stomach duct, ejection of clear drool, and a pale tongue with white fur. See ACID UPFLOW. [26: 328] [27: 411] [97: 299]

sweat 汗 *hàn*: The fluid that flows from the skin. See SWEATING.

sweating 汗 *hàn*: **1.** The expulsion of fluid through the skin. Sweating occurs in health as response to hot weather, heated environments, or strenuous physical activity. *The Magic Pivot* (*líng shū, wǔ lóng jīn yè bié*) states, "With hot summer weather and thick clothing, the interstices open; hence sweat passes out." From this, we can assume that the ancient Chinese understood that sweating has the function of dissipating body heat. It was posited in *The Inner Canon* (*nèi jīng*) that the HEART GOVERNS SWEAT. Heart blood is derived from fluids, and sweating drains the fluids; great sweating no only leads to excessive action to dissipate heat, but can also damage qi and the fluids, thereby damaging heart blood. Although sweat is said to be governed by the heart, the spleen is also closely associated with sweating since earth is the "mother of the myriad things," including sweat. Sweating occurs in sickness as a result of exterior evils, internal heat, or vacuous qi failing to contain fluids. In exterior patterns attributed to externally contracted evils, sweating or its absence is important in diagnosis. Wind-heat, for example, may cause sweating whereas wind-cold does not. In both cases, sweating is considered necessary for the expulsion of the evil from the body. In internal damage miscellaneous diseases, a major distinction is seen between spontaneous sweating and night sweating. Spontaneous sweating, which is a tendency to sweat in the daytime for no obvious cause, is attributed to yang qi vacuity, whereas night sweating, which is sweating at night that ceases on waking, is principally associated with yin vacuity. The precise nature of the sweating can provide more diagnostic detail. See entries listed below:

Sweating

Generalized
SPONTANEOUS SWEATING (*zì hàn*)
NIGHT SWEATING (*dào hàn*)
ABSENCE OF SWEATING (*wú hàn*)
PROFUSE SWEATING (*duō hàn*)
GREAT SWEATING (*dà hàn*)
DESERTION SWEATING (*tuō hàn*)
LEAKING SWEAT (*hàn lòu*)
EXPIRATION SWEATING (*jué hàn*)
SHIVER SWEATING (*zhàn hàn*)
YANG SWEATING (*yáng hàn*)
COLD SWEAT (*lěng hàn*)
OILY SWEAT (*yóu hàn*)
YELLOW SWEAT (*huáng hàn*)
Localized
GENITAL SWEATING (*yīn hàn*)
HEART SWEATING (*xīn hàn*)

HEMILATERAL SWEATING (*piān jù*)
SWEATING HANDS AND FEET (*shǒu zú hàn chū*)
SWEATING ARMPITS (*yè hàn*)
SWEATING HEAD (*tóu hàn*)
SWEATING BROW (*é hàn*)

See also CORPOREAL SOUL SWEATING. For methods to control sweating, see CONSTRAINING SWEAT; CONSTRAINING SWEAT AND SECURING THE EXTERIOR. **2.** *Synonym: promoting sweating; effusing sweat; diaphoresis (obs).* One of the EIGHT METHODS. Inducing perspiration as a method of resolving the exterior. It involves the use of acrid dissipating medicinals that promote outthrust and effusion to open and discharge the interstices and expel the evil from the body. Sweating is used to eliminate an evil from the skin and [body] hair before it enters the interior. This is the meaning of the line in *Elementary Questions* (*sù wèn, yīn yáng yìng xiàng dà lùn*) that states, "when it [an evil] is in the skin, it is made to effuse." Sweating is mainly used in exterior patterns such as the onset of external diseases and wind-damp and water swelling diseases, as well as in measles immediately preceding papular outthrust. Warm acrid exterior resolution treats cold patterns; cool acrid exterior resolution treats heat patterns. [92: No. 11-19]

sweating armpits 腋汗 *yè hàn*: Profuse sweating from the armpits; attributed to liver vacuity with heat or lesser yang (*shào yáng*) with heat. ☐MED☐ For liver vacuity with heat, supplement the liver and nourish the blood with variations of Six-Ingredient Rehmannia Pill (*liù wèi dì huáng wán*). For lesser yang with heat, use variations of Minor Bupleurum Decoction (*xiǎo chái hú tāng*) or Free Wanderer Powder (*xiāo yáo sǎn*). People with body odor frequently suffer from sweating armpits. See FOXY ODOR. [26: 745]

sweating brow 额汗 *é hàn*, 额头出汗 *é tóu chū hàn*, 额上汗出 *é shàng hàn chū*: Sweating only from the brow; most commonly seen in yang brightness (*yáng míng*) patterns with concurrent static blood and damp-heat. When heat lies depressed in the inner body and fails to discharge by effusion, it follows the channel upward. The sweating stops when heat abates. After major illness or in elderly patients suffering from panting, counterflow ascent of qi can also give rise to copious sweating of the brow. In such cases, it is a vacuity sign. In advanced stages of major disease with lassitude of spirit and cold limbs, diarrhea, and a faint fine pulse, the sudden appearance of a sweating brow is a critical sign of over-ascending yang with yin failing to hold onto yang and yin humor deserting with qi. [27: 389]

sweating hands and feet 手足汗 *shǒu zú hàn*: Clammy sweaty hands and feet. Sweating hands and feet is usually the manifestation of steaming of spleen-stomach dampness out to the extremities. If the hearts of the soles and palms are hot, it is attributable to yin depletion and blood vacuity. If the extremities are cold, it is ascribed to insufficiency of center yang. ☐MED☐ Yin-blood vacuity is treated with Four Agents Decoction (*sì wù tāng*) or Ophiopogon and Rehmannia Pill (*mài wèi dì huáng wán*), whereas insufficiency of center yang is treated with Center-Rectifying Decoction (*lǐ zhōng tāng*) plus mume (*wū méi*). If the condition persists, use Perfect Major Supplementation Decoction (*shí quán dà bǔ tāng*) plus schisandra (*wǔ wèi zǐ*). Topical: For sweating hands, decoct astragalus (*huáng qí*) 30 g, pueraria (*gé gēn*) 30 g, schizonepeta (*jīng jiè*) 9 g, and ledebouriella (*fáng fēng*) 9 g as a warm wash. For sweating feet, decoct alum (*bái fán*) 15 g and pueraria (*gé gēn*) 15 g as a foot bath. [26: 161]

sweating head 头汗 *tóu hàn*: Profuse sweating confined to the head. Sweating head is attributable to depleted water and effulgent fire, stomach heat seething upward, and dampness contending with yang. ☐MED☐ In depleted water and effulgent fire, it is treated by enriching yin and downbearing fire, using formulas such as Tangkuei Six Yellows Decoction (*dāng guī liù huáng tāng*). In stomach fire seething upward, it is treated by clearing and discharging stomach heat with Bamboo Leaf and Gypsum Decoction (*zhú yè shí gāo tāng*). When due to the damp evil contending with yang, it is treated by transforming dampness and warming the center, using Dampness-Overcoming Decoction (*shèng shī tāng*). Sweating from the head may also occur in block and repulsion, water chest bind, lesser yang (*shào yáng*) disease, panting in the elderly, and yang desertion in severe disease. [26: 906] [97: 164]

sweating of blood 汗血 *hàn xuè*: **1.** The putting forth of sweat tinged with blood. **2.** The putting forth of blood through the sweat pores. SPONTANEOUS BLEEDING OF THE FLESH.

sweat is the humor of the heart 汗为心液 *hàn wéi xīn yè*: See HEART GOVERNS SWEAT. [27: 61] [97: 226]

sweat macule 汗斑 *hàn bān*: PURPLE AND WHITE PATCH WIND.

sweep 豁 *huò*: Forceful elimination of evils, such as phlegm. See SWEEPING PHLEGM AND AROUSING THE BRAIN. ◇ Chin 豁 *huò*, clear, free, bright, broad, gape.

sweeping phlegm and arousing the brain 豁痰醒脑 *huò tán xǐng nǎo*: TRANSFORMING PHLEGM AND OPENING THE ORIFICES. [26: 169]

sweeping phlegm and opening the orifices 豁痰开窍 *huò tán kāi qiào*: TRANSFORMING PHLEGM AND OPENING THE ORIFICES.

sweet 甘 *gān*: See SWEETNESS.

sweetness 甘 *gān*: One of the FIVE FLAVORS. Sweetness enters the spleen; it can supplement and relax. See FIVE FLAVORS and FIVE FLAVOR ENTRIES.

sweetness enters the spleen 甘入脾 *gān rù pí*: Sweet things act upon the spleen. Agents that enter the spleen include ginseng (*rén shēn*), codonopsis (*dǎng shēn*), ovate atractylodes (*bái zhú*), poria (*fú líng*), licorice (*gān cǎo*), dioscorea (*shān yào*), astragalus (*huáng qí*), coix (*yì yǐ rén*), jujube (*dà zǎo*), barley sprout (*mài yá*), longan flesh (*lóng yǎn ròu*), malt sugar (*yí táng*), cimicifuga (*shēng má*), tangkuei (*dāng guī*), and star anise (*bā jiǎo huí xiāng*). The spleen is the source of qi and blood formation and the root of later heaven (i.e., the acquired constitution). These functions correspond in some measure to modern notions of production of energy from carbohydrates contained in sweet substances. [27: 62]

sweet taste in the mouth 口甜 *kǒu tián*: The subjective sensation of sweetness in the mouth; attributable either to spleen-stomach heat or to dual vacuity of spleen-stomach qi and yin. **Steaming spleen-stomach heat** gives rise to a sweet taste in the mouth associated with dry mouth with desire to drink, large food intake and rapid hungering, mouth and tongue sores, dry stool, yellow urine, red tongue with dry yellow fur, and a forceful rapid pulse. Spleen-stomach damp-heat is often observed in dispersion-thirst patients given to eating rich sweet and fatty foods. MED Clear heat and drain fire. For mild cases, use Yellow-Draining Powder (*xiè huáng sǎn*). If there are signs of bowel repletion, use variations of Rhubarb and Coptis Heart-Draining Decoction (*dà huáng huáng lián xiè xīn tāng*). **Dual vacuity of spleen-stomach qi and yin** gives rise to a sweet taste in the mouth associated with no thought of food and drink, dry mouth with no great desire for fluids, lassitude of spirit and lack of strength, stomach duct and abdominal distention, abnormal stool, a dry, slightly red tongue with little fur, and a weak fine pulse. *Elementary Questions* (*sù wèn, qí bìng lùn*) states, "When there is illness marked by sweet taste in the mouth,... this is a spillage of the five qi, and is called "splenic pure heat." MED Boost qi, fortify the spleen, and nourish stomach yin. Use Center-Supplementing Qi-Boosting Decoction (*bǔ zhōng yì qì tāng*) minus cimicifuga (*shēng má*) and bupleurum (*chái hú*), with the addition of basil (*luó lè*) and pueraria (*gé gēn*). Alternatively, use Seven-Ingredient Ovate Atractylodes Powder (*qī wèi bái zhú sǎn*) plus dioscorea (*shān yào*), dendrobium (*shí hú*), and lotus fruit/seed (*lián zǐ*). See TASTE IN THE MOUTH. [92: No. 82]

swelling 肿 *zhǒng*: Enlargement due to accumulation of water, blood, or pus. Localized swelling occurs with sores. Distinction is made between TOXIN SWELLING, which is swelling due to toxins and associated with welling-abscesses (*yōng*), flat-abscesses (*jū*), boils (*jié*), clove sores (*dīng chuāng*), and other sores, and WATER SWELLING, swelling due to water accumulation stemming from disease of the lung, spleen, and kidney, and including VACUITY SWELLING, REPLETION SWELLING, YIN WATER, YANG WATER, and WIND WATER, etc.

swelling and distention in pregnancy 妊娠肿胀 *rèn shēn zhǒng zhàng*: Swelling and distention of the limbs after the sixth month of pregnancy, attributed to spleen-kidney yang vacuity causing water-damp to collect and spill into the skin and flesh. See FULLNESS OF PREGNANCY; SWELLING OF PREGNANCY; PREGNANCY QI; BRITTLE FOOT; WRINKLY FOOT. [26: 341]

swelling of pregnancy 子肿 *zǐ zhǒng*: Mentioned in *The Gateway to Medicine* (*yī xué rù mén*). WATER SWELLING in pregnancy. Swelling of pregnancy tends to affect women suffering from constitutional spleen-kidney yang vacuity and usually occurs in the fifth or sixth month of pregnancy when, as the fetus becomes larger, the spleen's movement and transformation function breaks down and allow water to flood into the limbs. It affects the instep first, spreading up the low extremities and eventually to the whole body including the head and face. This is attended by short voidings of scant urine. It is caused by spleen vacuity, kidney vacuity, or qi stagnation. **Spleen vacuity** gives rise to swelling with fatigue and lack of strength, and distention and oppression in the stomach duct and abdomen. MED Fortify the spleen, promote qi transformation, and move water. Use Life-for-All Ovate Atractylodes Powder (*quán shēng bái zhú sǎn*). ACU Base treatment mainly on SP, ST, KI and back transport points. Main points: CV-9 (*shuǐ fēn*, Water Divide), ST-36 (*zú sān lǐ*, Leg Three Li), SP-9 (*yīn líng quán*, Yin Mound Spring), SP-6 (*sān yīn jiāo*, Three Yin Intersection), and KI-7 (*fù liū*, Recover Flow). For spleen vacuity, add BL-20 (*pí shū*, Spleen Transport), BL-21 (*wèi shū*, Stomach Transport), and LR-13 (*zhāng mén*, Camphorwood Gate); needle with supplementation and, if appropriate, moxa. **Kidney vacuity** patterns are characterized by aching limp lumbus and knees, and lack of warmth in the extremities. MED Warm yang, promote qi transformation, and move water using Poria (Hoelen) Five Powder (*wǔ líng sǎn*). ACU To the above main points, add BL-23 (*shèn shū*, Kidney Transport), KI-3 (*tài xī*, Great Ravine), and CV-4 (*guān yuán*, Pass Head); needle with supplementation and, if appropriate, moxa. **Qi stagnation** is marked by pronounced swelling of the head and face, and oppression in the chest and rib-side distention. MED Rectify qi, move stagnation, and disinhibit water using Aristolochia Stem Powder (*tiān xiān téng sǎn*). ACU To the above main points add CV-6 (*qì hǎi*, Sea of Qi), LR-3 (*tài chōng*, Supreme Surge), and BL-22 (*sān jiāo shū*, Triple Burner Transport); needle with even supplementation and drainage. Warning: strong stimulus should be avoided in pregnant women. [26: 56] [59: 118] [46: 596, 676]

swelling of the feet 足肿 *zú zhǒng*: See SWELLING OF THE FEET AND LOWER LEGS.

swelling of the feet and lower legs 足胻肿 *zú héng zhǒng*: A commonly observed form of water swelling, affecting the dorsum of the foot and the lower part of the lower leg. See WATER SWELLING. [26: 320]

swelter 薰蒸 *xūn zhēng*: Describes the behavior of damp-heat and its effect on organs.

swift digestion with rapid hungering 消谷善饥 *xiāo gǔ shàn jī*, 消谷喜饥 *xiāo gǔ xǐ jī*: Synonym: *increased eating and rapid hungering*. Increased appetite with recurrence of hunger sensation shortly after eating. Swift digestion with rapid hungering is the chief sign, but in itself is not necessarily an indication, of CENTER DISPERSION. If this gives rise to a in increase in food intake, it is called INCREASED EATING WITH RAPID HUNGERING. WMC observed in diabetes mellitus and hyperthyroidism. **Intense stomach fire,** which results from externally contracted dryness-heat or liver depression transforming into fire and invading the stomach, causes swift digestion and rapid hungering with emaciation, thirst, constipation, dry yellow tongue fur, red tongue, and a forceful slippery pulse. MED Clear heat and enrich yin. Use White Tiger Decoction Plus Ginseng (*bái hǔ jiā rén shēn tāng*) plus coptis (*huáng lián*), and dried/fresh rehmannia (*shēng dì huáng*). ACU Base treatment mainly on ST and LI. Select ST-44 (*nèi tíng*, Inner Court), LI-4 (*hé gǔ*, Union Valley), ST-36 (*zú sān lǐ*, Leg Three Li), and KI-6 (*zhào hǎi*, Shining Sea); needle with drainage. Selection of points according to causes: For externally contracted dryness-heat, add LI-11 (*qū chí*, Pool at the Bend) and LU-5 (*chǐ zé*, Cubit Marsh). For liver depression transforming into fire,

add LR-3 (*tài chōng*, Supreme Surge), LR-2 (*xíng jiān*, Moving Between), and GB-43 (*xiá xī*, Pinched Ravine), **Yang brightness blood amassment** causes swift digestion and rapid hungering accompanied by heat effusion without aversion to cold, dry throat and mouth, desire to wash the mouth but not to swallow fluids, forgetfulness, hard fullness in the lesser abdomen, uninhibited urination, black stool that is passed easily despite its hardness, dull lips and complexion, red tongue possibly with stasis macules, and a rapid bound sunken pulse. MED Expel amassed blood with Dead-On Decoction (*dǐ dàng tāng*) or Dead-On Pill (*dǐ dàng wán*). ACU Base treatment mainly on ST, SP, and LI. Select BL-17 (*gé shū*, Diaphragm Transport), ST-25 (*tiān shū*, Celestial Pivot), LI-6 (*piān lì*, Veering Passageway), ST-36 (*zú sān lǐ*, Leg Three Li), LI-4 (*hé gǔ*, Union Valley), SP-10 (*xuè hǎi*, Sea of Blood), and SP-6 (*sān yīn jiāo*, Three Yin Intersection); needle with even supplementation and drainage. See CENTER DISPERSION. [92: No. 194] [22: 302] [26: 482] [44: 561] [46: 596, 660] [75: 204]

swill diarrhea 飧泄 *sūn xiè*, 飧泻 *sūn xiè*: Diarrhea that is characterized by clean-looking stool containing some untransformed food and that often occurs shortly after eating. Swill diarrhea results from spleen-stomach qi and yang vacuity, or from wind, dampness, cold or heat invading the lung. MED Supplement the spleen and fortify the stomach with Ginseng, Poria (Hoelen), and Ovate Atractylodes Powder (*shēn líng bái zhú sǎn*). See WIND DIARRHEA; DAMP DIARRHEA, COLD DIARRHEA, and HEAT DIARRHEA. ◊ Chin 飧 *sun*, to soak cooked rice in water; cooked food; supper. The character is composed of 夕 *xì*, evening, and 食 *shí* food. [26: 750] [48: 391]

swollen feet 脚肿 *jiǎo zhǒng*: Swelling of the feet and ankles. See WATER SWELLING.

swollen welling-abscess 痈肿 *yōng zhǒng*: Any WELLING-ABSCESS (*yōng*) in the stage of swelling.

syrup 糖浆剂 *táng jiāng jì*: Syrup, made by boiling sugar cane in water and combining it with an equal amount of a strained, concentrated decoction of the formula constituents to provide a preparation especially suitable for children and for gentle treatment of acute diseases.

tablet 片 *piàn*: *Synonym: tablet preparation.* A medicinal preparation made by mixing a powder of ground medicinal materials with a formative medicinal and compressing them into a mold. Tablets are convenient to carry and use. They easily absorb dampness, so should be kept in a dry place. **Method**: Tablets may be hand or machine made. To make tablets by hand, the constituents are ground to a fine powders, and blended with flour and water paste or viscous rice water, pressed in a mold, and either oven-dried or left to dry in the shade. Less commonly, some of the constituents are boiled, and after straining off the dregs, the decoction is reduced to a paste, which is then mixed with the dry medicinals. See MEDICINAL PREPARATION. [27: 313]

tablet preparation 片剂 *piàn jì*: See TABLET.

tael 两 *liǎng*: LIANG.

tail bone 尾骨 *wěi gǔ*: Coccyx.

take drenched 冲服 *chōng fú*: Swallowing (powders, paste, or glue) mixed with several times the volume of cold, warm, or hot water or other fluid. Medicinals that should not or need not be decocted are taken drenched to facilitate swallowing. Some medicinals such as amber (*hǔ pò*), cinnabar (*zhū shā*), or notoginseng (*sān qī*) that are expensive or that should not be decocted are ground to a fine powder and mixed with warm water or an accompanying decoction and swallowed. Some gelatinous medicinals or mineral salts such as ass hide glue (*ē jiāo*), mirabilite (*máng xiāo*), or malt sugar (*yí táng*) can be dissolved in warm water or an accompanying decoction. [50: 320]

Tang 唐 *táng*: The name of a dynasty (A.D. 618–907).

tangled red-thread vessels 赤丝虬(蚪)脉 *chì sī qiú (qiú) mài*: *Synonyms: chaotic red-thread vessels; chaotic vessels in the white of the eye.* A disease pattern of the eye characterized by red vessels in the white of the eye that run in all directions like tangled threads. Tangled red-thread vessels are associated with dryness of the eyes and slight tearing and aversion to light. They are attributed to the enduring presence of evils causing stasis in the blood network vessels of the white of the eye. They are is observed in peppercorn sores, millet sores, eye strain, and long exposure to fumes or dust. WMC hyperemia of the bulbar conjunctiva as in chronic conjunctivitis. MED Dispel the evil and dissipate stasis. Compare RED VESSELS INVADING THE EYE. [26: 304] [27: 596] [97: 247]

taste in the mouth 口味 *kǒu wèi*: The taste experienced when there is nothing in the mouth. Changes in the taste in the mouth are of corroborative value in pattern identification. If the taste in the mouth is unaffected by illness, the mouth is said to be in harmony. This indicates that there is no heat in the interior. **Bitter** taste is the most commonly reported deviation from "harmony of mouth" and is attributed to bile. It is observed in lesser yang (*shào yáng*) disease and depressed liver-gallbladder heat. **Sweet** taste in the mouth is attributable either to spleen-stomach heat or to dual vacuity of spleen-stomach qi and yin. **Salty** taste, sometimes described as being "fishy," is ascribed to kidney vacuity. **Sour** taste in the mouth is a subjective feeling of sourness in the mouth, that in severe cases may be accompanied by a sour smell on the breath. It is attributed to liver heat, to spleen vacuity being exploited by wood, or to food stagnation. **Bland** taste in the mouth is diminished sense of taste. It is usually associated with no enjoyment in food and poor appetite. It is attributed to spleen-stomach vacuity or to dampness obstructing the center burner. See BITTER TASTE IN THE MOUTH; SWEET TASTE IN THE MOUTH; SOUR TASTE IN THE MOUTH; BLAND TASTE IN THE MOUTH. See also SLIMINESS IN THE MOUTH. [92: Nos. 81-85] [6: 134]

taste of urine in the mouth 口有尿味 *kǒu yǒu niào wèi*: See BLOCK AND REPULSION.

taxation 劳 *láo*: **1.** Physical exertion. **2.** Fatigue resulting from physical exertion. According to *Elementary Questions* (*sù wèn*), "taxation causes wearing of qi." **3.** Severe lasting wear and tear on the body by overexertion or lack of exercise, and in a wider context by intemperate living (including dietary irregularities and sexual intemperance), the seven affects (emotional imbalance), or enduring disease. The damage resulting from any of these factors is referred to as TAXATION FATIGUE or TAXATION DAMAGE (these terms also have another specific meanings; see TAXATION FATIGUE). The damage resulting from overexertion or lack of exercise is classically described in terms of the DAMAGE BY THE FIVE TAXATIONS (prolonged vision damages the blood; prolonged lying damages qi; prolonged sitting damages the flesh; prolonged standing damages the bones; and prolonged walking damages the sinews). Damage by excessive sexual activity is called SEXUAL TAXATION. The harmful effects of intemperate living and the seven affects are referred to as INTERNAL DAMAGE, and when they cause severe lasting wear and tear on the body, the resulting patterns are called VACUITY TAXATION or VACUITY DETRIMENT conditions. **4.** Consumption (corresponding to pulmonary tuberculosis in Western medicine), a contagious disease that causes gradual wasting away of the body. ◇ Chin 劳 *láo*, toil, fatigue. Note in the context of the fourth definition that the homophone 痨, consumption, is the same character with the addition of the illness signifier 疒. [26: 678] [97: 257]

taxation causes wearing of qi 劳则气耗 *láo zé qì hào*: Excessive taxation, panting, and excessive sweating can cause damage to qi, causing fatigue. [26: 679] [27: 146] [97: 257]

taxation cough 劳嗽 *láo sòu*, 劳咳 *láo ké*: Synonym: *vacuity taxation cough*; *taxation damage cough*. **1.** Cough occurring in severe vacuity patterns due to taxation fatigue, sexual and drinking intemperance. Taxation cough frequently manifests as lung-kidney yin vacuity flaming fire or lung-spleen vacuity cold. See also SPLEEN COUGH. **Lung-kidney yin vacuity flaming fire** taxation cough is characterized by signs of the lung being deprived of nourishment and of lung qi ascending counterflow, such as dry cough with scant phlegm, a hoarse cough, dry mouth and dry throat. This is accompanied by signs of effulgent yin vacuity fire such as postmeridian tidal heat [effusion], night sweating, and vexing heat in the five hearts. In this condition, heat easily stirs yin-blood and damages the network vessels of the lung so that the phlegm is flecked with blood. MED Treat with Fine Jade Paste (*qióng yù gāo*) or Six Gentlemen Metal and Water Brew (*jīn shuǐ liù jūn jiān*). ACU Base treatment mainly on LU and KI. Select BL-13 (*fèi shū*, Lung Transport), BL-43 (*gāo huāng shū*, Gao-Huang Transport), LU-5 (*chǐ zé*, Cubit Marsh), and KI-6 (*zhào hǎi*, Shining Sea); needle with supplementation. For phlegm flecked with blood, drain, LU-6 (*kǒng zuì*, Collection Hole), and LU-10 (*yú jì*, Fish Border). **Lung-spleen vacuity cold** taxation cough is characterized by enduring cough with copious phlegm that is easily expectorated, shortness of breath, sloppy stool, and aversion to cold. MED Treat with Supplemented Center-Rectifying Decoction (*jiā wèi lǐ zhōng tāng*). ACU Base treatment mainly on back transport points, LU, SP, and ST. Select BL-13 (*fèi shū*, Lung Transport), BL-20 (*pí shū*, Spleen Transport), LU-9 (*tài yuān*, Great Abyss), SP-3 (*tài bái*, Supreme White), CV-12 (*zhōng wǎn*, Center Stomach Duct), ST-40 (*fēng lóng*, Bountiful Bulge), and LI-4 (*hé gǔ*, Union Valley); needle with supplementation and add moxa. See SPLEEN

COUGH. **2.** The term taxation cough also includes, and sometimes specifically denotes, cough due to consumption, which is attributed to "worms gnawing the lungs." See CONSUMPTION and LUNG TAXATION. MED Use formulas such as Stemona Paste (*bǎi bù gāo*). ACU Base treatment mainly on LU and back transport points. Select LU-9 (*tài yuān*, Great Abyss), BL-13 (*fèi shū*, Lung Transport), BL-43 (*gāo huāng shū*, Gao-Huang Transport), LU-5 (*chǐ zé*, Cubit Marsh), ST-36 (*zú sān lǐ*, Leg Three Li), SP-6 (*sān yīn jiāo*, Three Yin Intersection), and KI-3 (*tài xī*, Great Ravine); needle with supplementation. See FIRE DEPRESSION COUGH. [97: 257] [26: 680] [92: No. 173] [34: 78] [46: 657] [113: 139]

taxation damage 劳伤 *láo shāng*: TAXATION FATIGUE. [26: 679]

taxation damage cough 劳伤咳嗽 *láo shāng ké sòu*: TAXATION COUGH. [26: 679]

taxation damage profuse menstruation 劳伤月经过多 *láo shāng yuè jīng guò duo*: Profuse menstruation (menorrhagia) occurring when taxation fatigue causes detriment to the thoroughfare (*chōng*) and controlling (*rèn*) vessels. Menstrual flow gradually increases and becomes persistent. It is dull and pale in color. Accompanying signs include withered-yellow facial complexion, physical fatigue and lack of strength, and in some cases sagging aching pain in the abdomen. MED Secure the thoroughfare (*chōng*) vessel and stanch bleeding with Thoroughfare-Quieting Decoction (*ān chōng tāng*). ACU Base treatment mainly on CV, SP, and ST. Select CV-6 (*qì hǎi*, Sea of Qi), SP-6 (*sān yīn jiāo*, Three Yin Intersection), SP-1 (*yǐn bái*, Hidden White), BL-20 (*pí shū*, Spleen Transport), ST-36 (*zú sān lǐ*, Leg Three Li), and SP-3 (*tài bái*, Supreme White); needle with supplementation and add moxa. [26: 679] [46: 688,689]

taxation detriment 劳损 *láo sǔn*: Any pattern caused by taxation which in turn causes vacuity detriment to yin-yang, qi-blood, or the organs. Taxation is the cause, whereas detriment is the resulting pattern. Taxation detriment is also used as a generic name for VACUITY TAXATION and VACUITY DETRIMENT. See also TAXATION FATIGUE. [26: 679]

taxation fatigue 劳倦 *láo juàn*: Synonym: *taxation damage*. **1.** Overexertion, intemperate living (including dietary irregularities and sexual intemperance), or the seven affects (emotional imbalance) as a cause of disease. **2.** A disease pattern resulting from taxation fatigue[1]. Overexertion, dietary irregularities, sexual intemperance, and affect damage tend to damage spleen qi and kidney essence; hence taxation fatigue is characterized by fatigue and laziness to speak, panting on exertion, heat vexation, spontaneous sweating, and heart palpitations. MED Use Center-Supplementing Qi-Boosting Decoction (*bǔ zhōng yì qì tāng*). For pronounced yin fire with heat agitation, add phellodendron (*huáng bǎi*) and dried/fresh rehmannia (*shēng dì huáng*) to supplement water and rescue yin. For vexation, combine the formula with Cinnabar Spirit-Quieting Pill (*zhū shā ān shén wán*) to drain fire and quiet the spirit. ACU Base treatment mainly on CV, SP, and ST. Select CV-6 (*qì hǎi*, Sea of Qi), BL-20 (*pí shū*, Spleen Transport), ST-36 (*zú sān lǐ*, Leg Three Li), CV-12 (*zhōng wǎn*, Center Stomach Duct), SP-6 (*sān yīn jiāo*, Three Yin Intersection), and SP-3 (*tài bái*, Supreme White); needle with supplementation and moxa if appropriate. For heat vexation and spontaneous sweating, add LI-4 (*hé gǔ*, Union Valley) and KI-7 (*fù liū*, Recover Flow). For heart vexation, add HT-7 (*shén mén*, Spirit Gate). See DAMAGE BY THE FIVE TAXATIONS and SEXUAL TAXATION. [26: 679] [25: 150] [27: 118] [46: 575,596]

taxation heat [effusion] 劳热 *láo rè*: HEAT EFFUSION in vacuity taxation patterns, attributable to qi-blood depletion or yang debilitation and yin vacuity. It takes the form of steaming bone taxation heat EFFUSION, and vexing heat in the five hearts. Accompanying signs differ according to the nature of the vacuity. See YIN VACUITY HEAT EFFUSION, YANG VACUITY HEAT EFFUSION, BLOOD VACUITY HEAT EFFUSION, and QI VACUITY HEAT EFFUSION. [26: 680] [27: 357] [97: 257]

taxation malaria 劳疟 *láo nüè*: **1.** Enduring malaria occurring when patients suffering from debilitation of right qi or enduring taxation detriment contract the evils that cause malaria. Taxation malaria is characterized by mild aversion to cold and mild heat effusion occurring in the day or at night, with attacks being brought on by taxation. Patients often suffer from qi vacuity copious sweating and reduced food intake. MED Supplement vacuity and terminate malaria, using Center-Supplementing Qi-Boosting Decoction (*bǔ zhōng yì qì tāng*) plus achyranthes (*niú xī*), processed flowery knotweed (*zhì hé shǒu wū*), and mume (*wū méi*). If there is pronounced vacuity heat and shortage of liquid characterized by a dry mouth and tongue, Bupleurum Decoction Minus Pinellia Plus Trichosanthes Root (*chái hú qù bàn xià jiā guā lóu tāng*) can be used. ACU Base treatment mainly on GV, PC, SI, ST, and back transport points. Select GV-14 (*dà zhuī*, Great Hammer), GV-13 (*táo dào*, Kiln Path), PC-5 (*jiān shǐ*, Intermediary Courier), SI-3 (*hòu xī*, Back Ravine), CV-12 (*zhōng wǎn*, Center Stomach Duct), ST-36 (*zú sān lǐ*, Leg Three Li), SP-2 (*dà dū*, Great Metropolis), BL-20 (*pí shū*, Spleen Transport), and BL-17 (*gé shū*, Diaphragm Transport); needle with supplementation and add moxa. For principles and

methods of treatment, see MALARIA. **2.** MOTHER-OF-MALARIA. [26: 679] [27: 359] [97: 257] [113: 171]

taxation relapse 劳复 *láo fù*: Relapse due to taxation. During recovery from an illness, before qi and blood have returned to normal or when residual heat is still present, physical exertion, affect damage, dietary or sexual intemperance can damage right qi and cause a relapse of the illness. [26: 679] [27: 122] [97: 431]

taxation steaming 劳蒸 *láo zhēng*: STEAMING DISEASE. [26: 680]

taxation strangury 劳淋 *láo lín*: Dribbling painful urination brought on by taxation fatigue. Distinction is made between spleen taxation and kidney taxation. MED Spleen taxation is treated by fortifying the spleen and boosting qi, using formulas such as Center-Supplementing Qi-Boosting Decoction (*bǔ zhōng yì qì tāng*) or Spleen-Returning Decoction (*guī pí tāng*) and their variations, whereas kidney taxation is treated by supporting vacuity and supplementing the kidney, using Six-Ingredient Rehmannia Pill (*liù wèi dì huáng wán*), and Golden Coffer Kidney Qi Pill (*jīn guì shèn qì wán*). ACU Base treatment mainly on the three yin channels of the foot and on alarm and back transport points of BL (CV-3 and BL-28). Main points: BL-28 (*páng guāng shū*, Bladder Transport), CV-3 (*zhōng jí*, Central Pole), SP-9 (*yīn líng quán*, Yin Mound Spring), KI-3 (*tài xī*, Great Ravine), and SP-6 (*sān yīn jiāo*, Three Yin Intersection) (moxa can be added at this last point). Selection of points according to pattern: For kidney taxation, add BL-23 (*shèn shū*, Kidney Transport), CV-4 (*guān yuán*, Pass Head), and KI-7 (*fù liū*, Recover Flow); needling with supplementation. For spleen taxation, add BL-20 (*pí shū*, Spleen Transport), CV-6 (*qì hǎi*, Sea of Qi), and ST-36 (*zú sān lǐ*, Leg Three Li); needle with supplementation and add moxa. [26: 679] [46: 674] [27: 425] [97: 257]

taxation timidity 劳怯 *láo què*: VACUITY TAXATION. [27: 358]

TB 三焦 *sān jiāo*: , 手少阳三焦经 *shǒu shào yáng sān jiāo jīng*: Abbreviation for the triple burner or the hand lesser yang (*shào yáng*) triple burner channel. [27: 22, 88] [97: 107]

tea 茶 *chá*: **1.** The dried leaves of the shrub *Camellia sinensis* (tea leaves) or the drink made by infusing tea leaves in hot water. **2.** Powders made loosely into cakes with binding medicinals which are prepared by brewing like tea, either with tea leaves or without. ◇ Eng from Du. *tee* (now *thee*), from the Minnan dialect of Chinese *té* akin to Mandarin Chinese *chá*. [27: 313] [26: 523]

tear hall 泪堂 *lèi táng*: The hole from which tears flow (i.e., the outlet of the lacrimal gland). Also called *tear orifice*.

tearing 流泪 *liú lèi*: *Synonym: lacrimation.* The discharge of tears other than for emotional reasons. A broad distinction is made between HEAT TEARING, COLD TEARING, and TEARING ON EXPOSURE TO WIND. In young children, crying without tearing is a sign of a relatively serious condition. [26: 478]

tearing on exposure to wind 迎风流泪 *yíng fēng liú lèi*: A sign of liver channel vacuity cold or liver channel wind-heat. Periodic tearing unassociated with exposure to wind may be due either to liver-kidney depletion or to effulgent yin vacuity fire.

tear orifice 泪窍 *lèi qiào*: *Synonym: tear hall.* The hole from which tears flow. ⟦WMC⟧ outlet of the lacrimal gland (punctum lacrimale, lacrimal point). [27: 65] [97: 367]

tears 泪 *lèi*: The humor of the liver. [97: 367]

tears are the humor of the liver 泪为肝液 *lèi wéi gān yè*: The liver opens at the eyes; hence tears are the humor of the liver. [27: 61]

teeth are the surplus of the bone 齿为骨之于 *chǐ wéi gǔ zhī yú*: The teeth are the product of a surplus qi of the bone, and since the kidney governs the bone, the teeth are considered to be related to the kidney qi. The growth and condition of the teeth are considered as a reflection of kidney qi. See SLOWNESS TO TEETHE; CHANGE OF TEETH; LOOSENING OF THE TEETH; DESICCATED TEETH; BLACK TEETH. [27: 53, 25]

teeth dry as desiccated bones 牙齿干燥如枯骨 *yá chǐ gān zào rú kū gǔ*: DESICCATED TEETH.

temple 颞颥 *niè rú*: *Synonym: greater yang.* The area medial to the eyebrow bone (superciliary arch), in front of the upper part of the ear. [26: 1009] [27: 64]

tendency to sleep 多寐 *duō mèi*, 多睡 *duō shuò*: SOMNOLENCE.

tender-red tongue 舌质嫩红 *shé zhí nèn hóng*: A tongue that is a pale soft red (pastel red) in color. It is a sign of severe vacuity.

tender-soft tongue 舌嫩 *shé nèn*: A tongue that looks smooth and tender like the flesh of a child. ◇ Eng tender-soft, 'tender' in the sense of soft and delicate, with the addition of '-soft' to prevent confusion with the sense of 'painful when pressed'.

tenesmus 里急后重 *lǐ jí hòu zhòng*: *Synonym: abdominal urgency and heaviness in the rectum.* The urgent desire to evacuate, with difficulty in defecation characterized by heaviness or pressure in the rectum. Tenesmus with stool containing pus and blood is a major sign of dysentery. ◇ Chin 里 *lǐ*, internal; 急 *jí*, urgency; 后 *hòu*, posterior, 重 *zhòng*, heaviness. Chinese expresses the notion of tenesmus as abdominal (literally internal) urgency and heaviness in the rectum (lit. posterior). [27: 363]

ten formula types 十剂 *shí jì*: Diffusing, freeing, supplementing, discharging, light, heavy, lubricating, astringent, dry, and moist formulas. [27: 305]

Ten Formula Types

DIFFUSING FORMULA 宣剂 (*xuān jì*)
FREEING FORMULA 通剂 (*tōng jì*)
SUPPLEMENTING FORMULA 补剂 (*bǔ jì*)
DISCHARGING FORMULA 泄剂 (*xiè jì*)
LIGHT FORMULA 轻剂 (*qīng jì*)
HEAVY FORMULA 重剂 (*zhòng jì*)
LUBRICATING FORMULA 滑剂 (*huá jì*)
ASTRINGENT FORMULA 涩剂 (*sè jì*)
DRY FORMULA 燥剂 (*zào jì*)
MOIST FORMULA 湿剂 (*shī jì*)

tennis elbow 网球肘 *wǎng qiú zhǒu*: ELBOW TAXATION. ◇ Chin 网球 *wǎng qiú*, tennis; 肘 *zhǒu*, elbow. The Chinese is a modern expression of Western origin.

ten-principle inspection of the complexion 望色十法 *wàng sè shí fǎ*: A method of evaluating the facial complexion according to ten paired principles: floating and sunken; clear and turbid; weak and strong; diffuse and intense; moist and perished. **Floating and sunken** (浮沉 *fú chén*): A floating complexion is one where the color appears to be in the skin; it signifies disease in the exterior. A sunken complexion is one where the color appears to be below the skin; it indicates that the disease is in the interior. A floating complexion that gradually becomes sunken indicates disease passing from the exterior into the interior. A sunken complexion that gradually becomes floating indicates disease passing from the interior out to the exterior. **Clear and turbid** (清浊 *qīng zhuó*): A clear complexion is clean and bright; it means that the disease is in yang. A turbid complexion is murky and dull; it means that the disease is in yin. A clear complexion that becomes turbid and a turbid complexion that becomes clear indicates disease movement from yang to yin or yin to yang. **Weak and strong** (微甚 *wēi shèn*): A weak complexion is pale-colored; it is associated with vacuity of right qi. A strong complexion is deep-colored; it signifies exuberant evil qi. A strong complexion changing to a weak complexion or vice-versa indicates repletion-vacuity conversion. **Diffuse and dense** (散抟 *sàn tuán*): A diffuse complexion is a dispersed complexion; it signifies illness about to resolve; a dense complexion is an unbroken complexion, and means a disease gradually gathering. A diffuse complexion becoming dense indicates that although the disease is of recent onset, it is gradually gathering; a dense complexion becoming diffuse indicates that although the illness is long standing, it is about to resolve. **Moist and perished** (泽夭 *zé yāo*): A moist complexion is one with a sheen; it signifies life. A perished complexion is a desiccated complexion; it signifies death. A perished complexion that becomes moist indicates the return of essence-spirit; a moist complexion that becomes perished indicates debilitation of qi and blood. The ten principles are helpful in assessing the development of a disease. However, they must be correlated with the five colors. For example, a red complexion means heat. A weak red complexion indicates vacuity heat, whereas a strong red complexion is repletion heat; a floating weak red complexion indicates vacuity heat in the exterior, while a deep weak red complexion indicated vacuity heat in the interior. [29: 39]

ten questions 十问 *shí wèn*: Inquiry into the following ten areas: (1) cold and heat; (2) sweating; (3) head and body; (4) stool and urine; (5) appetite; (6) chest; (7) hearing; (8) thirst; (9) previous illnesses; (10) cause [of present illness]. In addition, the practitioner should inquire into effectiveness of previous medication, menstruation in women, and smallpox and measles in children. [27: 187]

tension of the sinews 筋脉拘急 *jīn mài jū jí*: Tension of the sinews preventing normal bending and stretching. Sinew hypertonicity is mostly attributable to contraction of wind-cold in general vacuity, or to blood or liquid vacuity depriving the sinew vessels of nourishment. It is observed in LOCKJAW (*pò shāng fēng*), TETANY (*jìng*), IMPEDIMENT (*bì*), FRIGHT WIND (*jīng fēng*), and WIND STROKE (*zhòng fēng*). MED Use Five Accumulations Powder (*wǔ jī sǎn*) to dispel wind and dissipate cold or use Four Agents Decoction (*sì wù tāng*) to nourish blood and increase humor. ACU Needle the meeting point of the sinews, GB-34 (*yáng líng quán*, Yang Mound Spring), and add other points according to cause and location. [26: 741] [4: 150] [50: 1524]

ten strange pulses 十怪脉 *shí guài mài*: Ten critical pulse conditions, include the SEVEN STRANGE PULSES, i.e., *pecking sparrow pulse, leaking roof pulse, flicking stone pulse, untwining rope pulse, waving fish pulse, darting shrimp pulse,* and *seething cauldron pulse*, plus the three others: **Upturned knife pulse** 偃刀脉 (*yǎn dāo mài*): A pulse like a knife with the blade pointing upward, i.e., fine, stringlike, extremely tight. **Spinning bean pulse:** 转豆脉 (*zhuǎn dòu mài*): A pulse that comes and goes away elusive like a spinning bean. Also called a spinning pill pulse. **Frenzied sesame seed pulse:** 麻促脉 (*má cù mài*): A pulse that feels like sesame seeds under the finger, extremely fine and faint, and urgent, skipping and chaotic. [27: 199]

terminating lactation 回乳 *huí rǔ*, 断乳 *duàn rǔ*: A method of treatment used to stop the flow of milk. MED Preparea a decoction of stir-fried barley sprout (*mài yá*) and drink as tea. Decoct 80–100 g (some say only 60 g) per day, and take for 3–5 consecutive days. Some also claim that raw barley sprout should be used. If signs such distention and pain in the breasts, or lumps, or even a sensation of heat in the breast appear, dandelion (*pú gōng yīng*) can be added to clear heat and resolve toxin, and tangerine pip (*jú hé*), forsythia (*lián qiào*), and gizzard lining (*jī nèi jīn*) can be added to disperse stagnation to prevent the development of MAMMARY WELLING-ABSCESS. Alternatively, use No-Nursing-Worries Powder (*miǎn huái sǎn*) with the addition of barley sprout (*mài yá*), tangerine pip (*jú hé*), and crataegus (*shān zhā*). ACU Select GB-21 (*jiān jǐng*, Shoulder Well), ST-36 (*zú sān lǐ*, Leg Three Li), bilateral GB-37 (*guāng míng*, Bright Light), and bilateral GB-41 (*zú lín qì*, Foot Overlooking Tears); needle with drainage, and addg moxa at GB-37 and GB-41. [67: 333] [26: 260]

tertian malaria 间日疟 *jiān rì nüè*: MALARIA characterized by episodes occurring every other day. WMC tertian malaria, vivax malaria. ◇ Chin 间 *jiān*, interval; 日 *rì*, day; 疟 *nüè*, malaria. Malaria occurring with intervals of one day. Eng tertian, occurring every third day. [26: 709]

testicle 卵 *luǎn*, 阴卵 *yīn luǎn*, 睾 *gāo*, 睾丸 *gāo wán*: Either of the egg-shaped contents of the scrotum. *The Inner Canon* (*nèi jīng*) makes no comment about the function of the testicles, although it mentions them six times in the context of disease, e.g., *The Magic Pivot* (*líng shū, xié qì cáng fǔ bìng xíng*) states, "In disease of the small intestine, there is smaller-abdominal pain and pain in the lumbar spine referring to the testicles." [27: 26] [97: 292] [26: 787]

tetanic disease 痉病 *jìng bìng*: TETANY.

tetanic reversal 痉厥 *jìng jué*: Tetany accompanied by CLOUDING REVERSAL (loss of consciousness).

tetanus 破伤风 *pò shāng fēng*: LOCKJAW.

tetany 痉 *jìng*, 痓 *cì*: Severe spasm such as rigidity in the neck, clenched jaw, convulsions of the limbs, and arched-back rigidity. Repletion patterns are attributed to wind, cold, dampness, phlegm, or fire congesting the channels, whereas vacuity patterns occur when excessive sweating, loss of blood, or constitutional vacuity causes qi vacuity, shortage of blood, and insufficiency of the fluids, depriving the sinews of nourishment and allowing internal wind to stir. To resolve tetany, repletion patterns are treated primarily by dispelling wind and secondarily by supporting right qi, whereas vacuity patterns are treated primarily by boosting qi and nourishing the blood and secondarily by extinguishing wind. Distinction is made between SOFT TETANY and HARD TETANY, the former being distinguished from the latter by the presence of sweating and absence of aversion to cold. The terms YIN TETANY and YANG TETANY are synonymous with soft and hard tetany, or may denote tetany with and without counterflow cold of the limbs respectively. Tetany may occur as a signs of a variety of different diseases, including but not limited to tetanus (see LOCKJAW); occurring in infants and children, it is referred to as FRIGHT WIND. See FRIGHT and FRIGHT WIND. ◇ Eng from Gk. *tetanos*, rigid, stretched. [26: 672, 528, 428] [27: 631]

thick tongue fur 厚苔 *hòu tāi*: A thick tongue fur indicates the presence of an evil, usually dampness or phlegm. The thickening of the tongue fur means the advance of the evil, whereas its thinning marks regression. [6: 123]

thief sweating 盗汗 *dào hàn*: NIGHT SWEATING.

thigh 髀 *bì*, 股 *gǔ*: The upper section of the leg from the knee to the trunk; the thigh bone. *The Magic Pivot* (*líng shū, gǔ dù*) states, "[the distance] between the thighs is six inches and a half." ◇ Chin 髀 *bì* is composed of 卑, low, with 骨, the bone signifier, said to indicate that it is a bone of the lower body. In usage, it denotes the thigh in general, and especially the outer aspect. 股 *gǔ* also denotes the thigh, especially the inner aspect. [26: 690]

thigh bone 髀骨 *bì gǔ*: The bone of the upper leg. WMC femur.

thigh joint 髀关 *bì guān*: The area at the upper extremity of the thigh at the crease between the thigh and trunk. WMC hip joint. [97: 652] [27: 71] [25: 343] [46: 44]

thigh pivot 髀枢 *bì shū*: **1.** The prominence at the top of the lateral aspect of the thigh. WMC greater trochanter. **2.** The socket of the hip joint. WMC acetabulum. [25: 343] [26: 960] [27: 71] [97: 652]

thin tongue fur 薄苔 *bó tāi*: A tongue fur is thin if the underlying tongue surface shows through faintly. A thin white tongue fur may be normal, or may be a sign of initial-stage external contraction. Other thin furs are of pathological significance judged by their color and texture.

third yang channel 三阳 *sān yáng*: GREATER YANG CHANNEL.

third yin channel 三阴 *sān yīn*: GREATER YIN CHANNEL.

thirst 渴 *kě*, 口渴 *kǒu kě*: A sense of dryness in the mouth with a greater or lesser urge to drink. Thirst most commonly reflects insufficiency of yin fluids and/or the presence of heat that causes fluid loss through sweating, as observed in lung-stomach heat, yin vacuity, and blood vacuity. It may occur when water-damp, phlegm or static blood cause obstruction. It can also reflect impaired transportation of the essence of food and water due to spleen vacuity or in impaired transformation of fluids due to kidney vacuity. **Lung-stomach heat** thirst is characterized by desire for cold drinks and is associated with constipation, reddish urine, yellow tongue fur, and rapid pulse. MED Clear heat and drain fire with formulas such as Lung-Clearing Drink (*qīng fèi yǐn zi*), White Tiger Decoction (*bái hǔ tāng*), or one of the Qi-Coordinating Decoctions (*chéng qì tāng*). ACU Commonly used main points for all forms of thirst are Gold Liquid and Jade Humor (*jīn jīn yù yè*), Sea Source (*hǎi quán*), TB-2 (*yè mén*, Humor Gate), KI-6 (*zhào hǎi*, Shining Sea), and SP-6 (*sān yīn jiāo*, Three Yin Intersection), needle with supplementation. For lung-stomach heat, add LU-7 (*liè quē*, Broken Sequence), LU-5 (*chǐ zé*, Cubit Marsh), LI-11 (*qū chí*, Pool at the Bend), LI-4 (*hé gǔ*, Union Valley), ST-44 (*nèi tíng*, Inner Court), and ST-36 (*zú sān lǐ*, Leg Three Li), and needle with drainage. **Yin vacuity and diminished liquid** thirst is characterized by dry throat and mouth, heat vexation and upbearing fire flush, red lips, tongue with scant liquid, and a fine pulse. MED Nourish yin and engender liquid using formulas such as Humor-Increasing Decoction (*zēng yè tāng*), Five Juices Beverage (*wǔ zhī yǐn*), and Adenophora/Glehnia and Ophiopogon Decoction (*shā shēn mài dōng tāng*). ACU Use the main points for thirst described above, and add BL-23 (*shèn shū*, Kidney Transport), KI-3 (*tài xī*, Great Ravine), and KI-2 (*rán gǔ*, Blazing Valley), needling with supplementation. **Blood vacuity** thirst is most commonly observed after major blood loss and is attended by pale lips, bright white complexion, dizziness, pale tongue, and vacuous or scallion-stalk pulse. MED Supplement qi and boost the blood with formulas such as Tangkuei Blood-Supplementing Decoction (*dāng guī bǔ xuè tāng*) or Eight-Gem Decoction (*bā zhēn tāng*). ACU To the main points for thirst, add BL-20 (*pí shū*, Spleen Transport), BL-21 (*wèi shū*, Stomach Transport), LR-3 (*tài chōng*, Supreme Surge), ST-36 (*zú sān lǐ*, Leg Three Li), SP-10 (*xuè hǎi*, Sea of Blood), and BL-17 (*gé shū*, Diaphragm Transport), needling with supplementation. **Water-damp** thirst is characterized by thirst with no desire to drink, i.e., a thirst that is unquenched by drinking; it indicates not a lack of fluid in the body, but failure of fluids to reach the mouth. Thirst in such cases is associated with oppression in the chest, torpid intake, abdominal distention, swollen limbs, inhibited urination, slimy tongue fur, and a soggy pulse. MED Dry dampness and disinhibit water with formulas such as Stomach-Calming Poria (Hoelen) Five Decoction (*wèi líng tāng*) or Five-Peel Beverage (*wǔ pí yǐn*). [ACU] Add to the main points for thirst CV-9 (*shuǐ fēn*, Water Divide), CV-6 (*qì hǎi*, Sea of Qi), BL-22 (*sān jiāo shū*, Triple Burner Transport), ST-36 (*zú sān lǐ*, Leg Three Li), BL-20 (*pí shū*, Spleen Transport), and SP-9 (*yīn líng quán*, Yin Mound Spring), and needle with drainage. **Phlegm-rheum** thirst is associated with oppression in the chest, shortness of breath, heart palpitations, and ejection of phlegm-drool. [MED] Warm yang and transform rheum using formulas such as Poria (Hoelen), Cinnamon Twig, Ovate Atractylodes, and Licorice Decoction (*líng guì zhú gān tāng*). [ACU] To the main points for thirst add CV-12 (*zhōng wǎn*, Center Stomach Duct), ST-36 (*zú sān lǐ*, Leg Three Li), ST-40 (*fēng lóng*, Bountiful Bulge), LI-4 (*hé gǔ*, Union Valley), PC-6 (*nèi guān*, Inner Pass), and PC-4 (*xī mén*, Cleft Gate), and needle with supplementation and add moxa. **Blood stasis** thirst is characterized by thirst but with a desire only to wash the mouth rather than to swallow fluid and is attended by withered lips, purple tongue, and a rough pulse. Treat by quickening the blood and dispelling stasis with formulas like Peach Kernel and Carthamus Four Agents Decoction (*táo hóng sì wù tāng*) and House of Blood Stasis-Expelling Decoction (*xuè fǔ zhú yū tāng*). [ACU] To the main points for thirst add BL-17 (*gé shū*, Diaphragm Transport), SP-10 (*xuè hǎi*, Sea of Blood), CV-6 (*qì hǎi*, Sea of Qi), LI-4 (*hé gǔ*, Union Valley), and LR-3 (*tài chōng*, Supreme Surge); needle with even supplementation and drainage or prick to bleed with a three-edged needle. **Spleen vacuity** with impaired transportation of liquid causing thirst is characterized by desire for warm drinks and the intake of fluids in small amounts, and is attended by fatigued cumbersome limbs, clear urine, and sloppy stool. [MED] Fortify the spleen with formulas such as Center-Rectifying Decoction (*lǐ zhōng tāng*) and Seven-Ingredient Ovate Atractylodes Powder (*qī wèi bái zhú sǎn*). [ACU] To the main points for thirst add CV-12 (*zhōng wǎn*, Center Stomach Duct), BL-20 (*pí shū*, Spleen Transport), ST-36 (*zú sān lǐ*, Leg Three Li), SP-6 (*sān yīn jiāo*, Three Yin Intersection), and SP-4 (*gōng sūn*, Yellow Emperor), needling with supplementation and adding moxa. **Kidney yang debilitation** thirst is characterized by physical cold and aversion to cold, shortness of breath, swollen limbs, cold aching lumbus and legs, and long voidings of clear urine or dribbling urination, sunken pulse, and pale tongue. [MED] Warm yang and supplement the kidney using formulas such as True Warrior Decoction (*zhēn wǔ tāng*) or Golden Coffer Kidney Qi Pill (*jīn guì shèn qì wán*). Thirst with frequent intake of fluids, increased food intake, and copious urine is a

sign of dispersion-thirst. [ACU] To the main points for thirst add BL-23 (*shèn shū*, Kidney Transport), CV-4 (*guān yuán*, Pass Head), GV-4 (*mìng mén*, Life Gate), KI-3 (*tài xī*, Great Ravine), and KI-7 (*fù liū*, Recover Flow), needling with supplementation and adding moxa. [26: 667] [92: No. 88]

thirst with a liking for warm drinks 渴喜热饮 *kě xǐ rè yǐn*: See THIRST.

thirst with no desire to drink 渴不欲饮 *kě bù yù yǐn*: See THIRST.

Thirteen Ghost Points 十三鬼穴 *shí sān guǐ xué*: A group of points that originated from the Tang dynasty physician Sun Si-Miao's method for treating conditions such as mania, withdrawal, and epilepsy that were formerly attributed to demonic influence or possession. See Table 13.

13. Thirteen Ghost Points	
Point Name	Regular Name
Ghost Palace (*guǐ gōng*)	GV-26 (*rén zhōng*, Human Center)
Ghost Sincerity (*guǐ xìn*)	LU-11 (*shào shāng*, Lesser Shang)
Ghost Pile (*guǐ lěi*)	SP-1 (*yǐn bái*, Hidden White)
Ghost Heart (*guǐ xīn*)	PC-7 (*dà líng*, Great Mound)
Ghost Road (*guǐ lù*)	BL-62 (*shēn mài*, Extending Vessel)
Ghost Pillow (*guǐ zhěn*)	GV-16 (*fēng fǔ*, Wind Mansion)
Ghost Bed (*guǐ chuáng*)	ST-6 (*jiá chē*, Jawbone)
Ghost Market (*guǐ shì*)	CV-24 (*chéng jiāng*, Sauce Receptacle)
Ghost Cave (*guǐ kū*)	PC-8 (*láo gōng*, Palace of Toil)
Ghost Hall (*guǐ táng*)	GV-23 (*shàng xīng*, Upper Star)
Ghost Store (*guǐ cáng*)	CV-1 (*huì yīn*, Meeting of Yin)
Ghost Leg (*guǐ tuǐ*)	LI-11 (*qū chí*, Pool at the Bend)
Ghost Seal (*guǐ fēng*)	KI-1 (*yǒng quán*, Gushing Spring)

thoracic fullness 胸满 *xiōng mǎn*: FULLNESS IN THE CHEST.

thoracic glomus 胸痞 *xiōng pǐ*: GLOMUS IN THE CHEST.

thoracic impediment 胸痹 *xiōng bì*: CHEST IMPEDIMENT.

thoracic oppression 胸闷 *xiòng mèn*: OPPRESSION IN THE CHEST.

thoracic pain 胸痛 *xiōng tòng*: CHEST PAIN.

thoracic yang 胸阳 *xiōng yáng*: CHEST YANG.

thoroughfare vessel 冲脉 *chōng mài*: Abbreviation: Thoroughfare. *Synonym: penetrating vessel*. One of the EIGHT EXTRAORDINARY VESSELS. Pathway: The thoroughfare (*chōng*) vessel has a total of five paths. The first starts in the lower abdomen and emerges in the qi street, traveling up with the foot lesser yin (*shào yīn*) kidney channel and passing from the umbilicus to the chest, where it disperses between the ribs. The second path begins where the channel disperses in the chest. It runs up the throat and face, skirting the lips, and terminating in the nose. The third path emerges from the qi street in the lower abdomen at KI-11 (*héng gǔ*, Pubic Bone), then descends along the medial aspect of the thigh to the popliteal fossa. Continuing down along the medial margin of the tibia, it passes behind the medial malleolus before dispersing in the sole of the foot. The fourth branch diverges from ST-30 (*qì chōng*, Qi Thoroughfare) and descends obliquely down the lower extremity to the medial malleolus. It enters the heel, crosses the tarsal bones of the foot, and finally reaches the great toe. The fifth channel separates from the main course in the pelvic cavity and runs to the spine, which it then ascends. Functions: The thoroughfare (*chōng*) vessel is the sea of the major channels. It has a regulating effect on all twelve regular channels, and its main function is to regulate menstruation, for which reason it is sometimes called the "sea of blood." Signs: In women, uterine bleeding, miscarriage, menstrual block, menstrual irregularities, scant breast milk, lower abdominal pain, and blood ejection. In men, seminal emission, impotence, and conditions classed in Western medicine as prostatitis, urethritis, and orchitis. See UTERUS. ◇ Chin 冲 *chōng*, used in the simplified character set as a substitute for 衝, a thoroughfare; charge, thrust, surge upward; clash, crash. [26: 896] [6: 69] [27: 89] [97: 223]

thought 思 *sī*: One of the FIVE MINDS, associated with the spleen.

thought causes qi to bind 思则气结 *sī zé qì jié*: Excessive thought or cogitation can cause binding depression of spleen qi that affects normal splenic movement and transformation, causing glomus and fullness in the chest and stomach duct, poor appetite, abdominal distention, and thin stool. [27: 145] [97: 405]

thousand-day sore 千日疮 *qiān rì chuāng*: WART. [27: 585] [97: 31]

threaded ligation 挂线法 *guà xiàn fǎ*: A method of treating fistulas involving the threading of a medicated thread or fine shreds of elephant skin through the pathway of the fistula. This method makes use of the tensile strength of the thread to speed the degeneration of tissue to eventually open the fistula. [27: 268]

threatened miscarriage 先兆流产 *xiān zhào liú chǎn*: Lumbar and abdominal pain, sagging sensation, and bleeding from the vagina in pregnancy. In modern practice, a urine pregnancy test is routinely performed. See STIRRING FETUS. [26: 264] [44: 747]

three bars of the finger 指三关 *zhǐ sān guān*: The wind, qi, and life bars. See INFANT'S FINGER EXAMINATION. [6: 119]

three causes [of disease] 三因 *sān yīn*: Synonym: *three categories of cause*. External, internal, and neutral causes of disease. The term "three causes" was coined by Chen Wu-Ze in his *A Unified Treatise on Diseases, Patterns, and Remedies According to the Three Causes* (*sān yīn jí yī bìng zhèng fāng lùn*) published in A.D. 1174. External factors are the six excesses. Internal causes are the seven affects. Neutral causes (literally "non-external-internal") include eating too much or too little, taxation fatigue, knocks and falls, crushing, drowning, and animal, insect, and reptile injuries. [27: 105] [97: 15]

three dispersions 三消 *sān xiāo*: **1.** UPPER DISPERSION, CENTER DISPERSION, and LOWER DISPERSION. **2.** DISPERSION-THIRST, CENTER DISPERSION, and KIDNEY DISPERSION. See DISPERSION-THIRST. [26: 31] [27: 423] [97: 16]

three-edged needle 三棱针 *sān léng zhēn*: A thick needle with a sharp, three-edged tip used for letting blood. A three-edged needle is the modern equivalent of the *sharp-edged needle* among the *nine needles* in ancient times. The use of presterilized, disposable lancets has replaced the three-edged needle for bloodletting in many acupuncture clinics. See BLOODLETTING for instructions on how to use it. [26: 35] [80: 502]

three gems 三宝 *sān bǎo*: Synonym: *three mysteries*. Essence, qi, and spirit. [27: 82] [50: 48]

three grades 三品 *sān pǐn*: Three categories of medicinals of *The Divine Husbandman's Herbal Foundation Canon* (*shén nóng běn cǎo jīng*). Top-grade medicals are those that are nontoxic and can be taken for long periods of time without harming the body. Medium-grade medicinals are those that are nontoxic or not greatly toxic and can treat disease and supplement vacuity. Low grade medicinals are ones that are toxic or harsh in their effects, cannot be taken over long periods, and are used to dispel heat and cold evil qi or to break accumulations and gatherings. The classification system of *The Divine Husbandman's Herbal Foundation Canon* (*shén nóng běn cǎo jīng*) is now considered to lack precision and consistency, some medicinals marked as top grade, for example, being toxic. [26: 31]

three hairs 三毛 *sān máo*: The region just proximal to the base of the nail of the great toe, at which a number of hairs are often found growing. Not to be confused with TUFT OF HAIR. [27: 82] [97: 16]

Three Kingdoms 三国 *sān guó*: The name of a dynastic period (A.D. 220–280).

three mysteries 三奇 *sān qí*: THREE GEMS.

three positions and nine indicators 三部九候 *sān bù jiǔ hòu*: **1.** From *Elementary Questions* (*sù wèn, sān bù jiǔ hòu lùn*). An ancient pulse-taking scheme. The three positions are three areas on the head, upper limbs, and lower limbs, each area having three pulse points (indicators), which in most cases can be located by the acupuncture point located at the site. See the list below. Possibly owing to a change in mores, the less invasive practice of feeling only the wrist pulse replaced the system of taking the pulse at multiple points, which was probably no longer practiced by the Later Han (1st century A.D.). **2.** From *The Classic of Difficult Issues* (*nàn jīng, 18*). An ancient pulse-taking scheme. In the context of the wrist pulse, the inch, bar, cubit positions are the three positions, and the superficial level, mid-level, and deep level of each of these are the nine indicators. [50: 59] [27: 190] [97: 19]

Three Positions and Nine Indicators

Head
Greater Yang (*tài yáng*)
TB-21 (*ěr mén*, Ear Gate)
ST-4 (*dì cāng*, Earth Granary)
ST-5 (*dà yíng*, Great Reception)

Upper limbs
wrist pulse
HT-7 (*shén mén*, Spirit Gate)
LI-4 (*hé gǔ*, Union Valley)

Lower limbs
LR-10 (*zú wǔ lǐ*, Foot Five Li) in men and LR-3 (*tài chōng*, Supreme Surge) in women
SP-11 (*jī mén*, Winnower Gate)
ST-42 (*chōng yáng*, Surging Yang)
KI-3 (*tài xī*, Great Ravine)

---

three postpartum crises 产后三急 *chǎn hòu sān jí*: Three severe or critical conditions observed after giving birth: POSTPARTUM VOMITING, POSTPARTUM NIGHT SWEATING, and POSTPARTUM DIARRHEA. [26: 575] [27: 432]

three postpartum desertions 产后三脱 *chǎn hòu sān tuō*: Qi desertion, blood desertion, and desertion of the spirit after childbirth. Qi desertion is characterized by shortness of breath, blood desertion by flooding and spotting, and desertion of the spirit by raving and hallucination. [26: 575]

three postpartum diseases 产后三病 *chǎn hòu sān bìng*: POSTPARTUM TETANY, POSTPARTUM DEPRESSION AND VEILING, and POSTPARTUM DEFECATION DIFFICULTY. [26: 575]

three postpartum surges 产后三冲 *chǎn hòu sān chōng*: Upward surge of wasted blood from undischarged LOCHIA into the heart, lung, and stomach. See WASTED BLOOD SURGING INTO THE HEART; WASTED BLOOD SURGING INTO THE LUNG; WASTED BLOOD SURGING INTO THE STOMACH. [26: 575] [27: 542]

three worm diseases 三虫病 *sān chóng bìng*: From *The Origin and Indicators of Disease* (*zhū bìng yuán hòu lùn*). A generic term for LONGWORM DISEASE, REDWORM DISEASE, and PINWORM DISEASE. [26: 35]

three yang channels of the foot 足三阳经 *zú sān yáng jīng*: Of the twelve channels, the three that run on the anterior, lateral, and posterior face of the leg, i.e., the foot yang brightness (*yáng míng*) stomach channel, the foot lesser yang (*shào yáng*) gallbladder channel, and foot greater yang (*tài yáng*) bladder channel. These channels run from the head down the neck, back, and legs to the feet. [97: 269] [27: 85]

14.	Channels of the Hand and Foot	
Position	Yin channels (inside)	Yang channels (outside)
Hand Channels		
Front	Hand greater yin (*tài yīn*) LU	Hand yang brightness (*yáng míng*) LI
Middle	Hand reverting yin (*jué yīn*) PC	Hand lesser yang (*shào yáng*) LI
Rear	Hand lesser yin (*shào yīn*) HT	Hand greater yang (*tài yáng*) SI
Foot Channels		
Front	Foot greater yin (*tài yīn*) SP	Foot yang brightness (*yáng míng*) ST
Middle	Foot reverting yin (*jué yīn*) LR	Foot lesser yang (*shào yáng*) GB
Rear	Foot lesser yin (*shào yīn*) KI	Foot greater yang (*tài yáng*) BL

three yang channels of the hand 手三阳经 *shǒu sān yáng jīng*: Of the twelve channels, the three to run over the lateral aspect of the arm. They are the hand yang brightness (*yáng míng*) large intestine channel, the hand greater yang (*tài yáng*) small intestine channel, and the hand lesser yang (*shào yáng*) triple burner channel. [26: 159] [97: 104] [27: 85]

three yin channels of the foot 足三阴经 *zú sān yīn jīng*: Of the twelve channels, the three that pass along the medial aspect of the leg. They are the foot greater yin (*tài yīn*) spleen channel, the foot lesser yin (*shào yīn*) kidney channel, and the foot reverting yin (*jué yīn*) liver channel. They all start from the foot, and ascend the leg and abdomen to the chest. [97: 269] [27: 85]

three yin channels of the hand 手三阴经 *shǒu sān yīn jīng*: Of the twelve channels, the three that pass along the medial aspect of the arm. They are the hand greater yin (*tài yīn*) lung channel, the hand lesser yin (*shào yīn*) heart channel, and the hand reverting yin (*jué yīn*) pericardium channel. The all start from the chest and run out to the hands. [97: 104] [27: 85]

throat 咽喉 *yān hóu*throat, 咽 *yān*, 喉 *hóu*, 喉咙 *hóu lóng*: The cavity passing through the neck comprising the PHARYNX (upper part) and LARYNX (lower part). A red sore hot swollen throat or throat nodes (tonsils) indicate stomach or lung heat flaming upward; if yellowish white putrefaction speckles are also present, the cause is intense toxic heat. A dry red sore throat generally with slight swelling indicates effulgent yin vacuity fire. A pale red sore throat without the presence of heat or swelling may indicate vacuity fire floating upward. A slightly red sore swollen throat with grayish white putrefaction speckles or patches that are not easily removed may be diphtheria, which is attributable to scorching of lung-stomach yin liquid by dryness-heat. Diseases affecting the throat include: BABY MOTH; THROAT WIND; THROAT IMPEDIMENT; THROAT LICHEN; WELLING-ABSCESS OF THE THROAT; DIPHTHERIA. [26: 730] [27: 29] [97: 402] [50: 1085]

throat-entwining wind 缠喉风 *chán hóu fēng*: THROAT WIND in which the neck that is rigid as if entwined by a snake. Throat-entwining wind is attributed to accumulated heat in the bowels and viscera and wind-phlegm welling upward. There is redness, soreness, and swelling inside and outside the throat pass, with local numbness and itching that may spread as far as the anterior chest. The neck is rigid as if entwined by a snake. The swelling spreads deep down into the throat to the epiglottis and larynx, causing hasty labored breathing, phlegm rale, qi tightness in the chest and diaphragm, green-blue finger nails, vigorous heat [effusion] in the hearts of the palms, hypertonicity of the jaw, and difficulty in swallowing fluids. In severe cases, blockage of the throat can threaten death by asphyxiation. WMC parapharyngeal abscess; suppurative submaxillaritis. MED Resolve toxin and discharge heat; disperse swelling and disinhibit the throat. Use Scourge-Clearing Toxin-Vanquishing Beverage (*qīng wēn bài dú yǐn*). Modern methods may be necessary to maintain respiration. ACU Base treatment mainly on LI, LU,

and ST. Select LI-4 (*hé gǔ*, Union Valley), LI-11 (*qū chí*, Pool at the Bend), LU-5 (*chǐ zé*, Cubit Marsh), ST-44 (*nèi tíng*, Inner Court), CV-22 (*tiān tú*, Celestial Chimney), LU-10 (*yú jì*, Fish Border), ST-40 (*fēng lóng*, Bountiful Bulge), CV-24 (*chéng jiāng*, Sauce Receptacle), and ST-6 (*jiá chē*, Cheek Carriage); needle with drainage, and prick LU-11 (*shào shāng*, Lesser Shang), and LI-1 (*shāng yáng*, Shang Yang) to bleed. See THROAT WIND. [26: 998] [27: 498] [46: 597, 727] [14: 44]

throat impediment 喉痹 *hóu bì*: **1.** A generic name for swelling and soreness of the throat. Throat impediment is attributed generally either to externally contracted wind-heat or to yin vacuity. MED Wind-heat is treated with Lonicera and Forsythia Powder (*yín qiào sǎn*) plus isatis root (*bǎn lán gēn*), belamcanda (*shè gān*), and scrophularia (*xuán shēn*), whereas yin vacuity can be treated with Six-Ingredient Rehmannia Pill (*liù wèi dì huáng wán*). ACU For wind-heat, base treatment mainly on LU and LI. Select GB-20 (*fēng chí*, Wind Pool), LI-11 (*qū chí*, Pool at the Bend), GV-14 (*dà zhuī*, Great Hammer), LI-4 (*hé gǔ*, Union Valley), TB-1 (*guān chōng*, Passage Hub), and LU-5 (*chǐ zé*, Cubit Marsh); needle with drainage. Prick LU-11 (*shào shāng*, Lesser Shang) to bleed. For yin vacuity, base treatment mainly on KI and LU. Select KI-3 (*tài xī*, Great Ravine), KI-6 (*zhào hǎi*, Shining Sea), and LU-10 (*yú jì*, Fish Border); needle with even supplementation and drainage. For dry throat, add TB-2 (*yè mén*, Humor Gate). For pronounced sore swollen throat, prick LU-11 (*shào shāng*, Lesser Shang) to bleed. **2.** Critical swelling and soreness of the throat in which the throat becomes severely occluded. ◇ Chin 喉 *hóu*, larynx, throat; 痹 *bì*, blockage. [26: 732] [97: 618] [46: 726] [37: 470] [113: 505]

throat lichen 喉癣 *hóu xiǎn*: LICHEN (*xiǎn*) in the throat; so called because it appears as a moss or lichen growing in the throat. Throat lichen is attributable either to liver-kidney depletion or to stomach heat fuming the lung. It starts with a dry itchy, slightly sore throat that appears dark and gloomy in complexion, and is covered with red threads, like the veins of a Chinese flowering crabapple leaf (*hǎi táng yè*). Subsequently, the affected area begins to putrefy and take on the appearance of being coated with moss or lichen. Other signs include pain on swallowing that is mild in the morning, more pronounced in the evening, and most severe at night, and a hoarse voice. WMC membranous pharyngitis. **Liver-kidney depletion** causes throat lichen when it causes ascendant hyperactivity of the ministerial fire that in turn causes wear on lung yin. MED Enrich yin and downbear fire with Anemarrhena, Phellodendron, and Rehmannia Pill (*zhī bǎi dì huáng wán*) prepared as a decoction, or Four Agents Decoction (*sì* *wù tāng*) plus ligustrum (*nǔ zhēn zǐ*), scrophularia (*xuán shēn*), and ginseng (*rén shēn*), etc. **Stomach heat fuming the lung** results from excessive consumption of rich fatty fried foods and liquor that causes the accumulation of heat in the stomach. MED Clear heat and resolve toxin with Universal Aid Toxin-Dispersing Beverage (*pǔ jì xiāo dú yǐn*) or Diaphragm-Cooling Powder (*liáng gé sǎn*). [26: 733]

throat-locking wind 锁喉风 *suǒ hóu fēng*: THROAT WIND with clenched jaw. Throat-locking wind is caused by brewing lung-stomach heat with subsequent contraction of wind evil, which settles in the throat. There is soreness inside and outside the throat pass, with a red swelling as large as a hen's egg. There is oppression in the chest, short hasty breathing, difficulty in speaking and swallowing, jaw clenched tight as a lock, bad breath, constipation, and great heat [effusion] and aversion to cold. WMC peritonsillar abscess; retropharyngeal abscess. MED Course wind and clear heat; resolve toxin and disperse swelling. Use Throat-Clearing Diaphragm-Disinhibiting Decoction (*qīng yān lì gé tāng*) or allow Six Spirits Pill (*liù shén wán*) to dissolve in the mouth. When pus has formed, lance to drain, and insufflate Borneol and Borax Powder (*bīng péng sǎn*). [26: 964] [27: 498]

throat moth 喉蛾 *hóu é*: BABY MOTH.

throat node 喉核 *hóu hé*: The slightly protruding flesh between the front pharyngeal pillars (palatoglossal arch) and the rear pharyngeal pillars (palatopharyngeal arch). WMC (pharyngeal) tonsils. Swelling of the throat nodes is called NIPPLE MOTH, equivalent to tonsillitis in Western medicine. [26: 731] [27: 29] [97: 551]

throat pass 喉关 *hóu guān*: The constricted aperture between the mouth and throat at which the uvula is located. WMC isthmus faucium. ◇ Chin 喉 *hóu*, throat, larynx; 关 *guān*, mountain pass; bar; difficult juncture; shut, close. [27: 29] [97: 551]

throat wind 喉风 *hóu fēng*: A severe sudden soreness and swelling of the throat with labored breathing, discomfort in swallowing, phlegm-drool congestion, difficulty talking, and, in severe cases, there may be clenching of the jaw and stupor. Throat wind is caused by wind-heat with preexisting heat in the lung and stomach, with wind and fire fanning each other and binding to produce the sore throat. WMC peritonsillar abscess (quinsy); retropharyngeal abscess; acute epiglottitis, diphtheritic croup. Successive generations of physicians have distinguished different forms of the disease and used different names for them. Distinction is made between ACUTE THROAT WIND, PUTREFYING THROAT WIND, THROAT-LOCKING WIND, and THROAT-ENTWINING WIND. **Acute throat wind**

(also called *constricting throat wind*) is characterized by sudden swelling of the throat. **Putrefying throat wind** is marked by putrefaction and ulceration. **Throat-locking wind** is characterized by clenched jaw. **Throat-entwining wind** is characterized by rigidity of the neck as though it were entwined by a snake. See these entries. [27: 498] [26: 731] [27: 498] [97: 550]

throughflux diarrhea 洞泻 *dòng xiè*: **1.** Diarrhea after eating, with nontransformation of food. MED Warm the center with formulas such as Aconite Pill (*fù zǐ wán*) containing aconite (*fù zǐ*), mume (*wū méi*), dried ginger (*gān jiāng*), and coptis (*huáng lián*). ACU Base treatment mainly on CV, ST, and back transport points. Select CV-12 (*zhōng wǎn*, Center Stomach Duct), LR-13 (*zhāng mén*, Camphorwood Gate), ST-25 (*tiān shū*, Celestial Pivot), ST-36 (*zú sān lǐ*, Leg Three Li), BL-23 (*shèn shū*, Kidney Transport), CV-4 (*guān yuán*, Pass Head), CV-9 (*shuǐ fēn*, Water Divide), and CV-6 (*qì hǎi*, Sea of Qi). Needle with supplementation and use large amounts of moxa. **2.** SOGGY DIARRHEA. **3.** SPLEEN DIARRHEA. ◇ Chin 洞 *dòng*, hole, cave; pass through; 泻 *xiè*, drain. [26: 400] [27: 363] [97: 437]

thumb body-inch 拇指同身寸 *mǔ zhǐ tóng shēn cùn*: From *A Thousand Gold Pieces Prescriptions* (*qiān jīn yào fāng*). The distance between the transverse creases on the inside of the thumb as a standard method of calculating one body-inch. See BODY-INCH. [26: 364] [97: 334]

thumb-tack intradermal needle 揿钉型皮内针 *qìn dīng xíng pí nèi zhēn*: *Synonym: drawing-pin intradermal needle*. A small needle about 2–3 mm long, continuous with and perpendicular to a circle of wire that forms the head. Thumb-tack needles are mostly used in ear acupuncture or facial acupuncture, and are implanted into the skin using tweezers and then held in position with tape. See NEEDLE IMPLANTATION. [46: 506]

thunder head wind 雷头风 *léi tóu fēng*: A disease characterized by lumps and swellings of the head and face, sometimes accompanied by abhorrence of cold and vigorous heat [effusion] or by headache, and with a sound of thunder in the head. Thunder head wind is attributed to wind evil assailing from outside or to phlegm-heat engendering wind. MED Treat by clearing, diffusing, upbearing, and dissipating, using Clearing Invigoration Decoction (*qīng zhèn tāng*). When due to phlegm-heat, it can be treated with Phlegm-Expelling Pill (*qū tán wán*). If there is abhorrence of cold and vigorous heat [effusion], Schizonepeta and Ledebouriella Toxin-Vanquishing Powder (*jīng fáng bài dú sǎn*) can be used. See HEADACHE. [26: 773] [50: 1601] [27: 393] [97: 594]

thunderous rumbling in the intestines 肠中雷鸣 *cháng zhōng léi míng*: Severe RUMBLING INTESTINES.

thunder rampart 雷廓 *léi kuò*: See EIGHT RAMPARTS. [26: 24]

tian-gui 天癸 *tiān guǐ*: HEAVENLY TENTH. [26: 106]

tidal heat [effusion] 潮热 *cháo rè*: Heat effusion, sometimes only felt subjectively, occurring at regular intervals, usually in the afternoon or evening (POSTMERIDIAN TIDAL HEAT [EFFUSION]). Tidal heat effusion may form part of both vacuity and repletion patterns. **Yang brightness (*yáng míng*) bowel repletion** can cause tidal heat [effusion] at the stage of the disease when heat has abated somewhat but not fully. The yang brightness (*yáng míng*) tidal heat [effusion] is a specific form of postmeridian (p.m.) tidal heat [effusion] that is called *late afternoon tidal heat [effusion]* because it occurs at roughly 3–5 p.m. It differs from other tidal heat [effusion] occurring in other patterns by being a heightening of an otherwise constant heat effusion. It is associated with STREAMING SWEAT on the hands and feet, hard fullness and pain in the abdomen, constipation (sometimes HEAT BIND WITH CIRCUMFLUENCE), vexation and agitation, parched yellow tongue fur, and a sunken replete pulse. In severe cases, there may be clouded spirit and delirious raving. ⬚MED Use Major Qi-Coordinating Decoction (*dà chéng qì tāng*), Minor Qi-Coordinating Decoction (*xiǎo chéng qì tāng*), or Stomach-Regulating Qi-Coordinating Decoction (*tiáo wèi chéng qì tāng*). ⬚ACU Base treatment mainly on ST, LI, and GV. Select ST-44 (*nèi tíng*, Inner Court), LI-4 (*hé gǔ*, Union Valley), LI-11 (*qū chí*, Pool at the Bend), LI-6 (*piān lì*, Veering Passageway), ST-36 (*zú sān lǐ*, Leg Three Li), BL-25 (*dà cháng shū*, Large Intestine Transport), GV-14 (*dà zhuī*, Great Hammer), and PC-5 (*jiān shǐ*, Intermediary Courier); needle with drainage. **Yin vacuity blood depletion** causes postmeridian (p.m.) tidal heat [effusion], i.e., a tidal heat [effusion] in the afternoon, evening, or night. This is accompanied by heat in the heart of the palms and soles, heart vexation, insomnia, heart palpitations, night sweating, emaciation and haggard appearance, a red tongue with scant fur, and a fine rapid pulse. ⬚MED Enrich yin, nourish the blood, and clear heat. Use Bone-Clearing Powder (*qīng gǔ sǎn*) plus tangkuei (*dāng guī*) and white peony (*bái sháo yào*). ⬚ACU Base treatment mainly on the three yin channels of the foot, HT, and GV. Select KI-6 (*zhào hǎi*, Shining Sea), KI-2 (*rán gǔ*, Blazing Valley), SP-6 (*sān yīn jiāo*, Three Yin Intersection), HT-8 (*shào fǔ*, Lesser Mansion), HT-7 (*shén mén*, Spirit Gate), LU-10 (*yú jì*, Fish Border), GV-14 (*dà zhuī*, Great Hammer), and PC-5 (*jiān*

shǐ, Intermediary Courier); needle with even supplementation and drainage. **Spleen-stomach qi vacuity** causes morning tidal heat [effusion] that abates in the afternoon (or sometimes postmeridian tidal heat [effusion]), accompanied by shortage of qi, laziness to speak, lassitude of spirit, limp limbs, spontaneous sweating, bright white facial complexion, pale soft tongue, and a fine, vacuous, weak pulse. ⬚MED Eliminate heat with warmth and sweetness. Use Center-Supplementing Qi-Boosting Decoction (*bǔ zhōng yì qì tāng*). ⬚ACU Base treatment mainly on back transport points, CV, and GV. Select BL-20 (*pí shū*, Spleen Transport), BL-21 (*wèi shū*, Stomach Transport), CV-6 (*qì hǎi*, Sea of Qi), CV-12 (*zhōng wǎn*, Center Stomach Duct), ST-36 (*zú sān lǐ*, Leg Three Li), and GV-14 (*dà zhuī*, Great Hammer); needle with supplementation. **Summerheat-heat damaging qi** in children gives rise to a SUMMER INFIXATION with tidal heat [effusion] in children. It may take the form of heat effusion in the morning that cools in the evening or heat effusion in the evening that cools in the morning. This is associated with thirst with intake of fluid, vexation and agitation, torpid intake, lassitude of spirit, slimy tongue fur, and fine rapid pulse. ⬚MED Clear summerheat and boost qi with Wang's Summerheat-Clearing Qi-Boosting Decoction (*wáng shì qīng shǔ yì qì tāng*). ⬚ACU Base treatment mainly on PC, ST, LI, and GV. Select PC-6 (*nèi guān*, Inner Pass), LI-4 (*hé gǔ*, Union Valley), ST-36 (*zú sān lǐ*, Leg Three Li), and GV-14 (*dà zhuī*, Great Hammer); needle with drainage, and supplement CV-6 (*qì hǎi*, Sea of Qi), BL-20 (*pí shū*, Spleen Transport), and BL-21 (*wèi shū*, Stomach Transport). **Static blood** lying depressed in the inner body causes postmeridian tidal heat [effusion] with dry throat and mouth, washing the mouth with water but no desire to swallow it, concretion lump in the abdomen or a painful area on the body, a green-blue or purple tongue possibly bearing stasis macules, and a rough fine pulse. In severe cases, patients may have encrusted skin and dull black eyes. ⬚MED Quicken the blood, transform stasis, and clear heat. Use House of Blood Stasis-Expelling Decoction (*xuè fǔ zhú yū tāng*) plus rhubarb (*dà huáng*) and moutan (*mǔ dān pí*). ⬚ACU Base treatment mainly on SP, LR, and KI. Select BL-17 (*gé shū*, Diaphragm Transport), SP-10 (*xuè hǎi*, Sea of Blood), LI-4 (*hé gǔ*, Union Valley), LR-3 (*tài chōng*, Supreme Surge), SP-6 (*sān yīn jiāo*, Three Yin Intersection), KI-6 (*zhào hǎi*, Shining Sea), KI-2 (*rán gǔ*, Blazing Valley), and LR-2 (*xíng jiān*, Moving Between); needle with drainage. [26: 859] [27: 356] [97: 639] [92: No. 7] [46: 594, 657, 670] [113: 48]

tidal reddening of the cheeks 两颧潮红 *liǎng quán cháo hóng*, 面颊潮红 *miàn jiá cháo hóng*: See REDDENING OF THE CHEEKS.

tie 系 *xì*: See EYE TIE; HEART TIE; LUNG TIE.

ties of the five viscera home to the heart 五脏系皆属于心 *wǔ zàng xì jiē shǔ yú xīn*: The Gateway to Medicine (*yī xué rù mén*) states, "The ties of the five viscera connect with the heart; the heart connects with the ties of the five viscera. The tie of the heart is connected with the ties of the five viscera. It transports blood percolates marrow. Hence, disease among the five viscera first affects the heart..." The word "tie" may refer to blood vessels. [36: 67]

tiger's mouth 虎口 *hǔ kǒu*: The region between the first and second metacarpal bones, where LI-4 (*hé gǔ*, Union Valley) is located.

tiger's-whiskers clove sore 虎须疔 *hǔ xū dīng*: A CLOVE SORE at the corners of the mouth. See HUMAN CENTER CLOVE SORE. [27: 468]

tight pulse 紧脉 *jǐn mài*: A stringlike pulse that has marked forcefulness. "Stringlike" denotes a quality, whereas "tight" denotes a quality and a strength. A tight pulse is always stringlike, whereas a stringlike pulse is not necessarily tight. A tight pulse is associated with cold and pain. [27: 73] [97: 341]

tingling 麻 *má*: See NUMBNESS AND TINGLING. [92: No. 407]

tinnitus 耳鸣 *ěr míng*: Synonym: *sound of cicadas in the ear*. Unreal ringing, buzzing, or rushing sounds heard in the ears. Distinction is made between repletion and vacuity. Repletion patterns are attributed to ascendant counterflow of liver fire or phlegm fire. Vacuity patterns are attributed to depletion of kidney yin or center qi fall. In repletion patterns, tinnitus is of rapid onset and is characterized by the sound of frogs or of the tide. In vacuity patterns, it is like the sound of cicadas or a flute or pipe. **Liver fire** tinnitus is attended by headache, red eyes, dry mouth with bitter taste, vexation and agitation, irascibility, constipation, yellow tongue fur, and a rapid stringlike pulse. [MED] Clear and discharge liver fire using formulas such as Gentian Liver-Draining Decoction (*lóng dǎn xiè gān tāng*). [ACU] For treatment of repletion patterns, base treatment mainly on TB, GB, and SI, selecting TB-17 (*yì fēng*, Wind Screen), TB-3 (*zhōng zhǔ*, Central Islet), GB-2 (*tīng huì*, Auditory Convergence), SI-19 (*tīng gōng*, Auditory Palace), and GB-43 (*xiá xī*, Pinched Ravine) as the main points. For liver fire, combine these with LR-3 (*tài chōng*, Supreme Surge), LR-2 (*xíng jiān*, Moving Between), GB-34 (*yáng líng quán*, Yang Mound Spring), and KI-3 (*tài xī*, Great Ravine); needle with drainage. **Phlegm-fire** tinnitus is accompanied by oppression in the chest, copious phlegm, inhibited stool and urination, yellow slimy tongue fur, and a rapid stringlike pulse. [MED] Treat with Gallbladder-Warming

Decoction (*wēn dǎn tāng*) plus coptis (*huáng lián*) and trichosanthes (*guā lóu*). [ACU] Use the basic points for repletion combined with ST-40 (*fēng lóng*, Bountiful Bulge), CV-17 (*shān zhōng*, Chest Center), ST-44 (*nèi tíng*, Inner Court), LI-4 (*hé gǔ*, Union Valley), and LU-5 (*chǐ zé*, Cubit Marsh); needle with drainage. **Kidney vacuity** tinnitus, observed in vacuity patients and the elderly, takes the form of a fine thread-like sound that occurs frequently and is accompanied by limp aching lumbus and knees, enuresis, seminal emission, and a fine weak pulse that is forceless at the cubit (*chǐ*). [MED] Enrich yin and supplement the kidney with Six-Ingredient Rehmannia Pill (*liù wèi dì huáng wán*), and if there is also hyperactivity of yang with dizziness, loadstone (*cí shí*), tortoise plastron (*guī bǎn*), schisandra (*wǔ wèi zǐ*), and achyranthes (*niú xī*) should be added to subdue yang. [ACU] For treatment of vacuity patterns, base treatment mainly on TB and SI, selecting TB-17 (*yì fēng*, Wind Screen), SI-19 (*tīng gōng*, Auditory Palace), TB-3 (*zhōng zhǔ*, Central Islet), and TB-21 (*ěr mén*, Ear Gate) as the main points. To address the kidney yin vacuity, further needle with supplementation at BL-23 (*shèn shū*, Kidney Transport), CV-4 (*guān yuán*, Pass Head), and KI-3 (*tài xī*, Great Ravine). For kidney vacuity with yang hyperactivity, supplement KI-6 (*zhào hǎi*, Shining Sea), KI-2 (*rán gǔ*, Blazing Valley), and KI-3 (*tài xī*, Great Ravine); drain LR-3 (*tài chōng*, Supreme Surge), LR-2 (*xíng jiān*, Moving Between), and HT-7 (*shén mén*, Spirit Gate). **Qi vacuity** tinnitus is accompanied by fatigued limbs, reduced food intake, and sloppy stool. [MED] Supplement the center and boost qi with Center-Supplementing Qi-Boosting Decoction (*bǔ zhōng yì qì tāng*) plus cuscuta (*tù sī zǐ*). [ACU] Use the basic points for vacuity patterns combined with GV-20 (*bǎi huì*, Hundred Convergences), CV-6 (*qì hǎi*, Sea of Qi), ST-36 (*zú sān lǐ*, Leg Three Li), CV-12 (*zhōng wǎn*, Center Stomach Duct), and KI-3 (*tài xī*, Great Ravine); needle with supplementation and add moxa if appropriate. See also DEAFNESS. [26: 250] [27: 493] [97: 173] [46: 722] [37: 479]

tinted vision 视瞻有色 *shì zhān yǒu sè*: The sensation of a shadow in front of the eyes, which in severe cases may be green-blue or reddish yellow in color. It may precede CLEAR-EYE BLINDNESS. Tinted vision is attributed either to insufficiency of the liver and kidney or to phlegm-fire or damp-heat. [125: 278] [27: 505]

tip 标 *biāo*: See ROOT AND TIP.

tip-abscess 瘭疽 *biāo jū*: Synonyms: *biaoju*; *whitlow*; *flare-tip abscess*. A sore suddenly arising in the flesh, as big as a bean or as small as a millet seed, and, in severe cases, as big as a plum, with a root, starting as a red spot and subsequently turning black. A tip-abscess is associated with pain, and with a pain response in the heart. It can affect any part of the body, but most commonly occurs on the ventral aspect of the finger tips. [26: 901] [61: 306] [27: 466] [5: 930]

toad-egg menses 经如虾蟆子 *jīng rú hā má zǐ*: The passing of moles (fleshy masses) bearing the appearance of toad eggs during menstruation; occurs when the period is overdue and the patient suffers from drumlike distention of the abdomen. The patient may be comatose. WMC hydatiform mole (hydatic mole, grape mole). MED Treat by dual supplementation of qi and blood with Perfect Major Supplementation Decoction (*shí quán dà bǔ tāng*). [26: 814]

toad head scourge 虾蟆瘟 *há má wēn*: Massive head scourge with swelling around the neck spreading over the head, giving the appearance of a frog or toad. See MASSIVE HEAD SCOURGE. [27: 369] [97: 405]

toad skin 蛤蟆皮 *há má pí*: ENCRUSTED SKIN.

tofu tongue fur 腐苔 *fǔ tāi*: See BEAN CURD TONGUE FUR.

tongue 舌 *shé*: Synonyms: *orifice of the heart*; *magic root*. The soft fleshy process of the floor of the mouth used in chewing, swallowing, and tasting food. *The Magic Pivot (lín shū, mài dù)* says, "Heart qi flows through to the tongue; when the heart is harmony it can taste the five flavors." *The Magic Pivot (lín shū, yōu huì wú yén)* states, "The tongue is the moving part of the voice." Parts of the tongue include: tip of the tongue; root of the tongue; tongue margins; center of the tongue. Examination of the tongue constitutes a major element of diagnosis. See TONGUE EXAMINATION. [26: 264] [27: 28] [97: 193]

tongue blister 舌生泡 *shé shēng pào*: Synonym: *wind gan of the mouth*. A vesicle on the upper or lower surface of the tongue. Tongue blisters are attributed to spleen-kidney vacuity heat flaming upward or accumulated spleen-heart heat. **Spleen-kidney vacuity heat flaming upward** gives rise to red, white or yellow tongue blisters of different sizes, configured in strings of five or six. The pulse is vacuous and forceless. MED Nourish yin and clear heat. Use formulas such as Anemarrhena, Phellodendron, and Rehmannia Pill (*zhī bǎi dì huáng wán*) plus ovate atractylodes (*bái zhú*) and dioscorea (*shān yào*). Willow Flower Powder (*liǔ huā sǎn*) can be applied as an insufflation. **Accumulated spleen-heart heat** causes blisters forming configured strings of five or six on the upper surface of the tongue, that are painful, burst, and ulcerate. These are associated with a forceful surging pulse. MED Clear the heart and cool the diaphragm. Use formulas such as Diaphragm-Cooling Powder (*liáng gé sǎn*) for oral medica-

tion combined with an insufflation such as Tin-Like Powder (*xí lèi sǎn*). [26: 265] [44: 723]

tongue body 舌质 *shé zhí*, 舌体 *shé tǐ*: The tongue itself, in contradistinction to the tongue fur (coating). Examination of the tongue body focuses on the form, bearing, and color of the tongue. (1) **Tongue form:** Attention is paid to possible enlargement, shrinkage, red speckles and prickles, fissures, and mirror surface. (1a) Enlargement: A swollen tongue, with dental impressions on the margin, is known as an enlarged tongue, and indicates qi vacuity or the presence of water-damp. An enlarged tongue that is pale in color, with a white, glossy fur, indicates qi vacuity. With a slimy tongue fur, enlargement generally indicates damp or damp-heat. In Western medicine, tongue enlargement may be seen in myxedema, chronic nephritis, and chronic gastritis, and is thought to be due to hyperplasia of the connective tissue, tissue edema, or blood and lymphatic drainage disturbances. Enlargement is markedly different from a painful, swollen, red tongue, which characterizes an intense heat evil or heart fire flaming upward. (1b) Shrinkage: A thin, shrunken tongue indicates a yin liquid vacuity or a dual vacuity of yin and qi. A shrunken tongue due to damage to yin humor by exuberant heat is crimson in color and dry. In dual vacuity of qi and yin, the tongue is pale in color. The results of modern clinical observation show that shrinkage generally occurs in the latter stages of externally contracted heat (febrile) diseases, in conditions described in Western medicine as pulmonary tuberculosis, and in advanced-stage carcinoma. It is explained as atrophy of the lingual muscle and epithelium due to malnutrition. (1c) Red speckles and prickles: Red speckles and prickles appear on the tip or margins of the tongue and indicate exuberant heat. They occur in various external heat diseases, particularly yang brightness repletion heat patterns, and in conjunction with maculopapular eruptions. Speckles, prickles, and pain in the tongue may also occur in patients suffering from insomnia or constipation or in those working late at night. According to Western medicine, speckles and prickles are due to an increase in the size or number of fungiform papillae. (1d) Fissures: Fissures vary in depth and position. Occurring in conjunction with a dry tongue, they indicate fluid vacuity. They may also occur in exuberant heat patterns, in conjunction with a crimson tongue. Fissures are seen by Western medicine to be the result of mucosal atrophy, chiefly associated with chronic glossitis, and in 0.5% of cases to causes wholly unrelated to disease. (1e) Mirror tongue: A completely smooth tongue, free of liquid and fur, is sometimes referred to as a "mirror tongue" and indicates severe yin humor depletion. A smooth red or crimson tongue indicates damage to yin by intense heat. If pale in color, a smooth tongue indicates damage to both qi and yin. According to the results of recent clinical observation, the mirror tongue mostly occurs in the latter stages of glossitis, but may also be seen in vitamin B deficiency, anemia, and the latter stages of certain diseases. It is attributable to shrinkage of the filiform and fungiform papillae. (2) **Tongue bearing:** Morbid deviations from normal tongue bearing include stiffness, limpness, trembling, deviation, contraction, and worrying. (2a) Stiffness: If the tongue moves sluggishly, inhibiting speech, it is called a stiff tongue. This occurs in a number of serious diseases, such as heat entering the pericardium, phlegm confounding the orifices of the heart, phlegm obstructing the network vessels, and liver wind stirring in the inner body. Other signs are therefore decisive in determining the nature of the disease. In Western medicine, a stiff tongue generally indicates diseases of the central nervous system. (2b) Limpness: A tongue that is soft and floppy, moves with difficulty, and cannot be extended is known as a limp tongue. When limpness is due to intense heat or to yin humor depletion, the tongue is also red or crimson, and dry. In qi and blood depletion, it is limp and pale. In Western medicine, a limp tongue is seen as a sign of neurological diseases or lesions affecting the lingual muscle. (2c) Trembling: If the tongue trembles when it moves, the cause is ascendant hyperactivity of liver yang, internal wind stirred by exuberant heat, or qi vacuity. In the first two cases, the tongue is red or crimson, whereas in qi vacuity the tongue is pale. The results of modern clinical observation shows that trembling of the tongue occurs in high fever, hyperthyroidism, hypertension, and a number of neurological disorders. (2d) Deviation: In cases of wind stroke due to internal liver wind or phlegm obstructing the network vessels, the tongue often inclines to one side. Modern clinical observation associates a deviated tongue with disorders of the hypoglossal nerve or intracranial lesions. (2e) Contraction: Contraction of the tongue preventing extension is a critical sign in most cases. The cause is either damage to yin by extreme heat or fulminant yang qi desertion. A short frenulum due to congenital factors may also prevent extension. (2f) Worrying: Habitual extension of the tongue and licking of the lips is known as a worrying tongue. It is a sign of heat in the heart and spleen, and heralds the stirring of wind. It also occurs in mentally retarded children. (3) **Tongue color:** The normal color of the tongue is a pale red. In tongue diagnosis, the term "pale" denotes any color paler than normal, whereas "red" denotes a color deeper than normal. If considerably deeper in color, the term "crimson" is used. A "blue-green-purple" tongue is a red tongue with a

blue, or in pronounced cases, indigo hue. Changes in the color of the body of the tongue reflect the state of blood and qi and the severity of disease. In Western medicine, changes in the tongue color are explained by changes in blood chemistry, in the viscosity of the blood, and by hyperplasia or atrophy of the epithelial cells of the glossal mucosa. (3a) Pale Tongue: A pale tongue indicates vacuity qi and blood. A pale tongue that is enlarged and well-moistened, accompanying cold signs indicates yang qi vacuity. In Western medicine, a pale tongue is associated with the latter stages of schistosomiasis, chronic nephritis, cancer, and various forms of anemia, and is seen as the result of a reduction of red corpuscles, disturbance of protein metabolism, and tissue edema. (3b) Red tongue: A red tongue indicates heat, due to either vacuity or to repletion. A deep red tongue with a yellow fur indicates repletion heat (more at crimson below); a fresh tender-red (a pastel red) indicates vacuity heat. A red shrunken tongue indicates effulgent yin vacuity fire, and a red tongue with prickles indicates heat in the construction aspect. A dry red tongue indicates damage to stomach liquid, and a tongue that is red at the tip indicates heart fire flaming upward; and a tongue the is red at the margins indicates depressed liver-gallbladder heat. (3c) Crimson tongue: A crimson tongue is also associated with heat, but the added depth of color indicates that the heat is located in the construction or blood aspect. Red and crimson coloring of the tongue, according to modern clinical observation, is associated with heat effusion due to infection, burns, post-operative conditions, advanced carcinoma, hyperthyroidism, ascites due to cirrhosis of the liver, and tuberculosis. It is thought to be due to inflammation of the tongue causing dilation of the capillary vessels of the glossal mucosa. (3d) Purple tongue: Purple coloration indicates an impaired flow of blood and qi leading to congealing blood stasis. This is a part of either heat or cold patterns. A generalized blue-green-purple coloration indicates severe blood stasis. Purple macules indicate less severe or localized blood stasis. A glossy blue-green-purple tongue characterizes cold patterns caused by failure of yang qi to warm and move the blood. A reddish purple, dry tongue indicates binding blood stasis due to penetration of heat to the blood aspect. According to the results of modern clinical observation, a purple tongue is observed in cirrhosis of the liver, heart diseases, asthma, cholecystitis, ulcers, and gynecological diseases. It is associated with hemostasis of the blood in the orifice vein and superior vena cava. (4) **Correspondences between tongue surface sections and the organs:** Though subject to argument, some correspondence between parts of the tongue surface and the viscera is accepted. It is generally thought that the root of the tongue is related to the kidney, which in a sense is the root of the body. The center of the tongue's surface is said to reflect the condition of the spleen and stomach, which are at the body's center. The tip of the tongue reveals the condition of the heart. Agreement ends here. Some texts state that the condition of the liver and gallbladder is reflected on the sides of the tongue, and that the lung is reflected at the tip. In other sources, the left side of the tongue is assigned to the lung, and right side to the liver. A few other variations may also be found. In view of these inconsistencies, organ correspondences should always be correlated with data from the other examinations. See Table 15. [27: 177] [50: 549] [97: 194] [6: 119–122]

15. Correspondences Between Tongue Color and Disease		
Color	Febrile Disease	Other
Pale		Vacuity and cold patterns
Pale red	Exterior patterns	Normal color
Bright red	Heat entering the construction aspect	Effulgent yin vacuity fire
Crimson	Extreme construction aspect heat; heat entering the blood aspect	Effulgent yin vacuity fire
Purple	Extreme blood aspect heat; insufficiency of the fluids; bleeding and blood stasis	Deep purple: accumulation of static blood. Purple and glossy: cold patterns

tongue coating 舌苔 *shé tāi*: TONGUE FUR.

tongue examination 舌诊 *shé zhěn*: Inspection of the tongue and its fur (coating). The tongue examination provides some of the most important data for pattern identification. It can reveal the state of qi and blood, advance and regression of disease, the degree of heat and cold, and the depth of evil penetration. Changes in the appearance of the tongue are particularly pronounced in externally contracted heat (febrile) diseases and diseases of the stomach and spleen. However, in clinical practice, serious illnesses are not necessarily reflected in major changes in the appearance of the tongue. Furthermore, normal healthy individuals may show abnormal changes in the appearance of the tongue. Therefore, the data provided by the tongue examination must be carefully weighed against other signs and signs, the pulse, and the patient's history, before an accurate diagnosis can be made. Distinction is made between the TONGUE BODY and TONGUE FUR. Examination of the body of the

tongue involves observing color, form, and movement. Examination of the tongue fur involves observing color and nature. The body of the tongue is of greatest significance in judging the strength of right qi. It may also provide an indication of the severity of the condition, as in the case of a pale tongue, which indicates blood and qi vacuity, or a crimson tongue, which indicates yin vacuity or penetration of evil heat to the construction aspect. The tongue fur, though primarily an indicator of the severity of a disease, is sometimes a useful measure of the strength of right qi. This is true in the case of a thick slimy fur, which indicates exuberant damp turbidity, or a peeling fur, which indicates stomach qi vacuity or damage to yin humor. The moistness of the tongue sheds light on the state of the fluids. For these reasons, the tongue examination is of special importance in externally contracted heat (febrile) diseases. **Method**: When examining the tongue, the following four points should be kept in mind: (1) Light: The tongue examination should be conducted in adequately lit surroundings, with light shining directly into the mouth. Inadequate lighting may obscure color differences, such as the difference between yellow and white, or red and purple. (2) Stained fur: Some foods and medicines affect the color of the fur, and potentially the diagnosis. Milk and soybean milk stain the tongue fur white; coffee, tea, and tobacco leave brown stains; egg yolk, oranges, coptis (*huáng lián*), and ass hide glue (*ē jiāo*) leave yellow stains. Staining normally affects only the surface of the fur, and is washed away by saliva. If in doubt, the physician should ask the patient if anything that may have caused staining has been eaten. (3) The bearing of the tongue on extension: The patient should ensure that the tongue is relaxed and flat when extended. Forced or tense protraction may deepen the color of the tongue. (4) Miscellaneous factors: Consumption of rough foodstuffs or chewing gum may remove the tongue fur and deepen the color of the tongue body. Patients with missing teeth may tend to chew food on one side of the mouth, which may cause irregularities in fur distribution. In wind stroke patients, reduced mobility of the tongue may cause an increase in tongue fur. In patients tending to breathe through the mouth owing to nasal congestion or other factors, the surface of the tongue may be abnormally dry. Such changes in the tongue and tongue fur should not be taken to reflect internal morbidity. See TONGUE BODY and TONGUE FUR. [26: 606] [6: 119] [27: 177] [97: 194]

tongue fur 舌苔 *shě tāi*: Synonym: *tongue coating*. The normally whitish substances partially covering the upper side of the tongue. Healthy people have a thin layer of fur on their tongue, which is due to upward steaming of stomach qi.

Tongue furs are categorized as glossy, dry, thick, thin, clean, slimy, grimy, and peeling. (1) **Nature of the tongue fur:** It is important to observe how moist and how thick the tongue fur is, whether it is clean, slimy or grimy, and whether or not there are signs of peeling. (0a) Moistness: A healthy tongue is kept moist naturally by saliva. A tongue covered with a transparent or semitransparent film of fluid is described as having a glossy fur, and indicates damp-phlegm or cold-damp. Exuberant damp due to spleen vacuity is characterized by a slimy glossy fur in association with spleen-stomach signs of oppression in the chest, nausea, and diarrhea. Yang vacuity water flood is marked by a glossy white tongue fur, as well as signs of cold limbs and puffy swelling. A dry fur generally indicates heat. A tongue that is so dry that it looks rough, and feels dry or even prickly to the touch, is described as being "rough." It is mainly seen in external heat diseases and indicates damage to humor by exuberant heat. However, failure of fluids to reach the upper body in patients suffering from center phlegm-damp obstruction may also cause a dry fur. In such cases, the dryness is less severe; some degree of sliminess is present and the patient experiences thirst without any urge to drink. Western medical research shows that the moistness of the tongue depends on saliva secretion, viscosity, and evaporation speed. Dryness of the surface of the tongue is the most pronounced sign of dehydration. (0b) Thickness: The tongue fur is regarded as thin if the underlying tongue surface shows through faintly, whereas a thick fur is one that blots out the tongue surface completely. The thickness of the tongue fur is an index of evil exuberance, progression, and regression. A thick fur indicates a strong evil, whereas a thin fur indicates a weak evil. If the fur thickens the condition is advancing; if the fur thins, it is said to be transforming, and the condition is improving. Modern research shows that the thickness of the tongue fur is associated with the length of the filiform papillae. If the papillae are long, the tongue fur is thick; if short, the fur is thin. (0c) Clean, slimy, and grimy furs: An extremely fine fur with a grainy appearance is described as clean fur, and is a normal healthy fur. If the fur is thicker, appears as a layer of mucus covering the tongue, and no longer has its normal grainy appearance, it is described as slimy fur. If the mucus layer looks dirty, the terms grimy fur, slimy fur, or turbid slimy fur are used. A slimy fur indicates damp, phlegm, and food accumulations. These evils are said to be extremely strong when the slimy coating is "generalized," that is, covering the entire tongue. A slimy fur that covers only the center or the root of the tongue indicates a chronic condition, and does not transform (i.e., disappear) easily. A grimy slimy fur indicates, on

the one hand, the presence of turbid evils such as turbid damp and turbid phlegm, and on the other, stomach qi vacuity. In stomach qi vacuity, attention must be paid to safeguarding stomach qi when dispelling the evil. According to the findings of modern research, slimy tongue furs are attributed to an increase in the number of filiform papillae and their branches, and the collection of mucus, putrid matter, and sloughed epithelial cells between the papillae. (0d) Peeling: A patchy fur interspersed with mirror-like, furless areas is known as peeling fur. This generally indicates insufficiency of yin humor and vacuous stomach qi. A peeling fur that is nontransforming and slimy fur indicates nontransformed phlegm-damp and damage to yin humor and stomach qi, and suggests that the pattern is complex. A thick slimy fur that suddenly peels away completely indicates major damage to right qi. (1) **Color of the tongue fur:** (0a) White: The clinical significance of a white tongue fur is fourfold. A clean moist thin white fur is normal and healthy, but may also appear at the onset of sickness indicating that the evil has not yet entered the interior and right qi remains undamaged. A glossy white fur indicates cold; thin glossy white fur indicates external wind-cold or internal cold. A thick glossy white fur indicates cold-damp or cold-phlegm. A dry white fur indicates transformation of cold evil into heat. A thin, extremely dry white fur indicates insufficiency of fluids; thick dry fur indicates transformation of dampness into dryness. A white mealy fur with a red tongue body indicates impeded damp and deep-lying heat, which is treated by first transforming the damp to allow the heat to escape rather than with the excessive use of cool medicinals. A thick slimy white fur indicates phlegm damp, and is usually accompanied by a slimy sensation in the mouth, oppression in the chest, and torpid intake. Modern research suggests that a white tongue fur is essentially normal, and that a thick white fur is mainly associated with hypertrophy of the corneal layer of the filiform papillae for unknown reasons. See also ORAL PUTREFACTION and BEAN CURD TONGUE FUR. (0b) Yellow fur: A yellow fur usually signifies heat. Because heat patterns vary in severity and may involve different evils, different forms of yellow fur are distinguished. A thin dry yellow fur indicates damage to liquid by heat evil, posing the need to safeguard liquid. A slimy yellow fur usually indicates damp-heat. An "old yellow" (i.e., dark yellow) fur and a "burnt yellow" (i.e., blackish yellow) fur indicate binding of repletion heat. A mixed white and yellow fur indicates the initial stages of the transformation of cold into heat that is associated with evils entering the interior. Modern research suggests that yellow fur is associated with the infectious stage of inflammatory conditions and is mainly attributable to hypoplasia of the filiform papillae, coloring by bacteria, and localized manifestation of an inflammatory disease. (0c) Black fur: A black fur may occur in cold, heat, repletion, and vacuity patterns, but most commonly indicates an exuberant evil. A rough, dry, black fur, somewhat parched in appearance, together with a red or crimson tongue body, indicates damp-heat transforming into dryness or damage to yin by intense heat. Usually, a thick slimy black fur indicates a phlegm-damp complication. A glossy black fur signifies either gastric or kidney vacuity. A slimy yellow fur with a grayish black coating generally indicates an exuberant damp-heat evil. A mixed gray and white fur or a gray thin slimy glossy fur generally indicates cold-damp. Modern research shows that black fur is most often seen in acute pyogenic infections, such as toxemia, gangrenous appendicitis, peritonitis, and cholecystitis. However, it may also occur in diseases such as chronic bronchitis and uremia. It mostly corresponds to what Western medicine calls a black hairy fur. Opinions differ as to the exact causes of black fur. Explanations include: growth of bacteria after long administration of antibiotics, absorption by the tongue fur of iron present in blood from minor bleeding in the oral cavity, and high fever and loss of fluid. ◇ Chin 舌 *shé,* tongue; 苔 *tāi,* moss, lichen. [6: 122–25]

tongue is the sprout of the heart 舌为心苗 *shé wéi xīn miáo:* Synonym: *heart opens at the tongue.* [27: 37]

tongue margins 舌边 *shé biān:* The lateral edges of the tongue. The tongue margins can reflect the state of the liver and gallbladder. For example, red tongue margins indicate liver-gallbladder heat; speckles on the tongue margins indicate static blood amassment.

tongue mushroom 舌菌 *shé jùn:* TONGUE ROCK. [26: 267] [27: 482]

tongue rock 舌岩 *shé yán:* Synonym: *tongue mushroom.* A growth on the tongue like a bean or mushroom, with a big head and thin stalk. Tongue rock is attributed to seven-affect binding depression creating heat in the heart and spleen channels that transforms into fire and toxin. If enduring heat damages yin, it is red and ulcerated without skin, with continuous pain that is more severe in the evening than in the morning. WMC tumor of the tongue. MED In the early states, drain heart-spleen channel fire using Red-Abducting Powder (*dǎo chì sǎn*) plus coptis (*huáng lián*) and rhubarb (*dà huáng*). For damage to yin by enduring heat, treat by nourishing yin and clearing heat. Use Throat-Clearing Dryness-Moistening Decoction (*qīng yān rùn zào tāng*) plus

rhinoceros horn (*xī jiǎo*) and coptis (*huáng lián*). [26: 266] [96: 213] [27: 482]

tongue spirit 舌神 *shé shén:* The general vitality of the tongue manifest in its luxuriance or witheredness. A *luxuriant* tongue is fresh red in color and is able to move freely; it indicates sufficiency of liquid and humor, and a good chance of recovery from illness. A *withered* tongue is dull, dark, dry and withered; it indicates exhaustion of liquid and humor and a critical condition. Cao Bing-Zhang in his *Guide to Tongue Diagnosis* (*biàn shé zhǐ nán*) states, "If it (the tongue) is luxuriant and moist, liquid is sufficient; if dry and withered, liquid is lacking. Luxuriance indicates presence of spirit. As to spirit, [it means] agility and a fresh bright red. If it is present, [the patient] lives; if it is not, [the patient] dies. Brightness and glossiness with the color of blood is [a sign of] life; dryness and dullness without the color of blood is [a sign boding] death." [26: 266]

tooth 牙齿 *yá chǐ,* 牙 *yá,* 齿 *chǐ:* One of the hard bony appendages of the jaw, used for chewing food. In the infant, milk teeth (deciduous teeth) grow at the age of 6–7 months, and fall out at the age of 6–7 years; they are replaced by the permanent teeth in a process known as CHANGE OF TEETH. The teeth are located on the lesser yin (*shào yīn*) kidney channel. The *teeth are the surplus of the bone,* which is associated with the kidney (KIDNEY ENGENDERS BONE AND MARROW.) When the kidney is replete, the teeth are healthy and firm; kidney vacuity may be characterized by LOOSENING OF THE TEETH or DESICCATED TEETH. The foot yang brightness (*yáng míng*) channel enters the upper teeth, while the hand yang brightness channel enters the lower teeth. Tooth decay, for example, is often explained in terms of yang brightness heat. Among the seven gates, the teeth are the *door gate.* Diseases of or affecting the teeth and gums include: SLOWNESS TO TEETHE; TOOTHACHE; TOOTH DECAY; DRY TEETH; DESICCATED TEETH; PARCHED TEETH; GRINDING OF THE TEETH; TEETH. See also GUM. ◇ Chin 牙 *yá,* tooth, upper tooth, fang, tusk; 齿 *chǐ,* tooth, lower tooth, molar. [26: 132, 886]

toothache 牙痛 *yá tòng:* Pain felt in the teeth. Toothache is most commonly caused by tooth decay, a rotting away of the teeth, that the ancient Chinese ascribed to the work of "worms." Where decay is absent, Chinese medicine attributes toothache to wind-fire, wind-cold, stomach heat, kidney vacuity, or qi vacuity. **Wind-fire** (wind-heat) toothache is relieved by cold and is associated with painful swelling of the gums. It is exacerbated by exposure to heat or by eating hot spicy foods. Pain may relieved by coolness. The swelling may make eating difficult, and in some cases the cheeks are swollen and hot. Other signs include thirst, a red-tipped tongue with thin white fur or dry yellow fur, and rapid floating pulse. MED Oral: Course wind, clear heat, and relieve pain. Use variations of Lonicera and Forsythia Powder (*yín qiào sǎn*). Topical: Apply Mint and Refined Mirabilite Powder (*bò hé xuán míng sǎn*). ACU Base treatment for toothache mainly on ST and LI. Main points: ST-7 (*xià guān*, Below the Joint), LI-4 (*hé gǔ*, Union Valley), and ST-6 (*jiá chē*, Cheek Carriage). For wind-fire, add GB-20 (*fēng chí*, Wind Pool), TB-5 (*wài guān*, Outer Pass), and GV-14 (*dà zhuī*, Great Hammer); needle with drainage. If heat is exuberant, prick LU-11 (*shào shāng*, Lesser Shang) and LI-1 (*shāng yáng*, Shang Yang) to bleed. **Wind-cold** toothache is characterized by a pulling pain and is exacerbated by cold and relieved by the application of warmth. Other signs include periodic aversion to cold, absence of thirst, a thin white tongue fur, and a tight floating or a slow or moderate pulse. MED Oral: Course wind, dissipate cold, and relieve pain. Use Perilla Leaf Decoction (*sū yè tāng*). Topical: Apply Asarum Powder (*xì xīn sǎn*). ACU Add to the main points GB-20 (*fēng chí*, Wind Pool), TB-5 (*wài guān*, Outer Pass), and LU-7 (*liè quē*, Broken Sequence); needle with drainage and add moxa. **Stomach heat** toothache is toothache attributable to stomach fire ascending the hand and foot yang brightness (*yáng míng*) channels, which pass through the lower and upper jaws respectively. It is characterized by severe pain associated with bad breath, thirst, constipation, yellow tongue fur, and a stringlike pulse. MED Clear and discharge stomach fire with Sweet Dew Beverage (*gān lù yǐn*) or Stomach-Clearing Decoction (*qīng wèi tāng*). ACU Add to the main points ST-44 (*nèi tíng*, Inner Court) and ST-36 (*zú sān lǐ*, Leg Three Li); needle with drainage. **Kidney vacuity** toothache is vacuity fire toothache resulting from insufficiency of kidney yin with vacuity fire flaming upward. Kidney vacuity toothache is explained by the governing of the bone, and the teeth are the surplus of the bone. It is characterized by dull intermittent pain, absence of bad breath, a red-tipped tongue, and a fine pulse. In some cases, loosening of the teeth is also observed. MED Supplement kidney yin and drain liver fire using formulas such as Supplemented Six-Ingredient Rehmannia Pill (*jiā wèi liù wèi dì huáng wán*). ACU Needle with even supplementation and drainage or with supplementation at KI-3 (*tài xī*, Great Ravine) and KI-1 (*yǒng quán*, Gushing Spring); needle with drainage at LR-2 (*xíng jiān*, Moving Between) and the main points. **Qi vacuity** usually arises from taxation damage. It is a dull continuous toothache without markedly swollen gums or with swollen gums

that are not markedly red. Other signs include bright white facial complexion, shortage of qi, laziness to speak, faint low voice, fatigue and lack of strength, spontaneous sweating, heart palpitations, dizzy head, tinnitus, frequent voidings of clear urine, pale enlarged tongue with thin white tongue fur, and a weak vacuous or vacuous large pulse. MED Supplement qi and relieve pain. Use Center-Supplementing Qi-Boosting Decoction (*bǔ zhōng yì qì tāng*) plus cooked rehmannia (*shú dì huáng*), moutan (*mǔ dān pí*), poria (*fú líng*), and white peony (*bái sháo yào*). ACU Add to the main points ST-36 (*zú sān lǐ*, Leg Three Li), CV-6 (*qì hǎi*, Sea of Qi), BL-20 (*pí shū*, Spleen Transport), and BL-21 (*wèi shū*, Stomach Transport); needle with supplementation and add moxa. **Tooth decay** is observed in people who usually eat fat meat, fine grain, and strong flavors or sweet sugary things that get lodged between the teeth and fail to be removed by cleaning. Holes appear in the teeth with local blackening. The holes harbor food, further exacerbating the decay. Cold, hot, sour, and sweet foods can exacerbate the pain, as can inhalation of air. MED Clear heat and relieve pain. Topical: Grind zanthoxylum (*huā jiāo*) and limestone (*shí huī*) to a powder and blend with honey into pills. Apply by forcing pill material into the cavities. Other guidelines for the treatment of toothache are commonly applied. ACU Since the hand yang brightness (*yáng míng*) large intestine channel runs through the lower teeth, aching among the lower teeth can be treated mainly by large intestine channel points. Since the foot yang brightness (*yáng míng*) stomach channel passes through the upper teeth, aching among the upper teeth can be treated by stomach channel points. In addition, *The Magic Pivot* (*líng shū, zá bìng piān*) states, "Toothache without aversion to cold drinks is treated through the foot yang brightness (*yáng míng*); with aversion to cold drinks, it is treated through the hand yang brightness (*yáng míng*)." For toothache without discomfort when taking cold drinks, use ST-44 (*nèi tíng*, Inner Court) and ST-7 (*xià guān*, Below the Joint) as the main points; if there is discomfort, use LI-4 (*hé gǔ*, Union Valley). See TOOTH DECAY. [92: No. 126] [37: 473–4] [46: 725] [13: 704]

tooth bed 牙床 *yá chuáng*: CHEEK CARRIAGE BONE. [81: 564] [27: 65]

tooth carriage 牙车 *yá chē*: CHEEK CARRIAGE BONE. [81: 564]

tooth decay 齿齲 *chǐ qǔ*: Rotting of the teeth characterized by the cavities and toothache. Tooth decay is attributed to a lack of oral hygiene or to wind, phlegm, dampness and heat steaming in the hand and foot yang brightness (*yáng míng*) channels, which enter the lower and upper teeth respectively. MED Clear heat and relieve pain using Stomach-Clearing Powder (*qīng wèi sǎn*), Jade Lady Brew (*yù nǔ jiān*), or Coptis Gallbladder-Warming Decoction (*huáng lián wēn dǎn tāng*). Attention should be paid to oral hygiene. Wash mouth regularly with a decoction of lonicera (*jīn yín huā*), forsythia (*lián qiáo*), mint (*bò hé*), and raw licorice (*shēng gān cǎo*). ACU *Elementary Questions* (*sù wèn, miào cì lùn*) states, "For toothache, needle the hand yang brightness." Base treatment mainly on LI and ST. Select LI-4 (*hé gǔ*, Union Valley), LI-5 (*yáng xī*, Yang Ravine), ST-6 (*jiá chē*, Cheek Carriage), ST-44 (*nèi tíng*, Inner Court), and ST-7 (*xià guān*, Below the Joint); needle with drainage. To course wind, add GV-14 (*dà zhuī*, Great Hammer) and TB-5 (*wài guān*, Outer Pass). See TOOTHACHE. [26: 887] [97: 342] [50: 900] [25: 183] [46: 725]

topical eye medication 点眼 *diǎn yǎn*: **1.** A liquid, powder, or paste preparation (eye drops, eye powder, eye paste) applied to the eye or surrounding flesh. **2.** The application of a such a preparation. ◊ Chin 点 *diǎn*, dot, drop, dab; 眼 *yǎn*, eye. [125: 91]

topically applied paste 外敷膏剂 *wài fū gāo jì*: See MEDICINAL PASTE; PLASTER.

topsy-turvy speech 语言颠倒 *yǔ yán diān dǎo*: Speaking in garbled order. Observed in phlegm reversal headache.

torpid intake 纳呆 *nà dāi*: Synonym: *torpid stomach*. Impairment of the stomach's governing of intake (see STOMACH GOVERNS INTAKE). Torpid intake is attributable to spleen-stomach vacuity or to damp-heat obstruction and is characterized by indigestion and poor appetite, and in some cases by a sensation of bloating. See POOR APPETITE. ◊ Chin 纳 *nà*, receive; 呆 *dāi*, dull, torpid, feeble-minded. [27: 412]

torpid stomach 胃呆 *wèi dāi*: TORPID INTAKE.

torpid stomach intake 胃纳呆滞 *wèi nà dāi zhì*: See TORPID INTAKE.

tortoise back 龟背 *guī bèi*: Synonym: *hunchback*. A deformity in infants in which the spine curves outward giving the back the appearance of a tortoise's shell; hence the name. Turtle back is attributed to congenital insufficiency and/or poor nourishment after birth manifesting in spleen qi vacuity depriving the bones and governing of nourishment. [27: 436] [27: 463]

tortoise's-back phlegm 龟背痰 *guī bèi tán*: Flowing phlegm of the back. See FLOWING PHLEGM. [26: 921]

tortoise's head 龟头 *guī tóu*: YIN HEAD.

tortoise's head welling-abscess 龟头痈 *guī tóu yōng*: A condition in which the yin head (glans penis) becomes swollen and purple. MED Ap-

ply powdered calcined turtle shell (*duàn biē jiǎ*) blended with egg white (*jī zǐ bái*). [26: 624]

to treat disease, it is necessary to seek its root 治病必求于本 *zhì bìng bì qiú yú běn*: From *Elementary Questions* (*sù wèn, yīn yáng yìng xiàng lùn*). The first principle of treatment, whereby the cause or essential nature of disease rather than its manifestations are addressed. Treating disease by the root, or radical treatment, applies to most diseases and is divided into two forms: straight treatment and paradoxical treatment. Treating a disease by the tip, or signs treatment, represents an exception to this principle that applies under clearly defined conditions. See PRINCIPLE OF TREATMENT. [6: 242]

to treat wind, first treat the blood; when the blood moves, wind naturally disappears 治风先治血，血行风自灭 *zhì fēng xiān zhì xuè, xuè xíng fēng zì miè*: To nourish the blood is to enhance the elimination of wind. See DISPELLING WIND AND NOURISHING THE BLOOD. [26: 269]

toxicity 毒 *dú*: The quality of a medicinal that makes it cause illness or discomfort. [26: 355]

toxic qi 毒气 *dú qì*: PESTILENTIAL QI.

toxin 毒 *dú*: **1.** Any substance that that is harmful to the body when eaten or entering the body through a wound or through the skin, such as lacquer toxin or pitch toxin. The toxin of animals is called venom. See also TOXICITY. **2.** Any virulent evil qi, e.g., TOXIC QI, which denotes scourge epidemic qi; occasionally, a disease caused by such, e.g., SEASONAL TOXIN. **3.** Evil qi that causes painful reddening and swelling, suppuration, or weeping discharge. See HEAT TOXIN; DAMP TOXIN. **4.** A label for certain conditions of external medicine, e.g., CINNABAR TOXIN; INNOMINATE TOXIN SWELLING; BEND-CENTER TOXIN [SORE]; BIAN TOXIN (SORE); FETAL TOXIN. [96: 14] [97: 394]

toxin swelling 肿毒 *zhǒng dú*: Swelling due to the presence of toxin (heat toxin, damp toxin). See TOXIN. [96: 14]

tracking wind and expelling cold 搜风逐寒 *sōu fēng zhú hán*: A method of treatment used to address wind evil with cold evil and damp phlegm and static blood in the network vessels manifesting as pain in the sinews and bones of limbs. Minor Network-Quickening Elixir (*xiǎo huó luò dān*) is a representative wind-tracking cold-expelling formula. [27: 269] [97: 547]

transform 化 *huà*: *vb.* See TRANSFORMATION.

transformation 化 *huà*: (*vb.* transform). Change, usually of a gentle or gradual nature in relative contrast to *transmutation*, sudden or major change. Transformation implies progressive (productive) and regressive (destructive) change, and in the former case is frequently rendered as *formation*.

Hence, *fire formation* refers to the natural transformation of evils or yang qi into fire (progressive change), whereas *transforming phlegm* refers to a method of treatment to eliminate phlegm (i.e., regressive change). Transformation often specifically refers to digestion (which in modern medicine is called 消化 *xiāo huà*), e.g., NONTRANSFORMATION OF FOOD.

transformation into fire 化火 *huà huǒ*: A pathological change that results in a fire pattern. Excessive exuberance of the yang qi of the body, externally contracted evils (or stagnant qi, blood, phlegm, or food), seven-affect internal damage, and depletion of yin humor may all cause transformation into fire. (1) Extreme heat transforming into fire, as a result of excessive exuberance of the yang qi of the body. Under normal circumstances, yang qi nourishes the spirit and emolliates the sinews, warms the bowels and viscera and the whole body, and drives all physiological activity. Under such normal circumstances, yang qi is what is called the LESSER FIRE. But when yang qi becomes overexuberant, qi, blood, fluids, and essence are damaged. When this happens, yang qi becomes a damaging force that is known as VIGOROUS FIRE. Dan Xi described this as "Exuberant qi is fire." *Elementary Questions* (*sù wèn, yīn yáng yìng xiàng dà lùn*) explains the physiological and pathological significance of the "lesser fire" and the "vigorous fire" as follows: "The vigorous fire consumes qi, qi consumes the lesser fire; the vigorous fire dissipates qi, the lesser fire engenders qi." (2) Depressed evils transforming into fire. Externally contracted evils (wind, cold, dryness, dampness, etc.) may all enter the interior and become stagnant. With the yang qi of the body they then transform into heat or fire. Depressed cold transforms into heat, and depressed dampness transforms into fire. Pathological products of the body (such as phlegm-damp or static blood), food accumulations, and worm accumulations may also become depressed and transform into fire. The reason why depressed evils transform into fire is that they cause depression of yang qi. Depressed yang qi engenders heat and transforms into fire, causing an internal repletion heat bind. (3) Excesses among the five minds transforming into fire. Mental and emotional stimulus can cause imbalances of the yin and yang and the qi and blood of the body, which given rise to binding depression of qi dynamic, which in time transforms into heat. The most common clinical example of this is affect-mind depression preventing the normal free coursing of the liver and causing liver qi to become depressed and stagnant and transform into fire. This is called "liver fire". (4) Effulgent yin vacuity fire. When essence and blood are depleted or yin humor suffers major damage, the resulting yin vacuity give rise to yang hyperactivity, creat-

ing vacuity heat that engenders vacuity fire. Generally speaking, yin vacuity internal heat manifests in generalized signs, while effulgent yin vacuity fire is concentrated in a particular place, giving rise to local signs such as toothache, sore throat, steaming bone, or reddening of the cheeks. (5) Distinction is made between repletion and vacuity fire. Repletion fire mostly arises when depressed evils transform into fire; it is of rapid onset and tends follow a short course, and is characterized by vigorous heat [effusion], red face, thirst with a liking for cold things, short voidings of yellow urine, constipation, erosion and sores of the mouth, red tongue and red eyes, dry yellow tongue fur, and surging rapid pulse. In severe cases, there is clouded spirit and manic agitation. Vacuity fire arises from depletion of essence and blood; it tends to develop slowly and last for long time, and is characterized by vexing heat in the five hearts, in some cases steaming bone, post-meridian reddening of the cheeks, insomnia, night sweating, dry mouth and throat, dizziness and tinnitus, red tongue with scant fur, and a rapid fine pulse. Excess among the five minds transforming into fire can manifest in the form of repletion fire, as in LIVER FIRE FLAMING UPWARD; it can also manifest in the form of vacuity fire, as in EFFULGENT HEART FIRE. See REPLETION FIRE; VACUITY FIRE. [26: 168] [36: 280–281] [27: 138] [97: 109] [3: 53]

transformation into heat 化热 *huà rè*: *Synonym: heat formation.* The development of heat signs in externally contracted disease. In the initial-stage, external evils such as wind, cold, dryness, and dampness invade the body and give rise to an exterior cold pattern marked by aversion to cold and a thin white tongue fur. If the evil then penetrates the qi aspect, aversion to cold is replaced by aversion to heat, thirst, dry lips, heart vexation, constipation, reddish urine, a red tongue with yellow fur, and a rapid pulse. *On Warm Heat* (*wēn rè lùn*) states, "Cold damage evil lingers in the exterior, and then transforms into heat and enters the interior." Compare TRANSFORMATION INTO FIRE. [26: 169] [27: 138] [97: 109]

transforming dampness 化湿 *huà shī*: **1.** A method of treatment used to address dampness in the upper burner, in which aromatic medicinals are used. Damp evil in the exterior is treated by coursing the exterior and transforming dampness. Damp warmth seasonal epidemic with sore throat and oppression in the chest is treated by clearing heat and transforming dampness. See COURSING THE EXTERIOR AND TRANSFORMING DAMPNESS; CLEARING HEAT AND TRANSFORMING DAMPNESS. **2.** DISPELLING DAMPNESS. [26: 170] [27: 260]

transforming phlegm 化痰 *huà tán*: Any method of treatment used to eliminate phlegm gently. The method of transforming phlegm takes different forms depending on the location and cause of the phlegm pattern. **Lung:** Phlegm in the lung causing cough is treated by TRANSFORMING PHLEGM AND SUPPRESSING COUGH. Specific patterns are treated by specific methods. Externally contracted wind-cold causing nondiffusion of lung qi with nasal congestion, itchy throat, cough with copious phlegm, and thin white tongue fur is treated by DIFFUSING THE LUNG AND TRANSFORMING PHLEGM. Heat evil congesting the lung, reducing humor to phlegm, and characterized by cough, expectoration of thick yellow phlegm, red face, heat vexation, and a red tongue with yellow fur is treated by CLEARING HEAT AND TRANSFORMING PHLEGM. Warm dryness or insufficiency of lung yin causing dry cough and difficult expectoration of phlegm, and a red tongue with dry yellow fur is treated by MOISTENING THE LUNG AND TRANSFORMING PHLEGM. Lung-kidney yin vacuity with exuberant internal damp phlegm, characterized by cough and nausea, counterflow panting and copious phlegm, and cough especially pronounced at night, is treated by SUPPLEMENTING THE LUNG AND KIDNEY AND TRANSFORMING PHLEGM.

Transforming Phlegm

TRANSFORMING PHLEGM AND SUPPRESSING COUGH (*huà tán zhǐ ké*)

DIFFUSING THE LUNG AND TRANSFORMING PHLEGM (*xuān fèi huà tán*)

CLEARING HEAT AND TRANSFORMING PHLEGM (*qīng rè huà tán*)

MOISTENING THE LUNG AND TRANSFORMING PHLEGM (*rùn fèi huà tán*)

SUPPLEMENTING THE LUNG AND KIDNEY AND TRANSFORMING PHLEGM (*bǔ fèi huà tán*)

DRYING DAMPNESS AND TRANSFORMING PHLEGM (*zào shī huà tán*)

DISPELLING COLD AND TRANSFORMING PHLEGM (*qū hán huà tán*)

FORTIFYING THE SPLEEN, WARMING THE KIDNEY, AND TRANSFORMING PHLEGM (*jiàn pí, wēn shèn, huà tán*)

HARMONIZING THE STOMACH AND TRANSFORMING PHLEGM (*hé wèi huà tán*)

DISPERSING FOOD AND TRANSFORMING PHLEGM (*xiāo shí huà tán*)

TRANSFORMING PHLEGM AND OPENING THE ORIFICES (*huà tán kāi qiào*)

DISPELLING WIND AND TRANSFORMING PHLEGM (*qū fēng huà tán*)

DISPERSING PHLEGM AND SOFTENING HARDNESS (*xiāo tán ruǎn jiān*)

Spleen-stomach: Damp phlegm due to devitalization of spleen yang impairing normal movement and transformation, characterized by white easily expectorated phlegm, oppression in the chest and nausea, slimy glossy white tongue fur, and possibly dizziness and heart palpitations is treated by DRYING DAMPNESS AND TRANSFORMING PHLEGM. Cold phlegm arising from spleen-stomach yang vacuity and collection of cold rheum in the inner body characterized by ejection of thin clear phlegm, aversion to cold, lack of warmth in the extremities, and a slimy tongue fur is treated by DISPELLING COLD AND TRANSFORMING PHLEGM. Spleen-kidney yang vacuity with lung cold and phlegm obstruction characterized by physical cold and cold limbs, cold aching back and lumbus, cough with copious phlegm, enuresis accompanying acute cough, white tongue fur, and a slow sunken pulse is treated by FORTIFYING THE SPLEEN, WARMING THE KIDNEY, AND TRANSFORMING PHLEGM. Phlegm lodging in the stomach, characterized by signs such as vomiting and nausea, is treated by HARMONIZING THE STOMACH AND TRANSFORMING PHLEGM. Replete qi and exuberant phlegm causing cough and qi counterflow, oppression in the chest and copious phlegm, indigestion, distention and oppression in the stomach duct and abdomen, a slimy tongue, and a slippery pulse is treated by DISPERSING FOOD AND TRANSFORMING PHLEGM. **Heart:** Phlegm confounding the orifices of the heart is treated by TRANSFORMING PHLEGM AND OPENING THE ORIFICES. **Channels:** Phlegm scurrying through the channels, characterized by deviated mouth and eyes, stiff tongue, and impeded speech, is treated by DISPELLING WIND AND TRANSFORMING PHLEGM. Phlegm binding in masses, such as phlegm nodes, scrofula, and goiter, is treated by DISPERSING PHLEGM AND SOFTENING HARDNESS. See the entries listed below. [26: 169] [6: 263] [27: 271] [97: 109] [25: 64] [3: 84]

Phlegm-Transforming, Cough-Suppressing, Panting-Calming Medicinals

Phlegm-Transforming Medicinals

半夏 (*bàn xià*) pinellia (Pinelliae Tuber)

姜半夏 (*jiāng bàn xià*) ginger pinellia (Pinelliae Tuber cum Zingibere Praeparatum)

天南星 (*tiān nán xīng*) arisaema (Arisaematis Rhizoma)

胆星 (*dǎn xīng*) bile arisaema (Arisaematis Rhizoma cum Felle Bovis)

禹白附 (*yǔ bái fù*) giant typhonium tuber (Typhonii Gigantei Tuber)

关白附 (*guān bái fù*) Korean aconite (Aconiti Coreani Tuber)

白附子 (*bái fù zǐ*) aconite/typhonium (Aconiti Coreani seu Typhonii Gigantei Tuber)

白芥子 (*bái jiè zǐ*) white mustard (Brassicae Albae Semen)

芥子 (*jiè zǐ*) leaf mustard seed (Brassicac Junceae Semen)

皂荚 (*zào jiá*) gleditsia (Gleditsiae Fructus)

皂角刺 (*zào jiǎo cì*) gleditsia thorn (Gleditsiae Spina)

桔梗 (*jié gěng*) platycodon (Platycodonis Radix)

金沸草 (*jīn fèi cǎo*) inula (Inulae Caulis et Folium)

旋覆花 (*xuán fù huā*) inula flower (Inulae Flos)

白前 (*bái qián*) cynanchum (Cynanchi Baiqian Radix et Rhizoma)

前胡 (*qián hú*) peucedanum (Peucedani Radix)

栝楼 (*guā lóu*) trichosanthes (Trichosanthis Fructus)

栝楼子 (*guā lóu zǐ*) trichosanthes seed (Trichosanthis Semen)

栝楼皮 (*guā lóu pí*) trichosanthes rind (Trichosanthis Pericarpium)

川贝母 (*chuān bèi mǔ*) Sichuan fritillaria (Fritillariae Cirrhosae Bulbus)

浙贝母 (*zhè bèi mǔ*) Zhejiang fritillaria (Fritillariae Verticillatae Bulbus)

竹茹 (*zhú rú*) bamboo shavings (Bambusae Caulis in Taeniam)

天竹黄 (*tiān zhú huáng*) bamboo sugar (Bambusae Concretio Silicea)

竹沥 (*zhú lì*) dried bamboo sap (Bambusae Succus Exsiccatus)

海浮石 (*hǎi fú shí*) pumice (Pumex)

海蛤壳 (*hǎi gé ké*) clamshell (Cyclinae (seu Meretricis) Concha)

礞石 (*méng shí*) chlorite/mica (Chloriti seu Micae Lapis)

海藻 (*hǎi zǎo*) sargassum (Sargassi Herba)

昆布 (*kūn bù*) kelp (Algae Thallus)

海带 (*hǎi dài*) eelgrass (Zosterae Marinae Herba)

黄药子 (*huáng yào zǐ*) air potato (Dioscoreae Bulbiferae Tuber)

胖大海 (*pàng dà hài*) sterculia (Sterculiae Semen)

猪胆汁 (*zhū dǎn zhī*) pig's bile (Suis Bilis)

蔊菜 (*hān cài*) rorippa (Rorippae Herba seu Flos)

明党参 (*míng dǎng shēn*) changium root (Changii Radix)

罗汉果 (*luó hàn guǒ*) Grosvenor's momordica (Momordicae Grosvenori Fructus)

荸荠 (*bí qí*) water chestnut (Heleocharitis Cormus)

凤凰衣 (*fèng huáng yī*) chicken's egg membrane (Galli Membrana Ovi)

Cough-Suppressing Panting-Calming Medicinals

杏仁 (*xìng rén*) apricot kernel (Armeniacae Semen)

甜杏仁 (*tián xìng rén*) sweet apricot kernel (Armeniacae Semen Dulce)

巴旦杏仁 (*bā dàn xìng rén*) almond (Pruni Amygdali Semen)

白部 (*bǎi bù*) stemona (Stemonae Radix)

紫菀 (*zǐ wǎn*) aster (Asteris Radix et Rhizoma)

款冬花 (*kuǎn dōng huā*) tussilago (Tussilaginis Flos)

紫苏子 (*zǐ sū zǐ*) perilla seed (Perillae Fructus)

桑白皮 (*sāng bái pí*) mulberry root bark (Mori Radicis Cortex)

葶苈子 (*tíng lì zǐ*) tingli (Descurainiae seu Lepidii Semen)

枇杷叶 (*pí pá yè*) loquat leaf (Eriobotryae Folium)

马兜铃 (*mǎ dōu líng*) aristolochia fruit (Aristolochiae Fructus)

紫金牛 (*zǐ jīn niú*) Japanese ardisia (Ardisiae Japonicae Caulis et Folium)

白果 (*bái guǒ*) ginkgo (Ginkgo Semen)

洋金花 (*yáng jīn huā*) datura flower (Daturae Flos)

华山参 (*huá shān shēn*) physochlaina (Physochlainae Radix)

钟乳石 (*zhōng rǔ shí*) stalactite (Stalactitum)

钟乳粉 (*zhōng rǔ fěn*) powdered stalactite (Stalactitum Pulveratum)

满山红 (*mǎn shān hóng*) Daurian rhododendron (Rhododendri Daurici Folium)

鹅管石 (*é guǎn shí*) goose throat stone (Balanophyllia seu Stalactitum)

---

transforming phlegm and opening the orifices 化痰开窍 *huà tán kāi qiào*: *Synonyms: sweeping phlegm and opening the orifices; sweeping phlegm and arousing the brain; eliminating phlegm and opening the orifices.* To treat clouded spirit in phlegm patterns. Distinction is made between heat phlegm and cold phlegm. Heat phlegm 热痰 (*rè tán*) transforming phlegm and opening the orifices patterns are characterized by exuberant phlegm with rough breathing, clouded spirit and delirious speech, generalized heat [effusion], vexation and agitation, and a red tongue with yellow fur. MED Use Bovine Bezoar Pill (*niú huáng wán*) or Supreme Jewel Elixir (*zhì bǎo dān*). ACU Main points: ST-36 (*zú sān lǐ*, Leg Three Li), CV-22 (*tiān tú*, Celestial Chimney), ST-40 (*fēng lóng*, Bountiful Bulge), PC-6 (*nèi guān*, Inner Pass), PC-5 (*jiān shǐ*, Intermediary Courier), and GV-26 (*shuǐ gōu*, Water Trough). For heat phlegm, add LI-4 (*hé gǔ*, Union Valley), LI-11 (*qū chí*, Pool at the Bend), GV-14 (*dà zhuī*, Great Hammer); needle with drainage, and prick Twelve Well Points (*shí èr jǐng xué*) to bleed. Cold phlegm 寒痰 (*hán tán*) transforming phlegm and opening the orifices patterns are characterized by phlegm drool congestion, clouded spirit, green-blue or white face, cold extremities, and a sunken pulse. MED Use Liquid Storax Pill (*sū hé xiāng wán*). ACU To the main points given above add add CV-4 (*guān yuán*, Pass Head), GV-4 (*mìng mén*, Life Gate), and CV-8 (*shén què*, Spirit Gate Tower); needle with even supplementation and drainage and moxa (CV-8 can only be moxaed). See OPENING THE ORIFICES. [27: 276] [97: 110] [26: 169] [6: 266] [46: 597, 729, 731] [14: 54]

transforming phlegm and suppressing cough 化痰止咳 *huà tán zhǐ ké*: A method of treatment used to address cough and expectoration of phlegm using phlegm-transforming medicinals. Phlegm-transforming medicinals that are warm in nature and indicated for cold phlegm and damp phlegm include white mustard (*bái jiè zǐ*), arisaema (*tiān nán xīng*), pinellia (*bàn xià*), perilla seed (*sū zǐ*), perilla seed (*zǐ sū zǐ*), tangerine peel (*chén pí*), dried ginger (*gān jiāng*), and gleditsia (*zào jiá*). Phlegm-transforming medicinals that are cool in nature and indicated for heat phlegm and dryness phlegm include rorippa (*hān cài*), tingli (*tíng lì zǐ*), fritillaria (*bèi mǔ*), trichosanthes (*guā lóu*), arctium (*niú bàng zǐ*), wax gourd seed (*dōng guā zǐ*), and adenophora/glehnia (*shā shēn*). Medicinals more balanced in nature such as platycodon (*jié gěng*), apricot kernel (*xìng rén*), peucedanum (*qián hú*), aster (*zǐ wǎn*), and tussilago (*kuǎn dōng huā*) can be used for most kinds of phlegm. Among formulas, Minor Green-Blue Dragon Decoction (*xiǎo qīng lóng tāng*) treats cold phlegm, and Two Matured Ingredients Decoction (*èr chén tāng*) is effective for damp phlegm. Lonicera and Phragmites Mixture (*yín wěi hé jì*) may be used for heat phlegm, and Dryness-Clearing Lung-Rescuing Decoction (*qīng zào jiù fèi tāng*) treats dryness phlegm. Cough-Stopping Powder (*zhǐ sòu sǎn*) is a general phlegm-transforming cough-suppressing remedy. ACU Base treatment LU, SP, and ST. Select BL-13 (*fèi shū*, Lung Transport), LU-9 (*tài yuán*, Great Abyss), SP-3 (*tài bái*, Supreme White), CV-17 (*shān zhōng*, Chest Center), ST-36 (*zú sān lǐ*, Leg Three Li), ST-40 (*fēng lóng*, Bountiful Bulge), and LI-4 (*hé gǔ*, Union Valley); needle with drainage. See DISPELLING PHLEGM. [37: 274] [46: 653] [6: 263]

transforming stasis 化瘀 *huà yū*: See DISPELLING STASIS AND QUICKENING THE BLOOD. [6: 261] [27: 274]

transforming stasis and moving the blood 化瘀行血 *huà yū xíng xuè*: DISPELLING STASIS AND QUICKENING THE BLOOD.

transforming turbidity with aroma 芳香化浊 *fāng xiāng huà zhuó*: A method of treatment used to address damp turbidity brewing internally using aromatic dampness-transforming medicinals. Transforming turbidity with aroma is used to treat distention and oppression in the abdomen and stomach duct, with upflow nausea and de-

sire to vomit, thin sloppy stool, fatigue and lack of strength, and a slimy sensation and sweet taste in the mouth. MED Agastache/patchouli (*huò xiāng*) and eupatorium (*pèi lán*) are commonly used. If there is dizziness and distention in the head, a slimy white tongue fur, medicinals such as acorus (*shí chāng pú*), fresh lotus leaf (*xiān hé yè*), tangerine peel (*chén pí*), pro formula pinellia (*fǎ bàn xià*), and areca husk (*dà fù pí*) may be added. [50: 703]

Aromatic Dampness-Transforming Medicinals

苍术 (*cāng zhú*) atractylodes (Atractylodis Rhizoma)

厚朴 (*hòu pò*) magnolia bark (Magnoliae Cortex)

厚朴花 (*hòu pò huā*) magnolia flower[2] (Magnoliae Flos[2])

藿香 (*huò xiāng*) agastache/patchouli (Agastaches seu Pogostemi Herba)

佩兰 (*pèi lán*) eupatorium (Eupatorii Herba)

砂仁 (*shā rén*) amomum (Amomi Semen seu Fructus)

白豆蔻 (*bái dòu kòu*) cardamom (Amomi Cardamomi Fructus)

草豆蔻 (*cǎo dòu kòu*) Katsumada's galangal seed (Alpiniae Katsumadae Semen)

草果 (*cǎo guǒ*) tsaoko (Amomi Tsao-Ko Fructus)

石菖蒲 (*shí chāng pú*) acorus (Acori Rhizoma)

---

transmutation 变 *biàn*: Major, sudden, or untoward change. See TRANSFORMATION.

transmuted pattern 变证 *biàn zhèng*: Conversion of repletion into vacuity or a simple condition into a complex one because of inappropriate treatment (incorrect use of sweating, ejection, or precipitation, or use of supplementation in the treatment of repletion patterns) or insufficiency of right qi. For example, excessive use of sweat-effusing medicinals in the treatment of greater yang (*tài yáng*) cold damage patterns can cause detriment to heart yang and cause heart palpitations and fearful throbbing, and oppression in the chest. Another example is that of measles, where if papule outthrust is not complete, the papule toxin falls inward giving rise to a panting counterflow pattern. In both cases, the resulting condition is known as a transmuted pattern. [27: 222] [97: 372]

transport needling 输刺 *shū cì*: From *The Magic Pivot* (*líng shū, guān zhēn piān*). One of the NINE NEEDLING METHODS. Combining the five transport points with the back transport points. [27: 334]

transport point 俞穴 *shū xué*, 输穴 *shū xué*, 腧穴 *shū xué*: 1. Any acupuncture point. 2. Any of the FIVE TRANSPORT POINTS. ◇ Chin 俞 is the original form of the character, which in its meaning of transport came to be written with the cart signifier 车, and in the medical sense as here applied, with the flesh signifier 肉 simplified as 月.

transverse bone 横骨 *héng gǔ*: **1.** The small bone under the root of the tongue. WMC hyoid bone. **2.** *Synonym: covering bone.* The lower transverse bone. WMC pubic bone. [27: 68]

transverse insertion 横刺 *héng cì*: Insertion of an acupuncture needle at an angle of about 15°; it is applied to the head, chest, back, and abdomen, and on parts of the body with little flesh beneath the skin. A transverse insertion is also used in POINT JOINING, whereby the needle passes through two or more acupuncture points. [101: 32]

trauma 外伤 *wài shāng*: EXTERNAL INJURY.

treating disease before it arises 治未病 *zhì wèi bìng*: **1.** To prevent disease. *Elementary Questions* (*sù wèn, cì fǎ lùn*) states, "When right qi dwells within, evil cannot interfere, and toxic qi can be avoided." It offers suggestions for oral medication to prevent epidemics. **2.** To treat disease in its early stages. It is said that "the superior physician nips the bud." For example, recognition of dizzy head and vision, numbness of the thumb and middle finger, or twitching of the eyes and mouth is taken as a portent of of wind stroke as portends of wind stroke allows preventive treatment to be administered. **3.** To have a full grasp of the ways in which disease develops. Disease in the five viscera can undergo shifts that can be prevented by early treatment. The *Essential Prescriptions of the Golden Coffer* (*jīn guì yào lüè*) states, "Treating disease before it arises, means that when liver disease is observed and when it is known that liver disease passes to the spleen, the spleen can be made firm.... So is it with the other viscera." [27: 232]

treating cold with cold 寒因寒用 *rè yīn rè yòng*: From *Elementary Questions* (*sù wèn, zhì zhēn yào dà lùn*). A method of PARADOXICAL TREATMENT used to treat true internal heat and false external cold. In such cases, heat is true nature of the disease, and the cold is false. Hence, treatment involves the use of cool and cold medicinals. An example is when a patient presents great fever, great thirst, great sweating, and large surging pulse. and counterflow cold of the limbs. The counterflow cold of the limbs is a sign of false cold, while the other signs reflect true heat. This condition is treated with White Tiger Decoction (*bái hǔ tāng*) taken cold. In the *Elementary Questions* (*sù wèn, zhì zhēn yào dà lùn*), the term was originally written as "treating heat with cold", but was changed by later writers to align with *treating the stopped by stopping* and *treating the free by freeing.* [27: 236]

treating heat with heat 热因热用 *rè yīn rè yòng*: From *Elementary Questions* (*sù wèn, zhì zhēn yào dà lùn*). A method of PARADOXICAL

TREATMENT used to treat true internal cold and false external heat. In such cases, cold is the true nature of disease, and heat is false. Hence, treatment involves the use of warm and hot medicines. An example is when a patient presents counterflow cold of limbs, clear-food diarrhea, a deep fine pulse, and floating-red cheeks, vexation and agitation, and thirst with desire for cold drinks that is immediately allayed by drinking). The counterflow cold, clear-food diarrhea, and deep fine pulse are signs of true heat; the floating-red cheeks, vexation and agitation, and thirst with desire for cold drinks are signs of false cold. The condition is treated with Scallion Yang-Freeing Decoction (*bái tōng tāng*) taken cold. In the *Elementary Questions* (*sù wèn, zhì zhēn yào dà lùn*), the term was originally written as "treating cold with heat", but was changed by later writers to align with *treating the stopped by stopping* and *freeing the free by freeing.* [27: 235]

treating lower body disease through the upper body 下病取上 *xià bìng qǔ shàng*: From *Elementary Questions* (*sù wèn, wǔ cháng zhèng dà lùn*): "When the disease in lower body, treat it through the upper body." In acupuncture, this means treating disease of the lower by needling points on the upper body. For example, prolapse of the rectum can be treated by by needling GV-20 (*bǎi huì*, Hundred Convergences) at the vertex. In medicinal therapy, this means using medicinals that act from the upper body. For example, inhibited urination due to a dry lung that fails to move water manifesting in dry pharynx, vexation and thirst with a desire to drink, shortness of breath and rapid breathing, a thin yellow tongue tongue, and a rapid pulse can be treated through the upper burner with Lung-Clearing Drink (*qīng fèi yǐn zǐ*). [27: 237]

treating the free by freeing 通因通用 *tōng yīn tōng yòng*: From *Elementary Questions* (*sù wèn, zhì zhēn yào dà lùn*). A method of PARADOXICAL TREATMENT using freeing and disinhibiting agents to treat a disease patterns marked by freeness and disinhibition. For example, if food and drink accumulate and stagnate internally to give rise to glomus and oppression in the chest and stomach duct, distention and pain in the abdomen, no thought of food and drink, and diarrhea, then treatment must be to attack and expel the accumulation and stagnation using Unripe Bitter Orange Stagnation-Abducting Pill (*zhǐ shí dǎo zhì wán*). [27: 236]

treating the root 治本 *zhì běn*: Treating the cause or essential nature of disease. See PRINCIPLE OF TREATMENT. [6: 243]

treating the root and tip simultaneously 标本同治 *biāo běn tóng zhì*: *Synonym: simultane-*

ous treatment of the root and tip. See PRINCIPLE OF TREATMENT.

treating the stopped by stopping 塞因塞用 *sè yīn sāi yòng*: From *Elementary Questions* (*sù wèn, zhì zhēn yào dà lùn*). A method of PARADOXICAL TREATMENT using supplementing medicines to treat conditions marked by false obstruction and stoppage signs. An example is when a patient presents glomus and fullness in the chest and stomach duct that comes and goes and that likes pressure and warmth, as well as poor appetite, period vomiting, and pale tongue, and large vacuous pulse. The vacuity signs show that the glomus and oppression do not constitute a repletion pattern, but is caused spleen-stomach vacuity. Hence it is treated with Six Gentlemen Decoction (*liù jūn zǐ tāng*). ◇ Chin The first 塞 *sāi* refers to using stopping (astringent) medicinals; 因塞 *yīn sāi*, means 'because of' or 'in response to a pattern of stoppage'; 用 *yòng*, use. The phrase literally means 'using stopping in response to stoppage.' [27: 236] [102: 898]

treating the tip 治标 *zhì biāo*: A deviation from the normal practice of treating the root in the case of acute disease. For example, ascites is always the tip, never the root of the disease in which it appears, but by causing constipation and urine retention, and inhibiting respiration, initial treatment should aim to expel water before radical treatment (treatment that addresses the root) is prescribed. See PRINCIPLE OF TREATMENT. [6: 243]

treating upper body disease through the lower body 上病取下 *shàng bìng qǔ xià*: From *Elementary Questions* (*sù wèn, zhì zhēn yào dà lùn*): "When the disease is in the upper body, treat it through the lower body." In acupuncture, this means treating disease of the upper body by needling points on the lower body. For example, insomnia can be treated by needling ST-36 (*zú sān lǐ*, Leg Three Li), and dizzy head and vision can be treated by needling LR-3 (*tài chōng*, Supreme Surge). In medicinal therapy, it involves using medicinals that act from the lower body. For example, a patient suffering from dizzy head and vision, tinnitus, a feeling that as though he has fireworks exploding in his eyes, a yellow tongue fur and a rapid surging pulse can be given wine-steamed rhubarb (*dà huáng*) to provide light drainage. [27: 236]

treatment 治疗 *zhì liáo*: Any action serving or designed to eliminate or alleviate sickness. See PRINCIPLE OF TREATMENT; METHOD OF TREATMENT. [27: 458]

trembling tongue 舌颤 *shé chàn*: A tongue that trembles as it moves. A trembling tongue is observed in ascendant hyperactivity of liver yang, internal wind stirred by exuberant heat, or qi vacu-

ity. In the first two cases, the tongue is red or crimson, whereas in qi vacuity the tongue is pale. WMC According to modern clinical observation, a trembling tongue is seen in high fever, hyperthyroidism, hypertension, and certain nervous diseases. [6: 121]

triple burner 三焦 *sān jiāo*: One of the six bowels, comprising upper, middle, and lower burners. The hand lesser yang (*shào yáng*) triple burner channel passes through all three burners, linking up with many of the organs. The triple burner is an exterior organ, and its corresponding interior organ (for the purposes of acupuncture only) is the pericardium, to which it is connected by the hand reverting yin (*jué yīn*) pericardium channel. The nature of the triple burner has always been the subject of disagreement. The following three points, however, seem to be well established: (1) The triple burner refers to specific body areas: According to this view, the organs of the human body are distributed among three segments, referred to as the upper, middle, and lower burners. The upper burner includes the head and chest, the heart and the lung. The center burner corresponds to the upper abdomen (the area above the umbilicus) and includes the stomach and the spleen. The lower burner corresponds to the lower abdomen (inferior to the umbilicus) but includes the liver and kidney. (2) The triple burner represents the waterways: *Elementary Questions* (*sù wèn*) explains, "The triple burner holds the office of the sluices; it manifests as the waterways." This is interpreted to mean that the main functions of the triple burner are the processing of fluids by qi transformation and ensuring free flow through the waterways. As such, qi transformation in the triple burner is a global expression for the roles played by the lung, spleen, kidney, stomach, small intestine, large intestine, and bladder in regulating the body's water metabolism. *The Magic Pivot* (*líng shū*) states, "When the triple burner is open and permits effusion, it causes the five flavors of food to diffuse, nourishes the skin, makes the body firm, and keeps the [body] hair moistened, like the sprinkling of mist and dew. Such is the action of stomach qi." This fits the imagery of the phrase "the upper burner is like mist," which in practice refers to the diffusion of defense qi and distribution of fluids by the lung. *The Magic Pivot* (*líng shū*) states, "The center burner... strains off the waste and distills the fluids out of which the essence of grain and water is formed. This then flows upward into the lung channel where it is transformed into blood." This statement supports the phrase, "The center burner is like foam," which refers to the movement and formation of the essence of grain and water by the stomach and spleen, the source of blood formation. "In the middle burner, the

small intestine connects through to the bladder...
It transforms waste that is then sent down to the
large intestine... and distills the juices, sending
them down to the bladder." The intestines, kidney, and bladder are located in the lower burner.
The small intestine governs humor, the large intestine governs liquid, and the kidney governs the
opening and closing. Their combined functions explain the phrase "the lower burner is like a sluice."
(3) The triple burner is also a concept in pattern
identification; see TRIPLE BURNER PATTERN IDENTIFICATION. [6: 99] [26: 33]

triple burner channel 三焦经 *sān jiāo jīng*: See
HAND LESSER YANG TRIPLE BURNER CHANNEL.
[26: 24]

triple burner cough 三焦咳 *sān jiāo ké*: Cough
with abdominal fullness and no desire to eat or
drink.

triple burner governs the sluices 三焦主决渎
sān jiāo zhǔ jué dú: See TRIPLE BURNER. [27: 57]
[97: 20]

triple burner pattern identification 三焦辨证
sān jiāo biàn zhèng: A method of pattern identification developed in the Qing Dynasty by Wu Ju-
Tong of the warm disease school on the basis of the
experience of previous physicians. It divides warm
diseases according to stage of transmission through
the upper, middle, and lower burners. Diseases of
the upper burner include invasion of the lung by external evils, construction-aspect evil patterns, and
external evils penetrating the pericardium, which
for the most part correspond to initial-stage externally contracted heat (febrile) diseases. Diseases
of the center burner include gastrointestinal heat
bind and spleen-stomach damp-heat, which usually correspond to midstage externally contracted
heat diseases. Diseases of the lower burner include
such conditions as deep penetration of evils, wearing of kidney yin, insufficiency of liver blood, and
yin vacuity stirring wind, which correspond to the
advanced stages of externally contracted heat diseases. The concept of the three burners and the
triple burner method of pattern identification are
also used in diagnosing internal damage miscellaneous diseases, but to a much lesser degree and
in a less systematized way than that of externally
contracted heat diseases. [26: 34] [25: 14] [6: 100]
[27: 226]

triple burner repletion heat 三焦实热 *sān jiāo
shí rè*: **1.** Repletion heat in the upper burner
(heart and lung), center burner (spleen and stomach), or lower burner (liver and kidney). **2.** Qi-
aspect repletion heat. [27: 116] [97: 19]

triple burner vacuity cold 三焦虚寒 *sān jiāo
xū hán*: Vacuity cold in the upper burner (heart
and lung), center burner (spleen and stomach), or
lower burner (liver and kidney). [27: 116] [97: 19]

triple yang 三阳 *sān yáng*: A generic term for the
three yang channels.

triple-yang channel malaria 三阳经疟 *sān yáng
jīng nüè*: MALARIA developing in the three yang
channels. *Pathoconditions, Causes, Pulses, and
Treatments* (*zhèng yīn mài zhì*) states, "In malaria,
when cold is followed by heat and episodes are
regular, the episodes usually take place in the S4
watch (*sì shí*), S5 watch (*wǔ shí*), or S6 watch (*wèi
shí*). If there is one episode a day, this is lesser yang
(*shào yáng*); if there is one every other day, this is
yang brightness (*yáng míng*) or lesser yang (*shào
yáng*). [50: 59]

triple-yang combination disease 三阳合病 *sān
yáng hé bìng*: The simultaneous appearance of
greater yang (*tài yáng*), lesser yang (*shào yáng*),
and yang brightness (*yáng míng*) signs. *On Cold
Damage* (*shāng hán lùn, biàn yáng míng bìng mài
zhèng bìng zhì*) states, "Triple-yang combination
disease with a pulse floating and large, going beyond the bar, desire only to sleep, and sweating
as soon as the eyes are closed." "In triple-yang
disease with abdominal fullness, heavy body making it difficult to turn, insensitivity of the mouth,
grimy face, delirious speech, enuresis, and exacerbation of delirious speech by sweating." [26: 33]
[27: 221] [97: 19] [62: 902]

triple-yang disease 三阳病 *sān yáng bìng*: Synonym: *yang disease*.[1] Disease in any of the three
yang channels.

triple-yang headache 三阳头痛 *sān yáng tóu
tòng*: HEADACHE associated with one or more
of the three yang channels. See GREATER
YANG HEADACHE; YANG BRIGHTNESS HEADACHE;
LESSER YANG HEADACHE. See also HEADACHE.

triple yin 三阴 *sān yīn*: A generic term for the
three yin channels.

triple-yin disease 三阴病 *sān yīn bìng*: Synonym: *yin disease*.[1] Disease in any of the three
yang channels.

triple-yin headache 三阴头痛 *sān yīn tóu
tòng*: HEADACHE associated with one or more
of the three yin channels. See GREATER YIN
HEADACHE; LESSER YIN HEADACHE; REVERTING
YIN HEADACHE. See also HEADACHE.

triple-yin malaria 三阴疟 *sān yīn nüè*: **1.** QUARTAN MALARIA. MALARIA attributed to internal
vacuity of original qi and insecurity of defense qi
with the malarial evil lying latent in the three yin
channels; hence the name. Treat mainly by supporting right. **2.** Quartan malaria disease occurring before the winter solstice after exposure to
summerheat. **3.** MALARIA occurring in episodes
at night. See MALARIA. [26: 32] [27: 222] [97: 18]

trouser-bottom sore 裤口疮 *kù kǒu chuāng*: See
SHANK SORE.

trouser-bottom toxin sore 裤口毒 *kù kǒu dú*: See SHANK SORE.

true 真 *zhēn*: Pertaining to that upon which the health of the whole organism rests, in particular the kidney. For example, "true yin" and "true yang" refer to kidney yin and yang.

true cold and false heat 真寒假热 *zhēn hán jiǎ rè*: Any disease pattern presenting with signs of both heat and cold, in which the cold signs represent its essential nature, whereas the heat signs are deceptive. This accords with the principle that "extreme cold resembles heat." True cold and false heat is identified when reversal cold of the limbs, diarrhea containing untransformed food, or faint pulse verging on expiration are found occurring simultaneously with agitation, no aversion to cold, thirst with desire for warm fluids, upbearing fire flush, or sore pharynx. Here, the cold signs are caused by exuberant internal yin cold, whereas the false heat signs (agitation, upbearing fire flush, and sore pharynx) are attributable to vacuous yang floating upward. The principle of treatment applied in such cases is *treating heat with heat*. [27: 212] [97: 460] [6: 155]

true eye damage 真睛破损 *zhēn jīng pò sǔn*: Any fissuring, piercing, or other lesion of the eye due to external injury. ◇ Chin 真 *zhēn*, true; 睛 *jīng*, eye. The "true eye" means the physical eye.

true headache 真头痛 *zhēn tóu tòng*: Acute headache penetrating deep into the brain and reaching the vertex and accompanied by counterflow cold of the extremities up to the knees and elbows. A true headache is usually a critical sign, and is attributed to evils (some say wind-cold) invading the brain. MED Use Galenite Elixir (*hēi xí dān*) and large doses of Ginseng and Aconite Decoction (*shēn fù tāng*). ACU Either of the following methods can be used for emergency treatment of attacks: (1) Moxa GV-20 (*bǎi huì*, Hundred Convergences). (2) Moxa GV-20 (*bǎi huì*, Hundred Convergences), and BL-10 (*tiān zhù*, Celestial Pillar). See HEADACHE. [26: 504] [50: 1214] [113: 209]

true heart pain 真心痛 *zhēn xīn tòng*: A pattern described in *The Magic Pivot* (*líng shū, jué bìng*) in the following way; "In true heart pain, the hands and feet turn blue-green up to the joints and heart pain is severe. If it occurs at dawn, death ensues in the evening; if it occurs in the evening, death ensues at dawn." WMC According to the foregoing description, true heart pain corresponds to cardiodynia due to acute myocardiac infarction with circulatory failure. MED Return yang and stem counterflow; open the orifices with aroma; quicken the blood and transform stasis. Traditional medication is Liquid Storax Pill (*sū hé xiāng wán*) for emergency treatment and Ginseng and Aconite De-

coction (*shēn fù tāng*) plus aquilaria (*chén xiāng*) and notoginseng (*sān qī*). Compare HEART PAIN. ACU Base treatment mainly on CV, BL, and PC. Supplement CV-17 (*shān zhōng*, Chest Center), BL-15 (*xīn shū*, Heart Transport), BL-14 (*jué yīn shū*, Reverting Yin Transport), CV-14 (*jù què*, Great Tower Gate), PC-6 (*nèi guān*, Inner Pass), HT-5 (*tōng lǐ*, Connecting Li), PC-4 (*xī mén*, Cleft Gate), and ST-36 (*zú sān lǐ*, Leg Three Li); use large amounts of moxa at CV-4 (*guān yuán*, Pass Head), CV-6 (*qì hǎi*, Sea of Qi), BL-15 (*xīn shū*, Heart Transport), and BL-14 (*jué yīn shū*, Reverting Yin Transport). [14: 148] [26: 502] [97: 459] [46: 734] [15: 203] [42: 124] [37: 333]

true heat and false cold 真热假寒 *zhēn rè jiǎ hán*: Any disease presenting with signs of both heat and cold, in which the heat signs represent its essential nature, whereas the cold signs are deceptive. This follows the principle that "extreme heat resembles cold." True heat and false cold signs such as unsurfaced heat, reversal cold of the limbs, and even aversion to wind are found in combination with dry mouth, dry throat, thirst with desire for cold fluids, short voidings of reddish urine, hard stool, red tongue with slimy, yellow fur, and a forceful rapid pulse. The latter signs govern; the reversal cold of the limbs and aversion to cold are due to depressed heat in the interior preventing yang qi from reaching peripheral regions. The principle of treatment that applies in such cases is TREATING COLD WITH COLD. [6: 155] [27: 213] [97: 460]

true origin 真元 *zhēn yuán*: Original qi in its relationship to the kidney. Compare LOWER ORIGIN.

true origin vacuity panting 真元耗损喘 *zhēn yuán hào sǔn chuǎn*: PANTING due to a vacuous kidney failing to absorb qi. True origin vacuity panting usually develops from enduring panting and cough or as a result major illness. It is characterized by hasty panting with shortness of breath, with more exhalation than inhalation, and is accompanied by a tendency to sweat easily on exertion, thin body and lassitude of spirit, and in pronounced cases blue-green or purple lips and nails, heart palpitations, swelling of the limbs, rapid fine sunken pulse. In severe cases, critical signs such as counterflow cold of the limbs, red face, vexation and agitation, and discontinuity of breathing may be observed. MED True origin vacuity panting is treat by warming yang and banking up the origin, supplementing the kidney and promoting qi absorption. Use formulas such as Cinnamon Bark and Aconite Eight-Ingredient Pill (*guì fù bā wèi wán*), Metropolis Qi Pill (*dū qì wán*), Ginseng and Gecko Powder (*rén shēn gé jiè sǎn*), or Galenite Elixir (*hēi xí dān*). ACU Base treatment mainly on back transport points, CV, GV, KI and

LU. Select BL-13 (*fèi shū*, Lung Transport), Panting Stabilizer (*dìng chuǎn*), BL-43 (*gāo huāng shū*, Gao-Huang Transport), BL-23 (*shèn shū*, Kidney Transport), CV-4 (*guān yuán*, Pass Head), GV-4 (*mìng mén*, Life Gate), KI-3 (*tài xī*, Great Ravine), LU-9 (*tài yuān*, Great Abyss), and ST-36 (*zú sān lǐ*, Leg Three Li); needle with supplementation and large amounts of moxa. [26: 502] [113: 62] [37: 279] [14: 115]

true qi 真气 *zhēn qì*: **1.** Original qi or right qi. *The Inner Canon* (*nèi jīng*) states, "True qi is the product of that which is received from Heaven combined with grain qi, and which makes the body full." "Heaven" is explained as meaning congenital source qi. **2.** Heart qi. *Elementary Questions* (*sù wèn, píng rè bìng lùn*) states, " Heart qi ascends counterflow; hence the mouth is dry and bitter." [27: 78] [97: 459]

true repletion and false vacuity 真实假虚 *zhēn shí jiǎ xū*: Any disease pattern characterized by signs of both vacuity and repletion, in which the repletion signs represent its true nature, whereas the vacuity signs are deceptive. When damp-heat obstruction in the initial stage of nonicteric hepatitis presents such signs as fatigue and lack of strength, limpness and pain in the limbs, little thought of food and drink, and a soft soggy pulse, the condition may be wrongly identified as one of vacuity. Although there may be a spleen-stomach vacuity complication, the pattern of damp-heat obstruction is one of repletion. Careful examination will point to right diagnosis. Fatigue, lack of strength and weak limbs, together with oppression in the chest, abdominal distention, and a slimy tongue fur indicate encumbering damp rather than vacuity of original qi. If the tongue fur is yellow and slimy, and short voidings of reddish urine, the condition may be identified as one of damp-heat. Treatment should therefore aim to drain the repletion rather than to supplement the vacuity. [27: 215] [97: 460] [6: 159]

true vacuity and false repletion 真虚假实 *zhēn xū jiǎ shí*: Any disease pattern characterized by signs of both vacuity and repletion, in which the vacuity signs represent its true nature, whereas the repletion signs are deceptive. For example, vacuity panting that occurs when the kidney's function of governing qi absorption fails may be characterized by exuberant phlegm, panting and fullness, rapid breathing and inability to lie flat, as well as a slippery stringlike pulse, and a slimy tongue fur. These signs may easily be misinterpreted as repletion panting. Although there is lower body vacuity and upper body repletion, the pattern is, at root, one of vacuity. The exuberant phlegm congesting the upper body represents only the tip. Careful examination leads to the correct diagnosis. Respira-

tion is short, rapid, and distressed, hence different from the rough breathing and strident voice typifying repletion panting; the slippery, stringlike pulse has no strength when firm pressure is applied; and finally, although the tongue fur is slimy, the body of the tongue usually has a slightly blue-green or purple hue. These signs all indicate vacuity falsely presenting as repletion, and the additional presence of cold limbs and cold sweating on the head provide further confirmation that vacuity panting is the correct diagnosis. Treatment should focus on restoring qi absorption. Generally speaking, when faced with a confusing array of signs, all the information derived from the four examinations should be carefully synthesized, paying special attention to such factors as age, constitution, and duration of the disease. Misidentifying vacuity or repletion as its opposite or as a vacuity-repletion complex may lead to grave errors in treatment. [6: 159] [27: 215] [97: 460]

true visceral complexion 真脏色 *zhēn zàng sè*: One of five complexions of distinct color but desiccated, withered, and lacking in sheen, observed when visceral qi is bad and exposed. *Elementary Questions* (*sù wèn, wǔ zàng shēng chéng*) describes the true visceral complexions as follows: that of the liver as "green-blue as the color of new shoots of grass"; that of the spleen as "yellow like unripe bitter orange (*zhǐ shí*)"; that of the kidney as "black as as cinders"; that of the heart as "red as coagulated blood"; and that of the lung as "white as dry bones". Thus if the eyes and face and the whole body are dry and desiccated like yellow earth or like dried unripe bitter orange, this is the true visceral complexion of the spleen, indicating that the spleen and stomach are "wasted" (critically weakened); the true visceral color of spleen and stomach is thus "exposed" on the outside of the body. [50: 1215]

true visceral pulse 真脏脉 *zhēn zàng mài*: A pulse indicating that the true qi of, one or more of five viscera is bad and exposed; observed in critical stages of disease when the pulse is bereft of stomach, spirit, and root. *Elementary Questions* (*sù wèn, yù jī zhēn zàng lùn*) states, "When the true pulse of the liver appears... it feels awesome like a knife blade, like the string of a lute...When the true pulse of the heart appears, it is hard and contending, and feels like coix seeds coming one after the other... When the true pulse of the lung appears, it is large and vacuous, like feathers in the flesh... When the true pulse of the kidney appears, it is contending and expiring, flicking against the fingers.... When the true pulse of the spleen appears, it is weak, sometimes frequent, sometimes sparse.... The appearance of any visceral pulse means death and is beyond cure." [50: 1215]

true wind stroke 真中风 *zhēn zhòng fēng*: Sudden collapse with clouding loss of consciousness, in some cases with deviation of the eyes and mouth, hemiplegia, stiffness of the tongue impeding speech, and urinary and fecal stoppage, attributed to external wind. WMC cerebrovascular accident. MED Course and resolve wind evil. Use variations of Minor Life-Prolonging Decoction (*xiǎo xù mìng tāng*). For urinary and fecal stoppage in patients with exuberant qi and robust physique, treat by freeing and disinhibiting, uing formulas such as Three Transformations Decoction (*sān huà tāng*). If there are no six-channel external signs and no internal obstruction of stool and urine, and only deviated eyes and mouth, inhibited speech, or hemiplegia, the treatment should be to nourish the blood and dispel wind with variations of Large Gentian Decoction (*dà qín jiāo tāng*). Exuberant phlegm-drool congestion and clouding loss of consciousness constitute a block pattern, which must be first treated by opening the orifices, using formulas such as Supreme Jewel Elixir (*zhì bǎo dān*). Open mouth, limp hands, close eyes, enuresis, snoring, and copious sweating constitute a desertion pattern, which requires large amounts of Center-Rectifying Decoction (*lǐ zhōng tāng*) or Ginseng and Aconite Decoction (*shēn fù tāng*) to support right and stem desertion. ACU Base treatment mainly on BL, GB, and TB. Select GB-20 (*fēng chí*, Wind Pool), BL-11 (*dà zhù*, Great Shuttle), BL-12 (*fēng mén*, Wind Gate), TB-5 (*wài guān*, Outer Pass), LI-4 (*hé gǔ*, Union Valley), and LU-7 (*liè quē*, Broken Sequence); needle with drainage. Moxa may be added if necessary. Selection of points according to signs: For urinary and fecal stoppage, add ST-25 (*tiān shū*, Celestial Pivot), TB-6 (*zhī gōu*, Branch Ditch), SP-6 (*sān yīn jiāo*, Three Yin Intersection), BL-23 (*shèn shū*, Kidney Transport), CV-3 (*zhōng jí*, Central Pole), and BL-28 (*páng guāng shū*, Bladder Transport); needle with even supplementation and drainage. For deviated eyes and mouth or hemiplegia without obstruction of stool or urine, see HEMIPLEGIA and DEVIATED EYES AND MOUTH. For orifice block, add GV-26 (*shuǐ gōu*, Water Trough), GV-20 (*bǎi huì*, Hundred Convergences), PC-9 (*zhōng chōng*, Central Hub), LI-4 (*hé gǔ*, Union Valley), LR-2 (*xíng jiān*, Moving Between), and ST-40 (*fēng lóng*, Bountiful Bulge); needle with drainage. For desertion patterns, burn moxa cones at CV-4 (*guān yuán*, Pass Head), and CV-6 (*qì hǎi*, Sea of Qi), and apply moxibustion on salt or ginger at CV-8 (*shén què*, Spirit Gate Tower) until the sweating ceases, the limbs become warm, and pulse rises. See WIND STROKE. [26: 502] [27: 396] [97: 459] [113: 34] [46: 595] [50: 1214] [37: 338–340] [75: 63]

true yang 真阳 *zhēn yáng*: KIDNEY YANG.

true yin 真阴 *zhēn yīn*: KIDNEY YIN.

tube insertion 管针进针法 *guǎn zhēn jìn zhēn fǎ*, 管针法 *guǎn zhēn fǎ*: Insertion of acupuncture needles using a find tube as a guide. Tube insertion employs a thin stainless steel, glass, or plastic tubular guide into which a tailless needle (one without the end ring) is placed before insertion. Insertion tubes are approximately 4 mm shorter than the needles for which they are intended, thus exposing a consistent length of the needle handle when the tube and the needle tip are allowed to rest on the skin surface. The needle is gently tapped into the skin until the top of the needle handle is level with, or just below, the top of the tube. The guide tube is then removed and the needle inserted to the appropriate depth. This technique is most often used with long and/or fine needles, as well as in the treatment of children and sensitive adults. Practitioners who favor the use of insertion tubes often develop skill in manipulating the tube and the needle with one hand. Such skill allows acupuncture points to be palpated and located with the index finger of the left hand, whereas the tube and needle are prepared with the right hand. Care must be taken when practicing this technique that clean fields are not compromised. The practitioner must not come in contact with the body of the needle. [135: 6]

tuft of hair 聚毛 *jù máo*, 丛毛 *cóng máo*: The region just proximal to the first metatarsophalangeal articulation at which a tuft of hair is often found growing. Not to be confused with THREE HAIRS. [27: 73] [97: 619]

tugging and slackening 瘛瘲 *jì zòng*: *Synonyms: convulsions*; *tugging wind*. Alternating tensing and relaxation of the sinews, often observed in externally contracted heat (febrile) disease, epilepsy, and lockjaw. Tugging means a tensing and contraction, whereas slackening is a relaxation. Tugging and slackening together denote alternating contraction and relaxation of the sinews. In febrile disease, it is attributable to exuberant heat damaging yin with wind and fire exacerbating each other, and to congestion of phlegm fire. In summerheat disease with fatigued cumbersome limbs and copious sweating, it is a sign of damage to qi. In epilepsy and lockjaw, it is usually attributable to wind phlegm or phlegm heat. Tugging and slackening can also occur intermittently in spleen-stomach vacuity with vomiting and diarrhea, or in liver vacuity cold with rib-side pain and clouded or flowery vision. It is sometimes observed after blood loss. WMC clonic spasm. ◇ Chin 瘛 *jì* (*qì*, *chì*), tug, jerk; 瘲 *zòng*, relax. [26: 862] [97: 631] [27: 433]

tugging wind 抽风 *chōu fēng*: TUGGING AND SLACKENING. [27: 433]

tui-na 推拿 *tuī ná*: MASSAGE. [26: 604]

tumbled celestial pillar 天柱倒 *tiān zhù dǎo*: A bowed head. [27: 408] [97: 60]

tumor 瘤 *liú*: A growth on the surface of the body that is neither painful nor itchy. *The Origin and Indicators of Disease* (*zhū bìng yuán hòu lùn*) states, "A tumor is a sudden swelling in the skin and flesh that is as large as a plum at onset, growing gradually larger; it is neither painful nor itchy. It is not stiffly bound; rather it is lodged (留 *liú*) and does not dissipate, for which reason it is called 瘤 (*liú*). If untreated, it can become huge and will not be dispersed. It does not kill the person; care should be taken not to rupture them." WMC What is called a tumor in Chinese medicine is generally found to be a benign tumor in Western medicine. Distinctions are made between different kinds of tumor: QI TUMOR is soft and puffy (corresponds to neuroma cutis in modern medicine); BLOOD TUMOR is characterized by dilatation of blood vessels knotting together (corresponds to angioma); FLESH TUMOR is a spongy swelling like steamed bread that appears to well up from flesh (corresponds to lipoma); SINEW TUMOR is marked by "green-blue sinews" like a pile of knotted intertwined worms (varicose veins) and swells up from the sinews (corresponds to phlebangioma, varicosity, cavernous hemangioma and other shallow lesions); BONE TUMOR is stuck to the bone and is hard as stone (benign and malignant bone tumors); FATTY TUMOR is a tumor with a blue-black speck in the center from which from time to time a white substance like bean curd dregs can be squeezed, and which may suppurate, thus becoming a *suppurative tumor* (corresponds to a cystic tumor). See the individual entries. Compare ROCK, which normally corresponds to a malignant tumor in Western medicine. ◇ Chin 瘤 *liú* comprises the illness signifier 疒 with 留 *liú* to remain or become lodged, possibly indicating an understanding of the phenomena in terms of qi stagnation, blood stasis, etc. [96: 193] [26: 863]

turbid 浊 *zhuó*: (1) *adj.* murky; of the voice, unclear. (2) *n.* That which is turbid. Usually appears with the definite article as "the turbid." See TURBIDITY.

turbid evils harm the clear 浊邪害清 *zhuó xié hài qīng*: Damp turbidity and phlegm turbidity obstruct clear yang and cloud the clear orifices, causing clouded consciousness and poor hearing. [26: 897]

turbidity 浊 *zhuó*: 1. Turbid substances in the body. See TURBID YIN. 2. The quality of murkiness or dirtiness (of dampness or phlegm). See DAMP TURBIDITY; PHLEGM TURBIDITY; TURBID EVILS HARM THE CLEAR. 3. Murkiness of the urine or murky urethral discharge. See URINARY TUR-

BIDITY; ESSENCE TURBIDITY; WHITE TURBIDITY; RED TURBIDITY. [26: 897]

turbid orifices 浊窍 *zhuó qiào*: LOWER ORIFICES.

turbid qi 浊气 *zhuó qì*: 1. The turbid rich part of the essence of grain and water. *Elementary Questions* (*sù wèn, jīng mài bié lùn*) "Food enters the stomach, the turbid qi goes to the heart, and spreads essence to the vessels." 2. Cold evil. 3. Foul air, e.g., exhaled air or flatus. 4. Heavy matter as distinct from clear yang. *Elementary Questions* (*sù wèn, yīn yáng yìng xiàng dà lùn*) states, "Clear yang is heaven; turbid qi is earth." "When turbid qi is above, there is distention." [25: 237] [26: 897]

turbid qi goes to the heart 浊气归心 *zhuó qì guī xīn*: The turbid part of the essence of grain and water that goes to make blood, to be distributed around the body by the blood vessels, which are governed by the heart. [27: 80] [97: 436]

turbid slimy tongue fur 浊腻苔 *zhú nì tāi*: See SLIMY TONGUE FUR.

turbid urine 小便浑浊 *xiǎo biàn hún zhuó*: See URINARY TURBIDITY.

turbid water humor 水液混浊 *shuǐ yè hùn zhuó*: From *Elementary Questions* (*sù wèn, zhì zhēn yào dà lùn*), "All cramp, arched-back rigidity, and turbid water humors are ascribed to heat." Turbid urine. See URINARY TURBIDITY. [26: 152]

turbid qi failing to bear downward 浊气不降 *zhuó qì bù jiàng*: TURBID YIN FAILING TO BEAR DOWNWARD.

turbid yin 浊阴 *zhuó yīn*: Turbid substances within the body as distinct from clear substances referred to as clear yang. *Elementary Questions* (*sù wèn, yīn yáng yìng xiàng dà lùn*) states, "Clear yang issues from the upper orifices; turbid yin issues from the lower orifices. Clear yang effuses through the interstices; turbid yin pervades the five viscera. Clear yang fills the four limbs; turbid yin flows to the six bowels." From this, it can be seen that turbid yin refers to the waste products of the body discharged in the form of urine and stool. In some contexts, it also refers to the blood. See TURBID QI GOES TO THE HEART. [26: 897] [27: 81] [97: 463]

turbid yin failing to bear downward 浊阴不降 *zhuó yīn bù jiàng*: Synonym: *turbid qi failing to bear downward*. Breakdown of the spleen and stomach's function of moving and transforming grain and water, whereby grain and water do not move downward normally. The main signs are glomus and oppression in the chest, belching and hiccough, nausea and vomiting, and distention and fullness in the stomach duct and abdomen. Other signs include heavy-headedness and cumbersome body, no thought of food and drink, and scant urine and sloppy stool. MED Unripe

Bitter Orange and Ovate Atractylodes Pill (*zhǐ zhú wán*) or Stomach-Calming Powder (*píng wèi sǎn*). ACU Base treatment mainly on CV, ST, SP, and PC. Select CV-12 (*zhōng wǎn*, Center Stomach Duct), CV-10 (*xià wǎn*, Lower Stomach Duct), PC-6 (*nèi guān*, Inner Pass), ST-25 (*tiān shū*, Celestial Pivot), CV-6 (*qì hǎi*, Sea of Qi), ST-36 (*zú sān lǐ*, Leg Three Li), and SP-4 (*gōng sūn*, Yellow Emperor); needle with even supplementation and drainage or with supplementation. [57: 31] [46: 586, 602]

turtle-dove's tail 鸠尾 *jiū wěi*: The process at the lower end of the breastbone; so called by the similarity of shape. WMC xiphoid process or ensiform process. See BREASTBONE. [27: 68]

TV 冲脉 *chōng mài*: Abbreviation for thoroughfare (*chōng*) vessel. See THOROUGHFARE VESSEL.

twelve channel divergences 十二经别 *shí èr jīng bié*: Branches of each of the twelve channels that reach deeper parts of the body and then return to the primary channel. The divergences of the six yang channels return to the yang channel they branched from. The yin channel divergences connect to the channel with which they stand in exterior-interior relationship. For this reason, the twelve channel divergences have the function of complementing the main pathways by providing a link between the yin and the yang channels. [26: 814] [27: 92]

twelve channels 十二经脉 *shí èr jīng mài*: Synonym: *regular channels*. The channels that form the basic structure of the channel system. The twelve channels comprise six channels of the hand and six channels of the foot, each channel duplicated on both sides of the body. Each channel "homes" and "nets" to bowels and viscera that stand in interior-exterior relationship. See Table 16. The twelve channels have the function of interlinking the bowels and the viscera and providing a network of qi and blood by which the whole body is nourished. [27: 84]

16. The Twelve Channels	
Channel	Homes to
Hand greater yin (*tài yīn*) Foot greater yin (*tài yīn*)	Lung Spleen
Hand yang brightness (*yáng míng*) Foot yang brightness (*yáng míng*)	Large intestine Stomach
Hand reverting yin (*jué yīn*) Foot reverting yin (*jué yīn*)	Pericardium Liver
Hand lesser yang (*shào yáng*) Foot lesser yang (*shào yáng*)	Triple burner Gallbaldder
Hand lesser yin (*shào yín*) Foot lesser yin (*shào yín*)	Heart Kidney
Hand greater yang (*tài yáng*) Foot greater yang (*tài yáng*)	Small intestine Bladder

twelve channel sinews 十二经筋 *shí èr jīng jīn*: Sinews following the path of the channels, together filling the entire surface of the body. They are named after the channels (e.g., hand yang brightness channel sinews). Morbidity of the channel sinews includes impediment (*bì*), hypertonicity, and slackening. [27: 92] [97: 7]

twelve cutaneous regions 十二皮部 *shí èr pí bù*: Areas of the skin lying on and corresponding to the each of the twelve channels. [27: 94] [97: 7]

twelve formula types 十二剂 *shí èr jì*: **1.** The ten formula types plus cold formulas and hot formulas. **2.** The ten formula types plus upbearing and downbearing formulas.

twelve officials 十二官 *shí èr guān*: The twelve organs. [27: 32]

twelve source points 十二原穴 *shí èr yuán xué*: The source points of the twelve channels. See SOURCE POINT. [27: 101]

17. The Twelve Sources	
Entity	Point
Lung	LU-9 (*tài yuān*, Great Abyss)
Pericardium	PC-7 (*dà líng*, Great Mound)
Spleen	SP-3 (*tài bái*, Supreme White)
Kidney	KI-3 (*tài xī*, Great Ravine)
Gao	CV-15 (*jiū wěi*, Turtledove Tail)
Huang	CV-6 (*qì hǎi*, Sea of Qi)
Liver	LR-3 (*tài chōng*, Supreme Surge)

twelve sources 十二原 *shí èr yuán*: Twelve acupuncture points, two of which are each associated with the gao and the huang, and the other ten being associated with one of the five viscera. For example, The sources of the lung are the two LU-9 (*tài yuān*, Great Abyss) points on either side. See Table 17. *The Magic Pivot (líng shū, jiǔ zhēn shí èr yuán)* states, "When the five viscera are diseased, then use the twelve sources." The notion of the twelve sources is similar but not to be confused with that of the twelve source points of twelve channels (see SOURCE POINT). [26: 5]

twenty-eight pulses 二十八脉 *èr shí bā mài*: Twenty-eight commonly observed pulses listed by Li Shi-Cai. This list comprises the twenty-seven pulses of Li Shi-Zhen, with the addition of the racing pulse. The "twenty-eight pulses" still remains a standard list, but an additional large pulse is now often added. See the list below and PULSE CONDITION. [6: 137–145] [93: 15]

The Twenty-Eight Pulses

Floating 浮脉 *fú mài*: Superabundant under light pressure and insufficient under heavy pressure

Sunken 沉脉 *chén mài* Not felt under light pressure, and felt only under heavy pressure

Slow 迟脉 *chí mài*: Less than fours beats per respiration (less than 60 beats per minute)

Rapid 数脉 *shuò mài*: Over five beats per respiration (over 90 beats per minute); associated with heat (with repletion heat when forceful and vacuity heat when forceless)

Surging 洪脉 *hóng mài*: Extremely large, billowing like waves and arriving with a great force

Faint 微脉 *wēi mài*: Extremely fine and soft, and feels as if it is on the verge of expiry, barely detectable

Fine 细脉 *xì mài*: Like a fine but distinct thread

Scattered 散脉 *sàn mài*: Diffuse and floating without root

Vacuous 虚脉 *xū mài*: Forceless at all three positions, and feeling empty and vacuous under pressure

Replete 实脉 *shí mài*: Forceful at all three positions

Slippery 滑脉 *huá mài*: A smooth-flowing pulse classically described as "pearls rolling in a dish" or "small fish swimming"

Rough 涩脉 *sè mài*: The opposite of a slippery pulse, i.e., one that does not flow smoothly and that is classically described as "a knife lightly scraping bamboo"

Long 长脉 *cháng mài*: Can be felt beyond the inch and cubit positions

Short 短脉 *duǎn mài*: Felt only at the bar point

String-like 弦脉 *xián mài*: Feels like the string of a musical instrument

Scallion-stalk 芤脉 *kōu mài*: Floating and empty in the middle

Tight 紧脉 *jǐn mài*: String-like and forceful

Moderate 缓脉 *huǎn mài*: Three to four beats per respiration

Drum-skin 革脉 *gé mài*: String-like and empty in the middle

Firm 牢脉 *láo mài*: Forceful and feels as though "tied to the bone"

Weak 弱脉 *ruò mài*: A deep pulse without force

Soggy 濡脉 *rú mài*: A soft pulse lacking in force

Hidden 伏脉 *fú mài*: A pulse even deeper than the deep pulse; considerable pressure has to be applied in order to feel it

Stirred 动脉 *dòng mài*: A combination of the rapid, short, and slippery pulses

Racing 疾脉 *jí mài*: 7 or more beats per respiration

Skipping 促脉 *cù mài*: Rapid irregularly interrupted

Bound 结脉 *jié mài*: Slow irregularly interrupted

Intermittent 代脉 *dài mài*: Interrupted at regular intervals

---

twinge 酸 *suān*: An acute localized distressing sensation, as often experienced when insertion and manipulation of acupuncture needles results in "obtaining qi." Twinges are often shooting.

twirling 捻转法 *niǎn zhuǎn fǎ*: A method of needle manipulation whereby the practitioner grasps the handle of the needle between his thumb and forefinger and twists the needle first one way and then the other, in an arc between 180 and 360°. Avoid turning the needle in a single direction in order to prevent the needle from adhering to fibrous tissue and causing unnecessary pain. Rotating the needle rapidly in a wide arc drains; a narrow arc with slow motion supplements; a medium arc with medium speed produces even supplementation and drainage. The rotation method can be combined with the lifting and thrusting method described above. [46: 460]

twirling supplementation and drainage 捻转补泻 *niǎn zhuǎn bǔ xiè*: *Synonym: rotating supplementation and drainage.* A method of achieving supplementation or draining by rotating the needle between the thumb and index finger. Forward movement of the thumb and backward movement of the index finger making the needle rotate clockwise produces supplementing stimulus. Forward movement of the index finger and backward movement of the thumb making the needle rotate anticlockwise produces a draining needle stimulus. See NEEDLE MANIPULATION. [46: 469]

two-finger press needle insertion 挟持进针法 *jiā chí jìn zhēn fǎ*: A two-handed needle insertion technique whereby the handle of the needle is held by the fingers of one hand and the tip is held between the thumb and index finger of the other hand to guide it into the body. Method: The two-finger press needle insertion is performed in the following steps: (1) Hold the needle at the handle with the thumb and index finger of right hand, while the left thumb and forefinger support the shaft close to the tip with a small piece of sterile cotton. (2) Place the tip of the needle lightly on the surface of the skin over the point. (3) Insert the needle by exerting a quick, firm, downward thrust with both hands simultaneously. (4) Remove the cotton and continue to insert the needle until right depth has been reached. Application: The two-finger press is especially suited to the use of longer needles. This technique, in which two hands are used to guide the needle during insertion, provides stability over a greater portion of the length of the needle body. Longer needles are used where the flesh is thicker (such as the hips and legs), and for the special technique of POINT JOINING, which two points are connected by one needle. Proper clean needle technique requires that cotton be used around the base of the needle, as touching the body of the needle with the fingers poses the danger of infection. See NEEDLE INSERTION. [46: 460] [42: 25]

two-handed needle insertion 双手进针法 *shuāng shǒu jìn zhēn fǎ*: See NEEDLE INSERTION. [46: 460]

two intestines 二肠 *èr cháng*: The large and small intestines.

two turbidities 二浊 *èr zhuó*: RED AND WHITE TURBIDITY.

two yin 二阴 *èr yīn*: Anus and genitals. Compare LOWER ORIFICES. [27: 69, 90]

U

ulceration 糜烂 *mí làn,* 烂 *làn*: A disintegration of the skin (including what is known in modern medicine as mucosa) that easily suppurates; erosion. Compare PUTREFACTION.

ulceration of the eyelid rim 眼弦赤烂 *yǎn xián chì làn*: Synonym: *wind ulceration of the eyelid rim*. Erosion of palpebral margin with itching, soreness, and, in severe cases, loss of eyelashes. Attributable to damp-heat brewing in the spleen and stomach contending with subsequently contracted wind. WMC blepharitis marginalis. MED Dispel wind, clear heat, and eliminate dampness. Treatment depends on evil prevalence. If dampness is predominant, use Dampness-Eliminating Decoction (*chú shī tāng*). If wind prevails, use Bupleurum Powder (*chái hú sǎn*). If heat prevails, use Three Yellows Heart-Draining Decoction (*sān huáng xiè xīn tāng*). Egg Yolk Paste (*jī dàn huáng yóu gāo*), which is made by cooking egg yolks in oil and adding a pinch of ground processed smithsonite (*lú gān shí*) and borneol (*bīng piàn*), may be applied topically. ACU Moxa Thumb Bone Hollow (*dà gǔ kōng*), Little Finger Bone Hollow (*xiǎo gǔ kōng*), and GB-20 (*fēng chí*, Wind Pool), or needle with drainage. [26: 635] [113: 935] [27: 501] [97: 518]

umbilical damp 脐湿 *qí shī*: Synonym: *umbilical damp swelling*. A condition of wetness of and possible exudation from the umbilicus, sometimes with redness and swelling of the surrounding area after the umbilical cord has been shed. Umbilical damp is attributed to the invasion of water-damp due to improper care after removal of the cord. MED Disperse toxin. Dab dragon bone (*lóng gǔ*) or calcined oyster shell (*duàn mǔ lì*), and smithsonite (*lú gān shí*) onto the affected area. [26: 967]

umbilical damp swelling 脐湿肿 *qí shī zhǒng*: UMBILICAL DAMP SWELLING. [26: 967]

umbilical-level effusion 对脐发 *duì qí fā*: An EFFUSION, (a large welling-abscess or flat-abscess), at the level of the umbilicus. [27: 459] [97: 173]

umbilical sores 脐疮 *qí chuāng*: From *The Origin and Indicators of Disease* (*zhū bìng yuán hòu lùn*). A condition that usually develops from UMBILICAL DAMP. In mild cases, there is redness and swelling of the umbilicus; in severe cases, there is ulceration spreading all around the umbilicus exuding pus and water, and attended by heat effusion, vexation and agitation, red lips and dry mouth. MED Treat by clearing heat and resolving toxin, assisted by

coursing wind and relieving itch. Apply Indigo and Gold Powder (*qīng jīn sǎn*). In severe cases, administer Five-Ingredient Toxin-Dispersing Beverage (*wǔ wèi xiāo dú yǐn*). [26: 966] [96: 277]

umbilical wind 脐风 *qí fēng*: Synonym: *pursed mouth*. Lockjaw in neonates. Umbilical wind is characterized by clenched jaws, arched-back rigidity, and a peculiar grimace. In severe cases, facial complexion is green-blue, and there is hasty breathing. Attributable to unhygienic treatment or premature shedding of the umbilical cord. This disease has been almost largely eliminated by modern delivery methods. [26: 966] [27: 433] [97: 468]

umbilicus 脐 *qí*: Synonym: *navel*. The scar left by the umbilical cord. [26: 965]

unconstrained vacuous yang 虚阳不敛 *xū yáng bù liǎn*: VACUOUS YANG FLOATING UPWARD. [26: 629]

unctuous strangury 膏淋 *gāo lín*: STRANGURY with urine like rice water (water that rice has been washed in), snivel (nasal mucus), or animal fat. Distinction is made between vacuity and repletion. Vacuity虚 xū unctuous strangury patterns are usually attributed to spleen-kidney vacuity and are characterized by mild pain and absence of burning sensation, limp aching lumbus and knees, dizziness and tinnitus, shortness of breath, and fatigue. MED Supplement the spleen and kidney and promote astriction/ Use Center-Supplementing Qi-Boosting Decoction (*bǔ zhōng yì qì tāng*), Six-Ingredient Rehmannia Pill (*liù wèi dì huáng wán*), or Cuscuta Seed Pill (*tù sī zǐ wán*). ACU Base treatment mainly on the three yin channels of the foot and the alarm and back transport points of BL (CV-3 and BL-28). Main points: BL-28 (*páng guāng shū*, Bladder Transport), CV-3 (*zhōng jí*, Central Pole), SP-9 (*yīn líng quán*, Yin Mound Spring), LR-2 (*xíng jiān*, Moving Between), and KI-3 (*tài xī*, Great Ravine). For spleen-kidney vacuity, add BL-23 (*shèn shū*, Kidney Transport), BL-20 (*pí shū*, Spleen Transport), CV-4 (*guān yuán*, Pass Head), ST-36 (*zú sān lǐ*, Leg Three Li), and CV-6 (*qì hǎi*, Sea of Qi); needle with supplementation and add moxa. Repletion实 shí unctuous strangury patterns are attributed to damp-heat brewing in the lower burner and are characterized by pain and burning sensation on urination, heat effusion, lumbar pain, and headache. MED Clearing and transform damp-heat and separate the clear and eliminating the turbid. Use formulas such as Fish Poison Yam Clear-Turbid Separation Beverage (*bì xiè fēn qīng yǐn*) or Lygodium Spore Powder (*hǎi jīn shā sǎn*). ACU To the main points given above add LR-5 (*lǐ gōu*, Woodworm Canal), SP-6 (*sān yīn jiāo*, Three Yin Intersection), KI-7 (*fù liū*, Recover Flow), and LR-8 (*qū quán*, Spring at the Bend); needle with drainage. See STRANGURY PATTERNS. ◇ Chin 膏 *gāo*, paste, ointment; 淋 *lín*, dribble. [26: 826] [27: 425] [97: 629] [46: 674]

unfavorable measles pattern 麻疹逆证 *má zhěn nì zhèng*: Any manifestation of unfavorable turns in the development of measles that result from right vacuity and evil repletion in measles, e.g., signs such as inhibited eruption of papules, immediate disappearance of papules after eruption, or a dull purple coloration of the macules, signs such as vigorous heat [effusion], acute cough, rapid breathing with phlegm rale, flared nostrils and raised chest, green-blue or purple lips, and surging racing pulse. Such signs as a whole indicate heat toxin attacking the lung. Blackish purplish macules forming patches, and a dry crimson tongue with prickles indicate toxin penetrating construction-blood. Clouded spirit and TETANIC REVERSAL with convulsions indicate evil toxin falling inward to the pericardium. A somber white complexion with dull pale macules lacking a red flush with clouding spleen, limb reversal, white glossy tongue fur, and a faint sunken pulse indicate vacuity of original qi preventing the outthrust of evil. Also falling within the scope of unfavorable measles patterns are: a) the early disappearance of macules; b) the sudden disappearance of macules as they are erupting; c) failure of macules to disappear within the usual period with continuing vigorous heat [effusion]; d) the appearance of vigorous heat [effusion], cough, and diarrhea after the papules have disappeared. MED A general formula is Ephedra, Apricot Kernel, Licorice, and Gypsum Decoction (*má xìng gān shí tāng*) plus fritillaria (*bèi mǔ*), trichosanthes seed (*guā lóu zǐ*), dried bamboo sap (*zhú lì*), scutellaria (*huáng qín*), and lycium root bark (*dì gǔ pí*). For evil penetrating construction blood, use Rhinoceros Horn and Rehmannia Decoction (*xī jiǎo dì huáng tāng*) plus puccoon (*zǐ cǎo*) and isatis leaf (*dà qīng yè*). For evil entering the pericardium, use Peaceful Palace Bovine Bezoar Pill (*ān gōng niú huáng wán*) or Purple Snow (*zǐ xuě*). For original qi vacuity, use Center-Supplementing Qi-Boosting Decoction (*bǔ zhōng yì qì tāng*). [26: 587]

unfavorable pattern (sign) 逆证 *nì zhèng*: Compare FAVORABLE PATTERN (SIGN). [26: 495]

ungratifying defecation 便出不爽 *biàn chū bù shuǎng*, 排便不爽 *pái biàn bù shuǎng*: Defecation that leaves the patient with a feeling that the bowels have not been satisfactorily emptied; occurs in dysentery and other damp-heat patterns and in food stagnation and gastrointestinal accumulation. [29: 203]

ungratifying expectoration 咯痰不爽 *luò tán bù shuǎng*: Expectoration that fails to relieve discomfort in the chest; occurs in autumn dryness patterns and phlegm panting.

ungratifying menstruation 经行不爽 *jīng xíng bù shuǎng*: Absence of full menstrual flow. See SCANT MENSTRUATION. [27: 441]

ungratifying thought 神思不爽 *shén sī bù shuǎng*: A state of mind in which thinking is not creative or productive and is associated with dysphoria or unpleasant feelings; observed, for example, in gallbladder heat.

ungratifying urination 小便不爽 *xiǎo biàn bù shuǎng*: A feeling of incomplete urination; sometimes observed, for example, in binding depression of liver qi (see DRIBBLING URINARY BLOCK.)

unidirectional twirling 搓针 *cuō zhēn*: See NEEDLE TWISTING. [27: 333]

uninhibited stool 大便自利 *dà biàn zì lì*: Natural discharge of stool. The opposite of difficult defecation.

uninhibited urination 小便自利 *xiǎo biàn zì lì*: Normal voidings of urine.

united brightness of two yang 两阳合明 *liǎng yáng hé míng*: The yang brightness (*yáng míng*) channel. Yang brightness is the final stage in the development of yang qi, and is a continuation of greater yang (*tài yáng*) and lesser yang (*shào yáng*) and thus represents their combined radiance. See *opening, closing, and pivot*. [27: 91]

uniting point 合穴 *hé xué*: See TRANSPORT POINT. ◇ Chin 合 *hé*, merge, unite. The 五俞穴 *wǔ shū xué*, the five transports are named by analogy to five stages in the course of a river. 合穴 is the last point, where the river merges, or unites 合 the sea. [26: 290]

Uniting Points

LU-5 (*chǐ zé*, Cubit Marsh)
LI-11 (*qū chí*, Pool at the Bend)
ST-36 (*zú sān lǐ*, Leg Three Li)
SP-9 (*yīn líng quán*, Yin Mound Spring)
HT-3 (*shào hǎi*, Lesser Sea)
SI-8 (*xiǎo hǎi*, Small Sea)
BL-40 (*wěi zhōng*, Bend Center)
KI-10 (*yīn gǔ*, Yin Valley)
PC-3 (*qū zé*, Marsh at the Bend)
TB-10 (*tiān jǐng*, Celestial Well)
GB-34 (*yáng líng quán*, Yang Mound Spring)
LR-8 (*qū quán*, Spring at the Bend)

---

unlike treatment of like disease 同病异治 *tóng bìng yì zhì*: Using different methods to treat the same disease manifesting in different patterns in different people, in different places, or at different times. See DETERMINING TREATMENT BY PATTERNS IDENTIFIED; ACT(ION) ACCORDING TO TIME, PLACE, AND PERSON; PRINCIPLE OF TREATMENT. [27: 231]

unprocessed 生 *shēng*: (Of medicinals) not having been subject to processing of any kind, especially any that involves heating; uncooked.

unquiet sleep 夜卧不安 *yè wò bù ān*, 夜睡不安 *yè shuì bù ān*, 卧不安 *wò bù ān*, 睡眠不安 *shuì mián bù ān*, 睡眠不宁 *shuì mián bù níng*, 睡卧不宁 *shuì wò bù níng*: Inability to achieve a deep unbroken sleep. Unquiet sleep is observed in construction-aspect and other advanced-stage heat (febrile) disease patterns, GAN OF THE SPLEEN, HEART VACUITY, BLOOD VACUITY, DEPLETED WATER AND FLAMING FIRE, and ASCENDANT HYPERACTIVITY OF LIVER YANG. See also VEXATION AND AGITATION.

unquiet sleep due to stomach disharmony 胃不和卧不安 *wèi bù hé wò bù ān*: From *The Inner Canon* (*nèi jīng*). Inability to sleep well due to stomach counterflow panting. Unquiet sleep due to stomach disharmony arises when a strong stomach with large intake of food and a weak spleen result in stagnation in the "stomach domain" (stomach and intestines) and cause rheum and phlegm to form. [MED] Harmonize the stomach and dispel phlegm. Use Two Matured Ingredients Stomach-Calming Powder (*èr chén píng wèi sǎn*) plus acorus (*shí chāng pú*) and pumice (*hǎi fú shí*), or gardenia (*shān zhī zǐ*) and coptis (*huáng lián*). For hard bound stool, use Phlegm-Abducting Decoction (*dǎo tán tāng*). For stomach duct pain, use Phlegm-Rolling Pill (*gǔn tán wán*) or even Minor Stomach Elixir (*xiǎo wèi dān*). [ACU] Base treatment mainly on HT, CV, back transport points, and ST. Select Alert Spirit Quartet (*sì shén cōng*), HT-7 (*shén mén*, Spirit Gate), SP-6 (*sān yīn jiāo*, Three Yin Intersection), BL-21 (*wèi shū*, Stomach Transport), CV-12 (*zhōng wǎn*, Center Stomach Duct), ST-36 (*zú sān lǐ*, Leg Three Li), and PC-6 (*nèi guān*, Inner Pass); needle with drainage. [50: 1083] [46: 644] [37: 349]

unstop 通 *tōng*: See FREE.

unsurfaced heat 身热不（外）扬 *shēn rè bù (wài) yáng*: Generalized heat [effusion] in which heat is felt only by prolonged palpation; mostly due to binding of dampness and heat, where the dampness is blocked on the outside. Since the heat lies deep within the dampness it cannot easily be felt on the surface of the body. [27: 357]

untwining rope pulse 解索脉 *jiě suǒ mài*: See SEVEN STRANGE PULSES. [27: 199] [27: 199] [97: 605]

ununited fontanels 囟解 *xìn jiě*: UNUNITED SKULL. [97: 213]

ununited skull 解颅 *jiě lú*: Synonyms: *ununited fontanels*; *retarded closure of the fontanels*. The failure of the bones of the head to join together in infants. The bones of the skull harden at around the age of sixth months, and the anterior fontanel closes between the age of 12–18 months, whereas the posterior fontanel closes between the age of 1-3 months. Ununited skull is attributable to congenital insufficiency and depletion of kidney qi due to insufficiency of essence-blood in the parents. The signs are a taut shiny scalp with green-blue veins, bright white facial complexion, downward turned eyes, and poor mental development. [MED] Oral: Origin-Supporting Powder (*fú yuán sǎn*). Topical: Fontanel-Sealing Powder (*fēng xìn sǎn*), which comprises biota seed (*bǎi zǐ rén*), arisaema (*tiān nán xīng*), and ledebouriella (*fáng fēng*) in equal proportions, can be mixed with pig's bile and applied on gauze. [ACU] Select BL-23 (*shèn shū*, Kidney Transport), CV-6 (*qì hǎi*, Sea of Qi), BL-11 (*dà zhù*, Great Shuttle), SP-6 (*sān yīn jiāo*, Three Yin Intersection), KI-7 (*fù liū*, Recover Flow), and ST-36 (*zú sān lǐ*, Leg Three Li). [26: 802] [27: 437]

unyielding viscus 刚脏 *gāng zàng*: The liver. See LIVER IS THE UNYIELDING VISCUS.

upbear 升 *shēng*: vb. trans. rise; vb. intrans. raise or cause to rise.

upbearing and stirring 升动 *shēng dòng*: The movement of liver yang. When liver yin-blood (or liver-kidney yin humor) is depleted, upstirring of liver yang is unchecked. The resulting pattern is called ASCENDANT HYPERACTIVITY OF LIVER YANG. ◇ Chin 升 *shēng*, rise, bear upward; 动 *dòng*, move, stir.

upbearing [medicinals] can eliminate downbearing 升可去降 *shēng kě qù jiàng*: Upbearing medicinals (i.e., ones that ascend to the upper body and upbear yang) like cimicifuga (*shēng má*) and bupleurum (*chái hú*) treat qi vacuity fall patterns such as prolapse of the rectum or the vagina. See UPBEARING FORMULA.

upbearing fire flush 面红升火 *miàn hóng shēng huǒ*: A flushed complexion due to fire in the organs, e.g., heart fire flaming upward.

upbearing formula 升剂 *shēng jì*: One of the twelve kinds of formula. An example of an upbearing formula is Center-Supplementing Qi-Boosting Decoction (*bǔ zhōng yì qì tāng*), which contains, among others, the upbearing medicinals cimicifuga (*shēng má*) and bupleurum (*chái hú*) and treats prolapse of the rectum or vagina due to center qi fall. [27: 307]

upcast yang 戴阳 *dài yáng*: From *On Cold Damage* (*shāng hán lùn, biàn jué yīn bìng mài zhèng bìng zhì*). A critical disease pattern of true lower body cold and false upper body heat that arises when in debilitation of the lower origin, true yang floats astray and that is characterized by tidal reddening of the cheeks and attributable to vacuous yang floating upward. The tidal reddening is characterized by pale red patches, giving the cheeks the appearance of having been dabbed with rouge. Since the patches often constantly change location, this complexion is often described as a "floating red" facial complexion. It is a sign of false heat accompanied by other signs such as nosebleed and bleeding gums, sore swollen throat, and dry mouth. The true cold is reflected in counterflow cold of the lower limbs and long voidings of clear urine, and a moist black tongue fur. The pulse is large and floating, but vacuous and forceless. In severe cases, it is faint and fine, verging on expiration. **Comparison**: Upcast yang is similar to EXUBERANT YIN REPELLING YANG. Both are true cold and false heat. Upcast yang is lower body vacuity cold with false upper body heat, whereas exuberant yin repelling yang is true internal cold with false external heat. The two patterns cannot be categorically separated. ◇ Chin 戴 *dài*, to wear on the head; to look upward; 阳 *yáng*, the compliment of yin. [6: 117] [26: 933] [27: 431] [97: 650]

upcast eyes 戴眼 *dài yǎn*: A condition in which both eyes are fixed in an upturned direction; observed in greater yang (*tài yáng*) expiration patterns. *Elementary Questions* (*sù wèn, zhěn yào jīng zhōng lùn*) states, "The greater yang (*tài yáng*) vessel reaches its end with upcast eyes, arching [of the back], and tugging and slackening." It is also seen in child fright reversal and reverting yin (*jué yīn*) wind-phlegm obstruction patterns. ◇ Chin 戴 *dài*, to wear on the head; to look upward; 眼 *yǎn*, eye. [26: 933] [97: 657]

upflame 上炎 *shàng yán*: FLAME UPWARD.

upflaming heart fire 心火上炎 *xīn huǒ shàng yán*: HEART FIRE FLAMING UPWARD.

upflaming liver fire 肝火上炎 *gān huǒ shàng yán*: LIVER FIRE FLAMING UPWARD.

upflaming vacuity fire 虚火上炎 *xū huǒ shàng yán*: VACUITY FIRE FLAMING UPWARD.

upfloater 升浮药 *shēng fú yào*: Any medicinal that bears upward or floats, i.e., that acts on the upper body the surface of the body. See ³BEARING.

upflow nausea 泛恶 *fàn ě*: Desire to vomit either without vomiting or with upflow of clear drool into the mouth. See NAUSEA AND VOMITING. [27: 409] [97: 308]

uplift 升提 *shēng tí*: Synonym: *upraise*. Promote normal upbearing (of spleen qi and lifting prolapsed organs). "Upbearing eliminates down-bearing," e.g., center qi fall can be treated with Center-Supplementing Qi-Boosting Decoction (*bǔ zhōng yì qì tāng*), and downward fall of thoracic qi can be treated with Fall-Upbearing Decoction (*shēng xiàn tāng*). ◇ Chin 升 *shēng*, rise, bear upward; 提 *tí* lift.

uplifting center qi 升提中气 *shēng tí zhōng qì*: To treat center qi fall. Center qi, i.e., spleen qi, bears the essence of grain and water (nutrients) upward to the lung, which ensures their distribution to the organs and all parts of the body. When center qi falls, there is enduring diarrhea, prolapse of the rectum and uterus, or inhibited urination. The classic center-qi–uplifting formula is Center-Supplementing Qi-Boosting Decoction (*bǔ zhōng yì qì tāng*). ⟨ACU⟩ Base treatment mainly on back transport points, CV, GV, SP, and ST. Select GV-20 (*bǎi huì*, Hundred Convergences), CV-6 (*qì hǎi*, Sea of Qi), BL-43 (*gāo huāng shū*, Gao-Huang Transport), ST-36 (*zú sān lǐ*, Leg Three Li), BL-20 (*pí shū*, Spleen Transport), BL-21 (*wèi shū*, Stomach Transport), SP-3 (*tài bái*, Supreme White), and LU-9 (*tài yuān*, Great Abyss); needle with supplementation and moxa. [46: 594] [26: 165]

upper body 上 *shàng*: The upper part of the body (yang) as opposed to the lower body (yin); sometimes specifically denotes the upper burner.

upper body cold and lower body heat 上寒下热 *shàng hán xià rè*: **1.** A cold-heat complex in which cold evil is located in the upper body, characterized by aversion to cold, nausea, vomiting, and a white tongue fur, and heat evil in the lower body, characterized by abdominal distention, constipation, and reddish urine. **2.** Conditions in which there is a cold-natured disease in the upper body and an unrelated hot-natured disease in the lower, e.g., phlegm-rheum cough and panting in the upper body and heat strangury in the lower body. [26: 59] [27: 213] [97: 30]

upper body heat and lower body cold 上热下寒 *shàng rè xià hán*: **1.** A cold-heat complex characterized by the simultaneous presence of a heat pattern in the upper body and a cold pattern in the lower body. Such a complex may arise, for example, as a result of inappropriate precipitation creating a lower body cold pattern of persistent diarrhea with cold limbs, and a slow sunken pulse, and causing damage to liquids that encourages heat evil to rise upward to cause a sore throat and expectoration of yellow phlegm, possibly streaked with blood. **2.** Extreme vacuity of kidney yang creating exuberant yin cold in the lower body and causing vacuous yang to float upward to the upper body. See VACUOUS YANG FLOATING UPWARD. [26: 60] [27: 312] [97: 30]

upper burner 上焦 *shàng jiāo*: The upper part of the TRIPLE BURNER, comprising the heart and lung. [27: 22]

upper burner governs intake 上焦主纳 *shàng jiāo zhǔ nà*: The upper burner is responsible for the intake of air and food. [27: 58] [97: 30]

upper burner is like a mist 上焦如雾 *shàng jiāo rú wù*: The heart and lung, the two organs of the upper burner, distribute the nutrients around the body, as a nourishing dew settles from a mist. [27: 58] [97: 30]

upper dispersion 上消 *shàng xiāo*: Synonym: *lung dispersion*; A dispersion-thirst pattern characterized principally by thirst with taking of fluids, attributable to exuberant heart-stomach fire and upper burner dryness-heat. MED Moisten the lung and clear the stomach. Use White Tiger Decoction Plus Ginseng (*bái hǔ jiā rén shēn tāng*), Dispersion-Thirst Formula (*xiāo kě fāng*), or Ophiopogon and Asparagus Decoction (*èr dōng tāng*). ACU Base treatment mainly on LU and back transport points. Select BL-13 (*fèi shū*, Lung Transport), LI-4 (*hé gǔ*, Union Valley), LU-10 (*yú jì*, Fish Border), CV-23 (*lián quán*, Ridge Spring), KI-6 (*zhào hǎi*, Shining Sea), and SP-6 (*sān yīn jiāo*, Three Yin Intersection); needle with even supplementation and drainage. See DISPERSION-THIRST.[1] [26: 58] [27: 423] [97: 29] [37: 392]

upper gate tower 阙上 *què shàng*: The region above the gate tower, i.e., above the glabella. [27: 64]

upper orifices 上窍 *shàng qiào*: Synonym: *clear orifices*. The eyes, ears, nostrils, and mouth. [27: 27]

upper transverse bone 上横骨 *shàng héng gǔ*: The superior margin of the sternum. [27: 67]

upraise 升举 *shēng jǔ*: See UPLIFT.

upsurging yellow humor 黄液上冲 *huáng yè shàng chōng*: A condition characterized by the accumulation of yellow fluid in the wind wheel that can lead to protrusion of the eye surface and in some cases cover the pupil. Upsurging yellow humor is attributed to intense fire-heat toxin and is often seen in congealed fat screens or as a result of external injury. WMC hypopyon. MED Clear heat and resolve toxin using variations of Imperial Grace Rhinoceros Horn and Rehmannia Pill (*jú fāng xī jiāo dì huáng wán*). [26: 699]

upturned knife pulse 偃刀脉 *yǎn dāo mài*: See TEN STRANGE PULSES. [27: 199]

upward forcing of fetal qi 胎气上逼 *tāi qì shàng bī*: FETAL QI FORCING UPWARD.

urinary block 尿闭 *niào bì*: DRIBBLING URINARY BLOCK.

urinary incontinence 小便不禁 *xiǎo biàn bù jìn*, 小便失禁 *xiǎo biàn shī jìn*, 失溲 *shī sōu*: Invol-untary loss of urine, especially in the daytime. Urinary incontinence is involuntary loss of urine during the daytime as opposed to ENURESIS, which usually denotes loss of urine during sleep. Urinary incontinence most commonly occurs in vacuity patterns, but is sometimes observed in repletion heat patterns. **Insufficiency of the kidney origin** with vacuity cold in the lower burner causes urinary incontinence with clear urine. MED Warm the kidney and secure the bladder with Stream-Reducing Pill (*suō quán wán*). ACU Base treatment mainly on CV, back transport points, and KI. Select CV-4 (*guān yuán*, Pass Head), CV-3 (*zhōng jí*, Central Pole), BL-23 (*shèn shū*, Kidney Transport), BL-28 (*páng guāng shū*, Bladder Transport), KI-3 (*tài xī*, Great Ravine), BL-32 (*cì liáo*, Second Bone-Hole), and SP-6 (*sān yīn jiāo*, Three Yin Intersection); needle with supplementation and moxa. **Insufficiency of the lung and spleen** with vacuous qi failing to retain urine gives rise to urinary incontinence and frequent urination attended by cough, panting, qi timidity, lassitude of spirit and physical fatigue, reduced food intake, sloppy stool, abdominal distention after eating, pale tongue with white fur, and a rapid stringlike pulse. MED Supplement qi with formulas such as Center-Supplementing Qi-Boosting Decoction (*bǔ zhōng yì qì tāng*). ACU Base treatment mainly on CV, back transport points, GV, LU, SP, and ST. Select BL-13 (*fèi shū*, Lung Transport), BL-20 (*pí shū*, Spleen Transport), BL-43 (*gāo huāng shū*, Gao-Huang Transport), CV-6 (*qì hǎi*, Sea of Qi), GV-20 (*bǎi huì*, Hundred Convergences), CV-3 (*zhōng jí*, Central Pole), LU-9 (*tài yuān*, Great Abyss), SP-6 (*sān yīn jiāo*, Three Yin Intersection), and ST-36 (*zú sān lǐ*, Leg Three Li); needle with supplementation and moxa. **Frenetic stirring of bladder fire evil** can cause frequent urination and difficulty in retaining urine between voidings. MED Clear and disinhibit with Poria (Hoelen) Four Powder (*sì líng sǎn*) combined with Three Yellows Decoction (*sān huáng tāng*). ACU Base treatment mainly transport and alarm points of BL, and on SP. Select CV-3 (*zhōng jí*, Central Pole), SP-9 (*yīn líng quán*, Yin Mound Spring), SP-6 (*sān yīn jiāo*, Three Yin Intersection), BL-28 (*páng guāng shū*, Bladder Transport), and LR-2 (*xíng jiān*, Moving Between); needle with drainage. **Liver depression and binding heat** can cause urinary urgency and occasional scant involuntary losses of urine. MED Course the liver with variations of Supplemented Free Wanderer Powder (*jiā wèi xiāo yáo sǎn*) made into honey or water pills. ACU Base treatment mainly on PC, LR, SP, and CV. Select BL-18 (*gān shū*, Liver Transport), LR-3 (*tài chōng*, Supreme Surge), PC-6 (*nèi guān*, Inner Pass), SP-6 (*sān yīn jiāo*, Three Yin Intersection), GB-34 (*yáng* *líng quán,* Yang Mound Spring), KI-1 (*yǒng quán,* Gushing Spring), CV-3 (*zhōng jí,* Central Pole), and SP-9 (*yīn líng quán,* Yin Mound Spring); needle with drainage. **Incontinence with clouded spirit:** Wind stroke, externally contracted heat (febrile) disease, or epilepsy can cause urinary incontinence with clouded spirit, delirious speech, and rolled-back or forward-staring eyes. Such conditions are treated by emergency measures chosen according to presenting signs. See ENURESIS; URINE. [26: 75] [92: No. 227] [46: 596, 646, 700] [50: 141] [37: 378]

urinary stoppage 小便不通 *xiǎo biàn bù tōng:* DRIBBLING URINARY BLOCK.

urinary stoppage in pregnancy 妊娠小便不通 *rèn shēn xiǎo biàn bù tōng:* From *The Origin and Indicators of Disease* (*zhū bìng yuán hòu lùn*). Urinary stoppage due to pressure on the bladder in the latter stages of pregnancy; attributed to timidity of center qi or kidney qi vacuity with impairment of qi transformation and movement of water and inhibition of bladder action. **Qi vacuity** is attended by shortness of breath, heavy-headedness and dizziness. MED Supplement the center and raise the fetus with Center-Supplementing Qi-Boosting Decoction (*bǔ zhōng yì qì tāng*). **Kidney vacuity** is attended by fidgetiness, cold limbs and fear of cold, and dizzy head. MED Warm the kidney and support yang. Use Kidney Qi Pill (*shèn qì wán*). See also SHIFTED BLADDER. [26: 340]

urinary turbidity 溺浊 *niào zhuó:* Murkiness of the urine unassociated with inhibited urination or pain on urination. When the urine is white like rice water (泔 *gān,* water that rice has been rinsed in), the condition is called white turbidity. When the urine is red, it is called red turbidity. **White turbidity** is attributed to spleen-stomach damp-heat pouring down into the bladder, and is associated with fullness and oppression in the chest and stomach duct, dry mouth and thirst, yellow slimy tongue fur, and a rapid slippery pulse. If the condition persists, it may develop into insufficiency of the heart and spleen and into qi vacuity fall characterized by lassitude of spirit, lack of strength, white complexion, and a soft weak pulse. If there is insufficiency of kidney yin with vacuity fire, signs include heat vexation, dry pharynx, red tongue, and a fine rapid pulse. If there is insufficiency of kidney yang and lower origin vacuity cold, signs include white complexion, cold limbs, pale tongue, and a fine sunken pulse. White turbidity with pronounced stinging pain on voiding constitutes UNCTUOUS STRANGURY. MED For spleen-stomach damp-heat pouring down into the bladder, clear heat and disinhibit dampness using formulas like Fish Poison Yam Clear-Turbid Separation Beverage (*bì xiè fēn qīng yǐn*) and variations.

For qi vacuity fall, treat by nourishing the heart and fortifying the spleen, upbearing the clear, and promoting astriction using Center-Supplementing Qi-Boosting Decoction (*bǔ zhōng yì qì tāng*) or Origin-Securing Brew (*mì yuán jiān*). For kidney yin vacuity, treat by enriching yin and clearing heat with Anemarrhena and Phellodendron Eight-Ingredient Pill (*zhī bǎi bā wèi wán*) or Major Yin Supplementation Pill (*dà bǔ yīn wán*). For insufficiency of kidney yang, treat by warming the kidney and promoting astriction with Velvet Deerhorn Supplementing and Astringing Pill (*lù róng bǔ sè wán*). ACU For spleen-stomach damp-heat pouring down into the bladder, base treatment mainly on SP, LI, ST, CV, and back transport points. Select LI-4 (*hé gǔ,* Union Valley), ST-44 (*nèi tíng,* Inner Court), SP-9 (*yīn líng quán,* Yin Mound Spring), BL-28 (*páng guāng shū,* Bladder Transport), CV-3 (*zhōng jí,* Central Pole), SP-6 (*sān yīn jiāo,* Three Yin Intersection), and LR-8 (*qū quán,* Spring at the Bend); needle with drainage. See also BLOODY URINE; TURBIDITY. For enduring illness with qi vacuity fall, base treatment mainly on back transport points, CV, ST, and SP. Select BL-20 (*pí shū,* Spleen Transport), BL-15 (*xīn shū,* Heart Transport), CV-4 (*guān yuán,* Pass Head), CV-6 (*qì hǎi,* Sea of Qi), ST-36 (*zú sān lǐ,* Leg Three Li), and SP-6 (*sān yīn jiāo,* Three Yin Intersection); needle with supplementation. For kidney yin vacuity, base treatment mainly on KI and CV. Needle with supplementation at BL-23 (*shèn shū,* Kidney Transport), CV-4 (*guān yuán,* Pass Head), KI-3 (*tài xī,* Great Ravine), and KI-7 (*fù liū,* Recover Flow), and with drainage at KI-6 (*zhào hǎi,* Shining Sea), KI-2 (*rán gǔ,* Blazing Valley), and HT-8 (*shào fǔ,* Lesser Mansion). For kidney yang vacuity, base treatment mainly on KI, GV and CV. Select BL-23 (*shèn shū,* Kidney Transport), BL-20 (*pí shū,* Spleen Transport), GV-4 (*mìng mén,* Life Gate), CV-4 (*guān yuán,* Pass Head), and KI-3 (*tài xī,* Great Ravine); needle with supplementation and add moxa. **Red turbidity** is usually attributable to damp-heat in the lower burner scorching the blood aspect and damaging the network vessels. In the initial stage, it forms a repletion pattern which can be treated with the above formulas with judicious addition of fire-clearing blood-cooling medicinals. If the condition persists and causes heart channel vacuity heat or kidney qi vacuity, the same formulas may be used with the addition of heart-supplementing and kidney-boosting medicinals. WMC chyluria, urinary tract inflammation; tuberculosis; tumors; phosphaturia. ACU Base treatment mainly on SP, CV, LR, KI, and back transport points. Select SP-9 (*yīn líng quán,* Yin Mound Spring), BL-28 (*páng guāng shū,* Bladder Transport), CV-3 (*zhōng jí,* Central Pole), LR-8 (*qū quán,* Spring at the Bend), SP-6 (*sān yīn* *jiāo,* Three Yin Intersection), SP-10 (*xuè hǎi,* Sea of Blood), and KI-2 (*rán gǔ,* Blazing Valley); needle with drainage. For enduring illness with heart channel vacuity heat and kidney qi vacuity, add BL-15 (*xīn shū,* Heart Transport), BL-23 (*shèn shū,* Kidney Transport), HT-7 (*shén mén,* Spirit Gate), HT-8 (*shào fǔ,* Lesser Mansion), and KI-3 (*tài xī,* Great Ravine). [26: 757] [97: 323] [37: 374] [46: 588, 594, 597]

urinary urgency 尿急 *niào jí:* Increased frequency or urination; often referred to simply as urgency.

urine 小便 *xiǎo biàn,* 尿 *niào,* 小水 *xiǎo shuǐ,* 小溲 *xiǎo sōu,* 前溲 *qián sōu,* 溲 *sōu,* 水泉 *shuǐ quán,* 下泉 *xià quán:* Surplus body fluid discharged from the anterior yin. The production of urine involves the spleen's action of moving and transforming water-damp, the triple burner's regulation of the waterways, and the small intestine's separation of the clear and turbid, and in the final stage by kidney qi transformation. It is passed to the bladder by whose opening and closing action it can be stored and discharged at convenient times. The normal, healthy individual voids from four to six times a day, mostly during the daytime. **Appearance:** Urine is usually a pale yellow in color. Changes in color are usually associated with changes in volume (discussed below). *Yellow urine* or *reddish urine,* referring to urine darker than normal in color, is associated short scant voidings and indicates heat. Colorlessness of urine is associated with long copious voidings. Bloody urine without heat or pronounced pain may be due to spleen and kidney vacuity, vacuity fire, or damp-heat. Other signs must be correlated for accurate diagnosis. Murkiness of the urine is called URINARY TURBIDITY, a distinction being made between *red turbidity* and *white turbidity.* **Volume:** Urinary voidings marked by a long lasting stream of clear urine are called LONG VOIDINGS OF CLEAR URINE, and are a vacuity cold sign. Profuse urination (frequent copious voidings) is a sign of dispersion-thirst when accompanied by thirst, high fluid intake, and weight loss. Short scant voidings are normal in hot weather if fluids lost in sweating are not replaced by adequate fluid intake. SHORT VOIDINGS OF REDDISH URINE indicate heat. A gradual reduction of the amount of urine, leading to INHIBITED URINATION (scant urine with difficult urination) or DRIBBLING URINARY BLOCK with generalized puffy swelling is usually yang vacuity water flood arising when kidney yang is debilitated and fails to perform qi transformation and move water. Sudden urinary block (urine retention) together with foul-smelling urine, pain in the bladder, and heat effusion indicates repletion. **Frequency:** FREQUENT URINATION with clear urine or even incontinence indicates qi vacu-

ity. PROFUSE URINATION AT NIGHT, frequent urination at night, indicates vacuous kidney yang failing to secure and contain urine. Frequent short voidings of scant urine occurring in pregnancy indicates SHIFTED BLADDER and is attributable to qi vacuity. Frequent urination, urgency, and painful urination, often with blood or stones in the urine, constitute STRANGURY, which may be the result of qi vacuity, repletion heat, or damp-heat. See also SHIFTED BLADDER. **Lack of control:** ENURESIS (bedwetting) is usually attributable to insecurity of vacuous kidney qi. DRIBBLE AFTER VOIDING is a continuing dribble after urination has terminated (patients in such cases being unable to achieve a full stream of urine), and arises most commonly when debilitation of kidney qi leads to failure of the opening and closing action of the bladder. URINARY INCONTINENCE is usually due to vacuity and may be seen, for example, in wind stroke desertion patterns. **NB:** Western medicine establishes that the adult voids between 700 to 2000 ml per day. A daily volume in excess of 2500 ml is termed *polyuria* (excessive secretion of urine), and less than 500 ml is termed *oliguria* (diminished secretion of urine). *Anuria* (absence of urine) refers to a daily volume of less than 100 ml. [26: 75, 313] [80: 533] [56: 375] [29: 204] [6: 132] [92: No. 203]

Urine

Color
YELLOW URINE (*niào huáng*)
REDDISH URINE (*niào chì*)
STOOL IN THE URINE (*xiǎo biàn chū fèn*)

Volume
LONG VOIDINGS OF CLEAR URINE (*xiǎo biàn qīng cháng*)
SHORT VOIDINGS OF REDDISH URINE (*xiǎo biàn duǎn chì*)
INHIBITED URINATION (*xiǎo biàn bù lì*)
URINARY BLOCK (*niào bì*)
DRIBBLING URINARY BLOCK (*lóng bì*)

Frequency
FREQUENT URINATION (*niào pín*)
PROFUSE URINATION AT NIGHT (*yè niào*)

Lack of control
ENURESIS (*yí niào*)
DRIBBLE AFTER VOIDING (*niào hòu yú lì*)
URINARY INCONTINENCE (*xiǎo biàn bù jìn*)

Urinary diseases
URINARY TURBIDITY (*niào zhuó*)
STRANGURY (*lín*)

uterine cold infertility 胞寒不孕 *bāo hán bù yùn:* Inability to bear children due to kidney yang vacuity or wind-cold. Uterine cold infertility is usually associated with smaller-abdominal cold, physical cold and cold limbs, and delayed menstruation.

Insufficiency of kidney yang leads to infertility when it allows cold to arise internally and deprive the uterus of warmth. MED Treat insufficiency of kidney yang by warming the kidney and invigorating yang with Cinnamon Bark and Aconite Eight-Ingredient Pill (*guì fù bā wèi wán*). ACU Base treatment on back transport points, GV, CV, KI, and ST. Select BL-23 (*shèn shū,* Kidney Transport), GV-4 (*mìng mén,* Life Gate), CV-4 (*guān yuán,* Pass Head), KI-3 (*tài xī,* Great Ravine), CV-3 (*zhōng jí,* Central Pole), CV-7 (*yīn jiāo,* Yin Intersection), CV-2 (*qū gǔ,* Curved Bone), ST-29 (*guī lái,* Return), and KI-6 (*zhào hǎi,* Shining Sea); needle with supplementation and large amounts of moxa. **Wind-cold** can cause infertility when poor attention to health during menstruation allows wind-cold to settle in the uterus and prevent normal reception of essence (conception). MED Treat by warming the channels and assisting yang, warming the uterus and dispelling cold with Mugwort and Cyperus Palace-Warming Pill (*ài fù nuǎn gōng wán*). ACU Base treatment on GB, GV, CV, ST, and KI. Needle with drainage and moxa at GB-20 (*fēng chí,* Wind Pool), GV-20 (*bǎi huì,* Hundred Convergences), TB-5 (*wài guān,* Outer Pass), and LI-4 (*hé gǔ,* Union Valley), and with supplementation and large amounts of moxa at GV-4 (*mìng mén,* Life Gate), CV-4 (*guān yuán,* Pass Head), CV-3 (*zhōng jí,* Central Pole), ST-29 (*guī lái,* Return), CV-7 (*yīn jiāo,* Yin Intersection), and KI-6 (*zhào hǎi,* Shining Sea). [26: 452] [37: 416] [59: 100]

uterine network vessels 胞络 *bāo luò*: UTERINE VESSELS.

uterine obstruction 胞阻 *bāo zǔ: Synonym: pregnancy abdominal pain.* Smaller-abdominal pain during pregnancy; attributed to vacuity cold, blood vacuity, or qi depression causing inhibited movement of qi and blood, or blood vacuity depriving the uterine vessels of nourishment. **Vacuity cold** is characterized by smaller-abdominal cold pain that is relieved by warmth. MED Warm the channels and dissipate cold. Use Mugwort and Cyperus Palace-Warming Pill (*ài fù nuǎn gōng wán*). **Blood vacuity** is associated with headache, dizzy vision, and continuous smaller-abdominal pain that likes pressure. MED Nourish the blood, relieve pain, and quiet the fetus. Use Clove, Ass Hide Glue, and Mugwort Decoction (*dīng xiāng jiāo ài tāng*). **Qi depression** is smaller-abdominal pain with stomach duct and abdominal distention and fullness, vexation, agitation, and irascibility. MED Course the liver and resolve depression. Use Free Wanderer Powder (*xiāo yáo sǎn*). [26: 451]

uterine vessels 胞脉 *bāo mài: Synonym: uterine network vessels.* The vessels that supply the uterus, permit menstruation, and nourish the fetus. They include the uterine parts of the thoroughfare (*chōng*) and controlling (*rèn*) vessels. *Elementary Questions (sù wèn, píng rè bìng lùn)* states, "The uterine vessels home to the heart and net the uterus. When the menses come, the uterine vessel close." *The Magic Pivot (líng shū)* states, "The thoroughfare (*chōng*) and controlling (*rèn*) vessels start in the uterus." [27: 196] [97: 413] [24: 133]

uterus 子宫 *zǐ gōng: Synonym: womb.* One of the extraordinary organs whose main function is menstruation and childbearing, which are related to kidney essential qi, the thoroughfare (*chōng*) and controlling (*rèn*) vessels, and the heart, liver, and spleen. **Kidney essential qi:** Only when there is abundant essential qi can the female reproductive organs develop to maturity, ensuring proper menstruation and adequate conditions for conception and childbearing. In old age, the kidney essential qi grows weak and menstruation ceases; the reproductive function is then lost. *Elementary Questions (sù wèn)* states, "At the age of seven, the kidney qi of the female is strong, the teeth are replaced, and the hair is long. At the age of two sevens [i.e., fourteen], the "heavenly tenth" (*tiān guǐ*) arrives, controlling (*rèn*) vessel flows, and the thoroughfare (*chōng*) vessel fills, the menses come according to their times, and [she] can bear offspring... At seven sevens [i.e., the age of forty-two], the controlling (*rèn*) vessel empties, the thoroughfare (*chōng*) vessel weakens, *tián guǐ* is exhausted, the passages of the earth are cut, the body deteriorates, and she can no longer bear children." This statement highlights the key role of the essential qi of the kidney (kidney qi) in maintaining normal menstruation and the conditions for childbearing. **The thoroughfare and controlling vessels:** Both these vessels start from the uterus. The controlling (*rèn*) vessel joins with the three yin channels of the foot in the abdomen and regulates all the yin channels of the body. Thus it is sometimes referred to as "the sea of the yin channels." When there is an abundance of blood and qi in the twelve channels, it flows into the thoroughfare (*chōng*) and controlling (*rèn*) vessels, which control the flow into the uterus, permitting menstruation. Menstruation begins during puberty, when the essential qi of the kidney comes to fullness and the uterus develops. It was traditionally held that before the opening of the controlling (*rèn*) vessel and the full development of the thoroughfare (*chōng*) vessel, the menses would not start. At the age of about fifty, the thoroughfare (*chōng*) and controlling (*rèn*) vessels become vacuous as a result of the gradual debilitation of essential qi, causing menstrual irregularity, and finally, menopause. This represents the natural course of development, but disturbance of menstruation may occur at other times, owing to diseases of the thoroughfare (*chōng*) and controlling (*rèn*) vessels. **The heart, liver, and spleen:** The blood is governed by the heart, stored by the liver, and commanded by the spleen. The role of these organs with regard to the blood explains their connection with menstruation. If the liver fails to store blood or the spleen fails to command the blood, conditions such as profuse menstrual flow (menorrhagia), shortening of the menstrual cycle, prolonged menstrual periods, or flooding and spotting may occur. Such conditions are known as the liver and spleen failing to store and command the blood. Underproduction of blood resulting from diminished assimilation of the essence of grain and water in spleen vacuity conditions, or heart blood vacu-ity caused by mental and emotional disturbances, may lead to reduced menstrual flow, prolongation of the menstrual cycle, or even menstrual block, all of which fall under the general term of dual vacuity of heart and spleen. Mental depression may affect the liver's governing of free coursing, causing liver qi depression, which may also disrupt menstruation. ◇ Chin 子 *zǐ*, child, infant, son; 宫 *gōng*, palace. Infant's palace. [6: 99]

uvula 悬壅垂 *xuán yōng chuí*, 悬壅 *xuán yōng*, 帝（蒂）钟 *dì (dì) zhōng*, 帝（蒂）丁 *dì (dì) dīng*: The fleshy protuberance hanging down at the back of the palate. A disease of the uvula is FLYING FLAG WIND. ◇ Chin 悬 *xuán*, hang; 壅 *yōng*, congestion, swelling; 垂 *chuí*, hang. Eng uvula, from L. grape. [27: 30] [97: 442]

V

vacuity 虚 *xū*: Weakness, emptiness. See VACUITY AND REPLETION.

vacuity accumulation dysentery 虚积痢 *xū jī lì*: DYSENTERY in infants and children that develops when spleen-stomach vacuity dietary irregularities or excessive consumption of sweet or fatty foods causes a persistent accumulation. Vacuity accumulation dysentery is characterized by abdominal pain that likes pressure and tenesmus occurring any time during the day or night. MED It is treated by fortifying the spleen and boosting the stomach with Great Tranquility Pill (*dà ān wán*) combined with Saussurea and Coptis Pill (*xiāng lián wán*). ACU Base treatment mainly on LI, ST, CV, and back transport points. Select LI-4 (*hé gǔ*, Union Valley), ST-25 (*tiān shū*, Celestial Pivot), ST-37 (*shàng jù xū*, Upper Great Hollow), ST-36 (*zú sān lǐ*, Leg Three Li), Li Inner Court (*lǐ nèi tíng*), CV-21 (*xuán jī*, Jade Swivel), CV-12 (*zhōng wǎn*, Center Stomach Duct), BL-20 (*pí shū*, Spleen Transport), and BL-21 (*wèi shū*, Stomach Transport). Needle with supplementation and add moxa. [26: 631] [27: 214] [97: 513] [113: 18, 94] [46: 667]

vacuity and repletion 虚实 *xū shí*: Vacuity: emptiness or weakness. Repletion: fullness or strength. Vacuity is weakness of right qi, that is, the forces that maintain the health of the body and fight disease, whereas repletion is strength of evil qi or accumulation of physiological products within the body such as phlegm-rheum, water-damp, static blood, and stagnant qi. Vacuity patterns may be due to such causes as a weak constitution, damage to right qi either through enduring illness, loss of blood, seminal loss, and great sweating, or by invasion of an external evil (yang evils readily damaging yin humor and yin evils readily damaging yang qi). These causes are succinctly summed up in the phrase, "Where essential qi is despoliated, there is vacuity." Distinction is made between general insufficiencies of qi, blood, yin, and yang. Since these frequently affect specific organs, further distinction is made between such forms as heart yin vacuity, liver blood vacuity, kidney yang vacuity, and lung qi vacuity. Qi and yang vacuity are both forms of yang qi insufficiency, hence their clinical manifestations are similar. Signs include bright or somber white complexion, lassitude of spirit, lack of strength, spontaneous sweating, and low voice. Yang vacuity is characterized by pronounced cold signs. Blood vacuity denotes depletion of the blood and often occurs in conjunction with qi vacuity (dual vacuity of qi and blood) or with yin vacuity (dual vacuity of yin and blood). Yin vacuity refers to insufficiency of the yin humor, and is invariably characterized by signs of heat and dryness. See EXTERIOR VACUITY; INTERIOR VACUITY; VACUITY HEAT; VACUITY COLD. Repletion may be due to such factors as an invading evil, phlegm-rheum, water-damp, static blood, worm accumulations, and food accumulations. For this reason it is said, "Where evil qi is exuberant, there is repletion." Repletion patterns vary according to the nature of the evil and the organ affected. A common feature of repletion patterns is that they are associated with exuberant evil qi. Thus, when a heat evil is exuberant, a repletion heat pattern emerges; the presence of an exuberant cold evil gives rise to a repletion cold pattern; and exuberant phlegm gives rise to phlegm and drool congesting the upper body. It should be emphasized that repletion reflects not only the exuberance of an evil but also the strength of the body's reaction to it. This explains why rapid surging pulses, slippery stringlike pulses, and large replete pulses, which are all forceful at the deep level, are associated with repletion patterns. See EXTERIOR REPLETION; INTERIOR REPLETION; REPLETION HEAT; REPLETION COLD. For terms describing pathomechanisms that manifest in vacuity and repletion patterns, see EXUBERANCE AND DEBILITATION. ◊ Chin 虚 *xū*, empty, lacking, weak (originally written as 虍 *hū*, the conspicuous markings of a tiger's skin with 丘 *qiū*, hill, the two elements together signifying a "conspicuous hill"); 实 *shí*, full, solid, substantial, real, sincere, fruit, seed (originally 宀, a building, full of 贯, valuables). Vacuity and repletion are closely related to the terms insufficiency and superabundance respectively. In general, the latter are quantitative terms applied to specific entities within the body (blood, qi, yin, yang), whereas the former are comparatively qualitative terms that describe the same states in terms of their relationship to the whole body. [26: 630] [29: 286] [27: 217] [97: 514]

vacuity cold 虚寒 *xū hán*: A pattern of vacuity of right qi with cold (usually internal cold). The main manifestations are yellow face with little luster, poor appetite, upflow of clear drool into the mouth, physical cold and fear of cold, distention and pain in the stomach duct and abdomen that is relieved by warmth, heavy aching lumbus and back, long voidings of clear urine, thin stool, pale tongue with white fur, and a weak slow or moderate sunken pulse. In women there may be thin clear vaginal discharge. Vacuity cold is treated by warming yang and supplementing vacuity. [50: 1375]

vacuity cold of the lower origin 下元虚冷 *xià yuán xū lěng*: Cold due to insufficiency of the lower origin (the kidney). See LOWER ORIGIN.

vacuity constipation 虚秘 *xū bì*: CONSTIPATION due to vacuity of right. Vacuity constipation due to qi vacuity and yang qi vacuity is discussed under QI CONSTIPATION and COLD CONSTIPATION. Vacuity constipation is otherwise due to insufficiency of essence-blood in the elderly and due to postpartum blood vacuity and reduced liquid. [MED] Treat constipation in elderly and postpartum patients by boosting yin and nourishing the blood, and by engendering liquid and moistening the intestine. Use Four Agents Decoction (*sì wù tāng*) combined with Five Kernels Pill (*wǔ rén wán*), and by applying Honey Enema (*mì jiān dǎo fǎ*). [ACU] Base treatment on alarm, back transport, and lower uniting points of LI, on CV, ST, and SP, and on other back transport points. Select BL-25 (*dà cháng shū*, Large Intestine Transport), ST-25 (*tiān shū*, Celestial Pivot), ST-37 (*shàng jù xū*, Upper Great Hollow), BL-20 (*pí shū*, Spleen Transport), BL-21 (*wèi shū*, Stomach Transport), BL-17 (*gé shū*, Diaphragm Transport), KI-6 (*zhào hǎi*, Shining Sea), SP-6 (*sān yīn jiāo*, Three Yin Intersection), and ST-36 (*zú sān lǐ*, Leg Three Li); needle with supplementation. [26: 627] [97: 513] [46: 670] [37: 326]

vacuity desertion 虚脱 *xū tuō*: The manifestation of critical depletion of yin, yang, qi or blood occurring in enduring illness, as distinct from FULMINANT DESERTION, which occurs suddenly as with major blood loss or wind stroke. [WMC] heart, lung, liver, or kidney failure. See DESERTION. [27: 218]

vacuity desertion hiccough 虚脱呃 *xū tuō è*: Mentioned in *Systematized Patterns with Clear-Cut Treatments* (*lèi zhèng zhì cái, juàn sān*). HICCOUGH due to the true origin verging on the expiration. [MED] Use Yin-Rectifying Brew (*lǐ yīn jiān*), Major Origin-Supplementing Brew (*dà bǔ yuán jiān*), or Right-Restoring [Life Gate] Beverage (*yòu guī yǐn*). [ACU] Base treatment mainly on CV, GV, and PC. Select PC-6 (*nèi guān*, Inner Pass), CV-17 (*shān zhōng*, Chest Center), BL-17 (*gé shū*, Diaphragm Transport), ST-36 (*zú sān lǐ*, Leg Three Li), GV-26 (*shuǐ gōu*, Water Trough), GV-25 (*sù liáo*, White Bone-Hole), GV-20 (*bǎi huì*, Hundred Convergences), CV-4 (*guān yuán*, Pass Head), and KI-1 (*yǒng quán*, Gushing Spring). Needle with supplementation and large amounts of moxa. Apply moxa on salt or ginger at CV-8

(*shén què*, Spirit Gate Tower). See VACUITY HICCOUGH; HICCOUGH. [50: 1376] [46: 602, 658, 731] [113: 76]

vacuity detriment 虚损 *xū sǔn*: Any form of severe chronic insufficiency of yin-yang, qi-blood, and bowels and viscera, arising through internal damage by the seven affects, taxation fatigue, diet, excesses of drink and sex, or enduring illness. [WMC] observed in tuberculosis, anemia, leukemia, neurosis, and a wide range of chronic consumptive diseases. Distinction can be made between qi, blood, yang, and yin vacuity. **Qi vacuity** is mainly associated with lung-spleen vacuity detriment, which is characterized by lack of strength in the limbs, laziness to speak, shortness of breath at the slightest exertion, spontaneous sweating, and heart vexation. [MED] Use Center-Supplementing Qi-Boosting Decoction (*bǔ zhōng yì qì tāng*). **Blood vacuity** is associated with heart-liver vacuity detriment, which is characterized by blood ejection or bloody stool, flooding and spotting, and dizzy head and flowery vision. In severe cases, there may be DRY BLOOD CONSUMPTION. [MED] Use Four Agents Decoction (*sì wù tāng*) and Tangkuei Blood-Supplementing Decoction (*dāng guī bǔ xuè tāng*). If the vacuity is in the heart, use Spleen-Returning Decoction (*guī pí tāng*); if in the liver use Double Supreme Pill (*èr zhì wán*); if there is internal stasis, use Rhubarb and Wingless Cockroach Pill (*dà huáng zhè chóng wán*). **Yang vacuity** is mostly associated with spleen-kidney vacuity taxation with reduced intake of food and drink, thin sloppy stool sometimes with nontransformation of food, limp aching lumbus and knees, fatigue and lack of strength, fear of cold and cold limbs, impotence, seminal efflux, frequent long voidings of clear urine, somber white complexion, pale tongue with white fur, and a sunken fine or slow sunken pulse. [MED] Warm and supplement. For vacuity in the spleen, use Aconite Center-Rectifying Decoction (*fù zǐ lǐ zhōng tāng*); for vacuity in the kidney, use Cinnamon Bark and Aconite Eight-Ingredient Pill (*guì fù bā wèi wán*) or Right-Restoring [Life Gate] Pill (*yòu guī wán*). **Yin vacuity** is mostly seen in lung-kidney vacuity-detriment. Lung yin vacuity is marked by dry cough, expectoration of blood, dry mouth and throat, tidal heat [effusion], night sweating, tidal reddening of the cheeks, red tongue with little liquid, and a rapid fine pulse. Kidney yin vacuity is marked by limp aching lumbus and knees, dizzy head and tinnitus, seminal emission and premature ejaculation, sore throat, reddening of the cheeks, red tongue with little fur, and a sunken rapid fine pulse. [MED] Treat lung yin vacuity by nourishing yin and clearing the lung. Use variations of Adenophora/Glehnia and Ophiopogon Decoction (*shā shēn mài dōng tāng*). Treat kidney yin vacuity by enriching true yin with an additional fire downbearing action. Use Major Origin-Supplementing Brew (*dà bǔ yuán jiān*), Six-Ingredient Pill (*liù wèi wán*), or Major Yin Supplementation Pill (*dà bǔ yīn wán*). See VACUITY TAXATION; FIVE TAXATIONS; SIX EXTREMES; SEVEN DAMAGES. [26: 630]

vacuity-detriment taxation damage 虚损劳伤 *xū sǔn láo shāng*: VACUITY TAXATION.

vacuity diarrhea 虚泻 *xū xiè*: **1.** Sloppy DIARRHEA forming a vacuity pattern. Vacuity diarrhea is usually due to spleen-stomach vacuity and debilitation of kidney yang. It is associated with withered-yellow facial complexion, fatigue and lack of strength, low food intake, thin stool without sour malodor, a pale tender-soft tongue with white fur, and a vacuous pulse. [MED] Supplement the center and warm the kidney. Use Aconite Center-Rectifying Decoction (*fù zǐ lǐ zhōng tāng*), or Six Gentlemen Decoction (*liù jūn zǐ tāng*) combined with Four Spirits Pill (*sì shén wán*). [ACU] Base treatment mainly on the back transport and alarm points of the SP and ST. Select BL-20 (*pí shū*, Spleen Transport), BL-21 (*wèi shū*, Stomach Transport), CV-12 (*zhōng wǎn*, Center Stomach Duct), LR-13 (*zhāng mén*, Camphorwood Gate), ST-25 (*tiān shū*, Celestial Pivot), SP-4 (*gōng sūn*, Yellow Emperor), and ST-36 (*zú sān lǐ*, Leg Three Li); needle with supplementation and add moxa. Five Pillar Points (*wǔ zhù xué*), can also be moxaed. For debilitation of kidney yang, add BL-23 (*shèn shū*, Kidney Transport), CV-4 (*guān yuán*, Pass Head), and GV-4 (*mìng mén*, Life Gate). See SPLEEN-KIDNEY YANG VACUITY. **2.** A vacuous pulse with diarrhea, a sign of detriment to yin-blood. *Elementary Questions* (*sù wèn, yù bǎn lùn yào piān*) states, "Vacuity diarrhea is despoliation of the blood." [50: 1373] [46: 666] [37: 323]

vacuity distention 虚胀 *xū zhàng*: ABDOMINAL DISTENTION and fullness due to vacuity. Distinction is made between spleen-kidney yang vacuity and kidney yin vacuity. In spleen-kidney yang vacuity, abdominal fullness is accompanied by lassitude of spirit, torpid intake, fear of cold and cold limbs, somber white or withered-yellow facial complexion, pale tongue, and a fine pulse. In kidney yin vacuity, vacuity distention is attended by emaciation, soot black complexion, heart vexation, dry mouth, nosebleed and bleeding gums, short voidings of reddish urine, red or crimson tongue, and a rapid fine pulse. [MED] The spleen-kidney yang pattern is treated by fortifying the spleen and warming the kidney, promoting qi transformation and moving water. Aconite Center-Rectifying Decoction (*fù zǐ lǐ zhōng tāng*) combined with Poria (Hoelen) Five Powder (*wǔ líng sǎn*) is an appropriate formula. Golden Coffer Kidney Qi Pill (*jīn*

guì shèn qì wán) is an alternative. The kidney yin vacuity pattern is treated with enriching the liver and kidney and by cooling the blood and transforming stasis, an appropriate formula being All-the-Way-Through Brew (*yī guàn jiān*) combined with Infradiaphragmatic Stasis-Expelling Decoction (*gé xià zhú yū tāng*). [ACU] Base treatment mainly on PC, ST, back transport points, CV, SP, and KI. Main points: PC-6 (*nèi guān*, Inner Pass), ST-25 (*tiān shū*, Celestial Pivot), and ST-36 (*zú sān lǐ*, Leg Three Li). Selection of points according to pattern: For spleen-kidney yang vacuity, add CV-6 (*qì hǎi*, Sea of Qi), CV-4 (*guān yuán*, Pass Head), BL-20 (*pí shū*, Spleen Transport), BL-23 (*shèn shū*, Kidney Transport), GV-4 (*mìng mén*, Life Gate), and KI-7 (*fù liū*, Recover Flow), needling with supplementation and adding moxa. For kidney yin vacuity, add BL-23 (*shèn shū*, Kidney Transport), CV-4 (*guān yuán*, Pass Head), KI-6 (*zhào hǎi*, Shining Sea), KI-2 (*rán gǔ*, Blazing Valley), KI-10 (*yīn gǔ*, Yin Valley), and CV-6 (*qì hǎi*, Sea of Qi), needling with supplementation. [26: 629] [46: 602]

vacuity dysentery 虚痢 *xū lì*: DYSENTERY with vacuity signs. Dysentery is attributable to damp-heat and is characterized by blood and pus in the stool and by tenesmus. Occurring in weak patients or persisting for a long time so that it damages right qi, it may be attended by vacuity signs such as fatigue, milder abdominal pain, and straining to defecate. [MED] Treat by addressing both repletion and vacuity, using formulas such as Four Agents Decoction (*sì wù tāng*) plus cimicifuga (*shēng má*), cyperus (*xiāng fù zǐ*), and biota leaf (*cè bǎi yè*). For damage to essence through sexual intemperance causing dysentery, use Kidney Qi Pill (*shèn qì wán*). For vacuity taxation complicated by dysentery, use Saussurea and Coptis Pig's Stomach Pill (*xiāng lián zhū dǔ wán*). [ACU] Base treatment on ST, CV, and back transport points. Select ST-25 (*tiān shū*, Celestial Pivot), ST-37 (*shàng jù xū*, Upper Great Hollow), CV-12 (*zhōng wǎn*, Center Stomach Duct), BL-20 (*pí shū*, Spleen Transport), BL-21 (*wèi shū*, Stomach Transport), CV-4 (*guān yuán*, Pass Head), and CV-6 (*qì hǎi*, Sea of Qi); needle with supplementation. For abdominal pain, add SP-6 (*sān yīn jiāo*, Three Yin Intersection), and apply cross moxa (*shí zì jiǔ*). For damage to essence through sexual intemperance causing dysentery, add BL-23 (*shèn shū*, Kidney Transport), BL-52 (*zhì shì*, Will Chamber), KI-3 (*tài xī*, Great Ravine), and KI-7 (*fù liū*, Recover Flow). [26: 628] [46: 667] [113: 100]

vacuity epilepsy 虚痫 *xū xián*: EPILEPSY brought on by taxation. It tends to affect people who suffer from depression, and develops when vacuity following illness and repeated external contractions causes qi, blood, and phlegm accumulations. MED Supplement the kidney to treat the root; sweep phlegm to treat the tip. See root-securing right-supporting treatments for periods between fits under EPILEPSY. [26: 629]

vacuity evil 虚邪 *xū xié*: **1.** Any evil; so called because it exploits vacuity. **2.** One of the FIVE EVILS. An evil transmitted to an organ according to the mechanism that DISEASE OF THE MOTHER AFFECTS THE CHILD. [26: 627] [27: 108] [97: 512]

vacuity fall 虚陷 *xū xiàn*: A fall pattern occurring when a headed flat-abscess (*jū*) fails to heal owing to spleen-stomach vacuity and qi-blood depletion. In such patterns, the sore-opening is putrid and sloughing, although new flesh fails to grow. Vacuity fall is associated with heat effusion and aversion to cold, lassitude of spirit, torpid intake, abdominal pain and diarrhea. WMC toxemia. MED Supplement the stomach and spleen using Center-Supplementing Qi-Boosting Decoction (*bǔ zhōng yì qì tāng*) or Yang-Upbearing Stomach-Boosting Decoction (*shēng yáng yì wèi tāng*) and variations. See FALL PATTERN; HEADED FLAT-ABSCESS (*jū*). [26: 628] [96: 135]

vacuity fire 虚火 *xū huǒ*: **1.** Depletion of true yin causing low fever, tidal reddening of the face, vexing heat in the five hearts, steaming bone taxation heat [effusion], heart vexation and insomnia, night sweating, short voidings of reddish urine, dry mouth and throat, red tongue with scant fur, or a bare red tongue without fur, and a forceless rapid fine pulse. Vacuity fire is normally observed either in damage to yin in advanced-stage febrile disease or in yin vacuity TAXATION DETRIMENT. MED Enrich yin and drain fire according to the principle of "invigorating the governor water to restrain the brilliance of yang." Use formulas such as Anemarrhena, Phellodendron, and Rehmannia Pill (*zhī bǎi dì huáng wán*). ACU Base treatment mainly on KI and HT. Select BL-23 (*shèn shū*, Kidney Transport), KI-2 (*rán gǔ*, Blazing Valley), KI-6 (*zhào hǎi*, Shining Sea), KI-1 (*yǒng quán*, Gushing Spring), SP-6 (*sān yīn jiāo*, Three Yin Intersection), and HT-8 (*shào fǔ*, Lesser Mansion); needle with even supplementation and drainage. Selection of points according to signs: For heart vexation and insomnia, add HT-7 (*shén mén*, Spirit Gate). For night sweating, add SI-3 (*hòu xī*, Back Ravine) and HT-6 (*yīn xī*, Yin Cleft). For steaming bones, moxa ST-36 (*zú sān lǐ*, Leg Three Li) and BL-43 (*gāo huāng shū*, Gao-Huang Transport). The Four Flowers (*sì huā*) can also be moxaed. For steaming bone extreme heat, drain and then moxa GV-14 (*dà zhuī*, Great Hammer). **2.** False heat signs caused by exuberant yin repelling yang. See EXUBERANT YIN REPELLING YANG. [26: 626] [27: 216] [97: 512] [50: 1372] [46: 596] [14: 49, 178]

vacuity fire flaming upward 虚火上炎 *xū huǒ shàng yán*: Synonym: *upflaming vacuity fire*. Upper body heat signs due to kidney yin depletion and water failing to restrain fire. Signs include dry throat, sore throat, clouded head and dizzy vision, heart vexation and insomnia, tinnitus, forgetfulness, heat in the hearts of the palms and soles, soft red tongue, and fine pulse. Some patients may also display red eyes or mouth and tongue sores. Compare STIRRING OF THE MINISTERIAL FIRE. [26: 627] [27: 137] [97: 515]

vacuity fire rapid panting 虚火喘急 *xū huǒ chuǎn jí*: Rapid PANTING due to detriment to kidney yin and vacuity fire flaming upward in patients, usually children, suffering from weak constitutions or from residual heat after enduring illnesses. Other signs include tidal reddening of the cheeks, vexing heat in the five hearts, and dry lips and mouth. MED Enrich yin and downbear fire with formulas such as Metropolis Qi Pill (*dū qì wán*). ACU Base treatment mainly on KI, back transport points, and LU. Needle with supplementation at BL-23 (*shèn shū*, Kidney Transport), BL-13 (*fèi shū*, Lung Transport), BL-43 (*gāo huāng shū*, Gao-Huang Transport), KI-3 (*tài xī*, Great Ravine), and KI-6 (*zhào hǎi*, Shining Sea), and with drainage at LU-5 (*chǐ zé*, Cubit Marsh), Panting Stabilizer (*dìng chuǎn*), CV-17 (*shān zhōng*, Chest Center), and HT-8 (*shào fǔ*, Lesser Mansion). [26: 626] [37: 279]

vacuity glomus 虚痞 *xū pǐ*: GLOMUS (a localized subjective feeling of fullness and blockage in the chest or upper abdomen) attributed to debilitation of the spleen, stomach, heart, and kidney and depletion of yin, yang, qi, and blood, and traceable to irregular eating, excessive taxation fatigue, spleen-stomach vacuity cold with poor movement and transformation, and in some cases insufficiency of heart construction or debilitation of the life gate fire. Vacuity glomus is characterized by glomus and oppression when the stomach is empty and is accompanied by poor appetite, sloppy diarrhea, fear of cold and desire for warmth in the chest and abdomen, nontransformation of ingested food, belching of putrid gas, swallowing of upflowing acid, and, in severe cases, abdominal distention. MED Warm and supplement with formulas such as Center-Ordering Decoction (*zhì zhōng tāng*), Special Achievement Powder (*yì gōng sǎn*), Spleen-Returning Decoction (*guī pí tāng*), Stomach-Warming Beverage (*wēn wèi yǐn*), or Six-Ingredient Yang-Returning Beverage (*liù wèi huí yáng yǐn*). [26: 628]

vacuity heart pain 虚心痛 *xū xīn tòng*: PALPITATION HEART PAIN. [26: 626]

vacuity heat 虚热 *xū rè*: Heat due to insufficiency of yin humor. Vacuity heat is characterized by vexing heat in the five hearts, insomnia, steaming bone tidal heat [effusion], dry throat and mouth, smooth bare red tongue, and a rapid fine pulse. [MED] In treating vacuity heat, nourishing yin is of greater importance than clearing heat. Medicinals used include sweet wormwood (*qīng hāo*), baiwei (*bái wēi*), lanceolate stellaria (*yín chái hú*), lycium root bark (*dì gǔ pí*), anemarrhena (*zhī mǔ*), and phellodendron (*huáng bǎi*). A commonly used vacuity-heat–clearing formula is Sweet Wormwood and Turtle Shell Decoction (*qīng hāo biē jiǎ tāng*). [ACU] Base treatment mainly on KI. Needling with even supplementation and drainage or with drainage at KI-6 (*zhào hǎi*, Shining Sea), KI-2 (*rán gǔ*, Blazing Valley), and KI-1 (*yǒng quán*, Gushing Spring) can be used to treat vacuity heat. Needling with supplementation at KI-3 (*tài xī*, Great Ravine) and BL-23 (*shèn shū*, Kidney Transport) can be used to nourish yin. For insomnia, add HT-8 (*shào fǔ*, Lesser Mansion), LU-11 (*shào shāng*, Lesser Shang), HT-7 (*shén mén*, Spirit Gate), and SP-6 (*sān yīn jiāo*, Three Yin Intersection). For steaming bones, add moxa ST-36 (*zú sān lǐ*, Leg Three Li) and BL-43 (*gāo huāng shū*, Gao-Huang Transport). The Four Flowers (*sì huā*) can also be moxaed. For steaming bone extreme heat, drain and then moxa GV-14 (*dà zhuī*, Great Hammer). [6: 154] [50: 1374]

vacuity heat advanced menstruation 虚热经行先期 *xū rè jīng xíng xiān qī*: ADVANCED MENSTRUATION (i.e., premature arrival of periods) attributed to insufficiency of yin blood with vacuity heat harassing the thoroughfare (*chōng*) and controlling (*rèn*) vessels. The menstrual flow is scant, bright red, thick and sticky. Attending signs include reddening of the cheeks and heat in the palms and soles. [MED] Nourish yin and clear heat. Use formulas such as Lycium Root Bark Beverage (*dì gǔ pí yǐn*) and Rehmannia and Lycium Root Bark Decoction (*liǎng dì tāng*). [ACU] Base treatment mainly on CV, SP, and KI. Needle with supplementation at CV-4 (*guān yuán*, Pass Head), SP-10 (*xuè hǎi*, Sea of Blood), and SP-6 (*sān yīn jiāo*, Three Yin Intersection), and with drainage at KI-2 (*rán gǔ*, Blazing Valley) and HT-8 (*shào fǔ*, Lesser Mansion). [26: 6309] [97: 631]

vacuity hiccough 虚呃 *xū è*: HICCOUGH due to vacuity. Vacuity hiccough is mostly attributable to spleen-stomach vacuity cold and falls within the scope of COLD HICCOUGH. **Qi vacuity** can give rise to hiccough after major illness or after vomiting and diarrhea. Qi vacuity hiccough characterized by a faint sound, and is accompanied by discontinuous breathing (failure to catch one's breath). [MED] Treat by supplementation using Center-Supplementing Qi-Boosting Decoction (*bǔ zhōng yì qì tāng*) or Perfect Major Supplementation Decoction (*shí quán dà bǔ tāng*). **Liver-**

kidney yin vacuity hiccough, again, usually occurs after illness, and is a discontinuous hiccough associated with an upward surge of qi from below the umbilicus. [MED] Drain hidden heat in yin. Use Major Yin Supplementation Pill (*dà bǔ yīn wán*) or Kidney-Enriching Pill (*zī shèn wán*). Hiccough suddenly occurring in severe illness with sweating brow and a faint rough pulse is a sign that yang qi is on the verge of expiration, a critical pattern that requires swift action to warm yang with medicinals such as dried ginger (*gān jiāng*), evodia (*wú zhū yú*), ginseng (*rén shēn*), poria (*fú líng*), clove (*dīng xiāng*), persimmon calyx (*shì dì*), and aconite (*fù zǐ*). [ACU] Base treatment mainly on CV, ST, and PC. Main points: BL-17 (*gé shū*, Diaphragm Transport), PC-6 (*nèi guān*, Inner Pass), CV-17 (*shān zhōng*, Chest Center), and CV-6 (*qì hǎi*, Sea of Qi). Selection of points according to pattern: For qi vacuity, add CV-12 (*zhōng wǎn*, Center Stomach Duct) and ST-36 (*zú sān lǐ*, Leg Three Li). For liver-kidney yin vacuity, add BL-18 (*gān shū*, Liver Transport), BL-23 (*shèn shū*, Kidney Transport), and CV-4 (*guān yuán*, Pass Head). Needle with supplementation and add moxa. For hiccough due due to vacuity desertion of the true origin, see VACUITY DESERTION HICCOUGH. See HICCOUGH; COLD HICCOUGH. [26: 627] [37: 307] [46: 602, 658] [113: 76]

vacuity is treated by supplementing 虚者补之 *xū zhě bǔ zhī*: See DEBILITY IS TREATED BY SUPPLEMENTING. [26: 627] [27: 239] [97: 515]

vacuity is treated by supplementing the mother 虚者补其母 *xū zhě bǔ qí mǔ*: In the doctrine of the five phases, the treatment of vacuity or one organ or channel by supplementing the organ that engenders it. For example, water (kidney) engenders, or is the mother of, wood (liver). Liver vacuity is treated most effectively supplementing not only the liver but also the kidney. For liver vacuity fire characterized by insomnia, heart vexation and agitation, baking heat [effusion] in the head and face, and a forceless rapid fine pulse, the principle of enriching water to moisten wood can be used, i.e., supplementing kidney water to restrain the vacuity fire of the liver. [26: 627] [27: 246]

vacuity jaundice 虚黄 *xū huáng*: JAUNDICE with vacuity signs such as withered-yellow facial complexion, bland taste in the mouth, fearful throbbing, limp legs, mild heat effusion and aversion to cold, disfluent voidings of turbid urine, low food intake, sloppy stool, pale tongue, and a weak fine pulse. Vacuity jaundice develops as a result of enduring jaundice or spleen vacuity and blood depletion depriving the skin of nourishment. [MED] Support the vacuity and secure the root, taking care to avoid excessively cold formulas. Appropriate formulas include Tangkuei and Astragalus Center-Fortifying Decoction (*guī qí jiàn zhōng tāng*), Ginseng Construction-Nourishing Decoction (*rén shēn yǎng róng tāng*), and Eight-Ingredient Rehmannia Pill (*bā wèi dì huáng wán*). ACU Base treatment mainly on CV, back transport points, GB, ST, and SP. Select CV-12 (*zhōng wǎn*, Center Stomach Duct), CV-6 (*qì hǎi*, Sea of Qi), BL-20 (*pí shū*, Spleen Transport), BL-19 (*dǎn shū*, Gallbladder Transport), ST-36 (*zú sān lǐ*, Leg Three Li), SP-6 (*sān yīn jiāo*, Three Yin Intersection), and GB-34 (*yáng líng quán*, Yang Mound Spring). Needle with supplementation and add moxa. [26: 629] [46: 664] [37: 398] [?: 178]

vacuity macules 虚斑 *xū bān*: YIN MACULES. [26: 629]

vacuity malaria 虚疟 *xū nüè*: MALARIA occurring either when malaria evils are contracted in constitutional weakness or enduring malaria depletes original qi. Vacuity malaria is characterized by unpronounced heat effusion and aversion to cold, lack of strength in the extremities, reduced food intake, persistent spontaneous sweating, and a soft vacuous pulse. MED Nourish right and supplement vacuity with formulas such as Six Gentlemen Decoction (*liù jūn zǐ tāng*), Center-Supplementing Qi-Boosting Decoction (*bǔ zhōng yì qì tāng*), or Flowery Knotweed and Ginseng Beverage (*hé rén yǐn*). ACU Base treatment mainly on GV, PC, SI, ST, and KI. Select GV-14 (*dà zhuī*, Great Hammer), GV-13 (*táo dào*, Kiln Path), PC-5 (*jiān shǐ*, Intermediary Courier), SI-3 (*hòu xī*, Back Ravine), CV-12 (*zhōng wǎn*, Center Stomach Duct), ST-36 (*zú sān lǐ*, Leg Three Li), BL-20 (*pí shū*, Spleen Transport), and KI-3 (*tài xī*, Great Ravine). Needle with supplementation and add moxa. For principles and methods of treatment see MALARIA. [26: 630] [27: 359] [97: 513] [113: 171]

vacuity of the true origin in the lower body 真元下虚 *zhēn yuán xià xū*: Synonym: *exhaustion of the lower origin*. Severe kidney depletion, especially kidney yang. [27: 164]

vacuity panting 虚喘 *xū chuǎn*: PANTING attributed to lung qi vacuity and the kidney failing to absorb qi stemming from a weak constitution, from enduring panting, or from wear on the true origin through major illness. Vacuity panting is of gradual onset and chronic in nature. It is characterized shortness of breath with difficulty in catching one's breath, a condition brought on by physical movement; relief from discomfort comes when a deep breath can be drawn. See QI VACUITY PANTING; YIN VACUITY PANTING; TRUE ORIGIN VACUITY PANTING. [26: 629] [27: 216] [97: 514]

vacuity pattern 虚证 *xū zhèng*: Any disease pattern arising from weakness of the body's forces and absence of an evil. Vacuity patterns are attributed to insufficiencies of qi, blood, yin, and yang that arise from damage to right qi either through enduring illness, loss of blood, seminal loss, and great sweating, or by invasion of an external evil (yang evils readily damage yin humor and yin evils readily damage yang qi), constitutional weakness, or the wear and tear that comes with age. Since these insufficiencies frequently affect specific organs, further distinction is made between such forms as heart yin vacuity, liver blood vacuity, kidney yang vacuity, and lung qi vacuity. [27: 156]

vacuity phlegm 虚痰 *xū tán*: **1.** Any phlegm pattern due to vacuity of original qi. MED Boost qi and transform phlegm with Bupleurum and Peony Six Gentlemen Decoction (*chái sháo liù jūn zǐ tāng*). ACU Base treatment mainly on CV and ST. Select CV-4 (*guān yuán*, Pass Head), CV-6 (*qì hǎi*, Sea of Qi), CV-12 (*zhōng wǎn*, Center Stomach Duct), ST-36 (*zú sān lǐ*, Leg Three Li), and ST-40 (*fēng lóng*, Bountiful Bulge). Needle with supplementation and add moxa. **2.** COLD PHLEGM. [26: 629]

vacuity puffiness 虚浮 *xū fú*: **1.** Swelling of the outer body preceding distention in the inner body, with pale urine, unsolid stool, a withered-white facial complexion, low timid voice, and a forceless pulse faint fine pulse. **2.** VACUITY SWELLING. [111: 1248] [25: 264]

vacuity-repletion complex 虚实错杂 *xū shí cuò zá*: Any disease characterized by the presence of both vacuity and repletion signs. If a patient suffering from a cough expectorates thick, sticky phlegm and has a yellow tongue fur, the condition is one of phlegm-heat congesting the lung, which is a repletion pattern. If, at the same time, breathing is short and shallow, and becomes rapid at the slightest exertion, the patient is said to be suffering from insufficiency of lung qi, which is a vacuity pattern. The simultaneous existence of the repletion pattern and the vacuity pattern constitutes a vacuity-repletion complex. A further example is internal static blood obstruction, manifesting as abdominal glomus lump. If this repletion pattern occurs with signs of dual vacuity of yin and blood, characterized by emaciation, encrusted skin, and dark rings around the eyes, the patient is said to be suffering from a vacuity-repletion complex. Such patterns may be due to contraction of an external evil by patients ordinarily suffering from vacuity of right, or may be caused by an invading evil that both causes repletion and damages right. [6: 158]

vacuity stroke 虚中 *xū zhòng*: A pattern similar to WIND STROKE[1] characterized by bright white complexion, faint breath from the nose, stiff tongue and disfluent speech, deviation of the eyes and mouth, and hemiplegia, sometimes but not necessarily heralded by clouding collapse. Limp hands and open mouth constitutes a wind-stoke desertion pattern. It is attributed to constitutional weakness, physical taxation causing damage to qi and the spleen, and phlegm and qi congestion. It may also arise as a result of sexual intemperance causing detriment to essential qi. [MED] Treat primarily by boosting qi with Six Gentlemen Decoction (*liù jūn zǐ tāng*) or Center-Supplementing Qi-Boosting Decoction (*bǔ zhōng yì qì tāng*). Desertion patterns call for swift administration of large doses of ginseng (*rén shēn*) and astragalus (*huáng qí*). For sexual intemperance patterns use Pulse-Engendering Powder (*shēng mài sǎn*) plus tangkuei (*dāng guī*), cooked rehmannia (*shú dì huáng*), and velvet deerhorn (*lù róng*). [ACU] Base treatment mainly on GV and CV. Select GV-20 (*bǎi huì*, Hundred Convergences)ⓜ, CV-8 (*shén què*, Spirit Gate Tower)ⓜ, CV-4 (*guān yuán*, Pass Head)ⓜ, CV-6 (*qì hǎi*, Sea of Qi)ⓜ, PC-6 (*nèi guān*, Inner Pass), and LU-9 (*tài yuān*, Great Abyss) until the limbs become warm, the pulse rises and the patient's spirit-mind becomes clear, or just needle with supplementation with moxa. For stiff tongue and hemiplegia, see HEMIPLEGIA. For limp hands and open mouth etc., see desertion patterns under WIND-LIKE STROKE. For sexual intemperance, add BL-23 (*shèn shū*, Kidney Transport), KI-3 (*tài xī*, Great Ravine), BL-52 (*zhì shì*, Will Chamber), and GV-4 (*mìng mén*, Life Gate). [26: 627] [113: 34-8]

vacuity swelling 虚肿 *xū zhǒng*: WATER SWELLING attributable to vacuity; a form of YIN WATER. Vacuity swelling is essentially attributed to spleen and/or kidney vacuity (spleen failing to control water; kidney vacuity water flood; impaired kidney qi transformation; spleen-kidney debilitation). Vacuity swelling develops slowly, and is associated with signs such as weak breathing and low voice, pale dull completion, fatigue, diarrhea, fear of cold and cold limbs, forceless fine sunken pulse. [WMC] observed in chronic nephritis, hypothyroidism, menopausal syndrome, hypoproteinemia. [MED] See WATER SWELLING. [27: 418] [50: 1373][97: 512]

vacuity taxation 虚劳 *xū láo*: *Synonyms: vacuity-detriment taxation damage; taxation timidity.* Any pattern of severe vacuity (of qi, blood, or the organs), including notably steaming bone and consumption. The term comes from *Essential Prescriptions of the Golden Coffer* (*jīn guì yào lüè, xuè bì xū láo bìng mài zhèng bìng zhì*), and was explained in *The Origin and Indicators of Disease* (*zhū bìng yuán hòu lùn*) as referring to any of various qi, blood, or organ vacuity patterns on the one hand and contagious diseases such as steaming bone and corpse transmission (i.e., consumption) on the other. Since then, it has become

a convention to refer to the former patterns as VACUITY DETRIMENT, whereas the latter patterns are referred to as CONSUMPTION. Compare VACUITY DETRIMENT. [26: 628] [27: 385] [97: 512]

vacuity-taxation cough 虚劳咳嗽 *xū láo ké sòu*: See TAXATION COUGH. [26: 629]

vacuity-taxation lumbar pain 虚劳腰痛 *xū láo yāo tòng*: LUMBAR PAIN arising when taxation damage causes insufficiency of kidney qi and disturbs qi transformation. The pain spreads into the lesser abdomen and is accompanied by inhibited urination, and a sunken pulse. [MED] Use Cinnamon Bark and Aconite Eight-Ingredient Pill (*guì fù bā wèi wán*) combined with Astragalus Center-Fortifying Decoction (*huáng qí jiàn zhōng tāng*) and Major Yin Supplementation Pill (*dà bǔ yīn wán*). [ACU] Base treatment mainly on BL, GV, CV, and KI. Select BL-23 (*shèn shū*, Kidney Transport), GV-4 (*mìng mén*, Life Gate), KI-3 (*tài xī*, Great Ravine), CV-6 (*qì hǎi*, Sea of Qi), GV-3 (*yāo yáng guān*, Lumbar Yang Pass), BL-40 (*wěi zhōng*, Bend Center), ouch points (*ā shì xué*), and CV-4 (*guān yuán*, Pass Head); needle with supplementation and add moxa. [26: 629] [46: 633]

vacuity-taxation night sweating 虚劳盗汗 *xū láo dào hàn*: NIGHT SWEATING due to qi vacuity and yang weakness, to heart yang vacuity, to heart-kidney yang vacuity, or to yin blood vacuity. [MED] When due to qi vacuity and yang weakness, it can be treated with Oyster Shell Powder (*mǔ lì sǎn*) or Astragalus Center-Fortifying Decoction (*huáng qí jiàn zhōng tāng*). When due to heart yang vacuity, it can be treated with Biota Seed Decoction (*bǎi zǐ rén tāng*). When due to dual vacuity of the heart and kidney, use Heart-Kidney Pill (*xīn shèn wán*). Alternatively, use Spleen-Returning Decoction (*guī pí tāng*) combined with Six-Ingredient Rehmannia Pill (*liù wèi dì huáng wán*), adding oyster shell (*mǔ lì*), light wheat (*fú xiǎo mài*), and schisandra (*wǔ wèi zǐ*) if sweating is copious. For night sweating due to yin-blood vacuity, see YIN VACUITY NIGHT SWEATING. [ACU] Base treatment mainly on back transport points, KI, LI, and SI. Main points: LI-4 (*hé gǔ*, Union Valley), SI-3 (*hòu xī*, Back Ravine), and HT-6 (*yīn xī*, Yin Cleft). Selection of points according to pattern: For qi vacuity and yang weakness, add CV-6 (*qì hǎi*, Sea of Qi), CV-4 (*guān yuán*, Pass Head), and GV-4 (*mìng mén*, Life Gate). For heart yang vacuity, add BL-15 (*xīn shū*, Heart Transport), CV-14 (*jù què*, Great Tower Gate), PC-6 (*nèi guān*, Inner Pass), and HT-7 (*shén mén*, Spirit Gate). For heart-kidney yang vacuity, BL-15 (*xīn shū*, Heart Transport), BL-23 (*shèn shū*, Kidney Transport), CV-14 (*jù què*, Great Tower Gate), CV-4 (*guān yuán*, Pass Head), GV-4 (*mìng mén*, Life Gate), and PC-6 (*nèi guān*, Inner Pass). Needle with supplementation and add moxa for all three patterns. For night sweating due to yin-blood vacuity, see YIN VACUITY NIGHT SWEATING. [26: 629] [46: 602] [113: 18] [14: 175]

vacuity-taxation scant semen 虚劳精少 *xū láo jīng shǎo*: See SCANT SEMEN. [26: 629]

vacuity tetany 虚痉 *xū jìng*: TETANY (*jìng*) attributed to extreme qi and blood vacuity depriving the sinews of nourishment or to major loss of blood. Vacuity tetany is characterized by convulsions, clouded head and flowery vision, spontaneous sweating, lassitude of spirit, shortness of breath, pale tongue, and a fine stringlike pulse. MED Treat by boosting qi and supplementing the blood, supported by extinguishing wind. Appropriate formulas include Tangkuei Blood-Supplementing Decoction (*dāng guī bǔ xuè tāng*) or Eight-Gem Decoction (*bā zhēn tāng*) with the addition of uncaria (*gōu téng*) and scorpion tail (*xiē shāo*). ACU Base treatment mainly on back transport points, GV, SP, ST, and LR. Select BL-17 (*gé shū*, Diaphragm Transport), BL-20 (*pí shū*, Spleen Transport), ST-36 (*zú sān lǐ*, Leg Three Li), SP-6 (*sān yīn jiāo*, Three Yin Intersection), GV-20 (*bǎi huì*, Hundred Convergences), GV-16 (*fēng fǔ*, Wind Mansion), LR-3 (*tài chōng*, Supreme Surge), and GV-8 (*jīn suō*, Sinew Contraction); needle with supplementation and moxa if appropriate. [26: 628]

vacuity vexation 虚烦 *xū fán*: HEAT VEXATION due to vacuity fire harassing the inner body. Vacuity vexation is a feeling of unease and listlessness in the heart, accompanied by a condition that seems like distention but is not, food failing to be appetizing, and unquiet sleep, It occurs in febrile disease, either in the latter stages or or after sweating, ejection, or precipitation, when residual heat remains. MED Treat with Bamboo Leaf Decoction (*zhú yè tāng*) or Gardenia and Fermented Soybean Decoction (*zhī zǐ chǐ tāng*) and variations. See VEXATION. [26: 629] [27: 372] [97: 513]

vacuity vexation and sleeplessness 虚烦不得眠 *xū fán bù dé mián*: From *On Cold Damage* (*shāng hán lùn*). A feeling of uneasiness focused in the chest together with insomnia occurring in vacuity patterns. Distinction is made between qi vacuity, yang vacuity, yin vacuity, and residual heat. In qi vacuity it is accompanied by fatigue and lack of strength, reduced food intake, lassitude of spirit, dry mouth with low fluid intake and a soft soggy pulse, and is treated by supplementing qi. In yang vacuity, it is associated with cold limbs and fear of cold, and a slow sunken pulse, and is treated by warming supplementation. In yin vacuity, it is accompanied by dry mouth, red tongue, and a rapid fine pulse, and is treated by enriching yin and clearing fire. In residual heat harassing the inner

body occurring in the latter stages of febrile disease, it is associated with residual heat (effusion), dry mouth and tongue, and yellow or reddish urine, and is treated by clearing heat and eliminating vexation. ACU Base treatment mainly on HT and three yin channels of the foot. Main points: Alert Spirit Quartet (*sì shén cōng*), HT-7 (*shén mén*, Spirit Gate), BL-15 (*xīn shū*, Heart Transport), PC-6 (*nèi guān*, Inner Pass), and SP-6 (*sān yīn jiāo*, Three Yin Intersection). Selection of points according to pattern: For qi vacuity, add BL-20 (*pí shū*, Spleen Transport), ST-36 (*zú sān lǐ*, Leg Three Li), and CV-6 (*qì hǎi*, Sea of Qi), needling with supplementation and adding moxa. For yang vacuity, add CV-6 (*qì hǎi*, Sea of Qi), CV-4 (*guān yuán*, Pass Head), ST-36 (*zú sān lǐ*, Leg Three Li), and GV-20 (*bǎi huì*, Hundred Convergences), using both needles and moxa. For yin vacuity, needle with supplementation at BL-23 (*shèn shū*, Kidney Transport), KI-3 (*tài xī*, Great Ravine), and KI-6 (*zhào hǎi*, Shining Sea), and with drainage at the main points and HT-8 (*shào fǔ*, Lesser Mansion). For residual heat, add ST-41 (*jiě xī*, Ravine Divide), LI-4 (*hé gǔ*, Union Valley), LI-11 (*qū chí*, Pool at the Bend), ST-43 (*xiàn gǔ*, Sunken Valley), GB-39 (*xuán zhōng*, Suspended Bell), and ST-44 (*nèi tíng*, Inner Court), needling with drainage. See SLEEPLESSNESS. [26: 629] [14: 30, 49] [46: 644] [37: 346] [113: 145]

vacuity wind stirring internally 虚风内动 *xū fēng nèi dòng*: A WIND pattern attributable to yin vacuity or blood vacuity that arises when great sweating, great vomiting, great diarrhea, major loss of blood, or damage to yin in enduring illness with depletion of the fluids causes desiccation of the blood that deprives the sinews of nourishment and causes insufficiency of liver yin that leaves yang unsubdued and allows liver wind to scurry around internally. It may also occur when kidney-water failing to moisten liver-wood causes wind to harass the upper body. Vacuity wind stirring within is marked by dizziness, tremor, worm-like movement in the extremities, or clouding collapse. See LIVER WIND STIRRING INTERNALLY. [26: 627] [27: 139] [97: 515]

vacuity with repletion complication 虚中夹实 *xū zhōng jiā shí*: Any vacuity pattern with concurrent signs of an evil. For example, in blood dryness consumption, vacuity signs such as emaciation, dry skin, vexing heat in hearts of the palms and soles, and no thought of food and drink are observed in combination with repletion signs of blood stasis such as menstrual block, dark purple tongue, stasis speckles on the margins of the tongue, and a stringlike sunken pulse. [26: 627]

vacuous 虚 *xū*: Empty, not solid, weak. (1) Not solid, e.g., a vacuous pulse. (2) Of or relating to vacuity. See VACUITY AND REPLETION.

vacuous kidney failing to absorb qi 肾虚不纳气 *shèn xū bù nà qì*: KIDNEY FAILING TO ABSORB QI.

vacuous li 虚里 *xū lǐ*: *Synonym: apical pulse.* The place below the nipple at which a throbbing can be felt and said to be the collecting place of ancestral qi. Vacuous li corresponds in channel theory to the *great network vessel of the stomach,* and since stomach qi is a foundation of human life and is the source of ancestral qi in the chest, it reflects the state of ancestral qi and stomach qi. ◇ Chin 虚 *xū*, vacuous, empty, weak; 里 *lǐ*, area, township, village; unit of distance. Possibly from the Gk. *khylos*. [26: 627] [27: 193] [97: 513]

vacuous puffiness 浮虚 *fú xū*: *Synonym: qi swelling.*[3] From *Elementary Questions* (*sù wèn, liù yuán zhèng jì dà lùn*). WATER SWELLING in the interstices of the skin that springs back after being pressed. Compare VACUITY PUFFINESS; PUFFY SWELLING. [25: 265]

vacuous pulse 虚脉 *xū mài*: A forceless soft usually large pulse that feels empty. *The Pulse Canon* (*mài jīng*) states, "The vacuous pulse is slow, large, and soft, and feels under pressure to be insufficient and gapingly empty." It is also described as a combination of the floating, large, slow, and soft pulses. [26: 628]

vacuous qi failing to ensure containment 气虚不摄 *qì xū bù shè*: Qi failing to retain blood, fluids, essence etc., in the body, causing spontaneous sweating, seminal emission, diarrhea, enuresis, flooding and spotting, or blood in the stool. [26: 541] [27: 143]

vacuous yang floating upward 虚阳上浮 *xū yáng shàng fú*: **1.** EXUBERANT YIN REPELLING YANG. **2.** *Synonyms: unconstrained vacuous yang; solitary yang straying upward.* A pattern of tidal heat [effusion], tender-red complexion, dry mouth without thirst, and a vacuous rapid pulse arising when yang, deprived of support through essence-blood depletion, strays upward to the upper body. [26: 629]

vaginal discharge 带下 *dài xià*, 白带 *bái dài*: The emission of a viscid fluid via the vagina. Scant white vaginal discharge often occurs in healthy women. Only discharge that is profuse, bears an unnatural color, or gives off a malign odor is pathological. A copious clear white discharge without malodor is called white vaginal discharge and is caused by cold-damp pouring downward with spleen vacuity. A foul-smelling copious thick yellow discharge is called yellow vaginal discharge and is due to damp-heat pouring downward. A thick discharge that is white and red in color and bears

a faint fishy smell is called red vaginal discharge, and arises when depressed liver qi transforms into heat, which damages the network vessels of the uterus. Modern research shows that continued red vaginal discharge is in some cases a sign of cancer. Malodorous vaginal discharge like rice water (water in which rice has been washed), yellow-green like pus, or multicolored, and attended by pudendal itch and soreness is a sign of damp toxin. See entries listed below. ◇ Chin 带 *dài*, belt, sash, strap; 下 *xià*, down. In early medical texts, the term referred to women's diseases ("disease below the belt"); its specific use in denoting vaginal discharge may have been influenced by the interpretation of 带 as downward flow like an endless belt. [26: 599] [27: 444] [97: 391]

Vaginal Discharge

Classification by cause

SPLEEN VACUITY VAGINAL DISCHARGE (*pí xū dài xià*)

KIDNEY VACUITY VAGINAL DISCHARGE (*shèn xū dài xià*)

DAMP TOXIN VAGINAL DISCHARGE (*shī dú dài xià*)

LIVER CHANNEL DAMP-HEAT VAGINAL DISCHARGE (*gān jīng shī rè dài xià*)

Classification by color

WHITE VAGINAL DISCHARGE (*bái dài*)

GREEN-BLUE VAGINAL DISCHARGE (*qīng dài*)

YELLOW VAGINAL DISCHARGE (*huáng dài*)

BLACK VAGINAL DISCHARGE (*hēi xià*)

RED AND WHITE VAGINAL DISCHARGE (*chì bái dài*)

FIVE-COLORED VAGINAL DISCHARGE (*wǔ sè dài*)

WHITE FLOOD (*bái bēng*)

WHITE LEAK (*bái lòu*)

WHITE OOZE (*bái yín*)

vaginal flatus 阴吹 *yīn chuī*: From *Essential Prescriptions of the Golden Coffer* (*jīn guì yào lüè*). Expulsion of qi (gas) through the vagina. Vaginal flatulence is traditionally attributed to replete grain qi and the downward discharge stomach qi or to qi and blood vacuity with center qi fall. **Replete grain qi** causes vaginal flatus marked by a loud clear sound and continuous expulsions and is associated with constipation. MED Treat by moistening dryness and precipitation. Use Lard and Hair Brew (*gāo fà jiān*), which comprises pork lard (*zhū zhī gāo*) and hair (*xuè yú*). **Center qi fall** causes vaginal flatus with shortness of breath, laziness to speak, fatigue, and lack of strength. MED Supplement the center and boost qi. Use Perfect Major Supplementation Decoction (*shí quán dà bǔ tāng*) plus cimicifuga (*shēng má*) and bupleurum (*chái hú*). WMC flatus vaginalis.

Modern gynecology attributes flatus vaginalis to a number of causes: loosening of the vagina in childbirth allowing air to enter and accumulate before it is periodically expelled (e.g., when lying face downward or during physical exertion); carbohydrates resolving into gas in the vagina; deformities that cause intestinal flatus to be discharged through the vagina. These considerations may help to shed light on the traditional Chinese explanations. [26: 617] [67: 370]

vaginal protrusion 阴挺 *yīn tǐng*: YIN PROTRUSION.

vain straining 虚坐努责 *xū zuò nǔ zé*: Straining in vain to pass stool despite frequent desire to defecate. Vain straining occurs in damage to yin in enduring dysentery; it is more severe than tenesmus normally associated with dysentery. [26: 627] [50: 1377]

vein 青筋 *qīng jīn*, 筋 *jīn*, 筋脉 *jīn mài*: Blood vessels visible through the skin. ◇ Chin *qīng*, green, blue; *jīn*, sinew.

venter 胃脘 *wèi wǎn (guǎn)*: See STOMACH DUCT.

vertebra 脊椎骨 *jǐ zhuī gǔ*: Any of the bones forming part of the spine.

vertex 顶 *dǐng*: The top of the head. ⬚WMC vertex cranii.

vertex headache 巅顶头痛 *diān dǐng tóu tòng*: Synonym: *pain at the vertex*. Pain in the region of the vertex. The greater yang (*tài yáng*) channels meet at the vertex where they enter the brain. Pain at the vertex is usually a greater yang (*tài yáng*) disease. ⬚MED Use medicinals such as Chinese lovage (*gǎo běn*), ligusticum (*chuān xiōng*), notopterygium (*qiāng huó*), and duhuo (*dú huó*). ⬚ACU Select GV-20 (*bǎi huì*, Hundred Convergences), Alert Spirit Quartet (*sì shén cōng*), GV-21 (*qián dǐng*, Before the Vertex), GB-19 (*nǎo kōng*, Brain Hollow), GV-23 (*shàng xīng*, Upper Star), KI-1 (*yǒng quán*, Gushing Spring), LI-4 (*hé gǔ*, Union Valley), and LR-3 (*tài chōng*, Supreme Surge); needle with drainage. See HEADACHE. [26: 997] [113: 9] [46: 621] [14: 75]

vesicle 水（疱）泡 *shuǐ pào*: A BLISTER,[1] especially a small one.

vessel 脉 *mài*: Any pathway of the blood or of qi. *Elementary Questions* (*sù wèn, mài yào jīng wéi lùn*) states, "The vessels are the house of the blood." *The Magic Pivot* (*líng shū, jué qì*) states, "That which blocks [i.e., contains] construction qi and prevents it from going astray is the vessels." The vessels are intimately related to the heart; see HEART GOVERNS THE BLOOD AND VESSELS. ◇ Chin *mài*, vessel, related to 派 *pài* both in sound and in the meaning of branches of a river flowing apart and with the flesh signifier 肉 *ròu*, abbreviated to 月, depicting the ever ramifying system of vessels in the body. [26: 550]

vessel impediment 脉痹 *mài bì*: Synonym: *heat impediment*. IMPEDIMENT (*bì*) characterized by irregular heat effusion, palpable heat and pain in the flesh, and sometimes red patches on the skin; attributed to wind-damp stagnating in the vessels. Distinction is made between vacuity and repletion, the former being treated with Five Impediments Decoction (*wǔ bì tāng*) plus cinnamon twig (*guì zhī*), carthamus (*hóng huā*), root poria (*fú shén*), polygala (*yuǎn zhì*), and ophiopogon (*mài mén dōng*), and the latter with Ginseng Decoction (*rén shēn tāng*). [27: 404] [26: 551]

vessel opening 脉口 *mài kǒu*: Synonym: *qi opening*. The WRIST PULSE; so called because it is an "opening" in the body where the qi of the vessels can be felt. Also called qi opening for the same reason. ◇ Chin *mài*, vessel, pulse; *kǒu*, mouth, opening. See PULSE.

vessel qi 脉气 *mài qì*: CHANNEL QI.

vessel wilting 脉痿 *mài wěi*: Synonym: *heart wilting*. From *Elementary Questions* (*sù wèn, wěi lùn*). A WILTING (*wěi*) pattern attributed to heart qi heat with fire flaming upward and carrying qi and blood counterflow with it and causing emptiness of the blood vessels in the lower body. Since the heart governs the blood and vessels and both the heart and vessels are involved in this disease pattern, heart wilting is synonymous with vessel wilting. Signs include joints of the four limbs as if broken, inability to lift the limbs, and weakness in the lower leg preventing the patient from standing. ⬚MED Clear the heart and drain fire; nourish and quicken the blood with variations of Four Agents Decoction (*sì wù tāng*). ⬚ACU Base treatment on back transport points, HT, and GB. Needle with supplementation or with even supplementation and drainage at BL-20 (*pí shū*, Spleen Transport), LR-3 (*tài chōng*, Supreme Surge), BL-17 (*gé shū*, Diaphragm Transport), and BL-23 (*shèn shū*, Kidney Transport), and with drainage at BL-15 (*xīn shū*, Heart Transport), HT-8 (*shào fǔ*, Lesser Mansion), SI-1 (*shào zé*, Lesser Marsh), LU-9 (*tài yuān*, Great Abyss), GB-30 (*huán tiào*, Jumping Round), and GB-34 (*yáng líng quán*, Yang Mound Spring). See WILTING (*wěi*). [26: 551] [113: 242] [46: 638]

vexation 烦 *fán*: HEART VEXATION.

vexation and agitation 烦燥 *fán zào*: A subjective feeling of heat and disquietude in the chest (vexation) and objective fidgetiness of the limbs (agitation). Both signs may occur in vacuity, repletion, cold, and heat patterns. For example, when evils enter the interior, causing yang brightness (*yáng míng*) repletion heat, signs include high fever, thirst, vexation and oppression in the chest, fidgetiness of the extremities (yang brightness governs the four limbs). Heart vexation is often observed without agitation. Where heat sensations are pronounced, it is called HEAT VEXATION. Where vexation appears with thirst as a result of damage to liquid by exuberant heat, the term VEXATION AND THIRST is used. When vexation appears in the latter stages of febrile disease or after sweating (diaphoresis), ejection, or precipitation in the course of febrile disease when residual heat is still present, heat vexation in the chest with unquiet sleep is a sign of vacuity fire harassing the inner body, and in such cases is often referred to as VACUITY VEXATION. Vexation accompanied by a cold body and unconscious movement of the limbs, bodily fatigue and lassitude of spirit, dry mouth with intake of fluid, and a weak fine pulse is called AGITATED VEXATION. [27: 372] [27: 371] [97: 497]

vexation and thirst 烦渴 *fán kě*: A feeling of heat and disquietude focused in the chest and accompanied by a desire for fluids. See VEXATION AND AGITATION. [27: 372]

vexation of pregnancy 子烦 *zǐ fán*: HEART VEXATION occurring in pregnancy. Vexation of pregnancy is attributed to exploitation of the heart by fire-heat that results from a) insufficiency of yin-blood arising when the blood gathers to nourish the fetus or b) preexisting phlegm-rheum that is transformed into phlegm-heat by the action of depression, anger, anxiety, or thought. In the case of yin vacuity, there is vexing heat in five hearts and dry mouth, whereas in phlegm heat, there is dizziness, oppression in the stomach duct, nausea and vomiting, and copious phlegm. If there is pronounced liver depression, there is distending pain in both rib-sides. MED Yin vacuity patterns are treated by clearing heat, nourishing yin, and eliminating vexation with Coptis, Ass Hide Glue, and Egg Yolk Decoction (*huáng lián ē jiāo jī zǐ huáng tāng*). Phlegm-fire patterns are treated by clearing heat and flushing phlegm with Fritillaria and Trichosanthes Powder (*bèi mǔ guā lóu sǎn*). For liver depression, course the liver, resolve depression, and eliminate vexation with Moutan and Gardenia Free Wanderer Powder (*dān zhī xiāo yáo sǎn*). [26: 56] [27: 447] [97: 37] [24: 148]

vexing heat in the five hearts 五心烦热 *wǔ xīn fán rè*: Palpable heat in the palms of the hand, soles of the feet, and subjective feeling of heat in the chest. Vexing heat in the five hearts is observed in vacuity detriment and consumption, and arises from effulgent yin vacuity fire, vacuity heat failing to clear after illness, or internally depressed fire-heat. MED Nourish yin and abate heat effusion; clear heat and nourish yin; clear the liver and rectify the spleen. Use formulas such as Bone-Clearing Powder (*qīng gǔ sǎn*) or Free Wanderer Powder (*xiāo yáo sǎn*). For depressed fire, treat by

upbearing and effusing with Fire Depression Decoction (*huǒ yù tāng*). [26: 114]

vigorous fire 壮火 *zhuàng huǒ*: From *Elementary Questions* (*sù wèn, yīn yáng yìng xiàng dà lùn*). Pathological fire standing in opposition to the lesser fire, which is the healthy fire of physiological activity. Vigorous fire causes wear on right qi and affects physiological functions. [27: 59]

vigorous heat [effusion] 壮热 *zhuàng rè*: High fever occurring in repletion patterns and characteristic of qi-aspect heat in warm diseases. [27: 357] [97: 223]

viscera 脏腑 *zàng fǔ*: Plural of viscus. See BOWELS AND VISCERA.

visceral agitation 脏躁 *zàng zào*: From *Essential Prescriptions of the Golden Coffer* (*jīn guì yào lüè, fù rén zá bìng mài zhèng bìng zhì piān*). A paroxysmal mental disease most prevalent in women, heralded by melancholy and depression, illusions, emotionalism, and increased or diminished sensitivity. Attacks are characterized by vexation and oppression, rashness and impatience, sighing for no apparent reason, and sadness with an urge to weep. In severe cases, there may be convulsions, which, unlike those occurring in epilepsy, are accompanied by a white complexion or complete loss of consciousness. Visceral agitation falls into two basic patterns, heart spirit deprived of nourishment and insufficiency of the liver and kidney. WMC hysteria. **Heart spirit deprived of nourishment** arises when anxiety or thought damage the heart and excessive taxation fatigue damages the spleen. The resultant condition of dual damage to the heart and spleen and insufficiency of qi and blood deprives the heart spirit of nourishment. When the heart is deprived of nourishment, the heart spirit fails to be stored and spirit qi runs amok. Signs include devitalized essence-spirit, abstraction, sorrowfulness without apparent cause and abnormal laughing and crying. There may also be vexation, insomnia, profuse dreaming, susceptibility to fright, heart palpitations, lassitude of spirit, thirst, constipation, red tongue that may be soft in texture, and a weak fine or fine stringlike pulse. MED Enrich and supplement with sweet moist medicinals and nourishing and quieting the spirit. Use Licorice, Wheat, and Jujube Decoction (*gān mài dà zǎo tāng*) plus spiny jujube (*suān zǎo rén*), dried/fresh rehmannia (*shēng dì huáng*), and lily bulb (*bǎi hé*). ACU Base treatment mainly on HT, GV, and PC. Main points: GV-26 (*shuǐ gōu*, Water Trough), GV-20 (*bǎi huì*, Hundred Convergences), PC-6 (*nèi guān*, Inner Pass), and HT-7 (*shén mén*, Spirit Gate). For heart spirit deprived of nourishment, add BL-15 (*xīn shū*, Heart Transport), PC-8 (*láo gōng*, Palace of Toil), SP-10 (*xuè hǎi*, Sea of Blood), and SP-6 (*sān yīn jiāo*, Three

Yin Intersection); needle with supplementation. Selection of points according to signs: For abnormal laughing and weeping, add SI-3 (*hòu xī*, Back Ravine). For essence-spirit abstraction, add BL-15 (*xīn shū*, Heart Transport) and BL-47 (*hún mén*, Hun Gate). **Insufficiency of the liver and kidney** arises when childbirth or severe illness causes depletion of the blood, and can cause visceral agitation if the heart and liver are deprived of nourishment and effulgent qi and blood disquiet the heart spirit and prevent the ethereal soul from being stored. It is characterized by the similar heart spirit signs (insomnia, heart palpitations, susceptibility to fright) and heat signs (dry mouth, red tongue, dry stool) as the previous pattern. However, in addition there are distinctive kidney vacuity signs such as heat in the hearts of the palms and soles, tinnitus, and limp aching lumbus and knees, as well as liver vacuity signs such as vexation and irascibility. MED Treat insufficiency of the liver and kidney by enriching the kidney and clearing the liver and by nourishing the heart and quieting the spirit. Use Lily Bulb and Rehmannia Decoction (*bǎi hé dì huáng tāng*) combined with Water-Enriching Liver-Clearing Beverage (*zī shuǐ qīng gān yǐn*). If there are signs of binding depression of liver qi such as affect-mind depression, and oppression in the chest with qi counterflow, plum pit qi, and rib-side pain, use Free Wanderer Powder (*xiāo yáo sǎn*) or Bupleurum Liver-Coursing Powder (*chái hú shū gān sǎn*), adding moutan (*mǔ dān pí*) and gardenia (*shān zhī zǐ*) if the depression is transforming into fire. ACU Use the main points given above, and add PC-8 (*láo gōng*, Palace of Toil), CV-4 (*guān yuán*, Pass Head), KI-1 (*yǒng quán*, Gushing Spring), LR-3 (*tài chōng*, Supreme Surge), LR-2 (*xíng jiān*, Moving Between), and SP-6 (*sān yīn jiāo*, Three Yin Intersection); needle with even supplementation and drainage. For liver depression and qi stagnation, add TB-6 (*zhī gōu*, Branch Ditch), LR-3 (*tài chōng*, Supreme Surge), and LR-2 (*xíng jiān*, Moving Between); needle with drainage or with even supplementation and drainage. If there is transformation into fire, drain GB-43 (*xiá xī*, Pinched Ravine) and GB-34 (*yáng líng quán*, Yang Mound Spring). Selection of points according to signs: For oppression in the chest and counterflow qi, add CV-17 (*shān zhōng*, Chest Center) and ST-40 (*fēng lóng*, Bountiful Bulge). ◇ Chin *zàng*, viscus, explained in this context as referring to the heart viscus or the child's viscus (uterus); *zào*, agitation, said to refer to agitation of the blood due to damage to yin or to agitation, rashness, and impatience. [27: 395] [97: 471] [67: 398] [116: 37, 150] [113: 263] [37: 359] [37: 360, 402]

visceral impediment 五脏痹 *wǔ zàng bì*: IMPEDIMENTS OF THE FIVE VISCERA.

visceral manifestation 脏象 *zàng xiàng*: The manifestation of the activity of viscera and the bowels (and construction, defense, qi, blood, fluids, essence, and spirit) in outward signs; the Chinese medical physiology of the human body in which the viscera are understood to play a central role. [6: 78] [27: 36]

visceral stroke 中脏 *zhòng zàng*: The most severe form of wind stroke characterized by sudden clouding collapse, loss of speech, and inability to close the lips with drooling from the corners of the mouth. See WIND STROKE. [26: 142] [27: 396] [97: 79]

visceral toxin 脏毒 *zàng dú*: **1.** Dysentery attributed to toxin accumulated in the viscera. **2.** Distal bleeding (bleeding remote from the anus) due to accumulated heat toxin. MED Clear heat and resolve toxin with formulas such as Pig's Intestines and Coptis Pill (*zàng lián wán*). ACU Base treatment mainly on back transport points, ST, and BL. Select ST-25 (*tiān shū*, Celestial Pivot), BL-25 (*dà cháng shū*, Large Intestine Transport), ST-37 (*shàng jù xū*, Upper Great Hollow), BL-57 (*chéng shān*, Mountain Support), SP-10 (*xuè hǎi*, Sea of Blood), and SP-9 (*yīn líng quán*, Yin Mound Spring); needle with drainage. **3.** Hard painful swollen bleeding anus. MED Treat with Stomach-Clearing Powder (*qīng wèi sǎn*) or Gentian Liver-Draining Decoction (*lóng dǎn xiè gān tāng*). ACU Base treatment mainly on BL, SP, and empirical points. Select BL-32 (*cì liáo*, Second Bone-Hole), GV-1 (*cháng qiáng*, Long Strong), BL-35 (*huì yáng*, Meeting of Yang), BL-57 (*chéng shān*, Mountain Support), Two Whites (*èr bái*), SP-5 (*shāng qiū*, Shang Hill), and SP-6 (*sān yīn jiāo*, Three Yin Intersection); needle with drainage. **4.** ANAL WELLING-ABSCESS. [26: 997] [26: 835] [46: 739] [113: 111-113] [61: 231]

viscus 脏 *zàng*: Any of the five viscera (lung, kidney, liver, heart, and spleen). See BOWELS AND VISCERA. ◇ Chin The Chinese ideogram was originally written as 藏 *cáng* meaning to store, and was later distinguished by the addition of the flesh signifier 肉 (月). Eng *viscus* is the singular form, *viscera* the plural.

viscus of fire and water 水火之脏 *shuǐ huǒ zhī zàng*: The kidney. [27: 19] [97: 132]

viscus of wind and wood 风木之脏 *fēng mù zhī zàng*: The liver. The liver belongs to wood, and like wood thrives by orderly reaching. Just as trees are vulnerable to wind, so the liver is vulnerable to diseases characterized by spasm and itching attributed to wind. See LIVER. [27: 39]

visiting 客 *kè*: Occasional, seasonal, temporary.

visiting complexion 客色 *kè sè*: See RIGHT COMPLEXION.

visiting hostility 客忤 *kè wǔ*: See CHILD VISIT-ING HOSTILITY. [27: 437] [97: 434]

visual distortion 瞀 *mào*: Deranged, flowery vision.

visual examination 望诊 *wàng zhěn*: INSPECTION.

visual lining 视衣 *shì yī*: The inner surface of the eyeball. WMC retina. ◇ Chin 视 *shì*, see, look, visual; 衣 *yī*, clothing, coat, coating. [26: 592]

vital qi 生气 *shēng qì*: **1.** The qi developing in springtime that is vital to the growth of all things. **2.** Original qi. **3.** Loosely refers to the life force. [50: 421]

voice 声音 *shēng yīn*: See LISTENING AND SMELLING EXAMINATION.

vomiting (and retching) 呕吐 *ǒu tù*: Ejection of food through the mouth. The Chinese term is composed of two characters, 呕 *ǒu*, meaning retching (sound without matter), and 吐 *tù*, meaning ejection (matter without sound). However, the combined term, as the English *vomiting*, tends to exclude retching. While retching denotes a relative absence of expelled matter, "dry retching" (*gān ǒu*) denotes its complete absence. Vomiting and retching are the manifestations of stomach qi ascending counterflow, and like nausea may occur in almost any stomach pattern—stomach heat or cold, insufficiency of stomach yin, liver-stomach disharmony, or food damage, etc. Vomiting of ingested food that has remained for several hours without undergoing transformation is called STOMACH REFLUX. Very often this assumes a pattern of "vomiting in the morning of foods ingested in the evening," or "vomiting in the evening of foods ingested in the morning." Not only food but also clear water, bitter water, phlegm-drool, and roundworm may be vomited. See entries listed below. See also VOMITUS. [26: 845] [97: 420] [6: 127]

Vomiting

COLD VOMITING (*hán ǒu*)
HEAT VOMITING (*rè ǒu*)
PHLEGM VOMITING (*tán ǒu*)
FOOD ACCUMULATION VOMITING (*shí jī ǒu tù*)

QI VOMITING (*qì ǒu*)
VOMITING OF CLEAR WATER (*tù qīng shuǐ*)
BITTER VOMITING (*ǒu kǔ*)
ACID VOMITING (*tù suān*)
WATER COUNTERFLOW (*shuǐ nì*)
VOMITING OF PHLEGM-DROOL (*ǒu tù tán xián*)

---

vomiting of bile 呕胆 *ǒu dǎn*: BITTER VOMITING.

vomiting of bitter water 呕吐苦水 *ǒu tù kǔ shuǐ*: BITTER VOMITING.

vomiting of clear water 吐清水 *tù qīng shuǐ*: Bringing up of relatively clear water fluid from the stomach; observed in spleen-stomach vacuity cold, phlegm-rheum accumulation, lodged food failing to transform, and worm disease. For diagnosis and treatment, see COLD VOMITING; PHLEGM VOMITING; WATER COUNTERFLOW; FOOD ACCUMULATION VOMITING; ROUNDWORM VOMITING. [26: 259]

vomiting of phlegm-drool 呕吐痰涎 *ǒu tù tán xián*: VOMITING with vomitus containing copious phlegm-drool; observed in phlegm and phlegm-rheum patterns such as phlegm malaria, phlegm-rheum pregnancy vomiting, and wind-phlegm dizziness. Compare EJECTION OF FOAMY DROOL. [26: 845]

vomiting of phlegm-rheum 呕吐痰饮 *ǒu tù tán yǐn*: PHLEGM VOMITING. [26: 767]

vomiting pregnancy 妊娠呕吐 *rèn shēn ǒu tù*: MALIGN OBSTRUCTION.

vomitus 呕吐物 *ǒu tù wù*: The contents of the stomach expelled through the act of vomiting. Vomitus containing phlegm and water indicates stomach phlegm-rheum, and generally forms part of a cold pattern. Vomitus containing food without sour taste or malodor indicates vacuity cold or invasion of the stomach by liver qi. Vomitus with a sour taste and malodor indicates food accumulation, stomach heat, or liver-gallbladder damp-heat. Bitter, yellow vomitus generally indicates liver-gallbladder damp-heat. Vomiting of purplish black blood can only be diagnosed by taking account of other signs. [6: 127]

vulpine mounting 狐疝 *hú shàn*: FOXY MOUNTING. ◇ Eng *vulpine*, foxy.

waist as if girthed with rope 腰如绳束 *yāo rú shéng shù*: The sensation that the waist is bound tight with a cord or rope. Waist as if girthed with rope is attributable to disease of the girdling (*dài*) vessel or to liver channel damp-heat. **Qi binding in the girdling vessel** causes pain in the sinews and flesh around the waist and in the lumbus. There may be no other signs but these, and the tongue and pulse may be normal. MED Use Liver-Regulating Powder (*tiáo gān sǎn*). ACU Base treatment mainly on GIV, LR, CV, and PC. Select GB-26 (*dài mài*, Girdling Vessel), CV-6 (*qì hǎi*, Sea of Qi), PC-6 (*nèi guān*, Inner Pass), LI-4 (*hé gǔ*, Union Valley), and LR-3 (*tài chōng*, Supreme Surge); needle with drainage. **Liver channel damp-heat** signs include scorching stabbing pain in the skin, exacerbated by friction. The patient is afraid to move, and in severe cases is afraid to breathe deeply, cough, or sneeze; however, the pain may be relieved by pressure. In addition, there are signs of liver channel damp-heat such as rib-side pain, bitter taste in the mouth, red face, tinnitus, reddish urine possibly with painful voidings, constipation, yellow tongue fur that may be thick and slimy, and a stringlike, possibly rapid pulse. MED Clear and drain liver channel damp-heat with Gentian Liver-Draining Decoction (*lóng dǎn xiè gān tāng*). ACU Base treatment mainly on GB, LR, SP, and BL. Select GB-34 (*yáng líng quán*, Yang Mound Spring), GB-43 (*xiá xī*, Pinched Ravine), LR-2 (*xíng jiān*, Moving Between), SP-9 (*yīn líng quán*, Yin Mound Spring), BL-40 (*wěi zhōng*, Bend Center), BL-37 (*yīn mén*, Gate of Abundance); and GB-31 (*fēng shì*, Wind Market); needle with drainage. Selection of points according to signs: For rib-side pain, add LR-14 (*qī mén*, Cycle Gate), GB-24 (*rì yuè*, Sun and Moon), and TB-6 (*zhī gōu*, Branch Ditch). For tinnitus, add TB-17 (*yì fēng*, Wind Screen), GB-2 (*tīng huì*, Auditory Convergence), and TB-3 (*zhōng zhǔ*, Central Islet). For constipation, add BL-25 (*dà cháng shū*, Large Intestine Transport), ST-37 (*shàng jù xū*, Upper Great Hollow), CV-12 (*zhōng wǎn*, Center Stomach Duct), and CV-6 (*qì hǎi*, Sea of Qi). [37: 390] [4: 146] [92: No. 168] [46: 595]

walking bone 骺骨 *héng gǔ*: The larger of the two bones of the lower leg. WMC The tibia. [27: 71]

wandering knee wind 膝游风 *xī yóu fēng*: CRANE'S-KNEE WIND. [26: 891]

wandering wind 游风 *yóu fēng*: RED AND WHITE WANDERING WIND.

warm 温 *wēn*: **1.** *adj.* **1a.** Mildly hot. **1b.** Of a nature tending to create mild heat. See FOUR QI. **1c.** Of a nature tending to create heat effusion. See WARM DISEASE. **2.** *vb.* **2a.** (In physiology) to keep warm. **2b.** (Through treatment) to restore warmth to. See WARMING.

warm acrid exterior resolution 辛温解表 *xīn wēn jiě biǎo*: See RESOLVING THE EXTERIOR WITH WARMTH AND ACRIDITY.

warm disease 温病 *wēn bìng*: Any of various heat (febrile) diseases characterized by rapid onset and shifts, pronounced heat signs, and a tendency to form dryness and damage yin. **History:** The concept of warm disease was first mentioned in *The Inner Canon* (*nèi jīng*). For example, *Elementary Questions* (*sù wèn, shēng qì tōng tiān lùn*) states, "Damage by cold in winter necessarily engenders warm disease in the spring." Zhang Ji (Zhong-Jing) of the Han Dynasty in *On Cold Damage and Miscellaneous Diseases* (*shāng hán zá bìng lùn*) mentions warm disease, stating, for example, "Greater yang (*tài yáng*) disease with heat effusion and cough and without aversion to cold is warm disease. If sweating is applied, and there is generalized heat [effusion], this is wind warmth." However, the concept of warm disease was not central to his systematic presentation of externally contracted disease which placed the emphasis on wind and cold as the major causes of these diseases. Zhang Ji's theories centuries after in the Sung Dynasty were to become the focus of the cold damage school, whereas the concept of warm disease was to become the focus of a rival school, the warm disease school. In the Sui-Tang Period, *The Origin and Indicators of Disease* (*zhū bìng yuán hòu lùn*) mentions warm diseases, their causes, patterns, and major principles of treatment. Successive generations of doctors wrote about warm disease, and in the Ming Dynasty writings on the subject became more prolific. This development is attributable on the one hand to the opening up of the south of China where febrile diseases tended to be of a different nature than in the north, and on the other to pestilences arising as a result of wars. In this period, Wu You-Xing in *On Warm Epidemics* (*wēn yì lùn*) explained in detail the laws governing the origin, development and pattern identification of warm epidemics. Notably, he posed the etiological notion of a contagious *perverse qi* (戾气 *lì qì*). This notion represented a break away from the traditional conception of febrile diseases being caused by climatic influences (e.g., the wind and cold of the cold damage school), and made a great contribution to the foundation of the doctrine of warm diseases that developed later. In the Qing Dynasty, a comprehensive doctrine of warm diseases began to emerge. Ye Tian-Shi, in *On Warm Heat* (*wēn rè lùn*), introduced the four-aspect (construction, qi, construction, and blood) pattern identification system. Xue Xue, in *Systematized Identification of Damp-Heat* (*shī rè tiáo biàn*), described in detail damp-heat disease patterns. Wu Ju-Tong, in *Systematized Identification of Warm Diseases* (*wēn bìng tiáo biàn*), posed the notion of triple-burner pattern identification in the treatment of warm and damp-heat diseases. Finally, Wang Shi-Xiong, in *Warp and Weft of Warm Heat* (*wēn rè jīng wěi*), brought together all the theories of his predecessors in a complete doctrine of warm diseases. **Theory:** The doctrine of warm diseases considers warm disease to embrace all externally contracted heat (febrile) diseases. All such diseases have heat as a common feature and consequently they show a tendency toward dryness formation and a resultant damage to yin. Although the doctrine identifies many different diseases, the major classifications are wind warmth, damp warmth, and warm heat. (1) Wind warmth is characterized by heat effusion, and signs of exuberant lung or stomach heat such as cough, rapid breathing, flaring nostrils, and thirst. (2) Damp warmth is characterized by persistent heat effusion and signs of obstruction and stagnation caused by dampness, such as oppression in the chest, nausea, diminished appetite, abdominal distention, constipation or diarrhea, and slimy tongue fur. (3) Warm heat is characterized by high fever, red complexion, thirst, maculopapular eruptions, heart vexation and, in severe cases, clouded spirit. Defense, qi, construction, and blood are the four aspects used for identification and treatment of warm disease patterns. They are used to explain the origin and development of externally contracted heat (febrile) diseases; like the six channels of the doctrine of cold damage, they explain the degree of penetration, severity, and acuteness of diseases. In *On Warm Heat* (*wēn rè lùn*), Ye Tian-Shi states, "The general conception [of the doctrine of warm diseases] is that qi comes after defense and that blood comes after construction. When disease affects defense, sweating can be administered. Only when it reaches the qi aspect can qi-clearing treatment be prescribed. When it enters construction, treatment involves outthrusting heat to the qi aspect. Finally, when it reaches blood and causes depletion and frenetic movement, treatment involves cooling

and dissipating the blood." These lines represent the general outline of the four-aspect pattern identification and treatment system of the doctrine of warm diseases. See entries listed below. See also FOUR-ASPECT PATTERN IDENTIFICATION; TRIPLE BURNER PATTERN IDENTIFICATION. [27: 448] [97: 576] [26: 665] [6: 232]

Warm Disease

SPRING WARMTH (*chūn wēn*)
WIND WARMTH (*fēng wēn*)
SUMMERHEAT WARMTH (*shǔ wēn*)
LATENT SUMMERHEAT (*fú shǔ*)
DAMP WARMTH (*shī wēn*)
WINTER WARMTH (*dōng wēn*)
WARM EPIDEMIC (*wēn yì*)
WARM TOXIN (*wēn dú*)
WARM MALARIA (*wēn nüè*)
AUTUMN DRYNESS (*qiū wēn*)
LATENT QI WARM DISEASE (*fú qì wēn bìng*)
LATE EMERGENCE (*wǎn fā*)

---

warm dryness 温燥 *wēn zào*: Disease caused by contraction of the warm dryness evil and resultant scorching of pulmonary liquid; autumn dryness with marked heat signs. Warm dryness begins with headache, heat effusion, dry cough without phlegm, expectoration of thin sticky phlegm, qi counterflow panting, dry throat, sore throat, dry nose and lips, oppression in the chest and rib-side pain, tongue red at the margins with thin white tongue fur. ｜MED｜ Clear the lung and moisten dryness. Use Mulberry Leaf and Apricot Kernel Decoction (*sāng xìng tāng*) for mild cases and Dryness-Clearing Lung-Rescuing Decoction (*qīng zào jiù fèi tāng*) for severe cases. See AUTUMN DRYNESS; DRYNESS EVIL INVADING THE LUNG. [27: 352] [27: 353] [97: 576]

warm epidemic 温疫 *wēn yì*: SCOURGE EPIDEMIC.

warm evil 温邪 *wēn xié*: Any evil causing warm heat disease, including SPRING WARMTH, WIND WARMTH, SUMMERHEAT WARMTH, LATENT SUMMERHEAT, DAMP WARMTH, AUTUMN DRYNESS, WINTER WARMTH, WARM EPIDEMIC, WARM TOXIN, WARM MALARIA. *On Warm Heat* (*wēn rè lùn*) states, "Warm evil contracted in the upper body first invades the lung." [26: 664] [27: 115] [97: 575]

warm evil invading the lung 温邪犯肺 *wēn xié fàn fèi*: Warm heat disease characterized by cough, heat effusion, thirst, sometimes a sore swollen throat, a tongue that is red at the margins or tip, and a rapid floating pulse. ｜WMC｜ upper respiratory tract infection, acute bronchitis, or acute tonsillitis. [27: 159] [97: 578]

warm heat 温热 *wēn rè*: **1.** Warm evil. **2.** Warm disease characterized by the presence of heat signs and the absence of dampness signs. [27: 115] [97: 576]

warm heat disease 温热病 *wēn rè bìng*: **1.** Any WARM DISEASE or HEAT DISEASE. **2.** Warm disease pattern of wind combined with warmth. [26: 667]

Warming

WARMING THE CENTER AND DISSIPATING COLD (*wēn zhōng sàn hán*)

RETURNING YANG AND STEMMING COUNTER-FLOW (*huí yáng jiù nì*)

WARMING YANG AND DISINHIBITING WATER (*wēn yáng lì shuǐ*)

WARMING THE CHANNELS AND DISSIPATING COLD (*wēn jīng sàn hán*)

---

warming 温法 *wēn fǎ*: One of the EIGHT METHODS. The method of treating cold patterns. Warming involves the use of warm or hot medicinals to supplement yang qi and expel cold evil. Medicinals used in the method of warming are usually referred to as *interior-warming medicinals*. These are listed below. Warming is used in the treatment of interior cold patterns. (1) Cold evil invading the interior, and inhibiting yang qi, and causing retching and diarrhea, cold and pain in the stomach duct and abdomen, cold limbs and aversion to cold, and other signs of spleen-stomach vacuity and interior cold are treated by warming the center and dissipating cold. (2) Yang collapse with aversion to cold and curled-up lying posture, reversal cold of the four limbs, sweating, somber white complexion, and a faint fine pulse or rapid vacuous pulse is treated by returning yang and stemming counterflow. (3) Water-damp flood from yang qi vacuity, characterized by water swelling, is treated by warming yang and disinhibiting water.

Interior-Warming Medicinals

附子 (*fù zǐ*) aconite (Aconiti Tuber Laterale)

白附片 (*bái fù piàn*) white sliced aconite (Aconiti Tuber Laterale Album)

黑顺片 (*hēi shùn piàn*) black sliced aconite (Aconiti Tuber Laterale Denigratum)

熟附子 (*shú fù zǐ*) cooked aconite (Aconiti Tuber Laterale Conquitum)

咸附子 (*xián fù zǐ*) salted aconite (Aconiti Tuber Laterale Salsum)

川乌头 (*chuān wū tóu*) aconite main tuber (Aconiti Tuber)

草乌头 (*cǎo wū tóu*) wild aconite (Aconiti Tsao-Wu-Tou Tuber)

肉桂 (*ròu guì*) cinnamon bark (Cinnamomi Cortex)

干姜 (*gān jiāng*) dried ginger (Zingiberis Rhizoma Exsiccatum)

炮姜 (*páo jiāng*) blast-fried ginger (Zingiberis Rhizoma Tostum)

吴茱萸 (*wú zhū yú*) evodia (Evodiae Fructus)

细辛 (*xì xīn*) asarum (Asiasari Herba cum Radice)

花椒 (*huā jiāo*) zanthoxylum (Zanthoxyli Pericarpium)

高良姜 (*gāo liáng jiāng*) lesser galangal (Alpiniae Officinarum Rhizoma)

椒目 (*jiāo mù*) zanthoxylum seed (Zanthoxyli Semen)

丁香 (*dīng xiāng*) clove (Caryophylli Flos)

红豆蔻 (*hóng dòu kòu*) galangal fruit (Alpiniae Galangae Fructus)

母丁香 (*mǔ dīng xiāng*) clove fruit (Caryophylli Fructus)

胡椒 (*hú jiāo*) pepper (Piperis Fructus)

豆豉姜 (*dòu chǐ jiāng*) litsea (Litseae Rhizoma et Radix)

荜茇 (*bì bá*) long pepper (Piperis Longi Fructus)

荜澄茄 (*bì chéng qié*) cubeb (Cubebae Fructus)

茴香 (*huí xiāng*) fennel (Foeniculi Fructus)

八角茴香 (*bā jiǎo huí xiāng*) star anise (Anisi Stellati Fructus)

---

(4) Cold evil invading the channels, causing pain in the sinews and bones, and hypertonicity with inhibited bending and stretching is treated by freeing and warming the channels. In acumoxatherapy, warming is achieved through moxibustion. Warming methods are listed above, and warming medicinals are listed below. [6: 258] [27: 277] [97: 575]

warming and supplementing kidney yang 温补肾阳 *wēn bǔ shèn yáng*: WARMING AND SUPPLEMENTING THE LIFE GATE.

warming and supplementing the life gate 温补命门 *wēn bǔ mìng mén*: *Synonyms: warming and supplementing kidney yang; warming the kidney; warming the water viscus.* A method of treatment used to restore (spleen and) kidney yang qi in the treatment of insufficiency of the life gate fire with early morning diarrhea, abdominal pain and rumbling intestines, cold limbs, pale tongue with white fur, and slow sunken pulse. [MED] The method of warming and supplementing the life gate employs yang-invigorating fire-supplementing medicinals. Appropriate formulas include Four Spirits Pill (*sì shén wán*) and Right-Restoring [Life Gate] Pill (*yòu guī wán*). [ACU] Base treatment mainly on KI, GV, back transport points, and CV. Select BL-23 (*shèn shū*, Kidney Transport), GV-4 (*mìng mén*, Life Gate), CV-4 (*guān yuán*, Pass Head), and KI-3 (*tài xī*, Great Ravine); needle with supplementation and add moxa. [26: 665] [27: 263] [97: 578] [113: 14] [46: 588]

warming and transforming 温化 *wēn huà*: Warming and transforming is the principle for treating phlegm-rheum. *Essential Prescriptions of the Golden Coffer* (*jīn guì yào lüè*) states, "Disease of phlegm-rheum should be harmonized with warm medicinals." See WARMING YANG AND TRANSFORMING RHEUM, WARMING THE LUNG AND TRANSFORMING RHEUM, WARMING AND TRANSFORMING WATER-DAMP.

warming and transforming cold phlegm 温化寒痰 *wēn huà hán tán*: WARMING THE LUNG AND TRANSFORMING RHEUM.

warming and transforming cold rheum 温化寒饮 *wēn huà hán yǐn*: WARMING THE LUNG AND TRANSFORMING RHEUM.

warming and transforming static blood 温化祛瘀 *wēn huà qū yū*: See WARMING THE BLOOD.[2]

warming and transforming water-damp 温化水湿 *wēn huà shuǐ shī*: A method of treating PHLEGM-RHEUM, WATER SWELLING, IMPEDIMENT (*bì*) patterns and COLD-DAMP LEG QI arising when vacuous yang fails to transform water and dampness forms with cold. Warming and transforming water-damp uses hot acrid medicinals that warm and free yang qi, such as cinnamon twig (*guì zhī*) and aconite (*fù zǐ*), combined with an appropriate amount of dampness-disinhibiting medicinals such as poria (*fú líng*) and ovate atractylodes (*bái zhú*) to eliminate water-damp. Representative formulas include Fish Poison Yam Clear-Turbid Separation Beverage (*bì xiè fēn qīng yǐn*), Poria (Hoelen), Cinnamon Twig, Ovate Atractylodes, and Licorice Decoction (*líng guì zhú gān tāng*), Licorice, Dried Ginger, Poria (Hoelen), and Ovate Atractylodes Decoction (*gān cǎo gān jiāng fú líng bái zhú tāng*), Spleen-Firming Beverage (*shí pí yǐn*), and True Warrior Decoction (*zhēn wǔ tāng*). ACU Base treatment mainly on CV and back transport points. Select CV-9 (*shuǐ fēn*, Water Divide), CV-6 (*qì hǎi*, Sea of Qi), BL-20 (*pí shū*, Spleen Transport), BL-23 (*shèn shū*, Kidney Transport), ST-36 (*zú sān lǐ*, Leg Three Li), SP-6 (*sān yīn jiāo*, Three Yin Intersection), and BL-39 (*wěi yáng*, Bend Yang); needle with drainage and add moxa. Compare WARMING YANG AND DISINHIBITING DAMPNESS. [70: 336] [16: 515] [46: 597] [113: 19, 184]

warming heart yang 温心阳 *wēn xīn yáng*: A method of treatment used to address heart yang vacuity characterized by lassitude of spirit, dizziness, heart palpitations or fearful throbbing, and pronounced cold signs, such as gray or green-blue or purple complexion and reversal cold of the limbs. MED Formulas that warm heart yang include Cinnamon Twig, Licorice, Dragon Bone, and Oyster Shell Decoction (*guì zhī gān cǎo lóng gǔ mǔ lì tāng*) to which ginseng (*rén shēn*) and aconite (*fù zǐ*) can be added in severe cases. ACU Base treatment mainly on back transport points, CV, and HT. Select BL-15 (*xīn shū*, Heart Transport), CV-14 (*jù què*, Great Tower Gate), CV-17 (*shān zhōng*, Chest Center), and HT-7 (*shén mén*, Spirit Gate); needle with supplementation and add moxa. [6: 171]

warming the blood 温血 *wēn xuè*: A method of treatment used to address cold in the blood aspect. It includes warming and nourishing the blood aspect and warming and transforming static blood. **1. Warming and nourishing the blood aspect:** To treat flooding and spotting in females and blood ejection in males, with pale tongue, forceless vacuous pulse, and pale lusterless nails. MED Use formulas such as Perfect Major Supplementation Decoction (*shí quán dà bǔ tāng*). ACU Base treatment mainly on back transport points, SP, ST, and LR. Select BL-20 (*pí shū*, Spleen Transport), BL-21 (*wèi shū*, Stomach Transport), ST-36 (*zú sān lǐ*, Leg Three Li), SP-6 (*sān yīn jiāo*, Three Yin Intersection), and LR-3 (*tài chōng*, Supreme Surge); needle with supplementation and add moxa. **2. Warming and transforming static blood:** To treat cold-induced static blood manifesting in menstrual block or menstrual irregularities with dull pale menstrual flow, purple speckles on the tongue, and a tight sunken pulse. MED Agents that warm and transform static blood include tangkuei (*dāng guī*), white peony (*bái sháo yào*), ligusticum (*chuān xiōng*), cinnamon twig (*guì zhī*), moutan (*mǔ dān pí*), and fresh ginger (*shēng jiāng*). ACU Base treatment mainly on LR and SP. Select BL-17 (*gé shū*, Diaphragm Transport), SP-10 (*xuè hǎi*, Sea of Blood), LI-4 (*hé gǔ*, Union Valley), LR-3 (*tài chōng*, Supreme Surge), and SP-6 (*sān yīn jiāo*, Three Yin Intersection), as main points; needle with even supplementation and drainage and add moxa. For menstrual problems, add CV-3 (*zhōng jí*, Central Pole), SP-8 (*dì jī*, Earth's Crux), and ST-29 (*guī lái*, Return). See DISPELLING STASIS AND QUICKENING THE BLOOD. See also MENSTRUAL IRREGULARITIES; MENSTRUAL PAIN. [26: 663] [27: 274] [27: 274] [97: 575]

warming the center and dispelling cold 温中祛寒 *wēn zhōng qū hán*: WARMING THE CENTER AND DISSIPATING COLD. [26: 663] [27: 277] [97: 577]

warming the center and dissipating cold 温中散寒 *wēn zhōng sàn hán*: Synonym: *warming the center and dispelling cold*; *warming the spleen*. A method of treatment used to treat cold in constitutional yang vacuity, spleen-stomach vacuity cold, or external cold entering the interior, characterized by a moist white tongue fur, moderate soggy or slow sunken pulse, physical debilitation and fatigued spirit, aversion to cold, diarrhea, abdominal pain that likes pressure and heat, and stomach pain and vomiting of clear fluid. [MED] Treatment is based on center-warming medicinals such as dried ginger (*gān jiāng*), blast-fried ginger (*páo jiāng*), lesser galangal (*gāo liáng jiāng*), and zanthoxylum (*huā jiāo*), combined with medicinals that fortify the spleen and boost the stomach such as ovate atractylodes (*bái zhú*), poria (*fú líng*), and mix-fried licorice (*gān cǎo*). Where cold signs are particularly pronounced, yang-warming medicinals such as aconite (*fù zǐ*) and cinnamon bark (*ròu guì*) may be added. Great Rectifying Powder (*dà shùn sǎn*) dissipates cold and relieves pain. Center-Rectifying Pill (*lǐ zhōng wán*) warms the spleen and checks diarrhea, and Evodia Decoction (*wú zhū yú tāng*) warms the stomach and checks vomiting. [ACU] Base treatment mainly on CV and ST. Select as main points CV-12 (*zhōng wǎn*, Center Stomach Duct), CV-6 (*qì hǎi*, Sea of Qi), ST-36 (*zú sān lǐ*, Leg Three Li), BL-20 (*pí shū*, Spleen Transport), BL-21 (*wèi shū*, Stomach Transport), and CV-4 (*guān yuán*, Pass Head); needle with supplementation and add moxa. For pronounced diarrhea, moxa may be applied at the FIVE PILLAR POINTS, or the CROSS MOXA method can be used. Compare WARMING THE SPLEEN; WARMING THE STOMACH. [6: 256]

warming the channels and dispelling cold 温经祛寒 *wēn jīng qū hán*: WARMING THE CHANNELS AND DISSIPATING COLD. [27: 277] [97: 258]

warming the channels and dissipating cold 温经散寒 *wēn jīng sàn hán*: Synonym: *warming the channels and dispelling cold.* A method of treatment used to address wind-cold-damp impediment (*bì*) with pronounced cold signs, such as pain in the joints relieved by warmth and inhibited bending and stretching, using channel-warming medicinals such as aconite main tuber (*chuān wū tóu*), cinnamon twig (*guì zhī*), scorpion (*quán xiē*), and duhuo (*dú huó*). In cases with longer history, combinations include blood-quickening stasis-transforming medicinals as well as bone and sinew strengthening medicinals. Patients with weak constitutions may be given combinations that include blood-nourishing qi-boosting medicinals such as tangkuei (*dāng guī*), white peony (*bái sháo yào*), astragalus (*huáng qí*), and codonopsis (*dǎng shēn*). Commonly used channel-warming cold-dissipating formulas include Aconite Main Tuber Decoction (*wū tóu tāng*) and Tangkuei Counterflow Cold Decoction (*dāng guī sì nì tāng*). [ACU] Base treatment mainly on ouch points (*ā shì xué*), or select points on the affected channel. Use moxa, needle retention, or warm needle technique.

warming the gallbladder and quieting the spirit 温胆安神 *wēn dǎn ān shén*: A method of treatment used to address gallbladder vacuity causing vacuity vexation and insomnia. [MED] Gallbladder-Warming Decoction (*wēn dǎn tāng*). [50: 1567]

warming the kidney 温肾 *wēn shèn*: WARMING AND SUPPLEMENTING KIDNEY YANG. [27: 287]

warming the kidney and disinhibiting water 温肾利水 *wēn shèn lì shuǐ*: A method of treatment used to address kidney yang vacuity water swelling. When the kidney is vacuous, the transformative action is inhibited; hence water-damp collects internally causing swelling of the limbs, somber white complexion, cold aching lumbus, short voidings of urine, pale tongue with thin white fur, and sunken fine weak pulse. [MED] A representative kidney-warming water disinhibiting formula is Life Saver Kidney Qi Pill (*jì shēng shèn qì wán*). [ACU] Base treatment mainly on back transport points, CV, GV, and KI. Select BL-23 (*shèn shū*, Kidney Transport), GV-4 (*mìng mén*, Life Gate), CV-9 (*shuǐ fēn*, Water Divide), CV-6 (*qì hǎi*, Sea of Qi), KI-7 (*fù liū*, Recover Flow), ST-36 (*zú sān lǐ*, Leg Three Li), and SP-6 (*sān yīn jiāo*, Three Yin Intersection); needle with supplementation and add moxa. [26: 665] [113: 184, 186] [27: 261] [97: 578]

warming the kidney to promote qi absorption 温肾纳气 *wēn shèn nà qì*: See SUPPLEMENTING THE KIDNEY TO PROMOTE QI ABSORPTION. [6: 194]

warming the liver 暖肝 *nuǎn gān*: A method of treatment used to warm and supplement the liver and kidney and to move qi and expel cold in the treatment of liver-kidney yin cold with smaller-abdominal pain or mounting qi (*shàn qì*). A commonly used liver-warming formula is Liver-Warming Brew (*nuǎn gān jiān*). [26: 789]

warming the lung and expelling rheum 温肺逐饮 *wēn fèi zhú yǐn*: WARMING THE LUNG AND TRANSFORMING RHEUM. [25: 306]

warming the lung and transforming phlegm 温肺化痰 *wēn fèi huà tán*: WARMING THE LUNG AND TRANSFORMING RHEUM.

warming the lung and transforming rheum 温肺化饮 *wēn fèi huà yǐn*: Synonym: *warming the lung and expelling rheum*; *warming the lung and transforming phlegm*; *warming and transforming cold phlegm*; *warming and transforming cold rheum*. A method of treatment used to address cold rheum lying latent in the lung characterized by cough, counterflow panting with fullness that prevents the patient from lying down, copious foamy white phlegm, and swelling of the face and instep, occurring in episodes brought on by exposure to cold. [MED] A representative lung-warming rheum-transforming formula is Minor Green-Blue Dragon Decoction (*xiǎo qīng lóng tāng*). Others include Poria (Hoelen), Licorice, Schisandra, Ginger, and Asarum Decoction (*líng gān wǔ wèi jiāng xīn tāng*), Belamcanda and Ephedra Decoction (*shè gān má huáng tāng*) and Phlegm-Rheum Pill (*tán yǐn wán*). ACU Base treatment mainly on CV, ST, and LI. Select BL-13 (*fèi shū*, Lung Transport), LU-9 (*tài yuān*, Great Abyss), CV-12 (*zhōng wǎn*, Center Stomach Duct), ST-36 (*zú sān lǐ*, Leg Three Li), ST-40 (*fēng lóng*, Bountiful Bulge), and LI-4 (*hé gǔ*, Union Valley); needle with even supplementation and drainage and large amounts of moxa. See COLD RHEUM LYING LATENT IN THE LUNG; PHLEGM-RHEUM. [80: 151] [46: 653]

warming the spleen 温脾 *wēn pí*: A method of treatment used to address spleen vacuity cold, characterized by abdominal distention, reduced food intake, and possibly diarrhea or generalized water swelling, or, in women, copious thin white vaginal discharge. MED A representative spleen-warming formula is Center-Rectifying Decoction (*lǐ zhōng tāng*). ACU Base treatment mainly on CV, SP, and ST. Select CV-12 (*zhōng wǎn*, Center Stomach Duct), CV-6 (*qì hǎi*, Sea of Qi), ST-36 (*zú sān lǐ*, Leg Three Li), BL-20 (*pí shū*, Spleen Transport), BL-21 (*wèi shū*, Stomach Transport), SP-6 (*sān yīn jiāo*, Three Yin Intersection), and SP-4 (*gōng sūn*, Yellow Emperor); needle with supplementation and large amounts of moxa. Compare WARMING THE CENTER AND DISSIPATING COLD. [27: 278]

warming the stomach 暖胃 *nuǎn wèi*, 温胃 *wēn wèi*: A method of treatment used to address stomach cold, characterized by distention and cold pain exacerbated by drinking cold drinks, by vomiting of clear water, or vomiting after eating, and by a glossy white tongue fur and forceless fine sunken pulse. MED Stomach-warming medicinals include lesser galangal (*gāo liáng jiāng*), fresh ginger (*shēng jiāng*) or dried ginger (*gān jiāng*), evodia (*wú zhū yú*), aquilaria (*chén xiāng*), cyperus (*xiāng fù zǐ*), cinnamon twig (*guì zhī*), aconite (*fù zǐ*), and clove (*dīng xiāng*). Use Lesser Galangal and Cyperus Pill (*liáng fù wán*), Evodia Decoction (*wú zhū yú tāng*), or Clove Powder (*dīng xiāng sǎn*). ACU Base treatment mainly on CV and ST. Select CV-12 (*zhōng wǎn*, Center Stomach Duct), CV-6 (*qì hǎi*, Sea of Qi), ST-36 (*zú sān lǐ*, Leg Three Li), and BL-21 (*wèi shū*, Stomach Transport); needle with supplementation and large amounts of moxa. Compare WARMING THE CENTER AND DISSIPATING COLD. [27: 277] [57: 119]

warming the stomach and checking vomiting 温胃止呕 *wēn wèi zhǐ ǒu*: A method of treatment used to address vomiting due to stomach qi vacuity cold. See COLD VOMITING.

warming the stomach and dissipating cold 温胃散寒 *wēn wèi sàn hán*: WARMING THE STOMACH.

warming the stomach and fortifying the center 温胃健中 *wēn wèi jiàn zhōng*: A method of treatment used to address stomach qi vacuity cold with dull stomach duct pain that lessens after eating, vomiting of clear water, diarrhea, pale tongue, and fine pulse. MED A representative stomach-warming center-fortifying formula is Astragalus Center-Fortifying Decoction (*huáng qí jiàn zhōng tāng*). For pronounced cold, cooked aconite (*shú fù zǐ*), dried ginger (*gān jiāng*), evodia (*wú zhū yú*), lesser galangal (*gāo liáng jiāng*), and aquilaria (*chén xiāng*) can be used to dispel cold. ACU Base treatment mainly on CV, back transport points, and ST. Select CV-12 (*zhōng wǎn*, Center Stomach Duct), CV-6 (*qì hǎi*, Sea of Qi), CV-4 (*guān yuán*, Pass Head), ST-36 (*zú sān lǐ*, Leg Three Li), BL-20 (*pí shū*, Spleen Transport), and BL-21 (*wèi shū*, Stomach Transport); needle with supplementation and large amounts of moxa. [27: 279] [43: 271]

warming the water viscus 温水脏 *wēn shuǐ zàng*: Warming and supplementing the life gate fire. See WATER VISCUS. [27: 287]

warming yang and disinhibiting dampness 温阳利湿 *wēn yáng lì shī*: Synonym: *promoting qi transformation and disinhibiting water*. A method of treatment used to address yang qi obstructed by water-cold causing inhibited urination. When a patient has internal collection of water-damp and cold in the exterior, yang qi is blocked by water-cold, causing inhibited urination, headache, mild heat effusion, heart vexation, thirst, vomiting of ingested fluids, a slimy white tongue fur and a floating pulse. MED Use Poria (Hoelen) Five Powder (*wǔ líng sǎn*), which makes use of cinnamon twig (*guì zhī*) to warm yang and promote qi transformation, and Poria (Hoelen) Four Powder (*sì líng sǎn*) to move dampness and disinhibit water. ACU Base treatment mainly on CV, back transport points, SP, and ST. Select BL-11 (*dà zhù*, Great Shuttle), LI-4 (*hé gǔ*, Union Valley), CV-9 (*shuǐ fēn*, Water Divide), BL-22 (*sān jiāo shū*, Triple Burner Transport), SP-9 (*yīn líng quán*, Yin Mound Spring) and ST-36 (*zú sān lǐ*, Leg Three Li); needle with drainage. [50: 1567] [27: 261] [97: 578] [46: 597] [113: 19, 183]

warming yang and transforming rheum 温阳化饮 *wēn yáng huà yǐn*: A method of treatment used to address phlegm-rheum (FLOWING RHEUM) in the stomach and intestines marked by reduced appetite, emaciation in normally obese people, rumbling intestines, sloppy stool, heart palpitations, shortness of breath, and vomiting of foamy drool. [MED] Use formulas such as Poria (Hoelen), Cinnamon Twig, Ovate Atractylodes, and Licorice Decoction (*líng guì zhú gān tāng*) or Golden Coffer Kidney Qi Pill (*jīn guì shèn qì wán*). [ACU] Base treatment mainly on CV and ST. Select CV-12 (*zhōng wǎn*, Center Stomach Duct), ST-36 (*zú sān lǐ*, Leg Three Li), ST-40 (*fēng lóng*, Bountiful Bulge), BL-43 (*gāo huāng shū*, Gao-Huang Transport), ST-25 (*tiān shū*, Celestial Pivot), and CV-6 (*qì hǎi*, Sea of Qi); needle with supplementation and large amounts of moxa. [26: 766][46: 597]

warm malaria 温疟 *wēn nüè*: Synonym: *kidney channel malaria*. MALARIA characterized by generalized heat [effusion], with aversion to cold less pronounced than heat effusion, headache, thirst with taking of fluids, constipation and reddish urine, inhibited sweating, joint pain, red tongue with yellow fur, and a rapid stringlike pulse. Comparison: *Pure-heat malaria* is essentially the same as warm malaria, but differs in degree of severity. Warm malaria is characterized by heat effusion followed by aversion to cold, with pronounced heat effusion and mild aversion to cold. Pure-heat malaria is characterized by heat effusion without aversion to cold. [MED] Clear heat and resolve the flesh; dispel evil and interrupt malaria. Use White Tiger Decoction Plus Cinnamon Twig (*bái hǔ jiā guì zhī tāng*) plus sweet wormwood (*qīng hāo*) to dispel evil and interrupt malaria, and bupleurum (*chái hú*) to harmonize. [ACU] Base treatment mainly on GV, PC, SI, and LI. Select GV-14 (*dà zhuī*, Great Hammer), GV-13 (*táo dào*, Kiln Path), PC-5 (*jiān shǐ*, Intermediary Courier), SI-3 (*hòu xī*, Back Ravine), CV-12 (*zhōng wǎn*, Center Stomach Duct), and LI-4 (*hé gǔ*, Union Valley); needle with drainage. For principles and methods of treatment see MALARIA. [26: 666] [50: 1562] [27: 358] [97: 576] [37: 263]

warm needling 温针 *wēn zhēn*: Burning moxa on the handle of an acupuncture needle inserted in the body. This method, whereby the needle conducts the heat into the flesh, is appropriate for vacuity cold diseases and wind-damp impediment (*bì*) patterns. Method: Warm needling is done by first inserting the needle and placing a small piece of paper or aluminum foil around the needle. (Make a hole in the center of the piece of paper.) Moxa wool is then wrapped around the wire handle and lit. The paper will catch any ashes. The moxa is allowed to burn completely, and when no more heat radiates from the handle, the paper and moxa can be removed, and the needle withdrawn. One common practice is to snip a small cylindrical piece of moxa pole, and press a pointed object such as a pencil into the center of the cylinder, thus forming a hole that allows the moxa to be placed on the handle of the needle. This latter method is safer

and more convenient because the ash is firmer and less likely to fall from the handle. [27: 329] [97: 575]

warm opening 温开 *wēn kāi*: EXPELLING COLD AND OPENING THE ORIFICES.

warm precipitation 温下 *wēn xià*: A method of precipitation applied to cold-natured accumulation and stagnation forming interior repletion patterns often referred to as COLD BIND, and characterized by constipation, with abdominal fullness, cold extremities, white slimy tongue fur, and sunken stringlike or slow sunken pulse. [MED] Warm precipitation makes use of warm precipitating medicinals like croton (*bā dòu*), or uses warm or hot medicinals in combination with cold ones, such as aconite (*fù zǐ*) and asarum (*xì xīn*) with rhubarb (*dà huáng*). Representative formulas include Three Agents Emergency Pill (*sān wù bèi jí wán*) and Rhubarb and Aconite Decoction (*dà huáng fù zǐ tāng*). [ACU] Base treatment on the alarm, back transport, and lower uniting points of LI, and on CV, SP, KI, and other back transport points. Select BL-25 (*dà cháng shū*, Large Intestine Transport), ST-25 (*tiān shū*, Celestial Pivot), ST-37 (*shàng jù xū*, Upper Great Hollow), CV-6 (*qì hǎi*, Sea of Qi), KI-6 (*zhào hǎi*, Shining Sea), KI-18 (*shí guān*, Stone Pass), BL-23 (*shèn shū*, Kidney Transport), and CV-4 (*guān yuán*, Pass Head); needle with supplementation and add moxa. Apply moxa on salt or ginger at CV-8 (*shén què*, Spirit Gate Tower). [26: 663] [27: 265] [97: 575] [46: 671] [37: 325]

warmth 温 *wēn*: **1.** The quality or state of being warm. **2.** WARM EVIL. **3.** One of the FOUR QI (heat, cold, warmth, coolness) of medicinals, used in the treatment of cold patterns.

warm toxin 温毒 *wēn dú*: Synonym: *heat toxin; seasonal toxin*. Any febrile disease attributable to contraction of warm evil and heat toxin, usually occurring in the winter or spring. Warm toxin is characterized by sudden high fever and shivering, headache, nausea, vexation and agitation, thirst, red or crimson tongue with yellow fur, and a surging rapid pulse. As it continues its development, a red swollen head and face, swollen jowls, sore swollen throat with white putrescence, or maculopapular eruptions may be observed. [WMC] mumps, erysipelas of the head and face, scarlet fever, exanthematous typhus. [MED] Clear heat and resolve toxin with formulas such as Universal Aid Toxin-Dispersing Beverage (*pǔ jì xiāo dú yǐn*), Three Yellows and Gypsum Decoction (*sān huáng shí gāo tāng*), or Coptis Toxin-Resolving Decoction (*huáng lián jiě dú tāng*). If heat enters construction-blood, cool the blood and resolve toxin with Scourge-Clearing Toxin-Vanquishing Beverage (*qīng wēn bài dú yǐn*). [ACU] Base treatment mainly on LI, ST, and LU. Select GV-14 (*dà zhuī*, Great Hammer), LI-11 (*qū chí*, Pool at the Bend), LI-4 (*hé gǔ*, Union Valley), TB-5 (*wài guān*, Outer Pass), BL-40 (*wěi zhōng*, Bend Center), ST-43 (*xiàn gǔ*, Sunken Valley), and LU-10 (*yú jì*, Fish Border); needle with drainage, and prick the Twelve Well Points (*shí èr jīng xué*) to bleed. For heat entering yin blood, add SP-6 (*sān yīn jiāo*, Three Yin Intersection), SP-10 (*xuè hǎi*, Sea of Blood), LR-2 (*xíng jiān*, Moving Between), PC-7 (*dà líng*, Great Mound), and HT-7 (*shén mén*, Spirit Gate); needle with drainage or bloodletting. See MASSIVE HEAD SCOURGE; MUMPS. [26: 664] [27: 353] [97: 575] [46: 732]

Warring States 战国 *zhàn guó*: The name of a dynastic period (475–221 B.C.).

wart 疣 *yóu*, 疣疮 *yóu chuāng*: From *The Magic Pivot* (*líng shū, jīng mài*). A skin-colored, white or dirty yellowish nonsuppurating growth up to the size of a soybean, like the center of a daisy or similar flower in texture, dry and light in substance, slightly painful under pressure, tending to bleed easily when knocked or grazed, and occurring singly or multiply on the back, the back of the fingers, or scalp; attributed to wind evil contending in the skin or to liver vacuity and blood dryness and sinew qi lacking in luxuriance. WMC verruca vulgaris (common wart). MED Rub with chicken's gizzard lining (*jī nèi jīn*) or crushed brucea (*yā dǎn zǐ*). ACU Treat with moxa. [26: 401] [26: 80] [27: 485] [97: 427]

washing 洗 *xǐ*: To remove earth or unwanted parts by dipping, rubbing, or scrubbing in water. With the exception of flowers, whose active constituents are easily lost in water, most materials are washed before use. The main aim of washing is to remove earth: materials should not be left in water too long otherwise they lose their active constituents. Light, soft materials in particular should be washed as quickly as possible. See PROCESSING OF MEDICINALS. [27: 323]

wasted blood 败血 *bài xuè*: Static blood that has not been discharged from the body.

wasted blood surging into the heart 败血冲心 *bài xuè chōng xīn*: One of the THREE POSTPARTUM SURGES. Spirit-mind derangement, mania, or withdrawal stemming from RETENTION OF THE LOCHIA, and attributed to upsurge of retained LOCHIA. [26: 637]

wasted blood surging into the lung 败血冲肺 *bài xuè chōng fèi*: One of the THREE POSTPARTUM SURGES. A critical postpartum condition characterized by oppression in the chest, vexation and agitation, red face, rapid breathing, counterflow panting, or nosebleed. MED Treat with Two-Ingredient Ginseng and Sappan Beverage (*èr wèi shēn sū yǐn*), adding mirabilite (*máng xiāo*) in particularly severe cases. [26: 637]

wasted blood surging into the stomach 败血冲胃 *bài xuè chōng wèi*: One of the THREE POSTPARTUM SURGES. A postpartum condition of bloating, oppression, nausea, vomiting, abdominal fullness, distention, and pain attributed to retention and upsurge of the LOCHIA. MED Treat with Stomach-Calming Powder (*píng wèi sǎn*) or Return Again Elixir (*lái fù dān*). [26: 637]

water 水 *shuǐ*: **1.** The clear liquid of streams and rivers. **2.** Any form of fluid, in particular ingested fluids (such as in the expression SEA OF GRAIN AND WATER), and waste fluids or urine (as in *waterways*). **3.** Specifically, fluid accumulation refers to fluid accumulations in the form of water swelling attributable to morbidity of the lung, spleen, or kidney. Water in this context is often known as *water qi*. Distinction is made between YIN WATER and YANG WATER. Yin water patterns are ones of vacuity or cold patterns that develop slowly and are difficult to cure. Yang water patterns are ones of repletion or heat patterns that develop rapidly and can be eliminated swiftly. See WATER SWELLING. **4.** In the doctrine of the five phases, the water phase, to which the kidney corresponds. **5.** An alternate name for the kidney (and its corresponding bowel, the bladder), as in the phrase "water failing to moisten wood." [97: 130] [6: 28]

water by nature flows downward 水性流下 *shuǐ xìng liú xià*: The nature of water as described in the doctrine of the five phases. In the body, water-damp tends to flow downward causing diarrhea and fatigue and water swelling of the lower limbs. [26: 151] [27: 14] [97: 132]

water chest bind 水结胸 *shuǐ jié xiōng*: Synonym: *water qi chest bind*; *water-heat chest bind*. A condition attributed to water-rheum binding in the chest and rib-side, and characterized by pain and oppression in the chest and rib-side, a gurgling sound in the chest in response to pressing, fearful throbbing below the heart, and sweating from the head. MED Transform water-damp and quiet the heart spirit using formulas such as Minor Pinellia Decoction Plus Poria (Hoelen) (*xiǎo bàn xià jiā fú líng tāng*). ACU Base treatment mainly on CV, PC, LR, SP, and HT. Needle with drainage at PC-6 (*nèi guān*, Inner Pass), LR-3 (*tài chōng*, Supreme Surge), CV-17 (*shān zhōng*, Chest Center), CV-12 (*zhōng wǎn*, Center Stomach Duct), ST-36 (*zú sān lǐ*, Leg Three Li), SP-9 (*yīn líng quán*, Yin Mound Spring), BL-15 (*xīn shū*, Heart Transport) and HT-7 (*shén mén*, Spirit Gate). If rheum and heat bind to form a major chest bind, treat by opening bind and expelling water. See MAJOR CHEST BIND; CHEST BIND. [26: 153] [27: 376] [97: 133]

water-cold shooting into the lung 水寒射肺 *shuǐ hán shè fèi*: A pattern that occurs in patients suffering from phlegm-rheum or water swelling when they contract cold evil. Cold evil stirs the water-rheum and both evils rise into the lung counterflow, causing nondiffusion of lung qi. The chief signs are cough, hasty panting with inability to lie down and puffy swelling of the lower limbs. Other signs include copious thin white phlegm-drool, fullness and oppression in the chest and rib-side, distention and fullness in the lesser abdomen, cold pain in the lumbar region, cold knees and lower legs, and scant urine. In some cases, there may be aversion to cold with heat effusion, absence of sweating, and generalized pain. The tongue fur is thin, white, and glossy, or white and slimy. The pulse is tight and floating or tight and stringlike. [MED] Warm the lung and transform rheum; assist yang and disinhibit water. Use Minor Green-Blue Dragon Decoction (*xiǎo qīng lóng tāng*) combined with True Warrior Decoction (*zhēn wǔ tāng*). [ACU] Base treatment mainly on LU, ST, CV, and back transport points. Select BL-13 (*fèi shū*, Lung Transport), LU-9 (*tài yuān*, Great Abyss), ST-40 (*fēng lóng*, Bountiful Bulge), LI-4 (*hé gǔ*, Union Valley), CV-12 (*zhōng wǎn*, Center Stomach Duct), ST-36 (*zú sān lǐ*, Leg Three Li), and CV-17 (*shān zhōng*, Chest Center), to warm the lung and transform rheum, and select CV-9 (*shuǐ fēn*, Water Divide), CV-6 (*qì hǎi*, Sea of Qi), BL-23 (*shèn shū*, Kidney Transport), BL-20 (*pí shū*, Spleen Transport), BL-22 (*sān jiāo shū*, Triple Burner Transport), and SP-9 (*yīn líng quán*, Yin Mound Spring) to assist yang and disinhibit water; needle with supplementation and moxa. [26: 152] [27: 162] [97: 133] [57: 81] [46: 597, 653, 676] [4: 137]

water counterflow 水逆 *shuǐ nì*: From *On Cold Damage* (*shāng hán lùn, biàn tài yáng bìng mài zhèng bìng zhì*), which states, "Wind-damage with heat effusion failing to resolve in six or seven days, with heart vexation and exterior signs, thirst and drinking of water with immediate vomiting of water ingested is called "water counterflow." Later physicians referred to any vomiting of clear water or thirst and drinking of water with immediate vomiting of ingested water as "water counterflow." Counterflow water is attributed to the presence of deep-lying rheum. [MED] Free yang and disinhibit water with Poria (Hoelen) Five Powder (*wǔ líng sǎn*). If there is qi vacuity, use Six Gentlemen Decoction (*liù jūn zǐ tāng*) plus oven earth (*fú lóng gān*). [ACU] Base treatment mainly on BL, TB, CV, ST, and SP. Select BL-11 (*dà zhù*, Great Shuttle), BL-64 (*jīng gǔ*, Capital Bone), ST-36 (*zú sān lǐ*, Leg Three Li), TB-3 (*zhōng zhǔ*, Central Islet), PC-6 (*nèi guān*, Inner Pass), CV-6 (*qì hǎi*, Sea of Qi), CV-9 (*shuǐ fēn*, Water Divide), and SP-9 (*yīn líng quán*, Yin Mound Spring); needle with even supplementation and drainage or with drainage, and add moxa. For qi vacuity, supplement BL-20 (*pí shū*, Spleen Transport), and BL-21 (*wèi shū*, Stomach Transport). [27: 139] [97: 131] [46: 597, 602, 676] [75: 83]

water-damp 水湿 *shuǐ shī*: Any water or dampness as an actual or potential cause of disease. The term "water-damp" is commonly used in the context of the spleen, especially regarding its function of governing the movement and transformation of fluids and its intolerance of dampness.

water diarrhea 水泻 *shuǐ xiè*, 水泄 *shuǐ xiè*: Synonym: *outpour diarrhea*.
Diarrhea characterized by watery stool; observed in DAMP DIARRHEA, COLD DIARRHEA, and HEAT DIARRHEA. [26: 155]

water distention 水胀 *shuǐ zhàng*: **1.** WATER SWELLING. **2.** Abdominal distention with gradually developing water swelling. [26: 153] [27: 418] [97: 130]

water drum 水鼓 *shuǐ gǔ*: Synonyms: *water gu*; *water drum distention*. A disease pattern characterized by abdominal distention which gurgles when the patient moves. Water drum is usually caused by excessive consumption of liquor that impairs free coursing of the liver, with resultant liver depression damaging the spleen causing impaired movement and transformation that causes water-damp to collect. It is associated with a withered-yellow facial complexion, rib-side pain, red speckles on the body (spider nevi), and sometimes jaundice. In persistent cases, there is scant urine and generalized swelling that pits when pressed. [MED] Boost qi and supplement the blood; nourish yin and disinhibit urine. Use Spleen-Firming Beverage (*shí pí yǐn*) plus tangkuei (*dāng guī*) and toosendan (*chuān liàn zǐ*). For pronounced water-rheum, add cinnamon twig (*guì zhī*), polyporus (*zhū líng*), and alisma (*zé xiè*). Alternatively, use Stomach-Calming Poria (Hoelen) Five Decoction (*wèi líng tāng*) combined with Bupleurum Liver-Coursing Powder (*chái hú shū gān sǎn*). For persistent cases with generalized water swelling, apply the principle of attack followed by supplementation using water-expelling medicinals such as morning glory (*qiān niú zǐ*) and kansui (*gān suì*), combined with water-disinhibiting medicinals such as poria (*fú líng*), rice bean (*chì xiǎo dòu*), and plantago seed (*chē qián zǐ*), followed by regulating and supplementing formulas such as Poria (Hoelen) Five Powder (*wǔ líng sǎn*) or Four Gentlemen Decoction (*sì jūn zǐ tāng*). [ACU] Two groups of points may be applied. (1) CV-12 (*zhōng wǎn*, Center Stomach Duct), ST-25 (*tiān shū*, Celestial Pivot), ST-36 (*zú sān lǐ*, Leg Three Li), BL-20 (*pí shū*, Spleen Transport), CV-9 (*shuǐ fēn*, Water Divide), and ST-44 (*nèi tíng*, Inner Court). (2) SP-15 (*dà hèng*, Great Horizontal), CV-6 (*qì hǎi*, Sea of Qi), SP-6 (*sān yīn jiāo*, Three Yin Intersection), BL-20 (*pí shū*, Spleen Transport), CV-9 (*shuǐ fēn*, Water Divide), and ST-44 (*nèi tíng*, Inner Court). Alternate the groups and needle with drainage in treatments every 3–5 days. After needling, moxa CV-12 (*zhōng wǎn*, Center Stomach Duct), CV-4 (*guān yuán*, Pass Head), and bilateral SP-15 (*dà hèng*, Great Horizontal) for 30–60 minutes. [27: 414] [26: 153-4] [42: 194]

water drum distention 水臌 *shuǐ gǔ*: WATER DRUM.

water failing to help fire 水不济火 *shuǐ bù jì huǒ*: FIRE AND WATER FAILING TO AID EACH OTHER.

water failing to moisten wood 水不涵木 *shuǐ bù hán mù*: Kidney yin vacuity (water) causing insufficiency of liver yin (wood). In the five phases, the kidney belongs to water and the liver belongs to wood. Water failing to moisten wood manifests as low fever, dizziness, tinnitus, deafness, aching lumbus, seminal emission, and dry throat. When insufficiency of liver yin stirs internal wind, there may also be wriggling of the extremities or even jerking. See ENRICHING WATER TO MOISTEN WOOD. [26: 150]

water failing to transform into qi 水不化气 *shuǐ bù huà qì*: A disturbance of normal distribution and discharge of water in the body characterized by inhibited urination and water swelling. Normally, water (fluid in the body) is subject to qi transformation, in which the lung, spleen, and kidney are involved. When the transformative action of qi is impaired, and especially when kidney yang is vacuous, free flow through the waterways of the triple burner is jeopardized and water fails to turn into steam (transform into qi) and spread around the body. See QI TRANSFORMATION. [26: 150] [27: 142] [97: 132]

water-grinding 水飞 *shuǐ fēi*: Fine grinding of medicinal materials in water. **Method**: The materials are first roughly crushed. They are then placed in a porcelain mortar, covered with water, and ground until the grating sound of rough lumps ceases. At this point, more water is mixed in, and the water that contains suspended particles is poured off and reserved. More water and materials are added to the mortar, and the process is repeated. The reserved suspension is allowed to stand until the particles have settled, and the excess water is poured off. The remaining sludge is sun-dried, after which it is ready for use. This method is used for minerals and shells. Its advantage over dry grinding is that fine particles do not blow away or get lost, and that impurities dissolved in the water are (at least partly) removed. The

much finer power it produces makes for greater assimilation of orally taken medicinals and reduces irritation in topical applications. Cinnabar (*zhū shā*), talcum (*huá shí*), smithsonite (*lú gān shí*), and realgar (*xióng huáng*) are treated in this way for laryngeal insufflation, topical eye medication, or for coating pills. See WATER PROCESSING. [26: 151] [27: 323] [97: 130]

water gu 水蛊 *shuǐ gǔ*: From *The Origin and Indicators of Disease* (*zhū bìng yuán hòu lùn*). Abdominal distention due to the gathering of water toxin qi. See WATER DRUM. [26: 153] [97: 131]

water-heat chest bind 水热结胸 *shuǐ rè jié xiōng*: WATER CHEST BIND. [27: 276]

water mounting 水疝 *shuǐ shàn*: Painful swelling and periodic sweating of the scrotum attributed to water-damp pouring downward or to contraction of wind, cold, and damp evils. In some cases, the scrotum is greatly enlarged and translucent; sometimes there is itching and discharge of yellow fluid; sometimes pressing the abdomen produces a sound of water. ⌐WMC⌐ hydrocele of tunica vaginalis, scrotal hydrocele. ⌐MED⌐ Expel water and move qi using variations of Poria (Hoelen) Five Powder (*wǔ líng sǎn*) for mild cases, and Water Controller Yu Powder (*yǔ gōng sǎn*) for severe cases. ⌐ACU⌐ Base treatment mainly on LR, ST, and SP. Select LR-8 (*qū quán*, Spring at the Bend), ST-28 (*shuǐ dào*, Waterway), SP-9 (*yīn líng quán*, Yin Mound Spring), CV-3 (*zhōng jí*, Central Pole), LR-4 (*zhōng fēng*, Mound Center), and LR-1 (*dà dūn*, Large Pile); needle with drainage. Add moxa for cold patterns. [26: 150] [37: 456]

water panting 水喘 *shuǐ chuǎn*: Panting attributed to water-rheum invading the lung, and occurring when the kidney allows water to collect and the spleen fails to transform dampness and the resulting water qi ascends to the lung impairing depurative downbearing. Signs include qi counterflow rapid panting, oppression and fullness in the chest, abdominal distention, fearful throbbing, and swelling of the head, face, and limbs. ⌐MED⌐ Treatment can be directed at the root or tip according to need. To treat the tip, expel water and disinhibit dampness, and diffuse and downbear lung qi. To treat the root, move the spleen and warm the kidney. If panting precedes distention, focus treatment on the lung; if distention precedes panting, focus treatment on the spleen. Use Minor Green-Blue Dragon Decoction (*xiǎo qīng lóng tāng*) or tingli (*tíng lì zǐ*) and black jujube (*hēi zǎo*) to drain the lung. Use Poria (Hoelen), Cinnamon Twig, Ovate Atractylodes, and Licorice Decoction (*líng guì zhú gān tāng*), True Warrior Decoction (*zhēn wǔ tāng*), or Kidney Qi Pill (*shèn qì wán*) to move the spleen and warm the kidney. ⌐ACU⌐ If panting precedes distention, base treatment mainly on

LU, back transport points, and CV. Select Panting Stabilizer (*dìng chuǎn*), LU-7 (*liè quē*, Broken Sequence), LU-5 (*chǐ zé*, Cubit Marsh), BL-13 (*fèi shū*, Lung Transport), BL-22 (*sān jiāo shū*, Triple Burner Transport), CV-6 (*qì hǎi*, Sea of Qi), SP-9 (*yīn líng quán*, Yin Mound Spring), and ST-36 (*zú sān lǐ*, Leg Three Li); needle with drainage. If panting follows distention, base treatment mainly on back transport points, CV, GV, LU, and SP. Select BL-20 (*pí shū*, Spleen Transport), BL-13 (*fèi shū*, Lung Transport), BL-23 (*shèn shū*, Kidney Transport), BL-22 (*sān jiāo shū*, Triple Burner Transport), CV-12 (*zhōng wǎn*, Center Stomach Duct), PC-6 (*nèi guān*, Inner Pass), CV-6 (*qì hǎi*, Sea of Qi), CV-4 (*guān yuán*, Pass Head), Panting Stabilizer (*dìng chuǎn*), LU-5 (*chǐ zé*, Cubit Marsh), SP-9 (*yīn líng quán*, Yin Mound Spring) and ST-36 (*zú sān lǐ*, Leg Three Li); needle with supplementation and add moxa. [26: 153]

water pill 水丸 *shuǐ wán*, 水泛丸 *shuǐ fàn wán*: A preparation made by mixing the finely ground materials with cold water, yellow wine, vinegar, fresh herb juice, as the formula stipulates, before forming pills either by hand or by machine. [97: 130]

water processing 水制 *shuǐ zhì*: Any of various methods of treating medicinal materials with clean water to remove impurities, foreign bodies, unwanted elements (such as sand, earth, salt, unpleasant odors), to increase suppleness to facilitate cutting, to refine minerals, and to reduce toxicity. Methods must be carefully chosen to prevent loss of active constituents. See WASHING; STEEPING; LONG RINSING; COVERED MOISTENING; WATER-GRINDING. See PROCESSING OF MEDICINALS. [11: 15] [74: 5]

water qi 水气 *shuǐ qì*: Pathological excesses of water in the body and, specifically, water swelling provoked by it. The main cause is impairment of movement and transformation of water due to spleen-kidney yang vacuity. NB: "Qi" in the term "water qi" reflects the notion of water in this context as a pervasive (pathological) phenomenon. See WATER SWELLING. [26: 152] [27: 418, 113] [97: 130]

water qi chest bind 水气结胸 *shuǐ qì jié xiōng*: WATER CHEST BIND. [27: 376]

water qi intimidating the heart 水气凌心 *shuǐ qì líng xīn*: Upsurge of water qi causing disturbances of the heart. Spleen-yang vacuity and impairment of qi transformation causing water to be retained in the body and thereby causing water qi, which can manifest as phlegm-rheum or water swelling. When the water surges upward and lodges in the chest and diaphragm, it can cause devitalization of heart yang and disquieting of heart qi manifesting in the form of heart palpitations and hasty breathing. This is what is known as water qi intimidating the heart. The chief signs are heart palpitations, panting with inability to lie flat, generalized puffy swelling, and a bright white facial complexion. Other signs include flusteredness, lassitude of spirit and fatigue, fear of cold and cold limbs, and short voidings of scant clear urine. MED Warm yang and disinhibit water. Use True Warrior Decoction (*zhēn wǔ tāng*) or Poria (Hoelen) Five Powder (*wǔ líng sǎn*). ACU Base treatment mainly on CV, back transport points, HT, and PC. Select BL-15 (*xīn shū*, Heart Transport), PC-6 (*nèi guān*, Inner Pass), PC-4 (*xī mén*, Cleft Gate), HT-7 (*shén mén*, Spirit Gate), CV-17 (*shān zhōng*, Chest Center), CV-9 (*shuǐ fēn*, Water Divide), CV-6 (*qì hǎi*, Sea of Qi), BL-23 (*shèn shū*, Kidney Transport), BL-20 (*pí shū*, Spleen Transport), and SP-9 (*yīn líng quán*, Yin Mound Spring); needle with even supplementation and drainage or with drainage, and add moxa. [37: 335] [26: 152] [57: 53] [27: 149] [97: 139] [46: 597, 602, 676]

water rampart 水廓 *shuǐ kuò*: See EIGHT RAMPARTS. [26: 24] [27: 500] [97: 131]

water-rheum 水饮 *shuǐ yǐn*: Fluid exuded by diseased organs. Clear thin fluid is known as "water," whereas thin sticky fluid is known as "rheum." These differ in name and form, but are in essence the same; hence the compound term. [27: 381]

water-soaking sore 水渍疮 *shuǐ zì chuāng*: A sore, usually of the hand, attributable to long soaking in water and local friction. A water-soaking sore starts with swelling, white putrefaction, and wrinkling, that with continued friction and soaking becomes painful and itchy. WMC paddy field dermatitis. MED Treat by washing in a decoction of alum (*bái fán*). Indigo Powder (*qīng dài sǎn*) can be applied if the skin is ruptured. [26: 154]

water swelling 水肿 *shuǐ zhǒng*: Synonyms: water; water qi; water distention. Swelling of the flesh arising when organ dysfunction (spleen, kidney, lung) due to internal or external causes allows water to accumulate. Water swelling stands in contradistinction to toxin swelling, which denotes a localized swelling due to the local presence of toxin as in the case of welling-abscess (*yōng*), flat-abscess (*jū*), boils (*jié*), clove sores (*dīng chuāng*), and other sores. WMC cardiogenic edema, nephrotic edema, hepatogenic edema, nutritional edema, and endocrinologic edema. Water swelling patterns have been classified in different ways. For example, *Essential Prescriptions of the Golden Coffer* (*jīn guì yào lüè*) distinguishes between WIND WATER, SKIN WATER, REGULAR WATER, and STONE WATER. *Dan Xi's Experiential Methods* (*dān xī xīn fǎ*) differentiates yin water and yang water. A primary distinction exists between vacuity and repletion. **Vacuity** patterns are attributable to spleen-kidney yang vacuity preventing the normal movement and transformation of water-damp. MED Warm the kidney, fortify the spleen, boost qi, and free yang. Use formulas such as Spleen-Firming Beverage (*shí pí yǐn*) or Golden Coffer Kidney Qi Pill (*jīn guì shèn qì wán*). **Repletion** patterns are attributed to the invasion of external evils impairing diffusion of lung qi, the triple burner's governing of the sluices, or the qi transformation function of the bladder. MED Course wind, diffuse the lung, percolate dampness, and expel water. Use Spleen-Effusing Decoction (*yuè bì tāng*), Poria (Hoelen) Five Powder (*wǔ líng sǎn*), or Five-Peel Beverage (*wǔ pí yǐn*). Vacuity patterns often develop from repletion patterns and repletion patterns may arise in patients suffering from vacuity water swelling. Patients suffering from water swelling should control salt intake and avoid catching colds. Water swelling is variously labeled according to its nature. See YANG WATER; YIN WATER; WIND WATER; QI SWELLING; VACUOUS PUFFINESS; PUFFY SWELLING. It is also labeled according to location: see PUFFY FACE; SLEEPING SILKWORMS BENEATH THE EYES; SWELLING OF THE FEET; SWELLING OF THE FEET AND LOWER LEGS. See also YELLOW SWELLING; SWELLING OF PREGNANCY. Compare COLD DAMAGE WATER AMASSMENT PATTERN; TOXIN SWELLING; DISTENTION. ◇ Chin 水 *shuǐ*, water; 肿 *zhǒng*, swelling. In ancient times, it was referred to simply as *shuǐ*, water; the term 水肿 *shuǐ zhǒng* did not become popular until the Sui and Tang Dynasties. The Chinese term *shuǐ zhǒng* is used in Western medicine to render the term edema. "Water swelling" is preferred in the Chinese medical context because it reflects the notion of the waterways whose regulation is governed by the lung, distillation of water by the kidney (the water viscus), and the movement and transformation of water-damp by the spleen. The term edema, from the Greek *oidēma*, swelling, fails the make the notion of water explicit. [29: 653] [80: 504] [26: 154] [97: 130] [50: 351] [27: 418] [97: 512] [26: 712] [26: 616] [26: 456] [26: 181] [26: 191] [26: 483]

water toxin 水毒 *shuǐ dú*: A disease spoken of in ancient literature attributed to poisoning of water by malign worms at the source of rivers and said to be marked by aversion to cold, slight headache, pain in the eye sockets, heart vexation, rigidity of the joints of the lumbus and back, knee pain, desire only for sleep, and counterflow cold of the limbs up to the knees and elbows. Water toxin was also said to cause sores in the lower areas that are neither painful nor or itchy, and that suppurate and burst, dampness pouring downward, failure to eat, manic speech, and passage of bloody matter like a mashed liver. [26: 151]

water viscus 水脏 *shuǐ zàng*: The kidney. The kidney is sometimes referred to as the water viscus (e.g., in the phrase "warm the water viscus") because it is ascribed to water in the five phases and because it governs water. See KIDNEY GOVERNS WATER; VISCUS OF FIRE AND WATER.

water wheel 水轮 *shuǐ lún*: The pupil of the eye; related to the kidney. [27: 500, 65] [97: 130]

watery sniveling 鼽水 *qiú shuǐ*: SNIVELING NOSE.

waving fish pulse 鱼翔脉 *yú xiáng mài*: See SEVEN STRANGE PULSES. [27: 199] [27: 199] [97: 360]

waxing and waning of yin and yang 阴阳消长 *yīn yáng xiāo zhǎng*: Many yin-yang paired phenomena alternate their strength and prevalence. For example, daytime activity alternates with nighttime rest, and bursts of energy and enthusiasm are often followed by lethargy and disenchantment. [27: 4] [97: 235]

weak pulse 弱脉 *ruò mài*: A pulse that is sunken and without force. A weak pulse is associated with vacuity of qi and blood. [27: 195] [97: 552]

weak stomach malign obstruction 胃弱恶阻 *wèi ruò è zǔ*: Malign obstruction (vomiting in pregnancy) arising from spleen-stomach vacuity. In pregnancy, thoroughfare vessel qi is exuberant and in women suffering from spleen-stomach vacuity, it can impair stomach harmony and downbearing, causing oppression in the stomach duct and abdominal distention, vomiting and reduced food intake, or immediate vomiting of ingested food. MED Fortify the spleen and harmonize the stomach; regulate qi and check vomiting. An appropriate formula is Six Gentlemen Decoction (*liù jūn zǐ tāng*) with the addition of loquat leaf (*pí pá yè*), agastache/patchouli (*huò xiāng*), inula flower (*xuán fù huā*), amomum (*shā rén*), and bitter orange (*zhǐ ké*). ACU Base treatment mainly on CV, PC, SP, and back transport points. Select CV-12 (*zhōng wǎn*, Center Stomach Duct), PC-6 (*nèi guān*, Inner Pass), SP-4 (*gōng sūn*, Yellow Emperor), BL-20 (*pí shū*, Spleen Transport), BL-21 (*wèi shū*, Stomach Transport), and LR-13 (*zhāng mén*, Camphorwood Gate); needle with supplementation. [26: 437] [59: 117]

weak stomach qi 胃气弱 *wèi qì ruò*: Poor appetite; poor spleen-stomach function. See STOMACH QI.

weak wilting lumbus and knees 腰膝痿弱 *yāo xī wěi ruò*: LIMP WILTING LUMBUS AND KNEES.

wear 耗 *hào*: Describes gradual loss of, or damage to (the blood, fluids, etc.) associated with enduring illness. See EXUBERANCE AND DEBILITATION.

weeping canthus 漏睛 *lòu jīng*, 眦漏 *zì lòu*: A disease pattern characterized by discharge of pus from the canthus on application of pressure, or, in severe cases, a red hot swollen lump at the inner canthus that refuses pressure, and that turns into a sore or a fistula. Weeping canthus is attributed to depressed heat in the heart channel or wind-heat attacking the inner canthus. WMC dacryocystitis. MED Course wind, clear heat, drain fire, and resolve toxin. Take Three Yellows Decoction (*sān huáng tāng*) orally and apply Agreeable Golden Yellow Powder (*rú yì jīn huáng sǎn*) topically. [26: 823] [27: 501]

Wei 魏 *wèi*: The name of a dynasty (A.D. 220–265).

wei 痿 *wěi*: WILTING.

welling-abscess 痈 *yōng*: **1.** *Synonym: external welling-abscess*. A large suppuration in the flesh characterized by a painful swelling and redness that is clearly circumscribed, and that before rupturing is soft and characterized by a thin shiny skin. Before suppuration begins, it can be easily dispersed; when pus has formed, it easily ruptures; after rupture, it easily closes and heals. It may be associated with generalized heat [effusion], thirst, yellow tongue fur and a rapid pulse. WMC superficial abscess; cellulitis; acute purulent lymphadenitis. A welling-abscess results from congealing and stagnation of qi and blood arising when damp-heat and fire toxin block the channels. This pathomechanism can usually be traced to excessive consumption of rich foods or to toxin contracted through unclean wounds. The term welling-abscess is often used in contradistinction to FLAT-ABSCESS,[1] and the difference between them is pointed out in *The Inner Canon* (*nèi jīng*): "welling-abscesses are shallow and light; flat-absceses are deep and heavy; welling-abscess effuse from the six bowels; flat-abscess effuse from the five viscera." *Orthodox External Medicine* (*wài kē zhèng zōng*) explains the difference in greater detail: "welling-abscess means congestion; it is yang; it is ascribed to toxin of the six bowels prevailing in the outer; it appears suddenly and is floating [i.e., superficial or buoyant] and shallow. Because it originates from the yang aspect, and because yang qi is light, clear, and floating, it [the welling-abscess] rises high, easily swells, easily forms pus, easily putrefies, and easily closes, and does not damage the sinew and bone, and is easy to treat. Flat-abscess, meaning 疽 [obstruction; marsh], is yin; it is ascribed to toxin of the five viscera attacking the inner body; it develops slowly and its location is deep. Because it originates from the yin aspect, and because yin-blood is heavy and turbid, it [the flat-abscess] is sinking in nature, damages the sinew, erodes the bone, and is difficult to cure." **2.** *Synonym: internal welling-abscess.* A suppuration in the chest or abdomen affecting the organs; probably so called because it shares many of the

yang qualities of external welling-abscess, except for its location in the body. They include INTESTINAL WELLING-ABSCESS, PULMONARY WELLING-ABSCESS, LIVER WELLING-ABSCESS, and STOMACH WELLING-ABSCESS, which correspond roughly to appendicitis, pulmonary abscess, liver abscess, and pathologies of the stomach respectively in Western medicine. Compare FLAT-ABSCESS. ◇ Chin 痈 *yōng* is composed of the illness signifier 疒 with 雝 *yōng* formerly interchangeable with 壅 *yǒng*, *yǒng* meaning congestion. *Orthodox External Medicine* (*wài kē zhèng zōng, yōng jū mén*) states, "痈 means 壅." The character thus denotes a disease associated with congestion, reflecting the etiology. NB: The same character is now used in Western medicine to render the concept of carbuncle. The original definition in Chinese medicine is much wider. [26: 999] [96: 101]

welling-abscess of the liver 肝痈 *gān yōng*: A WELLING-ABSCESS (*yōng*) affecting the liver. It is attributed either to liver depression transforming into fire, qi stagnation and blood stasis, or to accumulated dampness engendering phlegm. It starts with dull pain at LR-14 (*qī mén*, Cycle Gate), followed by the gradual development of distending pain in the right rib-side that refuses pressure and prevents the patient from lying on the right side. There is often aversion to cold and heat effusion, and the pulse is wiry and rapid. As the condition progresses, the pain becomes more acute, and a persistent heat effusion is present. If it continues, unless successfully treated, it can burst, giving rise to coughing and vomiting of pus or the passage of pus in the stool. WMC hepatic abscess, suppurative cholecystitis and inflammation of the biliary tract, and hepatic echinococcosis. MED In the initial stage, when due to liver fire, clear the liver and drain fire with Bupleurum Liver-Coursing Powder (*chái hú shū gān sǎn*); when due to damp phlegm, rectify qi and transform phlegm using Qi-Clearing Phlegm-Transforming Pill (*qīng qì huà tán wán*) plus cyperus (*xiāng fù zǐ*), tangkuei (*dǎng guī*), and curcuma (*yù jīn*). When pus has formed, treat by clearing the liver and draining fire assisted by expelling pus; after rupture, add lung-clearing and intestine-clearing medicinals. For topical treatment, see INTESTINAL WELLING-ABSCESS. After healing, use Four Agents Decoction (*sì wù tāng*) for adjustment. [26: 333] [50: 784]

welling-abscess of the lung 肺痈 *fèi yōng*: PULMONARY WELLING-ABSCESS.

welling-abscess of the stomach 胃痈 *wèi yōng*: WELLING-ABSCESS OF THE STOMACH DUCT.

welling-abscess of the stomach duct 胃脘痈 *wèi wǎn (guǎn) yōng*: **1.** *Synonyms: welling-abscess of the stomach; stomach duct welling-abscess; stomach welling-abscess; internal welling-*

abscess of the stomach duct. A WELLING-ABSCESS (*yōng*) arising in the stomach duct. *The Gateway to Medicine* (*yī xué rù mén*) attributes it to "depressed fire arising from diet and the seven affects that becomes isolated by externally contracted cold qi, filling the stomach duct." It starts with dull pain and slight swelling at CV-12 (*zhōng wǎn*, Center Stomach Duct), a sunken fine stomach pulse, generalized heat [effusion], and dry skin. The local area becomes hard with pain stretching into the heart. Abatement of the heat effusion and pain are favorable signs; spreading of pus that causes the stomach and intestines to rot is an unfavorable sign. MED In the initial state, free the bowels and drain heat, move stasis and dissipate binds. Use Rhubarb and Moutan Decoction (*dà huáng mǔ dān pí tāng*). When pus has formed, move stasis and expel pus with medicinals such as rice bean (*chì xiǎo dòu*), coix (*yì yǐ rén*), fangji (*fáng jǐ*), and licorice (*gān cǎo*). After the pulse has been expelled, supplement qi with Center-Supplementing Qi-Boosting Decoction (*bǔ zhōng yì qì tāng*). **2.** An external welling-abscess (*yōng*) located at CV-12 (*zhōng wǎn*, Center Stomach Duct). For treatment, see EXTERNAL WELLING-ABSCESS. [26: 439] [50: 1081]

welling-abscess of the testicle 子痈 *zǐ yōng*: A WELLING-ABSCESS (*yōng*) growing on the testicle. Two patterns are observed: **Damp-heat pouring downward** and causing causing qi and blood to congeal and stagnate gives rise to welling-abscess of the testicle characterized by sudden swelling and heat in one side of the scrotum, shiny stretched skin of the scrotum, and acute pain and hard swelling of the testicle. After bursting and discharging thick yellow pus, it heals rapidly. WMC Suppurative orchitis. MED Clear heat and disinhibit dampness. Use Gentian Liver-Draining Decoction (*lóng dǎn xiè gān tāng*) plus tangerine pip (*jú hé*), litchee pit (*lì zhī hé*), and toosendan (*chuān liàn zǐ*). Topical: Golden Yellow Paste (*jīn huáng gāo*). **Yin vacuity and congealing phlegm-damp** gives rise to a welling-abscess of the testicle characterized by gradual swelling and hardening of the testicle, with mild pain, absence of heat and redness. It takes takes several months (or even up to two years) to begin suppurating, and after bursting, it discharges thin pus, and heals with difficulty. WMC tuberculosis of the testis. MED Enrich yin and eliminate dampness; transform stasis and free the network vessels. Use Yin-Enriching Dampness-Eliminating Decoction (*zī yī chú shī tāng*). [26: 57] [27: 462] [97: 37]

welling-abscess of the throat 喉痈 *hóu yōng*: A WELLING-ABSCESS (*yōng*) within the throat. Welling-abscess of the throat is attributable to disharmony among the organs and qi and blood and to wind evil lodging in the throat. It devel-

ops swiftly, often being associated with aversion to cold and high fever, phlegm-drool congestion, and labored breathing. WMC peritonsillar abscess (quinsy), retropharyngeal abscess. MED Course the exterior and resolve toxin; clear heat and disperse swelling. Use Throat-Clearing Diaphragm-Disinhibiting Decoction (*qīng yān lì gé tāng*) as oral medication and Borneol and Borax Powder (*bīng péng sǎn*) applied by insufflation. Lancing may be performed after formation of pus. A decoction of lonicera (*jīn yín huā*), mint (*bò hé*), licorice (*gān cǎo*), forsythia (*lián qiào*), and platycodon (*jié gěng*) can be used a mouthwash. [26: 733]

welling-abscess swelling 痈肿 *yōng zhǒng*: The swelling of WELLING-ABSCESS (*yōng*).

well point 井穴 *jǐng xué*: See TRANSPORT POINTS.

Western (Former) Han 西汉 *xī hàn*: The name of a dynasty (206 B.C.–A.D. 24).

Western Jin 西晋 *xī jìn*: The name of a dynasty (A.D. 265–316).

Western Wei 西魏 *xī wèi*: The name of a dynasty (A.D. 535–556).

Western Zhou 西周 *xī zhōu*: The name of a dynasty (approx. 11th cent. B.C. to 771 B.C.).

wet spreading sore 浸淫疮 *jìn yín chuāng*: A sore small sore that easily spreads by scratching. A wet spreading sore when first appearing on the skin is about the size of grain of millet. It itches incessantly, and when scratched, spreads very quickly. In severe cases, it is associated with generalized heat [effusion]. It is attributed to congealing stagnating heart fire and spleen dampness that after further contraction of external evil becomes depressed in the skin. WMC acute eczema and Engman's disease (dermatitis infectiosa eczematoides). MED Dispel wind and overcome dampness; clear heat and cool the blood. Oral: Take Wind-Dispersing Powder (*xiāo fēng sǎn*). Topical: Apply Indigo Powder (*qīng dài sǎn*) or Three Stones Powder (*sān shí sǎn*). Alternatively, use powdered coptis (*huáng lián*). [26: 480]

wheat-grain intradermal needle 麦粒型皮内针 *mài lì xíng pí nèi zhēn*: A small needle about 1 cm long, continuous with and in the same plane as a circle of wire that forms the head. A small intradermal needle with a handle the shape of a grain of wheat, used in the embedded needle method. A wheat-grain intradermal needle is inserted transversely into the skin to a depth of about 1 cm and the handle is then held flat against the skin by adhesive tape. See NEEDLE IMPLANTATION. [46: 506]

wheezing 哮 *xiāo*: Hasty rapid breathing with phlegm rale in the throat. *Indispensable Medical Reading* (*yī zōng bì dú*) states "Wheezing is similar to panting, but does not have as much opening of the mouth and expelling of air, and is characterized by a wheezy sound." *The Orthodox Tradition* *of Medicine* (*yī xué zhèng zhuàn*) states, "Hasty panting with frog rale in the throat is wheezing." See WHEEZING PATTERNS. [26: 525] [97: 465] [50: 1247]

wheezing and panting 哮喘 *xiāo chuǎn*: See WHEEZING. [26: 525] [27: 382] [97: 466] [50: 1247]

wheezing patterns 哮证 *xiāo zhèng*: Ailments characterized by paroxysmal phlegm rale and rapid panting. The phlegm rale is like the rasping sound of a saw, and in severe cases there is gaping mouth and raised shoulders, distended and protruding eyes, somber white facial complexion, and green-blue or purple lips and nails, with sweating as in desertion. Repeated attacks lead to debilitation of lung qi and wearing of the true origin. Wheezing patterns are treated by supplementing spleen and kidney, and, during attacks, by dispelling evil, diffusing and downbearing lung qi, flushing phlegm and calming panting. In vacuity-repletion complexes, treatment to support right and dispel evil can be given together. Wheezing patterns include the following: COLD WHEEZING; HEAT WHEEZING; SALT WHEEZING; PHLEGM WHEEZING; KIDNEY WHEEZING. Compare PANTING. [50: 1247]

when blood is despoliated, there is no sweat; when sweat is despoliated, there is no blood 夺血者无汗，夺汗者无血 *duó xuè zhǐ wú hàn, duó hàn zhě wú xuè*: From *The Magic Pivot* (*líng shū, yíng wèi shēng huì piān*). Because blood and sweat are of the same source, drastic loss of the blood reduces sweat, and drastic loss of sweat reduces the blood. For this reason, patients that have bled should not be allowed to sweat, and in patients that have sweated, nothing should be done that causes wear on the blood. See HEART GOVERNS SWEAT; HEART GOVERNS THE BLOOD AND VESSELS. [27: 243] [117: 169]

when cold prevails there is swelling 寒胜则浮 *hán shèng zé fú*: From *Elementary Questions* (*sù wèn, yin yáng yìn xiàng dà lùn*). When cold prevails, yang qi is insufficient. Congealing cold and stagnant qi affect the movement of blood and water-damp collects. The swelling associated in Western medicine with chronic nephritis is usually a pattern of cold qi and spleen-kidney yang vacuity. [26: 659] [27: 1141]

when dampness prevails, there is soft stool diarrhea 湿胜则濡泻 *shī shèng zé rú xiè*: Dampness causes diarrhea. The spleen is averse to dampness and likes dryness. Exuberant damp qi in the inner body obstructs spleen yang, impairing movement and transformation. Hence there is abdominal distention and oppression accompanied by diarrhea. [26: 925] [27: 141]

when dampness prevails, yang is debilitated 湿胜则阳微 *shī shèng zé yáng wēi*: Dampness damages yang qi. Dampness is a heavy, turbid, sticky evil, and obstructs the activity of yang qi, especially that of the spleen, causing a white complexion, oppression in the chest, abdominal distention, glomus and fullness, diarrhea, and, in severe cases, water swelling. In treating dampness, attention must be paid to safeguarding yang qi, to disinhibiting urine, and to avoiding excessive use of cold or cool medicinals. [26: 925] [27: 141]

when dryness prevails, there is aridity 燥胜则干 *zào shèng zé gān*: Dryness qi causes dry signs. Dryness qi causes damage to the fluids, causing dry mouth and nose, dry lusterless skin, dry cough without phlegm, short scant voidings of urine, and dry bound stool. ◇ Chin 燥 *zào* and 干 *gān* both mean dry(ness), and are usually translated by the same word in English. In actual fact, they differ slightly in meaning and usage. Among the six excesses is *zào*, also called dryness qi. This, when penetrating the body, gives rise to signs more commonly described with the term *gān* (here rendered as "aridity"). Thus, *zào* is a dryness-causing qi, whereas *gān* describes the manifestations of *zào*. [26: 932] [27: 141]

when evil qi is exuberant, there is repletion 邪气盛则实 *xié qì shèng zé shí*: From *Elementary Questions* (*sù wèn, tōng píng xū shí lùn*). In the course of disease, exuberance of evil qi and the violent reaction of right qi manifests as a repletion pattern. Vigorous heat effusion, absence of sweating, vexation and agitation, mania, abdominal pain that refuses pressure, constipation and reddish urine, and forceful slippery rapid pulse are all repletion signs attributable to exuberant evil qi. [26: 312] [27: 126] [97: 178]

when heat prevails, there is swelling 热胜则肿 *rè shèng zé zhǒng*: Prevalence of yang heat can cause local pain and swelling. When heat lies depressed in the flesh, skin, and interstices, then qi and blood become congested, causing sores characterized redness, swelling, heat, pain, and suppuration. [26: 874]

when qi is vacuous, there is cold 气虚则寒 *qì xū zé hán*: Insufficiency of yang qi gives rise to yin cold. When yang qi is insufficient, it fails to warm and nourish the bowels and viscera, and gives rise to signs such as aversion to cold and cold limbs, lassitude of the spirit and lack of strength, bland taste in the mouth and lack of thirst, white facial complexion and pale tongue, clear urine and sloppy stool, and a slow sunken pulse or fine weak pulse. *Elementary Questions* (*sù wèn, tiáo jīng lùn*) states, "When yang is vacuous, there is external cold." [26: 540] [27: 145] [97: 97]

when the kidney is full, marrow is replete 肾充则髓实 *shèn chōng zé suǐ shí*: See KIDNEY ENGENDERS BONE AND MARROW. [27: 53]

when there is stoppage, there is pain 不通则痛 *bù tōng zé tòng*: Pain arises when the free movement of qi and blood is inhibited, as in qi stagnation, blood stasis, and cold. [6: 166]

when the stomach is in disharmony, there is unquiet sleep 胃不和则卧不安 *wèi bù hé zé wò bù ān*: From *The Inner Canon* (*nèi jīng*). When the stomach is in disharmony as observed in phlegm-fire harassing the upper body or spleen-stomach vacuity, there may be poor sleep or insomnia. MED Harmonize the stomach, transform dampness, and dispel phlegm. Use formulas such as Two Matured Ingredients Stomach-Calming Powder (*èr chén píng wèi sǎn*) plus acorus (*shí chāng pú*) and pumice (*hǎi fú shí*), or plus gardenia (*shān zhī zǐ*) and coptis (*huáng lián*). If the stool is hard and bound, use Phlegm-Abducting Decoction (*dǎo tán tāng*); if there is stomach duct pain, use Phlegm-Rolling Pill (*gǔn tán wán*). ACU Base treatment mainly on HT, SP, ST, and CV. Main points: Alert Spirit Quartet (*sì shén cōng*), HT-7 (*shén mén*, Spirit Gate), SP-6 (*sān yīn jiāo*, Three Yin Intersection), CV-12 (*zhōng wǎn*, Center Stomach Duct), ST-36 (*zú sān lǐ*, Leg Three Li), ST-40 (*fēng lóng*, Bountiful Bulge), and PC-6 (*nèi guān*, Inner Pass). Selection of points according to cause: For phlegm-heat harassing the upper body, add LI-4 (*hé gǔ*, Union Valley) and LI-11 (*qū chí*, Pool at the Bend); needle with drainage. For spleen-stomach vacuity, add BL-20 (*pí shū*, Spleen Transport) and BL-21 (*wèi shū*, Stomach Transport); needle with supplementation. Selection of points according to signs: For hard bound stool, add ST-37 (*shàng jù xū*, Upper Great Hollow), SP-14 (*fù jié*, Abdominal Bind), and LI-4 (*hé gǔ*, Union Valley). For stomach duct pain, add LR-13 (*zhāng mén*, Camphorwood Gate), ST-34 (*liáng qiū*, Beam Hill), and SP-4 (*gōng sūn*, Yellow Emperor). [6: 135] [50: 1083] [46: 644, 660, 670] [37: 349]

when wind prevails, there is stirring 风胜则动 *fēng shèng zé dòng*: From *Elementary Questions* (*sù wèn, yīn yáng yìng xiàng dà lùn*). Wind evil can cause disease characterized by physical movement such as tremor, convulsions, deviated eyes and mouth, squint, arched-back rigidity, and clenched jaw, and apparent movement such as dizziness and wandering pain. See VISCUS OF WIND AND WOOD; LIVER. [26: 460]

when yang abates, yin hides 阳杀阴藏 *yáng shā yīn cáng*: From *Elementary Questions* (*sù wèn, yīn yáng yìng xiàng dà lùn*). Yin responds to a contraction, recession, or weakening of yang qi by a corresponding tendency to become latent or disappear. See YIN AND YANG ARE ROOTED IN EACH OTHER. ◇ Chin 杀 *shā*, kill, slaughter; abate, recede, weaken; draw off. [26: 716]

when yang arises, yin grows 阳生阴长 *yáng shēng yīn zhǎng*: From *Elementary Questions* (*sù wèn, yīn yáng yìng xiàng dà lùn*). Yin qi can only grow when yang qi has its normal power to work engendering transformations. See YIN AND YANG ARE ROOTED IN EACH OTHER. [26: 712] [27: 3] [97: 240]

when yang is exuberant, there is external heat 阳盛则外热 *yáng shèng zé wài rè*: External evils cause yang qi that defends the outer body to become exuberant and put up a fierce fight that manifests in heat effusion. *Elementary Questions* (*sù wèn, tiáo jīng lùn*) states, "When the upper burner is inhibited, the skin becomes tight, the interstices become blocked, the mysterious mansions [i.e., sweat pores] become stopped, and defense qi fails to be discharged; hence there is external heat." [26: 714] [27: 129] [97: 242]

when yang is vacuous, there is external cold 阳虚则外寒 *yáng xū zé wài hán*: From *Elementary Questions* (*sù wèn, tiáo jīng lùn*). Yang vacuity, i.e., qi vacuity or insufficiency of the life gate fire manifests in cold signs such as bright white facial complexion, aversion to cold, cold limbs, and tendency to catch colds. [26: 715] [27: 1300] [97: 242]

when yang network vessels are damaged, blood spills out 阳络伤则血外溢 *yáng luò shāng zé xuè wài yì*: When the yang network vessels (i.e., those of the upper or outer body) are damaged, there is bleeding. This refers to expectoration of blood, nosebleed, or bleeding gums due to damage to the network vessels by exuberant lung-stomach heat. [26: 717]

when yang prevails, there is heat 阳胜则热 *yáng shèng zé rè*: When yang qi is especially strong, febrile conditions develop. [26: 717] [27: 129]

when yang prevails, yin ails 阳胜则阴病 *yáng shèng zé yīn bìng*: From *Elementary Questions* (*sù wèn, yīn yáng yìng xiàng dà lùn*). Exuberant yang gives rise to illness involving damage to yin humor. See DAMAGE TO FLUIDS. [36: 23] [50: 651]

when yin is calm and yang is sound 阴平阳秘 *yīn píng yáng mì*: Health expressed in terms of yin and yang. When yin is undisturbed by hyperactive yang, it is calm. When yang is exuberant, it performs its normal securing function of protecting the body against external evils, and retaining yin essence in the body. *Elementary Questions* (*sù wèn, shēng qì tōng tiān lùn*) says, "When yin is calm and yang is sound, essence-spirit is in order." [26: 617]

when yin is exuberant, there is cold 阴盛则寒 *yīn shèng zé hán*: WHEN YIN PREVAILS, THERE IS COLD. [27: 129] [97: 236]

when yin is exuberant, there is internal cold
阴盛则内寒 *yáng shèng zé nèi hán*: When yin evil
is exuberant, the qi transformation of the bowels
and viscera is disturbed, there is congealing stagnation in the blood vessels, and cold-type pathoconditions such as water qi, phlegm-rheum, or swelling
and distention arise. *Elementary Questions* (*sù
wèn, tiáo jīng lùn*) states, "What is yin exuberance
engendering internal cold?... Reverse qi ascends
counterflow. Cold qi accumulates in the chest and
fails to drain away, and when it fails to drain away,
so warm qi disappears leaving only the cold and
the blood congeals causing stoppage in the vessels
and making the pulse large exuberant and rough;
hence this is center cold." See WHEN YIN PRE-
VAILS, THERE IS COLD. [50: 666] [26: 619] [27:
129] [97: 236]

when yin is vacuous, there is internal heat
阴虚则内热 *yīn xū zé nèi rè*: From *Elementary
Questions* (*sù wèn, tiáo jīng lùn*). **1.** (Originally) taxation fatigue damaging the spleen, causing spleen vacuity heat effusion. **2.** (Nowadays)
depletion of yin humor gives rise to internal heat
characterized by tidal heat [effusion], or vexing
heat in the five hearts, as well as night sweating,
dry mouth, red tongue, and a rapid fine pulse. [26:
619]

when yin prevails, there is cold 阴胜则寒 *yīn
shèng zé hán*: Synonym: *when yin is exuberant,
there is cold*. From *Elementary Questions* (*sù wèn,
yīn yáng yìng xìng dà lùn*). When yin qi prevails,
yang qi is debilitated; hence cold signs appear. See
WHEN YIN IS EXUBERANT, THERE IS INTERNAL
COLD. [26: 623]

when yin prevails, yang ails 阴胜则阳病 *yīn
shèng zé yáng bìng*: Exuberant yin gives rise to disease involving damage to the yang qi of the body.
[36: 23]

white 白 *bái*: **1.** The color of unsullied snow, or
any color approaching or tending toward it. In
the five phases, white is associated with metal,
an association that may derive from the color of
metals such as iron and silver. It possibly derives
from the purifying frost of autumn, although winter, the season of snow, is associated through water
with the color black. In the body, the white of the
eye, or qi wheel, is associated with lung-metal. In
the diagnosis of disease, a white (i.e., pale) complexion indicates vacuity or cold, whereas a white
tongue, if significant, indicates cold. White vaginal discharge is associated with spleen vacuity or
kidney vacuity. The associations of the color white
are thus related to those of purity and clearness
described in *Elementary Questions* (*sù wèn, zhì
zhēn yào dà lùn*): "all disease with watery humors
that are clear, pure, and cold is ascribed to cold."
2. The lung. In the term White-Draining Powder

(*xiè bái sǎn*), "white" refers to the lung. **3.** WHITE
TURBIDITY. [97: 154]

white crust 白疕 *bái bǐ*: Synonym: *snake lice*. A
skin disease characterized by red macules, papules
or plaque covered in scales. White crust affects
the extensor surface of the limbs, especially the elbows, knees, and shins, or the scalp and trunk,
often occurring symmetrically. It is attributed to
wind-cold invading from outside and the consequent disturbance of construction and defense, or
to wind-heat lying depressed in the skin for a long
time and transforming into dryness. WMC psoriasis. MED Dispel wind and moisten dryness;
clear heat and resolve toxin. Ledebouriella Sage-
Inspired Powder (*fáng fēng tōng shèng sǎn*) can
be given as oral medication. Apply Oxhide Lichen
Medicinal Paste (*niú pí xiǎn yào gāo*). ACU Base
treatment mainly on LI, SP, and ouch points (*ā
shì xué*). Select LI-4 (*hé gǔ*, Union Valley), LI-11
(*qū chí*, Pool at the Bend), SP-10 (*xuè hǎi*, Sea
of Blood), SP-6 (*sān yīn jiāo*, Three Yin Intersection), and ouch points (*ā shì xué*); needle with
drainage. In addition, the affected areas (ouch
points) can be tapped with a cutaneous needle
and cupped. They can be needled transversely
from several points on the periphery toward the
disease focus. Selection of supporting points according affected area: For the head, add LI-20
(*yíng xiāng*, Welcome Fragrance), GV-25 (*sù liáo*,
White Bone-Hole), TB-6 (*zhī gōu*, Branch Ditch),
and GB-20 (*fēng chí*, Wind Pool). For the upper limbs, add GB-20 (*fēng chí*, Wind Pool), TB-5
(*wài guān*, Outer Pass), and TB-6 (*zhī gōu*, Branch
Ditch). For the lower limbs, add ST-36 (*zú sān lǐ*,
Leg Three Li). Selection of points according to
signs: For pronounced itching, add Itch Reliever
(*zhǐ yǎng*) and GB-31 (*fēng shì*, Wind Market).
For blood dryness engendering wind, add BL-17
(*gé shū*, Diaphragm Transport) and BL-19 (*dǎn
shū*, Gallbladder Transport). If the condition has
been treated for a long time without success, prick
the veins behind the ears to let 1–3 drops of blood.
[26: 219] [15: 381] [113: 445]

white dry eye 白涩症 *bái sè zhèng*: Synonym:
white eye. Dryness of the eyes with blurring of the
vision without redness or swelling or other objective signs. White dry eye is attributed to vacuity
fire flaming upward that stems either from insufficiency of lung yin or from liver-kidney yin vacuity,
or to brewing damp-heat with deep-lying fire in the
qi aspect. MED For insufficiency of lung yin with
vacuity fire flaming upward, use Yin-Nourishing
Lung-Clearing Decoction (*yǎng yīn qīng fèi tāng*).
For liver-kidney yin vacuity with vacuity fire flaming upward, use Lycium Berry, Chrysanthemum,
and Rehmannia Pill (*qǐ jú dì huáng wán*) plus
tangkuei (*dāng guī*) and white peony (*bái sháo
yào*). For damp-heat, use variations of Three Ker-

nels Decoction (*sān rén tāng*) combined with Mulberry Root Bark Decoction (*sāng bái pí tāng*). [26: 228] [125: 187]

white dysentery 赤痢 *chì lì*: Dysentery characterized by pus in the stool. See DYSENTERY. [26: 226] [27: 360] [97: 155]

white eye 白眼 *bái yǎn*: WHITE DRY EYE. [26: 226]

white face 面白 *miàn bái*: WHITE FACIAL COMPLEXION.

white-face sand 白面痧 *bái miàn shā*: Erupting measles characterized by a somber white complexion, associated with improper eruption, cold limbs, and purple lips, and attributed to major depletion of center qi and nonmovement of spleen yang. Clinically, it is understood to be related to great sweating, diarrhea, or constitutional weakness. MED Treat by upraising and boosting qi with variations of Center-Supplementing Qi-Boosting Decoction (*bǔ zhōng yì qì tāng*). [26: 224]

white facial complexion 面色白 *miàn sè bái*: Synonym: *white face*. Any pale complexion, generally indicating cold or vacuity. Distinction is made between different forms of white: pale white means general pallor; bright white means pronounced lack of color observed, for example, when blood temporarily leaves the face; somber white is white with a tinge of gray or blue. A bright white complexion with facial vacuity edema generally indicates yang qi vacuity and occurs after massive bleeding, in chronic nephritis, or in WHEEZING AND PANTING patterns. A pale white lusterless complexion, together with general and facial emaciation, normally points to blood vacuity. *The Magic Pivot* (*líng shū*) states, "Blood desertion is characterized by a white, perished, and sheenless complexion." The sudden appearance of a somber white complexion in acute diseases is usually attributable to fulminant yang qi desertion. However, somber white may also be observed in cases of externally contracted wind-cold diseases characterized by aversion to cold, shivering, and severe abdominal pain due to interior cold. [6: 116] [92: 70]

white flesh 白肉 *bái ròu*: **1.** The white flesh of the palmar aspect of the hand and arm or plantar aspect of the foot in contradistinction to the RED FLESH, i.e., the sun-tanned flesh of the dorsal aspect. **2.** The outer layer of flesh that is white in color (fat). [25: 93] [27: 74]

white flood 白崩 *bái bēng*: Profuse white VAGINAL DISCHARGE of sudden onset. White flood is attributed to heart-spleen taxation damage from excessive anxiety and thought or to extreme vacuity cold taxation damaging the network vessels of the uterus. **Heart-spleen taxation damage** gives rise to white flood with heart palpitations,

shortness of breath, insomnia, and low food intake. MED Nourish the heart and quiet the spirit; fortify the spleen. Use Neutral Supplementing Heart-Settling Elixir (*píng bǔ zhèn xīn dān*). **Extreme vacuity cold taxation** gives rise to white flood with fatigue and lack of strength, physical cold and fear of cold, and cold in the smaller abdomen. MED Warm the channels and supplement vacuity. Combine sumac gallnut (*wǔ bèi zǐ*), psoralea (*bǔ gǔ zhī*), cistanche (*ròu cōng róng*), morinda (*bā jǐ tiān*), fenugreek (*hú lú bā*), poria (*fú líng*), calcined dragon bone (*duàn lóng gǔ*), and cinnabar (*zhū shā*), and make into pills with rice paste made by boiling rice in wine. Take 10 g at a time with warm wine or brine. ACU Base treatment mainly on the GIV, CV, back transport points, and SP. Main points: GB-26 (*dài mài*, Girdling Vessel), BL-30 (*bái huán shū*, White Ring Transport), CV-6 (*qì hǎi*, Sea of Qi), and SP-6 (*sān yīn jiāo*, Three Yin Intersection). Selection of points according to pattern: For heart-spleen taxation damage, add BL-20 (*pí shū*, Spleen Transport) BL-15 (*xīn shū*, Heart Transport), ST-36 (*zú sān lǐ*, Leg Three Li), SP-9 (*yīn líng quán*, Yin Mound Spring), and HT-7 (*shén mén*, Spirit Gate), needling with supplementation and adding moxa, and adding PC-6 (*nèi guān*, Inner Pass) and PC-4 (*xī mén*, Cleft Gate) for heart palpitations. For extreme vacuity cold taxation add BL-23 (*shèn shū*, Kidney Transport), BL-20 (*pí shū*, Spleen Transport), CV-4 (*guān yuán*, Pass Head), CV-3 (*zhōng jí*, Central Pole), and BL-32 (*cì liáo*, Second Bone-Hole), needling with supplementation and large amounts of moxa. [26: 226] [59: 87] [46: 689]

white lai 白癩 *bái lài*: A disease characterized by gradually whitening of areas of skin, numbness of the limbs, heat in the joints, lack of strength in the extremities, needling pain, hoarseness of the voice, and unclear vision. WMC tuberculoid leprosy. See PESTILENTIAL WIND. [26: 231]

white leak 白漏 *bái lòu*: From *A Thousand Gold Pieces Prescriptions* (*qiān jīn yào fāng*). A persistent watery thin white discharge from the vagina. MED Supplement the spleen and lung with Center-Supplementing Qi-Boosting Decoction (*bǔ zhōng yì qì tāng*) or Ginseng Construction-Nourishing Decoction (*rén shēn yǎng róng tāng*). ACU Base treatment mainly on GIV, CV, back transport points, and SP. Select GB-26 (*dài mài*, Girdling Vessel), BL-30 (*bái huán shū*, White Ring Transport), CV-6 (*qì hǎi*, Sea of Qi), SP-6 (*sān yīn jiāo*, Three Yin Intersection), BL-20 (*pí shū*, Spleen Transport), BL-13 (*fèi shū*, Lung Transport), ST-36 (*zú sān lǐ*, Leg Three Li), SP-9 (*yīn líng quán*, Yin Mound Spring), and LU-9 (*tài yuān*, Great Abyss). Needle with supplementation and add moxa. [26: 227]

white membrane invading the eye 白膜侵睛 *bái mó qīn jīng*: A disease of the eye characterized by the appearance of small gray-white vesicles at the border between the dark and white of the eye that gradually spreads into the dark of the eye. In severe cases, the vesicles join up, and after healing leave a nebulous screen. Other signs include aversion to light, pain, and tearing. The condition often repeatedly returns after clearing. It is caused by exuberant liver-lung heat or effulgent yin vacuity fire. WMC phlyctenular keratoconjunctivitis. MED Repletion patterns are treated by draining liver and lung fire with Gentian Liver-Draining Decoction (*lóng dǎn xiè gān tāng*) plus mulberry root bark (*sāng bái pí*), lycium root bark (*dì gǔ pí*), and scrophularia (*xuán shēn*). Effulgent yin vacuity fire patterns are treated by nourishing yin and clearing heat, using Yin-Nourishing Lung-Clearing Decoction (*yǎng yīn qīng fèi tāng*) plus abalone shell (*shí jué míng*) and fetid cassia (*jué míng zǐ*). [26: 228] [27: 503] [97: 157]

white of the eye 白睛 *bái jīng*, 白眼 *bái yǎn*, 白仁 *bái rén*: Synonym: *qi wheel*. The sclera and conjunctiva.

white ooze 白淫 *bái yín*: **1.** Semen in the urine or persistent vaginal discharge. **2.** Seminal efflux (i.e., loss of semen while awake), especially when severe. **3.** Severe seminal turbidity. [26: 225]

white patch 白癜 *bái diàn*: WHITE PATCH WIND.

white patch wind 白癜风 *bái diàn fēng*, 白驳风 *bái bó fēng*: Synonym: *white patch*. White patches on the skin attributed to disharmony of the blood arising when wind evil assails the exterior, causing the interstices to loose their tightness. White patch wind is most common in youth and the prime of life. It is characterized by creamy white macules of varying size, clearly distinguishable from the normal skin coloring. Any hair growing in the patches also turns white. Some of the patches have a brown or pale red papule in the center. The condition is associated with neither pain nor itching. It is of gradual onset, and often persists for a long period. WMC vitiligo. MED Dispel wind and overcome dampness; quicken the blood and rectify qi. Take White Patch Tablet (*bái bó piàn*) orally, and apply Psoralea Tincture (*bǔ gǔ zhī dīng*) topically. ACU The following two methods should be used in tandem. (1) Select ouch points (*ā shì xué*) as the main points, and tap lightly with a cutaneous needle and pole for 30 minutes once every other day. (2) Select distant points on the affected area: For the face, add LI-4 (*hé gǔ*, Union Valley). For the chest, add PC-6 (*nèi guān*, Inner Pass) and ST-36 (*zú sān lǐ*, Leg Three Li). For the abdomen, add SP-6 (*sān yīn jiāo*, Three Yin Intersection). For the lumbus and back, add BL-40 (*wěi zhōng*, Bend Center). Nee-

dle with even supplementation and drainage. [26: 230] [27: 473] [97: 156, 156] [42: 160]

white perverse crop 白鬎鬁 *bái là lì*: See BALD WHITE SCALP SORE; PERVERSE CROP.

white scaling wind 白屑风 *bái xiè fēng*: Synonym: *head-wind white scaling*. A scaling skin disease of the neck, which can spread over the face, nose, and ears. White scaling wind, is attributed to wind-heat that after invading the body through the pores, lies depressed for a long time and gives rise to blood dryness that deprives the skin of nourishment. It occurs after puberty, and is more common in males than females. The scales are easily removed by scratching or combing, and develop again. Sometimes some of the scales are yellow and oily, and crustlike. Sometimes there are itchy papules that produce a sticky or bloody fluid when scratched. The condition may be associated with hair loss in the affected areas. WMC seborrheic dermatitis; seborrheic ichthyosis. MED Dispel wind, moisten dryness, and clear heat. Take Wind-Dispersing Powder (*xiāo fēng sǎn*) orally, and rub on Flesh-Moistening Paste (*rùn jī gāo*) or Reversal Powder (*diān dǎo sǎn*) prepared as a wash with 1.5 g each of finely powdered raw rhubarb (*shēng dà huáng*) and sulfur (*shí liú huáng*) mixed into 100 ml. of limewash. [26: 225] [61: 369]

white tiger joint running 白虎历节 *bái hǔ lì jié*: See PAIN WIND; JOINT-RUNNING WIND.

white tongue fur 白苔 *bái tāi*: The clinical significance of a white tongue fur is fourfold. (1) Clean, moist, thin white fur is normal and healthy, but may also appear at the onset of sickness indicating that the evil has not yet entered the interior and right qi remains undamaged. (2) Glossy white fur indicates cold. If thin, it indicates external wind-cold or interior cold; if thick, it indicates cold-damp or cold-phlegm. (3) Dry white fur indicates transformation of cold evil into heat. An extremely dry thin white fur indicates insufficiency of fluids. A thick dry white fur indicates transformation of dampness into dryness. A mealy white fur with a red tongue body indicates "dampness trapping hidden heat," which is treated by first transforming the dampness to allow the heat to escape rather than with excessive use of cool medicinals. (4) Thick slimy white fur indicates phlegm-damp and is usually accompanied by a slimy sensation in the mouth, oppression in the chest, and torpid intake. White fur occurs in a variety of diseases. A thick white fur is mainly associated with hypertrophy of the corneal layer of the filiform papillae for unknown reasons. A white mold-like coating covering the tongue and the whole of the surface of the oral cavity, sometimes with small patches of mucosal erosion known as *erosion speckles*, is termed ORAL PUTREFACTION. A loose, crumblike fur is called a BEAN CURD FUR (tofu fur). These signs indicate the development of sweltering damp-heat in patterns of stomach vacuity and damage to yin. This generally occurs in enduring or serious illnesses and indicates complex patterns that are difficult to treat. [6: 124] [26: 223, 224, 229]

white turbidity 白浊 *bái zhuó*: **1.** Murky urine that is white in color. See URINARY TURBIDITY. **2.** Discharge of a murky white substance from the urethra, associated with inhibited urination with clear urine. See ESSENCE TURBIDITY. [26: 228] [56: 226] [97: 154]

white vaginal discharge 白带 *bái dài*: A discharge from the vagina of sticky white matter. White vaginal discharge is normal in some women, and may naturally increase before and after menstruation or during pregnancy. Only copious flow, especially when associated with abdominal pain or lumbar pain is viewed as pathological. White vaginal discharge is attributed to the girdling vessel failing to ensure retention, and insecurity of the controlling vessel resulting from spleen vacuity, liver depression and spleen vacuity, or damp-heat pouring downward. **Spleen vacuity** When due to spleen vacuity, white vaginal discharge is copious and associated with lassitude of spirit, yellow complexion, cold limbs, and sloppy stool. MED Fortify the spleen and eliminate dampness. Use Discharge-Ceasing Decoction (*wán dài tāng*). ACU Base treatment mainly on CV, GIV, SP, and ST. Select GB-26 (*dài mài*, Girdling Vessel), BL-30 (*bái huán shū*, White Ring Transport), BL-20 (*pí shū*, Spleen Transport), CV-6 (*qì hǎi*, Sea of Qi), SP-6 (*sān yīn jiāo*, Three Yin Intersection), ST-36 (*zú sān lǐ*, Leg Three Li), and SP-9 (*yīn líng quán*, Yin Mound Spring); needle with supplementation and add moxa. **Liver depression and spleen vacuity:** White vaginal discharge in patients with liver depression is sometime copious and sometimes scant. Other signs include mental problems, dizzy head, oppression in the chest, distention of the breasts. MED Course the liver and resolve depression. Use Free Wanderer Variant Powder (*jiā jiǎn xiāo yáo sǎn*). ACU Base treatment mainly on CV, GIV, SP, ST, and LR. Needle with supplementation at GB-26 (*dài mài*, Girdling Vessel), BL-30 (*bái huán shū*, White Ring Transport), CV-6 (*qì hǎi*, Sea of Qi), SP-6 (*sān yīn jiāo*, Three Yin Intersection), ST-36 (*zú sān lǐ*, Leg Three Li), and BL-20 (*pí shū*, Spleen Transport), and drainage at BL-18 (*gān shū*, Liver Transport), LR-3 (*tài chōng*, Supreme Surge), SP-9 (*yīn líng quán*, Yin Mound Spring); and LI-11 (*qū chí*, Pool at the Bend). **Damp-heat pouring downward:** White vaginal discharge due to damp-heat pouring downward has a fishy malodor. Other signs include pudendal itch, dizzy head, and fatigue. MED Clear heat and disinhibit dampness. Use Gentian Liver-Draining Decoction (*lóng dǎn xiè gān tāng*). ACU Base treatment mainly on CV, GIV, SP, and LR. Select GB-26 (*dài mài*, Girdling Vessel), BL-30 (*bái huán shū*, White Ring Transport), CV-6 (*qì hǎi*, Sea of Qi), SP-6 (*sān yīn jiāo*, Three Yin Intersection), SP-9 (*yīn líng quán*, Yin Mound Spring), LI-11 (*qū chí*, Pool at the Bend), and LR-2 (*xíng jiān*, Moving Between); needle with drainage. See SPLEEN VACUITY VAGINAL DISCHARGE; KIDNEY VACUITY VAGINAL DISCHARGE. [26: 225] [50: 431] [46: 597, 690] [37: 428] [113: 295]

white wandering wind 白游风 *bái yóu fēng*: See WANDERING WIND. [26: 226]

whiteworm disease 白虫病 *bái chóng bìng*: One of the NINE WORM DISEASES of *The Origin and Indicators of Disease* (*zhū bìng yuán hòu lùn*). INCH WHITEWORM.

whitlow 瘭疽 *biāo jū*: TIP-ABSCESS.

whooping cough 百日咳 *bǎi rì ké*: *Synonyms: cormorant cough; epidemic cough; hundred day cough; long-bout cough; hen cough.* A children's disease readily identifiable by the characteristic whoop of the cough. The whooping sound is similar to the sound made by a hen after laying an egg, hence the alternate name *hen cough*. Whooping cough is attributed to contraction of a seasonal evil, which causes phlegm turbidity to obstruct the airways and inhibit lung qi. If the cough continues, it can damage the network vessels of the lung and give rise to expectoration of blood. WMC pertussis. MED For initial-stage evil invading the lung, treat by transforming phlegm with warm acrid medicinals and by downbearing qi. Use Belamcanda and Ephedra Decoction (*shè gān má huáng tāng*). In the middle stage, where the evil is lodged in the lung, treat by clearing heat and diffusing the lung, using variations of Supplemented Ephedra, Apricot Kernel, Gypsum, and Licorice Decoction (*jiā wèi má xìng shí gān tāng*) or White-Draining Powder (*xiè bái sǎn*). Another formula is Cormorant Drool Pill (*lú cí xián wán*), containing cormorant's drool (*lú sī xián*), which is noted for its ability to treat cormorant cough and other types of cough. For enduring conditions causing lung-spleen vacuity, attention should be paid to supplementing the lung and spleen. ACU Base treatment mainly on LU, LI, and back transport points. Main points: LU-7 (*liè quē*, Broken Sequence), LI-4 (*hé gǔ*, Union Valley), BL-12 (*fēng mén*, Wind Gate), and BL-13 (*fèi shū*, Lung Transport). Selection of points according to stage of progression: For initial-stage evil invading the lung, add GB-20 (*fēng chí*, Wind Pool), and TB-5 (*wài guān*, Outer Pass), needling with drainage. For evil heat lodged in the lung, add GV-14 (*dà zhuī*, Great Hammer), GV-12 (*shēn zhù*, Body Pillar), LU-5 (*chǐ zé*, Cubit Marsh), and ST-40 (*fēng lóng*, Bountiful Bulge), needling with drainage. For spleen-lung vacuity in the late stage, add BL-20 (*pí shū*, Spleen Transport), LU-9 (*tài yuān*, Great Abyss), ST-36 (*zú sān lǐ*, Leg Three Li), and BL-43 (*gāo huāng shū*, Gao-Huang Transport), needling with supplementation. Selection of points according to signs: For expectoration of blood, add LU-3 (*tiān fǔ*, Celestial Storehouse) and GV-23 (*shàng xīng*, Upper Star). For reduced food intake and sloppy stool, add CV-12 (*zhōng wǎn*, Center Stomach Duct), ST-25 (*tiān shū*, Celestial Pivot), and CV-6 (*qì hǎi*, Sea of Qi). For lack of warmth in the extremities, add CV-4 (*guān yuán*, Pass Head). [26: 253]

wild-duck bones 鳧骨 *fú gǔ*: *The Golden Mirror of Medicine* (*yī zōng jīn jiàn, zhèng gǔ xīn fǎ yào zhǐ*) states, "The wild-duck bones are the side ribs of the lower chest." Modern sources say that these are the seventh, eighth, ninth and tenth ribs, which form the arch of the ribs. [26: 811]

wilting 痿 *wěi*: Synonyms: *atony* (*obs*); *wei* (*obs*). Weakness and limpness of the sinews that in severe cases prevents the lifting of the arms and legs accompanied by the sensation that the elbow, wrist, knee, and ankle are dislocated. In advanced cases, atrophy sets in. In clinical practice, the condition is mainly found to affect the legs, preventing the patient from walking, hence it is also called *crippling wilt*. Wilting patterns include withering and paralysis of the limbs in neonates and infants after high fever, which Western medicine attributes to poliomyelitis. WMC polyneuritis (multiple neuritis); acute myelitis; poliomyelitis; progressive myatrophy; myesthenia gravis; periodic paralysis; myodystrophy; hysterical paralysis. The pathomechanism of wilting has been explained in different ways over the centuries. *Elementary Questions* (*sù wèn, wěi lùn*) discusses five forms of wilting: SKIN AND [BODY] HAIR WILTING, due to lung qi scorching the lobes resulting from loss or unfulfilled hopes; VESSEL WILTING, due to heart qi heat that develops excessive sorrow and grief; SINEW WILTING, due to liver qi heat resulting from unfulfilled hopes, incontinent desires, and excessive sexual activity; FLESH WILTING, due to spleen qi heat resulting from being soaked with water, working with water, or living in damp places; BONE WILTING, due to kidney qi heat resulting from walking long distances and thirst after exposure to great heat. *The Inner Canon* (*nèi jīng*) also suggests that, at the time, the yang brightness was important in the treatment of wilting patterns, and that it was therefore important in the etiology. *Elementary Questions* (*sù wèn, wěi lùn*) explains this importance in the following way: "Yang brightness is the sea of the five viscera and six bowels, and governs the moistening of the ancestral sinews (see ANCESTRAL SINEW), which leash the bones and allow the hinges (i.e., the major joints) to move uninhibitedly. The thorough-

fare (*chōng*) vessel is the sea of the channel vessels; it governs irrigation of the ravines and valleys, and unites with the yang brightness at the ancestral sinews The yin and yang (the thoroughfare (*chōng*) vessel and yang brightness) converge at the ancestral sinews... They home to the girdling (*dài*) vessel and net the governing (*dū*) vessel. Thus, when yang brightness is vacuous, the ancestral sinews are slack and the girdling fails to conduct; hence the legs become wilted and useless." Over the centuries, wilting has generally been considered more commonly to be due to internal damage than to external evils, more commonly due to cold than heat, and more commonly to vacuity rather than to repletion. Nowadays, the view prevails that it is due to lung heat scorching the lobes, which spreads to the other viscera. When the heat affects the yang brightness (stomach) channel's ability to "moisten the ancestral sinew," the sinews are scorched by the heat and become wilted. Liver-kidney depletion also plays a role. When the kidney is depleted, the bones become desiccated and the marrow is reduced. When the kidney fails to nourish the liver, the sinews are deprived of nourishment. Liver-kidney depletion is considered to be sufficient in itself, without lung-stomach heat, to cause wilting. Wilting patterns, according to modern texts, primarily include lung heat with damage to liquid, soddening by damp-heat, spleen-stomach vacuity, and liver-kidney depletion. See also the entries listed below. **Lung heat with damage to liquid** during or after illness gives rise to sudden limpness of the limbs. It manifests as heat effusion, heart vexation, thirst, cough and dry pharynx, yellow or reddish urine, dry bound stool, a red tongue with yellow fur, and a fine rapid pulse. This is explained by warm heat invading the lung, which damages liquid. When liquid is insufficient, it cannot be distributed to all parts of the body, so that the sinews are deprived of nourishment. MED Clear heat and moisten dryness; nourish the lung and engender liquid. Use Dryness-Clearing Lung-Rescuing Decoction (*qīng zào jiù fèi tāng*). If poor appetite and dry mouth and pharynx are pronounced, this indicates damage to lung-stomach yin, which can be treated with Stomach-Boosting Decoction (*yì wèi tāng*). **Soddening by damp-heat** (i.e., saturation of the flesh by damp-heat) causes wilting characterized by heavy cumbersome limbs that are limp and lack strength, and that may be slightly swollen or numb. The lower limbs are most commonly affected. This is associated with a liking for coolness and fear of heat, in some cases with heat effusion. Other signs include glomus and oppression in the chest, inhibited voidings of reddish urine with stinging pain, a slimy yellow tongue fur, and a soggy rapid pulse. The heavy cumbersome and possibly slightly swollen limbs are explained by damp-heat soddening the flesh. The limp wilting limbs and numbness are explained by damp-heat soddening the vessels obstructing qi and blood. MED Clear heat and disinhibit dampness. Use variations of Mysterious Two Powder (*èr miào sǎn*). For pronounced heaviness and swelling, and white slimy tongue fur, add magnolia bark (*hòu pò*), poria (*fú líng*), and alisma (*zé xiè*). If damp-heat damages yin, causing emaciation, heat sensation in the lower limbs, heart vexation, a rapid fine pulse, and a tongue that is red at the tip or peeled clean of fur, remove atractylodes (*cāng zhú*) and add adenophora/glehnia (*shā shēn*), ophiopogon (*mài mén dōng*), dried/fresh rehmannia (*shēng dì huáng*), and trichosanthes root (*tiān huā fěn*) to clear heat and engender liquid. For pronounced signs of static blood obstruction such as numbness and inhibited movement of the joints with purple tongue and choppy pulse, add peach kernel (*táo rén*), carthamus (*hóng huā*), red peony (*chì sháo yào*), and cinnamon twig (*guì zhī*). **Spleen-stomach vacuity** gives rise to gradually worsening limpness and wilting of the limbs with reduced eating, sloppy stool, puffy face, lassitude of spirit and lack of strength, lusterless complexion, a thin white tongue fur, and a fine pulse. MED Fortify the spleen and boost qi. Use Ginseng, Poria (Hoelen), and Ovate Atractylodes Powder (*shēn líng bái zhú sǎn*). For fear of cold and cold limbs, add aconite (*fù zǐ*) and dried ginger (*gān jiāng*) to warm spleen yang. For dual vacuity of qi and blood due to enduring illness, add astragalus (*huáng qí*) and tangkuei (*dāng guī*). **Liver-kidney depletion** causes limp wilting lower limbs with limp aching lumbus. This condition develops slowly and is accompanied by dizziness, tinnitus, seminal emission, and in some cases enuresis and menstrual irregularities. The tongue is red with little fur, and the pulse is fine and rapid. Liver-kidney depletion causes insufficiency of essence blood which deprives the sinews of nourishment. MED Supplement the liver and kidney; enrich yin and clear heat. Use Hidden Tiger Pill (*hǔ qián wán*). For pronounced heat, remove cynomorium (*suǒ yáng*). For withered-yellow facial complexion, heart palpitations or fearful throbbing, pale red tongue, and a weak fine pulse, add codonopsis (*dǎng shēn*), astragalus (*huáng qí*), tangkuei (*dāng guī*), and millettia (*jī xuè téng*). For detriment to yin affecting yang in enduring illness, characterized by fear of cold, impotence, long voidings of clear urine, pale tongue with and a forceless fine sunken pulse, remove anemarrhena (*zhī mǔ*) and phellodendron (*huáng bǎi*), and add deerhorn flakes (*lù jiǎo xiè*), psoralea (*bǔ gǔ zhī*), epimedium (*yín yáng huò*), morinda (*bā jǐ tiān*), aconite (*fù zǐ*), and cinnamon bark (*ròu guì*). ACU Acupuncture and manipulation (*tuī ná*) provide effective complements

to treatment. Acupuncture treatment is based mainly on hand and foot yang brightness (*yáng míng*) LI-ST, to free channel qi and nourish the sinew and bone. The main points are: LI-10 (*shǒu sān lǐ*, Arm Three Li), CV-12 (*zhōng wǎn*, Center Stomach Duct), BL-21 (*wèi shū*, Stomach Transport), BL-20 (*pí shū*, Spleen Transport), ST-36 (*zú sān lǐ*, Leg Three Li), GB-34 (*yáng líng quán*, Yang Mound Spring), and SP-6 (*sān yīn jiāo*, Three Yin Intersection). On the upper limbs, add LI-15 (*jiān yú*, Shoulder Bone), LI-11 (*qū chí*, Pool at the Bend), LI-4 (*hé gǔ*, Union Valley), LI-5 (*yáng xī*, Yang Ravine), TB-5 (*wài guān*, Outer Pass), and SI-3 (*hòu xī*, Back Ravine). On the lower limbs, add GB-30 (*huán tiào*, Jumping Round), ST-31 (*bì guān*, Thigh Joint), ST-34 (*liáng qiū*, Beam Hill), GB-39 (*xuán zhōng*, Suspended Bell), and ST-41 (*jiě xī*, Ravine Divide). For variations according to pattern, see the entries listed below. See CHILD WILTING PATTERN. ◇ Chin 瘘 *wěi* is composed of the illness signifier 疒 with 委 *wěi*, probably used here as a simplification of 萎 *wěi*, wilt, wither. See the etymology of LUNG WILTING. [26: 770] [50: 1627] [80: 640] [9: 578] [106: 184–187] [39: 233] [46: 638] [113: 239]

Wilting (*wěi*)

BONE WILTING (*gū wěi*)
FLESH WILTING (*ròu wěi*)
SKIN AND HAIR WILTING (*pí máo wěi*)
SINEW WILTING (*jīn wěi*)
VESSEL WILTING (*mài wěi*)
DAMP-HEAT WILTING (*shī rè wěi*)
DAMP PHLEGM WILTING (*shī tán wěi*)
DRYNESS-HEAT WILTING (*zào rè wěi*)
BLOOD STASIS WILTING (*xuè yū wěi*)
BLOOD VACUITY WILTING (*xuè xū wěi*)
YIN VACUITY WILTING (*yīn xū wěi*)
QI VACUITY WILTING (*qì xū wěi*)
CHILD WILTING PATTERN (*xiǎo ér wěi zhèng*)

---

wilting-impediment 瘘痹 *wěi bì*: A general term denoting WILTING (*wěi*) and IMPEDIMENT (*bì*).

wilting pattern 瘘证 *wěi zhèng*: WILTING.

wind 风 *fēng*: **1.** One of the SIX QI; any natural movement of air. See AVERSION TO WIND; TEARING ON EXPOSURE TO WIND. **2.** *Synonym: wind evil.* One of the SIX EXCESSES; wind as a cause of disease, a yang evil. The nature of wind as an evil and its clinical manifestations are similar to those of the meteorological phenomenon from which it derives its name: it comes and goes quickly, moves swiftly, blows intermittently, and sways the branches of the trees. "Wind is swift and changeable," and its clinical manifestations as an evil have the following characteristics: **2a.** Rapid onset and swift changes in condition. **2b.** Convulsions, tremor, shaking of the head, dizziness, and wandering pain and itching. **2c.** Invasion of the upper part of the body and the exterior, e.g., the head (the uppermost part of the body), the lung (the uppermost of the major organs), and the skin and [body] hair. **2d.** Facial paralysis and hemiplegia. Note that although wind is associated with movement, by causing stiffness and clenched jaw, it can also be seen to have the power to check normal movement, as in facial paralysis. **3.** Internal wind, i.e., wind arising within the body by the following pathomechanisms: LIVER WIND STIRRING INTERNALLY, which occurs when liver yang and liver fire transform into wind, manifesting in dizziness, tremor, and convulsions; EXTREME HEAT ENGENDERING WIND, arising in externally contracted diseases such as FRIGHT WIND and manifesting in convulsions, stiffness of the neck, arched-back rigidity, etc.; BLOOD VACUITY ENGENDERING WIND, arising when great sweating, great vomiting, great diarrhea, major loss of blood, damage to yin in enduring illness, or kidney-water failing to moisten liver-wood causes desiccation of the blood that deprives the sinews of nourishment and insufficiency of liver yin that leaves yang unsubdued and allows liver wind to scurry around internally. Vacuity wind stirring within is marked by dizziness, tremor, worm-like movement in the extremities, or clouding collapse. See also VISCUS OF WIND AND WOOD; LIVER; FRIGHT WIND. **4.** Any of various diseases ascribed to wind or bearing attributes of wind; occurs in disease names such as LIP WIND, WHITE PATCH WIND, GOOSE-FOOT WIND, HEAD WIND, THUNDER HEAD WIND, CRANE'S-KNEE WIND, JOINT-RUNNING WIND, GREAT NUMBING WIND, SCROTAL WIND, CHILDBED WIND, WANDERING WIND, NIPPLE WIND, LOST HEART WIND, GREEN WIND INTERNAL OBSTRUCTION, and YELLOW WIND INTERNAL OBSTRUCTION. [26: 456] [27: 111] [97: 99] [6: 103]

wind and dampness contending with each other 风湿相搏 *fēng shī xiāng bó*: Interaction between wind and dampness evils after they have entered the body. Wind is a yang evil and mobile and penetrating; dampness is a yin evil, and tends to stagnate and impede the movement of qi and blood. When the two combine, they cause generalized pain in the joints and flesh. *On Cold Damage* (*shāng hán lùn*) states, "When wind and dampness contend with each other, the joints are affected by vexing and pulling pain that prevents bending and stretching and is exacerbated by touching. There is sweating, shortness of breath, inhibited urination, aversion to wind with disinclination to remove clothing, and in some cases mild generalized swelling. It is treated with Licorice and Aconite Decoction (*gān cǎo fù zǐ tāng*)." ACU Base treat-

ment mainly on GB, GV, TB, and LI. Select GB-20 (*fēng chí*, Wind Pool), GV-20 (*bǎi huì*, Hundred Convergences), TB-5 (*wài guān*, Outer Pass), LI-11 (*qū chí*, Pool at the Bend), LI-4 (*hé gǔ*, Union Valley), ST-36 (*zú sān lǐ*, Leg Three Li), and SP-9 (*yīn líng quán*, Yin Mound Spring), as the main points. Needle with drainage. [26: 462]

wind and fire fanning each other 风火相煽 *fēng huǒ xiāng shān*: Exuberant evil heat in febrile disease scorching the liver channel and causing internal stirring of liver wind characterized by clouded spirit and FRIGHT REVERSAL. [26: 456]

wind bar 风关 *fēng guān*: One of the THREE BARS OF THE FINGER. See INFANT'S FINGER EXAMINATION. [26: 463] [27: 177] [97: 99]

wind can overcome dampness 风能胜湿 *fēng néng shèng shī*: From *Elementary Questions* (*sù wèn, yìng yáng yìng xiàng dà lùn*): "wind overcomes dampness." In the natural environment, wind can dispel dampness; when the wind blows, things dry. In Chinese medicine, this analogy is used to explain the ability of wind-dispelling medicinals to treat dampness. Although in this context, wind refers to wind-dispelling medicinals (medicinals opposed to wind), rather than wind itself, it is observed that many wind medicinals are dry. Medicinals such as ledebouriella (*fáng fēng*), notopterygium (*qiāng huó*), duhuo (*dú huó*), ligusticum (*chuān xiōng*), Chinese lovage (*gǎo běn*), and vitex (*màn jīng zǐ*) are commonly used to overcome dampness. The ability of wind medicinals to overcome dampness is reflected in formula names such as Notopterygium Dampness-Overcoming Decoction (*qiāng huó shèng shī tāng*) and Bupleurum Dampness-Overcoming Decoction (*chái hú shèng shī tāng*). [77: 321]

wind choke 风懿 *fēng yì*: A condition occurring after sudden clouding with inability to recognize people, stiff tongue preventing speaking, and blockage of the throat sometimes attended by a characteristic "ee ee" sound. It falls within the scope of visceral stroke in wind stroke. [26: 463] [27: 397]

wind-cold 风寒 *fēng hán*: Wind and cold disease evils combined, manifesting pronounced aversion to cold with mild heat effusion, and such signs as headache, generalized pain, absence of sweating, nasal congestion and runny nose, cough, clear thin phlegm, absence of thirst. The tongue fur is glossy and white, and the pulse is floating and tight. Wind-cold is characterized by the presence of wind signs and pronounced cold signs, and therefore presents as an exterior cold pattern. [26: 458] [97: 115]

Wind-Cold–Dissipating Medicinals

麻黄 (*má huáng*) ephedra (Ephedrae Herba)

桂枝 (*guì zhī*) cinnamon twig (Cinnamomi Ramulus)

紫苏叶 (*zǐ sū yè*) perilla leaf (Perillae Folium)

紫苏 (*zǐ sū*) perilla (Perillae Folium, Caulis et Calyx)

生姜 (*shēng jiāng*) fresh ginger (Zingiberis Rhizoma Recens)

紫苏梗 (*zǐ sū gěng*) perilla stem (Perillae Caulis)

香薷 (*xiāng rú*) elsholtzia (Elsholtziae Herba)

姜皮 (*jiāng pí*) ginger skin (Zingiberis Rhizomatis Cortex)

荆芥 (*jīng jiè*) schizonepeta (Schizonepetae Herba et Flos)

防风 (*fáng fēng*) ledebouriella (Ledebouriellae Radix)

羌活 (*qiāng huó*) notopterygium (Notopterygii Rhizoma)

白芷 (*bái zhǐ*) angelica (Angelicae Dahuricae Radix)

藁本 (*gǎo běn*) Chinese lovage (Ligustici Sinensis Rhizoma et Radix)

苍耳子 (*cāng ěr zǐ*) xanthium (Xanthii Fructus)

辛夷 (*xīn yí*) magnolia flower[1] (Magnoliae Flos[1])

葱白 (*cōng bái*) scallion white (Allii Fistulosi Bulbus)

胡荽 (*hú suī*) coriander (Coriandri Herba cum Radice)

柽柳 (*chēng liǔ*) tamarisk (Tamaricis Ramulus et Folium)

---

wind-cold common cold 风寒感冒 *fēng hán gǎn mào*: Common cold due to contraction of wind-cold. The main signs are heat effusion, aversion to cold, headache, absence of sweating, nasal congestion, heavy voice, sneezing, itchy throat, cough, absence of thirst, a thin white tongue fur, and a tight floating pulse. MED Warm acrid exterior resolution. Use formulas such as Scallion and Fermented Soybean Decoction (*cōng chǐ tāng*) or Schizonepeta and Ledebouriella Toxin-Vanquishing Powder (*jīng fáng bài dú sǎn*). For pronounced exterior cold, add ephedra (*má huáng*) and cinnamon twig (*guì zhī*). For headache and aching joints, add angelica (*bái zhǐ*). For nasal congestion and heavy voice, add magnolia flower[1] (*xīn yí*), xanthium (*cāng ěr zǐ*), asarum (*xì xīn*), and chebule (*hē zǐ*). ACU Base treatment mainly on LI, LU, and BL. Main points: LU-7 (*liè quē*, Broken Sequence), LI-4 (*hé gǔ*, Union Valley), BL-12 (*fēng mén*, Wind Gate), and GB-20 (*fēng chí*, Wind Pool). For heat effusion, add GV-14 (*dà zhuī*, Great Hammer). For headache, add GV-20 (*bǎi huì*, Hundred Convergences), Greater Yang (*tài yáng*), and SI-3 (*hòu xī*, Back Ravine). For absence of sweating, add

KI-7 (*fù liū*, Recover Flow). For nasal congestion and runny nose, add LI-20 (*yíng xiāng*, Welcome Fragrance) and Hall of Impression (*yìn táng*). For cough, add BL-13 (*fèi shū*, Lung Transport), and BL-11 (*dà zhù*, Great Shuttle). Needle all points with drainage and add moxa. For back pain and generalized pain, cup BL-13 (*fèi shū*, Lung Transport), BL-12 (*fēng mén*, Wind Gate), and BL-11 (*dà zhù*, Great Shuttle). Alternatively, use push-cupping, from GV-14 (*dà zhuī*, Great Hammer) down to the lumbus and back, finally to leave the cup in place at BL-13 (*fèi shū*, Lung Transport) for 10–20 minutes. See WIND-COLD FETTERING THE LUNG. [27: 354] [97: 102] [80: 57]

wind-cold cough 风寒咳嗽 *fēng hán ké sòu*: COUGH attributed to wind-cold invading the lung, causing nondiffusion of lung qi. Wind-cold cough is associated with thin phlegm, nasal congestion and runny nose, heavy voice, headache, joint pain, heat effusion and aversion to cold without sweating, white tongue fur, and a floating pulse. MED Course wind and dissipate cold; diffuse lung qi. Use Inula Powder (*jīn fèi cǎo sǎn*) or Apricot Kernel and Perilla Powder (*xìng sū sǎn*). ACU Base treatment mainly on LU and LI. Select BL-13 (*fèi shū*, Lung Transport), LU-7 (*liè quē*, Broken Sequence), LI-4 (*hé gǔ*, Union Valley), BL-12 (*fēng mén*, Wind Gate), CV-22 (*tiān tú*, Celestial Chimney), and ST-40 (*fēng lóng*, Bountiful Bulge); needle with drainage and, if appropriate, add moxa. Apply moxibustion or fire cupping at BL-11 (*dà zhù*, Great Shuttle). [26: 458] [46: 652]

wind-cold-damp 风寒湿 *fēng hán shī*: A combination of wind, cold, and dampness evils. *Elementary Questions* (*sù wèn, bì lùn*) states, "When the wind, cold, and damp evils concur and combine, they give rise to IMPEDIMENT (*bì*)." See IMPEDIMENT. [27: 116]

wind-cold-damp impediment 风寒湿痹 *fēng hán shī bì*: IMPEDIMENT.[1] [26: 459]

wind-cold deafness 风寒耳聋 *fēng hán ěr lóng*: DEAFNESS attributed to wind-cold fettering the exterior, congealing in the channels, and blocking the ear orifices. Wind-cold deafness is associated with headache, aversion to cold, heat effusion, absence of sweating, nasal congestion, and tinnitus. MED Dispel cold with warm acrid medicinals; open the orifices and effuse sweat. Formulas such as Nine-Ingredient Notopterygium Decoction (*jiǔ wèi qiāng huó tāng*) may be used. ACU See DEAFNESS. [26: 458]

wind-cold dizziness 风寒眩晕 *fēng hán xuàn yūn*: DIZZINESS attributed to contraction of wind-cold. Distinction is made between wind evil dizziness and cold evil dizziness. **Wind evil dizziness** is dizziness associated with headache and frontal pain, vexing joint pain, generalized heat [effusion], copious sweating, qi ascent panting, vexation and agitation, and periodic dizzy spells. MED Dispel wind using formulas such as Notopterygium and Ledebouriella Decoction (*qiāng huó fáng fēng tāng*). ACU Base treatment mainly on GV, GB, and LI. Select GV-20 (*bǎi huì*, Hundred Convergences), GB-20 (*fēng chí*, Wind Pool), GV-16 (*fēng fǔ*, Wind Mansion), TB-5 (*wài guān*, Outer Pass), GB-15 (*tóu lín qì*, (Head) Overlooking Tears), TB-23 (*sī zhú kōng*, Silk Bamboo Hole), and LI-4 (*hé gǔ*, Union Valley); needle with drainage. **Cold evil dizziness** is periodic dizziness accompanied by generalized heat [effusion] without sweating, aversion to cold, hypertonicity, headache, generalized pain. MED Dispel cold using formulas such as Notopterygium Toxin-Vanquishing Decoction (*qiāng huó bài dú tāng*). ACU Base treatment mainly on GV, LU, and LI. Select GV-20 (*bǎi huì*, Hundred Convergences), GB-20 (*fēng chí*, Wind Pool), TB-5 (*wài guān*, Outer Pass), LI-4 (*hé gǔ*, Union Valley), and LU-7 (*liè quē*, Broken Sequence); needle with drainage and add moxa. [26: 459]

wind-cold fettering the exterior 风寒外束 *fēng hán wài shù*: WIND-COLD causing an exterior pattern. The main signs are headache, generalized pain, and aversion to wind. Other signs include absence of sweating, absence of thirst, cough with expectoration of clear thin phlegm, glossy white tongue fur, and a tight floating pulse. This pattern is one form a common cold can take. MED Resolve the exterior with warmth and acridity; dissipate wind-cold; diffuse lung qi. Use Ephedra Decoction (*má huáng tāng*) and its variations for cough, rapid breathing, and absence of sweating, and Tea-Blended Ligusticum (Cnidium Root) Powder (*chuān xiōng chá tiáo sǎn*) for especially severe headache. ACU Base treatment mainly on GB, LU, and LI. Select GB-20 (*fēng chí*, Wind Pool), LI-4 (*hé gǔ*, Union Valley), LU-7 (*liè quē*, Broken Sequence), and TB-5 (*wài guān*, Outer Pass); needle with drainage and add moxa. Selection of points according to signs: For headache, add GV-20 (*bǎi huì*, Hundred Convergences) and Greater Yang (*tài yáng*). For generalized pain, add BL-13 (*fèi shū*, Lung Transport) and BL-12 (*fēng mén*, Wind Gate), and cup BL-11 (*dà zhù*, Great Shuttle); alternatively, apply push-cupping from GV-14 (*dà zhuī*, Great Hammer) to the lumbus, and run back to BL-13 (*fèi shū*, Lung Transport), keeping the cup there for 20 minutes. For absence of sweating, add KI-7 (*fù liū*, Recover Flow) and BL-11 (*dà zhù*, Great Shuttle). See also WIND-COLD FETTERING THE LUNG.

wind-cold fettering the exterior panting 风寒外束喘 *fēng hán wài shù chuǎn*: See WIND-COLD RAPID PANTING. [26: 458] [46: 655]

wind-cold fettering the lung 风寒束肺 *fēng hán shù fèi*: Wind-cold invading the lung and causing nondiffusion of lung qi. The main signs are cough and aversion to cold. Other signs include nasal congestion and runny nose with clear snivel, itchy throat, and thin white phlegm. In some cases there may also be aversion to cold and slight heat effusion without sweating. The tongue fur is thin and white. The pulse is tight and floating. MED Effuse and dissipate wind-cold; diffuse the lung and suppress cough. Use Cough-Stopping Powder (*zhǐ sòu sǎn*). ACU Base treatment mainly on GB, LU, and LI. Select BL-13 (*fèi shū*, Lung Transport), GB-20 (*fēng chí*, Wind Pool), LU-7 (*liè quē*, Broken Sequence), LI-4 (*hé gǔ*, Union Valley), and TB-5 (*wài guān*, Outer Pass). Needle with drainage. **Analysis:** Externally contracted wind-cold affects the skin and [body] hair and then the lung. It causes nondiffusion of lung qi, which manifests as cough. The nose is the orifice of the lung and the throat is its gate, and when wind-cold impairs the lung's diffusion and depuration, there is nasal congestion with runny nose and clear snivel, and an itchy throat. When the evil settles in the lung-defense, defensive yang is obstructed, hence there is aversion to cold, and because of right qi's attempt to resist the evil, the ensuing fight between right and evil produces a slight heat effusion. The thin white tongue fur is a sign of evil invading the skin and [body] hair. The floating pulse is associated with the exterior, and a tight pulse is associated with cold. Hence a tight floating pulse indicates a wind-cold exterior pattern. **Comparison:** *Wind-heat invading the lung:* Wind-cold fettering the lung and wind-heat invading the lung are both external contractions. Wind-cold is characterized by pronounced aversion to cold and mild heat effusion, a thin white tongue fur, tight floating pulse, runny noise with clear snivel, and cough with thin clear white phlegm. Wind-heat is characterized by pronounced heat effusion with mild aversion to cold and wind, cough with thick yellow phlegm, nasal congestion with turbid yellow snivel, dry mouth, sore throat, a red-tipped tongue, white or yellow tongue fur, and a rapid floating pulse. *Wind-cold fettering the exterior:* Wind-cold fettering the lung and wind-cold fettering the exterior both involve wind-cold affecting the skin and [body] hair and the interstices. They differ by emphasis. Wind-cold fettering the exterior has cough as the main sign attended by exterior signs. Wind-cold fettering the exterior is marked principally by exterior signs, and has cough as a possible secondary sign. [26: 458] [116: 67] [57: 76]

wind-cold headache 风寒头痛 *fēng hán tóu tòng*: HEADACHE caused by wind-cold assailing from outside. Wind-cold headache is characterized by pain that may stretch to the nape and back, aversion to cold, pain in the joints, nasal congestion and runny nose, a thin white tongue fur, and a tight floating pulse. MED Course with and dissipate cold with Tea-Blended Ligusticum (Cnidium Root) Powder (*chuān xiōng chá tiáo sǎn*). ACU Base treatment mainly on points of the three yang channels, GV and LU. Select GB-20 (*fēng chí*, Wind Pool), GV-20 (*bǎi huì*, Hundred Convergences), Greater Yang (*tài yáng*), LI-4 (*hé gǔ*, Union Valley), LU-7 (*liè què*, Broken Sequence), and SI-3 (*hòu xī*, Back Ravine). Needle with even supplementation and drainage and, if appropriate, add moxa. For selection of points according to affected area, see HEADACHE. [26: 459] [46: 621] [37: 362]

wind-cold panting 风寒喘 *fēng hán chuǎn*: PANTING attributed to wind-cold fettering the exterior. See WIND-COLD RAPID PANTING. [26: 459]

wind-cold rapid panting 风寒喘急 *fēng hán chuǎn jí*: Synonym: *wind-cold panting*. PANTING attributed to externally contracted wind-cold lying depressed in the lung. MED If there is heat effusion and absence of swelling use Florid Canopy Powder (*huá gài sǎn*) to make the patient sweat. If there are also signs of lung vacuity, use Pulse-Engendering Powder (*shēng mài sǎn*) plus ephedra (*má huáng*), apricot kernel (*xìng rén*), pinellia (*bàn xià*), fresh ginger (*shēng jiāng*), and puccoon (*zǐ cǎo*) to "supplement and dissipate." ACU Base treatment mainly on LU, LI, and CV. Select BL-12 (*fēng mén*, Wind Gate), BL-13 (*fèi shū*, Lung Transport), Panting Stabilizer (*dìng chuǎn*), LU-7 (*liè què*, Broken Sequence), LU-5 (*chǐ zé*, Cubit Marsh), LI-4 (*hé gǔ*, Union Valley), and CV-17 (*shān zhōng*, Chest Center); needle with drainage and add moxa. For lung vacuity with wind-cold, add BL-43 (*gāo huāng shū*, Gao-Huang Transport) and CV-6 (*qì hǎi*, Sea of Qi), needling these two points with supplementation; if qi vacuity is pronounced, apply moxa. [26: 459]

wind-cold rib-side pain 风寒胁痛 *fēng hán xié tòng*: RIB-SIDE PAIN attributed to wind-cold evils lodged under the rib-side, and accompanied by heat effusion and aversion to cold, bitter taste in the mouth, dry retching, and a stringlike pulse. MED Treat by coursing and harmonizing with variations of Minor Bupleurum Decoction (*xiǎo chái hú tāng*). ACU Base treatment mainly on LU, LI, LR, and GB. Select GB-20 (*fēng chí*, Wind Pool), BL-12 (*fēng mén*, Wind Gate), LU-7 (*liè què*, Broken Sequence), LI-4 (*hé gǔ*, Union Valley), TB-5 (*wài guān*, Outer Pass), LR-14 (*qī mén*, Cycle Gate), TB-6 (*zhī gōu*, Branch Ditch), and GB-34 (*yáng líng quán*, Yang Mound Spring); needle with drainage and add moxa. See RIB-SIDE PAIN. [26: 458]

wind-cold toothache 风寒牙痛 *fēng hán yá tòng*: TOOTHACHE attributable to externally contracted wind-cold. See TOOTHACHE.

wind constipation 风秘 *fēng bì*: Dry bound stool and difficult defecation arising when wind contends with the lung and is transmitted to the large intestine, where it causes or exacerbates dryness of the fluids. Wind constipation is observed most commonly among the weak and elderly, and those predisposed to wind disease. MED Course wind, harmonize the blood, and moisten the intestines. Use formulas such as Hemp Seed Pill (*má rén wán*) or Intestine-Moistening Pill (*rùn cháng wán*). ACU Base treatment mainly on alarm, back transport, and lower uniting points of LI, and on LU. Select BL-25 (*dà cháng shū*, Large Intestine Transport), ST-25 (*tiān shū*, Celestial Pivot), ST-37 (*shàng jù xū*, Upper Great Hollow), BL-12 (*fēng mén*, Wind Gate), GB-20 (*fēng chí*, Wind Pool), LU-9 (*tài yuān*, Great Abyss), and LI-4 (*hé gǔ*, Union Valley); needle with drainage. [26: 458] [27: 366] [97: 99] [37: 327] [113: 102]

wind convulsions 风搐 *fēng chù*: 1. Shaking of the extremities attributable to exuberant heat and effulgent liver with stirring wind and phlegm congestion. The tremor prevents the holding of objects and impedes normal walking, and is attended by open eyes and mouth that continuously twitch, night heat effusion, generalized dryness and itching, and in some cases dizzy vision or arched-back rigidity. MED Calm the liver and extinguish wind. Use Antelope Horn and Uncaria Decoction (*líng jiǎo gōu téng tāng*). ACU Base treatment mainly on GV, LR, and GB. Select GV-20 (*bǎi huì*, Hundred Convergences), GV-16 (*fēng fǔ*, Wind Mansion), GB-20 (*fēng chí*, Wind Pool), LR-3 (*tài chōng*, Supreme Surge), GV-14 (*dà zhuī*, Great Hammer), LI-11 (*qū chí*, Pool at the Bend), SP-6 (*sān yīn jiāo*, Three Yin Intersection), KI-1 (*yǒng quán*, Gushing Spring), and ST-40 (*fēng lóng*, Bountiful Bulge); needle with drainage. Selection of points according to signs: For generalized dryness and itching, add SP-10 (*xuè hǎi*, Sea of Blood). For dizzy vision, add HT-5 (*tōng lǐ*, Connecting Li) and ST-41 (*jiě xī*, Ravine Divide). For arched-back rigidity, add GV-12 (*shēn zhù*, Body Pillar) and SI-3 (*hòu xī*, Back Ravine). 2. UMBILICAL WIND. [26: 460]

wind cough 风嗽 *fēng sòu*: WIND DAMAGE COUGH. [26: 461]

wind damage 伤风 *shāng fēng*: 1. From *Incisive Light on the Source of Miscellaneous Disease* (*zá bìng yuán liú xī zhú*). Common cold. 2. From *On Cold Damage* (*shāng hán lùn*). Greater yang (*tài yáng*) wind stroke. See WIND STROKE.[2] [26: 804] [27: 111] [97: 198]

wind damage cough 伤风咳嗽 *shāng fēng ké sòu*: *Synonym: wind cough.* COUGH due to wind evil damaging the lung. Wind damage cough is accompanied by aversion to cold and spontaneous sweating or aversion to cold and heat effusion, nasal congestion and runny nose, heavy voice, itchy throat, and a floating pulse. MED Course wind, diffuse the lung, transform phlegm, and relieve cough. Use formulas such as Cough-Stopping Powder (*zhǐ sòu sǎn*), Rough and Ready Three Decoction (*sān ào tāng*) and Inula Powder (*jīn fèi cǎo sǎn*). ACU Base treatment mainly on LU, LI, and GB. Select BL-13 (*fèi shū*, Lung Transport), LU-7 (*liè quē*, Broken Sequence), LI-4 (*hé gǔ*, Union Valley), GB-20 (*fēng chí*, Wind Pool), BL-12 (*fēng mén*, Wind Gate), CV-22 (*tiān tú*, Celestial Chimney), and ST-40 (*fēng lóng*, Bountiful Bulge); needle with drainage and moxa. [26: 804] [27: 116] [97: 100] [46: 597, 652]

wind-damp 风湿 *fēng shī*: **1.** Disease attributed to wind and dampness and characterized by pain in the joints; it falls within the category of IMPEDIMENT. WMC rheumatism. **2.** Wind and dampness evil in combination. [26: 462]

wind-damp headache 风湿头痛 *fēng shī tóu tòng*: HEADACHE due to wind evil assailing from outside and damp turbidity clouding the upper body. Wind-damp headache is characterized by headache with heavy head as if swathed (bag-over-the-head sensation), heavy cumbersome limbs, oppression in the chest and abdominal distention, nausea and torpid intake, dry mouth with little fluid intake, slimy tongue fur, and a soggy or floating moderate pulse. MED Dispel wind and transform dampness using formulas such as Notopterygium Dampness-Overcoming Decoction (*qiāng huó shèng shī tāng*). ACU Base treatment mainly on points of the three yang channels, GV, and ST. Select GB-20 (*fēng chí*, Wind Pool), GV-16 (*fēng fǔ*, Wind Mansion), GV-20 (*bǎi huì*, Hundred Convergences), Greater Yang (*tài yáng*), LI-4 (*hé gǔ*, Union Valley), LU-7 (*liè quē*, Broken Sequence), SI-3 (*hòu xī*, Back Ravine), SP-9 (*yīn líng quán*, Yin Mound Spring), ST-40 (*fēng lóng*, Bountiful Bulge), and ST-8 (*tóu wéi*, Head Corner); needle with drainage. For selection of points according to affected area, see HEADACHE. [26: 462] [46: 621] [37: 362]

wind-damp impediment 风湿痹 *fēng shī bì*: From *The Origin and Indicators of Disease* (*zhū bìng yuán hòu lùn*), which states, "When wind, cold, and damp evils concur and combine, they give rise to impediment. Impediment with more wind and damp qi than cold qi is wind-damp impediment." It is characterized by thickening of the skin, aching muscular pain. If it persists for a long time, voluntary physical movement may

be affected. MED Dispel wind and dampness. Use Erythrina Decoction (*hǎi tóng pí tāng*) or Notopterygium Dampness-Overcoming Decoction (*qiāng huó shèng shī tāng*). ACU The main points for dispelling wind and dampness are GB-20 (*fēng chí*, Wind Pool), GV-16 (*fēng fǔ*, Wind Mansion), BL-17 (*gé shū*, Diaphragm Transport), SP-10 (*xuè hǎi*, Sea of Blood), SP-6 (*sān yīn jiāo*, Three Yin Intersection), ST-36 (*zú sān lǐ*, Leg Three Li), SP-9 (*yīn líng quán*, Yin Mound Spring), and SP-5 (*shāng qiū*, Shang Hill); needle with drainage and add moxa. Warm needling or cutaneous needling may also be used. Points should also be selected according to affected area (see IMPEDIMENT). See WIND IMPEDIMENT; DAMP IMPEDIMENT. [50: 309] [46: 629] [113: 233]

wind-damp lumbar pain 风湿腰痛 *fēng shī yāo tòng*: LUMBAR PAIN that arises when, after lying in damp places and contracting wind, the evils stagnate in the channel. The contraction of wind and dampness is often encouraged by kidney vacuity. Wind-damp lumbar pain is characterized by hypertonicity of lumbus and back inhibiting movement, and a floating rough pulse. In some cases there may be heat effusion and aversion to wind, or swelling. MED Dispel wind and transform dampness with formulas such as Notopterygium Toxin-Vanquishing Decoction (*qiāng huó bài dú tāng*). ACU Base treatment mainly on BL, GV, SP, and GB. Select BL-23 (*shèn shū*, Kidney Transport), BL-40 (*wěi zhōng*, Bend Center), GV-3 (*yāo yáng guān*, Lumbar Yang Pass), ouch points (*ā shì xué*), GB-20 (*fēng chí*, Wind Pool), LI-11 (*qū chí*, Pool at the Bend), ST-36 (*zú sān lǐ*, Leg Three Li), and SP-9 (*yīn líng quán*, Yin Mound Spring). Needle with drainage. See LUMBAR PAIN. [26: 462]

wind diarrhea 风泻 *fēng xiè*: DIARRHEA characterized by discharge of clear water, attributed to contraction of wind evil, and accompanied by aversion to wind, spontaneous sweating, headache, heat effusion, and a floating pulse. MED Use atractylodes (*cāng zhú*) and ledebouriella (*fáng fēng*), or Schizonepeta and Ledebouriella Toxin-Vanquishing Powder (*jīng fáng bài dú sǎn*) plus tangerine peel (*chén pí*) and ovate atractylodes (*bái zhú*). ACU Base treatment mainly on GB, LI, CV, ST, and SP. Select GB-20 (*fēng chí*, Wind Pool), BL-12 (*fēng mén*, Wind Gate), LI-4 (*hé gǔ*, Union Valley), CV-12 (*zhōng wǎn*, Center Stomach Duct), ST-25 (*tiān shū*, Celestial Pivot), ST-36 (*zú sān lǐ*, Leg Three Li), and SP-9 (*yīn líng quán*, Yin Mound Spring); needle with drainage. [26: 463]

wind disablement 风痱 *fēng féi*: See DISABLEMENT. [26: 460] [27: 397] [97: 100]

wind dizziness 风眩 *fēng xuàn*: **1.** *Synonym: wind dizzy head.* DIZZINESS due to wind evil invading the brain in constitutional vacuity. Wind dizziness is characterized by dizzy head and vision, retching, limb pain, and, in severe cases, REVERSE-FLOW, and occurs at irregular intervals. ⸢MED⸣ Support right and dispel wind using formulas such as Ligusticum Powder (*chuān xiōng sǎn*) or Duhuo Powder (*dú huó sǎn*). ⸢ACU⸣ Base treatment mainly on GV, GB, ST, and SP. Needle with drainage at GB-20 (*fēng chí*, Wind Pool), GV-16 (*fēng fǔ*, Wind Mansion), GV-20 (*bǎi huì*, Hundred Convergences), and PC-6 (*nèi guān*, Inner Pass), and with supplementation at BL-20 (*pí shū*, Spleen Transport), CV-12 (*zhōng wǎn*, Center Stomach Duct), ST-36 (*zú sān lǐ*, Leg Three Li), and SP-6 (*sān yīn jiāo*, Three Yin Intersection). **2.** EPILEPSY. [26: 458]

wind dispersion 风消 *fēng xiāo*: A disease name mentioned in *Elementary Questions* (*sù wèn, yīn yáng biē lùn*) denoting heat effusion and general emaciation due to dissipation of the heart spirit through preoccupation and frustration. In women there may also be menstrual block or blood spillage, whereas in men there may be blood collapse and seminal loss. ⸢MED⸣ Course the liver and resolve depression; regulate and nourish the heart and spleen. Free Wanderer Powder (*xiāo yáo sǎn*) or Spleen-Returning Decoction (*guī pí tāng*) may be used. [26: 457]

wind dizzy head 风头眩 *fēng tóu xuàn*: WIND DIZZINESS.

wind dormant papules 风隐疹 *fēng yǐn zhěn*: See DORMANT PAPULES. [26: 463]

wind-dryness 风燥 *fēng zào*: Wind evil combining with dryness evil to cause disease; usually attributed to contraction of autumn dryness. Wind-dryness is characterized by headache, heat effusion, aversion to cold, absence of sweating, nasal congestion, dry lips and pharynx, dry skin, dry cough, chest and rib-side pain, a thin white dry tongue fur, and a rough floating pulse. [26: 463] [27: 116] [97: 100]

wind dysentery 风痢 *fēng lì*: DYSENTERY arising after contraction of wind evil; characterized by diarrhea turning into dysentery, rumbling intestines, abdominal pain, passage of pure blood, and tenesmus. [27: 394] [97: 100]

wind ear 风耳 *fēng ěr*: See PURULENT EAR. [26: 457]

wind epilepsy 风痫 *fēng xián*: **1.** EPILEPSY characterized by tremor of the extremities, shaking of the head, and clenched jaw. **2.** A condition occurring in febrile disease, equivalent to *fright wind*. **3.** Child epilepsy characterized by highly varied signs. **4.** Convulsions due to externally contracted wind evil. See EPILEPSY. [26: 462]

wind evil 风邪 *fēng xié*: WIND as disease-causing entity. See WIND.[2] [6: 103]

wind evil dizziness 风邪眩晕 *fēng xié xuàn yūn*: See WIND-COLD DIZZINESS. [26: 457]

wind evil assailing the exterior 风邪袭表 *fēng xié xí biǎo*: Wind-cold or wind-heat entering the body and giving rise to exterior patterns. [6: 196]

wind evil invading the lung 风邪犯肺 *fēng xié fàn fèi*: See WIND-COLD FETTERING THE LUNG; WIND-HEAT INVADING THE LUNG. [6: 174]

wind-fire 风火 *fēng huǒ*: Externally contracted wind and fire (heat) or externally contracted fire (heat) stirring internal wind. See WIND-HEAT; WIND AND FIRE FANNING EACH OTHER.

wind-fire eye 风火眼 *fēng huǒ yǎn*: Synonyms: *fire eye; wind-heat eye; wind-heat red eye.* Sore red dry eyes with aversion to light, copious discharge, and hot tears, sometimes accompanied by heat effusion and headache. Serious contagious cases caused by fulminant wind-heat with pronounced heat toxin signs are called *epidemic red eye.* ⸢WMC⸣ acute conjunctivitis. ⸢MED⸣ Course wind and clear heat. Use Wind-Expelling Heat-Dissipating Drink (*qū fēng sàn rè yǐn zi*). Dandelion (*pú gōng yīng*) can be decocted to make a steam-wash. ⸢ACU⸣ Base treatment mainly on BL, LI, and GB. Select GB-20 (*fēng chí*, Wind Pool), BL-1 (*jīng míng*, Bright Eyes), LI-4 (*hé gǔ*, Union Valley), LI-11 (*qū chí*, Pool at the Bend), and TB-5 (*wài guān*, Outer Pass); needle with drainage, and prick Greater Yang (*tài yáng*), GV-23 (*shàng xīng*, Upper Star), and LU-11 (*shào shāng*, Lesser Shang), to bleed. [26: 456] [46: 720] [37: 466]

wind-fire scrofula 风火疬 *fēng huǒ lì*: SCROFULA characterized shiny red swollen nodes on the neck, often below the ear, attributed to the gathering and binding of wind-heat possibly combined with liver-gallbladder fire. In severe cases, there may be heat effusion and aversion to cold and the nodes may be painful and suppurate. ⸢WMC⸣ acute lymphadenitis. ⸢MED⸣ Course wind, clear heat, and dissipate binds. Use a combination of bupleurum (*chái hú*), arctium (*niú bàng zǐ*), achyranthes (*niú xī*), unripe tangerine peel (*qīng pí*), ledebouriella (*fáng fēng*), trichosanthes root (*tiān huā fěn*), smooth greenbrier root (*tǔ fú líng*), shancigu (*shān cí gū*), pueraria (*gé gēn*), and prunella (*xià kū cǎo*). ⸢ACU⸣ Use the points given under SCROFULA, and needle with drainage at GV-20 (*bǎi huì*, Hundred Convergences), GB-20 (*fēng chí*, Wind Pool), TB-5 (*wài guān*, Outer Pass), GV-14 (*dà zhuī*, Great Hammer), LI-4 (*hé gǔ*, Union Valley), and ST-40 (*fēng lóng*, Bountiful Bulge); prick LU-11 (*shào shāng*, Lesser Shang) to bleed to course wind and dissipate fire. [26: 456]

wind-fire toothache 风火牙痛 *fēng huǒ yá tòng*: TOOTHACHE attributable to externally contracted wind-heat. See TOOTHACHE.

wind flat-abscess 风疽 *fēng jū*: A persistent sore occurring on the lower leg or ankle that is characterized by pain and itching and that exudes yellow fluid when ruptured and is attributed to damp-heat stagnating in the skin or in the blood and blood vessels. [WMC] chronic eczema. [MED] Clear and disinhibit dampness using Wind-Dispersing Powder (*xiāo fēng sǎn*) or Mysterious Three Pill (*sān miào wán*) as oral medication, and applying Indigo Powder (*qīng dài sǎn*) topically. [ACU] Base treatment mainly on GV, LI, ST, and SP. Needle with drainage at GV-14 (*dà zhuī*, Great Hammer), LI-11 (*qū chí*, Pool at the Bend), SP-9 (*yīn líng quán*, Yin Mound Spring), SP-6 (*sān yīn jiāo*, Three Yin Intersection), and with supplementation at BL-17 (*gé shū*, Diaphragm Transport), SP-10 (*xuè hǎi*, Sea of Blood), ST-36 (*zú sān lǐ*, Leg Three Li), and HT-7 (*shén mén*, Spirit Gate). Pricking and cupping may also be used. Selection of points according to signs: For pronounced itching, add HT-8 (*shào fǔ*, Lesser Mansion) and Itch Reliever (*zhǐ yǎng*). For pronounced dampness, add LI-4 (*hé gǔ*, Union Valley) and moxa. [26: 457]

wind gan 风疳 *fēng gān*: GAN OF THE LIVER. [26: 457]

wind gan of the mouth 口疳风 *kǒu gān fēng*: TONGUE BLISTER. [26: 61]

wind heart pain 风心痛 *fēng xīn tòng*: From *A Thousand Gold Pieces Prescriptions* (*qiān jīn yào fāng*). HEART PAIN attributable to wind-cold evil qi exploiting vacuity to cause internal disturbance, causing heart pain (stomach duct pain), rumbling and movement under the ribs, fullness in the chest, shortness of breath, and ejection of drool. [MED] Warm and dissipate using Cyperus and Perilla Powder (*xiāng sū sǎn*). [46: 596] [26: 456]

wind-heat 风热 *fēng rè*: Externally contracted wind and heat. A combination of wind and heat (or wind and fire) gives rise to heat signs pronounced heat effusion and mild aversion to cold, cough, thirst, tongue with red margins and tips, with slightly yelow fur, and a pulse that is floating and rapid. In severe cases, there may be dry mouth, red eye, sore throat, and spontaneous external bleeding. Compare WIND-FIRE. [26: 461] [27: 116] [97: 99]

Wind-Heat—Dissipating Medicinals

薄荷 (*bò hé*) mint (Menthae Herba)
牛蒡子 (*niú bàng zǐ*) arctium (Arctii Fructus)
蝉蜕 (*chán tuì*) cicada molting (Cicadae Periostracum)
淡豆豉 (*dàn dòu chǐ*) fermented soybean (Glycines Semen Fermentatum Insulsum)

大豆黄卷 (*dà dòu huáng juǎn*) dried soybean sprout (Glycines Semen Germinatum Exsiccatum)
桑叶 (*sāng yè*) mulberry leaf (Mori Folium)
菊花 (*jú huā*) chrysanthemum (Chrysanthemi Flos)
野菊花 (*yě jú huā*) wild chrysanthemum flower (Chrysanthemi Indicae seu Borealis Flos)
蔓荆子 (*màn jīng zǐ*) vitex (Viticis Fructus)
葛根 (*gé gēn*) pueraria (Puerariae Radix)
柴胡 (*chái hú*) bupleurum (Bupleuri Radix)
升麻 (*shēng má*) cimicifuga (Cimicifugae Rhizoma)
浮萍 (*fú píng*) duckweed (Lemnae Herba)
木贼 (*mù zéi*) equisetum (Equiseti Herba)

---

wind-heat common cold 风热感冒 *fēng rè gǎn mào*: A COMMON COLD due to contraction of wind-heat. Wind-heat common cold is characterized by heat effusion, headache, slight aversion to cold, spontaneous sweating, nasal congestion without snivel (nasal mucus), scorching sore throat, cough with thick yellow phlegm, thirst, red tongue with thin slightly yellowish white tongue fur, and a rapid floating pulse. [MED] Cool acrid exterior resolution. Use formulas such as Lonicera and Forsythia Powder (*yín qiào sǎn*). For nasal congestion without snivel, add xanthium (*cāng ěr zǐ*), angelica (*bái zhǐ*), mint (*bò hé*), and houttuynia (*yú xīng cǎo*). For scorching sore throat, add belamcanda (*shè gān*), isatis root (*bǎn lán gēn*), and scrophularia (*xuán shēn*). For cough with thick yellow phlegm, add fritillaria (*bèi mǔ*), scutellaria (*huáng qín*), apricot kernel (*xìng rén*), and peucedanum (*qián hú*). For thirst, add trichosanthes root (*tiān huā fěn*) and adenophora/glehnia (*shā shēn*). [ACU] Base treatment mainly on LU, LI, and TB. Main points: LU-10 (*yú jì*, Fish Border), GV-14 (*dà zhuī*, Great Hammer), LU-5 (*chǐ zé*, Cubit Marsh), LI-11 (*qū chí*, Pool at the Bend), ST-44 (*nèi tíng*, Inner Court), GB-20 (*fēng chí*, Wind Pool), and TB-5 (*wài guān;* Outer Pass). For headache, add GV-20 (*bǎi huì*, Hundred Convergences), Greater Yang (*tài yáng*), and SI-3 (*hòu xī*, Back Ravine). For spontaneous sweating, add LI-4 (*hé gǔ*, Union Valley) and KI-7 (*fù liū*, Recover Flow). For nasal congestion without snivel, add LI-20 (*yíng xiāng*, Welcome Fragrance) and Hall of Impression (*yìn táng*). For scorching sore throat, prick LU-11 (*shào shāng*, Lesser Shang) to bleed. For cough with thick yellow phlegm, add BL-13 (*fèi shū*, Lung Transport) LI-4 (*hé gǔ*, Union Valley), and LU-7 (*liè quē*, Broken Sequence). Needle with drainage at all points. See WIND-HEAT INVADING THE LUNG. [27: 354] [97: 102] [46: 650]

wind-heat cough 风热咳嗽 *fēng rè ké sòu*: COUGH attributed to wind-heat invading the lung impairing depuration of the lung. Attendant signs include thick phlegm, generalized heat [effusion], sweating, aversion to wind, dry mouth and sore throat, yellow snivel (nasal mucus), thin tongue fur, and a rapid floating pulse. MED Course wind and clear heat; diffuse lung qi. Variants of Mulberry Leaf and Chrysanthemum Beverage (*sāng jú yǐn*) or Lonicera and Forsythia Powder (*yín qiào sǎn*) can be used. ACU Base treatment mainly on LU and LI. Select BL-13 (*fèi shū*, Lung Transport), LU-5 (*chǐ zé*, Cubit Marsh), LU-7 (*liè quē*, Broken Sequence), GB-20 (*fēng chí*, Wind Pool), GV-14 (*dà zhuī*, Great Hammer), LI-4 (*hé gǔ*, Union Valley), and LI-11 (*qū chí*, Pool at the Bend); needle with drainage. For sore pharynx, prick LU-11 (*shào shāng*, Lesser Shang) to bleed. See COUGH. [26: 461] [46: 652] [37: 272]

wind-heat deafness 风热耳聋 *fēng rè ěr lóng*: DEAFNESS attributed to wind-heat attacking the upper body, inhibiting qi dynamic, and harassing the clear orifices. Wind-heat deafness is associated with headache, nasal congestion, ear pain, and tinnitus. MED Treat by coursing wind and clearing heat assisted by opening the orifices with aroma. Variants of Lonicera and Forsythia Powder (*yín qiào sǎn*) may be used. ACU See DEAFNESS. [26: 461] [97: 102]

wind-heat dizziness 风热眩晕 *fēng rè xuàn yūn*: DIZZINESS due to externally-contracted wind-heat congesting the upper body. Wind-heat dizziness is characterized by dizzy clouded vision or spinning dizziness that brings the patient near to falling over, a constrained feeling in the chest, and vomiting. MED Dispel wind and clear heat with Ledebouriella Sage-Inspired Powder (*fáng fēng tōng shèng sǎn*). ACU Base treatment mainly on GV, ST, GB, LU, and LI. Select GV-20 (*bǎi huì*, Hundred Convergences), ST-8 (*tóu wéi*, Head Corner), Hall of Impression (*yìn táng*), GB-20 (*fēng chí*, Wind Pool), TB-5 (*wài guān*, Outer Pass), LU-5 (*chǐ zé*, Cubit Marsh), LI-11 (*qū chí*, Pool at the Bend), LI-4 (*hé gǔ*, Union Valley), and GV-14 (*dà zhuī*, Great Hammer). Needle with drainage. For high fever, prick Ten Diffusing Points (*shí xuān*) to bleed. [26: 461] [46: 650]

wind-heat eye 风热眼 *fēng rè yǎn*: WIND-FIRE EYE. [26: 461] [27: 502] [97: 101]

wind-heat fright palpitations 风热惊悸 *fēng rè jīng jì*: FRIGHT PALPITATIONS that arises when wind evil invades to contend with heat congesting in the heart. MED Clear heat and stabilize fright using Bovine Bezoar Fright-Settling Pill (*niú huáng zhèn jīng wán*) or Red-Abducting Powder (*dǎo chì sǎn*) varied to take account of vacuity or repletion. ACU Base treatment mainly on HT, PC, GB, and LI. Select HT-7 (*shén mén*, Spirit Gate), PC-6 (*nèi guān*, Inner Pass), BL-15 (*xīn shū*, Heart Transport), PC-8 (*láo gōng*, Palace of Toil), HT-8

(*shào fǔ*, Lesser Mansion), GB-20 (*fēng chí*, Wind Pool), TB-5 (*wài guān*, Outer Pass), and LI-4 (*hé gǔ*, Union Valley); needle with drainage. For high fever, add GV-14 (*dà zhuī*, Great Hammer) and prick Ten Diffusing Points (*shí xuān*) to bleed. [26: 461]

wind-heat gan of the teeth and gums 风热牙疳 *fēng rè yá gān*: GAN OF THE TEETH AND GUMS characterized in the initial stages by sore red swollen gums, heat effusion, or alternating heat [effusion] and [aversion to] cold, and in more advanced stages by ulceration and bleeding, and in some cases constipation, and retching and vomiting. Wind-heat gan of the teeth and gums is attributed to evil heat surging upward to lodge in the teeth and gums, occurring when wind-heat contends with heat brewing in the yang brightness (*yáng míng*). MED Course wind and clear heat; drain fire and resolve toxin. Use Coptis Toxin-Resolving Decoction (*huáng lián jiě dú tāng*), Stomach-Clearing Powder (*qīng wèi sǎn*), or Jade Lady Brew (*yù nǚ jiān*), which can be decocted with lonicera (*jīn yín huā*), licorice (*gān cǎo*), and mint (*bò hé*) and used as a mouthwash. ACU Base treatment mainly on ST, LI, and GV. Select LI-4 (*hé gǔ*, Union Valley), ST-44 (*nèi tíng*, Inner Court), TB-5 (*wài guān*, Outer Pass), GB-20 (*fēng chí*, Wind Pool), and GV-14 (*dà zhuī*, Great Hammer). Needle with drainage. [26: 461] [97: 102]

wind-heat headache 风热头痛 *fēng rè tóu tòng*: HEADACHE due to wind-heat harassing the upper body. Wind-heat headache is usually associated with distention in the head, aversion to cold, and heat effusion, and may be attended by such signs as nasal congestion and runny nose, toothache, red sore swollen eyes, thirst with intake of fluid, or constipation and reddish urine. The tongue fur is thin and yellow, whereas the pulse is floating. MED Course wind and clear heat using formulas such as Clear Sky Paste (*qīng kōng gāo*) or Mulberry Leaf and Chrysanthemum Beverage (*sāng jú yǐn*). ACU Base treatment mainly on the three yang channels and GV. Select GB-20 (*fēng chí*, Wind Pool), GV-20 (*bǎi huì*, Hundred Convergences), Greater Yang (*tài yáng*), LI-4 (*hé gǔ*, Union Valley), LU-7 (*liè quē*, Broken Sequence), SI-3 (*hòu xī*, Back Ravine), GV-14 (*dà zhuī*, Great Hammer), and LI-11 (*qū chí*, Pool at the Bend), and needle with drainage. For selection of points according to affected area, see HEADACHE. [26: 461] [46: 621] [37: 362]

wind-heat invading the lung 风热犯肺 *fēng rè fàn fèi*: Externally contracted wind-heat entering the lung and hampering its normal diffusion and depuration. The chief signs are cough with thick yellow phlegm and slight aversion to wind and cold. Other signs include nasal congestion with runny nose and yellow turbid snivel, dry mouth and throat, red eyes, slight thirst, and generalized heat [effusion]. The tongue is red (or red at the tip) with a thin yellow tongue fur. The pulse is floating and rapid. MED Use Lonicera and Forsythia Powder (*yín qiào sǎn*) plus Zhejiang fritillaria (*zhè bèi mǔ*), apricot kernel (*xìng rén*), and peucedanum (*qián hú*). For pronounced heat, add gypsum (*shí gāo*). For pronounced sore throat, add scrophularia (*xuán shēn*), isatis root (*bǎn lán gēn*), or belamcanda (*shè gān*). ACU Base treatment mainly on LU, LI, and TB. Select BL-13 (*fèi shū*, Lung Transport), LI-4 (*hé gǔ*, Union Valley), LI-11 (*qū chí*, Pool at the Bend), LU-5 (*chǐ zé*, Cubit Marsh), TB-5 (*wài guān*, Outer Pass), and LU-10 (*yú jì*, Fish Border); needle with drainage. Selection of points according to signs: For nasal congestion, add LI-20 (*yíng xiāng*, Welcome Fragrance) and GV-23 (*shàng xīng*, Upper Star). For sore swollen throat, prick LU-11 (*shào shāng*, Lesser Shang) to bleed. **Analysis:** When wind-heat fetters the lung, it impairs diffusion and downbearing, hence the cough. Wind-heat scorches lung liquid to form phlegm, hence the phlegm is thick and yellow. The lung opens at the nose, and when lung qi fails to diffuse, the nasal orifices are inhibited, and the fluids are damaged by the wind-heat, hence nasal congestion with runny nose and yellow turbid snivel. When wind-heat evil harasses the upper body and damages the fluids, there is dry mouth and sore pharynx, slight thirst, and red eyes. When lung defense is affected by evil, defensive yang resists evil, hence heat effusion. At the same time, because defensive qi is depressed, there is slight aversion to wind and cold. Heat makes the tongue red. Wind-heat invading the exterior makes the tongue fur thin and yellow. The floating pulse is an exterior sign, while a rapid pulse indicates heat. **Comparison:** *Wind-cold fettering the lung:* Wind-heat invading the lung and wind-cold fettering the lung are both external contractions. Wind-heat invading the lung is marked by pronounced heat effusion and mild aversion to cold, a thin yellow tongue fur, and a rapid floating pulse. Wind-cold fettering the lung is characterized by pronounced aversion to cold and mild heat effusion, with a thin white tongue fur, and a tight floating pulse. *Dryness evil invading the lung:* Wind-heat invading the lung is marked by cough with thick yellow phlegm, generalized heat [effusion], aversion to cold, a red tongue with yellow fur, and a rapid floating pulse. Dryness evil invading the lung is characterized by dry cough with scant sticky phlegm, dry mouth and throat, aversion to cold and heat effusion, a red tongue with white fur, and a rapid pulse. *Heat evil congesting the lung:* Both wind-heat invading the lung and heat evil congesting the lung have cough

as the main sign. However, heat evil congesting the lung is marked by panting as well as cough, and high fever and much more pronounced heat signs. [57: 77] [116: 68] [29: 405]

wind-heat lumbar pain 风热腰痛 *fēng rè yāo tòng*: LUMBAR PAIN attributed to wind-heat invading the kidney channel. Wind-heat lumbar pain is characterized by acute pain that stretches into the legs and knees, thirst, and a rapid pulse. MED Course wind and clear heat with variations of Toxin-Vanquishing Powder (*bài dú sǎn*) or Minor Bupleurum Decoction (*xiǎo chái hú tāng*). ACU Base treatment mainly on BL, LU, LI, and GV. Select GB-20 (*fēng chí*, Wind Pool), GV-14 (*dà zhuī*, Great Hammer), LI-4 (*hé gǔ*, Union Valley), BL-23 (*shèn shū*, Kidney Transport), BL-40 (*wěi zhōng*, Bend Center), BL-54 (*zhì biān*, Sequential Limit), and ouch points (*ā shì xué*); needle with drainage. Prick LU-11 (*shào shāng*, Lesser Shang) to bleed (BL-40 may also be bled). See LUMBAR PAIN. [26: 461]

wind-heat red eye 风热赤眼 *fēng rè chì yǎn*, 风热目赤 *fēng rè mù chì*: WIND-FIRE EYE.

wind-heat sore 风热疮 *fēng rè chuāng*: A sore attributed to wind-heat lying depressed in the lung and effusing into the skin. Wind-heat sores start as papules on the limbs and chest and rib-side, which when scratched cause sores that exude fresh blood. WMC pityriasis rosea. MED Treat with Wind-Dispersing Powder (*xiāo fēng sǎn*) taken orally. ACU Base treatment mainly on GB, LU, LI, GV, and SP. Select GB-20 (*fēng chí*, Wind Pool), TB-5 (*wài guān*, Outer Pass), LU-5 (*chǐ zé*, Cubit Marsh), LI-4 (*hé gǔ*, Union Valley), LI-11 (*qū chí*, Pool at the Bend), GV-14 (*dà zhuī*, Great Hammer), SP-10 (*xuè hǎi*, Sea of Blood), SP-6 (*sān yīn jiāo*, Three Yin Intersection), GB-31 (*fēng shì*, Wind Market), HT-8 (*shào fǔ*, Lesser Mansion), and Itch Reliever (*zhǐ yǎng*); needle with drainage. [26: 461]

wind-heat throat impediment 风热喉痹 *fēng rè hóu bì*: THROAT IMPEDIMENT (a sore swollen throat with a feeling of blockage and difficulty swallowing) attributed to externally contracted wind-heat. Accompanying signs include heat effusion, cough, hoarse voice, thin yellow tongue fur, and a rapid floating pulse. MED Dispel wind, clear heat, and disinhibit the throat with Lonicera and Forsythia Powder (*yín qiào sǎn*) plus isatis root (*bǎn lán gēn*), belamcanda (*shè gān*), and scrophularia (*xuán shēn*). ACU Base treatment on LU and LI. Prick LU-11 (*shào shāng*, Lesser Shang) to bleed; select LI-4 (*hé gǔ*, Union Valley), LU-5 (*chǐ zé*, Cubit Marsh), LI-11 (*qū chí*, Pool at the Bend), PC-7 (*dà líng*, Great Mound), and ST-43 (*xiàn gǔ*, Sunken Valley), needling with drainage. For pronounced soreness, add SI-17 (*tiān róng*, Celestial

Countenance) and CV-22 (*tiān tú,* Celestial Chimney). See THROAT IMPEDIMENT. [46: 727] [113: 505] [27: 495]

wind impediment 风痹 *fēng bì: Synonym: moving impediment.* An IMPEDIMENT (*bì*) pattern attributed to wind-cold-damp invading the limbs and channels and characterized by wandering pain, which indicates that wind is the dominant evil. MED Treat primarily by dispelling wind and secondarily by dispelling cold and disinhibited dampness. Blood-supplementing medicinals are often used. Applicable formulas include Ledebouriella Decoction (*fáng fēng tāng*). ACU Main points: GB-20 (*fēng chí,* Wind Pool), GV-16 (*fēng fŭ,* Wind Mansion), BL-17 (*gé shū,* Diaphragm Transport), SP-10 (*xuè hăi,* Sea of Blood), and SP-6 (*sān yīn jiāo,* Three Yin Intersection). Apply a shallow needling with drainage, or tap with a cutaneous needle. For selection of points according to affected area, see IMPEDIMENT. Compare PAIN WIND. [27: 403] [97: 100]

wind-induced deviation 风起喎斜 *fēng qĭ wāi (kuāi) xié,* 风起喎偏 *fēng qĭ wāi (kuāi) piān,* 风引喎偏 *fēng yĭn wāi (kuāi) piān:* Deviation of the cheeks and mouth, inability to close the eyes fully, in some cases, with tremor, dizziness, seeing one as two (double vision), red eyes, and tearing, and, in severe cases, outward turning of the lower lid, squint, and hemiplegia. MED Dispel wind and free the network vessels using either Wind-Expelling Powder (*pái fēng săn*) or Face-Righting Decoction (*zhèng róng tāng*). ACU Base treatment mainly on GB, TB, LI, and ST. Select GB-20 (*fēng chí,* Wind Pool), TB-17 (*yì fēng,* Wind Screen), ST-4 (*dì cāng,* Earth Granary), ST-6 (*jiá chē,* Cheek Carriage), Pull Aright (*qiān zhèng*), LI-4 (*hé gŭ,* Union Valley), GB-14 (*yáng bái,* Yang White), BL-2 (*zăn zhú,* Bamboo Gathering), and ST-2 (*sì bái,* Four Whites) to dissipate wind and free the network vessels. In the early stages, use the point-joining method or oblique insertion; in advanced stages, use shallow needling supplementation. Selection of points according to signs: For dizziness, add LR-3 (*tài chōng,* Supreme Surge), GB-43 (*xiá xī,* Pinched Ravine), and KI-3 (*tài xī,* Great Ravine). For red eyes and tearing, add LR-2 (*xíng jiān,* Moving Between), BL-1 (*jīng míng,* Bright Eyes), and Greater Yang (*tài yáng*). [26: 458] [46: 720, 618] [27: 507]

wind lichen 风癣 *fēng xiăn:* LICHEN (*xiăn*) attributed to wind-cold settling in the skin and contending with qi and blood. Wind lichen is characterized by clearly circumscribed elevations of the skin that are round or oval in shape and scale when scratched. When they persist, the skin thickens. WMC tinea corporis. MED Topical: Lichen Medicinal Water (*xiăn yào shuĭ*) or Tinc-

ture of Golden Larch (root) Bark (*tŭ jĭn pí dīng*). ACU Base treatment mainly on LI, ST, GB and ouch points (*ā shì xué*). Pole ouch points (*ā shì xué*) (affected area) for 30–60 minutes. Select LI-11 (*qū chí,* Pool at the Bend), LI-4 (*hé gŭ,* Union Valley), ST-36 (*zú sān lĭ,* Leg Three Li), GB-20 (*fēng chí,* Wind Pool), and TB-5 (*wài guān,* Outer Pass); needle with drainage. For pronounced cold, use moxa. [26: 463] [50: 307] [42: 156] [46: 595]

wind-like stroke 类中风 *lèi zhòng fēng: Synonym: wind stroke.* **1.** WIND STROKE attributable to internal wind. Wind-like stroke arises when insufficiency of kidney yin, intense heart fire, and ascendant liver yang cause liver wind to stir or when congestion of damp phlegm transforms into heat and engenders wind. Other contributing factors include qi vacuity, qi counterflow, etc. Internal wind is the essential cause, although it may be brought on by external wind. The main signs are sudden clouding collapse that leaves the patient with hemiplegia, deviated eyes and mouth, and sluggish or difficult speech. In some cases, there is only deviation of the eyes and mouth. WMC cerebrovascular accident; Bell's palsy. Distinction is made between *channel and network stroke* and *bowel and visceral stroke.* **Channel and network stroke:** Deviated eyes and mouth, inhibited speech, and hemiplegia with no change in spirit-mind. MED If caused only by internal wind, it is treated by calming the liver and extinguishing wind with Liver-Settling Wind-Extinguishing Decoction (*zhèn gān xī fēng tāng*) or Gastrodia and Uncaria Beverage (*tiān má gōu téng yĭn*). If brought on by external wind, it can be treated by dispelling wind and freeing the network vessels and nourishing the blood and harmonizing construction, using formulas such as Pull Aright Powder (*qiān zhèng săn*) or Large Gentian Decoction (*dà qín jiāo tāng*). ACU Base treatment mainly on hand and foot yang brightness (*yáng míng*) LI/ST, assisted by greater yang (*tài yáng*) and lesser yang (*shào yáng*). The principle of treatment applied is to free the channels and regulate qi and blood. Main formula: LI-15 (*jiān yú,* Shoulder Bone), LI-11 (*qū chí,* Pool at the Bend), LI-4 (*hé gŭ,* Union Valley), TB-5 (*wài guān,* Outer Pass), GB-30 (*huán tiào,* Jumping Round), GB-34 (*yáng líng quán,* Yang Mound Spring), ST-42 (*chōng yáng,* Surging Yang), and BL-60 (*kūn lún,* Kunlun Mountains). In addition, one of the three following methods can be used. (1) First drain the unaffected side, then supplement the affected side. (2) Needle or moxa the two sides alternately. (3) Only needle the affected side, using a medium or strong stimulus. In enduring cases, needle and moxa on both sides to supplement. Selection of points according to causes: For liver wind stirring internally, add GV-20 (*băi huì,*

Hundred Convergences), GB-20 (*fēng chí,* Wind Pool), LR-3 (*tài chōng,* Supreme Surge), SP-6 (*sān yīn jiāo,* Three Yin Intersection), and KI-1 (*yǒng quán,* Gushing Spring). When external evil is contributory factor, add BL-17 (*gé shū,* Diaphragm Transport), BL-23 (*shèn shū,* Kidney Transport), BL-18 (*gān shū,* Liver Transport), GB-20 (*fēng chí,* Wind Pool), LR-3 (*tài chōng,* Supreme Surge), and SP-6 (*sān yīn jiāo,* Three Yin Intersection). Selection of points according to affected area: See HEMIPLEGIA. **Bowel and visceral stroke:** The main signs are sudden collapse and loss of consciousness. Distinction is made between BLOCK PATTERNS characterized by clenched jaw and clenched hands and DESERTION PATTERNS marked by open mouth, limp hand, open eyes, enuresis, snoring voice, and in some cases, by spontaneous sweating. (1) Block patterns: MED Diffuse the orifices and open the block with Supreme Jewel Elixir (*zhì bǎo dān*) or Liquid Storax Pill (*sū hé xiāng wán*) poured into the patient's mouth while he still unconscious; if necessary, first loosen tightly clenched jaws by rubbing Liquid Storax Pill or finely ground raw arisaema (*shēng nán xīng*) and borneol (*bīng piàn*) on the gums. Follow this with treatment to nourish yin and subdue yang, clear the liver and extinguish wind, and sweep phlegm with formulas such as Antelope Horn and Uncaria Decoction (*líng jiǎo gōu téng tāng*) or Phlegm-Abducting Decoction (*dǎo tán tāng*). ACU Base treatment mainly on GV, and Twelve Well Points (*shí èr jǐng xué*), supported by hand and foot reverting yin (*jué yīn*) PC/LR, and yang brightness (*yáng míng*) ST/LI channel points. Select Twelve Well Points (*shí èr jǐng xué*), GV-26 (*shuǐ gōu,* Water Trough), LR-3 (*tài chōng,* Supreme Surge), PC-8 (*láo gōng,* Palace of Toil), ST-40 (*fēng lóng,* Bountiful Bulge), and KI-1 (*yǒng quán,* Gushing Spring); needle with drainage or prick to bleed with a three-edged needle. Selection of points according to signs: For clenched jaw, add ST-6 (*jiá chē,* Cheek Carriage), ST-7 (*xià guān,* Below the Joint), and LI-4 (*hé gǔ,* Union Valley). For clenched hands, add PC-6 (*nèi guān,* Inner Pass), SI-3 (*hòu xī,* Back Ravine), and LI-4 (*hé gǔ,* Union Valley). (2) Desertion patterns: MED Use large doses of Ginseng and Aconite Decoction (*shēn fù tāng*) to support right and stem desertion. ACU Base treatment mainly on CV. Burn moxa cones at CV-4 (*guān yuán,* Pass Head), and CV-6 (*qì hǎi,* Sea of Qi), and apply moxibustion on salt or ginger at CV-8 (*shén què,* Spirit Gate Tower) until the sweating ceases, the limbs become warm, and pulse rises. Selection of points according to signs: For persistent sweating, add HT-6 (*yīn xī,* Yin Cleft), LI-4 (*hé gǔ,* Union Valley), and ST-36 (*zú sān lǐ,* Leg Three Li). For aftermath of wind stroke, see HEMIPLEGIA. **2.** Any of various diseases like wind stroke.

See FIRE STROKE; VACUITY STROKE; DAMPNESS STROKE; COLD STROKE; SUMMERHEAT STROKE; QI STROKE; FOOD STROKE; MALIGNITY STROKE. [26: 971] [80: 462] [46: 615] [113: 22]

wind malaria 风疟 *fēng nüè:* MALARIA attributed to contraction of wind due to excessive consumption of cold foods and beverages. Wind malaria is characterized by mild aversion to cold followed by pronounced heat effusion, headache, heat effusion and agitation. MED If there is aversion to wind without sweating, it is treated by coursing wind and resolving the exterior with Apricot Kernel and Perilla Powder (*xìng sū sǎn*) plus bupleurum (*chái hú*). If there is aversion to cold with sweating and heat vexation, it is treated by clearing heat and resolving the flesh with Cinnamon Twig Decoction (*guì zhī tāng*) plus scutellaria (*huáng qín*). ACU Base treatment mainly on GV, SI, PC, GV, and BL. Main points: GV-14 (*dà zhuī,* Great Hammer), GV-13 (*táo dào,* Kiln Path), SI-3 (*hòu xī,* Back Ravine), and PC-5 (*jiān shǐ,* Intermediary Courier). If there is aversion to wind without sweating, add BL-11 (*dà zhù,* Great Shuttle), BL-12 (*fēng mén,* Wind Gate), BL-13 (*fèi shū,* Lung Transport), and BL-64 (*jīng gǔ,* Capital Bone); needle with drainage and add moxa. If there is aversion to cold with sweating and heat vexation, add GB-20 (*fēng chí,* Wind Pool), BL-64 (*jīng gǔ,* Capital Bone), BL-62 (*shēn mài,* Extending Vessel), and ST-36 (*zú sān lǐ,* Leg Three Li); needle with drainage. For principles and methods of treatment, see MALARIA. [26: 460] [27: 358] [97: 99] [113: 170] [75: 46, 63]

wind medicinal 风药 *fēng yào:* Any medicinal that treats disease attributed to wind.

wind papules 风疹 *fēng zhěn:* **1.** WIND SAND. **2.** DORMANT PAPULES. [26: 458] [27: 370] [92: No. 410]

wind-phlegm 风痰 *fēng tán:* **1.** Disease pattern arising in patients ordinarily suffering from phlegm disease who contract wind evil or in whom wind-heat becomes depressed. **2.** Phlegm in the liver channel; characterized by a stringlike pulse, green-blue facial complexion, dizziness, fullness and oppression in the chest and rib-side, constipation and rough urination, periodic agitation and anger, and green-blue colored phlegm. According to *Dan Xi's Experiential Methods (dān xī xīn fǎ)* wind-phlegm should be treated with wind-phlegm medicinals such as aconite/typhonium (*bái fù zǐ*), gastrodia (*tiān má*), realgar (*xióng huáng*), bovine bezoar (*niú huáng*), old scutellaria (*kū qín*), silkworm (*bái jiāng cán*), and small gleditsia (*zhū yá zào*). [26: 460] [97: 100]

wind-phlegm dizziness 风痰眩晕 *fēng tán xuàn yūn:* DIZZINESS attributed to wind-phlegm congestion. Wind-phlegm dizziness is characterized by dizzy head and flowery vision, with headache, hypertonicity of the shoulder and back, heavy body, tendency to sleep, oppression in the chest, heart palpitations, and vomiting of phlegm-drool. MED Dispel wind and transform phlegm with formulas such as Pinellia, Ovate Atractylodes, and Gastrodia Decoction (*bàn xià bái zhú tiān má tāng*) or Gastrodia Pill (*tiān má wán*). ACU Base treatment mainly on GV, GB, LR, ST, and LI. Select GV-20 (*bǎi huì*, Hundred Convergences), GB-20 (*fēng chí*, Wind Pool), ST-8 (*tóu wéi*, Head Corner), Hall of Impression (*yìn táng*), CV-12 (*zhōng wǎn*, Center Stomach Duct), PC-6 (*nèi guān*, Inner Pass), LI-4 (*hé gǔ*, Union Valley), ST-40 (*fēng lóng*, Bountiful Bulge), LR-3 (*tài chōng*, Supreme Surge), and ST-41 (*jiě xī*, Ravine Divide); needle with drainage. [26: 460] [46: 619]

wind-phlegm headache 风痰头痛 *fēng tán tóu tòng*: HEADACHE attributed to wind-phlegm harassing the upper body. The headache is accompanied by dizziness, desire to keep the eyes closed, laziness to speak, fatigued heavy body, oppression in the chest, nausea, and in some cases, green-blue or yellow cheeks, or phlegm-drool ejection. MED Dispel wind and transform phlegm with formulas such as Pinellia, Ovate Atractylodes, and Gastrodia Decoction (*bàn xià bái zhú tiān má tāng*). ACU Base treatment mainly on CV, GB, ST, and LI. Select GV-20 (*bǎi huì*, Hundred Convergences), GB-20 (*fēng chí*, Wind Pool), PC-6 (*nèi guān*, Inner Pass) LI-4 (*hé gǔ*, Union Valley), CV-12 (*zhōng wǎn*, Center Stomach Duct), ST-40 (*fēng lóng*, Bountiful Bulge), ST-8 (*tóu wéi*, Head Corner), Greater Yang (*tài yáng*), LR-3 (*tài chōng*, Supreme Surge), and SP-9 (*yīn líng quán*, Yin Mound Spring); needle with drainage. For selection of points according to affected area, see HEADACHE. [26: 460] [37: 364] [46: 621]

wind qi stirring internally 风气内动 *fēng qì nèi dòng*: Dizziness, convulsions, and clouding collapse resulting from disturbances of the bowels and viscera when qi and blood flow chaotically counter to their normal direction and the sinews are deprived of nourishment. *Elementary Questions* (*sù wèn, yīn yáng yìng xiàng dà lùn*) states, "When wind prevails, there is stirring." *Elementary Questions* (*sù wèn, zhì zhēn yào dà lùn*) states, "all fulminant rigidity is ascribed to wind." [26: 458] [27: 153] [97: 101]

wind rampart 水廓 *fēng kuò*: See EIGHT RAMPARTS. [26: 24]

wind red sore 风赤疮痍 *fēng chì chuāng yí*: Synonym: *wind red sore disease*. A disease of the eyelid or eyelid rim characterized by redness, blisters, erosion, and soreness, itching, and ulceration. Wind red sore is caused by spleen-lung wind-heat, damp-heat congestion, or by wind-fire attacking

the upper body. **Spleen-lung wind-heat** patterns arise when wind-damp is contracted in the presence of damp-heat brewing in the stomach and spleen, so that wind, dampness, and heat bind in the eye. Such patterns are marked by swelling and itching, reddening of the skin, and a small number of papules exuding sticky fluid. MED Clear the spleen and lung and eliminate wind. Use Wind-Eliminating Spleen-Clearing Beverage (*chú fēng qīng pí yǐn*). **Wind-heat-damp toxin congestion** causes the eyes to be sore, swollen, and scorching hot with a cluster of vesicles (or pustules), which can rupture and ulcerate to give off a fishy odor and exude sticky fluid. MED Dispel wind and eliminate dampness; drain fire and resolve toxin. Use Dampness-Eliminating Decoction (*chú shī tāng*). The heat-clearing toxin-resolving power of this formula can be enhanced by adding smooth greenbrier root (*tǔ fú líng*), lonicera (*jīn yín huā*), dandelion (*pú gōng yīng*), and Yedo violet (*zǐ huā dì dīng*). **Wind-fire attacking the upper body:** An acute, severe form of wind red sore can arise when wind evil stirs heart fire and wind-fire attack the upper body and bind in the eyelid. The eyelid is swollen and red as if smeared with cinnabar, with unsufferable scorching pain, and with local necrosis and ulceration. When wind is prevalent, swelling is pronounced; when heat is prevalent, redness, heat, and pain are more pronounced. MED Clear heat, drain fire, and resolve toxin. Use the Universal Aid Toxin-Dispersing Beverage (*pǔ jì xiāo dú yǐn*) from *Medical Formulas Gathered and Explained* (*yī fāng jí jiě*). Topical: In all cases, Rub-On Medicinal Formula (*cā yào fāng*) can be applied to clear heat and resolve toxin, and to eliminate dampness and relieve pain. [26: 457] [125: 140]

wind red sore disease 风赤疮疾 *fēng chì chuāng jí*: WIND RED SORE.

wind sand 风痧 *fēng shā*: Synonym: *wind papules*. A contagious disease characterized by a papular eruption seen in children under five years of age in the winter and spring; attributed to externally contracted wind-heat lying depressed in the fleshy exterior and manifesting in small pale red papules that appear quickly and disappear without scaling or scarring. MED Clear heat and resolve the exterior with Lonicera and Forsythia Powder (*yín qiào sǎn*) with Five-Ingredient Toxin-Dispersing Beverage (*wǔ wèi xiāo dú yǐn*) plus cicada molting (*chán tuì*). [26: 459–460] [27: 370] [97: 100]

wind scrofula 风疬 *fēng lì*: Small itchy scrofula attributed to wind. See SCROFULA. [26: 463]

wind strike 中风 *zhòng fēng*: WIND STROKE.

wind stroke 中风 *zhòng fēng*: Synonym: *wind strike*. **1.** The sudden appearance of hemiplegia, deviated eyes and mouth, and impeded speech that may or may not start with sudden clouding collapse (loss of consciousness). In *The Inner Canon* (*nèi jīng*), the term *zhòng fēng* is used in the general sense of contracting wind evil, and terms such as MAJOR REVERSAL, SUDDEN REVERSAL, HEMILATERAL WITHERING, DISABLEMENT, and DEVIATED MOUTH most closely match what is now called wind stroke. It was Zhang Ji (Zhang Zhong-Jing) who in *Essential Prescriptions of the Golden Coffer* (*jīn guì yào lüè*) first used the term in the sense intended here. Zhang Ji attributed wind stroke to contraction of wind evil, and distinguished between network stroke, channel stroke, bowel stroke, and visceral stroke on the basis of signs: "When the evil is in the network [vessel], the skin is insensitive; when it is in the channels, [the body] is heavy and unwieldy; when it is in the bowels, [the patient] does not recognize people; when in the viscera, the tongue has difficulty in speaking and [the patient] drools at the mouth." Wind stroke continued to be attributed to external wind until the Northern Song (900–1127), when fire, phlegm, and vacuity also came to be identified as causes. In the Yuan Dynasty (1271–1368) Wang Lü (Wang An-Dao) made a clear distinction between TRUE WIND STROKE, i.e., wind stroke attributed to externally contracted wind and WIND-LIKE STROKE which is attributed to internal wind or other causes. In the Ming Dynasty, Li Zhong-Zi (Li Shi-Cai) made the distinction between block patterns and desertion patterns (see ahead). In the modern view, wind-like stroke is much more common, and usually only mild cases are ever considered to be true wind stroke, although external wind may trigger wind-like stroke. Wind-like is said to occur a) when depletion of yin essence or sudden anger causes hyperactivity of liver yang which stirs liver wind; b) when, owing to a predilection for rich, fatty foods, phlegm heat congests in the inner body and transforms into wind; c) when vacuity of qi and blood causes vacuity wind; or d) when a patient suffering from internal vacuity suddenly contracts external wind. Zhang Ji's distinctions between network, channel, bowel, and visceral stroke were never fully clarified, and modern texts tend to make only a dual distinction between channel and network stroke on the one hand and bowel and visceral stroke on the other. **Channel and network stroke** is marked by the sudden appearance of deviated eyes and mouth, hemiplegia, and difficulty in speech, or sometimes only numbness, without clouding collapse. **Bowel and visceral stroke** is marked by sudden clouding collapse that leaves the patient to regain consciousness with deviated eyes and mouth, hemiplegia, and sluggish or difficult speech or loss of speech. In other words, channel and network stroke is milder,

involving physical impairment, whereas bowel and visceral stroke is more severe and involves serious permanent impairment of mental faculties. Channel and network stroke is considered to be true wind stroke if there are signs such as aversion to cold, headache and body pains, and hypertonicity of the limbs; if not, like bowel and visceral stroke, it is considered to be wind-like stroke. In bowel and visceral stroke patterns, distinction is made between desertion and block patterns. **Desertion patterns** are those marked by open mouth, limp hands, open eyes, enuresis, snoring voice, and in some cases, by spontaneous sweating. **Block patterns** are those characterized by clenched jaw and clenched hands. Among block patterns, distinction is made between yin and yang. **Yin block** patterns are characterized by white lusterless complexion, inactivity and absence of heart vexation, lack of warmth in the extremities, dull moist lips, respiration characterized by the gurgling sound of phlegm, a dark tongue with slimy white fur and a sunken slippery or sunken moderate pulse. **Yang block** patterns are characterized by tidal reddening of the face, agitation, warm hands and feet, dry red lips, rough breathing, red tongue with yellow slimy tongue fur, and stringlike slippery or stringlike rapid pulse. WMC cerebrovascular accident (cerebral hemorrhage, cerebral embolism, cerebral thrombosis); cerebral angiospasm; toxic encephalopathy; facial paralysis. See TRUE WIND STROKE; WIND-LIKE STROKE. **2.** From *On Cold Damage* (*shāng hán lùn*). An external wind contraction, one type of greater yang *tài yáng* disease. *On Cold Damage* (*shāng hán lùn*) states, "Greater yang disease, with heat effusion, sweating, aversion to wind, and a pulse that is moderate, is called wind stroke." [26: 137] [27: 396] [97: 78] [80: 452]

wind stroke block pattern 中风闭证 *zhòng fēng bì zhèng*: See WIND-LIKE STROKE.

wind stroke desertion pattern 中风脱证 *zhòng fēng tuō zhèng*: See WIND-LIKE STROKE.

wind stroke in pregnancy 妊娠中风 *rèn shēn zhòng fēng*: From *The Origin and Indicators of Disease* (*zhū bìng yuán hòu lùn*). A disease due to strike by wind evil occurring in pregnancy when blood vacuity deprives the channels and network vessels and the bowels and viscera of nourishment. Channel and network vessel stroke is characterized by insensitivity of the skin, numbness of the extremities, deviated eyes and mouth, and, in severe cases, hemiplegia. Bowel and visceral stroke is marked by sudden collapse with phlegm-drool congestion and loss of consciousness. MED Supplement vacuity, quiet the fetus, and dispel wind. Use Modified Eight Agents Decoction (*zēng sǔn bā wù tāng*). For deviated eyes and mouth and stubborn impediment (*bì*), treat by nourishing the blood and dispelling wind, assisted by quieting the fetus. Use Fangji Powder (*fáng jǐ sǎn*). For sudden clouding collapse with phlegm-drool congestion, treat by tracking down wind, opening the orifices, and dispelling phlegm with Ledebouriella Powder (*fáng fēng sǎn*). For wind stroke with loss of voice, stiff limbs, and loss of consciousness, treat by dispelling wind and opening the orifices with Raw Rhinoceros Horn Powder (*shēng xī jiāo sǎn*). [26: 340] [56: 40]

wind taxation 风劳 *fēng láo*: VACUITY TAXATION disease with repeated contraction of wind evil. *The Wings of the Golden Coffer* (*jīn guì yì, fēng láo*) states, "Wind taxation patterns are characterized by steaming flesh and bone heat effusion, alternating heat [effusion] and [aversion to] cold, phlegm cough, night sweating, parched [body] hair, bad breath..." *The Great Peace Sagacious Benevolence Formulary* (*tài píng shèng huì fāng*) states, "In people with taxation damage, the interior and exterior are mostly vacuous, qi and blood are debilitated, and the interstices of the skin are loose and leaky, easily allowing wind evil to invade, which then either wanders through the skin or sinks to cause stagnation in the bowels and viscera, giving rise to a variety of different illnesses depending on the place affected." If the body is weak and there is reduced food intake, emaciation, inhibition of the sinews, pain in the hands and feet, then formulas such as Ledebouriella Powder (*fáng fēng sǎn*) can be used. If qi and blood are insufficient and the bowels and viscera are vacuous and damaged, and the patient has vexing pain in the joints, lack of strength in the lumbus and knees, emaciation, a withered-yellow facial complexion, frequent voidings of copious urine, and night sweating as soon as he sleeps, formulas such as Large Gentian and Turtle Shell Powder (*qín jiāo biē jiǎ sǎn*) can be used. [50: 303]

wind tetany 风痉 *fēng jìng*: **1.** TETANY (*jìng*) attributed to wind-cold-damp and characterized by repeated occurrence of signs similar to those of epilepsy such as sudden collapse, rigidity of the back, and clenched jaw. MED Dispel wind, dissipate cold, and transform dampness with formulas such as Minor Life-Prolonging Decoction (*xiǎo xù mìng tāng*). ACU Needle with drainage at GB-20 (*fēng chí*, Wind Pool), TB-5 (*wài guān*, Outer Pass), and GV-16 (*fēng fǔ*, Wind Mansion) to dispel wind; needle with supplementation and moxa at BL-23 (*shèn shū*, Kidney Transport), CV-4 (*guān yuán*, Pass Head), and GV-4 (*mìng mén*, Life Gate) to warm cold; and needle with even supplementation and drainage and apply moxa at ST-36 (*zú sān lǐ*, Leg Three Li), SP-9 (*yīn líng quán*, Yin Mound Spring), and SP-5 (*shāng qiū*, Shang Hill) to disinhibit dampness. Selection of points according to signs: For cold of the body and back, add GV-12 (*shēn zhù*, Body Pillar) and

SI-3 (*hòu xī*, Back Ravine). For clenched jaw, add ST-7 (*xià guān*, Below the Joint), ST-6 (*jiá chē*, Cheek Carriage), and LI-4 (*hé gǔ*, Union Valley). **2.** CHILDBED WIND. [26: 460] [46: 629]

wind tetany in pregnancy 妊娠风痉 *rèn shēn fēng jìng*: See EPILEPSY OF PREGNANCY. [26: 341]

wind ulceration of the eyelid rim 风弦赤烂 *fēng xián chì làn*: ULCERATION OF THE EYELID RIM. [26: 457]

wind warmth 风温 *fēng wēn*: **1.** A warm disease due to the contraction of wind warmth evil. Wind warmth usually occurs in winter or spring. At onset, the disease is in the lung and defense, and signs include generalized heat [effusion], cough, heart vexation, and thirst, but it easily makes an abnormal passage to the pericardium causing clouded spirit, delirious speech, and TETANIC REVERSAL with convulsions. MED When the evil is in the lung and defense, apply cool acrid exterior outthrust using Lonicera and Forsythia Powder (*yín qiào sǎn*), Ephedra, Apricot Kernel, Licorice, and Gypsum Decoction (*má xìng gān shí tāng*), or Thousand Gold Pieces Phragmites Decoction (*qiān jīn wěi jīng tāng*). For abnormal passage to the pericardium, clear construction and outthrust heat, and clear the heart and open the orifices. Use Construction-Clearing Decoction (*qīng yíng tāng*), Rhinoceros Horn and Rehmannia Decoction (*xī jiāo dì huáng tāng*), or Peaceful Palace Bovine Bezoar Pill (*ān gōng niú huáng wán*). See WARM DISEASE. **2.** From *On Cold Damage* (*shāng hán lùn*). Greater yang (*tài yáng*) disease with thirst and absence of aversion to cold that after sweating treatment gives way to scorching hot body, spontaneous sweating, heavy body and somnolence, and snoring from the nose. [26: 459] [27: 349] [97: 100]

wind warmth tetany 风温痉 *fēng wēn jìng*: An infantile TETANY pattern attributed to contraction of wind warmth. MED When accompanied by cough, it can be treated with Mulberry Leaf and Chrysanthemum Beverage (*sāng jú yǐn*). When there is clouded spirit and delirious speech, it is treated by opening the orifices with aroma, using Palace-Clearing Decoction (*qīng gōng tāng*) combined with Purple Snow Elixir (*zǐ xuě dān*). ACU Base treatment mainly on LU, LI, GV, and LR. Select BL-13 (*fèi shū*, Lung Transport), LU-7 (*liè quē*, Broken Sequence), LI-11 (*qū chí*, Pool at the Bend), LI-4 (*hé gǔ*, Union Valley), ST-44 (*nèi tíng*, Inner Court), GV-20 (*bǎi huì*, Hundred Convergences), GV-16 (*fēng fǔ*, Wind Mansion), LR-3 (*tài chōng*, Supreme Surge), and GV-8 (*jīn suō*, Sinew Contraction); needle with drainage. Selection of points according to signs: For high fever, add GV-14 (*dà zhuī*, Great Hammer), and prick Ten Diffusing Points (*shí xuān*) to bleed. For clouded spirit and delirious speech, add HT-7 (*shén* *mén,* Spirit Gate), and GV-26 (*shuǐ gōu,* Water Trough), and prick Twelve Well Points (*shí èr jǐng xué*) to bleed. Compare ACUTE FRIGHT WIND. [26: 459] [46: 651, 652, 733] [42: 188]

wind water 风水 *fēng shuǐ*: From *Elementary Questions* (*sù wèn, shuǐ rè xué lùn*). External wind contraction with water swelling. Signs include rapid onset, floating pulse, pain in the joints, heat effusion and aversion to cold, and swelling, particularly of the head and face (the upper part of the body being affected by wind evil). The disease is the result of impairment of lung qi's depurative downbearing by wind evil in patients suffering from spleen-kidney qi vacuity. ⟨MED⟩ Course wind, diffuse the lung, and disinhibit water using Spleen-Effusing Decoction (*yuè bì tāng*), Poria (Hoelen) Five Powder (*wǔ líng sǎn*), or Fangji and Astragalus Decoction (*fáng jǐ huáng qí tāng*). ⟨ACU⟩ Base treatment mainly on CV, back transport points, SP, ST, and GB. Select CV-9 (*shuǐ fēn,* Water Divide), CV-6 (*qì hǎi,* Sea of Qi), BL-22 (*sān jiāo shū,* Triple Burner Transport), ST-36 (*zú sān lǐ,* Leg Three Li), BL-13 (*fèi shū,* Lung Transport), BL-11 (*dà zhù,* Great Shuttle), GB-20 (*fēng chí,* Wind Pool), TB-5 (*wài guān,* Outer Pass), LI-4 (*hé gǔ,* Union Valley), LI-11 (*qū chí,* Pool at the Bend), SP-6 (*sān yīn jiāo,* Three Yin Intersection), and SP-9 (*yīn líng quán,* Yin Mound Spring); needle with drainage. Selection of points according to signs: For high fever, add GV-14 (*dà zhuī,* Great Hammer), and prick Ten Diffusing Points (*shí xuān*) to bleed. For swelling of the head and face, add GV-26 (*shuǐ gōu,* Water Trough) and GV-21 (*qián dǐng,* Before the Vertex). For headache and dizziness, add GB-20 (*fēng chí,* Wind Pool) and Greater Yang (*tài yáng*). See WATER SWELLING. [26: 456] [27: 419] [97: 99] [42: 120] [113: 182]

wind wheel 风轮 *fēng lún*: Cornea and iris; related to the liver. [27: 500, 65] [97: 99]

wind yang 风阳 *fēng yáng*: Wind as a yang evil; wind transforming from liver yang. See LIVER WIND STIRRING INTERNALLY.

wine 酒剂 *jiǔ jì*: WINE PREPARATION.

wine preparation 酒剂 *jiǔ jì*: Synonym: *wine.* Any preparation made by steeping medicinals in grain wine or liquor. **Method:** There are two methods of making wine preparations, cold steeping and hot steeping. (1) Cold steeping: The medicinal materials are cut, crushed, or ground, and steeped in white liquor (liquor distilled usually from sorghum or maize) or yellow wine (wine made from rice or millet) in a sealed large stone jar. The preparation is stirred each day, either with a ladle or by joggling the jar. When ready to drink, which is after a minimum of 30 days, but ideally for most wines much longer, the clear wine near the surface may be removed and strained to be made ready for drinking. Grubs are almost inevitably brought out from the materials by the liquor. It suffices that these should be filtered out in process of straining. Some formulas allow the materials to be reused. (2) Hot steeping: The materials and wine are placed in a receptacle and brought to the boil either in a steamer or double-boiler before they are placed in the jar to steep. In this method, the clear wine may be removed and strained for use after 15–20 days. Medicinal wines promote flow in the blood vessels, and are used in wind-damp impediment (*bì*) patterns (rheumatism) and other chronic conditions. [27: 311]

winter warmth 冬温 *dōng wēn*: From *On Cold Damage* (*shāng hán lùn, shāng hán lì*). A new contraction warm disease occurring in winter due to unseasonable warmth. Winter warmth is associated with the same disease shifts as wind warmth. See NEW CONTRACTION WARM DISEASE; WIND WARMTH. [26: 215] [27: 353]

wiry pulse 弦脉 *xián mài*: STRINGLIKE PULSE.

withdrawal 癫 *diān*: Synonym: *withdrawal disease.* Any pattern characterized by melancholy, indifferent expression, muttering soliloquy, abnormal laughing and weeping, hallucination and delusions, deranged speech, no sense of hygiene, no thought of food and drink, thin slimy tongue fur, and a slippery stringlike pulse; attributed to binding depression of phlegm and qi. ⟨MED⟩ Withdrawal is treated by rectifying qi and resolving depression, transforming phlegm, and opening the orifices. Suitable formulas include Coptis Gallbladder-Warming Decoction (*huáng lián wēn dǎn tāng*), Alum and Curcuma Pill (*bái jīn wán*), or Qi-Normalizing Phlegm-Abducting Decoction (*shùn qì dǎo tán tāng*), i.e., Phlegm-Abducting Decoction plus cyperus (*xiāng fù zǐ*), lindera (*wū yào*), aquilaria (*chén xiāng*), and saussurea (*mù xiāng*). For patients with dual vacuity of heart and spleen, Heart-Nourishing Decoction (*yǎng xīn tāng*) or Spleen-Returning Decoction (*guī pí tāng*) may be used. ⟨ACU⟩ Base treatment mainly on back transport points, HT, PC, LR, and SP. Needle with supplementation at BL-18 (*gān shū,* Liver Transport), BL-15 (*xīn shū,* Heart Transport), BL-20 (*pí shū,* Spleen Transport), ST-40 (*fēng lóng,* Bountiful Bulge), and SP-6 (*sān yīn jiāo,* Three Yin Intersection), and with drainage at HT-7 (*shén mén,* Spirit Gate), PC-7 (*dà líng,* Great Mound), LR-3 (*tài chōng,* Supreme Surge), and GV-20 (*bǎi huì,* Hundred Convergences). Selection of points according to signs: For abnormal laughing and crying, add PC-5 (*jiān shǐ,* Intermediary Courier) and PC-8 (*láo gōng,* Palace of Toil) (*guǐ kū,* Ghost Cave). For no thought of food and drink, add CV-12 (*zhōng wǎn,* Center Stomach Duct). For enduring withdrawal, the thirteen ghost points (*shí sān guǐ xuè*) can be needled. See MANIA AND WITHDRAWAL. Compare LOST HEART WIND. [26: 1005] [97: 660] [46: 642] [113: 153]

withdrawal disease 癲病 *diān bìng*: WITH-DRAWAL.

withered nose 鼻藁 *bí gǎo*: *Synonym: dried-meat nose.* Dryness and withering of the interior of the nose. Because the interior of the nose is dry and withered like cured meat, it is also called *dried-meat nose.* Withered nose is attributed to lung vacuity failing to nourish the nose. MED Use Dryness-Clearing Lung-Rescuing Decoction (*qīng zào jiù fèi tāng*) minus gypsum (*shí gāo*). WMC atrophic rhinitis. Compare BRAIN-GRIPPING SAND.

withered-yellow facial complexion 面色萎黄 *miàn sè wěi huáng*: A pale brownish yellow facial complexion, the color of withered leaves. A withered-yellow complexion is a lusterless brownish yellow facial complexion; it signifies vacuity or dampness. It is observed in the following situations: a) in spleen-stomach qi vacuity in conjunction with poor appetite, abdominal distention after eating, fatigue and lack of strength, shortage of qi and laziness to speak, sloppy stool, a pale tongue with white fur, and a weak moderate pulse; b) in spleen vacuity with damp obstruction with swelling of the face and limbs, cumbersome heavy limbs, reduced food intake, abdominal distention, fatigue and lack of strength, turbid heavy voice, scant urine and sloppy stool, pale enlarged tongue often with dental impression, glossy slimy tongue fur, and a forceless moderate pulse; c) in insufficiency of construction blood with pale lips and tongue, dizzy head and vision, heart palpitations and insomnia, numbness of the limbs, scant menstrual flow, delayed periods or menstrual block, shortness of breath and low voice, and a faint fine pulse. [92: No. 73] [97: 509]

withering of the helices 耳轮枯焦 *ěr lún kū jiāo*: Dry shriveled ears; in enduring or serious illness, a sign of qi and blood depletion and impending expiration of kidney qi when observed in the course of enduring sickness.

womb 子宫 *zǐ gōng*: UTERUS.

women's diseases 妇女疾病 *fù nǚ jí bìng*: See DISEASE.

wood 木 *mù*: (In the doctrine of the five phases) the phase associated with the season spring, the color green, the flavor sourness, and the color green-blue. In the body it is associated with liver and gallbladder and with related entities (eyes, sinews, and nails). [6: 29]

wood fire tormenting metal 木火刑金 *mù huǒ xíng jīn*: *Synonym: exuberant fire tormenting metal.* Liver fire affecting the lung. Wood in

the five phases is the liver, and metal is the lung. When liver fire becomes excessively effulgent, it can scorch lung yin, causing dry cough, chest and rib-side pain, heart vexation, bitter taste in the heart, red eyes, and, in severe cases, expectoration of blood. This is the manifestation of wood fire tormenting metal. MED Use White-Draining Powder (*xiè bái sǎn*) combined with Indigo and Clamshell Powder (*dài gé sǎn*) plus scutellaria (*huáng qín*), anemarrhena (*zhī mǔ*), platycodon (*jié gěng*), unripe tangerine peel (*qīng pí*), and tangerine peel (*chén pí*). ACU Base treatment mainly on LU and LR. Select BL-13 (*fèi shū*, Lung Transport), LU-5 (*chǐ zé*, Cubit Marsh), LU-10 (*yú jì*, Fish Border), LR-2 (*xíng jiān*, Moving Between), and GB-34 (*yáng líng quán*, Yang Mound Spring); needle with drainage. [26: 109] [27: 12] [97: 74] [46: 653]

worm 虫 *chóng*: Any small animal that can inhabit the body. Any worm such as roundworm, or ich whiteworm in the body. Attributable to unclean food or damp-heat. WMC Various parasites. See ROUNDWORM; INCH WHITEWORM; REDWORM; PINWORM; NINE WORM DISEASES; INVISIBLE WORM. [27: 122]

worm accumulation 虫积 *chóng jī*: FOOD ACCUMULATION due to worms in the digestive tract. Worm accumulation is characterized by yellow facial complexion, emaciation of the flesh, periodic vomiting of clear water or sour water, enlarged abdomen, and acute stomach duct pain and abdomen, sometimes specifically around the umbilicus. In some cases, there is a palpable accumulation lump. MED Expel worms and disperse accumulation using Worm-Transforming Pill (*huà chóng wán*), Myriad Applications Pill (*wàn yìng wán*), or Mume Pill (*wū méi wán*). ACU Base treatment mainly on back transport points and ST. Select BL-20 (*pí shū*, Spleen Transport), BL-25 (*dà cháng shū*, Large Intestine Transport), ST-36 (*zú sān lǐ*, Leg Three Li), Hundred Worm Nest (*bǎi chóng wō*), and CV-6 (*qì hǎi*, Sea of Qi)ⓜ; apply a strong needle stimulus and moxa. For palpable accumulation lump, needle at the head, middle and tail of the lump, and then burn 12 cones of moxa at the same three points; then moxa Glomus Root (*pǐ gēn*). [26: 959] [27: 416] [97: 183] [37: 320] [4: 159]

worm accumulation abdominal pain 虫积腹痛 *chong jī fù tòng*: ABDOMINAL PAIN due to worms in the stomach and intestine. Worm accumulation abdominal pain is associated with intermittent gripping pain, and in severe cases, with the vomiting of roundworm. Normally, there is clamoring stomach, predilection for strange foods, yellow face and emaciated flesh, worm macules on the face, blue speckles on the eyes, millet-shaped papules on the inside of the lips, and grinding of the teeth in sleep (bruxism). MED Expel worms and disperse accumulations with formulas such as Quisqualis Powder (*shǐ jūn zǐ sǎn*), Worm-Expelling Pill (*zhuī chóng wán*), and Worm-Transforming Pill (*huà chóng wán*). ACU Base treatment mainly on back transport points, ST, and empirical points. Select BL-20 (*pí shū*, Spleen Transport), BL-25 (*dà cháng shū*, Large Intestine Transport), ST-36 (*zú sān lǐ*, Leg Three Li), Hundred Worm Nest (*bǎi chóng wō*), and ST-4 (*dì cāng*, Earth Granary). Use a strong stimulus. [26: 959] [37: 320]

worm disease resembling epilepsy 虫病似痫 *chóng bìng sì xián*: Signs similar to those of epilepsy such as forward-staring eyes, clenched jaw preventing speech, loud shouting and crying, drool foaming at the mouth, white or green-blue facial complexion, and rigidity of the extremities. MED Use Bovine Bezoar Pill (*niú huáng wán*) taken with a decoction of chinaberry root bark (*kǔ liàn gēn pí*). Alternatively, use Mume Pill (*wū méi wán*) prepared as a decoction. WMC biliary ascariasis. [26: 958]

worm distention 虫胀 *chóng zhàng*: WORM DRUM. [26: 959]

worm drum 虫鼓 *chóng gǔ*: *Synonyms: worm drum distention*; WORM DISTENTION. Distention due to toxin binding in the stomach and intestines. Worm drum is distention associated with pain and accompanied by mild swelling of the four limbs, and ability to eat. There is often a strange craving to eat tea leaves, salt, and earth. There are red speckles or lines on the face as if eroded by worms. [26: 959]

worm drum distention 虫臌 *chóng gǔ*: WORM DRUM.

worm heart pain 虫心痛 *chóng xīn tòng*: From *A Thousand Gold Pieces Prescriptions* (*qiān jīn yào fāng*). Pain in the heart [region] due to worm accumulation in patients with spleen vacuity and tendency to excessive consumption of sweet fatty foods. Worm heart pain is an intermittent pain associated with the gathering of a swelling. Sometimes there are yellow-white patches on the face. The complexion is now green-blue, now white. There is also vomiting and the inability to eat. MED Kill the worms and attack the accumulation. Use Worm-Transforming Pill (*huà chóng wán*). [26: 958]

worm macule 虫斑 *chóng bān*: Grayish white patches on the skin in children; indicates roundworm infestation. [26: 959] [27: 486] [27: 183] [6: 117]

worrying tongue 弄舌 *nòng shé*: *Synonym: snake tongue*. See PROTRUSION AND WORRYING OF THE TONGUE. [6: 122]

wrap-boiling 包煎 *bāo jiān*: Boiling medicinals wrapped cloth. Highly sticky seeds such as plantago seed (*chē qián zǐ*) are wrap-boiled to prevent them sticking to the pot and burning. Some materials such as inula flower (*xuán fù huā*) are covered with a down that is hard to strain off and causes irritation to the throat if swallowed. Peach kernel (*táo rén*) pounded to a paste, as well as dragon bone (*lóng gǔ*) and oyster shell (*mǔ lì*), may be wrap-boiled to keep the decoction clear of unnecessary particles. [27: 319] [97: 163]

wrenched lumbus pain 闪挫腰痛 *shǎn cuò yāo tòng*: Lumbar pain attributable to lifting heavy weights or to twisting or falling. Wrenched lumbus pain is characterized by the inability to bend and stretch or or difficulty in turning, with any movement exacerbating pain. MED Quicken the blood and soothe the sinews. Use Four Agents Decoction (*sì wù tāng*) plus peach kernel (*táo rén*), carthamus (*hóng huā*), cyathula (*chuān niú xī*), cinnamon bark (*ròu guì*), corydalis (*yán hú suǒ*), frankincense (*rǔ xiāng*), and myrrh (*mò yào*). ACU Base treatment mainly on BL, GV, SP, and ouch points (*ā shì xué*). Select GV-26 (*rén zhōng*, Human Center), GV-3 (*yāo yáng guān*, Lumbar Yang Pass), BL-40 (*wěi zhōng*, Bend Center), BL-17 (*gé shū*, Diaphragm Transport), SP-10 (*xuè hǎi*, Sea of Blood), LR-3 (*tài chōng*, Supreme Surge), BL-32 (*cì liáo*, Second Bone-Hole), and ouch points (*ā shì xué*); needle with even supplementation and drainage. [26: 514] [27: 488] [97: 168] [46: 633] [37: 391] [113: 228]

wrinkly foot 皱脚 *zhòu jiǎo*: A form of swelling that occurs in late pregnancy, characterized by thick rough skin with a somber hue and not associated with any other discomforts. Wrinkly foot arises when the growing fetus inhibits qi dynamic. It usually disappears spontaneously after delivery. In women with qi-blood vacuity and insufficiency of the lower origin, with damp qi pouring downward to cause pain, it can be treated with Qi-Normalizing Blood-Nourishing Decoction (*shùn qì yǎng xuè tāng*). Compare BRITTLE FOOT; SWELLING AND DISTENTION IN PREGNANCY. [26: 892] [24: 156] [50: 1280]

wrist pulse 寸口 *cùn kǒu*: *Synonym: inch opening; qi opening; vessel opening*. The pulse felt on the inner (palmar) face of the wrist, at a location described in modern anatomy as the styloid process of the radius. The wrist pulse is divided into three sections: inch (*cùn*), bar (*guān*), and cubit (*chǐ*). It is generally agreed that, on the left wrist, the inch pulse reflects the heart, the bar reflects the liver, and the cubit reflects the kidney, whereas on the right wrist, the inch reflects the lung, the bar the spleen and stomach, and the cubit the life gate. See PULSE; THREE POSITIONS AND NINE INDICA-

TORS. ◇ Chin 寸 *cùn*, inch, *cun;* 口 *kǒu*, mouth, opening. [27: 188] [97: 90]

Wu 吴 *wú*: The name of a dynasty (A.D. 220–280).

X

Xia 夏 *xià*: The name of a dynastic period (approx. 21st cent. B.C.–16th cent. B.C.).

Y

YAL 阳维脉 *yáng wéi mài*: Abbreviation for the YANG LINKING VESSEL.

yang 阳 *yáng*: **1.** The bright, male, active principle that stands in complementary opposition to yin. See YIN AND YANG. **2.** The penis, as in terms such as "yang wilt" (阳痿 *yáng wěi*) and "yang matter failing to rise," (阳事不举 *yáng shì bù jǔ*), which both denote impotence. [26: 711] [97: 236]

yang bind 阳结 *yáng jié*: See HEAT BIND. [26: 717]

yang brightness 阳明 *yáng míng*: The hand yang brightness large intestine and foot yang brightness stomach channels. The yang brightness is the last stage in the development of yang qi. It is the innermost of the three yang channels, hence it is said that "yang brightness is the closedness." Yang brightness has copious qi and copious blood. [27: 91] [97: 237] [50: 643]

yang brightness blood amassment 阳明蓄血 *yáng míng xù xuè*: A disease pattern in which yang brightness (*yáng míng*) evil heat binds with preexisting static blood. Signs include forgetfulness and hard black stool that is easily passed. *On Cold Damage* (*shāng hán lùn*) states, "In yang brightness patterns, when the patient has forgetfulness, there must be blood amassment, the reason for this being the presence of enduring static blood; hence there is forgetfulness and stool that, though hard, is nevertheless easily passed, and that must be black. This is treated with Dead-On Decoction (*dǐ dàng tāng*)." [51: 344] [50: 649]

yang brightness bowel pattern 阳明腑证 *yáng míng fǔ zhèng*: A disease pattern arising when in externally contracted febrile disease, evil enters the yang brightness (*yáng míng*) channel, causing tidal heat [effusion], delirious speech, a hard, full, distended abdomen with pain that refuses pressure, constipation, burnt yellow or old yellow tongue fur, and a strong, sunken, replete pulse. This is often referred to as HEAT BINDING IN THE STOMACH AND INTESTINES or HEAT BIND. MED Treat by draining precipitation using cold bitter precipitants to flush the gastrointestinal heat accumulation. The principal formula is Major Qi-Coordinating Decoction (*dà chéng qì tāng*). See YANG BRIGHTNESS DISEASE. [26: 713] [71: 353] [6: 226]

yang brightness channel 阳明经 *yáng míng jīng*: See YANG BRIGHTNESS.

yang brightness channel pattern 阳明经证 *yáng míng jīng zhèng*: A disease arising when externally contracted evil enters the yang brightness (*yáng míng*) channel, causing great heat [effusion], great sweating, pronounced agitation, and a large, surging pulse. The four signs are collectively known as the *four greatnesses*. MED Clear heat and drain fire to safeguard liquid. Use White Tiger Decoction (*bái hǔ tāng*) as the basic formula, adding ginseng (*rén shēn*) to boost qi and engender liquid in cases of damage to both qi and yin. See YANG BRIGHTNESS DISEASE. [26: 713] [6: 226]

yang brightness disease 阳明病 *yáng míng bìng*: A disease arising when externally contracted evil enters the yang brightness (*yáng míng*) channel and exterior signs such as aversion to wind and cold give way to pronounced heat signs. Yang brightness disease is characterized by generalized heat [effusion], sweating and aversion to heat, agitation, and thirst, or, in more severe cases, abdominal fullness and pain, constipation, and, in severe cases, delirious mania. The tongue fur is usually dry and old yellow in color. The pulse is generally surging and large, slippery and rapid, or sunken, replete, and forceful. Yang brightness disease occurs in the exuberant heat effusion stage of externally contracted heat (febrile) diseases, and manifests, in terms of the eight principles, as interior heat or interior repletion. Yang brightness disease is divided into channel and bowel patterns depending on the presence of constipation. In yang brightness channel patterns, the stomach liquid is damaged by exuberant heat, although there is no heat bind in the yang brightness bowels (the stomach and large intestine). Yang brightness bowel patterns are so named because they arise when an evil binds with food accumulation or dry waste in the stomach or intestines, causing repletion heat. See YANG BRIGHTNESS BOWEL PATTERN; YANG BRIGHTNESS CHANNEL PATTERN. [6: 226] [27: 219] [97: 239]

yang brightness headache 阳明头痛 *yáng míng tóu tòng*: **1.** HEADACHE occurring in yang brightness (*yáng míng*) disease in cold damage, which is accompanied by generalized heat [effusion] with aversion not to cold but to heat. MED Use White Tiger Decoction (*bái hǔ tāng*) plus angelica (*bái zhǐ*), or formulas containing cimicifuga (*shēng má*), pueraria (*gé gēn*), gypsum (*shí gāo*), and angelica (*bái zhǐ*). ACU Select LI-4 (*hé gǔ*, Union Valley) and ST-42 (*chōng yáng*, Surging Yang); needle with drainage. **2.** HEADACHE on the pathway of the yang brightness (*yáng míng*) channel, i.e., on the forehead and sometimes stretching into the eyeballs. MED Treat with formulas containing angelica (*bái zhǐ*) and cimicifuga (*shēng má*) as conductors. ACU Select Hall of Impression (*yìn táng*), ST-8 (*tóu wéi*, Head Corner), LI-4 (*hé gǔ*, Union Valley), and ST-44 (*nèi tíng*, Inner Court). [26: 713] [113: 9] [4: 154]

yang channel 阳经 *yáng jīng*: Synonym: *yang vessel*. Any yang channel or vessel including the three yang channels of the hands and feet, i.e., greater yang (*tài yáng*), lesser yang (*shào yáng*), yang brightness (*yáng míng*), and the governing (*dū*) vessel, yang linking (*yáng wéi*), and yang springing (*yáng qiāo*) vessels. [27: 86]

yang collapse 亡阳 *wáng yáng*: Synonym: *yang desertion*. A disease pattern of critical debilitation of yang qi marked by sweating and cold skin and reversal cold of the limbs. The patient is apathetic or (rarely) agitated, and, in severe cases, his spirit is clouded. Either there is no thirst or there is a desire for warm fluids. The pulse is either hidden, sunken, fine and faint, or agitated and racing. The tongue is pale. MED Use large doses of Ginseng and Aconite Decoction (*shēn fù tāng*). ACU Base treatment mainly on CV and GV. Select GV-26 (*shuǐ gōu*, Water Trough), GV-25 (*sù liáo*, White Bone-Hole), PC-6 (*nèi guān*, Inner

Pass), GV-20 (*bǎi huì*, Hundred Convergences), CV-4 (*guān yuán*, Pass Head), ST-36 (*zú sān lǐ*, Leg Three Li) and KI-1 (*yǒng quán*, Gushing Spring); needle with supplementation or direct moxa. Apply moxa on salt or ginger at CV-8 (*shén què*, Spirit Gate Tower). [46: 730] [27: 206] [97: 33]

yang-collapse vacuity desertion 亡阳虚脱 *wáng yáng xū tuō*: See YANG COLLAPSE.

yang desertion 阳脱 *yáng tuó*: YANG COLLAPSE.

yang disease 阳病 *yáng bìng*: **1.** TRIPLE-YANG DISEASE. **2.** Any disease manifesting in a repletion pattern or heat pattern. [27: 348] [97: 238]

yang disease is treated through yin 阳病治阴 *yáng bìng zhì yīn*: **1.** The principle of treating damage to yin by exuberant yang heat. "When yang prevails, yin ails," and so that exuberant yang heat causes damage to yin fluids. Such patterns are treated by engendering liquid with cold sweet agents. **2.** Treating disease patterns associated with a yang channel by needling points on a yin channel. For example, foot yang brightness *yáng míng* channel vomiting and retching can be treated by needing PC-6 (*nèi guān*, Inner Pass) and LR-3 (*tài chōng*, Supreme Surge). See PRINCIPLE OF TREATMENT. [27: 237] [97: 240]

yang epilepsy 阳痫 *yáng xián*: EPILEPSY forming a yang pattern; usually attributed to phlegm heat settling in the heart and stomach, and characterized by convulsions, shrieking, generalized heat [effusion], floating pulse, upward staring eyes, worrying tongue, and shaking head. MED It is treated mainly with cold medicinals. ACU Use the general points given for fits under EPILEPSY, and further needle GV-14 (*dà zhuī*, Great Hammer), ST-44 (*nèi tíng*, Inner Court), and ST-45 (*lì duì*, Severe Mouth). Prick Twelve Well Points (*shí èr jǐng xué*) to bleed. [26: 717] [27: 427]

yang evil 阳邪 *yáng xié*: **1.** Any evil that is yang in nature, e.g., wind, summerheat, dryness, and fire. These evils have yang qualities like mobility (wind), heat (summerheat and fire), and absence of fluid (dryness). **2.** An evil invading any yang channel. [26: 713] [27: 110] [97: 237]

yang heat 阳热 *yáng rè*: Heat seen as a yang phenomenon.

yang is engendered by yin 阳生于阴 *yáng shēng yú yīn*: Yin is a prerequisite for the existence of yang, according to the principle of interdependence of yin and yang. In the human body, the production of yang qi, for example, is dependent on yin essence, blood, and fluids. See YIN AND YANG ARE ROOTED IN EACH OTHER. [26: 712] [27: 4]

yang jaundice 阳黄 *yáng huáng*: JAUNDICE attributable to contraction of external evils, damp-heat invading the liver and gallbladder, and resultant gallbladder heat causing bile to percolate through to the skin. Yang jaundice is a vivid yellow described as being like the color of tangerines; it is accompanied by heat effusion, thirst, urine the color of strong tea, constipation, abdominal distention, rib-side pain, slimy yellow tongue fur, and a rapid stringlike pulse. WMC acute infectious hepatitis; obstructive biliary tract diseases. MED Clear and disinhibit liver-gallbladder damp-heat with formulas such as Capillaris Decoction (*yīn chén hāo tāng*), Gardenia and Phellodendron Decoction (*zhī zǐ bǎi pí tāng*), Ephedra, Forsythia, and Rice Bean Decoction (*má huáng lián qiào chì xiǎo dòu tāng*), and Major Bupleurum Decoction (*dà chái hú tāng*), and with specific medicinals such as moneywort (*jīn qián cǎo*), hanging stonecrop (*shí zhǐ jiǎ*) (also called *shí zhǐ jiǎ*), bearded scutellaria (*bàn zhī lián*), schisandra (*wǔ wèi zǐ*), isatis root (*bǎn lán gēn*), and lesser hypericum (*dì ěr cǎo*) (also called *tián jī huáng*). ACU Base treatment mainly on GB and SP. Select BL-19 (*dǎn shū*, Gallbladder Transport), GB-34 (*yáng líng quán*, Yang Mound Spring), LR-3 (*tài chōng*, Supreme Surge), SP-9 (*yīn líng quán*, Yin Mound Spring), ST-44 (*nèi tíng*, Inner Court), and GV-9 (*zhì yáng*, Extremity of Yang); needle with drainage. Selection of points according to signs: If heat is predominant, add GV-14 (*dà zhuī*, Great Hammer) and LI-11 (*qū chí*, Pool at the Bend). If dampness is predominant, add SP-6 (*sān yīn jiāo*, Three Yin Intersection) and ST-36 (*zú sān lǐ*, Leg Three Li). For constipation, add TB-6 (*zhī gōu*, Branch Ditch). See also DAMP-HEAT JAUNDICE. [46: 664] [27: 207] [97: 238]

yang linking vessel 阳维脉 *yáng wéi mài*: One of the EIGHT EXTRAORDINARY VESSELS. **Abbreviation:** YAL. [6: 73]

yang macules 阳斑 *yáng bān*: Synonym: *yang-pattern macules*. MACULES occurring in repletion heat patterns due to externally contracted heat (febrile) disease. See MACULOPAPULAR ERUPTION. [26: 716]

yang network vessel 阳络 *yáng luò*: **1.** Network vessels in the surface of the body or ascending toward the upper body. **2.** Network vessels branching from the three yang channels of the hand and foot. **3.** The network vessels of the foot yang brightness (*yáng míng*) stomach channel. [26: 717]

yang pattern 阳证 *yáng zhèng*: **1.** Any exterior pattern, heat pattern, or repletion pattern, especially repletion heat characterized by signs such as heat effusion with aversion to cold, red facial complexion, headache, generalized heat [effusion] with a liking for coolness, manic agitation, dry cracked lips, vexation and thirst with taking of fluids, rough strident voice, rough breathing, constipation or foul smelling stool, abdominal pain that refuses pressure, short voidings of reddish urine, red tongue with dry yellow fur, and a forceful float-

ing, surging, rapid pulse. **2.** Of sores, the presentation of signs such as redness, swelling, hardness, and pain. Compare YIN PATTERN. [26: 718] [6: 160] [27: 111] [97: 237]

yang-pattern macules 阳证发斑 *yáng zhèng fā bān*: See YANG MACULES.

yang pattern resembling yin 阳证似阴 *yáng zhèng sì yīn*: Febrile disease developing to the extreme can manifest in false signs. When the root of a disease manifests as a yang pattern, the appearance of reversal cold in the limbs and sunken hidden pulse make it a yang pattern resembling yin. This is the same as TRUE HEAT AND FALSE COLD. [26: 719]

yang qi 阳气 *yáng qì*: **1.** Anything yang in nature, as complimentarily opposed to yin qi. **2.** The active or functional aspect of the body as complimentarily opposed to yin-blood or yin humor. See QI. [26: 714] [27: 2] [97: 237]

yang reversal 阳厥 *yáng jué*: **1.** From *Elementary Questions* (*sù wèn, bìng néng lùn*). A disease characterized by bursts of manic anger due to sudden stimulus. MED Use Iron Flakes Beverage (*shēng tiě luò yǐn*). See MANIA. **2.** Reversal counterflow of yang qi in the foot lesser yang (*shào yáng*) gallbladder channel. *The Magic Pivot* (*líng shū, jīng mài*) states, "The gallbladder foot lesser yang vessel,... when stirred [becomes affected by] disease [characterized by] bitter taste in the mouth, frequent sighing, heart and rib-side pain causing inability to turn over, and, in severe cases, a faint dusty complexion, general lack of sheen, and heat abnormally felt on the outside of the feet (under normal conditions, the sole is hotter than the dorsum of the foot). This is yang reversal." **3.** Heat reversal due extreme yang. See HEAT REVERSAL. [26: 716]

yang rigidity 阳强 *yáng qiáng*: Synonyms: *yin rigidity*; *yin protrusion*[1]; *rigid center*; *rigidity of the penis*; *persistent erection*. Abnormal persistent erection accompanied by tenderness of the penis and in some cases persistent discharge of semen. Yang rigidity is called RIGID CENTER especially when there is discharge of semen. **Liver-gallbladder repletion fire** gives rise to yang rigidity when it passes along the liver vessel to the ancestral sinew and scorches the genitals. The main signs are lasting erections and tenderness accompanied by rash temperament and red face. Secondary signs include dizziness, bitter taste in the mouth, and dry throat. MED Clear the liver and drain fire; enrich yin and soften hardness. Use Tangkuei, Gentian, and Aloe Pill (*dāng guī lóng huì wán*). ACU Base treatment mainly on LR and HT. Select BL-18 (*gān shū*, Liver Transport), LR-3 (*tài chōng*, Supreme Surge), HT-8 (*shào fǔ*, Lesser Mansion), ST-44 (*nèi tíng*, Inner Court), and HT-7 (*shén mén*, Spirit Gate); needle with drainage. **Liver-gallbladder damp-heat** gives rise to yang rigidity when it obstructs the liver vessel and blocks the network vessels of the penis. The signs are unabating erection and tenderness, accompanied by dizzy head and a feeling of distention of the brain, nausea, fullness and distention in the chest and abdomen, cumbersome fatigued limbs, bitter taste in the mouth, and scant yellow or reddish urine. |MED| Clear heat and disinhibit dampness; soften hardness and free binds. Gentian Liver-Draining Decoction (*lóng dǎn xiè gān tāng*) made into pills. |ACU| Base treatment mainly on LR, SP, and CV. Select LR-2 (*xíng jiān*, Moving Between), LR-3 (*tài chōng*, Supreme Surge), SP-9 (*yīn líng quán*, Yin Mound Spring), SP-6 (*sān yīn jiāo*, Three Yin Intersection), CV-3 (*zhōng jí*, Central Pole), and BL-28 (*páng guāng shū*, Bladder Transport); needle with drainage. **Yin vacuity with yang hyperactivity** yang rigidity arises when excessive sexual indulgence causes damage true yin so that it no longer constrains yang, and unrestrained yang causes invigoration of the ancestral sinew. In the past, it was also caused by excessive consumption of elixir minerals. The main signs are unabating erection with persistent discharge of semen. Secondary signs include dizzy head and tinnitus, limp aching lumus and knees, vexing heat in the five hearts, dry mouth, and night sweating. |MED| Enrich yin and clear heat; subdue hang and soften hardness. Use All-the-Way-Through Brew (*yī guàn jiān*). |ACU| Base treatment mainly on KI, LR, and CV. Select KI-3 (*tài xī*, Great Ravine), KI-5 (*shuǐ quán*, Water Spring), KI-6 (*zhào hǎi*, Shining Sea), LR-2 (*xíng jiān*, Moving Between), LR-3 (*tài chōng*, Supreme Surge), CV-3 (*zhōng jí*, Central Pole), and CV-2 (*qū gǔ*, Curved Bone); needle with even supplementation and drainage. Compare YIN PROTRACTION. [56: 65–68]

yang rising failure 阳事不举 *yáng shì bù jǔ* IMPOTENCE. [27: 427]

yang springing vessel 阳跷（跻）脉 *yáng qiāo (qiāo) mài*: One of the EIGHT EXTRAORDINARY VESSELS. **Abbreviation:** YAS. A vessel that runs from the heel up the outside of the leg and and trunk up to the eye, and that is responsible for the opening and closing of the eyes and for muscular movement in general. **Pathway:** The yang springing (*yáng qiāo*) vessel starts below the lateral malleolus at BL-62 (*shēn mài*, Extending Vessel) and runs up the lateral aspect of the trunk, gradually curving around posteriorly to the lateral aspect of the shoulder. It crosses over the shoulder to the front of the body, then runs up the neck, over the jaw, past the corners of the mouth to the inner canthus of the eye. From here it joins with the yin springing (*yīn qiāo*) vessel and the foot greater yang (*tài yáng*) bladder channel to run up the forehead and over the lateral aspect

of the head to GB-20 (*fēng chí*, Wind Pool) posterior to the mastoid process, before entering the brain at GV-16 (*fēng fǔ*, Wind Mansion). **Functions:** The main physiological functions of both the yang springing vessels (as the yin springing vessels) are to control the opening and closing of the eyes, control the ascent of fluids and the descent of qi, and to regulate muscular activity in general. **Signs:** Disease signs associated with the yang springing (*yáng qiāo*) vessel include eye diseases, dry and itching eyes, insomnia, lack of agility, lumbar pain, spasm along the lateral aspect of the lower extremity, with corresponding flaccidity along its medial aspect. Compare YIN SPRINGING VESSEL. [6: 69]

yang summerheat 阳暑 *yáng shǔ*: **1.** Summerheat damage from contraction of summerheat-heat through strenuous activity in the sun. Yang summerheat is characterized by headache, vexation and agitation, great heat [effusion], great thirst, great sweating, a floating pulse, and panting or shortness of breath. |MED| Clear summerheat using formulas such as White Tiger Decoction (*bái hǔ tāng*) or White Tiger Decoction Plus Ginseng (*bái hǔ jiā rén shēn tāng*). |ACU| Base treatment mainly on LI, BL, CV, and GV. Main points: PC-6 (*nèi guān*, Inner Pass), LI-4 (*hé gǔ*, Union Valley), and ST-36 (*zú sān lǐ*, Leg Three Li); needle with drainage. Selection of points according to signs: For headache, add GV-20 (*bǎi huì*, Hundred Convergences) and GB-20 (*fēng chí*, Wind Pool). For vexation and agitation, add HT-5 (*tōng lǐ*, Connecting Li) and HT-7 (*shén mén*, Spirit Gate). For great heat [effusion], add GV-14 (*dà zhuī*, Great Hammer) and LI-11 (*qū chí*, Pool at the Bend). For great thirst, add KI-6 (*zhào hǎi*, Shining Sea) and TB-2 (*yè mén*, Humor Gate). For great sweating, add KI-7 (*fù liū*, Recover Flow) and SI-3 (*hòu xī*, Back Ravine). **2.** SUMMERHEAT STROKE. [26: 717] [27: 249] [97: 238] [113: 48] [37: 486]

yang sweating 阳汗 *yáng hàn*: Synonym: *heat sweating*. *Jing-Yue's Complete Compendium* (*jǐng yuè quán shū, zá zhèng mó*) states, "Yang sweating is heat sweating... In yang-pattern spontaneous sweating or night sweating, if mere examination of the pulse and patterns reveals fire, or night heat effusion with vexation and thirst, or hot stool and liking for cold things, this is yang exuberance with yin vacuity. Tangkuei Six Yellows Decoction (*dāng guī liù huáng tāng*) is the first choice of treatment; Yin-Safeguarding Brew (*bǎo yīn jiān*) is also wondrously effectively. If there is mild fire in the yin aspect, use formulas like All Yin Brew (*yī yīn jiān*) or All Yin Variant Brew (*jiā jiǎn yī yīn jiān*). If there is disquieted heart fire, with vexation, agitation, and sweating, use formulas like Cinnabar Spirit-Quieting Pill (*zhū shā ān shén wán*), Celestial Emperor Heart-Supplementing Elixir (*tiān wáng bǔ xīn dān*), or Pulse-Engendering Powder (*shēng mài sǎn*). There is also a condition that is not yin vacuity, that arises simply because of sweltering internal heat that causes blood heat and profuse sweating. This is treated with Qi-Righting Decoction (*zhèng qì tāng*), Coptis and Peony Decoction (*huáng qín sháo yào tāng*), or Clearing Transforming Beverage (*qīng huà yǐn*)." [50: 643]

yang tetany 阳痉 *yáng jìng*: 1. HARD TETANY. 2. TETANY (*jìng*) without reversal cold of the limbs; usually caused by exuberant wind-heat. MED Clear heat, cool the blood, and dispel wind using formulas such as Antelope Horn Powder (*líng yáng jiǎo sǎn*). ACU Base treatment mainly on GV, LR, CV, and SP. Select GV-20 (*bǎi huì*, Hundred Convergences), GB-20 (*fēng chí*, Wind Pool), GV-16 (*fēng fǔ*, Wind Mansion), GV-14 (*dà zhuī*, Great Hammer), LI-11 (*qū chí*, Pool at the Bend), LR-3 (*tài chōng*, Supreme Surge), SP-10 (*xuè hǎi*, Sea of Blood), SP-6 (*sān yīn jiāo*, Three Yin Intersection), and KI-2 (*rán gǔ*, Blazing Valley); needle with drainage and prick the Ten Diffusing Points (*shí xuān*) to bleed. [26: 716]

yang vacuity 阳虚 *yáng xū*: The manifestation of insufficiency of yang qi; reduction in the warming and activating power of the body. Signs include fatigue and lack of strength, shortage of qi and laziness to speak, fear of cold, and cold limbs, spontaneous sweating, pale white complexion, long voidings of clear urine, sloppy stool, pale tender-soft tongue, and a large vacuous or faint fine pulse. Yang vacuity is treated by warming yang and boosting qi. [26: 715] [27: 206] [97: 238]

yang vacuity dizziness 阳虚眩晕 *yáng xū xuàn yūn*: DIZZINESS attributable to insufficiency of yang qi preventing clear yang from reaching the head. Vacuity dizziness may be accompanied by headache, aversion to cold, tinnitus, and deafness. In some cases, dizziness threatens loss of balance and is accompanied by shortness of breath, spontaneous sweating, cold extremities, and a fine sunken pulse. In some cases, there is dizziness on arising in the morning that quickly abates. MED Warm and supplement yang qi with Ginseng and Aconite Decoction (*shēn fù tāng*). ACU Base treatment mainly on GV and CV. Select GV-20 (*bǎi huì*, Hundred Convergences), GV-24 (*shén tíng*, Spirit Court), CV-6 (*qì hǎi*, Sea of Qi), CV-4 (*guān yuán*, Pass Head), and GV-4 (*mìng mén*, Life Gate); needle with supplementation and large amounts of moxa. Selection of points according to signs: For shortness of breath, add BL-13 (*fèi shū*, Lung Transport), BL-43 (*gāo huāng shū*, Gao-Huang Transport), and LU-9 (*tài yuān*, Great Abyss). For spontaneous sweating, add LI-4 (*hé gǔ*, Union Valley), and SI-3 (*hòu xī*, Back Ravine). [26: 715] [46: 602, 688]

yang vacuity headache 阳虚头痛 *yáng xū tóu tòng*: HEADACHE attributable to insufficiency of yang qi that fails to bear upward to the head. Yang vacuity headache is a dull headache accompanied aversion to light, fear of cold and cold limbs, fatigue and lack of strength, poor appetite, pale tongue, and a pulse that is faint or fine or sunken and slow or large, vacuous, and forceless. MED Supplement qi and support yang using Aconite Center-Rectifying Decoction (*fù zǐ lǐ zhōng tāng*), Ligusticum (Cnidium Root) and Atractylodes Decoction (*xiōng zhú tāng*), or Center-Supplementing Qi-Boosting Decoction (*bǔ zhōng yì qì tāng*). ACU Base treatment mainly on CV, GV, and ST. Select GV-20 (*bǎi huì*, Hundred Convergences), CV-6 (*qì hǎi*, Sea of Qi), CV-4 (*guān yuán*, Pass Head), GV-4 (*mìng mén*, Life Gate), ST-36 (*zú sān lǐ*, Leg Three Li), and BL-20 (*pí shū*, Spleen Transport); needle with supplementation and add moxa. For selection of points according to affected area, see HEADACHE. [26: 716]

yang vacuity heat effusion 阳虚发热 *yáng xū fā rè*: Vacuity heat due to debilitation of yang qi (debilitation of kidney yang or spleen-stomach qi vacuity). **Debilitation of kidney yang:** *Jing-Yue's Complete Compendium* (*jǐng yuè quán shū*) states, "In yang vacuity, too, there may be heat effusion. This is due to exhaustion of original yang and fire not returning to its source." It is characterized by heat effusion with vexation and agitation, pale red cheeks, thirst with desire but inability to drink, counterflow cold of the feet, clear white urine (lack of color), clear-food diarrhea, and a pulse that is sunken and fine or floating, rapid, and forceful, that feels about to dissipate when pressure is applied. MED Supplement the kidney and warm yang; return fire to its source. Use Cinnamon Bark and Aconite Eight-Ingredient Pill (*guì fù bā wèi wán*). **Spleen-stomach qi vacuity** arises from taxation fatigue and internal damage. Qi is yang, so qi vacuity heat effusion is a form of yang vacuity heat effusion. MED Supplement the center and boost yang qi. Use Center-Supplementing Qi-Boosting Decoction (*bǔ zhōng yì qì tāng*). [26: 715] [50: 650]

yang vacuity spontaneous sweating 阳虚自汗 *yáng xū zì hàn*: SPONTANEOUS SWEATING that arises in yang vacuity when the exterior becomes loose and the interstices become unsound, allowing sweat to be easily discharged. Accompanying signs include fear of cold, sweating associated with sensation of cold, fatigue, and a fine pulse. MED Warm yang and secure the exterior. Use Jade Wind-Barrier Powder (*yù píng fēng sǎn*) or Astragalus and Aconite Decoction (*qí fù tāng*). ACU Base treatment mainly on LU, CV, ST, LI, HT, and SI. Select LI-4 (*hé gǔ*, Union Valley), HT-6 (*yīn xī*, Yin Cleft), SI-3 (*hòu xī*, Back

Ravine), GV-20 (*bǎi huì*, Hundred Convergences), LU-9 (*tài yuān*, Great Abyss), LI-4 (*hé gǔ*, Union Valley), CV-6 (*qì hǎi*, Sea of Qi), and ST-36 (*zú sān lǐ*, Leg Three Li); needle with supplementation and add moxa. [26: 715] [46: 602] [14: 174]

yang vacuity water flood 阳虚水泛 *yáng xū shuǐ fàn*: WATER SWELLING or PHLEGM-RHEUM arising when spleen-kidney yang vacuity, especially kidney yang (life gate fire) vacuity fails in its warming and moving function and causes water to accumulate. *Indispensable Medical Reading* (*yī zōng bì dú*) states, "Although water is controlled by the spleen, in actual fact it is ruled by the kidney, which is the water viscus and the seat of original yang, the life gate. When the life gate fire is debilitated, it fails to restrain yin and to warm and nourish spleen-earth; yin is not subservient to yang, so that essence transforms into water. Hence most water swelling patterns can be ascribed to debilitation of fire." WMC edema in chronic nephritis, cardiac edema. MED For kidney yang vacuity, use Golden Coffer Kidney Qi Pill (*jīn guì shèn qì wán*). For spleen-kidney yang vacuity, combine the same formula with Spleen-Firming Beverage (*shí pí yǐn*). ACU Base treatment mainly on CV, back transport points, SP, and ST. Select CV-9 (*shuǐ fēn*, Water Divide), CV-6 (*qì hǎi*, Sea of Qi), ST-36 (*zú sān lǐ*, Leg Three Li), SP-6 (*sān yīn jiāo*, Three Yin Intersection), SP-9 (*yīn líng quán*, Yin Mound Spring), and BL-39 (*wěi yáng*, Bend Yang); needle with supplementation and add moxa. For kidney yang vacuity, add BL-23 (*shèn shū*, Kidney Transport), GV-4 (*mìng mén*, Life Gate), KI-7 (*fù liū*, Recover Flow), and KI-3 (*tài xī*, Great Ravine). For spleen yang vacuity, add CV-12 (*zhōng wǎn*, Center Stomach Duct), BL-20 (*pí shū*, Spleen Transport), and SP-4 (*gōng sūn*, Yellow Emperor). See KIDNEY VACUITY WATER FLOOD. [26: 715] [113: 184] [27: 127] [97: 241] [46: 676]

yang vacuity with yin exuberance 阳虚阴盛 *yáng xū yīn shèng*: Yang vacuity depriving the bowels and viscera of warmth and causing exuberant yin cold signs such as physical cold, cold limbs, phlegm-rheum, water swelling, and diarrhea. [26: 715]

yang water 阳水 *yáng shuǐ*: From *Dan Xi's Experiential Methods* (*dān xī xīn fǎ*). WATER SWELLING arising when water-damp and externally-contracted wind-cold cause nondiffusion of lung qi and triple burner congestion that prevents the free flow of water down to the bladder. Yang water is a repletion pattern characterized by swelling of the face first, and is attended by aversion to cold, heat effusion, cough, sore throat, rough voidings of red urine, constipation, abdominal fullness, and a slimy tongue fur, and rapid

pulse. MED Course wind, diffuse the lung, clear heat, and disinhibit water. Spleen-Effusing Decoction (*yuè bì tāng*). Add to this formula perilla seed (*zǐ sū zǐ*) and ledebouriella (*fáng fēng*) to course wind; duckweed (*fú píng*) and apricot kernel (*xìng rén*) to diffuse the lung; forsythia (*lián qiào*), platycodon (*jié gěng*), and fresh imperata (*xiān máo gēn*) to clear heat; and poria (*fú líng*) and alisma (*zé xiè*) to disinhibit water. ACU Base treatment mainly on CV, back transport points, ST and LI. Select CV-9 (*shuǐ fēn*, Water Divide), CV-6 (*qì hǎi*, Sea of Qi), BL-22 (*sān jiāo shū*, Triple Burner Transport), ST-36 (*zú sān lǐ*, Leg Three Li), BL-11 (*dà zhù*, Great Shuttle), BL-13 (*fèi shū*, Lung Transport), LI-4 (*hé gǔ*, Union Valley), GV-26 (*shuǐ gōu*, Water Trough), and LI-6 (*piān lì*, Veering Passageway); needle with drainage. Selection of points according to signs: For heat effusion and aversion to cold, add LI-11 (*qū chí*, Pool at the Bend), TB-5 (*wài guān*, Outer Pass), and GV-14 (*dà zhuī*, Great Hammer). For cough and sore pharynx, add LU-7 (*liè quē*, Broken Sequence), LU-5 (*chǐ zé*, Cubit Marsh), and KI-6 (*zhào hǎi*, Shining Sea), and prick LU-11 (*shào shāng*, Lesser Shang) to bleed. For swelling of the head and face, add GV-21 (*qián dǐng*, Before the Vertex). For constipation, add ST-25 (*tiān shū*, Celestial Pivot) and TB-6 (*zhī gōu*, Branch Ditch). For oppression and vexation in the chest, add PC-6 (*nèi guān*, Inner Pass) and KI-6 (*zhào hǎi*, Shining Sea). For abdominal fullness, add PC-6 (*nèi guān*, Inner Pass) and ST-25 (*tiān shū*, Celestial Pivot). See WATER. [26: 712] [27: 419] [97: 237] [80: 509] [46: 676] [113: 184]

yang wilt 阳萎 *yáng wěi*, 阳痿 *yáng wěi*: IMPOTENCE.

yang within yang 阳中之阳 *yáng zhōng zhī yáng*: The yang part of a yang phenomenon (i.e., an aspect of a yang phenomenon that is more yang than another aspect of the same phenomenon). For example, *Elementary Questions* (*sù wèn, jīn guì zhēn yán lùn*) states, "Calm dawn to midday is in the yang [part] of the day, and is the yang within yang." The morning falls in the daytime (yang) part of the day as opposed to nighttime (yin), and since during this period the sun grows stronger and higher, this is the yang part of the daytime, as opposed to the afternoon, which is the yin part of the daytime; hence the morning is an example of yang within yang. Compare YIN AND YANG ARE DIVISIBLE BUT INSEPARABLE. [26: 712] [27: 31] [97: 239]

yang within yin 阴中之阳 *yīn zhōng zhī yáng*: The yang aspect of a yin phenomenon. According to the principle that yin and yang are divisible but inseparable, all yang phenomena can be divided into yin and yang components, as can all yin phenomena. For instance, chest and abdomen are yin as opposed to the back, which is yang. However, the chest (upper part) is yang, whereas the abdomen (lower part) is yin. The chest is therefore the yang within yin. Compare YIN AND YANG ARE DIVISIBLE BUT INSEPARABLE. [26: 616] [27: 31] [97: 239]

yang vessel 阳脉 *yáng mài*: YANG CHANNEL.

YAS 阳跷（跷）脉 *yáng qiāo (qiāo) mài*: Abbreviation for the YANG SPRINGING VESSEL.

yawning 欠 *qiàn*, 呼欠 *hū qiàn*, 呵欠 *hē qiàn*, 欠伸 *qiàn shēn*, 失欠 *shī qiàn*: Noisy expulsion of breath after a short sharp inhalation associated with stretching; a sign of fatigue. Frequent yawning can be a sign of qi vacuity and yang debility, and in particular depletion of kidney qi. [26: 166]

yellow 黄 *huáng*: The color associated with earth in the five phases. The Chinese 黄 *huáng* includes shades is broader in meaning than the English 'yellow', including brown. See, for example, YELLOW OF THE EYE; YELLOW URINE.

yellow face 面黄 *miàn huáng*: YELLOW FACIAL COMPLEXION.

yellow facial complexion 面色黄 *miàn sè huáng*: *Synonym: yellow face.* A sign of dampness or vacuity. Yellowing of the sclerae and generalized yellowing of the skin indicate jaundice. Jaundice characterized by a vivid yellow (often described as the color of tangerines) indicates damp-heat and is called "yang yellow." Jaundice characterized by a dark yellow coloration is caused by cold-damp and is called "yin yellow." Yang yellow is seen mostly in cases described in Western medicine as acute icteric infectious hepatitis, acute cholecystitis, cholelithiasis, and toxic hepatitis; yin yellow occurs in cirrhosis of the liver and cancer of the head of the pancreas. A pale yellow skin that is dry and puffy, accompanied by pale lips but no yellowing of the sclerae, is referred to as withered-yellow, which is a vacuity yellow. The condition characterized by this complexion is sometimes called YELLOW SWELLING, and is normally caused by excessive loss of blood or depletion of blood and qi after major illnesses or by spleen-stomach damage resulting from intestinal parasites. It may thus be seen in diseases known in Western medicine as ankylostomiasis (hookworm infestation), anemia, and malnutrition due to poor assimilation. [6: 117]

yellow fat obstruction 黄油障 *huáng yóu zhàng*: YELLOW FAT PATTERN.

yellow fat pattern 黄油证 *huáng yóu zhèng*: *Synonym: yellow eye obstruction.* An eye disease that is attributed to damp-heat and in which the qi wheel appears to be filled with soft pale yellow fat. There is no pain, swelling, or blurring of vision; hence patients often do not seek treatment. It only occurs in old age. [26: 695]

yellowing 发黄 *fā huáng*: Yellowing of the skin and sometimes the white of the eye. See JAUNDICE.

yellowing of the eyes 目黄 *mù huáng*: Yellowing of the white of the eye (sclera), indicating jaundice.

yellow obesity 黄胖 *huáng pàng*: YELLOW SWELLING.

yellow of the eye 黄仁 *huáng rén*: The iris. So called because Chinese people's eyes are brown (see *yellow*). Also called *wind wheel*. [27: 65] [97: 503]

yellow sweat 黄汗 *huáng hàn*: From *Essential Prescriptions of the Golden Coffer* (*jīn guì yào lüè, shuǐ qì bìng mài zhèng bìng zhì*). A disease usually arising when immersion in water while sweating causes obstruction of construction and defense, or when depressed latent spleen-stomach damp-heat swelters the skin. It is characterized by yellow-colored watery sweat that stains clothing the color of the juice from boiled phellodendron (*huáng bǎi*), limpness of the lumbus and hip, heavy body, inhibited urination, and slow sunken pulse. Yellow sweat is attributed to the interaction of wind, water, dampness, and heat. When due to damp-heat damaging the blood aspect, there may also be sores. MED Harmonize construction and defense with formulas such as Cinnamon Twig Decoction Plus Astragalus (*guì zhī jiā huáng qí tāng*), or Astragalus, Peony, Cinnamon Twig, and Liquor Decoction (*qí sháo guì jiǔ tāng*) from *Essential Prescriptions of the Golden Coffer* (*jīn guì yào lüè*), which contains astragalus (*huáng qí*), peony (*sháo yào*), cinnamon twig (*guì zhī*), and liquor. NB: Yellow sweat was considered by Sun Si-Miao (581–682) in the Tang Dynasty to be a form of jaundice. Later medical books such as *The Level-Line of Pattern Identification and Treatment* (*zhèng zhì zhǔn shéng*) and *Pathoconditions, Causes, Pulses, and Treatments* (*zhèng yīn mài zhì*) treated yellow sweating with generalized swelling as water swelling and yellow sweating without generalized swelling as jaundice. [26: 695] [50: 1335] [27: 367] [97: 503] [80: 392] [49: 422]

yellow swelling 黄肿 *huáng zhǒng*: *Synonym: yellow obesity; strength desertion yellowing; food taxation gan yellowing.* Swelling of the face and ankles with a withered-yellow facial complexion, together with fatigued spirit and lack of strength. In some cases, it is associated with nausea and vomiting of yellow water, and a desire to eat uncooked rice, tea leaves, and coal. WMC hookworm infestation. [26: 697]

yellow tongue fur 黄苔 *huáng tāi*: A yellow fur usually signifies heat. Because heat patterns vary in severity and may involve different evils, different forms of yellow fur are distinguished. A thin dry yellow fur indicates damage to liquid by the heat evil, posing the need to safeguard liquid. A slimy yellow fur usually indicates damp-heat. An old yellow fur (dark yellow) and burnt yellow fur (blackish yellow) indicate binding of repletion heat. A mixed white and yellow fur indicates the initial stages of the transformation of cold into heat that occurs when evil passes into the interior. [26: 697] [6: 124]

yellow urine 尿黄 *niào huáng*: Urine a darker yellow than normal. See URINE.

yellow vaginal discharge 黄带 *huáng dài*: See LIVER CHANNEL DAMP-HEAT VAGINAL DISCHARGE; DAMP TOXIN VAGINAL DISCHARGE. [27: 445] [97: 503]

yellow-water sore 黄水疮 *huáng shuǐ chuāng*: A sore exuding yellow fluid. Yellow-water sores start with a red macule within which a millet-shaped vesicle develops that is painful and itchy. When the vesicle ruptures because of scratching, a yellow watery discharge escapes, after which the sore forms a scab and heals. It most commonly affects infants and children and occurs on the head, ears, and neck, easily spreading to other parts of the body. [WMC] impetigo herpetiformis. [MED] Dispel wind and overcome dampness; clear heat and cool the blood. Appropriate formulas include Cimicifuga Toxin-Dispersing Beverage (*shēng má xiāo dú yǐn*), and Scutellaria and Coptis Stomach-Clearing Decoction (*qín lián píng wèi tāng*). Indigo Powder (*qīng dài sǎn*) can be applied topically. [26: 694] [61: 398]

yellow wind 黄风 *huáng fēng*: **1.** HIGH-ALTITUDE WIND SPARROW-VISION INTERNAL OBSTRUCTION. **2.** YELLOW WIND INTERNAL OBSTRUCTION. [26: 696]

yellow wind internal obstruction 黄风内障 *huáng fēng nèi zhàng*: **Abbreviation:** yellow wind. A disease of the eye in which the pupil becomes enlarged and cloudy-turbid yellow. Yellow wind internal obstruction is a degeneration of GREEN WIND INTERNAL OBSTRUCTION that usually leads to blindness if treatment is unsuccessful. [26: 697]

YIL 阴维脉 *yīn wéi mài*: Abbreviation for the YIN LINKING VESSEL.

yin 阴 *yīn*: **1.** The dark, female, receptive principle that stands in complementary opposition to yang. **2.** Specifically the genitals or anus (the private, concealed parts of the body). For example, (二阴 *èr yīn*), "two yin," is a collective name for the genitals and anus, (阴头 *yīn tóu*), and "yin head," denotes the glans penis. [97: 229]

yin and yang 阴阳 *yīn yáng*: *Synonym:* *yin-yang*. Two mutually complementary and opposing principles in Chinese thought; one dark, female, receptive (yin), and the other bright, male, active (yang). The two principles categorize phenomena of like quality and relationship. The Chinese characters denoting yin and yang denote the dark side and light side of a mountain respectively, i.e., light and darkness. Many other phenomena are closely related to light and dark. For example, light is associated with heat, and darkness is associated with cold. Daytime is the warm, bright part of the day; nighttime is the cold, dark part of the day. Summer is the season of greatest light and heat; winter is the season of greatest darkness and cold. South is the position of greatest light and heat; north is the position of greatest darkness and cold. Daytime and summer are the times of activity; nighttime and winter are times of rest and quiescence. The upper and outer aspect of an object tends to receive sunlight; the inner and lower aspects of objects tend to be dark. Light (yang) is to darkness (yin) as heat is to cold, as day is to night, as summer is to winter, as north is to south, and as activity is to rest. Hence heat, daytime, summer, south, and activity are yang, while cold, night, winter, north, quiescence are yin.

18.	Yin-Yang in General Phenomena	
Phenomenon	Yang	Yin
Space	Heaven	Earth
Time	Day	Night
Season	Spring Summer	Autumn Winter
Sex	Male	Female
Temperature	Hot	Cold
Weight	Light	Heavy
Brightness	Light	Dark
Motion	Upward, outward	Downward, inward
	Evident motion	Relative stasis

YIN AND YANG ARE ROOTED IN EACH OTHER; they are interdependent. Light cannot exist without darkness, just as heat cannot exist without cold. Furthermore, an ebb and flow relationship is observed between many yin-yang phenomena. For example, as light increases, darkness wanes, and as heat increases, cold disappears. In addition, YIN AND YANG COUNTERBALANCE EACH OTHER. Cold can counteract heat, and heat can overcome cold. (NB: Here it is important to understand that while in Western thought, cold is defined as the absence of heat, and darkness as the absence of light, in Chinese thought, both members of each pair are equally "real" and therefore have the power to constrain each other.) Another important notion is that YIN AND YANG ARE DIVISIBLE BUT INSEPARABLE. Each yang phenomenon can (theoretically) be divided into yin and yang aspects. For example, light is yang in relation to darkness, which is yin. However, the sun is yang, whereas the moon is yin. Movement is yang in relation to quiescence, which is yin. Yet upward and outward movement is yang, whereas downward and inward movement is yin. Expansion is yang, while contraction is yin. Therefore, yin and yang are not fixed categories but relative ones. The basic concepts of yin and yang come into many aspects of Chinese medicine. This section explains concisely the application of the doctrine of yin and yang in the realm of physiology, pathology, diagnosis and treatment. **Structure of the body**: Chinese medicine sees the human body as a whole, the component parts of which may all be analyzed in terms of yin and yang. For an overview, see Table 19. For instance, the upper part of the body is yang and the lower part is yin; the exterior of the body is yang by contrast to the interior, which is yin. The surface of the body may be further divided, the abdominal surface being yin, and the back being yang. As to the organs, the viscera (liver, heart, spleen, lung, and kidney) are yin, and the bowels (the gallbladder, stomach, intestines, bladder, and triple burner) are yang. Each of the organs itself has a yin and a yang aspect: there is heart yin and heart yang, kidney yin and kidney yang. The two primary elements of the human body, blood and qi, may also be thus categorized, blood being yin and qi being yang. As to the channels, those passing over the back and the outer face of the limbs are yang, while those running through the surface of the abdomen and the inner face of the limbs are yin.

19. Yin-Yang in the Human Body	
Yang	Yin
Exterior, back	Interior, abdomen
Bowels Skin, body hair Qi and defense Agitation Strength	Viscera Bone, sinew Blood and construction Calm Weakness

Physiological functions: Yin and yang provide a general method of analyzing the functions of the human body. These are seen in terms of upbearing, downbearing, inward, and outward movement. Upbearing and outward movement are yang, while downbearing and inward are yin. These movements serve to explain the interactions between blood and qi, and the organs and channels. Physiological processes are explained in terms of the waxing and waning yin and yang. "Clear yang issues from the upper orifices, while turbid yin issues from the lower orifices; clear yang effuses [issues] through the interstices, while turbid yin

goes through [enters] the five viscera; clear yang fills the limbs, whereas turbid yin passes through the six bowels." That is to say, yang, the clear light qi of the body, ascends up to and out of the clear orifices, passing outward to the surface of the skin and strengthening the limbs, and how yin, the heavy turbid qi of the body, flows in the interior, its waste products being discharged through the anus and the urethra. The four movements are considered to be interdependent and mutually supporting. Thus *Elementary Questions* (*sù wèn, yīn yáng yìng xiàng dà lùn*) states, "Yin is in the inner body and protects yang; yang is in the outer body and moves yin." **Pathology:** In medicine, morbidity is explained in terms of yin-yang imbalance. Both evil and right qi can be analyzed in terms of yin and yang. There are both yin and yang evils. Yin evils cause a surfeit of yin, which manifests as a cold pattern; yang evils produce a surfeit of yang in the body characterized by repletion heat patterns. The "right," the body's health-maintaining forces, comprise two aspects, yang qi and yin humor. Yang qi vacuity is characterized by vacuity cold patterns, whereas yin humor vacuity is characterized by vacuity heat. A vast number of diseases can be summed up in the following four phrases: "When yin prevails, there is cold; when yang prevails, there is heat. When yang is vacuous, there is cold; when yin is vacuous, there is heat." The cause of these conditions is imbalance—surfeits or deficits—of either yin or yang. **Diagnosis:** Imbalance of yin and yang accounts for the emergence and development of disease. The essential nature of any disease may be analyzed in terms of yin and yang, despite the infinite number of possible clinical manifestations. Yin and yang form the basic principles of eight-principle pattern identification: exterior, heat, and repletion diseases being yang; interior, cold, and vacuity diseases being yin. *Elementary Questions* (*sù wèn*) states, "Proper diagnosis involves inspecting the appearance and feeling the pulse and first differentiating yin and yang." See Table 20.

20. Yin-Yang in Patterns & Pulses		
	Yang	Yin
Pattern	Exterior Repletion	Interior Vacuity
Pulse	Rapid Floating Slippery Replete Large & surging	Slow Deep Rough Vacuous Fine

Treatment: Because a surfeit of yin or yang is the primary cause of any disease, treatment must involve restoring the balance by reducing superabundance and supplying insufficiency. The nature and effect of medicinals may also be classified according to yin and yang. For example, cold, cool, rich, and moist medicinals are yin, whereas warm, hot, dry, and fierce medicinals are yang. Medicinals that are acrid and sweet in flavor are yang, while those that are salty, bitter, sour, or astringent in flavor are yin. Medicinals whose qi and flavor are bland and mild are yang, and those whose qi and flavor are strong are yin. Medicinals that upbear and effuse are yang in nature, and medicinals that contract and astringe are yin. Therefore, in diagnosis and treatment, it is necessary to identify yin-yang surfeits and deficits among the complex array of signs and determine the nature of the treatment. Medicinals must also be selected and used to make an appropriate combination of their yin and yang qualities. This means that a pattern due to a surfeit of yin or yang is one of repletion, and according to the principle of reducing superabundance, it is treated by the method of drainage. A pattern that is essentially the result of a deficit of either yin or yang is one of vacuity, and in accordance with the principle of supplying insufficiency, is treated by the method of supplementation. If yin is in surfeit, the problem is one of repletion cold, for which warm acrid yang medicinals should be used to dissipate the cold. If yang is in surfeit, the pattern is one of repletion-heat, requiring cold bitter heat-draining medicinals, which are yin in nature. If the pattern stems from an insufficiency of yin, yin-supplementing medicinals with a cooling and moistening effect are prescribed to nourish blood and fluids. Conditions stemming from a yang deficit manifest themselves as vacuity-cold, and are treated with yang medicinals, warm or hot medicinals, to warm and supplement yang qi. [26: 65] [27: 1] [97: 229] [6: 21]

yin and yang are divisible but inseparable 阴阳可分而不可离 *yīn yáng kě fēn ér bù kě lí*: The principle that although all phenomena can be divided into yin and yang, and each yin or yang phenomenon can be divided into yin and yang aspects, either phenomena of a pair that stands in a mutually dependent yin-yang relationship cannot be separated from the other without the loss of both. "Division" here means a cognitive distinction, whereas "separation" is the actual parting of the two. Yin and yang can be divided ad infinitum. For example, whereas motion is yang and stasis is yin, within motion there is a distinction between upward motion, which is yang, and downward motion, which is yin. Upward motion is yang within yang, whereas downward motion is yin within yang. However, though yin and yang can be differentiated in this way, they cannot be separated: the two are always interdependent and

therefore inseparable; one cannot exist without the other. [6: 23]

yin and yang are interdependent 阴阳相互依存 *yīn yáng xiāng hù yī cún*: See YIN AND YANG ARE ROOTED IN EACH OTHER.

yin and yang are rooted in each other 阴阳互根 *yīn yáng hù gēn*: Yin and yang are mutually dependent. "Yin is rooted in yang and yang is rooted in yin." The notion of interdependence means that neither phenomenon of a yin-yang pair can exist without the other. Yin exists by virtue of yang, and yang exists by virtue of yin. Light (yang) cannot exist without darkness (yin), and darkness cannot exist without light. Similarly, activity (yang) cannot exist without rest (yin). (**NB**: In modern Western thought, darkness and rest are defined by the absence of their opposites; in Chinese thought, both darkness and light, rest and activity are considered equally "real.") In medicine, the concept of interdependence of yin and yang is widely used in physiology, pathology, and treatment. Blood and qi, two fundamental elements of the human body, provide an example: blood is yin and qi is yang. It is said that "qi engenders blood," i.e., blood formation relies on the power of qi to move and transform food; "qi moves the blood," meaning that blood circulation relies on the warming and driving power of qi. Furthermore, "qi contains the blood," i.e., it keeps the blood within the vessels. The functions of engendering, moving, and containing the blood are summed up in the phrase, "qi is the commander of the blood." Conversely, qi is dependent on the provision of adequate nutrition by the blood; thus it is said that "qi has its abode in the blood," and "blood is the mother of qi." Because qi has the power to engender blood, treatment of blood vacuity involves dual supplementation of qi and blood. Massive bleeding, where qi deserts with the blood, is first treated by boosting qi, since blood-nourishing formulas should not be administered until qi is secured. Similarly, formulas used to treat qi vacuity often include blood-nourishing medicinals to enhance qi supplementation. Another example of the interdependence of yin and yang, seen in the development of diseases, is the principle that "detriment to yin affects yang" and "detriment to yang affects yin." Since "without yang, yin cannot be born," when yang vacuity reaches a certain point, the production of yin humor is affected, and yin also becomes vacuous. Most cases of what Western medicine calls chronic nephritis indicate yang vacuity, and are characterized by water swelling due to the inability of the kidney to transform fluids. However, when the yang vacuity reaches a certain point, fluid formation is affected and a yin vacuity pattern evolves. This demonstrates the principle that "detriment to yang affects yin." Similarly, yin vacuity, when reaching a certain peak, lead to simultaneous yang vacuity, since "without yin, yang cannot arise." What is termed hypertension in Western medicine usually corresponds to hyperactivity of yang caused by vacuity of yin. In severe cases, this condition may develop into a dual yin-yang vacuity, illustrating the principle that "detriment to yin affects yang." [6: 23] [27: 3] [97: 234]

yin and yang counterbalance each other 阴阳制约 *yīn yáng zhì yuē*: Yin and yang both prevent their complement from becoming disproportionately strong. When either pole weakens, the other may grow stronger. Thus in the body, when yin humor is depleted, yang qi appears relatively stronger, and manifests in the form of heat (vacuity heat). In the body, yin and yang counterbalance each other. A deficit of one naturally leads to a surfeit of the other, while a surfeit of one will weaken the other. In both cases, yin and yang no longer counterbalance each other, and disease arises as a result. In medicine, the notion of counterbalancing is widely applied in physiology, pathology, and therapy. In physiology, for example, liver yin counterbalances liver yang, preventing it from becoming too strong. If liver yin becomes insufficient and fails to counterbalance its complement, ascendant hyperactivity of liver yang develops. In the relationship of evils and the human body, yang evils invading the body will cause a surfeit of yang, which may lead to damage to yin humor and the emergence of a heat pattern. Conversely, a yin evil entering the body will lead to a surfeit of yin, causing damage to the body's yang qi and the emergence of a cold pattern. These processes are described in *Elementary Questions (sù wèn)* in the following way: "If yang abounds yin ails, and if yin abounds, yang ails; when yang prevails there is heat, and when yin prevails there is cold." In therapy, if a disease is caused by heat evil, it is treated with cool or cold medicinals according to the principle that "cold can counteract heat," meaning yin medicinals combat yang evils. Similarly, diseases caused by cold evil are treated with warm or hot medicinals, since "heat can overcome cold," i.e., yang medicinals can combat yin evils. This is summed up in a guiding principle of therapy, "heat is treated with cold; cold is treated with heat." It is most often applied in patterns of repletion characterized by a surfeit of either yin or yang. In conditions caused by deficit of yin or yang, the opposing complement is no longer kept in check and becomes disproportionately strong. If yin is vacuous, yang is no longer kept in check and its strength will grow out of proportion to that of yin. Such a condition is at root a yin vacuity, manifesting itself as vacuity heat. For this reason, treatment by draining fire and clearing heat alone

is not only ineffective but also detrimental to the patient's health. It is replaced by a method such as enriching yin and downbearing fire, or fostering yin and subduing yang, whereby clearing heat and draining fire are secondary to enriching yin. By supplementing yin, the yang surfeit will naturally diminish. This explains the principle "invigorate the governor of water to restrain the brilliance of yang." In the reverse situation, where yang is vacuous and fails to keep yin in check, there is exuberant internal yin cold, manifesting in such forms as clear-food diarrhea, fifth-watch diarrhea, and water swelling. Here, treatment should aim not simply at dissipating cold evil, but also at supplying the yang vacuity through such methods as assisting yang, boosting fire, and supplementing qi. This demonstrates the principle that "where warming is to no avail, fire is lacking" and "boost the source of fire to disperse the shroud of yin." It is important to note the difference between the natural ebb and flow of yin and yang and a surfeit of one or the other complement. WAXING AND WANING OF YIN AND YANG refers to their normal relationship in the human body, which is one of constant fluctuation, rather than a rigid, immutable balance. "When yin rises, yang ebbs," and "when yang swells, yin subsides." This constant fluctuation is apparent in all the body's functions, such as fluid production and metabolism, the role of the five viscera in storing essential qi, and the role of the six bowels in conveyance and transformation of food. By contrast, "deficit" and "surfeit" denote the disturbance of the normal relative balance and failure to rectify the imbalance immediately. This is known as imbalance of yin and yang, which is the underlying cause of all disease. [6: 24]

yin beating differently from yang 阴搏阳别 *yīn bó yáng bié*: A pulse description. *Elementary Questions (sù wèn)* states, "yin beating differently from yang means there is a child." There are two interpretations (1) According to Wang Bing of the Tang Dynasty, "yin" refers to the cubit pulse (*chǐ*); "yang" refers to the inch pulse (*cùn*). When the inch pulse beats more markedly than the cubit, this is called "yin contending differently from yang." (2) According to Zhang Jie-Bin of the Ming Dynasty, "yin" means the hand lesser yin or foot lesser yin: "The heart governs the blood and the kidney governs the uterus, so both these viscera are related to the fetus and pregnancy. 'Beating' means beating against the fingers. 'Differently from yang' means that the yin pulse beats against the fingers like yang evil, but it is slippery and uninhibited, so is not a pulse caused by evil. Here we see yang in yin, with signs of harmony. This is what is meant by yang beating differently from yin." [27: 201] [93: 577]

yin bind 阴结 *yīn jié*: **1.** Constipation attributed to spleen-kidney vacuity cold and characterized by the absence of bowel movements for many days despite desire to defecate, yet with the absence of fullness or distention. Yin bind is associated with a weak state of health, lack of warmth in the extremities, long voidings of clear urine, pale tongue with a thin white tongue fur, and a slow sunken pulse. See COLD CONSTIPATION. **2.** VACUITY CONSTIPATION. [26: 623] [27: 412] [97: 233]

yin-blood 阴血 *yīn xuè*: **1.** Blood considered as yin. **2.** Yin and blood as a combined entity. See YIN; BLOOD. [50: 653] [36: 287]

yin-blood depletion 阴血亏虚 *yīn xuè kuī xū*: Insufficiency of the blood or insufficiency yin and the blood. See YIN VACUITY; BLOOD VACUITY.

yin bulging 阴癀 *yīn tuí*: **1.** YIN PROTRUSION. **2.** MORBID PROMINENCE. [27: 454] [97: 233]

yin channel 阴经 *yīn jīng*: Synonym: *yin vessel*. Any of the three of the six channels labeled as yin, i.e., the greater yin (*tài yīn*), lesser yin (*shào yīn*), and reverting yin (*jué yīn*), as well as the controlling (*rèn*), thoroughfare (*chōng*), yin linking (*yīn wéi*), and yin springing (*yīn qiāo*) vessels. [27: 86]

¹**yin cold** 阴寒 *yīn hán*: Synonym: ²*yin cold*.² Cold seen as a yin phenomenon.

²**yin cold** 阴冷 *yīn lěng*: **1.** GENITAL COLD. **2.** ¹YIN COLD. [26: 617]

yin collapse 亡阴 *wáng yīn*: Synonyms: *yin desertion*; *fulminant desertion of yin humor*. A critical pattern of wearing of yin-blood. The chief signs are copious sweat, palpably hot skin, and warm limbs or reversal cold of the limbs with heat in the hearts of soles and palms. There is agitation or, in severe cases, clouded spirit. There is thirst with desire for cool fluids. Breathing is short and hasty with difficulty catching the breath. The tongue is dry and red, whereas the pulse is weak and rapid. MED Enrich yin and increase humor; nourish liquid and secure qi. Use large quantities of Pulse-Engendering Powder (*shēng mài sǎn*). Cornus (*shān zhū yú*), scutellaria (*huáng qín*), calcined dragon bone (*duàn lóng gǔ*), and calcined oyster shell (*duàn mǔ lì*) can also be used. ACU Base treatment mainly on CV and GV. Select GV-26 (*shuǐ gōu*, Water Trough), GV-25 (*sù liáo*, White Bone-Hole), PC-6 (*nèi guān*, Inner Pass), GV-20 (*bǎi huì*, Hundred Convergences), CV-4 (*guān yuán*, Pass Head), ST-36 (*zú sān lǐ*, Leg Three Li), and KI-1 (*yǒng quán*, Gushing Spring); needle with supplementation or direct moxa. Apply moxa on salt or ginger at CV-8 (*shén què*, Spirit Gate Tower). [26: 27] [27: 206] [97: 33] [57: 28]

yin-collapse vacuity desertion 亡阴虚脱 *wáng yīn xū tuō*: See YIN COLLAPSE. [46: 730]

yin desertion 阴脱 *yīn tuō*: **1.** PROLAPSE OF THE UTERUS. **2.** Failure of the yin door to close attributable to damage in childbirth or to physical strain. In some cases, there is painful swelling and difficult urination. MED Supplement qi and the blood with Perfect Major Supplementation Decoction (*shí quán dà bǔ tāng*). Cnidium seed (*shé chuáng zǐ*) and sumac gallnut (*wǔ bèi zǐ*) can be decocted as a steam-wash. **3.** Yin collapse. [26: 621] [27: 454] [97: 233] [29: 588]

yin disease 阴病 *yīn bìng*: **1.** TRIPLE-YIN DISEASE. **2.** Any disease manifesting as a vacuity pattern or cold pattern. [27: 348]

yin disease is treated through yang 阴病治阳 *yīn bìng zhì yáng* When exuberant yin cold damage yang qi, it should be treated by supporting yang. For example, water swelling with pale tongue and lips, low timid voice, lack of warmth in the extremities, inhibited urination or long voidings of clear urine, sloppy stool, and a deep slow pulse, can be treated by warming yang and fortifying the spleen and by moving qi and disinhibiting water, using Spleen-Firming Beverage (*shí pí yǐn*). **1.** Disease affecting a yin channel and be treated by needling points on yang channels. For example, for a hand greater yin *tài yīn* lung channel pattern of common cold and cough , points such as BL-11 (*dà zhù*, Great Shuttle) and BL-12 (*fēng mén*, Wind Gate) can be chosen. See PRINCIPLE OF TREATMENT. [26: 618] [27: 130] [97: 522]

yin door 阴户 *yīn hù*: Synonym: *yin gates*; *jade gates*; *jade door*; *birth gate*¹. The mouth of the vagina. WMC orificium vaginae. Compare BIRTH GATE. See POSTPARTUM FAILURE OF THE JADE DOOR TO HEAL; NONCLOSURE OF THE BIRTH GATE. [27: 69] [97: 229]

yin epilepsy 阴痫 *yīn xián*: EPILEPSY in which episodes are characterized by cold limbs, absence of shrieking, absence of convulsions, and a sunken pulse. Yin epilepsy develops when frequent episodes of yang epilepsy weaken the health, or when excessive precipitation causes damage to original qi. MED Supplement center qi, moisten dryness, and transform phlegm with Six Gentlemen Decoction (*liù jūn zǐ tāng*) plus dragon bone (*lóng gǔ*), oyster shell (*mǔ lì*), bupleurum (*chái hú*), cimicifuga (*shēng má*), bitter orange (*zhǐ ké*), bamboo shavings (*zhú rú*), acorus (*shí chāng pú*), polygala (*yuǎn zhì*), white peony (*bái sháo yào*), and schisandra (*wǔ wèi zǐ*). ACU See root-securing right-supporting treatments for remission periods (time between fits) under EPILEPSY. In addition, needle with supplementation and moxa at CV-12 (*zhōng wǎn*, Center Stomach Duct), CV-6 (*qì hǎi*, Sea of Qi), CV-4 (*guān yuán*, Pass Head), SP-6 (*sān yīn jiāo*, Three Yin Intersection), KI-2 (*rán gǔ*, Blazing Valley), and ST-36 (*zú sān lǐ*, Leg Three Li). [26: 624] [27: 69] [97: 229]

yin evil 阴邪 *yīn xié*: **1.** Any EVIL that is yin in nature, e.g., cold, dampness, phlegm. **2.** EVIL QI invading a yin channel. [27: 110] [97: 229]

yin exuberance with yang debilitation 阴盛阳衰 *yīn shèng yáng shuāi*: Exuberant yin cold with resulting debilitation of yang qi. In practice, this generally refers to water-damp damaging yang or to excessive use of cold or cool medicinals. [27: 127] [27: 127]

yin exuberance with yang vacuity 阴盛阳虚 *yīn shèng yáng xū*: Exuberant internal yin cold with resulting debilitation of yang qi characterized by signs such as aversion to cold, cold limbs, diarrhea, water swelling, and pale glossy tongue. A pulse that is small at the superficial level and replete and large at the deep level reflects the yang vacuity and yin cold respectively. [26: 619]

yin fire 阴火 *yīn huǒ*: **1.** Fire engendered by diet, taxation fatigue, or joy, anger, anxiety, and thought. **2.** Heart fire. [26: 616] [50: 652]

yin flat-abscess 阴疽 *yīn jū*: **1.** A FLAT-ABSCESS (*jū*) characterized by yin cold signs. **2.** A genital sore. [97: 231]

yin head 阴头 *yīn tóu*: Synonym: *glans penis*; *balanus*; *tortoise's head*. The cap-shaped expansion that forms the head of the penis.

yin head welling-abscess 阴头痈 *yīn tóu yōng*: TORTOISE'S HEAD WELLING-ABSCESS. [26: 624]

yin humor 阴液 *yīn yè*: Essence, blood, liquid, and humor, viewed as yin-natured entities in contrast to yang qi. [26: 619] [27: 77] [97: 232]

yin is engendered by yang 阴生于阳 *yīn shēng yú yáng*: According to the principle of yin-yang interdependence, if there is no yang, yin has not the wherewithal to arise. In the body, essence-blood and fluids rely on the transporting and constraining action of yang qi to perform their functions. [26: 617]

yin jaundice 阴黄 *yīn huáng*: JAUNDICE characterized by somber withered-yellow facial complexion, torpid stomach, abdominal distention, lassitude of spirit, lack of strength, dull rib-side pain, short voidings of scant urine, unsolid stool, pale tongue with slimy tongue fur, and a sunken slow fine pulse. When this is the result of cold-damp, it is characterized by reduced food intake, oppression in the stomach duct, or even abdominal distention. When due to spleen vacuity and blood depletion, additional signs include dry skin, heart palpitations, and shortness of breath. When due to accumulation of static blood, there is a painful concretion under the left rib-side, and spider nevi. Yin jaundice sometimes develops from yang jaundice. MED Cold-damp patterns are treated by warming the center, fortifying the spleen and transforming dampness with formulas such as Capillaris, Atractylodes, and Aconite Decoction (*yīn*

chén zhú fù tāng). Spleen vacuity and blood depletion is treated by fortifying the spleen and warming the center and by boosting qi and nourishing the blood, using formulas such as Astragalus Center-Fortifying Decoction (*huáng qí jiàn zhōng tāng*). Blood stasis accumulation is treated by quickening blood, transforming stasis and abating jaundice with Infradiaphragmatic Stasis-Expelling Decoction (*gé xià zhú yū tāng*). ACU Base treatment mainly on ST, SP, and back transport points. Select BL-20 (*pí shū*, Spleen Transport), BL-19 (*dǎn shū*, Gallbladder Transport), ST-36 (*zú sān lǐ*, Leg Three Li), SP-6 (*sān yīn jiāo*, Three Yin Intersection), and GB-34 (*yáng líng quán*, Yang Mound Spring); needle with supplementation and add moxa. Selection of points according to signs: For lassitude of spirit and lack of strength, add CV-4 (*guān yuán*, Pass Head), GV-4 (*mìng mén*, Life Gate), and CV-6 (*qì hǎi*, Sea of Qi). For abdominal distention, add LR-13 (*zhāng mén*, Camphorwood Gate) and SP-4 (*gōng sūn*, Yellow Emperor). For dull pain in the rib-side, add SP-6 (*sān yīn jiāo*, Three Yin Intersection) and CV-6 (*qì hǎi*, Sea of Qi). For sloppy diarrhea, add ST-25 (*tiān shū*, Celestial Pivot), and CV-4 (*guān yuán*, Pass Head). [26: 621] [106: 247] [46: 664] [27: 207] [80: 398]

yin lichen 阴癣 *yīn xiǎn*: LICHEN (*xiǎn*) of the anterior and posterior yin, i.e., the anus and genitals, and surrounding areas; attributed to wind-heat-damp invading the skin. It starts with papules or small vesicles that gradually spread to form clearly circumscribed patches that are covered with thin scales. WMC tinea cruris. MED Apply No.1 Lichen Medicinal Water (*yī hào xiǎn yào shuǐ*) or realgar (*xióng huáng*) (12 g) steeped in 100 ml old vinegar. ACU Base treatment mainly on BL, LI, SP, ST, and LR. Select a number of points from the following: BL-12 (*fēng mén*, Wind Gate), BL-18 (*gān shū*, Liver Transport), BL-40 (*wěi zhōng*, Bend Center), LI-11 (*qū chí*, Pool at the Bend), SP-9 (*yīn líng quán*, Yin Mound Spring), BL-20 (*pí shū*, Spleen Transport), SP-6 (*sān yīn jiāo*, Three Yin Intersection), ST-44 (*nèi tíng*, Inner Court), LR-2 (*xíng jiān*, Moving Between), and GB-34 (*yáng líng quán*, Yang Mound Spring); needle with drainage. [26: 626] [46: 597] [42: 155]

yin linking vessel 阴维脉 *yīn wéi mài*: One of the EIGHT EXTRAORDINARY VESSELS. **Abbreviation:** YIL.

yin macules 阴斑 *yīn bān*: Synonyms: *vacuity macules*; *yin-pattern macules*. MACULES occurring in vacuity cold patterns, arising when constitutional vacuity and deep-lying cold or inappropriate use of cold medicinals causes exuberant internal yin cold and causes rootless fire to spread to the exterior. Yin macules are pale red and indistinct, and in some cases occur in a small number on the chest only. They are accompanied by counterflow cold of the extremities, unpronounced thirst, clear-food diarrhea, and a faint sunken pulse. The tongue bears a glossy white fur or may be enlarged with a glossy black fur. [26: 621]

yin mounting 阴疝 *yīn shàn*: **1.** A MOUNTING disease characterized by acute pain of the testicles and genitals attributed to cold evil invading the liver channel. ⟨MED⟩ Warm and transform; move qi. Use Liver-Warming Brew (*nuǎn gān jiān*). ⟨ACU⟩ Base treatment mainly on LR, SP, and CV. Select CV-3 (*zhōng jí*, Central Pole), LR-8 (*qū quán*, Spring at the Bend), LR-2 (*xíng jiān*, Moving Between), LR-3 (*tài chōng*, Supreme Surge), KI-10 (*yīn gǔ*, Yin Valley), LR-1 (*dà dūn*, Large Pile), SP-6 (*sān yīn jiāo*, Three Yin Intersection), and KI-3 (*tài xī*, Great Ravine); needle with drainage and adding moxa. Alternatively, apply direct moxa at LR-3 (*tài chōng*, Supreme Surge) and LR-1 (*dà dūn*, Large Pile). **2.** A generic term for PROMINENT MOUNTING, COLD MOUNTING, and REVERSAL MOUNTING. [26: 618]

yin of the thigh 阴股 *yīn gǔ*, 股阴 *gǔ yīn*: The inside (yin side) of the thigh. *The Magic Pivot* (*líng shū, jīng mài*) states, "The liver foot reverting yin (*jué yīn*) vessel... ascends in the inner face of the back of the knee, follows the yin of the thigh [upward], and enters the [region of the pubic] hair. [25: 193]

yin organs 阴器 *yīn qì*: The external genitals. The yin organs are traversed by the foot reverting yin (*jué yīn*) liver channel, and their development and functioning is related to the strength and weakness of kidney qi. Diseases of the yin organs are often treated through the liver and kidney. [27: 26] [97: 233]

yin pattern 阴证 *yīn zhèng*: **1.** Any interior, cold, or vacuity pattern, e.g., somber white or dark dull complexion, curled-up lying posture, cold limbs, inactivity and tendency to talk little, low faint voice, faint weak breathing, shortness of breath and lack of strength, reduced food intake, bland taste in the mouth, absence of vexation and thirst or desire for warm drinks, sloppy stool, long voidings of clear urine, abdominal pain that likes pressure, pale enlarged tongue, glossy slimy tongue fur, and a forceless sunken slow fine pulse. **2.** A pattern in which sores of any kind present with broad roots, with paleness of the skin in the affected area, and with absence of heat, swelling, redness and pain. Compare YANG PATTERN. [26: 625]

yin-pattern cold damage 阴证伤寒 *yīn zhèng shāng hán*: COLD DAMAGE affecting any of the three yin channels. ⟨MED⟩ Greater yin (*tài yīn*) cold strike is treated with Stomach-Calming Poria (Hoelen) Five Decoction (*wèi líng tāng*) or Aconite

Center-Rectifying Decoction (*fù zǐ lǐ zhōng tāng*). Lesser yin (*shào yīn*) is treated with formulas like True Warrior Decoction (*zhēn wǔ tāng*). Reverting yin (*jué yīn*) is treated with formulas such as Tangkuei Counterflow Cold Decoction (*dāng guī sì nì tāng*) or Vessel-Freeing Counterflow Cold Decoction (*tōng mài sì nì tāng*). [26: 625]

yin-pattern macules 阴证发斑 *yīn zhèng fā bān*: YIN MACULES. [26: 621]

yin pattern resembling yang 阴证似阳 *yīn zhèng sì yáng*: The appearance of heat signs in disease of a cold nature developing to a critical stage. When a disease is at root a yin pattern, the appearance of red face, thirst, flailing of the arms and legs, and a large floating pulse is described as a yin pattern resembling yang. This is the same as TRUE COLD AND FALSE HEAT. [26: 625]

yin pile 阴痔 *yīn zhì*: Any protrusion of flesh from female genitals. ⟨WMC⟩ prolapse of the uterus; submucosal myoma of the uterus. **Liver depression or damp-heat** causes yin pile with a flow of yellow water from the vagina. ⟨MED⟩ Resolve depression, clear heat, and disinhibit dampness. Use Gentian Liver-Draining Decoction (*lóng dǎn xiè gān tāng*) or Moutan and Gardenia Free Wanderer Powder (*dān zhī xiāo yáo sǎn*). ⟨ACU⟩ Base treatment mainly on GV, LR, GB, SP, ST, and LI. Select GV-20 (*bǎi huì*, Hundred Convergences), GB-28 (*wéi dào*, Linking Path), KI-12 (*dà hè*, Great Manifestation), LR-3 (*tài chōng*, Supreme Surge), LR-2 (*xíng jiān*, Moving Between), SP-9 (*yīn líng quán*, Yin Mound Spring), LR-8 (*qū quán*, Spring at the Bend), SP-6 (*sān yīn jiāo*, Three Yin Intersection), LI-4 (*hé gǔ*, Union Valley), and ST-36 (*zú sān lǐ*, Leg Three Li); needle with drainage. The nonchannel points Infant's Palace (*zǐ gōng*) and Holding the Uterus (*wéi bāo*) can both be used for prolapse of the uterus due to any cause. **Spleen vacuity** causes yin pile characterized by a flow of white water from the vagina. ⟨MED⟩ Fortify the spleen and boost qi. Use Center-Supplementing Qi-Boosting Decoction (*bǔ zhōng yì qì tāng*) or Spleen-Returning Decoction (*guī pí tāng*). ⟨ACU⟩ Base treatment mainly on GV, CV, and SP. Select GV-20 (*bǎi huì*, Hundred Convergences), CV-6 (*qì hǎi*, Sea of Qi), BL-20 (*pí shū*, Spleen Transport), BL-21 (*wèi shū*, Stomach Transport), LR-13 (*zhāng mén*, Camphorwood Gate), GB-28 (*wéi dào*, Linking Path), KI-12 (*dà hè*, Great Manifestation), and SP-6 (*sān yīn jiāo*, Three Yin Intersection); needle with supplementation and moxa. A steam-wash can be prepared by stewing seven aconite main tuber (*chuān wū tóu*) in vinegar. See PILE; YIN PROTRUSION; PROLAPSE OF THE UTERUS. [26: 619] [4: 118] [46: 595, 597] [113: 322] [37: 436]

yin protraction 阴纵 *yīn zòng*: *Synonym: yin protrusion*[1]. A condition characterized by a tendency to erections of the penis of abnormally long duration (lasting hours or days) or swelling of the penis that gives the appearance of a partial erection. It is caused by liver channel damp-heat. MED Oral: Minor Bupleurum Decoction (*xiǎo chái hú tāng*) plus coptis (*huáng lián*) and phellodendron (*huáng bǎi*). Alternatively, use Bupleurum Dampness-Overcoming Decoction (*chái hú shèng shī tāng*) or Gentian Liver-Draining Decoction (*lóng dǎn xiè gān tāng*). In severe cases, use Three-in-One Qi-Coordinating Decoction (*sān yī chéng qì tāng*). Topical: Make a decoction of impure mirabilite (*pò xiāo*) and schizonepeta (*jīng jiè*), to wash and soak the affected area. If the swelling and protrusion is alleviated but a hard lump remains, treat with unripe tangerine peel (*qīng pí*), combined with wind-dissipating medicinals. See also YIN PROTRUSION. Compare RIGID CENTER. [26: 625] [97: 230] [50: 654]

yin protrusion 阴挺 *yīn tǐng*: 1. RIGID CENTER. 2. YANG RIGIDITY. 3. YIN PROTRACTION. 4. *Synonyms: vaginal protrusion; eggplant disease; eggplant yin; yin bulging.* A women's disease characterized by heaviness, sagging, and swelling of the anterior yin or the hanging of the interior outside the body. Yin protrusion is usually the result of center qi fall or insufficiency of kidney qi, if not due to holding the breath and straining in childbirth. The center qi fall pattern is one of vacuity and includes signs such as a sagging sensation in the abdomen, heart palpitations, shortness of breath, lassitude of spirit, vaginal discharge, and a floating vacuous pulse. Kidney vacuity is identified by the presence of limp aching lumbus and knees. If there is redness, swelling, and a exudation of yellow water, as is often the case when friction causes damage, the pattern is considered to be one of damp-heat pouring downward; this condition may also be identified by a burning sensation on urination, heart vexation, spontaneous sweating, a dry mouth with bitter taste, and a slippery rapid pulse. WMC prolapse of the uterus, cystocele, colpocele. MED For center qi fall, treat by supplementing vacuity and raising the fall using Center-Supplementing Qi-Boosting Decoction (*bǔ zhōng yì qì tāng*) with extra cimicifuga (*shēng má*) and mix-fried astragalus (*huáng qí*). For kidney vacuity, treat by supplementing the kidney and boosting qi with Major Origin-Supplementing Brew (*dà bǔ yuán jiān*). If protruding parts have become swollen and exude yellow water, and if voidings are rough with reddish urine, use Gentian Liver-Draining Decoction (*lóng dǎn xiè gān tāng*) and variations. For topical treatment, decoct mume (*wū méi*) and cnidium seed (*shé chuáng zǐ*) as a wash. ACU Base treatment on CV and GV. Main points: CV-4 (*guān yuán*, Pass Head), CV-6 (*qì hǎi*, Sea of Qi), GV-20 (*bǎi huì*, Hundred Conver-

gences), and Infant's Palace (*zǐ gōng*). For qi vacuity fall, add ST-36 (*zú sān lǐ*, Leg Three Li) and SP-6 (*sān yīn jiāo*, Three Yin Intersection); needle with supplementation and add moxa. For kidney vacuity, add KI-12 (*dà hè*, Great Manifestation), and KI-6 (*zhào hǎi*, Shining Sea), needling with supplementation and adding moxa. For damp-heat pouring downward, add LI-11 (*qū chí*, Pool at the Bend), LI-4 (*hé gǔ*, Union Valley), ST-36 (*zú sān lǐ*, Leg Three Li), and SP-9 (*yīn líng quán*, Yin Mound Spring); needle with drainage. ◇ Chin 阴 *yīn*, yin (complement of yang), yin (i.e., private) parts; 挺 *tǐng*, stick up or forward, protrude, project, describing the erect or quasi-erect state of the penis and prolapse of the uterus. Note that *eggplant disease* and *eggplant yin* describing the pathological condition in females derive from the similarity in appearance of a prolapsed uterus to a an eggplant. [26: 618] [46: 694]

yin qi 阴气 *yīn qì*: The opposite of yang qi. Yin and yang are the complementary and opposite poles of phenomena. Yin qi and yang qi are yin and yang viewed as complementary and opposing forces. Yin denotes physical substrata as opposed to function. It denotes the qi of the five viscera as opposed to that of the bowels. It denotes construction qi as opposed to defense qi. It denotes inward and downward movement, suppressive action, weakening, and that which is heavy and turbid. See YIN; QI. [26: 618] [27: 2] [97: 229]

yin rigidity 阴强 *yīn qiáng*: YANG RIGIDITY. [56: 65]

yin sac 阴囊 *yīn náng*: SCROTUM.

scrotal itch 阴囊瘙痒 *yīn náng sāo yǎng*: SCROTAL ITCH.

yin sore 阴疮 *yīn chuāng*: 1. A diffusely swollen painful sore below the cheek on the left or right, accompanied by generalized heat [effusion] and aversion to cold. 2. A sore in the female pudenda. 3. A sore or flat-abscess (*jū*) manifesting as a yin pattern. 4. BEDSORE. [50: 654] [61: 299]

yin springing vessel 阴跷（跻）脉 *yīn qiāo (qiāo) mài*: One of the EIGHT EXTRAORDINARY VESSELS. Abbreviation: YIS. Pathway: The yin linking (*yīn wéi*) originates at KI-6 (*zhào hǎi*, Shining Sea) below the medial malleolus, runs up the medial aspect of the leg, penetrates the genital region and then continues internally up the abdomen and chest to emerge in the supraclavicular fossa at ST-12 (*quē pén*, Empty Basin). It proceeds up the throat, passing in front of ST-12 (*quē pén*, Empty Basin), then continues up the medial aspect of the cheek to the inner canthus, where it joins the foot greater yang (*tài yáng*) bladder and yang springing channels to ascend over the head and enter the brain. Functions: The main physiological functions of both the yin (as also the yang) springing vessels are to control the opening and closing of the eyes, control the ascent of fluids and the descent of qi, and to regulate muscular activity in general. **Signs:** Disease signs associated with the yin springing (*yīn qiāo*) vessels include: eye diseases, heavy sensation of the eyelids or inability to open the eyes, clouding sleep, watery eyes, lower abdominal pain, pain along the waist extending into the genitals, hernia, vaginal discharge, and tightness and spasms along the medial aspect of the lower limb, with corresponding flaccidity along its lateral aspect. [6: 69]

yin summerheat 阴暑 *yīn shǔ*: A summerheat pattern attributed to exposure to wind or drafts or to excessive consumption of cold drinks in the hot summer months. When cold invades the FLESHY EXTERIOR, there is heat effusion, headache, aversion to cold, sweating, and generalized pain; this is treated by warming and dissipating with formulas such as Origin-Boosting Powder (*yì yuán sǎn*). When cold damages the viscera, there is vomiting, diarrhea, abdominal pain; this is treated by warming the center with formulas such as Agastache/Patchouli Qi-Righting Tablet (*huò xiāng zhèng qì piàn*). [ACU] Base treatment mainly on PC, LI, ST, and CV. Main points: PC-6 (*nèi guān*, Inner Pass), LI-4 (*hé gǔ*, Union Valley), and ST-36 (*zú sān lǐ*, Leg Three Li). Selection of points according to pattern: For cold assailing the fleshy exterior, select GV-20 (*bǎi huì*, Hundred Convergences), GB-20 (*fēng chí*, Wind Pool), TB-5 (*wài guān*, Outer Pass), LU-7 (*liè quē*, Broken Sequence), LI-11 (*qū chí*, Pool at the Bend), and GB-34 (*yáng líng quán*, Yang Mound Spring), needling with drainage and adding moxa. For cold damaging the viscera, select CV-12 (*zhōng wǎn*, Center Stomach Duct), CV-4 (*guān yuán*, Pass Head), CV-6 (*qì hǎi*, Sea of Qi), and ST-25 (*tiān shū*, Celestial Pivot), needling with supplementation and adding moxa. [26: 623] [113: 47] [37: 486]

yin sweating 阴汗 *yīn hàn*: 1. Synonym: *genital sweating*. Sweating of the external genitals and surrounding area. Yin sweating due to liver channel damp-heat is associated with cold of the genitals relieved by warmth, animal odor, reddish urine, and impotence. Damp-heat pouring downward can also occur in combination with liver-kidney depletion. When due to kidney yang vacuity, there is copious sweating of the scrotum with fear of cold and cold limbs, and limp aching lumbus and knees. Other signs include unhard erection, seminal efflux, premature ejaculation, and long voidings of clear urine. The tongue is moist, pale, and enlarged with dental impressions; the pulse is sunken and slow. [MED] Liver channel damp-heat is treated by draining, clearing, and disinhibiting, using Gentian Liver-Draining Decoction (*lóng dǎn xiè gān tāng*). Since "wind can overcome dampness," one or two wind medicinals such as schizo-

nepeta (*jīng jiè*) or ledebouriella (*fáng fēng*) may be added. Tangkuei, Gentian, and Aloe Pill (*dāng guī lóng huì wán*) and Mysterious Two Powder (Pill) (*èr miào sǎn* (*wán*)) are also effective. For clammy scrotum, dab on powdered calcined smithsonite (*lú gān shí*). Litharge (*mì tuó sēng*) is also effective. Damp-heat pouring downward with signs of liver-kidney depletion is treated by supplementing the liver and kidney, and clearing heat and dispelling dampness. Use Six-Ingredient Rehmannia Decoction (*liù wèi dì huáng tāng*) plus phellodendron (*huáng bǎi*) and white peony (*bái sháo yào*). Kidney yang vacuity is treated by warming supplementing, as with Kidney-Quieting Pill (*ān shèn wán*). [ACU] For liver channel damp-heat, use LR-2 (*xíng jiān*, Moving Between), GB-43 (*xiá xī*, Pinched Ravine), GB-34 (*yáng líng quán*, Yang Mound Spring), SP-9 (*yīn líng quán*, Yin Mound Spring), LI-4 (*hé gǔ*, Union Valley), and KI-7 (*fù liū*, Recover Flow), needling with drainage. For damp-heat pouring downward with signs of liver-kidney depletion, needle with supplementation or with even supplementation and drainage at BL-18 (*gān shū*, Liver Transport), BL-23 (*shèn shū*, Kidney Transport), LR-3 (*tài chōng*, Supreme Surge), and KI-3 (*tài xī*, Great Ravine), and with drainage at CV-3 (*zhōng jí*, Central Pole), SP-9 (*yīn líng quán*, Yin Mound Spring), SP-6 (*sān yīn jiāo*, Three Yin Intersection), and KI-7 (*fù liū*, Recover Flow). For kidney vacuity and yang debilitation, use CV-4 (*guān yuán*, Pass Head), GV-4 (*mìng mén*, Life Gate), BL-23 (*shèn shū*, Kidney Transport), KI-3 (*tài xī*, Great Ravine), CV-6 (*qì hǎi*, Sea of Qi), and HT-6 (*yīn xī*, Yin Cleft), needling with supplementation and adding moxa. **2.** Sweating due to debilitated yang and exuberant yin. [MED] Support right and warm yang. Use Ginseng Center-Fortifying Decoction (*rén shēn jiàn zhōng tāng*) (Minor Center-Fortifying Decoction (*xiǎo jiàn zhōng tāng*), with the addition of ginseng (*rén shēn*)). Ginseng and Aconite Decoction (*shēn fù tāng*), or Six-Ingredient Yang-Returning Beverage (*liù wèi huí yáng yǐn*). [ACU] Base treatment mainly on CV, GV, back transport points, LI, HT, and SI. Select LI-4 (*hé gǔ*, Union Valley), HT-6 (*yīn xī*, Yin Cleft), SI-3 (*hòu xī*, Back Ravine), CV-6 (*qì hǎi*, Sea of Qi), CV-4 (*guān yuán*, Pass Head), ST-36 (*zú sān lǐ*, Leg Three Li), BL-23 (*shèn shū*, Kidney Transport), GV-4 (*mìng mén*, Life Gate), and BL-20 (*pí shū*, Spleen Transport); needle with supplementation and, if appropriate, moxa. [26: 617] [27: 350] [97: 232] [50: 653] [113: 18] [46: 587, 597, 599, 678] [56: 149]

yin tetany 阴痉 *yīn jìng*: 1. SOFT TETANY. 2. TETANIC DISEASE with counterflow cold of the limbs. [MED] Warm yang and dispel the evil using formulas such as Ovate Atractylodes Powder (*bái zhú sǎn*). [ACU] Base treatment mainly on

GV, LR, and KI. Select GV-20 (*bǎi huì*, Hundred Convergences), KI-1 (*yǒng quán*, Gushing Spring), LR-3 (*tài chōng*, Supreme Surge), GV-16 (*fēng fǔ*, Wind Mansion), GV-8 (*jīn suō*, Sinew Contraction), KI-3 (*tài xī*, Great Ravine), ST-36 (*zú sān lǐ*, Leg Three Li), BL-23 (*shèn shū*, Kidney Transport), and GV-4 (*mìng mén*, Life Gate); needle with supplementation and add moxa. [26: 621] [42: 187]

yin-type weather 阴天 *yīn tiān*: Weather bearing yin qualities, i.e., dull, cloudy, damp weather.

yin vacuity 阴虚 *yīn xū*: The manifestation of insufficiency of the yin aspect and depletion of liquid and blood. When yin is vacuous, internal heat arises; hence there is low fever, heat in the hearts of the palms and soles, postmeridian heat effusion, emaciation, night sweating, dry mouth and throat, short voidings of reddish urine, red tongue with little or no fur, and a forceless fine rapid pulse. Yin vacuity may be focused in any of the five viscera, especially in the kidney. See LIVER YIN VACUITY; HEART YIN VACUITY; SPLEEN YIN VACUITY; LUNG YIN VACUITY; KIDNEY YIN VACUITY. [26: 619] [27: 206] [97: 232]

yin vacuity blood heat 阴虚血热 *yīn xū xuè rè*: Heat in the blood owing to yin vacuity and in some cases also nurtured by externally contracted heat evil. [92: No. 313]

yin vacuity headache 阴虚头痛 *yīn xū tóu tòng*: HEADACHE caused by yin vacuity stirring fire. Yin vacuity headache is accompanied by heat vexation, red face and upbearing fire flush, insomnia, red tongue, and a fine stringlike rapid pulse. MED Enrich yin and downbear fire with Anemarrhena and Phellodendron Eight-Ingredient Pill (*zhī bǎi bā wèi wán*) or Jade Lady Brew (*yù nǚ jiān*). If effulgent fire signs are not pronounced, use Six-Ingredient Rehmannia Pill (*liù wèi dì huáng wán*), Four Agents Decoction (*sì wù tāng*), or Left-Restoring [Kidney Yin] Pill (*zuǒ guī wán*). ACU For yin vacuity with stirring fire, base treatment mainly on back transport points, KI, and HT. Supplement GV-20 (*bǎi huì*, Hundred Convergences), BL-2 (*zǎn zhú*, Bamboo Gathering), Fish's Lumbus (*yú yāo*), SP-6 (*sān yīn jiāo*, Three Yin Intersection), BL-23 (*shèn shū*, Kidney Transport), BL-18 (*gān shū*, Liver Transport), and KI-3 (*tài xī*, Great Ravine); drain KI-2 (*rán gǔ*, Blazing Valley), HT-7 (*shén mén*, Spirit Gate), and HT-8 (*shào fǔ*, Lesser Mansion). For yin vacuity without effulgent fire, use the same formula as above, but remove KI-2 (*rán gǔ*, Blazing Valley), HT-7 (*shén mén*, Spirit Gate), and HT-8 (*shào fǔ*, Lesser Mansion), and add BL-20 (*pí shū*, Spleen Transport), BL-17 (*gé shū*, Diaphragm Transport), and ST-36 (*zú sān lǐ*, Leg Three Li), needling with supplemen-

tation. Selection of points according to affected area, see HEADACHE. [26: 620] [37: 364] [46: 396]

yin vacuity heat effusion 阴虚发热 *yīn xū fā rè*: HEAT EFFUSION due to depletion of essence, blood, and fluids. Yin vacuity heat effusion may take the form of postmeridian heat effusion (occurring sometime after midday), steaming bone heat effusion (appearing to emanate from the bones), or vexing heat in the five hearts (heat or sensation of heat the hearts of the palms and soles and the heart of the chest). Yin vacuity heat effusion is associated with emaciation, night sweating, dry mouth, red tongue, and a rapid fine pulse. It is seen in a wide variety of enduring sicknesses. MED Enrich yin and nourish the blood to abate the vacuity heat. Use Major Yin Supplementation Pill (*dà bǔ yīn wán*) or Six-Ingredient Rehmannia Pill (*liù wèi dì huáng wán*). ACU Base treatment mainly on KI, PC, and HT. Select KI-6 (*zhào hǎi*, Shining Sea), KI-2 (*rán gǔ*, Blazing Valley), LU-10 (*yú jì*, Fish Border), HT-8 (*shào fǔ*, Lesser Mansion), PC-8 (*láo gōng*, Palace of Toil), KI-1 (*yǒng quán*, Gushing Spring), and HT-7 (*shén mén*, Spirit Gate); needle with even supplementation and drainage. For night sweating, add HT-6 (*yīn xī*, Yin Cleft), SI-3 (*hòu xī*, Back Ravine), and LI-4 (*hé gǔ*, Union Valley); [26: 620] [46: 597]

yin vacuity fire effulgence 阴虚火旺 *yīn xū huǒ wàng*: See EFFULGENT YIN VACUITY FIRE.

yin vacuity lung dryness 阴虚肺燥 *yīn xū fēi zào*: LUNG DRYNESS due to yin vacuity. The lung is the delicate viscus, and is susceptible to scorching by fire, especially effulgent yin vacuity fire, which manifests in dryness and pronounced vacuity. The main signs are dry cough without phlegm, blood-flecked phlegm, sore throat, hoarse voice, pale red tongue with little fur, and a rapid floating pulse. WMC observed in pulmonary tuberculosis, and chronic laryngitis or pharyngitis. MED Use Adenophora/Glehnia and Ophiopogon Decoction (*shā shēn mài dōng tāng*). For acute dry cough, add Sichuan fritillaria (*chuān bèi mǔ*), apricot kernel (*xìng rén*), and steamed stemona (*bǎi bù*). For blood-flecked phlegm, add moutan (*mǔ dān pí*), gardenia (*shān zhī zǐ*), and lotus root node (*ǒu jié*). For sore throat, add scrophularia (*xuán shēn*). ACU Base treatment mainly on back transport points, LU, KI, ST, and SP. Select BL-13 (*fèi shū*, Lung Transport), BL-43 (*gāo huāng shū*, Gao-Huang Transport), LU-5 (*chǐ zé*, Cubit Marsh), KI-6 (*zhào hǎi*, Shining Sea), BL-21 (*wèi shū*, Stomach Transport), ST-36 (*zú sān lǐ*, Leg Three Li), and SP-6 (*sān yīn jiāo*, Three Yin Intersection). Needle with supplementation. ACU Base treatment mainly on LU, back transport points, and KI. Select LU-9 (*tài yuān*, Great Abyss), BL-13 (*fèi shū*, Lung Transport), BL-43 (*gāo huāng shū*, Gao-Huang Transport), LU-5 (*chǐ zé*, Cubit Marsh), SP-6 (*sān yīn jiāo*, Three Yin Intersection), KI-6 (*zhào hǎi*, Shining Sea), and KI-3 (*tài xī*, Great Ravine); needle with supplementation. Selection of points according to signs: For sore pharynx, prick LU-11 (*shào shāng*, Lesser Shang) to bleed. For blood-flecked phlegm, add LU-10 (*yú jì*, Fish Border) and LU-6 (*kǒng zuì*, Collection Hole). [26: 620] [27: 161] [97: 236]

yin vacuity night sweating 阴虚盗汗 *yīn xū dào hàn*: Yin vacuity heat causing the discharge of the humor of the heart (sweat). In this pattern, night sweating is accompanied by heat vexation, dry mouth, and a rapid fine pulse. MED Nourish yin and clear heat using Six-Ingredient Rehmannia Pill (*liù wèi dì huáng wán*) plus white peony (*bái sháo yào*), ophiopogon (*mài mén dōng*), schisandra (*wǔ wèi zǐ*), and lycium root bark (*dì gǔ pí*). For effulgent fire, use Tangkuei Six Yellows Decoction (*dāng guī liù huáng tāng*). ACU Base treatment mainly on KI, LI, SI, and HT. Select LI-4 (*hé gǔ*, Union Valley), SI-3 (*hòu xī*, Back Ravine), HT-6 (*yīn xī*, Yin Cleft), BL-13 (*fèi shū*, Lung Transport), BL-23 (*shèn shū*, Kidney Transport), KI-3 (*tài xī*, Great Ravine), KI-6 (*zhào hǎi*, Shining Sea), KI-2 (*rán gǔ*, Blazing Valley), and SP-6 (*sān yīn jiāo*, Three Yin Intersection); needle with supplementation. See NIGHT SWEATING. [26: 620] [46: 602] [113: 18] [14: 175]

yin vacuity panting 阴虚喘 *yīn xū chuǎn*: PANTING due to yin vacuity with floating yang. Yin vacuity panting stems from yin-blood depletion or kidney vacuity, which deprives yang qi of its support and causes it to surge upward. During episodes of panting, the patient experiences qi surging up from below the umbilicus. Other signs include tidal heat [effusion] and night sweating. MED Enrich yin and nourish the blood; supplement the kidney and boost yin. Use formulas such as Four Agents Decoction (*sì wù tāng*), Pulse-Engendering Variant Powder (*jiā jiǎn shēng mài sǎn*), Ophiopogon and Rehmannia Pill (*mài wèi dì huáng wán*), and Placenta Great Creation Pill (*hé chē dà zào wán*), adding medicinals that subdue yang and promote qi absorption if necessary. ACU Base treatment mainly on back transport points, LU, and KI. Select BL-23 (*shèn shū*, Kidney Transport), KI-3 (*tài xī*, Great Ravine), KI-6 (*zhào hǎi*, Shining Sea), BL-13 (*fèi shū*, Lung Transport), Panting Stabilizer (*dìng chuǎn*), BL-43 (*gāo huāng shū*, Gao-Huang Transport), LU-5 (*chǐ zé*, Cubit Marsh), CV-17 (*shān zhōng*, Chest Center), and LU-9 (*tài yuān*, Great Abyss); needle with supplementation. For tidal heat [effusion], add GV-14 (*dà zhuī*, Great Hammer) and PC-5 (*jiān shǐ*, Intermediary Courier). For night sweating, add SI-3 (*hòu xī*, Back Ravine) and HT-6 (*yīn xī*, Yin Cleft). [26: 620] [46: 655]

yin vacuity stomach duct pain 阴虚胃脘痛 *yīn xū wèi wǎn (guǎn) tòng*: See INTERNAL DAMAGE STOMACH DUCT PAIN.

yin vacuity throat impediment 阴虚喉痹 *yīn xū hóu bì*: THROAT IMPEDIMENT (sore throat with difficulty swallowing) attributable to yin vacuity. When due to liver-kidney yin vacuity, signs include tinnitus, night sweating, and limp aching lumbus and knees. When due to damage to the lung-stomach yin by dryness, it is characterized by dry throat, dry lips, and cough without phlegm. WMC chronic pharyngitis. MED Liver kidney-yin vacuity is treated by enriching yin and downbearing fire with formulas such as Anemarrhena, Phellodendron, and Rehmannia Pill (*zhī bǎi dì huáng wán*). Damage to lung-stomach yin is treated by moistening the lung and nourishing yin with formulas such as Yin-Nourishing Lung-Clearing Decoction (*yǎng yīn qīng fèi tāng*) and Dryness-Clearing Lung-Rescuing Decoction (*qīng zào jiù fèi tāng*). ACU For liver-kidney yin vacuity, base treatment mainly on KI and LU. Needle with supplementation at BL-18 (*gān shū*, Liver Transport), BL-23 (*shèn shū*, Kidney Transport), SP-6 (*sān yīn jiāo*, Three Yin Intersection), KI-3 (*tài xī*, Great Ravine), KI-6 (*zhào hǎi*, Shining Sea), and KI-2 (*rán gǔ*, Blazing Valley), and with drainage at LU-10 (*yú jì*, Fish Border), KI-1 (*yǒng quán*, Gushing Spring), and TB-1 (*guān chōng*, Passage Hub). For damage to lung-stomach yin, base treatment mainly on back transport points, LU, ST, and KI. Select BL-13 (*fèi shū*, Lung Transport), BL-43 (*gāo huāng shū*, Gao-Huang Transport), BL-21 (*wèi shū*, Stomach Transport), LU-5 (*chǐ zé*, Cubit Marsh), KI-6 (*zhào hǎi*, Shining Sea), ST-36 (*zú sān lǐ*, Leg Three Li), and ST-44 (*nèi tíng*, Inner Court). Selection of points according to signs: For dry pharynx, add TB-2 (*yè mén*, Humor Gate). For pronounced soreness, prick LU-11 (*shào shāng*, Lesser Shang) to bleed. [26: 620] [27: 496] [97: 236] [46: 727] [113: 506]

yin vacuity throat lichen 阴虚喉癣 *yīn xū hóu xiǎn*: THROAT LICHEN due to yin vacuity. See THROAT LICHEN. [26: 620] [27: 497] [97: 236]

yin vacuity tidal heat [effusion] 阴虚潮热 *yīn xū cháo rè*: TIDAL HEAT EFFUSION due to yin vacuity, as opposed to yang brightness (*yáng míng*) interior repletion patterns. See TIDAL HEAT [EFFUSION].

yin vacuity wilting 阴虚痿 *yīn xū wěi*: WILTING (*wěi*) (weakness and limpness of the sinews) arising when enduring illness or sexual intemperance cause insufficiency of the liver and kidney and effulgent yin vacuity fire which damage the sinew and bones. MED Enrich yin and clear fire; supplement the liver and kidney. An appropriate formula is Hidden Tiger Pill (*hǔ qián wán*). ACU Use the basic treatments given under WILTING, and add KI-3 (*tài xī*, Great Ravine), KI-2 (*rán gǔ*, Blazing Valley), KI-6 (*zhào hǎi*, Shining Sea), SP-6 (*sān yīn jiāo*, Three Yin Intersection), LR-3 (*tài chōng*, Supreme Surge), and HT-8 (*shào fǔ*, Lesser Mansion), needling with supplementation. [26: 620]

yin vacuity with floating yang 阴虚阳浮 *yīn xū yáng fú*: Insufficiency of true yin and liquid-blood depletion causing yang qi to stray to the upper body, and causing dizziness, tidal reddening of the face, red eyes, dry sore throat, and toothache. [26: 620]

yin vacuity with yang hyperactivity 阴虚阳亢 *yīn xū yáng kàng*: Essence-blood or fluid depletion causing a yin-yang imbalance in which yang becomes unrestrained and exuberant. Yang hyperactivity exacerbates depletion of fluid so that a vicious circle is set in motion. Yin vacuity with yang hyperactivity is characterized by tidal heat [effusion], reddening of the cheeks, night sweating, vexing heat in the five hearts, coughing of blood, emaciation, dry red tongue, and rapid fine pulse. In some cases, there is insomnia, vexation, agitation, and irascibility, or seminal emission and excessive libido. MED Foster yin and subdue yang. Use Gastrodia and Uncaria Beverage (*tiān má gōu téng yīn*) or Liver-Settling Wind-Extinguishing Decoction (*zhèn gān xī fēng tāng*). ACU Base treatment mainly on KI, LR, and HT, needling with supplementation at BL-23 (*shèn shū*, Kidney Transport), SP-6 (*sān yīn jiāo*, Three Yin Intersection), KI-6 (*zhào hǎi*, Shining Sea), and KI-2 (*rán gǔ*, Blazing Valley), and with drainage at GB-20 (*fēng chí*, Wind Pool), LI-11 (*qū chí*, Pool at the Bend), KI-1 (*yǒng quán*, Gushing Spring), LR-3 (*tài chōng*, Supreme Surge), and HT-8 (*shào fǔ*, Lesser Mansion). Selection of points according to signs: For tidal heat [effusion], add PC-8 (*láo gōng*, Palace of Toil), needling with drainage. For night sweating, add SI-3 (*hòu xī*, Back Ravine) and HT-6 (*yīn xī*, Yin Cleft), needling with drainage. For coughing of blood, add LU-10 (*yú jì*, Fish Border), and LU-6 (*kǒng zuì*, Collection Hole), needling with drainage. For insomnia, add Alert Spirit Quartet (*sì shén cōng*) and HT-7 (*shén mén*, Spirit Gate), needling with drainage. For seminal emission, add HT-7 (*shén mén*, Spirit Gate), PC-7 (*dà líng*, Great Mound), CV-4 (*guān yuán*, Pass Head), and BL-52 (*zhì shì*, Will Chamber), needling with drainage. [26: 620] [46: 596] [37: 338]

yin vessel 阴脉 *yīn mài*: YIN CHANNEL.

yin water 阴水 *yīn shuǐ*: From *Dan Xi's Experiential Methods* (*dān xī xīn fǎ*) WATER SWELLING attributed to devitalized spleen yang and debilitated kidney yang failing to move and transform water, and characterized by swelling of face and instep, or by swelling of the lower limbs first.

The swelling pits under pressure, and is associated with oppression in the chest, reduced food intake, cold limbs, lassitude of spirit, sloppy stool, scant urine, heavy body and aching lumbus, an enlarged tongue with white fur, and a sunken slow weak pulse. Yin water is so named because it includes vacuity and cold patterns. MED Fortify the spleen, warm the kidney, free yang, and transform dampness. For devitalization of spleen yang, warm spleen yang and control water-damp. Use Spleen-Firming Beverage (*shí pí yǐn*). Add ginseng (*rén shēn*) and astragalus (*huáng qí*) for pronounced qi vacuity; add cinnamon twig (*guì zhī*) and alisma (*zé xiè*) for scant urine. For debilitation of kidney yang, treat by warming kidney and dissipating cold and by moving qi and disinhibiting water with True Warrior Decoction (*zhēn wǔ tāng*) combined with Poria (Hoelen) Five Powder (*wǔ líng sǎn*); add fenugreek (*hú lú bā*), morinda (*bā jǐ tiān*), and cinnamon bark (*ròu guì*) for pronounced vacuity cold signs. ACU Base treatment mainly on CV, back transport points, SP, and ST. Select CV-9 (*shuǐ fēn*, Water Divide), CV-6 (*qì hǎi*, Sea of Qi), BL-22 (*sān jiāo shū*, Triple Burner Transport), SP-6 (*sān yīn jiāo*, Three Yin Intersection), BL-39 (*wěi yáng*, Bend Yang), SP-9 (*yīn líng quán*, Yin Mound Spring), and ST-36 (*zú sān lǐ*, Leg Three Li), needling with supplementation and adding moxa. Selection of points according to pattern: For devitalization of spleen yang, add BL-20 (*pí shū*, Spleen Transport), CV-12 (*zhōng wǎn*, Center Stomach Duct), and LR-13 (*zhāng mén*, Camphorwood Gate). For debilitation of kidney yang, add BL-23 (*shèn shū*, Kidney Transport), GV-4 (*mìng mén*, Life Gate), KI-3 (*tài xī*, Great Ravine), and KI-7 (*fù liū*, Recover Flow). Selection of points according to signs: For swelling of the upper limbs, add LI-6 (*piān lì*, Veering Passageway). For swelling of the lower limbs, add SP-9 (*yīn líng quán*, Yin Mound Spring). For swelling of insteps, add GB-41 (*zú lín qì*, Foot Overlooking Tears). For oppression in the chest and reduced food intake, add CV-12 (*zhōng wǎn*, Center Stomach Duct), PC-6 (*nèi guān*, Inner Pass), and ST-25 (*tiān shū*, Celestial Pivot). For sloppy diarrhea, add ST-25 (*tiān shū*, Celestial Pivot). [26: 616] [27: 419] [97: 229] [46: 676] [113: 184]

yin within yang 阳中之阴 *yáng zhōng zhī yīn*: The yin part of yang phenomenon (i.e., a phenomenon that is yang in relation to others). For example, the upper body is yang and the lower body is yin, whereas the back of the body is yang and the front is yin. The chest is therefore the yin within yang. *Elementary Questions* (*sù wèn, jīn guì zhēn yán lùn*) states, "Midday to dusk is in the yang [part] of the day, and is the yin within yang." This is to say, the afternoon falls in daytime (yang) as opposed to nighttime (yin), and being the decline of daytime, it is their the yin part; hence, the afternoon is one example of yin within yang. Compare YIN AND YANG ARE DIVISIBLE BUT INSEPARABLE. [26: 712]

yin within yin 阴中之阴 *yīn zhōng zhī yīn*: The yin aspect of a yin phenomenon. According to the principle that yin and yang are divisible but inseparable, all yang phenomena can be divided into yin and yang components, as can all yin phenomena. For instance, chest and abdomen are yin as opposed to the back, which is yang. However, the chest (upper part) is yang, whereas the abdomen (lower part) is yin. The abdomen is thus the yin within yin. Compare YIN AND YANG ARE DIVISIBLE BUT INSEPARABLE. [26: 616]

yin-yang 阴阳 *yīn yáng*: YIN AND YANG.

yin-yang disharmony 阴阳失调 *yīn yáng shī tiáo*: Imbalance between any yin and yang elements of the body and evils within the body. *Elementary Questions* (*sù wèn, yīn yáng yìng xiàng dà lùn*) sums up the essence of yin-yang disharmony as follows, "When yin prevails, yang ails; when yang prevails, yin ails. When yang prevails, there is heat; when yin prevails, there is cold." Yin and yang can fall out of harmony in more than one way. When the counterbalancing principle observed in ebb and flow breaks down, a surfeit of one pole means a deficit of the other. A fierce sun parches the land, and a long winter shortens the summer. Likewise, a deficit of one complement is often observed with a surfeit of the other, as a lack of warmth manifests as cold. Sometimes, when interdependence breaks down, a deficit of one complement can lead to a deficit of the other. For example, absence of rest can make incessant activity unproductive. Since both evils and aspects of the body may be classified according to yin and yang, both health and disease may be viewed in terms of yin and yang. When the yin and yang elements within the body and between the body and the environment are in balance, the body is healthy. When any aspect of the balance is upset, disease arises. When a person is healthy, the principle of interdependence and mutual counterbalancing of yin and yang operates. A morbid imbalance is seen in terms of a failure of these relationships, or in terms of the mutual convertibility of yin and yang. [26: 621]

YIS 阴跷（蹻）脉 *yīn qiāo (qiāo) mài*: Abbreviation for the YIN SPRINGING VESSEL.

Yuan 元 *yuán*: The name of a dynasty (A.D. 1274–1368).

Z

Zhou 周 *zhōu*: The name of a dynasty (approx. 11th cent.–221 B.C.).

zi 字 *zì*: A unit of measure equal to four qian. The term "zi" occurs in the formula names Wind-Expelling One Zi Powder (*qū fēng yī zì sǎn*) and One Zi Decoction (*yī zì tāng*).

Appendix I: Weights and Measures

21.	Weights in Different Dynasties	
Dynasty	Date	Grams/liang
Zhou	1066–221 B.C.	14.18
Qin	221–206 B.C.	16.14
Western Han	206 B.C.–23 A.D.	16.14
Eastern Han	25– 220	13.92
Wei	220–265	13.92
Jin	265–420	13.92
Liu Sung, Nan Qi Liang	420–589 (Southern Dynasties)	20.88 13.92
Chen		13.92
Northern Wei Northern Qi	386–581 (Northern Dynasties)	13.92 27.84
Northern Zhou		15.66
Sui (Kaihuang) Sui (Daye)	581–618	41.76 13.92
Tang	618–907	37.30
Five Dynasties	907–960	37.30
Song	960–1279	37.30
Yuan	1279–1368	37.30
Ming	1368–1644	37.30
Qing	1644–1911	37.30

22.	Measures in Different Dynasties	
Dynasty	Date	Ml./sheng
Zhou	1066–221 B.C.	193.7
Qin	221–206 B.C.	342.5
Western Han	206 B.C.–23 A.D.	342.5
Eastern Han	25–220	198.1
Wei	220–265	202.3
Jin	265–420	202.3
Liu Sung, Nan Qi Liang	420–589 (Southern Dynasties)	297.2 198.1
Chen		198.1
Northern Wei Northern Qi	386–581 (Northern Dynasties)	396.3 396.3
Northern Zhou		210.5
Sui (Kaihuang) Sui (Daye)	581–618	594.4 198.1
Tang	618–907	594.4
Five Dynasties	907–960	594.4
Song	960–1279	664.1
Yuan	1279–1368	948.8
Ming	1368–1644	1073.7
Qing	1644–1911	1035.5

23. Weights Conversion Table	
Unit	Grams
1 jin 斤	500.0g
1 liang 两	31.25g
1 qian 钱	3.125g
1 fen 分	0.3125g

Appendix II: A Classified List of Medicinals

Medicinals are here presented in thematic order of functional class. For each entry, the English name is followed by Chinese, Pinyin, and Latin pharmaceutical name.

Warm Acrid Exterior-Resolving Agents 辛温解表药

ephedra 麻黄 *má huáng* Ephedrae Herba
cinnamon twig 桂枝 *guì zhī* Cinnamomi Ramulus
perilla leaf 紫苏叶 *zǐ sū yè* Perillae Folium
perilla 紫苏 *zǐ sū* Perillae Folium, Caulis et Calyx
fresh ginger 生姜 *shēng jiāng* Zingiberis Rhizoma Recens
perilla stem 紫苏梗 *zǐ sū gěng* Perillae Caulis
elsholtzia 香薷 *xiāng rú* Elsholtziae Herba
ginger skin 姜皮 *jiāng pí* Zingiberis Rhizomatis Cortex
schizonepeta 荆芥 *jīng jiè* Schizonepetae Herba et Flos
ledebouriella 防风 *fáng fēng* Ledebouriellae Radix
notopterygium 羌活 *qiāng huó* Notopterygii Rhizoma
angelica 白芷 *bái zhǐ* Angelicae Dahuricae Radix
Chinese lovage 藁本 *gǎo běn* Ligustici Sinensis Rhizoma et Radix
xanthium 苍耳子 *cāng ěr zǐ* Xanthii Fructus
magnolia flower[1] 辛夷 *xīn yí* Magnoliae Flos[1]
scallion white 葱白 *cōng bái* Allii Fistulosi Bulbus
coriander 胡荽 *hú suī* Coriandri Herba cum Radice
tamarisk 柽柳 *chēng liǔ* Tamaricis Ramulus et Folium

Cool Acrid Exterior-Resolving Agents 辛温解表药

mint 薄荷 *bò hé* Menthae Herba
arctium 牛蒡子 *niú bàng zǐ* Arctii Fructus
cicada molting 蝉蜕 *chán tuì* Cicadae Periostracum
fermented soybean 淡豆豉 *dàn dòu chǐ* Glycines Semen Fermentatum Insulsum
dried soybean sprout 大豆黄卷 *dà dòu huáng juǎn* Glycines Semen Germinatum Exsiccatum
mulberry leaf 桑叶 *sāng yè* Mori Folium
chrysanthemum 菊花 *jú huā* Chrysanthemi Flos
wild chrysanthemum flower 野菊花 *yě jú huā* Chrysanthemi Indicae seu Borealis Flos
vitex 蔓荆子 *màn jīng zǐ* Viticis Fructus
pueraria 葛根 *gé gēn* Puerariae Radix
bupleurum 柴胡 *chái hú* Bupleuri Radix
cimicifuga 升麻 *shēng má* Cimicifugae Rhizoma
duckweed 浮萍 *fú píng* Lemnae Herba
equisetum 木贼 *mù zéi* Equiseti Herba

Heat-Clearing Medicinals 清热药

Heat-Clearing Fire-Draining Medicinals

清热泻火药

gypsum 石膏 *shí gāo* Gypsum
crude gypsum 生石膏 *shēng shí gāo* Gypsum Crudum
anemarrhena 知母 *zhī mǔ* Anemarrhenae Rhizoma
phragmites 芦根 *lú gēn* Phragmititis Rhizoma
fresh phragmites 鲜芦根 *xiān lú gēn* Phragmititis Rhizoma Recens
trichosanthes root 天花粉 *tiān huā fěn* Trichosanthis Radix
gardenia 山栀子 *shān zhī zǐ* Gardeniae Fructus
prunella 夏枯草 *xià kū cǎo* Prunellae Spica
bamboo leaf (lophatherum) 淡竹叶 *dàn zhú yè* Lophatheri Folium
bamboo leaf 竹叶 *zhú yè* Bambusae Folium
glauberite 寒水石 *hán shuǐ shí* Gypsum seu Calcitum
dayflower 鸭跖草 *yā zhí cǎo* Commelinae Herba
buddleia 密蒙花 *mì méng huā* Buddleiae Flos
celosia 青葙子 *qīng xiāng zǐ* Celosiae Argenteae Semen
watermelon 西瓜 *xī guā* Citrulli Fructus
watermelon rind 西瓜皮 *xī guā pí* Citrulli Exocarpium
watermelon frost 西瓜霜 *xī guā shuāng* Mirabiliti et Citrulli Praeparatio

Heat-Clearing Dampness-Drying Medicinals 清热燥湿药

scutellaria 黄芩 *huáng qín* Scutellariae Radix
coptis 黄连 *huáng lián* Coptidis Rhizoma
phellodendron 黄柏 *huáng bǎi* Phellodendri Cortex
gentian 龙胆 *lóng dǎn* Gentianae Radix
flavescent sophora 苦参 *kǔ shēn* Sophorae Flavescentis Radix
meadow rue 马尾连 *mǎ wěi lián* Thalictri Rhizoma et Radix
mahonia 十大功劳叶 *shí dà gōng láo yè* Mahoniae Folium

Heat-Clearing Blood-Cooling Medicinals 清热凉血药

rhinoceros horn 犀角 *xī jiǎo* Rhinocerotis Cornu
water buffalo horn 水牛角 *shuǐ niú jiǎo* Bubali Cornu
dried rehmannia 干地黄 *gān dì huáng* Rehmanniae Radix Exsiccata
fresh rehmannia 鲜地黄 *xiān dì huáng* Rehmanniae Radix Recens
scrophularia 玄参 *xuán shēn* Scrophulariae Radix
moutan 牡丹皮 *mǔ dān pí* Moutan Radicis Cortex

red peony 赤芍药 *chì sháo yào* Paeoniae Radix Rubra

moutan 牡丹皮 *mǔ dān pí* Moutan Radicis Cortex

red peony 赤芍药 *chì sháo yào* Paeoniae Radix Rubra

puccoon 紫草 *zǐ cǎo* Lithospermi, Macrotomiae, seu Onosmatis Radix

Heat-Clearing Toxin-Resolving Medicinals 清热解毒

lonicera 金银花 *jīn yín huā* Lonicerae Flos

lonicera stem and leaf 忍冬藤 *rěn dōng téng* Lonicerae Caulis et Folium

forsythia 连翘 *lián qiào* Forsythiae Fructus

dandelion 蒲公英 *pú gōng yīng* Taraxaci Herba cum Radice

Yedo violet 紫花地丁 *zǐ huā dì dīng* Violae Yedoensis Herba cum Radice

violet 地丁 *dì dīng* Violae Herba cum Radice

isatis leaf 大青叶 *dà qīng yè* Isatidis Folium

isatis root 板蓝根 *bǎn lán gēn* Isatidis Radix

indigo 青黛 *qīng dài* Indigo Pulverata Levis

andrographis 穿心莲 *chuān xīn lián* Andrographidis Herba

bovine bezoar 牛黄 *niú huáng* Bovis Bezoar

paris 蚤休 *zǎo xiū* Paridis Rhizoma

Chinese lobelia 半边莲 *bàn biān lián* Lobeliae Chinensis Herba cum Radice

bistort 拳参 *quán shēn* Polygoni Bistortae Rhizoma

hanging stonecrop 石指甲 *shí zhǐ jiǎ* Sedi Sarmentosi Herba

smooth greenbrier root 土茯苓 *tǔ fú líng* Smilacis Glabrae Rhizoma

houttuynia 鱼腥草 *yú xīng cǎo* Houttuyniae Herba cum Radice

belamcanda 射干 *shè gān* Belamcandae Rhizoma

bushy sophora 山豆根 *shān dòu gēn* Sophorae Subprostratae Radix

puffball 马勃 *mǎ bó* Lasiosphaera seu Calvatia

purslane 马齿苋 *mǎ chǐ xiàn* Portulacae Herba

pulsatilla 白头翁 *bái tóu wēng* Pulsatillae Radix

ash 秦皮 *qín pí* Fraxini Cortex

brucea 鸦胆子 *yā dǎn zǐ* Bruceae Fructus

sargentodoxa 大血藤 *dà xuè téng* Sargentodoxae Caulis

baijiang 败酱草 *bài jiàng cǎo* Baijiang Herba cum Radice

heterophyllous patrinia 墓头回 *mù tóu huí* Patriniae Heterophyllae Radix

bái huā shé shé cǎo 白花蛇舌草 *hedyotis* Hedyotis Herba

bear's gall 熊胆 *xióng dǎn* Ursi Fel

ampelopsis 白蔹 *bái liǎn* Ampelopsis Radix

dictamnus 白鲜皮 *bái xiān pí* Dictamni Radicis Cortex

rhaponticum/echinops 漏芦 *lòu lú* Rhapontici seu Echinopis Radix

shancigu 山慈姑 *shān cí gū* Shancigu Bulbus

Chinese ilex leaf 冬青叶 *dōng qīng yè* Ilicis Chinensis Folium

wild buckwheat root 天荞麦根 *tiān qiáo mài gēn* Fagopyri Cymosi Radix et Rhizoma

humifuse euphorbia 地锦草 *dì jǐn cǎo* Euphorbiae Humifusae Herba

bending bugle 白毛夏枯草 *bái máo xià kū cǎo* Ajugae Decumbentis Herba

Spanish needles 鬼针草 *guǐ zhēn cǎo* Bidentis Bipinnatae Herba

mung bean seed-coat 绿豆皮 *lǜ dòu pí* Phaseoli Aurei Testa

climbing groundsel 千里光 *qiān lǐ guāng* Senecionis Scandentis Herba

Japanese hop 葎草 *lǜ cǎo* Humuli Scandentis Herba

saxifrage 虎耳草 *hǔ ěr cǎo* Saxifragae Herba

lesser hypericum 地耳草 *dì ěr cǎo* Hyperici Japonici Herba

pretty swertia 青叶胆 *qīng yè dǎn* Swertiae Pulchellae Herba

prayer-beads 鸡骨草 *jī gǔ cǎo* Abri Cantoniensis Herba cum Radice

sarcandra 九节茶 *jiǔ jié chá* Sarcandrae Ramulus et Folium

bearded scutellaria 半枝莲 *bàn zhī lián* Scutellariae Barbatae Herba

semiaquilegia tuber 天葵子 *tiān kuí zǐ* Semiaquilegiae Tuber

black nightshade 龙葵 *lóng kuí* Solani Nigri Herba

climbing nightshade 白毛藤 *bái máo téng* Solani Lyrati Herba

snake strawberry 蛇莓 *shé méi* Duchesneae Herba

phoenix-tail fern 凤尾草 *fèng wěi cǎo* Pteridis Multifidi Herba

serissa 白马骨 *bái mǎ gǔ* Serissae Herba

Chinese silverweed 委陵菜 *wěi líng cài* Potentillae Chinensis Radix seu Herba cum Radice

globeflower 金莲花 *jīn lián huā* Trollii Flos

lantern plant calyx 挂金灯 *guà jīn dēng* Physalis Alkekengi Calyx

devil's tongue 蒟蒻 *jǔ ruò* Amorphophalli Tuber

lantern plant 酸浆 *suān jiāng* Physalis Alkekengi Herba

tinospora tuber 金果榄 *jīn guǒ lǎn* Tinosporae Tuber

Chinese olive 橄榄 *gǎn lǎn* Canarii Albi Fructus

rohdea root 万年青根 *wàn nián qīng gēn* Rohdeae Rhizoma et Radix

unripe chebule 藏青果 *zàng qīng guǒ* Chebulae Fructus Immaturus

Vacuity-Heat–Clearing Medicinals 清虚热药

sweet wormwood 青蒿 *qīng hāo* Artemisiae Apiaceae seu Annuae Herba

baiwei 白薇 *bái wēi* Cynanchi Baiwei Radix

lycium root bark 地骨皮 *dì gǔ pí* Lycii Radicis Cortex

lanceolate stellaria 银柴胡 *yín chái hú* Stellariae Lanceolatae Radix

picrorhiza 胡黄连 *hú huáng lián* Picrorhizae Rhizoma

Draining Precipitation Medicinals 泻下药

Attacking precipitants 攻下药

rhubarb 大黄 *dà huáng* Rhei Rhizoma

raw rhubarb 生大黄 *shēng dà huáng* Rhei Rhizoma Crudum

refined mirabilite 玄明粉 *xuán míng fěn* Mirabilitum Depuratum

impure mirabilite 朴硝 *pò xiāo* Mirabilitum Non-Purum

mirabilite 芒硝 *máng xiāo* Mirabilitum

senna 番泻叶 *fān xiè yè* Sennae Folium

aloe 芦荟 *lú huì* Aloe

croton 巴豆 *bā dòu* Crotonis Semen

croton frost 巴豆霜 *bā dòu shuāng* Crotonis Seminis Pulvis

Moist Precipitants 润下药

hemp seed 火麻仁 *huǒ má rén* Cannabis Semen

bush cherry kernel 郁李仁 *yù lǐ rén* Pruni Japonicae Semen

Water-Expelling Medicinals 逐水药

kansui 甘遂 *gān suì* Kansui Radix

caper spurge seed 续随子 *xù suí zǐ* Euphorbiae Lathyridis Semen

euphorbia/knoxia 大戟 *dà jǐ* Euphorbiae seu Knoxiae Radix

genkwa 芫花 *yuán huā* Daphnes Genkwa Flos

morning glory 牵牛子 *qiān niú zǐ* Pharbitidis Semen

phytolacca 商陆 *shāng lù* Phytolaccae Radix

caper spurge seed 续随子 *xù suí zǐ* Euphorbiae Lathyridis Semen

Wind-Damp–Dispelling Medicinals 祛风湿药

duhuo 独活 *dú huó* Angelicae Duhuo Radix

clematis 威灵仙 *wēi líng xiān* Clematidis Radix

fangji 防己 *fáng jǐ* Fangji Radix

, includes the following items woody fangji 木防己 *mù fáng jǐ* Cocculi Radix

mealy fangji 粉防己 *fěn fáng jǐ* Stephaniae Tetrandrae Radix

northern fangji 汉中防己 *hàn zhōng fáng jǐ* Aristolochiae Heterophyllae Radix

southern fangji 广防己 *guǎng fáng jǐ* Aristolochiae Fangchi Radix

large gentian 秦艽 *qín jiāo* Gentianae Macrophyllae Radix

siegesbeckia 豨莶 *xī xiān* Siegesbeckiae Herba

clerodendron 臭梧桐 *chòu wú tóng* Clerodendri Folium

chaenomeles 木瓜 *mù guā* Chaenomelis Fructus

star jasmine stem 络石藤 *luò shí téng* Trachelospermi Caulis

paniculate cynanchum 徐长卿 *xú cháng qīng* Cynanchi Paniculati Herba cum Radice

mulberry twig 桑枝 *sāng zhī* Mori Ramulus

mistletoe 桑寄生 *sāng jì shēng* Loranthi seu Visci Ramus

acanthopanax 五加皮 *wǔ jiā pí* Acanthopanacis Radicis Cortex

dog's bone 狗骨 *gǒu gǔ* Canis Os

tiger bone 虎骨 *hǔ gǔ* Tigris Os

leopard's bone 豹骨 *bào gǔ* Leopardi Os

krait/agkistrodon 白花蛇 *bái huā shé* Bungarus seu Agkistrodon

agkistrodon 蕲蛇 *qí shé* Agkistrodon

erythrina 海桐皮 *hǎi tóng pí* Erythrinae Cortex

black-striped snake 乌蛇 *wū shé* Zaocys

snake slough 蛇蜕 *shé tuì* Serpentis Exuviae

silkworm droppings 原蚕沙 *yuán cán shā* Bombycis Excrementum

kadsura pepper stem 海风藤 *hǎi fēng téng* Piperis Kadsurae Caulis

mollissima 寻骨风 *xún gǔ fēng* Aristolochiae Mollissimae Rhizoma seu Herba

homalomena 千年健 *qiān nián jiàn* Homalomenae Rhizoma

knotty pine wood 松节 *sōng jié* Pini Lignum Nodi

Orient vine 青风藤 *qīng fēng téng* Sinomenii seu Sabiae Caulis et Rhizoma

Japanese dioscorea 穿山龙 *chuān shān lóng* Dioscoreae Nipponicae Rhizoma

thunder god vine 雷公藤 *léi gōng téng* Tripterygii Wilfordi Radix, Folium et Flos

Jilong corydalis 夏天无 *xià tiān wú* Corydalis Decumbentis Tuber et Herba

ground pine 伸筋草 *shēn jīn cǎo* Lycopodii Clavati Herba cum Radice

Chinese tinospora 伸筋藤 *shēn jīn téng* Tinosporae Sinensis Caulis

cranesbill 老鹳草 *lǎo guàn cǎo* Geranii Herba

pyrola 鹿衔草 *lù xián cǎo* Pyrolae Herba

Aromatic Dampness-Transforming Medicinals 芳香化浊药

atractylodes 苍术 *cāng zhú* Atractylodis Rhizoma

magnolia bark 厚朴 *hòu pò* Magnoliae Cortex

magnolia flower[2] 厚朴花 *hòu pò huā* Magnoliae Flos[2]

agastache/patchouli 藿香 *huò xiāng* Agastaches seu Pogostemi Herba

eupatorium 佩兰 *pèi lán* Eupatorii Herba

amomum 砂仁 *shā rén* Amomi Semen seu Fructus

cardamom 白豆蔻 *bái dòu kòu* Amomi Cardamomi Fructus

Katsumada's galangal seed 草豆蔻 *cǎo dòu kòu* Alpiniae Katsumadae Semen

tsaoko 草果 *cǎo guǒ* Amomi Tsao-Ko Fructus

acorus 石菖蒲 *shí chāng pú* Acori Rhizoma

Water-Disinhibiting Dampness-Percolating Medicinals 利水渗湿药

poria 茯苓 *fú líng* Poria

poria skin 茯苓皮 *fú líng pí* Poriae Cortex

polyporus 猪苓 *zhū líng* Polyporus

alisma 泽泻 *zé xiè* Alismatis Rhizoma

coix 薏苡仁 *yì yǐ rén* Coicis Semen

coix root 薏苡根 *yì yǐ gēn* Coicis Radix

plantago 车前 *chē qián* Plantaginis Herba

plantago seed 车前子 *chē qián zǐ* Plantaginis Semen

talcum 滑石 *huá shí* Talcum

mutong 木通 *mù tōng* Mutong Caulis

rice-paper plant pith 通草 *tōng cǎo* Tetrapanacis Medulla

juncus 灯心草 *dēng xīn cǎo* Junci Medulla

dichondra 小金钱草 *xiǎo jīn qián cǎo* Dichondrae Herba

moneywort 金钱草 *jīn qián cǎo* Jinqiancao Herba

lygodium spore 海金沙 *hǎi jīn shā* Lygodii Spora

pyrrosia 石韦 *shí wéi* Pyrrosiae Folium

kochia 地肤子 *dì fū zǐ* Kochiae Fructus

knotgrass 萹蓄 *biǎn xù* Polygoni Avicularis Herba

dianthus 瞿麦 *qū mài* Dianthi Herba

fish poison yam 萆薢 *bì xiè* Dioscoreae Hypoglaucae Rhizoma

capillaris 茵陈蒿 *yīn chén hāo* Artemisiae Capillaris Herba

bottle gourd 壶芦 *hú lú* Lagenariae Depressae Fructus

wax gourd seed 冬瓜子 *dōng guā zǐ* Benincasae Semen

wax gourd rind 冬瓜皮 *dōng guā pí* Benincasae Exocarpium

rice bean 赤小豆 *chì xiǎo dòu* Phaseoli Calcarati Semen

sun spurge 泽漆 *zé qī* Euphorbiae Helioscopiae Herba

corn silk 玉米须 *yù mǐ xū* Mays Stylus

mallow seed 冬葵子 *dōng kuí zǐ* Malvae Verticillatae Semen

mole cricket 蝼蛄 *lóu gū* Gryllotalpa

lesser hypericum 地耳草 *dì ěr cǎo* Hyperici Japonici Herba

bushy knotweed 虎杖 *hǔ zhàng* Polygoni Cuspidati Rhizoma

Interior-Warming Medicinals 温里药

aconite 附子 *fù zǐ* Aconiti Tuber Laterale

white sliced aconite 白附片 *bái fù piàn* Aconiti Tuber Laterale Album

black sliced aconite 黑顺片 *hēi shùn piàn* Aconiti Tuber Laterale Denigratum

cooked aconite 熟附子 *shú fù zǐ* Aconiti Tuber Laterale Conquitum

salted aconite 咸附子 *xián fù zǐ* Aconiti Tuber Laterale Salsum

aconite main tuber 川乌头 *chuān wū tóu* Aconiti Tuber

wild aconite 草乌头 *cǎo wū tóu* Aconiti Tsao-Wu-Tou Tuber

cinnamon bark 肉桂 *ròu guì* Cinnamomi Cortex

dried ginger 干姜 *gān jiāng* Zingiberis Rhizoma Exsiccatum

blast-fried ginger 炮姜 *pào jiāng* Zingiberis Rhizoma Tostum

evodia 吴茱萸 *wú zhū yú* Evodiae Fructus

asarum 细辛 *xì xīn* Asiasari Herba cum Radice

zanthoxylum 花椒 *huā jiāo* Zanthoxyli Pericarpium

lesser galangal 高良姜 *gāo liáng jiāng* Alpiniae Officinarum Rhizoma

zanthoxylum seed 椒目 *jiāo mù* Zanthoxyli Semen

clove 丁香 *dīng xiāng* Caryophylli Flos

galangal fruit 红豆蔻 *hóng dòu kòu* Alpiniae Galangae Fructus

clove fruit 母丁香 *mǔ dīng xiāng* Caryophylli Fructus

pepper 胡椒 *hú jiāo* Piperis Fructus

litsea 豆豉姜 *dòu chǐ jiāng* Litseae Rhizoma et Radix

long pepper 荜茇 *bì bá* Piperis Longi Fructus

cubeb 荜澄茄 *bì chéng qié* Cubebae Fructus

fennel 茴香 *huí xiāng* Foeniculi Fructus

star anise 八角茴香 *bā jiǎo huí xiāng* Anisi Stellati Fructus

Qi-Rectifying Medicinals 理气药

tangerine peel 陈皮 *chén pí* Citri Exocarpium

white tangerine peel 橘白 *jú bái* Citri Exocarpium Album

red tangerine peel 橘红 *jú hóng* Citri Exocarpium Rubrum

tangerine pip 橘核 *jú hé* Citri Semen

tangerine pith 橘络 *jú luò* Citri Fructus Fasciculus Vascularis

tangerine leaf 橘叶 *jú yè* Citri Folium

Huazhou pomelo rind 化橘红 *huà jú hóng* Citri Grandis Exocarpium Rubrum

unripe tangerine peel 青皮 *qīng pí* Citri Exocarpium Immaturum

bitter orange 枳壳 *zhǐ ké* Aurantii Fructus

unripe bitter orange 枳实 *zhǐ shí* Aurantii Fructus Immaturus

toosendan 川楝子 *chuān liàn zǐ* Toosendan Fructus

litchee pit 荔枝核 *lì zhī hé* Litchi Semen

cyperus 香附子 *xiāng fù zǐ* Cyperi Rhizoma

saussurea 木香 *mù xiāng* Saussureae (seu Vladimiriae) Radix

Sichuan saussurea 川木香 *chuān mù xiāng* Vladimiriae Souliei Radix

costusroot 广木香 *guǎng mù xiāng* Saussureae Radix

vladimiria 青木香 *qīng mù xiāng* Vladimiriae Radix
lindera 乌药 *wū yào* Linderae Radix
Chinese chive 薤白 *xiè bái* Allii Bulbus
sandalwood 檀香 *tán xiāng* Santali Lignum
aquilaria 沉香 *chén xiāng* Aquilariae Lignum
persimmon calyx 柿蒂 *shì dì* Kaki Calyx
nardostachys 甘松 *gān sōng* Nardostachydis Rhizoma et Radix
Buddha's hand 佛手柑 *fó shǒu gān* Citri Sarcodactylidis Fructus
Buddha's hand flower 佛手花 *fó shǒu huā* Citri Sarcodactylidis Flos
sword bean pod 刀豆壳 *dāo dòu ké* Canavaliae Legumen
horse chestnut 娑罗子 *suō luó zǐ* Aesculi Fructus
akebia 八月札 *bā yuè zhá* Akebiae Fructus
rose 玫瑰花 *méi guī huā* Rosae Flos
mume flower 梅花 *méi huā* Mume Flos
stinkbug 九香虫 *jiǔ xiāng chóng* Aspongopus

Food-Dispersing Medicinals 消食药

crataegus 山楂 *shān zhā* Crataegi Fructus
medicated leaven 神麴 *shén qū* Massa Medicata Fermentata
Fujian leaven 建神麴 *jiàn shén qū* Massa Medicata Fermentata Fujianensis
barley sprout 麦芽 *mài yá* Hordei Fructus Germinatus
rice sprout 谷芽 *gǔ yá* Oryzae Fructus Germinatus
radish seed 莱菔子 *lái fú zǐ* Raphani Semen
gizzard lining 鸡内金 *jī nèi jīn* Galli Gigerii Endothelium

Worm-Expelling Medicinals 驱虫药

quisqualis 使君子 *shǐ jūn zǐ* Quisqualis Fructus
chinaberry (root) bark 苦楝皮 *kǔ liàn pí* Meliae Cortex (Radicis)
areca 槟榔 *bīng láng* Arecae Semen
areca husk 大腹皮 *dà fù pí* Arecae Pericarpium
pumpkin seed 南瓜子 *nán guā zǐ* Cucurbitae Semen
omphalia 雷丸 *léi wán* Omphalia
carpesium seed 鹤虱 *hè shī* Carpesii Fructus
torreya 榧子 *fěi zǐ* Torreyae Semen
elm cake 芜荑 *wú yí* Ulmi Fructus Praeparatio
aspidium 贯众 *guàn zhòng* Aspidii Rhizoma

Blood-Stanching Medicinals 止血药

cirsium 大蓟 *dà jì* Cirsii Herba seu Radix
cephalanoplos 小蓟 *xiǎo jì* Cephalanoploris Herba seu Radix
sanguisorba 地榆 *dì yú* Sanguisorbae Radix
ramie 苎麻根 *zhù má gēn* Boehmeriae Radix
imperata 白茅根 *bái máo gēn* Imperatae Rhizoma
sophora flower 槐花 *huái huā* Sophorae Flos

biota leaf 侧柏叶 *cè bǎi yè* Biotae Folium
dock root 羊蹄根 *yáng tí gēn* Rumicis Radix Recens
beauty-berry leaf 紫珠 *zǐ zhū* Callicarpae Folium
agrimony 仙鹤草 *xiān hè cǎo* Agrimoniae Herba
bletilla 白及 *bái jí* Bletillae Tuber
trachycarpus 棕榈皮 *zōng lǘ pí* Trachycarpi Stipulae Fibra
weed soot 百草霜 *bǎi cǎo shuāng* Herbarum Ustarum Fuligo
lotus root node 藕节 *ǒu jié* Nelumbinis Rhizomatis Nodus
copperleaf 铁苋 *tiě xiàn* Acalyphae Herba
notoginseng 三七 *sān qī* Notoginseng Radix
charred hair 血余炭 *xuè yú tàn* Hominis Crinis Carbonisatus
madder 茜草根 *qiàn cǎo gēn* Rubiae Radix
typha pollen 蒲黄 *pú huáng* Typhae Pollen
ophicalcite 花蕊石 *huā ruǐ shí* Ophicalcitum
selaginella 卷柏 *juǎn bǎi* Selaginellae Herba
oven earth 伏龙肝 *fú lóng gān* Terra Flava Usta

Stasis-Dispelling Blood-Quickening Medicinals 祛瘀活血药

ligusticum 川芎 *chuān xiōng* Ligustici Rhizoma
frankincense 乳香 *rǔ xiāng* Olibanum
myrrh 没药 *mò yào* Myrrha
raw myrrh 生没药 *shēng mò yào* Myrrha Cruda
corydalis 延胡索 *yán hú suǒ* Corydalis Tuber
curcuma 郁金 *yù jīn* Curcumae Tuber
turmeric 姜黄 *jiāng huáng* Curcumae Longae Rhizoma
zedoary 莪术 *é zhú* Zedoariae Rhizoma
sparganium 三棱 *sān léng* Sparganii Rhizoma
salvia 丹参 *dān shēn* Salviae Miltiorrhizae Radix
bushy knotweed 虎杖 *hǔ zhàng* Polygoni Cuspidati Rhizoma
leonurus 益母草 *yì mǔ cǎo* Leonuri Herba
leonurus fruit 茺蔚子 *chōng wèi zǐ* Leonuri Fructus
millettia 鸡血藤 *jī xuè téng* Millettiae Radix et Caulis
peach kernel 桃仁 *táo rén* Persicae Semen
carthamus 红花 *hóng huā* Carthami Flos
saffron 藏红花 *zàng hóng huā* Croci Stigma
flying squirrel's droppings 五灵脂 *wǔ líng zhī* Trogopteri seu Pteromydis Excrementum
achyranthes 牛膝 *niú xī* Achyranthis Bidentatae Radix
native achyranthes 土牛膝 *tǔ niú xī* Achyranthis Radix
pangolin scales 穿山甲 *chuān shān jiǎ* Manitis Squama
wingless cockroach 蟅虫 *zhè chóng* Eupolyphaga seu Opisthoplatia
leech 水蛭 *shuǐ zhì* Hirudo seu Whitmania
tabanus 虻虫 *méng chóng* Tabanus

dalbergia 降真香 *jiàng zhēn xiāng* Dalbergiae Lignum

lycopus 泽兰 *zé lán* Lycopi Herba

China tea rose 月季花 *yuè jì huā* Rosae Chinensis Flos et Fructus

campsis flower 凌霄花 *líng xiāo huā* Campsitis Flos

pyrite 自然铜 *zì rán tóng* Pyritum

vaccaria 王不留行 *wáng bù liú xíng* Vaccariae Semen

anomalous artemisia 刘寄奴 *liú jì nú* Artemisiae Anomalae Herba

sappan 苏木 *sū mù* Sappan Lignum

lacquer 干漆 *gān qī* Lacca Exsiccata

hairy holly root 毛冬青 *máo dōng qīng* Ilicis Pubescentis Radix

hairy holly root   verbena 马鞭草 *mǎ biān cǎo* Verbenae Herba (cum Radice)

centella 积雪草 *jī xuě cǎo* Centellae Herb (cum Radice)

Chinese sage 石见穿 *shí jiàn chuān* Salviae Chinensis Herba

bat's droppings 夜明砂 *yè míng shā* Vespertilionis Excrementum

spindle tree wings 鬼箭羽 *guǐ jiàn yǔ* Euonymi Lignum Suberalatum

dung beetle 蜣螂 *qiāng láng* Catharsius

Phlegm-Transforming, Cough-Suppressing, Panting-Calming Medicinals 化痰止咳平喘

Phlegm-Transforming Medicinals 化痰

pinellia 半夏 *bàn xià* Pinelliae Tuber

ginger pinellia 姜半夏 *jiāng bàn xià* Pinelliae Tuber cum Zingibere Praeparatum

arisaema 天南星 *tiān nán xīng* Arisaematis Rhizoma

bile arisaema 胆星 *dǎn xīng* Arisaematis Rhizoma cum Felle Bovis

giant typhonium tuber 禹白附 *yǔ bái fù* Typhonii Gigantei Tuber

Korean aconite 关白附 *guān bái fù* Aconiti Coreani Tuber

aconite/typhonium 白附子 *bái fù zǐ* Aconiti Coreani seu Typhonii Gigantei Tuber

white mustard 白芥子 *bái jiè zǐ* Brassicae Albae Semen

leaf mustard seed 芥子 *jiè zǐ* Brassicae Junceae Semen

gleditsia 皂荚 *zào jiá* Gleditsiae Fructus

gleditsia thorn 皂角刺 *zào jiǎo cì* Gleditsiae Spina

platycodon 桔梗 *jié gěng* Platycodonis Radix

inula 金沸草 *jīn fèi cǎo* Inulae Caulis et Folium

inula flower 旋覆花 *xuán fù huā* Inulae Flos

cynanchum 白前 *bái qián* Cynanchi Baiqian Radix et Rhizoma

peucedanum 前胡 *qián hú* Peucedani Radix

trichosanthes 栝楼 *guā lóu* Trichosanthis Fructus

trichosanthes seed 栝楼子 *guā lóu zǐ* Trichosanthis Semen

trichosanthes rind 栝楼皮 *guā lóu pí* Trichosanthis Pericarpium

Sichuan fritillaria 川贝母 *chuān bèi mǔ* Fritillariae Cirrhosae Bulbus

Zhejiang fritillaria 浙贝母 *zhè bèi mǔ* Fritillariae Verticillatae Bulbus

bamboo shavings 竹茹 *zhú rú* Bambusae Caulis in Taeniam

bamboo sugar 天竹黄 *tiān zhú huáng* Bambusae Concretio Silicea

dried bamboo sap 竹沥 *zhú lì* Bambusae Succus Exsiccatus

pumice 海浮石 *hǎi fú shí* Pumex

clamshell 海蛤壳 *hǎi gé ké* Cyclinae (seu Meretricis) Concha

chlorite/mica 礞石 *méng shí* Chloriti seu Micae Lapis

sargassum 海藻 *hǎi zǎo* Sargassi Herba

kelp 昆布 *kūn bù* Algae Thallus

eelgrass 海带 *hǎi dài* Zosterae Marinae Herba

air potato 黄药子 *huáng yào zǐ* Dioscoreae Bulbiferae Tuber

sterculia 胖大海 *pàng dà hài* Sterculiae Semen

pig's bile 猪胆汁 *zhū dǎn zhī* Suis Bilis

rorippa 薸菜 *hān cài* Rorippae Herba seu Flos

changium root 明党参 *míng dǎng shēn* Changii Radix

Grosvenor's momordica 罗汉果 *luó hàn guǒ* Momordicae Grosvenori Fructus

water chestnut 荸荠 *bí qí* Heleocharitis Cormus

chicken's egg membrane 凤凰衣 *fèng huáng yī* Galli Membrana Ovi

Cough-Suppressing Panting-Calming Medicinals 止咳化痰药

apricot kernel 杏仁 *xìng rén* Armeniacae Semen

sweet apricot kernel 甜杏仁 *tián xìng rén* Armeniacae Semen Dulce

almond 巴旦杏仁 *bā dàn xìng rén* Pruni Amygdali Semen

stemona 百部 *bǎi bù* Stemonae Radix

aster 紫菀 *zǐ wǎn* Asteris Radix et Rhizoma

tussilago 款冬花 *kuǎn dōng huā* Tussilaginis Flos

perilla seed 紫苏子 *zǐ sū zǐ* Perillae Fructus

mulberry root bark 桑白皮 *sāng bái pí* Mori Radicis Cortex

tingli 葶苈子 *tíng lì zǐ* Descurainiae seu Lepidii Semen

loquat leaf 枇杷叶 *pí pá yè* Eriobotryae Folium

aristolochia fruit 马兜铃 *mǎ dōu líng* Aristolochiae Fructus

Japanese ardisia 紫金牛 *zǐ jīn niú* Ardisiae Japonicae Caulis et Folium

ginkgo 白果 *bái guǒ* Ginkgo Semen

datura flower 洋金花 *yáng jīn huā* Daturae Flos

physochlaina 华山参 *huá shān shēn* Physochlainae Radix

stalactite 钟乳石 *zhōng rǔ shí* Stalactitum

powdered stalactite 钟乳粉 *zhōng rǔ fěn* Stalactitum Pulveratum

Daurian rhododendron 满山红 *mǎn shān hóng* Rhododendri Daurici Folium

goose throat stone 鹅管石 *é guǎn shí* Balanophyllia seu Stalactitum

Spirit-Quieting Medicinals 安神药

Heavy settling spirit-quieting medicinals 重镇安神药

cinnabar 朱砂 *zhū shā* Cinnabaris

loadstone 磁石 *cí shí* Magnetitum

dragon bone 龙骨 *lóng gǔ* Mastodi Ossis Fossilia

dragon tooth 龙齿 *lóng chǐ* Mastodi Dentis Fossilia

oyster shell 牡蛎 *mǔ lì* Ostreae Concha

amber 琥珀 *hǔ pò* Succinum

mother-of-pearl 珍珠母 *zhēn zhū mǔ* Concha Margaritifera

pearl 珍珠 *zhēn zhū* Margarita

amethyst/fluorite 紫石英 *zǐ shí yīng* Amethystum seu Fluoritum

Heart-nourishing spirit-quieting medicinals 养心安神药

spiny jujube 酸枣仁 *suān zǎo rén* Ziziphi Spinosi Semen

biota seed 柏子仁 *bǎi zǐ rén* Biotae Semen

polygala 远志 *yuǎn zhì* Polygalae Radix

root poria 茯神 *fú shén* Poria cum Pini Radice

flowery knotweed stem 夜交藤 *yè jiāo téng* Polygoni Multiflori Caulis

longan flesh 龙眼肉 *lóng yǎn ròu* Longanae Arillus

lotus fruit/seed 莲子 *lián zǐ* Nelumbinis Fructus seu Semen

schisandra 五味子 *wǔ wèi zǐ* Schisandrae Fructus

silk tree bark 合欢皮 *hé huān pí* Albizziae Cortex

dwarf magnolia 夜合花 *yè hé huā* Magnoliae Coco Flos

ganoderma 灵芝 *líng zhī* Ganoderma

Liver-Calming Wind-Extinguishing Medicinals 平肝熄风药

antelope horn 羚羊角 *líng yáng jiǎo* Antelopis Cornu

goral horn 山羊角 *shān yáng jiǎo* Naemorhedi Goral Cornu

abalone shell 石决明 *shí jué míng* Haliotidis Concha

oyster shell 牡蛎 *mǔ lì* Ostreae Concha

crude oyster shell 生牡蛎 *shēng mǔ lì* Ostreae Concha Cruda

pearl 珍珠 *zhēn zhū* Margarita

mother-of-pearl 珍珠母 *zhēn zhū mǔ* Concha Margaritifera

hawksbill shell 玳瑁 *dài mào* Eretmochelydis Carapax

purple cowrie 紫贝 *zǐ bèi* Mauritiae, Erosariae seu Cypraeae Testa

hematite 代赭石 *dài zhě shí* Haematitum

uncaria 钩藤 *gōu téng* Uncariae Ramulus cum Unco

gastrodia 天麻 *tiān má* Gastrodiae Rhizoma

tribulus 刺蒺藜 *cì jí lí* Tribuli Fructus

black soybean 黑大豆 *hēi dà dòu* Glycines Semen Atrum

scorpion 全蝎 *quán xiē* Buthus

centipede 蜈蚣 *wú gōng* Scolopendra

silkworm 白僵蚕 *bái jiāng cán* Bombyx Batryticatus

earthworm 地龙 *dì lóng* Lumbricus

iron flakes 铁落 *tiě luò* Ferri Frusta

Orifice-Opening Medicinals 开窍药

musk 麝香 *shè xiāng* Moschus

borneol 冰片 *bīng piàn* Borneolum

liquid storax 苏合香 *sū hé xiāng* Styrax Liquidus

acorus 石菖蒲 *shí chāng pú* Acori Rhizoma

Supplementing Medicinals 补气药

Qi-Supplementing Medicinals

ginseng 人参 *rén shēn* Ginseng Radix

red ginseng 红参 *hóng shēn* Ginseng Radix Rubra

Korean ginseng 高丽参 *gāo lì shēn* Ginseng Radix Coreensis

American ginseng 西洋参 *xī yáng shēn* Panacis Quinquefolii Radix

codonopsis 党参 *dǎng shēn* Codonopsitis Radix

pseudostellaria 太子参 *tài zǐ shēn* Pseudostellariae Radix

astragalus 黄芪 *huáng qí* Astragali (seu Hedysari) Radix

ovate atractylodes 白术 *bái zhú* Atractylodis Ovatae Rhizoma

dioscorea 山药 *shān yào* Dioscoreae Rhizoma

lablab 扁豆 *biǎn dòu* Lablab Semen'

licorice 甘草 *gān cǎo* Glycyrrhizae Radix

jujube 大枣 *dà zǎo* Ziziphi Fructus

malt sugar 饴糖 *yí táng* Granorum Saccharon

honey 蜜 *mì* Mel

Yang-Supplementing Medicinals 补阳药

velvet deerhorn 鹿茸 *lù róng* Cervi Cornu Parvum

deerhorn 鹿角 *lù jiǎo* Cervi Cornu

deerhorn glue 鹿角胶 *lù jiǎo jiāo* Cervi Gelatinum Cornu

degelatinated deerhorn 鹿角霜 *lù jiǎo shuāng* Cervi Cornu Degelatinatum

dog's penis 牡狗阴茎 *mǔ gǒu yīn jīng* Canis Penis

placenta 紫河车 *zǐ hé chē* Hominis Placenta

gecko 蛤蚧 *gé jiè* Gekko

cordyceps 冬虫夏草 *dōng chóng xià cǎo* Cordyceps

walnut 胡桃仁 *hú táo rén* Juglandis Semen

cistanche 肉苁蓉 *ròu cōng róng* Cistanches Caulis
cynomorium 锁阳 *suǒ yáng* Cynomorii Caulis
morinda 巴戟天 *bā jǐ tiān* Morindae Radix
epimedium 淫羊藿 *yín yáng huò* Epimedii Herba
curculigo 仙茅 *xiān máo* Curculiginis Rhizoma
eucommia 杜仲 *dù zhòng* Eucommiae Cortex
dipsacus 续断 *xù duàn* Dipsaci Radix
cibotium 狗脊 *gǒu jǐ* Cibotii Rhizoma
drynaria 骨碎补 *gǔ suì bǔ* Drynariae Rhizoma
psoralea 补骨脂 *bǔ gǔ zhī* Psoraleae Semen
alpinia 益智仁 *yì zhì rén* Alpiniae Oxyphyllae Fructus
complanate astragalus seed 沙苑子 *shā yuàn zǐ* Astragali Complanati Semen
cuscuta 菟丝子 *tù sī zǐ* Cuscutae Semen
Chinese leek 韭菜 *jiǔ cài* Allii Tuberosi Folium
Chinese leek seed 韭子 *jiǔ zǐ* Allii Tuberosi Semen
fenugreek 胡芦巴 *hú lú bā* Foeni-Graeci Semen
actinolite 阳起石 *yáng qǐ shí* Actinolitum

Blood-Supplementing Medicinals 补血药

tangkuei 当归 *dāng guī* Angelicae Sinensis Radix
cooked rehmannia 熟地黄 *shú dì huáng* Rehmanniae Radix Conquita
flowery knotweed 何首乌 *hé shǒu wū* Polygoni Multiflori Radix
flowery knotweed stem 夜交藤 *yè jiāo téng* Polygoni Multiflori Caulis
white peony 白芍药 *bái sháo yào* Paeoniae Radix Alba
ass hide glue 阿胶 *ē jiāo* Asini Corii Gelatinum
longan flesh 龙眼肉 *lóng yǎn ròu* Longanae Arillus
millettia 鸡血藤 *jī xuè téng* Millettiae Radix et Caulis

Yin-Supplementing Medicinals 补阴药

glehnia 北沙参 *běi shā shēn* Glehniae Radix
adenophora 南沙参 *nán shā shēn* Adenophorae Radix
adenophora/glehnia 沙参 *shā shēn* Adenophorae seu Glehniae Radix
ophiopogon 麦门冬 *mài mén dōng* Ophiopogonis Tuber
asparagus 天门冬 *tiān mén dōng* Asparagi Tuber
dendrobium 石斛 *shí hú* Dendrobii Caulis
Solomon's seal 玉竹 *yù zhú* Polygonati Yuzhu Rhizoma
polygonatum 黄精 *huáng jīng* Polygonati Huangjing Rhizoma
lily bulb 百合 *bǎi hé* Lilii Bulbus
lycium berry 枸杞子 *gǒu qǐ zǐ* Lycii Fructus
mulberry 桑椹 *sāng shèn* Mori Fructus
eclipta 墨旱莲 *mò hàn lián* Ecliptae Herba
ligustrum 女贞子 *nǚ zhēn zǐ* Ligustri Fructus
tortoise plastron 龟版 *guī bǎn* Testudinis Plastrum
tortoise plastron glue 龟版胶 *guī bǎn jiāo* Testudinis Plastri Gelatinum
turtle shell 鳖甲 *biē jiǎ* Amydae Carapax

turtle shell glue 鳖甲胶 *biē jiǎ jiāo* Amydae Carapacis Gelatinum
black sesame 黑脂麻 *hēi zhī má* Sesami Semen Atrum

Astringent Medicinals 收涩药

schisandra 五味子 *wǔ wèi zǐ* Schisandrae Fructus
mume 乌梅 *wū méi* Mume Fructus
sumac gallnut 五倍子 *wǔ bèi zǐ* Rhois Galla
light wheat 浮小麦 *fú xiǎo mài* Tritici Semen Leve
ephedra root 麻黄根 *má huáng gēn* Ephedrae Radix
glutinous rice root 糯稻根须 *nuò dào gēn xū* Oryzae Glutinosae Rhizoma et Radix
pomegranate rind 石榴皮 *shí liú pí* Granati Pericarpium
chebule 诃子 *hē zǐ* Chebulae Fructus
nutmeg 肉豆蔻 *ròu dòu kòu* Myristicae Semen
halloysite 赤石脂 *chì shí zhī* Halloysitum Rubrum
limonite 禹余粮 *yǔ yú liáng* Limonitum
poppy husk 罂粟壳 *yīng sù ké* Papaveris Pericarpium
lotus seed 莲肉 *lián ròu* Nelumbinis Semen
lotus fruit/seed 莲子 *lián zǐ* Nelumbinis Fructus seu Semen
lotus receptacle 莲房 *lián fáng* Nelumbinis Receptaculum
lotus stamen 莲须 *lián xū* Nelumbinis Stamen
euryale 芡实 *qiàn shí* Euryales Semen
cornus 山茱萸 *shān zhū yú* Corni Fructus
Cherokee rose fruit 金樱子 *jīn yīng zǐ* Rosae Laevigatae Fructus
mantis egg-case 桑螵蛸 *sāng piāo xiāo* Mantidis Oötheca
rubus 覆盆子 *fù pén zǐ* Rubi Fructus
cuttlefish bone 海螵蛸 *hǎi piāo xiāo* Sepiae seu Sepiellae Os
hedgehog's pelt 刺猬皮 *cì wèi pí* Erinacei Pellis

Ejection Medicinals 涌吐药

melon stalk 瓜蒂 *guā dì* Cucumeris Melonis Pedicellus
dichroa 常山 *cháng shān* Dichroae Radix
dichroa leaf 蜀漆 *shǔ qī* Dichroae Folium
chalcanthite 胆矾 *dǎn fán* Chalcanthitum
veratrum 藜芦 *lí lú* Veratri Radix et Rhizoma
ginseng top 人参芦 *rén shēn lú* Ginseng Rhizoma
gleditsia 皂荚 *zào jiá* Gleditsiae Fructus

Medicinals for External Use 外用药

sulfur 石硫黄 *shí liú huáng* Sulphur
realgar 雄黄 *xióng huáng* Realgar
orpiment 雌黄 *cī huáng* Auripigmentum
arsenic 砒石 *pī shí* Arsenicum
calomel 轻粉 *qīng fěn* Calomelas
upborne elixir 升丹 *shēng dān* Sublimatum Triplex

minium 铅丹 *qiān dān* Minium
litharge 密陀僧 *mì tuó sēng* Lithargyrum
smithsonite 炉甘石 *lú gān shí* Smithsonitum
borax 硼砂 *péng shā* Borax
alum 白矾 *bái fán* Alumen
melanterite 绿矾 *lù fán* Melanteritum
limestone 石灰 *shí huī* Calx
niter 硝石 *xiāo shí* Nitrum
sal ammoniac 硇砂 *náo shā* Sal Ammoniacum
Japanese ranunculus 毛茛 *máo gèn* Ranunculi
  Japonici Herba et Radix
garlic 大蒜 *dà suàn* Allii Sativi Bulbus
mylabris 斑蝥 *bān máo* Mylabris
toad venom 蟾酥 *chán sū* Bufonis Venenum
nux vomica 马钱子 *mǎ qián zǐ* Nux-Vomicae Semen
momordica 木鳖子 *mù biē zǐ* Momordicae Semen
cnidium seed 蛇床子 *shé chuáng zǐ* Cnidii Monnieri Fructus
hornet's nest 露蜂房 *lù fēng fáng* Vespae Nidus
cotton rose 木芙蓉花 *mù fú róng huā* Hibisci Mutabilis Flos

cotton rose leaf 木芙蓉叶 *mù fú róng yè* Hibisci
  Mutabilis Folium
hydnocarpus 大风子 *dà fēng zǐ* Hydnocarpi Semen
rose-of-Sharon root bark 木槿皮 *mù jǐn pí* Hibisci
  Syriaci Radicis Cortex
golden larch (root) bark 土荆皮 *tǔ jīng pí* Pseudolaricis Kaempferi Cortex (Radicis)
rose-of-Sharon 木槿花 *mù jǐn huā* Hibisci Syriaci
  Flos
loofah 丝瓜络 *sī guā luò* Luffae Fasciculus Vascularis
Chinese wolfsbane 狼毒 *láng dú* Stellerae seu Euphorbiae Radix
dragon's blood 血竭 *xuè jié* Daemonoropis Draconis Resina
camphor 樟脑 *zhāng nǎo* Camphora
rosin 松香 *sōng xiāng* Pini Resina
cutch 孩儿茶 *hái ér chá* Catechu
ark shell 瓦楞子 *wǎ léng zǐ* Arcae Concha
house lizard 壁虎 *bì hǔ* Gekko Swinhoana
elephant's hide 象皮 *xiàng pí* Elephantis Corium
insect wax 虫白腊 *chóng bái là* Ericeri Pelae Cera

Appendix III: A Classified List of Formulas

Exterior-Resolving Formulas 解表剂

Resolve the exterior with warmth and acridity 辛温解表

Scallion and Fermented Soybean Decoction 葱豉汤 *cōng chǐ tāng*

Major Notopterygium Decoction 大羌活汤 *dà qiāng huó tāng*

Major Green-Blue Dragon Decoction 大青龙汤 *dà qīng lóng tāng*

Pueraria Decoction 葛根汤 *gé gēn tāng*

Cinnamon Twig Decoction Plus Pueraria 桂枝加葛根汤 *guì zhī jiā gé gēn tāng*

Cinnamon Twig Decoction Plus Magnolia Bark and Apricot Kernel 桂枝加厚朴杏仁汤 *guì zhī jiā hòu pò xìng rén tāng*

Cinnamon Twig Decoction Plus Peony 桂枝加芍药汤 *guì zhī jiā sháo yào tāng*

Cinnamon Twig Decoction 桂枝汤 *guì zhī tāng*

Book of Life Scallion and Fermented Soybean Decoction 活人葱豉汤 *huó rén cōng chǐ tāng*

Book of Life Renewal Elsholtzia Powder 活人香薷散 *huó rén xiāng rú yǐn*

Supplemented Cyperus and Perilla Powder 加味香苏散 *jiā wèi xiāng sū sǎn*

Schizonepeta and Ledebouriella Toxin-Vanquishing Powder 荆防败毒散 *jīng fáng bài dú sǎn*

Schizonepeta and Ledebouriella Decoction 荆防汤 *jīng fáng tāng*

Nine-Ingredient Notopterygium Decoction 九味羌活汤 *jiǔ wèi qiāng huó tāng*

Scallion with Root Decoction 连须葱白汤 *lián xū cōng bái tāng*

Six-Ingredient Elsholtzia Beverage 六味香薷饮 *liù wèi xiāng rú yǐn*

Ephedra Decoction Plus Ovate Atractylodes 麻黄加术汤 *má huáng jiā zhú tāng*

Ephedra Decoction 麻黄汤 *má huáng tāng*

Ephedra, Apricot Kernel, Coix, and Licorice Decoction 麻杏薏甘汤 *má xìng yì gān tāng*

Rough and Ready Three Decoction 三拗汤 *sān ào tāng*

Three-Agent Elsholtzia Powder 三物香薷饮 *sān wù xiāng rú yǐn*

Wondrous Atractylodes Powder 神术散 *shén zhú sǎn*

Four-Ingredient Elsholtzia Beverage 四味香薷饮 *sì wèi xiāng rú yǐn*

Five Agents Elsholtzia Beverage 五物香薷饮 *wǔ wù xiāng rú yǐn*

Elsholtzia Powder 香薷散 *xiāng rú sǎn*

Elsholtzia Decoction 香薷汤 *xiāng rú tāng*

Cyperus and Perilla Powder 香苏散 *xiāng sū sǎn*

Yang Dawn Decoction 阳旦汤 *yáng dàn*

Resolve the exterior with coolness and acridity 辛凉解表

Bupleurum and Pueraria Flesh-Resolving Decoction 柴葛解肌汤 *chái gé jiě jī tāng*

Scallion, Fermented Soybean, and Platycodon Decoction 葱豉桔梗汤 *cōng chǐ jié gěng tāng*

Duckweed and Scutellaria Decoction 浮萍黄芩汤 *fú píng huáng qín tāng*

Pueraria Flesh-Resolving Decoction 干葛解肌汤 *gān gé jiě jī tāng*

Common Cold Formula 2 感冒二方 *gǎn mào èr fāng*

Supplemented Ephedra, Apricot Kernel, Gypsum, and Licorice Decoction 加味麻杏石甘汤 *jiā wèi má xìng shí gān tāng*

Ephedra, Apricot Kernel, Licorice, and Gypsum Decoction 麻杏甘石汤 *má xìng gān shí tāng*, also called Ephedra, Apricot Kernel, Gypsum, and Licorice Decoction (*má xìng shí gān tāng*), and Ephedra, Apricot Kernel, Gypsum, and Licorice Decoction (*má huáng xìng rén shí gāo gān cǎo tāng*)

Notopterygium and Isatis Root Decoction 羌蓝汤 *qiāng lán tāng*

Mulberry Leaf and Chrysanthemum Beverage 桑菊饮 *sāng jú yǐn*

Cimicifuga and Pueraria Decoction 升麻葛根汤 *shēng má gé gēn tāng*

Iron Flute Pill 铁笛丸 *tiě dí wán*

Broken Flute Pill 响声破笛丸 *xiǎng shēng pò dí wán*

Newly Supplemented Elsholtzia Beverage 新加香薷饮 *xīn jiā xiāng rú yǐn*

Toxin-Diffusing Exterior-Effusing Decoction 宣毒发表汤 *xuān dú fā biǎo tāng*

Lonicera, Forsythia, and Puffball Powder 银翘马勃散 *yín qiào mǎ bó sǎn*

Lonicera and Forsythia Powder 银翘散 *yín qiào sǎn*

Lonicera and Forsythia Decoction 银翘汤 *yín qiào tāng*

Spleen-Effusing Decoction 越婢汤 *yuè bì tāng*

Bamboo Leaf, Tamarisk, and Arctium Decoction 竹叶柳蒡汤 *zhú yè liǔ bàng tāng*

Enrich yin and resolve the exterior 滋阴解表

Tangkuei and Pueraria Decoction 归葛汤 *guī gé tāng*

Solomon's Seal Variant Decoction 加减葳蕤汤 *jiā jiǎn wēi ruí tāng*

Scallion White Seven-Ingredient Beverage 葱白七味饮 *cōng bái qī wèi yǐn* (nourishes the blood and resolves the exterior)

**Assist yang and resolve the exterior
助阳解表**

Ephedra, Aconite, and Licorice Decoction 麻黄附子甘草汤 *má huáng fù zǐ gān cǎo tāng*

Ephedra, Aconite, and Asarum Decoction 麻黄附子细辛汤 *má huáng fù zǐ xì xīn tāng*

Renewal Powder 再造散 *zài zào sǎn*

**Boosting qi and resolve the exterior
益气解表**

Old Rice Granary Powder 仓廪散 *cāng lǐn sǎn*

Ginseng Toxin-Vanquishing Powder 人参败毒散 *rén shēn bài dú sǎn*

Ginseng and Perilla Beverage 参苏饮 *shēn sū yǐn*

Ten-Ingredient Elsholtzia Beverage 十味香薷饮 *shí wèi xiāng rú yǐn*

Resolve both exterior and interior 表里双解

Major Bupleurum Decoction 大柴胡汤 *dà chái hú tāng*

Ledebouriella Sage-Inspired Powder 防风通圣散 *fáng fēng tōng shèng sǎn*

Cinnamon Twig Decoction Plus Rhubarb 桂枝加大黄汤 *guì zhī jiā dà huáng tāng*

Magnolia Bark Seven Agents Decoction 厚朴七物汤 *hòu pò qī wù tāng*

Three Yellows and Gypsum Decoction 三黄石膏汤 *sān huáng shí gāo tāng*

Gypsum Decoction 石膏汤 *shí gāo tāng*

Five Accumulations Powder 五积散 *wǔ jī sǎn*

Heat-Clearing Formulas 清热剂

Clear qi-aspect heat 清气分热

White Tiger Decoction Plus Rehmannia 白虎加地黄汤 *bái hǔ jiā dì huáng tāng*

White Tiger Decoction Plus Cinnamon Twig 白虎加桂枝汤 *bái hǔ jiā guì zhī tāng*

White Tiger Decoction Plus Ginseng 白虎加人参汤 *bái hǔ jiā rén shēn tāng*

White Tiger Decoction 白虎汤 *bái hǔ tāng*

Counterflow-Settling White Tiger Decoction 镇逆白虎汤 *zhèn nì bái hǔ tāng*

Gardenia and Fermented Soybean Decoction 栀子豉汤 *zhī zǐ chǐ tāng*

Gardenia, Licorice, and Fermented Soybean Decoction 栀子甘草豉汤 *zhī zǐ gān cǎo chǐ tāng*

Gardenia and Magnolia Bark Decoction 栀子厚朴汤 *zhī zǐ hòu pò tāng*

Gardenia, Fresh Ginger, and Fermented Soybean Decoction 栀子生姜豉汤 *zhī zǐ shēng jiāng chǐ tāng*

Bamboo Leaf and Gypsum Decoction 竹叶石膏汤 *zhú yè shí gāo tāng*

**Clear construction and cool the blood
清营凉血**

Jade Lady Variant Brew 加减玉女煎 *jiā jiǎn yù nǚ jiān*

Schizonepeta and Scutellaria Four Agents Decoction 荆芩四物汤 *jīng qín sì wù tāng*

Scutellaria and Coptis Four Agents Decoction 芩连四物汤 *qín lián sì wù tāng*

Palace-Clearing Decoction 清宫汤 *qīng gōng tāng*

Construction-Clearing Decoction 清营汤 *qīng yíng tāng*

Three Yellows Four Agents Decoction 三黄四物汤 *sān huáng sì wù tāng*

Four Agents Decoction Plus Scutellaria and Coptis 四物加黄芩黄连汤 *sì wù jiā huáng qín huáng lián tāng*

Rhinoceros Horn and Rehmannia Network-Clearing Beverage 犀地清络饮 *xī dì qīng luò yǐn*

Rhinoceros Horn and Rehmannia Decoction 犀角地黄汤 *xī jiǎo dì huáng tāng*

Premature Periods Decoction 先期汤 *xiān qí tāng*

Eye Stasis Formula 瘀血灌眼睛方 *yū xuè guàn yǎn jīng fāng*

Clear both qi and construction 气营两清

Black Paste (Formula) 黑膏（方）*hēi gāo (fāng)*

Macule-Transforming Decoction 化斑汤 *huà bān tāng*

Scourge-Clearing Toxin-Vanquishing Beverage 清瘟败毒饮 *qīng wēn bài dú yǐn*

Clear heat and resolve summerheat 清热解暑

Jasper Jade Powder 碧玉散 *bì yù sǎn*

Cinnamon and Poria (Hoelen) Sweet Dew Beverage 桂苓甘露饮 *guì líng gān lù yǐn*

Mint Powder 鸡苏散 *jī sū sǎn*

Li's Summerheat-Clearing Qi-Boosting Decoction 李氏清暑益气汤 *lǐ shì qīng shǔ yì qì tāng*

Six-to-One Powder 六一散 *liù yī sǎn*

Network-Clearing Beverage 清络饮 *qīng luò yǐn*

Summerheat-Clearing Qi-Boosting Decoction 清暑益气汤 *qīng shǔ yì qì tāng*

Wang's Summerheat-Clearing Qi-Boosting Decoction 王氏清暑益气汤 *wáng shì qīng shǔ yì qì tāng*

Origin-Boosting Powder 益元散 *yì yuán sǎn*

Clear heat and resolve toxin 清热解毒

Isatis Root and Leaf Decoction 板蓝大青汤 *bǎn lán dà qīng tāng*

Common Cold Fever-Abating Granules 感冒退热冲剂 *gǎn mào tuì rè chōng jì*

Macule-Transforming Toxin-Resolving Decoction 化斑解毒汤 *huà bān jiě dú tāng*

Coptis Toxin-Resolving Decoction 黄连解毒汤 *huáng lián jiě dú tāng*

Heat-Resolving Blood-Dissipating Decoction 解热散血汤 *jiě rè sàn xuè tāng*

Diphtheria Mixture 抗白喉合剂 *kàng bái hóu hé jì*

Universal Aid Toxin-Dispersing Beverage 普济消毒饮 *pǔ jì xiāo dú yǐn*

Universal Aid Toxin-Dispersing Beverage Minus Cimicifuga, Bupleurum, Scutellaria, & Coptis 普济消毒饮去升麻柴胡黄芩黄连方 *pǔ jì xiāo dú yǐn qù shēng má chái hú huáng qín huáng lián*

Clearing Resolution Tablet 清解片 *qīng jiě piàn*

Brightness Pill 宣明丸 *xuān míng wán*

Scrophularia Toxin-Resolving Decoction 玄参解毒汤 *xuán shēn jiě dú tāng*

Scrophularia and Cimicifuga Decoction 玄参升麻汤 *xuán shēn shēng má tāng*

Lonicera and Scutellaria Tablet 银黄片 *yín huáng piàn*

Encephalitis Formula 治乙脑方 *zhì yǐ nǎo fāng*

Clear and Quiet Pill 清宁丸 *qīng níng wán*

Clear organ heat 清脏腑热

Pulsatilla Decoction 白头翁汤 *bái tóu wēng tāng*

Bupleurum Liver-Clearing Powder 柴胡清肝散 *chái hú qīng gān sǎn*

Tangkuei, Gentian, and Aloe Pill 当归龙荟丸 *dāng guī lóng huì wán*

Red-Abducting Powder 导赤散 *dǎo chì sǎn*

Deafness Pill 耳聋丸 *ěr lóng wán*

Licorice and Gardenia Decoction 甘草栀子汤 *gān cǎo zhī zǐ tāng*

Sweet Dew Beverage 甘露饮 *gān lù yǐn*

Pueraria, Scutellaria, and Coptis Decoction 葛根黄芩黄连汤 *gé gēn huáng qín huáng lián tāng*

Coptis and Goat's Liver Pill 黄连羊肝丸 *huáng lián yáng gān wán*

Scutellaria Decoction 黄芩汤 *huáng qín tāng*

Supplemented Pulsatilla Decoction 加味白头翁汤 *jiā wèi bái tóu wēng tāng*

Bacillary Dysentery Herbal Formula 菌痢草药方 *jùn lì cǎo yào fāng*

Coptis and Aconite Six-to-One Decoction 连附六一汤 *lián fù liù yī tāng*

Diaphragm-Cooling Forsythia Powder 凉膈连翘散 *liáng gé lián qiào sǎn*

Diaphragm-Cooling Powder 凉膈散 *liáng gé sǎn*

Gentian Liver-Draining Decoction 龙胆泻肝汤 *lóng dǎn xiè gān tāng*

Lung-Clearing Drink 清肺饮子 *qīng fèi yǐn zǐ*

Stomach-Clearing Powder 清胃散 *qīng wèi sǎn*

Heart-Clearing Lotus Seed Beverage 清心莲子饮 *qīng xīn lián zǐ yǐn*

Dizziness-Clearing Beverage 清眩饮 *qīng xuàn yǐn*

Pancreas-Clearing Formula No.2 清胰二号 *qīng yí èr hào*

Pancreas-Clearing Formula No.1 清胰一号 *qīng yí yī hào*

Peony Decoction 芍药汤 *sháo yào tāng*

Heat-Abating Powder 退热散 *tuì rè sǎn*

Rhinoceros Horn Powder 犀角散 *xī jiǎo sǎn*

Saussurea and Coptis Pill 香连丸 *xiāng lián wán*

White-Draining Powder 泻白散 *xiè bái sǎn*

Liver-Draining Spirit-Quieting Pill 泻肝安神丸 *xiè gān ān shén wán*

Yellow-Draining Powder 泻黄散 *xiè huáng sǎn*

Spleen-Draining Powder 泻脾散 *xiè pí sǎn*

Green-Blue–Draining Pill 泻青丸 *xiè qīng wán*

Heart-Draining Decoction 泻心汤 *xiè xīn tāng*

Jade Lady Brew 玉女煎 *yù nǚ jiān*

Anemarrhena Beverage 知母饮 *zhī mǔ yǐn*

Gardenia and Phellodendron Decoction 栀子柏皮汤 *zhī zǐ bǎi pí tāng*

Bamboo Leaf Decoction 竹叶汤 *zhú yè tāng*

Left-Running Metal Pill 左金丸 *zuǒ jīn wán*

Clear vacuity heat 清虚热

Tangkuei Six Yellows Decoction 当归六黄汤 *dāng guī liù huáng tāng*

Lycium Root Bark Beverage 地骨皮饮 *dì gǔ pí yǐn*

Rehmannia and Lycium Root Bark Decoction 两地汤 *liǎng dì tāng*

Large Gentian and Turtle Shell Powder 秦艽鳖甲散 *qín jiāo biē jiǎ sǎn*

Large Gentian Emaciation Decoction 秦艽扶羸汤 *qín jiāo fú léi tāng*

Bone-Clearing Powder 清骨散 *qīng gǔ sǎn*

Sweet Wormwood and Turtle Shell Decoction 青蒿鳖甲汤 *qīng hāo biē jiǎ tāng*

Channel-Clearing (Menses-Clearing) Decoction (Powder) 清经汤（散）*qīng jīng tāng (sǎn)*

Anemarrhena, Phellodendron, and Rehmannia Pill 知柏地黄丸 *zhī bǎi dì huáng wán*

Yin-Enriching Fire-Downbearing Decoction 滋阴降火汤 *zī yīn jiàng huǒ tāng*

Precipitant Formulas 泻下剂

Cold precipitation 寒下

White Tiger Qi-Coordinating Decoction 白虎承气汤 *bái hǔ chéng qì tāng*

Major Qi-Coordinating Decoction 大承气汤 *dà chéng qì tāng*

Major Chest Bind Decoction 大陷胸汤 *dà xiàn xiōng tāng*

Major Chest Bind Pill 大陷胸丸 *dà xiàn xiōng wán*

Red-Abducting Qi-Coordinating Decoction 导赤承气汤 *dǎo chì chéng qì tāng*

Compound Formula Major Qi-Coordinating Decoction 复方大承气汤 *fù fāng dà chéng qì tāng*

Magnolia Bark Three Agents Decoction 厚朴三物汤 *hòu pò sān wù tāng*

Three-in-One Qi-Coordinating Decoction 三一承气汤 *sān yī chéng qì tāng*

Stomach-Regulating Qi-Coordinating Decoction 调胃承气汤 *tiáo wèi chéng qì tāng*

Minor Qi-Coordinating Decoction 小承气汤 *xiǎo chéng qì tāng*

White-Diffusing Qi-Coordinating Decoction 宣白承气汤 *xuān bái chéng qì tāng*

Warm precipitation 温下

Pinellia and Sulfur Pill 半硫丸 *bàn liú wán*

Rhubarb and Aconite Decoction 大黄附子汤 *dà huáng fù zǐ tāng*

Three Agents White Powder 三物白散 *sān wù bái sǎn*

Three Agents Emergency Pill 三物备急丸 *sān wù bèi jí wán*

Three Agents Little White Powder 三物小白散 *sān wù xiǎo bái sǎn*

Spleen-Warming Decoction 温脾汤 *wēn pí tāng*

Moist precipitation 润下

Toilette Pill 更衣丸 *gēng yī wán*

Ferry Brew 济川煎 *jì chuān jiān*

Hemp Seed Pill 麻子仁丸 *má zǐ rén wán*

Intestine-Moistening Decoction 润肠汤 *rùn cháng tāng*

Intestine-Moistening Pill 润肠丸 *rùn cháng wán*

Five Kernels Decoction 五仁汤 *wǔ rén tāng*

Five Kernels Pill 五仁丸 *wǔ rén wán*

Simultaneous supplementation and attack 攻补兼施

Qi-Coordinating Construction-Nourishing Decoction 承气养营汤 *chéng qì yǎng yíng tāng*

Yellow Dragon Decoction 黄龙汤 *huáng lóng tāng*

Newly Supplemented Yellow Dragon Decoction 新加黄龙汤 *xīn jiā huáng lóng tāng*

Jade Candle Powder 玉烛散 *yù zhú sǎn*

Humor-Increasing Qi-Coordinating Decoction 增液承气汤 *zēng yè chéng qì tāng*

Expel water 逐水

Fangji, Zanthoxylum, Tingli, and Rhubarb Pill 己椒苈黄丸 *jǐ jiāo lì huáng wán*

Radish Seed and Magnolia Bark Bind-Freeing Decoction 莱朴通结汤 *lái pò tōng jié tāng*

Three Flowers Spirit Protection Pill 三花神佑丸 *sān huā shén yòu wán*

Ten Jujubes Decoction 十枣汤 *shí zǎo tāng*

Caper Spurge Seed Pill 续随子丸 *xù suí zǐ wán*

Water Controller Yu Powder 禹功散 *yǔ gōng sǎn*

Boats and Carts Pill 舟车丸 *zhōu chē (jū) wán*

Young Dragon Pill 子龙丸 *zǐ lóng wán*

Harmonizing Formulas 和解剂

Harmonize lesser yang 和解少阳

Bupleurum Decoction Plus Bitter Orange and Platycodon 柴胡枳桔汤 *chái hú zhǐ jié tāng*

Minor Bupleurum Decoction 小柴胡汤 *xiǎo chái hú tāng*

Bupleurum, Cinnamon Twig, and Dried Ginger Decoction 柴胡桂枝干姜汤 *chái hú guì zhī gān jiāng tāng*

Harmonize the liver and stomach 调和肝脾

Bupleurum Liver-Coursing Powder 柴胡疏肝散 *chái hú shū gān sǎn*

Bupleurum and Peony Six Gentlemen Decoction 柴芍六君子汤 *chái sháo liù jūn zǐ tāng*

Moutan and Gardenia Free Wanderer Powder 丹栀逍遥散 *dān zhī xiāo yáo sǎn*

Black Free Wanderer Powder 黑逍遥散 *hēi xiāo yáo sǎn*

Counterflow Cold Powder 四逆散 *sì nì sǎn*

Pain and Diarrhea Formula 痛泻要方 *tòng xiè yào fāng*

Fifth and Sixth Heavenly Stem Pill 戊己丸 *wù jǐ wán*

Free Wanderer Powder 逍遥散 *xiāo yáo sǎn*

Harmonize the stomach and intestines 调和胃肠

Pinellia Heart-Draining Decoction 半夏泻心汤 *bàn xià xiè xīn tāng*

Licorice Heart-Draining Decoction 甘草泻心汤 *gān cǎo xiè xīn tāng*

Coptis Decoction 黄连汤 *huáng lián tāng*

Fresh Ginger Heart-Draining Decoction 生姜泻心汤 *shēng jiāng xiè xīn tāng*

Sudden Smile Pill 失笑丸 *shī xiào wán*

Control malaria 治疟

Bupleurum Membrane-Source–Opening Beverage 柴胡达原饮 *chái hú dá yuán yǐn*

Membrane-Source–Opening Beverage 达原饮 *dá yuán yǐn*

Malaria-Interrupting Seven-Jewel Beverage 截疟七宝饮 *jié nüè qī bǎo yǐn*

Seven-Jewel Powder 七宝散 *qī bǎo sǎn*

Spleen-Clearing Beverage 清脾饮 *qīng pí yǐn*

Dampness-Dispelling Formulas 祛湿剂

Dry dampness and harmonize the stomach 燥湿和胃

Priceless Qi-Righting Powder 不换金正气散 *bù huàn jīn zhèng qì sǎn*

Bupleurum Stomach-Calming Decoction 柴平汤 *chái píng tāng*

Second Variant Qi-Righting Powder 二加减正气散 *èr jiā jiǎn zhèng qì sǎn*

Pueraria Flower Liquor-Resolving Decoction 葛花解醒汤 *gé huā jiě chéng tāng*

Agastache/Patchouli Qi-Righting Powder 藿香正气散 *huò xiāng zhèng qì sǎn*

Six Harmonizations Decoction 六和汤 *liù hé tāng*

Stomach-Calming Powder 平胃散 *píng wèi sǎn*

Wondrous Atractylodes Powder 神术散 *shén zhú sǎn*

Summerheat-Damp Qi-Righting Pill 暑湿正气丸 *shǔ shī zhèng qì wán*

Fourth Variant Qi-Righting Powder 四加减正气散 *sì jiā jiǎn zhèng qì sǎn*

Amomum Splenic Beverage 缩脾饮 *suō pí yǐn*

Stomach-Calming Poria (Hoelen) Five Decoction 胃苓汤 *wèi líng tāng*

Fifth Variant Qi-Righting Powder 五加减正气散 *wǔ jiā jiǎn zhèng qì sǎn*

Xu's Wondrous Atractylodes Powder 许学士神术散 *xǔ xué shì shén zhú sǎn*

First Variant Qi-Righting Powder 一加减正气散 *yī jiā jiǎn zhèng qì sǎn*

Enchanted Land Jade Shavings 醉乡玉屑 *zuì xiāng yù xiè*

Clear heat and dispel dampness 清热祛湿

Eight Corrections Powder 八正散 *bā zhèng sǎn*

Fish Poison Yam Dampness-Percolating Decoction 萆薢渗湿汤 *bì xiè shèn shī tāng*

Silkworm Droppings Decoction 蚕矢汤 *cán shǐ tāng*

Biliary Calculus Decoction 胆道排石汤 *dǎn dào pái shí tāng*

Tangkuei Pain-Assuaging Decoction 当归拈痛汤 *dāng guī niān tòng tāng*

Mysterious Two Powder (Pill) 二妙散（丸）*èr miào sǎn (wán)*

Poria (Hoelen) Skin Decoction 茯苓皮汤 *fú líng pí tāng*

Aconite Heart-Draining Decoction 附子泻心汤 *fù zǐ xiè xīn tāng*

Hepatolith Formula 肝胆管结石方 *gān dǎn guǎn jié shí fāng*

Sweet Dew Toxin-Dispersing Elixir 甘露消毒丹 *gān lù xiāo dú dān*

Sweet Wormwood and Scutellaria Gallbladder-Clearing Decoction 蒿芩清胆汤 *hāo qín qīng dǎn tāng*

Amber Powder 琥珀散 *hǔ pò sǎn*

Stone-Transforming Powder 化石散 *huà shí sǎn*

Yin-Forming Brew 化阴煎 *huà yīn jiān*

Jaundice Capillaris Granules 黄疸茵陈冲剂 *huáng dǎn yīn chén chōng jì*

Scutellaria and Talcum Decoction 黄芩滑石汤 *huáng qín huá shí tāng*

Agastache/Patchouli, Magnolia Bark, Pinellia, and Poria (Hoelen) Decoction 藿朴夏苓汤 *huò pò xià líng tāng*

Woody Fangji Variant Decoction 加减木防己汤 *jiā jiǎn mù fáng jǐ tāng*

Gallbladder-Disinhibiting Stone-Expelling Tablet 利胆排石片 *lì dǎn pái shí piàn*

Gallbladder-Disinhibiting Jaundice-Abating Decoction 利胆退黄汤 *lì dǎn tuì huáng tāng*

Coptis and Magnolia Bark Beverage 连朴饮 *lián pò yǐn*

Mutong Powder 木通散 *mù tōng sǎn*

Stone-Expelling Decoction 排石汤 *pái shí tāng*

Gallbladder-Clearing Dampness-Disinhibiting Decoction 清胆利湿汤 *qīng dǎn lì shī tāng*

Liver-Clearing Dampness-Percolating Decoction 清肝渗湿汤 *qīng gān shèn shī tāng*

Green-Blue Unicorn Pill 青麟丸 *qīng lín wán*

Clear and Quiet Pill 清宁丸 *qīng níng wán*

Third Variant Qi-Righting Powder 三加减正气散 *sān jiā jiǎn zhèng qì sǎn*

Golden Three Decoction 三金汤 *sān jīn tāng*

Mysterious Three Powder 三妙散 *sān miào sǎn*

Mysterious Three Pill 三妙丸 *sān miào wán*

Three Kernels Decoction 三仁汤 *sān rén tāng*

Pyrrosia Powder 石苇散 *shí wéi sǎn*

Mysterious Four Pill 四妙丸 *sì miào wán*

Five Stranguries Powder 五淋散 *wǔ lín sǎn*

Five Wiltings Decoction 五痿汤 *wǔ wěi tāng*

Whiteness-Dispersing Beverage 消白饮 *xiāo bái yǐn*

Dampness-Draining Decoction 泻湿汤 *xiè shī tāng*

Coix and Bamboo Leaf Powder 薏苡竹叶散 *yì yǐ zhú yè sǎn*

Capillaris Decoction 茵陈蒿汤 *yīn chén hāo tāng*

Capillaris and Poria (Hoelen) Five Powder 茵陈五苓散 *yīn chén wǔ líng sǎn*

Center Fullness Separating and Dispersing Pill 中满分消丸 *zhōng mǎn fēn xiāo wán*

Kidney-Enriching Pill 滋肾丸 *zī shèn wán*

Disinhibit water and percolate dampness 利水渗湿

Ovate Atractylodes Powder 白术散 *bái zhú sǎn*

Spring Pond Decoction 春泽汤 *chūn zé tāng*

Water-Abducting Poria (Hoelen) Decoction 导水茯苓汤 *dǎo shuǐ fú líng tāng*

Fangji and Poria (Hoelen) Decoction 防己茯苓汤 *fáng jǐ fú líng tāng*

Fangji and Astragalus Decoction 防己黄芪汤 *fáng jǐ huáng qí tāng*

Thorough Clearing Beverage 廓清饮 *kuò qīng yǐn*

Oyster Shell and Alisma Powder 牡蛎泽泻散 *mǔ lì zé xiè sǎn*

Woody Fangji Decoction 木防己汤 *mù fáng jǐ tāng*

Poria (Hoelen) Four Powder 四苓散 *sì líng sǎn*

Poria (Hoelen) Five Powder 五苓散 *wǔ líng sǎn*

Five-Peel Powder (Beverage) 五皮散（饮）*wǔ pí sǎn (yǐn)*

Polyporus Decoction 猪苓汤 *zhū líng tāng*

Warm and transform water-damp 温化水湿

Fish Poison Yam Clear-Turbid Separation Beverage 萆薢分清饮 *bì xiè fēn qīng yǐn*

Poria (Hoelen) and Licorice Decoction 茯苓甘草汤 *fú líng gān cǎo tāng*

Licorice, Dried Ginger, Poria (Hoelen), and Ovate Atractylodes Decoction 甘草干姜茯苓白术汤 *gān cǎo gān jiāng fú líng bái zhú tāng*

Cockcrow Powder 鸡鸣散 *jī míng sǎn*

Rectifying Poria (Hoelen) Decoction 理苓汤 *lǐ líng tāng*

Poria (Hoelen), Cinnamon Twig, Ovate Atractylodes, and Licorice Decoction 苓桂术甘汤 *líng guì zhú gān tāng*

Kidney Fixity Decoction 肾着汤 *shèn zhuó tāng*

Spleen-Firming Beverage 实脾饮 *shí pí yǐn*

True Warrior Decoction 真武汤 *zhēn wǔ tāng*

Ovate Atractylodes and Aconite Decoction 术附汤 *zhú fù tāng*

Fenugreek Powder 胡芦巴散 *hú lú bā sǎn*

Fenugreek Pill 葫芦巴丸 *hú lú bā wán*

Chaenomeles and Achyranthes Pill 木瓜牛膝丸 *mù guā niú xī wán*

Pain-Relieving Pill 定痛丸 *dìng tòng wán*

Dispel wind and overcome dampness 祛风胜湿

Baiwei Pill 白薇丸 *bái wēi wán*

Ovate Atractylodes and Aconite Decoction 白术附子汤 *bái zhú fù zǐ tāng*

Hundred and One Formulas Impediment-Alleviating Decoction 百一蠲痹汤 *bǎi yī juān bì tāng*

Leopard's Bone and Chaenomelis Wine 豹骨木瓜酒 *bào gǔ mù guā jiǔ*

Cheng's Impediment-Alleviating Decoction 程氏蠲痹汤 *chéng shì juàn bì tāng*

Dampness-Eliminating Impediment-Alleviating Decoction 除湿蠲痹汤 *chú shī juān bì tāng*

Damp-Eliminating Decoction 除湿汤 *chú shī tāng*

Major Network-Quickening Elixir 大活络丹 *dà huó luò dān*

Fangji Decoction 防己汤 *fáng jǐ tāng*

Siegesbeckia and Clerodendron Wind-Damp Tablet 风湿豨桐片 *fēng shī xī tóng piàn*

Licorice and Aconite Decoction 甘草附子汤 *gān cǎo fù zǐ tāng*

Cinnamon Twig and Aconite Decoction 桂枝附子汤 *guì zhī fù zǐ tāng*

Cinnamon Twig Decoction Plus Ovate Atractylodes and Aconite 桂枝加术附汤 *guì zhī jiā zhú fù tāng*

Statesman Wine 国公酒 *guó gōng jiǔ*

Erythrina Wine 海桐皮酒 *hǎi tóng pí jiǔ*

Network-Quickening Elixir 活络丹 *huó luò dān*

Impediment-Alleviating Decoction 蠲痹汤 *juān bì tāng*

Notopterygium Dampness-Eliminating Decoction 羌活除湿汤 *qiāng huó chú shī tāng*

Notopterygium Dampness-Overcoming Decoction 羌活胜湿汤 *qiāng huó shèng shī tāng*

Three Impediment Decoction 三痹汤 *sān bì tāng*

Mulberry Twig and Bushy Knotweed Decoction 桑枝虎杖汤 *sāng zhī hǔ zhàng tāng*

Upper, Middle, and Lower Body General-Use Wind Pain Formula 上中下通用痛风方 *shàng zhōng xià tōng yòng tòng fēng fāng*

Statesman Shi's Wine-Steeped Formula 史国公浸酒方 *shǐ guó gōng jìn jiǔ fāng*

Five Impediments Decoction 五痹汤 *wǔ bì tāng*

Siegesbeckia and Clerodendron Pill 豨桐丸 *xī tóng wán*

Minor Network-Quickening Elixir 小活络丹 *xiǎo huó luò dān*

Coix Decoction 薏苡仁汤 *yì yǐ rén tāng*

Duhuo and Mistletoe Decoction 独活寄生汤 *dú huó jì shēng tāng*

Sinew-Soothing Decoction 舒筋汤 *shū jīn tāng*

Dryness-Moistening Formulas 润燥剂

Moisten dryness by light diffusion 轻宣润燥

Forsythia and Mint Decoction 翘荷汤 *qiào hé tāng*

Dryness-Clearing Lung-Rescuing Decoction 清燥救肺汤 *qīng zào jiù fèi tāng*

Mulberry Leaf and Apricot Kernel Decoction 桑杏汤 *sāng xìng tāng*

Apricot Kernel and Perilla Powder 杏苏散 *xìng sū sǎn*

Enrich yin and moisten dryness 滋阴润燥

Lily Bulb Metal-Securing Decoction 百合固金汤 *bǎi hé gù jīn tāng*

Lily Bulb and Tussilago Paste 百花膏 *bǎi huā gāo*

Ass Hide Glue Decoction 补肺阿胶汤 *bǔ fèi ē jiāo tāng*

Ass Hide Glue Powder 阿胶散 *ē jiāo sǎn*

Ass Hide Glue Decoction 阿胶汤 *ē jiāo tāng*

Astragalus Decoction 黄芪汤 *huáng qí tāng*

Blood-Quickening Dryness-Moistening Liquid-Engendering Powder 活血润燥生津散 *huó xuè rùn zào shēng jīn sǎn*

Coptis and Mume Decoction 连梅汤 *lián méi tāng*

Ophiopogon Decoction 麦门冬汤 *mài mén dōng tāng*

Throat-Clearing Construction-Nourishing Decoction 清咽养营汤 *qīng yān yǎng yíng tang*

Fine Jade Paste 琼玉膏 *qióng yù gāo*

Dryness-Moistening Fetus-Quieting Decoction 润燥安胎汤 *rùn zào ān tāi tāng*

Adenophora/Glehnia and Ophiopogon Decoction 沙参麦冬汤 *shā shēn mài dōng tāng*

Four-Yin Decoction 四阴汤 *sì yīn tāng*

Five Juices Beverage 五汁饮 *wǔ zhī yǐn*

Dispersion-Thirst Formula 消渴方 *xiāo kě fāng*

Stomach-Nourishing Decoction 养胃汤 *yǎng wèi tāng*

Yin-Nourishing Lung-Clearing Decoction 养阴清肺汤 *yǎng yīn qīng fèi tāng*

Stomach-Boosting Decoction 益胃汤 *yì wèi tāng*

Jade Humor Decoction 玉液汤 *yù yè tāng*

Humor-Increasing Decoction 增液汤 *zēng yè tāng*

Interior-Warming Formulas 温里剂

Warm the center and dispel cold 温中散寒

Major Center-Fortifying Decoction 大建中汤 *dà jiàn zhōng tāng*

Tangkuei Center-Fortifying Decoction 当归建中汤 *dāng guī jiàn zhōng tāng*

Clove and Cinnamon Powder 丁桂散 *dīng guì sǎn*

Clove and Evodia Center-Rectifying Decoction 丁萸理中汤 *dīng yú lǐ zhōng tāng*

Aconite and Cinnamon Center-Rectifying Pill 附桂理中丸 *fù guì lǐ zhōng wán*

Aconite and Rice Decoction 附子粳米汤 *fù zǐ gēng mǐ tāng*

Aconite Center-Rectifying Pill 附子理中丸 *fù zǐ lǐ zhōng wán*

Licorice and Dried Ginger Decoction 甘草干姜汤 *gān cǎo gān jiāng tāng*

Cinnamon and Aconite Center-Rectifying Decoction 桂附理中汤 *guì fù lǐ zhōng tāng*

Cinnamon Twig Decoction Plus Extra Cinnamon 桂枝加桂汤 *guì zhī jiā guì tāng*

Cinnamon Twig and Ginseng Decoction 桂枝人参汤 *guì zhī rén shēn tāng*

Magnolia Bark Center-Warming Decoction 厚朴温中汤 *hòu pò wēn zhōng tāng*

Astragalus Center-Fortifying Decoction 黄芪建中汤 *huáng qí jiàn zhōng tāng*

Nine Pains Pill 九痛丸 *jiǔ tòng wán*

Yin-Rectifying Brew 理阴煎 *lǐ yīn jiān*

Center-Rectifying Decoction 理中汤 *lǐ zhōng tāng*

Center-Rectifying Pill 理中丸 *lǐ zhōng wán*

Ginseng Decoction 人参汤 *rén shēn tāng*

Stomach Gate Brew 胃关煎 *wèi guān jiān*

Channel-Warming (Menses-Warming) Decoction 温经汤 *wēn jīng tāng*

Evodia Decoction with Aconite Decoction 吴茱萸加附子汤 *wú zhū yú jiā fù zǐ tāng*

Evodia Decoction 吴茱萸汤 *wú zhū yú tāng*

Minor Center-Fortifying Decoction 小建中汤 *xiǎo jiàn zhōng tāng*

Capillaris Counterflow Cold Decoction 茵陈四逆汤 *yīn chén sì nì tāng*

Capillaris, Atractylodes, and Aconite Decoction 茵陈术附汤 *yīn chén zhú fù tāng*

Unripe Bitter Orange Center-Rectifying Pill 枳实理中丸 *zhǐ shí lǐ zhōng wán*

Center-Ordering Decoction 治中汤 *zhì zhōng tāng*

Cold-Dispelling Fright-Assuaging Decoction 逐寒荡惊汤 *zhú hán dàng jīng tāng*

Return yang and stem counterflow 回阳救逆

Scallion Yang-Freeing Decoction Plus Pig's Bile 白通加猪胆汁汤 *bái tōng jiā zhū dǎn zhī tāng*

Scallion Yang-Freeing Decoction 白通汤 *bái tōng tāng*

Great Rectifying Powder 大顺散 *dà shùn sǎn*

Pure Ginseng Decoction 独参汤 *dú shēn tāng*

Poria (Hoelen) Counterflow Cold Decoction 茯苓四逆汤 *fú líng sì nì tāng*

Galenite Elixir 黑锡丹 *hēi xí dān*

Yang-Returning Root-Reviving Decoction 回阳返本汤 *huí yáng fǎn běn tāng*

Yang-Returning Emergency Decoction 回阳救急汤 *huí yáng jiù jí tāng*

Millet Water Powder 浆水散 *jiāng shuǐ sǎn*

Astragalus and Aconite Decoction 芪附汤 *qí fù tāng*

Ginseng, Aconite, Dragon Bone, and Oyster Shell Decoction 参附龙牡汤 *shēn fù lóng mǔ tāng*

Ginseng and Aconite Decoction 参附汤 *shēn fù tāng*

Counterflow Cold Decoction Plus Ginseng 四逆加人参汤 *sì nì jiā rén shēn tāng*

Counterflow Cold Decoction 四逆汤 *sì nì tāng*

Vessel-Freeing Counterflow Cold Decoction 通脉四逆汤 *tōng mài sì nì tāng*

Origin-Boosting Decoction 益元汤 *yì yuán tāng*

Yang-Righting Powder 正阳散 *zhèng yáng sǎn*

Warm the channels and dissipate cold 温经散寒

Tangkuei Counterflow Cold Decoction Plus Evodia and Fresh Ginger 当归四逆加吴茱萸生姜汤 *dāng guī sì nì jiā wú zhū yú shēng jiāng tāng*

Tangkuei Counterflow Cold Decoction 当归四逆汤 *dāng guī sì nì tāng*

Astragalus and Cinnamon Twig Five Agents Decoction 黄芪桂枝五物汤 *huáng qí guì zhī wǔ wù tāng*

Aconite Main Tuber and Cinnamon Twig Decoction 乌头桂枝汤 *wū tóu guì zhī tāng*

Aconite Main Tuber Decoction 乌头汤 *wū tóu tāng*

Qi-Rectifying Formulas 理气剂

Move qi 行气

Pinellia and Magnolia Bark Decoction 半夏厚朴汤 *bàn xià hòu pò tāng*

Intestinal Adhesion Decoction 肠粘连缓解汤 *cháng zhān lián huǎn jiě tāng*

Birth-Hastening Beverage 催生饮 *cuī shēng yǐn*

Qi-Abducting Decoction 导气汤 *dǎo qì tāng*

Trichosanthes, Chinese Chive, and White Liquor Decoction 栝楼薤白白酒汤 *guā lóu xiè bái bái jiǔ tāng*

Trichosanthes, Chinese Chive, and Pinellia Decoction 栝楼薤白半夏汤 *guā lóu xiè bái bàn xià tāng*

Trichosanthes and Unripe Bitter Orange Decoction 栝楼枳实汤 *guā lóu zhǐ shí tāng*

Magnolia Bark, Fresh Ginger, Pinellia, Licorice, and Ginseng Decoction 厚朴生姜半夏甘草人参汤 *hòu pò shēng jiāng bàn xià gān cǎo rén shēn tāng*

Liver-Transforming Brew 化肝煎 *huà gān jiān*

Life Saver Tangerine Pip Pill 济生橘核丸 *jì shēng jú hé wán*

Supplemented Lindera Decoction 加味乌药汤 *jiā wèi wū yào tāng*

Toosendan Powder 金铃子散 *jīn líng zǐ sǎn*

Tangerine Pip Pill 橘核丸 *jú hé wán*

Lesser Galangal and Cyperus Pill 良附丸 *liáng fù wán*

Six Milled Ingredients Decoction 六磨汤 *liù mò tāng*

Saussurea Qi-Normalizing Powder 木香顺气散 *mù xiāng shùn qì sǎn*

Saussurea Qi-Normalizing Pill 木香顺气丸 *mù xiāng shùn qì wán*

Liver-Warming Brew 暖肝煎 *nuǎn gān jiān*

Qi-Discharging Beverage 排气饮 *pái qì yǐn*

Diaphragm-Arousing Powder 启膈散 *qǐ gé sǎn*

Gallbladder-Clearing Qi-Moving Decoction 清胆行气汤 *qīng dǎn xíng qì tāng*

Three-Option Anise Pill 三层茴香丸 *sān céng huí xiāng wán*

Ten Fragrances Pill 十香丸 *shí xiāng wán*

Liver-Coursing Depression-Resolving Decoction 疏肝解郁汤 *shū gān jiě yù tāng*

Liver-Soothing Pill 舒肝丸 *shū gān wán*

Qi-Smoothing Powder 舒气散 *shū qì sǎn*

Four Milled Ingredients Beverage 四磨饮 *sì mò yǐn*

Four-Seven Decoction 四七汤 *sì qī tāng*

Tiantai Lindera Powder 天台乌药散 *tiān tái wū yào sǎn*

Liver-Regulating Powder 调肝散 *tiáo gān sǎn*

Channel-Freeing Network-Quickening Decoction 通经活络汤 *tōng jīng huó luò tāng*

Lindera Powder 乌药散 *wū yào sǎn*

Lindera Decoction 乌药汤 *wū yào tāng*

Five Milled Ingredients Drink 五磨饮子 *wǔ mò yǐn zǐ*

Saussurea and Magnolia Bark Pill 香朴丸 *xiāng pò wán*

Saussurea and Amomum Stomach-Calming Pill 香砂平胃丸 *xiāng shā píng wèi wán*

Depression-Overcoming Pill 越鞠丸 *yuè jú wán*

Qi-Righting Lindera and Cyperus Powder 正气天香散 *zhèng qì tiān xiāng sǎn*

Bitter Orange Powder 枳壳散 *zhǐ ké sǎn*

Unripe Bitter Orange, Chinese Chive, and Cinnamon Twig Decoction 枳实薤白桂枝汤 *zhǐ shí xiè bái guì zhī tāng*

Perilla Leaf Fetus-Quieting Beverage 紫苏安胎饮 *zǐ sū ān tāi yǐn*

Downbear counterflow and check vomiting 降逆止呕

Major Pinellia Decoction 大半夏汤 *dà bàn xià tāng*

Clove and Persimmon Decoction 丁香柿蒂汤 *dīng xiāng shì dì tāng*

Dried Ginger, Ginseng, and Pinellia Pill 干姜人参半夏丸 *gān jiāng rén shén bàn xià wán*

Life Saver Tangerine Peel and Bamboo Shavings Decoction 济生橘皮竹茹汤 *jì shēng jú pí zhú rú tāng*

Tangerine Peel and Bamboo Shavings Decoction 橘皮竹茹汤 *jú pí zhú rú tāng*

Imperata and Pueraria Decoction 茅葛汤 *máo gé tāng*

Scutellaria, Coptis, Tangerine Peel, and Bamboo Shavings Decoction 芩连橘茹汤 *qíng lián jú rú tāng*

Persimmon Decoction 柿蒂汤 *shì dì tāng*

Gingerless Clove and Persimmon Powder 柿钱散 *shì qián sǎn*

Minor Pinellia Decoction 小半夏汤 *xiǎo bàn xià tāng*

Inula and Hematite Decoction 旋覆花代赭石汤 *xuán fù huā dài zhě shí tāng*

Bamboo Shavings Decoction 竹茹汤 *zhú rú tāng*

Downbear qi and calm panting 降气平喘

Panting-Stabilizing Decoction 定喘汤 *dìng chuǎn tāng*

Nine-Ingredient Center-Rectifying Decoction 九味理中汤 *jiǔ wèi lǐ zhōng tāng*

Codonopsis and Hematite Qi-Settling Decoction 参赭镇气汤 *shēn zhě zhèn qì tnag1*

Perilla Seed Qi-Downbearing Decoction 苏子降气汤 *sū zǐ jiàng qì tāng*

Abductive Dispersion and Accumulation-Transforming Formulas 消导化积剂

Disperse food and abduct stagnation 消食导滞

Infant-Safeguarding Red Powder 保赤散 *bǎo chì sǎn*

Harmony-Preserving Pill 保和丸 *bǎo hé wán*

Great Tranquility Pill 大安丸 *dà ān wán*

Spleen-Fortifying Pill 健脾丸 *jiàn pí wán*

Tangerine Peel, Pinellia, Unripe Bitter Orange, and Ovate Atractylodes Pill 橘半枳术丸 *jú bàn zhǐ zhú wán*

Saussurea and Areca Pill 木香槟榔丸 *mù xiāng bīng láng wán*

Saussurea Stagnation-Abducting Pill 木香导滞丸 *mù xiāng dǎo zhì wán*

Spleen-Arousing Pill 启脾散 *qǐ pí sǎn*

Medicated Leaven, Barley Sprout, Unripe Bitter Orange, and Ovate Atractylodes Pill 麯麦枳术丸 *qū mài zhǐ zhú wán*

Medicated Leaven, Barley Sprout, Unripe Bitter Orange, and Ovate Atractylodes Pill 麯蘖枳术丸 *qū niè zhǐ zhú wán*

Ginseng Spleen-Arousing Pill 人参启脾丸 *rén shēn qǐ pí wán*

Three Yellows Bitter Orange and Ovate Atractylodes Pill 三黄枳术丸 *sān huáng zhǐ zhú wán*

Three Dispersers Beverage 三消饮 *sān xiāo yǐn*

Saussurea, Amomum, Unripe Bitter Orange, and Ovate Atractylodes Pill 香砂枳术丸 *xiāng shā zhǐ zhú wán*

Glomus-Dispersing Asafetida Pill 消痞阿魏丸 *xiāo pǐ ē wèi wán*

Minor Center-Warming Pill 小温中丸 *xiǎo wēn zhōng wán*

Crataegus and Medicated Leaven Stomach-Calming Powder 楂麯平胃散 *zhā qū píng wèi sǎn*

Unripe Bitter Orange Stagnation-Abducting Pill 枳实导滞丸 *zhǐ shí dǎo zhì wán*

Unripe Bitter Orange and Glomus-Dispersing Pill 枳实消痞丸 *zhǐ shí xiāo pǐ wán*

Unripe Bitter Orange and Ovate Atractylodes Pill 枳术丸 *zhǐ zhú wán*

Disperse goiter, scrofula, and phlegm nodes 消瘿瘰痰核

Offensive Dispersion Harmonizing and Softening Decoction 攻消和解软坚汤 *gōng xiāo hé jiě ruǎn jiān tāng*

Sargassum Jade Flask Decoction 海藻玉壶汤 *hǎi zǎo yù hú tāng*

Scrofula Internal Dispersion Pill 内消瘰疬丸 *nèi xiāo luǒ lì wán*

Scutellaria and Coptis Two Matured Ingredients Decoction 芩连二陈汤 *qín lián èr chén tāng*

Scutellaria, Coptis, Anemarrhena, and Fritillaria Pill 芩连二母丸 *qín lián èr mǔ wán*

Swelling-Dispersing Hardness-Breaking Decoction 散肿溃坚汤 *sàn zhǒng kuì jiān tāng*

Four Seas Depression-Soothing Pill 四海舒郁丸 *sì hǎi shū yù wán*

Rhinoceros Bezoar Pill 犀黄丸 *xī huáng wán*

Prunella Paste 夏枯草膏 *xià kū cǎo gāo*

Prunella Decoction 夏枯草汤 *xià kū cǎo tāng*

Cyperus and Fritillaria Construction-Nourishing Decoction 香贝养营汤 *xiāng bèi yǎng yíng tāng*

Scrofula-Dispersing Pill 消瘰丸 *xiāo luǒ wán*

Goiter-Dispersing Decoction 消瘿汤 *xiāo yǐng tāng*

Minor Golden Elixir 小金丹 *xiǎo jīn dān*

Disperse concretions, conglomerations, accumulations and gatherings 消癥瘕积聚

Turtle Shell Decocted Pill 鳖甲煎丸 *biē jiǎ jiān wán*

Turtle Shell Drink 鳖甲饮子 *biē jiǎ yǐn zǐ*

Cinnamon Twig and Poria (Hoelen) Pill 桂枝茯苓丸 *guì zhī fú líng wán*

Moutan Powder 牡丹皮散 *mǔ dān pí sǎn*

Sparganium Decoction 三棱汤 *sān léng tāng*

Niter and Alum Powder 硝石矾石散 *xiāo shí fán shí sǎn*

Worm-Expelling Formulas 驱虫剂

Stemona Enema 百部灌肠剂 *bǎi bù guàn cháng jì*

Cloth Bag Pill 布袋丸 *bù dài wán*

Wood-Quelling Pill 伐木丸 *fá mù wán*

Chubby Child Pill 肥儿丸 *féi ér wán*

Torreya and Aspidium Decoction 榧子贯众汤 *fěi zǐ guàn zhòng tāng*

Licorice, Processed Galenite, and Honey Decoction 甘草粉蜜汤 *gān cǎo fěn mì tāng*

Worm-Transforming Pill 化虫丸 *huà chóng wán*

Center-Rectifying Roundworm-Quieting Powder 理中安蛔散 *lǐ zhōng ān huí sǎn*

Picrorhiza and Mume Roundworm-Quieting Decoction 连梅安蛔汤 *lián méi ān huí tāng*

Roundworm-Expelling Decoction No.2 驱蛔汤二号 *qū huí tāng èr hào*

Tapeworm-Expelling Decoction 驱绦汤 *qū tāo tāng*

Quisqualis and Rhubarb Powder 使君子大黄粉 *shǐ jūn zǐ dà huáng fěn*

Quisqualis Powder 使君子散 *shǐ jūn zǐ sǎn*

Myriad Applications Pill 万应丸 *wàn yìng wán*

Mume Pill 乌梅丸 *wū méi wán*

Jujube and Melanterite Pill 枣矾丸 *zǎo fán wán*

Abdominal Worm Formula 治腹内虫方 *zhì fù nèi chóng fāng*

Worm-Expelling Pill 追虫丸 *zhuī chóng wán*

Blood-Rectifying Formulas 理血剂

See "Supplement the blood" under Supplementing Formulas

Dispel stasis and quicken the blood 祛瘀活血

Eight Pinches Powder 八厘散 *bā lí sǎn*

Yang-Supplementing Five-Returning Decoction 补阳还五汤 *bǔ yáng huán wǔ tāng*

Bupleurum and Asarum Decoction 柴胡细辛汤 *chái hú xì xīn tāng*

Rhubarb and Wingless Cockroach Pill 大黄蟅虫丸 *dà huáng zhè chóng wán*

Substitute Dead-On Pill 代抵当丸 *dài dǐ dàng wán*

Salvia Beverage 丹参饮 *dān shēn yǐn*

Tangkuei Blood-Quickening Decoction 当归活血汤 *dāng guī huó xuè tāng*

Dead-On Decoction 抵当汤 *dǐ dàng tāng*

Dead-On Pill 抵当丸 *dǐ dàng wán*

Life-Clutching Elixir 夺命丹 *duó mìng dān*

Origin-Restorative Blood-Quickening Decoction 复元活血汤 *fù yuán huó xuè tāng*

Infradiaphragmatic Stasis-Expelling Decoction 膈下逐瘀汤 *gé xià zhú yū tāng*

Ectopic Pregnancy Formula No.II 宫外孕二号方 *gōng wài yùn èr hào fāng*

Coronary No.2 冠心二号 *guàn xīn èr hào*

Overdue Beverage 过期饮 *guò qī yǐn*

Network-Quickening Efficacious Elixir 活络效灵丹 *huó luò xiào líng dān*

Bone-Joining Elixir 接骨丹 *jiē gǔ dān*

Mother's Rescue Elixir 救母丹 *jiù mǔ dān*

Seven Pinches Powder 七厘散 *qī lí sǎn*

Three Yellow Jewels Wax Pill 三黄宝腊丸 *sān huáng bǎo là wán*

Three Yellows Wax Pill 三黄腊丸 *sān huáng là wán*

Bind-Dissipating Pain-Relieving Decoction 散结定疼汤 *sàn jié dìng téng tāng*

Lesser Abdomen Stasis-Expelling Decoction 少腹逐瘀汤 *shào fù zhú yū tāng*

Generalized Pain Stasis-Expelling Decoction 身痛逐瘀汤 *shēn tòng zhú yū tāng*

Engendering Transformation Decoction 生化汤 *shēng huà tāng*

Sudden Smile Powder 失笑散 *shī xiào sǎn*

Instant Relief Powder 手拈散 *shǒu niān sǎn*

Sinew-Soothing Blood-Quickening Tablet 舒筋活血片 *shū jīn huó xuè piàn*

Four Stems Decoction 四藤汤 *sì téng tāng*

Peach Kernel Qi-Coordinating Decoction 桃核承气汤 *táo hé chéng qì tāng*

Peach Kernel and Carthamus Four Agents Decoction 桃红四物汤 *táo hóng sì wù tāng*

Peach Kernel Qi-Coordinating Decoction 桃仁承气汤 *táo rén chéng qì tāng*

Orifice-Freeing Blood-Quickening Decoction 通窍活血汤 *tōng qiào huó xuè tāng*

Stasis-Freeing Brew 通瘀煎 *tōng yū jiān*

Stasis-Precipitating Decoction 下瘀血汤 *xià yū xuè tāng*

House of Blood Stasis-Expelling Decoction 血府逐瘀汤 *xuè fǔ zhú yū tāng*

Corydalis Decoction 延胡索汤 *yán hú suǒ tāng*

Leonurus (Motherwort) Metal-Overcoming Elixir 益母胜金丹 *yì mǔ shèng jīn dān*

Stanch bleeding 止血

Bletilla Mixture 白及合剂 *bái jí hé jì*

Bletilla and Loquat Pill 白及枇杷丸 *bái jí pí pá wán*

Biota Leaf Decoction 柏叶汤 *bǎi yè tāng*

Ophicalcite Powder 花蕊石散 *huā ruǐ shí sǎn*

Sophora Flower Powder 槐花散 *huái huā sǎn*

Sophora Fruit Pill 槐角丸 *huái jiǎo wán*

Yellow Earth Decoction 黄土汤 *huáng tǔ tāng*

Blood Cough Formula 咳血方 *ké xuè fāng*

Blood-Cooling Rehmannia Decoction 凉血地黄汤 *liáng xuè dì huáng tāng*

Blood-Quieting Decoction 宁血汤 *níng xuè tāng*

Ten Cinders Powder (Pill) 十灰散（丸）*shí huī sǎn (wán)*

Four Fresh Agents Pill 四生丸 *sì shēng wán*

Cephalanoplos Drink 小蓟饮子 *xiǎo jì yǐn zǐ*

Pig's Intestines and Coptis Pill 脏连丸 *zàng lián wán*

Blood-Stanching Powder 止血粉 *zhǐ xuè fěn*

Blood-Stanching Decoction 止血汤 *zhǐ xuè tāng*

Pig's Intestine Pill 猪脏丸 *zhū zàng wán*

Phlegm-Dispelling Formulas 祛痰剂

Dry dampness and transform phlegm 燥湿化痰

Pinellia and Poria (Hoelen) Decoction 半夏茯苓汤 *bàn xià fú líng tāng*

Phlegm-Abducting Decoction 导痰汤 *dǎo tán tāng*

Two Matured Ingredients Decoction 二陈汤 *èr chén tāng*

Six Gentlemen Metal and Water Brew 金水六君煎 *jīn shuǐ liù jūn jiān*

Six Quietings Brew 六安煎 *liù ān jiān*

Calming Matured Ingredients Decoction 平陈汤 *píng chén tāng*

Gallbladder-Warming Decoction 温胆汤 *wēn dǎn tāng*

Saussurea and Amomum Two Matured Ingredients Decoction 香砂二陈汤 *xiāng shā èr chén tāng*

Pathfinder Poria (Hoelen) Pill 指迷茯苓丸 *zhǐ mí fú líng wán*

Diffuse the lung and transform phlegm 宣肺化痰

Florid Canopy Powder 华盖散 *huá gài sǎn*

Inula Powder 金沸草散 *jīn fèi cǎo sǎn*

Wind-Damage Cough Swill-Down Pill 伤风咳嗽吞剂 *shāng fēng ké sòu tūn jì*

Diffusing-Freeing Lung-Rectifying Pill 通宣理肺丸 *tōng xuān lǐ fèi wán*

Cough-Stopping Powder 止嗽散 *zhǐ sòu sǎn*

Clear heat and transform phlegm 清热化痰

Bupleurum Chest Bind Decoction 柴胡陷胸汤 *chái hú xiàn xiōng tāng*

Indigo and Clamshell Powder 黛蛤散 *dài gé sǎn*

Anemarrhena and Fritillaria Powder 二母散 *èr mǔ sǎn*

Licorice and Platycodon Decoction 甘桔汤 *gān jié tāng*

Phlegm-Rolling Pill 滚痰丸 *gǔn tán wán*

Platycodon Decoction 桔梗汤 *jié gěng tāng*

Cormorant Drool Pill 鸬鹚涎丸 *lú cí xián wán*

Chlorite/Mica Phlegm-Rolling Pill 礞石滚痰丸 *méng shí gǔn tán wán*

Bronchitis Tablet 气管炎片 *qì guǎn yán piàn*

Scutellaria, Stemona, and Salvia Elixir 芩部丹 *qín bù dān*

Lung-Clearing Phlegm-Transforming Pill 清肺化痰丸 *qīng fèi huà tán wán*

Lung-Clearing Decoction 清肺汤 *qīng fèi tāng*

Metal-Clearing Phlegm-Transforming Decoction 清金化痰汤 *qīng jīn huà tán tāng*

Qi-Clearing Phlegm-Transforming Pill 清气化痰丸 *qīng qì huà tán wán*

Mulberry Root Bark Decoction 桑白皮汤 *sāng bái pí tāng*

Tingli and Jujube Lung-Draining Decoction 葶苈大枣泻肺汤 *tíng lì dà zǎo xiè fèi tāng*

Minor Chest Bind Decoction 小陷胸汤 *xiǎo xiàn xiōng tāng*

Snow Soup Decoction 雪羹汤 *xuě gēng tāng*

Cough-Suppressing Phlegm-Transforming Panting-Stabilizing Pill 止嗽化痰定喘丸 *zhǐ sòu huà tán dìng chuǎn wán*

Bamboo Sap Phlegm-Outthrusting Pill 竹沥达痰丸 *zhú lì dá tán wán*

Warm the lung and transform rheum (phlegm) 温肺化饮（痰）

Cold Wheezing Pill 冷哮丸 *lěng xiāo wán*

Center-Rectifying Phlegm-Transforming Pill 理中化痰丸 *lǐ zhōng huà tán wán*

Poria (Hoelen), Licorice, Schisandra, Ginger, and Asarum Decoction 苓甘五味姜辛汤 *líng gān wǔ wèi jiāng xīn tāng*

Belamcanda and Ephedra Decoction 射干麻黄汤 *shè gān má huáng tāng*

Phlegm-Rheum Pill 痰饮丸 *tán yǐn wán*

Lung-Warming Nose-Drying Elixir 温肺止流丹 *wēn fèi zhǐ liú dān*

Minor Green-Blue Dragon Decoction Plus Gypsum 小青龙加石膏汤 *xiǎo qīng lóng jiā shí gāo tāng*

Minor Green-Blue Dragon Decoction 小青龙汤 *xiǎo qīng lóng tāng*

Spleen-Effusing Decoction Plus Pinellia 越婢加半夏汤 *yuè bì jiā bàn xià tāng*

Moisten the lung and transform phlegm 润肺化痰

Fritillaria and Trichosanthes Powder 贝母栝蒌散 *bèi mǔ guā lóu sǎn*

Lung-Moistening Powder 润肺散 *rùn fèi sǎn*

Aster Decoction 紫菀汤 *zǐ wǎn tāng*

Control wind and transform phlegm 治风化痰

Pinellia, Ovate Atractylodes, and Gastrodia Decoction 半夏白术天麻汤 *bàn xià bái zhú tiān má tāng*

Priceless Elixir 不换金丹 *bù huàn jīn dān*

Major Wind Arousal Decoction 大醒风汤 *dà xǐng fēng tāng*

Uncaria Powder 钩藤散 *gōu téng sǎn*

Qingzhou White Pill 青州白丸子 *qīng zhōu bái wán zǐ*

Three Raw Agents Beverage 三生饮 *sān shēng yǐn*

Arisaema Pill 天南星丸 *tiān nán xīng wán*

Arisaema and Saussurea Decoction 星香汤 *xīng xiāng tāng*

Normalize qi and transform phlegm 顺气化痰

Three-Seed Filial Devotion Decoction 三子养亲汤 *sān zǐ yǎng qīn tāng*

Qi-Normalizing Phlegm-Abducting Decoction 顺气导痰汤 *shùn qì dǎo tán tāng*

Qi-Normalizing Food-Dispersing Phlegm-Transforming Pill 顺气消食化痰丸 *shùn qì xiāo shí huà tán wán*

Spirit-Quieting Formulas 安神剂

Quiet the spirit with heavy settlers 重镇安神

Bupleurum Decoction Plus Dragon Bone and Oyster Shell 柴胡加龙骨牡蛎汤 *chái hú jiā lóng gǔ mǔ lì tāng*

Loadstone and Cinnabar Pill 磁朱丸 *cí zhū wán*

Cinnamon Twig Decoction Plus Dragon Bone and Oyster Shell 桂枝加龙骨牡蛎汤 *guì zhī jiā lóng gǔ mǔ lì tāng*

Cinnamon Twig Counterflow-Stemming Decoction 桂枝救逆汤 *guì zhī jiù nì tāng*

Amber Spirit-Quieting Decoction 琥珀安神汤 *hǔ pò ān shén tāng*

Sagacious Confucius' Pillow Elixir 孔圣枕中丹 *kǒng shèng zhěn zhōng dān*

Confucius' Pillow Powder 孔子枕中散 *kǒng zǐ zhěn zhōng sǎn*

Medicated Leaven Pill 神麯丸 *shén qū wán*

Iron Flakes Beverage 生铁落饮 *shēng tiě luò yǐn*

Polygala Pill 远志丸 *yuǎn zhì wán*

Mother-of-Pearl Pill 珍珠母丸 *zhēn zhū mǔ wán*

Pillow Elixir 枕中丹 *zhěn zhōng dān*

Cinnabar Spirit-Quieting Pill 朱砂安神丸 *zhū shā ān shén wán*

Nourish the heart and quiet the spirit 养心安神

Spirit-Quieting Mind-Stabilizing Pill 安神定志丸 *ān shén dìng zhì wán*

Spirit-Quieting Pill 安神丸 *ān shén wán*

Biota Seed Heart-Nourishing Pill 柏子养心丸 *bǎi zǐ yǎng xīn wán*

Mind-Stabilizing Pill 定志丸 *dìng zhì wán*

Ass Hide Glue and Coptis Decoction 阿胶黄连汤 *ē jiāo huáng lián tāng*

Licorice, Wheat, and Jujube Decoction 甘草小麦大枣汤 *gān cǎo xiǎo mài dà zǎo tāng*

Licorice, Wheat, and Jujube Decoction 甘麦大枣汤 *gān mài dà zǎo tāng*

Coptis and Ass Hide Glue Decoction 黄连阿胶汤 *huáng lián ē jiāo tāng*

Supplemented Mind-Stabilizing Pill 加味定志丸 *jiā wèi dìng zhì wán*

Peaceful Interaction Pill 交泰丸 *jiāo tài wán*

Mysterious Fragrance Powder 妙香散 *miào xiāng sǎn*

Enriching Ginseng Tablet 人参滋补片 *rén shēn zī bǔ piàn*

Heaven, Human, and Earth Marrow-Retaining Elixir 三才封髓丹 *sān cái fēng suǐ dān*

Spiny Jujube Decoction 酸枣仁汤 *suān zǎo rén tāng*

Celestial Emperor Heart-Supplementing Elixir 天王补心丹 *tiān wáng bǔ xīn dān*

Heart-Nourishing Decoction 养心汤 *yǎng xīn tāng*

Enriching Supplementation Tablet 滋补片 *zī bǔ piàn*

Other spirit-quieting formulas 其他安神剂

Pinellia and Broomcorn Millet Decoction 半夏秫米汤 *bàn xià shú mǐ tāng*

Pinellia Decoction 半夏汤 *bàn xià tāng*

Coptis Gallbladder-Warming Decoction 黄连温胆汤 *huáng lián wēn dǎn tāng*

Supplemented Gallbladder-Warming Decoction 加味温胆汤 *jiā wèi wēn dǎn tāng*

Ten-Ingredient Gallbladder-Warming Decoction 十味温胆汤 *shí wèi wēn dǎn tāng*

Eleven-Ingredient Gallbladder-Warming Decoction 十一味温胆汤 *shí yī wèi wēn dǎn tāng*

Wind-Dispelling Formulas 祛风剂

Course and dissipate external wind 疏散外风
Xanthium Powder 苍耳散 *cāng ěr sǎn*
Xanthium Powder 苍耳子散 *cāng ěr zǐ sǎn*
Wind-Eliminating Boosting Decoction 除风益损汤 *chú fēng yì sǔn tāng*
Tea-Blended Ligusticum (Cnidium Root) Powder 川芎茶调散 *chuān xiōng chá tiáo sǎn*
Large Gentian Decoction 大秦艽汤 *dà qín jiāo tāng*
Hou's Black Powder 侯氏黑散 *hóu shì hēi sǎn*
Agastache/Patchouli and Pig's Bile Pill 藿胆丸 *huò dǎn wán*
Tea-Blended Chrysanthemum Powder 菊花茶调散 *jú huā chá tiáo sǎn*
Fetid Cassia Powder 决明子散 *jué míng zǐ sǎn*
Eye Brightener Clear-Raising Pill 明目上清丸 *míng mù shàng qīng wán*
Upper-Body-Clearing Pain-Alleviating Decoction 清上蠲痛汤 *qīng shàng juān tòng tāng*
Wind-Expelling Heat-Dissipating Drink 驱风散热饮子 *qū fēng sàn rè yǐn zi*
Abalone Shell Powder 石决明散 *shí jué míng sǎn*
Wind-Coursing Blood-Nourishing Decoction 疏风养血汤 *shū fēng yǎng xuè tāng*
Heart-Washing Powder 洗心散 *xǐ xīn sǎn*
Wind-Dispersing Powder 消风散 *xiāo fēng sǎn*
Wind-Dispersing Blood-Nourishing Decoction 消风养血汤 *xiāo fēng yǎng xuè tāng*
Minor Life-Prolonging Decoction 小续命汤 *xiǎo xù mìng tāng*
Magnolia Flower Powder 辛夷散 *xīn yí sǎn*
Liver-Repairing Decoction 修肝汤 *xiū gān tāng*

Calm and extinguish internal wind 平熄内风
Major Wind-Stabilizing Pill 大定风珠 *dà dìng fēng zhū*
Rehmannia Drink 地黄饮子 *dì huáng yǐn zi*
Ass Hide Glue and Egg Yolk Decoction 阿胶鸡子黄汤 *ē jiāo jī zǐ huáng tāng*
Uncaria Decoction 钩藤汤 *gōu téng tāng*
Sweeping Down Decoction 建瓴汤 *jiàn líng tāng*
Antelope Horn and Uncaria Decoction 羚角钩藤汤 *líng jiǎo gōu téng tāng*
Antelope Horn Decoction 羚羊角汤 *líng yáng jiǎo tāng*
Triple-Armored Pulse-Restorative Decoction 三甲复脉汤 *sān jiǎ fù mài tāng*
Gastrodia and Uncaria Beverage 天麻钩藤饮 *tiān má gōu téng yǐn*
Liver-Settling Wind-Extinguishing Decoction 镇肝熄风汤 *zhèn gān xī fēng tāng*

Dispel wind and resolve tetany 祛风解痉
Pursing Wind Powder 撮风散 *cuò fēng sǎn*
Uncaria Beverage 钩藤饮 *gōu téng yǐn*
Antelope Horn Powder 羚羊角散 *líng yáng jiǎo sǎn*
Pull Aright Powder 牵正散 *qiān zhèng sǎn*

Five-Tigers-Chasing-the-Wind Powder 五虎追风散 *wǔ hǔ zhuī fēng sǎn*
True Jade Powder 玉真散 *yù zhēn sǎn*
Tetany-Relieving Powder 止痉散 *zhǐ jìng sǎn*

Orifice-Opening Formulas 开窍剂

Clear heat and open the orifices 清热开窍
Peaceful Palace Bovine Bezoar Pill 安宫牛黄丸 *ān gōng niú huáng wán*
Dragon-Embracing Pill 抱龙丸 *bào lóng wán*
Amber Dragon-Embracing Pill 琥珀抱龙丸 *hǔ pò bào lóng wán*
Fright-Cooling Pill 凉惊丸 *liáng jīng wán*
Bovine Bezoar Dragon-Embracing Pill 牛黄抱龙丸 *niú huáng bào lóng wán*
Bovine Bezoar Heart-Clearing Pill 牛黄清心丸 *niú huáng qīng xīn wán*
Spirit-Like Rhinoceros Horn Elixir 神犀丹 *shén xī dān*
Children's Return-of-Spring Elixir 小儿回春丹 *xiǎo ér huí chūn dān*
Troop-Marching Powder 行军散 *xíng jūn sǎn*
Xingnaojing 醒脑静 *xǐng nǎo jìng*
Supreme Jewel Elixir 至宝丹 *zhì bǎo dān*
Purple Snow Elixir 紫雪丹 *zǐ xuě dān*

Expel cold and open the orifices 逐寒开窍
Coronary Liquid Storax Pill 冠心苏合丸 *guān xīn sū hé wán*
Red Spirit Elixir 红灵丹 *hóng líng dān*
Liquid Storax Pill 苏合香丸 *sū hé xiāng wán*
Gate-Freeing Powder 通关散 *tōng guān sǎn*
Sleeping Dragon Elixir 卧龙丹 *wò lóng dān*
Warlord's Troop-Marching Powder 武侯行军散 *wǔ hóu xíng jūn sǎn*
Jade Pivot Elixir 玉枢丹 *yù shū dān*
Zhuge's Troop-Marching Powder 诸葛行军散 *zhū gě xíng jūn sǎn*
Purple Gold Powder 紫金粉 *zǐ jīn fěn*

Transform phlegm and open the orifices 化痰开窍
Phlegm-Flushing Decoction 涤痰汤 *dí tán tāng*
Mania and Withdrawal Pill 癫狂丸 *diān kuáng wán*
Fit-Settling Pill 定痫丸 *dìng xián wán*
Return-of-Spring Elixir 回春丹 *huí chūn dān*

Supplementing Formulas 补益剂

Supplement qi 补气
Origin-Preserving Decoction 保元汤 *bǎo yuán tāng*
Lung-Supplementing Decoction 补肺汤 *bǔ fèi tāng*
Center-Supplementing Qi-Boosting Decoction 补中益气汤 *bǔ zhōng yì qì tāng*
Origin-Lifting Brew 举元煎 *jǔ yuán jiān*

Six Gentlemen Decoction 六君子汤 liù jūn zǐ tāng

Wondrous Six Powder 六神散 liù shén sǎn

Seven-Ingredient Ovate Atractylodes Powder 七味白术散 qī wèi bái zhú sǎn

Ginseng and Gecko Powder 人参蛤蚧散 rén shēn gé jiè sǎn

Ginseng and Walnut Decoction 人参胡桃汤 rén shēn hú táo tāng

Ginseng Spleen-Fortifying Pill 人参健脾丸 rén shēn jiàn pí wán

Ginseng with Gecko Powder 参蚧散 shēn jiè sǎn

Ginseng, Poria (Hoelen), and Ovate Atractylodes Powder 参苓白术散 shēn líng bái zhú sǎn

Fall-Upbearing Decoction 升陷汤 shēng xiàn tāng

Yang-Upbearing Stomach-Boosting Decoction 升阳益胃汤 shēng yáng yì wèi tāng

Qi-Normalizing Center-Harmonizing Decoction 顺气和中汤 shùn qì hé zhōng tāng

Four Gentlemen Decoction 四君子汤 sì jūn zǐ tāng

Saussurea and Amomum Six Gentlemen Decoction 香砂六君子汤 xiāng shā liù jūn zǐ tāng

Saussurea and Amomum Six Gentlemen Pill 香砂六君子丸 xiāng shā liù jūn zǐ wán

Special Achievement Powder 异功散 yì gōng sǎn

Qi-Boosting Sharp and Bright Decoction 益气聪明汤 yì qì cōng míng tāng

Life-Promoting Pill 资生丸 zī shēng wán

Supplement the blood 补血

Mugwort and Cyperus Palace-Warming Pill 艾附暖宫丸 ài fù nuǎn gōng wán

Fetus-Quieting Qi-Harmonizing Beverage 安胎和气饮 ān tāi hé qì yǐn

Liver-Supplementing Decoction 补肝汤 bǔ gān tāng

Construction-Supplementing Decoction 补荣汤 bǔ róng tāng

Major Construction Brew 大营煎 dà yíng jiān

Tangkuei and Peony Powder 当归芍药散 dāng guī sháo yào sǎn

Tangkuei, Fresh Ginger, and Goat Meat Decoction 当归生姜羊肉汤 dāng guī shēng jiāng yáng ròu tāng

Ass Hide Glue Four Agents Decoction 阿胶四物汤 ē jiāo sì wù tāng

Pulse-Restorative Decoction 复脉汤 fù mài tāng

Tangkuei, Peony, and Rehmannia Decoction 归芍地黄汤 guī sháo dì huáng tāng

Pulse-Restorative Variant Decoction 加减复脉汤 jiā jiǎn fù mài tāng

Supplemented Tangkuei and Peony Powder 加味当归芍药散 jiā wèi dāng guī sháo yào sǎn

Four Agents Decoction 四物汤 sì wù tāng

Supplemented Four Agents Decoction Formula 四物汤加味方 sì wù tāng jiā wèi fāng

Child-Delivering Elixir 送子丹 sòng zǐ dān

Celestial Fluid Lactation-Promoting Beverage 下乳天浆饮 xià rǔ tiān jiāng yǐn

Minor Construction Brew 小营煎 xiǎo yíng jiān

Honey-Fried Licorice Decoction 炙甘草汤 zhì gān cǎo tāng

Ramie (Boehmeria) Decoction 苎根汤 zhù gēn tāng

Dryness-Enriching Construction-Nourishing Decoction 滋燥养营汤 zī zào yǎng yíng tāng

Supplement both qi and the blood 气血双补

Fetus-Quieting Beverage 安胎饮 ān tāi yǐn

Eight-Gem Decoction 八珍汤 bā zhēn tāng

Eight-Gem Leonurus (Motherwort) Pill 八珍益母丸 bā zhēn yì mǔ wán

Carefree Pregnancy Formula 保产无忧方 bǎo chǎn wú yōu fāng

Abdomen-Quieting Decoction 肠宁汤 cháng níng tāng

Tangkuei Blood-Supplementing Decoction 当归补血汤 dāng guī bǔ xuè tāng

Tangkuei and Goat Meat Decoction 当归羊肉汤 dāng guī yáng ròu tāng

Spleen-Returning Decoction 归脾汤 guī pí tāng

Tangkuei and Astragalus Center-Fortifying Decoction 归芪建中汤 guī qí jiàn zhōng tāng

Tangkuei and Peony Six Gentlemen Pill 归芍六君丸 guī sháo liù jūn wán

Flowery Knotweed and Ginseng Beverage 何人饮 hé rén yǐn

Ginseng Construction-Nourishing Decoction (Pill) 人参养荣汤（丸）rén shēn yǎng róng tāng (wán)

Sagacious Cure Decoction 圣愈汤 shèng yù tāng

Perfect Major Supplementation Decoction 十全大补汤 shí quán dà bǔ tāng

Dioscorea Pill 薯蓣丸 shǔ yù wán

Rock of Taishan Fetus-Quieting Powder 泰山磐石散 tài shān pán shí sǎn

Lactation Elixir 通乳丹 tōng rǔ dān

Black Chicken and White Phoenix Pill 乌鸡白凤丸 wū jī bái fèng wán

Fetus-Turning Formula 转胎方 zhuǎn tāi fāng

Supplement yang 补阳

Eight-Ingredient Rehmannia Pill 八味地黄丸 bā wèi dì huáng wán

Striped Dragon Pill 斑龙丸 bān lóng wán

Kidney-Supplementing Thoroughfare-Securing Pill 补肾固冲丸 bǔ shèn gù chōng wán

Two Immortals Decoction 二仙汤 èr xiān tāng

Hyperosteogeny Pill 骨质增生丸 gǔ zhí zēng shēng wán

Tortoise Plastron and Deerhorn Two Immortals Glue 龟鹿二仙胶 guī lù èr xiān jiāo

Cinnamon Bark and Aconite Eight-Ingredient Pill 桂附八味丸 guì fù bā wèi wán

Cinnamon Twig and Licorice Decoction 桂枝甘草汤 guì zhī gān cǎo tāng

Eight-Ingredient Placenta Pill 河车八味丸 hé chē bā wèi wán

Water-Transforming Seed-Planting Decoction 化水种子汤 huà shuǐ zhòng zǐ tāng

Life Saver Kidney Qi Pill 济生肾气丸 *jì shēng shèn qì wán*

Supplemented Metal Strength Pill 加味金刚丸 *jiā wèi jīn gāng wán*

Supplemented Kidney Qi Pill 加味肾气丸 *jiā wèi shèn qì wán*

Lumbus-Fortifying Pill 健腰丸 *jiàn yāo wán*

Internal Supplementation Pill 内补丸 *nèi bǔ wán*

Whole Deer Pill 全鹿丸 *quán lù wán*

Kidney Qi Pill 肾气丸 *shèn qì wán*

Ten Supplements Pill 十补丸 *shí bǔ wán*

Right-Restoring [Life Gate] Pill 右归丸 *yòu guī wán*

Right-Restoring [Life Gate] Beverage 右归饮 *yòu guī yǐn*

Earth-Rescuing Fetus-Securing Decoction 援土固胎汤 *yuán tǔ gù tāi tāng*

Procreation Elixir 赞育丹 *zàn yù dān*

Supplement yin 补阴

Eight Immortals Longevity Pill 八仙长寿丸 *bā xiān cháng shòu wán*

Kidney-Supplementing Sinew-Strengthening Decoction 补肾壮筋汤 *bǔ shèn zhuàng jīn tāng*

Major Yin Supplementation Pill 大补阴丸 *dà bǔ yīn wán*

Great Creation Pill 大造丸 *dà zào wán*

Rehmannia Pill 地黄丸 *dì huáng wán*

Rehmannia Drink 地黄饮子 *dì huáng yǐn zǐ*

Metropolis Qi Pill 都气丸 *dū qì wán*

Deafness Left-Benefiting Loadstone Pill 耳聋左慈丸 *ěr lóng zuǒ cí wán*

Double-Armored Pulse-Restorative Decoction 二甲复脉汤 *èr jiǎ fù mài tāng*

Double Supreme Pill 二至丸 *èr zhì wán*

Rejuvenation Elixir 还少丹 *huán shào dān*

Steady Gait Hidden Tiger Pill 健步虎潜丸 *jiàn bù hǔ qián wán*

Six-Ingredient Rehmannia Pill 六味地黄丸 *liù wèi dì huáng wán*

Ophiopogon and Rehmannia Pill 麦味地黄丸 *mài wèi dì huáng wán*

Eye Brightener Rehmannia Pill 明目地黄丸 *míng mù dì huáng wán*

Seven-Jewel Beard-Blackening Elixir 七宝美髯丹 *qī bǎo měi rán dān*

Lycium Berry, Chrysanthemum, and Rehmannia Decoction 杞菊地黄汤 *qǐ jú dì huáng tāng*

Lycium Berry, Chrysanthemum, and Rehmannia Pill 杞菊地黄丸 *qǐ jú dì huáng wán*

Mulberry Paste 桑椹子膏 *sāng shèn zǐ gāo*

Dendrobium Eye Brightener Pill 石斛明目丸 *shí hú míng mù wán*

Dendrobium Night Vision Pill 石斛夜光丸 *shí hú yè guāng wán*

Fetal Longevity Pill 寿胎丸 *shòu tāi wán*

Mulberry Paste 文武膏 *wén wǔ tāng*

Five-Seed Kidney-Supplementing Pill 五子补肾丸 *wǔ zǐ bǔ shèn wán*

Five-Seed Progeny Pill 五子衍宗丸 *wǔ zǐ yǎn zōng wán*

All-the-Way-Through Brew 一贯煎 *yī guàn jiān*

Single-Armored Pulse-Restorative Decoction 一甲复脉汤 *yī jiǎ fù mài tāng*

Moonlight Pill 月华丸 *yuè huá wán*

Long Vistas Pill Variant Formula 驻景丸加减方 *zhù jǐng wán jiā jiǎn fāng*

Water-Enriching Liver-Clearing Beverage 滋水清肝饮 *zī shuǐ qīng gān yǐn*

Yin-Enriching Major Supplementation Pill 滋阴大补丸 *zī yīn dà bǔ wán*

Left-Restoring [Kidney Yin] Pill 左归丸 *zuǒ guī wán*

Left-Restoring [Kidney Yin] Beverage 左归饮 *zuǒ guī yǐn*

Enrich yin and boost qi 滋阴益气

Ginseng Root-Securing Pill 人参固本丸 *rén shēn gù běn wán*

Ginseng and Astragalus Powder 人参黄芪散 *rén shēn huáng qí sǎn*

Heaven, Human, and Earth Decoction 三才汤 *sān cǎi tāng*

Pulse-Engendering Powder 生脉散 *shēng mài sǎn*

Wherewithal-to-Bear Pill 所以载丸 *suǒ yǐ zài wán*

Securing and Astringing Formulas 固涩剂

Constrain sweat and secure the exterior 敛汗固表

Biota Seed Pill 柏子仁丸 *bǎi zǐ rén wán*

Oyster Shell Powder 牡蛎散 *mǔ lì sǎn*

Jade Wind-Barrier Powder 玉屏风散 *yù píng fēng sǎn*

Perspiration-Checking Powder 止汗散 *zhǐ hàn sǎn*

Astringe the intestines and stem desertion 涩肠固脱

Halloysite and Limonite Decoction 赤石脂禹余粮汤 *chì shí zhī yǔ yú liáng tāng*

Pure Yang True Man Viscus-Nourishing Decoction 纯阳真人养脏汤 *chún yáng zhēn rén yǎng zàng tāng*

Major Peach Blossom Decoction 大桃花汤 *dà táo huā tāng*

Sanguisorba Pill 地榆丸 *dì yú wán*

Two Spirits Pill 二神丸 *èr shén wán*

Spleen-Kidney Supplementation Pill 脾肾双补丸 *pí shèn shuāng bǔ wán*

Four Spirits Pill 四神丸 *sì shén wán*

Peach Blossom Decoction 桃花汤 *táo huā tāng*

Yellow-Boosting Powder 益黄散 *yì huáng sǎn*

True Man Viscus-Nourishing Decoction 真人养脏汤 *zhēn rén yǎng zàng tāng*

Carriage-Halting Pill 驻车丸 *zhù chē wán*

Astringe essence and check seminal emission and enuresis 涩精止遗

Poria (Hoelen) and Cuscuta Elixir 茯菟丹 *fú tù dān*

Unctuous Strangury Decoction 膏淋汤 *gāo lín tāng*

Dyke-Strengthening Pill 巩堤丸 *gǒng tí wán*

Bladder-Securing Decoction 固脬汤 *gù pāo tāng*

True-Securing Pill 固真丸 *gù zhēn wán*

Immediate Aid Pill 既济丸 *jì jì wán*

Golden Lock Essence-Securing Pill 金锁固精丸 *jīn suǒ gù jīng wán*

Origin-Securing Brew 秘元煎 *mì yuán jiān*

Mantis Egg-Case Powder 桑螵蛸散 *sāng piāo xiāo sǎn*

Land and Water Two Immortals Elixir 水陆二仙丹 *shuǐ lù èr xiān dān*

Song-Shi Pig's Stomach Pill 松石猪肚丸 *sōng shí zhū dǔ wán*

Stream-Reducing Pill 缩泉丸 *suō quán wán*

Cuscuta Seed Pill 菟丝子丸 *tù sī zǐ wán*

Powerful Happiness Pill 威喜丸 *wēi xǐ wán*

Pig's Stomach Pill 猪肚丸 *zhū dǔ wán*

Stem flooding and check discharge 固崩止带

White Discharge Tablet 白带片 *bái dài piàn*

Well-Tried Flooding Formula 崩证极验方 *bēng zhèng jí yàn fāng*

Biota Leaf and Toona Bark Pill 侧柏樗皮丸 *cè bǎi shū pí wán*

Sanguisorba Powder 地榆散 *dì yú sǎn*

Clove, Ass Hide Glue, and Mugwort Decoction 丁香胶艾汤 *dīng xiāng jiāo ài tāng*

Precipitation-Checking Decoction 断下汤 *duàn xià tāng*

Root-Securing Flood-Stanching Decoction 固本止崩汤 *gù běn zhǐ bēng tāng*

Thoroughfare-Securing Decoction 固冲汤 *gù chōng tāng*

Menses-Securing Pill 固经丸 *gù jīng wán*

Supplemented Yellow Earth Decoction 加味黄土汤 *jiā wèi huáng tǔ tāng*

Ass Hide Glue and Mugwort Decoction 胶艾汤 *jiāo ài tāng*

Deerhorn and Cuscuta Pill 鹿角菟丝丸 *lù jiǎo tù sī wán*

Discharge-Clearing Decoction 清带汤 *qīng dài tāng*

Heat-Clearing Channel-Securing (Menses-Securing) Decoction 清热固经汤 *qīng rè gù jīng tāng*

Heat-Clearing Uterine Bleeding Decoction 清热止崩汤 *qīng rè zhǐ bēng tāng*

Discharge-Ceasing Decoction 完带汤 *wán dài tāng*

Transforming Yellow Decoction 易黄汤 *yì huáng tāng*

Discharge-Curing Pill 愈带丸 *yù dài wán*

Discharge-Checking Tablet 止带片 *zhǐ dài piàn*

Kidney-Enriching Thoroughfare-Securing Decoction 滋肾固冲汤 *zī shèn gù chōng tāng*

Constrain the lung and suppress cough 敛肺止咳

Panting-Stabilizing Powder 定喘散 *dìng chuān sǎn*

Nine Immortals Elixir 九仙丹 *jiǔ xiān dān*

Nine Immortals Powder 九仙散 *jiǔ xiān sǎn*

Schisandra Decoction 五味子汤 *wǔ wèi zǐ tāng*

One Dose Powder 一服散 *yī fú sǎn*

Ejection Formulas 涌吐剂

Repletion patterns 实证

Sagacious Two Powder 二圣散 *èr shèng sǎn*

Melon Stalk Powder 瓜蒂散 *guā dì sǎn*

Emergency Drool-Thinning Powder 急救稀涎散 *jí jiù xī xián sǎn*

Sagacious Three Powder 三圣散 *sān shèng sǎn*

Drool-Thinning Powder 稀涎散 *xī xián sǎn*

Mechanical Ejection Brine 盐汤探吐方 *yán tāng tàn tù fāng*

Vacuity patterns 虚证

Ginseng Tops Beverage 参芦饮 *shēn lú yǐn*

Oral Formulas for Welling-Abscesses and Sores 痈疡剂

Internal welling-abscess 内痈

Rice Bean and Tangkuei Powder 赤小豆当归散 *chì xiǎo dòu dāng guī sǎn*

Rhubarb and Moutan Decoction 大黄牡丹皮汤 *dà huáng mǔ dān pí tāng*

Red Brocade Tablet 锦红片 *jǐn hóng piàn*

Appendix Stasis-Transforming Decoction 阑尾化瘀汤 *lán wěi huà yū tāng*

Appendix Clearing and Transforming Decoction 阑尾清化汤 *lán wěi qīng huà tāng*

Appendix-Clearing and Resolving Decoction 阑尾清解汤 *lán wěi qīng jiě tāng*

Intestine-Clearing Beverage 清肠饮 *qīng cháng yǐn*

Phragmites Stem Decoction 苇茎汤 *wěi jīng tāng*

Coix, Aconite, and Baijiang Powder 薏苡附子败酱散 *yì yǐ fù zǐ bài jiàng sǎn*

Pyothorax Formula 治脓胸方 *zhì nóng xiōng fāng*

External sores—yang patterns 外疡阳证

Sore-Toxin Pill 疮毒丸 *chuāng dú wán*

Spare-the-Knife Powder 代刀散 *dài dāo sǎn*

Trichosanthes and Arctium Decoction 瓜蒌牛蒡汤 *guā lóu niú bàng tāng*

Forsythia, Lonicera, and Bolbostemma Brew 连翘金贝煎 *lián qiào jīn bèi jiān*

Six Spirits Pill 六神丸 *liù shén wán*

Internal Coursing Coptis Decoction 内疏黄连汤 *nèi shū huáng lián tāng*

Bovine Bezoar Awake to Relief Pill 牛黄醒消丸 *niú huáng xǐng xiāo wán*

Mysterious Four Decoction 四妙汤 *sì miào tāng*

Mysterious Four Resting Hero Decoction 四妙勇安汤 *sì miào yǒng ān tāng*

Pus-Outthrusting Powder 透脓散 *tòu nóng sǎn*

Internal Expression and Pain-Relieving Decoction 托里定痛汤 *tuō lǐ dìng tòng tāng*

Internal Expression Pus-Expelling Decoction 托里透脓汤 *tuō lǐ tòu nóng tāng*

Internal Expression Toxin-Dispersing Powder 托里消毒散 *tuō lǐ xiāo dú sǎn*

External Medicine Toad Venom Pill 外科蟾酥丸 *wài kē chán sū wán*

Five-Jewel Powder 五宝散 *wǔ bǎo sǎn*

Five Spirits Decoction 五神汤 *wǔ shén tāng*

Five-Ingredient Toxin-Dispersing Beverage 五味消毒饮 *wǔ wèi xiāo dú yǐn*

Immortal Formula Life-Giving Beverage 仙方活命饮 *xiān fāng huó mìng yǐn*

Sore-Healing Beverage 消疮饮 *xiāo chuāng yǐn*

Hemorrhoid-Dispersing Beverage 消痔饮 *xiāo zhì yǐn*

Medical Insights Pus-Outthrusting Powder 心悟透脓散 *xīn wù tòu nóng sǎn*

Awake to Dispersion Pill 醒消丸 *xǐng xiāo wán*

External sores—yin patterns 外疡阴证

Unlimited Efficacy Elixir 万灵丹 *wàn líng dān*

Harmonious Yang Decoction 阳和汤 *yáng hé tāng*

Formulas for External Use 外用剂

Internal medicine formulas for external use 内科外用剂

Kansui Powder 甘遂散 *gān suì sǎn*

Melon Stalk Wonder Powder 瓜蒂神妙散 *guā dì shén miào sǎn*

Melon Pedicel Powder 瓜丁散 *guā dīng sǎn*

Fire and Water Hexagram Granules 坎离砂 *kǎn lí shā*

Sulfur and Scallion Topical Application 硫葱敷剂 *liú cōng fū jì*

Navel-Warming Paste 暖脐膏 *nuǎn qí gāo*

Wheezing and Panting External Application Formula 哮喘敷治方 *xiāo chuǎn fū zhì fāng*

Eye, ear, nose, and throat formulas for external use 眼耳喉鼻科外用剂

Eight-Jewel Eye Medication 八宝眼药 *bā bǎo yǎn yào*

Bai Jing-Yu's Eye Medication 白敬宇眼药 *bái jìng yǔ yǎn yào*

Bai's Eye Medication 白氏眼药 *bái shì yǎn yào*

Borneol and Borax Powder 冰硼散 *bīng péng sǎn*

Bright and Glorious Elixir 光明丹 *guāng míng dān*

Obstruction-Abrading Spirit Light Paste 磨障灵光膏 *mó zhàng líng guāng gāo*

Arsenic and Jujube Powder 砒枣散 *pī zǎo sǎn*

Indigo Powder 青黛散 *qīng dài sǎn*

Tin-Like Powder 锡类散 *xí lèi sǎn*

Pearl and Bezoar Powder 珠黄散 *zhū huáng sǎn*

Nasal Insufflation Jasper Clouds Powder 嗜鼻碧云散 *xiù bí bì yún sǎn*

External medicine formulas for external use 外科外用剂

Eight-Jewel Elixir 八宝丹 *bā bǎo dān*

Leukoplakia No.3 Medicinal Paste 白斑二号药膏 *bái bān èr hào yào gāo*

Leukoplakia Wash 白斑洗剂 *bái bān xǐ jì*

Leukoplakia No.1 Medicinal Paste 白斑一号药膏 *bái bān yī hào yào gāo*

White Downborne Elixir 白降丹 *bái jiàng dān*

Fire-Repelling Elixir 避火丹 *bì huǒ dān*

Reversal Powder 颠倒散 *diān dǎo sǎn*

Compound Formula Coptis Paste 复方黄连膏 *fù fāng huáng lián gāo*

Cinnamon Twig and Musk Powder 桂麝散 *guì shè sǎn*

Black Tiger Elixir 黑虎丹 *hēi hǔ dān*

Red Upborne Elixir 红升丹 *hóng shēng dān*

Scutellaria Decoction Wash Formula 黄芩汤洗方 *huáng qín tāng xǐ fāng*

Yang-Returning Jade Dragon Paste 回阳玉龙膏 *huí yáng yù lóng gāo*

Paper Plaster 夹纸膏 *jiā zhǐ gāo*

Golden Yellow Powder 金黄散 *jīn huáng sǎn*

Nine-to-One Elixir 九一丹 *jiǔ yī dān*

Alum Hemorrhoid-Desiccating Powder 枯痔散 *kū zhì sǎn*

Flavescent Sophora Decoction 苦参汤 *kǔ shēn tāng*

Thoroughly Pounded Paste 千捶膏 *qiān chuí gāo*

Cool Clearing Paste 清凉膏 *qīng liáng gāo*

Agreeable Golden Yellow Powder 如意金黄散 *rú yì jīn huáng sǎn*

Three Yellows Wash Preparation 三黄洗剂 *sān huáng xǐ jì*

Three-Shot Gun 三品一条枪 *sān pǐn yī tiáo qiāng*

Cnidium Seed Powder 蛇床子散 *shé chuáng zǐ sǎn*

Flesh-Engendering Powder 生肌散 *shēng jī sǎn*

Flesh-Engendering Jade and Red Paste 生肌玉红膏 *shēng jī yù hóng gāo*

Sumac Gallnut Powder 五倍子散 *wǔ bèi zǐ sǎn*

Five-to-Five Elixir 五五丹 *wǔ wǔ dān*

Harmonious Yang Decongealing Plaster 阳和解凝膏 *yáng hé jiě níng gāo*

Curled Dock Root Powder 羊蹄根散 *yáng tí gēn sǎn*

Gone-in-One-Sweep 一扫光 *yī sǎo guāng*

Jade and Red Paste 玉红膏 *yù hóng gāo*

Jade Dew Powder 玉露散 *yù lù sǎn*

Wind-Smoothing Powder 熨风散 *yùn fēng sǎn*

External injuries formulas for external use 伤科外用剂

Eight Immortals Free Wanderer Decoction 八仙逍遥汤 *bā xiān xiāo yáo tāng*

Pain-Relieving Paste 定痛膏 *dìng tòng gāo*

Dog Skin Plaster 狗皮膏 *gǒu pí gāo*

Erythrina Decoction 海桐皮汤 *hǎi tóng pí tāng*

Sagacious Incised Wound Powder 如圣金刀散 *rú shèng jīn dāo sǎn*

Stasis-Dissipating Injury Decoction 散瘀和伤汤 *sàn yū hé shāng tāng*

Dampness Damage Pain-Relieving Plaster 伤湿止痛膏 *shāng shī zhǐ tòng gāo*

Sinew-Soothing Blood-Quickening Wash Formula 舒筋活血洗方 *shū jīn huó xuè xǐ fāng*

Peach Blossom Powder 桃花散 *táo huā sǎn*

Litharge Paste 陀僧膏 *tuó sēng gāo*

Topical Bone-Joining Powder 外敷接骨散 *wài fū jiē gǔ sǎn*

Myriad Applications Paste 万应膏 *wàn yìng gāo*

Five Yellows Powder 五黄散 *wǔ huáng sǎn*

Bone-Righting Hot Pack 正骨烫药 *zhèng gǔ tàng yào*

Blood-Stanching Powder 止血散 *zhǐ xuè sǎn*

Cercis Powder 紫荆皮散 *zǐ jīng pí sǎn*

Purple Clouds Plaster 紫云膏 *zǐ yún gāo*

Gynecological formulas for external use 妇科外用剂

Trichomonas Cleansing Pill 霉滴净丸 *méi dī jīng wán*

Cnidium Seed Rinse 蛇床子冲洗剂 *shé chuáng zǐ chōng xǐ jì*

Cancer Formulas 治癌剂

Air Potato Wine 黄药子酒 *huáng yào zǐ jiǔ*

Gate-Opening Powder 开关散 *kāi guān sǎn*

Earthworm, House Lizard, and Three Gallbladders Powder 龙虎三胆散 *lóng hǔ sān dǎn sǎn*

Esophageal Cancer No.2 Formula 食道癌二号方 *shí dào ái èr hào fāng*

Esophageal Cancer No.1 Formula 食道癌一号方 *shí dào ái yī hào fāng*

Origin-Regulating Kidney Qi Pill 调元肾气丸 *tiáo yuán shèn qì tāng*

Arsenic-Jujube Powder 信枣散 *xìn zǎo sǎn*

Appendix IV: A Classified List of Acupuncture Points

Hand Great Yīn Lung Channel

LU-1 中府 *zhōng fǔ*, Central Treasury
LU-2 云门 *yún mén*, Cloud Gate
LU-3 天府 *tiān fǔ*, Celestial Storehouse
LU-4 侠白 *xiá bái*, Guarding White
LU-5 尺泽 *chǐ zé*, Cubit Marsh
LU-6 孔最 *kǒng zuì*, Collection Hole
LU-7 列缺 *liè quē*, Broken Sequence
LU-8 经渠 *jīng qú*, Channel Ditch
LU-9 太渊 *tài yuān*, Great Abyss
LU-10 鱼际 *yú jì*, Fish Border
LU-11 少商 *shào shāng*, Lesser Shang

Hand Yáng Brightness Large Intestine Channel

LI-1 商阳 *shāng yáng*, Shang Yang
LI-2 二间 *èr jiān*, Second Space
LI-3 三间 *sān jiān*, Third Space
LI-4 合谷 *hé gǔ*, Union Valley
LI-5 阳溪 *yáng xī*, Yang Ravine
LI-6 偏历 *piān lì*, Veering Passageway
LI-7 温溜 *wēn liū*, Warm Dwelling
LI-8 下廉 *xià lián*, Lower Ridge
LI-9 上廉 *shàng lián*, Upper Ridge
LI-10 手三里 *shǒu sān lǐ*, Arm Three Li
LI-11 曲池 *qū chí*, Pool at the Bend
LI-12 肘髎 *zhǒu liáo*, Elbow Bone-Hole
LI-13 手五里 *shǒu wǔ lǐ*, (Arm) Five Li
LI-14 臂臑 *bì nào*, Upper Arm
LI-15 肩髃 *jiān yú*, Shoulder Bone
LI-16 巨骨 *jù gǔ*, Great Bone
LI-17 天鼎 *tiān dǐng*, Celestial Tripod
LI-18 扶突 *fú tú*, Protuberance Assistant
LI-19 禾髎 *hé liáo*, Grain Bone-Hole
LI-20 迎香 *yíng xiāng*, Welcome Fragrance

Foot Yáng Brightness Stomach Channel

ST-1 承泣 *chéng qì*, Tear Container
ST-2 四白 *sì bái*, Four Whites
ST-3 巨髎 *jù liáo*, Great Bone-Hole
ST-4 地仓 *dì cāng*, Earth Granary
ST-5 大迎 *dà yíng*, Great Reception
ST-6 颊车 *jiá chē*, Cheek Carriage
ST-7 下关 *xià guān*, Below the Joint
ST-8 头维 *tóu wéi*, Head Corner
ST-9 人迎 *rén yíng*, Man's Prognosis
ST-10 水突 *shuǐ tú*, Water Prominence
ST-11 气舍 *qì shè*, Qi Abode
ST-12 缺盆 *quē pén*, Empty Basin
ST-13 气户 *qì hù*, Qi Door
ST-14 库房 *kù fáng*, Storeroom
ST-15 屋翳 *wū yì*, Roof
ST-16 膺窗 *yīng chuāng*, Breast Window
ST-17 乳中 *rǔ zhōng*, Breast Center

ST-18 乳根 *rǔ gēn*, Breast Root
ST-19 不容 *bù róng*, Not Contained
ST-20 承满 *chéng mǎn*, Assuming Fullness
ST-21 梁门 *liáng mén*, Beam Gate
ST-22 关门 *guān mén*, Pass Gate
ST-23 太乙 *tài yǐ*, Supreme Unity
ST-24 滑肉门 *huá ròu mén*, Slippery Flesh Gate
ST-25 天枢 *tiān shū*, Celestial Pivot
ST-26 外陵 *wài líng*, Outer Mound
ST-27 大巨 *dà jù*, Great Gigantic
ST-28 水道 *shuǐ dào*, Waterway
ST-29 归来 *guī lái*, Return
ST-30 气冲 *qì chōng*, Qi Thoroughfare
ST-31 髀关 *bì guān*, Thigh Joint
ST-32 伏兔 *fú tù*, Crouching Rabbit
ST-33 阴市 *yīn shì*, Yin Market
ST-34 梁丘 *liáng qiū*, Beam Hill
ST-35 犊鼻 *dú bí*, Calf's Nose
ST-36 足三里 *zú sān lǐ*, Leg Three Li
ST-37 上巨虚 *shàng jù xū*, Upper Great Hollow
ST-38 条口 *tiáo kǒu*, Ribbon Opening
ST-39 下巨虚 *xià jù xū*, Lower Great Hollow
ST-40 丰隆 *fēng lóng*, Bountiful Bulge
ST-41 解溪 *jiě xī*, Ravine Divide
ST-42 冲阳 *chōng yáng*, Surging Yang
ST-43 陷谷 *xiàn gǔ*, Sunken Valley
ST-44 内庭 *nèi tíng*, Inner Court
ST-45 厉兑 *lì duì*, Severe Mouth

Foot Greater Yīn Spleen Channel

SP-1 隐白 *yǐn bái*, Hidden White
SP-2 大都 *dà dū*, Great Metropolis
SP-3 太白 *tài bái*, Supreme White
SP-4 公孙 *gōng sūn*, Yellow Emperor
SP-5 商丘 *shāng qiū*, Shang Hill
SP-6 三阴交 *sān yīn jiāo*, Three Yin Intersection
SP-7 漏谷 *lòu gǔ*, Leaking Valley
SP-8 地机 *dì jī*, Earth's Crux
SP-9 阴陵泉 *yīn líng quán*, Yin Mound Spring
SP-10 血海 *xuè hǎi*, Sea of Blood
SP-11 箕门 *jī mén*, Winnower Gate
SP-12 冲门 *chōng mén*, Surging Gate
SP-13 府舍 *fǔ shè*, Bowel Abode
SP-14 腹结 *fù jié*, Abdominal Bind
SP-15 大横 *dà hèng*, Great Horizontal
SP-16 腹哀 *fù āi*, Abdominal Lament
SP-17 食窦 *shí dòu*, Food Hole
SP-18 天溪 *tiān xī*, Celestial Ravine
SP-19 胸乡 *xiōng xiāng*, Chest Village
SP-20 周荣 *zhōu róng*, All-Round Flourishing
SP-21 大包 *dà bāo*, Great Embracement

Hand Lesser Yīn Heart Channel

HT-1 极泉 *jí quán*, Highest Spring
HT-2 青灵 *qīng líng*, Green-Blue Spirit

HT-3 少海 *shào hǎi*, Lesser Sea
HT-4 灵道 *líng dào*, Spirit Pathway
HT-5 通里 *tōng lǐ*, Connecting Li
HT-6 阴郄 *yīn xī*, Yin Cleft
HT-7 神门 *shén mén*, Spirit Gate
HT-8 少府 *shào fǔ*, Lesser Mansion
HT-9 少冲 *shào chōng*, Lesser Surge

Hand Greater Yang Small Intestine Channel

SI-1 少泽 *shào zé*, Lesser Marsh
SI-2 前谷 *qián gǔ*, Front Valley
SI-3 后溪 *hòu xī*, Back Ravine
SI-4 腕骨 *wàn gǔ*, Wrist Bone
SI-5 阳谷 *yáng gǔ*, Yang Valley
SI-6 养老 *yǎng lǎo*, Nursing the Aged
SI-7 支正 *zhī zhèng*, Branch to the Correct
SI-8 小海 *xiǎo hǎi*, Small Sea
SI-9 肩贞 *jiān zhēn*, True Shoulder
SI-10 臑俞 *nào shū*, Upper Arm Transport
SI-11 天宗 *tiān zōng*, Celestial Gathering
SI-12 秉风 *bǐng fēng*, Grasping the Wind
SI-13 曲垣 *qū yuán*, Crooked Wall
SI-14 肩外俞 *jiān wài shū*, Outer Shoulder Transport
SI-15 肩中俞 *jiān zhōng shū*, Central Shoulder Transport
SI-16 天窗 *tiān chuāng*, Celestial Window
SI-17 天容 *tiān róng*, Celestial Countenance
SI-18 颧髎 *quán liáo*, Cheek Bone-Hole
SI-19 听宫 *tīng gōng*, Auditory Palace

Foot Greater Yang Bladder Channel

BL-1 睛明 *jīng míng*, Bright Eyes
BL-2 攒竹 *zǎn zhú*, Bamboo Gathering
BL-3 眉冲 *méi chōng*, Eyebrow Ascension
BL-4 曲差 *qū chā*, Deviating Turn
BL-5 五处 *wǔ chù*, Fifth Place
BL-6 承光 *chéng guāng*, Light Guard
BL-7 通天 *tōng tiān*, Celestial Connection
BL-8 络却 *luò què*, Declining Connection
BL-9 玉枕 *yù zhěn*, Jade Pillow
BL-10 天柱 *tiān zhù*, Celestial Pillar
BL-11 大杼 *dà zhù*, Great Shuttle
BL-12 风门 *fēng mén*, Wind Gate
BL-13 肺俞 *fèi shū*, Lung Transport
BL-14 厥阴俞 *jué yīn shū*, Reverting Yin Transport
BL-15 心俞 *xīn shū*, Heart Transport
BL-16 督俞 *dū shū*, Governing Transport
BL-17 膈俞 *gé shū*, Diaphragm Transport
BL-18 肝俞 *gān shū*, Liver Transport
BL-19 胆俞 *dǎn shū*, Gallbladder Transport
BL-20 脾俞 *pí shū*, Spleen Transport
BL-21 胃俞 *wèi shū*, Stomach Transport
BL-22 三焦俞 *sān jiāo shū*, Triple Burner Transport
BL-23 肾俞 *shèn shū*, Kidney Transport
BL-24 气海俞 *qì hǎi shū*, Sea-of-Qi Transport

BL-25 大肠俞 *dà cháng shū*, Large Intestine Transport
BL-26 关元俞 *guān yuán shū*, Pass Head Transport
BL-27 小肠俞 *xiǎo cháng shū*, Small Intestine Transport
BL-28 膀胱俞 *páng guāng shū*, Bladder Transport
BL-29 中膂俞 *zhōng lǚ shū*, Central Backbone Transport
BL-30 白环俞 *bái huán shū*, White Ring Transport
BL-31 上髎 *shàng liáo*, Upper Bone-Hole
BL-32 次髎 *cì liáo*, Second Bone-Hole
BL-33 中髎 *zhōng liáo*, Central Bone-Hole
BL-34 下髎 *xià liáo*, Lower Bone-Hole
BL-35 会阳 *huì yáng*, Meeting of Yang
BL-36 承扶 *chéng fú*, Support
BL-37 殷门 *yīn mén*, Gate of Abundance
BL-38 浮郄 *fú xī*, Superficial Cleft
BL-39 委阳 *wěi yáng*, Bend Yang
BL-40 委中 *wěi zhōng*, Bend Center
BL-41 附分 *fù fēn*, Attached Branch
BL-42 魄户 *pò hù*, Po Door
BL-43 膏肓俞 *gāo huāng shū*, Gao Huang Transport
BL-44 神堂 *shén táng*, Spirit Hall
BL-45 谚譆 *yī xǐ*, Yi Xi
BL-46 膈关 *gé guān*, Diaphragm Pass
BL-47 魂门 *hún mén*, Hun Gate
BL-48 阳纲 *yáng gāng*, Yang Headrope
BL-49 意舍 *yì shè*, Reflection Abode
BL-50 胃仓 *wèi cāng*, Stomach Granary
BL-51 肓门 *huāng mén*, Huang Gate
BL-52 志室 *zhì shì*, Will Chamber
BL-53 胞肓 *bāo huāng*, Bladder Huang
BL-54 秩边 *zhì biān*, Sequential Limit
BL-55 合阳 *hé yáng*, Yang Union
BL-56 承筋 *chéng jīn*, Sinew Support
BL-57 承山 *chéng shān*, Mountain Support
BL-58 飞扬 *fēi yáng*, Taking Flight
BL-59 跗阳 *fū yáng*, Instep Yang
BL-60 昆仑 *kūn lún*, Kunlun Mountains
BL-61 仆参 *pú cān*, Subservient Visitor
BL-62 申脉 *shēn mài*, Extending Vessel
BL-63 金门 *jīn mén*, Metal Gate
BL-64 京骨 *jīng gǔ*, Capital Bone
BL-65 束骨 *shù gǔ*, Bundle Bone
BL-66 通谷 (足) *tōng gǔ (zú)*, (Foot) Valley Passage
BL-67 至阴 *zhì yīn*, Reaching Yin

Foot Lesser Yin Kidney Channel

KI-1 涌泉 *yǒng quán*, Gushing Spring
KI-2 然谷 *rán gǔ*, Blazing Valley
KI-3 太溪 *tài xī*, Great Ravine
KI-4 大钟 *dà zhōng*, Large Goblet
KI-5 水泉 *shuǐ quán*, Water Spring
KI-6 照海 *zhào hǎi*, Shining Sea
KI-7 复溜 *fù liū*, Recover Flow
KI-8 交信 *jiāo xìn*, Intersection Reach

KI-9 筑宾 *zhú bīn*, Guest House
KI-10 阴谷 *yīn gǔ*, Yin Valley
KI-11 横骨 *héng gǔ*, Pubic Bone
KI-12 大赫 *dà hè*, Great Manifestation
KI-13 气穴 *qì xué*, Qi Point
KI-14 四满 *sì mǎn*, Fourfold Fullness
KI-15 中注 *zhōng zhù*, Central Flow
KI-16 肓俞 *huāng shū*, Huang Transport
KI-17 商曲 *shāng qū*, Shang Bend
KI-18 石关 *shí guān*, Stone Pass
KI-19 阴都 *yīn dū*, Yin Metropolis
KI-20 通谷（腹）*tōng gǔ (fù)*, Open Valley
KI-21 幽门 *yōu mén*, Dark Gate
KI-22 步廊 *bù láng*, Corridor Walk
KI-23 神封 *shén fēng*, Spirit Seal
KI-24 灵墟 *líng xū*, Spirit Ruins
KI-25 神藏 *shén cáng*, Spirit Storehouse
KI-26 彧中 *yù zhōng*, Lively Center
KI-27 俞府 *shū fǔ*, Transport Mansion

Hand Reverting Yin Pericardium Channel

PC-1 天池 *tiān chí*, Celestial Pool
PC-2 天泉 *tiān quán*, Celestial Spring
PC-3 曲泽 *qū zé*, Marsh at the Bend
PC-4 郄门 *xī mén*, Cleft Gate
PC-5 间使 *jiān shǐ*, Intermediary Courier
PC-6 内关 *nèi guān*, Inner Pass
PC-7 大陵 *dà líng*, Great Mound
PC-8 劳宫 *láo gōng*, Palace of Toil
PC-9 中冲 *zhōng chōng*, Central Hub

Hand Lesser Yang Triple Burner Channel

TB-1 关冲 *guān chōng*, Passage Hub
TB-2 液门 *yè mén*, Humor Gate
TB-3 中渚 *zhōng zhǔ*, Central Islet
TB-4 阳池 *yáng chí*, Yang Pool
TB-5 外关 *wài guān*, Outer Pass
TB-6 支沟 *zhī gōu*, Branch Ditch
TB-7 会宗 *huì zōng*, Convergence and Gathering
TB-8 三阳络 *sān yáng luò*, Three Yang Connection
TB-9 四渎 *sì dú*, Four Rivers
TB-10 天井 *tiān jǐng*, Celestial Well
TB-11 清冷渊 *qīng lěng yuān*, Clear Cold Abyss
TB-12 消泺 *xiāo luò*, Dispersing Riverbed
TB-13 臑会 *nào huì*, Upper Arm Convergence
TB-14 肩髎 *jiān liáo*, Shoulder Bone-Hole
TB-15 天髎 *tiān liáo*, Celestial Bone-Hole
TB-16 天牖 *tiān yǒu*, Celestial Window
TB-17 翳风 *yì fēng*, Wind Screen
TB-18 瘈脉 *qì mài*, Tugging Vessel
TB-19 颅息 *lú xī*, Skull Rest
TB-20 角孙 *jiǎo sūn*, Angle Vertex
TB-21 耳门 *ěr mén*, Ear Gate
TB-22 和髎 *hé liáo*, Harmony Bone-Hole
TB-23 丝竹空 *sī zhú kōng*, Silk Bamboo Hole

Foot Lesser Yang Gallbladder Channel

GB-1 瞳子髎 *tóng zǐ liáo*, Pupil Bone-Hole

GB-2 听会 *tīng huì*, Auditory Convergence
GB-3 上关 *shàng guān*, Upper Gate
GB-4 颔厌 *hàn yàn*, Forehead Fullness
GB-5 悬颅 *xuán lú*, Suspended Skull
GB-6 悬厘 *xuán lí*, Suspended Tuft
GB-7 曲鬓 *qū bìn*, Temporal Hairline Curve
GB-8 率谷 *shuài gǔ*, Valley Lead
GB-9 天冲 *tiān chòng*, Celestial Hub
GB-10 浮白 *fú bái*, Floating White
GB-11 头窍阴 *tóu qiào yīn*, Head Orifice Yin
GB-12 完骨 *wán gǔ*, Completion Bone
GB-13 本神 *běn shén*, Root Spirit
GB-14 阳白 *yáng bái*, Yang White
GB-15 （头）临泣 *tóu lín qì*, (Head) Overlooking Tears
GB-16 目窗 *mù chuāng*, Eye Window
GB-17 正营 *zhèng yíng*, Upright Construction
GB-18 承灵 *chéng líng*, Spirit Support
GB-19 脑空 *nǎo kōng*, Brain Hollow
GB-20 风池 *fēng chí*, Wind Pool
GB-21 肩井 *jiān jǐng*, Shoulder Well
GB-22 渊腋 *yuān yè*, Armpit Abyss
GB-23 辄筋 *zhé jīn*, Sinew Seat
GB-24 日月 *rì yuè*, Sun and Moon
GB-25 京门 *jīng mén*, Capital Gate
GB-26 带脉 *dài mài*, Girdling Vessel
GB-27 五枢 *wǔ shū*, Fifth Pivot
GB-28 维道 *wéi dào*, Linking Path
GB-29 居髎 *jū liáo*, Squatting Bone-Hole
GB-30 环跳 *huán tiào*, Jumping Round
GB-31 风市 *fēng shì*, Wind Market
GB-32 中渎 *zhōng dú*, Central River
GB-33 膝阳关 *xī yáng guān*, Knee Yang Joint
GB-34 阳陵泉 *yáng líng quán*, Yang Mound Spring
GB-35 阳交 *yáng jiāo*, Yang Intersection
GB-36 外丘 *wài qiū*, Outer Hill
GB-37 光明 *guāng míng*, Bright Light
GB-38 阳辅 *yáng fǔ*, Yang Assistance
GB-39 悬钟 *xuán zhōng*, Suspended Bell
GB-40 丘墟 *qiū xū*, Hill Ruins
GB-41 足临泣 *zú lín qì*, Foot Overlooking Tears
GB-42 地五会 *dì wǔ huì*, Earth Fivefold Convergence
GB-43 侠溪 *xiá xī*, Pinched Ravine
GB-44 足窍阴 *zú qiào yīn*, Foot Orifice Yin

Foot Reverting Yin Liver Channel

LR-1 大敦 *dà dūn*, Large Pile
LR-2 行间 *xíng jiān*, Moving Between
LR-3 太冲 *tài chōng*, Supreme Surge
LR-4 中封 *zhōng fēng*, Mound Center
LR-5 蠡沟 *lí gōu*, Woodworm Canal
LR-6 中都 *zhōng dū*, Central Metropolis
LR-7 膝关 *xī guān*, Knee Joint
LR-8 曲泉 *qū quán*, Spring at the Bend
LR-9 阴包 *yīn bāo*, Yin Bladder
LR-10 足五里 *zú wǔ lǐ*, Foot Five Li

LR-11 阴廉 *yīn lián,* Yin Corner
LR-12 急脉 *jí mài,* Urgent Pulse
LR-13 章门 *zhāng mén,* Camphorwood Gate
LR-14 期门 *qī mén,* Cycle Gate

Controlling Vessel

CV-1 会阴 *huì yīn,* Meeting of Yin
CV-2 曲骨 *qū gǔ,* Curved Bone
CV-3 中极 *zhōng jí,* Central Pole
CV-4 关元 *guān yuán,* Pass Head
CV-5 石门 *shí mén,* Stone Gate
CV-6 气海 *qì hǎi,* Sea of Qi
CV-7 阴交 *yīn jiāo,* Yin Intersection
CV-8 神阙 *shén què,* Spirit Gate Tower
CV-9 水分 *shuǐ fēn,* Water Divide
CV-10 下脘 *xià wǎn,* Lower Stomach Duct
CV-11 建里 *jiàn lǐ,* Interior Strengthening
CV-12 中脘 *zhōng wǎn,* Central Stomach Duct
CV-13 上脘 *shàng wǎn,* Upper Stomach Duct
CV-14 巨阙 *jù què,* Great Tower Gate
CV-15 鸠尾 *jiū wěi,* Turtledove Tail
CV-16 中庭 *zhōng tíng,* Center Palace
CV-17 膻中 *shān zhōng,* Chest Center
CV-18 玉堂 *yù táng,* Jade Hall
CV-19 紫宫 *zǐ gōng,* Purple Palace
CV-20 华盖 *huá gài,* Florid Canopy
CV-21 璇玑 *xuán jī,* Jade Swivel
CV-22 天突 *tiān tú,* Celestial Chimney
CV-23 廉泉 *lián quán,* Ridge Spring
CV-24 承浆 *chéng jiāng,* Sauce Receptacle

Governing Vessel

GV-1 长强 *cháng qiáng,* Long Strong
GV-2 腰俞 *yāo shū,* Lumbar Transport
GV-3 腰阳关 *yāo yáng guān,* Lumbar Yang Pass
GV-4 命门 *mìng mén,* Life Gate
GV-5 悬枢 *xuán shū,* Suspended Pivot
GV-6 脊中 *jǐ zhōng,* Spinal Center
GV-7 中枢 *zhōng shū,* Central Pivot
GV-8 筋缩 *jīn suō,* Sinew Contraction
GV-9 至阳 *zhì yáng,* Extremity of Yang
GV-10 灵台 *líng tái,* Spirit Tower
GV-11 神道 *shén dào,* Spirit Path
GV-12 身柱 *shēn zhù,* Body Pillar
GV-13 陶道 *táo dào,* Kiln Path
GV-14 大椎 *dà zhuī,* Great Hammer
GV-15 哑门 *yǎ mén,* Mute's Gate
GV-16 风府 *fēng fǔ,* Wind Mansion
GV-17 脑户 *nǎo hù,* Brain's Door
GV-18 强间 *qiáng jiān,* Unyielding Space
GV-19 后顶 *hòu dǐng,* Behind the Vertex
GV-20 百会 *bǎi huì,* Hundred Convergences
GV-21 前顶 *qián dǐng,* Before the Vertex
GV-22 囟会 *xìn huì,* Fontanel Meeting
GV-23 上星 *shàng xīng,* Upper Star
GV-24 神庭 *shén tíng,* Spirit Court
GV-25 素髎 *sù liáo,* White Bone-Hole
GV-26 水沟 *shuǐ gōu,* Water Trough
GV-27 兑端 *duì duān,* Extremity of the Mouth
GV-28 龈交 *yín jiāo,* Gum Intersection

References

[1] 《三百种医籍录》. 台北：启业书局，1986.
[2] 《中医伤科学》. 台北：启业书局，1978.
[3] 《风火痰瘀论》. 台北：启业书局，1989.
[4] 《针灸配穴》. 台北：启业书局，1981.

二画

[5] 丁光迪主编，隋·巢元方. 《诸病源候论校注》. 北京：人民卫生出版社，1992.

三画

[6] 上海中医学院. 《中医学基础》. 香港：商务印书馆香港分馆，1995.
[7] 上海中医学院. 《妇产科学》. 香港：商务印书馆，1976.
[8] 上海中医学院中医文献研究所. 《中国医籍字典》. 南昌：江西科学技术出版社，1989.
[9] 山东中医学院、河北中医学院校释. 《黄帝内经素问校释》. 人民卫生出版社，北京：1992.
[10] 广州中医学院汉英常用中医词汇编写组. 《汉英常用中医词汇》. (Chinese-English Glossary of Common Terms in Traditional Chinese Medicine). 香港：三联书店，1982.
[11] 马兴民. 《新编中药炮制法》. 西安：陕西科学技术出版社，1980.
[12] 马建中. 《温热病篇新解》. 台北：国立中医药研究所，1993.

四画

[13] 王立早主编. 《中国针灸处方大成》. 南昌：江西科学技术出版社，1990.
[14] 王岱主编. 《针灸处方学》. 北京：北京出版社，1990.
[15] 王振坤、肖淑春编著. 《现代针灸临床聚英》. 北京：中医古籍出版社，1987.
[16] 王绵之、许济群主编. 《方剂学》. 台北：知音出版社，1997；原版：许济群、王绵之主编. 北京：人民卫生出版社，1995.
[17] 王德鉴主编. 《中医耳鼻喉科学》. 台北：知音出版社，1990；原版：北京：人民卫生出版社，1987.
[18] 天津科学技术出版社总纂. 《金元四大家医学全书（上、下）》. 天津：天津科学技术出版社，1994.
[19] 中文大辞典编纂委员会. 《中文大辞典》. 台北：中国文化大学出版部，1992.
[20] 中医大辞典编辑委员会. 《中医大辞典·外科骨伤五官科分册》. 北京：人民卫生出版社，1987.
[21] 中医大辞典编辑委员会. 《中医大辞典·中药分册》. 北京：人民卫生出版社，1982.
[22] 中医大辞典编辑委员会. 《中医大典·内科分册》. 北京：人民卫生出版社，1987.
[23] 中医大辞典编辑委员会. 《中医大辞典·医史文献分册》. 北京：人民卫生出版社，1981.
[24] 中医大辞典编辑委员会. 《中医大辞典·妇科儿科分册》. 北京：人民卫生出版社，1980.
[25] 中医大辞典编辑委员会. 《中医大辞典·基础理论分册》. 北京：人民卫生出版社，1982.
[26] 中国中医研究院、广州中医学院主编. 《实用中医辞典》. 台北：知音出版社，1992；原版：中医研究院、广州医学院合编，《简明中医辞典》. 北京：人民卫生出版社，1979.
[27] 中医研究院、广东中医学院合编. 《中医常用术语集注》. 台北：王家出版社，1985；原版：《中医名词术语词典》. 香港：商务印书馆，1975.
[28] 中医研究院中药研究所、北京药品生物检定所编. 《中药炮制经验集成》. 北京：人民卫生出版社，1963.
[29] 邓铁涛主编. 《中医诊断学》. 知音出版社，台北：1989；原版：北京：人民卫生出版社，1987.
[30] 邓铁涛主编. 《实用中医诊断学》. 上海：上海科学技术出版社，1988.
[31] 丹波元简. 《素问识·素问绍识、灵枢识、难经疏证》. 北京：人民卫生出版社，1984.
[32] 丹波元坚、丹波元简. 《伤寒广要、药治通义、救急选方、脉学辑要》. 北京：人民卫生出版社，1983.
[33] 丹波元胤编. 《中医医籍考》. 北京：人民卫生出版社，1956.

五画

[34] 田润芝主编. 《脏腑辨证用药规律》. 太原：山西科学技术出版社，1994.
[35] 汉英医学大词典编纂委员会. 《汉英医学大词典》. 北京：人民卫生出版社，1987.
[36] 印会河、张伯讷主编. 《中医基础理论》. 台北：知音出版社，1990；原版：北京：人民卫生出版社，1989.

六画

[37] 刘汉银编著. 《实用针灸大全》. 北京：北京出版社，1988.
[38] 江克明、包明蕙编著. 《简明方剂辞典》. 上海：上海科学技术出版社，1991.
[39] 江育仁主编. 《中医儿科学》. 台北：知音出版社，1989；原版：北京：人民卫生出版社，1987.
[40] 朱江等编. 《实用针灸治疗表解》. 北京：中医古籍出版社，1994.
[41] 孙孝洪. 《中医治疗学原理》. 台北：知音出版社，1990.
[42] 孙学全编. 《针灸临床问答》. 济南：山东科学技术出版社，1987.
[43] 孙国杰、涂晋文主编. 《中医治疗学》. 北京：中国医药科技出版社，1990.

[44] 创医会学术部主编.《汉方用语大辞典》. 东京：燎原株式会社， 1984.

七画

[45] 杨大春、赵成祐、刘方英.《脏腑证治》. 天津：天津科学技术出版社， 1981.

[46] 杨甲三主编.《针灸学(上、下)》. 台北：知音出版社， 1990；原版：北京：人民卫生出版社， 1985.

[47] 杨志一.《中医学诊断释义》. 台北：文光图书有限公司， 1981.

[48] 杨华森主编.《简明中医字典》. 贵州：贵州人民出版社， 1983.

[49] 李克光主编.《金匮要略》. 台北：知音出版社， 1990；原版：北京：人民卫生出版社， 1989.

[50] 李经纬、区永欣等主编.《中医大辞典》. 北京：人民卫生出版社， 1995.

[51] 李培生主编.《伤寒论》. 台北：知音出版社， 1979；原版：北京：人民卫生出版社， 1987.

[52] 李箱主编.《温病学辞典》. 北京：中医古籍出版社， 1991.

[53] 吴克潜.《病源辞典》. 香港：实用书局， 1965；原版：上海：大众书局， 1937.

[54] 清·吴谦等编.《医宗金鉴》. 台北：新文丰出版公司， 1985.

[55] 吴成中主编.《中医证候诊断治疗学》. 北京：人民卫生出版社， 1983.

[56] 冷方南主编.《中医男科临床治疗学》. 台北：知音出版社， 1992.

[57] 冷方南主编.《中医证候辨治轨范》. 北京：人民卫生出版社， 1989.

[58] 邱洪钟.《医学与人类文化》. 长沙：湖南科学技术出版社， 1993.

[59] 何志韶主编.《妇人针方九集》. 台北：知音出版社， 1993.

[60] 余海若.《实用中医内科表典》. 北京：中国科学技术出版社， 1993.

[61] 明·陈实功.《外科正宗》. 台北：世一书局， 1988.

[62] 陈亦人主编.《伤寒论译释》. 上海：上海科学技术出版社，第三版1992 (第一版1959).

[63] 陈西河编.《中医名词辞典》. 台北：五洲出版社， 1978.

[64] 陈贵廷、杨思澍主编.《实用中西医结核诊断治疗学》. 北京：中国医药科技出版社， 1991.

八画

[65] 林华森.《中医外科学》. 台北：迅雷出版社， 1989.

[66] 清·林佩琴.《类证治裁》. 台北，新文丰出版公司：1980.

[67] 罗元慨主编.《中医妇科学》. 台北：知音出版社， 1989.

[68] 罗荣汉.《医用古汉语基础》. 重庆：重庆出版社， 1991.

[69] 欧明.《汉英中医词典》. (Chinese-English Dictionary of Traditional Chinese Medicine). 香港：三联书店， 1988.

[70] 杨维杰等编.《实用中医治法学》. 台北：乐群出版社， 1985.

[71] 国医编辑社编辑.《伤寒论新注》. 台北：文光图书有限公司， 1979.

[72] 武春发、张安桢主编.《中医骨伤科学(上、下)》. 台北：知音出版社， 1992.

[73] 府强主编.《实用针灸疗法临床大全》. 北京：中国医药出版社， 1991.

[74] 河南省卫生厅.《河南省中药材规范》. 郑州：河南科学技术出版社， 1974.

[75] 单玉堂著.《伤寒论针灸配穴选注》. 台北：启业书局， 1986.

[76] 周楣生著，黄时泰、张载义译.《针灸穴名释义》. 合肥：安徽科学技术出版社， 1985.

[77] 禹侯编，清·汪昂原著.《医方集解》. 台北：志远书局， 1990.

[78] 张成国.《灸法、拔罐及放血疗法》. 台中：中国医药学院出版组， 1985.

[79] 张大千主编.《中国针灸大词典》. 北京：北京体育学院出版社， 1998.

[80] 张伯臾主编.《中医内科学》. 台北：知音出版社， 1989；原版：北京：人民卫生出版社， 1988.

[81] 张登本、武长春主编.《内经辞典》. 北京：人民卫生出版社， 1990.

[82] 张贤哲、蔡贵花.《中药炮制学》. 台中：中国医药学院， 1984.

[83] 孟澍江主编.《温病学》. 台北：知音出版社， 1991.

[84] 孟澍江、沈凤阁编.《温病学概要》. 厦门：厦门大学海外函授学院， 1982.

九画

[85] 索延昌.《新脾胃论》. 台北：启业书局， 1987；原版：太原，山西科学教育出版社， 1986.

[86] 清·姚止庵.《素问经注节解》. 北京：人民卫生出版社， 1963.

[87] 清·段玉裁，注汉·许慎撰.《说文解字注》. 台北：黎明文化事业股份有限公司， 1994.

[88] 段德森.《实用古汉语虚词》. 太原：山西教育出版社， 1990.

[89] 帅学忠等编.《汉英双解常用中医名辞术语》. 长沙：湖南科学技术出版社， 1981.

[90] 赵金铎主编.《中医证候诊断治疗学》. 台北：启业书局， 1986.

[91] 赵金铎主编.《中医证候鉴别诊断学》. 北京：人民卫生出版社， 1987.

[92] 赵金铎主编.《中医症状鉴别诊断学》. 北京：人民卫生出版社， 1985.

[93] 赵恩俭.《中医脉诊学》. 天津：天津科学技术出版社， 1990.

[94] 侯天印、王春华编著.《痰证论》. 北京：人民军医出版社， 1989.

十画

[95] 清·唐容川.《血证论》. 台北：五洲出版社， 1984.

[96] 顾伯康主编.《中医外科学》. 台北：知音出版社， 1989；原版：北京：人民卫生出版社， 1987.

[97] 徐元贞等.《中医词释》. 郑州：河南科学技术出版社， 1983.

[98] 徐轩、陈国.《干祖望谈"走黄"与"乳蛾"》. 江苏中医，1992 年第 2 期 35(083) 页.

[99] 徐荣庆等.《针灸学概要》. 厦门：厦门大学海外函授学院， 1981.

[100] 徐楚江主编.《中药炮制学》. 上海：上海科学技术出版社， 1985.

[101] 陆寿康、胡伯虎、张兆发.《图说针刺手法一百二十种》. 台北：知音出版社， 1994.

[102] 郭霭春主编.《黄帝内经词典》. 天津：天津科学技术出版社， 1991.

十一画

[103] 曹炳章编.《中国医学大成》. 上海：上海科学技术出版社， 1988.

[104] 黄三元.《中医方剂学新编》. 台北：八德教育文化出版社， 1984.

[105] 黄云台编.《医用古汉语字典》. 南宁：广西科学技术出版社， 1992.

[106] 黄文东等.《中医内科学》. 厦门：厦门大学海外函授学院， 1982.

[107] 黄三元编审.《中医难字字典》. 台北：八德教育文化出版社， 1990.

[108] 黄明堂校勘，明·杨继洲著.《针灸大成》. 台北：文光图书有限公司， 1987.

[109] 黄维三.《针灸科学》. 台北：国立编译馆， 1985.

[110] 黄进辉编，清·汪昂原著.《医方集解》. 台北：昭人出版社， 1982.

[111] 谢观.《中国医学大辞典》. 北京：中华书店（据 1921 商务印书馆版影印）1988.

[112] 隋·巢元方.《诸病源侯论》. 台北：国立中国医药研究所， 1981.

[113] 萧少卿.《中国针灸处方学》. 台北：启业书局， 1989.

十二画

[114] 湖南省卫生厅.《湖南省中药材规范》. 长沙：湖南科学技术出版社， 1983.

[115] 游士勋、张锦清.《实用中医方剂学》. 台北：乐群文化事业公司， 1983.

[116] 程绍恩、夏洪生主编.《中医证候诊断治疗学》. 北京：北京科学技术出版社， 1993.

[117] 程士德主编.《内经》. 台北：知音出版社， 1990.

[118] 傅延龄主编.《伤寒论研究大辞典》. 济南：山东科学技术出版社， 1994.

[119] 傅瘦生等校注，陈修园著.《灵素集注节要》. 福州：福建科学技术出版社， 1984.

十三画

[120] 裘沛然、丁光迪主编.《中医各家学说》. 台北：知音出版社， 1993；原版：北京：人民卫生出版社， 1992.

[121] 赖天松主编.《临床方剂手册》. 北京：人民卫生出版社， 1992.

十四画

[122] 蔡鸿祺.《中医诊断学表解》. 台北：志远书局， 1990.

[123] 蔡济舟.《针灸学重点整理》. 台北：志远书局， 1991.

[124] 甄志亚主编.《中国医学史》. 台北：知音出版社， 1994.

[125] 廖品正主编.《中医眼科学》. 台北：知音出版社， 1993.

十八画

[126] 颜正华主编.《中药学（上、下)》. 台北：知音出版社， 1991.

[127] 颜道铭编著.《伤科古今汇编》. 台北：启业书局， 1990.

[128] 魏迺杰 (Nigel Wiseman).《汉英英汉中医词典》. 长沙：湖南科技出版社， 1995.

Non-Chinese Works

[129] Kleinman, Arthur, *Patients and Healers in the Context of Culture: An Exploration of the Borderland between Anthropology, Medicine, and Psychiatry*. Berkeley: University of California Press, 1980.

[130] Unschuld, P.U., *Medicine in China: A History of Ideas*. Berkeley: University of California Press, 1985.

[131] Unschuld, P.U., *Medicine in China: Nan-Ching, the Classic of Difficult Issues*, Berkeley: University of California Press, 1986.

[132] Unschuld, P.U., *Chinese Medicine*, Munich: C.H. Beck, 1997.

[133] Wiseman, Nigel, with Ken Boss, *Glossary of Chinese Medical Terms and Acupuncture Points*. Brookline: Paradigm Publications, 1990.

[134] Wiseman, Nigel （魏迺杰）, *English-Chinese Chinese-English Dictionary of Chinese Medicine*. Changsha: Hunan Science and Technology Press, 1995.

[135] Ellis A, Wiseman, N., Boss, K., *Fundamentals of Chinese Acupuncture*. Brookline: Paradigm Publications, 1988.

Index

This index allows all English entry terms to be accessed by Pinyin-Chinese. For example, by looking up *shèn yán* 肾岩 in this index, the reader will be given English term "kidney rock," which is the entry under which this item appears in the body of the text.

The names of medicinals and formulas appearing in the main body of the text in their English names with parenthesized Pinyin can be accessed in the index by English and Pinyin-Chinese; medicinals can also be accessed by Latin pharmaceutical names which are capitalized. Acupuncture point names, which appear in the text in alphanumeric code with parenthesized Pinyin and English, can be accessed their alphanumeric code, Pinyin-Chinese, and English names.

The index also includes classical texts such as *The Inner Canon* (*nèi jīng*) and *On Cold Damage* (*shāng hán lùn*). These can be accessed by the Pinyin-Chinese title or by the English translation. Modern source texts used in the creation of this dictionary are given under References (preceding pages).

*   indicates a Western medical term.

[1,2]   after a drug name indicates that this name serves for two drugs.

ā shì xué 阿是穴, a-shi point, 11

ā shì xué 阿是穴, ouch point, 422

ā shì xué 阿是穴, ouch points, 11, 39, 44, 53, 63, 70, 76, 80, 105, 113–115, 118, 142, 221, 260, 295, 327, 332, 370, 403, 422, 425, 442, 453, 484, 515, 567, 571, 585, 651, 662, 674, 676, 684, 688, 689, 696

aristolochia fruit, *mǎ dōu líng* 马兜铃, Aristolochiae Fructus, 95, 624, 725

Aristolochia Stem Powder, *tiān xiān téng sǎn* 天仙藤散, 454, 601

Aristolochiae Fangchi Radix, *guǎng fáng jǐ* 广防己, southern fangji, 139, 722

Aristolochiae Fructus, *mǎ dōu líng* 马兜铃, aristolochia fruit, 95, 624, 725

Aristolochiae Heterophyllae Radix, *hàn zhōng fáng jǐ* 汉中防己, northern fangji, 139, 154, 722

Aristolochiae Mollissimae Rhizoma seu Herba, *xún gǔ fēng* 寻骨风, mollissima, 139, 722

abalone shell, *shí jué míng* 石决明, Haliotidis Concha, 53, 54, 230, 495, 511, 538, 676, 726

Abalone Shell Powder, *shí jué míng sǎn* 石决明散, 195, 500, 740

Abdomen-Quieting Decoction, *cháng níng tāng* 肠宁汤, 447, 741

Abdominal Worm Formula, *zhì fù nèi chóng fāng* 治腹内虫方, 737

Abri Cantoniensis Herba cum Radice, *jī gǔ cǎo* 鸡骨草, prayer-beads, 68, 721

abscess of the iliac fossa*, 342

abscess*

  alveolar, 323

  hepatic, 670

  parapharyngeal, 611

  perianal, 9

  periappendicular, 318

  peritonsillar, 612, 671

  pulmonary, 469

  retropharyngeal, 6, 612, 671

  superficial, 670

abscesses*, 187

Acalyphae Herba, *tiě xiàn* 铁苋, copperleaf, 724

Acanthopanacis Radicis Cortex, *wǔ jiā pí* 五加皮, acanthopanax, 139, 722

acanthopanax, *wǔ jiā pí* 五加皮, Acanthopanacis Radicis Cortex, 139, 722

accident*

  cerebrovascular, 433, 631, 689

Account of Medicine (*yī shù*) 医述, 1826 (Qīng), Chéng Wén-Yòu 程文囿, 366

acetabulum*, 607

achyranthes, *niú xī* 牛膝, Achyranthis Bidentatae Radix, 36, 45, 78, 138, 154, 328, 352, 390, 415, 485, 503, 548, 604, 614, 685, 724

Achyranthis Bidentatae Radix, *niú xī* 牛膝, achyranthes, 36, 45, 78, 138, 154, 328, 352, 390, 415, 485, 503, 548, 604, 614, 685, 724

Achyranthis Radix, *tǔ niú xī* 土牛膝, native achyranthes, 138, 459, 724

acne rosacea*, 149

acne*, 5

aconite, *fù zǐ* 附子, Aconiti Tuber Laterale, 12, 23, 26, 83, 84, 97, 182, 183, 217, 228, 242, 247, 272, 292, 293, 332, 335, 341, 343, 393, 402, 405, 426, 438, 456, 467, 469, 474, 480, 489, 504, 526, 529, 556, 564, 596, 612, 649, 660–664, 679, 723

aconite, *xián fù zǐ* 咸附子, Aconiti Tuber Laterale Salsum, 311

Aconite and Cinnamon Center-Rectifying Pill, *fù guì lǐ zhōng wán* 附桂理中丸, 734

Aconite and Rice Decoction, *fù zǐ gēng mǐ tāng* 附子粳米汤, 734

Aconite Center-Rectifying Decoction, *fù zǐ lǐ zhōng tāng* 附子理中汤, 29, 46, 62, 80, 85, 86, 124, 145, 151, 247, 559, 564, 646, 647, 702, 711

Aconite Center-Rectifying Pill, *fù zǐ lǐ zhōng wán* 附子理中丸, 425, 734

Aconite Heart-Draining Decoction, *fù zǐ xiè xīn tāng* 附子泻心汤, 733

aconite main tuber, *chuān wū tóu* 川乌头, Aconiti Tuber, 97, 242, 400, 411, 527, 660, 662, 711, 723

Aconite Main Tuber and Cinnamon Twig Decoction, *wū tóu guì zhī tāng* 乌头桂枝汤, 735

Aconite Main Tuber and Halloysite Pill, *wū tóu chì shí zhī wán* 乌头赤石脂丸, 58

Aconite Main Tuber Brew, *wū tóu jiān* 乌头煎, 505

Aconite Main Tuber Decoction, *wū tóu tāng* 乌头汤, 662, 735

Aconite Pill, *fù zǐ wán* 附子丸, 612

aconite/typhonium, *bái fù zǐ* 白附子, Aconiti Coreani seu Typhonii Gigantei Tuber, 140, 623, 690, 725

Aconiti Coreani seu Typhonii Gigantei Tuber, *bái fù zǐ* 白附子, aconite/typhonium, 140, 623, 690, 725

Aconiti Coreani Tuber, *guān bái fù* 关白附, Korean aconite, 623, 725

Aconiti Tsao-Wu-Tou Tuber, *cǎo wū tóu* 草乌头, wild aconite, 411, 660, 723

Aconiti Tsao-Wu-Tou Tuber Crudum, *shēng cǎo wū* 生草乌, raw wild aconite, 460

Aconiti Tuber, *chuān wū tóu* 川乌头, aconite main tuber, 97, 242, 400, 411, 527, 660, 662, 711, 723

Aconiti Tuber Laterale, *fù zǐ* 附子, aconite, 12, 23, 26, 83, 84, 97, 182, 183, 217, 228, 242, 247, 272, 292, 293, 332, 335, 341, 343, 393, 402, 405, 426, 438, 456, 467, 469, 474, 480, 489, 504, 526, 529, 556, 564, 596, 612, 649, 660–664, 679, 723

Aconiti Tuber Laterale Album, *bái fù piàn* 白附片, white sliced aconite, 660, 723

Aconiti Tuber Laterale Conquitum, *shú fù zǐ* 熟附子, cooked aconite, 11, 48, 660, 663, 723

Aconiti Tuber Laterale Denigratum, *hēi shùn piàn* 黑顺片, black sliced aconite, 660, 723

Aconiti Tuber Laterale Parvum, *cè zǐ* 侧子, small aconite, 97

Aconiti Tuber Laterale Salsum, *xián fù zǐ* 咸附子, salted aconite, 311, 367, 660, 723

Aconiti Tuber Laterale Tianxiong, *tiān xióng* 天雄, tianxiong aconite, 23, 97

Acori Rhizoma, *shí chāng pú* 石菖蒲, acorus, 10, 122, 222, 223, 331, 420, 433, 476, 526, 540, 541, 625, 638, 673, 709, 722, 726

acorus, *shí chāng pú* 石菖蒲, Acori Rhizoma, 10, 122, 222, 223, 331, 420, 433, 476, 526, 540, 541, 625, 638, 673, 709, 722, 726

Acorus and Curcuma Decoction, *chāng pú yù jīn tāng* 菖蒲郁金汤, 434

actinolite, *yáng qǐ shí* 阳起石, Actinolitum, 53, 511, 593, 727

Actinolitum, *yáng qǐ shí* 阳起石, actinolite, 53, 511, 593, 727

acute bronchitis*, 438, 659

acute conjunctivitis*, 685

acute enteritis*, 77, 588

acute epiglottitis*, 612

acute icteric hepatitis*, 111

acute infectious hepatitis*, 700

acute lymphadenitis*, 685

acute myelitis*, 678

acute purulent lymphadenitis*, 670

acute tonsillitis*, 659

adenophora, *nán shā shēn* 南沙参, Adenophorae Radix, 593, 727

adenophora/glehnia, *shā shēn* 沙参, Adenophorae seu Glehniae Radix, 88, 108, 175, 310, 395, 398, 416, 515, 565, 581, 589, 593, 625, 679, 686, 727

Adenophora/Glehnia and Ophiopogon Decoction, *shā shēn mài dōng tāng* 沙参麦冬汤, 72, 108, 181, 237, 387, 398, 416, 607, 646, 714, 734

Adenophorae Radix, *nán shā shēn* 南沙参, adenophora, 593, 727

Adenophorae seu Glehniae Radix, *shā shēn* 沙参, adenophora/glehnia, 88, 108, 175, 310, 395, 398, 416, 515, 565, 581, 589, 593, 625, 679, 686, 727

adenocarcinoma of the breast*, 385, 386

adenoma*

thyroid, 243

Aesculi Fructus, *suō luó zǐ* 娑罗子, horse chestnut, 493, 724

agastache/patchouli, *huò xiāng* 藿香, Agastaches seu Pogostemi Herba, 7, 10, 66, 82, 121, 143, 153, 167, 384, 401, 457, 587, 588, 625, 669, 722

Agastache/Patchouli and Pig's Bile Pill, *huò dǎn wán* 藿胆丸, 740

Agastache/Patchouli Qi-Righting Powder, *huò xiāng zhèng qì sǎn* 藿香正气散, 77, 152, 153, 218, 539, 580, 732

Agastache/Patchouli Qi-Righting Tablet, *huò xiāng zhèng qì piàn* 藿香正气片, 588, 713

Agastache/Patchouli, Magnolia Bark, Pinellia, and Poria (Hoelen) Decoction, *huò pò xià líng tāng* 藿朴夏苓汤, 23, 118, 410, 733

Agastache/Patchouli, Pinellia, and Poria (Hoelen) Decoction, *huò pò xià líng tāng* 藿朴夏苓汤, 539

Agastaches seu Pogostemi Herba, *huò xiāng* 藿香, agastache/patchouli, 7, 10, 66, 82, 121, 143, 153, 167, 384, 401, 457, 587, 588, 625, 669, 722

Agelena, *cǎo zhī zhū* 草蜘蛛, agelena, 298

agelena, *cǎo zhī zhū* 草蜘蛛, Agelena, 298

Agelena and Hornet's Nest Pill, *zhī fēng wán* 蜘蜂丸, 298

Agkistrodon, *qí shé* 蕲蛇, agkistrodon, 139, 722

agkistrodon, *qí shé* 蕲蛇, Agkistrodon, 139, 722

Agreeable Birth-Hastening Powder, *cuī shēng rú yì sǎn* 催生如意散, 128

Agreeable Golden Yellow Powder, *rú yì jīn huáng sǎn* 如意金黄散, 497, 585, 670, 744

Agrimoniae Herba, *xiān hè cǎo* 仙鹤草, agrimony, 298, 502, 519, 569, 724

Agrimoniae Rhizoma Pullulatum, *xiān hè cǎo gēn yá* 仙鹤草根芽, agrimony root sprout, 183

agrimony, *xiān hè cǎo* 仙鹤草, Agrimoniae Herba, 298, 502, 519, 569, 724

agrimony root sprout, *xiān hè cǎo gēn yá* 仙鹤草根芽, Agrimoniae Rhizoma Pullulatum, 183

ài fǔ 嗳腐, belching of putrid qi, 17

ài fù nuǎn gōng wán 艾附暖宫丸, Mugwort and Cyperus Palace-Warming Pill, 643, 741

ài jiǔ 艾灸, moxa, 401

ài jiǔ bǔ xiè 艾灸补泻, moxibustion supplementing and draining, 403

ài juǎn 艾卷, moxa roll, 402

ài qì 嗳气, belching, 17

ài qì 嗳气, eructation, 178

ài qì fǔ chòu 嗳气腐臭, putrid belching, 474

ài tiáo 艾条, moxa pole, 402

ài tiáo 艾条, moxa stick, 402

ài tiáo jiǔ 艾条灸, poling, 446

ài yè 艾叶, moxa, 401

ài yè 艾叶 mugwort, Artemisiae Argyi Folium, 401, 402, 468, 569

ài yè tàn 艾叶炭 charred mugwort, Artemisiae Argyi Folium Carbonisatum, 38, 331, 488

ài zhù 艾炷, moxa cone, 401

Ailanthi Altissimae Radicis Cortex, *shū gēn bái pí* 樗根白皮, ailanthus root bark, 572

ailanthus root bark, *shū gēn bái pí* 樗根白皮, Ailanthi Altissimae Radicis Cortex, 572

Ailanthus Root Bark Pill, *shū shù pí pí* 樗树根皮丸, 572

air potato, *huáng yào zǐ* 黄药子, Dioscoreae Bulbiferae Tuber, 544, 624, 725

Air Potato Wine, *huáng yào zǐ jiǔ* 黄药子酒, 745

Ajugae Decumbentis Herba, *bái máo xià kū cǎo* 白毛夏枯草, bending bugle, 68, 721

akebia, *bā yuè zhá* 八月札, Akebiae Fructus, 19, 493, 724

Akebiae Fructus, *bā yuè zhá* 八月札, akebia, 19, 493, 724

Albizziae Cortex, *hé huān pí* 合欢皮, silk tree bark, 491, 537, 726

Albizziae Flos, *hé huān huā* 合欢花, silk tree flower, 234, 310

alcoholic cirrhosis*, 149

Alert Spirit Quartet, *sì shén cōng* 四神聪, 11, 25, 178, 236, 259, 261, 271, 333, 365, 413, 457, 506, 520, 537, 638, 652, 654, 673, 716

Aleuritis Seminis Oleum, *tóng yóu* 桐油, tung-oil, 445

Algae Thallus, *kūn bù* 昆布, kelp, 30, 141, 243, 544, 624, 725

alisma, *zé xiè* 泽泻, Alismatis Rhizoma, 21, 30, 47, 56, 136, 224, 230, 238, 243, 390, 394, 397, 410, 434, 463, 666, 679, 703, 716, 723

Alisma Decoction, *zé xiè tāng* 泽泻汤, 87

Alismatis Rhizoma, *zé xiè* 泽泻, alisma, 21, 30, 47, 56, 136, 224, 230, 238, 243, 390, 394, 397, 410, 434, 463, 666, 679, 703, 716, 723

All Yin Brew, *yī yīn jiān* 一阴煎, 450, 701

All Yin Variant Brew, *jiā jiǎn yī yīn jiān* 加减一阴煎, 701

All-the-Way-Through Brew, *yī guàn jiān* 一贯煎, 144, 151, 228, 244, 256, 310, 314, 467, 647, 701, 742

allergic rhinitis*, 543

Allii Bulbus, *xiè bái* 薤白, Chinese chive, 398, 493, 724

Allii Fistulosi Bulbus, *cōng bái* 葱白, scallion white, 176, 422, 500, 502, 681, 720

Allii Fistulosi Bulbus cum Radice, *lián xū cōng bái* 连须葱白, scallion white with root, 228, 502

Allii Fistulosi Herbae Succus, *cōng zhī* 葱汁, scallion juice, 307

Allii Sativi Bulbi Succus, *suàn zhī* 蒜汁, garlic juice, 307

Allii Sativi Bulbus, *dà suàn* 大蒜, garlic, 111, 183, 445, 728

Allii Sativi Bulbus Pulpatus, *suàn ní* 蒜泥, mashed garlic, 388, 389

Allii Tuberosi Folium, *jiǔ cài* 韭菜, Chinese leek, 241, 593, 727

Allii Tuberosi Semen, *jiǔ zǐ* 韭子, Chinese leek seed, 593, 727

almond, *bā dàn xìng rén* 巴旦杏仁, Pruni Amygdali Semen, 624, 725

Aloe, *lú huì* 芦荟, aloe, 459, 460, 722

aloe, *lú huì* 芦荟, Aloe, 459, 460, 722

Aloe Gan-Dispersing Beverage, *lú huì xiāo gān yǐn* 芦荟消疳饮, 236

alopecia areata*, 243

alpinia, *yì zhì rén* 益智仁, Alpiniae Oxyphyllae Fructus, 12, 177, 223, 335, 454, 496, 593, 727

Alpiniae Galangae Fructus, *hóng dòu kòu* 红豆蔻, galangal fruit, 660, 723

Alpiniae Katsumadae Semen, *cǎo dòu kòu* 草豆蔻, Katsumada's galangal seed, 66, 105, 625, 722

Alpiniae Officinarum Rhizoma, *gāo liáng jiāng* 高良姜, lesser galangal, 84, 581, 660, 662, 663, 723

Alpiniae Oxyphyllae Fructus, *yì zhì rén* 益智仁, alpinia, 12, 177, 223, 335, 454, 496, 593, 727

alum, *bái fán* 白矾, Alumen, 53, 154, 225, 244, 383, 395, 401, 464, 466, 497, 599, 668, 728

Alum and Curcuma Pill, *bái jīn wán* 白金丸, 434, 694

Alum Hemorrhoid-Desiccating Powder, *kū zhì sǎn* 枯痔散, 290, 565, 744

Alumen, *bái fán* 白矾, alum, 53, 154, 225, 244, 383, 395, 401, 464, 466, 497, 599, 668, 728

Alumen Calcinatum, *kū fán* 枯矾, calcined alum, 221, 226, 412, 468

amber, *hǔ pò* 琥珀, Succinum, 153, 230, 262, 433, 490, 602, 726

Amber Dragon-Embracing Pill, *hǔ pò bào lóng wán* 琥珀抱龙丸, 740

Amber Powder, *hǔ pò sǎn* 琥珀散, 34, 35, 733

Amber Spirit-Quieting Decoction, *hǔ pò ān shén tāng* 琥珀安神汤, 739

amebic dysentery*, 28, 250

American ginseng, *xī yáng shēn* 西洋参, Panacis Quinquefolii Radix, 175, 593, 726

amethyst/fluorite, *zǐ shí yīng* 紫石英, Amethystum seu Fluoritum, 467, 490, 519, 526, 726

Amethystum seu Fluoritum, *zǐ shí yīng* 紫石英, amethyst/fluorite, 467, 490, 519, 526, 726

Amomi Cardamomi Fructus, *bái dòu kòu* 白豆蔻, cardamom, 153, 167, 224, 434, 625, 722

Amomi Cardamomi Semen, *kòu rén* 蔻仁, cardamom kernel, 401

Amomi Semen seu Fructus, *shā rén* 砂仁, amomum, 10, 45, 80, 103, 105, 141, 224, 257, 437, 443, 450, 454, 512, 561, 564, 625, 669, 722

amomum, *shā rén* 砂仁, Amomi Semen seu Fructus, 10, 45, 80, 103, 105, 141, 224, 257, 437, 443, 450, 454, 512, 561, 564, 625, 669, 722

Amomum Splenic Beverage, *suō pí yǐn* 缩脾饮, 348, 732

Amorphophalli Tuber, *jǔ ruò* 蒟蒻, devil's tongue, 68, 721

ampelopsis, *bái liǎn* 白蔹, Ampelopsis Radix, 68, 721

Ampelopsis Radix, *bái liǎn* 白蔹, ampelopsis, 68, 721

Amydae Carapacis Gelatinum, *biē jiǎ jiāo* 鳖甲胶, turtle shell glue, 243, 593, 727

Amydae Carapax, *biē jiǎ* 鳖甲, turtle shell, 72, 98, 175, 176, 218, 277, 336, 352, 399, 460, 544, 593, 597, 727

Amydae Carapax Calcinatus, *duàn biē jiǎ* 煅鳖甲, calcined turtle shell, 621

Amydae Sanguis, *biē xuè* 鳖血, turtle's blood, 397

ān 安, quiet, 490

ān chōng tāng 安冲汤, Thoroughfare-Quieting Decoction, 603

ān gōng niú huáng wán 安宫牛黄丸, Peaceful Palace Bovine Bezoar Pill, 6, 65, 69, 73, 88, 197, 202, 364, 426, 437, 450, 637, 693, 740

ān huí sǎn 安蛔散, Roundworm-Quieting Powder, 510

ān hún tāng 安魂汤, Soul-Quieting Decoction, 60

ān mián 安眠, Quiet Sleep, 83, 281, 409

ān shén 安神, quieting the spirit, 490

ān shén dìng zhì wán 安神定志丸, Spirit-Quieting Mind-Stabilizing Pill, 230, 268, 538, 739

ān shén shēng huà tāng 安神生化汤, Spirit-Quieting Engendering Transformation Decoction, 455

ān shén wán 安神丸, Spirit-Quieting Pill, 491, 739

ān shèn wán 安肾丸, Kidney-Quieting Pill, 325, 713

ān tāi 安胎, quieting the fetus, 490

ān tāi hé qì yǐn 安胎和气饮, Fetus-Quieting Qi-Harmonizing Beverage, 741

ān tāi yǐn 安胎饮, Fetus-Quieting Beverage, 741

ān wèi yǐn 安胃饮, Stomach-Quieting Beverage, 280

ān xīn 安心, quieting the heart, 490

ān zhōng 安中, quieting the center, 490

àn jié fǎ 按截法, damming method, 109

àn jīng 暗经, surreptitious menstruation, 598

àn mó 按摩, massage, 387

andrographis, *chuān xīn lián* 穿心莲, Andrographidis Herba, 67, 69, 111, 721

Andrographidis Herba, *chuān xīn lián* 穿心莲, andrographis, 67, 69, 111, 721

anemarrhena, *zhī mǔ* 知母, Anemarrhenae Rhizoma, 65, 67, 71, 104, 127, 154, 176, 239, 281, 282, 326, 331, 388, 397, 422, 456, 495, 527, 546, 589, 649, 679, 695, 720

Anemarrhena and Fritillaria Cough-Quieting Decoction, *èr mǔ níng sòu tāng* 二母宁嗽汤, 216

Anemarrhena and Fritillaria Powder, *èr mǔ sǎn* 二母散, 738

Anemarrhena and Phellodendron Eight-Ingredient Pill, *zhī bǎi bā wèi wán* 知柏八味丸, 147, 176, 288, 296, 330, 331, 355, 476, 583, 641, 714

Anemarrhena and Phellodendron Four Agents Decoction, *zhī bǎi sì wù tāng* 知柏四物汤, 38

Anemarrhena Beverage, *zhī mǔ yǐn* 知母饮, 731

Anemarrhena, Phellodendron, and Rehmannia Decoction, *zhī bǎi dì huáng tāng* 知柏地黄汤, 36

Anemarrhena, Phellodendron, and Rehmannia Pill, *zhī bǎi dì huáng wán* 知柏地黄丸, 14, 33, 41, 76, 104, 167, 181, 230, 292, 294, 336, 415, 474, 495, 512, 547, 566, 574, 597, 611, 615, 648, 715, 731

Anemarrhenae Rhizoma, *zhī mǔ* 知母, anemarrhena, 65, 67, 71, 104, 127, 154, 176, 239, 281, 282, 326, 331, 388, 397, 422, 456, 495, 527, 546, 589, 649, 679, 695, 720

anemia*, 162, 194, 261, 272, 290, 616, 646, 704

aplastic, 30

angelica, *bái zhǐ* 白芷, Angelicae Dahuricae Radix, 55, 102, 103, 116, 315, 339, 546, 681, 686, 699, 720

Angelicae Dahuricae Radix, *bái zhǐ* 白芷, angelica, 55, 102, 103, 116, 315, 339, 546, 681, 686, 699, 720

Angelicae Duhuo Radix, *dú huó* 独活, duhuo, 45, 55, 102, 139, 154, 247, 326, 328, 546, 654, 662, 680, 722

Angelicae Sinensis Radicis Corpus, *dāng guī shēn* 当归身, tangkuei body, 256

Angelicae Sinensis Radicis Extremitas, *dāng guī wěi* 当归尾, tangkuei tails, 27, 439

Angelicae Sinensis Radicis Tenuis, *dāng guī xū* 当归须, tangkuei fine root, 356, 390

Angelicae Sinensis Radix, *dāng guī* 当归, tangkuei, 17, 19, 28, 34, 37, 39, 58, 60, 93, 95, 103, 104, 116, 120, 139, 140, 154, 161, 172, 175, 227, 234, 259, 272, 309, 310, 315, 338, 352, 386, 390, 391, 398, 415, 428, 431, 448, 449, 467, 493, 495, 503, 516, 526, 588, 593, 595, 600, 613, 651, 661, 662, 666, 670, 674, 679, 727

Angelicae Sinensis Radix Pinguis, *yóu dāng guī* 油当归, oily tangkuei, 399

angiitis*

thrombotic, 540

angina pectoris*, 268, 270

angina*

Vincent's, 474

angioedema*, 494

angioma of the neck*, 30

angioma*, 37, 632

angiospasm*
    cerebral, 692
Anisi Stellati Fructus, *bā jiǎo huí xiāng* 八角茴香,
    star anise, 222, 600, 660, 723
ankylostomiasis*, 194, 704
Annotated Cold Damage (*zhù jiě shāng hán lùn*) 注
    解伤寒论, 1144 (Jīn), Chéng Wú-Jǐ 成无己, 583
anomalous artemisia, *liú jì nú* 刘寄奴, Artemisiae
    Anomalae Herba, 138, 725
antelope horn, *líng yáng jiǎo* 羚羊角, Antelopis
    Cornu, 54, 56, 65, 93, 209, 245, 526, 591, 726
Antelope Horn and Uncaria Decoction, *líng jiǎo gōu*
    téng tāng 羚角钩藤汤, 53, 73, 364, 683, 690, 740
Antelope Horn and Uncaria Decoction, *líng jiǎo gōu*
    téng tāng 羚角钩藤汤, 51
Antelope Horn Decoction, *líng yáng jiǎo tāng* 羚羊
    角汤, 740
Antelope Horn Powder, *líng yáng jiǎo sǎn* 羚羊角
    散, 178, 702, 740
Antelopis Cornu, *líng yáng jiǎo* 羚羊角, antelope
    horn, 54, 56, 65, 93, 209, 245, 526, 591, 726
Anti-Turbidity Root-Securing Pill, *zhì zhuó gù běn*
    wán 治浊固本丸, 179
ào nóng 懊憹, anguish, 9
aorta*, 272
aphonia*
    spastic, 586
aphthous stomatitis*, 400
appendicitis*, 318
Appendix Clearing and Transforming Decoction, *lán*
    wěi qīng huà tāng 阑尾清化汤, 743
Appendix Point, *lán wěi xué* 阑尾穴, 318
Appendix Stasis-Transforming Decoction, *lán wěi*
    huà yū tāng 阑尾化瘀汤, 743
Appendix-Clearing and Resolving Decoction, *lán wěi*
    qīng jiě tāng 阑尾清解汤, 743
apricot kernel, *xìng rén* 杏仁, Armeniacae Semen,
    56, 72, 82, 95, 127–129, 201, 228, 246, 368, 376,
    398, 399, 410, 434, 513, 527, 571, 624, 625, 683,
    686, 688, 703, 714, 725
Apricot Kernel and Perilla Powder, *xìng sū sǎn* 杏
    苏散, 12, 86, 102, 129, 405, 681, 690, 734
aqueous humor*, 551
aquilaria, *chén xiāng* 沉香, Aquilariae Lignum, 214,
    262, 417, 493, 512, 629, 663, 694, 724
Aquilaria and Asafetida Pill, *chén xiāng ē wèi wán*
    沉香阿魏丸, 515
aquilaria leaven, *chén xiāng qū* 沉香麯, Aquilariae
    Ligni Massa, 388
Aquilaria Powder, *chén xiāng sǎn* 沉香散, 149, 485
Aquilaria Qi-Downbearing Decoction, *chén xiāng*
    jiàng qì tāng 沉香降气汤, 362, 478, 484
Aquilaria Stomach-Warming Pill, *chén xiāng wēn*
    wèi wán 沉香温胃丸, 86
Aquilariae Ligni Massa, *chén xiāng qū* 沉香麯, aquilaria
    leaven, 388
Aquilariae Lignum, *chén xiāng* 沉香, aquilaria, 214,
    262, 417, 493, 512, 629, 663, 694, 724

Aranea, *zhī zhū* 蜘蛛, spider, 98
Arcae Concha, *wǎ léng zǐ* 瓦楞子, ark shell, 59, 478,
    581, 728
Arcae Concha Calcinata, *duàn wǎ léng zǐ* 煅瓦楞子,
    calcined ark shell, 257
arch*
    superciliary, 191
Arctii Fructus, *niú bàng zǐ* 牛蒡子, arctium, 103,
    184, 214, 368, 422, 459, 501, 548, 625, 685, 686,
    720
arctium, *niú bàng zǐ* 牛蒡子, Arctii Fructus, 103,
    184, 214, 368, 422, 459, 501, 548, 625, 685, 686,
    720
Arctium Flesh-Resolving Decoction, *niú bàng jiě jī*
    tāng 牛蒡解肌汤, 187
Ardisiae Japonicae Caulis et Folium, *zǐ jīn niú* 紫金
    牛, Japanese ardisia, 624, 725
areca, *bīng láng* 槟榔, Arecae Semen, 115, 141, 154,
    183, 216, 298, 317, 510, 512, 572, 588, 724
areca husk, *dà fù pí* 大腹皮, Arecae Pericarpium,
    153, 183, 454, 625, 724
Arecae Pericarpium, *dà fù pí* 大腹皮, areca husk,
    153, 183, 454, 625, 724
Arecae Semen, *bīng láng* 槟榔, areca, 115, 141, 154,
    183, 216, 298, 317, 510, 512, 572, 588, 724
arisaema, *tiān nán xīng* 天南星, Arisaematis Rhi-
    zoma, 97, 572, 623, 625, 638, 725
Arisaema and Saussurea Decoction, *xīng xiāng tāng*
    星香汤, 739
Arisaema Pill, *tiān nán xīng wán* 天南星丸, 739
Arisaematis Rhizoma, *tiān nán xīng* 天南星, arisaema,
    97, 572, 623, 625, 638, 725
Arisaematis Rhizoma Crudum, *shēng nán xīng* 生南
    星, raw arisaema, 243, 439, 460, 690
Arisaematis Rhizoma cum Felle Bovis, *dǎn xīng* 胆
    星, bile arisaema, 60, 84, 140, 178, 214, 448, 453,
    541, 623, 725
Arisaematis Rhizoma cum Felle Bovis, *dǎn xīng* 胆
    星, bile arisaema [root], 417
ark shell, *wǎ léng zǐ* 瓦楞子, Arcae Concha, 59, 478,
    581, 728
Armeniacae Semen, *xìng rén* 杏仁, apricot kernel,
    56, 72, 82, 95, 127–129, 201, 228, 246, 368, 376,
    398, 399, 410, 434, 513, 527, 571, 624, 625, 683,
    686, 688, 703, 714, 725
Armeniacae Semen Amarum, *kǔ xìng rén* 苦杏仁,
    bitter apricot kernel, 458
Armeniacae Semen Dulce, *tián xìng rén* 甜杏仁,
    sweet apricot kernel, 624, 725
arrhythmia*, 261, 270
arsenic, *pī shí* 砒石, Arsenicum, 98, 727
Arsenic and Jujube Powder, *pī zǎo sǎn* 砒枣散, 744
Arsenic-Jujube Powder, *xìn zǎo sǎn* 信枣散, 745
Arsenicum, *pī shí* 砒石, arsenic, 98, 727
Arsenicum Sublimatum, *pī shuāng* 砒霜, sublimed
    arsenic, 411
Artemisiae Anomalae Herba, *liú jì nú* 刘寄奴, anoma-
    lous artemisia, 138, 725

Artemisiae Apiaceae seu Annuae Herba, *qīng hāo* 青蒿, sweet wormwood, 68, 69, 72, 255, 277, 281, 282, 587, 649, 664, 721

Artemisiae Argyi Folium, *ài yè* 艾叶, mugwort, 401, 402, 468, 569

Artemisiae Argyi Folium Carbonisatum, *ài yè tàn* 艾叶炭, charred mugwort, 38, 331, 488

Artemisiae Capillaris Herba, *yīn chén hāo* 茵陈蒿, capillaris, 69, 116, 136, 198, 357, 589, 723

Artemisiae Cinae Flos et Folium, *shān dào nián hāo* 山道年蒿, Levant wormseed flower and leaf, 183, 509

arteriosclerosis*, 297, 584

arthritis*, 295
    rheumatic, 82, 280
    rheumatoid, 82, 280

asafetida, *ē wèi* 阿魏, Asafoetida, 243

Asafoetida, *ē wèi* 阿魏, asafetida, 243

asarum, *xì xīn* 细辛, Asiasari Herba cum Radice, 11, 17, 55, 243, 262, 311, 326, 343, 405, 438, 660, 664, 681, 723

Asarum Powder, *xì xīn sǎn* 细辛散, 620

ascariasis*
    biliary, 509, 696

ascites*, 28, 150, 182, 616

ash, *qín pí* 秦皮, Fraxini Cortex, 68, 338, 721

Asiasari Herba cum Radice, *xì xīn* 细辛, asarum, 11, 17, 55, 243, 262, 311, 326, 343, 405, 438, 660, 664, 681, 723

Asini Corii Gelatini Pilula, *ē jiāo zhū* 阿胶珠, ass hide glue pellets, 573

Asini Corii Gelatinum, *ē jiāo* 阿胶, ass hide glue, 31, 37, 38, 58, 70, 161, 243, 256, 390, 488, 519, 526, 537, 557, 569, 574, 593, 595, 597, 602, 617, 727

Asparagi Tuber, *tiān mén dōng* 天门冬, asparagus, 88, 336, 385, 409, 495, 593, 597, 727

asparagus, *tiān mén dōng* 天门冬, Asparagi Tuber, 88, 336, 385, 409, 495, 593, 597, 727

asphyxia*, 193

Aspidii Rhizoma, *guàn zhòng* 贯众, aspidium, 183, 445, 724

aspidium, *guàn zhòng* 贯众, Aspidii Rhizoma, 183, 445, 724

Aspongopus, *jiǔ xiāng chóng* 九香虫, stinkbug, 493, 724

ass hide glue, *ē jiāo* 阿胶, Asini Corii Gelatinum, 31, 37, 38, 58, 70, 161, 243, 256, 390, 488, 519, 526, 537, 557, 569, 574, 593, 595, 597, 602, 617, 727

Ass Hide Glue and Coptis Decoction, *ē jiāo huáng lián tāng* 阿胶黄连汤, 739

Ass Hide Glue and Egg Yolk Decoction, *ē jiāo jī zǐ huáng tāng* 阿胶鸡子黄汤, 740

Ass Hide Glue and Mugwort Decoction, *jiāo ài tāng* 胶艾汤, 743

Ass Hide Glue and Mugwort Four Agents Decoction, *jiāo ài sì wù tāng* 胶艾四物汤, 212, 574

Ass Hide Glue Decoction, *bǔ fèi ē jiāo tāng* 补肺阿胶汤, 469, 734

Ass Hide Glue Decoction, *ē jiāo tāng* 阿胶汤, 734

Ass Hide Glue Four Agents Decoction, *ē jiāo sì wù tāng* 阿胶四物汤, 741

ass hide glue pellets, *ē jiāo zhū* 阿胶珠, Asini Corii Gelatini Pilula, 573

Ass Hide Glue Powder, *ē jiāo sǎn* 阿胶散, 41, 734

aster, *zǐ wǎn* 紫菀, Asteris Radix et Rhizoma, 95, 267, 397, 434, 624, 625, 725

Aster Decoction, *zǐ wǎn tāng* 紫菀汤, 267, 739

Asteris Radix et Rhizoma, *zǐ wǎn* 紫菀, aster, 95, 267, 397, 434, 624, 625, 725

asthma*, 616
    acute attacks of, 428
    bronchial, 280, 435, 438

Astragali (seu Hedysari) Radix, *huáng qí* 黄芪, astragalus, 11, 17, 40, 45, 47, 95, 161, 196, 223, 227, 267, 270, 315, 328, 329, 333, 378, 391, 397, 426, 456, 466, 486, 488, 527, 556, 572, 581, 593–595, 599, 600, 651, 662, 679, 704, 712, 716, 726

Astragali (seu Hedysari) Radix Cruda, *shēng huáng qí* 生黄芪, raw astragalus, 259

Astragali Complanati Semen, *shā yuàn zǐ* 沙苑子, complanate astragalus seed, 11, 297, 584, 593, 727

astragalus, *huáng qí* 黄芪, Astragali (seu Hedysari) Radix, 11, 17, 40, 45, 47, 95, 161, 196, 223, 227, 267, 270, 315, 328, 329, 333, 378, 391, 397, 426, 456, 466, 486, 488, 527, 556, 572, 581, 593–595, 599, 600, 651, 662, 679, 704, 712, 716, 726

Astragalus and Aconite Decoction, *qí fù tāng* 芪附汤, 702, 735

Astragalus and Cinnamon Twig Five Agents Decoction, *huáng qí guì zhī wǔ wù tāng* 黄芪桂枝五物汤, 32, 417, 454, 735

Astragalus Center-Fortifying Decoction, *huáng qí jiàn zhōng tāng* 黄芪建中汤, 217, 251, 314, 427, 529, 566, 581, 651, 663, 710, 735

Astragalus Decoction, *huáng qí tāng* 黄芪汤, 477, 734

Astragalus, Peony, Cinnamon Twig, and Liquor Decoction, *qí sháo guì jiǔ tāng* 芪芍桂酒汤, 704

atherosclerosis*
    cerebral, 355, 365

athlete's foot*, 221

atractylodes, *cāng zhú* 苍术, Atractylodis Rhizoma, 55, 63, 66, 93, 115, 116, 153, 154, 240, 287, 291, 319, 401, 410, 418, 430, 441, 457, 587, 625, 679, 684, 722

Atractylodes and Cyperus Phlegm-Abducting Pill, *cāng fù dǎo tán wán* 苍附导痰丸, 435

Atractylodes Dampness-Eliminating Decoction, *cāng zhú chú shī tāng* 苍术除湿汤, 247

Atractylodes White Tiger Decoction, *cāng zhú bái hǔ tāng* 苍术白虎汤, 113, 591

Atractylodis Ovatae Rhizoma, *bái zhú* 白术, ovate atractylodes, 12, 17, 50, 84, 93, 116, 139, 141, 153, 154, 223, 224, 227, 240, 256, 257, 272, 315, 319, 390, 393, 450, 463, 486, 563, 564, 573, 574, 593–596, 600, 615, 661, 662, 684, 726

Atractylodis Rhizoma, *cāng zhú* 苍术, atractylodes, 55, 63, 66, 93, 115, 116, 153, 154, 240, 287, 291, 319, 401, 410, 418, 430, 441, 457, 587, 625, 679, 684, 722

atrophy*
   optic, 64

Aurantii Fructus, *zhǐ ké* 枳壳, bitter orange, 19, 47, 50, 153, 217, 234, 317, 318, 415, 421, 437, 439, 466, 477, 483, 493, 538, 573, 588, 669, 709, 723

Aurantii Fructus Immaturus, *zhǐ shí* 枳实, unripe bitter orange, 17, 50, 72, 98, 141, 216, 217, 255, 257, 276, 357, 417, 419, 434, 459, 493, 544, 564, 630, 723

Auripigmentum, *cí huáng* 雌黄, orpiment, 727

Awake to Dispersion Pill, *xǐng xiāo wán* 醒消丸, 259, 744

Awake-From-Wind Decoction, *shěng fēng tāng* 省风汤, 417

Axioms of Medicine (*yī mén fǎ lǜ*) 医门法律, 1658, Qīng, Yù Chāng 喻昌, 582

bā bǎo dān 八宝丹, Eight-Jewel Elixir, 744

bā bǎo yǎn yào 八宝眼药, Eight-Jewel Eye Medication, 744

bā dàn xìng rén 巴旦杏仁 almond, Pruni Amygdali Semen, 624, 725

bā dòu 巴豆 croton, Crotonis Semen, 98, 182, 411, 460, 464, 527, 664, 722

bā dòu shuāng 巴豆霜 croton frost, Crotonis Seminis Pulvis, 231, 460, 722

bā fǎ 八法, eight methods, 169

bā fēng 八风, Eight Winds, 80, 112, 115, 221, 289, 540

bā gāng 八纲, eight principles, 169

bā gāng biàn zhèng 八纲辨证, eight-principle pattern identification, 169

bā huì xué 八会穴, eight meeting points, 169

bā jǐ tiān 巴戟天 morinda, Morindae Radix, 222, 310, 332, 400, 529, 593, 675, 679, 716, 727

bā jiǎo huí xiāng 八角茴香 star anise, Anisi Stellati Fructus, 222, 600, 660, 723

bā kuò 八廓, eight ramparts, 169

bā lí sǎn 八厘散, Eight Pinches Powder, 737

bā liáo 八髎, BL-31 through BL-34, Eight Bone-Holes, 45, 297

bā mài jiāo huì xué 八脉交会穴, confluence points of the eight vessels, 92

bā mài jiāo huì xué 八脉交会穴, master points of the eight vessels, 387

bā wèi dì huáng wán 八味地黄丸, Eight-Ingredient Rehmannia Pill, 47, 228, 650, 741

bā wèi wán 八味丸, Eight-Ingredient Pill, 229, 425

bā wù tāng 八物汤, Eight Agents Decoction, 157

bā xiān cháng shòu wán 八仙长寿丸, Eight Immortals Longevity Pill, 742

bā xiān xiāo yáo tāng 八仙逍遥汤, Eight Immortals Free Wanderer Decoction, 744

bā xié 八邪, Eight Evils, 231, 244, 289, 540

bā yuè zhá 八月札 akebia, Akebiae Fructus, 19, 493, 724

bā zhēn tāng 八珍汤, Eight-Gem Decoction, 36, 159, 161, 162, 172, 289, 312, 370, 426, 450, 451, 453, 457, 485, 488, 503, 594, 595, 607, 652, 741

bā zhēn yì mǔ wán 八珍益母丸, Eight-Gem Leonurus (Motherwort) Pill, 741

bā zhèng sǎn 八正散, Eight Corrections Powder, 21, 22, 68, 69, 148, 229, 283, 302, 583, 733

bā zhù sǎn 八柱散, Five Pillars Powder, 168

bá guàn fǎ 拔罐法, cupping, 106

bá zhēn 拔针, needle extraction, 406

bá zhēn 拔针, needle removal, 407

Bacillary Dysentery Herbal Formula, *jùn lì cǎo yào fāng* 菌痢草药方, 731

bacillary dysentery*, 28, 250, 278

bacillary enteritis*, 278

Back of the Ball, *qiú hòu* 球后, 521, 568, 586

bacterial food poisoning*, 278

Bai Jing-Yu's Eye Medication, *bái jìng yǔ yǎn yào* 白敬宇眼药, 744

Bai's Eye Medication, *bái shì yǎn yào* 白氏眼药, 744

bái 白, white, 674

bái bān èr hào yào gāo 白斑二号药膏, Leukoplakia No.3 Medicinal Paste, 744

bái bān xǐ jì 白斑洗剂, Leukoplakia Wash, 744

bái bān yī hào yào gāo 白斑一号药膏, Leukoplakia No.1 Medicinal Paste, 744

bái bēng 白崩, white flood, 675

bái bǐ 白疕, white crust, 674

bái bó fēng 白驳风, white patch wind, 676

bái bó piàn 白驳片, White Patch Tablet, 676

bái chóng bìng 白虫病, whiteworm disease, 677

bái dài 白带, vaginal discharge, 653

bái dài 白带, white vaginal discharge, 677

bái dài piàn 白带片, White Discharge Tablet, 743

bái diàn 白癜, white patch, 676

bái diàn fēng 白癜风, white patch wind, 676

bái dòu kòu 白豆蔻 cardamom, Amomi Cardamomi Fructus, 153, 167, 224, 434, 625, 722

bái fán 白矾 alum, Alumen, 53, 154, 225, 244, 383, 395, 401, 464, 466, 497, 599, 668, 728

bái fú líng 白茯苓 white poria, Poria Alba, 141, 394

bái fù piàn 白附片 white sliced aconite, Aconiti Tuber Laterale Album, 660, 723

bái fù zǐ 白附子 aconite/typhonium, Aconiti Coreani seu Typhonii Gigantei Tuber, 140, 623, 690, 725

bái guǒ 白果 ginkgo, Ginkgo Semen, 57, 624, 725

bái guǒ ké 白果壳 ginkgo husk, Ginkgo Testa, 241

bái guǒ zhòng dú 白果中毒 ginkgo poisoning, 241

bái hóu 白喉, diphtheria, 129

bái hú jiāo 白胡椒 white pepper, Piperis Fructus Albicatus, 402

bái hǔ chéng qì tāng 白虎承气汤, White Tiger Qi-Coordinating Decoction, 731

bái hǔ jiā dì huáng tāng 白虎加地黄汤, White Tiger Decoction Plus Rehmannia, 730 *bái hǔ jiā guì zhī tāng* 白虎加桂枝汤, White Tiger Decoction Plus Cinnamon Twig, 664, 730

bái hǔ jiā rén shēn tāng 白虎加人参汤, White Tiger Decoction Plus Ginseng, 455, 588, 591, 601, 640, 701, 730

bái hǔ lì jié 白虎历节, white tiger joint running, 676

bái hǔ tāng 白虎汤, White Tiger Decoction, 54, 71, 73, 202, 203, 281, 283, 431, 505, 589, 591, 607, 626, 698, 699, 701, 730

bái huā shé 白花蛇 krait/agkistrodon, Bungarus seu Agkistrodon, 139, 722

bái huán shū 白环俞, BL-30, White Ring Transport, 57, 94, 118, 160, 241, 330, 334, 353, 418, 435, 497, 522, 563, 675, 677, 747

bái jí 白及 bletilla, Bletillae Tuber, 449, 502, 569, 724

bái jí hé jì 白及合剂, Bletilla Mixture, 738

bái jí pí pá wán 白及枇杷丸, Bletilla and Loquat Pill, 738

bái jiāng cán 白僵蚕 silkworm, Bombyx Batryticatus, 5, 54, 74, 76, 140, 150, 167, 456, 526, 690, 726

bái jiàng dān 白降丹, White Downborne Elixir, 744

bái jiàng dān 白降丹 white downborne elixir, Praeparatio Sublimata Alba, 171, 383

bái jiè zǐ 白芥子 white mustard, Brassicae Albae Semen, 104, 388, 389, 433, 434, 438, 624, 625, 725

bái jīn wán 白金丸, Alum and Curcuma Pill, 434, 694

bái jīng 白睛, white of the eye, 676

bái jīng luàn mài 白睛乱脉, chaotic vessels in the white of the eye, 56

bái jìng yǔ yǎn yào 白敬宇眼药, Bai Jing-Yu's Eye Medication, 744

bái là lì 白鬎鬁, white perverse crop, 676

bái lài 白癞, white lai, 675

bái liǎn 白蔹 ampelopsis, Ampelopsis Radix, 68, 721

bái lòu 白漏, white leak, 675

bái mǎ gǔ 白马骨 serissa, Serissae Herba, 68, 721

bái máo gēn 白茅根 imperata, Imperatae Rhizoma, 106, 130, 277, 390, 566, 569, 724

bái máo huā 白茅花 imperata flower, Imperatae Flos, 414, 415

bái máo téng 白毛藤 climbing nightshade, Solani Lyrati Herba, 68, 721

bái máo xià kū cǎo 白毛夏枯草 bending bugle, Ajugae Decumbentis Herba, 68, 721

bái miàn shā 白面痧, white-face sand, 675

bái mó qīn jīng 白膜侵睛, white membrane invading the eye, 676

bái péi 白痦, miliaria alba, 395

bái qián 白前 cynanchum, Cynanchi Baiqian Radix et Rhizoma, 624, 725

bái rén 白仁, white of the eye, 676

bái ròu 白肉, white flesh, 675

bái sè zhèng 白涩症, white dry eye, 674

bái shā táng 白沙糖 white sugar, Saccharon Granulatum Album, 45

bái sháo yào 白芍药 white peony, Paeoniae Radix Alba, 17, 19, 28, 36, 37, 39, 95, 103, 116, 140, 154, 172, 175–177, 227, 246, 256, 259, 309, 310, 315, 352, 363, 390, 391, 397, 416, 425, 428, 495, 498, 502, 516, 537, 546, 548, 566, 567, 580, 588, 593, 613, 620, 661, 662, 674, 709, 713, 715, 727

bái shí yīng 白石英 white quartz, Quartz Album, 53

bái shì yǎn yào 白氏眼药, Bai's Eye Medication, 744

bái sū pí 白苏皮 white perilla bark, Perillae Albae Cortex, 66

bái sū yè 白苏叶 white perilla leaf, Perillae Albae Folium, 47

bái sū zǐ 白苏子 white perilla seed, Perillae Albae Semen, 17, 64, 145

bái tāi 白苔, white tongue fur, 676

bái tōng jiā zhū dǎn zhī tāng 白通加猪胆汁汤, Scallion Yang-Freeing Decoction Plus Pig's Bile, 735

bái tōng tāng 白通汤, Scallion Yang-Freeing Decoction, 626, 735

bái tóu wēng 白头翁 pulsatilla, Pulsatillae Radix, 68, 338, 352, 721

bái tóu wēng tāng 白头翁汤, Pulsatilla Decoction, 28, 110, 177, 197, 278, 338, 343, 731

bái tū 白秃, bald white scalp sore, 16

bái tū chuāng 白秃疮, bald white scalp sore, 16

bái wēi 白薇 baiwei, Cynanchi Baiwei Radix, 68, 72, 177, 277, 281, 282, 511, 649, 721

bái wēi tāng 白薇汤, Baiwei Decoction, 33

bái wēi wán 白薇丸, Baiwei Pill, 734

bái xiān pí 白鲜皮 dictamnus, Dictamni Radicis Cortex, 68, 116, 430, 468, 721

bái xiè fēng 白屑风, white scaling wind, 676

bái yǎn 白眼, white eye, 675

bái yǎn 白眼, white of the eye, 676

bái yín 白淫, white ooze, 676

bái yóu fēng 白游风, white wandering wind, 677

bái yù gāo 白玉膏, White Jade Plaster, 528

bái zhǐ 白芷 angelica, Angelicae Dahuricae Radix, 55, 102, 103, 116, 315, 339, 546, 681, 686, 699, 720

bái zhú 白术 ovate atractylodes, Atractylodis Ovatae Rhizoma, 12, 17, 50, 84, 93, 116, 139, 141, 153, 154, 223, 224, 227, 240, 256, 257, 272, 315, 319, 390, 393, 450, 463, 486, 563, 564, 573, 574, 593–596, 600, 615, 661, 662, 684, 726

bái zhú fù zǐ tāng 白术附子汤, Ovate Atractylodes and Aconite Decoction, 342, 734

bái zhú sǎn 白术散, Ovate Atractylodes Powder, 713, 733

bái zhuó 白浊, white turbidity, 677

bǎi bù 百部 stemona, Stemonae Radix, 95, 183, 445, 468, 624, 714, 725

bǎi bù gāo 百部膏, Stemona Paste, 603

bǎi bù guàn cháng jì 百部灌肠剂, Stemona Enema, 737

bǎi bù qīng jīn tāng 百部清金汤, Stemona Metal-Clearing Decoction, 97 *bǎi cǎo shuāng* 百草霜 weed soot, Herbarum Ustarum Fuligo, 724

bǎi chóng rù ěr 百虫入耳, insects in the ear, 307

bǎi chóng wō 百虫窝, Hundred Worm Nest, 64, 183, 426, 509, 510, 522, 549, 695, 696

bǎi hé 百合 lily bulb, Lilii Bulbus, 175, 416, 467, 539, 593, 597, 655, 727

bǎi hé dì huáng tāng 百合地黄汤, Lily Bulb and Rehmannia Decoction, 656

bǎi hé gù fèi tāng 百合固肺汤, Lily Bulb Lung-Securing Decoction, 277, 291, 374

bǎi hé gù jīn tāng 百合固金汤, Lily Bulb Metal-Securing Decoction, 158, 162, 172, 336, 368, 377, 380, 547, 734

bǎi huā gāo 百花膏, Lily Bulb and Tussilago Paste, 734

bǎi huì 百会, GV-20, Hundred Convergences, 27, 29, 32, 33, 38, 41, 50, 53, 55, 69, 71, 73, 74, 83, 86, 89, 92, 103, 119, 146, 155, 156, 160, 161, 168, 174–178, 196, 199, 203, 212, 218, 219, 225, 226, 231–233, 245, 251, 256, 259, 260, 287–289, 292, 296, 297, 310, 316, 318, 329, 331, 336, 345, 355, 362, 364–366, 384, 386, 409, 434, 442, 448, 451–453, 456–458, 465, 466, 478–480, 482, 485–488, 493, 501, 504, 506, 515, 516, 520, 544, 559, 570, 572, 585, 589–591, 595, 614, 626, 629, 631, 639, 640, 643, 646, 651, 652, 654, 655, 680–687, 690, 691, 693, 694, 699, 701–703, 709, 711–714, 749

bǎi láo 百劳, Hundred Taxations, 142, 277, 393, 442, 515, 544

bǎi rì ké 百日咳, hundred-day cough, 293

bǎi rì ké 百日咳, whooping cough, 677

bǎi yè tāng 柏叶汤, Biota Leaf Decoction, 738

bǎi yī juān bì tāng 百一蠲痹汤, Hundred and One Formulas Impediment-Alleviating Decoction, 734

bǎi zǐ rén 柏子仁 biota seed, Biotae Semen, 28, 230, 262, 433, 490, 526, 537, 597, 638, 726

bǎi zǐ rén tāng 柏子仁汤, Biota Seed Decoction, 651

bǎi zǐ rén wán 柏子仁丸, Biota Seed Pill, 742

bǎi zǐ yǎng xīn wán 柏子养心丸, Biota Seed Heart-Nourishing Pill, 416, 524, 739

bǎi zuì ké 百晬咳, hundred-day cough, 293

bǎi zuì sòu 百晬嗽, hundred-day cough, 293

bài dú sǎn 败毒散, Toxin-Vanquishing Powder, 517, 688

bài jiàng cǎo 败酱草 baijiang, Baijiang Herba cum Radice, 68, 721

bài xuè 败血, wasted blood, 665

bài xuè chōng fèi 败血冲肺, wasted blood surging into the lung, 665

bài xuè chōng wèi 败血冲胃, wasted blood surging into the stomach, 665

bài xuè chōng xīn 败血冲心, wasted blood surging into the heart, 665

baijiang, *bài jiàng cǎo* 败酱草, Baijiang Herba cum Radice, 68, 721

Baijiang Herba cum Radice, *bài jiàng cǎo* 败酱草, baijiang, 68, 721

baiwei, *bái wēi* 白薇, Cynanchi Baiwei Radix, 68, 72, 177, 277, 281, 282, 511, 649, 721

Baiwei Decoction, *bái wēi tāng* 白薇汤, 33

Baiwei Pill, *bái wēi wán* 白薇丸, 734

Balanophyllia seu Stalactitum, *é guǎn shí* 鹅管石, goose throat stone, 460, 624, 726

Bald Sores Oil, *tū chuāng yóu* 秃疮油, 16

bamboo leaf, *zhú yè* 竹叶, Bambusae Folium, 67, 720

bamboo leaf (lophatherum), *dàn zhú yè* 淡竹叶, Lophatheri Folium, 66, 67, 108, 261, 263, 387, 463, 720

Bamboo Leaf and Astragalus Decoction, *zhú yè huáng qí tāng* 竹叶黄芪汤, 259

Bamboo Leaf and Gypsum Decoction, *zhú yè shí gāo tāng* 竹叶石膏汤, 108, 155, 157, 221, 284, 415, 499, 558, 590, 599, 730

Bamboo Leaf Decoction, *dàn zhú yè tāng* 淡竹叶汤, 457

Bamboo Leaf Decoction, *zhú yè tāng* 竹叶汤, 458, 652, 731

Bamboo Leaf, Tamarisk, and Arctium Decoction, *zhú yè liǔ bàng tāng* 竹叶柳蒡汤, 422, 729

Bamboo Sap Phlegm-Outthrusting Pill, *zhú lì dá tán wán* 竹沥达痰丸, 738

bamboo shavings, *zhú rú* 竹茹, Bambusae Caulis in Taeniam, 20, 256, 257, 434, 440, 526, 574, 577, 578, 624, 709, 725

Bamboo Shavings Decoction, *zhú rú tāng* 竹茹汤, 284, 736

bamboo sugar, *tiān zhú huáng* 天竹黄, Bambusae Concretio Silicea, 140, 214, 541, 624, 725

Bambusae Caulis in Taeniam, *zhú rú* 竹茹, bamboo shavings, 20, 256, 257, 434, 440, 526, 574, 577, 578, 624, 709, 725

Bambusae Concretio Silicea, *tiān zhú huáng* 天竹黄, bamboo sugar, 140, 214, 541, 624, 725

Bambusae Folium, *zhú yè* 竹叶, bamboo leaf, 67, 720

Bambusae Succus Exsiccatus, *zhú lì* 竹沥, dried bamboo sap, 84, 116, 178, 282, 434, 448, 624, 637, 725

bān 斑, macule, 382

bān hén jiǔ 瘢痕灸, scarring moxibustion, 514

bān lóng wán 斑龙丸, Striped Dragon Pill, 523, 741

bān máo 斑蝥 mylabris, Mylabris, 98, 388, 574, 728

bān zhěn 斑疹, maculopapular eruption, 382

bǎn chǐ 板齿, front teeth, 231

bǎn lán dà qīng tāng 板蓝大青汤, Isatis Root and Leaf Decoction, 730

bǎn lán gēn 板蓝根 isatis root, Isatidis Radix, 64, 67, 70, 214, 357, 387, 388, 501, 611, 686, 688, 700, 721

bàn biān lián 半边莲 Chinese lobelia, Lobeliae Chinensis Herba cum Radice, 68, 721

bàn biǎo bàn lǐ zhèng 半表半里证, half exterior half interior pattern, 252

bàn biǎo bàn lǐ zhèng 半表半里证, midstage pattern, 394

bàn chǎn 半产, miscarriage, 396

bàn huáng wán 半黄丸, Pinellia and Scutellaria Pill, 280, 438

bàn liú wán 半硫丸, Pinellia and Sulfur Pill, 78, 338, 731

bàn shēn bù suí 半身不随, hemiplegia, 289

bàn shēn bù suì 半身不遂, hemiplegia, 289

bàn shēn má mù 半身麻木, half-body numbness, 251

bàn xià 半夏 pinellia, Pinelliae Tuber, 20, 63, 66, 84, 93, 98, 136, 141, 146, 153, 157, 230, 255–257, 259, 287, 343, 367, 372, 418, 434, 457, 527, 538, 572, 577, 578, 596, 623, 625, 683, 725

bàn xià bái zhú tiān má tāng 半夏白术天麻汤, Pinellia, Ovate Atractylodes, and Gastrodia Decoction, 98, 115, 287, 440, 691, 739

bàn xià fú líng tāng 半夏茯苓汤, Pinellia and Poria (Hoelen) Decoction, 738

bàn xià gān jiāng sǎn 半夏干姜散, Pinellia and Dried Ginger Powder, 156

bàn xià hòu pò tāng 半夏厚朴汤, Pinellia and Magnolia Bark Decoction, 19, 123, 735

bàn xià qū 半夏麴 pinellia leaven, Pinelliae Massa Fermentata, 201, 388

bàn xià shú mǐ tāng 半夏秫米汤, Pinellia and Broomcorn Millet Decoction, 739

bàn xià tāng 半夏汤, Pinellia Decoction, 739

bàn xià xiè xīn tāng 半夏泻心汤, Pinellia Heart-Draining Decoction, 242, 257, 732

bàn zhī lián 半枝莲 bearded scutellaria, Scutellariae Barbatae Herba, 68, 76, 700, 721

bàng 镑, flaking, 209

bāo bì 胞痹, bladder impediment, 22

bāo hán bù yùn 胞寒不孕, uterine cold infertility, 642

bāo huāng 胞肓, BL-53, Bladder Huang, 253, 747

bāo jiān 包煎, wrap-boiling, 696

bāo luò 胞络, uterine network vessels, 643

bāo mài 胞脉, uterine vessels, 643

bāo yī 胞衣, afterbirth, 7

bāo yī bù xià 胞衣不下, retention of the afterbirth, 503

bāo zǔ 胞阻, uterine obstruction, 643

bǎo ān wàn líng dān 保安万灵丹, Safeguard Unlimited Efficacy Elixir, 417, 431

bǎo chǎn wú yōu fāng 保产无忧方, Carefree Pregnancy Formula, 385, 741

bǎo chì sǎn 保赤散, Infant-Safeguarding Red Powder, 736

bǎo hé wán 保和丸, Harmony-Preserving Pill, 2, 3, 15, 19, 141, 143, 157, 197, 199, 215–218, 231, 238, 395, 549, 557, 578, 736

bǎo yīn jiān 保阴煎, Yin-Safeguarding Brew, 31, 199, 431, 574, 701

bǎo yuán tāng 保元汤, Origin-Preserving Decoction, 58, 267, 272, 274, 566, 740

bào 暴, fulminant, 232

bào bēng 暴崩, fulminant flooding, 233

bào biāo 报标, heralding tip, 290

bào diǎn 报点, heralding speckle, 290

bào gǔ 豹骨 leopard's bone, Leopardi Os, 139, 722

bào gǔ mù guā jiǔ 豹骨木瓜酒, Leopard's Bone and Chaenomelis Wine, 734

bào hūn 暴昏, fulminant clouding, 232

bào jué 暴厥, fulminant reversal, 233

bào lóng 暴聋, sudden deafness, 586

bào lóng wán 抱龙丸, Dragon-Embracing Pill, 6, 70, 437, 740

bào lún hong 抱轮红, red areola surrounding the dark of the eye, 494

bào máng 暴盲, sudden blindness, 586

bào tóu huǒ dān 抱头火丹, head fire cinnabar, 259

bào tuō 暴脱, fulminant desertion, 232

bào yīn 暴瘖, sudden loss of voice, 586

bào zhù 暴注, fulminant downpour, 233

barley sprout, *mài yá* 麦芽, Hordei Fructus Germinatus, 23, 141, 216, 217, 420, 450, 479, 499, 564, 573, 600, 606, 724

basil, *luó lè* 罗勒, Basilici Herba, 600

Basil Drink, *lán xiāng yǐn zǐ* 兰香饮子, 539, 565

Basilici Herba, *luó lè* 罗勒, basil, 600

bat's droppings, *yè míng shā* 夜明砂, Vespertilionis Excrementum, 139, 291, 725

bean curd dregs, *dòu fǔ zhā* 豆腐渣, Glycines Lactis Residuum, 104

bear's gall, *xióng dǎn* 熊胆, Ursi Fel, 68, 721

bearded scutellaria, *bàn zhī lián* 半枝莲, Scutellariae Barbatae Herba, 68, 76, 700, 721

beauty-berry leaf, *zǐ zhū* 紫珠, Callicarpae Folium, 724

beef marrow, *niú gǔ suǐ* 牛骨髓, Medulla Bovis, 45

bēi 悲, sorrow, 548

bēi zé qì xiāo 悲则气消, sorrow causes qi to disperse, 548

běi cháo 北朝, Northern Dynasties, 414

běi qí 北齐, Northern Qi, 414

běi shā shēn 北沙参 glehnia, Glehniae Radix, 175, 256, 593, 597, 727

běi sòng 北宋, Northern Song, 414

běi wèi 北魏, Northern Wei, 414

běi zhōu 北周, Northern Zhou, 414

bèi 背, back, 14

bèi 焙, stone-baking, 581

bèi hán 背寒, cold back, 77

bèi mǔ 贝母 fritillaria, Fritillariae Bulbus, 30, 120, 230, 398, 434, 544, 625, 637, 686

bèi mǔ guā lóu sǎn 贝母栝蒌散, Fritillaria and Trichosanthes Powder, 156, 203, 398, 655, 739

bèi rè 背热, hot back, 292

bèi shū 背俞, associated point, 11

bèi shū 背俞, back associated point, 14

bèi shū 背俞, back transport point, 15

bèi tòng 背痛, back pain, 14

bèi wù hán 背恶寒, aversion to cold in the back, 13

belamcanda, *shè gān* 射干, Belamcandae Rhizoma, 68, 368, 480, 611, 686, 688, 721

Belamcanda and Ephedra Decoction, *shè gān má huáng tāng* 射干麻黄汤, 87, 663, 677, 739

Belamcandae Rhizoma, *shè gān* 射干, belamcanda, 68, 368, 480, 611, 686, 688, 721

Bell's palsy*, 125, 689

bēn mén 贲门, rushing gate, 510

bēn tún 奔豚, running piglet, 510

bēn tún tāng 奔豚汤, Running Piglet Decoction, 510

běn cǎo 本草, bencao, 17

běn cǎo 本草, herbal foundation, 290

běn cǎo 本草, pen-ts'ao, 430

běn cǎo bèi yào 本草备要 (*Essential Herbal Foundation*), 1694 (Qīng), Wāng Áng 汪昂, 290

běn cǎo gāng mù 本草纲目 (*Comprehensive Herbal Foundation*), 1590 (Míng), Lǐ Shí-Zhēn 李时珍, 49, 204, 290

běn jié 本节, base joint, 16

běn jīng xuǎn xué 本经选穴, selection of same-channel points, 523

běn shén 本神, GB-13, Root Spirit, 748

bending bugle, *bái máo xià kū cǎo* 白毛夏枯草, Ajugae Decumbentis Herba, 68, 721

bēng lòu 崩漏, flooding and spotting, 211

bēng zhèng jí yàn fāng 崩证极验方, Well-Tried Flooding Formula, 743

bēng zhōng 崩中, flooding, 211

benign tumor the mammary glands*, 385

Benincasae Exocarpium, *dōng guā pí* 冬瓜皮, wax gourd rind, 136, 723

Benincasae Semen, *dōng guā zǐ* 冬瓜子, wax gourd seed, 136, 282, 625, 723

beriberi*, 112, 154, 342

bī zhēn fǎ 逼针法, needle-driving method, 406

bí 鼻, nose, 414

bí chì 鼻赤, red nose, 496

bí gān 鼻疳, gan of the nose, 238

bí gǎo 鼻藁, withered nose, 695

bí gǎo là 鼻藁腊, dried-meat nose, 149

bí liáng 鼻梁, nose pillar, 415

bí miáo 鼻苗, nasal inoculation, 405

bí míng 鼻鸣, noisy nose, 412

bí nì chuāng 鼻䘌疮, invisible worm sore of the nose, 319

bí nǜ 鼻衄, nosebleed, 414

bí qí 荸荠 water chestnut, Heleocharitis Cormus, 624, 725

bí qiào 鼻窍, nasal orifices, 405

bí qiú 鼻鼽, sniveling nose, 543

bí sāi bù tōng 鼻塞不通, nasal congestion, 405

bí sè 鼻塞, nasal congestion, 405

bí shān 鼻煽, flaring nostrils, 209

bí suān 鼻痠, sour-sore nose, 548

bí suì 鼻隧, nasal passages, 405

bí tōng 鼻通, 1, 543

bí wèng 鼻齆, nasal congestion, 405

bí xī ròu 鼻瘜肉, nasal polyp, 405

bí yuān 鼻渊, deep-source nasal congestion, 120

bí zhì 鼻痔, nose pile, 415

bí zhì 鼻窒, nasal congestion, 405

bí zhù 鼻柱, nose beam, 414

bì 闭, block, 24

bì 痹, bi, 18

bì 痹, impediment, 295

bì 髀, thigh, 607

bì 蔽, shelter, 529

bì bá 荜茇 long pepper, Piperis Longi Fructus, 660, 723

bì chéng qié 荜澄茄 cubeb, Cubebae Fructus, 660, 723

bì gǔ 髀骨, femur, 197

bì gǔ 髀骨, thigh bone, 607

bì guān 髀关, ST-31, Thigh Joint, 61, 222, 679, 746

bì guān 髀关, thigh joint, 607

bì hǔ 壁虎 house lizard, Gekko Swinhoana, 728

bì huì 辟秽, repelling foulness, 498

bì huǒ dān 避火丹, Fire-Repelling Elixir, 744

bì lóng 闭癃, dribbling urinary block, 148

bì nào 臂臑, LI-14, Upper Arm, 142, 341, 515, 520, 746

bì shū 髀枢, thigh pivot, 607

bì wēn dān 辟瘟丹, Scourge-Repelling Elixir, 171

bì wēn sǎn 避瘟散, Scourge-Averting Powder, 590

bì xiè 萆薢 fish poison yam, Dioscoreae Hypoglaucae Rhizoma, 21, 45, 116, 136, 328, 516, 584, 723

bì xiè fēn qīng yǐn 萆薢分清饮, Fish Poison Yam Clear-Turbid Separation Beverage, 637, 641, 661, 733

bì xiè huà dú tāng 萆薢化毒汤, Fish Poison Yam Toxin-Transforming Decoction, 187, 528

bì xiè shèn shī tāng 萆薢渗湿汤, Fish Poison Yam Dampness-Percolating Decoction, 8, 116, 117, 221, 241, 468, 528, 733

bì xīn gǔ 蔽心骨, heart-covering bone, 261

bì yù sǎn 碧玉散, Jasper Jade Powder, 730

bì zhèng 闭证, block pattern, 24

bì zhèng 痹证, impediment pattern, 296

biān tóu fēng 边头风, side head wind, 531

biǎn dòu 扁豆 lablab, Lablab Semen, 563, 564, 593, 726

biǎn dòu huā 扁豆花 lablab flower, Lablab Flos, 69

biǎn dòu yè 扁豆叶 lablab leaf, Lablab Folium, 61

biǎn xù 萹蓄 knotgrass, Polygoni Avicularis Herba, 21, 69, 136, 723

biàn 变, transmutation, 625

biàn bì 便闭, fecal block, 196

biàn bì 便秘, constipation, 94

biàn chū bù shuǎng 便出不爽, ungratifying defecation, 637

biàn dú 便毒, bian toxin [sore], 18

biàn huà 变化, mutation, 403

biàn nán 便难, difficult defecation, 126

biàn niào qīng lì 便溺清利, clear uninhibited stool and urine, 72

biàn shé zhǐ nán 辨舌指南 (*Guide to Tongue Diagnosis*), 1920 (Republic), Cáo Bǐng-Zhāng 曹炳章, 619

biàn táng 便溏, sloppy stool, 540

biàn xuè 便血, blood in the stool, 32

biàn xuè 便血, bloody stool, 40

biàn zhèng 辨证, pattern identification, 429

biàn zhèng 变证, transmuted pattern, 625

biàn zhèng lùn zhì 辨证论治, determining treatment by patterns identified, 124

biàn zhèng lùn zhì 辨证论治, identifying patterns and determining treatment, 295

biàn zhèng qiú yīn 辨证求因, identifying patterns and seeking the causes, 295

biàn zhèng qiú yīn 辨证求因, seeking the cause from patterns identified, 519

biàn zhèng shī zhì 辨证施治, identifying patterns and administering treatment, 295

biāo 标, tip, 614

biāo běn 标本, root and tip, 508

biāo běn tóng zhì 标本同治, treating the root and tip simultaneously, 626

biāo jū 瘭疽, biaoju, 18

biāo jū 瘭疽, tip-abscess, 614

biāo jū 瘭疽, whitlow, 677

biāo jū 熛疽, flare-tip abscess, 209

biāo yōu fù 标幽赋 (*Song to Elucidate Mysteries*), Jīn-Yuán (1115–1368), Dòu Jié 窦杰 [Hàn-Qīng 汉卿], 225, 419

biāo 表, exterior, 183

biāo hán 表寒, exterior cold, 184

biāo hán lǐ rè 表寒里热, exterior cold and interior heat, 184

biāo lǐ 表里, exterior and interior, 183

biāo lǐ jīng xuǎn xué 表里经选穴, selection of interior-exterior–related channel points, 520

biāo lǐ shuāng jiě 表里双解, dual resolution of both exterior and interior, 159

biāo lǐ shuāng jiě 表里双解, resolving both exterior and interior, 500

biāo lǐ tóng bìng 表里同病, dual disease of the interior and exterior, 158

biāo qì bù gù 表气不固, insecurity of exterior qi, 307

biāo rè 表热, exterior heat, 184

biāo rè chuán lǐ 表热传里, exterior heat passing into the interior, 184

biāo rè lǐ hán 表热里寒, exterior heat and interior cold, 184

biāo shí 表实, exterior repletion, 185

biāo shí lǐ xū 表实里虚, exterior repletion and interior vacuity, 185

biāo xū 表虚, exterior vacuity, 185

biāo xū lǐ shí 表虚里实, exterior vacuity and interior repletion, 185

biāo zhèng 表证, exterior pattern, 184

Bidentis Bipinnatae Herba, *guǐ zhēn cǎo* 鬼针草, Spanish needles, 68, 721

biē jiǎ 鳖甲 turtle shell, Amydae Carapax, 72, 98, 175, 176, 218, 277, 336, 352, 399, 460, 544, 593, 597, 727

biē jiǎ dì huáng tāng 鳖甲地黄汤, Turtle Shell and Rehmannia Decoction, 97

biē jiǎ jiān wán 鳖甲煎丸, Turtle Shell Decocted Pill, 26, 138, 140, 737

biē jiǎ jiāo 鳖甲胶 turtle shell glue, Amydae Carapacis Gelatinum, 243, 593, 727

biē jiǎ sǎn 鳖甲散, Turtle Shell Powder, 237, 363

biē jiǎ yǐn zǐ 鳖甲饮子, Turtle Shell Drink, 737

biē xuè 鳖血 turtle's blood, Amydae Sanguis, 397

bié luò 别络, diverging network vessel, 143

bile arisaema, *dǎn xīng* 胆星, Arisaematis Rhizoma cum Felle Bovis, 60, 84, 140, 178, 214, 448, 453, 541, 623, 725

bile arisaema [root], *dǎn xīng* 胆星, Arisaematis Rhizoma cum Felle Bovis, 417

Biliary Calculus Decoction, *dǎn dào pái shí tāng* 胆道排石汤, 182, 544, 733

biliary tract diseases*
obstructive, 700

biliary tract infections*, 357

Bin-Hu Sphygmology (*bīn hú mài xué*) 濒湖脉学, 1564 (Míng), Lǐ Shí-Zhēn 李时珍 [Bīn-Hú 濒湖], 367, 461, 471, 492, 509, 592

bīn hú mài xué 濒湖脉学 (*Bin-Hu Sphygmology*), 1564 (Míng), Lǐ Shí-Zhēn 李时珍 [Bīn-Hú 濒湖], 367, 461, 471, 492, 509, 592

bìn gǔ 鬓骨, side-lock bone, 531

Bind-Dissipating Pain-Relieving Decoction, *sàn jié dìng téng tāng* 散结定疼汤, 300, 737

bīng láng 槟榔 areca, Arecae Semen, 115, 141, 154, 183, 216, 298, 317, 510, 512, 572, 588, 724

bīng péng sǎn 冰硼散, Borneol and Borax Powder, 6, 440, 612, 671, 744

bīng piàn 冰片 borneol, Borneolum, 5, 51, 243, 389, 398, 405, 420, 458, 636, 690, 726

bīng sī sǎn 冰螄散, Borneol and Freshwater Snail Powder, 32

bǐng fēng 秉风, SI-12, Grasping the Wind, 220, 253, 254, 747

bǐng huǒ 丙火, S3-fire, 511

bìng 病, disease, 130

bìng 病, illness, 295

bìng 病, morbid, 399

bìng bìng 并病, dragover disease, 146

bìng jī 病机, pathomechanism, 429

bìng jī shí jiǔ tiáo 病机十九条, nineteen pathomechanisms, 411

bìng mài 病脉, morbid pulse, 399

bìng sè 病色, morbid complexion, 399

bìng tuí 病癀, morbid prominence, 399

bìng xié 病邪, disease evil, 135

bìng xié biàn zhèng 病邪辨证, disease-evil pattern identification, 135

bìng zhèng 病证, disease pattern, 135

biota leaf, *cè bǎi yè* 侧柏叶, Biotae Folium, 36, 70, 569, 647, 724

Biota Leaf and Toona Bark Pill, *cè bǎi shū pí wán* 侧柏樗皮丸, 743

Biota Leaf Decoction, *bǎi yè tāng* 柏叶汤, 738

biota seed, *băi zĭ rén* 柏子仁, Biotae Semen, 28, 230, 262, 433, 490, 526, 537, 597, 638, 726

Biota Seed Decoction, *băi zĭ rén tāng* 柏子仁汤, 651

Biota Seed Heart-Nourishing Pill, *băi zĭ yăng xīn wán* 柏子养心丸, 416, 524, 739

Biota Seed Pill, *băi zĭ rén wán* 柏子仁丸, 742

Biotae Folium, *cè băi yè* 侧柏叶, biota leaf, 36, 70, 569, 647, 724

Biotae Semen, *băi zĭ rén* 柏子仁, biota seed, 28, 230, 262, 433, 490, 526, 537, 597, 638, 726

Birth-Hastening Beverage, *cuī shēng yĭn* 催生饮, 128, 735

bistort, *quán shēn* 拳参, Polygoni Bistortae Rhizoma, 68, 721

bitter apricot kernel, *kŭ xìng rén* 苦杏仁, Armeniacae Semen Amarum, 458

bitter bamboo leaf, *kŭ zhú yè* 苦竹叶, Pleioblasti Folium, 259, 430

bitter orange, *zhĭ ké* 枳壳, Aurantii Fructus, 19, 47, 50, 153, 217, 234, 317, 318, 415, 421, 437, 439, 466, 477, 483, 493, 538, 573, 588, 669, 709, 723

Bitter Orange and Tangerine Peel Decoction, *zhĭ jú tāng* 枳橘汤, 481

Bitter Orange Powder, *zhĭ ké săn* 枳壳散, 736

BL-1, *jīng míng* 睛明, Bright Eyes, 27, 64, 89, 93, 150, 181, 195, 222, 291, 320, 395, 406, 495, 500, 520, 549, 568, 585, 586, 685, 689, 747

BL-2, *zăn zhú* 攒竹, Bamboo Gathering, 27, 62, 93, 125, 140, 150, 192, 194, 195, 259, 260, 289, 290, 331, 349, 395, 406, 500, 521, 568, 586, 689, 714, 747

BL-3, *méi chōng* 眉冲, Eyebrow Ascension, 747

BL-4, *qū chā* 曲差, Deviating Turn, 747

BL-5, *wŭ chù* 五处, Fifth Place, 520, 747

BL-6, *chéng guāng* 承光, Light Guard, 747

BL-7, *tōng tiān* 通天, Celestial Connection, 120, 520, 747

BL-8, *luò què* 络却, Declining Connection, 747

BL-9, *yù zhĕn* 玉枕, Jade Pillow, 259, 747

BL-10, *tiān zhù* 天柱, Celestial Pillar, 89, 105, 120, 168, 247, 259, 629, 747

BL-11, *dà zhù* 大杼, Great Shuttle, 45, 78, 84, 86, 105, 155, 184, 185, 226, 252, 391, 501, 517, 580, 589, 631, 638, 663, 666, 681, 682, 690, 694, 703, 709, 747

BL-12, *fēng mén* 风门, Wind Gate, 12, 78, 84, 87, 91, 113, 119, 155, 184, 185, 281, 285, 374, 422, 443, 501, 517, 547, 586, 631, 677, 681–684, 690, 709, 710, 747

BL-13, *fèi shū* 肺俞, Lung Transport, 5, 12, 13, 15, 65, 70, 72, 78, 83, 84, 86–89, 91, 92, 95–97, 99, 109, 128, 129, 142, 146, 155, 156, 158, 161, 163, 169, 184, 185, 201, 203, 224, 228, 237, 257, 261, 267–269, 277, 280–282, 285, 291, 292, 301, 336, 341, 348, 356, 368, 372, 374, 378–380, 393, 398, 409, 415, 416, 434, 435, 438, 439, 441, 443, 453, 467, 477, 481, 486, 489, 506, 515, 517, 535, 547, 550, 562, 571, 572, 595–597, 603, 625, 630, 640,

648, 663, 666, 668, 675, 677, 681–684, 686–688, 690, 693–695, 702, 703, 714, 715, 747

BL-14, *jué yīn shū* 厥阴俞, Reverting Yin Transport, 58, 59, 89, 91, 228, 230, 236, 265, 268, 427, 452, 629, 747

BL-15, *xīn shū* 心俞, Heart Transport, 11, 15, 33, 38, 39, 58, 59, 81, 87, 89, 91, 129, 147, 153, 159, 160, 162, 180, 222, 223, 228, 230, 232, 235, 236, 261, 263–274, 281, 282, 294, 296, 297, 301, 308, 333, 335, 336, 345, 386, 392, 410, 413, 416, 418, 427, 434, 436, 437, 448–452, 457, 461, 467, 484, 488, 514, 518, 521, 524–526, 537, 538, 551, 572, 594, 595, 597, 629, 641, 642, 651, 652, 654–656, 661, 665, 668, 675, 687, 694, 747

BL-16, *dū shū* 督俞, Governing Transport, 747

BL-17, *gé shū* 膈俞, Diaphragm Transport, 4, 15, 24, 26–30, 32–41, 53, 58, 59, 63, 64, 72, 73, 82, 87, 99, 118, 123, 127, 138–140, 145, 149, 152, 159, 161, 162, 164, 168, 169, 175, 212, 223, 227, 228, 230, 251, 256, 260, 261, 265–269, 271–274, 279, 280, 288, 291, 292, 297, 332, 333, 336, 339, 348, 349, 352, 356, 359, 362, 366, 390, 393, 410, 415, 416, 422, 426, 438, 445, 447, 449–454, 456–458, 461, 462, 475, 480, 482–484, 493, 499, 503, 511, 516, 522, 533, 534, 537, 540, 552, 563, 566, 568, 570, 571, 586, 591, 596, 597, 601, 604, 607, 608, 613, 646, 649, 652, 654, 661, 674, 684, 686, 689, 690, 696, 714, 747

BL-18, *gān shū* 肝俞, Liver Transport, 11, 15, 16, 19, 20, 24, 26, 29, 33, 35, 53, 58, 60, 61, 64, 89, 91, 103, 119, 123, 140, 151, 152, 157, 162, 164, 175, 189, 195, 202, 218, 223, 225, 227, 233, 235, 256, 266, 288, 291, 292, 296, 297, 310, 336, 347, 352, 353, 355–362, 365, 366, 384, 385, 390, 392, 393, 399, 406, 445, 452, 453, 462, 475, 477–479, 493, 495, 497, 499, 500, 511, 515, 533, 534, 538, 547, 549, 552, 554, 566, 568, 569, 571, 586, 597, 640, 649, 677, 690, 694, 700, 710, 713–715, 747

BL-19, *dăn shū* 胆俞, Gallbladder Transport, 15, 66, 89, 91, 151, 195, 230, 234–236, 268, 297, 349, 357, 538, 564, 650, 674, 700, 710, 747

BL-20, *pí shū* 脾俞, Spleen Transport, 1, 3–5, 15, 26–29, 32, 33, 36–41, 47, 55, 58, 59, 61–64, 66, 73, 78–81, 83, 84, 86, 91, 94, 97, 109, 115, 117–119, 127, 128, 145, 149–151, 156, 159–164, 174, 175, 177, 183, 196, 197, 199, 210–212, 215–217, 223, 224, 227, 228, 234, 235, 237, 240, 251, 256, 257, 261, 265, 267–272, 274, 278, 282, 288, 291, 296, 301, 308–310, 312, 314, 316, 318–320, 325, 332–335, 339, 340, 349, 352, 359, 361, 365, 366, 370, 378, 379, 384, 390, 393, 395, 399–401, 410, 415, 416, 418, 425–427, 434–436, 441, 443, 445, 447, 449–458, 461, 465, 477, 484–487, 489, 490, 493, 497–499, 503, 513, 514, 516, 524, 525, 529, 534, 537, 547, 549–551, 554, 555, 557–559, 561–566, 575, 578, 579, 581, 586, 589, 594–597, 600, 603, 604, 607, 608, 613, 620, 636, 639–641, 645–647, 650, 652, 654, 661–663, 666–669, 673, 675,

Index   766

677–679, 685, 694–696, 702, 703, 710, 711, 713, 714, 716, 747

BL-21, *wèi shū* 胃俞, Stomach Transport, 1, 3, 4, 15, 17, 27, 29, 33, 37–41, 47, 55, 73, 80, 84, 87–89, 91, 97, 127, 128, 156, 161, 164, 174, 175, 197, 199, 215, 216, 218, 223, 224, 237, 251, 256, 257, 309, 312, 314, 316, 333, 339, 349, 359, 361, 370, 379, 415, 416, 418, 447, 449, 457, 477, 486, 487, 489, 499, 503, 537, 557, 561–565, 575, 577–579, 581, 595–597, 600, 607, 613, 620, 638, 639, 645–647, 661–663, 666, 669, 673, 679, 711, 714, 715, 747

BL-22, *sān jiāo shū* 三焦俞, Triple Burner Transport, 15, 22, 37, 87, 91, 117, 149, 152, 182, 224, 228, 269, 301, 302, 334, 379, 449, 453, 457, 485, 537, 559, 601, 608, 663, 666, 668, 694, 703, 716, 747

BL-23, *shèn shū* 肾俞, Kidney Transport, 4, 11, 15, 16, 22, 23, 26, 27, 29, 36, 39, 41, 45, 47, 59–61, 64, 78, 80–86, 88, 89, 91, 94, 96, 105, 114, 115, 117, 119, 127, 137, 140, 147, 149, 151, 152, 156–158, 160, 163, 164, 167–169, 174, 175, 177, 180, 196, 199, 210, 222, 224, 225, 227–230, 239, 240, 256, 263, 265, 266, 268, 283, 288, 291, 292, 294, 296, 297, 301, 302, 308, 310, 312, 314, 318, 325, 326, 329, 331–337, 340, 342, 345, 347–349, 352, 355, 359, 360, 366, 368–370, 374, 379, 381, 385, 393, 401, 406, 410, 413, 415, 425, 426, 434, 449, 452–454, 456, 457, 461, 462, 465–467, 474, 477, 482, 484, 489, 495, 497, 500, 513, 515, 516, 518, 521, 523–525, 529, 534, 537, 538, 542, 547, 549, 559, 563, 567–569, 571, 579, 584, 586, 594–597, 600, 604, 607, 608, 612, 614, 630, 631, 636, 638, 640–643, 647–649, 651, 652, 654, 660–662, 664, 666, 668, 675, 684, 688, 690, 693, 703, 713–716, 747

BL-24, *qì hǎi shū* 气海俞, Sea-of-Qi Transport, 747

BL-25, *dà cháng shū* 大肠俞, Large Intestine Transport, 3, 15, 40, 61, 72, 77, 78, 83, 89, 91, 117, 128, 183, 196, 215, 216, 277, 284, 289, 290, 298, 318, 335, 338–340, 390, 415, 426, 434, 444, 449, 465, 466, 477, 480, 493, 509, 570, 585, 589, 613, 646, 656, 658, 664, 683, 695, 696, 747

BL-26, *guān yuán shū* 关元俞, Pass Head Transport, 747

BL-27, *xiǎo cháng shū* 小肠俞, Small Intestine Transport, 15, 36, 41, 89, 91, 509, 542, 747

BL-28, *páng guāng shū* 膀胱俞, Bladder Transport, 15, 21–23, 36, 68, 69, 82, 86, 91, 149, 177, 180, 229, 283, 301, 302, 308, 449, 465, 485, 529, 533, 541, 542, 582, 597, 604, 631, 636, 640, 641, 701, 747

BL-29, *zhōng lǚ shū* 中膂俞, Central Backbone Transport, 747

BL-30, *bái huán shū* 白环俞, White Ring Transport, 57, 94, 118, 160, 241, 330, 334, 353, 418, 435, 497, 522, 563, 675, 677, 747

BL-31 through BL-34, *bā liáo* 八髎, Eight Bone-Holes, 45, 297

BL-31, *shàng liáo* 上髎, Upper Bone-Hole, 220, 747

BL-32, *cì liáo* 次髎, Second Bone-Hole, 35, 40, 89, 94, 160, 177, 284, 289, 330, 334, 444, 480, 571, 640, 656, 675, 696, 747

BL-33, *zhōng liáo* 中髎, Central Bone-Hole, 747

BL-34, *xià liáo* 下髎, Lower Bone-Hole, 118, 220, 241, 424, 468, 747

BL-35, *huì yáng* 会阳, Meeting of Yang, 41, 289, 493, 557, 656, 747

BL-36, *chéng fú* 承扶, Support, 137, 252, 567, 747

BL-37, *yīn mén* 殷门, Gate of Abundance, 61, 111, 370, 658, 747

BL-38, *fú xī* 浮郄, Superficial Cleft, 747

BL-39, *wěi yáng* 委阳, Bend Yang, 22, 117, 369, 449, 582, 661, 703, 716, 747

BL-40, *wěi zhōng* 委中, Bend Center, 4, 5, 11, 14, 15, 17, 25, 34, 36, 39, 44, 62, 63, 70, 73, 75, 80, 89, 99, 111, 113–115, 137, 145, 152, 154, 160, 225, 292, 296, 302, 327, 330, 332, 336, 337, 342, 347, 369, 370, 382, 415, 422, 427, 450, 453, 455, 462, 484, 540, 546, 559, 566, 567, 571, 589, 590, 597, 637, 651, 658, 665, 676, 684, 688, 696, 710, 747

BL-41, *fù fēn* 附分, Attached Branch, 747

BL-42, *pò hù* 魄户, Po Door, 747

BL-43, *gāo huāng shū* 膏肓俞, Gao Huang Transport, 747

BL-43, *gāo huāng shū* 膏肓俞, Gao-Huang Transport, 15, 72, 83, 87, 88, 95, 97, 146, 156, 158, 161, 163, 169, 201, 237, 251, 267, 282, 291, 336, 372, 374, 378–380, 398, 409, 415, 416, 441, 467, 486, 489, 515, 524, 572, 595–597, 603, 630, 639, 640, 648, 649, 664, 678, 683, 702, 714, 715

BL-44, *shén táng* 神堂, Spirit Hall, 747

BL-45, *yī xǐ* 谚譆, Yi Xi, 747

BL-46, *gé guān* 膈关, Diaphragm Pass, 164, 747

BL-47, *hún mén* 魂门, Hun Gate, 656, 747

BL-48, *yáng gāng* 阳纲, Yang Headrope, 747

BL-49, *yì shè* 意舍, Reflection Abode, 747

BL-50, *wèi cāng* 胃仓, Stomach Granary, 747

BL-51, *huāng mén* 肓门, Huang Gate, 169, 747

BL-52, *jīng gōng* 精宫, Palace of Essence, 296, 310, 514, 518, 524

BL-52, *zhì shì* 志室, Will Chamber, 4, 89, 97, 148, 160, 222, 266, 288, 294, 308, 332, 333, 336, 347, 352, 360, 453, 461, 513, 518, 521, 524, 525, 569, 584, 594, 597, 647, 651, 716, 747

BL-53, *bāo huāng* 胞肓, Bladder Huang, 253, 747

BL-54, *zhì biān* 秩边, Sequential Limit, 89, 137, 290, 480, 567, 688, 747

BL-55, *hé yáng* 合阳, Yang Union, 747

BL-56, *chéng jīn* 承筋, Sinew Support, 747

BL-57, *chéng shān* 承山, Mountain Support, 40, 61, 62, 89, 154, 178, 196, 284, 289, 318, 319, 342, 347, 382, 390, 446, 456–458, 465, 466, 480, 493, 522, 530, 589–591, 656, 747

BL-58, *fēi yáng* 飞扬, Taking Flight, 90, 290, 408, 453, 480, 747

BL-59, *fū yáng* 跗阳, Instep Yang, 747

BL-60, *kūn lún* 昆仑, Kunlun Mountains, 14, 21, 22, 34, 61, 80, 105, 114, 137, 160, 221, 231, 247, 288, 289, 296, 330, 332, 336, 342, 347, 366, 370, 382, 503, 519, 521, 567, 591, 689, 747

BL-61, *pú cān* 仆参, Subservient Visitor, 747

BL-62, *shēn mài* 申脉, Extending Vessel, 90, 93, 178, 255, 288, 296, 330, 341, 366, 425, 440, 519, 567, 690, 701, 747

BL-63, *jīn mén* 金门, Metal Gate, 425, 747

BL-64, *jīng gǔ* 京骨, Capital Bone, 90, 185, 247, 255, 341, 370, 391, 440, 548, 666, 690, 747

BL-65, *shù gǔ* 束骨, Bundle Bone, 89, 259, 747

BL-66, *tōng gǔ (zú)* 通谷（足）, (Foot) Valley Passage, 747

BL-67, *zhì yīn* 至阴, Reaching Yin, 82, 128, 219, 385, 420, 747

Black Chicken and White Phoenix Pill, *wū jī bái fèng wán* 乌鸡白凤丸, 741

Black Cloth Paste, *hēi bù gāo* 黑布膏, 171

Black Free Wanderer Powder, *hēi xiāo yáo sǎn* 黑逍遥散, 352, 566, 732

black jujube, *hēi zǎo* 黑枣, Ziziphi Fructus Ater, 667

black nightshade, *lóng kuí* 龙葵, Solani Nigri Herba, 68, 721

Black Paste (Formula), *hēi gāo (fāng)* 黑膏（方）, 730

Black Paste (Formula), *hēi gāo (fāng)* 黑膏（方）, 65

black sesame, *hēi zhī má* 黑脂麻, Sesami Semen Atrum, 28, 108, 127, 398, 593, 727

black sliced aconite, *hēi shùn piàn* 黑顺片, Aconiti Tuber Laterale Denigratum, 660, 723

black soybean, *hēi dà dòu* 黑大豆, Glycines Semen Atrum, 54, 108, 726

Black Tiger Elixir, *hēi hǔ dān* 黑虎丹, 528, 744

black-striped snake, *wū shé* 乌蛇, Zaocys, 139, 722

Bladder-Securing Decoction, *gù pāo tāng* 固脬汤, 743

Bladder-Securing Pill, *gù pāo wán* 固脬丸, 465

blast-fried ginger, *páo jiāng* 炮姜, Zingiberis Rhizoma Tostum, 26, 139, 199, 417, 431, 503, 556, 562, 564, 569, 660, 662

blast-fried ginger, *pào jiāng* 炮姜, Zingiberis Rhizoma Tostum, 723

blepharitis marginalis*, 636

bletilla, *bái jí* 白及, Bletillae Tuber, 449, 502, 569, 724

Bletilla and Loquat Pill, *bái jí pí pá wán* 白及枇杷丸, 738

Bletilla Mixture, *bái jí hé jì* 白及合剂, 738

Bletillae Tuber, *bái jí* 白及, bletilla, 449, 502, 569, 724

Blood Cough Formula, *ké xuè fāng* 咳血方, 738

Blood Depression Decoction, *xuè yù tāng* 血郁汤, 27

blood fluke infestation*, 28

blood flukes*, 250

Blood-Boosting Intestine-Moistening Pill, *yì xuè rùn cháng wán* 益血润肠丸, 127

Blood-Cooling Dryness-Moistening Beverage, *liáng xuè rùn zào yǐn* 凉血润燥饮, 173

Blood-Cooling Four Agents Decoction, *liáng xuè sì wù tāng* 凉血四物汤, 149

Blood-Cooling Rehmannia Decoction, *liáng xuè dì huáng tāng* 凉血地黄汤, 25, 29, 32, 284, 290, 317, 566, 738

Blood-Nourishing Skin-Moistening Beverage, *yǎng xuè rùn fū yǐn* 养血润肤饮, 173

Blood-Nourishing Tangkuei and Rehmannia Decoction, *yǎng xuè dāng guī dì huáng tāng* 养血当归地黄汤, 568

Blood-Quickening Decoction, *huó xuè tāng* 活血汤, 570

Blood-Quickening Dryness-Moistening Liquid-Engendering Powder, *huó xuè rùn zào shēng jīn sǎn* 活血润燥生津散, 734

Blood-Quickening Stasis-Dissipating Decoction, *huó xuè sàn yū tāng* 活血散瘀汤, 18, 315

Blood-Quieting Decoction, *níng xuè tāng* 宁血汤, 738

Blood-Stanching Decoction, *zhǐ xuè tāng* 止血汤, 738

Blood-Stanching Powder, *zhǐ xuè fěn* 止血粉, 738

Blood-Stanching Powder, *zhǐ xuè sǎn* 止血散, 745

Blood-Supplementing Sinew-Enhancing Pill, *bǔ xuè róng jīn wán* 补血荣筋丸, 40, 534

bō tāi 剥苔, peeling fur, 429

bó jué 薄厥, sudden reversal, 586

bó tāi 薄苔, thin tongue fur, 607

bò hé 薄荷 mint, Menthae Herba, 7, 17, 69, 103, 130, 143, 176, 184, 368, 414, 422, 463, 497, 501, 548, 621, 671, 686, 687, 720

bò hé xuán míng sǎn 薄荷玄明散, Mint and Refined Mirabilite Powder, 620

Boats and Carts Pill, *zhōu chē (jū) wán* 舟车丸, 151, 182, 732

Boehmeriae Radix, *zhù má gēn* 苎麻根, ramie, 724

boil*, 44

bolbosteema, *tǔ bèi mǔ* 土贝母, Bolbosteematis Tuber, 291

Bolbosteematis Tuber, *tǔ bèi mǔ* 土贝母, bolbosteema, 291

Bombycis Excrementum, *yuán cán shā* 原蚕沙, silkworm droppings, 139, 722

Bombyx Batryticatus, *bái jiāng cán* 白僵蚕, silkworm, 5, 54, 74, 76, 140, 150, 167, 456, 526, 690, 726

bone tumor*, 632

Bone-Clearing Powder, *qīng gǔ sǎn* 清骨散, 72, 572, 613, 655, 731

Bone-Joining Elixir, *jiē gǔ dān* 接骨丹, 737

Bone-Opening Powder, *kāi gǔ sǎn* 开骨散, 195

Bone-Righting Hot Pack, *zhèng gǔ tàng yào* 正骨烫药, 745

Bone-Righting Purple Gold Elixir, *zhèng gǔ zǐ jīn dān* 正骨紫金丹, 45, 337

Book of Life Renewal Elsholtzia Powder, *huó rén xiāng rú yǐn* 活人香薷散, 729

Book of Life Scallion and Fermented Soybean Decoction, *huó rén cōng chǐ tāng* 活人葱豉汤, 729

Borax, *péng shā* 硼砂, borax, 53, 291, 383, 728

borax, *péng shā* 硼砂, Borax, 53, 291, 383, 728

borneol, *bīng piàn* 冰片, Borneolum, 5, 51, 243, 389, 398, 405, 420, 458, 636, 690, 726

Borneol and Borax Powder, *bīng péng sǎn* 冰硼散, 6, 440, 612, 671, 744

Borneol and Freshwater Snail Powder, *bīng sī sǎn* 冰蛳散, 32

Borneolum, *bīng piàn* 冰片, borneol, 5, 51, 243, 389, 398, 405, 420, 458, 636, 690, 726

bottle gourd, *hú lú* 壶芦, Lagenariae Depressae Fructus, 136, 723

bovine bezoar, *niú huáng* 牛黄, Bovis Bezoar, 67, 98, 153, 458, 690, 721

Bovine Bezoar Awake to Relief Pill, *niú huáng xǐng xiāo wán* 牛黄醒消丸, 743

Bovine Bezoar Dragon-Embracing Pill, *niú huáng bào lóng wán* 牛黄抱龙丸, 569, 591, 740

Bovine Bezoar Fright-Settling Pill, *niú huáng zhèn jīng wán* 牛黄镇惊丸, 687

Bovine Bezoar Heart-Clearing Pill, *niú huáng qīng xīn wán* 牛黄清心丸, 88, 203, 264, 343, 538, 740

Bovine Bezoar Pill, *niú huáng wán* 牛黄丸, 624, 696

Bovine Bezoar Upper-Body-Clearing Pill, *niú huáng shàng qīng wán* 牛黄上清丸, 319

Bovis Bezoar, *niú huáng* 牛黄, bovine bezoar, 67, 98, 153, 458, 690, 721

Bovis Cornus Os, *niú jiǎo sāi* 牛角腮, ox horn bone, 519, 569

Bovis Vesica Fellea, *niú dǎn* 牛胆, ox's gallbladder, 82

brain tumor*, 260

brandy nose*, 149

Brassicae Albae Semen, *bái jiè zǐ* 白芥子, white mustard, 104, 388, 389, 433, 434, 438, 624, 625, 725

Brassicae Junceae Semen, *jiè zǐ* 芥子, leaf mustard seed, 624, 725

Bright and Glorious Elixir, *guāng míng dān* 光明丹, 744

Brightness Pill, *xuān míng wán* 宣明丸, 730

Broken Flute Pill, *xiǎng shēng pò dí wán* 响声破笛丸, 729

bronchial asthma*, 435

bronchiectasis*, 469

Bronchitis Tablet, *qì guǎn yán piàn* 气管炎片, 738

bronchitis*, 280, 349
    acute, 438, 659
    chronic, 115, 120, 434, 435, 584

bronchodilatation*, 434

brucea, *yā dǎn zǐ* 鸦胆子, Bruceae Fructus, 68, 183, 445, 665, 721

Bruceae Fructus, *yā dǎn zǐ* 鸦胆子, brucea, 68, 183, 445, 665, 721

bǔ 补, supplement, 592

bǔ fǎ 补法, supplementation, 592

bǔ fèi ē jiāo tāng 补肺阿胶汤, Ass Hide Glue Decoction, 469, 734

bǔ fèi tāng 补肺汤, Lung-Supplementing Decoction, 47, 163, 378, 379, 740

bǔ gān sǎn 补肝散, Liver-Supplementing Powder, 157, 359

bǔ gān tāng 补肝汤, Liver-Supplementing Decoction, 266, 352, 741

bǔ gǔ zhī 补骨脂 psoralea, Psoraleae Semen, 12, 45, 229, 297, 332, 335, 343, 370, 393, 397, 593, 596, 675, 679, 727

bǔ gǔ zhī dīng 补骨脂酊, Psoralea Tincture, 676

bǔ huǒ shēng tǔ 补火生土, supplementing fire to engender earth, 594

bǔ jì 补剂, supplementing formula, 594

bǔ kě qù ruò 补可去弱, supplementing [medicinals] can eliminate weakness, 595

bǔ pí 补脾, supplementing the spleen, 596

bǔ pí yì fèi 补脾益肺, supplementing the spleen to boost the lung, 596

bǔ pí yì qì 补脾益气, supplementing the spleen and boosting qi, 596

bǔ qì 补气, supplementing qi, 594

bǔ qì gù biǎo 补气固表, supplementing qi and securing the exterior, 595

bǔ qì jiàn pí 补气健脾, supplementing qi and fortifying the spleen, 595

bǔ qì jiě biǎo 补气解表, supplementing qi and resolving the exterior, 595

bǔ qì jiě yūn tāng 补气解晕汤, Qi-Supplementing Dizziness-Resolving Decoction, 448

bǔ qì shè xuè 补气摄血, supplementing qi and containing the blood, 595

bǔ qì tōng pāo yǐn 补气通胞饮, Qi-Supplementing Bladder-Freeing Beverage, 452

bǔ qì yùn pí tāng 补气运脾汤, Qi-Supplementing Spleen-Moving Decoction, 164

bǔ qì zhǐ xuè 补气止血, supplementing qi and stanching bleeding, 595

bǔ róng tāng 补荣汤, Construction-Supplementing Decoction, 27, 741

bǔ shèn 补肾, supplementing the kidney, 596

bǔ shèn gù chōng wán 补肾固冲丸, Kidney-Supplementing Thoroughfare-Securing Pill, 741

bǔ shèn nà qì 补肾纳气, supplementing the kidney to promote qi absorption, 596

bǔ shèn yáng 补肾阳, supplementing kidney yang, 594

bǔ shèn yīn 补肾阴, supplementing kidney yin, 594

bǔ shèn zhuàng jīn tāng 补肾壮筋汤, Kidney-Supplementing Sinew-Strengthening Decoction, 742

bǔ tuō 补托, supplemental expression, 592

bǔ xīn dān 补心丹, Heart-Supplementing Elixir, 265, 272, 274, 333, 537, 541

bǔ xīn qì 补心气, supplementing heart qi, 594

bǔ xīn tāng 补心汤, Heart-Supplementing Decoction, 497

bǔ xuè 补血, supplementing the blood, 595

bǔ xuè róng jīn wán 补血荣筋丸, Blood-Supplementing Sinew-Enhancing Pill, 40, 534

bǔ yáng 补阳, supplementing yang, 596

bǔ yáng huán wǔ tāng 补阳还五汤, Yang-Supplementing Five-Returning Decoction, 289, 454, 568, 737

bǔ yì fèi qì 补益肺气, boosting (and supplementing) lung qi, 47

bǔ yì fèi shèn huà tán 补益肺肾化痰, supplementing the lung and kidney and transforming phlegm, 596

bǔ yīn 补阴, supplementing yin, 597

bǔ yīn wán 补阴丸, Yin-Supplementing Pill, 40

bǔ zhōng yì qì 补中益气, supplementing the center and boosting qi, 596

bǔ zhōng yì qì tāng 补中益气汤, Center-Supplementing Qi-Boosting Decoction, 41, 55, 73, 119, 120, 122, 127, 148, 150, 161, 171, 174, 177, 251, 283, 287, 289, 291, 302, 309, 311, 312, 317, 338, 346, 348, 370, 388, 399, 412, 449, 456, 465, 466, 469, 485, 487–489, 525, 537, 541, 562–566, 595, 596, 600, 604, 613, 614, 620, 636–641, 646, 648–651, 671, 675, 702, 711, 712, 740

bù dài wán 布袋丸, Cloth Bag Pill, 737

bù dé mián 不得眠, sleeplessness, 536

bù dé wò 不得卧, sleeplessness, 536

bù gēng yī 不更衣, not to change one's clothes, 415

bù gù 不固, insecurity, 307

bù hé 不和, disharmony, 135

bù huàn jīn dān 不换金丹, Priceless Elixir, 739

bù huàn jīn zhèng qì sǎn 不换金正气散, Priceless Qi-Righting Powder, 80, 109, 114, 154, 177, 394, 732

bù jǔ 不举, failure to rise, 195

bù láng 步廊, KI-22, Corridor Walk, 748

bù lì 不利, inhibition, 302

bù mèi 不寐, sleeplessness, 536

bù mèng ér yí 不梦而遗, seminal emission without dreaming, 525

bù nèi wài yīn 不内外因, neutral cause [of disease], 409

bù néng shǔn rǔ 不能吮乳, inability to suckle, 298

bù néng yuǎn shì 不能远视, nearsightedness, 406

bù qǐ 不起, failure to rise, 195

bù róng 不容, ST-19, Not Contained, 746

bù shí 不食, inability to eat, 298

bù sī yǐn shí 不思饮食, no thought of food and drink, 415

bù suì 不遂, -plegia, 445

bù tōng 不通, blockage, 24

bù tōng 不通, stoppage, 582

bù tōng zé tòng 不通则痛, when there is stoppage, there is pain, 673

bù xǐng rén shì 不省人事, loss of consciousness, 367

bù yù yǐn shí 不欲饮食, no desire for food and drink, 412

bù yùn 不孕, infertility, 300

bù zhèn 不振, devitalization, 125

bù zhī jī bǎo 不知饥饱, not knowing hunger or satiety, 415

bù zhī jī è 不知饥饿, obliviousness of hunger and satiety, 418

bù zhī rén 不知人, inability to recognize people, 298

bù zú 不足, insufficiency, 309

Bubali Cornu, *shuǐ niú jiǎo* 水牛角, water buffalo horn, 67, 720

buchnera, *guǐ yǔ jiàn* 鬼羽箭, Buchnerae Herba, 98

Buchnerae Herba, *guǐ yǔ jiàn* 鬼羽箭, buchnera, 98

Buddha's hand, *fó shǒu gān* 佛手柑, Citri Sarcodactylidis Fructus, 103, 490, 493, 724

Buddha's hand flower, *fó shǒu huā* 佛手花, Citri Sarcodactylidis Flos, 223, 493, 724

buddleia, *mì méng huā* 密蒙花, Buddleiae Flos, 67, 720

Buddleiae Flos, *mì méng huā* 密蒙花, buddleia, 67, 720

Bufonis Venenum, *chán sū* 蟾酥, toad venom, 728

Bungarus seu Agkistrodon, *bái huā shé* 白花蛇, krait/agkistrodon, 139, 722

Bupleuri Radix, *chái hú* 柴胡, bupleurum, 19, 20, 55, 103, 120, 223, 227, 234, 255, 256, 317, 344, 357, 359, 392, 397, 454, 455, 464, 466, 483, 490, 493, 546, 574, 600, 638, 653, 664, 685, 686, 690, 709, 720

bupleurum, *chái hú* 柴胡, Bupleuri Radix, 19, 20, 55, 103, 120, 223, 227, 234, 255, 256, 317, 344, 357, 359, 392, 397, 454, 455, 464, 466, 483, 490, 493, 546, 574, 600, 638, 653, 664, 685, 686, 690, 709, 720

Bupleurum and Asarum Decoction, *chái hú xì xīn tāng* 柴胡细辛汤, 737

Bupleurum and Cinnamon Twig Decoction, *chái hú guì zhī tāng* 柴胡桂枝汤, 344

Bupleurum and Peony Six Gentlemen Decoction, *chái sháo liù jūn zǐ tāng* 柴芍六君子汤, 435, 568, 650, 732

Bupleurum and Pueraria Flesh-Resolving Decoction, *chái gé jiě jī tāng* 柴葛解肌汤, 455, 502, 729

Bupleurum Chest Bind Decoction, *chái hú xiàn xiōng tāng* 柴胡陷胸汤, 738

Bupleurum Dampness-Overcoming Decoction, *chái hú shèng shī tāng* 柴胡胜湿汤, 240, 680, 712

Bupleurum Decoction Minus Pinellia Plus Trichosanthes Root, *chái hú qù bàn xià jiā guā lóu tāng* 柴胡去半夏加栝楼汤, 604

Bupleurum Decoction Plus Bitter Orange and Platycodon, *chái hú zhǐ jié tāng* 柴胡枳桔汤, 732

Bupleurum Decoction Plus Dragon Bone and Oyster Shell, *chái hú jiā lóng gǔ mǔ lì tāng* 柴胡加龙骨牡蛎汤, 739

Bupleurum Drink, *chái hú yǐn zǐ* 柴胡饮子, 353

Bupleurum Gallbladder-Clearing Decoction, *chái hú qīng dǎn tāng* 柴胡清胆汤, 20

Bupleurum Liver-Clearing Beverage, *chái hú qīng gān yǐn* 柴胡清肝饮, 155, 238, 483

Bupleurum Liver-Clearing Decoction, *chái hú qīng gān tāng* 柴胡清肝汤, 533, 549

Bupleurum Liver-Clearing Powder, *chái hú qīng gān sǎn* 柴胡清肝散, 731

Bupleurum Liver-Coursing Powder, *chái hú shū gān sǎn* 柴胡疏肝散, 19, 57, 103, 149, 151, 223, 302, 343, 359, 361, 362, 393, 445, 462, 466, 478, 479, 483, 502, 554, 656, 666, 670, 732

Bupleurum Membrane-Source–Opening Beverage, *chái hú dá yuán yǐn* 柴胡达原饮, 732

Bupleurum Powder, *chái hú sǎn* 柴胡散, 363, 636

Bupleurum Stomach-Calming Brew, *chái píng jiān* 柴平煎, 113, 439

Bupleurum Stomach-Calming Decoction, *chái píng tāng* 柴平汤, 732

Bupleurum White Tiger Decoction, *chái hú bái hǔ tāng* 柴胡白虎汤, 590

Bupleurum, Cinnamon Twig, and Dried Ginger Decoction, *chái hú guì jiāng tāng* 柴胡桂姜汤, 197

Bupleurum, Cinnamon Twig, and Dried Ginger Decoction, *chái hú guì zhī gān jiāng tāng* 柴胡桂枝干姜汤, 732

Bupleurum, Cinnamon Twig, and Dried Ginger, *chái hú guì jiāng tāng* 柴胡桂姜汤, 82

bursitis*

    radiohumoral, 171

bush cherry kernel, *yù lǐ rén* 郁李仁, Pruni Japonicae Semen, 460, 462, 722

bushy knotweed, *hǔ zhàng* 虎杖, Polygoni Cuspidati Rhizoma, 136, 138, 357, 540, 723, 724

bushy sophora, *shān dòu gēn* 山豆根, Sophorae Subprostratae Radix, 68, 420, 721

Buthi Caudex, *xiē shāo* 蝎梢, scorpion tail, 562, 652

Buthus, *quán xiē* 全蝎, scorpion, 54, 56, 74, 140, 146, 150, 417, 526, 541, 662, 726

bèi jí qiān jīn yào fāng 备急千金要方 (*Thousand Gold Pieces Prescriptions for Emergencies*), 7th century (Táng), Sūn Sī-Miǎo 孙思邈, 243

bái huā shé shé cǎo, *hedyotis* 白花蛇舌草, Hedyotis Herba, 68, 721

bāo xū rú qiú 胞虚如球, eyelid vacuous as a ball, 192

cā yào fāng 擦药方, Rub-On Medicinal Formula, 691

cachexia, 529

Cai Song-Ding's Difficult Delivery Formula, *cài sōng dīng nán chǎn fāng* 蔡松汀难产方, 128

cài sōng dīng nán chǎn fāng 蔡松汀难产方, Cai Song-Ding's Difficult Delivery Formula, 128

calcaneus*, 288

calcined alum, *kū fán* 枯矾, Alumen Calcinatum, 221, 226, 412, 468

calcined ark shell, *duàn wǎ léng zǐ* 煅瓦楞子, Arcae Concha Calcinata, 257

calcined cuttlefish bone, *duàn wū zéi gǔ* 煅乌贼骨, Sepiae seu Sepiellae Os Calcinatum, 57, 334

calcined dragon bone, *duàn lóng gǔ* 煅龙骨, Mastodi Ossis Fossilia Calcinata, 95, 176, 267, 333, 566, 675, 709

calcined oyster shell, *duàn mǔ lì* 煅牡蛎, Ostreae Concha Calcinata, 57, 95, 176, 334, 636, 709

calcined turtle shell, *duàn biē jiǎ* 煅鳖甲, Amydae Carapax Calcinatus, 621

calculus*

    urinary, 21, 148, 582, 583

    vesical, 582

Callicarpae Folium, *zǐ zhū* 紫珠, beauty-berry leaf, 724

Callorhini seu Phocae Testis et Penis, *hǎi gǒu shèn* 海狗肾, seal's genitals, 511

Calming Matured Ingredients Decoction, *píng chén tāng* 平陈汤, 738

calomel, *qīng fěn* 轻粉, Calomelas, 98, 319, 412, 727

Calomelas, *qīng fěn* 轻粉, calomel, 98, 319, 412, 727

Calx, *shí huī* 石灰, limestone, 569, 620, 728

camphor, *zhāng nǎo* 樟脑, Camphora, 389, 398, 728

Camphora, *zhāng nǎo* 樟脑, camphor, 389, 398, 728

campsis flower, *líng xiāo huā* 凌霄花, Campsitis Flos, 138, 725

Campsitis Flos, *líng xiāo huā* 凌霄花, campsis flower, 138, 725

cán dēng fù míng 残灯复明, last flicker of the lamp, 340

cán shǐ tāng 蚕矢汤, Silkworm Droppings Decoction, 733

Canarii Albi Fructus, *gǎn lǎn* 橄榄, Chinese olive, 68, 721

Canavaliae Legumen, *dāo dòu ké* 刀豆壳, sword bean pod, 724

Canavaliae Semen, *dāo dòu* 刀豆, sword bean, 493

cancer, 616

cancer of the head of the pancreas*, 193

cancer of the lip*, 76

cāng ěr sǎn 苍耳散, Xanthium Powder, 740

cāng ěr zǐ 苍耳子 xanthium, Xanthii Fructus, 120, 121, 681, 686, 720

cāng ěr zǐ sǎn 苍耳子散, Xanthium Powder, 120, 740

cāng fù dǎo tán wán 苍附导痰丸, Atractylodes and Cyperus Phlegm-Abducting Pill, 435

cāng lǐn sǎn 仓廪散, Old Rice Granary Powder, 730

cāng lǐn zhī guān 仓廪之官, office of the granaries, 419

cāng zhú 苍术 atractylodes, Atractylodis Rhizoma, 55, 63, 66, 93, 115, 116, 153, 154, 240, 287, 291, 319, 401, 410, 418, 430, 441, 457, 587, 625, 679, 684, 722

cāng zhú bái hǔ tāng 苍术白虎汤, Atractylodes White Tiger Decoction, 113, 591

cāng zhú chú shī tāng 苍术除湿汤, Atractylodes Dampness-Eliminating Decoction, 247

Canis Os, *gǒu gǔ* 狗骨, dog's bone, 139, 722

Canis Penis, *mǔ gǒu yīn jīng* 牡狗阴茎, dog's penis, 593, 726

Cannabis Semen, *huǒ má rén* 火麻仁, hemp seed, 72, 399, 415, 449, 460, 462, 722

Canon of the Golden Coffer and Jade Sheath (jīn guì yù hán jīng) 金匮玉函经, Eastern Han, Zhāng Jī 张机 [Zhòng-Jǐng 仲景], 380

cāo tāi 糙苔, rough tongue fur, 509

cáo zá 嘈杂, clamoring stomach, 63

cǎo dòu kòu 草豆蔻 Katsumada's galangal seed, Alpiniae Katsumadae Semen, 66, 105, 625, 722

cǎo guǒ 草果 tsaoko, Amomi Tsao-Ko Fructus, 45, 113, 217, 317, 574, 625, 722

cǎo wū tóu 草乌头 wild aconite, Aconiti Tsao-Wu-Tou Tuber, 411, 660, 723

cǎo xié fēng 草鞋风, straw-shoe wind, 584

cǎo yào 草药, herbal medicinal, 290

cǎo zhī zhū 草蜘蛛 agelena, Agelena, 298

caper spurge seed, *xù suí zǐ* 续随子, Euphorbiae Lathyridis Semen, 460, 722

Caper Spurge Seed Pill, *xù suí zǐ wán* 续随子丸, 732

capillaris, *yīn chén hāo* 茵陈蒿, Artemisiae Capillaris Herba, 69, 116, 136, 198, 357, 589, 723

Capillaris and Poria (Hoelen) Five Powder, *yīn chén wǔ líng sǎn* 茵陈五苓散, 495, 564, 733

Capillaris Counterflow Cold Decoction, *yīn chén sì nì tāng* 茵陈四逆汤, 735

Capillaris Decoction, *yīn chén hāo tāng* 茵陈蒿汤, 66, 69, 70, 79, 111, 112, 151, 198, 357, 570, 700, 733

Capillaris, Atractylodes, and Aconite Decoction, *yīn chén zhú fù tāng* 茵陈术附汤, 710, 735

Caprae seu Ovis Renes, *yáng shèn* 羊肾, goat's kidney, 333

caput medusae*, 466

carcinoma of the penis*, 330

carcinoma*, 530, 616

cardamom, *bái dòu kòu* 白豆蔻, Amomi Cardamomi Fructus, 153, 167, 224, 434, 625, 722

cardamom kernel, *kòu rén* 蔻仁, Amomi Cardamomi Semen, 401

cardiac failure*, 193, 270, 428

cardialgia*, 268

cardiodynia*, 268, 629

cardiopulumonary failure*
    chronic, 326

cardiovascular disease*, 34, 262

Carefree Pregnancy Formula, *bǎo chǎn wú yōu fāng* 保产无忧方, 385, 741

Carp Soup, *lǐ yú tāng* 鲤鱼汤, 232

Carpesii Fructus, *hè shī* 鹤虱, carpesium seed, 183, 445, 468, 724

carpesium seed, *hè shī* 鹤虱, Carpesii Fructus, 183, 445, 468, 724

Carriage-Halting Pill, *zhù chē wán* 驻车丸, 174, 312, 742

Carthami Flos, *hóng huā* 红花, carthamus, 34, 59, 98, 137, 138, 140, 181, 182, 227, 244, 352, 388, 431, 451, 493, 503, 512, 571, 654, 679, 696, 724

carthamus, *hóng huā* 红花, Carthami Flos, 34, 59, 98, 137, 138, 140, 181, 182, 227, 244, 352, 388, 431, 451, 493, 503, 512, 571, 654, 679, 696, 724

Caryophylli Flos, *dīng xiāng* 丁香, clove, 82, 146, 157, 217, 224, 316, 393, 411, 443, 463, 649, 660, 663, 723

Caryophylli Fructus, *mǔ dīng xiāng* 母丁香, clove fruit, 660, 723

Cassiae Torae Semen, *jué míng zǐ* 决明子, fetid cassia, 459, 676

cataract*, 76

Catechu, *hái ér chá* 孩儿茶, cutch, 368, 728

Catharsius, *qiāng láng* 蜣螂, dung beetle, 138, 139, 725

cè bǎi shù pí wán 侧柏樗皮丸, Biota Leaf and Toona Bark Pill, 743

cè bǎi yè 侧柏叶 biota leaf, Biotae Folium, 36, 70, 569, 647, 724

cè zǐ 侧子 small aconite, Aconiti Tuber Laterale Parvum, 97

Celestial Emperor Heart-Supplementing Elixir, *tiān wáng bǔ xīn dān* 天王补心丹, 37, 244, 261, 266, 336, 525, 537, 701, 739

Celestial Fluid Lactation-Promoting Beverage, *xià rǔ tiān jiāng yǐn* 下乳天浆饮, 741

cellulitis of the breast*, 169
    necrotic, 169

cellulitis*, 187, 670
    palpebral, 62

celosia, *qīng xiāng zǐ* 青葙子, Celosiae Argenteae Semen, 67, 720

Celosiae Argenteae Semen, *qīng xiāng zǐ* 青葙子, celosia, 67, 720

centella, *jī xuě cǎo* 积雪草, Centellae Herb (cum Radice), 139, 725

Centellae Herb (cum Radice), *jī xuě cǎo* 积雪草, centella, 139, 725

Center Fullness Separating and Dispersing Decoction, *zhōng mǎn fēn xiāo tāng* 中满分消汤, 80

Center Fullness Separating and Dispersing Pill, *zhōng mǎn fēn xiāo wán* 中满分消丸, 151, 278, 733

Center-Clearing Decoction, *qīng zhōng tāng* 清中汤, 186, 314, 442

Center-Fortifying Decoctions, *jiàn zhōng tāng* 建中汤, 555

Center-Ordering Decoction, *zhì zhōng tāng* 治中汤, 3, 77, 216, 648, 735

Center-Rectifying Decoction, *lǐ zhōng tāng* 理中汤, 1, 61, 77, 79, 80, 82, 85, 87, 156, 198, 217, 316, 339, 457, 489, 510, 555, 561, 562, 599, 608, 631, 663, 735

Center-Rectifying Phlegm-Transforming Pill, *lǐ zhōng huà tán wán* 理中化痰丸, 136, 738

Center-Rectifying Pill, *lǐ zhōng wán* 理中丸, 84, 247, 314, 564, 662, 735

Center-Rectifying Roundworm-Quieting Decoction, *lǐ zhōng ān huí tāng* 理中安蛔汤, 509

Center-Rectifying Roundworm-Quieting Powder, *lǐ zhōng ān huí sǎn* 理中安蛔散, 737

Center-Supplementing Qi-Boosting Decoction, *bǔ zhōng yì qì tāng* 补中益气汤, 41, 55, 73, 119, 120,

122, 127, 148, 150, 161, 171, 174, 177, 251, 283, 287, 289, 291, 302, 309, 311, 312, 317, 338, 346, 348, 370, 388, 399, 412, 449, 456, 465, 466, 469, 485, 487–489, 525, 537, 541, 562–566, 595, 596, 600, 604, 613, 614, 620, 636–641, 646, 648–651, 671, 675, 702, 711, 712, 740

centipeda, *é bù shí cǎo* 鹅不食草, Centipedae Herba cum Radice, 310, 405

Centipedae Herba cum Radice, *é bù shí cǎo* 鹅不食草, centipeda, 310, 405

centipede, *wú gōng* 蜈蚣, Scolopendra, 54, 74, 98, 140, 146, 434, 726

Central Eminence, *zhōng kuí* 中魁, 164, 579

Central Spring, *zhōng quán* 中泉, 61

Central Treasury Canon (zhōng zàng jīng) 中藏经, 2nd century (Eastern Hàn), attributed to Huà Tuó 华佗 (?), 86, 205

Cephalanoploris Herba seu Radix, *xiǎo jì* 小蓟, cephalanoplos, 21, 30, 34, 70, 569, 724

cephalanoplos, *xiǎo jì* 小蓟, Cephalanoploris Herba seu Radix, 21, 30, 34, 70, 569, 724

Cephalanoplos Drink, *xiǎo jì yǐn zǐ* 小蓟饮子, 22, 30, 36, 41, 738

Cera Aurea, *huáng là* 黄腊, yellow wax, 57

Cercis Powder, *zǐ jīng pí sǎn* 紫荆皮散, 745

cerebral angiospasm*, 692

cerebral hemorrhage*, 44, 586

cerebrovascular accident, 692

cerebrovascular accident*, 433, 631, 689

cerebrovascular spasm*, 44, 586

Cervi Cornu, *lù jiǎo* 鹿角, deerhorn, 17, 310, 570, 593, 596, 726

Cervi Cornu Degelatinatum, *lù jiǎo shuāng* 鹿角霜, degelatinated deerhorn, 593, 726

Cervi Cornu in Frustis, *lù jiǎo xiè* 鹿角屑, deerhorn flakes, 679

Cervi Cornu Parvum, *lù róng* 鹿茸, velvet deerhorn, 45, 229, 511, 593, 651, 726

Cervi Gelatinum Cornu, *lù jiǎo jiāo* 鹿角胶, deerhorn glue, 222, 243, 332, 466, 541, 572, 593, 726

cestodiasis*, 298

chā jīng 差经, deviated menstruation, 125

chá 茶, tea, 604

chaenomeles, *mù guā* 木瓜, Chaenomelis Fructus, 139, 154, 363, 452, 454, 548, 722

Chaenomeles and Achyranthes Pill, *mù guā niú xī wán* 木瓜牛膝丸, 80, 733

Chaenomeles Decoction, *mù guā tāng* 木瓜汤, 61

Chaenomelis Fructus, *mù guā* 木瓜, chaenomeles, 139, 154, 363, 452, 454, 548, 722

chái gé jiě jī tāng 柴葛解肌汤, Bupleurum and Pueraria Flesh-Resolving Decoction, 455, 502, 729

chái hú 柴胡 bupleurum, Bupleuri Radix, 19, 20, 55, 103, 120, 223, 227, 234, 255, 256, 317, 344, 357, 359, 392, 397, 454, 455, 464, 466, 483, 490, 493, 546, 574, 600, 638, 653, 664, 685, 686, 690, 709, 720

chái hú bái hǔ tāng 柴胡白虎汤, Bupleurum White Tiger Decoction, 590

chái hú dá yuán yǐn 柴胡达原饮, Bupleurum Membrane-Source–Opening Beverage, 732

chái hú guì jiāng tāng 柴胡桂姜汤, Bupleurum, Cinnamon Twig, and Dried Ginger, 82

chái hú guì jiāng tāng 柴胡桂姜汤, Bupleurum, Cinnamon Twig, and Dried Ginger Decoction, 197

chái hú guì zhī gān jiāng tāng 柴胡桂枝干姜汤, Bupleurum, Cinnamon Twig, and Dried Ginger Decoction, 732

chái hú guì zhī tāng 柴胡桂枝汤, Bupleurum and Cinnamon Twig Decoction, 344

chái hú jiā lóng gǔ mǔ lì tāng 柴胡加龙骨牡蛎汤, Bupleurum Decoction Plus Dragon Bone and Oyster Shell, 739

chái hú qīng dǎn tāng 柴胡清胆汤, Bupleurum Gallbladder-Clearing Decoction, 20

chái hú qīng gān sǎn 柴胡清肝散, Bupleurum Liver-Clearing Powder, 731

chái hú qīng gān tāng 柴胡清肝汤, Bupleurum Liver-Clearing Decoction, 533, 549

chái hú qīng gān yǐn 柴胡清肝饮, Bupleurum Liver-Clearing Beverage, 155, 238, 483

chái hú qù bàn xià jiā guā lóu tāng 柴胡去半夏加栝楼汤, Bupleurum Decoction Minus Pinellia Plus Trichosanthes Root, 604

chái hú sǎn 柴胡散, Bupleurum Powder, 363, 636

chái hú shèng shī tāng 柴胡胜湿汤, Bupleurum Dampness-Overcoming Decoction, 240, 680, 712

chái hú shū gān sǎn 柴胡疏肝散, Bupleurum Liver-Coursing Powder, 19, 57, 103, 149, 151, 223, 302, 343, 359, 361, 362, 393, 445, 462, 466, 478, 479, 483, 502, 554, 656, 666, 670, 732

chái hú xì xīn tāng 柴胡细辛汤, Bupleurum and Asarum Decoction, 737

chái hú xiàn xiōng tāng 柴胡陷胸汤, Bupleurum Chest Bind Decoction, 738

chái hú yǐn zǐ 柴胡饮子, Bupleurum Drink, 353

chái hú zhǐ jié tāng 柴胡枳桔汤, Bupleurum Decoction Plus Bitter Orange and Platycodon, 732

chái píng jiān 柴平煎, Bupleurum Stomach-Calming Brew, 113, 439

chái píng tāng 柴平汤, Bupleurum Stomach-Calming Decoction, 732

chái sháo liù jūn zǐ tāng 柴芍六君子汤, Bupleurum and Peony Six Gentlemen Decoction, 435, 568, 650, 732

chalazion*, 439

chalcanthite, *dǎn fán* 胆矾, Chalcanthitum, 170, 727

Chalcanthitum, *dǎn fán* 胆矾, chalcanthite, 170, 727

chān yāo shé dān 缠腰蛇丹, girdling snake cinnabar, 241

chán hóu fēng 缠喉风, throat-entwining wind, 611

chán sū 蟾酥 toad venom, Bufonis Venenum, 728

chán sū wán 蟾酥丸, Toad Venom Pill, 315

chán tuì 蝉蜕 cicada molting, Cicadae Periostracum, 128–130, 338, 368, 422, 430, 686, 691, 720 *chán yāo huǒ dān* 缠腰火丹, girdling fire cinnabar, 241

chǎn 产, birth, 19

chǎn 产, childbirth, 60

chǎn 产, delivery, 122

chǎn hòu 产后, postpartum, 447

chǎn hòu bì zhèng 产后痹证, postpartum impediment pattern, 452

chǎn hòu bìng jìng 产后病痉, postpartum tetany, 455

chǎn hòu bù yǔ 产后不语, postpartum loss of speech, 453

chǎn hòu chì zhòng 产后瘛瘲, postpartum tugging and slackening, 456

chǎn hòu chū xuè 产后出血, postpartum bleeding, 448

chǎn hòu chuāng yáng 产后疮疡, postpartum sore, 455

chǎn hòu dà biàn nán 产后大便难, postpartum defecation difficulty, 448

chǎn hòu dào hàn 产后盗汗, postpartum night sweating, 454

chǎn hòu è lù bù xià 产后恶露不下, postpartum retention of the lochia, 455

chǎn hòu fā rè 产后发热, postpartum heat effusion, 449

chǎn hòu fú zhǒng 产后浮肿, postpartum puffy swelling, 454

chǎn hòu fù tòng 产後腹痛, afterpains, 7

chǎn hòu fù tòng 产后腹痛, postpartum abdominal pain, 447

chǎn hòu fù zhàng ǒu tù 产后腹胀呕吐, postpartum abdominal distention and vomiting, 447

chǎn hòu hán rè 产后寒热, postpartum heat [effusion] and [aversion to] cold, 452

chǎn hòu jiāo cháng bìng 产后交肠病, postpartum communicating bowels, 448

chǎn hòu jīng jì 产后惊悸, postpartum fright heart palpitations, 451

chǎn hòu jū luán 产后拘挛, postpartum hypertonicity, 452

chǎn hòu kǒu kě 产后口渴, postpartum thirst, 456

chǎn hòu lèi zhòng fēng 产后类中风, postpartum wind-like stroke, 457

chǎn hòu liú zhù 产后流注, postpartum streaming sore, 455

chǎn hòu ǒu tù 产后呕吐, postpartum vomiting, 457

chǎn hòu pǐ mǎn 产后痞满, postpartum glomus and fullness, 451

chǎn hòu piàn shēn téng tòng 产后遍身疼痛, postpartum generalized pain, 451

chǎn hòu qì chuǎn 产后气喘, postpartum panting, 454

chǎn hòu rǔ zhī zì chū 产后乳汁自出, postpartum loss of breast milk, 453

chǎn hòu sān bìng 产后三病, three postpartum diseases, 610

chǎn hòu sān chōng 产后三冲, three postpartum surges, 610

chǎn hòu sān jí 产后三急, three postpartum crises, 610

chǎn hòu sān tuō 产后三脱, three postpartum desertions, 610

chǎn hòu shāng shí 产后伤食, postpartum food damage, 450

chǎn hòu shuǐ zhǒng 产后水肿, postpartum water swelling, 457

chǎn hòu sì zhī xū zhǒng 产后四肢虚肿, postpartum vacuity swelling of the limbs, 456

chǎn hòu tān huàn 产后瘫痪, postpartum paralysis, 454

chǎn hòu tóu tòng 产后头痛, postpartum headache, 451

chǎn hòu wán gǔ bù huà 产后完谷不化, postpartum nontransformation of food, 454

chǎn hòu wàng yán wàng jiàn 产后妄言妄见, postpartum raving and hallucination, 454

chǎn hòu xiǎo biàn bù lì 产后小便不利, postpartum inhibited urination, 452

chǎn hòu xiè xiè 产后泄泻, postpartum diarrhea, 449

chǎn hòu xīn bāo luò tòng 产后心包络痛, postpartum pericardiac network [vessel] pain, 454

chǎn hòu xīn tòng 产后心痛, postpartum heart pain, 451

chǎn hòu xū fán 产后虚烦, postpartum vacuity vexation, 456

chǎn hòu xuè bēng 产后血崩, postpartum flooding, 450

chǎn hòu xuè yūn 产后血晕, postpartum blood dizziness, 448

chǎn hòu yāo tòng 产后腰痛, postpartum lumbar pain, 453

chǎn hòu yí niào 产后遗尿, postpartum enuresis, 449

chǎn hòu yù hù bù liǎn 产后玉户不敛, postpartum failure of the jade door to heal, 449

chǎn hòu yù mào 产后郁冒, postpartum depression and veiling, 449

chǎn hòu yīn 产后瘖, postpartum loss of voice, 453

chǎn hòu zhà hán zhà rè 产后乍寒乍热, postpartum sudden bouts of heat [effusion] and [aversion] to cold, 455

chǎn hòu zhēng chōng 产后怔忡, postpartum fearful throbbing, 449

chǎn hòu zhòng fēng 产后中风, postpartum wind stroke, 458

chǎn hòu zhòng shǔ 产后中暑, postpartum summer-heat stroke, 455

chǎn hòu zhuàng rè 产后壮热, postpartum vigorous heat [effusion], 457

chǎn mén 产门, birth gate, 19

chǎn mén bù bì 产门不闭, nonclosure of the birth gate, 412

chāng pú yù jīn tāng 菖蒲郁金汤, Acorus and Curcuma Decoction, 434

cháng 肠, intestine, 319

cháng bì 肠痹, intestinal impediment, 317

cháng chóng bìng 长虫病, longworm disease, 367

cháng fēng 肠风, intestinal wind, 318

cháng fēng biàn xuè 肠风便血, intestinal wind bleeding, 319

cháng fēng xià xuè 肠风下血, intestinal wind bleeding, 319

cháng mài 长脉, long pulse, 367

cháng míng 肠鸣, borborygmus, 48

cháng míng 肠鸣, rumbling intestines, 510

cháng míng lù lù 肠鸣漉漉, gurgling intestines, 250

cháng níng tāng 肠宁汤, Abdomen-Quieting Decoction, 447, 741

cháng pì 肠澼, intestinal afflux, 317

cháng pì 肠癖, intestinal aggregation, 317

cháng qiáng 长强, GV-1, Long Strong, 29, 40, 74, 89, 174, 196, 220, 244, 284, 289, 297, 318, 319, 390, 408, 465, 466, 480, 493, 522, 550, 656, 749

cháng shān 常山 dichroa, Dichroae Radix, 97, 170, 317, 464, 727

cháng wèi bù hé 肠胃不和, gastrointestinal disharmony, 240

cháng wèi jī zhì 肠胃积滞, gastrointestinal accumulation, 239

cháng xià 长夏, long summer, 367

cháng xū huá tuō 肠虚滑脱, intestinal vacuity efflux desertion, 317

cháng yè kuī hào 肠液亏耗, intestinal humor depletion, 317

cháng yōng 肠痈, intestinal welling-abscess, 318

cháng zào biàn bì 肠燥便秘, intestinal dryness constipation, 317

cháng zào biàn jiān 肠燥便艰, intestinal dryness with difficult defecation, 317

cháng zhān lián huǎn jiě tāng 肠粘连缓解汤, Intestinal Adhesion Decoction, 735

cháng zhōng léi míng 肠中雷鸣, thunderous rumbling in the intestines, 613

Changii Radix, *míng dǎng shēn* 明党参, changium root, 624, 725

changium root, *míng dǎng shēn* 明党参, Changii Radix, 624, 725

Channel-Clearing (Menses-Clearing) Decoction (Powder), *qīng jīng tāng* (*sǎn*) 清经汤（散）, 731

Channel-Clearing Decoction, *qīng jīng tāng* 清经汤, 31

Channel-Freeing Network-Quickening Decoction, *tōng jīng huó luò tāng* 通经活络汤, 736

Channel-Freeing Stagnation-Abducting Decoction, *tōng jīng dǎo zhì tāng* 通经导滞汤, 571

Channel-Regulating Powder, *tiáo jīng sǎn* 调经散, 456

Channel-Warming (Menses-Warming) Decoction, *wēn jīng tāng* 温经汤, 26, 93, 326, 735

cháo rè 潮热, tidal heat [effusion], 613

chǎo 炒, stir-frying, 573

chǎo jiāo 炒焦, scorch-frying, 514

chǎo tàn 炒炭, char-frying, 56

charred crataegus, *shān zhā tàn* 山楂炭, Crataegi Fructus Carbonisatus, 139

charred eucommia, *dù zhòng tàn* 杜仲炭, Eucommiae Cortex Carbonisatus, 331, 572

charred gardenia, *hēi shān zhī zǐ* 黑山栀子, Gardeniae Fructus Carbonisatus, 120, 459

charred hair, *xuè yú tàn* 血余炭, Hominis Crinis Carbonisatus, 567, 724

charred mugwort, *ài yè tàn* 艾叶炭, Artemisiae Argyi Folium Carbonisatum, 38, 331, 488

charred phellodendron, *huáng bǎi tàn* 黄柏炭, Phellodendri Cortex Carbonisatus, 546

charred schizonepeta, *jīng jiè tàn* 荆芥炭, Schizonepetae Herba et Flos Carbonisatae, 586

charred sophora fruit, *huái jiǎo tàn* 槐角炭, Sophorae Fructus Carbonisatus, 317

chē qián 车前 plantago, Plantaginis Herba, 21, 69, 136, 463, 503, 723

chē qián zǐ 车前子 plantago seed, Plantaginis Semen, 36, 69, 116, 136, 229, 497, 666, 696, 723

chè tòng 掣痛, pulling pain, 469

Chebulae Fructus, *hē zǐ* 诃子, chebule, 80, 95, 201, 291, 316, 318, 449, 466, 518, 681, 727

Chebulae Fructus Immaturus, *zàng qīng guǒ* 藏青果, unripe chebule, 68, 721

chebule, *hē zǐ* 诃子, Chebulae Fructus, 80, 95, 201, 291, 316, 318, 449, 466, 518, 681, 727

Chebule Powder, *hē lí lè sǎn* 诃黎勒散, 479

Chebule Powder, *hē zǐ sǎn* 诃子散, 168

chén 陈, Chen, 57

chén 臣, minister, 396

chén jiàng yào 沉降药, downsinker, 146

chén mài 沉脉, deep pulse, 120

chén mài 沉脉, sunken pulse, 592

chén pí 陈皮 tangerine peel, Citri Exocarpium, 5, 20, 38, 47, 80, 128, 129, 141, 153, 224, 230, 234, 256, 257, 272, 315, 317, 318, 401, 410, 418, 421, 430, 439, 454, 457, 475, 483, 493, 499, 542, 563, 577, 578, 581, 596, 625, 684, 695, 723

chén xiāng 沉香 aquilaria, Aquilariae Lignum, 214, 262, 417, 493, 512, 629, 663, 694, 724

chén xiāng ē wèi wán 沉香阿魏丸, Aquilaria and Asafetida Pill, 515

chén xiāng jiàng qì tāng 沉香降气汤, Aquilaria Qi-Downbearing Decoction, 362, 478, 484

chén xiāng qū 沉香麯 aquilaria leaven, Aquilariae Ligni Massa, 388

chén xiāng sǎn 沉香散, Aquilaria Powder, 149, 485

chén xiāng wēn wèi wán 沉香温胃丸, Aquilaria Stomach-Warming Pill, 86

chén xiè 晨泄, early morning diarrhea, 166

chén zhòng 沉重, heaviness, 286

chén zhòng 沉重, heavy, 286

chén zōng pí 陈棕皮 old trachycarpus, Trachycarpi Stipulae Fibra Veta, 53

Cheng's Impediment-Alleviating Decoction, *chéng shì juàn bì tāng* 程氏蠲痹汤, 734

chēng liǔ 柽柳 tamarisk, Tamaricis Ramulus et Folium, 422, 501, 681, 720

chéng fú 承扶, BL-36, Support, 137, 252, 567, 747

chéng guāng 承光, BL-6, Light Guard, 747

chéng jiāng 承浆, CV-24, Sauce Receptacle, 189, 194, 222, 366, 400, 401, 521, 611, 749

chéng jiāng 承浆, sauce receptacle, 512

chéng jiāng dīng 承浆疔, sauce receptacle clove sore, 512

chéng jīn 承筋, BL-56, Sinew Support, 747

chéng líng 承灵, GB-18, Spirit Support, 748

chéng mǎn 承满, ST-20, Assuming Fullness, 746

chéng qì 承泣, ST-1, Tear Container, 64, 89, 406, 495, 585, 586, 746

chéng qì tāng 承气汤, Qi-Coordinating Decoctions, 79, 172, 190, 505, 607

chéng qì yǎng yíng tāng 承气养营汤, Qi-Coordinating Construction-Nourishing Decoction, 732

chéng shān 承山, BL-57, Mountain Support, 40, 61, 62, 89, 154, 178, 196, 284, 289, 318, 319, 342, 347, 382, 390, 446, 456–458, 465, 466, 480, 493, 522, 530, 589–591, 656, 747

chéng shì juàn bì tāng 程氏蠲痹汤, Cheng's Impediment-Alleviating Decoction, 734

Cherokee rose fruit, *jīn yīng zǐ* 金樱子, Rosae Laevigatae Fructus, 12, 308, 496, 518, 727

chī dāi 痴呆, feeble-mindedness, 197

chí mài 迟脉, slow pulse, 541

chǐ 尺, cubit, 105

chǐ 齿, teeth, 619

chǐ bǐng jiǔ 豉饼灸, moxibustion on fermented bean cake, 402

chǐ chí 齿迟, slowness to teethe, 541

chǐ fū 尺肤, cubit skin, 106

chǐ gǎo 齿槁, desiccated teeth, 124

chǐ gēng 齿更, change of teeth, 55

chǐ hēi 齿黑, black teeth, 21

chǐ jiāo 齿焦, parched teeth, 428

chǐ mài 尺脉, cubit pulse, 106

chǐ nǜ 齿衄, bleeding gums, 23

chǐ nǜ 齿衄, spontaneous bleeding of the gums, 566

chǐ qǔ 齿龋, tooth decay, 620

chǐ wéi gǔ zhī yú 齿为骨之于, teeth are the surplus of the bone, 605

chǐ xiè 齿齘, grinding of the teeth, 249

chǐ yín jié bàn 齿龈结瓣, petalled gums, 431

chǐ zào 齿燥, dry teeth, 157

chǐ zé 尺泽, LU-5, Cubit Marsh, 12–15, 22, 44, 70, 72, 88, 89, 91, 95–97, 103, 106, 109, 115, 119, 129, 142, 145–147, 149, 155, 156, 158, 163, 176, 184, 190, 201–203, 230, 237, 261, 267, 269, 277, 280–283, 285, 289, 291, 292, 295, 301, 336, 342, 343, 348, 366, 368, 372, 374, 378–380, 393, 398, 409, 415, 416, 418, 435–439, 443, 448, 458, 467, 501, 506, 520, 521, 530, 535, 547, 571, 572, 586, 587, 596, 597, 601, 603, 607, 611, 614, 637, 648, 668, 677, 683, 686–688, 695, 703, 714, 715, 746

chì 赤, red, 494

chì 炽, intense heat, 310

chì bái dài xià 赤白带下, red and white vaginal discharge, 494

chì bái lì 赤白痢, red and white dysentery, 494

chì bái ròu jì 赤白肉际, border of the red and white flesh, 48

chì bái yóu fēng 赤白游风, red and white wandering wind, 494

chì bái zhuó 赤白浊, red and white turbidity, 494

chì bí 赤鼻, red nose, 496

chì chóng 赤虫, redworm, 497

chì chóng bìng 赤虫病, redworm disease, 497

chì dài 赤带, red vaginal discharge, 497

chì dài bào lún 赤带抱轮, red areola surrounding the dark of the eye, 494

chì lì 赤痢, red dysentery, 495

chì lì 赤痢, white dysentery, 675

chì mài qīn jīng 赤脉侵睛, red vessels invading the eye, 497

chì mài qīn jīng 赤脉传睛, red vessels spreading across the eye, 497

chì miàn fēng 赤面风, red face wind, 495

chì ròu 赤肉, red flesh, 496

chì sháo yào 赤芍药 red peony, Paeoniae Radix Rubra, 17, 30, 34, 58, 67, 70, 116, 137, 139, 140, 150, 181, 227, 386, 390, 395, 430, 462, 463, 467, 497, 548, 679, 721

chì shí zhī 赤石脂 halloysite, Halloysitum Rubrum, 12, 177, 196, 242, 318, 411, 518, 519, 727

chì shí zhī yǔ yú liáng tāng 赤石脂禹余粮汤, Halloysite and Limonite Decoction, 742

chì shuǐ xuán zhū 赤水玄珠 (*Mysterious Pearl of Red Water*), 1584 (Míng), Sūn Yī-Kuí 孙一奎, 123, 583

chì sī luàn mài 赤丝乱脉, chaotic red-thread vessels, 56

chì sī qiú (qiú) mài 赤丝虬(虬)脉, tangled red-thread vessels, 602

chì xiǎo dòu 赤小豆 rice bean, Phaseoli Calcarati Semen, 40, 136, 164, 666, 671, 723

chì xiǎo dòu dāng guī sǎn 赤小豆当归散, Rice Bean and Tangkuei Powder, 743

chì yán chuāng 赤炎疮, red flaming sore, 496

chì yóu dān 赤游丹, red wandering cinnabar, 497

chì yóu dān dú 赤游丹毒, red wandering cinnabar toxin, 497

chì yóu fēng 赤游风, red wandering wind, 497

chì zhuó 赤浊, red turbidity, 496

chicken's egg membrane, *fèng huáng yī* 凤凰衣, Galli Membrana Ovi, 624, 725

child's urine, *tóng biàn* 童便, Infantis Urina, 201, 567

Child-Curing Powder, *liáo ér sǎn* 疗儿散, 503

Child-Delivering Elixir, *sòng zǐ dān* 送子丹, 741

Children's Diseases: Remedies and Sources (*xiǎo ér bìng yuán fāng lùn*) 小儿病源方论, 1254 (Sòng), Chén Wén-Zhōng 陈文中, 48

Children's Return-of-Spring Elixir, *xiǎo ér huí chūn dān* 小儿回春丹, 740

China tea rose, *yuè jì huā* 月季花, Rosae Chinensis Flos et Fructus, 138, 725 chinaberry (root) bark, *kŭ liàn pí* 苦楝皮, Meliae Cortex (Radicis), 183, 724

chinaberry root bark, *kŭ liàn gēn pí* 苦楝根皮, Meliae Radicis Cortex, 183, 509, 510, 696

Chinaberry Root Bark Paste, *kŭ liàn gāo* 苦楝膏, 16

Chinese chive, *xiè bái* 薤白, Allii Bulbus, 398, 493, 724

Chinese ilex leaf, *dōng qīng yè* 冬青叶, Ilicis Chinensis Folium, 68, 721

Chinese leek, *jiŭ cài* 韭菜, Allii Tuberosi Folium, 241, 593, 727

Chinese leek seed, *jiŭ zĭ* 韭子, Allii Tuberosi Semen, 593, 727

Chinese Leek Seed Pill, *jiā jiŭ zĭ wán* 家韭子丸, 177

Chinese lobelia, *bàn biān lián* 半边莲, Lobeliae Chinensis Herba cum Radice, 68, 721

Chinese lovage, *gǎo běn* 藁本, Ligustici Sinensis Rhizoma et Radix, 55, 103, 654, 680, 681, 720

Chinese olive, *gǎn lǎn* 橄榄, Canarii Albi Fructus, 68, 721

Chinese sage, *shí jiàn chuān* 石见穿, Salviae Chinensis Herba, 139, 725

Chinese silverweed, *wěi líng cài* 委陵菜, Potentillae Chinensis Radix seu Herba cum Radice, 68, 721

Chinese tinospora, *shēn jīn téng* 伸筋藤, Tinosporae Sinensis Caulis, 140, 722

Chinese wolfsbane, *láng dú* 狼毒, Stellerae seu Euphorbiae Radix, 411, 728

Chinese Wolfsbane Paste, *láng dú gāo* 狼毒膏, 154, 516

chlorite/mica, *méng shí* 礞石, Chloriti seu Micae Lapis, 12, 53, 214, 291, 624, 725

Chlorite/Mica Phlegm-Rolling Pill, *méng shí gǔn tán wán* 礞石滚痰丸, 12, 214, 282, 386, 437, 539, 738

Chloriti seu Micae Lapis, *méng shí* 礞石, chlorite/mica, 12, 53, 214, 291, 624, 725

cholangitis*
    pyoegenic, 363

cholecystitis*, 110, 284, 616
    acute, 193
    suppurative, 363, 670

cholelithiasis*, 110

cholera*, 61, 77, 109

chong jī fù tòng 虫积腹痛, worm accumulation abdominal pain, 695

chōng 冲, drench, 148

chōng fú 冲服, take drenched, 602

chōng hé gāo 冲和膏, Harmonious Flow Paste, 116

chōng jì 冲剂, soluble granules, 545

chōng mài 冲脉, TV, 633

chōng mài 冲脉, penetrating vessel, 430

chōng mài 冲脉, thoroughfare vessel, 609

chōng mén 冲门, SP-12, Surging Gate, 35, 57, 221, 233, 241, 746

chōng rèn bù gù 冲任不固, insecurity of the thoroughfare and controlling vessels, 308

chōng rèn kōng xū 冲任空虚, emptiness of the thoroughfare and controlling vessels, 173

chōng rèn sǔn shāng 冲任损伤, damage to the thoroughfare and controlling vessels, 108

chōng wèi zĭ 茺蔚子 leonurus fruit, Leonuri Fructus, 138, 484, 724

chōng yáng 冲阳, ST-42, Surging Yang, 90, 222, 289, 548, 610, 689, 699, 746

chóng 虫, worm, 695

chóng bái là 虫白腊 insect wax, Ericeri Pelae Cera, 728

chóng bān 虫斑, worm macule, 696

chóng bìng sì xián 虫病似痫, worm disease resembling epilepsy, 696

chóng gǔ 崇骨, Lofty Bone, 8, 384

chóng gǔ 虫鼓, worm drum, 696

chóng gǔ 虫臌, worm drum distention, 696

chóng jī 虫积, worm accumulation, 695

chóng lèi 虫类, chong product, 61

chóng rù ěr 虫入耳, insects in the ear, 307

chóng xīn tòng 虫心痛, worm heart pain, 696

chóng zhàng 虫胀, worm distention, 696

chōu chù 抽搐, convulsions, 99

chōu fēng 抽风, tugging wind, 631

chōu xīn yǐn 抽薪饮, Firewood-Raking Beverage, 54, 179

chòu 臭, malodorous, 384

chòu qì 臭气, bad odor, 15

chòu qì 臭气, malodor, 384

chòu tián luó 臭田螺, fetid water snail, 199

chòu wú tóng 臭梧桐 clerodendron, Clerodendri Folium, 139, 722

chronic bronchitis*, 115, 120, 434, 435, 584

chronic conjunctivitis*, 602

chronic diarrhea*, 334

chronic dysentery*, 339

chronic eczema*, 154

chronic enteritis*, 339, 483

chronic gastritis*, 63, 483, 615

chronic indigestion*, 237

chronic laryngitis*, 714

chronic nephritis*, 334, 615, 616, 651, 703

chronic pharyngitis*, 714, 715

chronic rhinitis*, 120, 378

chronic tonsillitis*, 581

Chrysanthemi Flos, *jú huā* 菊花, chrysanthemum, 53, 104, 130, 225, 230, 394, 420, 497, 526, 686, 720

Chrysanthemi Folium, *jú huā yè* 菊花叶, chrysanthemum leaf, 104

Chrysanthemi Indicae seu Borealis Flos, *yě jú huā* 野菊花, wild chrysanthemum flower, 686, 720

chrysanthemum, *jú huā* 菊花, Chrysanthemi Flos, 53, 104, 130, 225, 230, 394, 420, 497, 526, 686, 720

chrysanthemum leaf, *jú huā yè* 菊花叶, Chrysanthemi Folium, 104

chū xuè 出血, bleed, 23

chū xuè 出血, bleeding, 23

chū zhēn 出针, needle extraction, 406

chū zhēn 出针, needle removal, 407

chú 除, eliminate, 171

chú fēng qīng pí yǐn 除风清脾饮, Wind-Eliminating Spleen-Clearing Beverage, 395, 691

chú fēng yì sǔn tāng 除风益损汤, Wind-Eliminating Boosting Decoction, 740

chú shī juān bì tāng 除湿蠲痹汤, Dampness-Eliminating Impediment-Alleviating Decoction, 112, 347, 734

chú shī tāng 除湿汤, Damp-Eliminating Decoction, 734

chú shī tāng 除湿汤, Dampness-Eliminating Decoction, 109, 636, 691

chú shī wèi líng tāng 除湿胃苓汤, Dampness-Eliminating Stomach-Calming Poria (Hoelen) Five Decoction, 112, 116, 173, 241, 441

chú tán kài qiào 除痰开窍, eliminating phlegm and opening the orifices, 171

chù nuò 搐搦, convulsions, 99

chù zhěn 触诊, body palpation, 41

chù zhěn 触诊, palpation, 427

chuǎi 腨, calf, 53

chuān bèi mǔ 川贝母 Sichuan fritillaria, Fritillariae Cirrhosae Bulbus, 175, 282, 480, 624, 714, 725

chuān huái tán 穿踝痰, ankle-boring phlegm, 9

chuān huáng lián 川黄连 Sichuan coptis, Coptidis Rhizoma Sichuanensis, 439

chuān lián zhǐ ké tāng 川连枳壳汤, Sichuan Coptis and Bitter Orange Decoction, 199

chuān liàn zǐ 川楝子 toosendan, Toosendan Fructus, 19, 103, 183, 256, 310, 334, 343, 390, 400, 483, 493, 509, 542, 581, 589, 666, 671, 723

chuān mù xiāng 川木香 Sichuan saussurea, Vladimiriae Souliei Radix, 493, 723

chuān niú xī 川牛膝 cyathula, Cyathulae Radix, 97, 116, 150, 251, 448, 467, 516, 696

chuān shān jiǎ 穿山甲 pangolin scales, Manitis Squama, 34, 50, 137, 138, 182, 227, 315, 398, 419, 513, 516, 724

chuān shān lóng 穿山龙 Japanese dioscorea, Dioscoreae Nipponicae Rhizoma, 140, 722

chuān wū tóu 川乌头 aconite main tuber, Aconiti Tuber, 97, 242, 400, 411, 527, 660, 662, 711, 723

chuān xīn lián 穿心莲 andrographis, Andrographidis Herba, 67, 69, 111, 721

chuān xiōng 川芎 ligusticum, Ligustici Rhizoma, 11, 55, 58, 93, 102, 115, 116, 137–140, 227, 247, 259, 309, 315, 317, 390, 391, 398, 418, 428, 431, 448, 480, 503, 586, 654, 661, 680, 724

chuān xiōng chá tiáo sǎn 川芎茶调散, Tea-Blended Ligusticum (Cnidium Root) Powder, 682, 683, 740

chuān xiōng sǎn 川芎散, Ligusticum Powder, 685

chuán 传, pass, 428

chuán biàn 传变, passage and transmutation, 428

chuán biàn 传变, shift, 529

chuán dǎo zhī guān 传导之官, office of conveyance, 419

chuán jīng 传经, channel passage, 56

chuán shī 传尸, corpse transmission, 100

chuǎn 喘, dyspnea, 165

chuǎn 喘, panting, 427

chuǎn cù 喘促, hasty panting, 258

chuǎn míng 喘鸣, panting with rale, 428

chuǎn nì 喘逆, panting counterflow, 428

chuǎn sì jūn zǐ tāng 喘四君子汤, Four Gentlemen Panting Decoction, 269, 487, 489

chuǎn xī 喘息, Panting, 439

chuāng 疮, sore, 545

chuāng dú 疮毒, sore-toxin, 548

chuāng dú wán 疮毒丸, Sore-Toxin Pill, 743

chuāng kǒu 疮口, sore-opening, 546

chuāng yáng 疮疡, sore, 545

Chubby Child Pill, *féi ér wán* 肥儿丸, 60, 238, 509, 549, 557, 737

chuī 吹, insufflate, 310

chuī bí 吹鼻, nasal insufflation, 405

chuī hóu sǎn 吹喉散, Throat Insufflation Powder, 310

chuī huā xiǎn 吹花癣, blown blossom lichen, 41

chuī nǎi 吹奶, breast blowing, 50

chuī rǔ 吹乳, breast blowing, 50

chuī yào 吹药, insufflation, 310

chuí lián yì 垂帘翳, falling curtain screen, 195

chūn qiū 春秋, Spring and Autumn, 567

chūn wēn 春温, spring warmth, 568

chūn zé tāng 春泽汤, Spring Pond Decoction, 733

chún 唇, lip, 348

chún fēng 唇风, lip wind, 348

chún gān 唇干, dry lips, 154

chún jiāo 唇焦, parched lips, 428

chún liè 唇裂, cracked lips, 104

chún yáng zhēn rén yǎng zàng tāng 纯阳真人养脏汤, Pure Yang True Man Viscus-Nourishing Decoction, 174, 196, 742

chún zào 唇燥, dry lips, 154

chún zào liè 唇燥裂, cracked dry lips, 104

chyluria*, 641

cí huáng 雌黄 orpiment, Auripigmentum, 727

cí shí 磁石 loadstone, Magnetitum, 53, 225, 230, 287, 288, 490, 511, 525, 526, 538, 539, 585, 614, 726

cí zhū wán 磁朱丸, Loadstone and Cinnabar Pill, 230, 287, 526, 739

cì 刺, needle, 406

cì 痓, tetany, 606

cì jí lí 刺蒺藜 tribulus, Tribuli Fructus, 5, 53, 54, 234, 308, 320, 461, 518, 726

cì liáo 次髎, BL-32, Second Bone-Hole, 35, 40, 89, 94, 160, 177, 284, 289, 330, 334, 444, 480, 571, 640, 656, 675, 696, 747

cì luò bá guàn 刺络拔罐, pricking and cupping, 463

cì tòng 刺痛, stabbing pain, 569

cì tòng 刺痛, stinging pain, 573

cì wèi pí 刺猬皮 hedgehog's pelt, Erinacei Pellis, 98, 518, 727

cì xuè bá guàn 刺血拔罐, pricking and cupping, 463

Cibotii Rhizoma, *gǒu jǐ* 狗脊, cibotium, 593, 727

cibotium, *gǒu jǐ* 狗脊, Cibotii Rhizoma, 593, 727

cicada molting, *chán tuì* 蝉蜕, Cicadae Periostracum, 128–130, 338, 368, 422, 430, 686, 691, 720

Cicadae Periostracum, *chán tuì* 蝉蜕, cicada molting, 128–130, 338, 368, 422, 430, 686, 691, 720

cimicifuga, *shēng má* 升麻, Cimicifugae Rhizoma, 17, 55, 334, 338, 339, 415, 454, 466, 546, 600, 638, 647, 653, 686, 699, 709, 712, 720

Cimicifuga and Pueraria Decoction, *shēng má gé gēn tāng* 升麻葛根汤, 198, 422, 729

Cimicifuga Paste, *shēng má gāo* 升麻膏, 384

Cimicifuga Toxin-Dispersing Beverage, *shēng má xiāo dú yǐn* 升麻消毒饮, 705

Cimicifugae Rhizoma, *shēng má* 升麻, cimicifuga, 17, 55, 334, 338, 339, 415, 454, 466, 546, 600, 638, 647, 653, 686, 699, 709, 712, 720

cinnabar, *zhū shā* 朱砂, Cinnabaris, 148, 230, 249, 262, 287, 288, 383, 392, 490, 524, 526, 585, 602, 667, 675, 726

cinnabar root poria, *zhū fú shén* 朱茯神, Poria cum Pini Radice et Cinnabare, 433

Cinnabar Spirit-Quieting Pill, *zhū shā ān shén wán* 朱砂安神丸, 39, 61, 274, 310, 525, 537, 538, 604, 701, 739

Cinnabaris, *zhū shā* 朱砂, cinnabar, 148, 230, 249, 262, 287, 288, 383, 392, 490, 524, 526, 585, 602, 667, 675, 726

Cinnamomi Cortex, *ròu guì* 肉桂, cinnamon bark, 48, 81, 84, 98, 182, 196, 243, 316, 326, 331, 332, 335, 338, 393, 411, 425, 428, 450, 467, 488, 489, 502–504, 526, 562, 564, 596, 660, 662, 679, 696, 716, 723

Cinnamomi Cortex Rasus, *guì xīn* 桂心, shaved cinnamon bark, 242, 343

Cinnamomi Cortex Tubiformis, *guān guì* 官桂, quilled cinnamon, 45, 328

Cinnamomi Ramulus, *guì zhī* 桂枝, cinnamon twig, 11, 12, 17, 103, 136, 140, 184, 217, 218, 228, 246, 255, 391, 427, 438, 500–502, 526, 581, 654, 661–663, 666, 679, 681, 704, 716, 720

Cinnamon and Aconite Center-Rectifying Decoction, *guì fù lǐ zhōng tāng* 桂附理中汤, 734

Cinnamon and Poria (Hoelen) Sweet Dew Beverage, *guì líng gān lù yǐn* 桂苓甘露饮, 730

cinnamon bark, *ròu guì* 肉桂, Cinnamomi Cortex, 48, 81, 84, 98, 182, 196, 243, 316, 326, 331, 332, 335, 338, 393, 411, 425, 428, 450, 467, 488, 489, 502–504, 526, 562, 564, 596, 660, 662, 679, 696, 716, 723

Cinnamon Bark and Aconite Eight-Ingredient Pill, *guì fù bā wèi wán* 桂附八味丸, 174, 180, 288, 335, 369, 466, 579, 596, 629, 643, 646, 651, 702, 741

Cinnamon Bark and Musk Powder, *guì shè sǎn* 桂麝散, 243

cinnamon twig, *guì zhī* 桂枝, Cinnamomi Ramulus, 11, 12, 17, 103, 136, 140, 184, 217, 218, 228, 246, 255, 391, 427, 438, 500–502, 526, 581, 654, 661–663, 666, 679, 681, 704, 716, 720

Cinnamon Twig and Aconite Decoction, *guì zhī fù zǐ tāng* 桂枝附子汤, 734

Cinnamon Twig and Ginseng Decoction, *guì zhī rén shēn tāng* 桂枝人参汤, 532, 735

Cinnamon Twig and Licorice Decoction, *guì zhī gān cǎo tāng* 桂枝甘草汤, 427, 741

Cinnamon Twig and Musk Powder, *guì shè sǎn* 桂麝散, 210, 744

Cinnamon Twig and Poria (Hoelen) Pill, *guì zhī fú líng wán* 桂枝茯苓丸, 32, 140, 737

Cinnamon Twig Counterflow-Stemming Decoction, *guì zhī jiù nì tāng* 桂枝救逆汤, 739

Cinnamon Twig Decoction Plus Aconite, *guì zhī jiā fù zǐ tāng* 桂枝加附子汤, 145, 341, 529

Cinnamon Twig Decoction Plus Astragalus, *guì zhī jiā huáng qí tāng* 桂枝加黄芪汤, 704

Cinnamon Twig Decoction Plus Dragon Bone and Oyster Shell, *guì zhī jiā lóng gǔ mǔ lì tāng* 桂枝加龙骨牡蛎汤, 739

Cinnamon Twig Decoction Plus Extra Cinnamon, *guì zhī jiā guì tāng* 桂枝加桂汤, 510, 735

Cinnamon Twig Decoction Plus Magnolia Bark and Apricot Kernel, *guì zhī jiā hòu pò xìng rén tāng* 桂枝加厚朴杏仁汤, 729

Cinnamon Twig Decoction Plus Ovate Atractylodes and Aconite, *guì zhī jiā zhú fù tāng* 桂枝加术附汤, 734

Cinnamon Twig Decoction Plus Peony, *guì zhī jiā sháo yào tāng* 桂枝加芍药汤, 729

Cinnamon Twig Decoction Plus Pueraria, *guì zhī jiā gé gēn tāng* 桂枝加葛根汤, 729

Cinnamon Twig Decoction Plus Rhubarb, *guì zhī jiā dà huáng tāng* 桂枝加大黄汤, 730

Cinnamon Twig Decoction Plus Tangkuei, *guì zhī jiā dāng guī tāng* 桂枝加当归汤, 528

Cinnamon Twig Decoction, *guì zhī tāng* 桂枝汤, 95, 185, 246, 247, 255, 341, 458, 500, 502, 690, 729

Cinnamon Twig, Licorice, Dragon Bone, and Oyster Shell Decoction, *guì zhī gān cǎo lóng gǔ mǔ lì tāng* 桂枝甘草龙骨牡蛎汤, 269, 274, 661

Cinnamon Twig, Peony, and Anemarrhena Decoction, *guì zhī sháo yào zhī mǔ tāng* 桂枝芍药知母汤, 280

cirrhosis of the liver*, 150, 182, 193, 194, 250, 290, 616

cirrhosis*
  alcoholic, 149

Cirsii Herba seu Radix, *dà jì* 大蓟, cirsium, 569, 724

cirsium, *dà jì* 大蓟, Cirsii Herba seu Radix, 569, 724

cistanche, *ròu cōng róng* 肉苁蓉, Cistanches Caulis, 78, 222, 298, 310, 332, 338, 367, 511, 593, 596, 675, 727

Cistanche Pill, *ròu cōng róng wán* 肉苁蓉丸, 86, 506

Cistanches Caulis, *ròu cōng róng* 肉苁蓉, cistanche, 78, 222, 298, 310, 332, 338, 367, 511, 593, 596, 675, 727

Citri Exocarpium, *chén pí* 陈皮, tangerine peel, 5, 20, 38, 47, 80, 128, 129, 141, 153, 224, 230, 234, 256, 257, 272, 315, 317, 318, 401, 410, 418, 421, 430, 439, 454, 457, 475, 483, 493, 499, 542, 563, 577, 578, 581, 596, 625, 684, 695, 723

Citri Exocarpium Album, *jú bái* 橘白, white tangerine peel, 493, 723

Citri Exocarpium Immaturum, *qīng pí* 青皮, unripe tangerine peel, 19, 50, 55, 217, 223, 234, 262, 363, 397, 475, 478, 483, 490, 493, 546, 574, 685, 695, 712, 723

Citri Exocarpium Rubrum, *jú hóng* 橘红, red tangerine peel, 95, 136, 448, 493, 723

Citri Folium, *jú yè* 橘叶, tangerine leaf, 493, 723

Citri Fructus Fasciculus Vascularis, *jú luò* 橘络, tangerine pith, 417, 493, 723

Citri Grandis Exocarpium Rubrum, *huà jú hóng* 化橘红, Huazhou pomelo rind, 493, 723

Citri Sarcodactylidis Flos, *fó shǒu huā* 佛手花, Buddha's hand flower, 223, 493, 724

Citri Sarcodactylidis Fructus, *fó shǒu gān* 佛手柑, Buddha's hand, 103, 490, 493, 724

Citri Semen, *jú hé* 橘核, tangerine pip, 19, 291, 385, 493, 606, 671, 723

Citrulli Exocarpium, *xī guā pí* 西瓜皮, watermelon rind, 67, 589, 720

Citrulli Fructus, *xī guā* 西瓜, watermelon, 67, 231, 720

clamshell, *hǎi gé ké* 海蛤壳, Cyclinae (seu Meretricis) Concha, 30, 511, 624, 725

clamshell powder, *gé fěn* 蛤粉, Cyclinae (seu Meretricis) Concha Pulverata, 319

clamshell powder, *hǎi gé fěn* 海蛤粉, Cyclinae (seu Meretricis) Concha Pulverata, 243, 573

Classic of Difficult Issues (*nàn jīng*) 难经, 1st century, Eastern Hàn, 2, 15, 78, 120, 125, 143, 179, 195, 204, 208, 270, 329, 346, 360, 377, 378, 411, 561, 610

Classified Canon (*lèi jīng*) 类经, 1604 (Míng), Zhāng Jiè-Bīn 张介宾 [Jǐng-Yuè 景岳], 100, 311

Clear and Quiet Pill, *qīng níng wán* 清宁丸, 731, 733

Clear Rationale of Cold Damage (*shāng hán míng lǐ lùn*) 伤寒明理论, 1156 (Jīn), Chéng Wú-Jǐ 成无己, 308

Clear Sea Pill, *qīng hǎi wán* 清海丸, 360

Clear Sky Paste, *qīng kōng gāo* 清空膏, 111, 287, 288, 687

Clearing Invigoration Decoction, *qīng zhèn tāng* 清震汤, 612

Clearing Resolution Tablet, *qīng jiě piàn* 清解片, 730

Clearing Transforming Beverage, *qīng huà yǐn* 清化饮, 349, 702

Clematidis Radix, *wēi líng xiān* 威灵仙, clematis, 45, 139, 227, 722

clematis, *wēi líng xiān* 威灵仙, Clematidis Radix, 45, 139, 227, 722

Clematis Pill, *wēi líng xiān wán* 威灵仙丸, 477

Clerodendri Folium, *chòu wú tóng* 臭梧桐, clerodendron, 139, 722

clerodendron, *chòu wú tóng* 臭梧桐, Clerodendri Folium, 139, 722

Clever Powder, *xīng xīng sǎn* 惺惺散, 61

climbing groundsel, *qiān lǐ guāng* 千里光, Senecionis Scandentis Herba, 68, 721

climbing nightshade, *bái máo téng* 白毛藤, Solani Lyrati Herba, 68, 721

Clinical Guide with Case Histories (*lín zhèng zhǐ nán yī àn*) 临证指南医案, 1766 (Qīng), Yè Guì 叶桂 [Tiān-Shì 天士], 322, 364, 512

Cloth Bag Pill, *bù dài wán* 布袋丸, 737

clove, *dīng xiāng* 丁香, Caryophylli Flos, 82, 146, 157, 217, 224, 316, 393, 411, 443, 463, 649, 660, 663, 723

Clove and Aquilaria Diaphragm-Freeing Decoction, *dīng chén tòu gé tāng* 丁沉透膈汤, 490, 579

Clove and Cinnamon Powder, *dīng guì sǎn* 丁桂散, 402, 734

Clove and Evodia Center-Rectifying Decoction, *dīng yú lǐ zhōng tāng* 丁萸理中汤, 489, 734

Clove and Persimmon Decoction, *dīng xiāng shì dì tāng* 丁香柿蒂汤, 145, 578, 736

clove fruit, *mǔ dīng xiāng* 母丁香, Caryophylli Fructus, 660, 723

Clove Powder, *dīng xiāng sǎn* 丁香散, 82, 663

Clove, Ass Hide Glue, and Mugwort Decoction, *dīng xiāng jiāo ài tāng* 丁香胶艾汤, 643, 743

Cnidii Monnieri Fructus, *shé chuáng zǐ* 蛇床子, cnidium seed, 116, 225, 424, 468, 516, 709, 712, 728

cnidium seed, *shé chuáng zǐ* 蛇床子, Cnidii Monnieri Fructus, 116, 225, 424, 468, 516, 709, 712, 728

Cnidium Seed Powder, *shé chuáng zǐ sǎn* 蛇床子散, 112, 240, 468, 513, 516, 744

Cnidium Seed Rinse, *shé chuáng zǐ chōng xǐ jì* 蛇床子冲洗剂, 745

Cocculi Radix, *mù fáng jǐ* 木防己, woody fangji, 139, 722

Cockcrow Powder, *jī míng sǎn* 鸡鸣散, 112, 342, 733

codonopsis, *dǎng shēn* 党参, Codonopsitis Radix, 11, 12, 17, 47, 84, 141, 161, 175, 223, 227, 255, 270, 315, 329, 378, 454, 466, 486, 504, 526, 556, 563, 574, 593–596, 600, 662, 679, 726

Codonopsis and Hematite Qi-Settling Decoction, *shēn zhě zhèn qì tnag1* 参赭镇气汤, 736

Codonopsitis Radix, *dǎng shēn* 党参, codonopsis, 11, 12, 17, 47, 84, 141, 161, 175, 223, 227, 255, 270, 315, 329, 378, 454, 466, 486, 504, 526, 556, 563, 574, 593–596, 600, 662, 679, 726

Coicis Radix, *yì yǐ gēn* 薏苡根, coix root, 136, 723

Coicis Semen, *yì yǐ rén* 薏苡仁, coix, 69, 84, 98, 136, 223, 251, 434, 600, 671, 723

coix, *yì yǐ rén* 薏苡仁, Coicis Semen, 69, 84, 98, 136, 223, 251, 434, 600, 671, 723

Coix and Bamboo Leaf Powder, *yì yǐ zhú yè sǎn* 薏苡竹叶散, 733

Coix Decoction, *yì yǐ rén tāng* 薏苡仁汤, 734

coix root, *yì yǐ gēn* 薏苡根, Coicis Radix, 136, 723

Coix, Aconite, and Baijiang Powder, *yì yǐ fù zǐ bài jiàng sǎn* 薏苡附子败酱散, 318, 743

Cold Damage Life-for-All Collection (shāng hán quán shēng jí) 伤寒全生集, Míng, Táo Jié-Ān 陶节庵, 24

Cold Wheezing Pill, *lěng xiāo wán* 冷哮丸, 136, 738

Cold-Dispelling Fright-Assuaging Decoction, *zhú hán dàng jīng tāng* 逐寒荡惊汤, 735

colitis*, 338
 ulcerative, 28

Colocasiae Tuber Exsiccatum, *qīng yù nǎi gān* 青芋苏干, dried taro, 544

color blindness*, 519

colpocele*, 712

colpomycosis*, 468

comedones*, 5

Coming and Going Decoction, *qù lái tāng* 去来汤, 91

Commelinae Herba, *yā zhí cǎo* 鸭跖草, dayflower, 67, 69, 720

Common Cold Fever-Abating Granules, *gǎn mào tuì rè chōng jì* 感冒退热冲剂, 730

Common Cold Formula 2, *gǎn mào èr fāng* 感冒二方, 729

common dysosma, *guǐ jiù* 鬼臼, Dysosmae Versipellis Rhizoma, 503

complanate astragalus seed, *shā yuàn zǐ* 沙苑子, Astragali Complanati Semen, 11, 297, 584, 593, 727

Complementarity Decoction, *jì jì tāng* 既济汤, 22

Complete Compendium of Medical Works, Ancient and Modern (gǔ jīn yī tǒng dà quán) 古今医统大全, 1556 (Míng), Xú Chūn-Fǔ 徐春甫, 548

Compound Formula Coptis Paste, *fù fāng huáng lián gāo* 复方黄连膏, 744

Compound Formula Major Qi-Coordinating Decoction, *fù fāng dà chéng qì tāng* 复方大承气汤, 731

Comprehensive Herbal Foundation (běn cǎo gāng mù) 本草纲目, 1590 (Míng), Lǐ Shí-Zhēn 李时珍, 49, 204, 290

Construction-Clearing Decoction, *qīng yíng tāng* 清营汤, 65, 69, 202, 388, 431, 455, 589, 591, 693, 730

Construction-Cooling Qi-Clearing Decoction, *liáng yíng qīng qì tāng* 凉营清气汤, 178

Construction-Enriching Network-Quickening Decoction, *zī róng huó luò tāng* 滋荣活络汤, 457

Construction-Enriching Qi-Boosting Spirit-Returning Decoction, *zī róng yì qì fù shén tāng* 滋荣益气复神汤, 455

Construction-Harmonizing Hardness-Dissipating Pill, *hé róng sàn jiān wán* 和荣散坚丸, 367

Construction-Nourishing Kidney-Invigorating Decoction, *yǎng róng zhuàng shèn tāng* 养荣壮肾汤, 453

Construction-Regulating Beverage, *tiáo yíng yǐn* 调营饮, 151, 467

Construction-Supplementing Decoction, *bǔ róng tāng* 补荣汤, 27, 741

Concha Margaritifera, *zhēn zhū mǔ* 珍珠母, mother-of-pearl, 53, 54, 230, 434, 490, 526, 538, 539, 585, 726

Concretion-Transforming Return-to-Life Elixir, *huà zhēng huí shēng dān* 化癥回生丹, 26

Confucian Filiality (rú mén shì qīn) 儒门事亲, Jīn (1115–1234), Zhāng Cóng-Zhèng 张从正 [Zǐ-Hé 子和], 181

Confucius' Pillow Powder, *kǒng zǐ zhěn zhōng sǎn* 孔子枕中散, 739

cōng bái 葱白 scallion white, Allii Fistulosi Bulbus, 176, 422, 500, 502, 681, 720

cōng bái qī wèi yǐn 葱白七味饮, Scallion White Seven-Ingredient Beverage, 416, 729

cōng chǐ jié gěng tāng 葱豉桔梗汤, Scallion, Fermented Soybean, and Platycodon Decoction, 729

cōng chǐ tāng 葱豉汤, Scallion and Fermented Soybean Decoction, 12, 681, 729

cōng zhī 葱汁 scallion juice, Allii Fistulosi Herbae Succus, 307

cóng máo 丛毛, tuft of hair, 631

cóng wài cè nèi 从外测内, judging the inside from the outside, 323

cóng zhì 从治, coacting treatment, 76

congestion*
 ciliary, 494

conjunctivitis*
 acute, 685
 chronic, 602
 follicular, 395
 phlyctenular, 394

convulsions*
 infantile, 230

cooked aconite, *shú fù zǐ* 熟附子, Aconiti Tuber Laterale Conquitum, 11, 48, 660, 663, 723

cooked rehmannia, *shú dì huáng* 熟地黄, Rehmanniae Radix Conquita, 28, 37, 39, 47, 88, 140, 161, 175, 225, 298, 310, 333, 458, 459, 467, 504, 526, 537, 570, 584, 593, 595, 596, 620, 651, 727

Cool Clearing Beverage, *qīng liáng yǐn* 清凉饮, 104

Cool Clearing Paste, *qīng liáng gāo* 清凉膏, 744

Cool Clearing Sweet Dew Beverage, *qīng liáng gān lù yǐn* 清凉甘露饮, 76

copperleaf, *tiě xiàn* 铁苋, Acalyphae Herba, 724

Coptidis Rhizoma, *huáng lián* 黄连, coptis, 20, 30, 65–67, 69, 70, 81, 82, 116, 141, 146, 153, 154, 230, 243, 256, 257, 261–263, 281, 317, 338, 358, 387, 390, 417, 421, 434, 440, 459, 462, 466, 474, 500, 510, 524, 526, 539, 541, 569, 574, 577, 578, 587, 589, 601, 612, 614, 617, 619, 638, 671, 673, 712, 720

Coptidis Rhizoma Sichuanensis, *chuān huáng lián* 川黄连, Sichuan coptis, 439

coptis, *huáng lián* 黄连, Coptidis Rhizoma, 20, 30, 65–67, 69, 70, 81, 82, 116, 141, 146, 153, 154, 230, 243, 256, 257, 261–263, 281, 317, 338, 358, 387, 390, 417, 421, 434, 440, 459, 462, 466, 474, 500, 510, 524, 526, 539, 541, 569, 574, 577, 578, 587,

589, 601, 612, 614, 617, 619, 638, 671, 673, 712, 720

Coptis and Aconite Six-to-One Decoction, *lián fù liù yī tāng* 连附六一汤, 731

Coptis and Ass Hide Glue Decoction, *huáng lián ē jiāo tāng* 黄连阿胶汤, 28, 230, 263, 268, 345, 525, 537, 538, 739

Coptis and Elsholtzia Powder, *huáng lián xiāng rú sǎn* 黄连香薷散, 276, 588

Coptis and Goat's Liver Pill, *huáng lián yáng gān wán* 黄连羊肝丸, 731

Coptis and Magnolia Bark Beverage, *lián pò yǐn* 连朴饮, 66, 118, 276, 539, 733

Coptis and Mume Decoction, *lián méi tāng* 连梅汤, 734

Coptis and Peony Decoction, *huáng qín sháo yào tāng* 黄芩芍药汤, 702

Coptis and Pig's Stomach Pill, *huáng lián zhū dǔ wán* 黄连猪肚丸, 508

Coptis and Pueraria Flower Pill, *gé huáng wán* 葛黄丸, 502

Coptis Decoction, *huáng lián tāng* 黄连汤, 732

Coptis Gallbladder-Warming Decoction, *huáng lián wēn dǎn tāng* 黄连温胆汤, 20, 24, 230, 269, 436, 539, 621, 694, 739

Coptis Paste, *huáng lián gāo* 黄连膏, 283, 533

Coptis Phlegm-Transforming Beverage, *huáng lián huà tán yǐn* 黄连化痰饮, 277

Coptis Pill, *huáng lián wán* 黄连丸, 40, 82, 284

Coptis Powder, *huáng lián sǎn* 黄连散, 154

Coptis Toxin-Resolving Decoction, *huáng lián jiě dú tāng* 黄连解毒汤, 6, 51, 63, 70, 75, 76, 81, 168, 197, 202, 214, 221, 259, 285, 315, 338, 445, 533, 566, 664, 687, 730

Coptis, Ass Hide Glue, and Egg Yolk Decoction, *huáng lián ē jiāo jī zǐ huáng tāng* 黄连阿胶鸡子黄汤, 284, 413, 467, 538, 655

Cordyceps, *dōng chóng xià cǎo* 冬虫夏草, cordyceps, 593, 726

cordyceps, *dōng chóng xià cǎo* 冬虫夏草, Cordyceps, 593, 726

coriander, *hú suī* 胡荽, Coriandri Herba cum Radice, 387, 422, 542, 681, 720

Coriandri Herba cum Radice, *hú suī* 胡荽, coriander, 387, 422, 542, 681, 720

Cormorant Drool Pill, *lú cí xián wán* 鸬鹚涎丸, 677, 738

cormorant's drool, *lú sī xián* 鸬鹚涎, Phalacrocoracis Saliva, 677

corn silk, *yù mǐ xū* 玉米须, Mays Stylus, 136, 723

cornea*, 118

Corni Fructus, *shān zhū yú* 山茱萸, cornus, 11, 39, 47, 96, 175, 176, 310, 336, 352, 458, 467, 504, 518, 526, 548, 596, 709, 727

cornus, *shān zhū yú* 山茱萸, Corni Fructus, 11, 39, 47, 96, 175, 176, 310, 336, 352, 458, 467, 504, 518, 526, 548, 596, 709, 727

coronary heart disease*, 58

Coronary Liquid Storax Pill, *guàn xīn sū hé wán* 冠心苏合丸, 300, 740

Coronary No.2, *guàn xīn èr hào* 冠心二号, 265, 484, 737

corydalis, *yán hú suǒ* 延胡索, Corydalis Tuber, 19, 103, 137, 138, 227, 361, 363, 397, 431, 464, 493, 561, 574, 581, 696, 724

Corydalis Decoction, *yán hú suǒ tāng* 延胡索汤, 738

Corydalis Decumbentis Tuber et Herba, *xià tiān wú* 夏天无, Jilong corydalis, 140, 722

Corydalis Tuber, *yán hú suǒ* 延胡索, corydalis, 19, 103, 137, 138, 227, 361, 363, 397, 431, 464, 493, 561, 574, 581, 696, 724

costusroot, *guǎng mù xiāng* 广木香, Saussureae Radix, 490, 493, 723

cotton rose, *mù fú róng huā* 木芙蓉花, Hibisci Mutabilis Flos, 728

cotton rose leaf, *mù fú róng yè* 木芙蓉叶, Hibisci Mutabilis Folium, 104, 728

còu lǐ 腠理, interstice, 317

Cough-Stopping Powder, *zhǐ sòu sǎn* 止嗽散, 84, 99, 129, 625, 682, 684, 738

Cough-Suppressing Phlegm-Transforming Panting-Stabilizing Pill, *zhǐ sòu huà tán dìng chuǎn wán* 止嗽化痰定喘丸, 738

Counterflow Cold Decoction Plus Ginseng, *sì nì jiā rén shēn tāng* 四逆加人参汤, 84, 735

Counterflow Cold Decoction, *sì nì tāng* 四逆汤, 74, 77, 85, 87, 130, 292, 345, 488, 504, 505, 735

Counterflow Cold Powder, *sì nì sǎn* 四逆散, 19, 103, 123, 283, 297, 361, 362, 475, 483, 505, 732

Counterflow-Settling White Tiger Decoction, *zhèn nì bái hǔ tāng* 镇逆白虎汤, 730

Coursing and Piercing Drink, *shū záo yǐn zǐ* 疏凿饮子, 302

cracked nipple*, 412

Crane Top, *hè dǐng* 鹤顶, 521

cranesbill, *lǎo guàn cǎo* 老鹳草, Geranii Herba, 140, 722

Crataegi Fructus, *shān zhā* 山楂, crataegus, 107, 141, 216, 217, 418, 420, 450, 499, 514, 548, 573, 606, 724

Crataegi Fructus Carbonisatus, *shān zhā tàn* 山楂炭, charred crataegus, 139

crataegus, *shān zhā* 山楂, Crataegi Fructus, 107, 141, 216, 217, 418, 420, 450, 499, 514, 548, 573, 606, 724

Crataegus and Medicated Leaven Stomach-Calming Powder, *zhā qū píng wèi sǎn* 楂麴平胃散, 736

Crick in the Neck Point, *luò zhěn xué* 落枕穴, 105

Croci Stigma, *zàng hóng huā* 藏红花, saffron, 98, 138, 387, 724

cross moxa, *shí zì jiǔ* 十字灸, 80, 109, 647

croton, *bā dòu* 巴豆, Crotonis Semen, 98, 182, 411, 460, 464, 527, 664, 722

croton frost, *bā dòu shuāng* 巴豆霜, Crotonis Seminis Pulvis, 231, 460, 722

Crotonis Semen, *bā dòu* 巴豆, croton, 98, 182, 411, 460, 464, 527, 664, 722

Crotonis Seminis Pulvis, *bā dòu shuāng* 巴豆霜, croton frost, 231, 460, 722

croup*

  diphtheritic, 612

crude abalone shell, *shēng shí jué míng* 生石决明, Haliotidis Concha Cruda, 146, 225, 585

crude dragon bone, *shēng lóng gǔ* 生龙骨, Mastodi Ossis Fossilia Cruda, 225, 585

crude gypsum, *shēng shí gāo* 生石膏, Gypsum Crudum, 67, 422, 720

crude oyster shell, *shēng mǔ lì* 生牡蛎, Ostreae Concha Cruda, 54, 146, 225, 256, 726

cù chǎo 醋炒, stir-frying with vinegar, 574

cù mài 促脉, skipping pulse, 536

cù pào fāng 醋泡方, Vinegar Soaking Formula, 11, 221, 244

cù zhì 醋炙, mix-frying with vinegar, 397

cuàn 篡, perineum, 430

cuàn tòng 窜痛, scurrying pain, 517

cubeb, *bì chéng qié* 荜澄茄, Cubebae Fructus, 660, 723

Cubebae Fructus, *bì chéng qié* 荜澄茄, cubeb, 660, 723

Cucumeris Melonis Pedicellus, *guā dì* 瓜蒂, melon stalk, 170, 727

Cucurbitae Semen, *nán guā zǐ* 南瓜子, pumpkin seed, 183, 298, 724

cuī rǔ 催乳, promoting lactation, 467

cuī shēng rú yì sǎn 催生如意散, Agreeable Birth-Hastening Powder, 128

cuī shēng yǐn 催生饮, Birth-Hastening Beverage, 128, 735

cuì 淬, calcining and quenching, 53

cuì cì 焠刺, red-hot needling, 496

cuì jiǎo 脆脚, brittle foot, 50

cùn 寸, body-inch, 41

cùn 寸, cun, 106

cùn 寸, inch, 298

cùn bái chóng 寸白虫, inch whiteworm, 298

cùn kǒu 寸口, inch opening, 298

cùn kǒu 寸口, wrist pulse, 696

cuō kōng lǐ xiàn 撮空理线, groping in the air and pulling at invisible strings, 249

cuō kǒu 撮口, pursed mouth, 474

cuō zhēn 搓针, needle twisting, 408

cuō zhēn 搓针, unidirectional twirling, 637

cuó chuāng 痤疮, pimples, 444

cuó fèi 痤痱, pock pimples, 445

cuò 锉, 剉, grating, 245

cuò fēng sǎn 撮风散, Pursing Wind Powder, 740

cuò jīng 错经, crossed menstruation, 105

Curculiginis Rhizoma, *xiān máo* 仙茅, curculigo, 335, 593, 596, 727

curculigo, *xiān máo* 仙茅, Curculiginis Rhizoma, 335, 593, 596, 727

curcuma, *yù jīn* 郁金, Curcumae Tuber, 19, 27, 138, 223, 234, 262, 356, 357, 385, 393, 411, 434, 475, 480, 483, 493, 538, 586, 670, 724

Curcumae Longae Rhizoma, *jiāng huáng* 姜黄, tureric, 138, 427, 724

Curcumae Tuber, *yù jīn* 郁金, curcuma, 19, 27, 138, 223, 234, 262, 356, 357, 385, 393, 411, 434, 475, 480, 483, 493, 538, 586, 670, 724

Curled Dock Root Powder, *yáng tí gēn sǎn* 羊蹄根散, 744

cuscuta, *tù sī zǐ* 菟丝子, Cuscutae Semen, 310, 518, 529, 572, 593, 614, 727

Cuscuta Seed Pill, *tù sī zǐ wán* 菟丝子丸, 180, 523, 636, 743

Cuscutae Semen, *tù sī zǐ* 菟丝子, cuscuta, 310, 518, 529, 572, 593, 614, 727

cutch, *hái ér chá* 孩儿茶, Catechu, 368, 728

cuttlefish bone, *hǎi piāo xiāo* 海螵蛸, Sepiae seu Sepiellae Os, 478, 502, 511, 518, 572, 581, 727

CV-1, *huì yīn* 会阴, Meeting of Yin, 98, 244, 297, 749

CV-2, *qū gǔ* 曲骨, Curved Bone, 221, 297, 308, 332, 453, 497, 522, 643, 701, 749

CV-3, *zhōng jí* 中极, Central Pole, 7, 8, 21–23, 26, 33–36, 68, 69, 71, 80, 84, 86, 89, 91, 93, 94, 111, 112, 118, 149, 151, 177, 180, 199, 219–221, 227, 229, 240, 241, 282, 283, 297, 300–302, 308, 317, 331, 332, 353, 393, 424, 431, 447, 449–451, 456, 457, 465, 468, 483–485, 497, 503, 516, 518, 522, 533, 541, 542, 582, 589, 597, 604, 631, 636, 640, 641, 643, 661, 667, 675, 701, 711, 713, 749

CV-4, *guān yuán* 关元, Pass Head, 1, 3, 4, 8, 22, 23, 26, 28–33, 35, 36, 38, 39, 41, 45, 47, 51, 58, 59, 64, 71, 73, 74, 78–87, 89, 91, 94, 105, 109, 111, 119, 127, 128, 149, 152, 160, 161, 163, 168, 174, 175, 177, 180, 189, 196, 199, 210–212, 216, 217, 219–222, 224, 226–229, 231–233, 239, 240, 251, 263, 266, 267, 269–272, 274, 287–291, 296, 297, 300–302, 308, 309, 312, 314, 318, 319, 325, 329, 331–336, 338, 340, 342, 343, 345, 349, 352, 353, 360, 369, 370, 379, 380, 393, 418, 425, 426, 430, 435, 447–450, 452–454, 457, 461, 465–467, 477–479, 482, 487–489, 497, 499, 503, 504, 511, 513, 516, 518, 521–525, 529, 541–543, 549, 557, 559, 563, 564, 570, 578, 579, 586, 594, 595, 597, 600, 604, 608, 612, 614, 625, 629–631, 636, 640, 641, 643, 646, 647, 649–652, 656, 660, 662–664, 667, 668, 675, 678, 690, 693, 699, 702, 709, 710, 712, 713, 716, 749

CV-5, *shí mén* 石门, Stone Gate, 8, 91, 431, 749

CV-6, *qì hǎi* 气海, Sea of Qi, 1, 3, 4, 14, 15, 17, 22–24, 26–28, 31, 33–38, 40, 41, 47, 55, 57–59, 61, 62, 64, 71, 73, 74, 77, 78, 80–87, 94, 97, 105, 109, 111, 114–119, 127, 136, 139, 141, 151, 153, 157, 159–164, 168, 174, 177, 186, 194, 196, 197, 199, 212, 215–218, 223, 224, 226–231, 233–235, 240, 241, 247, 251, 257, 261, 265, 267, 269–272, 274, 278, 279, 287, 296, 297, 300–302, 309, 314, 318,

329, 331, 333, 334, 336, 338–340, 343, 349, 353, 355, 356, 370, 378, 379, 393, 395, 410, 418, 425, 426, 431, 433, 435, 438–440, 442, 447–454, 456, 457, 461, 465–467, 475, 477–481, 483–490, 497, 498, 503, 504, 517, 522–525, 529, 537, 541, 542, 547, 555, 557–559, 561–565, 570, 579–581, 586, 589, 590, 594–596, 601, 603, 604, 608, 612–614, 620, 629, 631, 633, 636, 638–641, 647, 649–652, 658, 661–664, 666–668, 675, 677, 678, 683, 690, 694, 695, 702, 703, 709–713, 716, 749

CV-7, *yīn jiāo* 阴交, Yin Intersection, 27, 332, 643, 749

CV-8, *shén què* 神阙, Spirit Gate Tower, 74, 77, 78, 82–86, 105, 127, 152, 168, 212, 231, 232, 289, 314, 338, 342, 425, 448, 453, 489, 504, 521, 625, 631, 646, 651, 664, 690, 699, 709, 749

CV-9, *shuǐ fēn* 水分, Water Divide, 37, 105, 109, 117, 168, 182, 224, 228, 301, 334, 335, 379, 418, 457, 485, 537, 559, 600, 608, 612, 661–663, 666–668, 694, 703, 716, 749

CV-10, *xià wǎn* 下脘, Lower Stomach Duct, 2–4, 15, 141, 157, 186, 197, 207, 215–217, 237, 239, 302, 316, 426, 450, 499, 557, 564, 578, 633, 749

CV-11, *jiàn lǐ* 建里, Interior Strengthening, 152, 749

CV-12, *zhōng wǎn* 中脘, Center Stomach Duct, 2–4, 6, 8, 17, 20, 28, 29, 32, 38, 41, 54, 55, 59, 61–64, 66, 70, 73, 77, 79–89, 94, 99, 109–111, 113–115, 117–119, 127, 136, 141, 142, 145, 151–153, 156, 157, 161, 163, 164, 168, 174, 186, 189, 196, 203, 207, 210–212, 215–218, 222–224, 230, 235, 237, 240, 242, 247, 251, 252, 256, 257, 260, 268, 272, 278, 284, 287, 291, 301, 302, 309, 312, 314, 318, 325, 339, 340, 343, 349, 358, 361, 362, 383, 390, 394–396, 401, 403, 410, 414, 418, 425, 433–443, 445, 447, 448, 450, 457, 462, 477–480, 482, 487, 488, 490, 498, 503, 506, 509, 510, 521, 522, 537, 539, 540, 549–551, 554, 555, 557–559, 561–566, 571, 575, 577–581, 585, 587–589, 591, 595, 596, 603, 604, 608, 612–614, 633, 638, 645, 647, 649, 650, 658, 662–669, 671, 673, 678, 679, 684, 685, 691, 694, 703, 709, 713, 716, 749

CV-13, *shàng wǎn* 上脘, Upper Stomach Duct, 4, 29, 87, 157, 222, 252, 390, 436, 578, 749

CV-14, *jù què* 巨阙, Great Tower Gate, 8, 39, 58, 59, 81, 91, 159, 160, 207, 223, 232, 261, 263, 265–267, 269–271, 273, 274, 280, 294, 297, 301, 336, 343, 410, 427, 451, 452, 488, 499, 537, 538, 594, 595, 629, 651, 661, 749

CV-15, *jiū wěi* 鸠尾, Turtledove Tail, 178, 408, 434, 440, 482, 749

CV-16, *zhōng tíng* 中庭, Center Palace, 749

CV-17, *dàn zhōng* 膻中, Chest Center, 89, 91

CV-17, *shān zhōng* 膻中, Chest Center, 8, 13, 19, 25, 26, 33, 34, 58, 64, 72, 81, 82, 87, 115, 118, 123, 127, 139, 141, 142, 146, 153, 156, 158, 164, 186, 202, 210, 223, 227, 228, 230, 235, 253, 261, 263, 265, 266, 269, 273, 274, 277, 280, 285, 302, 343, 349, 366, 379, 383, 385, 386, 418, 426, 427, 433–

435, 437, 438, 443, 445, 448, 452, 462, 475, 477, 478, 480, 482–484, 499, 506, 513, 522, 537, 539, 570, 571, 578, 581, 587, 588, 614, 625, 629, 646, 648, 649, 656, 661, 665, 666, 668, 683, 715, 749

CV-18, *yù táng* 玉堂, Jade Hall, 749

CV-19, *zǐ gōng* 紫宫, Purple Palace, 749

CV-20, *huá gài* 华盖, Florid Canopy, 749

CV-21, *xuán jī* 璇玑, Jade Swivel, 15, 141, 145, 186, 197, 215, 218, 224, 426, 499, 564, 578, 645, 749

CV-22, *tiān tú* 天突, Celestial Chimney, 13, 14, 19, 30, 87, 92, 93, 109, 115, 123, 129, 153, 156, 158, 164, 210, 277, 282, 291, 292, 368, 398, 433, 435, 439, 440, 443, 445, 477, 480, 506, 521, 522, 544, 547, 611, 624, 681, 684, 689, 749

CV-23, *lián quán* 廉泉, Ridge Spring, 89, 125, 140, 289, 291, 292, 294, 368, 521, 552, 573, 640, 749

CV-24, *chéng jiāng* 承浆, Sauce Receptacle, 189, 194, 222, 366, 400, 401, 521, 611, 749

cyathula, *chuān niú xī* 川牛膝, Cyathulae Radix, 97, 116, 150, 251, 448, 467, 516, 696

Cyathulae Radix, *chuān niú xī* 川牛膝, cyathula, 97, 116, 150, 251, 448, 467, 516, 696

Cyclinae (seu Meretricis) Concha, *hǎi gé ké* 海蛤壳, clamshell, 30, 511, 624, 725

Cyclinae (seu Meretricis) Concha Pulverata, *gé fěn* 蛤粉, clamshell powder, 319

Cyclinae (seu Meretricis) Concha Pulverata, *hǎi gé fěn* 海蛤粉, clamshell powder, 243, 573

Cynanchi Baiqian Radix et Rhizoma, *bái qián* 白前, cynanchum, 624, 725

Cynanchi Baiwei Radix, *bái wēi* 白薇, baiwei, 68, 72, 177, 277, 281, 282, 511, 649, 721

Cynanchi Paniculati Herba cum Radice, *xú cháng qīng* 徐长卿, paniculate cynanchum, 139, 722

cynanchum, *bái qián* 白前, Cynanchi Baiqian Radix et Rhizoma, 624, 725

Cynomorii Caulis, *suǒ yáng* 锁阳, cynomorium, 310, 593, 679, 727

cynomorium, *suǒ yáng* 锁阳, Cynomorii Caulis, 310, 593, 679, 727

Cyperi Rhizoma, *xiāng fù zǐ* 香附子, cyperus, 19, 93, 103, 115, 201, 227, 384, 397, 418, 426, 428, 433, 457, 474, 475, 478, 480, 483, 493, 538, 574, 581, 647, 663, 670, 694, 723

cyperus, *xiāng fù zǐ* 香附子, Cyperi Rhizoma, 19, 93, 103, 115, 201, 227, 384, 397, 418, 426, 428, 433, 457, 474, 475, 478, 480, 483, 493, 538, 574, 581, 647, 663, 670, 694, 723

Cyperus and Fritillaria Construction-Nourishing Decoction, *xiāng bèi yǎng yíng tāng* 香贝养营汤, 737

Cyperus and Perilla Powder, *xiāng sū sǎn* 香苏散, 480, 686, 729

cystolith*, 582

cystocele*, 712

dā shǒu 搭手, reachable sore, 492

dá yù tāng 达郁汤, Depression-Freeing Decoction, 297

dá yuán yǐn 达原饮, Membrane-Source–Opening Beverage, 177, 514, 732

dà ān wán 大安丸, Great Tranquility Pill, 564, 645, 736

dà bàn xià tāng 大半夏汤, Major Pinellia Decoction, 87, 443, 579, 736

dà bāo 大包, SP-21, Great Embracement, 26, 118, 248, 408, 746

dà biàn 大便, stool, 582

dà biàn bì 大便闭, fecal block, 196

dà biàn bù tōng 大便不通, fecal stoppage, 197

dà biàn gān jié 大便干结, dry bound stool, 152

dà biàn hēi sè 大便黑色, black stool, 21

dà biàn jiān nán 大便艰难, difficult defecation, 126

dà biàn kùn nán 大便困难, difficult defecation, 126

dà biàn nóng xuè 大便脓血, stool containing pus and blood, 582

dà biàn pái chū kùn nán 大便排出困难, difficult defecation, 126

dà biàn shī jìn 大便失禁, fecal incontinence, 196

dà biàn suí shǐ qì ér chū 大便随矢气而出, discharge of stool with flatus, 130

dà biàn zào jié 大便燥结, dry bound stool, 152

dà biàn zì lì 大便自利, uninhibited stool, 637

dà bǔ yīn wán 大补阴丸, Major Yin Supplementation Pill, 213, 296, 330, 461, 512, 571, 597, 641, 647, 649, 651, 714, 742

dà bǔ yuán jiān 大补元煎, Major Origin-Supplementing Brew, 178, 296, 332, 369, 466, 482, 487, 646, 647, 712

dà chái hú tāng 大柴胡汤, Major Bupleurum Decoction, 3, 110, 255, 344, 357, 439, 700, 730

dà cháng 大肠, LI, 345

dà cháng 大肠, large intestine, 340

dà cháng bìng 大肠病, large intestinal disease, 339

dà cháng hán jié 大肠寒结, large intestinal cold bind, 338

dà cháng jīng 大肠经, large intestine channel, 340

dà cháng ké 大肠咳, large intestinal cough, 338

dà cháng rè jié 大肠热结, large intestinal heat bind, 339

dà cháng shī rè 大肠湿热, large intestinal damp-heat, 338

dà cháng shū 大肠俞, BL-25, Large Intestine Transport, 3, 15, 40, 61, 72, 77, 78, 83, 89, 91, 117, 128, 183, 196, 215, 216, 277, 284, 289, 290, 298, 318, 335, 338–340, 390, 415, 426, 434, 444, 449, 465, 466, 477, 480, 493, 509, 570, 585, 589, 613, 646, 656, 658, 664, 683, 695, 696, 747

dà cháng xū 大肠虚, large intestinal vacuity, 339

dà cháng xū hán 大肠虚寒, large intestinal vacuity cold, 339

dà cháng yè kuī 大肠液亏, large intestinal humor depletion, 339

dà cháng yīn xū zào jié 大肠阴虚燥结, large intestinal yin vacuity dryness bind, 340

dà cháng yōng 大肠痈, large intestinal welling-abscess, 340

dà cháng zhàng 大肠胀, large intestinal distention, 339

dà cháng zhě, chuán dǎo zhī guān yě, biàn huà chū yān 大肠者，传导之官也，变化出焉, large intestine holds the office of conveyance, whence mutation emanates, 340

dà cháng zhǔ chuán dǎo 大肠主传导, large intestine governs conveyance, 340

dà cháng zhǔ chuán huà zāo pò 大肠主传化糟粕, large intestine governs transformation and conveyance of waste, 340

dà cháng zhǔ jīn 大肠主津, large intestine governs liquid, 340

dà chéng qì tāng 大承气汤, Major Qi-Coordinating Decoction, 2, 12, 24, 73, 84, 276, 280, 283, 290, 386, 426, 459, 504, 532, 542, 613, 698, 731

dà dìng fēng zhū 大定风珠, Major Wind-Stabilizing Pill, 74, 176, 456, 569, 740

dà dòu huáng juǎn 大豆黄卷 dried soybean sprout, Glycines Semen Germinatum Exsiccatum, 686, 720

dà dū 大都, SP-2, Great Metropolis, 54, 61, 212, 233, 281, 395, 487, 489, 604, 746

dà dūn 大敦, LR-1, Large Pile, 31, 41, 83, 86, 111, 169, 177, 220, 226, 355, 362, 420, 424, 448, 478, 504, 506, 511, 542, 667, 711, 748

dà fán kě 大烦渴, great vexing thirst, 248

dà fáng fēng tāng 大防风汤, Major Ledebouriella Decoction, 104, 530

dà fēn 大分, major divide, 383

dà fēng 大风, great wind, 248

dà fēng 大风, leprosy, 343

dà fēng è jí 大风恶疾, leprosy, 343

dà fēng è jí 大风恶疾, malign disease of great wind, 384

dà fēng zǐ 大风子 hydnocarpus, Hydnocarpi Semen, 244, 728

dà fù 大腹, greater abdomen, 245

dà fù pí 大腹皮 areca husk, Arecae Pericarpium, 153, 183, 454, 625, 724

dà gǔ kōng 大骨空, Thumb Bone Hollow, 93, 195, 500, 586, 636

dà hàn 大汗, great sweating, 248

dà hàn chū 大汗出, great sweating, 248

dà hè 大赫, KI-12, Great Manifestation, 57, 160, 308, 330, 331, 333, 336, 466, 518, 524, 525, 582, 711, 712, 748

dà héng 大横, SP-15, Great Horizontal, 28, 64, 77, 83, 85, 183, 479, 509, 667, 746

dà huáng 大黄 rhubarb, Rhei Rhizoma, 7, 17, 19, 24, 34, 50, 51, 72, 84, 93, 130, 182, 215, 255, 261, 281, 298, 311, 357, 390, 397, 434, 445, 459, 460, 502, 544, 548, 573, 577, 613, 619, 627, 664, 722

dà huáng dāng guī sǎn 大黄当归散, Rhubarb and Tangkuei Powder, 33

dà huáng fù zǐ tāng 大黄附子汤, Rhubarb and Aconite Decoction, 24, 311, 664, 731 *dà huáng gān cǎo tāng* 大黄甘草汤, Rhubarb and Licorice Decoction, 284

dà huáng huáng lián xiè xīn tāng 大黄黄连泻心汤, Rhubarb and Coptis Heart-Draining Decoction, 600

dà huáng mǔ dān pí tāng 大黄牡丹皮汤, Rhubarb and Moutan Decoction, 318, 671, 743

dà huáng mǔ dān tāng 大黄牡丹汤, Rhubarb and Moutan Decoction, 459

dà huáng xiāo shí tāng 大黄硝石汤, Rhubarb and Niter Decoction, 111

dà huáng zhè chóng wán 大黄䗪虫丸, Rhubarb and Wingless Cockroach Pill, 24, 34, 152, 173, 646, 737

dà huó luò dān 大活络丹, Major Network-Quickening Elixir, 289, 734

dà jǐ 大戟 euphorbia/knoxia, Euphorbiae seu Knoxiae Radix, 97, 182, 438, 460, 574, 722

dà jì 大蓟 cirsium, Cirsii Herba seu Radix, 569, 724

dà jiàn zhōng tāng 大建中汤, Major Center-Fortifying Decoction, 734

dà jié xiōng 大结胸, major chest bind, 383

dà jīng 大经, main channel, 383

dà jù 大巨, ST-27, Great Gigantic, 746

dà jué 大厥, major reversal, 383

dà lián qiào yǐn 大连翘饮, Major Forsythia Beverage, 198

dà líng 大陵, PC-7, Great Mound, 15, 25, 30, 43, 63, 70, 90, 99, 147, 155, 156, 244, 277, 282, 285, 288, 289, 330, 333, 356, 383, 386, 410, 413, 427, 434, 436, 467, 525, 538, 548, 552, 570, 587, 665, 688, 694, 716, 748

dà má fēng 大麻风, great numbing wind, 248

dà má fēng 大麻风, leprosy, 343

dà mài 大脉, large pulse, 340

dà qī qì tāng 大七气汤, Major Seven Qi Decoction, 149, 325, 475, 479

dà qì 大气, great qi, 248

dà qiāng huó tāng 大羌活汤, Major Notopterygium Decoction, 729

dà qín jiāo tāng 大秦艽汤, Large Gentian Decoction, 289, 631, 689, 740

dà qīng lóng tāng 大青龙汤, Major Green-Blue Dragon Decoction, 246, 550, 729

dà qīng yè 大青叶 isatis leaf, Isatidis Folium, 67, 70, 146, 420, 422, 450, 459, 547, 637, 721

dà rè 大热, great heat [effusion], 247

dà shùn sǎn 大顺散, Great Rectifying Powder, 74, 662, 735

dà sōu 大溲, stool, 582

dà suàn 大蒜 garlic, Allii Sativi Bulbus, 111, 183, 445, 728

dà táo huā tāng 大桃花汤, Major Peach Blossom Decoction, 318, 742

dà tóu wēn 大头瘟, massive head scourge, 387

dà xiàn xiōng tāng 大陷胸汤, Major Chest Bind Decoction, 283, 383, 731

dà xiàn xiōng wán 大陷胸丸, Major Chest Bind Pill, 731

dà xǐng fēng tāng 大醒风汤, Major Wind Arousal Decoction, 739

dà xuè téng 大血藤 sargentodoxa, Sargentodoxae Caulis, 68, 721

dà yán mì tāng 大岩蜜汤, Great Rock Honey Decoction, 451, 452, 454

dà yíng 大迎, ST-5, Great Reception, 142, 220, 222, 515, 521, 610, 746

dà yíng jiān 大营煎, Major Construction Brew, 26, 741

dà zǎo 大枣 jujube, Ziziphi Fructus, 11, 96, 217, 255, 358, 499, 580, 593, 600, 726

dà zào wán 大造丸, Great Creation Pill, 147, 742

dà zhōng 大钟, KI-4, Large Goblet, 197, 222, 408, 747

dà zhù 大杼, BL-11, Great Shuttle, 45, 78, 84, 86, 105, 155, 184, 185, 226, 252, 391, 501, 517, 580, 589, 631, 638, 663, 666, 681, 682, 690, 694, 703, 709, 747

dà zhuī 大椎, GV-14, Great Hammer, 6, 8, 25, 29, 44, 61–63, 65, 66, 69–71, 74–76, 82, 91, 103, 105, 111–113, 117–120, 129, 145, 146, 155, 156, 158, 161, 166, 168, 174, 184, 192, 194, 197, 201, 203, 219, 220, 222, 231, 235, 245, 247, 252–255, 260, 277–283, 285, 291, 292, 301, 317, 318, 339, 342, 349, 357, 364, 366, 368, 374, 383, 391, 394, 399, 403, 405, 406, 418, 427, 439, 444, 450, 451, 455, 458, 474, 501, 508, 515, 516, 521, 529, 544, 546, 547, 550, 561, 569, 570, 572, 585, 586, 588–591, 595, 604, 611, 613, 620, 621, 624, 648–650, 664, 665, 677, 681–683, 685–688, 690, 693, 694, 699–703, 715, 749

dà zì 大眦, inner canthus, 303

dacryocystitis*, 670

Daemonoropis Draconis Resina, *xuè jié* 血竭, dragon's blood, 728

dāi bìng 呆病, dementia, 122

dài 带, discharge, 130

dài dāo sǎn 代刀散, Spare-the-Knife Powder, 743

dài dǐ dàng wán 代抵当丸, Substitute Dead-On Pill, 37, 149, 542, 737

dài gé sǎn 黛蛤散, Indigo and Clamshell Powder, 101, 277, 695, 738

dài mài 带脉, GB-26, Girdling Vessel, 57, 93, 94, 118, 160, 241, 242, 330, 334, 353, 418, 435, 497, 522, 563, 658, 675, 677, 748

dài mài 带脉, GIV, 242

dài mài 带脉, girdling vessel, 241

dài mài 代脉, intermittent pulse, 312

dài mài 代脉, regularly interrupted pulse, 497

dài mào 玳瑁 hawksbill shell, Eretmochelydis Carapax, 54, 726

dài xià 带下, vaginal discharge, 653

dài yǎn 戴眼, upcast eyes, 639

dài yáng 戴阳, dai yang, 108

dài yáng 戴阳, upcast yang, 639

dài zhě shí 代赭石 hematite, Haematitum, 53, 54, 98, 146, 460, 578, 585, 726 dalbergia, *jiàng zhēn xiāng* 降真香, Dalbergiae Lignum, 27, 138, 512, 725

Dalbergiae Lignum, *jiàng zhēn xiāng* 降真香, dalbergia, 27, 138, 512, 725

Damp Depression Decoction, *shī yù tāng* 湿郁汤, 109

Damp-Eliminating Decoction, *chú shī tāng* 除湿汤, 734

Dampness Damage Pain-Relieving Plaster, *shāng shī zhǐ tòng gāo* 伤湿止痛膏, 745

dampness trapping hidden heat, 676

Dampness-Draining Decoction, *xiè shī tāng* 泻湿汤, 733

Dampness-Eliminating Decoction, *chú shī tāng* 除湿汤, 109, 636, 691

Dampness-Eliminating Impediment-Alleviating Decoction, *chú shī juān bì tāng* 除湿蠲痹汤, 112, 347, 734

Dampness-Eliminating Stomach-Calming Poria (Hoelen) Five Decoction, *chú shī wèi líng tāng* 除湿胃苓汤, 112, 116, 173, 241, 441

Dampness-Overcoming Decoction, *shèng shī tāng* 胜湿汤, 599

Dan Xi's Experiential Methods (*dān xī xīn fǎ*) 丹溪心法, 1481 (Yuán), Zhū Zhèn-Hēng 朱震亨 [Dān-Xī 丹溪], 123, 201, 216, 359, 439, 668, 690, 703, 716

dān 丹, elixir, 171

dān 瘅, pure heat, 473

dān chǎo 单炒, plain stir-frying, 445

dān dú 丹毒, cinnabar toxin, 62

dān fù gǔ 单腹鼓, simple abdominal drum, 532

dān fù zhàng 单腹胀, simple abdominal distention, 532

dān fù zhàng dà 单腹胀大, simple abdominal distention, 532

dān gǔ 单鼓, simple drum, 532

dān shā 丹痧, cinnabar sand, 62

dān shēn 丹参 salvia, Salviae Miltiorrhizae Radix, 17, 20, 28, 34, 37, 137, 138, 227, 262, 493, 516, 526, 540, 586, 724

dān shēn yǐn 丹参饮, Salvia Beverage, 300, 484, 737

dān shì bǔ xiè shǒu fǎ 单式补泻手法, simple supplementation and drainage manipulation, 532

dān shǒu jìn zhēn fǎ 单手进针法, single-handed needle insertion, 534

dān tián 丹田, cinnabar field, 62

dān xī xīn fǎ 丹溪心法 (*Dan Xi's Experiential Methods*), 1481 (Yuán), Zhū Zhèn-Hēng 朱震亨 [Dān-Xī 丹溪], 123, 201, 216, 359, 439, 668, 690, 703, 716

dān xíng 单行, going alone, 243

dān zhī xiāo yáo sǎn 丹栀逍遥散, Moutan and Gardenia Free Wanderer Powder, 19, 29, 31, 143, 177, 353, 354, 393, 453, 462, 502, 586, 655, 711, 732

dǎn 胆, GB, 240

dǎn 胆, gallbladder, 234

dǎn bìng 胆病, gallbladder disease, 234

dǎn dān 胆瘅, gallbladder pure heat, 235

dǎn dào pái shí tāng 胆道排石汤, Biliary Calculus Decoction, 182, 544, 733

dǎn fán 胆矾 chalcanthite, Chalcanthitum, 170, 727

dǎn fēng dú qì 胆风毒气, gallbladder wind toxin qi, 236

dǎn huáng 胆黄, gallbladder jaundice, 235

dǎn huǒ bù dé wò 胆火不得卧, gallbladder fire sleeplessness, 234

dǎn huǒ wàng shèng 胆火旺盛, effulgent gallbladder fire, 168

dǎn jīng 胆经, gallbladder channel, 234

dǎn ké 胆咳, gallbladder cough, 234

dǎn qì bù zú 胆气不足, insufficiency of gallbladder qi, 309

dǎn qì xū 胆气虚, gallbladder qi vacuity, 235

dǎn qì xū hán 胆气虚寒, gallbladder qi vacuity cold, 235

dǎn qì xū qiè 胆气虚怯, gallbladder qi vacuity and timidity, 235

dǎn qiè 胆怯, gallbladder timidity, 236

dǎn qiè yì jīng 胆怯易惊, gallbladder timidity and susceptibility to fright, 236

dǎn rè 胆热, gallbladder heat, 234

dǎn rè duō shuì 胆热多睡, gallbladder heat profuse sleeping, 235

dǎn shí 胆实, gallbladder repletion, 235

dǎn shū 胆俞, BL-19, Gallbladder Transport, 15, 66, 89, 91, 151, 195, 230, 234–236, 268, 297, 349, 357, 538, 564, 650, 674, 700, 710, 747

dǎn wú jué duàn 胆无决断, gallbladder lacking decisiveness, 235

dǎn xīng 胆星 bile arisaema [root], Arisaematis Rhizoma cum Felle Bovis, 417

dǎn xīng 胆星 bile arisaema, Arisaematis Rhizoma cum Felle Bovis, 60, 84, 140, 178, 214, 448, 453, 541, 623, 725

dǎn xū 胆虚, gallbladder vacuity, 236

dǎn xū bù dé mián 胆虚不得眠, gallbladder vacuity sleeplessness, 236

dǎn xū qì qiè 胆虚气怯, gallbladder vacuity and qi timidity, 236

dǎn zhàng 胆胀, gallbladder distention, 234

dǎn zhě, zhōng zhèng zhī guān, jué duàn chū yān 胆者，中正之官，决断出焉, gallbladder holds the office of justice, from which decision emanates, 235

dǎn zhǔ jué duàn 胆主决断, gallbladder governs decision, 234

dàn 淡, bland, 23

dàn 淡, blandness, 23

dàn dài wú wèi 但代无胃, intermittent only, without stomach, 312

dàn dòu chǐ 淡豆豉 fermented soybean, Glycines Semen Fermentatum Insulsum, 70, 130, 176, 184, 402, 410, 481, 501, 686, 720

dàn nüè 瘅疟, pure-heat malaria, 473

dàn shèn lì shī 淡渗利湿, disinhibiting dampness by bland percolation, 136

dàn xián wú wèi 但弦无胃, stringlike only, without stomach, 584

dàn yù mèi 但欲寐, desire only to sleep, 124

dàn zhōng 膻中, CV-17, Chest Center, 89, 91

dàn zhú yè 淡竹叶 bamboo leaf (lophatherum), Lophatheri Folium, 66, 67, 108, 261, 263, 387, 463, 720

dàn zhú yè tāng 淡竹叶汤, Bamboo Leaf Decoction, 457

dandelion, *pú gōng yīng* 蒲公英, Taraxaci Herba cum Radice, 17, 67, 69, 70, 93, 120, 214, 282, 386, 440, 459, 501, 606, 685, 691, 721

dāng guī 当归 tangkuei, Angelicae Sinensis Radix, 17, 19, 28, 34, 37, 39, 58, 60, 93, 95, 103, 104, 116, 120, 139, 140, 154, 161, 172, 175, 227, 234, 259, 272, 309, 310, 315, 338, 352, 386, 390, 391, 398, 415, 428, 431, 448, 449, 467, 493, 495, 503, 516, 526, 588, 593, 595, 600, 613, 651, 661, 662, 666, 670, 674, 679, 727

dāng guī bǔ xuè tāng 当归补血汤, Tangkuei Blood-Supplementing Decoction, 25, 37–39, 152, 161, 171, 457, 566, 607, 646, 652, 741

dāng guī dì huáng yǐn 当归地黄饮, Tangkuei and Rehmannia Beverage, 332, 333

dāng guī huó xuè tāng 当归活血汤, Tangkuei Blood-Quickening Decoction, 737

dāng guī jiàn zhōng tāng 当归建中汤, Tangkuei Center-Fortifying Decoction, 38, 39, 94, 477, 734

dāng guī liù huáng tāng 当归六黄汤, Tangkuei Six Yellows Decoction, 40, 95, 176, 410, 599, 701, 715, 731

dāng guī lóng huì wán 当归龙荟丸, Tangkuei, Gentian, and Aloe Pill, 158, 278, 297, 356, 365, 459, 549, 552, 566, 700, 713, 731

dāng guī niān tòng tāng 当归拈痛汤, Tangkuei Pain-Assuaging Decoction, 342, 347, 733

dāng guī sǎn 当归散, Tangkuei Powder, 571

dāng guī sháo yào sǎn 当归芍药散, Tangkuei and Peony Powder, 741

dāng guī shēn 当归身 tangkuei body, Angelicae Sinensis Radicis Corpus, 256

dāng guī shēng jiāng yáng ròu tāng 当归生姜羊肉汤, Tangkuei, Fresh Ginger, and Goat Meat Decoction, 741

dāng guī sì nì jiā wú zhū yú shēng jiāng tāng 当归四逆加吴茱萸生姜汤, Tangkuei Counterflow Cold Decoction Plus Evodia and Fresh Ginger, 735

dāng guī sì nì tāng 当归四逆汤, Tangkuei Counterflow Cold Decoction, 50, 85, 228, 231, 343, 504, 662, 711, 735

dāng guī tāng 当归汤, Tangkuei Decoction, 32

dāng guī wěi 当归尾 tangkuei tails, Angelicae Sinensis Radicis Extremitas, 27, 439

dāng guī xū 当归须 tangkuei fine root, Angelicae Sinensis Radicis Tenuis, 356, 390

dāng guī yáng ròu tāng 当归羊肉汤, Tangkuei and Goat Meat Decoction, 741

dāng guī yǐn 当归饮, Tangkuei Beverage, 468

dāng guī yǐn zǐ 当归饮子, Tangkuei Drink, 117, 145, 422

dǎng shēn 党参 codonopsis, Codonopsitis Radix, 11, 12, 17, 47, 84, 141, 161, 175, 223, 227, 255, 270, 315, 329, 378, 454, 466, 486, 504, 526, 556, 563, 574, 593–596, 600, 662, 679, 726

dàng dí 荡涤, flush, 214

dàng dí wán tán 荡涤顽痰, flushing stubborn phlegm, 214

dāo dòu 刀豆 sword bean, Canavaliae Semen, 493

dāo dòu ké 刀豆壳 sword bean pod, Canavaliae Legumen, 724

dǎo 导, abduct, 2

dǎo 捣, crushing, 105

dǎo 捣, pounding, 458

dǎo chì chéng qì tāng 导赤承气汤, Red-Abducting Qi-Coordinating Decoction, 731

dǎo chì sǎn 导赤散, Red-Abducting Powder, 36, 41, 189, 230, 238, 263, 264, 281, 283, 284, 400, 541, 542, 583, 619, 687, 731

dǎo jiù 捣臼, pounding, 458

dǎo qì tāng 导气汤, Qi-Abducting Decoction, 226, 481, 735

dǎo shuǐ fú líng tāng 导水茯苓汤, Water-Abducting Poria (Hoelen) Decoction, 733

dǎo tán tāng 导痰汤, Phlegm-Abducting Decoction, 81, 88, 192, 203, 433–435, 438, 439, 441, 442, 638, 673, 690, 738

dǎo zhēn 捣针, needle pounding, 407

dào hàn 盗汗, night sweating, 409

dào hàn 盗汗, thief sweating, 607

dào jié quán máo 倒睫拳毛, ingrown eyelash, 300

dào jīng 倒经, inverted menstruation, 319

Daphnes Genkwa Flos, *yuán huā* 芫花, genkwa, 44, 97, 182, 460, 574, 722

Dark-Gate–Freeing Decoction, *tōng yōu tāng* 通幽汤, 164

datura flower, *yáng jīn huā* 洋金花, Daturae Flos, 624, 725

Daturae Flos, *yáng jīn huā* 洋金花, datura flower, 624, 725

Daurian rhododendron, *mǎn shān hóng* 满山红, Rhododendri Daurici Folium, 624, 726

dayflower, *yā zhí cǎo* 鸭跖草, Commelinae Herba, 67, 69, 720

dé qì 得气, obtaining qi, 419

dé shén 得神, spiritedness, 551

Dead-On Decoction, *dǐ dàng tāng* 抵当汤, 25, 78, 601, 698, 737

Dead-On Pill, *dǐ dàng wán* 抵当丸, 24, 28, 78, 182, 601, 737

deaf-mutism, 541

Deafness Left-Benefiting Loadstone Pill, *ěr lóng zuǒ cí wán* 耳聋左慈丸, 119, 329, 742

Deafness Pill, *ěr lóng wán* 耳聋丸, 731

Deep-Source Decoction, *qǔ yuān tāng* 取渊汤, 120

deerhorn, *lù jiǎo* 鹿角, Cervi Cornu, 17, 310, 570, 593, 596, 726

Deerhorn and Cuscuta Pill, *lù jiǎo tù sī wán* 鹿角菟丝丸, 743

deerhorn flakes, *lù jiǎo xiè* 鹿角屑, Cervi Cornu in Frustis, 679

deerhorn glue, *lù jiǎo jiāo* 鹿角胶, Cervi Gelatinum Cornu, 222, 243, 332, 466, 541, 572, 593, 726

Deerhorn Major Supplementation Decoction, *lù róng dà bǔ tāng* 鹿茸大补汤, 333

Deerhorn Powder, *lù jiǎo sǎn* 鹿角散, 17

degelatinated deerhorn, *lù jiǎo shuāng* 鹿角霜, Cervi Cornu Degelatinatum, 593, 726

dementia*, 433

Dementia-Shifting Elixir, *zhuǎn dāi dān* 转呆丹, 122

Dendrobii Caulis, *shí hú* 石斛, dendrobium, 65, 174, 175, 395, 511, 565, 581, 589, 593, 597, 600, 727

dendrobium, *shí hú* 石斛, Dendrobii Caulis, 65, 174, 175, 395, 511, 565, 581, 589, 593, 597, 600, 727

Dendrobium Eye Brightener Pill, *shí hú míng mù wán* 石斛明目丸, 742

Dendrobium Night Vision Pill, *shí hú yè guāng wán* 石斛夜光丸, 742

dēng xīn cǎo 灯心草 juncus, Junci Medulla, 53, 60, 136, 262, 263, 723

Depression-Freeing Decoction, *dá yù tāng* 达郁汤, 297

Depression-Opening Jade-Planting Decoction, *kāi yù zhòng yù tāng* 开郁种玉汤, 353

Depression-Overcoming Pill, *yuè jú wán* 越鞠丸, 19, 244, 736

dermatitis rhus*, 338

dermatitis*, 112
  allergic, 496
  drug-induced, 496
  infectiosa eczematoides, 671
  paddy field, 668
  seborrheic, 676

dermatomycosis microsporina*, 473

dermatomyositis*, 210

Descurainiae seu Lepidii Semen, *tíng lì zǐ* 葶苈子, tingli, 12, 70, 130, 232, 282, 438, 624, 625, 667, 725

Desertion-Stemming Mother-Reviving Decoction, *jiù tuō huó mǔ tāng* 救脱活母汤, 454

detachment*
  retinal, 586

devil's tongue, *jǔ ruò* 蒟蒻, Amorphophalli Tuber, 68, 721

dí 涤, flush, 214

dí tán 涤痰, flushing phlegm, 214

dí tán tāng 涤痰汤, Phlegm-Flushing Decoction, 93, 740

dǐ dàng tāng 抵当汤, Dead-On Decoction, 25, 78, 601, 698, 737

dǐ dàng wán 抵当丸, Dead-On Pill, 24, 28, 78, 182, 601, 737

dì bù 地部, earth level, 167

dì cāng 地仓, ST-4, Earth Granary, 73, 89, 125, 140, 183, 254, 289, 426, 446, 509, 610, 689, 696, 746

dì dǎn 地胆 oil beetle, Meloë, 98

dì dīng 地丁 violet, Violae Herba cum Radice, 67, 588, 721

dì ěr cǎo 地耳草 lesser hypericum, Hyperici Japonici Herba, 68, 136, 700, 721, 723

dì fū zǐ 地肤子 kochia, Kochiae Fructus, 116, 136, 225, 395, 424, 513, 516, 723

dì gǔ pí 地骨皮 lycium root bark, Lycii Radicis Cortex, 68, 72, 106, 175, 244, 277, 281, 282, 388, 391, 394, 450, 495, 637, 649, 676, 715, 721

dì gǔ pí yǐn 地骨皮饮, Lycium Root Bark Beverage, 31, 391, 649, 731

dì huáng 地黄 rehmannia, Rehmanniae Radix, 172, 175, 176, 336, 352, 398, 455, 464

dì huáng sǎn 地黄散, Rehmannia Powder, 403

dì huáng wán 地黄丸, Rehmannia Pill, 742

dì huáng yǐn zǐ 地黄饮子, Rehmannia Drink, 289, 368, 740, 742

dì jī 地机, SP-8, Earth's Crux, 26, 31, 34–36, 94, 212, 227, 233, 279, 300, 353, 393, 431, 447, 450, 451, 483, 484, 503, 520, 540, 661, 746

dì jǐn cǎo 地锦草 humifuse euphorbia, Euphorbiae Humifusae Herba, 68, 111, 721

dì kuò 地廓, earth rampart, 167

dì lóng 地龙 earthworm, Lumbricus, 53, 54, 74, 146, 516, 526, 569, 726

dì qí sǎn 的奇散, Truly Wondrous Powder, 449

dì wǔ huì 地五会, GB-42, Earth Fivefold Convergence, 748

dì yú 地榆 sanguisorba, Sanguisorbae Radix, 28, 30, 51, 338, 548, 569, 724

dì yú sǎn 地榆散, Sanguisorba Powder, 462, 743

dì yú wán 地榆丸, Sanguisorba Pill, 742

dì (dì) dīng 帝（蒂）丁, uvula, 644

dì (dì) zhōng 帝（蒂）钟, uvula, 644

dioscorea, *shān yào* 山药, Dioscoreae Rhizoma, 12, 47, 141, 175, 223, 251, 267, 308, 496, 504, 563, 564, 572, 574, 593, 596, 600, 615, 726

Dioscorea Pill, *shǔ yù wán* 薯蓣丸, 741

Dioscoreae Bulbiferae Tuber, *huáng yào zǐ* 黄药子, air potato, 544, 624, 725

Dioscoreae Hypoglaucae Rhizoma, *bì xiè* 萆薢, fish poison yam, 21, 45, 116, 136, 328, 516, 584, 723

Dioscoreae Nipponicae Rhizoma, *chuān shān lóng* 穿山龙, Japanese dioscorea, 140, 722

Dioscoreae Rhizoma, *shān yào* 山药, dioscorea, 12, 47, 141, 175, 223, 251, 267, 308, 496, 504, 563, 564, 572, 574, 593, 596, 600, 615, 726

diabetes*
  insipidus, 142
  mellitus, 142

diān 癫, withdrawal, 694

diān bìng 癫病, withdrawal disease, 695

diān dǎo sǎn 颠倒散, Reversal Powder, 5, 149, 676, 744

diān dǐng tòng 巅顶痛, pain at the vertex, 424

diān dǐng tóu tòng 巅顶头痛, vertex headache, 654

diān kuáng 癫狂, mania and withdrawal, 386

diān kuáng wán 癫狂丸, Mania and Withdrawal Pill, 740

diān xián 癫痫, epilepsy, 178

diǎn cì chū xuè 点刺出血, prick to bleed, 463

diǎn cì fàng xuè 点刺放血, prick to bleed, 463

diǎn yǎn 点眼, topical eye medication, 621

diàn zhēn 电针, electroacupuncture, 171

diàn zhēn liáo fǎ 电针疗法, electroacupuncture, 171

Dianthi Herba, *qū mài* 瞿麦, dianthus, 21, 69, 98, 136, 723

dianthus, *qū mài* 瞿麦, Dianthi Herba, 21, 69, 98, 136, 723

diào 掉, shaking, 528

diào jiǎo shā 吊脚痧, leg-hoisting sand, 342

Diaphragm-Arousing Powder, *qǐ gé sǎn* 启膈散, 164, 735

Diaphragm-Cooling Forsythia Powder, *liáng gé lián qiào sǎn* 凉膈连翘散, 731

Diaphragm-Cooling Powder, *liáng gé sǎn* 凉膈散, 15, 76, 166, 201, 203, 261, 277, 280, 283, 459, 548, 612, 615, 731

diarrhea*
chronic, 334

dichondra, *xiǎo jīn qián cǎo* 小金钱草, Dichondrae Herba, 136, 723

Dichondrae Herba, *xiǎo jīn qián cǎo* 小金钱草, dichondra, 136, 723

dichroa, *cháng shān* 常山, Dichroae Radix, 97, 170, 317, 464, 727

dichroa leaf, *shǔ qī* 蜀漆, Dichroae Folium, 170, 197, 510, 727

Dichroae Folium, *shǔ qī* 蜀漆, dichroa leaf, 170, 197, 510, 727

Dichroae Radix, *cháng shān* 常山, dichroa, 97, 170, 317, 464, 727

Dictamni Radicis Cortex, *bái xiān pí* 白鲜皮, dictamnus, 68, 116, 430, 468, 721

dictamnus, *bái xiān pí* 白鲜皮, Dictamni Radicis Cortex, 68, 116, 430, 468, 721

dié dǎ 跌打, knocks and falls, 337

Diffusing-Freeing Lung-Rectifying Pill, *tōng xuān lǐ fèi wán* 通宣理肺丸, 738

dīng chén tòu gé tāng 丁沉透膈汤, Clove and Aquilaria Diaphragm-Freeing Decoction, 490, 579

dīng chuāng 疔疮, clove sore, 75

dīng chuāng zǒu huáng 疔疮走黄, clove sore running yellow, 75

dīng ěr 聍耳, ceruminal congestion, 55

dīng guì sǎn 丁桂散, Clove and Cinnamon Powder, 402, 734

dīng huǒ 丁火, S4-fire, 511

dīng xiāng 丁香 clove, Caryophylli Flos, 82, 146, 157, 217, 224, 316, 393, 411, 443, 463, 649, 660, 663, 723

dīng xiāng jiāo ài tāng 丁香胶艾汤, Clove, Ass Hide Glue, and Mugwort Decoction, 643, 743

dīng xiāng sǎn 丁香散, Clove Powder, 82, 663

dīng xiāng shì dì tāng 丁香柿蒂汤, Clove and Persimmon Decoction, 145, 578, 736

dīng yú lǐ zhōng tāng 丁萸理中汤, Clove and Evodia Center-Rectifying Decoction, 489, 734

dǐng 顶, vertex, 654

dìng 锭, lozenge, 369

dìng chuǎn 定喘, Panting Stabilizer, 83, 87, 142, 146, 202, 203, 228, 281, 285, 343, 379, 434, 441, 443, 489, 550, 596, 630, 648, 668, 683, 715

dìng chuǎn 定喘, stabilizing panting, 569

dìng chuǎn sǎn 定喘散, Panting-Stabilizing Powder, 743

dìng chuǎn tāng 定喘汤, Panting-Stabilizing Decoction, 146, 285, 736

dìng fēng 定风, stabilizing wind, 569

dìng jì 锭剂, lozenge preparation, 369

dìng jīng tāng 定经汤, Menses-Stabilizing Decoction, 385, 393

dìng tòng gāo 定痛膏, Pain-Relieving Paste, 744

dìng tòng wán 定痛丸, Pain-Relieving Pill, 733

dìng xián wán 定痫丸, Fit-Settling Pill, 19, 178, 434, 740

dìng zhèn wán 定振丸, Tremor-Stabilizing Pill, 365

dìng zhì 定志, stabilizing the mind, 569

dìng zhì wán 定志丸, Mind-Stabilizing Pill, 147, 297, 406, 739

Diphtheria Mixture, *kàng bái hóu hé jì* 抗白喉合剂, 730

Dipsaci Radix, *xù duàn* 续断, dipsacus, 251, 352, 453, 593, 727

dipsacus, *xù duàn* 续断, Dipsaci Radix, 251, 352, 453, 593, 727

Dipsacus Pill, *xù duàn wán* 续断丸, 347

Discharge-Ceasing Decoction, *wán dài tāng* 完带汤, 563, 677, 743

Discharge-Checking Formula, *zhǐ dài fāng* 止带方, 118

Discharge-Checking Tablet, *zhǐ dài piàn* 止带片, 57, 743

Discharge-Clearing Decoction, *qīng dài tāng* 清带汤, 743

Discharge-Curing Pill, *yù dài wán* 愈带丸, 743

Dispersion-Thirst Formula, *xiāo kě fāng* 消渴方, 640, 734

Divine Husbandman's Herbal Foundation Canon (shén nóng běn cǎo jīng) 神农本草经, 241, 290, 609

Dizziness-Clearing Beverage, *qīng xuàn yǐn* 清眩饮, 731

dock root, *yáng tí gēn* 羊蹄根, Rumicis Radix Recens, 724

Dog Skin Plaster, *gǒu pí gāo* 狗皮膏, 744

dog's bone, *gǒu gǔ* 狗骨, Canis Os, 139, 722

dog's penis, *mǔ gǒu yīn jīng* 牡狗阴茎, Canis Penis, 593, 726

dōng chóng xià cǎo 冬虫夏草 cordyceps, Cordyceps, 593, 726

dōng fāng yī xué 东方医学, Oriental medicine, 421

dōng guā pí 冬瓜皮 wax gourd rind, Benincasae Exocarpium, 136, 723

dōng guā zǐ 冬瓜子 wax gourd seed, Benincasae Semen, 136, 282, 625, 723

dōng hàn 东汉, Eastern (Later), 167

dōng jìn 东晋, Eastern Jin, 167

dōng kuí zǐ 冬葵子 mallow seed, Malvae Verticillatae Semen, 98, 136, 370, 582, 723

dōng qīng yè 冬青叶 Chinese ilex leaf, Ilicis Chinensis Folium, 68, 721

dōng wèi 东魏, Eastern Wei, 167

dōng wēn 冬温, winter warmth, 694

dōng yī 东医, Eastern medicine, 167

dōng zhōu 东周, Eastern Zhou, 167

dòng 动, stirring, 574

dòng chuāng 冻疮, frostbite, 231

dòng mài 动脉, stirred pulse, 574

dòng tài 动态, bearing, 16

dòng xiè 洞泻, throughflux diarrhea, 612

dòu 痘, pox, 458

dòu chǐ jiāng 豆豉姜 litsea, Litseae Rhizoma et Radix, 410, 500, 660, 723

dòu chuāng 痘疮, pox, 458

dòu fǔ zhā 豆腐渣 bean curd dregs, Glycines Lactis Residuum, 104

dòu kòu wán 豆蔻丸, Tsaoko Pill, 77, 314, 581

dòu zhěn fāng 痘疹方论 (*On Pox Formulas*), 1518 (Míng), Cài Wéi-Fán 蔡维藩, 59

Double Resolution Sage-Inspired Powder, *shuāng jiě tōng shèng sǎn* 双解通圣散, 330

Double Supreme Pill, *èr zhì wán* 二至丸, 336, 365, 528, 646, 742

double vision*, 519

Double-Armored Pulse-Restorative Decoction, *èr jiǎ fù mài tāng* 二甲复脉汤, 742

dragon bone, *lóng gǔ* 龙骨, Mastodi Ossis Fossilia, 11, 53, 183, 230, 308, 409, 433, 449, 461, 490, 504, 518, 524–526, 537, 572, 585, 636, 696, 709, 726

dragon tooth, *lóng chǐ* 龙齿, Mastodi Dentis Fossilia, 490, 525, 526, 538, 539, 726

dragon's blood, *xuè jié* 血竭, Daemonoropis Draconis Resina, 728

Dragon-Embracing Pill, *bào lóng wán* 抱龙丸, 6, 70, 437, 740

dried bamboo sap, *zhú lì* 竹沥 Bambusae Succus Exsiccatus, 84, 116, 178, 282, 434, 448, 624, 637, 725

Dried Bamboo Sap Phlegm-Moving Pill, *zhú lì yùn tán wán* 竹沥运痰丸, 433

dried ginger, *gān jiāng* 干姜, Zingiberis Rhizoma Exsiccatum, 5, 12, 23, 84, 94, 98, 128, 136, 182, 196, 228, 242, 257, 272, 292, 293, 343, 345, 393, 425, 426, 438, 455, 456, 463, 469, 504, 612, 625, 649, 660, 662, 663, 679, 723

Dried Ginger, Ginseng, and Pinellia Pill, *gān jiāng rén shén bàn xià wán* 干姜人参半夏丸, 736

dried persimmon, *shì bǐng* 柿饼, Kaki Fructus Exsiccatus, 231

dried rehmannia, *gān dì huáng* 干地黄, Rehmanniae Radix Exsiccata, 20, 67, 256, 526, 557, 720

dried soybean sprout, *dà dòu huáng juǎn* 大豆黄卷, Glycines Semen Germinatum Exsiccatum, 686, 720

dried taro, *qīng yù nǎi gān* 青芋艿干, Colocasiae Tuber Exsiccatum, 544

dried/fresh rehmannia, *shēng dì huáng* 生地黄, Rehmanniae Radix Exsiccata seu Recens, 19, 28, 30, 65, 70, 88, 108, 116, 122, 154, 174–176, 256, 259, 277, 298, 310, 390, 391, 399, 415, 416, 422, 450, 462, 467, 495, 508, 516, 519, 526, 577, 581, 584, 586, 595, 597, 601, 604, 655, 679

Drool-Controlling Elixir, *kòng xián dān* 控涎丹, 88, 182, 433, 434, 438, 442, 506

Drool-Thinning Powder, *xī xián sǎn* 稀涎散, 170, 743

drynaria, *gǔ suì bǔ* 骨碎补, Drynariae Rhizoma, 45, 367, 593, 727

Drynariae Rhizoma, *gǔ suì bǔ* 骨碎补, drynaria, 45, 367, 593, 727

Dryness-Clearing Lung-Rescuing Decoction, *qīng zào jiù fèi tāng* 清燥救肺汤, 49, 66, 72, 155, 156, 161, 291, 348, 366, 379, 398, 625, 659, 678, 695, 715, 734

Dryness-Enriching Construction-Nourishing Decoction, *zī zào yǎng yíng tāng* 滋燥养营汤, 28, 741

Dryness-Moistening Fetus-Quieting Decoction, *rùn zào ān tāi tāng* 润燥安胎汤, 734

dū lū 嘟噜, dulu, 163

dū mài 督脉, GV, 250

dū mài 督脉, governing vessel, 244

dū qì wán 都气丸, Metropolis Qi Pill, 325, 379, 629, 648, 742

dū shí shàn jī 多食善饥, increased eating with rapid hungering, 298

dū shí yì jī 多食易饥, increased eating with rapid hungering, 298

dū shū 督俞, BL-16, Governing Transport, 747

dú 毒, toxicity, 621

dú 毒, toxin, 621

dú bí 犊鼻, ST-35, Calf's Nose, 337, 520, 746

dú huó 独活 duhuo, Angelicae Duhuo Radix, 45, 55, 102, 139, 154, 247, 326, 328, 546, 654, 662, 680, 722

dú huó gé gēn tāng 独活葛根汤, Duhuo and Pueraria Decoction, 254

dú huó jì shēng tāng 独活寄生汤, Duhuo and Mistletoe Decoction, 104, 140, 315, 337, 347, 370, 734

dú huó sǎn 独活散, Duhuo Powder, 685

dú qì 毒气, toxic qi, 621

dú shēn tāng 独参汤, Pure Ginseng Decoction, 27, 29, 33, 40, 233, 448, 478, 482, 489, 527, 586, 595, 735 *dú shèng sǎn* 独圣散, Single Sage Powder, 582

dú yīn 独阴, Solitary Yin, 128, 503, 542

dú yǔ 独语, soliloquy, 544

dù 肚, belly, 17

dù 炖, stewing, 572

dù jīng chuāng 妒精疮, begrudging semen sore, 17

dù rǔ 妒乳, begrudging milk, 17

dù zhòng 杜仲 eucommia, Eucommiae Cortex, 106, 251, 310, 328, 453, 485, 488, 593, 727

dù zhòng tàn 杜仲炭 charred eucommia, Eucommiae Cortex Carbonisatus, 331, 572

dù zi 肚子, belly, 17

duǎn mài 短脉, short pulse, 530

duǎn qì 短气, shortness of breath, 530

duàn 煅, calcination, 53

duàn biē jiǎ 煅鳖甲 calcined turtle shell, Amydae Carapax Calcinatus, 621

duàn cún xìng 煅存性, nature-preservative calcination, 405

duàn hóng wán 断红丸, Redness-Severing Pill, 143

duàn lóng gǔ 煅龙骨 calcined dragon bone, Mastodi Ossis Fossilia Calcinata, 95, 176, 267, 333, 566, 675, 709

duàn mǔ lì 煅牡蛎 calcined oyster shell, Ostreae Concha Calcinata, 57, 95, 176, 334, 636, 709

duàn rǔ 断乳, terminate lactation, 606

duàn wǎ léng zǐ 煅瓦楞子 calcined ark shell, Arcae Concha Calcinata, 257

duàn wū zéi gǔ 煅乌贼骨 calcined cuttlefish bone, Sepiae seu Sepiellae Os Calcinatum, 57, 334

duàn xià tāng 断下汤 Precipitation-Checking Decoction, 743

Duchesneae Herba, *shé méi* 蛇莓, snake strawberry, 68, 721

duckweed, *fú píng* 浮萍, Lemnae Herba, 130, 228, 686, 703, 720

Duckweed and Scutellaria Decoction, *fú píng huáng qín tāng* 浮萍黄芩汤, 729

duhuo, *dú huó* 独活, Angelicae Duhuo Radix, 45, 55, 102, 139, 154, 247, 326, 328, 546, 654, 662, 680, 722

Duhuo and Mistletoe Decoction, *dú huó jì shēng tāng* 独活寄生汤, 104, 140, 315, 337, 347, 370, 734

Duhuo and Pueraria Decoction, *dú huó gé gēn tāng* 独活葛根汤, 254

Duhuo Powder, *dú huó sǎn* 独活散, 685

duī shā là lì 堆沙鬎鬁, sand-heap perverse crop, 512

duì duān 兑端, GV-27, Extremity of the Mouth, 21, 415, 749

duì gǔ 兑骨, protuberant bone, 468

duì kǒu 对口, mouth-level nape flat-abscess, 400

duì qí fā 对脐发, umbilical-level effusion, 636

duì xīn fā 对心发, heart-level effusion, 266

duì zhèng xuǎn xué 对症选穴, selection of pathocondition points, 521

dùn 炖, double-boiling, 145

dùn ké 顿咳, long-bout cough, 366

dùn sòu 顿嗽, long-bout cough, 366

dung beetle, *qiāng láng* 蜣螂, Catharsius, 138, 139, 725

duō hàn 多汗, profuse sweating, 465

duō mèi 多寐, tendency to sleep, 605

duō mèng 多梦, profuse dreaming, 465

duō shuò 多睡, tendency to sleep, 605

duó 夺, despoliate, 124

duó mìng dān 夺命丹 Life-Clutching Elixir, 454, 455, 737

duó mìng sǎn 夺命散, Life-Clutching Powder, 448

duó xuè zhě wú hàn, duó hàn zhě wú xuè 夺血者无汗, 夺汗者无血, when blood is despoliated, there is no sweat; when sweat is despoliated, there is no blood, 672

dwarf elm bark, *yú bái pí* 榆白皮, Ulmi Pumilae Cortex, 370

dwarf magnolia, *yè hé huā* 夜合花, Magnoliae Coco Flos, 491, 726

Dyke-Strengthening Pill, *gǒng tí wán* 巩堤丸, 23, 743

dysentery*, 338

    amebic, 28, 250

    bacillary, 28, 110, 250, 278

    chronic, 110, 339

    toxic, 177

dysfunctional metrorrhagia*, 162

Dysosmae Versipellis Rhizoma, *guǐ jiù* 鬼臼, common dysosma, 503

dysphonia*, 291

dyspnea*, 428

ē jiāo 阿胶 ass hide glue, Asini Corii Gelatinum, 31, 37, 38, 58, 70, 161, 243, 256, 390, 488, 519, 526, 537, 557, 569, 574, 593, 595, 597, 602, 617, 727

ē jiāo huáng lián tāng 阿胶黄连汤, Ass Hide Glue and Coptis Decoction, 739

ē jiāo jī zǐ huáng tāng 阿胶鸡子黄汤, Ass Hide Glue and Egg Yolk Decoction, 740

ē jiāo sǎn 阿胶散, Ass Hide Glue Powder, 41, 734

ē jiāo sì wù tāng 阿胶四物汤, Ass Hide Glue Four Agents Decoction, 741

ē jiāo tāng 阿胶汤, Ass Hide Glue Decoction, 734

ē jiāo zhū 阿胶珠 ass hide glue pellets, Asini Corii Gelatini Pilula, 573

ē wèi 阿魏 asafetida, Asafoetida, 243

é 额, forehead, 222

é bù shí cǎo 鹅不食草 centipeda, Centipedae Herba cum Radice, 310, 405

é guǎn shí 鹅管石 goose throat stone, Balanophyllia seu Stalactitum, 460, 624, 726

é hàn 额汗, sweating brow, 599

é huáng sǎn 鹅黄散, Gosling Yellow Powder, 494

é kǒu chuāng 鹅口疮, goose-mouth sore, 244

é lú 额颅, forehead, 222

é shàng hàn chū 额上汗出, sweating brow, 599

é tóu chū hàn 额头出汗, sweating brow, 599

é xìn 额囟, forehead fontanel, 222

é zhǎng fēng 鹅掌风, goose-foot wind, 244

é zhǎo (zhuǎ) feng 鹅爪风, goose-claw wind, 244

é zhú 莪术 zedoary, Zedoariae Rhizoma, 34, 98, 116, 138, 182, 385, 544, 574, 724

é zǐ 蛾子, baby moth, 14

ě xīn 恶心, nausea, 405

ě xǐn ǒu tù 恶心呕吐, nausea and vomiting, 406

è 恶, malign, 384

è chuāng 恶疮, malign sore, 384

è lù 恶露, lochia, 366

è lù bù duàn 恶露不断, persistent flow of lochia, 430

è lù bù jìn 恶露不尽, persistent flow of lochia, 430

è lù bù xià 恶露不下, retention of the lochia, 503

è nì 呃逆, hiccough, 290

è ròu 恶肉, malign flesh, 384

è sè 恶色, malign complexion, 384

è xuè 恶血, malign blood, 384

è zǔ 恶阻, malign obstruction, 384

è zǔ 恶阻, morning sickness, 399

Earth-Rescuing Fetus-Securing Decoction, *yuán tǔ gù tāi tāng* 援土固胎汤, 742

earthworm, *dì lóng* 地龙, Lumbricus, 53, 54, 74, 146, 516, 526, 569, 726

Earthworm, House Lizard, and Three Gallbladders Powder, *lóng hǔ sān dǎn sǎn* 龙虎三胆散, 745

echinococcosis*

hepatic, 363, 670

eclampsia*, 178

eclipta, *mò hàn lián* 墨旱莲, Ecliptae Herba, 37, 88, 172, 225, 277, 336, 352, 388, 415, 467, 548, 569, 586, 593, 597, 727

Ecliptae Herba, *mò hàn lián* 墨旱莲, eclipta, 37, 88, 172, 225, 277, 336, 352, 388, 415, 467, 548, 569, 586, 593, 597, 727

Ectopic Pregnancy Formula No.II, *gōng wài yùn èr hào fāng* 宫外孕二号方, 737

eczema of the nose*, 319

eczema rhagadiforme*, 244

eczema*, 112, 117

acute, 671

chronic, 154, 686

ectopic, 225

infantile, 586

papular, 395

scrotal, 516

edema*, 668, 703

angioneurotic, 494

cardiac, 703

cardiogenic, 668

endocrinologic, 668

hepatogenic, 668

nephrotic, 668

nutritional, 668

Quincke's, 494

throat, 6

wandering, 494

eelgrass, *hǎi dài* 海带, Zosterae Marinae Herba, 624, 725

egg white, *jī zǐ bái* 鸡子白, Galli Albumen, 621

egg yolk, *jī zǐ huáng* 鸡子黄, Galli Vitellus, 17, 176, 256

Egg Yolk Paste, *jī dàn4 huáng yóu gāo* 鸡蛋黄油膏, 636

Eight Agents Decoction, *bā wù tāng* 八物汤, 157

Eight Corrections Powder, *bā zhèng sǎn* 八正散, 21, 22, 68, 69, 148, 229, 283, 302, 583, 733

Eight Evils, *bā xié* 八邪, 231, 244, 289, 540

Eight Immortals Free Wanderer Decoction, *bā xiān xiāo yáo tāng* 八仙逍遥汤, 744

Eight Immortals Longevity Pill, *bā xiān cháng shòu wán* 八仙长寿丸, 742

Eight Pinches Powder, *bā lí sǎn* 八厘散, 737

Eight Winds, *bā fēng* 八风, 80, 112, 115, 221, 289, 540

Eight-Gem Decoction, *bā zhēn tāng* 八珍汤, 36, 159, 161, 162, 172, 289, 312, 370, 426, 450, 451, 453, 457, 485, 488, 503, 594, 595, 607, 652, 741

Eight-Gem Leonurus (Motherwort) Pill, *bā zhēn yì mǔ wán* 八珍益母丸, 741

Eight-Ingredient Pill, *bā wèi wán* 八味丸, 229, 425

Eight-Ingredient Placenta Pill, *hé chē bā wèi wán* 河车八味丸, 741

Eight-Ingredient Rehmannia Pill, *bā wèi dì huáng wán* 八味地黄丸, 47, 228, 650, 741

Eight-Jewel Elixir, *bā bǎo dān* 八宝丹, 744

Eight-Jewel Eye Medication, *bā bǎo yǎn yào* 八宝眼药, 744

Elaboration of the Fourteen Channels (*shí sì jīng fā huī*) 十四经发挥, 1341 (Yuán), Huá Shòu 滑寿 [Bó-Rén 伯仁], 226

Elementary Questions (*sù wèn*) 素问, first part of *huáng dì nèi jīng* 黄帝内经, 4, 13, 19–22, 25, 31, 47, 49, 53, 55–58, 67, 76–78, 80, 82, 85, 93, 100, 108, 114, 120, 123, 142, 144, 163, 171, 173, 179, 180, 185, 190, 200, 204, 205, 207–209, 213, 214, 216, 221, 229, 232, 233, 235, 251, 260, 263–265, 270, 272, 281, 283, 284, 286, 288, 295, 307, 308, 311, 313, 316–319, 327–331, 336, 340, 347, 341, 343, 349–351, 356, 358–361, 364, 367, 371, 373–379, 383, 384, 395, 400, 404, 408, 411, 419–421, 425, 428, 431, 444, 461, 469, 472, 473, 486, 488, 495, 498–499, 505, 506, 508, 514, 515, 525, 527, 529, 534–536, 543, 551–554, 557, 558, 560, 561, 578, 581–583, 586, 587, 592, 599, 600, 602, 610, 621, 622, 626–627, 630, 632, 639, 643, 647, 653–655, 658, 672–674, 678, 680, 681, 685, 691, 694, 700, 703, 706, 708, 716, 717

Elephant Skin Paste, *xiàng pí gāo* 象皮膏, 100

elephant's hide, *xiàng pí* 象皮, Elephantis Corium, 728

Elephantis Corium, *xiàng pí* 象皮, elephant's hide, 728

Eleven-Ingredient Gallbladder-Warming Decoction, *shí yī wèi wēn dǎn tāng* 十一味温胆汤, 739

elm cake, *wú yí* 芜荑, Ulmi Fructus Praeparatio, 183, 724

elsholtzia, *xiāng rú* 香薷, Elsholtziae Herba, 69, 587, 681, 720

Elsholtzia Beverage, *xiāng rú yǐn* 香薷饮, 18, 588, 590

Elsholtzia Decoction, *xiāng rú tāng* 香薷汤, 729

Elsholtzia Powder, *xiāng rú sǎn* 香薷散, 729

Elsholtziae Herba, *xiāng rú* 香薷, elsholtzia, 69, 587, 681, 720

embolism*

  amniotic, 448

  cerebral, 692

Emergency Drool-Thinning Powder, *jí jiù xī xián sǎn* 急救稀涎散, 440, 743

Emergency Standby Remedies (*zhǒu hòu bèi jí fāng*) 肘后备急方, Gě Hóng 葛洪 (281–341, Jìn) 281–341, 58, 83, 106, 384

emesis gravidarum*, 384

emphysema, 58

emphysema*, 280

  pulmonary, 120, 334, 428, 434

Engendering Transformation Decoction, *shēng huà tāng* 生化汤, 182, 300, 447–450, 454, 455, 457, 503, 737

encephalitis B*, 3, 433

Encephalitis Formula, *zhì yǐ nǎo fāng* 治乙脑方, 731

encephalitis*, 10

  epidemic, 433, 591

encephalopathy*

  toxic, 692

Enchanted Land Jade Shavings, *zuì xiāng yù xiè* 醉乡玉屑, 732

endemic goiter*, 243

endocrine disturbances*, 444

Engman's disease*, 671

enlargement of the thyroid gland*, 243

  tubercular, 243

Enriching Ginseng Tablet, *rén shēn zī bǔ piàn* 人参滋补片, 739

Enriching Supplementation Tablet, *zī bǔ piàn* 滋补片, 739

Enriching the Meaning of the Wine of Medicine (*yī chún shèng yì*) 医醇賸义, 1863 (Qīng), Fèi Bó-Xióng 费伯雄, 363

ensiform process*, 633

enteritis*

  acute, 77, 588

  bacillary, 278

  chronic, 339, 483

ephedra, *má huáng* 麻黄, Ephedrae Herba, 5, 17, 70, 103, 128, 129, 184, 228, 243, 246, 247, 346, 391, 438, 460, 500–502, 681, 683, 720

Ephedra Decoction Plus Ovate Atractylodes, *má huáng jiā zhú tāng* 麻黄加术汤, 729

Ephedra Decoction, *má huáng tāng* 麻黄汤, 3, 83, 184, 185, 246, 247, 346, 372, 502, 682, 729

Ephedra Panting-Stabilizing Decoction, *má huáng dìng chuǎn tāng* 麻黄定喘丸, 281

ephedra root, *má huáng gēn* 麻黄根, Ephedrae Radix, 11, 518, 727

Ephedra, Aconite, and Asarum Decoction, *má huáng fù zǐ xì xīn tāng* 麻黄附子细辛汤, 325, 345, 730

Ephedra, Aconite, and Licorice Decoction, *má huáng fù zǐ gān cǎo tāng* 麻黄附子甘草汤, 729

Ephedra, Apricot Kernel, Coix, and Licorice Decoction, *má xìng yì gān tāng* 麻杏薏甘汤, 729

Ephedra, Apricot Kernel, Gypsum, and Licorice Decoction, *má huáng xìng rén shí gāo gān cǎo tāng* 麻黄杏仁石膏甘草汤, 246, 729

Ephedra, Apricot Kernel, Licorice, and Gypsum Decoction, *má huáng xìng rén gān cǎo shí gāo tāng* 麻黄杏仁甘草石膏汤, 247

Ephedra, Apricot Kernel, Licorice, and Gypsum Decoction, *má xìng gān shí tāng* 麻杏甘石汤, 388, 637, 693, 729

Ephedra, Forsythia, and Rice Bean Decoction, *má huáng lián qiào chì xiǎo dòu tāng* 麻黄连翘赤小豆汤, 700

Ephedrae Herba, *má huáng* 麻黄, ephedra, 5, 17, 70, 103, 128, 129, 184, 228, 243, 246, 247, 346, 391, 438, 460, 500–502, 681, 683, 720

Ephedrae Radix, *má huáng gēn* 麻黄根, ephedra root, 11, 518, 727

epicondylitis*

  external humeral, 171

  radiohumeral, 171

epigastric pain*, 576

epiglottis*, 50

epiglottitis*

  acute, 612

epilepsy*, 433

Epimedii Herba, *yín yáng huò* 淫羊藿, epimedium, 298, 335, 397, 593, 596, 679, 727

epimedium, *yín yáng huò* 淫羊藿, Epimedii Herba, 298, 335, 397, 593, 596, 679, 727

epiphysitis*, 45

Equiseti Herba, *mù zéi* 木贼, equisetum, 686, 720

equisetum, *mù zéi* 木贼, Equiseti Herba, 686, 720

ér zhěn tòng 儿枕痛, infant's-pillow pain, 300

ěr 耳, ear, 166

ěr chì 耳赤, red ears, 495

ěr jiān 耳尖, Tip of the Ear, 585

ěr jùn 耳菌, ear mushroom, 166

ěr kuì 耳聩, deafness, 118

ěr kuò 耳廓, auricle, 12

ěr lóng 耳聋, deafness, 118

ěr lóng wán 耳聋丸, Deafness Pill, 731

ěr lóng zuǒ cí wán 耳聋左慈丸, Deafness Left-Benefiting Loadstone Pill, 119, 329, 742

ěr lún 耳轮, helix, 288

ěr lún kū jiāo 耳轮枯焦, withering of the helices, 695

ěr mén 耳门, TB-21, Ear Gate, 119, 166, 167, 260, 474, 488, 521, 610, 614, 748

ěr mén 耳门, ear gate, 166

ěr míng 耳鸣, tinnitus, 614

ěr nǜ 耳衄, spontaneous bleeding of the ear, 565

ěr qián qǐ ròu 耳前起肉, fleshy protuberance before the ear, 211

ěr tòng 耳痛, ear pain, 166

ěr xùn 耳蕈, ear mushroom, 166

ěr yǎng 耳痒, itchy ear, 320

ěr zhēn 耳针, ear acupuncture, 166

ěr zhēn liǎo fǎ 耳针疗法, ear acupuncture, 166

ěr zhì 耳痔, ear pile, 167

ěr zhū 耳珠, pearl of the ear, 429

ěr zuò chán míng 耳作蝉鸣, sound of cicadas in the ear, 548

èr bái 二白, Two Whites, 289, 656

èr biàn qīng lì 二便清利, clear uninhibited stool and urine, 72

èr cháng 二肠, two intestines, 635

èr chén píng wèi sǎn 二陈平胃散, Two Matured Ingredients Stomach-Calming Powder, 638, 673

èr chén tāng 二陈汤, Two Matured Ingredients Decoction, 101, 115, 116, 128, 153, 199, 216, 217, 240, 257, 400, 417, 419, 434, 435, 437, 439–443, 453, 457, 515, 625, 738

èr dōng tāng 二冬汤, Ophiopogon and Asparagus Decoction, 348, 366, 640

èr jiā jiǎn zhèng qì sǎn 二加减正气散, Second Variant Qi-Righting Powder, 732

èr jiǎ fù mài tāng 二甲复脉汤, Double-Armored Pulse-Restorative Decoction, 742

èr jiān 二间, LI-2, Second Space, 31, 414, 415, 520, 547, 746

èr miào sǎn 二妙散, Mysterious Two Powder, 337, 425, 489, 679

èr miào sǎn (wán) 二妙散（丸）, Mysterious Two Powder (Pill), 713, 733

èr miào wán 二妙丸, Mysterious Two Pill, 8, 40, 116, 117, 347

èr mǔ níng sòu tāng 二母宁嗽汤, Anemarrhena and Fritillaria Cough-Quieting Decoction, 216

èr mǔ sǎn 二母散, Anemarrhena and Fritillaria Powder, 738

èr shén wán 二神丸, Two Spirits Pill, 742

èr shèng sǎn 二圣散, Sagacious Two Powder, 743

èr shí bā mài 二十八脉, twenty-eight pulses, 633

èr wèi bá dú sǎn 二味拔毒散, Two-Ingredient Toxin-Drawing Powder, 395

èr wèi shēn sū yǐn 二味参苏饮, Two-Ingredient Ginseng and Sappan Beverage, 665

èr xiān tāng 二仙汤, Two Immortals Decoction, 741

èr yáng 二阳, second yang channel, 517

èr yīn 二阴, second yin channel, 517

èr yīn 二阴, two yin, 635

èr zhì wán 二至丸, Double Supreme Pill, 336, 365, 528, 646, 742

èr zhuó 二浊, two turbidities, 635

Eretmochelydis Carapax, *dài mào* 玳瑁, hawksbill shell, 54, 726

Ericeri Pelae Cera, *chóng bái là* 虫白腊, insect wax, 728

Erinacei Pellis, *cì wèi pí* 刺猬皮, hedgehog's pelt, 98, 518, 727

Eriobotryae Folium, *pí pá yè* 枇杷叶, loquat leaf, 65, 95, 387, 480, 624, 669, 725

erysipelas*, 299, 664

erythrina, *hǎi tóng pí* 海桐皮, Erythrinae Cortex, 116, 138, 139, 722

Erythrina Decoction, *hǎi tóng pí tāng* 海桐皮汤, 45, 684, 744

Erythrina Wine, *hǎi tóng pí jiǔ* 海桐皮酒, 734

Erythrinae Cortex, *hǎi tóng pí* 海桐皮, erythrina, 116, 138, 139, 722

Esophageal Cancer No.1 Formula, *shí dào ái yī hào fāng* 食道癌一号方, 745

Esophageal Cancer No.2 Formula, *shí dào ái èr hào fāng* 食道癌二号方, 745

Essence-Containing Pill, *mì jīng wán* 秘精丸, 112, 525

Essence-Nourishing Jade-Planting Decoction, *yǎng jīng zhòng yù tāng* 养精种玉汤, 39

Essential Herbal Foundation (*běn cǎo bèi yào*) 本草备要, 1694 (Qīng), Wāng Áng 汪昂, 290

Essential Prescriptions of the Golden Coffer (*jīn guì yào lüè*) 金匮要略, full title *jīn guì yào lüè fāng lùn* 金匮要略方论, 1, 3, 20, 34, 58, 120, 124, 152, 173, 194, 197, 204, 209, 273, 292, 306, 308, 318, 322, 334, 349, 350, 360, 363, 379, 384, 449, 469, 498, 526, 529, 535, 536, 564, 626, 651, 653, 655, 661, 668, 692, 704

Essential Rhymes for Patterns and Treatment (*zhèng zhì yào jué*) 证治要诀, Míng (1368–1644), Dài Sī-Gōng 戴思恭 [Yuán-Lǐ 原礼], 529

Essential Secrets from Outside the Metropolis (*wài tái mì yào*) 外台秘要, 752 (Táng), Wáng Táo 王焘, 142

etiology*, 429

eucommia, *dù zhòng* 杜仲, Eucommiae Cortex, 106, 251, 310, 328, 453, 485, 488, 593, 727

Eucommiae Cortex, *dù zhòng* 杜仲, eucommia, 106, 251, 310, 328, 453, 485, 488, 593, 727

Eucommiae Cortex Carbonisatus, *dù zhòng tàn* 杜仲炭, charred eucommia, 331, 572

Euonymi Lignum Suberalatum, *guǐ jiàn yǔ* 鬼箭羽, spindle tree wings, 139, 338, 725

Eupatorii Herba, *pèi lán* 佩兰, eupatorium, 7, 10, 66, 401, 434, 587, 588, 625, 722

eupatorium, *pèi lán* 佩兰, Eupatorii Herba, 7, 10, 66, 401, 434, 587, 588, 625, 722

euphorbia/knoxia, *dà jǐ* 大戟, Euphorbiae seu Knoxiae Radix, 97, 182, 438, 460, 574, 722

Euphorbiae Helioscopiae Herba, *zé qī* 泽漆, sun spurge, 136, 723

Euphorbiae Humifusae Herba, *dì jǐn cǎo* 地锦草, humifuse euphorbia, 68, 111, 721

Euphorbiae Lathyridis Semen, *xù suí zǐ* 续随子, caper spurge seed, 460, 722

Euphorbiae seu Knoxiae Radix, *dà jǐ* 大戟, euphorbia/knoxia, 97, 182, 438, 460, 574, 722

Eupolyphaga seu Opisthoplatia, *zhè chóng* 蟅虫, wingless cockroach, 34, 50, 138, 182, 540, 724

euryale, *qiàn shí* 芡实, Euryales Semen, 11, 12, 57, 308, 334, 496, 518, 727

Euryales Semen, *qiàn shí* 芡实, euryale, 11, 12, 57, 308, 334, 496, 518, 727

evodia, *wú zhū yú* 吴茱萸, Evodiae Fructus, 84, 256, 343, 363, 400, 447, 450, 506, 542, 561, 578, 581, 649, 660, 663, 723

Evodia Decoction with Aconite Decoction, *wú zhū yú jiā fù zǐ tāng* 吴茱萸加附子汤, 735

Evodia Decoction, *wú zhū yú tāng* 吴茱萸汤, 81, 83, 87, 156, 170, 343, 506, 578, 662, 663, 735

Evodiae Fructus, *wú zhū yú* 吴茱萸, evodia, 84, 256, 343, 363, 400, 447, 450, 506, 542, 561, 578, 581, 649, 660, 663, 723

exanthematous typhus*, 25

External Medicine Toad Venom Pill, *wài kē chán sū wán* 外科蟾酥丸, 744

Eye Brightener Clear-Raising Pill, *míng mù shàng qīng wán* 明目上清丸, 740

Eye Brightener Rehmannia Pill, *míng mù dì huáng wán* 明目地黄丸, 249, 742

Eye of the Knee, *xī yǎn* 膝眼, 104, 137, 296, 337, 521, 567

Eye Stasis Formula, *yū xuè guàn yǎn jīng fāng* 瘀血灌眼睛方, 730

fā 发, effuse, 168

fā 发, effusion, 168

fā bèi 发背, effusion of the back, 168

fā gān 伐肝, quelling the liver, 490

fā hàn 发汗, effusing sweat, 168

fā hàn 发汗, promoting sweat, 467

fā huáng 发黄, yellowing, 704

fā mù wán 伐木丸, Wood-Quelling Pill, 737

fā nǎo 发脑, effusion of the brain, 169

fā rè 发热, fever, 199

fā rè 发热, heat effusion, 278

fā rǔ 发乳, effusion of the breast, 169

fā yí 发颐, jowl effusion, 323

fā zuò 发作, attack, 12

fā zuò 发作, episode, 178

fá lì 乏力, lack of strength, 338

fǎ bàn xià 法半夏 pro formula pinellia, Pinelliae Tuber Pro Formula Praeparatum, 625

fà 发, hair, 251

fà bái 发白, graying of the hair, 245

fà chí 发迟, slowness to grow hair, 540

fà kū 发枯, dry hair, 153

fà luò 发落, hair loss, 251

fà wéi xuè zhī yú 发为血之馀, hair [of the head] is the surplus of the blood, 251

Face-Righting Decoction, *zhèng róng tāng* 正容汤, 568, 569, 689

Facial Pain No.1 Formula, *miàn tòng yī hào fāng* 面痛一号方, 194

Facial Pain No.2 Formula, *miàn tòng èr hào fāng* 面痛二号方, 194

Facial Pain No.3 Formula, *miàn tòng sān hào fāng* 面痛三号方, 194

Facial Pain No.4 Formula, *miàn tòng sì hào fāng* 面痛四号方, 194

facial paralysis*, 125

Fagopyri Cymosi Radix et Rhizoma, *tiān qiáo mài gēn* 天荞麦根, wild buckwheat root, 68, 469, 721

Fall-Upbearing Decoction, *shēng xiàn tāng* 升陷汤, 639, 741

Falling Flower Brew, *tuō huā jiān* 脱花煎, 503

Family Secret Lung-Moistening Beverage, *jiā mì rùn fèi yǐn* 家秘润肺饮, 372

Family Secret Lung-Warming Decoction, *jiā mì wēn fèi tāng* 家秘温肺汤, 372

Family Secret White-Draining Powder, *jiā mì xiè bái sǎn* 家秘泻白散, 292, 372, 376

fān 蕃, borderland, 48

fān huā zhì 翻花痔, everted-flower hemorrhoids, 180

fān wèi 翻胃, stomach reflux, 579

fān xiè yè 番泻叶 senna, Sennae Folium, 84, 460, 722

fán fán 烦, vexation, 654

fán 燔, blaze, 23

fán kě 烦渴, vexation and thirst, 655

fán rè 烦热, heart vexation, 273

fán rè 烦热, heat vexation, 284

fán zào 烦燥, vexation and agitation, 654

fǎn guān mài 反关脉, dorsal styloid pulse, 145

fǎn guān mài 反关脉, pulse on the back of the wrist, 473

fǎn wèi 反胃, stomach reflux, 579

fǎn zhì 反治, paradoxical treatment, 428

fàn 犯, invade, 319

fàn 泛, flood, 211

fàn ě 泛恶, upflow nausea, 639

fàn suān 泛酸, acid upflow, 4

fāng 方, formula, 223

fāng jì 方剂, formula, 223

fāng xiāng 芳香, aromatic, 10

fāng xiāng huà zhuó 芳香化浊, transforming turbidity with aroma, 625

fáng fēng 防风 ledebouriella, Ledebouriellae Radix, 11, 14, 55, 102, 103, 115, 139, 167, 184, 191, 240, 244, 319, 370, 424, 430, 439, 500–502, 527, 548, 599, 638, 680, 681, 684, 685, 703, 713, 720

fáng fēng sǎn 防风散, Ledebouriella Powder, 693

fáng fēng tāng 防风汤, Ledebouriella Decoction, 689

fáng fēng tōng shèng sǎn 防风通圣散, Ledebouriella Sage-Inspired Powder, 395, 476, 496, 546, 674, 687, 730

fáng jǐ 防己 fangji, Fangji Radix, 84, 139, 227, 671, 722

fáng jǐ fú líng tāng 防己茯苓汤, Fangji and Poria (Hoelen) Decoction, 536, 733

fáng jǐ huáng qí tāng 防己黄芪汤, Fangji and Astragalus Decoction, 114, 694, 733 *fáng jǐ sǎn* 防己散, Fangji Powder, 693

fáng jǐ tāng 防己汤, Fangji Decoction, 734

fáng jǐ yǐn 防己饮, Fangji Beverage, 112

fáng shì láo shāng 房室劳伤, sexual taxation, 528

fàng xuè 放血, bloodletting, 32

fangji, *fáng jǐ* 防己, Fangji Radix, 84, 139, 227, 671, 722

Fangji and Astragalus Decoction, *fáng jǐ huáng qí tāng* 防己黄芪汤, 114, 694, 733

Fangji and Poria (Hoelen) Decoction, *fáng jǐ fú líng tāng* 防己茯苓汤, 536, 733

Fangji Beverage, *fáng jǐ yǐn* 防己饮, 112

Fangji Decoction, *fáng jǐ tāng* 防己汤, 734

Fangji Powder, *fáng jǐ sǎn* 防己散, 693

Fangji Radix, *fáng jǐ* 防己, fangji, 84, 139, 227, 671, 722

Fangji, Zanthoxylum, Tingli, and Rhubarb Pill, *jǐ jiāo lì huáng wán* 己椒苈黄丸, 732

Fat Oil Paste, *féi yóu gāo* 肥油膏, 196

Fat Qi Pill, *féi qì wán* 肥气丸, 195

favus*, 196

fēi mén 飞门, flying gates, 214

fēi shī 飞尸, flying corpse, 214

fēi yáng 飞扬, BL-58, Taking Flight, 90, 290, 408, 453, 480, 747

fēi yáng hóu 飞扬喉, flying throat, 214

féi 痱, disablement, 130

féi cháng 腓肠, calf, 53

féi chuāng 肥疮, fat sore, 195

féi chuāng 痱疮, prickly heat, 463

féi dú 痱毒, prickly heat toxin, 463

féi ér wán 肥儿丸, Chubby Child Pill, 60, 238, 509, 549, 557, 737

féi gān 肥疳, fat gan, 195

féi nào 腓腨, calf, 53

féi pàng 肥胖, obesity, 418

féi pàng bù yùn 肥胖不孕, obesity infertility, 418

féi qì 肥气, fat qi, 195

féi qì wán 肥气丸, Fat Qi Pill, 195

féi rē gān 肥热疳, fat heat gan, 195

féi yóu gāo 肥油膏, Fat Oil Paste, 196

féi zǐ 榧子 torreya, Torreyae Semen, 183, 509, 724

féi zǐ guàn zhòng tāng 榧子贯众汤, Torreya and Aspidium Decoction, 737

fèi 肺, LU, 369

fèi 肺, lung, 371

fèi 肺, pulmonary, 469

fèi bì 肺痹, lung impediment, 376

fèi bì 肺痹, pulmonary impediment, 469

fèi bì chuǎn ké 肺闭喘咳, lung block panting and cough, 371

fèi bìng 肺病, lung disease, 372

fèi cáng pò 肺藏魄, lung stores the corporeal soul, 378

fèi cháng bù zú 肺常不足, lung is often in insufficiency, 376

fèi cháo bǎi mài 肺朝百脉, lung faces the hundred vessels, 374

fèi fēng 肺风, lung wind, 380

fèi fēng fěn cì 肺风粉刺, lung wind acne, 380

fèi gān 肺疳, gan of the lung, 238

fèi gān 肺疳, pulmonary gan, 469

fèi hé dà cháng 肺合大肠, lung is connected with the large intestine, 376

fèi hé pí máo 肺合皮毛, lung is connected with the skin and [body] hair, 376

fèi hé pí yě, qí róng máo yě 肺合皮也，其荣毛也, lung is connected with the skin; its luxuriance is the [body] hair, 376

fèi huǒ 肺火, lung fire, 374

fèi jī 肺积, lung accumulation, 371

fèi jīn 肺金, lung-metal, 377

fèi jīn 肺津, liquid of the lung, 348

fèi jīn 肺津, pulmonary liquid, 469

fèi jīn bù bù 肺津不布, nondistribution of pulmonary liquid, 413

fèi jīng 肺经, lung channel, 372

fèi jīng ké sòu 肺经咳嗽, lung channel cough, 372

fèi kāi qiào yú bí 肺开窍于鼻, lung opens at the nose, 377

fèi ké 肺咳, lung cough, 372

fèi láo 肺劳, lung taxation, 378

fèi láo 肺痨, pulmonary consumption, 469

fèi luò sǔn shāng 肺络损伤, damage to the network vessels of the lung, 108

fèi mài fú 肺脉浮, lung pulse is floating, 378

fèi qì 肺气, lung qi, 378

fèi qì bì sè 肺气闭塞, lung qi block, 378

fèi qì bù lì 肺气不利, inhibition of lung qi, 303

fèi qì bù xuān 肺气不宣, nondiffusion of lung qi, 413

fèi qì nì 肺气逆, counterflow lung qi, 102

fèi qì shàng nì 肝气上逆, liver qi ascending counterflow, 361

fèi qì shàng nì 肺气上逆, lung qi ascending counterflow, 378

fèi qì tōng yú bí 肺气通于鼻, lung qi flows to the nose, 378

fèi qì xū 肺气虚, lung qi vacuity, 378

fèi qì yīn liǎng xū 肺气阴两虚, dual vacuity of lung qi and yin, 160

fèi qiào 肺窍, orifices of the lung, 421

fèi rè 肺热, lung heat, 375

fèi rè ké sòu 肺热咳嗽, lung heat cough, 376

fèi rè yè jiāo 肺热叶焦, lung heat scorching the lobes, 376

fèi shàn 肺疝, lung mounting, 377

fèi shàn 肺疝, pulmonary mounting, 469

fèi shèn liǎng xū 肺肾两虚, dual vacuity of the lung and kidney, 162

fèi shèn tóng yuán 肺肾同源, lung and kidney are of the same source, 371

fèi shèn tóng zhì 肺肾同治, combined treatment of lung and kidney, 88

fèi shèn xiāng shēng 肺肾相生, lung and kidney are mutually engendering, 371 *fèi shèn yīn xū* 肺肾阴虚, lung-kidney yin vacuity, 377

fèi shēng pí máo 肺生皮毛, lung engenders the skin and [body] hair, 373

fèi shī qīng sù 肺失清肃, impaired depurative downbearing of the lung, 295

fèi shī qīng sù 肺失清肃, impaired lung depuration, 295

fèi shī qīng sù 肺失清肃, impaired pulmonary depuration, 295

fèi shī sù jiàng 肺失肃降, impaired depurative downbearing of the lung, 295

fèi shí 肺实, lung repletion, 378

fèi shū 肺俞, BL-13, Lung Transport, 5, 12, 13, 15, 65, 70, 72, 78, 83, 84, 86–89, 91, 92, 95–97, 99, 109, 128, 129, 142, 146, 155, 156, 158, 161, 163, 169, 184, 185, 201, 203, 224, 228, 237, 257, 261, 267–269, 277, 280–282, 285, 291, 292, 301, 336, 341, 348, 356, 368, 372, 374, 378–380, 393, 398, 409, 415, 416, 434, 435, 438, 439, 441, 443, 453, 467, 477, 481, 486, 489, 506, 515, 517, 535, 547, 550, 562, 571, 572, 595–597, 603, 625, 630, 640, 648, 663, 666, 668, 675, 677, 681–684, 686–688, 690, 693–695, 702, 703, 714, 715, 747

fèi shuǐ 肺水, lung water, 379

fèi wéi huá gài 肺为华盖, lung is the florid canopy, 377

fèi wéi jiāo zàng 肺为娇脏, lung is the delicate viscus, 377

fèi wéi qì zhī zhǔ, shèn wéi qì zhī gēn 肺为气之主，肾为气之根, lung is the governor of qi, kidney is the root of qi, 377

fèi wéi shuǐ zhī shàng yuán 肺为水之上源, lung is the upper source of water, 377

fèi wéi tì 肺为涕, lung forms snivel, 374

fèi wéi zhù tán zhī qì 肺为贮痰之器, lung is the receptacle that holds phlegm, 377

fèi wěi 肺痿, lung wilting, 379

fèi wěi 肺痿, pulmonary wilting, 469

fèi wěi 肺萎, lung wilting, 379

fèi wèi huǒ yán chuǎn 肺胃火炎喘, lung-stomach flaming fire panting, 378

fèi wèi rè shèng 肺胃热盛, exuberant lung-stomach heat, 189

fèi wù hán 肺恶寒, lung is averse to cold, 376

fèi xì 肺系, lung tie, 379

fèi xián 肺痫, pulmonary epilepsy, 469

fèi xiāo 肺消, lung dispersion, 373

fèi xiāo 肺消, pulmonary dispersion, 469

fèi xié xié tòng 肺邪胁痛, lung evil rib-side pain, 373

fèi xū 肺虚, lung vacuity, 379

fèi xū chuǎn jí 肺虚喘急, lung vacuity rapid panting, 379

fèi xū ké sòu 肺虚咳嗽, lung vacuity cough, 379

fèi yáng xū 肺阳虚, lung yang vacuity, 380

fèi yīn 肺阴, lung yin, 380

fèi yīn xū 肺阴虚, lung yin vacuity, 380

fèi yōng 肺痈, pulmonary welling-abscess, 469

fèi yōng 肺痈, welling-abscess of the lung, 670

fèi yōng bù dé wò 肺壅不得卧, lung congestion sleeplessness, 372

fèi yǔ dà cháng xiāng biǎo lǐ 肺与大肠相表里, lung and large intestine stand in interior-exterior relationship, 371

fèi zào 肺燥, lung dryness, 373

fèi zào ké sòu 肺燥咳嗽, lung dryness cough, 373

fèi zhàng 肺胀, pulmonary distention, 469

fèi zhě, xiàng fù zhī guān yě, zhì jié chū yān 肺者，相傅之官也，治节出焉, lung holds the office of assistant, whence management and regulation emanate, 376

fèi zhǔ bí 肺主鼻, lung governs the nose, 375

fèi zhǔ pí máo 肺主皮毛, lung governs the skin and [body] hair, 375

fèi zhǔ qì 肺主气, lung governs qi, 374

fèi zhǔ shēng 肺主声, lung governs the voice, 375

fèi zhǔ sù jiàng 肺主肃降, lung governs depurative downbearing, 374

fèi zhǔ tōng tiáo shuǐ dào 肺主通调水道, lung governs regulation of the waterways, 375

fèi zhǔ xíng shuǐ 肺主行水, lung governs movement of water, 374

fèi zhǔ xíng shuǐ 肺主行水, lung governs the movement of water, 375

fèi zhǔ xuān sàn 肺主宣散, lung governs diffusion, 374

fèi zhǔ yī shēn zhī biǎo 肺主一身之表, lung governs the exterior of the entire body, 375

fèi zhǔ zhì jié 肺主治节, lung governs management and regulation, 374

fèi zi 痱子, prickly heat, 463

fèi, qí huá zài máo 肺，其华在毛, lung, its bloom is in the [body] hair, 377

femur*, 607

fēn 分, candareen, 54

fēn 分, fen, 197

fēn cì 分刺, divide needling, 144

fēn dàn 分诞, birth, 19

fēn dàn 分诞, childbirth, 60

fēn dàn 分诞, delivery, 122

fēn jiě 分解, birth, 19

fēn jiě 分解, childbirth, 60

fēn jiě 分解, delivery, 122

fēn miǎn 分娩, birth, 19

fēn miǎn 分娩, childbirth, 60

fēn miǎn 分娩, delivery, 122

fēn qīng bié zhuó 分清别浊, separating the clear and the turbid, 525

fēn ròu 分肉, divided flesh, 144

fén 焚, deflagrate, 121

fěn cì 粉刺, acne, 5

fěn fáng jǐ 粉防己 mealy fangji, Stephaniae Tetrandrae Radix, 139, 722

fěn liú 粉瘤, mealy tumor, 387

fēng 风, wind, 679

fēng bì 风痹, wind impediment, 689

fēng bì 风秘, wind constipation, 683

fēng chí 风池, GB-20, Wind Pool, 8, 11, 14, 50, 53, 60–63, 66, 69, 73, 74, 87, 89, 91–93, 99, 103, 105, 119, 120, 125, 129, 139, 140, 145, 146, 150, 155, 158, 166, 167, 169, 175, 176, 178, 181, 184, 185, 192, 194, 195, 203, 218, 225, 235, 247, 255, 256, 259, 260, 279, 287, 288, 290–292, 301, 310, 319, 320, 337, 341, 342, 344, 349, 355, 359, 362, 364–366, 368, 370, 374, 386, 391, 395, 405, 406, 415, 416, 442, 448, 450–452, 454–458, 462, 468, 474, 478, 495, 499, 501, 508, 515–517, 521, 530, 544, 546, 547, 568, 569, 580, 585, 586, 591, 611, 620, 631, 636, 643, 674, 677, 680–691, 693, 694, 701, 702, 713, 716, 748

fēng chì chuāng jí 风赤疮疾, wind red sore disease, 691

fēng chì chuāng yí 风赤疮痍, wind red sore, 691

fēng chù 风搐, wind convulsions, 683

fēng ěr 风耳, wind ear, 685

fēng féi 风痱, wind disablement, 684

fēng fǔ 风府, GV-16, Wind Mansion, 14, 69, 71, 74, 86, 105, 125, 156, 160, 178, 194, 226, 245, 247, 255, 259, 260, 287, 316, 329, 331, 336, 344, 366, 391, 414, 415, 434, 451, 452, 456, 458, 501, 506, 573, 652, 682–685, 689, 693, 701, 702, 714, 749

fēng gān 风疳, wind gan, 686

fēng guān 风关, wind bar, 680

fēng hán 风寒, wind-cold, 680

fēng hán chuǎn 风寒喘, wind-cold panting, 683

fēng hán chuǎn jí 风寒喘急, wind-cold rapid panting, 683

fēng hán ěr lóng 风寒耳聋, wind-cold deafness, 681

fēng hán gǎn mào 风寒感冒, wind-cold common cold, 681

fēng hán ké sòu 风寒咳嗽, wind-cold cough, 681

fēng hán shī 风寒湿, wind-cold-damp, 681

fēng hán shī bì 风寒湿痹, wind-cold-damp impediment, 681

fēng hán shù fèi 风寒束肺, wind-cold fettering the lung, 682

fēng hán tóu tòng 风寒头痛, wind-cold headache, 682

fēng hán wài shù 风寒外束, wind-cold fettering the exterior, 682

fēng hán wài shù chuǎn 风寒外束喘, wind-cold fettering the exterior panting, 682

fēng hán xié tòng 风寒胁痛, wind-cold rib-side pain, 683

fēng hán xuàn yūn 风寒眩晕, wind-cold dizziness, 681

fēng hán yá tòng 风寒牙痛, wind-cold toothache, 683

fēng huà xiāo 风化硝 mirabilite efflorescence, MirabilitEfflorescentia, 401

fēng huǒ 风火, wind-fire, 685

fēng huǒ lì 风火疬, wind-fire scrofula, 685

fēng huǒ xiāng shān 风火相煽, mutual fanning of wind and fire, 404

fēng huǒ xiāng shān 风火相煽, wind and fire fanning each other, 680

fēng huǒ yá tòng 风火牙痛, wind-fire toothache, 685

fēng huǒ yǎn 风火眼, wind-fire eye, 685

fēng jìng 风痉, wind tetany, 693

fēng jū 风疽, wind flat-abscess, 686

fēng kuò 水廓, wind rampart, 691

fēng láo 风劳, wind taxation, 693

fēng lì 风痢, wind dysentery, 685

fēng lì 风疬, wind scrofula, 691

fēng lóng 丰隆, ST-40, Bountiful Bulge, 4, 6, 14, 15, 58, 59, 63, 65, 70, 74, 78, 84, 87, 88, 90, 99, 109, 115, 116, 119, 123, 129, 136, 140–142, 153, 178, 186, 192, 203, 210, 216, 223, 224, 230, 235, 240, 247, 251, 257, 260, 269, 277, 280–282, 285, 287, 288, 291, 297, 301, 386, 394, 400, 408, 418, 425, 433–443, 445, 448, 457, 477, 478, 499, 507, 511, 515, 537, 539, 540, 544, 550, 562, 565, 568, 578, 588, 591, 596, 603, 608, 611, 614, 624, 625, 631, 650, 656, 663, 664, 666, 673, 677, 681, 683–685, 690, 691, 694, 746

fēng lún 风轮, wind wheel, 694

fēng mén 风门, BL-12, Wind Gate, 12, 78, 84, 87, 91, 113, 119, 155, 184, 185, 281, 285, 374, 422, 443, 501, 517, 547, 586, 631, 677, 681–684, 690, 709, 710, 747

fēng mù zhī zàng 风木之脏, viscus of wind and wood, 656

fēng néng shèng shī 风能胜湿, wind can overcome dampness, 680

fēng nüè 风疟, wind malaria, 690

fēng qǐ wāi (kuāi) xié 风起㖞斜, wind-induced deviation, 689

fēng qǐ (kuāi) piān 风起㖞偏, wind-induced deviation, 689

fēng qì nèi dòng 风气内动, wind qi stirring internally, 691

fēng rè 风热, wind-heat, 686

fēng rè chì yǎn 风热赤眼, wind-heat red eye, 688

fēng rè chuāng 风热疮, wind-heat sore, 688

fēng rè ěr lóng 风热耳聋, wind-heat deafness, 687

fēng rè fàn fèi 风热犯肺, wind-heat invading the lung, 687

fēng rè gǎn mào 风热感冒, wind-heat common cold, 686

fēng rè hóu bì 风热喉痹, wind-heat throat impediment, 688

fēng rè jīng jì 风热惊悸, wind-heat fright palpitations, 687

fēng rè ké sòu 风热咳嗽, wind-heat cough, 686

fēng rè mù chì 风热目赤, wind-heat red eye, 688

fēng rè tóu tòng 风热头痛, wind-heat headache, 687

fēng rè xuàn yuān 风热眩晕, wind-heat dizziness, 687

fēng rè yá gān 风热牙疳, wind-heat gan of the teeth and gums, 687

fēng rè yǎn 风热眼, wind-heat eye, 687

fēng rè yāo tòng 风热腰痛, wind-heat lumbar pain, 688

fēng shā 风痧, wind sand, 691

fēng shèng zé dòng 风胜则动, when wind prevails, there is stirring, 673

fēng shī 风湿, rheumatism, 506

fēng shī 风湿, wind-damp, 684

fēng shī bì 风湿痹, wind-damp impediment, 684

fēng shī tóu tòng 风湿头痛, wind-damp headache, 684

fēng shī xī tóng piàn 风湿豨桐片, Siegesbeckia and Clerodendron Wind-Damp Tablet, 734

fēng shī xiāng bó 风湿相搏, mutual contention of wind and dampness, 403

fēng shī xiāng bó 风湿相搏, wind and dampness contending with each other, 680

fēng shī yāo tòng 风湿腰痛, wind-damp lumbar pain, 684

fēng shì 风市, GB-31, Wind Market, 28, 47, 104, 139, 145, 154, 289, 342, 370, 418, 532, 591, 658, 674, 688, 748

fēng shuǐ 风水, wind water, 694

fēng sòu 风嗽, wind cough, 683

fēng suǐ dān 封髓丹, Marrow-Sealing Elixir, 94

fēng tán 风痰, wind-phlegm, 690

fēng tán tóu tòng 风痰头痛, wind-phlegm headache, 691

fēng tán xuàn yūn 风痰眩晕, wind-phlegm dizziness, 690

fēng tóu xuàn 风头眩, wind dizzy head, 685

fēng wēn 风温, wind warmth, 693

fēng wēn jìng 风温痉, wind warmth tetany, 693

fēng xián 风痫, wind epilepsy, 685

fēng xián chì làn 风弦赤烂, wind ulceration of the eyelid rim, 693

fēng xiǎn 风癣, wind lichen, 689

fēng xiāo 风消, wind dispersion, 685

fēng xié 风邪, wind evil, 685

fēng xié fàn fèi 风邪犯肺, wind evil invading the lung, 685

fēng xié xí biǎo 风邪袭表, wind evil assailing the exterior, 685

fēng xié xuàn yūn 风邪眩晕, wind evil dizziness, 685

fēng xiè 风泻, wind diarrhea, 684

fēng xīn tòng 风心痛, wind heart pain, 686

fēng xìn sǎn 封囟散, Fontanel-Sealing Powder, 638

fēng xuàn 风眩, wind dizziness, 684

fēng yáng 风阳, wind yang, 694

fēng yào 风药, wind medicinal, 690

fēng yì 风懿, wind choke, 680

fēng yǐn zhěn 风隐疹, wind dormant papules, 685

fēng yǐn (kuāi) piàn 风引喎偏, wind-induced deviation, 689

fēng yóu gāo 疯油膏, Ill-Wind Oil Paste, 422

fēng zào 风燥, wind-dryness, 685

fēng zhěn 风疹, wind papules, 690

fēng zhěn kuài 风疹块, papular wind lumps, 428

fèng huáng yī 凤凰衣 chicken's egg membrane, Galli Membrana Ovi, 624, 725

fèng wěi cǎo 凤尾草 phoenix-tail fern, Pteridis Multifidi Herba, 68, 69, 721

fèng xiān huā 凤仙花 garden balsam flower, Impatientis Balsaminae Flos, 11

fennel, *huí xiāng* 茴香, Foeniculi Fructus, 83, 343, 397, 400, 447, 542, 660, 723

fenugreek, *hú lú bā* 胡芦巴, Foeni-Graeci Semen, 83, 335, 343, 400, 593, 675, 716, 727

Fenugreek Pill, *hú lú bā wán* 葫芦巴丸, 80, 733

Fenugreek Powder, *hú lú bā sǎn* 胡芦巴散, 733

fermented soybean, *dàn dòu chǐ* 淡豆豉, Glycines Semen Fermentatum Insulsum, 70, 130, 176, 184, 402, 410, 481, 501, 686, 720

Ferri Frusta, *tiě luò* 铁落, iron flakes, 54, 526, 585, 726

Ferry Brew, *jì chuān jiān* 济川煎, 50, 127, 732

Fetal Longevity Pill, *shòu tāi wán* 寿胎丸, 199, 331, 574, 742

Fetal Origin Beverage, *tāi yuán yǐn* 胎元饮, 38, 199, 574

fetid cassia, *jué míng zǐ* 决明子, Cassiae Torae Semen, 459, 676

Fetid Cassia Powder, *jué míng zǐ sǎn* 决明子散, 740

Fetus-Quieting Beverage, *ān tāi yǐn* 安胎饮, 741

Fetus-Quieting Qi-Harmonizing Beverage, *ān tāi hé qì yǐn* 安胎和气饮, 741

Fetus-Turning Formula, *zhuǎn tāi fāng* 转胎方, 384, 741

fever
  high, 279

fibula*, 11, 422

Fifth and Sixth Heavenly Stem Pill, *wù jǐ wán* 戊己丸, 109, 732

Fifth Variant Qi-Righting Powder, *wǔ jiā jiǎn zhèng qì sǎn* 五加减正气散, 732

filariasis*, 583

Fine Jade Paste, *qióng yù gāo* 琼玉膏, 603, 734

Fire and Water Hexagram Granules, *kǎn lí shā* 坎离砂, 744

Fire Depression Decoction, *huǒ yù tāng* 火郁汤, 655

Fire-Dissipating Decoction, *sàn huǒ tāng* 散火汤, 110

Fire-Draining Lung-Clearing Decoction, *xiè huǒ qīng fèi tāng* 泻火清肺汤, 281

Fire-Repelling Elixir, *bì huǒ dān* 避火丹, 744

Firewood-Raking Beverage, *chōu xīn yǐn* 抽薪饮, 54, 179

Firewood-Removing Beverage, *xǐ xīn yǐn* 徙薪饮, 29

First Variant Qi-Righting Powder, *yī jiā jiǎn zhèng qì sǎn* 一加减正气散, 732

fish poison yam, *bì xiè* 萆薢, Dioscoreae Hypoglaucae Rhizoma, 21, 45, 116, 136, 328, 516, 584, 723

Fish Poison Yam Clear-Turbid Separation Beverage, *bì xiè fēn qīng yǐn* 萆薢分清饮, 637, 641, 661, 733

Fish Poison Yam Dampness-Percolating Decoction, *bì xiè shèn shī tāng* 萆薢渗湿汤, 8, 116, 117, 221, 241, 468, 528, 733

Fish Poison Yam Toxin-Transforming Decoction, *bì xiè huà dú tāng* 萆薢化毒汤, 187, 528

Fish's Lumbus, *yú yāo* 鱼腰, 150, 259, 714

fissure of nipple*, 412

fistula*
  rectovaginal, 448

Fit-Settling Pill, *dìng xián wán* 定痫丸, 19, 178, 434, 740

Five Accumulations Powder, *wǔ jī sǎn* 五积散, 80, 82, 104, 186, 216, 516, 606, 730

Five Agents Elsholtzia Beverage, *wǔ wù xiāng rú yǐn* 五物香薷饮, 729

Five Grains Return-of-Spring Elixir, *wǔ lì huí chūn dān* 五粒回春丹, 171

Five Happinesses Toxin-Transforming Elixir, *wǔ fú huà dú dān* 五福化毒丹, 238

Five Impediments Decoction, *wǔ bì tāng* 五痹汤, 45, 210, 328, 358, 654, 734

Five Juices Beverage, *wǔ zhī yǐn* 五汁饮, 607, 734

Five Juices Center-Quieting Beverage, *wǔ zhī ān zhōng yǐn* 五汁安中饮, 164

Five Kernels Decoction, *wǔ rén tāng* 五仁汤, 732

Five Kernels Pill, *wǔ rén wán* 五仁丸, 399, 646, 732

Five Milled Ingredients Drink, *wǔ mò yǐn zi* 五磨饮子, 426, 736

Five Pillar Points, *wǔ zhù xué* 五柱穴, 2, 5, 61, 73, 562, 647

Five Pillars Powder, *bā zhù sǎn* 八柱散, 168

Five Spirits Decoction, *wǔ shén tāng* 五神汤, 744

Five Stranguries Powder, *wǔ lín sǎn* 五淋散, 283, 583, 733

Five Tigers Decoction, *wǔ hǔ tāng* 五虎汤, 443

Five Wiltings Decoction, *wǔ wěi tāng* 五痿汤, 733

Five Yellows Powder, *wǔ huáng sǎn* 五黄散, 745

Five-Ingredient Toxin-Dispersing Beverage, *wǔ wèi xiāo dú yǐn* 五味消毒饮, 75, 76, 636, 691, 744

Five-Jewel Powder, *wǔ bǎo sǎn* 五宝散, 586, 744

Five-Peel Beverage, *wǔ pí yǐn* 五皮饮, 153, 239, 608, 669

Five-Peel Powder (Beverage), *wǔ pí sǎn (yǐn)* 五皮散（饮）, 733

Five-Peel Powder, *wǔ pí sǎn* 五皮散, 136

Five-Seed Kidney-Supplementing Pill, *wǔ zǐ bǔ shèn wán* 五子补肾丸, 742

Five-Seed Progeny Pill, *wǔ zǐ yǎn zōng wán* 五子衍宗丸, 461, 523, 742

Five-Tigers-Chasing-the-Wind Powder, *wǔ hǔ zhuī fēng sǎn* 五虎追风散, 74, 140, 366, 740

Five-to-Five Elixir, *wǔ wǔ dān* 五五丹, 187, 259, 492, 744

Fixed Impediment Empirical Formula, *zhuó bì yàn fāng* 着痹验方, 138

flatus vaginalis*, 653

flavescent sophora, *kǔ shēn* 苦参, Sophorae Flavescentis Radix, 66, 67, 116, 225, 338, 353, 395, 424, 468, 720

Flavescent Sophora Decoction, *kǔ shēn tāng* 苦参汤, 744

Flesh-Engendering Jade and Red Paste, *shēng jī yù hóng gāo* 生肌玉红膏, 17, 187, 231, 259, 412, 540, 565, 744

Flesh-Engendering Powder, *shēng jī sǎn* 生肌散, 187, 259, 385, 528, 540, 565, 744

Flesh-Moistening Paste, *rùn jī gāo* 润肌膏, 586, 676

Florid Canopy Powder, *huá gài sǎn* 华盖散, 83, 683, 738

flowery knotweed, *hé shǒu wū* 何首乌, Polygoni Multiflori Radix, 28, 37, 127, 172, 175, 245, 309, 336, 352, 467, 593, 595, 727

Flowery Knotweed and Ginseng Beverage, *hé rén yǐn* 何人饮, 174, 650, 741

Flowery Knotweed Life-Extending Elixir, *shǒu wū yán shòu dān* 首乌延寿丹, 245, 251

flowery knotweed stem, *yè jiāo téng* 夜交藤, Polygoni Multiflori Caulis, 490, 537, 593, 726, 727

flu*
  intestinal, 143

flying squirrel's droppings, *wǔ líng zhī* 五灵脂, Trogopteri seu Pteromydis Excrementum, 137, 138, 397, 411, 448, 467, 574, 724

fó shǒu gān 佛手柑 Buddha's hand, Citri Sarcodactylidis Fructus, 103, 490, 493, 724

fó shǒu huā 佛手花 Buddha's hand flower, Citri Sarcodactylidis Flos, 223, 493, 724

fó shǒu sǎn 佛手散, Hand-of-Buddha Powder, 35, 451

Foeni-Graeci Semen, *hú lú bā* 胡芦巴, fenugreek, 83, 335, 343, 400, 593, 675, 716, 727

Foeniculi Fructus, *huí xiāng* 茴香, fennel, 83, 343, 397, 400, 447, 542, 660, 723

Fontanel-Sealing Powder, *fēng xìn sǎn* 封囟散, 638

Food Denial Powder, *kāi jìn sǎn* 开噤散, 217

Food Depression Decoction, *shí yù tāng* 食郁汤, 217

food poisoning*
  bacillary, 109, 588
  bacterial, 278

forsythia, *lián qiáo* 连翘, Forsythiae Fructus, 310, 422, 621

forsythia, *lián qiào* 连翘, Forsythiae Fructus, 20, 65, 67, 69, 70, 118, 130, 141, 189, 214, 234, 263, 303, 315, 387, 388, 412, 430, 439, 450, 463, 497, 501, 548, 606, 671, 703, 721

Forsythia and Mint Decoction, *qiào hé tāng* 翘荷汤, 734

Forsythia Drink, *lián qiào yǐn zi* 连翘饮子, 497

Forsythia Powder, *lián qiào sǎn* 连翘散, 17

Forsythia, Lonicera, and Bolbosteema Brew, *lián qiào jīn bèi jiān* 连翘金贝煎, 743

Forsythiae Fructus, *lián qiào* 连翘, forsythia, 310, 422, 621

Forsythiae Fructus, *lián qiào* 连翘, forsythia, 20, 65, 67, 69, 70, 118, 130, 141, 189, 214, 234, 263, 303, 315, 387, 388, 412, 430, 439, 450, 463, 497, 501, 548, 606, 671, 703, 721

Fortunellae Fructus, *jīn jú* 金橘, kumquat, 363

fossa, popliteal*, 336

Four Agents Decoction Plus Scutellaria and Coptis, *sì wù jiā huáng qín huáng lián tāng* 四物加黄芩黄连汤, 730

Four Agents Decoction, *sì wù tāng* 四物汤, 30, 37–40, 152, 153, 167, 243, 251, 261, 266, 288, 320, 322, 352, 370, 390, 391, 451, 452, 455, 456, 466, 474, 484, 595, 599, 606, 612, 646, 647, 654, 670, 696, 714, 715, 741

Four Agents Depression-Transforming Decoction, *sì wù huà yù tāng* 四物化郁汤, 27

Four Animals Decoction, *sì shòu yǐn* 四兽饮, 399

Four Colors Powder, *sì sè sǎn* 四色散, 63, 198

Four Flowers, *sì huā* 四花, 26, 227, 648, 649

Four Fresh Agents Pill, *sì shēng wán* 四生丸, 738

Four Gentlemen Decoction, *sì jūn zǐ tāng* 四君子汤, 172, 178, 223, 228, 267, 401, 486, 488, 562, 563, 594–596, 666, 741

Four Gentlemen Panting Decoction, *chuǎn sì jūn zǐ tāng* 喘四君子汤, 269, 487, 489

Four Milled Ingredients Beverage, *sì mò yǐn* 四磨饮, 481, 482, 736

Four Milled Ingredients Decoction, *sì mò tāng* 四磨汤, 477

Four Seams, *sì fèng* 四缝, 60, 61, 237, 239, 522, 557

Four Seas Depression-Soothing Pill, *sì hǎi shū yù wán* 四海舒郁丸, 244, 480, 737

Four Spirits Pill, *sì shén wán* 四神丸, 312, 325, 335, 647, 660, 742

Four Stems Decoction, *sì téng tāng* 四藤汤, 737

Four Yin Brew, *sì yīn jiān* 四阴煎, 416

Four-Ingredient Elsholtzia Beverage, *sì wèi xiāng rú yǐn* 四味香薷饮, 729

Four-Seven Decoction, *sì qī tāng* 四七汤, 19, 157, 256, 736

Four-Yin Decoction, *sì yīn tāng* 四阴汤, 734

Fourth Variant Qi-Righting Powder, *sì jiā jiǎn zhèng qì sǎn* 四加减正气散, 732

frankincense, *rǔ xiāng* 乳香, Olibanum, 104, 137, 138, 503, 540, 574, 696, 724

Fraxini Cortex, *qín pí* 秦皮, ash, 68, 338, 721

Free Wanderer Powder, *xiāo yáo sǎn* 逍遥散, 19, 103, 202, 223, 229, 256, 315, 358, 362, 367, 385, 386, 393, 412, 478, 480, 482, 484, 493, 497, 513, 515, 524, 599, 643, 655, 656, 685, 732

Free Wanderer Variant Powder, *jiā jiǎn xiāo yáo sǎn* 加减逍遥散, 677

fresh bamboo leaf (lophatherum), *xiān zhú yè* 鲜竹叶, Lophatheri Folium Recens, 589

fresh flowery knotweed, *xiān shǒu wū* 鲜首乌, Polygoni Multiflori Radix Recens, 399

fresh gardenia, *shēng shān zhī* 生山栀, Gardeniae Fructus Recens, 116

fresh ginger, *shēng jiāng* 生姜, Zingiberis Rhizoma Recens, 11, 70, 84, 95, 128, 201, 230, 243, 255, 256, 319, 343, 358, 397, 417, 426, 443, 448, 454, 464, 500–502, 527, 547, 574, 578, 581, 661, 663, 681, 683, 720

Fresh Ginger Heart-Draining Decoction, *shēng jiāng xiè xīn tāng* 生姜泻心汤, 732

fresh imperata, *xiān máo gēn* 鲜茅根, Imperatae Rhizoma Recens, 30, 703

fresh lotus leaf, *xiān hé yè* 鲜荷叶, Nelumbinis Folium Recens, 625

fresh phragmites, *xiān lú gēn* 鲜芦根, Phragmititis Rhizoma Recens, 67, 282, 720

fresh rehmannia, *xiān dì huáng* 鲜地黄, Rehmanniae Radix Recens, 67, 116, 720

Fright-Cooling Pill, *liáng jīng wán* 凉惊丸, 740

Fright-Disinhibiting Pill, *lì jīng wán* 利惊丸, 6

fritillaria, *bèi mǔ* 贝母, Fritillariae Bulbus, 30, 120, 230, 398, 434, 544, 625, 637, 686

Fritillaria and Trichosanthes Powder, *bèi mǔ guā lóu sǎn* 贝母栝蒌散, 156, 203, 398, 655, 739

Fritillariae Bulbus, *bèi mǔ* 贝母, fritillaria, 30, 120, 230, 398, 434, 544, 625, 637, 686

Fritillariae Cirrhosae Bulbus, *chuān bèi mǔ* 川贝母, Sichuan fritillaria, 175, 282, 480, 624, 714, 725

Fritillariae Verticillatae Bulbus, *zhè bèi mǔ* 浙贝母, Zhejiang fritillaria, 70, 385, 387, 544, 624, 688, 725

fū chǎo 麸炒, bran-frying, 50

fū chǎo 麸炒, stir-frying with bran, 573

fū yáng 跗阳, BL-59, Instep Yang, 747

fū yáng mài 跗阳脉, instep yang pulse, 309

fú 浮, floating, 211

fú 伏, deep-lying, 120

fú 伏, latent, 341

fú 扶, support, 597

fú bái 浮白, GB-10, Floating White, 219, 748

fú gǔ 凫骨, wild-duck bones, 678

fú liáng 伏梁, deep-lying beam, 120

fú líng 茯苓 poria, Poria, 17, 47, 66, 84, 93, 136, 141, 157, 223, 224, 234, 236, 256, 257, 315, 401, 418, 428, 434, 454, 456, 457, 486, 499, 563, 587, 594, 596, 600, 620, 649, 661, 662, 666, 675, 679, 703, 723

fú líng gān cǎo tāng 茯苓甘草汤, Poria (Hoelen) and Licorice Decoction, 733

fú líng guì zhī gān cǎo dà zào tāng 茯苓桂枝甘草大枣汤, Poria (Hoelen), Cinnamon Twig, Licorice, and Jujube Decoction, 510

fú líng pí 茯苓皮 poria skin, Poriae Cortex, 5, 116, 136, 153, 723

fú líng pí tāng 茯苓皮汤, Poria (Hoelen) Skin Decoction, 733

fú líng sì nì tāng 茯苓四逆汤, Poria (Hoelen) Counterflow Cold Decoction, 735

fú líng tāng 茯苓汤, Poria (Hoelen) Decoction, 82

fú lóng gān 伏龙肝 oven earth, Terra Flava Usta, 311, 556, 569, 573, 666, 724

fú luò 浮络, superficial network vessel, 592

fú mài 浮脉, floating pulse, 211

fú mài 伏脉, hidden pulse, 291

fú píng 浮萍 duckweed, Lemnae Herba, 130, 228, 686, 703, 720

fú píng huáng qín tāng 浮萍黄芩汤, Duckweed and Scutellaria Decoction, 729

fú qì 伏气, latent qi, 341

fú qì wēn bìng 伏气温病, latent qi warm disease, 341

fú rè 浮热, floating heat, 211

fú rè 浮热, floating heat [effusion], 211

fú shén 茯神 root poria, Poria cum Pini Radice, 60, 122, 256, 262, 392, 490, 654, 726

fú shén sǎn 茯神散, Root Poria Powder, 235

fú shǔ 伏暑, latent summerheat, 341

fú tú 扶突, LI-18, Protuberance Assistant, 129, 291, 378, 521, 746

fú tù 伏兔, ST-32, Crouching Rabbit, 222, 342, 520, 746

fú tù dān 茯菟丹, Poria (Hoelen) and Cuscuta Elixir, 742

fú xī 浮郄, BL-38, Superficial Cleft, 747

fú xiǎo mài 浮小麦 light wheat, Tritici Semen Leve, 95, 410, 518, 651, 727

fú xū 浮虚, vacuous puffiness, 653

fú yǐn 伏饮, deep-lying rheum, 120

fú yuán sǎn 扶元散, Origin-Supporting Powder, 638

fú zhèng jiě biǎo 扶正解表, supporting right and resolving the exterior, 597

fú zhèng qū xié 扶正祛邪, supporting right and dispelling evil, 597

fú zhǒng 浮肿, puffy swelling, 469

fǔ 府, dwelling place, 163

fǔ 府, house, 293

fǔ 辅, support, 597

fǔ 腐, putrefaction, 474

fǔ 腑, bowel, 48

fǔ chòu 腐臭, putrid smell, 474

fǔ dǐ chōu xīn 釜底抽薪, raking the firewood from beneath the cauldron, 492

fǔ fèi mài 釜沸脉, seething cauldron pulse, 519

fǔ gǔ 辅骨, assisting bone, 11

fǔ làn 腐烂, putrefaction, 474

fǔ shè 府舍, SP-13, Bowel Abode, 221, 746

fǔ tāi 腐苔, bean curd tongue fur, 16

fǔ tāi 腐苔, tofu tongue fur, 615

fǔ xiōng tāng 抚芎汤, Fuuzhou Ligusticum Decoction, 439

fù 腹, abdomen, 1

fù āi 腹哀, SP-16, Abdominal Lament, 746

fù bǐng jiǔ 附饼灸, moxibustion on aconite cake, 402

fù fāng dà chéng qì tāng 复方大承气汤, Compound Formula Major Qi-Coordinating Decoction, 731

fù fāng huáng lián gāo 复方黄连膏, Compound Formula Coptis Paste, 744

fù fēn 附分, BL-41, Attached Branch, 747

fù gǔ jū 附骨疽, bone-clinging flat-abscess, 44

fù gǔ jū 贴骨疽, bone-clinging tumor, 44

fù guì lǐ zhōng wán 附桂理中丸, Aconite and Cinnamon Center-Rectifying Pill, 734

fù jié 腹结, SP-14, Abdominal Bind, 2, 72, 127, 164, 277, 298, 318, 339, 544, 585, 673, 746

fù kē jí bìng 妇科疾病, gynecological diseases, 250

fù liào chǎo 副料炒, stir-frying with adjuvants, 573

fù liū 复溜, KI-7, Recover Flow, 47, 86, 95, 114, 128, 174, 184, 185, 199, 211, 224, 228, 240, 266, 288, 297, 302, 308, 331, 333, 334, 348, 358, 370, 393, 425, 450, 453, 461, 514, 518, 521, 522, 524, 547, 550, 559, 563, 569, 589, 590, 594, 597, 600, 604, 608, 637, 638, 641, 647, 662, 681, 682, 686, 701, 703, 713, 716, 747

fù lù qīng jīn 腹露青筋, prominent green-blue abdominal veins, 466

fù mài tāng 复脉汤, Pulse-Restorative Decoction, 156, 283, 741

fù mǎn 腹满, abdominal fullness, 1

fù míng sǎn 复明散, Light-Restoring Powder, 519

fù nǚ jí bìng 妇女疾病, women's diseases, 695

fù pén zǐ 覆盆子 rubus, Rubi Fructus, 12, 229, 496, 518, 548, 727

fù tòng 腹痛, abdominal pain, 2

fù yuán huó xuè tāng 复元活血汤, Origin-Restorative Blood-Quickening Decoction, 45, 118, 138, 337, 737

fù yuán tōng qì sǎn 复元通气散, Origin-Restoring Qi-Freeing Powder, 316, 454

fù zhàng 腹胀, abdominal distention, 1

fù zhàng mǎn 腹胀满, abdominal fullness, 1

fù zhōng jiǎo tòng 腹中绞痛, gripping pain in the abdomen, 249

fù zǐ 附子 aconite, Aconiti Tuber Laterale, 12, 23, 26, 83, 84, 97, 182, 183, 217, 228, 242, 247, 272, 292, 293, 332, 335, 341, 343, 393, 402, 405, 426, 438, 456, 467, 469, 474, 480, 489, 504, 526, 529, 556, 564, 596, 612, 649, 660–664, 679, 723

fù zǐ gēng mǐ tāng 附子粳米汤, Aconite and Rice Decoction, 734

fù zǐ lǐ zhōng tāng 附子理中汤, Aconite Center-Rectifying Decoction, 29, 46, 62, 80, 85, 86, 124, 145, 151, 247, 559, 564, 646, 647, 702, 711

fù zǐ lǐ zhōng wán 附子理中丸, Aconite Center-Rectifying Pill, 425, 734

fù zǐ wán 附子丸, Aconite Pill, 612

fù zǐ xiè xīn tāng 附子泻心汤, Aconite Heart-Draining Decoction, 733

Fujian leaven, *jiàn shén qū* 建神麴, Massa Medicata Fermentata Fujianensis, 141, 724

furuncle*, 44

furuncles*
   multiple, 445

furunculosis*, 445

Fuuzhou Ligusticum Decoction, *fǔ xiōng tāng* 抚芎汤, 439

fù rén liáng fāng 妇人良方 (*Good Remedies for Women*), 1237 (Sòng), Chén Zì-Míng 陈自明, 454

fēn bié qīng zhuó 分别清浊, separate the clear and the turbid, 525

gā yá 嘎牙, grinding of the teeth, 249

gài gǔ 盖骨, covering bone, 104

galangal fruit, *hóng dòu kòu* 红豆蔻, Alpiniae Galangae Fructus, 660, 723

galenite, *qiān* 铅, Galenitum, 467, 526

Galenite Elixir, *hēi xí dān* 黑锡丹, 330, 335, 526, 629, 735

Galenitum, *qiān* 铅, galenite, 467, 526

Galenitum Praeparatum, *qiān fěn* 铅粉, processed galenite, 98, 445

Gallbladder-Clearing Dampness-Disinhibiting Decoction, *qīng dǎn lì shī tāng* 清胆利湿汤, 733

Gallbladder-Clearing Decoction, *qīng dǎn tāng* 清胆汤, 476

Gallbladder-Clearing Qi-Moving Decoction, *qīng dǎn xíng qì tāng* 清胆行气汤, 735

Gallbladder-Disinhibiting Jaundice-Abating Decoction, *lì dǎn tuì huáng tāng* 利胆退黄汤, 733

Gallbladder-Disinhibiting Stone-Expelling Tablet, *lì dǎn pái shí piàn* 利胆排石片, 733

Gallbladder-Warming Decoction, *wēn dǎn tāng* 温胆汤, 70, 123, 223, 230, 236, 358, 417, 418, 437, 537, 539, 541, 578, 614, 662, 738

Galli Albumen, *jī zǐ bái* 鸡子白, egg white, 621

Galli Gigerii Endothelium, *jī nèi jīn* 鸡内金, gizzard lining, 141, 216, 385, 420, 544, 582, 606, 665, 724

Galli Membrana Ovi, *fèng huáng yī* 凤凰衣, chicken's egg membrane, 624, 725

Galli Vitellus, *jī zǐ huáng* 鸡子黄, egg yolk, 17, 176, 256

gallstones*, 110

gān 干, stem, 572

gān 甘, sweet, 600

gān 甘, sweetness, 600

gān 肝, LR, 369

gān 肝, liver, 351

gān 疳, gan, 236

gān 干, dry, 152

gān bì 肝痹, liver impediment, 358

gān bìng 肝病, liver disease, 354

gān cáng hún 肝藏魂, liver stores the ethereal soul, 363

gān cáng xuè 肝藏血, liver stores the blood, 363

gān cǎo 甘草 licorice, Glycyrrhizae Radix, 11, 17, 20, 47, 84, 108, 110, 115, 129, 141, 154, 161, 192, 214, 223, 227, 228, 230, 241, 255, 256, 259, 263, 285, 292, 315, 343, 378, 387, 390, 392, 394, 416, 430, 455, 463, 464, 486, 495, 498, 504, 526, 548, 556, 567, 580, 589, 593–595, 600, 662, 671, 687, 726

gān cǎo 炙甘草 mix-fried licorice, mix-fried Glycyrrhizae Radix, 270

gān cǎo fěn mì tāng 甘草粉蜜汤, Licorice, Processed Galenite, and Honey Decoction, 737

gān cǎo fù zǐ tāng 甘草附子汤, Licorice and Aconite Decoction, 680, 734

gān cǎo gān jiāng fú líng bái zhú tāng 甘草干姜茯苓白术汤, Licorice, Dried Ginger, Poria (Hoelen), and Ovate Atractylodes Decoction, 661, 733

gān cǎo gān jiāng tāng 甘草干姜汤, Licorice and Dried Ginger Decoction, 380, 734

gān cǎo tāng 甘草汤, Licorice Decoction, 527

gān cǎo xiǎo mài dà zǎo tāng 甘草小麦大枣汤, Licorice, Wheat, and Jujube Decoction, 739

gān cǎo xiè xīn tāng 甘草泻心汤, Licorice Heart-Draining Decoction, 732

gān cǎo zhī zǐ tāng 甘草栀子汤, Licorice and Gardenia Decoction, 731

gān cháng yǒu yú 肝常有馀, liver is often in superabundance, 359

gān chuāng 疳疮, gan sore, 238

gān dǎn guǎn jié shí fāng 肝胆管结石方, Hepatolith Formula, 733

gān dǎn shī rè 肝胆湿热, liver-gallbladder damp-heat, 356

gān dì huáng 干地黄 dried rehmannia, Rehmanniae Radix Exsiccata, 20, 67, 256, 526, 557, 720

gān dú yǎn 疳毒眼, gan toxin eye, 239

gān fēng 肝风, liver wind, 364

gān fēng nèi dòng 肝风内动, liver wind stirring internally, 364

gān gān 肝疳, gan of the liver, 238

gān gé jiě jī tāng 干葛解肌汤, Pueraria Flesh-Resolving Decoction, 729

gān hán 肝寒, liver cold, 353

gān hán zī rùn 甘寒滋润, enriching and moistening with cold sweet medicinals, 175

gān hé dǎn 肝合胆, liver is connected with the gallbladder, 359

gān hé jīn 肝合筋, liver is connected with the sinews, 359

gān huǎn tāng 甘缓汤, Sweet Relief Decoction, 480

gān huǒ 肝火, liver fire, 355

gān huǒ bù dé wò 肝火不得卧, liver fire sleeplessness, 356

gān huǒ fàn fèi 肝火犯肺, liver fire invading the lung, 356

gān huǒ shàng yán 肝火上炎, liver fire flaming upward, 355

gān huǒ shàng yán 肝火上炎, upflaming liver fire, 639

gān huǒ xuàn yūn 肝火眩晕, liver fire dizziness, 355

gān huò luàn 干霍乱, dry cholera, 152

gān jī 肝积, liver accumulation, 351

gān jī 疳积, gan accumulation, 237

gān jí 疳疾, gan disease, 237

gān jí shàng mù 疳疾上目, gan disease ascending to the eye, 237

gān jiāng 干姜 dried ginger, Zingiberis Rhizoma Exsiccatum, 5, 12, 23, 84, 94, 98, 128, 136, 182, 196, 228, 242, 257, 272, 292, 293, 343, 345, 393, 425,

426, 438, 455, 456, 463, 469, 504, 612, 625, 649, 660, 662, 663, 679, 723

gān jiāng rén shēn bàn xià wán 干姜人参半夏丸, Dried Ginger, Ginseng, and Pinellia Pill, 736

gān jiǎo qì 干脚气, dry leg qi, 154

gān jié tāng 甘桔汤, Licorice and Platycodon Decoction, 203, 738

gān jīng 肝经, liver channel, 352

gān jīng ké sòu 肝经咳嗽, liver channel cough, 352

gān jīng shī rè dài xià 肝经湿热带下, liver channel damp-heat vaginal discharge, 352

gān jīng shí huǒ 肝经实火, liver channel repletion fire, 353

gān jué 肝厥, liver reversal, 362

gān jué tóu tòng 肝厥头痛, liver reversal headache, 362

gān kāi qiào yú mù 肝开窍于目, liver opens at the eyes, 360

gān ké 肝咳, liver cough, 353

gān kě 疳渴, gan thirst, 239

gān kū 干枯, desiccation, 124

gān láo 肝劳, liver taxation, 363

gān láo 疳痨, gan consumption, 237

gān lì 疳痢, gan dysentery, 237

gān lù xiāo dú dān 甘露消毒丹, Sweet Dew Toxin-Dispersing Elixir, 66, 69, 70, 117, 118, 167, 177, 297, 539, 733

gān lù yǐn 甘露饮, Sweet Dew Beverage, 239, 367, 547, 620, 731

gān mài dà zǎo tāng 甘麦大枣汤, Licorice, Wheat, and Jujube Decoction, 655, 739

gān mài xián 肝脉弦, liver pulse is stringlike, 360

gān mù 肝木, liver-wood, 365

gān mù chéng pí 肝木乘脾, liver-wood exploiting the spleen, 365

gān nì 疳䘌, invisible gan worms, 319

gān nì tóu tòng 肝逆头痛, liver counterflow headache, 353

gān ǒu 干呕, dry retching, 156

gān pí bù hé 肝脾不和, liver-spleen disharmony, 362

gān pí liǎng xū 肝脾两虚, dual vacuity of the liver and spleen, 162

gān qī 干漆 lacquer, Lacca Exsiccata, 97, 138, 725

gān qì 肝气, liver qi, 360

gān qì bù hé 肝气不和, disharmony of liver qi, 135

gān qì bù shū 肝气不舒, constrained liver qi, 95

gān qì bù zú 肝气不足, insufficiency of liver qi, 310

gān qì fàn pí 肝气犯脾, liver qi invading the spleen, 361

gān qì fàn wèi 肝气犯胃, liver qi invading the stomach, 361

gān qì nì 肝气逆, counterflow liver qi, 102

gān qì tōng yú mù 肝气通于目, liver qi flows to the eyes, 361

gān qì xié tòng 肝气胁痛, liver qi rib-side pain, 362

gān qì xū 肝气虚, liver qi vacuity, 362

gān qì yù 肝气郁, depressed liver qi, 123

gān qì yù 肝气郁, liver qi depression, 361

gān qì yù jié 肝气郁结, binding depression of liver qi, 18

gān qì, gān yáng, gān xuè, gān yīn 肝气，肝阳，肝血，肝阴, liver qi, liver yang, liver blood, and liver yin, 361

gān rè 肝热, liver heat, 358

gān rè 疳热, gan heat effusion, 237

gān rè è zǔ 肝热恶阻, liver heat malign obstruction, 358

gān rè zì hàn 肝热自汗, liver heat spontaneous sweating, 358

gān rù pí 甘入脾, sweetness enters the spleen, 600

gān shèn jīng xuè kuī sǔn 肝肾精血亏损, liver-kidney essence-blood depletion, 360

gān shèn jīng xuè kuī xū 肝肾精血亏虚, liver-kidney essence-blood depletion, 360

gān shèn kuī sǔn 肝肾亏损, liver-kidney depletion, 359

gān shèn kuī sǔn tòng jīng 肝肾亏损痛经, liver-kidney depletion menstrual pain, 359

gān shèn tóng yuán 肝肾同源, liver and kidney are of the same source, 352

gān shèn xiāng shēng 肝肾相生, liver and kidney are mutually engendering, 352

gān shèn yīn xū 肝肾阴虚, liver-kidney yin vacuity, 360

gān shèn yīn xū bēng lòu 肝肾阴虚崩漏, liver-kidney yin vacuity flooding and spotting, 360

gān shēng yú zuǒ 肝生于左, liver lives on the left, 360

gān shí 肝实, liver repletion, 362

gān shòu xuè ér néng shì 肝受血而能视, liver receives blood and there is vision, 362

gān shū 肝俞, BL-18, Liver Transport, 11, 15, 16, 19, 20, 24, 26, 29, 33, 35, 53, 58, 60, 61, 64, 89, 91, 103, 119, 123, 140, 151, 152, 157, 162, 164, 175, 189, 195, 202, 218, 223, 225, 227, 233, 235, 256, 266, 288, 291, 292, 296, 297, 310, 336, 347, 352, 353, 355–362, 365, 366, 384, 385, 390, 392, 393, 399, 406, 445, 452, 453, 462, 475, 477–479, 493, 495, 497, 499, 500, 511, 515, 533, 534, 538, 547, 549, 552, 554, 566, 568, 569, 571, 586, 597, 640, 649, 677, 690, 694, 700, 710, 713–715, 747

gān shuǐ 肝水, liver water, 363

gān sōng 甘松 nardostachys, Nardostachydis Rhizoma et Radix, 493, 724

gān suì 甘遂 kansui, Kansui Radix, 171, 182, 438, 460, 464, 508, 574, 666, 722

gān suì sǎn 甘遂散, Kansui Powder, 744

gān wéi gāng zàng 肝为刚脏, liver is the unyielding viscus, 359

gān wéi lèi 肝为泪, liver forms tears, 356

gān wěi 肝痿, liver wilting, 363

gān wèi bù hé 肝胃不和, liver-stomach disharmony, 362

gān wèi qì tòng 肝胃气痛, liver-stomach qi pain, 362

gān wēn chú (dà) rè 甘温除（大）热, eliminating (great) heat with warmth and sweetness, 171 *gān wù fēng* 肝恶风, liver is averse to wind, 359

gān xiǎn 干癣, dry lichen, 154

gān xiàn 干陷, dry fall, 152

gān xié tòng 干胁痛, dry rib-side pain, 157

gān xiè 疳泻, gan diarrhea, 237

gān xū 肝虚, liver vacuity, 363

gān xū què mù nèi zhàng 肝虚雀目内障, liver vacuity sparrow-vision internal obstruction, 363

gān xuè 肝血, liver blood, 352

gān xuè bù zú 肝血不足, insufficiency of liver blood, 310

gān xuè bù zú xié tòng 肝血不足胁痛, insufficiency of liver blood rib-side pain, 310

gān xuè láo 干血痨, dry blood consumption, 152

gān xuè xū 肝血虚, liver blood vacuity, 352

gān yǎn 疳眼, eye gan, 192

gān yáng 肝阳, liver yang, 365

gān yáng huà fēng 肝阳化风, liver yang transforming into wind, 365

gān yáng huà huǒ 肝阳化火, liver yang transforming into fire, 365

gān yáng piān wàng 肝阳偏旺, effulgent liver yang, 168

gān yáng shàng kàng 肝阳上亢, ascendant liver yang, 11

gān yáng shàng yàng 肝阳上亢, ascendant hyperactivity of liver yang, 10

gān yáng tóu tòng 肝阳头痛, liver yang headache, 365

gān yáng xuàn yūn 肝阳眩晕, liver yang dizziness, 365

gān yīn 肝阴, liver yin, 365

gān yīn bù zú 肝阴不足, insufficiency of liver yin, 310

gān yīn xū 肝阴虚, liver yin vacuity, 365

gān yōng 肝痈, liver welling-abscess, 363

gān yōng 肝痈, welling-abscess of the liver, 670

gān yǔ dǎn xiāng biǎo lǐ 肝与胆相表里, liver and gallbladder stand in interior-exterior relationship, 352

gān yù 肝郁, depressed liver, 123

gān yù 肝郁, liver depression, 353

gān yù bù yùn 肝郁不孕, liver depression infertility, 353

gān yù huà huǒ 肝郁化火, liver depression transforming into fire, 354

gān yù jīng xíng hòu qī 肝郁经行后期, liver depression delayed menstruation, 353

gān yù jīng xíng xiān qī 肝郁经行先期, liver depression advanced menstruation, 353

gān yù pí xū 肝郁脾虚, liver depression and spleen vacuity, 353

gān yù xié tòng 肝郁胁痛, liver depression rib-side pain, 353

gān zhàng 肝胀, liver distention, 355

gān zhě, jiāng jūn zhī guān, móu lǜ chū yān 肝者，将军之官，谋虑出焉, liver holds the office of general, whence strategies emanate, 358

gān zhě, pí jí zhī běn 肝者，罢极之本, liver is the root of resistance to fatigue, 359

gān zhèng 疳证, gan pattern, 238

gān zhǒng zhàng 疳肿胀, gan swelling and distention, 238

gān zhǔ jīn 肝主筋, liver governs the sinews, 358

gān zhǔ jīng 肝主惊, liver governs fright, 357

gān zhǔ móu lǜ 肝主谋虑, liver governs the making of strategies, 358

gān zhǔ mù 肝主目, liver governs the eyes, 357

gān zhǔ shēng fā 肝主升发, liver governs upbearing effusion, 358

gān zhǔ shū xiè 肝主疏泄, liver governs free coursing, 357

gān zhǔ xuè hǎi 肝主血海, liver governs the sea of blood, 358

gān zhǔ yùn dòng 肝主运动, liver governs physical movement, 357

gān zhuó 肝着, liver fixity, 356

gān, qí huá zài zhǎo 肝，其华在爪, liver, its bloom is in the nails, 359

gān, tǐ yīn ér yòng yáng 肝，体阴而用阳, liver is yin in substance and yang in function, 359

gǎn 感, contraction, 97

gǎn lǎn 橄榄 Chinese olive, Canarii Albi Fructus, 68, 721

gǎn mào 感冒, common cold, 91

gǎn mào èr fāng 感冒二方, Common Cold Formula 2, 729

gǎn mào tóu tòng 感冒头痛, common cold headache, 92

gǎn mào tuì rè chōng jì 感冒退热冲剂, Common Cold Fever-Abating Granules, 730

gāng cì (jìng) 刚痉, hard tetany, 254

gāng jìng 刚痉, hard tetany, 254

gāng liè 肛裂, splitting of the anus, 565

gāng lòu 肛漏, anal fistula, 8

gāng mén 肛门, anus, 9

gāng mén yōng 肛门痈, anal welling-abscess, 9

gāng zàng 刚脏, unyielding viscus, 638

Ganoderma, *líng zhī* 灵芝, ganoderma, 491, 726

ganoderma, *líng zhī* 灵芝, Ganoderma, 491, 726

gāo 膏, gao, 239

gāo 膏, paste, 429

gāo 睪, testicle, 606

gāo fà jiān 膏发煎, Lard and Hair Brew, 653

gāo fēng què mù nèi zhàng 高风雀目内障, high-altitude wind sparrow-vision internal obstruction, 291

gāo huāng 膏肓, gao-huang, 239

gāo huāng shū 膏肓俞, BL-43, Gao-Huang Transport, 15, 72, 83, 87, 88, 95, 97, 146, 156, 158, 161, 163, 169, 201, 237, 251, 267, 282, 291, 336, 372, 374, 378–380, 398, 409, 415, 416, 441, 467, 486, 489, 515, 524, 572, 595–597, 603, 630, 639, 640, 648, 649, 664, 678, 683, 702, 714, 715, 747

gāo jì 膏剂, paste preparation, 429

gāo lì shēn 高丽参 Korean ginseng, Ginseng Radix Coreensis, 593, 726

gāo liáng hòu wèi 膏粱厚味, fat meat, fine grain, and strong flavors, 195

gāo liáng jiāng 高良姜 lesser galangal, Alpiniae Officinarum Rhizoma, 84, 581, 660, 662, 663, 723

gāo lín 膏淋, unctuous strangury, 636

gāo lín tāng 膏淋汤, Unctuous Strangury Decoction, 743

gāo wán 睾丸, testicle, 606

gāo yào 膏药, plaster, 445

gāo zī 膏滋, rich paste, 507

gǎo běn 藁本 Chinese lovage, Ligustici Sinensis Rhizoma et Radix, 55, 103, 654, 680, 681, 720

garden balsam flower, *fèng xiān huā* 凤仙花, Impatientis Balsaminae Flos, 11

gardenia, *shān zhī zǐ* 山栀子, Gardeniae Fructus, 20, 21, 67, 69–71, 81, 105, 116, 189, 230, 238, 263, 303, 310, 357, 386, 390, 414, 439, 462, 493, 500, 501, 526, 538, 539, 547, 548, 574, 577, 588, 589, 638, 656, 673, 714, 720

gardenia, *zhī zǐ* 栀子, Gardeniae Fructus, 524

Gardenia and Coptis Two Matured Ingredients Decoction, *zhī lián èr chén tāng* 栀连二陈汤, 4, 211, 443

Gardenia and Fermented Soybean Decoction, *zhī zǐ chǐ tāng* 栀子豉汤, 71, 284, 303, 652, 730

Gardenia and Magnolia Bark Decoction, *zhī zǐ hòu pò tāng* 栀子厚朴汤, 730

Gardenia and Phellodendron Decoction, *zhī zǐ bǎi pí tāng* 栀子柏皮汤, 198, 700, 731

Gardenia and Rhubarb Decoction, *zhī zǐ dà huáng tāng* 栀子大黄汤, 349

gardenia husk, *shān zhī pí* 山栀皮, Gardeniae Epicarpium, 234

Gardenia Liver-Clearing Decoction, *zhī zǐ qīng gān tāng* 栀子清肝汤, 166, 244

Gardenia, Fresh Ginger, and Fermented Soybean Decoction, *zhī zǐ shēng jiāng chǐ tāng* 栀子生姜豉汤, 730

Gardenia, Licorice, and Fermented Soybean Decoction, *zhī zǐ gān cǎo chǐ tāng* 栀子甘草豉汤, 730

Gardeniae Epicarpium, *shān zhī pí* 山栀皮, gardenia husk, 234

Gardeniae Fructus, *shān zhī zǐ* 山栀子, gardenia, 20, 21, 67, 69–71, 81, 105, 116, 189, 230, 238, 263, 303, 310, 357, 386, 390, 414, 439, 462, 493, 500, 501, 526, 538, 539, 547, 548, 574, 577, 588, 589, 638, 656, 673, 714, 720

Gardeniae Fructus, *zhī zǐ* 栀子, gardenia, 524

Gardeniae Fructus Carbonisatus, *hēi shān zhī zǐ* 黑山栀子, charred gardenia, 120, 459

Gardeniae Fructus Recens, *shēng shān zhī* 生山栀, fresh gardenia, 116

garlic, *dà suàn* 大蒜, Allii Sativi Bulbus, 111, 183, 445, 728

garlic juice, *suàn zhī* 蒜汁, Allii Sativi Bulbi Succus, 307

gastric neurosis*, 580

gastric ulcer*, 483

gastritis*, 218
  acute, 143, 284, 499
  chronic, 63, 123, 483, 615

gastrodia, *tiān má* 天麻, Gastrodiae Rhizoma, 53, 54, 56, 225, 257, 417, 690, 726

Gastrodia and Astragalus Decoction, *shēng má huáng qí tāng* 升麻黄芪汤, 15

Gastrodia and Uncaria Beverage, *tiān má gōu téng yǐn* 天麻钩藤饮, 11, 178, 292, 365, 417, 526, 568, 574, 689, 716, 740

Gastrodia Pill, *tiān má wán* 天麻丸, 691

Gastrodiae Rhizoma, *tiān má* 天麻, gastrodia, 53, 54, 56, 225, 257, 417, 690, 726

gastroenteritis*
  acute, 61, 254

Gate-Freeing Powder, *tōng guān sǎn* 通关散, 740

Gate-Opening Powder, *kāi guān sǎn* 开关散, 745

Gateway to Medicine (*yī xué rù mén*) 医学入门, 1515 (Míng), Lǐ Yán 李延, 317, 435, 550, 600, 614, 671

GB-1, *tóng zǐ liáo* 瞳子髎, Pupil Bone-Hole, 64, 93, 150, 195, 252, 320, 395, 495, 520, 568, 748

GB-2, *tīng huì* 听会, Auditory Convergence, 75, 89, 119, 160, 166, 167, 296, 320, 330, 336, 348, 474, 521, 566, 614, 658, 748

GB-3, *shàng guān* 上关, Upper Gate, 194, 222, 253, 748

GB-4, *hàn yàn* 颔厌, Forehead Fullness, 235, 365, 748

GB-5, *xuán lú* 悬颅, Suspended Skull, 748

GB-6, *xuán lí* 悬厘, Suspended Tuft, 222, 253, 748

GB-7, *qū bìn* 曲鬓, Temporal Hairline Curve, 219, 748

GB-8, *shuài gǔ* 率谷, Valley Lead, 89, 219, 258, 260, 288, 344, 506, 519, 748

GB-9, *tiān chòng* 天冲, Celestial Hub, 748

GB-10, *fú bái* 浮白, Floating White, 219, 748

GB-11, *tóu qiào yīn* 头窍阴, Head Orifice Yin, 219, 748

GB-12, *wán gǔ* 完骨, Completion Bone, 219, 247, 748

GB-13, *běn shén* 本神, Root Spirit, 748

GB-14, *yáng bái* 阳白, Yang White, 89, 125, 140, 150, 194, 253, 258, 520, 586, 689, 748

GB-15, *tóu lín qì* (头)临泣, (Head) Overlooking Tears, 150, 219, 495, 520, 682, 748

GB-16, *mù chuāng* 目窗, Eye Window, 748

GB-17, *zhèng yíng* 正营, Upright Construction, 748

GB-18, *chéng líng* 承灵, Spirit Support, 748

GB-19, *nǎo kōng* 脑空, Brain Hollow, 120, 331, 365, 654, 748

GB-20, *fēng chí* 风池, Wind Pool, 8, 11, 14, 50, 53, 60–63, 66, 69, 73, 74, 87, 89, 91–93, 99, 103, 105, 119, 120, 125, 129, 139, 140, 145, 146, 150, 155, 158, 166, 167, 169, 175, 176, 178, 181, 184, 185, 192, 194, 195, 203, 218, 225, 235, 247, 255, 256,

259, 260, 279, 287, 288, 290–292, 301, 310, 319, 320, 337, 341, 342, 344, 349, 355, 359, 362, 364–366, 368, 370, 374, 386, 391, 395, 405, 406, 415, 416, 442, 448, 450–452, 454–458, 462, 468, 474, 478, 495, 499, 501, 508, 515–517, 521, 530, 544, 546, 547, 568, 569, 580, 585, 586, 591, 611, 620, 631, 636, 643, 674, 677, 680–691, 693, 694, 701, 702, 713, 716, 748

GB-21, *jiān jǐng* 肩井, Shoulder Well, 61, 128, 142, 253, 307, 385, 386, 503, 515, 530, 606, 748

GB-22, *yuān yè* 渊腋, Armpit Abyss, 748

GB-23, *zhé jīn* 辄筋, Sinew Seat, 748

GB-24, *rì yuè* 日月, Sun and Moon, 8, 20, 88, 91, 112, 219, 235, 302, 357, 480, 590, 658, 748

GB-25, *jīng mén* 京门, Capital Gate, 8, 91, 291, 461, 748

GB-26, *dài mài* 带脉, Girdling Vessel, 57, 93, 94, 118, 160, 241, 242, 330, 334, 353, 418, 435, 497, 522, 563, 658, 675, 677, 748

GB-27, *wǔ shū* 五枢, Fifth Pivot, 242, 748

GB-28, *wéi dào* 维道, Linking Path, 242, 711, 748

GB-29, *jū liáo* 居髎, Squatting Bone-Hole, 296, 748

GB-30, *huán tiào* 环跳, Jumping Round, 47, 61, 89, 104, 137, 212, 219, 220, 289, 296, 323, 382, 410, 418, 567, 654, 679, 689, 748

GB-31, *fēng shì* 风市, Wind Market, 28, 47, 104, 139, 145, 154, 289, 342, 370, 418, 532, 591, 658, 674, 688, 748

GB-32, *zhōng dú* 中渎, Central River, 19, 89, 519, 748

GB-33, *xī yáng guān* 膝阳关, Knee Yang Joint, 61, 104, 137, 154, 296, 337, 521, 567, 748

GB-34, *yáng líng quán* 阳陵泉, Yang Mound Spring, 3, 4, 6, 11, 14, 19, 20, 26, 30, 31, 47, 51, 57, 61, 66, 75, 80, 88, 89, 93, 104, 110, 112, 115, 118, 120, 123, 127, 138, 139, 147, 151, 154, 157, 158, 164, 166, 167, 169, 178, 194, 202, 203, 215–217, 229, 230, 234–236, 240, 241, 256, 257, 263, 268, 269, 281, 288, 289, 293, 296, 297, 302, 310, 314, 330, 337, 342, 349, 355–359, 361, 362, 366, 369, 374, 382, 393, 395, 445, 450, 452, 453, 456–458, 462, 474, 475, 478, 480, 482–485, 504, 511, 516, 519–522, 530, 534, 538, 540, 546, 554, 561, 564, 586, 587, 589–591, 597, 606, 614, 637, 641, 650, 654, 656, 658, 679, 683, 689, 695, 700, 710, 713, 748

GB-35, *yáng jiāo* 阳交, Yang Intersection, 748

GB-36, *wài qiū* 外丘, Outer Hill, 748

GB-37, *guāng míng* 光明, Bright Light, 64, 90, 291, 406, 408, 495, 549, 586, 606, 748

GB-38, *yáng fǔ* 阳辅, Yang Assistance, 20, 61, 142, 515, 748

GB-39, *jué gǔ* 绝骨, Severed Bone, 11, 197, 310, 331, 508

GB-39, *xuán zhōng* 悬钟, Suspended Bell, 47, 61, 80, 89, 105, 112, 115, 120, 138, 154, 160, 289, 296, 329–331, 336, 342, 540, 652, 679, 748

GB-40, *qiū xū* 丘墟, Hill Ruins, 3, 4, 19, 20, 90, 118, 137, 189, 215, 216, 236, 255, 296, 342, 344, 355, 394, 446, 474, 521, 538, 548, 567, 748

GB-41, *zú lín qì* 足临泣, Foot Overlooking Tears, 8, 33, 75, 89, 90, 93, 112, 142, 162, 195, 220, 221, 231, 320, 386, 474, 500, 515, 606, 716, 748

GB-42, *dì wǔ huì* 地五会, Earth Fivefold Convergence, 748

GB-43, *xiá xī* 侠溪, Pinched Ravine, 11, 20, 66, 93, 119, 147, 158, 167, 175, 176, 235, 240, 241, 263, 281, 292, 337, 344, 355, 356, 359, 364–366, 462, 495, 511, 519, 538, 568, 585, 601, 614, 656, 658, 689, 713, 748

GB-44, *zú qiào yīn* 足窍阴, Foot Orifice Yin, 75, 147, 148, 220, 333, 413, 420, 521, 538, 546, 748

gé 膈, diaphragm, 125

gé bǐng jiǔ 隔饼灸, moxibustion on cake, 402

gé fěn 蛤粉 clamshell powder, Cyclinae (seu Meretricis) Concha Pulverata, 319

gé fěn chǎo 蛤粉炒, stir-frying with clamshell powder, 573

gé gēn 葛根 pueraria, Puerariae Radix, 47, 55, 103, 176, 214, 246, 346, 422, 501, 599, 600, 685, 686, 699, 720

gé gēn huáng qín huáng lián tāng 葛根黄芩黄连汤, Pueraria, Scutellaria, and Coptis Decoction, 731

gé gēn qín lián tāng 葛根芩连汤, Pueraria, Scutellaria, and Coptis Decoction, 110, 278

gé gēn tāng 葛根汤, Pueraria Decoction, 73, 105, 729

gé guān 膈关, BL-46, Diaphragm Pass, 164, 747

gé huā 葛花 pueraria flower, Puerariae Flos, 415

gé huā jiě chéng tāng 葛花解酲汤, Pueraria Flower Liquor-Resolving Decoction, 257, 348, 349, 732

gé huáng wán 葛黄丸, Coptis and Pueraria Flower Pill, 502

gé jiāng jiǔ 隔姜灸, moxibustion on ginger, 402

gé jiè 蛤蚧 gecko, Gekko, 511, 526, 593, 726

gé mài 革脉, drumskin pulse, 152

gé shū 膈俞, BL-17, Diaphragm Transport, 4, 15, 24, 26–30, 32–41, 53, 58, 59, 63, 64, 72, 73, 82, 87, 99, 118, 123, 127, 138–140, 145, 149, 152, 159, 161, 162, 164, 168, 169, 175, 212, 223, 227, 228, 230, 251, 256, 260, 261, 265–269, 271–274, 279, 280, 288, 291, 292, 297, 332, 333, 336, 339, 348, 349, 352, 356, 359, 362, 366, 390, 393, 410, 415, 416, 422, 426, 438, 445, 447, 449–454, 456–458, 461, 462, 475, 480, 482–484, 493, 499, 503, 511, 516, 522, 533, 534, 537, 540, 552, 563, 566, 568, 570, 571, 586, 591, 596, 597, 601, 604, 607, 608, 613, 646, 649, 652, 654, 661, 674, 684, 686, 689, 690, 696, 714, 747

gé shuǐ dùn 隔水炖, double-boiling, 145

gé tán 膈痰, diaphragm phlegm, 125

gé xià zhú yū tāng 膈下逐瘀汤, Infradiaphragmatic Stasis-Expelling Decoction, 24, 26, 35, 36, 152, 570, 647, 710, 737

gé xiāo 膈消, diaphragmatic dispersion, 125

gé yáng 格阳, repelled yang, 498

gecko, *gé jiè* 蛤蚧, Gekko, 511, 526, 593, 726

Gekko, *gé jiè* 蛤蚧, gecko, 511, 526, 593, 726

Gekko Swinhoana, *bì hǔ* 壁虎, house lizard, 728

Gelsemii Herba, *gōu wěn* 钩吻, yellow jessamine, 97

gēn gǔ 跟骨, heel bone, 288

gén suàn jiǔ 隔蒜灸, moxibustion on garlic, 402

gén yán jiǔ 隔盐灸, moxibustion on salt, 403

Generalized Pain Stasis-Expelling Decoction, *shēn tòng zhú yū tāng* 身痛逐瘀汤, 138, 737

gēng jīn 庚金, S7-metal, 511

gēng yī wán 更衣丸, Toilette Pill, 459, 732

genkwa, *yuán huā* 芫花, Daphnes Genkwa Flos, 44, 97, 182, 460, 574, 722

gentian, *lóng dǎn* 龙胆, Gentianae Radix, 19, 66, 67, 357, 459, 720

Gentian Liver-Draining Decoction, *lóng dǎn xiè gān tāng* 龙胆泻肝汤, 20, 63, 66, 73, 93, 104, 111, 112, 119, 147, 166, 167, 172, 200, 235, 241, 297, 352, 355, 356, 359, 365, 412, 415, 424, 462, 468, 474, 495, 497, 511, 516, 533, 538–540, 566, 614, 656, 658, 671, 676, 677, 701, 711–713, 731

Gentianae Macrophyllae Radix, *qín jiāo* 秦艽, large gentian, 72, 139, 167, 263, 451, 722

Gentianae Radix, *lóng dǎn* 龙胆, gentian, 19, 66, 67, 357, 459, 720

Geranii Herba, *lǎo guàn cǎo* 老鹳草, cranesbill, 140, 722

giant typhonium tuber, *yǔ bái fù* 禹白附, Typhonii Gigantei Tuber, 623, 725

ginger, *jiāng* 姜, Zingiberis Rhizoma, 154, 217

Ginger and Aconite Decoction, *jiāng fù tāng* 姜附汤, 80, 81, 86

ginger juice, *jiāng zhī* 姜汁, Zingiberis Rhizomatis Succus, 116, 448

ginger pinellia, *jiāng bàn xià* 姜半夏, Pinelliae Tuber cum Zingibere Praeparatum, 47, 97, 257, 317, 421, 623, 725

ginger skin, *jiāng pí* 姜皮, Zingiberis Rhizomatis Cortex, 153, 262, 681, 720

Gingerless Clove and Persimmon Powder, *shì qián sǎn* 柿钱散, 736

ginkgo, *bái guǒ* 白果, Ginkgo Semen, 57, 624, 725

ginkgo husk, *bái guǒ ké* 白果壳, Ginkgo Testa, 241

Ginkgo Semen, *bái guǒ* 白果, ginkgo, 57, 624, 725

Ginkgo Testa, *bái guǒ ké* 白果壳, ginkgo husk, 241

ginseng, *rén shēn* 人参, Ginseng Radix, 47, 84, 183, 223, 236, 251, 255, 259, 270, 325, 334, 345, 384, 392, 395, 411, 448, 450, 455–457, 480, 495, 499, 503, 504, 525, 527, 572, 593–595, 600, 612, 649, 651, 661, 698, 713, 716, 726

Ginseng and Aconite Decoction, *shēn fù tāng* 参附汤, 27, 59, 62, 83, 84, 232, 335, 448, 629, 631, 690, 699, 702, 713, 735

Ginseng and Astragalus Powder, *rén shēn huáng qí sǎn* 人参黄芪散, 175, 742

Ginseng and Gecko Powder, *rén shēn gé jiè sǎn* 人参蛤蚧散, 629, 741

Ginseng and Perilla Beverage, *shēn sū yǐn* 参苏饮, 47, 51, 428, 517, 730

Ginseng and Walnut Decoction, *rén shēn hú táo tāng* 人参胡桃汤, 741

Ginseng Center-Fortifying Decoction, *rén shēn jiàn zhōng tāng* 人参建中汤, 713

Ginseng Construction-Nourishing Decoction (Pill), *rén shēn yǎng róng tāng* (*wán*) 人参养荣汤 (丸), 540

Ginseng Construction-Nourishing Decoction (Pill), *rén-shēn yǎng róng tāng* (*wán*) 人参养荣汤 (丸), 741

Ginseng Construction-Nourishing Decoction, *rén shēn yǎng róng tāng* 人参养荣汤, 26, 27, 32, 38, 40, 116, 143, 150, 174, 213, 271, 449, 456, 461, 650, 675

Ginseng Decoction, *rén shēn tāng* 人参汤, 654, 735

Ginseng Lung-Clearing Decoction, *rén shēn qīng fèi tāng* 人参清肺汤, 143

Ginseng Radix, *rén shēn* 人参, ginseng, 47, 84, 183, 223, 236, 251, 255, 259, 270, 325, 334, 345, 384, 392, 395, 411, 448, 450, 455–457, 480, 495, 499, 503, 504, 525, 527, 572, 593–595, 600, 612, 649, 651, 661, 698, 713, 716, 726

Ginseng Radix Coreensis, *gāo lì shēn* 高丽参, Korean ginseng, 593, 726

Ginseng Radix Rubra, *hóng shēn* 红参, red ginseng, 593, 726

Ginseng Rhizoma, *rén shēn lú* 人参芦, ginseng top, 170, 511, 727

Ginseng Root-Securing Pill, *rén shēn gù běn wán* 人参固本丸, 175, 378, 742

Ginseng Spleen-Arousing Pill, *rén shēn qǐ pí wán* 人参启脾丸, 736

Ginseng Spleen-Fortifying Pill, *rén shēn jiàn pí wán* 人参健脾丸, 741

Ginseng Spleen-Returning Pill, *rén shēn guī pí wán* 人参归脾丸, 271

Ginseng Stomach Wind Decoction, *rén shēn wèi fēng tāng* 人参胃风汤, 318

ginseng top, *rén shēn lú* 人参芦, Ginseng Rhizoma, 170, 511, 727

Ginseng Tops Beverage, *shēn lú yǐn* 参芦饮, 170, 743

Ginseng Toxin-Vanquishing Powder, *rén shēn bài dú sǎn* 人参败毒散, 258, 730

Ginseng with Gecko Powder, *shēn jiè sǎn* 参蛤散, 335, 741

Ginseng, Aconite, Dragon Bone, and Oyster Shell Decoction, *shēn fù lóng mǔ tāng* 参附龙牡汤, 59, 232, 735

Ginseng, Poria (Hoelen), and Ovate Atractylodes Powder, *shēn líng bái zhú sǎn* 参苓白术散, 163, 197, 237, 238, 393, 395, 486, 557, 558, 562–565, 601, 679, 741

gizzard lining, *jī nèi jīn* 鸡内金, Galli Gigerii Endothelium, 141, 216, 385, 420, 544, 582, 606, 665, 724

glabella*, 252

glauberite, *hán shuǐ shí* 寒水石, Gypsum seu Calcitum, 17, 67, 720

glaucoma*, 249, 260, 494

gleditsia, *zào jiá* 皂荚, Gleditsiae Fructus, 5, 170, 214, 244, 405, 419, 434, 624, 625, 725, 727

Gleditsia and Flavescent Sophora Pill, *zào jiǎo kǔ shēn wán* 皂角苦参丸, 395

gleditsia thorn, *zào jiǎo cì* 皂角刺, Gleditsiae Spina, 315, 398, 516, 624, 725

Gleditsiae Fructus, *zào jiá* 皂荚, gleditsia, 5, 170, 214, 244, 405, 419, 434, 624, 625, 725, 727

Gleditsiae Fructus Parvus, *zhū yá zào* 猪牙皂, small gleditsia, 243, 690

Gleditsiae Spina, *zào jiǎo cì* 皂角刺, gleditsia thorn, 315, 398, 516, 624, 725

glehnia, *běi shā shēn* 北沙参, Glehniae Radix, 175, 256, 593, 597, 727

Glehniae Radix, *běi shā shēn* 北沙参, glehnia, 175, 256, 593, 597, 727

globeflower, *jīn lián huā* 金莲花, Trollii Flos, 68, 721

globus hystericus*, 445

Glomus Qi Pill, *pǐ qì wán* 痞气丸, 242

Glomus Root, *pǐ gēn* 痞根, 24, 26, 34, 138, 215, 384, 399, 544, 695

Glomus-Dispersing Asafetida Pill, *xiāo pǐ ē wèi wán* 消痞阿魏丸, 736

glutinous rice, *nuò mǐ* 糯米, Oryzae Glutinosae Semen, 251

glutinous rice root, *nuò dào gēn xū* 糯稻根须, Oryzae Glutinosae Rhizoma et Radix, 95, 410, 518, 727

Glycines Lactis Residuum, *dòu fǔ zhā* 豆腐渣, bean curd dregs, 104

Glycines Semen Atrum, *hēi dà dòu* 黑大豆, black soybean, 54, 108, 726

Glycines Semen Fermentatum Insulsum, *dàn dòu chǐ* 淡豆豉, fermented soybean, 70, 130, 176, 184, 402, 410, 481, 501, 686, 720

Glycines Semen Germinatum Exsiccatum, *dà dòu huáng juǎn* 大豆黄卷, dried soybean sprout, 686, 720

glycosuria*, 142

Glycyrrhizae Radix, *gān cǎo* 甘草, licorice, 11, 17, 20, 47, 84, 108, 110, 115, 129, 141, 154, 161, 192, 214, 223, 227, 228, 230, 241, 255, 256, 259, 263, 285, 292, 315, 343, 378, 387, 390, 392, 394, 416, 430, 455, 463, 464, 486, 495, 498, 504, 526, 548, 556, 567, 580, 589, 593–595, 600, 662, 671, 687, 726

Glycyrrhizae Radix Cruda, *shēng gān cǎo* 生甘草, raw licorice, 17, 116, 175, 263, 310, 422, 439, 499, 516, 621

goat's kidney, *yáng shèn* 羊肾, Caprae seu Ovis Renes, 333

goiter*
    endemic, 480

Goiter-Dispersing Decoction, *xiāo yǐng tāng* 消瘿汤, 737

Gold Liquid and Jade Humor, *jīn jīn yù yè* 金津玉液, 37, 125, 160, 174, 186, 284, 289, 336, 348, 455, 456, 573, 587, 607

Golden Coffer Kidney Qi Pill, *jīn guì shèn qì wán* 金匮肾气丸, 24, 36, 44, 86, 117, 148, 163, 240, 265, 331, 334, 415, 440, 461, 523, 529, 569, 604, 608, 647, 664, 669, 703

golden larch (root) bark, *tǔ jīng pí* 土荆皮, Pseudolaricis Kaempferi Cortex (Radicis), 41, 728

Golden Lock Essence-Securing Pill, *jīn suǒ gù jīng wán* 金锁固精丸, 11, 12, 147, 308, 461, 518, 524, 743

Golden Mirror of Medicine (*yī zōng jīn jiàn*) 医宗金鉴, 1742 (Qīng), Wú Qiān 吴谦 ed., 17, 60, 232, 259, 386, 395, 461, 482, 678

Golden Three Decoction, *sān jīn tāng* 三金汤, 733

Golden Yellow Paste, *jīn huáng gāo* 金黄膏, 323, 528, 671

Golden Yellow Powder, *jīn huáng sǎn* 金黄散, 187, 259, 386, 494, 540, 744

Gone-in-One-Sweep, *yī sǎo guāng* 一扫光, 744

gōng 宫, palace, 426

gōng 攻, attack, 12

gōng 攻, offensive treatment, 419

gōng bǔ jiān shī 攻补兼施, simultaneous supplementation and attack, 532

gōng kuì 攻溃, offensive bursting, 419

gōng lǐ bù yuǎn hán 攻里不远寒, interior attack does not shun cold, 311

gōng sūn 公孙, SP-4, Yellow Emperor, 3, 4, 28, 63, 77, 81, 83, 85–87, 90, 92, 141, 156, 164, 186, 197, 215, 216, 218, 314, 349, 353, 358, 362, 408, 425, 426, 437, 442, 443, 478, 487, 490, 499, 510, 519, 522, 551, 557–559, 562, 564, 565, 571, 575, 577–579, 608, 633, 647, 663, 669, 673, 703, 710, 746

gōng tán 攻痰, attacking phlegm, 12

gōng wài yùn èr hào fāng 宫外孕二号方, Ectopic Pregnancy Formula No.II, 737

gōng xiāo hé jiě ruǎn jiān tāng 攻消和解软坚汤, Offensive Dispersion Harmonizing and Softening Decoction, 737

gōng xiào 功效, action, 5

gǒng tí wán 巩堤丸, Dyke-Strengthening Pill, 23, 743

Good Remedies for Women (*fù rén liáng fāng*) 妇人良方, 1237 (Sòng), Chén Zì-Míng 陈自明, 454

goose throat stone, *é guǎn shí* 鹅管石, Balanophyllia seu Stalactitum, 460, 624, 726

goral horn, *shān yáng jiǎo* 山羊角, Naemorhedi Goral Cornu, 54, 726

Gosling Yellow Powder, *é huáng sǎn* 鹅黄散, 494

gōu gē fǎ 钩割法, hooking and cutting, 292

gōu téng 钩藤 uncaria, Uncariae Ramulus cum Unco, 7, 53, 54, 65, 146, 176, 225, 230, 452, 453, 526, 562, 591, 652, 726

gōu téng sǎn 钩藤散, Uncaria Powder, 292, 739

gōu téng tāng 钩藤汤, Uncaria Decoction, 740

gōu téng yǐn 钩藤饮, Uncaria Beverage, 140, 279, 740

gōu wěn 钩吻 yellow jessamine, Gelsemii Herba, 97

gǒu gǔ 狗骨 dog's bone, Canis Os, 139, 722

gǒu jǐ 狗脊 cibotium, Cibotii Rhizoma, 593, 727

gǒu pí gāo 狗皮膏, Dog Skin Plaster, 744

gǒu qǐ zǐ 枸杞子 lycium berry, Lycii Fructus, 19, 28, 37, 88, 104, 172, 175, 225, 256, 310, 333, 352, 458, 467, 541, 584, 593, 595, 727

gòu 垢, grimy, 249

gout*, 82, 280

Granati Pericarpium, *shí liú pí* 石榴皮, pomegranate rind, 183, 298, 318, 445, 518, 727

Granorum Saccharon, *yí táng* 饴糖, malt sugar, 148, 511, 580, 593, 600, 602, 726

granulated sugar, *shā táng* 沙糖, Saccharon Granulatum, 511

grape mole*, 615

Great Compendium of Acupuncture and Moxibustion (*zhēn jiǔ dà chéng*) 针灸大成, 1601 (Míng), Yáng Jì-Zhōu 杨继洲, 225

Great Compendium of External Medicine (*wài kē dà chéng*) 外科大成, 1665 (Qīng), Qí Kūn 祁坤, 303, 528

Great Creation Pill, *dà zào wán* 大造丸, 147, 742

Great Peace Sagacious Benevolence Formulary (*tài píng shèng huì fāng*) 太平圣惠方, 992 (Sòng), Wáng Huái-Yǐn 王怀隐 et. al. ed., 363, 508, 693

Great Rectifying Powder, *dà shùn sǎn* 大顺散, 74, 662, 735

Great Rock Honey Decoction, *dà yán mì tāng* 大岩蜜汤, 451, 452, 454

Great Tranquility Pill, *dà ān wán* 大安丸, 564, 645, 736

great trochanter*, 607

Greater Yang, *tài yáng* 太阳, 11, 50, 62, 63, 79, 88, 89, 92, 111, 129, 181, 194, 217, 247, 258, 260, 287, 288, 301, 320, 344, 365, 395, 435, 437, 440, 462, 478, 495, 506, 520, 568, 586, 610, 681–687, 689, 691, 694

Green Wind Antelope Horn Beverage, *lǜ fēng líng yáng yǐn* 绿风羚羊饮, 248, 249

Green-Blue Unicorn Pill, *qīng lín wán* 青麟丸, 733

Green-Blue–Draining Half-and-Half Decoction, *xiè qīng gè bàn tāng* 泻清各半汤, 353, 401

Green-Blue–Draining Pill, *xiè qīng wán* 泻青丸, 6, 51, 359, 731

groove*
    mentolabial, 512

Grosvenor's momordica, *luó hàn guǒ* 罗汉果, Momordicae Grosvenori Fructus, 624, 725

ground pine, *shēn jīn cǎo* 伸筋草, Lycopodii Clavati Herba cum Radice, 140, 569, 722

Gryllotalpa, *lóu gū* 蝼蛄, mole cricket, 98, 136, 723

gū yáng shàng yuè 孤阳上越, solitary yang straying upward, 545

gǔ 骨, bone, 44

gǔ 鼓, drum distention, 150

gǔ 臌, drum distention, 150

gǔ 蛊, gu, 249

gǔ 股, thigh, 607

gǔ bì 骨痹, bone impediment, 45

gǔ cáo fēng 骨槽风, bone trough wind, 46

gǔ dú 蛊毒, gu toxin, 250

gǔ dù 骨度, bone standard, 45

gǔ gān 骨疳, gan of the bone, 237

gǔ gěng 骨鲠, bones stuck in the throat, 45

gǔ jié 骨节, joint, 322

gǔ jié téng tòng 骨节疼痛, joint pain, 322

gǔ jīn yī tǒng dà quán 古今医统大全 (*Complete Compendium of Medical Works, Ancient and Modern*), 1556 (Míng), Xú Chūn-Fǔ 徐春甫, 548

gǔ jū 骨疽, bone flat-abscess, 45

gǔ liú 骨瘤, bone tumor, 46

gǔ shāng 骨伤, bone damage, 44

gǔ shí 骨蚀, bone erosion, 44

gǔ suān 骨酸, aching bones, 3

gǔ suì bǔ 骨碎补 drynaria, Drynariae Rhizoma, 45, 367, 593, 727

gǔ tòng 骨痛, bone pain, 45

gǔ wěi 骨痿, bone wilting, 46

gǔ yá 谷芽 rice sprout, Oryzae Fructus Germinatus, 23, 141, 420, 499, 563, 724

gǔ yīn 股阴, yin of the thigh, 711

gǔ zhàng 鼓胀, drum distention, 150

gǔ zhàng 臌胀, drum distention, 150

gǔ zhàng 蛊胀, gu distention, 250

gǔ zhé 骨折, bone fracture, 45

gǔ zhēng 骨蒸, steaming bone, 572

gǔ zhēng cháo rè 骨蒸潮热, steaming bone tidal heat [effusion], 572

gǔ zhí zēng shēng wán 骨质增生丸, Hyperosteogeny Pill, 741

gù 固, secure, 517

gù 固, stem, 572

gù běn wán 固本丸, Root-Securing Pill, 325

gù běn zhǐ bēng tāng 固本止崩汤, Root-Securing Flood-Stanching Decoction, 212, 743

gù bēng zhǐ dài 固崩止带, stemming flooding and checking (vaginal) discharge, 572

gù cháng wán 固肠丸, Intestine-Securing Pill, 168

gù chōng tāng 固冲汤, Thoroughfare-Securing Decoction, 478, 743

gù jīng 固经, securing the menses, 519

gù jīng 固精, securing essence, 518

gù jīng wán 固经丸, Menses-Securing Pill, 572, 743

gù pāo tāng 固脬汤, Bladder-Securing Decoction, 743

gù pāo wán 固脬丸, Bladder-Securing Pill, 465

gù sè fǎ 固涩法, securing and astriction, 517

gù shèn nà qì 固肾纳气, securing the kidney to promote qi absorption, 519

gù shèn sè jīng 固肾涩精, securing the kidney and astringing essence, 518

gù yīn jiān 固阴煎, Yin-Securing Brew, 331, 332, 369, 393

gù zhēn tāng 固真汤, True-Securing Decoction, 122

gù zhēn wán 固真丸, True-Securing Pill, 743

guā dì 瓜蒂 melon stalk, Cucumeris Melonis Pedicellus, 170, 727

guā dì sǎn 瓜蒂散, Melon Stalk Powder, 128, 170, 254, 743

guā dì shén miào sǎn 瓜蒂神妙散, Melon Stalk Wonder Powder, 744

guā dīng sǎn 瓜丁散, Melon Pedicel Powder, 744

guā fǎ 刮法, needle scratching, 407

guā lóu 栝楼 trichosanthes, Trichosanthis Fructus, 201, 230, 282, 376, 388, 398, 399, 614, 624, 625, 725

guā lóu guì zhī tāng 栝楼桂枝汤 Trichosanthes and Cinnamon Twig Decoction, 544

guā lóu niú bàng tāng 瓜蒌牛蒡汤, Trichosanthes and Arctium Decoction, 386, 743

guā lóu pí 栝楼皮 trichosanthes rind, Trichosanthis Pericarpium, 70, 107, 624, 725

guā lóu rén shuāng 栝楼仁霜 trichosanthes seed frost, Trichosanthis Seminis Pulvis, 127, 231

guā lóu xiè bái bái jiǔ tāng 栝楼薤白白酒汤, Trichosanthes, Chinese Chive, and White Liquor Decoction, 58, 228, 273, 735

guā lóu xiè bái bàn xià tāng 栝楼薤白半夏汤, Trichosanthes, Chinese Chive, and Pinellia Decoction, 58, 59, 735

guā lóu zhǐ shí tāng 栝楼枳实汤, Trichosanthes and Unripe Bitter Orange Decoction, 735

guā lóu zǐ 栝楼子 trichosanthes seed, Trichosanthis Semen, 372, 399, 624, 637, 725

guā shā 刮痧, gua-sha, 249

guā shā 刮痧, sand scraping, 512

guà jīn dēng 挂金灯 lantern plant calyx, Physalis Alkekengi Calyx, 68, 721

guà xiàn fǎ 挂线法, threaded ligation, 609

guān 关, bar, 16

guān 关, pass, 428

guān bái fù 关白附 Korean aconite, Aconiti Coreani Tuber, 623, 725

guān chōng 关冲, TB-1, Passage Hub, 14, 152, 167, 384, 394, 403, 420, 547, 590, 611, 715, 748

guān gé 关格, block and repulsion, 24

guān guì 官桂 quilled cinnamon, Cinnamomi Cortex Tubiformis, 45, 328

guān jié 关节, joint, 322

guān mén 关门, ST-22, Pass Gate, 746

guān xīn sū hé wán 冠心苏合丸, Coronary Liquid Storax Pill, 300, 740

guān yuán 关元, CV-4, Pass Head, 1, 3, 4, 8, 22, 23, 26, 28–33, 35, 36, 38, 39, 41, 45, 47, 51, 58, 59, 64, 71, 73, 74, 78–87, 89, 91, 94, 105, 109, 111, 119, 127, 128, 149, 152, 160, 161, 163, 168, 174, 175, 177, 180, 189, 196, 199, 210–212, 216, 217, 219–222, 224, 226–229, 231–233, 239, 240, 251, 263, 266, 267, 269–272, 274, 287–291, 296, 297, 300–302, 308, 309, 312, 314, 318, 319, 325, 329, 331–336, 338, 340, 342, 343, 345, 349, 352, 353, 360, 369, 370, 379, 380, 393, 418, 425, 426, 430, 435, 447–450, 452–454, 457, 461, 465–467, 477–479, 482, 487–489, 497, 499, 503, 504, 511, 513, 516, 518, 521–525, 529, 541–543, 549, 557, 559, 563, 564, 570, 578, 579, 586, 594, 595, 597, 600, 604, 608, 612, 614, 625, 629–631, 636, 640, 641, 643, 646, 647, 649–652, 656, 660, 662–664, 667, 668, 675, 678, 690, 693, 699, 702, 709, 710, 712, 713, 716, 749

guān yuán shū 关元俞, BL-26, Pass Head Transport, 747

guǎn zhēn fǎ 管针法, tube insertion, 631

guǎn zhēn jìn zhēn fǎ 管针进针法, tube insertion, 631

guàn xīn èr hào 冠心二号, Coronary No.2, 265, 484, 737

guàn zhòng 贯众 aspidium, Aspidii Rhizoma, 183, 445, 724

guāng míng 光明, GB-37, Bright Light, 64, 90, 291, 406, 408, 495, 549, 586, 606, 748

guāng míng dān 光明丹, Bright and Glorious Elixir, 744

guǎng fáng jǐ 广防己 southern fangji, Aristolochiae Fangchi Radix, 139, 722

guǎng míng 广明, broad and bright, 51

guǎng mù xiāng 广木香 costusroot, Saussureae Radix, 490, 493, 723

guǎng wēn yì lùn 广温疫论 (*On Warm Epidemics Expanded*), 1722 (Qīng), Dài Tiān-Zhāng 戴天章, 53, 349, 350

guī 归, return, 504

guī bǎn 龟版 tortoise plastron, Testudinis Plastrum, 53, 98, 175, 176, 310, 336, 352, 511, 524, 526, 593, 597, 614, 727

guī bǎn jiāo 龟版胶 tortoise plastron glue, Testudinis Plastri Gelatinum, 243, 593, 727

guī bèi 龟背, hunchback, 293

guī bèi 龟背, tortoise back, 621

guī bèi tán 龟背痰, tortoise's-back phlegm, 621

guī gé tāng 归葛汤, Tangkuei and Pueraria Decoction, 729

guī jīng 归经, channel entry, 56

guī lái 归来, ST-29, Return, 26, 35, 36, 94, 226, 300, 332, 447, 483, 484, 524, 643, 661, 746

guī lù èr xiān jiāo 龟鹿二仙胶, Tortoise Plastron and Deerhorn Two Immortals Glue, 741

guī pí tāng 归脾汤, Spleen-Returning Decoction, 32, 37–39, 41, 161, 162, 211, 223, 251, 265, 268, 271, 272, 289, 296, 311, 367, 409, 417, 427, 453, 461, 489, 502, 537, 551, 556, 561, 562, 595, 604, 646, 648, 651, 685, 694, 711, 741

guī pí wán 归脾丸, Spleen-Returning Pill, 348

guī qí jiàn zhōng tāng 归芪建中汤, Tangkuei and Astragalus Center-Fortifying Decoction, 650, 741

guī sháo dì huáng tāng 归芍地黄汤, Tangkuei, Peony, and Rehmannia Decoction, 741

guī sháo liù jūn wán 归芍六君丸, Tangkuei and Peony Six Gentlemen Pill, 741 *guī shū wán* 龟樗丸, Tortoise Plastron and Ailanthus Bark Pill, 115

guī tóu 龟头, tortoise's head, 621

guī tóu yōng 龟头痈, tortoise's head welling-abscess, 621

guī jiàn yǔ 鬼箭羽 spindle tree wings, Euonymi Lignum Suberalatum, 139, 338, 725

guī jiù 鬼臼 common dysosma, Dysosmae Versipellis Rhizoma, 503

guī mén 鬼门, ghost gate, 241

guī shì tóu 鬼舐头, demon-licked head, 122

guī shuǐ 癸水, S10-water, 511

guī yán 鬼言, ghost talk, 241

guī yǔ jiàn 鬼羽箭 buchnera, Buchnerae Herba, 98

guī zhēn cǎo 鬼针草 Spanish needles, Bidentis Bipinnatae Herba, 68, 721

guī zhù 鬼注, demonic influx, 122

guì fù bā wèi wán 桂附八味丸, Cinnamon Bark and Aconite Eight-Ingredient Pill, 174, 180, 288, 335, 369, 466, 579, 596, 629, 643, 646, 651, 702, 741

guì fù lǐ zhōng tāng 桂附理中汤, Cinnamon and Aconite Center-Rectifying Decoction, 734

guì líng gān lù yǐn 桂苓甘露饮 Cinnamon and Poria (Hoelen) Sweet Dew Beverage, 730

guì shè sǎn 桂麝散, Cinnamon Bark and Musk Powder, 243

guì shè sǎn 桂麝散, Cinnamon Twig and Musk Powder, 210, 744

guì xīn 桂心 shaved cinnamon bark, Cinnamomi Cortex Rasus, 242, 343

guì zhī 桂枝 cinnamon twig, Cinnamomi Ramulus, 11, 12, 17, 103, 136, 140, 184, 217, 218, 228, 246, 255, 391, 427, 438, 500–502, 526, 581, 654, 661–663, 666, 679, 681, 704, 716, 720

guì zhī fú líng wán 桂枝茯苓丸, Cinnamon Twig and Poria (Hoelen) Pill, 32, 140, 737

guì zhī fù zǐ tāng 桂枝附子汤, Cinnamon Twig and Aconite Decoction, 734

guì zhī gān cǎo lóng gǔ mǔ lì tāng 桂枝甘草龙骨牡蛎汤, Cinnamon Twig, Licorice, Dragon Bone, and Oyster Shell Decoction, 269, 274, 661

guì zhī gān cǎo tāng 桂枝甘草汤, Cinnamon Twig and Licorice Decoction, 427, 741

guì zhī jiā dà huáng tāng 桂枝加大黄汤, Cinnamon Twig Decoction Plus Rhubarb, 730

guì zhī jiā dāng guī tāng 桂枝加当归汤, Cinnamon Twig Decoction Plus Tangkuei, 528

guì zhī jiā fù zǐ tāng 桂枝加附子汤, Cinnamon Twig Decoction Plus Aconite, 145, 341, 529

guì zhī jiā gé gēn tāng 桂枝加葛根汤, Cinnamon Twig Decoction Plus Pueraria, 729

guì zhī jiā guì tāng 桂枝加桂汤, Cinnamon Twig Decoction Plus Extra Cinnamon, 510, 735

guì zhī jiā hòu pò xìng rén tāng 桂枝加厚朴杏仁汤, Cinnamon Twig Decoction Plus Magnolia Bark and Apricot Kernel, 729

guì zhī jiā huáng qí tāng 桂枝加黄芪汤, Cinnamon Twig Decoction Plus Astragalus, 704

guì zhī jiā lóng gǔ mǔ lì tāng 桂枝加龙骨牡蛎汤, Cinnamon Twig Decoction Plus Dragon Bone and Oyster Shell, 739

guì zhī jiā sháo yào tāng 桂枝加芍药汤, Cinnamon Twig Decoction Plus Peony, 729

guì zhī jiā zhú fù tāng 桂枝加术附汤, Cinnamon Twig Decoction Plus Ovate Atractylodes and Aconite, 734

guì zhī jiù nì tāng 桂枝救逆汤, Cinnamon Twig Counterflow-Stemming Decoction, 739

guì zhī rén shēn tāng 桂枝人参汤, Cinnamon Twig and Ginseng Decoction, 532, 735

guì zhī sháo yào zhī mǔ tāng 桂枝芍药知母汤, Cinnamon Twig, Peony, and Anemarrhena Decoction, 280

guì zhī tāng 桂枝汤, Cinnamon Twig Decoction, 95, 185, 246, 247, 255, 341, 458, 500, 502, 690, 729

Guide to Tongue Diagnosis (*biàn shé zhǐ nán*) 辨舌指南, 1920 (Republic), Cáo Bǐng-Zhāng 曹炳章, 619

gǔn tán wán 滚痰丸, Phlegm-Rolling Pill, 115, 436, 439, 565, 638, 673, 738

guó gōng jiǔ 国公酒, Statesman Wine, 734

guò qī yǐn 过期饮, Overdue Beverage, 35, 36, 737

GV-1, *cháng qiáng* 长强, Long Strong, 29, 40, 74, 89, 174, 196, 220, 244, 284, 289, 297, 318, 319, 390, 408, 465, 466, 480, 493, 522, 550, 656, 749

GV-2, *yāo shū* 腰俞, Lumbar Transport, 749

GV-3, *yāo yáng guān* 腰阳关, Lumbar Yang Pass, 11, 14, 15, 39, 80, 114, 115, 137, 160, 296, 302, 326, 330, 332, 336, 347, 366, 370, 453, 462, 521, 559, 567, 571, 597, 651, 684, 696, 749

GV-4, *mìng mén* 命门, Life Gate, 4, 14, 22, 23, 26, 35, 36, 45, 61, 64, 80–86, 94, 105, 151, 160, 163, 164, 168, 174, 180, 196, 199, 210, 211, 224, 229, 240, 263, 266, 267, 269, 272, 274, 288, 291, 296, 297, 301, 308, 312, 325, 327, 329, 331–335, 337, 340, 342, 345, 347, 369, 379, 380, 425, 426, 449, 452, 453, 461, 465, 466, 488, 489, 506, 514, 518, 521, 524, 549, 559, 564, 569, 579, 594, 596, 608, 625, 630, 641, 643, 647, 651, 660, 662, 693, 702, 703, 710, 713, 714, 716, 749

GV-5, *xuán shū* 悬枢, Suspended Pivot, 749

GV-6, *jǐ zhōng* 脊中, Spinal Center, 749

GV-7, *zhōng shū* 中枢, Central Pivot, 749

GV-8, *jīn suō* 筋缩, Sinew Contraction, 74, 86, 117, 168, 178, 316, 366, 437, 456, 591, 652, 693, 714, 749

GV-9, *zhì yáng* 至阳, Extremity of Yang, 151, 174, 349, 384, 564, 700, 749

GV-10, *líng tái* 灵台, Spirit Tower, 44, 75, 427, 749

GV-11, *shén dào* 神道, Spirit Path, 749

GV-12, *shēn zhù* 身柱, Body Pillar, 14, 15, 61, 74, 75, 201, 296, 366, 383, 427, 677, 683, 693, 749

GV-13, *táo dào* 陶道, Kiln Path, 8, 82, 197, 219, 383, 384, 394, 399, 439, 550, 590, 604, 650, 664, 690, 749

GV-14, *dà zhuī* 大椎, Great Hammer, 6, 8, 25, 29, 44, 61–63, 65, 66, 69–71, 74–76, 82, 91, 103, 105, 111–113, 117–120, 129, 145, 146, 155, 156, 158, 161, 166, 168, 174, 184, 192, 194, 197, 201, 203, 219, 220, 222, 231, 235, 245, 247, 252–255, 260, 277–283, 285, 291, 292, 301, 317, 318, 339, 342, 349, 357, 364, 366, 368, 374, 383, 391, 394, 399, 403, 405, 406, 418, 427, 439, 444, 450, 451, 455, 458, 474, 501, 508, 515, 516, 521, 529, 544, 546, 547, 550, 561, 569, 570, 572, 585, 586, 588–591, 595, 604, 611, 613, 620, 621, 624, 648–650, 664, 665, 677, 681–683, 685–688, 690, 693, 694, 699–703, 715, 749

GV-15, *yǎ mén* 哑门, Mute's Gate, 291, 368, 410, 573, 749

GV-16, *fēng fǔ* 风府, Wind Mansion, 14, 69, 71, 74, 86, 105, 125, 156, 160, 178, 194, 226, 245, 247, 255, 259, 260, 287, 316, 329, 331, 336, 344, 366, 391, 414, 415, 434, 451, 452, 456, 458, 501, 506, 573, 652, 682–685, 689, 693, 701, 702, 714, 749

GV-17, *nǎo hù* 脑户, Brain's Door, 50, 749

GV-18, *qiáng jiān* 强间, Unyielding Space, 749

GV-19, *hòu dǐng* 后顶, Behind the Vertex, 749

GV-20, *bǎi huì* 百会, Hundred Convergences, 27, 29, 32, 33, 38, 41, 50, 53, 55, 69, 71, 73, 74, 83, 86, 89, 92, 103, 119, 146, 155, 156, 160, 161, 168, 174–178, 196, 199, 203, 212, 218, 219, 225, 226, 231–233, 245, 251, 256, 259, 260, 287–289, 292, 296, 297, 310, 316, 318, 329, 331, 336, 345, 355, 362, 364–366, 384, 386, 409, 434, 442, 448, 451–453, 456–458, 465, 466, 478–480, 482, 485–488, 493, 501, 504, 506, 515, 516, 520, 544, 559, 570, 572, 585, 589–591, 595, 614, 626, 629, 631, 639, 640, 643, 646, 651, 652, 654, 655, 680–687, 690, 691, 693, 694, 699, 701–703, 709, 711–714, 749

GV-21, *qián dǐng* 前顶, Before the Vertex, 586, 654, 694, 703, 749

GV-22, *xìn huì* 囟会, Fontanel Meeting, 50, 260, 415, 749

GV-23, *shàng xīng* 上星, Upper Star, 50, 62, 92, 120, 258, 260, 320, 348, 379, 405, 414, 415, 478, 495, 521, 544, 586, 654, 678, 685, 688, 749

GV-24, *shén tíng* 神庭, Spirit Court, 192, 219, 222, 702, 749

GV-25, *sù liáo* 素髎, White Bone-Hole, 32, 33, 212, 232, 478, 504, 521, 646, 674, 699, 709, 749

GV-26, *rén zhōng* 人中, Human Center, 6, 14, 15, 19, 32, 63, 88, 178, 231, 232, 301, 394, 408, 420, 434, 437, 448, 454, 458, 696

GV-26, *shuǐ gōu* 水沟, Water Trough, 4, 6, 33, 69, 71, 74, 75, 86, 117, 118, 147, 156, 178, 203, 212, 218, 260, 263, 281, 282, 296, 343, 366, 384, 386, 392, 400, 437, 442, 478, 482, 485, 504, 521, 522, 567, 589, 590, 624, 631, 646, 655, 690, 694, 699, 703, 709, 749

GV-27, *duì duān* 兑端, Extremity of the Mouth, 21, 415, 749

GV-28, *yín jiāo* 龈交, Gum Intersection, 749

Gypsum, *shí gāo* 石膏, gypsum, 49, 53, 65, 67, 70, 71, 110, 239, 259, 281, 319, 339, 412, 439, 460, 500, 546, 577, 588, 589, 688, 695, 699, 720

gypsum, *shí gāo* 石膏, Gypsum, 49, 53, 65, 67, 70, 71, 110, 239, 259, 281, 319, 339, 412, 439, 460, 500, 546, 577, 588, 589, 688, 695, 699, 720

Gypsum and Anemarrhena Decoction, *shí gāo zhī mǔ tāng* 石膏知母汤, 587

Gypsum and Apricot-Leaved Adenophora Decoction, *shí zǐ jì ní tāng* 石子荠苨汤, 508

Gypsum Crudum, *shēng shí gāo* 生石膏, crude gypsum, 67, 422, 720

Gypsum Decoction, *shí gāo tāng* 石膏汤, 730

Gypsum seu Calcitum, *hán shuǐ shí* 寒水石, glauberite, 17, 67, 720

há má pí 蛤蟆皮, toad skin, 615

há má wēn 虾蟆瘟, toad head scourge, 615

Haematitum, *dài zhě shí* 代赭石, hematite, 53, 54, 98, 146, 460, 578, 585, 726

hái ér chá 孩儿茶 cutch, Catechu, 368, 728

hái guān 骸关, knee joint, 337

hǎi dài 海带 eelgrass, Zosterae Marinae Herba, 624, 725

hǎi fēng téng 海风藤 kadsura pepper stem, Piperis Kadsurae Caulis, 139, 722

hǎi fú shí 海浮石 pumice, Pumex, 201, 291, 419, 511, 624, 638, 673, 725

hǎi gé fěn 海蛤粉 clamshell powder, Cyclinae (seu Meretricis) Concha Pulverata, 243, 573

hǎi gé ké 海蛤壳 clamshell, Cyclinae (seu Meretricis) Concha, 30, 511, 624, 725

hǎi gǒu shèn 海狗肾 seal's genitals, Callorhini seu Phocae Testis et Penis, 511

hǎi jīn shā 海金沙 lygodium spore, Lygodii Spora, 136, 369, 723

hǎi jīn shā sǎn 海金沙散, Lygodium Spore Powder, 637

hǎi piāo xiāo 海螵蛸 cuttlefish bone, Sepiae seu Sepiellae Os, 478, 502, 511, 518, 572, 581, 727

hǎi quán 海泉, Sea Source, 37, 158, 174, 348, 607

hǎi tóng pí 海桐皮 erythrina, Erythrinae Cortex, 116, 138, 139, 722

hǎi tóng pí jiǔ 海桐皮酒, Erythrina Wine, 734

hǎi tóng pí tāng 海桐皮汤, Erythrina Decoction, 45, 684, 744

hǎi zǎo 海藻 sargassum, Sargassi Herba, 30, 141, 243, 367, 511, 544, 624, 725

hǎi zǎo yù hú tāng 海藻玉壶汤, Sargassum Jade Flask Decoction, 19, 141, 210, 243, 244, 480, 544, 737

hair, *xuè yú* 血余, Hominis Crinis, 653

hairy holly root, *máo dōng qīng* 毛冬青, Ilicis Pubescentis Radix, 138, 725

Haliotidis Concha, *shí jué míng* 石决明, abalone shell, 53, 54, 230, 495, 511, 538, 676, 726

Haliotidis Concha Cruda, *shēng shí jué míng* 生石决明, crude abalone shell, 146, 225, 585

Hall of Impression, *yìn táng* 印堂, 6, 83, 89, 92, 120, 149, 281, 349, 409, 448, 543, 681, 686, 687, 691, 699

halloysite, *chì shí zhī* 赤石脂, Halloysitum Rubrum, 12, 177, 196, 242, 318, 411, 518, 519, 727

Halloysite and Limonite Decoction, *chì shí zhī yǔ yú liáng tāng* 赤石脂禹余粮汤, 742

Halloysitum Rubrum, *chì shí zhī* 赤石脂, halloysite, 12, 177, 196, 242, 318, 411, 518, 519, 727

hān cài 蔊菜 rorippa, Rorippae Herba seu Flos, 624, 625, 725

hán 寒, cold, 76

hán bāo huǒ 寒包火, cold enveloping fire, 81

hán bāo rè 寒包热, cold enveloping heat, 81

hán bì 寒痹, cold impediment, 82

hán chuǎn 寒喘, cold panting, 83

hán è 寒呃, cold hiccough, 82

hán gé 寒膈, cold occlusion, 83

hán huò luàn 寒霍乱, cold cholera, 77

hán jī fù tòng 寒积腹痛, cold accumulation abdominal pain, 77

hán jì 寒剂, cold formula, 81

hán jié 寒结, cold bind, 77

hán jié xiōng 寒结胸, cold chest bind, 77

hán jìng 寒痉, cold tetany, 86

hán jué 寒厥, cold reversal, 85

hán jué xīn tòng 寒厥心痛, cold reversal heart pain, 85

hán kě qù rè 寒可去热, cold [medicinals] can eliminate heat, 82

hán lěng fù tòng 寒冷腹痛, cold abdominal pain, 77

hán lì 寒痢, cold dysentery, 80

hán níng gān mài 寒凝肝脉, cold congealing in the liver vessel, 78

hán nüè 寒疟, cold malaria, 82

hán ǒu 寒呕, cold vomiting, 86

hán pì 寒癖, cold aggregation, 77

hán qì fù tòng 寒气腹痛, cold qi abdominal pain, 85

hán qì níng zhì 寒气凝滞, congealing cold and stagnant qi, 93

hán rè 寒热, alternating fever and chills, 8

hán rè 寒热, alternating heat [effusion] and [aversion to] cold, 8

hán rè 寒热, cold and heat, 77

hán rè 寒热, heat [effusion] and [aversion to] cold, 279

hán rè cuò zá 寒热错杂, cold-heat complex, 81

hán rè wǎng lái 寒热往来, alternating fever and chills, 8

hán rè wǎng lái 寒热往来, alternating heat [effusion] and [aversion to] cold, 8

hán shàn 寒疝, cold mounting, 82

hán shāng xíng 寒伤形, cold damages the physical body, 79

hán shèng zé fú 寒胜则浮, when cold prevails there is swelling, 672

hán shī 寒湿, cold-damp, 79

hán shī jiǎo qì 寒湿脚气, cold-damp leg qi, 80

hán shī jiǔ bì 寒湿久痹, cold-damp enduring impediment, 79

hán shī kùn pí 寒湿困脾, cold-damp encumbering the spleen, 79

hán shī níng zhì jīng bì 寒湿凝滞经闭, congealing cold-damp menstrual block, 93

hán shī níng zhì tòng jīng 寒湿凝滞痛经, congealing cold-damp menstrual pain, 94

hán shī tóu tòng 寒湿头痛, cold-damp headache, 79

hán shī xuàn yūn 寒湿眩晕, cold-damp dizziness, 79

hán shī yāo tòng 寒湿腰痛, cold-damp lumbar pain, 80

hán shī zhōng zǔ 寒湿中阻, cold-damp obstructing the center, 80

hán shí 寒实, cold repletion, 85

hán shí 寒实, repletion cold, 498

hán shí jié xiōng 寒实结胸, cold repletion chest bind, 85

hán shuǐ shí 寒水石 glauberite, Gypsum seu Calcitum, 17, 67, 720

hán sòu 寒嗽, cold cough, 78

hán tán 寒痰, cold phlegm, 84

hán tán zǔ fèi 寒痰阻肺, cold phlegm obstructing the lung, 84

hán tù 寒吐, cold vomiting, 86

hán wú fàn hán 寒无犯寒, do not use cold against cold, 144

hán xià 寒下, cold precipitation, 84

hán xián 寒痫, cold epilepsy, 81

hán xié 寒邪, cold evil, 81

hán xié fàn wèi 寒邪犯胃, cold evil invading the stomach, 81

hán xié xuàn yūn 寒邪眩晕, cold evil dizziness, 81

hán xiè 寒泄, cold diarrhea, 80

hán xiè 寒泻, cold diarrhea, 80

hán xīn tòng 寒心痛, cold heart pain, 81

hán yè tí 寒夜啼, cold night crying, 83

hán yǐn 寒饮, cold rheum, 85

hán yǐn fú fèi 寒饮伏肺, cold rheum lying latent in the lung, 85

hán zé qì shōu 寒则气收, cold causes qi to contract, 77

hán zé shōu yǐn 寒则收引, cold causes contracture and tension, 77

hán zhàn 寒战, shivering, 529

hán zhàng 寒胀, cold distention, 80

hán zhě rè zhī 寒者热之, cold is treated with heat, 82

hán zhèng 寒证, cold pattern, 83

hán zhì gān mài 寒滞肝脉, cold stagnating in the liver vessel, 85

hán zhòng 寒中, cold stroke, 86

hàn 汗, sweat, 598

hàn 汗, sweating, 598

hàn 汉, Han, 252

hàn 颔, submandibular region, 585

hàn bān 汗斑, sweat macule, 599

hàn chū rú yóu 汗出如油, putting forth oily sweat, 474

hàn duō 汗多, copious sweat, 99

hàn fǎ 汗法, diaphoresis, 125

hàn fāng 汉方, kampo, 324

hàn wéi xīn yè 汗为心液, sweat is the humor of the heart, 599

hàn xuè 汗血, sweating of blood, 599

hàn yàn 颔厌, GB-4, Forehead Fullness, 235, 365, 748

hàn zhōng fáng jǐ 汉中防己 northern fangji, Aristolochiae Heterophyllae Radix, 139, 154, 722

Hand-of-Buddha Powder, *fó shǒu sǎn* 佛手散, 35, 451

hanging stonecrop, *shí zhǐ jiǎ* 石指甲, Sedi Sarmentosi Herba, 68, 357, 700, 721

hāo qín qīng dǎn tāng 蒿芩清胆汤, Sweet Wormwood and Scutellaria Gallbladder-Clearing Decoction, 235, 538, 587, 733

háo zhēn 毫针, filiform needle, 200

hào 耗, wear, 669

Harmonious Flow Paste, *chōng hé gāo* 冲和膏, 116

Harmonious Yang Decoction, *yáng hé tāng* 阳和汤, 44, 46, 213, 259, 315, 540, 744

Harmonious Yang Decongealing Plaster, *yáng hé jiě níng gāo* 阳和解凝膏, 45, 46, 210, 243, 259, 315, 744

Harmony-Preserving Pill, *bǎo hé wán* 保和丸, 2, 3, 15, 19, 141, 143, 157, 197, 199, 215–218, 231, 238, 395, 549, 557, 578, 736

hawksbill shell, *dài mào* 玳瑁, Eretmochelydis Carapax, 54, 726

hē lí lè sǎn 诃黎勒散, Chebule Powder, 479

hē qiàn 呵欠, yawning, 704

hē zǐ 诃子 chebule, Chebulae Fructus, 80, 95, 201, 291, 316, 318, 449, 466, 518, 681, 727

hē zǐ sǎn 诃子散, Chebule Powder, 168

hé 和, harmonize, 255

hé 核, node, 412

hé 颌, jaw corner, 322

hé bìng 合病, combination disease, 88

hé chē bā wèi wán 河车八味丸, Eight-Ingredient Placenta Pill, 741

hé chē dà zào wán 河车大造丸, Placenta Great Creation Pill, 310, 379, 715

hé chē wán 河车丸, Placenta Pill, 178

hé fǎ 和法, harmonization, 255

hé gān 和肝, harmonizing the liver, 256

hé gàn 髑骭, breastbone, 50

hé gǔ 合谷, LI-4, Union Valley, 1, 2, 4–6, 8, 11, 12, 14, 15, 24, 26, 28–30, 33–35, 39, 40, 44, 47, 50, 59, 60, 62–66, 69–73, 75–80, 82–91, 93, 95, 96, 99, 103, 105, 109–115, 117–120, 125, 127–129, 136, 138–141, 145, 146, 149–153, 155, 158, 164, 166, 167, 171, 174, 178, 182–186, 189, 190, 192, 194, 197, 202, 203, 216–218, 224, 225, 227, 228, 231, 239–241, 244, 247, 257, 259–261, 269, 272, 276–278, 280–285, 287–291, 294, 295, 298, 301, 302, 312, 318–320, 337–339, 341, 347, 348, 356, 358, 366, 368, 374, 382, 384, 386, 395, 400, 401, 403, 405, 410, 414–416, 418, 422, 426, 427, 433–439, 441–443, 445, 448–452, 454–458, 462, 463, 466, 471, 475, 477, 480, 482–485, 489, 493, 495, 499, 501, 503, 504, 506, 509, 511, 515, 517, 519–522, 530, 539, 540, 543, 544, 546–548, 550, 560, 562, 563, 565, 566, 568, 569, 571, 572, 577–580, 585–591, 595, 597, 601, 603, 604, 607, 608, 610, 611, 613, 614, 620, 621, 624, 625, 631, 640, 641, 643, 645, 651, 652, 654, 658, 661, 663–666, 673, 674, 676, 677, 679–691, 693, 694, 699, 701–703, 711–715, 746

hé huān huā 合欢花 silk tree flower, Albizziae Flos, 234, 310

hé huān pí 合欢皮 silk tree bark, Albizziae Cortex, 491, 537, 726

hé jiě 和解, harmonize, 255

hé jiě bàn biǎo bàn lǐ 和解半表半里, harmonizing midstage patterns, 255

hé jiě bàn biǎo bàn lǐ 和解半表半里, midstage harmonization, 394

hé jiě biǎo lǐ 和解表里, harmonizing the exterior and interior, 256

hé jiě fǎ 和解法, harmonization, 255

hé jiě shào yáng 和解少阳, harmonizing lesser yang, 255

hé liáo 和髎, TB-22, Harmony Bone-Hole, 748

hé liáo 禾髎, LI-19, Grain Bone-Hole, 45, 219, 400, 401, 415, 746

hé rén yǐn 何人饮, Flowery Knotweed and Ginseng Beverage, 174, 650, 741

hé róng sàn jiān wán 和荣散坚丸, Construction-Harmonizing Hardness-Dissipating Pill, 367

hé shǒu wū 何首乌 flowery knotweed, Polygoni Multiflori Radix, 28, 37, 127, 172, 175, 245, 309, 336, 352, 467, 593, 595, 727

hé wèi 和胃, gastric harmonization, 239

hé wèi 和胃, harmonizing the stomach, 257

hé wèi huà tán 和胃化痰, harmonizing the stomach and transforming phlegm, 257

hé wèi jiě chéng 和胃解酲, harmonizing the stomach and resolving liquor, 257

hé wèi lǐ qì 和胃理气, harmonizing the stomach and rectifying qi, 257

hé wèi xǐng jiǔ 和胃醒酒, harmonizing the stomach and restoring soberness, 257

hé wèi zhǐ ǒu 和胃止呕, harmonizing the stomach and checking vomiting, 257

hé xué 合穴, uniting point, 637

hé xuè xī fēng 和血熄风, harmonizing the blood and extinguishing wind, 256

hé yáng 合阳, BL-55, Yang Union, 747

hé yè 荷叶 lotus leaf, Nelumbinis Folium, 569

hé zhōng 和中, harmonizing the center, 256

hè dǐng 鹤顶, Crane Top, 521

hè shī 鹤虱 carpesium seed, Carpesii Fructus, 183, 445, 468, 724 *hè wèi jiàng qì* 和胃降气, harmonizing the stomach and downbearing qi, 257

hè xī fēng 鹤膝风, crane's-knee wind, 104

hè xī tán 鹤膝痰, crane's-knee phlegm, 104

headache*
 nervous, 260
 odontogenic, 202
 otogenic, 202
 vascular, 202, 260

heart disease*, 265
 coronary, 58, 265
 pulmogenic, 120, 193

heart failure*, 124, 270, 646

Heart-Clearing Lotus Seed Beverage, *qīng xīn lián zǐ yǐn* 清心莲子饮, 147, 731

Heart-Draining Decoction, *xiè xīn tāng* 泻心汤, 29, 189, 263, 281, 294, 459, 552, 731

Heart-Draining Red-Abducting Decoction, *xiè xīn dǎo chì tāng* 泻心导赤汤, 237

Heart-Kidney Pill, *xīn shèn wán* 心肾丸, 651

Heart-Nourishing Decoction, *yǎng xīn tāng* 养心汤, 270, 451, 594, 694, 739

Heart-Supplementing Decoction, *bǔ xīn tāng* 补心汤, 497

Heart-Supplementing Elixir, *bǔ xīn dān* 补心丹, 265, 272, 274, 333, 537, 541

Heart-Washing Powder, *xǐ xīn sǎn* 洗心散, 202, 740

Heat Depression Decoction, *rè yù tāng* 热郁汤, 278

Heat-Abating Powder, *tuì rè sǎn* 退热散, 731

Heat-Clearing Channel-Securing (Menses-Securing) Decoction, *qīng rè gù jīng tāng* 清热固经汤, 31, 743

Heat-Clearing Uterine Bleeding Decoction, *qīng rè zhǐ bēng tāng* 清热止崩汤, 743

Heat-Resolving Blood-Dissipating Decoction, *jiě rè sàn xuè tāng* 解热散血汤, 730

Heaven, Human, and Earth Decoction, *sān cái tāng* 三才汤, 742

Heaven, Human, and Earth Marrow-Retaining Elixir, *sān cái fēng suǐ dān* 三才封髓丹, 524, 739

hedgehog's pelt, *cì wèi pí* 刺猬皮, Erinacei Pellis, 98, 518, 727

hedyotis 白花蛇舌草 *bái huā shé shé cǎo*, Hedyotis Herba, 68, 721

Hedyotis Herba, *hedyotis* 白花蛇舌草, *bái huā shé shé cǎo*, 68, 721

hēi 黑, black, 20

hēi bù gāo 黑布膏, Black Cloth Paste, 171

hēi dà dòu 黑大豆 black soybean, Glycines Semen Atrum, 54, 108, 726

hēi dài 黑带, black vaginal discharge, 21

hēi dǎn 黑疸, black jaundice, 20

hēi gāo (fāng) 黑膏（方）, Black Paste (Formula), 65, 730

hēi hǔ dān 黑虎丹, Black Tiger Elixir, 528, 744

hēi jīng 黑睛, dark of the eye, 118

hēi jīng qīng lán 白睛青蓝, blue whites of the eye, 41

hēi shān zhī zǐ 黑山栀子 charred gardenia, Gardeniae Fructus Carbonisatus, 120, 459

hēi shùn piàn 黑顺片 black sliced aconite, Aconiti Tuber Laterale Denigratum, 660, 723

hēi tāi 黑苔, black tongue fur, 21

hēi tóu fěn cì 黑头粉刺, blackhead, 20

hēi xí dān 黑锡丹, Galenite Elixir, 330, 335, 526, 629, 735

hēi xiāo yáo sǎn 黑逍遥散, Black Free Wanderer Powder, 352, 566, 732

hēi zǎo 黑枣 black jujube, Ziziphi Fructus Ater, 667

hēi zhī má 黑脂麻 black sesame, Sesami Semen Atrum, 28, 108, 127, 398, 593, 727

hēi zhì 黑痣, black mole, 21

hēi zhū 黑珠, dark of the eye, 118

Heleocharitis Cormus, *bí qí* 荸荠, water chestnut, 624, 725

hemangioma of the neck*, 243

hemangioma*
 cavernous, 632

hematite, *dài zhě shí* 代赭石, Haematitum, 53, 54, 98, 146, 460, 578, 585, 726

hematoma of testis*, 399

Hemilateral Headache Decoction, *sàn piān tāng* 散偏汤, 288

hemorrhage*
 cerebral, 44, 586, 692
 retinal, 586
 subarachnoid, 44, 586

hemorrhagic shock*, 478

Hemorrhoid-Dispersing Beverage, *xiāo zhì yǐn* 消痔饮, 744

hemp seed, *huǒ má rén* 火麻仁, Cannabis Semen, 72, 399, 415, 449, 460, 462, 722

Hemp Seed Pill, *má rén wán* 麻仁丸, 72, 542, 683

Hemp Seed Pill, *má zǐ rén wán* 麻子仁丸, 399, 584, 732

héng cì 横刺, transverse insertion, 626

héng gǔ 横骨, KI-11, Pubic Bone, 609, 748

héng gǔ 横骨, transverse bone, 626

héng gǔ 骺骨, walking bone, 658

héng xián 横痃, bubo sore, 51

hepatic odor, 53

hepatitis*, 284
 acute icteric, 111
 acute icteric infectious, 193
 acute infectious, 700
 hepatitis, 193
 icteric, 357

Hepatolith Formula, *gān dǎn guǎn jié shí fāng* 肝胆管结石方, 733

hepatosplenomegaly*, 34

Herbarum Ustarum Fuligo, *bǎi cǎo shuāng* 百草霜, weed soot, 724

hernia*
 inguinal, 399

herpes zoster*, 241

heterophyllous patrinia, *mù tóu huí* 墓头回, Patriniae Heterophyllae Radix, 68, 721

heterotopic pregnancy*, 34

Hibisci Mutabilis Flos, *mù fú róng huā* 木芙蓉花, cotton rose, 728

Hibisci Mutabilis Folium, *mù fú róng yè* 木芙蓉叶, cotton rose leaf, 104, 728

Hibisci Syriaci Flos, *mù jǐn huā* 木槿花, rose-of-Sharon, 728

Hibisci Syriaci Radicis Cortex, *mù jǐn pí* 木槿皮, rose-of-Sharon root bark, 728

Hidden Tiger Pill, *hǔ qián wán* 虎潜丸, 47, 337, 679, 715

hidradenitis*, 463

hip joint*, 607

Hirudo seu Whitmania, *shuǐ zhì* 水蛭, leech, 98, 138, 724

Holding the Uterus, *wéi bāo* 维胞, 711

homalomena, *qiān nián jiàn* 千年健, Homalomenae Rhizoma, 139, 722

Homalomenae Rhizoma, *qiān nián jiàn* 千年健, homalomena, 139, 722

Hominis Crinis, *xuè yú* 血余, hair, 653

Hominis Crinis Carbonisatus, *xuè yú tàn* 血余炭, charred hair, 567, 724

Hominis Placenta, *zǐ hé chē* 紫河车, placenta, 222, 298, 310, 511, 593, 726

honey, *mì* 蜜, Mel, 201, 399, 449, 593, 726

Honey Enema, *mì jiān dǎo fǎ* 蜜煎导法, 542, 646

honey tree fruit, *zhǐ jǔ zǐ* 枳椇子, Hoveniae Fructus seu Semen, 415

Honey-Fried Licorice Decoction, *zhì gān cǎo tāng* 炙甘草汤, 59, 159, 160, 269, 270, 594, 741

honeycomb ringworm*, 196

hōng rè 烘热, baking heat [effusion], 15

hóng 红, red, 494

hóng cǎi 虹彩, iris, 320

hóng chì xuè sī 红赤血丝, red blood threads, 494

hóng dòu kòu 红豆蔻 galangal fruit, Alpiniae Galangae Fructus, 660, 723

hóng huā 红花 carthamus, Carthami Flos, 34, 59, 98, 137, 138, 140, 181, 182, 227, 244, 352, 388, 431, 451, 493, 503, 512, 571, 654, 679, 696, 724

hóng líng dān 红灵丹, Red Spirit Elixir, 740

hóng líng jiǔ 红灵酒, Red Spirit Wine, 231

hóng lǚ chì hén 红缕赤痕, red thread mark, 496

hóng mài 洪脉, surging pulse, 598

hóng shēn 红参 red ginseng, Ginseng Radix Rubra, 593, 726

hóng shēng 红升 red upborne elixir, Hydrogyrum Oxydatum Crudum Rubrum, 171

hóng shēng dān 红升丹, Red Upborne Elixir, 385, 744

hóng sī dīng 红丝疔, red-thread clove sore, 496

hóng yóu gāo 红油膏, Red Oil Paste, 17

hookworm infestation*, 704

hookworm*, 704

Hordei Fructus Germinatus, *mài yá* 麦芽, barley sprout, 23, 141, 216, 217, 420, 450, 479, 499, 564, 573, 600, 606, 724

hornet's nest, *lù fēng fáng* 露蜂房, Vespae Nidus, 298, 449, 728

horse chestnut, *suō luó zǐ* 娑罗子, Aesculi Fructus, 493, 724

Hou's Black Powder, *hóu shì hēi sǎn* 侯氏黑散, 740

hóu 喉, larynx, 340

hóu 喉, throat, 611

hóu bì 喉痹, throat impediment, 611

hóu é 喉蛾, throat moth, 612

hóu fēng 喉风, throat wind, 612

hóu guān 喉关, throat pass, 612

hóu hé 喉核, throat node, 612

hóu lóng 喉咙, throat, 611

hóu lóng tòng 喉咙痛, sore throat, 547

hóu shì hēi sǎn 侯氏黑散, Hou's Black Powder, 740

hóu xiǎn 喉癣, throat lichen, 611

hóu yān gān zào 喉咽干燥, dry throat, 157

hóu yǎng 喉痒, itchy throat, 321

hóu yōng 喉痈, welling-abscess of the throat, 671

hóu zhōng yǒu shuǐ jī shēng 喉中有水鸡声, frog rale in the throat, 231

hòu dǐng 后顶, GV-19, Behind the Vertex, 749

hòu hàn 后汉, Later Han, 341

hòu jìn 后晋, Later Jin, 341

hòu liáng 后梁, Later Liang, 341

hòu pò 厚朴 magnolia bark, Magnoliae Cortex, 10, 66, 72, 98, 103, 153, 217, 223, 224, 246, 276, 287, 363, 397, 401, 421, 430, 441, 459, 587, 625, 679, 722

hòu pò huā 厚朴花 magnolia flower[2], Magnoliae Flos[2], 625, 722

hòu pò qī wù tāng 厚朴七物汤, Magnolia Bark Seven Agents Decoction, 500, 730

hòu pò sān wù tāng 厚朴三物汤, Magnolia Bark Three Agents Decoction, 500, 731

hòu pò shēng jiāng bàn xià gān cǎo rén shēn tāng 厚朴生姜半夏甘草人参汤, Magnolia Bark, Fresh Ginger, Pinellia, Licorice, and Ginseng Decoction, 1, 339, 735

hòu pò wēn zhōng tāng 厚朴温中汤, Magnolia Bark Center-Warming Decoction, 1, 85, 339, 561, 735

hòu tāi 厚苔, thick tongue fur, 607

hòu táng 后唐, Later Tang, 341

hòu tiān 后天, acquired constitution, 5

hòu tiān 后天, later heaven, 341

hòu tiān zhī běn 后天之本, root of later heaven, 508

hòu tóu tòng 后头痛, posterior headache, 447

hòu xī 后溪, SI-3, Back Ravine, 8, 40, 50, 61, 74, 82, 83, 89, 90, 92, 93, 95, 105, 113, 114, 138, 174, 178, 185, 194, 197, 240, 244, 247, 255, 260, 269, 272, 275, 281, 287, 289, 295, 317, 336, 341, 342, 358, 366, 383, 391, 394, 399, 409, 410, 415, 439, 440, 454, 489, 506, 508, 519–521, 530, 540, 542, 544, 572, 588–591, 595, 597, 604, 648, 650, 651,

656, 664, 679, 681, 683, 684, 686, 687, 690, 693, 701–703, 713–716, 747

hòu xià 后下, add at end, 7

hòu xià 后下, end addition, 173

hòu yīn 后阴, posterior yin, 447

hòu zhōu 后周, Later Zhou, 341

house lizard, *bì hǔ* 壁虎, Gekko Swinhoana, 728

House of Blood Stasis-Expelling Decoction, *xuè fǔ zhú yū tāng* 血府逐瘀汤, 34, 35, 59, 230, 260, 273, 297, 417, 484, 570, 571, 586, 608, 613, 738

houttuynia, *yú xīng cǎo* 鱼腥草, Houttuyniae Herba cum Radice, 64, 68, 69, 118, 282, 388, 469, 686, 721

Houttuyniae Herba cum Radice, *yú xīng cǎo* 鱼腥草, houttuynia, 64, 68, 69, 118, 282, 388, 469, 686, 721

Hoveniae Fructus seu Semen, *zhǐ jù zǐ* 枳椇子, honey tree fruit, 415

HT-1, *jí quán* 极泉, Highest Spring, 746

HT-2, *qīng líng* 青灵, Green-Blue Spirit, 540, 746

HT-3, *shào hǎi* 少海, Lesser Sea, 138, 142, 515, 540, 637, 747

HT-4, *líng dào* 灵道, Spirit Pathway, 747

HT-5, *tōng lǐ* 通里, Connecting Li, 39, 58, 69, 71, 90, 140, 223, 230, 268, 289, 294, 302, 365, 383, 408, 427, 449, 451, 455, 521, 538, 540, 572, 573, 589, 597, 629, 683, 701, 747

HT-6, *yīn xī* 阴郄, Yin Cleft, 40, 72, 95, 97, 176, 210, 237, 269, 272, 275, 336, 341, 410, 448, 454, 463, 489, 521, 572, 589, 590, 595, 597, 648, 651, 690, 702, 713–716, 747

HT-7, *shén mén* 神门, Spirit Gate, 5, 6, 11, 19, 25, 29–31, 35, 39, 41, 43, 58, 75, 87–91, 99, 113, 117, 123, 129, 147, 153, 155, 159, 160, 162, 168, 177, 178, 180, 203, 210, 223, 230, 232, 235, 236, 261, 263–272, 274, 275, 281, 282, 294, 296, 297, 301, 302, 308, 330, 331, 333, 335, 336, 345, 365, 386, 392, 410, 413, 416, 418, 420, 434, 436, 437, 448, 449, 451, 452, 457, 461, 467, 478, 484, 488, 514, 521, 524–526, 537, 548, 551, 572, 589–591, 594, 597, 604, 610, 613, 614, 638, 642, 648, 649, 651, 652, 655, 661, 665, 668, 673, 675, 686, 687, 694, 700, 701, 714, 716, 747

HT-8, *shào fǔ* 少府, Lesser Mansion, 29, 65, 74, 117, 123, 147, 155, 156, 168, 180, 203, 241, 244, 261, 263, 264, 269, 281, 282, 292, 294, 296, 332, 333, 336, 364, 386, 391, 392, 400, 401, 415, 416, 436, 437, 456, 495, 516, 524, 542, 567, 572, 597, 613, 641, 642, 648, 649, 652, 654, 686–688, 700, 714, 716, 747

HT-9, *shào chōng* 少冲, Lesser Surge, 25, 65, 73, 99, 147, 263, 264, 281, 294, 400, 420, 437, 455, 538, 547, 585, 747

hū qiàn 呼欠, yawning, 704

hū xī 呼吸, breathing, 50

hū xī 呼吸, respiration, 502

hū xī bǔ xiè 呼吸补泻, respiratory supplementation and drainage, 502

hú chòu 狐臭, foxy odor, 226

hú huáng lián 胡黄连 picrorhiza, Picrorhizae Rhizoma, 68, 391, 722

hú jiāo 胡椒 pepper, Piperis Fructus, 94, 226, 660, 723

hú lú 壶芦 bottle gourd, Lagenariae Depressae Fructus, 136, 723

hú lú bā 胡芦巴 fenugreek, Foeni-Graeci Semen, 83, 335, 343, 400, 593, 675, 716, 727

hú lú bā sǎn 胡芦巴散 Fenugreek Powder, 733

hú lú bā wán 葫芦巴丸 Fenugreek Pill, 80, 733

hú shàn 狐疝, foxy mounting, 226

hú shàn 狐疝, vulpine mounting, 657

hú suī 胡荽 coriander, Coriandri Herba cum Radice, 387, 422, 542, 681, 720

hú táo rén 胡桃仁 walnut, Juglandis Semen, 97, 467, 526, 593, 596, 726

hǔ ěr cǎo 虎耳草 saxifrage, Saxifragae Herba, 68, 721

hǔ gǔ 虎骨 tiger bone, Tigris Os, 45, 139, 397, 722

hǔ gǔ jiāo 虎骨胶 tiger bone glue, Tigris Gelatinum Ossis, 243

hǔ gǔ sǎn 虎骨散, Tiger Bone Powder, 45

hǔ gǔ sì jīn wán 虎骨四斤丸, Tiger Bone Four Jin Pill, 337

hǔ kǒu 虎口, tiger's mouth, 614

hǔ pò 琥珀 amber, Succinum, 153, 230, 262, 433, 490, 602, 726

hǔ pò ān shén tāng 琥珀安神汤, Amber Spirit-Quieting Decoction, 739

hǔ pò bào lóng wán 琥珀抱龙丸, Amber Dragon-Embracing Pill, 740

hǔ pò sǎn 琥珀散, Amber Powder, 34, 35, 733

hǔ qián wán 虎潜丸, Hidden Tiger Pill, 47, 337, 679, 715

hǔ xū dīng 虎须疔, tiger's-whiskers clove sore, 614

hǔ zhàng 虎杖 bushy knotweed, Polygoni Cuspidati Rhizoma, 136, 138, 357, 540, 723, 724

hù mén 户门, door gate, 145

Hua Tuo's Wind-Healing Powder, *huá tuó yù fēng sǎn* 华陀愈风散, 60, 458

huā jiāo 花椒 zanthoxylum, Zanthoxyli Pericarpium, 225, 242, 320, 405, 468, 513, 620, 660, 662, 723

huā jiāo gēn 花椒根 zanthoxylum root, Zanthoxyli Radix, 36

huā ruǐ shí 花蕊石 ophicalcite, Ophicalcitum, 548, 724

huā ruǐ shí sǎn 花蕊石散 ophicalcite, Ophicalcite Powder, 738

huá 滑, efflux, 167

huá cháng 滑肠, lubricate the intestines, 369

huá gài 华盖, CV-20, Florid Canopy, 749

huá gài sǎn 华盖散, Florid Canopy Powder, 83, 683, 738

huá jì 滑剂, lubricating formula, 369

huá jīng 滑精, seminal efflux, 524

huá kě qù zhuó 滑可去着, lubricating [medicinals] can eliminate fixity, 370

huá mài 滑脉, slippery pulse, 539

huá ròu mén 滑肉门, ST-24, Slippery Flesh Gate, 746

huá shān shēn 华山参 physochlaina, Physochlainae Radix, 624, 725

huá shí 滑石 talcum, Talcum, 17, 21, 22, 66, 69, 93, 115, 136, 463, 573, 667, 723

huá tāi 滑苔, glossy tongue fur, 243

huá tāi 滑胎, habitual miscarriage, 251

huá tuō 滑脱, efflux desertion, 168

huá tuó jiá jǐ xué 华佗夹脊穴, Hua Tuo's paravertebral points, 293

huá tuó yù fēng sǎn 华陀愈风散, Hua Tuo's Wind-Healing Powder, 60, 458

huá xiè 滑泄, efflux diarrhea, 168

huà 化, formation, 223

huà 化, transform, 621

huà 化, transformation, 621

huà bān jiě dú tāng 化斑解毒汤, Macule-Transforming Toxin-Resolving Decoction, 338, 730

huà bān tāng 化斑汤, Macule-Transforming Decoction, 422, 730

huà chóng wán 化虫丸, Worm-Transforming Pill, 64, 172, 426, 445, 509, 695, 696, 737

huà gān jiān 化肝煎, Liver-Transforming Brew, 33, 314, 735

huà huǒ 化火, fire formation, 202

huà huǒ 化火, transformation into fire, 622

huà jú hóng 化橘红 Huazhou pomelo rind, Citri Grandis Exocarpium Rubrum, 493, 723

huà qì lì shī 化气利湿, promoting qi transformation and disinhibiting water, 467

huà rè 化热, heat formation, 280

huà rè 化热, transformation into heat, 622

huà shī 化湿, transforming dampness, 622

huà shí sǎn 化石散, Stone-Transforming Powder, 733

huà shuǐ zhòng zǐ tāng 化水种子汤, Water-Transforming Seed-Planting Decoction, 741

huà tán 化痰, transforming phlegm, 622

huà tán kāi qiào 化痰开窍, transforming phlegm and opening the orifices, 624

huà tán zhǐ ké 化痰止咳, transforming phlegm and suppressing cough, 625

huà yīn jiān 化阴煎, Yin-Forming Brew, 733

huà yū 化瘀, transforming stasis, 625

huà yū xíng xuè 化瘀行血, transforming stasis and moving the blood, 625

huà zhēng huí shēng dān 化癥回生丹, Concretion-Transforming Return-to-Life Elixir, 26

huái huā 槐花 sophora flower, Sophorae Flos, 466, 566, 567, 569, 724

huái huā sǎn 槐花散, Sophora Flower Powder, 40, 117, 738

huái jiǎo tàn 槐角炭 charred sophora fruit, Sophorae Fructus Carbonisatus, 317

huái jiǎo wán 槐角丸, Sophora Fruit Pill, 318, 738

huái shēn 怀娠, pregnancy, 460

huái yùn 怀孕, pregnancy, 460

huái zhī 槐枝 sophora twigs, Sophorae Ramulus, 196

huán shào dān 还少丹, Rejuvenation Elixir, 297, 742

huán tiào 环跳, GB-30, Jumping Round, 47, 61, 89, 104, 137, 212, 219, 220, 289, 296, 323, 382, 410, 418, 567, 654, 679, 689, 748

huán tiào liú tán 环跳流痰, Jumping-Round flowing phlegm, 323

huǎn jí 缓急, relaxing tension, 498

huǎn jí zhǐ tòng 缓急止痛, relaxing tension and relieving pain, 498

huǎn mài 缓脉, moderate pulse, 398

huǎn zé zhì běn 缓则治本, in moderate (chronic) conditions treat root, 303

huàn chǐ 换齿, change of teeth, 55

huāng 肓, huang, 293

huāng mén 肓门, BL-51, Huang Gate, 169, 747

huāng mó 肓膜, huang membrane, 293

huāng shū 肓俞, KI-16, Huang Transport, 28, 748

huáng 黄, yellow, 704

huáng bǎi 黄柏 phellodendron, Phellodendri Cortex, 17, 66, 67, 69, 70, 81, 94, 104, 106, 116, 127, 153, 154, 176, 281, 282, 319, 338, 352, 357, 397, 424, 449, 456, 514, 527, 604, 649, 679, 704, 712, 713, 720

huáng bǎi mò 黄柏末 powdered phellodendron, Phellodendri Cortex Pulveratus, 330, 331

huáng bǎi tàn 黄柏炭 charred phellodendron, Phellodendri Cortex Carbonisatus, 546

huáng dài 黄带, yellow vaginal discharge, 705

huáng dǎn 黄疸, jaundice, 322

huáng dǎn yīn chén chōng jì 黄疸茵陈冲剂, Jaundice Capillaris Granules, 733

huáng fēng 黄风, yellow wind, 705

huáng fēng nèi zhàng 黄风内障, yellow wind internal obstruction, 705

huáng hàn 黄汗, yellow sweat, 704

huáng jīng 黄精 polygonatum, Polygonati Huangjing Rhizoma, 593, 727

huáng là 黄腊 yellow wax, Cera Aurea, 57

huáng lián 黄连 coptis, Coptidis Rhizoma, 20, 30, 65–67, 69, 70, 81, 82, 116, 141, 146, 153, 154, 230, 243, 256, 257, 261–263, 281, 317, 338, 358, 387, 390, 417, 421, 434, 440, 459, 462, 466, 474, 500, 510, 524, 526, 539, 541, 569, 574, 577, 578, 587, 589, 601, 612, 614, 617, 619, 638, 671, 673, 712, 720

huáng lián ē jiāo jī zǐ huáng tāng 黄连阿胶鸡子黄汤, Coptis, Ass Hide Glue, and Egg Yolk Decoction, 284, 413, 467, 538, 655

huáng lián ē jiāo tāng 黄连阿胶汤, Coptis and Ass Hide Glue Decoction, 28, 230, 263, 268, 345, 525, 537, 538, 739

huáng lián gāo 黄连膏, Coptis Paste, 283, 533

huáng lián huà tán yǐn 黄连化痰饮, Coptis Phlegm-Transforming Beverage, 277

huáng lián jiě dú tāng 黄连解毒汤, Coptis Toxin-Resolving Decoction, 6, 51, 63, 70, 75, 76, 81, 168,

197, 202, 214, 221, 259, 285, 315, 338, 445, 533, 566, 664, 687, 730

huáng lián sǎn 黄连散, Coptis Powder, 154

huáng lián tāng 黄连汤, Coptis Decoction, 732

huáng lián wán 黄连丸, Coptis Pill, 40, 82, 284

huáng lián wēn dǎn tāng 黄连温胆汤, Coptis Gallbladder-Warming Decoction, 20, 24, 230, 269, 436, 539, 621, 694, 739

huáng lián xiāng rú sǎn 黄连香薷散, Coptis and Elsholtzia Powder, 276, 588

huáng lián yáng gān wán 黄连羊肝丸, Coptis and Goat's Liver Pill, 731

huáng lián zhū dǔ wán 黄连猪肚丸, Coptis and Pig's Stomach Pill, 508

huáng lóng tāng 黄龙汤, Yellow Dragon Decoction, 24, 532, 732

huáng páng 黄胖, yellow obesity, 704

huáng qí 黄芪 astragalus, Astragali (seu Hedysari) Radix, 11, 17, 40, 45, 47, 95, 161, 196, 223, 227, 267, 270, 315, 328, 329, 333, 378, 391, 397, 426, 456, 466, 486, 488, 527, 556, 572, 581, 593–595, 599, 600, 651, 662, 679, 704, 712, 716, 726

huáng qí guì zhī wǔ wù tāng 黄芪桂枝五物汤, Astragalus and Cinnamon Twig Five Agents Decoction, 32, 417, 454, 735

huáng qí jiàn zhōng tāng 黄芪建中汤, Astragalus Center-Fortifying Decoction, 217, 251, 314, 427, 529, 566, 581, 651, 663, 710, 735

huáng qí tāng 黄芪汤, Astragalus Decoction, 477, 734

huáng qín 黄芩 scutellaria, Scutellariae Radix, 20, 30, 65–67, 70, 81, 82, 115, 116, 153, 189, 191, 199, 230, 243, 255, 257, 259, 282, 303, 310, 317, 319, 338, 339, 357, 358, 372, 386, 388, 390, 394, 397, 414, 419, 421, 428, 439, 440, 457, 459, 466, 500, 501, 527, 538, 548, 569, 577, 587, 588, 637, 686, 690, 695, 709, 720

huáng qín huá shí tāng 黄芩滑石汤, Scutellaria and Talcum Decoction, 733

huáng qín sháo yào tāng 黄芩芍药汤, Coptis and Peony Decoction, 702

huáng qín tāng 黄芩汤, Scutellaria Decoction, 71, 278, 731

huáng qín tāng xǐ fāng 黄芩汤洗方, Scutellaria Decoction Wash Formula, 744

huáng rén 黄仁, iris, 320

huáng rén 黄仁, yellow of the eye, 704

huáng shēng 黄升 yellow upborne elixir, Hydrogyrum Oxydatum Crudum Aureum, 445

huáng shuǐ chuāng 黄水疮, yellow-water sore, 705

huáng tāi 黄苔, yellow tongue fur, 704

huáng tǔ tāng 黄土汤, Yellow Earth Decoction, 28, 143, 314, 556, 738

huáng yào zǐ 黄药子 air potato, Dioscoreae Bulbiferae Tuber, 544, 624, 725

huáng yào zǐ jiǔ 黄药子酒, Air Potato Wine, 745

huáng yè shàng chōng 黄液上冲, upsurging yellow humor, 640

huáng yóu zhàng 黄油障, yellow fat obstruction, 704

huáng yóu zhèng 黄油证, yellow fat pattern, 704

huáng zhǒng 黄肿, yellow swelling, 704

huǎng hū 恍惚, abstraction, 3

Huazhou pomelo rind, *huà jú hóng* 化橘红, Citri Grandis Exocarpium Rubrum, 493, 723

huī zhǐ jiǎ 灰指甲, ashen nail, 11

huí 回, return, 504

huí cháng 回肠, large intestine, 340

huí chóng 蛔虫, roundworm, 509

huí chóng bìng 蛔虫病, roundworm disease, 509

huí chóng bìng 蚘虫病, roundworm disease, 509

huí chūn dān 回春丹, Return-of-Spring Elixir, 740

huí dòng wèi wǎn (guǎn) tòng 蚘动胃脘痛, roundworm stomach duct pain, 509

huí gān 蛔疳, roundworm gan, 509

huí guāng fǎn zhào 回光反照, last radiance of the setting sun, 340

huí jué 蛔厥, roundworm reversal, 509

huí rǔ 回乳, terminating lactation, 606

huí xiāng 茴香 fennel, Foeniculi Fructus, 83, 343, 397, 400, 447, 542, 660, 723

huí yáng fǎn běn tāng 回阳返本汤, Yang-Returning Root-Reviving Decoction, 735

huí yáng jiǔ zhēn 回阳九针, nine needles for returning yang, 410

huí yáng jiù jí tāng 回阳救急汤, Yang-Returning Emergency Decoction, 735

huí yáng jiù nì 回阳救逆, returning yang and stemming counterflow, 504

huí yáng yù lóng gāo 回阳玉龙膏, Yang-Returning Jade Dragon Paste, 104, 744

huì chòu 秽臭, foul smell, 225

huì xué 会穴, meeting point, 389

huì yáng 会阳, BL-35, Meeting of Yang, 41, 289, 493, 557, 656, 747

huì yīn 会阴, CV-1, Meeting of Yin, 98, 244, 297, 749

huì yīn 会阴, meeting of yin, 389

huì yīn 会阴, perineum, 430

huì zhuó 秽浊, foul turbidity, 225

huì zōng 会宗, TB-7, Convergence and Gathering, 748

humifuse euphorbia, *dì jǐn cǎo* 地锦草, Euphorbiae Humifusae Herba, 68, 111, 721

humor*
  aqueous, 551
  vitreous, 551

Humor-Increasing Decoction, *zēng yè tāng* 增液汤, 108, 127, 298, 416, 597, 607, 734

Humor-Increasing Qi-Coordinating Decoction, *zēng yè chéng qì tāng* 增液承气汤, 298, 532, 732

Humuli Scandentis Herba, *lǜ cǎo* 葎草, Japanese hop, 68, 721

hūn 昏, cloud, 74

hūn jué 昏厥, clouding reversal, 75

hūn mí (bù xǐng) 昏迷（不醒）, coma, 88

hūn shuì 昏睡, clouding sleep, 75

hūn shuì 昏睡, hypersomnia, 294

hún 魂, ethereal soul, 180

hún mén 魂门, BL-47, Hun Gate, 656, 747

hùn jīng zhàng 混睛障, murky eye obstruction, 403

Hundred and One Formulas Impediment-Alleviating Decoction, *bǎi yī juān bì tāng* 百一蠲痹汤, 734

Hundred Taxations, *bǎi láo* 百劳, 142, 277, 393, 442, 515, 544

Hundred Worm Nest, *bǎi chóng wō* 百虫窝, 64, 183, 426, 509, 510, 522, 549, 695, 696

huó 活, quicken, 490

huó luò 活络, quickening the network vessels, 490

huó luò dān 活络丹, Network-Quickening Elixir, 734

huó luò liú qì yǐn 活络流气饮, Network-Quickening Qi Flow Beverage, 249

huó luò xiào líng dān 活络效灵丹, Network-Quickening Efficacious Elixir, 737

huó rén cōng chǐ tāng 活人葱豉汤, Book of Life Scallion and Fermented Soybean Decoction, 729

huó rén xiāng rú yǐn 活人香薷散, Book of Life Renewal Elsholtzia Powder, 729

huó xuè 活血, quickening the blood, 490

huó xuè huà yū 活血化瘀, quickening the blood and transforming stasis, 490

huó xuè qū yū 活血祛瘀, quickening the blood and dispelling stasis, 490

huó xuè rùn zào shēng jīn sǎn 活血润燥生津散, Blood-Quickening Dryness-Moistening Liquid-Engendering Powder, 734

huó xuè sàn yū tāng 活血散瘀汤, Blood-Quickening Stasis-Dissipating Decoction, 18, 315

huó xuè shēng xīn 活血生新, quickening the blood and engendering the new, 490

huó xuè tāng 活血汤, Blood-Quickening Decoction, 570

huǒ 火, fire, 200

huǒ bǔ huǒ xiè 火补火泻, fire supplementation and fire drainage, 203

huǒ bù shēng tǔ 火不生土, fire failing to engender earth, 202

huǒ chuǎn 火喘, fire panting, 203

huǒ dài chuāng 火带疮, fire-girdle sore, 202

huǒ dān 火丹, fire cinnabar, 201

huǒ dān jiǎo 火丹脚, fire cinnabar leg, 201

huǒ gān 火疳, fire gan, 202

huǒ guàn 火罐, fire cup, 201

huǒ guàn 火罐, fire cupping, 201

huǒ ké 火咳, fire cough, 201

huǒ kuò 火廓, fire rampart, 203

huǒ má rén 火麻仁 hemp seed, Cannabis Semen, 72, 399, 415, 449, 460, 462, 722

huǒ rè 火热, fire heat, 202

huǒ rè tóu tòng 火热头痛, fire heat headache, 202

huǒ shāng fēng 火伤风, fire wind damage, 203

huǒ shèng xíng jīn 火盛刑金, exuberant fire tormenting metal, 189

huǒ shuǐ gòng zhì 水火共制, fire and water processing, 201

huǒ sòu 火嗽, fire cough, 201

huǒ tán 火痰, fire phlegm, 203

huǒ tóu tòng 火头痛, fire headache, 202

huǒ xiàn 火陷, fire fall, 202

huǒ xiè 火泄, fire diarrhea, 202

huǒ xiè 火泻, fire diarrhea, 202

huǒ xīn tòng 火心痛, fire heart pain, 202

huǒ xìng shàng yán 火性上炎, fire by nature flames upward, 201

huǒ yǎn 火眼, fire eye, 202

huǒ yù 火郁, fire depression, 201

huǒ yù chuǎn 火郁喘, fire depression panting, 202

huǒ yù sòu 火郁嗽, fire depression cough, 201

huǒ yù tāng 火郁汤, Fire Depression Decoction, 655

huǒ zhēn 火针, fire needle, 202

huǒ zhēn 火针, fire needling, 202

huǒ zhēn liáo fǎ 火针疗法, fire needling, 202

huǒ zhì 火制, fire processing, 203

huǒ zhòng 火中, fire stroke, 203

huò 豁, sweep, 599

huò dǎn wán 藿胆丸, Agastache/Patchouli and Pig's Bile Pill, 740

huò luàn 霍乱, cholera, 61

huò luàn 霍乱, sudden turmoil, 587

huò luàn zhuǎn jīn 霍乱转筋, cholera cramps, 61

huò pò xià líng tāng 藿朴夏苓汤, Agastache/Patchouli, Magnolia Bark, Pinellia, and Poria (Hoelen) Decoction, 23, 118, 410, 733

huò pò xià líng tāng 藿朴夏苓汤, Agastache/Patchouli, Pinellia, and Poria (Hoelen) Decoction, 539

huò tán kāi qiào 豁痰开窍, sweeping phlegm and opening the orifices, 599

huò tán xǐng nǎo 豁痰醒脑, sweeping phlegm and arousing the brain, 599

huò xiāng 藿香 agastache/patchouli, Agastaches seu Pogostemi Herba, 7, 10, 66, 82, 121, 143, 153, 167, 384, 401, 457, 587, 588, 625, 669, 722

huò xiāng zhèng qì piàn 藿香正气片, Agastache/Patchouli Qi-Righting Tablet, 588, 713

huò xiāng zhèng qì sǎn 藿香正气散, Agastache/Patchouli Qi-Righting Powder, 77, 152, 153, 218, 539, 580, 732

hydatic mole*, 615

hydatiform mole*, 615

Hydnocarpi Semen, *dà fēng zǐ* 大风子, hydnocarpus, 244, 728

hydnocarpus, *dà fēng zǐ* 大风子, Hydnocarpi Semen, 244, 728

Hydrargyrum, *shuǐ yín* 水银, mercury, 98, 171, 383, 411

hydrocele of tunica vaginalis*, 667

hydrocele*, 399
scrotal, 667

hydrocephalus*, 51

Hydrogyrum Oxydatum Crudum Aureum, *huáng shēng* 黄升, yellow upborne elixir, 445

Hydrogyrum Oxydatum Crudum Rubrum, *hóng shēng* 红升, red upborne elixir, 171 hydrothorax*, 182

hyoid bone*, 626

hyperadrenocorticalism*, 194

hyperemia of the bulbar conjunctiva*, 602

hyperemia*
ciliary, 497

Hyperici Japonici Herba, *dì ěr cǎo* 地耳草, lesser hypericum, 68, 136, 700, 721, 723

hyperlipemia*, 297

hyperopia*, 195

Hyperosteogeny Pill, *gǔ zhí zēng shēng wán* 骨质增生丸, 741

hyperplasia of the mammary glands*, 385

hyperplasia of the prostate in old age*, 148

hypersomnia*, 306

hypertension*, 10, 123, 290, 297, 336, 355, 365, 443, 444, 584, 616, 627, 708

hyperthyroidism*, 261, 336, 616, 627

hyphema*, 33

hypoadrenocorticism*, 142

hypochondriac pain*, 228

hypochondrium*, 507

hypoproteinemia*, 651

hypopyon*, 640

hypothyroidism*, 444, 651

hysterical paralysis*, 678

hán shù 含漱, mouth wash, 401

ichthyosis*
seborrheic, 676

ileocecal valve*, 515

ileotyphus*, 118

iliac fossa*, 342

Ilicis Chinensis Folium, *dōng qīng yè* 冬青叶, Chinese ilex leaf, 68, 721

Ilicis Pubescentis Radix, *máo dōng qīng* 毛冬青, hairy holly root, 138, 725

ilium*, 291

Ill-Wind Oil Paste, *fēng yóu gāo* 疯油膏, 422

Immediate Aid Pill, *jì jì wán* 既济丸, 743

Immortal Formula Life-Giving Beverage, *xiān fāng huó mìng yǐn* 仙方活命饮, 62, 187, 259, 386, 427, 585, 744

Impatientis Balsaminae Flos, *fèng xiān huā* 凤仙花, garden balsam flower, 11

Impediment-Alleviating Decoction, *juān bì tāng* 蠲痹汤, 14, 84, 734

Impediment-Diffusing Decoction, *xuān bì tāng* 宣痹汤, 547

imperata, *bái máo gēn* 白茅根, Imperatae Rhizoma, 106, 130, 277, 390, 566, 569, 724

Imperata and Pueraria Decoction, *máo gé tāng* 茅葛汤, 736

imperata flower, *bái máo huā* 白茅花, Imperatae Flos, 414, 415

Imperatae Flos, *bái máo huā* 白茅花, imperata flower, 414, 415

Imperatae Rhizoma, *bái máo gēn* 白茅根, imperata, 106, 130, 277, 390, 566, 569, 724

Imperatae Rhizoma Recens, *xiān máo gēn* 鲜茅根, fresh imperata, 30, 703

Imperial Garden Qi-Evening Powder, *yù yuàn yún qì sǎn* 御苑匀气散, 238

Imperial Grace Rhinoceros Horn and Rehmannia Pill, *jú fāng xī jiǎo dì huáng wán* 局方犀角地黄丸, 640

impetigo herpetiformis*, 705

impure mirabilite, *pò xiāo* 朴硝, Mirabilitum Non-Purum, 310

impure mirabilite, *pò xiāo* 朴硝, Mirabilitum Non-Purum, 44, 411, 460, 712, 722

incarcerated placenta*, 503

Incisive Light on the Source of Miscellaneous Disease (*zá bìng yuán liú xī zhú*) 杂病源流犀烛, 1773 (Qīng), Shěn Jīn-Áo 沈金鳌, 45, 191, 683

indigestion*, 218
chronic, 237

indigo, *qīng dài* 青黛, Indigo Pulverata Levis, 67, 201, 319, 419, 721

Indigo and Clamshell Pill, *qīng gé wán* 青蛤丸, 356

Indigo and Clamshell Powder, *dài gé sǎn* 黛蛤散, 101, 277, 695, 738

Indigo and Gold Powder, *qīng jīn sǎn* 青金散, 636

Indigo Paste, *qīng dài gāo* 青黛膏, 445

Indigo Powder, *qīng dài sǎn* 青黛散, 59, 117, 225, 238, 338, 516, 546, 586, 668, 671, 686, 705, 744

Indigo Pulverata Levis, *qīng dài* 青黛, indigo, 67, 201, 319, 419, 721

indigo residue, *lán diàn* 蓝靛, Indigonis Residuum, 497

Indigonis Residuum, *lán diàn* 蓝靛, indigo residue, 497

Indispensable Medical Reading (*yī zōng bì dú*) 医宗必读, 1637 (Míng), Lǐ Zhōng-Zǐ 李中梓 [Shì-Cái 士材], 380, 671, 703

Infant's Palace, *zǐ gōng* 子宫, 39, 332, 466, 711, 712

Infant-Safeguarding Red Powder, *bǎo chì sǎn* 保赤散, 736

infantile convulsions*, 230

infantile paralysis*, 541

Infantis Urina, *tóng biàn* 童便, child's urine, 201, 567

infestation*
parasite, 237

Infradiaphragmatic Stasis-Expelling Decoction, *gé xià zhú yū tāng* 膈下逐瘀汤, 24, 26, 35, 36, 152, 570, 647, 710, 737

Inner Canon (*nèi jīng*) 内经, full title *huáng dì nèi jīng* 黄帝内经, 46, 100, 108, 149, 178, 206, 208, 244, 264, 265, 298, 322, 324, 326, 341, 346, 349, 367, 371, 376, 377, 421, 459, 477, 505, 520, 534, 535, 549, 551, 560, 598, 606, 630, 638, 658, 670, 673, 678, 692

Inner Welcome Fragrance, *nèi yíng xiāng* 内迎香, 586

insect wax, *chóng bái là* 虫白腊, Ericeri Pelae Cera, 728

Insomnia, *shī mián* 失眠, 333

Instant Relief Powder, *shǒu niān sǎn* 手拈散, 571, 737

intercostal neuralgia*, 58

Internal Coursing Coptis Decoction, *nèi shū huáng lián tāng* 内疏黄连汤, 187, 303, 315, 743

Internal Expression and Pain-Relieving Decoction, *tuō lǐ dìng tòng tāng* 托里定痛汤, 744

Internal Expression Pus-Expelling Decoction, *tuō lǐ tòu nóng tāng* 托里透脓汤, 116, 744

Internal Expression Toxin-Dispersing Powder, *tuō lǐ xiāo dú sǎn* 托里消毒散, 9, 153, 259, 744

Internal Supplementation Pill, *nèi bǔ wán* 内补丸, 333, 742

Intestinal Adhesion Decoction, *cháng zhān lián huǎn jiě tāng* 肠粘连缓解汤, 735

Intestine-Clearing Beverage, *qīng cháng yǐn* 清肠饮, 743

Intestine-Moistening Decoction, *rùn cháng tāng* 润肠汤, 315, 565, 732

Intestine-Moistening Pill, *rùn cháng wán* 润肠丸, 399, 683, 732

Intestine-Securing Pill, *gù cháng wán* 固肠丸, 168

inula, *jīn fèi cǎo* 金沸草, Inulae Caulis et Folium, 624, 725

Inula and Hematite Decoction, *xuán fù huā dài zhě shí tāng* 旋覆花代赭石汤, 445, 499, 578, 736

Inula Decoction, *xuán fù huā tāng* 旋覆花汤, 356

inula flower, *xuán fù huā* 旋覆花, Inulae Flos, 17, 145, 146, 394, 578, 624, 669, 696, 725

Inula Powder, *jīn fèi cǎo sǎn* 金沸草散, 681, 684, 738

Inulae Caulis et Folium, *jīn fèi cǎo* 金沸草, inula, 624, 725

Inulae Flos, *xuán fù huā* 旋覆花, inula flower, 17, 145, 146, 394, 578, 624, 669, 696, 725

iridoptosis*, 104

iron flakes, *tiě luò* 铁落, Ferri Frusta, 54, 526, 585, 726

Iron Flakes Beverage, *shēng tiě luò yǐn* 生铁落饮, 386, 437, 700, 739

Iron Flute Pill, *tiě dí wán* 铁笛丸, 729

Isatidis Folium, *dà qīng yè* 大青叶, isatis leaf, 67, 70, 146, 420, 422, 450, 459, 547, 637, 721

Isatidis Radix, *bǎn lán gēn* 板蓝根, isatis root, 64, 67, 70, 214, 357, 387, 388, 501, 611, 686, 688, 700, 721

isatis leaf, *dà qīng yè* 大青叶, Isatidis Folium, 67, 70, 146, 420, 422, 450, 459, 547, 637, 721

isatis root, *bǎn lán gēn* 板蓝根, Isatidis Radix, 64, 67, 70, 214, 357, 387, 388, 501, 611, 686, 688, 700, 721

Isatis Root and Leaf Decoction, *bǎn lán dà qīng tāng* 板蓝大青汤, 730

ischium*, 517

isthmus faucium*, 612

Itch Reliever, *zhǐ yǎng xué* 止痒穴, 145

Itch Reliever, *zhǐ yǎng* 止痒, 113, 117, 422, 516, 522, 561, 591, 674, 686, 688

Itch-Soothing Decoction, *tā yǎng tāng* 塌痒汤, 241

Jade and Red Paste, *yù hóng gāo* 玉红膏, 744

Jade Candle Powder, *yù zhú sǎn* 玉烛散, 28, 732

Jade Countenance Pill, *yù róng wán* 玉容丸, 226

Jade Dew Powder, *yù lù sǎn* 玉露散, 187, 494, 540, 744

Jade Flask Pill, *yù hú wán* 玉壶丸, 478

Jade Humor Decoction, *yù yè tāng* 玉液汤, 734

Jade Lady Brew, *yù nǚ jiān* 玉女煎, 172, 190, 202, 239, 414, 431, 566, 577, 621, 687, 714, 731

Jade Lady Variant Brew, *jiā jiǎn yù nǚ jiān* 加减玉女煎, 730

Jade Pivot Elixir, *yù shū dān* 玉枢丹, 152, 171, 578, 590, 740

Jade Spring Powder, *yù quán sǎn* 玉泉散, 455

Jade Wind-Barrier Powder, *yù píng fēng sǎn* 玉屏风散, 95, 378, 489, 527, 702, 742

Japanese ardisia, *zǐ jīn niú* 紫金牛, Ardisiae Japonicae Caulis et Folium, 624, 725

Japanese dioscorea, *chuān shān lóng* 穿山龙, Dioscoreae Nipponicae Rhizoma, 140, 722

Japanese hop, *lǜ cǎo* 葎草, Humuli Scandentis Herba, 68, 721

Japanese ranunculus, *máo gèn* 毛茛, Ranunculi Japonici Herba et Radix, 388, 728

Jasper Jade Powder, *bì yù sǎn* 碧玉散, 730

Jaundice Capillaris Granules, *huáng dǎn yīn chén chōng jì* 黄疸茵陈冲剂, 733

jī 积, accumulation, 3

jī 肌, flesh, 210

jī bì 肌痹, flesh impediment, 210

jī biǎo 肌表, fleshy exterior, 211

jī bù yù shí 饥不欲食, no desire to eat despite hunger, 412

jī còu 肌腠, interstices of the flesh, 317

jī dàn4 huáng yóu gāo 鸡蛋黄油膏, Egg Yolk Paste, 636

jī fū bù rén 肌肤不仁, insensitivity of the skin, 308

jī fū jiǎ cuò 肌肤甲错, encrusted skin, 173

jī fū jiǎ cuò 肌肤甲错, incrusted skin, 299

jī fū má mù 肌肤麻木, numbness and tingling of the skin, 416

jī gǔ cǎo 鸡骨草 prayer-beads, Abri Cantoniensis Herba cum Radice, 68, 721

jī ké 鸡咳, hen cough, 290

jī lěng wèi wǎn (guǎn) tòng 积冷胃脘痛, accumulated cold stomach duct pain, 3

jī mén 箕门, SP-11, Winnower Gate, 520, 610, 746

jī míng sǎn 鸡鸣散, Cockcrow Powder, 112, 342, 733

jī nèi jīn 鸡内金 gizzard lining, Galli Gigerii Endothelium, 141, 216, 385, 420, 544, 582, 606, 665, 724

jī nǜ 肌衄, spontaneous bleeding of the flesh, 566

jī rè wèi wăn (guăn) tòng 积热胃脘痛, accumulated heat stomach duct pain, 3

jī ròu bù rén 肌肉不仁, insensitivity of the flesh, 308

jī sū săn 鸡苏散, Mint Powder, 730

jī xiōng 鸡胸, chicken breast, 59

jī xiōng 鸡胸, pigeon chest, 444

jī xuě căo 积雪草 centella, Centellae Herb (cum Radice), 139, 725

jī xuè téng 鸡血藤 millettia, Millettiae Radix et Caulis, 37, 137, 138, 352, 484, 516, 593, 679, 724, 727

jī yăn 鸡眼, corn, 99

jī zhuă (zhăo) fēng 鸡爪风, chicken's-claw wind, 60

jī zĭ bái 鸡子白 egg white, Galli Albumen, 621

jī zĭ huáng 鸡子黄 egg yolk, Galli Vitellus, 17, 176, 256

jí 疾, disease, 130

jí bìng 疾病, disease, 130

jí hóu fēng 急喉风, acute throat wind, 6

jí huáng 急黄, acute jaundice, 6

jí jīng fēng 急惊风, acute fright wind, 6

jí jiù xī xián săn 急救稀涎散, Emergency Drool-Thinning Powder, 440, 743

jí mài 急脉, LR-12, Urgent Pulse, 51, 297, 504, 749

jí mài 疾脉, racing pulse, 492

jí quán 极泉, HT-1, Highest Spring, 746

jí rán hán chū 溅然汗出, streaming sweat, 584

jí xià cún yīn 急下存阴, emergency precipitation to preserve yin, 172

jí xú bŭ xiè 疾徐补泻, quick and slow supplementation and drainage, 490

jí zào yì nù 急燥易怒, rashness, impatience, and irascibility, 492

jí zé zhì biāo 急则治标, in acute conditions treat the tip, 298

jĭ gān 脊疳, gan of the spine, 238

jĭ jiāo lì huáng wán 己椒苈黄丸, Fangji, Zanthoxylum, Tingli, and Rhubarb Pill, 732

jĭ tŭ 己土, S6-earth, 511

jĭ zhōng 脊中, GV-6, Spinal Center, 749

jĭ zhuī gŭ 脊椎骨, vertebra, 654

jì chuān jiān 济川煎, Ferry Brew, 50, 127, 732

jì jì tāng 既济汤, Complementarity Decoction, 22

jì jì wán 既济丸, Immediate Aid Pill, 743

jì kŏu 忌口, dietary contraindications, 126

jì lè 季肋, free ribs, 229

jì shēng jú hé wán 济生橘核丸, Life Saver Tangerine Pip Pill, 467, 735

jì shēng jú pí zhú rú tāng 济生橘皮竹茹汤, Life Saver Tangerine Peel and Bamboo Shavings Decoction, 736

jì shēng shèn qì wán 济生肾气丸, Life Saver Kidney Qi Pill, 22, 148, 151, 302, 335, 542, 662, 742

jì xié 季肋, free ribs, 229

jì xié tòng 季肋痛, free-rib pain, 228

jì xīn tòng 悸心痛, palpitation heart pain, 427

jì xíng 剂型, medicinal preparation, 389

jì zòng 瘛瘲, tugging and slackening, 631

jiā 痂, crust, 105

jiā 痂, scab, 512

jiā chí jìn zhēn fă 夹持进针法, skin-pinching needle insertion, 535

jiā chí jìn zhēn fă 挟持进针法, two-finger press needle insertion, 634

jiā jí 夹脊, Paravertebrals, 89

jiā jiăn fù mài tāng 加减复脉汤, Pulse-Restorative Variant Decoction, 741

jiā jiăn mù fáng jĭ táng 加减木防己汤, Woody Fangji Variant Decoction, 733

jiā jiăn shēng mài săn 加减生脉散, Pulse-Engendering Variant Powder, 456, 591, 715

jiā jiăn wēi ruí tāng 加减葳蕤汤, Solomon's Seal Variant Decoction, 176, 729

jiā jiăn xiāo yáo săn 加减逍遥散, Free Wanderer Variant Powder, 677

jiā jiăn yī yīn jiān 加减一阴煎, All Yin Variant Brew, 701

jiā jiăn yù nǚ jiān 加减玉女煎, Jade Lady Variant Brew, 730

jiā jiăn zhĭ zhú tāng 加减枳术汤, Unripe Bitter Orange and Ovate Atractylodes Variant Decoction, 562

jiā jiŭ zĭ wán 家韭子丸, Chinese Leek Seed Pill, 177

jiā mì rùn fèi yĭn 家秘润肺饮, Family Secret Lung-Moistening Beverage, 372

jiā mì wēn fèi tāng 家秘温肺汤, Family Secret Lung-Warming Decoction, 372

jiā mì xiè bái săn 家秘泻白散, Family Secret White-Draining Powder, 292, 372, 376

jiā wèi bái tóu wēng tāng 加味白头翁汤, Supplemented Pulsatilla Decoction, 731

jiā wèi cāng zhú gāo 加味苍术膏, Supplemented Atractylodes Paste, 173

jiā wèi dāng guī sháo yào săn 加味当归芍药散, Supplemented Tangkuei and Peony Powder, 741

jiā wèi dìng zhì wán 加味定志丸, Supplemented Mind-Stabilizing Pill, 739

jiā wèi èr miào săn 加味二妙散, Supplemented Mysterious Two Powder, 111, 112, 337

jiā wèi huáng tŭ tāng 加味黄土汤, Supplemented Yellow Earth Decoction, 743

jiā wèi jīn gāng wán 加味金刚丸, Supplemented Metal Strength Pill, 742

jiā wèi lĭ zhōng tāng 加味理中汤, Supplemented Center-Rectifying Decoction, 603

jiā wèi liù wèi dì huáng wán 加味六味地黄丸, Supplemented Six-Ingredient Rehmannia Pill, 226, 620

jiā wèi má xìng shí gān tāng 加味麻杏石甘汤, Supplemented Ephedra, Apricot Kernel, Gypsum, and Licorice Decoction, 189, 303, 677, 729

jiā wèi sān ào tāng 加味三拗汤, Supplemented Rough and Ready Three Decoction, 83

jiā wèi shèn qì wán 加味肾气丸, Supplemented Kidney Qi Pill, 742 *jiā wèi wēn dǎn tāng* 加味温胆汤, Supplemented Gallbladder-Warming Decoction, 739

jiā wèi wū yào tāng 加味乌药汤, Supplemented Lindera Decoction, 484, 735

jiā wèi xiāng sū sǎn 加味香苏散, Supplemented Cyperus and Perilla Powder, 729

jiā wèi xiāo yáo sǎn 加味逍遥散, Supplemented Free Wanderer Powder, 123, 640

jiā wèi xiè bái sǎn 加味泻白散, Supplemented White-Draining Powder, 469

jiā zhǐ gāo 夹纸膏, Paper Plaster, 744

jiá chē 颊车, ST-6, Cheek Carriage, 73, 89, 125, 140, 178, 189, 194, 222, 289, 366, 403, 446, 485, 521, 522, 611, 620, 621, 689, 690, 693, 746

jiá chē 颊车, cheek carriage, 57

jiá chē gǔ 颊车骨, cheek carriage bone, 57

jiá cuò 夹错, complex, 92

jiá nǎo fēng 夹脑风, brain-squeezing wind, 50

jiá zá 夹杂, complex, 92

jiǎ 瘕, conglomeration, 94

jiǎ 胛, scapula, 514

jiǎ 胛, shoulder blade, 530

jiǎ cuò 甲错, encrusted skin, 173

jiǎ cuò 甲错, incrusted skin, 299

jiǎ mù 甲木, S1-wood, 511

jiǎ shén 假神, false spiritedness, 195

jiān 煎, brew, 50

jiān 煎, decoct, 119

jiān 肩, shoulder, 530

jiān 坚, hardness, 254

jiān bǎng 肩膀, shoulder, 530

jiān bǎng tòng 肩膀痛, shoulder pain, 530

jiān bèi tòng 肩背痛, shoulder and back pain, 530

jiān jì 煎剂, decoction, 119

jiān jiē jiǔ 间接灸, indirect moxibustion, 299

jiān jǐng 肩井, GB-21, Shoulder Well, 61, 128, 142, 253, 307, 385, 386, 503, 515, 530, 606, 748

jiān jué 煎厥, boiling reversal, 44

jiān liáo 肩髎, TB-14, Shoulder Bone-Hole, 61, 89, 137, 289, 295, 342, 521, 530, 567, 748

jiān qián, Shoulder Front, 530

jiān rì nüè 间日疟, tertian malaria, 606

jiān shǐ 间使, PC-5, Intermediary Courier, 8, 19, 25, 71, 74, 82, 89, 113, 174, 197, 269, 282, 294, 317, 336, 378, 383, 386, 394, 396, 399, 416, 434, 439, 440, 442, 445, 482, 497, 521, 544, 572, 590, 604, 613, 624, 650, 664, 690, 694, 715, 748

jiān tòng 肩痛, shoulder pain, 530

jiān wài shū 肩外俞, SI-14, Outer Shoulder Transport, 105, 747

jiān xī 肩息, raised-shoulder breathing, 492

jiān yīn 坚阴, consolidating yin, 94

jiān yú 肩髃, LI-15, Shoulder Bone, 61, 137, 289, 295, 341, 418, 521, 530, 567, 679, 689, 746

jiān zhēn 肩贞, SI-9, True Shoulder, 137, 341, 530, 567, 747

jiān zhōng shū 肩中俞, SI-15, Central Shoulder Transport, 747

jiǎn chún 茧唇, cocoon lip, 76

jiàn 健, fortify, 223

jiàn bù hǔ qián wán 健步虎潜丸, Steady Gait Hidden Tiger Pill, 742

jiàn gǔ 楗骨, bolt bone, 44

jiàn lǐ 建里, CV-11, Interior Strengthening, 152, 749

jiàn líng tāng 建瓴汤, Sweeping Down Decoction, 53, 740

jiàn pí 健脾, fortifying the spleen, 223

jiàn pí 健脾, splenic fortification, 565

jiàn pí hé wèi 健脾和胃, fortifying the spleen and harmonizing the stomach, 224

jiàn pí huà tán 健脾化痰, fortifying the spleen and transforming phlegm, 224

jiàn pí lì shī 健脾利湿, fortifying the spleen and disinhibiting dampness, 224

jiàn pí lì shuǐ 健脾利水, fortifying the spleen and disinhibiting water, 224

jiàn pí shèn shī 健脾渗湿, fortifying the spleen and percolating dampness, 224

jiàn pí shū gān 健脾疏肝, fortifying the spleen and coursing the liver, 223

jiàn pí wán 健脾丸, Spleen-Fortifying Pill, 141, 224, 736

jiàn pí wēn shèn huà tán 健脾温肾化痰, fortifying the spleen, warming the kidney, and transforming phlegm, 224

jiàn pí yì qì 健脾益气, fortifying the spleen and boosting qi, 223

jiàn shén qū 建神麴 Fujian leaven, Massa Medicata Fermentata Fujianensis, 141, 724

jiàn wàng 健忘, forgetfulness, 222

jiàn wàng 健忘, poor memory, 447

jiàn wèi 健胃, fortifying the stomach, 224

jiàn yāo wán 健腰丸, Lumbus-Fortifying Pill, 742

jiàn zhōng 健中, fortifying the center, 223

jiàn zhōng tāng 建中汤, Center-Fortifying Decoctions, 555

jiāng 姜 ginger, Zingiberis Rhizoma, 154, 217

jiāng bàn xià 姜半夏 ginger pinellia, Pinelliae Tuber cum Zingibere Praeparatum, 47, 97, 257, 317, 421, 623, 725

jiāng fù tāng 姜附汤, Ginger and Aconite Decoction, 80, 81, 86

jiāng huáng 姜黄 tureric, Curcumae Longae Rhizoma, 138, 427, 724

jiāng jūn zhī guān 将军之官, office of general, 419

jiāng pí 姜皮 ginger skin, Zingiberis Rhizomatis Cortex, 153, 262, 681, 720

jiāng shuǐ sǎn 浆水散, Millet Water Powder, 735

jiāng zhī 姜汁 ginger juice, Zingiberis Rhizomatis Succus, 116, 448

jiāng zhī chǎo 姜汁炒, stir-frying with ginger juice, 574

jiāng zhì 姜炙, mix-frying with ginger, 397

jiàng 降, downbear, 145

jiàng 绛, crimson, 105

jiàng jì 降剂, downbearing formula, 145

jiàng kě qù shēng 降可去升, downbearing [medicinals] can eliminate upbearing, 145

jiàng nì píng chuǎn 降逆平喘, downbearing qi and calming panting, 146

jiàng nì xià qì 降逆下气, downbearing counterflow and precipitating qi, 145

jiàng nì zhǐ ǒu 降逆止呕, downbearing counterflow and checking vomiting, 145

jiàng qì 降气, downbearing qi, 146

jiàng zhēn xiāng 降真香 dalbergia, Dalbergiae Lignum, 27, 138, 512, 725

jiāo 焦, parch, 428

jiāo 胶, gelatin, 240

jiāo 胶, glue, 243

jiāo ài sì wù tāng 胶艾四物汤, Ass Hide Glue and Mugwort Four Agents Decoction, 212, 574

jiāo ài tāng 胶艾汤, Ass Hide Glue and Mugwort Decoction, 743

jiāo bǐng jiǔ 椒饼灸, moxibustion on pepper cake, 402

jiāo chā qǔ xué 交叉取穴, selection of contralateral points, 519

jiāo cháng 交肠, communicating bowels, 92

jiāo chuāng 椒疮, peppercorn sore, 430

jiāo gǔ 交骨, interlocking bones, 311

jiāo gǔ bù kāi 交骨不开, failure of the interlocking bones to open, 194

jiāo huì xué 交会穴, intersection point, 317

jiāo jiē chū xuè 交接出血, intercourse bleeding, 310

jiāo jié chū xuè 交结出血, intercourse bleeding, 310

jiāo mù 椒目 zanthoxylum seed, Zanthoxyli Semen, 660, 723

jiāo tài wán 交泰丸, Peaceful Interaction Pill, 413, 467, 538, 739

jiāo tōng xīn shèn 交通心肾, promoting heart-kidney interaction, 467

jiāo tōng xīn shèn 交通心肾, promoting interaction of the heart and kidney, 467

jiāo xìn 交信, KI-8, Intersection Reach, 747

jiǎo cháng shā 绞肠痧, intestine-gripping sand, 319

jiǎo gēn tòng 脚跟痛, heel pain, 288

jiǎo gōng fǎn zhāng 角弓反张, arched-back rigidity, 10

jiǎo qì 脚气, leg qi, 342

jiǎo qì chōng xīn 脚气冲心, leg qi surging into the heart, 343

jiǎo qì chuāng 脚气疮, foot qi sore, 221

jiǎo qì gōng xīn 脚气攻心, leg qi attacking the heart, 342

jiǎo qì rù xīn 脚气入心, leg qi entering the heart, 342

jiǎo shī qì 脚湿气, foot damp qi, 218

jiǎo sūn 角孙, TB-20, Angle Vertex, 500, 748

jiǎo tòng 绞痛, gripping pain, 249

jiǎo yā mí làn 脚丫糜烂, eroding foot, 178

jiǎo zhǒng 脚肿, swollen feet, 601

jiē gǔ dān 接骨丹, Bone-Joining Elixir, 737

jié 结, bind, 18

jié 结, bound, 48

jié 疖, boil, 44

jié 竭, exhaust, 181

jié dài (mài) 结代（脉）, bound or intermittent (pulse), 48

jié gēn liáo fǎ 截根疗法, root-severing therapy, 508

jié gěng 桔梗 platycodon, Platycodonis Radix, 5, 47, 56, 128, 129, 175, 199, 227, 315, 338, 368, 388, 392, 394, 414, 422, 546, 549, 624, 625, 671, 695, 703, 725

jié gěng tāng 桔梗汤, Platycodon Decoction, 261, 469, 738

jié hé 结核, node, 412

jié hóu 结喉, laryngeal prominence, 340

jié jiā 结痂, crust, 105

jié mài 结脉, bound pulse, 48

jié nüè 截疟, interrupting malaria, 317

jié nüè qī bǎo yǐn 截疟七宝饮, Malaria-Interrupting Seven-Jewel Beverage, 317, 732

jié xiōng 结胸, chest bind, 57

jié yáng 结阳, binding in yang, 19

jié yīn 结阴, binding in yin, 19

jié zhǒng 疖肿, boil swelling, 44

jiě 解, resolve, 500

jiě biǎo 解表, exterior resolution, 185

jiě biǎo 解表, resolving the exterior, 500

jiě jī 解肌, resolving the flesh, 502

jiě jìng 解痉, resolving tetany, 500

jiě kě 解渴, allaying thirst, 8

jiě lú 解颅, ununited skull, 638

jiě rè sàn xuè tāng 解热散血汤, Heat-Resolving Blood-Dissipating Decoction, 730

jiě suǒ mài 解索脉, untwining rope pulse, 638

jiě xī 解溪, ST-41, Ravine Divide, 80, 90, 99, 112, 115, 137, 153, 192, 223, 258, 296, 309, 342, 395, 433, 434, 436, 441, 519, 520, 567, 652, 679, 683, 691, 746

jiě yù 解郁, resolving depression, 500

jiè 疥, scab, 512

jiè chuāng 疥疮, scab, 512

jiè zǐ 芥子 leaf mustard seed, Brassicae Junceae Semen, 624, 725

Jilong corydalis, *xià tiān wú* 夏天无, Corydalis Decumbentis Tuber et Herba, 140, 722

jīn 金, Jin, 322

jīn 金, metal, 394

jīn 筋, sinew, 532

jīn 筋, vein, 654

jīn 津, liquid, 348

jīn 斤, catty, 54

jīn 斤, jin, 322

jīn bì 筋痹, sinew impediment, 533

jīn bù shàng chéng 津不上承, liquid failing to bear upward, 348

jīn chuāng 金疮, incised wound, 298

jīn chuāng 金创, incised wound, 298

jīn chuāng fēng 金疮风, incised-wound tetany, 298

jīn fèi cǎo 金沸草 inula, Inulae Caulis et Folium, 624, 725

jīn fèi cǎo sǎn 金沸草散, Inula Powder, 681, 684, 738

jīn gān 金疳, metal gan, 394

jīn gān 筋疳, gan of the sinew, 238

jīn gān 筋疳, sinew gan, 533

jīn gāng wán 金刚丸, Metal Strength Pill, 47

jīn gǔ téng tòng 筋骨疼痛, sinew and bone pain, 533

jīn guì shèn qì wán 金匮肾气丸, Golden Coffer Kidney Qi Pill, 24, 36, 44, 86, 117, 148, 163, 240, 265, 331, 334, 415, 440, 461, 523, 529, 569, 604, 608, 647, 664, 669, 703

jīn guì yào lüè 金匮要略 (*Essential Prescriptions of the Golden Coffer*), full title *jīn guì yào lüè fāng lùn* 金匮要略方论, 1, 3, 20, 34, 58, 120, 124, 152, 173, 194, 197, 204, 209, 273, 292, 306, 308, 318, 322, 334, 349, 350, 360, 363, 379, 384, 449, 469, 498, 526, 529, 535, 536, 564, 626, 651, 653, 655, 661, 668, 692, 704

jīn guì yì 金匮翼 (*Wings of the Golden Coffer*), 1768 (Qīng), Lóng Zài-Jīng 龙在泾, 693

jīn guǒ lǎn 金果榄 tinospora tuber, Tinosporae Tuber, 68, 721

jīn huǎn 筋缓, slack sinews, 536

jīn huáng gāo 金黄膏, Golden Yellow Paste, 323, 528, 671

jīn huáng sǎn 金黄散, Golden Yellow Powder, 187, 259, 386, 494, 540, 744

jīn jīn yù yè 金津玉液, Gold Liquid and Jade Humor, 37, 125, 160, 174, 186, 284, 289, 336, 348, 455, 456, 573, 587, 607

jīn jú 金橘 kumquat, Fortunellae Fructus, 363

jīn lì 筋疠, sinew scrofula, 533

jīn lián huā 金莲花 globeflower, Trollii Flos, 68, 721

jīn líng zǐ sǎn 金铃子散, Toosendan Powder, 19, 27, 280, 354, 478, 483, 735

jīn liú 筋瘤, sinew tumor, 533

jīn luò 筋络, sinew network vessel, 533

jīn mài 筋脉, sinew, 532

jīn mài 筋脉, sinew vessel, 534

jīn mài 筋脉, vein, 654

jīn mén 金门, BL-63, Metal Gate, 425, 747

jīn mó 筋膜, sinew membrane, 533

jīn mài jū jí 筋脉拘急, hypertonicity of the sinews, 294

jīn mài jū jí 筋脉拘急, tension of the sinews, 606

jīn pò bù míng 金破不鸣, broken metal failing to sound, 51

jīn qì 津气, liquid qi, 348

jīn qián cǎo 金钱草 moneywort, Jinqiancao Herba, 21, 136, 369, 544, 582, 700, 723

jīn qián xiǎn 金钱癣, coin lichen, 76

jīn shàn 筋疝, sinew mounting, 533

jīn shí bù míng 金实不鸣, replete metal failing to sound, 498

jīn shuǐ liù jūn jiān 金水六君煎, Six Gentlemen Metal and Water Brew, 63, 440, 596, 603, 738

jīn shuǐ xiāng shēng 金水相生, metal and water engender each other, 394

jīn shuǐ xiāng shēng 金水相生, mutual engendering of metal and water, 404

jīn suō 筋缩, GV-8, Sinew Contraction, 74, 86, 117, 168, 178, 316, 366, 437, 456, 591, 652, 693, 714, 749

jīn suǒ gù jīng wán 金锁固精丸, Golden Lock Essence-Securing Pill, 11, 12, 147, 308, 461, 518, 524, 743

jīn tì ròu rùn (shùn) 筋惕肉瞤, jerking sinews and twitching flesh, 322

jīn tòng 筋痛, sinew pain, 533

jīn wěi 筋痿, sinew wilting, 534

jīn yè 津液, fluids, 213

jīn yè bù zú 津液不足, insufficiency of fluids, 309

jīn yè sǔn shāng 津液损伤, damage to fluids, 108

jīn yín huā 金银花 lonicera, Lonicerae Flos, 17, 28, 64, 67, 69, 70, 118, 130, 143, 189, 214, 282, 303, 315, 338, 386–388, 412, 422, 450, 459, 463, 501, 621, 671, 687, 691, 721

jīn yīng zǐ 金樱子 Cherokee rose fruit, Rosae Laevigatae Fructus, 12, 308, 496, 518, 727

jīn yīng 筋瘿, sinew goiter, 533

jīn zhī fǔ 筋之府, house of the sinews, 293

jīn hóng piàn 锦红片, Red Brocade Tablet, 743

jīn hóu fēng 紧喉风, constricting throat wind, 96

jīn mài 紧脉, tight pulse, 614

jìn 晋, Jin, 322

jìn bù xuǎn xué 近部选穴, selection of local points, 520

jìn kǒu lì 噤口痢, food-denying dysentery, 217

jìn pào 浸泡, soaking, 544

jìn pào 浸泡, steeping, 572

jìn shí 进食, increasing food intake, 298

jìn xuè 近血, proximal bleeding, 468

jìn yín chuāng 浸淫疮, wet spreading sore, 671

jìn zhēn 进针, needle insertion, 406

Jing-Yue's Complete Compendium (jǐng yuè quán shū) 景岳全书, 1624 (Míng), Zhāng Jiè-Bīn 张介宾 [Jǐng-Yuè 景岳], 123, 324, 427, 469, 524, 701, 702

jīng 经, channel, 55

jīng 惊, fright, 229

jīng 精, essence, 178

jīng 精, semen, 523

jīng bì 经闭, amenorrhea, 8

jīng bì 经闭, menstrual block, 389

jīng bié 经别, channel divergence, 55

jīng chù 惊搐, fright convulsions, 230

jīng cì 经刺, channel needling, 56

jīng duàn 经断, menopause, 389

jīng fáng 精房, essence chamber, 179

jīng fáng bài dú sǎn 荆防败毒散, Schizonepeta and Ledebouriella Toxin-Vanquishing Powder, 62, 91, 145, 184, 187, 303, 449, 502, 612, 681, 684, 729

jīng fáng sì wù tāng 荆防四物汤, Schizonepeta and Ledebouriella Four Agents Decoction, 452 *jīng fáng tāng* 荆防汤, Schizonepeta and Ledebouriella Decoction, 729

jīng fēng 惊风, fright wind, 230

jīng fēng bā hòu 惊风八候, eight signs of fright wind, 170

jīng fēng sì zhèng 惊风四证, four patterns of fright wind, 226

jīng fǔ 精府, house of essence, 293

jīng gōng 精宫, BL-52, Palace of Essence, 296, 310, 514, 518, 524

jīng gōng 精宫, palace of essence, 426

jīng gǔ 京骨, BL-64, Capital Bone, 90, 185, 247, 255, 341, 370, 391, 440, 548, 666, 690, 747

jīng guān 精关, essence gate, 179

jīng guān bù gù 精关不固, insecurity of the essence gate, 308

jīng hán 精寒, seminal cold, 523

jīng hòu tù nǜ 经后吐衄, postmenstrual blood ejection and spontaneous external bleeding, 447

jīng jì 惊悸, fright palpitations, 230

jīng jiè 荆芥 schizonepeta, Schizonepetae Herba et Flos, 102, 184, 244, 338, 412, 422, 430, 449, 497, 500–502, 548, 599, 681, 712, 713, 720

jīng jiè suì 荆芥穗 schizonepeta spike, Schizonepetae Flos, 320, 439, 549

jīng jiè tàn 荆芥炭 charred schizonepeta, Schizonepetae Herba et Flos Carbonisatae, 586

jīng jīn 经筋, channel sinew, 56

jīng jué 经绝, menopause, 389

jīng jué 惊厥, fright reversal, 230

jīng kē 精窠, nest of essence, 408

jīng kuáng 惊狂, fright mania, 230

jīng lái chéng kuài 经来成块, clotted menstrual flow, 74

jīng lái fā kuáng 经来发狂, menstrual mania, 392

jīng lái fā rè 经来发热, menstrual heat effusion, 390

jīng lái fú zhǒng 经来浮肿, menstrual puffy swelling, 392

jīng lái ǒu tù 经来呕吐, menstrual vomiting, 393

jīng lái sè dàn 经来色淡, pale menstrual flow, 426

jīng lái zǐ sè 经来紫色, purple menstrual flow, 474

jīng lěng 精冷, seminal cold, 523

jīng lián 睛帘, iris, 320

jīng lòu 经漏, menstrual spotting, 393

jīng luàn 经乱, chaotic menstruation, 56

jīng luò 经络, channels and network vessels, 56

jīng luò cè dìng yí 经络测定仪, meridiometer, 393

jīng luò xué shuō 经络学说, channel theory, 56

jīng luò zhī qì 经络之气, channel [and network] qi, 55

jīng mài 经脉, channel, 55

jīng mài zhī hǎi 经脉之海, sea of the channels, 517

jīng mén 京门, GB-25, Capital Gate, 8, 91, 291, 461, 748

jīng míng 睛明, BL-1, Bright Eyes, 27, 64, 89, 93, 150, 181, 195, 222, 291, 320, 395, 406, 495, 500, 520, 549, 568, 585, 586, 685, 689, 747

jīng míng zhī fǔ 精明之府, house of bright essence, 293

jīng péi 晶痦, miliaria crystallina, 395

jīng qī yán cháng 经期延长, prolonged menstruation, 466

jīng qì 经气, channel qi, 56

jīng qì 精气, essential qi, 180

jīng qián biàn xuè 经前便血, premenstrual bloody stool, 462

jīng qián ǒu tù 经前呕吐, premenstrual vomiting, 463

jīng qián qī jǐn zhāng zōng hé zhèng 经前期紧张综合症, premenstrual syndrome, 462

jīng qiáng 茎强, persistent erection, 430

jīng qiáng 茎强, rigidity of the penis, 508

jīng qín sì wù tāng 荆芩四物汤, Schizonepeta and Scutellaria Four Agents Decoction, 730

jīng qú 经渠, LU-8, Channel Ditch, 207, 291, 368, 746

jīng rè 惊热, fright heat [effusion], 230

jīng rú hā má zǐ 经如虾蟆子, toad-egg menses, 615

jīng shǎo 精少, scant semen, 513

jīng shén 精神, essence-spirit, 179

jīng shì 精室, essence chamber, 179

jīng shuǐ duàn jué 经水断绝, menopause, 389

jīng suǐ xū kuī 精髓虚亏, essence-marrow depletion, 179

jīng wài qí xué 经外奇穴, nonchannel point, 412

jīng wài xué 经外穴, nonchannel point, 412

jīng xián 惊痫, fright epilepsy, 230

jīng xíng biàn xuè 经行便血, menstrual bloody stool, 390

jīng xíng bù lì 经行不利, inhibited menstruation, 301

jīng xíng bù shuǎng 经行不爽, ungratifying menstruation, 637

jīng xíng fā rè 经行发热, menstrual heat effusion, 390

jīng xíng fù tòng 经行腹痛, menstrual abdominal pain, 389

jīng xíng hòu qī 经行后期, delayed menstruation, 121

jīng xíng nǜ xuè 经行衄血, menstrual spontaneous external bleeding, 392

jīng xíng tù xuè 经行吐血, menstrual blood ejection, 390

jīng xíng xiān hòu wú dìng qī 经行先后无定期, menstruation at irregular intervals, 393

jīng xíng xiān qī 经行先期, advanced menstruation, 7

jīng xué 经穴, channel point, 56

jīng xué 经穴, river point, 508

jīng xuè 经血, menstrual blood, 390

jīng xuè 精血, essence-blood, 179

jīng xuè bù jué 经血水不绝, persistent menstrual flow, 431

jīng xuè bù zú 精血不足, insufficiency of essence-blood, 309

jīng xuè tóng yuán 精血同源, essence and blood are of the same source, 179 *jīng yè dà xiè* 精液大泄, great seminal discharge, 248

jīng zé qì luàn 惊则气乱, fright causes derangement of qi, 229

jīng zhuó 精浊, essence turbidity, 179

jǐng gǔ 颈骨, neck bone, 406

jǐng xiàng fǎn zhāng 颈项反张, arched rigidity of the neck, 10

jǐng xiàng 颈项, neck, 406

jǐng xué 井穴, well point, 671

jīng yuè quán shū 景岳全书 (*Jing-Yue's Complete Compendium*), 1624 (Míng), Zhāng Jiè-Bīn 张介宾 [Jǐng-Yuè 景岳], 123, 324, 427, 469, 524, 701, 702

jìng 痉, tetany, 606

jìng bìng 痉病, tetanic disease, 606

jìng fǔ 净腑, clean bowel, 64

jìng jué 痉厥, tetanic reversal, 606

jìng luán 痉挛, spasm, 550

jìng miàn shé 镜面舌, mirror tongue, 396

jìng tāi 净苔, clean tongue fur, 64

Jinqiancao Herba, *jīn qián cǎo* 金钱草, moneywort, 21, 136, 369, 544, 582, 700, 723

jiū wěi 鸠尾, CV-15, Turtledove Tail, 178, 408, 434, 440, 482, 749

jiū wěi 鸠尾, turtle-dove's tail, 633

jiǔ 久, enduring, 173

jiǔ cài 韭菜 Chinese leek, Allii Tuberosi Folium, 241, 593, 727

jiǔ chóng bìng 九虫病, nine worm diseases, 412

jiǔ cì 九刺, nine needling methods, 410

jiǔ dǎn 酒疸, liquor jaundice, 349

jiǔ fǎ 灸法, moxibustion, 402

jiǔ huáng dǎn 酒黄疸, liquor jaundice, 349

jiǔ jì 酒剂, wine, 694

jiǔ jì 酒剂, wine preparation, 694

jiǔ jié chá 九节茶 sarcandra, Sarcandrae Ramulus et Folium, 68, 721

jiǔ ké 久咳, enduring cough, 173

jiǔ lì 久痢, enduring dysentery, 174

jiǔ liù bǔ xiè 九六补血, nine and six supplementation and drainage, 410

jiǔ nüè 久疟, enduring malaria, 174

jiǔ pǐ 酒癖, drinker's aggregation, 149

jiǔ qiào 九窍, nine orifices, 411

jiǔ tòng rù luò 久痛入络, enduring pain entering the network vessels, 174

jiǔ tòng wán 九痛丸, Nine Pains Pill, 182, 735

jiǔ wèi lǐ zhōng tāng 九味理中汤, Nine-Ingredient Center-Rectifying Decoction, 83, 736

jiǔ wèi qiāng huó tāng 九味羌活汤, Nine-Ingredient Notopterygium Decoction, 119, 586, 681, 729

jiǔ xiān dān 九仙丹, Nine Immortals Elixir, 743

jiǔ xiān sǎn 九仙散, Nine Immortals Powder, 96, 743

jiǔ xiāng chóng 九香虫 stinkbug, Aspongopus, 493, 724

jiǔ xiè 久泄, enduring diarrhea, 174

jiǔ xiè huá tuō 久泄滑脱, enduring diarrhea efflux desertion, 174

jiǔ yī dān 九一丹, Nine-to-One Elixir, 17, 187, 492, 528, 744

jiǔ zhā 酒齇, drinker's nose, 149

jiǔ zhēn 九针, nine needles, 410

jiǔ zhēng 酒癥, drinker's concretion, 149

jiǔ zhì 酒炙, mix-frying with wine, 397

jiǔ zǐ 韭子 Chinese leek seed, Allii Tuberosi Semen, 593, 727

jiù 救, stem, 572

jiù mǔ dān 救母丹, Mother's Rescue Elixir, 737

jiù tuō huó mǔ tāng 救脱活母汤, Desertion-Stemming Mother-Reviving Decoction, 454

jū jū 疽, flat-abscess, 209

jū jí 拘急, hypertonicity, 294

jū liáo 居髎, GB-29, Squatting Bone-Hole, 296, 748

jū luán 拘挛, hypertonicity, 294

jú bái 橘白 white tangerine peel, Citri Exocarpium Album, 493, 723

jú bàn zhǐ zhú wán 橘半枳术丸, Tangerine Peel, Pinellia, Unripe Bitter Orange, and Ovate Atractylodes Pill, 736

jú bù qǔ xué 局部取穴, selection of local points, 520

jú bù xué wèi 局部穴位, local point, 366

jú fāng xī jiǎo dì huáng wán 局方犀角地黄丸, Imperial Grace Rhinoceros Horn and Rehmannia Pill, 640

jú hé 橘核 tangerine pip, Citri Semen, 19, 291, 385, 493, 606, 671, 723

jú hé wán 橘核丸, Tangerine Pip Pill, 51, 111, 399, 511, 735

jú hóng 橘红 red tangerine peel, Citri Exocarpium Rubrum, 95, 136, 448, 493, 723

jú huā 菊花 chrysanthemum, Chrysanthemi Flos, 53, 104, 130, 225, 230, 394, 420, 497, 526, 686, 720

jú huā chá tiáo sǎn 菊花茶调散, Tea-Blended Chrysanthemum Powder, 740

jú huā yè 菊花叶 chrysanthemum leaf, Chrysanthemi Folium, 104

jú luò 橘络 tangerine pith, Citri Fructus Fasciculus Vascularis, 417, 493, 723

jú pí jiān wán 橘皮煎丸, Tangerine Peel Decocted Pill, 485

jú pí zhú rú tāng 橘皮竹茹汤, Tangerine Peel and Bamboo Shavings Decoction, 156, 280, 736

jú xìng wán 橘杏丸, Tangerine Peel and Apricot Kernel Pill, 477

jú yè 橘叶 tangerine leaf, Citri Folium, 493, 723

jǔ ruò 蒟蒻 devil's tongue, Amorphophalli Tuber, 68, 721

jǔ yuán jiān 举元煎, Origin-Lifting Brew, 199, 430, 487–489, 574, 740

jù 聚, gathering, 240

jù àn 拒按, refuse pressure, 497

jù cì 巨刺, grande piqûre, 245

jù cì 巨刺, great needling, 248

jù fēn 巨分, grand cleft, 245

jù gǔ 巨骨, LI-16, Great Bone, 61, 90, 530, 746

jù gǔ 巨骨, clavicle, 64

jù liáo 巨髎, ST-3, Great Bone-Hole, 45, 521, 746

jù máo 聚毛, tuft of hair, 631

jù què 巨阙, CV-14, Great Tower Gate, 8, 39, 58, 59, 81, 91, 159, 160, 207, 223, 232, 261, 263, 265–267, 269–271, 273, 274, 280, 294, 297, 301, 336, 343, 410, 427, 451, 452, 488, 499, 537, 538, 594, 595, 629, 651, 661, 749

juān bì tāng 蠲痹汤, Impediment-Alleviating Decoction, 14, 84, 734

juǎn bǎi 卷柏 selaginella, Selaginellae Herba, 724

juàn dài 倦怠, fatigue, 195

juàn dài fá lì 倦怠乏力, fatigue and lack of strength, 195

jué 绝, expire, 183

jué 厥, reversal, 504

jué gǔ 绝骨, GB-39, Severed Bone, 11, 197, 310, 331, 508

jué hàn 绝汗, expiration sweating, 183

jué lè 橛肋, peg ribs, 430

jué míng zǐ 决明子 fetid cassia, Cassiae Torae Semen, 459, 676

jué míng zǐ sǎn 决明子散, Fetid Cassia Powder, 740

jué nì 厥逆, reverse-flow, 505

jué nì tóu tòng 厥逆头痛, reverse-flow headache, 505

jué shàn 厥疝, reversal mounting, 505

jué tóu tòng 厥头痛, reversal headache, 505

jué tuō 厥脱, reversal desertion, 505

jué xīn tòng 厥心痛, reversal heart pain, 505

jué yīn 厥阴, reverting yin, 506

jué yīn bìng 厥阴病, reverting yin disease, 506

jué yīn huà fēng 厥阴化风, reverting yin transforming into wind, 506

jué yīn jīng 厥阴经, reverting yin channel, 506

jué yīn shū 厥阴俞, BL-14, Reverting Yin Transport, 58, 59, 89, 91, 228, 230, 236, 265, 268, 427, 452, 629, 747

jué yīn tóu tòng 厥阴头痛, reverting yin headache, 506

jué zhèng 厥证, reversal pattern, 505

Juglandis Semen, *hú táo rén* 胡桃仁, walnut, 97, 467, 526, 593, 596, 726

jujube, *dà zǎo* 大枣, Ziziphi Fructus, 11, 96, 217, 255, 358, 499, 580, 593, 600, 726

Jujube and Melanterite Pill, *zǎo fán wán* 枣矾丸, 737

jujube paste, *zǎo ní* 枣泥, Ziziphi Fructus Pasta, 251

jūn chén zuǒ shǐ 君臣佐使, medicinal roles, 389

jūn chén zuǒ shǐ 君臣佐使, sovereign, minister, assistant, and courier, 549

jūn huǒ 君火, sovereign fire, 549

jūn zhǔ zhī guān 君主之官, office of monarch, 419

jùn 峻, drastic, 147

jùn lì cǎo yào fāng 菌痢草药方, Bacillary Dysentery Herbal Formula, 731

Junci Medulla, *dēng xīn cǎo* 灯心草, juncus, 53, 60, 136, 262, 263, 723

juncus, *dēng xīn cǎo* 灯心草, Junci Medulla, 53, 60, 136, 262, 263, 723

jīn guì yù hán jīng 金匮玉函经 (*Canon of the Golden Coffer and Jade Sheath*), Eastern Han, Zhāng Jī 张机 [Zhòng-Jīng 仲景], 380

jīng yàn xué 经验穴, empirical points, 172

jūn 君, sovereign, 549

kǎ tán 咯痰, expectoration of phlegm, 181

kǎ xuè 咯血, expectoration of blood, 181

kǎ xuè 咯血, hacking of blood, 251

kà xuè 喀血, hacking of blood, 251

kadsura pepper stem, *hǎi fēng téng* 海风藤, Piperis Kadsurae Caulis, 139, 722

kāi gǔ sǎn 开骨散, Bone-Opening Powder, 195

kāi guān sǎn 开关散, Gate-Opening Powder, 745

kāi hé bǔ xiè 开阖补泻, open and closed supplementation and drainage, 419

kāi jìn sǎn 开噤散, Food Denial Powder, 217

kāi qiào 开窍, opening the orifices, 420

kāi qiào 开窍, orifice opening, 421

kāi qiào tōng shén 开窍通神, opening the orifices and freeing the spirit, 420

kāi qiào xǐng shén 开窍醒神, opening the orifices and arousing the spirit, 420

kāi wèi 开胃, opening the stomach, 420

kāi wèi jìn shí 开胃进食, opening the stomach and increasing food intake, 420

kāi xiè 开泄, opening and discharging, 420

kāi yù zhòng yù tāng 开郁种玉汤, Depression-Opening Jade-Planting Decoction, 353

kāi, hé, shū 开、合、枢, opening, closing, and pivot, 420

Kaki Calyx, *shì dì* 柿蒂, persimmon calyx, 493, 499, 649, 724

Kaki Fructus Exsiccatus, *shì bǐng* 柿饼, dried persimmon, 231

Kaki Saccharum, *shì shuāng* 柿霜, persimmon frost, 231

Kalimeridis Herba et Radix, *mǎ lán* 马兰, kalimeris, 542

kalimeris, *mǎ lán* 马兰, Kalimeridis Herba et Radix, 542

kǎn lí shā 坎离砂, Fire and Water Hexagram Granules, 744

kàng 亢, hyperactivity, 294

kàng bái hóu hé jì 抗白喉合剂, Diphtheria Mixture, 730

kansui, *gān suì* 甘遂, Kansui Radix, 171, 182, 438, 460, 464, 508, 574, 666, 722

Kansui Powder, *gān suì sǎn* 甘遂散, 744

Kansui Radix, *gān suì* 甘遂, kansui, 171, 182, 438, 460, 464, 508, 574, 666, 722

Katsumada's galangal seed, *cǎo dòu kòu* 草豆蔻, Alpiniae Katsumadae Semen, 66, 105, 625, 722

kē gǔ 髁骨, hip bone, 291

ké chuǎn 咳喘, cough and panting, 101

ké nì shàng qì 咳逆上气, counterflow qi ascent cough, 102

ké sòu 咳嗽, cough, 100

ké sòu xuè 咳嗽血, coughing of blood, 101

ké xuè 咳血, coughing of blood, 101

ké xuè fāng 咳血方, Blood Cough Formula, 738

kě 渴, thirst, 607

kě bù yù yǐn 渴不欲饮, thirst with no desire to drink, 608

kě xǐ rè yǐn 渴喜热饮, thirst with a liking for warm drinks, 608

kè 客, visiting, 656

kè sè 客色, visiting complexion, 656

kè wǔ 客忤, visiting hostility, 657

keloma*, 384

kelp, *kūn bù* 昆布, Algae Thallus, 30, 141, 243, 544, 624, 725

kěn tāi 揹苔, generalized slimy tongue fur, 240

keratitis*
  interstitial, 403
  parenchymatous, 403
  suppurative, 93

keratoconjunctivitis*
  phlyctenular, 676

keratomalacia*, 60

KI-1, *yǒng quán* 涌泉, Gushing Spring, 6, 32, 33, 47, 53, 63, 74, 81, 88, 123, 156, 160, 176, 178, 203, 212, 225, 231, 232, 256, 282, 283, 289, 292, 294, 319, 320, 331, 333, 336, 337, 343, 345, 364, 366, 384, 391, 401, 410, 413, 415, 420, 425, 437, 448, 452, 456, 458, 467, 478, 495, 504, 506, 511, 534, 537, 547, 566–568, 572, 597, 620, 641, 646, 648, 649, 654, 656, 683, 690, 699, 709, 714–716, 747

KI-2, *rán gǔ* 然谷, Blazing Valley, 16, 28–31, 36, 72, 76, 97, 99, 122, 152, 156, 158, 160, 161, 164, 168, 174–176, 180, 199, 203, 220, 229, 237, 277, 282, 283, 292, 294, 296, 332, 336, 348, 349, 360, 390, 391, 393, 410, 455, 456, 461, 462, 535, 552, 566, 567, 572, 582, 591, 597, 607, 613, 614, 641, 642, 647–649, 702, 709, 714–716, 747

KI-3, *tài xī* 太溪, Great Ravine, 4, 11, 14, 23, 26, 28–31, 36, 41, 43, 45, 47, 54, 59, 61, 69, 70, 72, 84, 86, 88–90, 95–97, 105, 111, 117, 119, 123, 128, 151, 152, 154–156, 158, 160, 161, 163, 164, 167, 168, 174–177, 180, 197, 199, 201, 203, 222, 225, 229, 230, 237, 239, 256, 260, 263, 266–268, 275, 277, 282, 283, 285, 288–292, 294, 296, 302, 308, 310, 312, 314, 320, 327, 329, 331–337, 345, 347, 349, 352, 355, 360, 364–366, 368–370, 378–381, 391, 393, 398, 401, 410, 413, 415, 416, 425, 426, 449, 450, 453, 456, 461, 462, 465–467, 474, 485, 495, 500, 513, 515, 518, 521–525, 529, 547–549, 552, 559, 566, 567, 569, 570, 579, 580, 582, 584–586, 591, 594, 596, 597, 600, 603, 604, 607, 608, 610, 611, 614, 620, 630, 636, 640–643, 647–652, 660, 689, 701, 703, 711, 713–716, 747

KI-4, *dà zhōng* 大钟, Large Goblet, 197, 222, 408, 747

KI-5, *shuǐ quán* 水泉, Water Spring, 31, 160, 332, 333, 393, 701, 747

KI-6, *zhào hǎi* 照海, Shining Sea, 12–14, 28–31, 47, 59, 60, 69, 71, 72, 78, 88, 90, 91, 93, 95–97, 111, 119, 122, 127–129, 148, 152, 154–156, 158, 160, 161, 163, 164, 168, 174–176, 178, 180, 186, 201–203, 226, 229, 235, 237, 239, 256, 267, 268, 275, 277, 282, 283, 285, 288–292, 294, 296, 299, 302, 314, 319, 320, 331–333, 336, 337, 339, 348, 349, 355, 360, 365, 368, 369, 372, 374, 378–380, 390, 391, 398, 401, 409, 410, 415, 416, 425, 438, 446, 450, 452, 455–457, 461, 462, 466, 468, 495, 516, 521, 524, 525, 535, 537, 538, 547, 552, 565–569, 572, 577, 580–582, 585, 587–589, 591, 596, 597, 601, 603, 607, 611, 613, 614, 640, 641, 643, 646–649, 652, 664, 701, 703, 712, 714–716, 747

KI-7, *fù liū* 复溜, Recover Flow, 47, 86, 95, 114, 128, 174, 184, 185, 199, 211, 224, 228, 240, 266, 288, 297, 302, 308, 331, 333, 334, 348, 358, 370, 393, 425, 450, 453, 461, 514, 518, 521, 522, 524, 547, 550, 559, 563, 569, 589, 590, 594, 597, 600, 604, 608, 637, 638, 641, 647, 662, 681, 682, 686, 701, 703, 713, 716, 747

KI-8, *jiāo xìn* 交信, Intersection Reach, 747

KI-9, *zhú bīn* 筑宾, Guest House, 28, 75, 748

KI-10, *yīn gǔ* 阴谷, Yin Valley, 22, 41, 149, 289, 301, 302, 360, 431, 453, 461, 589, 637, 647, 711, 748

KI-11, *héng gǔ* 横骨, Pubic Bone, 609, 748

KI-12, *dà hè* 大赫, Great Manifestation, 57, 160, 308, 330, 331, 333, 336, 466, 518, 524, 525, 582, 711, 712, 748

KI-13, *qì xué* 气穴, Qi Point, 26, 35, 36, 38, 57, 217, 331, 353, 418, 479, 484, 748

KI-14, *sì mǎn* 四满, Fourfold Fullness, 34, 35, 748

KI-15, *zhōng zhù* 中注, Central Flow, 748

KI-16, *huāng shū* 肓俞, Huang Transport, 28, 748

KI-17, *shāng qū* 商曲, Shang Bend, 748

KI-18, *shí guān* 石关, Stone Pass, 78, 664, 748

KI-19, *yīn dū* 阴都, Yin Metropolis, 748

KI-20, *tōng gǔ (fù)* 通谷 (腹), Open Valley, 748

KI-21, *yōu mén* 幽门, Dark Gate, 748

KI-22, *bù láng* 步廊, Corridor Walk, 748

KI-23, *shén fēng* 神封, Spirit Seal, 748

KI-24, *líng xū* 灵墟, Spirit Ruins, 748

KI-25, *shén cáng* 神藏, Spirit Storehouse, 748

KI-26, *yù zhōng* 彧中, Lively Center, 748

KI-27, *shū fǔ* 俞府, Transport Mansion, 748

kidney failure*, 124, 646

Kidney Fixity Decoction, *shèn zhuó tāng* 肾着汤, 22, 326, 425, 733

Kidney Qi Pill, *shèn qì wán* 肾气丸, 46, 379, 441, 452, 512, 641, 647, 667, 742

Kidney-Enriching Gate-Opening Pill, *zī shèn tōng guān wán* 滋肾通关丸, 203

Kidney-Enriching Pill, *zī shèn wán* 滋肾丸, 122, 649, 733

Kidney-Enriching Thoroughfare-Securing Decoction, *zī shèn gù chōng tāng* 滋肾固冲汤, 743

Kidney-Quieting Pill, *ān shèn wán* 安肾丸, 325, 713

Kidney-Settling Abalone Shell Pill, *zhèn shèn jué míng wán* 镇肾决明丸, 104

Kidney-Supplementing Sinew-Strengthening Decoction, *bǔ shèn zhuàng jīn tāng* 补肾壮筋汤, 742

Kidney-Supplementing Thoroughfare-Securing Pill, *bǔ shèn gù chōng wán* 补肾固冲丸, 741

knotgrass, *biǎn xù* 萹蓄, Polygoni Avicularis Herba, 21, 69, 136, 723

knotty pine wood, *sōng jié* 松节, Pini Lignum Nodi, 139, 722

kochia, *dì fū zǐ* 地肤子, Kochiae Fructus, 116, 136, 225, 395, 424, 513, 516, 723

Kochiae Fructus, *dì fū zǐ* 地肤子, kochia, 116, 136, 225, 395, 424, 513, 516, 723

kōng tòng 空痛, empty pain, 173

kǒng 恐, fear, 196

kǒng shèng zhěn zhōng dān 孔圣枕中丹, Sagacious Confucius' Pillow Elixir, 739

kǒng xué 孔穴, acupuncture point, 6

kǒng zé qì xià 恐则气下, fear causes qi to precipitate, 196

kǒng zǐ zhěn zhōng sǎn 孔子枕中散, Confucius' Pillow Powder, 739

kǒng zuì 孔最, LU-6, Collection Hole, 30, 70, 73, 97, 156, 277, 281, 290, 372, 379, 393, 520, 570, 603, 715, 716, 746

kòng nǎo shā 控脑痧, brain-gripping sand, 49

kòng xián dān 控涎丹, Drool-Controlling Elixir, 88, 182, 433, 434, 438, 442, 506

Korean aconite, *guān bái fù* 关白附, Aconiti Coreani Tuber, 623, 725

Korean ginseng, *gāo lì shēn* 高丽参, Ginseng Radix Coreensis, 593, 726

kōu mài 芤脉, scallion-stalk pulse, 513

kǒu 口, mouth, 400

kǒu bù kě 口不渴, absence of thirst, 3

kǒu chòu 口臭, bad breath, 15

kǒu chuāng 口疮, mouth sore, 400

kǒu dàn 口淡, bland taste in the mouth, 23

kǒu gān 口疳, gan of the mouth, 238

kǒu gān 口疳, oral gan, 421

kǒu gān 口干, dry mouth, 154

kǒu gān fēng 口疳风, wind gan of the mouth, 686

kǒu jìn 口噤, clenched jaw, 73

kǒu kāi mù hé 口开目合, open mouth and closed eyes, 421

kǒu kě 口渴, thirst, 607

kǒu kǔ 口苦, bitter taste in the mouth, 20

kǒu mí 口糜, oral putrefaction, 421

kǒu nì 口腻, sliminess in the mouth, 539

kǒu pì 口僻, deviated mouth, 125

kǒu shé chuāng 口舌疮, sore of the mouth or tongue, 546

kǒu shé shēng chuāng 口舌生疮, mouth and tongue sores, 400

kǒu shé shēng chuāng 口舌生疮, sore of the mouth or tongue, 546

kǒu suān 口酸, sour taste in the mouth, 549

kǒu tián 口甜, sweet taste in the mouth, 600

kǒu wāi (kuāi) 口喎, deviated mouth, 125

kǒu wèi 口味, taste in the mouth, 602

kǒu xián 口咸, salty taste in the mouth, 511

kǒu yǎn wāi (kuāi) xié 口眼喎斜, deviated eyes and mouth, 125

kǒu yǒu niào wèi 口有尿味, taste of urine in the mouth, 602

kǒu zào 口燥, dry mouth, 154

kǒu zhōng hé 口中和, harmony of mouth, 258

kòu rén 蔻仁 cardamom kernel, Amomi Cardamomi Semen, 401

krait/agkistrodon, *bái huā shé* 白花蛇, Bungarus seu Agkistrodon, 139, 722

kū 枯, desiccated, 124

kū 枯, desiccation, 124

kū fán 枯矾 calcined alum, Alumen Calcinatum, 221, 226, 412, 468

kū péi 枯痦, dry miliaria, 154

kū qín 枯芩 old scutellaria, Scutellariae Radix Veta, 690

kū zhì fǎ 枯痔法, hemorrhoid desiccation, 290

kū zhì sǎn 枯痔散, Alum Hemorrhoid-Desiccating Powder, 290, 565, 744

kǔ 苦, bitter, 20

kǔ 苦, bitterness, 20

kǔ hán qīng qì 苦寒清气, clearing qi with coldness and bitterness, 71

kǔ hán zào shī 苦寒燥湿, drying dampness with cold and bitterness, 153

kǔ liàn gāo 苦楝膏, Chinaberry Root Bark Paste, 16

kǔ liàn gēn pí 苦楝根皮 chinaberry root bark, Meliae Radicis Cortex, 183, 509, 510, 696

kǔ liàn pí 苦楝皮 chinaberry (root) bark, Meliae Cortex (Radicis), 183, 724

kǔ rù xīn 苦入心, bitterness enters the heart, 20

kǔ shēn 苦参 flavescent sophora, Sophorae Flavescentis Radix, 66, 67, 116, 225, 338, 353, 395, 424, 468, 720

kǔ shēn tāng 苦参汤, Flavescent Sophora Decoction, 744

kǔ wēn zào shī 苦温燥湿, drying dampness with warmth and bitterness, 153

kǔ xìng rén 苦杏仁 bitter apricot kernel, Armeniacae Semen Amarum, 458

kǔ zhú yè 苦竹叶 bitter bamboo leaf, Pleioblasti Folium, 259, 430

kù fáng 库房, ST-14, Storeroom, 746

kù kǒu chuāng 裤口疮, trouser-bottom sore, 628

kù kǒu dú 裤口毒, trouser-bottom toxin sore, 629

kuà gǔ 胯骨, hip bone, 291

kuà gǔ 跨骨, hip bone, 291

kuà gǔ 骻骨, hip bone, 291

kuān xiōng 宽胸, loosening the chest, 367

kuān zhōng 宽中, loosening the center, 367

kuǎn dōng huā 款冬花 tussilago, Tussilaginis Flos, 56, 95, 267, 434, 464, 527, 624, 625, 725 *kuáng* 狂, mania, 386

kuáng xié 狂邪, mania evil, 387

kuáng zào 狂躁, manic agitation, 387

kuī 亏, depletion, 122

kuí zǐ sǎn 葵子散, Mallow Seed Powder, 369

kumquat, *jīn jú* 金橘, Fortunellae Fructus, 363

kūn bù 昆布 kelp, Algae Thallus, 30, 141, 243, 544, 624, 725

kūn lún 昆仑, BL-60, Kunlun Mountains, 14, 21, 22, 34, 61, 80, 105, 114, 137, 160, 221, 231, 247, 288, 289, 296, 330, 332, 336, 342, 347, 366, 370, 382, 503, 519, 521, 567, 591, 689, 747

kùn 困, cumbersome, 106

kùn 困, encumbrance, 173

kuò qīng yǐn 廓清饮, Thorough Clearing Beverage, 733

là lí 腊梨, perverse crop, 431

là lì 瘌痢, perverse crop, 431

là lì 鬎鬁, perverse crop, 431

lablab, *biǎn dòu* 扁豆, Lablab Semen, 563, 564, 593, 726

Lablab Flos, *biǎn dòu huā* 扁豆花, lablab flower, 69

lablab flower, *biǎn dòu huā* 扁豆花, Lablab Flos, 69

Lablab Folium, *biǎn dòu yè* 扁豆叶, lablab leaf, 61

lablab leaf, *biǎn dòu yè* 扁豆叶, Lablab Folium, 61

Lablab Semen, *biǎn dòu* 扁豆, lablab, 563, 564, 593, 726

Lacca Exsiccata, *gān qī* 干漆, lacquer, 97, 138, 725

lacquer, *gān qī* 干漆, Lacca Exsiccata, 97, 138, 725

lacrimal gland*, 604

lacrimal point*, 605

Lactation Elixir, *tōng rǔ dān* 通乳丹, 513, 741

lactigo*, 586

Lagenariae Depressae Fructus, *hú lú* 壶芦, bottle gourd, 136, 723

lái fú 莱菔 radish, Raphani Radix, 527

lái fú zǐ 莱菔子 radish seed, Raphani Semen, 5, 141, 216, 418, 512, 589, 724

lái fù dān 来复丹, Return Again Elixir, 330, 443, 590, 665

lái pò tōng jié tāng 莱朴通结汤, Radish Seed and Magnolia Bark Bind-Freeing Decoction, 732

lài 癞, lai, 338

lài chuāng 癞疮, lai sore, 338

lài dà fēng 癞大风, lai great wind, 338

lài dà fēng 癞大风, leprosy, 343

lài tóu chuāng 癞头疮, lai scalp sore, 338

lán diàn 蓝靛 indigo residue, Indigonis Residuum, 497

lán mén 阑门, screen gate, 515

lán shì mì cáng 兰室秘藏 (*Secret Treasure of the Orchid Chamber*), 1276, Lǐ Gǎo 李杲 [Dōng-Yuán 东垣], 393

lán wěi huà yū tāng 阑尾化瘀汤, Appendix Stasis-Transforming Decoction, 743

lán wěi qīng huà tāng 阑尾清化汤, Appendix Clearing and Transforming Decoction, 743

lán wěi qīng jiě tāng 阑尾清解汤, Appendix-Clearing and Resolving Decoction, 743

lán wěi xué 阑尾穴, Appendix Point, 318

lán xiāng yǐn zǐ 兰香饮子, Basil Drink, 539, 565

lǎn yán 懒言, laziness to speak, 341

làn 烂, rot, 508

làn 烂, ulceration, 636

làn hóu fēng 烂喉风, putrefying throat wind, 474

làn hóu shā 烂喉痧, putrefying throat sand, 474

làn jiǎo 烂脚, foot rot, 221

làn jiǎo yā 烂脚丫, foot rot, 221

lanceolate stellaria, *yín chái hú* 银柴胡, Stellariae Lanceolatae Radix, 68, 72, 281, 282, 649, 722

Land and Water Two Immortals Elixir, *shuǐ lù èr xiān dān* 水陆二仙丹, 743

láng dú 狼毒 Chinese wolfsbane, Stellerae seu Euphorbiae Radix, 411, 728

láng dú gāo 狼毒膏, Chinese Wolfsbane Paste, 154, 516

lantern plant, *suān jiāng* 酸浆, Physalis Alkekengi Herba, 68, 721

lantern plant calyx, *guà jīn dēng* 挂金灯, Physalis Alkekengi Calyx, 68, 721

láo 劳, taxation, 602

láo fù 劳复, taxation relapse, 604

láo gōng 劳宫, PC-8, Palace of Toil, 31, 33, 40, 65, 69, 74, 88, 89, 118, 123, 147, 194, 202, 203, 241, 244, 261, 263, 264, 277, 281, 284, 289, 290, 294, 333, 343, 364, 386, 390, 392, 393, 400, 413, 420, 437, 440, 450, 452, 467, 483, 522, 537, 538, 552, 566, 567, 589, 590, 655, 656, 687, 690, 694, 714, 716, 748

láo juàn 劳倦, taxation fatigue, 603

láo ké 劳咳, taxation cough, 603

láo lín 劳淋, taxation strangury, 604

láo mài 牢脉, confined pulse, 92

láo mài 牢脉, firm pulse, 203

láo nüè 劳疟, taxation malaria, 604

láo què 劳怯, taxation timidity, 604

láo rè 劳热, taxation heat [effusion], 604

láo shāng 劳伤, taxation damage, 603

láo shāng ké sòu 劳伤咳嗽, taxation damage cough, 603

láo shāng yuè jīng guò duo 劳伤月经过多, taxation damage profuse menstruation, 603

láo sòu 劳嗽, taxation cough, 603

láo sǔn 劳损, taxation detriment, 603

láo zé qì hào 劳则气耗, taxation causes wearing of qi, 603

láo zhài 痨瘵, consumption, 96

láo zhēng 劳蒸, taxation steaming, 604

lǎo guàn cǎo 老鹳草 cranesbill, Geranii Herba, 140, 722

lǎo shǔ chuāng 老鼠疮, mouse sores, 400

lǎo tán 老痰, old phlegm, 419

Lard and Hair Brew, *gāo fà jiān* 膏发膏, 653

large gentian, *qín jiāo* 秦艽, Gentianae Macrophyllae Radix, 72, 139, 167, 263, 451, 722

Large Gentian and Rehmannia Decoction, *qín jiāo dì huáng tāng* 秦艽地黄汤, 535

Large Gentian and Turtle Shell Powder, *qín jiāo biē jiǎ sǎn* 秦艽鳖甲散, 176, 572, 693, 731

Large Gentian Decoction, *dà qín jiāo tāng* 大秦艽汤, 289, 631, 689, 740

Large Gentian Emaciation Decoction, *qín jiāo fú léi tāng* 秦艽扶赢汤, 731

laryngitis*, 349, 368
  acute, 586
  chronic, 714

Lasiosphaera seu Calvatia, *mǎ bó* 马勃, puffball, 68, 721

leaf mustard seed, *jiè zǐ* 芥子, Brassicae Junceae Semen, 624, 725

ledebouriella, *fáng fēng* 防风, Ledebouriellae Radix, 11, 14, 55, 102, 103, 115, 139, 167, 184, 191, 240, 244, 319, 370, 424, 430, 439, 500–502, 527, 548, 599, 638, 680, 681, 684, 685, 703, 713, 720

Ledebouriella Decoction, *fáng fēng tāng* 防风汤, 689

Ledebouriella Powder, *fáng fēng sǎn* 防风散, 693

Ledebouriella Sage-Inspired Powder, *fáng fēng tōng shèng sǎn* 防风通圣散, 395, 476, 496, 546, 674, 687, 730

Ledebouriellae Radix, *fáng fēng* 防风, ledebouriella, 11, 14, 55, 102, 103, 115, 139, 167, 184, 191, 240, 244, 319, 370, 424, 430, 439, 500–502, 527, 548, 599, 638, 680, 681, 684, 685, 703, 713, 720

leech, *shuǐ zhì* 水蛭, Hirudo seu Whitmania, 98, 138, 724

Left-Restoring [Kidney Yin] Beverage, *zuǒ guī yǐn* 左归饮, 369, 594, 742

Left-Restoring [Kidney Yin] Pill, *zuǒ guī wán* 左归丸, 160, 256, 310, 329, 331, 332, 352, 360, 524, 528, 714, 742

Left-Running Metal Pill, *zuǒ jīn wán* 左金丸, 4, 19, 20, 24, 63, 202, 362, 461, 478, 549, 578, 731

léi gōng téng 雷公藤 thunder god vinc, Tripterygii Wilfordi Radix, Folium et Flos, 140, 722

léi kuò 雷廓, thunder rampart, 613

léi tóu fēng 雷头风, thunder head wind, 612

léi wán 雷丸 omphalia, Omphalia, 183, 445, 724

lèi 泪, tears, 605

lèi jīng 类经 (*Classified Canon*), 1604 (Míng), Zhāng Jiè-Bīn 张介宾 [Jǐng-Yuè 景岳], 100, 311

lèi jīng fù yì 类经附翼 (*Wings to the Classified Canon*), 1624 (Míng), Zhāng Jiè-Bīn 张介宾 (Jǐng-Yuè 景岳), 20

lèi qiào 泪窍, tear orifice, 605

lèi rè 泪热, hot tears, 293

lèi táng 泪堂, tear hall, 604

lèi wéi gān yè 泪为肝液, tears are the humor of the liver, 605

lèi zhèng zhì cái 类证治裁 (*Systematized Patterns with Clear-Cut Treatments*), 1839 (Qīng), Lín Pèi-Qín 林佩琴, 172, 362, 646

lèi zhòng fēng 类中风, wind-like stroke, 689

Lemnae Herba, *fú píng* 浮萍, duckweed, 130, 228, 686, 703, 720

lěng 冷, cold, 77

lěng bì 冷秘, cold constipation, 78

lěng gān 冷疳, cold gan, 81

lěng hàn 冷汗, cold sweating, 86

lěng jiǔ 冷灸, cold moxibustion, 83

lěng lèi 冷泪, cold tearing, 86

lěng lín 冷淋, cold strangury, 86

lěng lú yī huà 冷庐医话 (*Medical Discussions of the Cold Shack*), 1897 (Qīng), Lù Yǐ-Tián 陆以湉, 538

lěng rè gān 冷热疳, cold-heat gan, 81

lěng tòng 冷痛, cold pain, 83

lěng xiāo 冷哮, cold wheezing, 87

lěng xiāo wán 冷哮丸, Cold Wheezing Pill, 136, 738

lěng xīn tòng 冷心痛, cold heart pain, 81

Leonuri Fructus, *chōng wèi zǐ* 茺蔚子, leonurus fruit, 138, 484, 724

Leonuri Herba, *yì mǔ cǎo* 益母草, leonurus, 34, 94, 137, 138, 431, 448, 724

leonurus, *yì mǔ cǎo* 益母草, Leonuri Herba, 34, 94, 137, 138, 431, 448, 724

Leonurus (Motherwort) Metal-Overcoming Elixir, *yì mǔ shèng jīn dān* 益母胜金丹, 738

Leonurus (Motherwort) Paste, *yì mǔ cǎo gāo* 益母草膏, 35

leonurus fruit, *chōng wèi zǐ* 茺蔚子, Leonuri Fructus, 138, 484, 724

leopard's bone, *bào gǔ* 豹骨, Leopardi Os, 139, 722

Leopard's Bone and Chaenomelis Wine, *bào gǔ mù guā jiǔ* 豹骨木瓜酒, 734

Leopardi Os, *bào gǔ* 豹骨, leopard's bone, 139, 722

leprosy*
  tuberculoid, 675

leptospirosis*, 118

Lesser Abdomen Stasis-Expelling Decoction, *shào fù zhú yū tāng* 少腹逐瘀汤, 26, 32, 35, 36, 94, 737

lesser galangal, *gāo liáng jiāng* 高良姜, Alpiniae Officinarum Rhizoma, 84, 581, 660, 662, 663, 723

Lesser Galangal and Cyperus Pill, *liáng fù wán* 良附丸, 84, 314, 580, 663, 735

lesser hypericum, *dì ěr cǎo* 地耳草, Hyperici Japonici Herba, 68, 136, 700, 721, 723

leukemia*, 30, 646

Leukoplakia No.1 Medicinal Paste, *bái bān yī hào yào gāo* 白斑一号药膏, 744

Leukoplakia No.3 Medicinal Paste, *bái bān èr hào yào gāo* 白斑二号药膏, 744

Leukoplakia Wash, *bái bān xǐ jì* 白斑洗剂, 744

Levant wormseed flower and leaf, *shān dào nián hāo* 山道年蒿, Artemisiae Cinae Flos et Folium, 183, 509

Level-Line of Pattern Identification and Treatment (*zhèng zhì zhǔn shéng*) 证治准绳, 1602 (Míng), Wáng Kěn-Táng 王肯堂, 299, 368, 384, 557, 568, 704

Level-Line of Pediatrics (*yòu kē zhǔn shéng*) 幼科准绳, full title *yòu kē zhèng zhì zhǔn shéng* 幼科证治准绳, 81, 82

Li Inner Court, *lǐ nèi tíng* 里内庭, 2, 3, 15, 141, 157, 186, 197, 215–217, 224, 227, 316, 395, 426, 450, 451, 499, 558, 564, 578, 645

Li's Summerheat-Clearing Qi-Boosting Decoction, *lǐ shì qīng shǔ yì qì tāng* 李氏清暑益气汤, 488, 730

LI-1, *shāng yáng* 商阳, Shang Yang, 14, 63, 75, 103, 112, 129, 147, 158, 184, 190, 277, 281, 283, 374, 398, 420, 438, 520, 546, 547, 561, 590, 611, 620, 746

LI-2, *èr jiān* 二间, Second Space, 31, 414, 415, 520, 547, 746

LI-3, *sān jiān* 三间, Third Space, 746

LI-4, *hé gǔ* 合谷, Union Valley, 1, 2, 4–6, 8, 11, 12, 14, 15, 24, 26, 28–30, 33–35, 39, 40, 44, 47, 50, 59, 60, 62–66, 69–73, 75–80, 82–91, 93, 95, 96, 99, 103, 105, 109–115, 117–120, 125, 127–129, 136, 138–141, 145, 146, 149–153, 155, 158, 164, 166, 167, 171, 174, 178, 182–186, 189, 190, 192, 194, 197, 202, 203, 216–218, 224, 225, 227, 228, 231, 239–241, 244, 247, 257, 259–261, 269, 272, 276–278, 280–285, 287–291, 294, 295, 298, 301, 302, 312, 318–320, 337–339, 341, 347, 348, 356, 358, 366, 368, 374, 382, 384, 386, 395, 400, 401, 403, 405, 410, 414–416, 418, 422, 426, 427, 433–439, 441–443, 445, 448–452, 454–458, 462, 463, 466, 471, 475, 477, 480, 482–485, 489, 493, 495, 499, 501, 503, 504, 506, 509, 511, 515, 517, 519–522, 530, 539, 540, 543, 544, 546–548, 550, 560, 562, 563, 565, 566, 568, 569, 571, 572, 577–580, 585–591, 595, 597, 601, 603, 604, 607, 608, 610, 611, 613, 614, 620, 621, 624, 625, 631, 640, 641, 643, 645, 651, 652, 654, 658, 661, 663–666, 673, 674, 676, 677, 679–691, 693, 694, 699, 701–703, 711–715, 746

LI-5, *yáng xī* 阳溪, Yang Ravine, 137, 296, 520, 521, 567, 621, 679, 746

LI-6, *piān lì* 偏历, Veering Passageway, 90, 182, 301, 408, 601, 613, 703, 716, 746

LI-7, *wēn liū* 温溜, Warm Dwelling, 386, 746

LI-8, *xià lián* 下廉, Lower Ridge, 542, 746

LI-9, *shàng lián* 上廉, Upper Ridge, 746

LI-10, *shǒu sān lǐ* 手三里, Arm Three Li, 103, 139, 142, 171, 211, 515, 520, 540, 679, 746

LI-11, *qū chí* 曲池, Pool at the Bend, 2, 5, 6, 8, 13–16, 22, 25, 29–31, 39, 40, 44, 60–63, 65, 66, 69–76, 89, 91, 99, 103, 105, 109–113, 117, 118, 120, 127, 129, 137–140, 146, 147, 149, 151, 155, 156, 158, 167, 168, 171, 174, 178, 184, 186, 190, 197, 201, 203, 216, 225, 235, 239, 241, 244, 260, 276–278, 280–285, 287–292, 294, 295, 298, 301, 302, 318–320, 337–339, 341, 342, 347, 349, 357, 364, 366, 370, 374, 380, 382–384, 386, 390, 394, 398, 403, 405, 422, 426, 427, 434, 437–439, 443, 450, 455, 457, 458, 462, 466, 493, 501, 516, 520–522, 530, 540, 544, 546, 547, 560, 567, 569, 578, 579, 585–591, 601, 607, 611, 613, 624, 637, 652, 665, 673, 674, 677, 679, 680, 683–689, 693, 694, 700–703, 710, 712, 713, 716, 746

LI-12, *zhǒu liáo* 肘髎, Elbow Bone-Hole, 520, 746

LI-13, *shǒu wǔ lǐ* 手五里, (Arm) Five Li, 746

LI-14, *bì nào* 臂臑, Upper Arm, 142, 341, 515, 520, 746

LI-15, *jiān yú* 肩髃, Shoulder Bone, 61, 137, 289, 295, 341, 418, 521, 530, 567, 679, 689, 746

LI-16, *jù gǔ* 巨骨, Great Bone, 61, 90, 530, 746

LI-17, *tiān dǐng* 天鼎, Celestial Tripod, 30, 129, 210, 480, 746

LI-18, *fú tú* 扶突, Protuberance Assistant, 129, 291, 378, 521, 746

LI-19, *hé liáo* 禾髎, Grain Bone-Hole, 45, 219, 400, 401, 415, 746

LI-20, *yíng xiāng* 迎香, Welcome Fragrance, 5, 75, 89, 92, 120, 149, 194, 260, 348, 378, 405, 521, 522, 543, 674, 681, 686, 688, 746

lí hēi 黧黑, soot black, 545

lí lú 藜芦 veratrum, Veratri Radix et Rhizoma, 98, 170, 727

lí pí 梨皮 pear peel, Pyri Exocarpium, 398

lǐ 理, rectify, 493

lǐ 里, interior, 311

lǐ gōu 蠡沟, LR-5, Woodworm Canal, 19–21, 35, 36, 51, 90, 111, 255, 353, 355, 395, 468, 481, 484, 522, 637, 748

lǐ gōu 蠡沟, LV-5, Woodworm Canal, 408

lǐ hán 里寒, interior cold, 311

lǐ jí hòu zhòng 里急后重, abdominal urgency and heaviness in the rectum, 2

lǐ jí hòu zhòng 里急后重, tenesmus, 605

lǐ líng tāng 理苓汤, Rectifying Poria (Hoelen) Decoction, 733

lǐ nèi tíng 里内庭, Li Inner Court, 2, 3, 15, 141, 157, 186, 197, 215–217, 224, 227, 316, 395, 426, 450, 451, 499, 558, 564, 578, 645

lǐ qì 理气, rectifying qi, 493

lǐ qì hé wèi 理气和胃, rectifying qi and harmonizing the stomach, 494

lǐ qì hé yíng 理气和营, rectifying qi and harmonizing construction, 493

lǐ qì jiàng tán tāng 理气降痰汤, Qi-Rectifying Phlegm-Downbearing Decoction, 439

lǐ rè 里热, interior heat, 311

lǐ shí 里实, interior repletion, 311

lǐ shì qīng shǔ yì qì tāng 李氏清暑益气汤, Li's Summerheat-Clearing Qi-Boosting Decoction, 488, 730

lǐ xū 里虚, interior vacuity, 311

lǐ xuè 理血, rectifying the blood, 494

lǐ yīn jiān 理阴煎, Yin-Rectifying Brew, 63, 82, 425, 646, 735

lǐ yú tāng 鲤鱼汤, Carp Soup, 232

lǐ zhèng 里证, interior pattern, 311

lǐ zhōng 理中, rectifying the center, 494

lǐ zhōng ān huí sǎn 理中安蛔散, Center-Rectifying Roundworm-Quieting Powder, 737

lǐ zhōng ān huí tāng 理中安蛔汤, Center-Rectifying Roundworm-Quieting Decoction, 509

lǐ zhōng huà tán wán 理中化痰丸, Center-Rectifying Phlegm-Transforming Pill, 136, 738

lǐ zhōng tāng 理中汤, Center-Rectifying Decoction, 1, 61, 77, 79, 80, 82, 85, 87, 156, 198, 217, 316, 339, 457, 489, 510, 555, 561, 562, 599, 608, 631, 663, 735

lǐ zhōng wán 理中丸, Center-Rectifying Pill, 84, 247, 314, 564, 662, 735

lì 利, disinhibit, 135

lì 疠, pestilence, 431

lì chí 立迟, slowness to stand, 541

lì dǎn pái shí piàn 利胆排石片, Gallbladder-Disinhibiting Stone-Expelling Tablet, 733

lì dǎn tuì huáng tāng 利胆退黄汤, Gallbladder-Disinhibiting Jaundice-Abating Decoction, 733

lì duì 厉兑, ST-45, Severe Mouth, 148, 186, 189, 268, 269, 279, 281, 283, 314, 333, 413–415, 420, 520, 538, 577, 699, 746

lì fēng 疠风, leprosy, 343

lì fēng 疠风, pestilential wind, 431

lì jí 痢疾, dysentery, 163

lì jié 历节, joint-running wind, 322

lì jié fēng 历节风, joint-running wind, 322

lì jīng wán 利惊丸, Fright-Disinhibiting Pill, 6

lì qì 利气, disinhibiting qi, 136

lì qì 疠气, pestilential qi, 431

lì qì 戾气, perverse qi, 431

lì shī 利湿, disinhibiting dampness, 135

lì shuǐ 利水, disinhibiting water, 136

lì shuǐ shèn shī 利水渗湿, disinhibiting water and percolating dampness, 136

lì xiāng sǎn 荔香散, Litchee Pit and Fennel Powder, 481

lì zhī 荔枝 litchee, Litchi Fructus, 548

lì zhī hé 荔枝核 litchee pit, Litchi Semen, 291, 493, 671, 723

lián 廉, face, 193

lián chuāng 臁疮, shank sore, 528

lián fáng 莲房 lotus receptacle, Nelumbinis Receptaculum, 518, 727

lián fù liù yī tāng 连附六一汤, Coptis and Aconite Six-to-One Decoction, 731

lián méi ān huí tāng 连梅安蛔汤, Picrorhiza and Mume Roundworm-Quieting Decoction, 737

lián méi tāng 连梅汤, Coptis and Mume Decoction, 734

lián pí fú líng 连皮茯苓 poria with skin, Poria cum Cortice, 228

lián pò yǐn 连朴饮, Coptis and Magnolia Bark Beverage, 66, 118, 276, 539, 733

lián qiáo 连翘 forsythia, Forsythiae Fructus, 310, 422, 621

lián qiào 连翘 forsythia, Forsythiae Fructus, 20, 65, 67, 69, 70, 118, 130, 141, 189, 214, 234, 263, 303, 315, 387, 388, 412, 430, 439, 450, 463, 497, 501, 548, 606, 671, 703, 721

lián qiào jīn bèi jiān 连翘金贝煎, Forsythia, Lonicera, and Bolbosteema Brew, 743

lián qiào sǎn 连翘散, Forsythia Powder, 17

lián qiào yǐn zǐ 连翘饮子, Forsythia Drink, 497

lián quán 廉泉, CV-23, Ridge Spring, 89, 125, 140, 289, 291, 292, 294, 368, 521, 552, 573, 640, 749

lián ròu 莲肉 lotus seed, Nelumbinis Semen, 12, 518, 727

lián xū 莲须 lotus stamen, Nelumbinis Stamen, 11, 308, 496, 518, 727

lián xū cōng bái 连须葱白 scallion white with root, Allii Fistulosi Bulbus cum Radice, 228, 502

lián xū cōng bái tāng 连须葱白汤, Scallion with Root Decoction, 729

lián zǐ 莲子 lotus fruit/seed, Nelumbinis Fructus seu Semen, 490, 518, 525, 600, 726, 727

lián zǐ xīn 莲子心 lotus embryo, Nelumbinis Embryo, 263

liǎn 敛, constrain, 95

liǎn fèi 敛肺, constraining the lung, 95

liǎn fèi zhǐ ké 敛肺止咳, constraining the lung and suppressing cough, 95

liǎn hàn 敛汗, constraining sweat, 95

liǎn hàn gù biǎo 敛汗固表, constraining sweat and securing the exterior, 95

liǎn yīn 敛阴, constraining yin, 96

liáng 凉, cool, 99

liáng 凉, coolness, 99

liáng 梁, Liang, 345

liáng fù wán 良附丸, Lesser Galangal and Cyperus Pill, 84, 314, 580, 663, 735

liáng gé lián qiào sǎn 凉膈连翘散, Diaphragm-Cooling Forsythia Powder, 731

liáng gé sǎn 凉膈散, Diaphragm-Cooling Powder, 15, 76, 166, 201, 203, 261, 277, 280, 283, 459, 548, 612, 615, 731

liáng jīng wán 凉惊丸, Fright-Cooling Pill, 740

liáng kāi 凉开, cool opening, 99

liáng mén 梁门, ST-21, Beam Gate, 80, 87, 111, 164, 168, 207, 215, 217, 218, 224, 521, 580, 581, 746

liáng qiū 梁丘, ST-34, Beam Hill, 29, 73, 104, 137, 186, 215, 218, 296, 337, 386, 390, 520, 521, 567, 673, 679, 746

liáng xuè 凉血, cooling the blood, 99

liáng xuè dì huáng tāng 凉血地黄汤, Blood-Cooling Rehmannia Decoction, 25, 29, 32, 284, 290, 317, 566, 738

liáng xuè rùn zào yǐn 凉血润燥饮, Blood-Cooling Dryness-Moistening Beverage, 173

liáng xuè sàn xuè 凉血散血, cooling and dissipating the blood, 99

liáng xuè sì wù tāng 凉血四物汤, Blood-Cooling Four Agents Decoction, 149

liáng yíng qīng qì tāng 凉营清气汤, Construction-Cooling Qi-Clearing Decoction, 178

liáng zào 凉燥, cool dryness, 99

liáng zào 凉燥, cooling dryness, 99

liǎng 两, liang, 345

liǎng 两, tael, 602

liǎng dì tāng 两地汤, Rehmannia and Lycium Root Bark Decoction, 31, 360, 649, 731

liǎng gǎn 两感, double contraction, 145

liǎng quán cháo hóng 两颧潮红, tidal reddening of the cheeks, 613

liǎng quán fā chì 两颧发赤, reddening of the cheeks, 494

liǎng yáng hé míng 两阳合明, united brightness of two yang, 637

liáo 辽, Liao, 345

liáo 髎, bone-hole, 45

liáo ér sǎn 疗儿散, Child-Curing Powder, 503

Lichen Medicinal Water, *xiǎn yào shuǐ* 癣药水, 689

licorice, *gān cǎo* 甘草, Glycyrrhizae Radix, 11, 17, 20, 47, 84, 108, 110, 115, 129, 141, 154, 161, 192, 214, 223, 227, 228, 230, 241, 255, 256, 259, 263, 285, 292, 315, 343, 378, 387, 390, 392, 394, 416, 430, 455, 463, 464, 486, 495, 498, 504, 526, 548, 556, 567, 580, 589, 593–595, 600, 662, 671, 687, 726

Licorice and Aconite Decoction, *gān cǎo fù zǐ tāng* 甘草附子汤, 680, 734

Licorice and Dried Ginger Decoction, *gān cǎo gān jiāng tāng* 甘草干姜汤, 380, 734

Licorice and Gardenia Decoction, *gān cǎo zhī zǐ tāng* 甘草栀子汤, 731

Licorice and Platycodon Decoction, *gān jié tāng* 甘桔汤, 203, 738

Licorice Decoction, *gān cǎo tāng* 甘草汤, 527

Licorice Heart-Draining Decoction, *gān cǎo xiè xīn tāng* 甘草泻心汤, 732

Licorice, Dried Ginger, Poria (Hoelen), and Ovate Atractylodes Decoction, *gān cǎo gān jiāng fú líng bái zhú tāng* 甘草干姜茯苓白术汤, 661, 733

Licorice, Processed Galenite, and Honey Decoction, *gān cǎo fěn mì tāng* 甘草粉蜜汤, 737

Licorice, Wheat, and Jujube Decoction, *gān cǎo xiǎo mài dà zǎo tāng* 甘草小麦大枣汤, 739

Licorice, Wheat, and Jujube Decoction, *gān mài dà zǎo tāng* 甘麦大枣汤, 655, 739

liè quē 列缺, LU-7, Broken Sequence, 12, 22, 50, 60, 65, 70, 73, 78, 84, 86–89, 91, 93, 96, 99, 103, 105, 111, 119, 120, 128, 129, 142, 145, 146, 155, 182, 184–186, 202, 203, 218, 225, 259, 260, 280, 281, 285, 291, 301, 342, 368, 374, 383, 405, 408, 415, 416, 438, 443, 448, 451, 452, 458, 477, 481, 501, 517, 519, 520, 522, 530, 544, 547, 586, 607, 620, 631, 668, 677, 681–684, 686, 687, 693, 703, 713, 746

Life Saver Kidney Qi Pill, *jì shēng shèn qì wán* 济生肾气丸, 22, 148, 151, 302, 335, 542, 662, 742

Life Saver Tangerine Peel and Bamboo Shavings Decoction, *jì shēng jú pí zhú rú tāng* 济生橘皮竹茹汤, 736

Life Saver Tangerine Pip Pill, *jì shēng jú hé wán* 济生橘核丸, 467, 735

Life-Clutching Elixir, *duó mìng dān* 夺命丹, 454, 455, 737

Life-Clutching Powder, *duó mìng sǎn* 夺命散, 448

Life-for-All Compendium of External Medicine, Patterns and Treatment (*wài kē zhèng zhì quán shēng jí*) 外科证治全生集, 1740 (Qīng), Wáng Wéi-Dé 王维德 [Hóng-Xù 洪绪], 46

Life-for-All Ovate Atractylodes Powder, *quán shēng bái zhú sǎn* 全生白术散, 50, 461, 600

Life-Promoting Pill, *zī shēng wán* 资生丸, 741

light wheat, *fú xiǎo mài* 浮小麦, Tritici Semen Leve, 95, 410, 518, 651, 727

Light-Restoring Powder, *fù míng sǎn* 复明散, 519

Ligustici Rhizoma, *chuān xiōng* 川芎, ligusticum, 11, 55, 58, 93, 102, 115, 116, 137–140, 227, 247, 259, 309, 315, 317, 390, 391, 398, 418, 428, 431, 448, 480, 503, 586, 654, 661, 680, 724

Ligustici Sinensis Rhizoma et Radix, *gǎo běn* 藁本, Chinese lovage, 55, 103, 654, 680, 681, 720

ligusticum, *chuān xiōng* 川芎, Ligustici Rhizoma, 11, 55, 58, 93, 102, 115, 116, 137–140, 227, 247, 259, 309, 315, 317, 390, 391, 398, 418, 428, 431, 448, 480, 503, 586, 654, 661, 680, 724

Ligusticum (Cnidium Root) and Atractylodes Decoction, *xiōng zhú tāng* 芎术汤, 702

Ligusticum and Asarum Decoction, *xiōng xīn tāng* 芎辛汤, 79, 435

Ligusticum and Asarum Phlegm-Abducting Decoction, *xiōng xīn dǎo tán tāng* 芎辛导痰汤, 260, 440

Ligusticum and Tangkuei Powder, *xiōng guī sǎn* 芎归散, 453

Ligusticum Powder, *chuān xiōng sǎn* 川芎散, 685

Ligustri Fructus, *nǚ zhēn zǐ* 女贞子, ligustrum, 88, 175, 336, 352, 467, 504, 526, 584, 593, 597, 612, 727

ligustrum, *nǚ zhēn zǐ* 女贞子, Ligustri Fructus, 88, 175, 336, 352, 467, 504, 526, 584, 593, 597, 612, 727

Lilii Bulbus, *bǎi hé* 百合, lily bulb, 175, 416, 467, 539, 593, 597, 655, 727

lily bulb, *bǎi hé* 百合, Lilii Bulbus, 175, 416, 467, 539, 593, 597, 655, 727

Lily Bulb and Rehmannia Decoction, *bǎi hé dì huáng tāng* 百合地黄汤, 656

Lily Bulb and Tussilago Paste, *bǎi huā gāo* 百花膏, 734

Lily Bulb Lung-Securing Decoction, *bǎi hé gù fèi tāng* 百合固肺汤, 277, 291, 374

Lily Bulb Metal-Securing Decoction, *bǎi hé gù jīn tāng* 百合固金汤, 158, 162, 172, 336, 368, 377, 380, 547, 734

limestone, *shí huī* 石灰, Calx, 569, 620, 728

limonite, *yǔ yú liáng* 禹余粮, Limonitum, 12, 318, 518, 519, 727

Limonitum, *yǔ yú liáng* 禹余粮, limonite, 12, 318, 518, 519, 727 *lín* 淋, strangury, 583

lín jìn bù wèi xuǎn xué 邻近部位选穴, selection of adjacent points, 519

lín zhèng zhǐ nán yī àn 临证指南医案 (*Clinical Guide with Case Histories*), 1766 (Qīng), Yè Guì 叶桂 [Tiān-Shì 天士], 322, 364, 512

lín zhuó 淋浊, strangury-turbidity, 583

lindera, *wū yào* 乌药, Linderae Radix, 19, 83, 103, 493, 572, 694, 724

Lindera Decoction, *wū yào tāng* 乌药汤, 736

Lindera Powder, *wū yào sǎn* 乌药散, 736

Linderae Radix, *wū yào* 乌药, lindera, 19, 83, 103, 493, 572, 694, 724

líng 凌, intimidate, 319

líng dào 灵道, HT-4, Spirit Pathway, 747

líng gān wǔ wèi jiāng xīn tāng 苓甘五味姜辛汤, Poria (Hoelen), Licorice, Schisandra, Ginger, and Asarum Decoction, 84, 380, 663, 738

líng gēn 灵根, magic root, 383

líng guì zhú gān tāng 苓桂术甘汤, Poria (Hoelen), Cinnamon Twig, Ovate Atractylodes, and Licorice Decoction, 87, 230, 269, 440, 441, 443, 537, 608, 661, 664, 667, 733

líng jiǎo gōu téng tāng 羚角钩藤汤, Antelope Horn and Uncaria Decoction, 53, 73, 364, 683, 690, 740

líng shū 灵枢 (*Magic Pivot*), second part of *huáng dì nèi jīng* 黄帝内经, 3, 10, 20, 43, 45, 48, 49, 56–58, 72, 96, 100, 120, 121, 124–126, 130, 143, 144, 180, 189, 190, 192, 193, 195, 204, 205, 213, 226, 244, 245, 252–254, 260, 264, 268, 310, 311, 329, 339, 358, 360, 361, 363, 370, 375, 377, 400, 409, 410, 469, 479, 485, 504, 505, 533, 548, 551, 553, 554, 556, 560, 561, 576, 598, 606, 607, 615, 620, 625, 627, 629, 633, 643, 654, 665, 672, 675, 700, 711

líng tái 灵台, GV-10, Spirit Tower, 44, 75, 427, 749

líng xiāo huā 凌霄花 campsis flower, Campsitis Flos, 138, 725

líng xū 灵墟, KI-24, Spirit Ruins, 748

líng yáng jiǎo 羚羊角 antelope horn, Antelopis Cornu, 54, 56, 65, 93, 209, 245, 526, 591, 726

líng yáng jiǎo sǎn 羚羊角散, Antelope Horn Powder, 178, 702, 740

líng yáng jiǎo tāng 羚羊角汤, Antelope Horn Decoction, 740

líng yào 灵药, magic medicine, 383

líng yī 铃医, bell healer, 17

líng zhī 灵芝 ganoderma, Ganoderma, 491, 726

lìng jiān 另煎, separate decoction, 525

lipoma, 211

lipoma*, 632

liquid storax, *sū hé xiāng* 苏合香, Styrax Liquidus, 10, 420, 485, 726

Liquid Storax Pill, *sū hé xiāng wán* 苏合香丸, 74, 86, 88, 152, 182, 228, 300, 384, 394, 590, 624, 629, 690, 740

liquidambar fruit, *lù lù tōng* 路路通, Liquidambaris Fructus, 19, 386, 417

Liquidambaris Fructus, *lù lù tōng* 路路通, liquidambar fruit, 19, 386, 417

litchee, *lì zhī* 荔枝, Litchi Fructus, 548

litchee pit, *lì zhī hé* 荔枝核, Litchi Semen, 291, 493, 671, 723

Litchee Pit and Fennel Powder, *lì xiāng sǎn* 荔香散, 481

Litchi Fructus, *lì zhī* 荔枝, litchee, 548

Litchi Semen, *lì zhī hé* 荔枝核, litchee pit, 291, 493, 671, 723

litharge, *mì tuó sēng* 密陀僧, Lithargyrum, 411, 713, 728

Litharge Paste, *tuó sēng gāo* 陀僧膏, 298, 745

Litharge Powder, *mì tuó sēng sǎn* 密陀僧散, 226, 474

Lithargyrum, *mì tuó sēng* 密陀僧, litharge, 411, 713, 728

Lithospermi, Macrotomiae, seu Onosmatis Radix, *zǐ cǎo* 紫草, puccoon, 30, 67, 387, 459, 637, 683, 721

litsea, *dòu chǐ jiāng* 豆豉姜, Litseae Rhizoma et Radix, 410, 500, 660, 723

Litseae Rhizoma et Radix, *dòu chǐ jiāng* 豆豉姜, litsea, 410, 500, 660, 723

Little Finger Bone Hollow, *xiǎo gǔ kōng* 小骨空, 93, 195, 500, 586, 636

liú 瘤, tumor, 632

liú 留, lodge, 366

liú bí tì 流鼻涕, runny nose, 510

liú cōng fū jì 硫葱敷剂, Sulfur and Scallion Topical Application, 744

liú guàn fǎ 留罐法, retained cupping, 502

liú huǒ 流火, fire flow, 202

liú jì nú 刘寄奴 anomalous artemisia, Artemisiae Anomalae Herba, 138, 725

liú lèi 流泪, lacrimation, 338

liú lèi 流泪, tearing, 605

liú liàn 留恋, linger, 348

liú qì yǐn zǐ 流气饮子, Qi Flow Drink, 481

liú tán 流痰, flowing phlegm, 212

liú xián 流涎, drooling, 150

liú yǐn 流饮, flowing rheum, 213

liú yǐn 留饮, lodged rheum, 366

liú zhēn 留针, needle retention, 407

liú zhù 流注, streaming sore, 584

liǔ huā sǎn 柳花散, Willow Flower Powder, 615

liù ān jiān 六安煎, Six Quietings Brew, 738

liù fǔ 六腑, six bowels, 534

liù hé tāng 六和汤, Six Harmonizations Decoction, 591, 732

liù jí 六极, six extremes, 535

liù jīng biàn zhèng 六经辨证, six-channel pattern identification, 534

liù jīng xíng zhèng 六经形证, six-channel patterns, 534

liù jūn zǐ tāng 六君子汤, Six Gentlemen Decoction, 63, 115, 146, 153, 163, 199, 215, 378, 440, 441, 486, 489, 537, 549, 562–564, 627, 647, 650, 651, 666, 669, 709, 740 *liù mò tāng* 六磨汤, Six Milled Ingredients Decoction, 127, 130, 479, 735

liù qì 六气, six qi, 535

liù shén sǎn 六神散, Wondrous Six Powder, 740

liù shén wán 六神丸, Six Spirits Pill, 612, 743

liù wèi dì huáng tāng 六味地黄汤, Six-Ingredient Rehmannia Decoction, 27, 36, 95, 309, 332, 713

liù wèi dì huáng wán 六味地黄丸, Six-Ingredient Rehmannia Pill, 9, 104, 105, 151, 153, 156–158, 177, 181, 198, 203, 222, 229, 238, 239, 251, 288, 291, 314, 319, 327, 331–333, 336, 360, 367, 369, 401, 409, 426, 453, 462, 497, 502, 515, 528, 538, 540, 541, 566, 567, 569, 594, 599, 604, 611, 614, 636, 651, 714, 715, 742

liù wèi huí yáng yǐn 六味回阳饮, Six-Ingredient Yang-Returning Beverage, 648, 713

liù wèi tāng 六味汤, Six-Ingredient Decoction, 547

liù wèi wán 六味丸, Six-Ingredient Pill, 217, 331, 647

liù wèi xiāng rú yǐn 六味香薷饮, Six-Ingredient Elsholtzia Beverage, 587, 591, 729

liù yī sǎn 六一散, Six-to-One Powder, 71, 221, 418, 587–590, 730

liù yín 六淫, six excesses, 535

liù yù 六郁, six depressions, 535

liù zhù yǐn 六柱饮, Six Pillars Beverage, 196

liver abscess*, 363

liver failure*, 124, 646

Liver-Clearing Aloe Pill, *qīng gān lú huì wán* 清肝芦荟丸, 243, 533, 534

Liver-Clearing Channel-Conducting Decoction, *qīng gān yǐn jīng tāng* 清乾引经汤, 390

Liver-Clearing Dampness-Percolating Decoction, *qīng gān shèn shī tāng* 清肝渗湿汤, 733

Liver-Coursing Depression-Resolving Decoction, *shū gān jiě yù tāng* 疏肝解郁汤, 353, 736

Liver-Coursing Powder, *shū gān sǎn* 疏肝散, 356

Liver-Draining Spirit-Quieting Pill, *xiè gān ān shén wán* 泻肝安神丸, 731

Liver-Regulating Decoction, *tiáo gān tāng* 调肝汤, 360

Liver-Regulating Powder, *tiáo gān sǎn* 调肝散, 658, 736

Liver-Repairing Decoction, *xiū gān tāng* 修肝汤, 740

Liver-Settling Wind-Extinguishing Decoction, *zhèn gān xī fēng tāng* 镇肝熄风汤, 53, 364, 689, 716, 740

Liver-Soothing Pill, *shū gān wán* 舒肝丸, 102, 736

Liver-Supplementing Decoction, *bǔ gān tāng* 补肝汤, 266, 352, 741

Liver-Supplementing Powder, *bǔ gān sǎn* 补肝散, 157, 359

Liver-Transforming Brew, *huà gān jiān* 化肝煎, 33, 314, 735

Liver-Warming Brew, *nuǎn gān jiān* 暖肝煎, 85, 355, 662, 711, 735

loadstone, *cí shí* 磁石, Magnetitum, 53, 225, 230, 287, 288, 490, 511, 525, 526, 538, 539, 585, 614, 726

Loadstone and Cinnabar Pill, *cí zhū wán* 磁朱丸, 230, 287, 526, 739

Lobeliae Chinensis Herba cum Radice, *bàn biān lián* 半边莲, Chinese lobelia, 68, 721

lochioschesis*, 503

lochiostasis*, 503

Lofty Bone, *chóng gǔ* 崇骨, 8, 384

long pepper, *bì bá* 荜茇, Piperis Longi Fructus, 660, 723

Long Vistas Pill Variant Formula, *zhù jǐng wán jiā jiǎn fāng* 驻景丸加减方, 64, 742

Long Vistas Pill, *zhù jǐng wán* 驻景丸, 406

lóng bì 癃闭, dribbling urinary block, 148

lóng chǐ 龙齿 dragon tooth, Mastodi Dentis Fossilia, 490, 525, 526, 538, 539, 726

lóng dǎn 龙胆 gentian, Gentianae Radix, 19, 66, 67, 357, 459, 720

lóng dǎn xiè gān tāng 龙胆泻肝汤, Gentian Liver-Draining Decoction, 20, 63, 66, 73, 93, 104, 111, 112, 119, 147, 166, 167, 172, 200, 235, 241, 297, 352, 355, 356, 359, 365, 412, 415, 424, 462, 468, 474, 495, 497, 511, 516, 533, 538–540, 566, 614, 656, 658, 671, 676, 677, 701, 711–713, 731

lóng gǔ 龙骨 dragon bone, Mastodi Ossis Fossilia, 11, 53, 183, 230, 308, 409, 433, 449, 461, 490, 504, 518, 524–526, 537, 572, 585, 636, 696, 709, 726

lóng hǔ sān dǎn sǎn 龙虎三胆散, Earthworm, House Lizard, and Three Gallbladders Powder, 745

lóng kuí 龙葵 black nightshade, Solani Nigri Herba, 68, 721

lóng léi zhī huǒ 龙雷之火, dragon and thunder fire, 146

lóng quán dīng 龙泉疔, dragon-spring clove sore, 146

lóng yǎn hé 龙眼核 longan pit, Longanae Semen, 226

lóng yǎn ròu 龙眼肉 longan flesh, Longanae Arillus, 37, 490, 593, 595, 600, 726, 727

lóng zhēng 笼蒸, basket-steam, 16

longan flesh, *lóng yǎn ròu* 龙眼肉, Longanae Arillus, 37, 490, 593, 595, 600, 726, 727

longan pit, *lóng yǎn hé* 龙眼核, Longanae Semen, 226

Longanae Arillus, *lóng yǎn ròu* 龙眼肉, longan flesh, 37, 490, 593, 595, 600, 726, 727

Longanae Semen, *lóng yǎn hé* 龙眼核, longan pit, 226

lonicera, *jīn yín huā* 金银花, Lonicerae Flos, 17, 28, 64, 67, 69, 70, 118, 130, 143, 189, 214, 282, 303, 315, 338, 386–388, 412, 422, 450, 459, 463, 501, 621, 671, 687, 691, 721

Lonicera and Forsythia Decoction, *yín qiào tāng* 银翘汤, 729

Lonicera and Forsythia Powder, *yín qiào sǎn* 银翘散, 59, 69, 91, 103, 118, 178, 184, 320, 387, 469, 501, 547, 586, 591, 611, 620, 686–688, 691, 693, 729

Lonicera and Phragmites Mixture, *yín wěi hé jì* 银苇合剂, 282, 625

Lonicera and Scutellaria Tablet, *yín huáng piàn* 银黄片, 731

lonicera stem and leaf, *rěn dōng téng* 忍冬藤, Lonicerae Caulis et Folium, 67, 116, 540, 721

Lonicera, Forsythia, and Puffball Powder, *yín qiào mǎ bó sǎn* 银翘马勃散, 729

Lonicerae Caulis et Folium, *rěn dōng téng* 忍冬藤, lonicera stem and leaf, 67, 116, 540, 721

Lonicerae Flos, *jīn yín huā* 金银花, lonicera, 17, 28, 64, 67, 69, 70, 118, 130, 143, 189, 214, 282, 303, 315, 338, 386–388, 412, 422, 450, 459, 463, 501, 621, 671, 687, 691, 721

loofah, *sī guā luò* 丝瓜络, Luffae Fasciculus Vascularis, 417, 569, 589, 728

Lophatheri Folium, *dàn zhú yè* 淡竹叶, bamboo leaf (lophatherum), 66, 67, 108, 261, 263, 387, 463, 720

Lophatheri Folium Immaturum, *zhú yè xīn* 竹叶心, tender bamboo leaf (lophatherum), 65

Lophatheri Folium Recens, *xiān zhú yè* 鲜竹叶, fresh bamboo leaf (lophatherum), 589

loquat leaf, *pí pá yè* 枇杷叶, Eriobotryae Folium, 65, 95, 387, 480, 624, 669, 725

Loquat Leaf Lung-Clearing Beverage, *pí pá qīng fèi yǐn* 枇杷清肺饮, 5

Loranthi seu Visci Ramus, *sāng jì shēng* 桑寄生, mistletoe, 139, 297, 352, 370, 456, 488, 722

lotus embryo, *lián zǐ xīn* 莲子心, Nelumbinis Embryo, 263

lotus fruit, *shí lián zǐ* 石莲子, Nelumbinis Fructus, 82

lotus fruit/seed, *lián zǐ* 莲子, Nelumbinis Fructus seu Semen, 490, 518, 525, 600, 726, 727

lotus leaf, *hé yè* 荷叶, Nelumbinis Folium, 569

lotus receptacle, *lián fáng* 莲房, Nelumbinis Receptaculum, 518, 727

lotus root node, *ǒu jié* 藕节, Nelumbinis Rhizomatis Nodus, 277, 714, 724

lotus seed, *lián ròu* 莲肉, Nelumbinis Semen, 12, 518, 727

lotus stamen, *lián xū* 莲须, Nelumbinis Stamen, 11, 308, 496, 518, 727

lóu gū 蝼蛄 mole cricket, Gryllotalpa, 98, 136, 723

lòu chuāng 漏疮, fistula, 204

lòu gǔ 漏谷, SP-7, Leaking Valley, 746

lòu hàn 漏汗, leaking sweat, 341

lòu jiān fēng 漏肩风, leaky shoulder wind, 341

lòu jīng 漏睛, weeping canthus, 669

lòu lú 漏芦 rhaponticum/echinops, Rhapontici seu Echinopis Radix, 68, 227, 384, 386, 721

lòu xià 漏下, spotting, 567

low back pain*, 370

LR-1, *dà dūn* 大敦, Large Pile, 31, 41, 83, 86, 111, 169, 177, 220, 226, 355, 362, 420, 424, 448, 478, 504, 506, 511, 542, 667, 711, 748

LR-2, *xíng jiān* 行间, Moving Between, 3, 4, 11, 14, 19–21, 29–32, 34–36, 40, 61, 66, 69, 72, 74, 84, 86, 93, 97, 99, 117, 119, 120, 123, 127, 147, 155, 158, 164, 167, 176, 194, 203, 218, 225, 229, 231, 233, 235, 240, 241, 263, 281, 283, 291, 292, 297, 310, 319, 349, 353, 355, 356, 358, 359, 365, 384, 386, 390–393, 403, 415, 424, 436, 437, 442, 445, 450, 462, 477, 480–485, 495, 497, 504, 511, 533, 534, 538, 542, 547, 549, 552, 566, 567, 570, 582, 586, 601, 613, 614, 620, 631, 636, 640, 656, 658, 665, 677, 689, 695, 701, 710, 711, 713, 748

LR-3, *tài chōng* 太冲, Supreme Surge, 4, 6, 11, 14, 19, 20, 24–26, 28–37, 39, 40, 43, 53, 57–59, 61, 62, 64, 66, 69–72, 74, 82, 89, 90, 94, 99, 103, 109, 111, 118, 119, 123, 127, 128, 138, 140, 146, 147, 151, 152, 156–158, 161, 162, 164, 167, 175, 176, 178, 194, 201, 202, 210, 212, 215, 217, 218, 223, 225–230, 233–235, 241, 251, 256, 257, 259, 261, 266, 269, 273, 274, 279, 280, 284, 288, 290–292, 294, 296, 297, 300, 302, 314, 316, 319, 320, 333, 336, 337, 347–349, 352, 353, 355–362, 364–366, 382, 385, 390–393, 403, 415, 416, 424, 426, 434, 437, 438, 442, 447–449, 451–454, 456–458, 462, 468, 475, 477–485, 490, 493, 495, 499, 503, 504, 506, 511, 513, 515, 516, 524, 533, 534, 537, 538, 540, 548, 552, 554, 561, 564, 566–570, 579, 581, 585, 586, 591, 596, 597, 601, 607, 608, 610, 613, 614, 627, 640, 652, 654, 656, 658, 661, 665, 677, 683, 689–691, 693, 694, 696, 699–702, 711, 713, 714, 716, 748

LR-4, *zhōng fēng* 中封, Mound Center, 61, 511, 542, 667, 748

LR-5, *lǐ gōu* 蠡沟, Woodworm Canal, 19–21, 35, 36, 51, 90, 111, 255, 353, 355, 395, 468, 481, 484, 522, 637, 748

LR-6, *zhōng dū* 中都, Central Metropolis, 19, 296, 431, 481, 748

LR-7, *xī guān* 膝关, Knee Joint, 337, 748

LR-8, *qū quán* 曲泉, Spring at the Bend, 28, 69, 111, 226, 256, 283, 289, 297, 300, 320, 337, 365, 403, 415, 447, 452, 456, 457, 468, 484, 487, 489, 506, 516, 566, 568, 637, 641, 667, 711, 748

LR-9, *yīn bāo* 阴包, Yin Bladder, 748

LR-10, *zú wǔ lǐ* 足五里, Foot Five Li, 610, 748

LR-11, *yīn lián* 阴廉, Yin Corner, 749

LR-12, *jí mài* 急脉, Urgent Pulse, 51, 297, 504, 749

LR-13, *zhāng mén* 章门, Camphorwood Gate, 1, 4, 8, 19, 37, 61, 62, 64, 78–80, 91, 109, 114, 151, 156, 161–163, 174, 196, 197, 217, 220, 233, 237, 242, 256, 271, 272, 301, 312, 314, 318, 325, 340, 349, 361, 384, 399, 401, 410, 418, 436, 479, 482, 487, 498, 499, 509, 521, 522, 537, 544, 554, 555, 557, 558, 561–565, 579, 581, 588, 596, 600, 612, 647, 669, 673, 710, 711, 716, 749

LR-14, *qī mén* 期门, Cycle Gate, 8, 19, 29, 34, 57, 88, 91, 112, 123, 157, 181, 215, 219, 223, 228, 234, 235, 256, 257, 279, 302, 310, 314, 352, 355, 357, 361–363, 374, 386, 390, 462, 478–480, 482, 483, 493, 571, 590, 658, 670, 683, 749

LU-1, *zhōng fǔ* 中府, Central Treasury, 8, 91, 142, 203, 219, 261, 439, 587, 746

LU-2, *yún mén* 云门, Cloud Gate, 746

LU-3, *tiān fǔ* 天府, Celestial Storehouse, 414, 678, 746

LU-4, *xiá bái* 侠白, Guarding White, 520, 746

LU-5, *chǐ zé* 尺泽, Cubit Marsh, 12–15, 22, 44, 70, 72, 88, 89, 91, 95–97, 103, 106, 109, 115, 119, 129, 142, 145–147, 149, 155, 156, 158, 163, 176, 184, 190, 201–203, 230, 237, 261, 267, 269, 277, 280–283, 285, 289, 291, 292, 295, 301, 336, 342, 343, 348, 366, 368, 372, 374, 378–380, 393, 398, 409, 415, 416, 418, 435–439, 443, 448, 458, 467, 501, 506, 520, 521, 530, 535, 547, 571, 572, 586, 587, 596, 597, 601, 603, 607, 611, 614, 637, 648, 668, 677, 683, 686–688, 695, 703, 714, 715, 746

LU-6, *kǒng zuì* 孔最, Collection Hole, 30, 70, 73, 97, 156, 277, 281, 290, 372, 379, 393, 520, 570, 603, 715, 716, 746

LU-7, *liè quē* 列缺, Broken Sequence, 12, 22, 50, 60, 65, 70, 73, 78, 84, 86–89, 91, 93, 96, 99, 103, 105, 111, 119, 120, 128, 129, 142, 145, 146, 155, 182, 184–186, 202, 203, 218, 225, 259, 260, 280, 281, 285, 291, 301, 342, 368, 374, 383, 405, 408, 415, 416, 438, 443, 448, 451, 452, 458, 477, 481, 501, 517, 519, 520, 522, 530, 544, 547, 586, 607, 620, 631, 668, 677, 681–684, 686, 687, 693, 703, 713, 746

LU-8, *jīng qú* 经渠, Channel Ditch, 207, 291, 368, 746

LU-9, *tài yuān* 太渊, Great Abyss, 30, 43, 47, 70, 72, 83, 90, 92, 96, 97, 109, 146, 161, 163, 177, 207, 216, 224, 228, 237, 251, 257, 267, 301, 368, 378–380, 435, 441, 453, 467, 477, 486, 489, 515, 520, 530, 548, 550, 562, 570, 571, 589, 590, 595, 596, 603, 625, 630, 633, 639, 640, 651, 654, 663, 666, 675, 678, 683, 702, 703, 714, 715, 746

LU-10, *yú jì* 鱼际, Fish Border, 14, 65, 70, 72, 91, 97, 147, 156, 158, 176, 184, 190, 201, 207, 237, 277, 280, 281, 285, 291, 292, 336, 356, 374, 393, 416, 501, 520, 547, 572, 603, 611, 613, 640, 665, 686, 688, 695, 714–716, 746

LU-11, *shào shāng* 少商, Lesser Shang, 5, 14, 62, 63, 66, 73, 90, 92, 103, 129, 147, 149, 156, 158, 184, 190, 201–203, 207, 216, 237, 261, 277, 280–283, 285, 291, 301, 348, 374, 378, 386, 394, 405, 414–416, 420, 438, 495, 501, 515, 519, 520, 522, 547, 569, 611, 620, 649, 685–688, 703, 715, 746

lú cí xián wán 鸬鹚涎丸, Cormorant Drool Pill, 677, 738

lú gān shí 炉甘石 smithsonite, Smithsonitum, 53, 636, 667, 713, 728

lú gēn 芦根 phragmites, Phragmititis Rhizoma, 64, 67, 69, 70, 358, 577, 720

lú huì 芦荟 aloe, Aloe, 459, 460, 722

lú huì xiāo gān yǐn 芦荟消疳饮, Aloe Gan-Dispersing Beverage, 236

lú sī xián 鸬鹚涎 cormorant's drool, Phalacrocoracis Saliva, 677

lú xī 颅息, TB-19, Skull Rest, 748

lù 露, dew, 125

lù 露, distillate, 143

lù cí ké 鹭鹚咳, cormorant cough, 99

lù fēng fáng 露蜂房 hornet's nest, Vespae Nidus, 298, 449, 728

lù jì 露剂, distillate, 143

lù jiǎo 鹿角 deerhorn, Cervi Cornu, 17, 310, 570, 593, 596, 726

lù jiǎo jiāo 鹿角胶 deerhorn glue, Cervi Gelatinum Cornu, 222, 243, 332, 466, 541, 572, 593, 726

lù jiǎo sǎn 鹿角散, Deerhorn Powder, 17

lù jiǎo shuāng 鹿角霜 degelatinated deerhorn, Cervi Cornu Degelatinatum, 593, 726

lù jiǎo tù sī wán 鹿角菟丝丸, Deerhorn and Cuscuta Pill, 743

lù jiǎo xiè 鹿角屑 deerhorn flakes, Cervi Cornu in Frustis, 679

lù lù tōng 路路通 liquidambar fruit, Liquidambaris Fructus, 19, 386, 417

lù róng 鹿茸 velvet deerhorn, Cervi Cornu Parvum, 45, 229, 511, 593, 651, 726

lù róng bǔ sè wán 鹿茸补涩丸, Velvet Deerhorn Supplementing and Astringing Pill, 641

lù róng dà bǔ tāng 鹿茸大补汤, Deerhorn Major Supplementation Decoction, 333

lù róng sì jīn wán 鹿茸四斤丸, Velvet Deerhorn Four Jin Pill, 337

lù róng wán 鹿茸丸, Velvet Deerhorn Pill, 508

lù si ké 鹭鹚咳, heron cough, 290

lù xián cǎo 鹿衔草 pyrola, Pyrolae Herba, 140, 722

lǘ zuǐ fēng 驴嘴风, donkey's-mouth wind, 144

lǚ 膂, paravertebral sinews, 428

lǚ gǔ 膂骨, spinal column, 550

lǚ gǔ 膂骨, spine bone, 550

lǚ jīn 膂筋, paravertebral sinews, 428

lǜ cǎo 葎草 Japanese hop, Humuli Scandentis Herba, 68, 721

lǜ dòu 绿豆 mung bean, Phaseoli Aurei Semen, 463, 527

lǜ dòu pí 绿豆皮 mung bean seed-coat, Phaseoli Aurei Testa, 68, 95, 721

lǜ fán 绿矾 melanterite, Melanteritum, 383, 728

lǜ fēng 绿风, green wind, 249

lǜ fēng líng yáng yǐn 绿风羚羊饮, Green Wind Antelope Horn Beverage, 248, 249

lǜ fēng nèi zhàng 绿风内障, green wind internal obstruction, 249

lǜ shuǐ guàn zhū 绿水灌珠, green water pouring into the eye, 249

luǎn 卵, testicle, 606

luǎn suō 卵缩, retracted testicles, 504

luffa stem, *sī guā* 丝瓜藤, Luffae Caulis, 121

Luffa Stem Powder, *tiān luó sǎn* 天罗散, 121

Luffae Caulis, *sī guā* 丝瓜藤, luffa stem, 121

Luffae Fasciculus Vascularis, *sī guā luò* 丝瓜络, loofah, 417, 569, 589, 728

lumbago*, 370

Lumbar Eye, *yāo yǎn* 腰眼, 360

Lumbar Rub Elixir, *mó yāo dān* 摩腰丹, 80

Lumbricus, *dì lóng* 地龙, earthworm, 53, 54, 74, 146, 516, 526, 569, 726

Lumbus-Fortifying Pill, *jiàn yāo wán* 健腰丸, 742

Lumbus-Lightening Decoction, *qīng yāo tāng* 轻腰汤, 326

lung failure*, 124, 646

Lung-Clearing Beverage, *qīng fèi yǐn* 清肺饮, 22, 443

Lung-Clearing Decoction, *qīng fèi tāng* 清肺汤, 535, 738

Lung-Clearing Drink, *qīng fèi yǐn zǐ* 清肺饮子, 148, 607, 626, 731

Lung-Clearing Phlegm-Transforming Pill, *qīng fèi huà tán wán* 清肺化痰丸, 738

Lung-Moistening Powder, *rùn fèi sǎn* 润肺散, 739

Lung-Supplementing Decoction, *bǔ fèi tāng* 补肺汤, 47, 163, 378, 379, 740

Lung-Warming Nose-Drying Elixir, *wēn fèi zhǐ liú dān* 温肺止流丹, 739

luó hàn guǒ 罗汉果 Grosvenor's momordica, Momordicae Grosvenori Fructus, 624, 725

luó lè 罗勒 basil, Basilici Herba, 600

luǒ lì 瘰疬, scrofula, 515

luò 络, connect, 94

luò 络, net, 408

luò cì 络刺, network vessel pricking, 409

luò huā shēng zhōu 落花生粥, Peanut Gruel, 420

luò mài 络脉, network vessel, 409

luò què 络却, BL-8, Declining Connection, 747

luò shí téng 络石藤 star jasmine stem, Trachelospermi Caulis, 139, 256, 722

luò shǔ 络属, netting and homing, 408

luò tán bù shuǎng 咯痰不爽, ungratifying expectoration, 637

luò xué 络穴, network point, 408

luò zhěn 落枕, crick in the neck, 105

luò zhěn xué 落枕穴, Crick in the Neck Point, 105

LV-5, *lǐ gōu* 蠡沟, Woodworm Canal, 408

Lycii Fructus, *gǒu qǐ zǐ* 枸杞子, lycium berry, 19, 28, 37, 88, 104, 172, 175, 225, 256, 310, 333, 352, 458, 467, 541, 584, 593, 595, 727

Lycii Radicis Cortex, *dì gǔ pí* 地骨皮, lycium root bark, 68, 72, 106, 175, 244, 277, 281, 282, 388, 391, 394, 450, 495, 637, 649, 676, 715, 721

lycium berry, *gǒu qǐ zǐ* 枸杞子, Lycii Fructus, 19, 28, 37, 88, 104, 172, 175, 225, 256, 310, 333, 352, 458, 467, 541, 584, 593, 595, 727

Lycium Berry, Chrysanthemum, and Rehmannia Decoction, *qǐ jú dì huáng tāng* 杞菊地黄汤, 742

Lycium Berry, Chrysanthemum, and Rehmannia Pill, *qǐ jú dì huáng wán* 杞菊地黄丸, 11, 38, 64, 86, 119, 144, 175, 195, 336, 352, 365, 674, 742

lycium root bark, *dì gǔ pí* 地骨皮, Lycii Radicis Cortex, 68, 72, 106, 175, 244, 277, 281, 282, 388, 391, 394, 450, 495, 637, 649, 676, 715, 721

Lycium Root Bark Beverage, *dì gǔ pí yǐn* 地骨皮饮, 31, 391, 649, 731

Lycopi Herba, *zé lán* 泽兰, lycopus, 34, 116, 137, 138, 356, 725

Lycopodii Clavati Herba cum Radice, *shēn jīn cǎo* 伸筋草, ground pine, 140, 569, 722

lycopus, *zé lán* 泽兰, Lycopi Herba, 34, 116, 137, 138, 356, 725

Lygodii Spora, *hǎi jīn shā* 海金沙, lygodium spore, 136, 369, 723

lygodium spore, *hǎi jīn shā* 海金沙, Lygodii Spora, 136, 369, 723

Lygodium Spore Powder, *hǎi jīn shā sǎn* 海金沙散, 637

lymphadenectasis*, 51

lymphadenhypertrophy*, 544

lymphadenitis*, 515

    acute, 685

    acute purulent, 670

má 麻, tingling, 614

má cù mài 麻促脉, frenzied sesame seed pulse, 229

má dú rù yíng 麻毒入营, measles toxin entering construction, 388

má dú xiàn fèi 麻毒陷肺, measles toxin falling into the lung, 388

má fēng 麻风, leprosy, 343

má fēng 麻风, numbing wind, 416

má huáng 麻黄 ephedra, Ephedrae Herba, 5, 17, 70, 103, 128, 129, 184, 228, 243, 246, 247, 346, 391, 438, 460, 500–502, 681, 683, 720

má huáng dìng chuǎn tāng 麻黄定喘丸, Ephedra Panting-Stabilizing Decoction, 281

má huáng fù zǐ gān cǎo tāng 麻黄附子甘草汤, Ephedra, Aconite, and Licorice Decoction, 729

má huáng fù zǐ xì xīn tāng 麻黄附子细辛汤, Ephedra, Aconite, and Asarum Decoction, 325, 345, 730

má huáng gēn 麻黄根 ephedra root, Ephedrae Radix, 11, 518, 727

má huáng jiā zhú tāng 麻黄加术汤, Ephedra Decoction Plus Ovate Atractylodes, 729

má huáng lián qiào chì xiǎo dòu tāng 麻黄连翘赤小豆汤, Ephedra, Forsythia, and Rice Bean Decoction, 700

má huáng tāng 麻黄汤, Ephedra Decoction, 3, 83, 184, 185, 246, 247, 346, 372, 502, 682, 729

má huáng xìng rén gān cǎo shí gāo tāng 麻黄杏仁甘草石膏汤, Ephedra, Apricot Kernel, Licorice, and Gypsum Decoction, 247

má huáng xìng rén shí gāo gān cǎo tāng 麻黄杏仁石膏甘草汤, Ephedra, Apricot Kernel, Gypsum, and Licorice Decoction, 729

má mù 麻木, numbness and tingling, 416

má rén wán 麻仁丸, Hemp Seed Pill, 72, 542, 683

má xìng gān shí tāng 麻杏甘石汤, Ephedra, Apricot Kernel, Gypsum, and Licorice Decoction, 246, 729

má xìng gān shí tāng 麻杏甘石汤, Ephedra, Apricot Kernel, Licorice, and Gypsum Decoction, 388, 637, 693, 729

má yóu 麻油 sesame oil, Sesami Seminis Oleum, 51

má zhěn 麻疹, measles, 387

má zhěn bì zhèng 麻疹闭证, measles block pattern, 387

má zhěn hóu tòng 麻疹喉痛, sore throat in measles, 547

má zhěn nì zhèng 麻疹逆证, unfavorable measles pattern, 637

má zhěn shī yīn 麻疹失音, loss of voice in measles, 368

má zhěn shùn zhèng 麻疹顺证, favorable measles pattern, 196

má zhěn xiǎn zhèng 麻疹险证, critical measles pattern, 105

má zǐ rén wán 麻子仁丸, Hemp Seed Pill, 399, 584, 732

mǎ biān cǎo 马鞭草 verbena, Verbenae Herba (cum Radice), 138, 725

mǎ bó 马勃 puffball, Lasiosphaera seu Calvatia, 68, 721

mǎ chǐ xiàn 马齿苋 purslane, Portulacae Herba, 68, 111, 338, 445, 516, 721

mǎ dān yáng tiān xīng shí èr xué 马丹阳天星十二穴, Ma Dan-Yang's twelve heavenly star points, 382

mǎ dāo xiá yǐng 马刀侠瘿, saber and pearl-string lumps, 511

mǎ dōu líng 马兜铃 aristolochia fruit, Aristolochiae Fructus, 95, 624, 725

mǎ lán 马兰 kalimeris, Kalimeridis Herba et Radix, 542

mǎ qián zǐ 马钱子 nux vomica, Nux-Vomicae Semen, 97, 397, 728

mǎ wěi lián 马尾连 meadow rue, Thalictri Rhizoma et Radix, 67, 720

Macule-Transforming Decoction, *huà bān tāng* 化斑汤, 422, 730

Macule-Transforming Toxin-Resolving Decoction, *huà bān jiě dú tāng* 化斑解毒汤, 338, 730

Madaio dock root, *tǔ dà huáng* 土大黄, Rumicis Madaio Radix, 116, 569

madder, *qiàn cǎo gēn* 茜草根, Rubiae Radix, 20, 34, 70, 97, 390, 493, 512, 572, 724

Magic Pivot (líng shū) 灵枢, second part of *huáng dì nèi jīng* 黄帝内经, 3, 10, 20, 43, 45, 48, 49, 56–58, 72, 96, 100, 120, 121, 124–126, 130, 143, 144, 180, 189, 190, 192, 193, 195, 204, 205, 213, 226, 244, 245, 252–254, 260, 264, 268, 310, 311, 329, 339, 358, 360, 361, 363, 370, 375, 377, 400, 409, 410, 469, 479, 485, 504, 505, 533, 548, 551, 553, 554, 556, 560, 561, 576, 598, 606, 607, 615, 620, 625, 627, 629, 633, 643, 654, 665, 672, 675, 700, 711

Magnetitum, *cí shí* 磁石, loadstone, 53, 225, 230, 287, 288, 490, 511, 525, 526, 538, 539, 585, 614, 726

magnolia bark, *hòu pò* 厚朴, Magnoliae Cortex, 10, 66, 72, 98, 103, 153, 217, 223, 224, 246, 276, 287, 363, 397, 401, 421, 430, 441, 459, 587, 625, 679, 722

Magnolia Bark Center-Warming Decoction, *hòu pò wēn zhōng tāng* 厚朴温中汤, 1, 85, 339, 561, 735

Magnolia Bark Seven Agents Decoction, *hòu pò qī wù tāng* 厚朴七物汤, 500, 730

Magnolia Bark Three Agents Decoction, *hòu pò sān wù tāng* 厚朴三物汤, 500, 731

Magnolia Bark, Fresh Ginger, Pinellia, Licorice, and Ginseng Decoction, *hòu pò shēng jiāng bàn xià gān cǎo rén shēn tāng* 厚朴生姜半夏甘草人参汤, 1, 339, 735

Magnolia Flower Lung-Clearing Powder, *xīn yí qīng fèi sǎn* 辛夷清肺散, 283

Magnolia Flower Powder, *xīn yí sǎn* 辛夷散, 120, 405, 543, 740

magnolia flower[1], *xīn yí* 辛夷, Magnoliae Flos[1], 120, 129, 405, 681, 720

magnolia flower[2], *hòu pò huā* 厚朴花, Magnoliae Flos[2], 625, 722

Magnoliae Coco Flos, *yè hé huā* 夜合花, dwarf magnolia, 491, 726

Magnoliae Cortex, *hòu pò* 厚朴, magnolia bark, 10, 66, 72, 98, 103, 153, 217, 223, 224, 246, 276, 287, 363, 397, 401, 421, 430, 441, 459, 587, 625, 679, 722

Magnoliae Flos[1], *xīn yí* 辛夷, magnolia flower[1], 120, 129, 405, 681, 720

Magnoliae Flos[2], *hòu pò huā* 厚朴花, magnolia flower[2], 625, 722

mahonia, *shí dà gōng láo yè* 十大功劳叶, Mahoniae Folium, 67, 720

Mahoniae Folium, *shí dà gōng láo yè* 十大功劳叶, mahonia, 67, 720

mái xiàn liáo fǎ 埋线疗法, catgut embedding, 54

mái zhēn 埋针, needle embedding, 406

mái zhēn 埋针, needle implantation, 406

mài 脉, pulse, 470

mài 脉, vessel, 654

mài bì 脉痹, vessel impediment, 654

mài bó 脉搏, pulse, 470

mài gēn 脉根, Vessel's Root, 540

mài jīng 脉经 (*Pulse Canon*), 3rd century, Western Jìn, Wáng Shú-Hé 王叔和, 48, 236, 351, 371, 554, 653

mài kǒu 脉口, vessel opening, 654

mài lì xíng pí nèi zhēn 麦粒型皮内针, wheat-grain intradermal needle, 671

mài mén dōng 麦门冬 ophiopogon, Ophiopogonis Tuber, 47, 88, 95, 104, 108, 174–176, 227, 256, 259, 298, 310, 325, 358, 368, 394, 398, 399, 409, 416, 457, 467, 495, 508, 515, 526, 541, 565, 569, 577, 581, 589, 593, 597, 654, 679, 715, 727

mài mén dōng tāng 麦门冬汤, Ophiopogon Decoction, 379, 581, 734

mài mén dōng yǐn zǐ 麦门冬饮子, Ophiopogon Drink, 447

mài qì 脉气, vessel qi, 654

mài wēi yù jué 脉微欲绝, faint pulse verging on expiration, 195

mài wěi 脉痿, vessel wilting, 654

mài wèi dì huáng wán 麦味地黄丸, Ophiopogon and Rehmannia Pill, 101, 163, 599, 715, 742

mài wú wèi qì 脉无胃气, pulse bereft of stomach qi, 470

mài xiàng 脉象, pulse, 470

mài xiàng 脉象, pulse condition, 470

mài yá 麦芽 barley sprout, Hordei Fructus Germinatus, 23, 141, 216, 217, 420, 450, 479, 499, 564, 573, 600, 606, 724

mài zhěn 脉诊, pulse examination, 472

Major Bupleurum Decoction, *dà chái hú tāng* 大柴胡汤, 3, 110, 255, 344, 357, 439, 700, 730

Major Center-Fortifying Decoction, *dà jiàn zhōng tāng* 大建中汤, 734

Major Chest Bind Decoction, *dà xiàn xiōng tāng* 大陷胸汤, 283, 383, 731

Major Chest Bind Pill, *dà xiàn xiōng wán* 大陷胸丸, 731

Major Construction Brew, *dà yíng jiān* 大营煎, 26, 741

Major Forsythia Beverage, *dà lián qiào yǐn* 大连翘饮, 198

Major Green-Blue Dragon Decoction, *dà qīng lóng tāng* 大青龙汤, 246, 550, 729

Major Ledebouriella Decoction, *dà fáng fēng tāng* 大防风汤, 104, 530

Major Network-Quickening Elixir, *dà huó luò dān* 大活络丹, 289, 734

Major Notopterygium Decoction, *dà qiāng huó tāng* 大羌活汤, 729

Major Origin-Supplementing Brew, *dà bǔ yuán jiān* 大补元煎, 178, 296, 332, 369, 466, 482, 487, 646, 647, 712

Major Peach Blossom Decoction, *dà táo huā tāng* 大桃花汤, 318, 742

Major Pinellia Decoction, *dà bàn xià tāng* 大半夏汤, 87, 443, 579, 736

Major Qi-Coordinating Decoction, *dà chéng qì tāng* 大承气汤, 2, 12, 24, 73, 84, 276, 280, 283, 290, 386, 426, 459, 504, 532, 542, 613, 698, 731

Major Seven Qi Decoction, *dà qī qì tāng* 大七气汤, 149, 325, 475, 479

Major Wind Arousal Decoction, *dà xǐng fēng tāng* 大醒风汤, 739

Major Wind-Stabilizing Pill, *dà dìng fēng zhū* 大定风珠, 74, 176, 456, 569, 740

Major Yin Supplementation Pill, *dà bǔ yīn wán* 大补阴丸, 213, 296, 330, 461, 512, 571, 597, 641, 647, 649, 651, 714, 742

Malaria Gate, *nüè mén* 疟门, 8

malaria*, 399
  cerebral, 439
  quartan, 490
  tertian, 606
  vivax, 606

Malaria-Interrupting Seven-Jewel Beverage, *jié nüè qī bǎo yǐn* 截疟七宝饮, 317, 732

mallow seed, *dōng kuí zǐ* 冬葵子, Malvae Verticillatae Semen, 98, 136, 370, 582, 723

Mallow Seed Powder, *kuí zǐ sǎn* 葵子散, 369

malnutrition*, 194, 704

malt sugar, *yí táng* 饴糖, Granorum Saccharon, 148, 511, 580, 593, 600, 602, 726

Malvae Verticillatae Semen, *dōng kuí zǐ* 冬葵子, mallow seed, 98, 136, 370, 582, 723

mǎn 满, fullness, 231

mǎn shān hóng 满山红 Daurian rhododendron, Rhododendri Daurici Folium, 624, 726

màn jīn fēng 慢惊风, chronic fright wind, 61

màn jīng zǐ 蔓荆子 vitex, Viticis Fructus, 17, 55, 420, 488, 680, 686, 720

màn pí fēng 慢脾风, chronic spleen wind, 62

màn zhǒng 漫肿, diffuse swelling, 128

mandible*, 57

máng xiāo 芒硝 mirabilite, Mirabilitum, 17, 34, 84, 98, 148, 182, 231, 255, 261, 276, 298, 419, 459, 460, 544, 548, 602, 665, 722

Mania and Withdrawal Pill, *diān kuáng wán* 癫狂丸, 740

Manitis Squama, *chuān shān jiǎ* 穿山甲, pangolin scales, 34, 50, 137, 138, 182, 227, 315, 398, 419, 513, 516, 724

Mantidis Oötheca, *sāng piāo xiāo* 桑螵蛸, mantis egg-case, 11, 12, 177, 229, 308, 496, 511, 518, 727

mantis egg-case, *sāng piāo xiāo* 桑螵蛸, Mantidis Oötheca, 11, 12, 177, 229, 308, 496, 511, 518, 727

Mantis Egg-Case Powder, *sāng piāo xiāo sǎn* 桑螵蛸散, 12, 148, 174, 176, 177, 308, 449, 465, 496, 518, 743

máo cì 毛刺, hair needling, 251

máo dōng qīng 毛冬青 hairy holly root, Ilicis Pubescentis Radix, 138, 725

máo gé tāng 茅葛汤, Imperata and Pueraria Decoction, 736

máo gèn 毛茛 Japanese ranunculus, Ranunculi Japonici Herba et Radix, 388, 728

mào 瞀, visual distortion, 657

Margarita, *zhēn zhū* 珍珠, pearl, 54, 249, 490, 726

Marrow-Engendering Unicorn-Fostering Elixir, *shēng suǐ yù lín dān* 生髓育麟丹, 513

Marrow-Sealing Elixir, *fēng suǐ dān* 封髓丹, 94

mashed garlic, *suàn ní* 蒜泥, Allii Sativi Bulbus Pulpatus, 388, 389

Massa Medicata Fermentata, *shén qū* 神麯, medicated leaven, 141, 216, 223, 287, 388, 418, 450, 499, 514, 573, 724

Massa Medicata Fermentata Fujianensis, *jiàn shén qū* 建神麯, Fujian leaven, 141, 724

mastitis*
   acute, 386
Mastodi Dentis Fossilia, *lóng chǐ* 龙齿, dragon tooth, 490, 525, 526, 538, 539, 726
Mastodi Ossis Fossilia, *lóng gǔ* 龙骨, dragon bone, 11, 53, 183, 230, 308, 409, 433, 449, 461, 490, 504, 518, 524–526, 537, 572, 585, 636, 696, 709, 726
Mastodi Ossis Fossilia Calcinata, *duàn lóng gǔ* 煅龙骨, calcined dragon bone, 95, 176, 267, 333, 566, 675, 709
Mastodi Ossis Fossilia Cruda, *shēng lóng gǔ* 生龙骨, crude dragon bone, 225, 585
mastoid process*, 92
Matchless Dioscorea Pill, *wú bǐ shān yào wán* 无比山药丸, 41
Mauritiae, Erosariae seu Cypraeae Testa, *zǐ bèi* 紫贝, purple cowrie, 54, 726
Mays Stylus, *yù mǐ xū* 玉米须, corn silk, 136, 723
meadow rue, *mǎ wěi lián* 马尾连, Thalictri Rhizoma et Radix, 67, 720
mealy fangji, *fěn fáng jǐ* 粉防己, Stephaniae Tetrandrae Radix, 139, 722
measles pneumonia*, 388
measles*, 25
Mechanical Ejection Brine, *yán tāng tàn tù fāng* 盐汤探吐方, 743
Medical Discussions of the Cold Shack (*lěng lú yī huà*) 冷庐医话, 1897 (Qīng), Lù Yǐ-Tián 陆以湉, 538
Medical Formulas Gathered and Explained (*yī fāng jí jiě*) 医方集解, 1682 (Qīng), Wāng Áng 汪昂, 691
Medical Insights (*yī xué xīn wù*) 医学心悟, 1732 (Qīng), Chéng Guó-Péng 程国彭, 245, 587
Medical Insights Pus-Outthrusting Powder, *xīn wù tòu nóng sǎn* 心悟透脓散, 744
Medical Remedies Researched (*yī fāng kǎo*) 医方考, 1584 (Míng), Wú Kūn 吴昆, 553
medicated leaven, *shén qū* 神麯, Massa Medicata Fermentata, 141, 216, 223, 287, 388, 418, 450, 499, 514, 573, 724
Medicated Leaven and Atractylodes Pill, *qū zhú wán* 麯术丸, 4, 63
Medicated Leaven Pill, *shén qū wán* 神麯丸, 739
Medicated Leaven, Barley Sprout, Unripe Bitter Orange, and Ovate Atractylodes Pill, *qū mài zhǐ zhú wán* 麯麦枳术丸, 736
Medicated Leaven, Barley Sprout, Unripe Bitter Orange, and Ovate Atractylodes Pill, *qū niè zhǐ zhú wán* 麯蘖枳术丸, 736
Medulla Bovis, *niú gǔ suǐ* 牛骨髓, beef marrow, 45
méi chōng 眉冲, BL-3, Eyebrow Ascension, 747
méi dī jìng wán 霉滴净丸, Trichomonas Cleansing Pill, 745
méi guī huā 玫瑰花 rose, Rosae Flos, 493, 724
méi hé qì 梅核气, plum-pit qi, 445
méi huā 梅花 mume flower, Mume Flos, 493, 724
méi huā zhēn 梅花针, plum-blossom needle, 445

méi léng gǔ 眉棱骨, eyebrow bone, 191
méi léng gǔ tòng 眉棱骨痛, eyebrow bone pain, 191
Mel, *mì* 蜜, honey, 201, 399, 449, 593, 726
melanterite, *lǜ fán* 绿矾, Melanteritum, 383, 728
Melanteritum, *lǜ fán* 绿矾, melanterite, 383, 728
Meliae Cortex (Radicis), *kǔ liàn pí* 苦楝皮, chinaberry (root) bark, 183, 724
Meliae Radicis Cortex, *kǔ liàn gēn pí* 苦楝根皮, chinaberry root bark, 183, 509, 510, 696
Melon Pedicel Powder, *guā dīng sǎn* 瓜丁散, 744
melon stalk, *guā dì* 瓜蒂, Cucumeris Melonis Pedicellus, 170, 727
Melon Stalk Powder, *guā dì sǎn* 瓜蒂散, 128, 170, 254, 743
Melon Stalk Wonder Powder, *guā dì shén miào sǎn* 瓜蒂神妙散, 744
Meloë, *dì dǎn* 地胆, oil beetle, 98
Membrane-Source–Opening Beverage, *dá yuán yǐn* 达原饮, 177, 514, 732
membranous pharyngitis*, 611
mèn rùn 闷润, covered moistening, 104
méng 蒙, cloud, 74
méng chóng 虻虫 tabanus, Tabanus, 98, 138, 724
méng shí 礞石 chlorite/mica, Chloriti seu Micae Lapis, 12, 53, 214, 291, 624, 725
méng shí gǔn tán wán 礞石滚痰丸, Chlorite/Mica Phlegm-Rolling Pill, 12, 214, 282, 386, 437, 539, 738
mèng jiāo 梦交, dreaming of intercourse, 148
mèng yí 梦遗, dream emission, 147
mèng yì 梦呓, sleep talking, 539
mèng yóu 梦游, sleep walking, 539
mèng zhōng yì yǔ 梦中呓语, dream talking, 148
meningitis*, 10
Menses-Securing Pill, *gù jīng wán* 固经丸, 572, 743
Menses-Stabilizing Decoction, *dìng jīng tāng* 定经汤, 385, 393
menstrual disorders*, 34, 336
menstruation*
   vicarious, 102, 390, 392
Menstruation-Normalizing Decoction, *shùn jīng tāng* 顺经汤, 390
Menthae Herba, *bò hé* 薄荷, mint, 7, 17, 69, 103, 130, 143, 176, 184, 368, 414, 422, 463, 497, 501, 548, 621, 671, 686, 687, 720
mentolabial groove*, 512
mercury, *shuǐ yín* 水银, Hydrargyrum, 98, 171, 383, 411
Mercury and Apricot Kernel Carefree Powder, *yín xìng wú yōu sǎn* 银杏无忧散, 468
metabolism*, 486
Metal Strength Pill, *jīn gāng wán* 金刚丸, 47
Metal-Clearing Phlegm-Transforming Decoction, *qīng jīn huà tán tāng* 清金化痰汤, 356, 738
Metropolis Qi Pill, *dū qì wán* 都气丸, 325, 379, 629, 648, 742
metrorrhagia*, 212
   dysfunctional, 162

mí 迷, confound, 93

mí làn 糜烂, erosion, 178

mí làn 糜烂, ulceration, 636

mǐ chǎo 米炒, stir-frying with rice, 574

mì 蜜 honey, Mel, 201, 399, 449, 593, 726

mì bié qīng zhuó 泌别清浊, separation of the clear and the turbid, 525

mì fāng 秘方, secret formula, 517

mì jiān dǎo fǎ 蜜煎导法, Honey Enema, 542, 646

mì jīng wán 秘精丸, Essence-Containing Pill, 112, 525

mì méng huā 密蒙花 buddleia, Buddleiae Flos, 67, 720

mì tuó sēng 密陀僧 litharge, Lithargyrum, 411, 713, 728

mì tuó sēng sǎn 密陀僧散, Litharge Powder, 226, 474

mì wán 蜜丸, honey pill, 292

mì yuán jiān 秘元煎, Origin-Securing Brew, 180, 369, 525, 641, 743

mì zhì 蜜炙, mix-frying with honey, 397

miǎn huái sǎn 免怀散, No-Nursing-Worries Powder, 606

miǎn shēn 免身, birth, 19

miǎn shēn 免身, childbirth, 60

miǎn shēn 免身, delivery, 122

miàn 面, face, 193

miàn bái 面白, white face, 675

miàn chì 面赤, red face, 495

miàn fú 面浮, puffy face, 469

miàn gòu 面垢, grimy face, 249

miàn hēi 面黑, black face, 20

miàn hóng 面红, red face, 495

miàn hóng shēng huǒ 面红升火, upbearing fire flush, 638

miàn huáng 面黄, yellow face, 704

miàn jiá cháo hóng 面颊潮红, malar flush, 383

miàn jiá cháo hóng 面颊潮红, tidal reddening of the cheeks, 613

miàn mù fú zhǒng 面目浮种, puffy swelling of the face and eyes, 469

miàn qīng 面青, green-blue face, 248

miàn sè 面色, facial complexion, 193

miàn sè bái 面色白, white facial complexion, 675

miàn sè bù huá 面色不华, lusterless facial complexion, 381

miàn sè cāng bái 面色苍白, somber white facial complexion, 545

miàn sè dàn bái 面色淡白, pale white facial complexion, 426

miàn sè fú hóng 面色浮红, floating-red facial complexion, 211

miàn sè hēi 面色黑, black facial complexion, 20

miàn sè hóng 面色红, red facial complexion, 496

miàn sè huáng 面色黄, yellow facial complexion, 704

miàn sè huǎng bái 面色㿠白, bright white facial complexion, 50

miàn sè qīng 面色青, green-blue facial complexion, 248

miàn sè wěi huáng 面色萎黄, withered-yellow facial complexion, 695

miàn tòng 面痛, facial pain, 194

miàn tòng èr hào fāng 面痛二号方, Facial Pain No.2 Formula, 194

miàn tòng sān hào fāng 面痛三号方, Facial Pain No.3 Formula, 194

miàn tòng sì hào fāng 面痛四号方, Facial Pain No.4 Formula, 194

miàn tòng yī hào fāng 面痛一号方, Facial Pain No.1 Formula, 194

miàn wáng 面王, king of face, 336

miào xiāng sǎn 妙香散, Mysterious Fragrance Powder, 147, 427, 525, 739

migraine*, 260

Millet Water Powder, *jiāng shuǐ sǎn* 浆水散, 735

millettia, *jī xuè téng* 鸡血藤, Millettiae Radix et Caulis, 37, 137, 138, 352, 484, 516, 593, 679, 724, 727

Millettiae Radix et Caulis, *jī xuè téng* 鸡血藤, millettia, 37, 137, 138, 352, 484, 516, 593, 679, 724, 727

mín jiān yào 民间药, folk medicinal, 214

Mind-Stabilizing Pill, *dìng zhì wán* 定志丸, 147, 297, 406, 739

míng 明, Ming, 396

míng dǎng shēn 明党参 changium root, Changii Radix, 624, 725

míng mù 明目, brightening the eyes, 50

míng mù dì huáng wán 明目地黄丸, Eye Brightener Rehmannia Pill, 249, 742

míng mù shàng qīng wán 明目上清丸, Eye Brightener Clear-Raising Pill, 740

míng táng 明堂, bright hall, 50

mìng guān 命关, life bar, 345

mìng huǒ 命火, life fire, 345

mìng huǒ bù zú 命火不足, insufficiency of the life fire, 310

mìng mén 命门, GV-4, Life Gate, 4, 14, 22, 23, 26, 35, 36, 45, 61, 64, 80–86, 94, 105, 151, 160, 163, 164, 168, 174, 180, 196, 199, 210, 211, 224, 229, 240, 263, 266, 267, 269, 272, 274, 288, 291, 296, 297, 301, 308, 312, 325, 327, 329, 331–335, 337, 340, 342, 345, 347, 369, 379, 380, 425, 426, 449, 452, 453, 461, 465, 466, 488, 489, 506, 514, 518, 521, 524, 549, 559, 564, 569, 579, 594, 596, 608, 625, 630, 641, 643, 647, 651, 660, 662, 693, 702, 703, 710, 713, 714, 716, 749

mìng mén 命门, life gate, 346

mìng mén huǒ shuāi 命门火衰, debilitation of the life gate fire, 119

mìng mén huǒ wàng 命门火旺, effulgent life gate fire, 168

mìng mén zhī huǒ 命门之火, life gate fire, 346

Minium, *qiān dān* 铅丹, minium, 728

minium, *qiān dān* 铅丹, Minium, 728

Minor Bupleurum Decoction, *xiǎo chái hú tāng* 小柴胡汤, 20, 57, 255, 279, 284, 344, 362, 394, 449, 599, 683, 688, 712, 732

Minor Center-Fortifying Decoction, *xiǎo jiàn zhōng tāng* 小建中汤, 217, 487, 488, 581, 713, 735

Minor Center-Warming Pill, *xiǎo wēn zhōng wán* 小温中丸, 736

Minor Chest Bind Decoction, *xiǎo xiàn xiōng tāng* 小陷胸汤, 189, 277, 303, 396, 738

Minor Construction Brew, *xiǎo yíng jiān* 小营煎, 94, 741

Minor Golden Elixir, *xiǎo jīn dān* 小金丹, 259, 737

Minor Green-Blue Dragon Decoction Plus Gypsum, *xiǎo qīng lóng jiā shí gāo tāng* 小青龙加石膏汤, 441, 469, 739

Minor Green-Blue Dragon Decoction, *xiǎo qīng lóng tāng* 小青龙汤, 78, 85, 120, 170, 246, 373, 438, 468, 550, 625, 663, 666, 667, 739

Minor Life-Prolonging Decoction, *xiǎo xù mìng tāng* 小续命汤, 45, 456, 568, 631, 693, 740

Minor Network-Quickening Elixir, *xiǎo huó luò dān* 小活络丹, 14, 621, 734

Minor Pinellia Decoction Plus Poria (Hoelen), *xiǎo bàn xià jiā fú líng tāng* 小半夏加茯苓汤, 87, 442, 578, 665

Minor Pinellia Decoction, *xiǎo bàn xià tāng* 小半夏汤, 736

Minor Qi-Coordinating Decoction, *xiǎo chéng qì tāng* 小承气汤, 84, 127, 239, 426, 459, 499, 613, 731

Minor Stomach Elixir, *xiǎo wèi dān* 小胃丹, 442, 638

mint, *bò hé* 薄荷, Menthae Herba, 7, 17, 69, 103, 130, 143, 176, 184, 368, 414, 422, 463, 497, 501, 548, 621, 671, 686, 687, 720

Mint and Refined Mirabilite Powder, *bò hé xuán míng sǎn* 薄荷玄明散, 620

Mint Powder, *jī sū sǎn* 鸡苏散, 730

MirabilitEfflorescentia, *fēng huà xiāo* 风化硝, mirabilite efflorescence, 401

mirabilite, *máng xiāo* 芒硝, Mirabilitum, 17, 34, 84, 98, 148, 182, 231, 255, 261, 276, 298, 419, 459, 460, 544, 548, 602, 665, 722

mirabilite efflorescence, *fēng huà xiāo* 风化硝, MirabilitEfflorescentia, 401

Mirabiliti et Citrulli Praeparatio, *xī guā shuāng* 西瓜霜, watermelon frost, 67, 720

Mirabilitum, *máng xiāo* 芒硝, mirabilite, 17, 34, 84, 98, 148, 182, 231, 255, 261, 276, 298, 419, 459, 460, 544, 548, 602, 665, 722

Mirabilitum Depuratum, *xuán míng fěn* 玄明粉, refined mirabilite, 44, 460, 722

Mirabilitum Non-Purum, *pò xiāo* 朴硝, impure mirabilite, 310

Mirabilitum Non-Purum, *pò xiāo* 朴硝, impure mirabilite, 44, 411, 460, 712, 722

mistletoe, *sāng jì shēng* 桑寄生, Loranthi seu Visci Ramus, 139, 297, 352, 370, 456, 488, 722

Misty Decoction, *yīn yūn tāng* 氤氲汤, 395

miù cì 缪刺, cross needling, 105

mix-fried Glycyrrhizae Radix, *gān cǎo* 炙甘草, mix-fried licorice, 270

mix-fried licorice, *gān cǎo* 炙甘草, mix-fried Glycyrrhizae Radix, 270

mó 磨, grinding, 249

mó yāo dān 摩腰丹, Lumbar Rub Elixir, 80

mó yuán 膜原, membrane source, 389

mó zhàng líng guāng gāo 磨障灵光膏, Obstruction-Abrading Spirit Light Paste, 744

mó zhàng líng guāng gāo 磨障灵光高, Obstruction-Abrading Spirit Light Paste, 181, 403

mò hàn lián 墨旱莲 eclipta, Ecliptae Herba, 37, 88, 172, 225, 277, 336, 352, 388, 415, 467, 548, 569, 586, 593, 597, 727

mò yào 没药 myrrh, Myrrha, 137, 138, 451, 503, 540, 574, 696, 724

Modified Eight Agents Decoction, *zēng sǔn bā wù tāng* 增损八物汤, 692

mole cricket, *lóu gū* 蝼蛄, Gryllotalpa, 98, 136, 723

mole*
   hydatic, 615
   hydatiform, 615

mollissima, *xún gǔ fēng* 寻骨风, Aristolochiae Mollissimae Rhizoma seu Herba, 139, 722

momordica, *mù biē zǐ* 木鳖子, Momordicae Semen, 728

Momordicae Grosvenori Fructus, *luó hàn guǒ* 罗汉果, Grosvenor's momordica, 624, 725

Momordicae Semen, *mù biē zǐ* 木鳖子, momordica, 728

moneywort, *jīn qián cǎo* 金钱草, Jinqiancao Herba, 21, 136, 369, 544, 582, 700, 723

Moonlight Pill, *yuè huá wán* 月华丸, 379, 742

Mori Folium, *sāng yè* 桑叶, mulberry leaf, 103, 107, 184, 420, 501, 526, 591, 686, 720

Mori Fructus, *sāng shèn* 桑椹, mulberry, 37, 172, 352, 593, 597, 727

Mori Radicis Cortex, *sāng bái pí* 桑白皮, mulberry root bark, 64, 70, 153, 199, 228, 282, 388, 394, 624, 676, 725

Mori Ramulus, *sāng zhī* 桑枝, mulberry twig, 116, 139, 263, 722

morinda, *bā jǐ tiān* 巴戟天, Morindae Radix, 222, 310, 332, 400, 529, 593, 675, 679, 716, 727

Morindae Radix, *bā jǐ tiān* 巴戟天, morinda, 222, 310, 332, 400, 529, 593, 675, 679, 716, 727

morning glory, *qiān niú zǐ* 牵牛子, Pharbitidis Semen, 98, 171, 182, 215, 411, 438, 445, 460, 666, 722

morning sickness*, 384

Moschus, *shè xiāng* 麝香, musk, 98, 243, 392, 398, 420, 449, 726

Mother's Rescue Elixir, *jiù mǔ dān* 救母丹, 737

mother-of-pearl, *zhēn zhū mǔ* 珍珠母, Concha Margaritifera, 53, 54, 230, 434, 490, 526, 538, 539, 585, 726

Index   848

Mother-of-Pearl Pill, *zhēn zhū mǔ wán* 珍珠母丸, 365, 739

moutan, *mǔ dān pí* 牡丹皮, Moutan Radicis Cortex, 20, 30, 47, 67, 70, 93, 97, 116, 120, 137, 140, 176, 263, 390, 412, 422, 428, 450, 459, 493, 495, 526, 529, 540, 547, 586, 591, 613, 620, 656, 661, 714, 720, 721

Moutan and Gardenia Free Wanderer Powder, *dān zhī xiāo yáo sǎn* 丹栀逍遥散, 19, 29, 31, 143, 177, 353, 354, 393, 453, 462, 502, 586, 655, 711, 732

Moutan Powder, *mǔ dān pí sǎn* 牡丹皮散, 737

Moutan Radicis Cortex, *mǔ dān pí* 牡丹皮, moutan, 20, 30, 47, 67, 70, 93, 97, 116, 120, 137, 140, 176, 263, 390, 412, 422, 428, 450, 459, 493, 495, 526, 529, 540, 547, 586, 591, 613, 620, 656, 661, 714, 720, 721

Moxibustion Triangle, *sān jiǎo jiǔ* 三角灸, 226

mǔ bìng jí zǐ 母病及子, disease of the mother affects the child, 135

mǔ dān pí 牡丹皮 moutan, Moutan Radicis Cortex, 20, 30, 47, 67, 70, 93, 97, 116, 120, 137, 140, 176, 263, 390, 412, 422, 428, 450, 459, 493, 495, 526, 529, 540, 547, 586, 591, 613, 620, 656, 661, 714, 720, 721

mǔ dān pí sǎn 牡丹皮散, Moutan Powder, 737

mǔ dīng xiāng 母丁香 clove fruit, Caryophylli Fructus, 660, 723

mǔ gǒu yīn jīng 牡狗阴茎 dog's penis, Canis Penis, 593, 726

mǔ lì 牡蛎 oyster shell, Ostreae Concha, 11, 53, 54, 95, 176, 177, 183, 230, 308, 409, 433, 460, 461, 490, 495, 504, 511, 518, 524–526, 537, 544, 572, 585, 651, 696, 709, 726

mǔ lì sǎn 牡蛎散, Oyster Shell Powder, 11, 95, 595, 651, 742

mǔ lì wán 牡蛎丸, Oyster Shell Pill, 177

mǔ lì zé xiè sǎn 牡蛎泽泻散, Oyster Shell and Alisma Powder, 733

mǔ nüè 牡疟, male malaria, 384

mǔ zhǐ tóng shēn cùn 拇指同身寸, thumb body-inch, 612

mù 木, numbness, 416

mù 木, wood, 695

mù 目, eye, 190

mù bāo 目胞, eyelid, 192

mù biē zǐ 木鳖子 momordica, Momordicae Semen, 728

mù chì 目赤, red eyes, 495

mù chì 目赤, reddening of the eyes, 495

mù chuāng 目窗, GB-16, Eye Window, 748

mù fáng jǐ 木防己 woody fangji, Cocculi Radix, 139, 722

mù fáng jǐ tāng 木防己汤, Woody Fangji Decoction, 120, 468, 733

mù fēi xuè 目飞血, blood flying to the eye, 30

mù fú róng huā 木芙蓉花 cotton rose, Hibisci Mutabilis Flos, 728

mù fú róng yè 木芙蓉叶 cotton rose leaf, Hibisci Mutabilis Folium, 104, 728

mù gān sè 目干涩, dry eyes, 152

mù guā 木瓜 chaenomeles, Chaenomelis Fructus, 139, 154, 363, 452, 454, 548, 722

mù guā niú xī wán 木瓜牛膝丸, Chaenomeles and Achyranthes Pill, 80, 733

mù guā tāng 木瓜汤, Chaenomeles Decoction, 61,

mù huā 目花, flowery vision, 212

mù huáng 目黄, yellowing of the eyes, 704

mù hūn 目昏, clouded vision, 75

mù huǒ xíng jīn 木火刑金, wood fire tormenting metal, 695

mù jǐn huā 木槿花 rose-of-Sharon, Hibisci Syriaci Flos, 728

mù jǐn pí 木槿皮 rose-of-Sharon root bark, Hibisci Syriaci Radicis Cortex, 728

mù kē 目窠, eye nest, 192

mù kē shàng wēi zhǒng 目窠上微肿, slight swelling of the eye nest, 539

mù piān shì 目偏视, squint, 568

mù tōng 木通 mutong, Mutong Caulis, 21, 69, 110, 136, 154, 263, 387, 395, 457, 723

mù tōng sǎn 木通散, Mutong Powder, 452, 733

mù tòng 目痛, eye pain, 192

mù tóu huí 墓头回 heterophyllous patrinia, Patriniae Heterophyllae Radix, 68, 721

mù xì 目系, eye tie, 192

mù xià yǒu wò cán 目下有卧蚕, sleeping silkworms beneath the eyes, 536

mù xián 目弦, eyelid rim, 192

mù xiāng 木香 saussurea, Saussureae (seu Vladimiriae) Radix, 38, 47, 80, 141, 223, 257, 317, 318, 338, 361, 384, 392, 398, 454, 480, 483, 493, 581, 588, 596, 694, 723

mù xiāng bīng láng wán 木香槟榔丸, Saussurea and Areca Pill, 217, 240, 277, 426, 481, 549, 736

mù xiāng dǎo zhì wán 木香导滞丸, Saussurea Stagnation-Abducting Pill, 736

mù xiāng liú qì yǐn 木香流气饮, Saussurea Qi Flow Beverage, 116, 481

mù xiāng pò qì sǎn 木香破气散, Saussurea Qi-Breaking Powder, 481

mù xiāng shùn qì sǎn 木香顺气散, Saussurea Qi-Normalizing Powder, 735

mù xiāng shùn qì tāng 木香顺气汤, Saussurea Qi-Normalizing Decoction, 19, 483

mù xiāng shùn qì wán 木香顺气丸, Saussurea Qi-Normalizing Pill, 735

mù xiāng tiáo qì sǎn 木香调气散, Saussurea Qi-Regulating Powder, 74, 480

mù xuàn 目眩, dizzy vision, 144

mù xué 募穴, alarm point, 7

mù xué 募穴, mustering point, 403

mù yǎng 目痒, itchy eyes, 320

mù yì 目翳, eye screen, 192

mù yù huà fēng 木郁化风, depressed wood transforming into wind, 123 *mù yù huà huǒ* 木郁化火, depressed wood transforming into fire, 123

mù zéi 木贼 equisetum, Equiseti Herba, 686, 720

mù zhū piān xié 目珠偏斜, squint, 568

mugwort, *ài yè* 艾叶, Artemisiae Argyi Folium, 401, 402, 468, 569

Mugwort and Cyperus Palace-Warming Pill, *ài fù nuǎn gōng wán* 艾附暖宫丸, 643, 741

mulberry, *sāng shèn* 桑椹, Mori Fructus, 37, 172, 352, 593, 597, 727

mulberry leaf, *sāng yè* 桑叶, Mori Folium, 103, 107, 184, 420, 501, 526, 591, 686, 720

Mulberry Leaf and Apricot Kernel Decoction, *sāng xìng tāng* 桑杏汤, 12, 101, 128, 155, 156, 158, 181, 398, 659, 734

Mulberry Leaf and Chrysanthemum Beverage, *sāng jú yǐn* 桑菊饮, 91, 103, 158, 184, 203, 291, 405, 414, 501, 687, 693, 729

Mulberry Paste, *sāng shèn zǐ gāo* 桑椹子膏, 245, 742

Mulberry Paste, *wén wǔ tāng* 文武膏, 742

mulberry root bark, *sāng bái pí* 桑白皮, Mori Radicis Cortex, 64, 70, 153, 199, 228, 282, 388, 394, 624, 676, 725

Mulberry Root Bark Decoction, *sāng bái pí tāng* 桑白皮汤, 285, 438, 675, 738

mulberry twig, *sāng zhī* 桑枝, Mori Ramulus, 116, 139, 263, 722

Mulberry Twig and Bushy Knotweed Decoction, *sāng zhī hǔ zhàng tāng* 桑枝虎杖汤, 734

multiflora rose root, *qiáng wēi gēn* 蔷薇根, Rosae Multiflorae Radix, 401

multiple neuritis*, 678

mume, *wū méi* 乌梅, Mume Fructus, 80, 82, 417, 462, 510, 518, 548, 599, 604, 612, 712, 727

Mume Flos, *méi huā* 梅花, mume flower, 493, 724

mume flower, *méi huā* 梅花, Mume Flos, 493, 724

Mume Fructus, *wū méi* 乌梅, mume, 80, 82, 417, 462, 510, 518, 548, 599, 604, 612, 712, 727

Mume Pill, *wū méi wán* 乌梅丸, 64, 228, 509, 510, 695, 696, 737

mumps*, 664

mung bean, *lǜ dòu* 绿豆, Phaseoli Aurei Semen, 463, 527

mung bean seed-coat, *lǜ dòu pí* 绿豆皮, Phaseoli Aurei Testa, 68, 95, 721

musk, *shè xiāng* 麝香, Moschus, 98, 243, 392, 398, 420, 449, 726

mutong, *mù tōng* 木通, Mutong Caulis, 21, 69, 110, 136, 154, 263, 387, 395, 457, 723

Mutong Caulis, *mù tōng* 木通, mutong, 21, 69, 110, 136, 154, 263, 387, 395, 457, 723

Mutong Powder, *mù tōng sǎn* 木通散, 452, 733

myatrophy*
  progressive, 678

mydystrophy*, 60

myelitis*, 148
  acute, 678

myesthenia gravis*, 678

Mylabris, *bān máo* 斑蝥, mylabris, 98, 388, 574, 728

mylabris, *bān máo* 斑蝥, Mylabris, 98, 388, 574, 728

myodystrophy*, 541, 678

myofibroma*, 211

myoma*
  submucosal of uterus, 711

Myriad Applications Paste, *wàn yìng gāo* 万应膏, 745

Myriad Applications Pill, *wàn yìng wán* 万应丸, 509, 695, 737

Myristicae Semen, *ròu dòu kòu* 肉豆蔻, nutmeg, 12, 80, 141, 316, 318, 454, 508, 518, 727

myrrh, *mò yào* 没药, Myrrha, 137, 138, 451, 503, 540, 574, 696, 724

Myrrha, *mò yào* 没药, myrrh, 137, 138, 451, 503, 540, 574, 696, 724

Myrrha Cruda, *shēng mò yào* 生没药, raw myrrh, 138, 724

Mysterious Four Decoction, *sì miào tāng* 四妙汤, 743

Mysterious Four Pill, *sì miào wán* 四妙丸, 733

Mysterious Four Resting Hero Decoction, *sì miào yǒng ān tāng* 四妙勇安汤, 540, 743

Mysterious Fragrance Powder, *miào xiāng sǎn* 妙香散, 147, 427, 525, 739

Mysterious Pearl of Red Water (chì shuǐ xuán zhū) 赤水玄珠, 1584 (Míng), Sūn Yī-Kuí 孙一奎, 123, 583

Mysterious Three Pill, *sān miào wán* 三妙丸, 225, 528, 686, 733

Mysterious Three Powder, *sān miào sǎn* 三妙散, 45, 117, 733

Mysterious Two Pill, *èr miào wán* 二妙丸, 8, 40, 116, 117, 347

Mysterious Two Powder (Pill), *èr miào sǎn (wán)* 二妙散(丸), 713, 733

Mysterious Two Powder, *èr miào sǎn* 二妙散, 337, 425, 489, 679

myxedema*, 615

nà dāi 纳呆, torpid intake, 621

nà gǔ bù xiāng 纳谷不香, no pleasure in eating, 413

nà gǔ bù xīn 纳谷不馨, no pleasure in eating, 413

nà gǔ jiǎn tuì 纳谷减退, reduced food intake, 496

nà qì 纳气, qi absorption, 475

nà shǎo 纳少, reduced food intake, 496

nà shí 纳食, increase food intake, 298

Naemorhedi Goral Cornu, *shān yáng jiǎo* 山羊角, goral horn, 54, 726

nǎi xiǎn 奶癣, suckling lichen, 585

nán běi cháo 南北朝, Northern and Southern Dynasties, 414

nán chǎn 难产, difficult delivery, 128

nán cháo 南朝, Southern Dynasties, 549

nán guā zǐ 南瓜子 pumpkin seed, Cucurbitae Semen, 183, 298, 724

nán kē jí bìng 男科疾病, andriatric diseases, 9

nán shā shēn 南沙参 adenophora, Adenophorae Radix, 593, 727

nán shēng jí bìng 男生疾病, men's diseases, 389

nán sòng 南宋, Southern Song, 549

nàn jīng 难经 (*Classic of Difficult Issues*), 1st century, Eastern Hàn, 2, 15, 78, 120, 125, 143, 179, 195, 204, 208, 270, 329, 346, 360, 377, 378, 411, 561, 610

náng suō 囊缩, retracted scrotum, 504

náng tuō 囊脱, sloughing scrotum, 540

náng yōng 囊痈, scrotal welling-abscess, 516

náo chóng 蛲虫, pinworm, 444

náo chóng bìng 蛲虫病, pinworm disease, 444

náo jū 脑疽, flat-abscess of the brain, 210

náo shā 硇砂 sal ammoniac, Sal Ammoniacum, 98, 728

náo shā jiān wán 硇砂煎丸, Sal Ammoniac Decocted Pill, 77

náo shā sǎn 硇砂散, Sal Ammoniac Powder, 166

nǎo 脑, brain, 49

nǎo fēng 脑风, brain wind, 50

nǎo gān 脑疳, gan of the brain, 237

nǎo hù 脑户, GV-17, Brain's Door, 50, 749

nǎo kōng 脑空, GB-19, Brain Hollow, 120, 331, 365, 654, 748

nǎo lòu 脑漏, brain leak, 50

nǎo suǐ bù zú 脑髓不足, insufficiency of the brain marrow, 310

nǎo wéi suǐ zhī hǎi 脑为髓之海, brain is the sea of marrow, 49

nǎo wéi yuán shén zhī fǔ 脑为元神之府, brain is the house of the original spirit, 49

nào huì 臑会, TB-13, Upper Arm Convergence, 30, 210, 480, 748

nào shū 臑俞, SI-10, Upper Arm Transport, 295, 342, 521, 530, 747

Nardostachydis Rhizoma et Radix, *gān sōng* 甘松, nardostachys, 493, 724

nardostachys, *gān sōng* 甘松, Nardostachydis Rhizoma et Radix, 493, 724

Nasal Insufflation Jasper Clouds Powder, *xiù bí bì yún sǎn* 嗅鼻碧云散, 744

native achyranthes, *tǔ niú xī* 土牛膝, Achyranthis Radix, 138, 459, 724

Navel-Warming Paste, *nuǎn qí gāo* 暖脐膏, 744

navicular bone*, 23

nèi 内, inner body, 303

nèi 内, internal, 312

nèi bì 内闭, internal block, 312

nèi bì hūn jué 内闭昏厥, internal block clouding reversal, 312

nèi bǔ wán 内补丸, Internal Supplementation Pill, 333, 742

nèi chuī 内吹, internal blowing, 312

nèi chuī rǔ yōng 内吹乳痈, internal blowing mammary welling-abscess, 312

nèi fēng 内风, internal wind, 317

nèi fú gāo jì 内服膏剂, orally taken paste, 421

nèi guān 内关, PC-6, Inner Pass, 1, 3, 4, 11, 17, 19, 20, 24, 25, 29, 31–33, 35, 39, 47, 53, 57, 58, 62–64, 69–74, 77, 80–83, 85–93, 103, 109, 111, 114, 117, 118, 123, 129, 138, 141, 145, 151, 153, 156–160, 178, 186, 189, 194, 201–203, 210–212, 215–218, 223–225, 227–230, 232–236, 241, 242, 247, 255–257, 260, 261, 263–269, 271–274, 276, 278, 280, 284, 287, 288, 294, 296, 297, 301, 302, 308, 314, 318, 333, 335, 336, 339, 343, 349, 353, 355, 356, 358, 359, 361, 362, 366, 379, 383–386, 390, 392–394, 401, 406, 408, 410, 413, 426, 427, 433–440, 442, 443, 445–449, 451–453, 455, 457, 462, 475, 477–485, 487, 488, 490, 493, 498, 499, 504, 510, 513, 522, 524, 526, 533, 537–540, 551, 552, 554, 555, 561, 562, 565, 569–572, 575, 577–581, 585–591, 597, 608, 613, 624, 629, 633, 638, 640, 646, 647, 649, 651, 652, 655, 658, 665, 666, 668, 669, 673, 675, 676, 685, 687, 690, 691, 699, 701, 703, 709, 713, 716, 748

nèi hán 内寒, internal cold, 313

nèi huǒ (rè) 内火（热）, internal fire (heat), 315

nèi jīng 内经 (*Inner Canon*), full title *huáng dì nèi jīng* 黄帝内经, 46, 100, 108, 149, 178, 206, 208, 244, 264, 265, 298, 322, 324, 326, 341, 346, 349, 367, 371, 376, 377, 421, 459, 477, 505, 520, 534, 535, 549, 551, 560, 598, 606, 630, 638, 658, 670, 673, 678, 692

nèi rè 内热, internal heat, 316

nèi shāng 内伤, internal damage, 313

nèi shāng 内伤, internal injury, 316

nèi shāng bù dé wò 内伤不得卧, internal damage sleeplessness, 313

nèi shāng qī qíng 内伤七情, affect damage, 7

nèi shāng qī qíng 内伤七情, internal damage by the seven affects, 313

nèi shāng tóu tòng 内伤头痛, internal damage headache, 313

nèi shāng wèi wǎn (guǎn) tòng 内伤胃脘痛, internal damage stomach duct pain, 314

nèi shāng yāo tòng 内伤腰痛, internal damage lumbar pain, 313

nèi shāng yǐn shí jìng 内伤饮食痉, internal food damage tetany, 316

nèi shāng zá bìng 内伤杂病, internal damage miscellaneous diseases, 313

nèi shī 内湿, internal dampness, 314

nèi shū huáng lián tāng 内疏黄连汤, Internal Coursing Coptis Decoction, 187, 303, 315, 743

nèi sǔn 内损, internal injury, 316

nèi tíng 内庭, ST-44, Inner Court, 2, 4, 5, 8, 14, 15, 28–31, 63, 66, 70–73, 87, 89, 91, 109–112, 127, 129, 149, 158, 164, 168, 175, 186, 189, 190, 194, 197, 202, 203, 217, 239, 241, 276–284, 288, 290, 292, 294, 299, 302, 312, 314, 338, 342, 349, 358, 382, 386, 390, 395, 400, 414, 415, 426, 436, 437, 439, 442, 443, 448, 455, 499, 504, 515, 519, 520, 546, 547, 560, 564, 566, 567, 570, 577, 578, 580, 581, 585, 586, 588, 589, 601, 607, 611, 613, 614,

620, 621, 641, 652, 667, 686, 687, 693, 699, 700, 710, 715, 746

nèi tuō 内托, internal expression, 315

nèi xiàn 内陷, inward fall, 320

nèi xiāo 内消, internal dispersion, 315

nèi xiāo luǒ lì wán 内消瘰疬丸, Scrofula Internal Dispersion Pill, 141, 544, 737

nèi yīn 内因, internal cause [of disease], 312

nèi yíng xiāng 内迎香, Inner Welcome Fragrance, 586

nèi yōng 内痈, internal welling-abscess, 316

nèi zào 内燥, internal dryness, 315

nèi zhàng 内障, internal obstruction, 316

Nelumbinis Embryo, *lián zǐ xīn* 莲子心, lotus embryo, 263

Nelumbinis Folium, *hé yè* 荷叶, lotus leaf, 569

Nelumbinis Folium Recens, *xiān hé yè* 鲜荷叶, fresh lotus leaf, 625

Nelumbinis Fructus, *shí lián zǐ* 石莲子, lotus fruit, 82

Nelumbinis Fructus seu Semen, *lián zǐ* 莲子, lotus fruit/seed, 490, 518, 525, 600, 726, 727

Nelumbinis Receptaculum, *lián fáng* 莲房, lotus receptacle, 518, 727

Nelumbinis Rhizomatis Nodus, *ǒu jié* 藕节, lotus root node, 277, 714, 724

Nelumbinis Semen, *lián ròu* 莲肉, lotus seed, 12, 518, 727

Nelumbinis Stamen, *lián xū* 莲须, lotus stamen, 11, 308, 496, 518, 727

néng jìn qiè yuǎn 能近怯远, nearsightedness, 406

néng yuǎn qiè jìn 能远怯近, farsightedness, 195

neoplasm of the ear*
  benign, 166

nephritis*
  chronic, 334, 615, 616, 651, 707

nervous disorders*, 262

Network-Clearing Beverage, *qīng luò yǐn* 清络饮, 69, 730

Network-Quickening Efficacious Elixir, *huó luò xiào líng dān* 活络效灵丹, 737

Network-Quickening Elixir, *huó luò dān* 活络丹, 734

Network-Quickening Qi Flow Beverage, *huó luò liú qì yǐn* 活络流气饮, 249

neuralgia
  intercostal*, 58

neurasthenia sexualis*, 334

neuritis*
  multiple, 678
  optic, 586

neurodermatitis*, 154, 422, 516

neurological disease*, 616

neurosis*, 123, 261, 270, 272, 336
  gastric, 499, 580
  gastrointestinal, 483

Neutral Supplementing Heart-Settling Elixir, *píng bǔ zhèn xīn dān* 平补镇心丹, 230, 675

New Tangerine Peel and Bamboo Shavings Decoction, *xīn zhì jú pí zhú rú tāng* 新制橘皮竹茹汤, 72

Newly Supplemented Elsholtzia Beverage, *xīn jiā xiāng rú yǐn* 新加香薷饮, 591, 729

Newly Supplemented Yellow Dragon Decoction, *xīn jiā huáng lóng tāng* 新加黄龙汤, 732

nì 逆, counterflow, 102

nì 蜃, invisible worm, 319

nì chuán xīn bāo 逆传心包, abnormal passage to the pericardium, 3

nì chuāng 蜃疮, invisible worm sore, 319

nì jīng 逆经, counterflow menstruation, 102

nì liú wǎn zhōu 逆流挽舟, hauling the boat upstream, 258

nì tāi 腻苔, slimy tongue fur, 539

nì zhèng 逆证, unfavorable pattern (sign), 637

nì zhì 逆治, counteracting treatment, 102

niān tòng tāng 拈痛汤, Pain-Assuaging Decoction, 347

nián hàn 黏汗, sticky sweat, 572

niǎn zhēn 捻针, needle twirling, 408

niǎn zhuǎn bǔ xiè 捻转补泻, rotating supplementation and drainage, 508

niǎn zhuǎn bǔ xiè 捻转补泻, twirling supplementation and drainage, 634

niǎn zhuǎn fǎ 捻转法, twirling, 634

niào 尿, urine, 642

niào bì 尿闭, urinary block, 640

niào chì 尿赤, dark-colored urine, 118

niào chì 尿赤, reddish urine, 495

niào chuáng 尿床, bedwetting, 17

niào duō 尿多, copious urine, 99

niào duō 尿多, polyuria, 446

niào hòu yú lì 尿后余沥, dribble after voiding, 148

niào hòu yú lì 尿后余沥, post-voiding dribble, 458

niào huáng 尿黄, yellow urine, 705

niào jí 尿急, urinary urgency, 642

niào lái 小儿遗尿, child enuresis, 60

niào lái 尿来, child bedwetting, 60

niào pín 尿频, frequent urination, 229

niào shǎo 尿少, scant urine, 514

niào tòng 尿痛, painful urination, 424

niào xuè 尿血, blood in the urine, 32

niào xuè 尿血, bloody urine, 41

niào xuè 尿血, hematuria, 288

niào xuè 溺血, bloody urine, 41

niào zhuó 溺浊, urinary turbidity, 641

niē jǐ 捏脊, spine pinching, 550

niè chǐ 啮齿, bruxism, 51

niè chǐ 啮齿, grinding of the teeth, 249

niè chǐ 囓齿, grinding of the teeth, 249

niè rú 颞颥, temple, 605

Nine Immortals Elixir, *jiǔ xiān dān* 九仙丹, 743

Nine Immortals Powder, *jiǔ xiān sǎn* 九仙散, 96, 743

Nine Pains Pill, *jiǔ tòng wán* 九痛丸, 182, 735

Nine-Ingredient Center-Rectifying Decoction, *jiǔ wèi lǐ zhōng tāng* 九味理中汤, 83, 736

Nine-Ingredient Notopterygium Decoction, *jiǔ wèi qiāng huó tāng* 九味羌活汤, 119, 586, 681, 729

Nine-to-One Elixir, *jiǔ yī dān* 九一丹, 17, 187, 492, 528, 744

níng 凝, congealing, 93

níng xuè tāng 宁血汤, Blood-Quieting Decoction, 738

níng zhī yì 凝脂翳, congealed-fat screen, 93

niter, *xiāo shí* 硝石, Nitrum, 214, 383, 458, 544, 728

Niter and Alum Powder, *xiāo shí fán shí sǎn* 硝石矾石散, 21, 737

Nitrum, *xiāo shí* 硝石, niter, 214, 383, 458, 544, 728

Nitrum Dentatum, *yá xiāo* 牙硝, tooth niter, 411

niú bàng jiě jī tāng 牛蒡解肌汤, Arctium Flesh-Resolving Decoction, 187

niú bàng zǐ 牛蒡子 arctium, Arctii Fructus, 103, 184, 214, 368, 422, 459, 501, 548, 625, 685, 686, 720

niú dǎn 牛胆 ox's gallbladder, Bovis Vesica Fellea, 82

niú huáng 牛黄 bovine bezoar, Bovis Bezoar, 67, 98, 153, 458, 690, 721

niú huáng bào lóng wán 牛黄抱龙丸, Bovine Bezoar Dragon-Embracing Pill, 569, 591, 740

niú huáng qīng xīn wán 牛黄清心丸, Bovine Bezoar Heart-Clearing Pill, 88, 203, 264, 343, 538, 740

niú huáng shàng qīng wán 牛黄上清丸, Bovine Bezoar Upper-Body-Clearing Pill, 319

niú huáng wán 牛黄丸, Bovine Bezoar Pill, 624, 696

niú huáng xǐng xiāo wán 牛黄醒消丸, Bovine Bezoar Awake to Relief Pill, 743

niú huáng zhèn jīng wán 牛黄镇惊丸, Bovine Bezoar Fright-Settling Pill, 687

niú jiǎo sāi 牛角腮 ox horn bone, Bovis Cornus Os, 519, 569

niú pí xiǎn 牛皮癣, oxhide lichen, 422

niú pí xiǎn yào gāo 牛皮癣药膏, Oxhide Lichen Medicinal Paste, 674

niú xī 牛膝 achyranthes, Achyranthis Bidentatae Radix, 36, 45, 78, 138, 154, 328, 352, 390, 415, 485, 503, 548, 604, 614, 685, 724

niǔ shāng 扭伤, sprain, 567

niú gǔ suǐ 牛骨髓 beef marrow, Medulla Bovis, 45

No-Nursing-Worries Powder, *miǎn huái sǎn* 免怀散, 606

No.1 Lichen Medicinal Water, *yī hào xiǎn yào shuǐ* 一号癣药水, 710

nòng shé 弄舌, worrying tongue, 696

northern fangji, *hàn zhōng fáng jǐ* 汉中防己, Aristolochiae Heterophyllae Radix, 139, 154, 722

notoginseng, *sān qī* 三七, Notoginseng Radix, 34, 137, 139, 540, 569, 602, 629, 724

Notoginseng Radix, *sān qī* 三七, notoginseng, 34, 137, 139, 540, 569, 602, 629, 724

Notopterygii Rhizoma, *qiāng huó* 羌活, notopterygium, 11, 14, 22, 55, 102, 103, 116, 139, 154, 184, 191, 240, 247, 500–502, 546, 562, 654, 680, 681, 720

notopterygium, *qiāng huó* 羌活, Notopterygii Rhizoma, 11, 14, 22, 55, 102, 103, 116, 139, 154, 184, 191, 240, 247, 500–502, 546, 562, 654, 680, 681, 720

Notopterygium and Aconite Decoction, *qiāng huó fù zǐ tāng* 羌活附子汤, 506

Notopterygium and Isatis Root Decoction, *qiāng lán tāng* 羌蓝汤, 729

Notopterygium and Ledebouriella Decoction, *qiāng huó fáng fēng tāng* 羌活防风汤, 682

Notopterygium Dampness-Eliminating Decoction, *qiāng huó chú shī tāng* 羌活除湿汤, 734

Notopterygium Dampness-Overcoming Decoction, *qiāng huó shèng shī tāng* 羌活胜湿汤, 14, 79, 103, 114, 287, 530, 588, 680, 684, 734

Notopterygium Toxin-Vanquishing Decoction, *qiāng huó bài dú tāng* 羌活败毒汤, 682, 684

Notopterygium, Arctium, Dandelion, and Mint Decoction, *qiāng bàng pú bò tāng* 羌蒡蒲薄汤, 501

nǔ ròu 胬肉, excrescence, 181

nǔ ròu 胬肉, outcrop, 422

nǔ ròu pān jīng 胬肉攀睛, excrescence creeping over the eye, 181

nù 怒, anger, 9

nù qì shāng gan 怒气伤肝, anger damages the liver, 9

nù qì shāng gan 怒气伤肝, damage to the liver by anger, 108

nù shāng gān 怒伤肝, anger damages the liver, 9

nù shāng gān 怒伤肝, damage to the liver by anger, 108

nù zé qì shàng 怒则气上, anger causes qi to rise, 9

nǚ zhēn zǐ 女贞子 ligustrum, Ligustri Fructus, 88, 175, 336, 352, 467, 504, 526, 584, 593, 597, 612, 727

nǜ xuè 衄血, spontaneous external bleeding, 567

nuǎn gān 暖肝, warming the liver, 662

nuǎn gān jiān 暖肝煎, Liver-Warming Brew, 85, 355, 662, 711, 735

nuǎn qí gāo 暖脐膏, Navel-Warming Paste, 744

nuǎn wèi 暖胃, warming the stomach, 663

nüè jí 疟疾, malaria, 383

nüè mén 疟门, Malaria Gate, 8

nüè mǔ 疟母, mother-of-malaria, 399

nueroma cutis*, 632

nuò dào gēn xū 糯稻根须 glutinous rice root, Oryzae Glutinosae Rhizoma et Radix, 95, 410, 518, 727

nuò mǐ 糯米 glutinous rice, Oryzae Glutinosae Semen, 251

nutmeg, *ròu dòu kòu* 肉豆蔻, Myristicae Semen, 12, 80, 141, 316, 318, 454, 508, 518, 727

nutritional disturbance*, 261

nux vomica, *mǎ qián zǐ* 马钱子, Nux-Vomicae Semen, 97, 397, 728

Nux-Vomicae Semen, *mǎ qián zǐ* 马钱子, nux vomica, 97, 397, 728

obesity*, 297

obstruction*
  ascaris intestinal, 509

Obstruction-Abrading Spirit Light Paste, *mó zhàng líng guāng gāo* 磨障灵光高, 181, 403

Obstruction-Abrading Spirit Light Paste, *mó zhàng líng guāng gāo* 磨障灵光膏, 744

occipital bone*, 444

odor*
  hepatic, 53

Offensive Dispersion Harmonizing and Softening Decoction, *gōng xiāo hé jiě ruǎn jiān tāng* 攻消和解软坚汤, 737

oil beetle, *dì dǎn* 地胆, Meloë, 98

oily tangkuei, *yóu dāng guī* 油当归, Angelicae Sinensis Radix Pinguis, 399

Old Hermit Agastache/Patchouli Pill, *qí shòu huò xiāng wán* 奇授藿香丸, 121

Old Rice Granary Powder, *cāng lǐn sǎn* 仓廪散, 730

old scutellaria, *kū qín* 枯芩, Scutellariae Radix Veta, 690

old trachycarpus, *chén zōng pí* 陈棕皮, Trachycarpi Stipulae Fibra Veta, 53

Olibanum, *rǔ xiāng* 乳香, frankincense, 104, 137, 138, 503, 540, 574, 696, 724

Omphalia, *léi wán* 雷丸, omphalia, 183, 445, 724

omphalia, *léi wán* 雷丸, Omphalia, 183, 445, 724

On Blood Patterns (xuè zhèng lùn) 血证论, 1884 (Qīng), Táng Róng-Chuān 唐容川, 152, 181

On Cold Damage (shāng hán lùn) 伤寒论, Eastern Hàn, Zhāng Jī 张机 [Zhòng-Jīng 仲景], 9, 20, 25, 57, 78, 152, 157, 186, 242, 246, 247, 249, 254, 276, 279, 306, 322, 341, 344, 345, 383, 396, 412, 415, 427, 505, 506, 509, 510, 532, 534, 545, 567, 576, 583, 584, 628, 639, 652, 666, 680, 683, 692–694, 698

On Cold Damage and Miscellaneous Diseases (shāng hán zá bìng lùn) 伤寒杂病论, Eastern Hàn, Zhāng Jī 张机 [Zhòng-Jīng 仲景], 318, 658

On Pox Formulas (dòu zhěn fāng) 痘疹方论, 1518 (Míng), Cài Wéi-Fán 蔡维藩, 59

On Warm Epidemics (wēn yì lùn) 温疫论, 1642 (Míng), Wú Yǒu-Xìng 吴有性 [Yòu-Kě 又可], 276, 658

On Warm Epidemics Expanded (guǎng wēn yì lùn) 广温疫论, 1722 (Qīng), Dài Tiān-Zhāng 戴天章, 53, 349, 350

On Warm Heat (wēn rè lùn) 温热论, 1746, Qīng, Gù Jǐng-Wén 顾景文, 186, 279, 382, 581, 622, 659

One Dose Powder, *yī fú sǎn* 一服散, 743

One Zi Decoction, *yǐ zì tāng* 乙字汤, 718

One-Packet Red Bayberry Powder, *yáng méi yī jì sǎn* 杨梅一剂散, 494

ophicalcite, *huā ruǐ shí* 花蕊石, Ophicalcitum, 548, 724

Ophicalcite Powder, *huā ruǐ shí sǎn* 花蕊石散, 738

Ophicalcitum, *huā ruǐ shí* 花蕊石, ophicalcite, 548, 724

ophiopogon, *mài mén dōng* 麦门冬, Ophiopogonis Tuber, 47, 88, 95, 104, 108, 174–176, 227, 256, 259, 298, 310, 325, 358, 368, 394, 398, 399, 409, 416, 457, 467, 495, 508, 515, 526, 541, 565, 569, 577, 581, 589, 593, 597, 654, 679, 715, 727

Ophiopogon and Asparagus Decoction, *èr dōng tāng* 二冬汤, 348, 366, 640

Ophiopogon and Rehmannia Pill, *mài wèi dì huáng wán* 麦味地黄丸, 101, 163, 599, 715, 742

Ophiopogon Decoction, *mài mén dōng tāng* 麦门冬汤, 379, 581, 734

Ophiopogon Drink, *mài mén dōng yǐn zǐ* 麦门冬饮子, 447

Ophiopogonis Tuber, *mài mén dōng* 麦门冬, ophiopogon, 47, 88, 95, 104, 108, 174–176, 227, 256, 259, 298, 310, 325, 358, 368, 394, 398, 399, 409, 416, 457, 467, 495, 508, 515, 526, 541, 565, 569, 577, 581, 589, 593, 597, 654, 679, 715, 727

opisthotonos*, 10

optic atrophy*, 64

optic nerve*, 192

orchitis*, 399
  supperative, 671

Orient vine, *qīng fēng téng* 青风藤, Sinomenii seu Sabiae Caulis et Rhizoma, 139, 722

Orifice-Freeing Blood-Quickening Decoction, *tōng qiào huó xuè tāng* 通窍活血汤, 571, 738

orificium uteri*, 300

orificium vaginae*, 709

Origin and Indicators of Disease (zhū bìng yuán hòu lùn) 诸病源候论, 610 (Suí), Cháo Yuán-Fāng 巢元方, 6, 51, 122, 149, 150, 154, 178, 189, 298, 302, 311, 363, 367, 370, 412, 444, 451, 485, 497, 513, 526, 572, 583, 610, 632, 636, 641, 651, 658, 667, 677, 684, 692

Origin-Boosting Decoction, *yì yuán tāng* 益元汤, 735

Origin-Boosting Powder, *yì yuán sǎn* 益元散, 36, 179, 590, 713, 730

Origin-Lifting Brew, *jǔ yuán jiān* 举元煎, 199, 430, 487–489, 574, 740

Origin-Preserving Decoction, *bǎo yuán tāng* 保元汤, 58, 267, 272, 274, 566, 740

Origin-Regulating Kidney Qi Pill, *tiáo yuán shèn qì tāng* 调元肾气丸, 745

Origin-Restorative Blood-Quickening Decoction, *fù yuán huó xuè tāng* 复元活血汤, 45, 118, 138, 337, 737

Origin-Restoring Qi-Freeing Powder, *fù yuán tōng qì sǎn* 复元通气散, 316, 454

Origin-Securing Brew, *mì yuán jiān* 秘元煎, 180, 369, 525, 641, 743

Origin-Supporting Powder, *fú yuán sǎn* 扶元散, 638

orpiment, *cī huáng* 雌黄, Auripigmentum, 727

Orthodox External Medicine (wài kē zhèng zōng) 外科正宗, 1617 (Qīng), Chén Shí-Gōng 陈实功, 210, 670

Orthodox Tradition of Medicine (*yī xué zhèng zhuàn*) 医学正传, 1515 (Míng), Yú Tuán 虞抟, 231, 428, 672

Oryzae Fructus Germinatus, *gǔ yá* 谷芽, rice sprout, 23, 141, 420, 499, 563, 724

Oryzae Glutinosae Rhizoma et Radix, *nuò dào gēn xū* 糯稻根须, glutinous rice root, 95, 410, 518, 727

Oryzae Glutinosae Semen, *nuò mǐ* 糯米, glutinous rice, 251

osteochondritis*, 45

osteomyletis of the mandible*, 323

osteomylitis*
  pyogenic, 44

Ostreae Concha, *mǔ lì* 牡蛎, oyster shell, 11, 53, 54, 95, 176, 177, 183, 230, 308, 409, 433, 460, 461, 490, 495, 504, 511, 518, 524–526, 537, 544, 572, 585, 651, 696, 709, 726

Ostreae Concha Calcinata, *duàn mǔ lì* 煅牡蛎, calcined oyster shell, 57, 95, 176, 334, 636, 709

Ostreae Concha Cruda, *shēng mǔ lì* 生牡蛎, crude oyster shell, 54, 146, 225, 256, 726

otitis media*
  suppurative, 474

otolith, *yú nǎo shí* 鱼脑石, Pseudosciaenae Otolithum, 310, 405

otogenic vertigo*, 443

ǒu 呕, retching, 502

ǒu dǎn 呕胆, vomiting of bile, 657

ǒu jié 藕节 lotus root node, Nelumbinis Rhizomatis Nodus, 277, 714, 724

ǒu kǔ 呕苦, bitter vomiting, 20

ǒu tù 呕吐, vomiting (and retching), 657

ǒu tù kǔ shuǐ 呕吐苦水, vomiting of bitter water, 657

ǒu tù tán xián 呕吐痰涎, vomiting of phlegm-drool, 657

ǒu tù tán yǐn 呕吐痰饮, vomiting of phlegm-rheum, 657

ǒu tù wù 呕吐物, vomitus, 657

ǒu xuè 呕血, retching of blood, 502

ouch points, *ā shì xué* 阿是穴, 11, 39, 44, 53, 63, 70, 76, 80, 105, 113–115, 118, 142, 221, 260, 295, 327, 332, 370, 403, 422, 425, 442, 453, 484, 515, 567, 571, 585, 651, 662, 674, 676, 684, 688, 689, 696

ovate atractylodes, *bái zhú* 白术, Atractylodis Ovatae Rhizoma, 12, 17, 50, 84, 93, 116, 139, 141, 153, 154, 223, 224, 227, 240, 256, 257, 272, 315, 319, 390, 393, 450, 463, 486, 563, 564, 573, 574, 593–596, 600, 615, 661, 662, 684, 726

Ovate Atractylodes and Aconite Decoction, *bái zhú fù zǐ tāng* 白术附子汤, 342, 734

Ovate Atractylodes and Aconite Decoction, *zhú fù tāng* 术附汤, 80, 588, 733

Ovate Atractylodes Powder, *bái zhú sǎn* 白术散, 713, 733

oven earth, *fú lóng gān* 伏龙肝, Terra Flava Usta, 311, 556, 569, 573, 666, 724

Overdue Beverage, *guò qī yǐn* 过期饮, 35, 36, 737

ox horn bone, *niú jiǎo sāi* 牛角腮, Bovis Cornus Os, 519, 569

ox's gallbladder, *niú dǎn* 牛胆, Bovis Vesica Fellea, 82

Oxhide Lichen Medicinal Paste, *niú pí xiǎn yào gāo* 牛皮癣药膏, 674

oyster shell, *mǔ lì* 牡蛎, Ostreae Concha, 11, 53, 54, 95, 176, 177, 183, 230, 308, 409, 433, 460, 461, 490, 495, 504, 511, 518, 524–526, 537, 544, 572, 585, 651, 696, 709, 726

Oyster Shell and Alisma Powder, *mǔ lì zé xiè sǎn* 牡蛎泽泻散, 733

Oyster Shell Pill, *mǔ lì wán* 牡蛎丸, 177

Oyster Shell Powder, *mǔ lì sǎn* 牡蛎散, 11, 95, 595, 651, 742

pà fēng 怕风, fear of wind, 196

pà lěng 怕冷, fear of cold, 196

paddy field dermatitis*, 668

Paeoniae Radix, *sháo yào* 芍药, peony, 11, 72, 255, 319, 493, 500, 704

Paeoniae Radix Alba, *bái sháo yào* 白芍药, white peony, 17, 19, 28, 36, 37, 39, 95, 103, 116, 140, 154, 172, 175–177, 227, 246, 256, 259, 309, 310, 315, 352, 363, 390, 391, 397, 416, 425, 428, 495, 498, 502, 516, 537, 546, 548, 566, 567, 580, 588, 593, 613, 620, 661, 662, 674, 709, 713, 715, 727

Paeoniae Radix Alba Cruda, *shēng bái sháo yào* 生白芍药, raw white peony, 256

Paeoniae Radix Rubra, *chì sháo yào* 赤芍药, red peony, 17, 30, 34, 58, 67, 70, 116, 137, 139, 140, 150, 181, 227, 386, 390, 395, 430, 462, 463, 467, 497, 548, 679, 721

pái 排, expel, 181

pái biàn bù shuǎng 排便不爽, ungratifying defecation, 637

pái biàn kùn nán 排便困难, difficult defecation, 126

pái fēng sǎn 排风散, Wind-Expelling Powder, 689

pái nóng 排脓, expelling pus, 182

pái nóng tuō dú 排脓托毒, expelling pus and expressing toxin, 182

pái qì 排气, passing of flatus, 429

pái qì yǐn 排气饮, Qi-Discharging Beverage, 735

pái shí 排石, expelling stones, 182

pái shí tāng 排石汤, Stone-Expelling Decoction, 733

pái tuō 排托, expel, 181

pái zhēn 排针, needle extraction, 406

pái zhēn 排针, needle removal, 407

Pain and Diarrhea Formula, *tòng xiè yào fāng* 痛泻要方, 19, 256, 361, 479, 732

pain*
  wandering, 517

Pain-Assuaging Decoction, *niān tòng tāng* 拈痛汤, 347

Pain-Chasing Powder, *qū tòng sǎn* 趋痛散, 451

Pain-Relieving Paste, *dìng tòng gāo* 定痛膏, 744

Pain-Relieving Pill, *dìng tòng wán* 定痛丸, 733

Palace-Clearing Decoction, *qīng gōng tāng* 清宫汤, 71, 294, 693, 730

Palace-Opening Pill, *qǐ gōng wán* 启宫丸, 418

palsy*

  Bell's, 689

Panacis Quinquefolii Radix, *xī yáng shēn* 西洋参, American ginseng, 175, 593, 726

Pancreas-Clearing Formula No.1, *qīng yí yī hào* 清胰一号, 731

Pancreas-Clearing Formula No.2, *qīng yí èr hào* 清胰二号, 731

Pancreas-Enriching Beverage, *zī cuì yǐn* 滋膵饮, 369

pancreatitis*, 284

páng guāng 膀胱, bladder, 21

páng guāng bì 膀胱痹, bladder impediment, 22

páng guāng bìng 膀胱病, bladder disease, 22

páng guāng jīng 膀胱经, BL, 20

páng guāng jīng 膀胱经, bladder channel, 21

páng guāng ké 膀胱咳, bladder cough, 21

páng guāng qì bì 膀胱气闭, bladder qi block, 22

páng guāng qì huà bù lì 膀胱气化不利, inhibited bladder qi transformation, 301

páng guāng qì huà shī sī 膀胱气化失司, bladder qi transformation failure, 22

páng guāng shī rè 膀胱湿热, bladder damp-heat, 21

páng guāng shī rè niào xuè 膀胱湿热尿血, bladder damp-heat bloody urine, 21

páng guāng shū 膀胱俞, BL-28, Bladder Transport, 15, 21–23, 36, 68, 69, 82, 86, 91, 149, 177, 180, 229, 283, 301, 302, 308, 449, 465, 485, 529, 533, 541, 542, 582, 597, 604, 631, 636, 640, 641, 701, 747

páng guāng xū hán 膀胱虚寒, bladder vacuity cold, 23

páng guāng zhàng 膀胱胀, bladder distention, 22

páng guāng zhě, zhōu dū zhī guān, jīn yè cáng yān 膀胱者，州都之官，津液藏焉, bladder holds the office of the river island; it stores fluids, 22

páng guāng zhǔ cáng jīn yè 膀胱主藏津液, bladder governs fluid storage, 22

pàng dà hǎi 胖大海 sterculia, Sterculiae Semen, 291, 368

pàng dà hài 胖大海 sterculia, Sterculiae Semen, 624, 725

pangolin scales, *chuān shān jiǎ* 穿山甲, Manitis Squama, 34, 50, 137, 138, 182, 227, 315, 398, 419, 513, 516, 724

paniculate cynanchum, *xú cháng qīng* 徐长卿, Cynanchi Paniculati Herba cum Radice, 139, 722

pannus*

  trachomatous corneal, 195

Panting Stabilizer, *dìng chuǎn* 定喘, 83, 87, 142, 146, 202, 203, 228, 281, 285, 343, 379, 434, 441, 443, 489, 550, 596, 630, 648, 668, 683, 715

Panting, *chuǎn xī* 喘息, 439

Panting-Stabilizing Decoction, *dìng chuǎn tāng* 定喘汤, 146, 285, 736

Panting-Stabilizing Powder, *dìng chuǎn sǎn* 定喘散, 743

pāo bì 脬痹, bladder impediment, 22

pāo qì bù gù 脬气不固, insecurity of bladder qi, 307

páo 炮, blast-frying, 23

páo jiāng 炮姜 blast-fried ginger, Zingiberis Rhizoma Tostum, 26, 139, 199, 417, 431, 503, 556, 562, 564, 569, 660, 662, 723

páo shé 匏舌, gourd tongue, 244

páo zhì 炮制, processing, 464

páo zhì 炮制, processing of medicinals, 464

páo zhì 炮炙, processing, 464

páo zhì 炮炙, processing of medicinals, 464

Papaveris Pericarpium, *yīng sù ké* 罂粟壳, poppy husk, 12, 95, 318, 518, 727

Paper Plaster, *jiā zhǐ gāo* 夹纸膏, 744

papilloma*

  intracanalicular, 566

papular eczema*, 395

paracholera*, 77, 109

paralysis*

  hysterical, 678

  infantile, 541

  periodic, 678

paranasal sinusitis*, 543

parasite infestation*, 237

parasites, 695

paratyphoid*, 118

Paravertebrals, *jiā jí* 夹脊, 89

Paridis Rhizoma, *zǎo xiū* 蚤休, paris, 67, 721

paris, *zǎo xiū* 蚤休, Paridis Rhizoma, 67, 721

Pathfinder Poria (Hoelen) Pill, *zhǐ mí fú líng wán* 指迷茯苓丸, 14, 439, 441, 738

Pathoconditions, Causes, Pulses, and Treatments (*zhèng yīn mài zhì*) 症因脉治, 1641 (Míng), Qín Jīng-Míng 秦景明, 58, 313, 356, 372, 628, 704

Patriniae Heterophyllae Radix, *mù tóu huí* 墓头回, heterophyllous patrinia, 68, 721

PC-1, *tiān chí* 天池, Celestial Pool, 216, 220, 748

PC-2, *tiān quán* 天泉, Celestial Spring, 748

PC-3, *qū zé* 曲泽, Marsh at the Bend, 25, 30, 34, 65, 70, 99, 289, 455, 540, 589, 590, 637, 748

PC-4, *xī mén* 郄门, Cleft Gate, 29, 30, 58, 70, 89, 129, 265, 268, 294, 314, 343, 390, 416, 427, 440, 452, 522, 538, 566, 567, 570, 608, 629, 668, 675, 748

PC-5, *jiān shǐ* 间使, Intermediary Courier, 8, 19, 25, 71, 74, 82, 89, 113, 174, 197, 269, 282, 294, 317, 336, 378, 383, 386, 394, 396, 399, 416, 434, 439, 440, 442, 445, 482, 497, 521, 544, 572, 590, 604, 613, 624, 650, 664, 690, 694, 715, 748

PC-6, *nèi guān* 内关, Inner Pass, 1, 3, 4, 11, 17, 19, 20, 24, 25, 29, 31–33, 35, 39, 47, 53, 57, 58, 62–64, 69–74, 77, 80–83, 85–93, 103, 109, 111, 114, 117, 118, 123, 129, 138, 141, 145, 151, 153, 156–160, 178, 186, 189, 194, 201–203, 210–212, 215–218, 223–225, 227–230, 232–236, 241, 242, 247, 255–257, 260, 261, 263–269, 271–274, 276, 278, 280,

284, 287, 288, 294, 296, 297, 301, 302, 308, 314, 318, 333, 335, 336, 339, 343, 349, 353, 355, 356, 358, 359, 361, 362, 366, 379, 383–386, 390, 392–394, 401, 406, 408, 410, 413, 426, 427, 433–440, 442, 443, 445–449, 451–453, 455, 457, 462, 475, 477–485, 487, 488, 490, 493, 498, 499, 504, 510, 513, 522, 524, 526, 533, 537–540, 551, 552, 554, 555, 561, 562, 565, 569–572, 575, 577–581, 585–591, 597, 608, 613, 624, 629, 633, 638, 640, 646, 647, 649, 651, 652, 655, 658, 665, 666, 668, 669, 673, 675, 676, 685, 687, 690, 691, 699, 701, 703, 709, 713, 716, 748

PC-7, *dà líng* 大陵, Great Mound, 15, 25, 30, 43, 63, 70, 90, 99, 147, 155, 156, 244, 277, 282, 285, 288, 289, 330, 333, 356, 383, 386, 410, 413, 427, 434, 436, 467, 525, 538, 548, 552, 570, 587, 665, 688, 694, 716, 748

PC-8, *láo gōng* 劳宫, Palace of Toil, 31, 33, 40, 65, 69, 74, 88, 89, 118, 123, 147, 194, 202, 203, 241, 244, 261, 263, 264, 277, 281, 284, 289, 290, 294, 333, 343, 364, 386, 390, 392, 393, 400, 413, 420, 437, 440, 450, 452, 467, 483, 522, 537, 538, 552, 566, 567, 589, 590, 655, 656, 687, 690, 694, 714, 716, 748

PC-9, *zhōng chōng* 中冲, Central Hub, 25, 65, 73, 99, 147, 203, 218, 263, 281, 294, 384, 400, 408, 420, 427, 437, 442, 455, 485, 567, 589, 590, 631, 748

Peaceful Interaction Pill, *jiāo tài wán* 交泰丸, 413, 467, 538, 739

Peaceful Palace Bovine Bezoar Pill, *ān gōng niú huáng wán* 安宫牛黄丸, 6, 65, 69, 73, 88, 197, 202, 364, 426, 437, 450, 637, 693, 740

Peach Blossom Decoction, *táo huā tāng* 桃花汤, 174, 742

Peach Blossom Powder, *táo huā sǎn* 桃花散, 25, 330, 745

peach kernel, *táo rén* 桃仁, Persicae Semen, 20, 27, 34, 50, 59, 137–140, 182, 227, 356, 415, 428, 451, 512, 513, 571, 588, 679, 696, 724

Peach Kernel and Carthamus Brew, *táo rén hóng huā jiān* 桃仁红花煎, 269, 273, 484

Peach Kernel and Carthamus Four Agents Decoction, *táo hóng sì wù tāng* 桃红四物汤, 24, 34, 36, 37, 138, 316, 540, 608, 738

Peach Kernel Qi-Coordinating Decoction, *táo hé chéng qì tāng* 桃核承气汤, 24, 25, 36, 78, 182, 245, 316, 570, 571, 738

Peach Kernel Qi-Coordinating Decoction, *táo rén chéng qì tāng* 桃仁承气汤, 34, 738

Peanut Gruel, *luò huā shēng zhōu* 落花生粥, 420

pear peel, *lí pí* 梨皮, Pyri Exocarpium, 398

pearl, *zhēn zhū* 珍珠, Margarita, 54, 249, 490, 726

Pearl and Bezoar Powder, *zhū huáng sǎn* 珠黄散, 744

Pearl Powder, *zhēn zhū sǎn* 真珠散, 32

pectus carinatum*, 59

pectus gallinatum*, 59

péi 痦, miliaria, 395

péi tǔ 培土, banking up earth, 16

péi tǔ shēng jīn 培土生金, banking up earth to engender metal, 16

péi tǔ zhì shuǐ 培土制水, banking up earth to dam water, 16

pèi lán 佩兰 eupatorium, Eupatorii Herba, 7, 10, 66, 401, 434, 587, 588, 625, 722

pèi xué 配穴, point combination, 445

pelade*, 243

pemphigus*, 285

péng shā 硼砂 borax, Borax, 53, 291, 383, 728

pèng zhuàng sǔn shāng 碰撞损伤, impact injury, 295

peony, *sháo yào* 芍药, Paeoniae Radix, 11, 72, 255, 319, 493, 500, 704

Peony and Licorice Decoction, *sháo yào gān cǎo tāng* 芍药甘草汤, 415

Peony Decoction, *sháo yào tāng* 芍药汤, 110, 426, 731

pepper, *hú jiāo* 胡椒, Piperis Fructus, 94, 226, 660, 723

Perfect Major Supplementation Decoction, *shí quán dà bǔ tāng* 十全大补汤, 26, 27, 40, 198, 412, 449, 451, 453, 503, 528, 540, 599, 615, 649, 653, 661, 709, 741

perilla, *zǐ sū* 紫苏, Perillae Folium, Caulis et Calyx, 128, 256, 681, 720

Perilla Fruit Qi-Downbearing Decoction, *sū zǐ jiàng qì tāng* 苏子降气汤, 439, 477

perilla leaf, *zǐ sū yè* 紫苏叶, Perillae Folium, 82, 103, 107, 176, 184, 454, 500, 501, 502, 547, 577, 681, 720

perilla leaf, *zǐ sū* 紫苏, Perillae Folium, Caulis et Calyx, 449

Perilla Leaf Decoction, *sū yè tāng* 苏叶汤, 620

Perilla Leaf Fetus-Quieting Beverage, *zǐ sū ān tāi yǐn* 紫苏安胎饮, 736

perilla seed, *sū zǐ* 苏子, Perillae Semen, 625

perilla seed, *zǐ sū zǐ* 紫苏子, Perillae Fructus, 145, 146, 439, 624, 625, 703, 725

Perilla Seed and Apricot Seed Decoction, *sū zǐ xìng zǐ tāng* 苏子杏子汤, 372

Perilla Seed and Tingli Phlegm-Rolling Pill, *sū tíng gǔn tán wán* 苏葶滚痰丸, 441

Perilla Seed Qi-Downbearing Decoction, *sū zǐ jiàng qì tāng* 苏子降气汤, 145, 362, 477, 736

perilla stem, *zǐ sū gěng* 紫苏梗, Perillae Caulis, 19, 386, 540, 681, 720

Perillae Albae Cortex, *bái sū pí* 白苏皮, white perilla bark, 66

Perillae Albae Folium, *bái sū yè* 白苏叶, white perilla leaf, 47

Perillae Albae Semen, *bái sū zǐ* 白苏子, white perilla seed, 17, 64, 145

Perillae Caulis, *zǐ sū gěng* 紫苏梗, perilla stem, 19, 386, 540, 681, 720

Perillae Folium, *zǐ sū yè* 紫苏叶, perilla, 502

Perillae Folium, *zǐ sū yè* 紫苏叶, perilla leaf, 82, 103, 107, 176, 184, 454, 500, 501, 547, 577, 681, 720

Perillae Folium, Caulis et Calyx, *zǐ sū* 紫苏, perilla, 128, 256, 681, 720

Perillae Folium, Caulis et Calyx, *zǐ sū* 紫苏, perilla leaf, 449

Perillae Fructus, *zǐ sū zǐ* 紫苏子, perilla seed, 145, 146, 439, 624, 625, 703, 725

Perillae Semen, *sū zǐ* 苏子, perilla seed, 625

periodic paralysis*, 678

periodontitis*, 239

peritonitis*
   tubercular, 150

Persicae Semen, *táo rén* 桃仁, peach kernel, 20, 27, 34, 50, 59, 137–140, 182, 227, 356, 415, 428, 451, 512, 513, 571, 588, 679, 696, 724

persimmon calyx, *shì dì* 柿蒂, Kaki Calyx, 493, 499, 649, 724

Persimmon Decoction, *shì dì tāng* 柿蒂汤, 736

persimmon frost, *shì shuāng* 柿霜, Kaki Saccharum, 231

Perspiration-Checking Powder, *zhǐ hàn sǎn* 止汗散, 454, 742

pertussis*, 677

Peucedani Radix, *qián hú* 前胡, peucedanum, 5, 47, 64, 624, 625, 686, 688, 725

peucedanum, *qián hú* 前胡, Peucedani Radix, 5, 47, 64, 624, 625, 686, 688, 725

Phalacrocoracis Saliva, *lú sī xián* 鸬鹚涎, cormorant's drool, 677

Pharbitidis Semen, *qiān niú zǐ* 牵牛子, morning glory, 98, 171, 182, 215, 411, 438, 445, 460, 666, 722

pharyngitis*
   chronic, 714, 715
   membranous, 611

pharynx*
   laryngeal part of, 340
   oral part of, 432

Phaseoli Aurei Semen, *lǜ dòu* 绿豆, mung bean, 463, 527

Phaseoli Aurei Testa, *lǜ dòu pí* 绿豆皮, mung bean seed-coat, 68, 95, 721

Phaseoli Calcarati Semen, *chì xiǎo dòu* 赤小豆, rice bean, 40, 136, 164, 666, 671, 723

Phellodendri Cortex, *huáng bǎi* 黄柏, phellodendron, 17, 66, 67, 69, 70, 81, 94, 104, 106, 116, 127, 153, 154, 176, 281, 282, 319, 338, 352, 357, 397, 424, 449, 456, 514, 527, 604, 649, 679, 704, 712, 713, 720

Phellodendri Cortex Carbonisatus, *huáng bǎi tàn* 黄柏炭, charred phellodendron, 546

Phellodendri Cortex Pulveratus, *huáng bǎi mò* 黄柏末, powdered phellodendron, 330, 331

phellodendron, *huáng bǎi* 黄柏, Phellodendri Cortex, 17, 66, 67, 69, 70, 81, 94, 104, 106, 116, 127, 153, 154, 176, 281, 282, 319, 338, 352, 357, 397, 424, 449, 456, 514, 527, 604, 649, 679, 704, 712, 713, 720

phlebangioma*, 534, 632

Phlegm Depression Decoction, *tán yù tāng* 痰郁汤, 435

Phlegm-Abducting Decoction, *dǎo tán tāng* 导痰汤, 81, 88, 192, 203, 433–435, 438, 439, 441, 442, 638, 673, 690, 738

Phlegm-Expelling Pill, *qū tán wán* 祛痰丸, 612

Phlegm-Flushing Decoction, *dí tán tāng* 涤痰汤, 93, 740

Phlegm-Rheum Pill, *tán yǐn wán* 痰饮丸, 224, 663, 739

Phlegm-Rolling Pill, *gǔn tán wán* 滚痰丸, 115, 436, 439, 565, 638, 673, 738

phoenix-tail fern, *fèng wěi cǎo* 凤尾草, Pteridis Multifidi Herba, 68, 69, 721

phosphaturia*, 641

phragmites, *lú gēn* 芦根, Phragmititis Rhizoma, 64, 67, 69, 70, 358, 577, 720

Phragmites Stem Decoction, *wěi jīng tāng* 苇茎汤, 743

Phragmititis Rhizoma, *lú gēn* 芦根, phragmites, 64, 67, 69, 70, 358, 577, 720

Phragmititis Rhizoma Recens, *xiān lú gēn* 鲜芦根, fresh phragmites, 67, 282, 720

Physalis Alkekengi Calyx, *guà jīn dēng* 挂金灯, lantern plant calyx, 68, 721

Physalis Alkekengi Herba, *suān jiāng* 酸浆, lantern plant, 68, 721

physochlaina, *huá shān shēn* 华山参, Physochlainae Radix, 624, 725

Physochlainae Radix, *huá shān shēn* 华山参, physochlaina, 624, 725

phytolacca, *shāng lù* 商陆, Phytolaccae Radix, 460, 574, 722

Phytolaccae Radix, *shāng lù* 商陆, phytolacca, 460, 574, 722

pī shí 砒石 arsenic, Arsenicum, 98, 727

pī shuāng 砒霜 sublimed arsenic, Arsenicum Sublimatum, 411

pī zǎo sǎn 砒枣散, Arsenic and Jujube Powder, 744

pí 脾, SP, 549

pí 脾, spleen, 552

pí 脾, splenic, 565

pí 皮, cutaneous, 106

pí 皮, skin, 535

pí bì 脾痹, spleen impediment, 558

pí bì 皮痹, skin impediment, 535

pí bìng 脾病, spleen disease, 555

pí bù 皮部, cutaneous region, 106

pí bù tǒng xuè 脾不统血, blood management failure, 32

pí bù tǒng xuè 脾不统血, spleen failing to manage the blood, 556

pí bù tǒng xuè 脾不统血, splenic blood management failure, 565

pí cáng yì 脾藏意, spleen stores reflection, 561

pí cáng yíng 脾藏营, spleen stores construction, 561

pí chóng bìng 脾虫病, spleen worm disease, 564

pí dān 脾瘅, splenic pure heat, 565

pí fèi liǎng xū 脾肺两虚, dual vacuity of the spleen and lung, 163

pí fèi qì xū 脾肺气虚, spleen-lung qi vacuity, 560

pí fū 皮肤, cutaneous, 106

pí fū 皮肤, skin, 535

pí fū má mù 皮肤麻木, numbness and tingling of the skin, 416

pí fū zhēn 皮肤针, cutaneous needle, 106

pí gān 脾疳, gan of the spleen, 238

pí gān 脾疳, spleen gan, 557

pí hé wèi 脾合胃, spleen is connected with the stomach, 558

pí jī 脾积, spleen accumulation, 554

pí jīng 脾经, spleen channel, 554

pí jīng ké sòu 脾经咳嗽, spleen channel cough, 554

pí juàn 疲倦, fatigue, 195

pí kāi qiào yú kǒu 脾开窍于口, spleen opens at the mouth, 560

pí ké 脾咳, spleen cough, 554

pí láo 脾劳, spleen taxation, 561

pí mài huǎn 脾脉缓, spleen pulse is moderate, 560

pí máo 皮毛, skin and [body] hair, 535

pí máo wěi 皮毛痿, skin and [body] hair wilting, 535

pí nèi zhēn 皮内针, intradermal needle, 319

pí pá qīng fèi yǐn 枇杷清肺饮, Loquat Leaf Lung-Clearing Beverage, 5

pí pá yè 枇杷叶 loquat leaf, Eriobotryae Folium, 65, 95, 387, 480, 624, 669, 725

pí qì 脾气, spleen qi, 560

pí qì bù shēng 脾气不升, nonupbearing of spleen qi, 413

pí qì bù shū 脾气不舒, constrained spleen qi, 95

pí qì bù zú 脾气不足, insufficiency of spleen qi, 310

pí qì tōng yú kǒu 脾气通于口, spleen qi flows to the mouth, 560

pí qì xià xiàn 脾气下陷, spleen qi fall, 560

pí qì xū 脾气虚, spleen qi vacuity, 560

pí qì xū ruò 脾气虚弱, spleen qi vacuity, 560

pí qì zhǔ shēng 脾气主升, spleen qi governs upbearing, 560

pí rè 脾热, spleen heat, 558

pí rè duō xián 脾热多涎, spleen heat copious drool, 558

pí sè cāng huáng 皮色苍黄, somber yellow skin, 545

pí shèn shuāng bǔ wán 脾肾双补丸, Spleen-Kidney Supplementation Pill, 742

pí shèn yáng xū 脾肾阳虚, spleen-kidney yang vacuity, 559

pí shī gān yù 脾湿肝郁, spleen dampness and liver depression, 554

pí shī jiàn yùn 脾失健运, impairment of splenic movement and transformation, 295

pí shī jiàn yùn 脾失健运, spleen failing to move and transform, 557

pí shī jiàn yùn 脾失健运, splenic movement and transformation failure, 565

pí shū 脾俞, BL-20, Spleen Transport, 1, 3–5, 15, 26–29, 32, 33, 36–41, 47, 55, 58, 59, 61–64, 66, 73, 78–81, 83, 84, 86, 91, 94, 97, 109, 115, 117–119, 127, 128, 145, 149–151, 156, 159–164, 174, 175, 177, 183, 196, 197, 199, 210–212, 215–217, 223, 224, 227, 228, 234, 235, 237, 240, 251, 256, 257, 261, 265, 267–272, 274, 278, 282, 288, 291, 296, 301, 308–310, 312, 314, 316, 318–320, 325, 332–335, 339, 340, 349, 352, 359, 361, 365, 366, 370, 378, 379, 384, 390, 393, 395, 399–401, 410, 415, 416, 418, 425–427, 434–436, 441, 443, 445, 447, 449–458, 461, 465, 477, 484–487, 489, 490, 493, 497–499, 503, 513, 514, 516, 524, 525, 529, 534, 537, 547, 549–551, 554, 555, 557–559, 561–566, 575, 578, 579, 581, 586, 589, 594–597, 600, 603, 604, 607, 608, 613, 620, 636, 639–641, 645–647, 650, 652, 654, 661–663, 666–669, 673, 675, 677–679, 685, 694–696, 702, 703, 710, 711, 713, 714, 716, 747

pí shuǐ 脾水, spleen water, 564

pí shuǐ 皮水, skin water, 536

pí tǒng xuè 脾统血, spleen manages the blood, 559

pí tǔ 脾土, spleen-earth, 556

pí tǔ yì mù 培土抑木, banking up earth and repressing wood, 16

pí wéi hòu tiān zhī běn 脾为后天之本, spleen is the root of later heaven, 559

pí wéi shēng huà qì xuè zhī yuán 脾为生化气血之源, spleen is the source of qi and blood formation, 559

pí wéi shēng huà zhī yuán 脾为生化之源, spleen is the source of engendering transformation, 559

pí wéi shēng tán zhī yuán 脾为生痰之源, spleen is the source of phlegm formation, 559

pí wéi xián 脾为涎, spleen forms drool, 557

pí wěi 脾痿, spleen wilting, 564

pí wèi bù hé 脾胃不和, spleen-stomach disharmony, 561

pí wèi qì xū 脾胃气虚, spleen-stomach qi vacuity, 561

pí wèi shī rè 脾胃湿热, spleen-stomach damp-heat, 560

pí wèi xū hán 脾胃虚寒, spleen-stomach vacuity cold, 561

pí wèi xū hán wèi wǎn (guǎn) tòng 脾胃虚寒胃脘痛, spleen-stomach vacuity cold stomach duct pain, 561

pí wèi xū ruò 脾胃虚弱, spleen-stomach vacuity, 561

pí wèi yáng xū 脾胃阳虚, spleen-stomach yang vacuity, 561

pí wèi yīn xū 脾胃阴虚, spleen-stomach yin vacuity, 561

pí wèi zhě, cāng lǐn zhī gān, wǔ wèi chū yān 脾胃者，仓廪之官，五味出焉, spleen and stomach hold the office of the granaries, whence the five flavors emanate, 554 *pí wù shī* 脾恶湿, spleen is averse to dampness, 558

pí xiāo 脾消, spleen dispersion, 556

pí xiāo 脾消, splenic dispersion, 565

pí xiè 脾泄, spleen diarrhea, 555

pí xiè 脾泻, spleen diarrhea, 555

pí xū 脾虚, spleen vacuity, 561

pí xū dài xià 脾虚带下, spleen vacuity vaginal discharge, 563

pí xū duō xián 脾虚多涎, spleen vacuity copious drool, 562

pí xū fèi ruò 脾虚肺弱, spleen-lung vacuity, 559

pí xū fù zhàng 脾虚腹胀, spleen vacuity abdominal distention, 562

pí xū hán 脾虚寒, spleen vacuity cold, 562

pí xū huáng 脾虚发黄, spleen vacuity yellowing, 564

pí xū jiā shí 脾虚夹食, spleen vacuity with food damage, 563

pí xū jīng bì 脾虚经闭, spleen vacuity menstrual block, 562

pí xū jiǔ sòu 脾虚久嗽, spleen vacuity enduring cough, 562

pí xū ǒu tù 脾虚呕吐, spleen vacuity vomiting, 563

pí xū qì zhì 脾虚气滞, spleen vacuity qi stagnation, 563

pí xū rú qiú 脾虚如球, spleen vacuous as a ball, 564

pí xū shēng fēng 脾虚生风, spleen vacuity engendering wind, 562

pí xū shī kùn 脾虚湿困, spleen vacuity with damp encumbrance, 563

pí xū xiè xiè 脾虚泄泻, spleen vacuity diarrhea, 562

pí xū zì hàn 脾虚自汗, spleen vacuity spontaneous sweating, 563

pí yáng 脾阳, spleen yang, 564

pí yáng bù zhèn 脾阳不振, devitalized spleen yang, 125

pí yáng xū 脾阳虚, spleen yang vacuity, 564

pí yīn 脾阴, spleen yin, 564

pí yīn xū 脾阴虚, spleen yin vacuity, 564

pí yǔ wèi xiāng biǎo lǐ 脾与胃相表里, spleen and stomach stand in interior-exterior relationship, 554

pí yuē 脾约, straitened spleen, 583

pí yuē má rén wán 脾约麻仁丸, Straitened Spleen Hemp Seed Pill, 289

pí zhàng 脾胀, spleen distention, 556

pí zhī dà luò 脾之大络, great network vessel of the spleen, 248

pí zhǔ hòu tiān 脾主后天, spleen governs later heaven, 557

pí zhǔ jī ròu 脾主肌肉, spleen governs the flesh, 558

pí zhǔ jī ròu, sì zhī 脾主肌肉、四肢, spleen governs the flesh and limbs, 558

pí zhǔ kǒu 脾主口, spleen governs the mouth, 558

pí zhǔ shēng qīng 脾主升清, spleen governs upbearing of the clear, 558

pí zhǔ sì zhī 脾主四肢, spleen governs the four limbs, 558

pí zhǔ wèi wèi xíng qí jīn yè 脾主为胃行其津液, spleen governs movement of stomach liquid, 558

pí zhǔ yùn huà 脾主运化, spleen governs movement and transformation, 557

pí zhǔ zhōng tǔ 脾主中土, spleen governs center-earth, 557

pí zhǔ zhōng zhōu 脾主中州, spleen governs the central region, 558

pí, qí huá zài chún sì bái 脾，其华在唇四白, spleen, its bloom is in the four whites of the lips, 559

pǐ 痞, glomus, 242

pǐ gēn 痞根, Glomus Root, 24, 26, 34, 138, 215, 384, 399, 544, 695

pǐ kuài 痞块, glomus lump, 242

pǐ qì 痞气, glomus qi, 242

pǐ qì wán 痞气丸, Glomus Qi Pill, 242

pǐ sè 痞塞, glomus blockage, 242

pì 癖, aggregation, 7

pì 僻, pi, 444

pì náng 澼囊, afflux pouch, 7

piān fēng 偏风, hemilateral wind, 289

piān jù 偏沮, hemilateral sweating, 288

piān kū 偏枯, hemilateral withering, 289

piān lì 偏历, LI-6, Veering Passageway, 90, 182, 301, 408, 601, 613, 703, 716, 746

piān shèng 偏胜, surfeit, 598

piān shí 偏食, partiality for certain foods, 428

piān shì yóu nì hòu wèi 偏嗜油腻厚味, predilection for greasy and rich foods, 460

piān shuāi 偏衰, deficit, 121

piān tóu fēng 偏头风, hemilateral head wind, 288

piān tóu tòng 偏头痛, hemilateral headache, 288

piān zhuì 偏坠, hemilateral sagging, 288

piān zhuì 偏坠, sagging of one testicle, 511

pián zhī 胼胝, callus, 53

piàn 片, tablet, 602

piàn jì 片剂, tablet preparation, 602

piāo 漂, long rinsing, 367

picrorhiza, *hú huáng lián* 胡黄连, Picrorhizae Rhizoma, 68, 391, 722

Picrorhiza and Mume Roundworm-Quieting Decoction, *lián méi ān huí tāng* 连梅安蛔汤, 737

Picrorhizae Rhizoma, *hú huáng lián* 胡黄连, picrorhiza, 68, 391, 722

pig's bile, *zhū dǎn zhī* 猪胆汁, Suis Bilis, 624, 725

Pig's Intestine Pill, *zhū zàng wán* 猪脏丸, 738

Pig's Intestines and Coptis Pill, *zàng lián wán* 脏连丸, 143, 290, 656, 738

pig's liver, *zhū gān* 猪肝, Suis Iecur, 291

pig's spine marrow, *zhū jǐ suǐ* 猪脊髓, Suis Spinae Medulla, 64, 333

Pig's Stomach Pill, *zhū dǔ wán* 猪肚丸, 122, 743

pig's thyroid gland, *zhū yè* 猪靥, Suis Glandula Thyroidea, 30, 243

pigmentary degeneration of retina*, 291, 549

Pillow Elixir, *zhěn zhōng dān* 枕中丹, 739

pìn nüè 牝疟, female malaria, 197

pinellia, *bàn xià* 半夏, Pinelliae Tuber, 20, 63, 66, 84, 93, 98, 136, 141, 146, 153, 157, 230, 255–257, 259, 287, 343, 367, 372, 418, 434, 457, 527, 538, 572, 577, 578, 596, 623, 625, 683, 725

Pinellia and Broomcorn Millet Decoction, *bàn xià shú mǐ tāng* 半夏秫米汤, 739

Pinellia and Dried Ginger Powder, *bàn xià gān jiāng sǎn* 半夏干姜散, 156

Pinellia and Magnolia Bark Decoction, *bàn xià hòu pò tāng* 半夏厚朴汤, 19, 123, 735

Pinellia and Poria (Hoelen) Decoction, *bàn xià fú líng tāng* 半夏茯苓汤, 738

Pinellia and Scutellaria Pill, *bàn huáng wán* 半黄丸, 280, 438

Pinellia and Sulfur Pill, *bàn liú wán* 半硫丸, 78, 338, 731

Pinellia Decoction, *bàn xià tāng* 半夏汤, 739

Pinellia Heart-Draining Decoction, *bàn xià xiè xīn tāng* 半夏泻心汤, 242, 257, 732

pinellia leaven, *bàn xià qū* 半夏麴, Pinelliae Massa Fermentata, 201, 388

Pinellia, Ovate Atractylodes, and Gastrodia Decoction, *bàn xià bái zhú tiān má tāng* 半夏白术天麻汤, 98, 115, 287, 440, 691, 739

Pinelliae Massa Fermentata, *bàn xià qū* 半夏麴, pinellia leaven, 201, 388

Pinelliae Tuber, *bàn xià* 半夏, pinellia, 20, 63, 66, 84, 93, 98, 136, 141, 146, 153, 157, 230, 255–257, 259, 287, 343, 367, 372, 418, 434, 457, 527, 538, 572, 577, 578, 596, 623, 625, 683, 725

Pinelliae Tuber Crudum, *shēng bàn xià* 生半夏, raw pinellia, 243, 464

Pinelliae Tuber cum Zingibere Praeparatum, *jiāng bàn xià* 姜半夏, ginger pinellia, 47, 97, 257, 317, 421, 623, 725

Pinelliae Tuber Pro Formula Praeparatum, *fǎ bàn xià* 法半夏, pro formula pinellia, 625

píng 平, calm, 53

píng bǔ píng xiè 平补平泻, even supplementation and drainage, 180

píng bǔ píng xiè 平补平泻, neutral supplementation and drainage, 409

píng bǔ zhèn xīn dān 平补镇心丹, Neutral Supplementing Heart-Settling Elixir, 230, 675

píng chén tāng 平陈汤, Calming Matured Ingredients Decoction, 738

píng chuǎn 平喘, calming panting, 53

píng dàn 平旦, calm dawn, 53

píng gān qián yáng 平肝潜阳, calming the liver and subduing yang, 54

píng gān xī fēng 平肝熄风, calming the liver and extinguishing wind, 53

píng gān zhǐ tòng 平肝止痛, calming the liver and relieving pain, 54

píng wèi sǎn 平胃散, Stomach-Calming Powder, 19, 109, 114, 153, 154, 197, 216, 218, 257, 384, 395, 418, 435, 498, 539, 563, 633, 665, 732

píng xī 平息, calm breathing, 53

píng xī nèi fēng 平熄内风, calming and extinguishing internal wind, 53

píng yì 屏翳, perineum, 430

Pini Lignum Nodi, *sōng jié* 松节, knotty pine wood, 139, 722

Pini Resina, *sōng xiāng* 松香, rosin, 728

Piperis Fructus, *hú jiāo* 胡椒, pepper, 94, 226, 660, 723

Piperis Fructus Albicatus, *bái hú jiāo* 白胡椒, white pepper, 402

Piperis Kadsurae Caulis, *hǎi fēng téng* 海风藤, kadsura pepper stem, 139, 722

Piperis Longi Fructus, *bì bá* 荜茇, long pepper, 660, 723

Piscis Vesica Aeris, *yú biào* 鱼鳔, swim bladder, 333

pityriasis of the face*, 41

pityriasis rosea*, 688

pityriasis versicolor*, 473

Pivot of External Medicine (wài kē shū yào) 外科枢要, 1571 (Míng), Xuē Jǐ 薛己 [Lì-Zhāi 立斋], 46

placenta, *zǐ hé chē* 紫河车, Hominis Placenta, 222, 298, 310, 511, 593, 726

Placenta Great Creation Pill, *hé chē dà zào wán* 河车大造丸, 310, 379, 715

Placenta Pill, *hé chē wán* 河车丸, 178

Plantaginis Herba, *chē qián* 车前, plantago, 21, 69, 136, 463, 503, 723

Plantaginis Semen, *chē qián zǐ* 车前子, plantago seed, 36, 69, 116, 136, 229, 497, 666, 696, 723

plantago, *chē qián* 车前, Plantaginis Herba, 21, 69, 136, 463, 503, 723

plantago seed, *chē qián zǐ* 车前子, Plantaginis Semen, 36, 69, 116, 136, 229, 497, 666, 696, 723

platycodon, *jié gěng* 桔梗, Platycodonis Radix, 5, 47, 56, 128, 129, 175, 199, 227, 315, 338, 368, 388, 392, 394, 414, 422, 546, 549, 624, 625, 671, 695, 703, 725

Platycodon Decoction, *jié gěng tāng* 桔梗汤, 261, 469, 738

Platycodonis Radix, *jié gěng* 桔梗, platycodon, 5, 47, 56, 128, 129, 175, 199, 227, 315, 338, 368, 388, 392, 394, 414, 422, 546, 549, 624, 625, 671, 695, 703, 725

Pleioblasti Folium, *kǔ zhú yè* 苦竹叶, bitter bamboo leaf, 259, 430

pleurisy*, 58

pneumonia, 372

pneumonia*, 58, 280, 438

pò 魄, animal soul, 9

pò 魄, corporeal soul, 100

pò 迫, distress, 143

pò hàn 魄汗, corporeal soul sweating, 100

pò hù 魄户, BL-42, Po Door, 747

pò jiǒng (jùn) tuō ròu 破䐃脱肉, loss of bulk and shedding of flesh, 367

pò mén 魄门, corporeal soul gate, 100

pò qì 破气, breaking qi, 50

pò shāng fēng 破伤风, lockjaw, 366

pò shāng fēng 破伤风, tetanus, 606

pò xiāo 朴硝 impure mirabilite, Mirabilitum Non-Purum, 310

pò xiāo 朴硝 impure mirabilite, Mirabilitum Non-Purum, 44, 411, 460, 712, 722

pò xuè 破血, breaking blood, 50

pò yū xiāo zhēng 破瘀消癥, breaking stasis and dispersing concretions, 50

pomegranate rind, *shí liú pí* 石榴皮, Granati Pericarpium, 183, 298, 318, 445, 518, 727

poliomyelitis*, 60, 678

polygala, *yuǎn zhì* 远志, Polygalae Radix, 20, 60, 222, 331, 392, 433, 476, 490, 540, 557, 654, 709, 726

Polygala Pill, *yuǎn zhì wán* 远志丸, 739

Polygalae Radix, *yuǎn zhì* 远志, polygala, 20, 60, 222, 331, 392, 433, 476, 490, 540, 557, 654, 709, 726

Polygonati Huangjing Rhizoma, *huáng jīng* 黄精, polygonatum, 593, 727

Polygonati Yuzhu Rhizoma, *yù zhú* 玉竹, Solomon's seal, 88, 108, 175, 176, 581, 593, 597, 727

polygonatum, *huáng jīng* 黄精, Polygonati Huangjing Rhizoma, 593, 727

Polygoni Avicularis Herba, *biǎn xù* 萹蓄, knotgrass, 21, 69, 136, 723

Polygoni Bistortae Rhizoma, *quán shēn* 拳参, bistort, 68, 721

Polygoni Cuspidati Rhizoma, *hǔ zhàng* 虎杖, bushy knotweed, 136, 138, 357, 540, 723, 724

Polygoni Multiflori Caulis, *yè jiāo téng* 夜交藤, flowery knotweed stem, 490, 537, 593, 726, 727

Polygoni Multiflori Radix, *hé shǒu wū* 何首乌, flowery knotweed, 28, 37, 127, 172, 175, 245, 309, 336, 352, 467, 593, 595, 727

Polygoni Multiflori Radix Praeparatum, *zhì hé shǒu wū* 制何首乌, processed flowery knotweed, 604

Polygoni Multiflori Radix Recens, *xiān shǒu wū* 鲜首乌, fresh flowery knotweed, 399

polyneuritis*, 678

Polyporus, *zhū líng* 猪苓, polyporus, 21, 136, 153, 224, 230, 390, 410, 434, 666, 723

polyporus, *zhū líng* 猪苓, Polyporus, 21, 136, 153, 224, 230, 390, 410, 434, 666, 723

Polyporus Decoction, *zhū líng tāng* 猪苓汤, 176, 467, 541, 733

Polyporus Pill, *zhū líng wán* 猪苓丸, 434

Polyporus Powder, *zhū líng sǎn* 猪苓散, 239

polyps*, 378

polyuria*, 99

poppy husk, *yīng sù ké* 罂粟壳, Papaveris Pericarpium, 12, 95, 318, 518, 727

Poria, *fú líng* 茯苓, poria, 17, 47, 66, 84, 93, 136, 141, 157, 223, 224, 234, 236, 256, 257, 315, 401, 418, 428, 434, 454, 456, 457, 486, 499, 563, 587, 594, 596, 600, 620, 649, 661, 662, 666, 675, 679, 703, 723

poria, *fú líng* 茯苓, Poria, 17, 47, 66, 84, 93, 136, 141, 157, 223, 224, 234, 236, 256, 257, 315, 401, 418, 428, 434, 454, 456, 457, 486, 499, 563, 587, 594, 596, 600, 620, 649, 661, 662, 666, 675, 679, 703, 723

Poria (Hoelen) and Cuscuta Elixir, *fú tù dān* 茯菟丹, 742

Poria (Hoelen) and Licorice Decoction, *fú líng gān cǎo tāng* 茯苓甘草汤, 733

Poria (Hoelen) Counterflow Cold Decoction, *fú líng sì nì tāng* 茯苓四逆汤, 735

Poria (Hoelen) Decoction, *fú líng tāng* 茯苓汤, 82

Poria (Hoelen) Five Powder, *wǔ líng sǎn* 五苓散, 79, 110, 117, 136, 151, 170, 179, 224, 232, 245, 348, 400, 541, 588, 600, 647, 663, 666–669, 694, 716, 733

Poria (Hoelen) Four Powder, *sì líng sǎn* 四苓散, 640, 663, 733

Poria (Hoelen) Skin Decoction, *fú líng pí tāng* 茯苓皮汤, 733

Poria (Hoelen), Cinnamon Twig, Licorice, and Jujube Decoction, *fú líng guì zhī gān cǎo dà zào tāng* 茯苓桂枝甘草大枣汤, 510

Poria (Hoelen), Cinnamon Twig, Ovate Atractylodes, and Licorice Decoction, *líng guì zhú gān tāng* 苓桂术甘汤, 87, 230, 269, 440, 441, 443, 537, 608, 661, 664, 667, 733

Poria (Hoelen), Licorice, Schisandra, Ginger, and Asarum Decoction, *líng gān wǔ wèi jiāng xīn tāng* 苓甘五味姜辛汤, 84, 380, 663, 738

Poria Alba, *bái fú líng* 白茯苓, white poria, 141, 394

Poria cum Cortice, *lián pí fú líng* 连皮茯苓, poria with skin, 228

Poria cum Pini Radice, *fú shén* 茯神, root poria, 60, 122, 256, 262, 392, 490, 654, 726

Poria cum Pini Radice et Cinnabare, *zhū fú shén* 朱茯神, cinnabar root poria, 433

poria skin, *fú líng pí* 茯苓皮, Poriae Cortex, 5, 116, 136, 153, 723

poria with skin, *lián pí fú líng* 连皮茯苓, Poria cum Cortice, 228

Poriae Cortex, *fú líng pí* 茯苓皮, poria skin, 5, 116, 136, 153, 723

pork lard, *zhū zhī gāo* 猪脂膏, Suis Adeps, 653

Portulacae Herba, *mǎ chǐ xiàn* 马齿苋, purslane, 68, 111, 338, 445, 516, 721

Potentillae Chinensis Radix seu Herba cum Radice, *wěi líng cài* 委陵菜, Chinese silverweed, 68, 721

powdered phellodendron, *huáng bǎi mò* 黄柏末, Phellodendri Cortex Pulveratus, 330, 331

powdered stalactite, *zhōng rǔ fěn* 钟乳粉, Stalactitum Pulveratum, 624, 726

Powerful Happiness Pill, *wēi xǐ wán* 威喜丸, 743

Praeparatio Sublimata Alba, *bái jiàng dān* 白降丹, white downborne elixir, 171, 383

prayer-beads, *jī gǔ cǎo* 鸡骨草, Abri Cantoniensis Herba cum Radice, 68, 721

Precipitation-Checking Decoction, *duàn xià tāng* 断下汤, 743

Premature Periods Decoction, *xiān qí tāng* 先期汤, 730

presbyopia*, 195

pretty swertia, *qīng yè dǎn* 青叶胆, Swertiae Pulchellae Herba, 68, 721

Priceless Elixir, *bù huàn jīn dān* 不换金丹, 739

Priceless Qi-Righting Powder, *bù huàn jīn zhèng qì sǎn* 不换金正气散, 80, 109, 114, 154, 177, 394, 732

pro formula pinellia, *fǎ bàn xià* 法半夏, Pinelliae Tuber Pro Formula Praeparatum, 625

process*
  ensiform, 633
  mastoid, 92
  xiphoid, 633

processed flowery knotweed, *zhì hé shǒu wū* 制何首乌, Polygoni Multiflori Radix Praeparatum, 604

processed galenite, *qiān fěn* 铅粉, Galenitum Praeparatum, 98, 445

processus styloideus ulnae*, 468

Procreation Elixir, *zàn yù dān* 赞育丹, 296, 742

progressive myatrophy*, 678

prolapse of the uterus*, 711, 712

Prolonging Life and Preserving the Origin (*shòu shì bǎo yuán*) 寿世保元, 17th century (Míng), Gōng Tíng-Xián 龚廷贤, 199

prostatitis*, 583

prunella, *xià kū cǎo* 夏枯草, Prunellae Spica, 67, 141, 385, 459, 526, 538, 544, 685, 720

Prunella Decoction, *xià kū cǎo tāng* 夏枯草汤, 737

Prunella Paste, *xià kū cǎo gāo* 夏枯草膏, 737

Prunellae Spica, *xià kū cǎo* 夏枯草, prunella, 67, 141, 385, 459, 526, 538, 544, 685, 720

Pruni Amygdali Semen, *bā dàn xìng rén* 巴旦杏仁, almond, 624, 725

Pruni Japonicae Semen, *yù lǐ rén* 郁李仁, bush cherry kernel, 460, 462, 722

prurigo*, 395

Pseudolaricis Kaempferi Cortex (Radicis), *tǔ jīng pí* 土荆皮, golden larch (root) bark, 41, 728

Pseudosciaenae Otolithum, *yú nǎo shí* 鱼脑石, otolith, 310, 405

pseudostellaria, *tài zǐ shēn* 太子参, Pseudostellariae Radix, 108, 175, 593, 726

Pseudostellariae Radix, *tài zǐ shēn* 太子参, pseudostellaria, 108, 175, 593, 726

psoralea, *bǔ gǔ zhī* 补骨脂, Psoraleae Semen, 12, 45, 229, 297, 332, 335, 343, 370, 393, 397, 593, 596, 675, 679, 727

Psoralea Tincture, *bǔ gǔ zhī dīng* 补骨脂酊, 676

Psoraleae Semen, *bǔ gǔ zhī* 补骨脂, psoralea, 12, 45, 229, 297, 332, 335, 343, 370, 393, 397, 593, 596, 675, 679, 727

psoriasis*, 674

Pteridis Multifidi Herba, *fèng wěi cǎo* 凤尾草, phoenix-tail fern, 68, 69, 721

pterygium*, 181

ptyalocele*
  sublingual, 440

pú cān 仆参, BL-61, Subservient Visitor, 747

pú gōng yīng 蒲公英 dandelion, Taraxaci Herba cum Radice, 17, 67, 69, 70, 93, 120, 214, 282, 386, 440, 459, 501, 606, 685, 691, 721

pú huáng 蒲黄 typha pollen, Typhae Pollen, 21, 30, 34, 56, 59, 137, 139, 464, 567, 569, 724

pǔ jì fāng 普济方 (*Universal Aid Formulary*), 1406 (Míng), Téng Hóng 滕弘 et al. ed., 281

pǔ jì xiāo dú yǐn 普济消毒饮, Universal Aid Toxin-Dispersing Beverage, 63, 323, 387, 403, 612, 664, 691, 730

pǔ jì xiāo dú yǐn qù shēng má chái hú huáng qín huáng lián fāng 普济消毒饮去升麻柴胡黄芩黄连方, Universal Aid Toxin-Dispersing Beverage Minus Cimicifuga, Bupleurum, Scutellaria, & Coptis, 730

pubic bone*, 369, 626

puccoon, *zǐ cǎo* 紫草, Lithospermi, Macrotomiae, seu Onosmatis Radix, 30, 67, 387, 459, 637, 683, 721

pueraria, *gé gēn* 葛根, Puerariae Radix, 47, 55, 103, 176, 214, 246, 346, 422, 501, 599, 600, 685, 686, 699, 720

Pueraria Decoction, *gé gēn tāng* 葛根汤, 73, 105, 729

Pueraria Flesh-Resolving Decoction, *gān gé jiě jī tāng* 干葛解肌汤, 729

pueraria flower, *gé huā* 葛花, Puerariae Flos, 415

Pueraria Flower Liquor-Resolving Decoction, *gé huā jiě chéng tāng* 葛花解酲汤, 257, 348, 349, 732

Pueraria, Scutellaria, and Coptis Decoction, *gé gēn huáng qín huáng lián tāng* 葛根黄芩黄连汤, 731

Pueraria, Scutellaria, and Coptis Decoction, *gé gēn qín lián tāng* 葛根芩连汤, 110, 278

Puerariae Flos, *gé huā* 葛花, pueraria flower, 415

Puerariae Radix, *gé gēn* 葛根, pueraria, 47, 55, 103, 176, 214, 246, 346, 422, 501, 599, 600, 685, 686, 699, 720

puffball, *mǎ bó* 马勃, Lasiosphaera seu Calvatia, 68, 721

Pull Aright Powder, *qiān zhèng sǎn* 牵正散, 125, 140, 689, 740

Pull Aright, *qiān zhèng* 牵正, 125, 689

pulmogenic heart disease*, 120, 193

pulmonary emphysema*, 120

pulmonary tuberculosis*, 97, 237, 380, 530, 615

pulsatilla, *bái tóu wēng* 白头翁, Pulsatillae Radix, 68, 338, 352, 721

Pulsatilla Decoction, *bái tóu wēng tāng* 白头翁汤, 28, 110, 177, 197, 278, 338, 343, 731

Pulsatillae Radix, *bái tóu wēng* 白头翁, pulsatilla, 68, 338, 352, 721

Pulse Canon (*mài jīng*) 脉经, 3rd century, Western Jìn, Wáng Shú-Hé 王叔和, 48, 236, 351, 371, 554, 653

Pulse-Engendering Powder, *shēng mài sǎn* 生脉散, 47, 59, 161, 175, 239, 265, 272, 376, 428, 455, 469, 502, 586, 651, 683, 702, 709, 742

Pulse-Engendering Variant Powder, *jiā jiǎn shēng mài sǎn* 加减生脉散, 456, 591, 715

Pulse-Restorative Decoction, *fù mài tāng* 复脉汤, 156, 283, 741

Pulse-Restorative Variant Decoction, *jiā jiǎn fù mài tāng* 加减复脉汤, 741

Pumex, *hǎi fú shí* 海浮石, pumice, 201, 291, 419, 511, 624, 638, 673, 725

pumice, *hǎi fú shí* 海浮石, Pumex, 201, 291, 419, 511, 624, 638, 673, 725

pumpkin seed, *nán guā zǐ* 南瓜子, Cucurbitae Semen, 183, 298, 724

punctum lacrimale*, 605

Pure Ginseng Decoction, *dú shēn tāng* 独参汤, 27, 29, 33, 40, 233, 448, 478, 482, 489, 527, 586, 595, 735

Pure Yang True Man Viscus-Nourishing Decoction, *chún yáng zhēn rén yǎng zàng tāng* 纯阳真人养脏汤, 174, 196, 742

Purple Clouds Plaster, *zǐ yún gāo* 紫云膏, 745

purple cowrie, *zǐ bèi* 紫贝, Mauritiae, Erosariae seu Cypraeae Testa, 54, 726

Purple Gold Powder, *zǐ jīn fěn* 紫金粉, 740

Purple Snow Elixir, *zǐ xuě dān* 紫雪丹, 65, 69, 88, 156, 171, 177, 202, 394, 589, 693, 740

Purple Snow Powder, *zǐ xuě sǎn* 紫雪散, 198

Purple Snow, *zǐ xuě* 紫雪, 450, 637

purpura*, 162
  anaphylactoid, 30
  thrombocytopenic, 30

Pursing Wind Powder, *cuò fēng sǎn* 撮风散, 740

purslane, *mǎ chǐ xiàn* 马齿苋, Portulacae Herba, 68, 111, 338, 445, 516, 721

Pus-Outthrusting Powder, *tòu nóng sǎn* 透脓散, 187, 323, 744

pylorus*, 118

Pyothorax Formula, *zhì nóng xiōng fāng* 治脓胸方, 743

Pyri Exocarpium, *lí pí* 梨皮, pear peel, 398

pyrite, *zì rán tóng* 自然铜, Pyritum, 53, 138, 725

Pyritum, *zì rán tóng* 自然铜, pyrite, 53, 138, 725

pyrola, *lù xián cǎo* 鹿衔草, Pyrolae Herba, 140, 722

Pyrolae Herba, *lù xián cǎo* 鹿衔草, pyrola, 140, 722

pyrrosia, *shí wéi* 石韦, Pyrrosiae Folium, 69, 107, 136, 723

Pyrrosia Powder, *shí wéi sǎn* 石苇散, 21, 68, 544, 733

Pyrrosiae Folium, *shí wéi* 石韦, pyrrosia, 69, 107, 136, 723

Qi Depression Decoction, *qì yù tāng* 气郁汤, 64, 480

Qi Flow Drink, *liú qì yǐn zǐ* 流气饮子, 481

Qi Gate, *qì mén* 气门, 226, 353

Qi Goiter, *qì yǐng* 气瘿, 210, 480

Qi-Abducting Decoction, *dǎo qì tāng* 导气汤, 226, 481, 735

Qi-Boosting Sharp and Bright Decoction, *yì qì cōng míng tāng* 益气聪明汤, 741

Qi-Boosting Strangury-Checking Decoction, *yì qì zhǐ lín tāng* 益气止淋汤, 583

Qi-Boosting Urine-Abducting Decoction, *yì qì dǎo niào tāng* 益气导尿汤, 529

Qi-Clearing Phlegm-Transforming Pill, *qīng qì huà tán wán* 清气化痰丸, 70, 282, 670, 738

Qi-Coordinating Construction-Nourishing Decoction, *chéng qì yǎng yíng tāng* 承气养营汤, 732

Qi-Coordinating Decoctions, *chéng qì tāng* 承气汤, 79, 172, 190, 505, 607

Qi-Discharging Beverage, *pái qì yǐn* 排气饮, 735

Qi-Freeing Hardness-Dissipating Pill, *tōng qì sàn jiān wán* 通气散坚丸, 486

Qi-Normalizing Blood-Nourishing Decoction, *shùn qì yǎng xuè tāng* 顺气养血汤, 696

Qi-Normalizing Center-Harmonizing Decoction, *shùn qì hé zhōng tāng* 顺气和中汤, 741

Qi-Normalizing Food-Dispersing Phlegm-Transforming Pill, *shùn qì xiāo shí huà tán wán* 顺气消食化痰丸, 141, 739

Qi-Normalizing Phlegm-Abducting Decoction, *shùn qì dǎo tán tāng* 顺气导痰汤, 414, 694, 739

Qi-Rectifying Phlegm-Downbearing Decoction, *lǐ qì jiàng tán tāng* 理气降痰汤, 439

Qi-Righting Decoction, *zhèng qì tāng* 正气汤, 702

Qi-Righting Lindera and Cyperus Powder, *zhèng qì tiān xiāng sǎn* 正气天香散, 736

Qi-Smoothing Powder, *shū qì sǎn* 舒气散, 736

Qi-Supplementing Bladder-Freeing Beverage, *bǔ qì tōng pāo yǐn* 补气通胞饮, 452

Qi-Supplementing Dizziness-Resolving Decoction, *bǔ qì jiě yūn tāng* 补气解晕汤, 448

Qi-Supplementing Spleen-Moving Decoction, *bǔ qì yùn pí tāng* 补气运脾汤, 164

qī bǎo měi rán dān 七宝美髯丹, Seven-Jewel Beard-Blackening Elixir, 4, 742

qī bǎo sǎn 七宝散, Seven-Jewel Powder, 500, 732

qī chōng mén 七冲门, seven gates, 527

qī chuāng 漆疮, lacquer sore, 338

qī guài mài 七怪脉, seven strange pulses, 527

qī lí sǎn 七厘散, Seven Pinches Powder, 137, 138, 337, 737

qī mén 期门, LR-14, Cycle Gate, 8, 19, 29, 34, 57, 88, 91, 112, 123, 157, 181, 215, 219, 223, 228, 234, 235, 256, 257, 279, 302, 310, 314, 352, 355, 357, 361–363, 374, 386, 390, 462, 478–480, 482, 483, 493, 571, 590, 658, 670, 683, 749

qī qì tāng 七气汤, Seven Qi Decoction, 485

qī qiào 七窍, seven orifices, 527

qī qíng 七情, seven affects, 526

qī qíng 七情, seven relations, 527

qī qíng nèi shāng 七情内伤, internal damage by the seven affects, 313

qī shāng 七伤, seven damages, 526

qī wèi bái zhú sǎn 七味白术散, Seven-Ingredient Ovate Atractylodes Powder, 600, 608, 741

qī xīng zhēn 七星针, seven-star needle, 527

qī yǎo 漆咬, lacquer bite, 338

qī zhēn sǎn 七珍散, Seven-Gem Powder, 453

qī zhì xiāng fù wán 七制香附丸, Sevenfold Processed Cyperus Pill, 36, 484

qí 脐, navel, 406

qí 脐, umbilicus, 636

qí 齐, Qi, 475

qí chuāng 脐疮, umbilical sores, 636

qí fēng 脐风, umbilical wind, 636

qí fù tāng 芪附汤, Astragalus and Aconite Decoction, 702, 735

qí fù tòng 脐腹痛, pain in the umbilical region, 425

qí gǔ 岐骨, bone juncture, 45

qí héng zhī fǔ 奇恒之腑, extraordinary organ, 188

qí huáng 岐黄, Qi Bo and the Yellow Emperor, 477

qí jīng 奇经, extraordinary vessel, 188

qí jīng bā mài 奇经八脉, eight extraordinary vessels, 169

qí sháo guì jiǔ tāng 芪芍桂酒汤, Astragalus, Peony, Cinnamon Twig, and Liquor Decoction, 704

qí shé 蕲蛇 agkistrodon, Agkistrodon, 139, 722

qí shī 脐湿, umbilical damp, 636

qí shī zhǒng 脐湿肿, umbilical damp swelling, 636

qí shòu huò xiāng wán 奇授藿香丸, Old Hermit Agastache/Patchouli Pill, 121

qí tú 脐突, protrusion of the umbilicus, 468

qǐ bì 启闭, opening blocks, 420

qǐ gé sǎn 启膈散, Diaphragm-Arousing Powder, 164, 735

qǐ gōng wán 启宫丸, Palace-Opening Pill, 418

qǐ jú dì huáng tāng 杞菊地黄汤, Lycium Berry, Chrysanthemum, and Rehmannia Decoction, 742

qǐ jú dì huáng wán 杞菊地黄丸, Lycium Berry, Chrysanthemum, and Rehmannia Pill, 11, 38, 64, 86, 119, 144, 175, 195, 336, 352, 365, 674, 742

qǐ pí sǎn 启脾散, Spleen-Arousing Pill, 736

qǐ pí wán 启脾丸, Spleen-Arousing Pill, 197

qǐ zhēn 起针, needle extraction, 406

qì 气, ch'i, 59

qì 气, qi, 475

qì bì 气闭, qi block, 476

qì bì 气痹, qi impediment, 481

qì bì 气秘, qi constipation, 477

qì bì ěr lóng 气闭耳聋, qi block deafness, 476

qì bìng zhèng hòu 气病证候, qi disease pattern, 479

qì bù guì gēn 气不归根, qi not homing to its root, 481

qì chōng 气冲, ST-30, Qi Thoroughfare, 35, 57, 111, 212, 222, 226, 233, 241, 424, 435, 450, 484, 503, 609, 746

qì chuǎn 气喘, panting, 427

qì cū 气粗, rough breathing, 509

qì cù 气促, hasty breathing, 258

qì dào 气道, pathway of qi, 429

qì duǎn 气短, shortness of breath, 530

qì è 气呃, qi hiccough, 480

qì fèn 气分, qi aspect, 476

qì fèn chū rè 气分初热, initial-stage qi-aspect heat, 303

qì fèn dà rè 气分大热, great heat in the qi aspect, 247

qì fèn zhèng 气分证, qi-aspect pattern, 476

qì gān 气疳, qi gan, 480

qì gé 气膈, qi occlusion, 481

qì gōng 气功, qi cultivation, 477

qì gōng 气功, qi-gong, 480

qì gǔ 气鼓, qi drum, 479

qì gǔ 气臌, qi drum distention, 479

qì guān 气关, qi bar, 476

qì guǎn yán piàn 气管炎片, Bronchitis Tablet, 738

qì hǎi 气海, CV-6, Sea of Qi, 1, 3, 4, 14, 15, 17, 22–24, 26–28, 31, 33–38, 40, 41, 47, 55, 57–59, 61, 62, 64, 71, 73, 74, 77, 78, 80–87, 94, 97, 105, 109, 111, 114–119, 127, 136, 139, 141, 151, 153, 157, 159–164, 168, 174, 177, 186, 194, 196, 197, 199, 212, 215–218, 223, 224, 226–231, 233–235, 240, 241, 247, 251, 257, 261, 265, 267, 269–272, 274, 278, 279, 287, 296, 297, 300–302, 309, 314, 318, 329, 331, 333, 334, 336, 338–340, 343, 349, 353, 355, 356, 370, 378, 379, 393, 395, 410, 418, 425, 426, 431, 433, 435, 438–440, 442, 447–454, 456, 457, 461, 465–467, 475, 477–481, 483–490, 497, 498, 503, 504, 517, 522–525, 529, 537, 541, 542, 547, 555, 557–559, 561–565, 570, 579–581, 586, 589, 590, 594–596, 601, 603, 604, 608, 612–614, 620, 629, 631, 633, 636, 638–641, 647, 649–652, 658, 661–664, 666–668, 675, 677, 678, 683, 690, 694, 695, 702, 703, 709–713, 716, 749

qì hǎi 气海, sea of qi, 517

qì hǎi shū 气海俞, BL-24, Sea-of-Qi Transport, 747

qì hù 气户, ST-13, Qi Door, 39, 254, 332, 746

qì huà 气化, qi transformation, 486

qì jī 气积, qi accumulation, 475

qì jī 气机, qi dynamic, 479

qì jī bù lì 气机不利, inhibited qi dynamic, 301

qì jiē 气街, qi street, 485

qì jié fù tòng 气结腹痛, qi bind abdominal pain, 476

qì jué 气厥, qi reversal, 482

qì kǒu 气口, qi opening, 481

qì kuài 气块, qi lump, 481

qì lì 气痢, qi dysentery, 479

qì lì 气疬, qi scrofula, 482

qì lín 气淋, qi strangury, 484

qì liú 气瘤, qi tumor, 486

qì lún 气轮, qi wheel, 490

qì mài 瘈脉, TB-18, Tugging Vessel, 748

qì mén 气门, Qi Gate, 226, 353

qì mén 气门, qi gate, 480

qì nì 气逆, qi counterflow, 477

qì ǒu 气呕, qi vomiting, 489

qì pǐ 气痞, qi glomus, 480

qì qiè 气怯, qi timidity, 485

qì shàn 气疝, qi mounting, 481

qì shàng chōng xīn 气上冲心, qi surging up into the heart, 485

qì shàng nì 气上逆, counterflow qi ascent, 102

qì shǎo 气少, qi shortage, 482

qì shè 气舍, ST-11, Qi Abode, 746

qì shēn fā rè 气虚身热, qi vacuity generalized heat [effusion], 488

qì sòu 气嗽, qi cough, 477

qì suí xuè tuō 气随血脱, qi deserting with the blood, 478

qì tāi 气胎, qi fetus, 480

qì tán 气痰, qi phlegm, 482

qì tòng 气痛, qi pain, 481

qì tuō 气脱, qi desertion, 479

qì wéi xuè zhī shuài 气为血之帅, qi is the commander of the blood, 481

qì wèi 气味, qi and flavor, 475

qì xiàn 气陷, qi fall, 480

qì xiàn xiè xiè 气陷泄泻, qi fall diarrhea, 480

qì xiè 气泄, qi diarrhea, 479

qì xiè 气泻, qi diarrhea, 479

qì xū 气虚, qi vacuity, 486

qì xū bēng lòu 气虚崩漏, qi vacuity flooding and spotting, 487

qì xū bì 气虚痹, qi vacuity impediment, 488

qì xū bù shè 气虚不摄, vacuous qi failing to ensure containment, 653

qì xū chuǎn 气虚喘, qi vacuity panting, 489

qì xū ěr lóng 气虚耳聋, qi vacuity deafness, 487

qì xū ěr míng 气虚耳鸣, qi vacuity tinnitus, 489

qì xū fā rè 气虚发热, qi vacuity heat effusion, 488

qì xū fù tòng 气虚腹痛, qi vacuity abdominal pain, 486

qì xū huá tāi 气虚滑胎, qi vacuity habitual miscarriage, 488

qì xū jīng xíng xiān qī 气虚经行先期, qi vacuity advanced menstruation, 487

qì xū rè 气虚热, qi vacuity heat, 488

qì xū tóu tòng 气虚头痛, qi vacuity headache, 488

qì xū wěi 气虚痿, qi vacuity wilting, 489

qì xū xià xiàn 气虚下陷, qi vacuity fall, 487

qì xū xīn jì 气虚心悸, qi vacuity heart palpitations, 488

qì xū xuàn yūn 气虚眩晕, qi vacuity dizziness, 487

qì xū yuè jīng guò duō 气虚月经过多, qi vacuity profuse menstruation, 489

qì xū zé hán 气虚则寒, when qi is vacuous, there is cold, 672

qì xū zhōng mǎn 气虚中满, qi vacuity center fullness, 487

qì xū zì hàn 气虚自汗, qi vacuity spontaneous sweating, 489

qì xué 气穴, KI-13, Qi Point, 26, 35, 36, 38, 57, 217, 331, 353, 418, 479, 484, 748

qì xuè 气血, qi-blood, 476

qì xuè biàn zhèng 气血辨证, qi-blood pattern identification, 476

qì xuè chōng hé 气血冲和, harmonious flow of qi and blood, 255

qì xuè jù xū 气血俱虚, dual vacuity of qi and blood, 160

qì xuè liǎng fán 气血两燔, blazing of both qi and blood, 23

qì xuè liǎng fán 气血两燔, qi and blood both ablaze, 475

qì xuè shī tiáo 气血失调, disharmony of qi and blood, 135

qì xuè shuāng bǔ 气血双补, dual supplementation of qi and blood, 159

qì xuè shuāng bǔ 气血双补, supplementing both qi and blood, 594

qì xuè tán shí biàn zhèng 气血痰食辨证, qi, blood, phlegm, and food pattern identification, 476

qì xuè xū ruò tòng jīng 气血虚弱痛经, qi-blood vacuity menstrual pain, 477

qì yì 气翳, qi screen, 482

qì yīn liǎng shāng 气阴两伤, damage to both qi and yin, 108

qì yīn liǎng xū 气阴两虚, dual vacuity of qi and yin, 161

qì yíng liǎng fán 气营两燔, blazing of both qi and construction, 23

qì yíng liǎng fán 气营两燔, qi and construction both ablaze, 475

qì yíng liǎng qīng 气营两清, clearing both qi and construction, 65

qì yíng liǎng qīng 气营两清, dual clearing of both qi and construction, 158

qì yíng tóng bìng 气营同病, dual disease of qi and construction, 158

qì yǐng 气瘿, Qi Goiter, 210, 480

qì yǐng 气瘿, qi goiter, 480

qì yǒu yú biàn shì huǒ 气有余便是火, superabundance of qi gives rise to fire, 592

qì yù 气郁, qi depression, 478

qì yù tāng 气郁汤, Qi Depression Decoction, 64, 480

qì yù wǎn tòng 气郁脘痛, qi depression stomach duct pain, 478

qì yù xié tòng 气郁胁痛, qi depression rib-side pain, 478

qì yù xuàn yūn 气郁眩晕, qi depression dizziness, 478

qì yù xuè bēng 气郁血崩, qi depression flooding, 478

qì zhàng 气胀, qi distention, 479

qì zhì 气痔, qi hemorrhoids, 480

qì zhì 气滞, qi stagnation, 482

qì zhì fù tòng 气滞腹痛, qi stagnation abdominal pain, 483

qì zhì jīng xíng hòu qī 气滞经行后期, qi stagnation delayed menstruation, 484

qì zhì tòng jīng 气滞痛经, qi stagnation menstrual pain, 484

qì zhì xuè yū 气滞血瘀, qi stagnation and blood stasis, 483

qì zhì xuè yū jīng bì 气滞血瘀经闭, qi stagnation blood stasis menstrual block, 484

qì zhì xuè yū xīn jì 气滞血瘀心悸, qi stagnation blood stasis heart palpitations, 483

qì zhì yāo tòng 气滞腰痛, qi stagnation lumbar pain, 484

qì zhǒng 气肿, qi swelling, 485

qì zhòng 气中, qi stroke, 485

qiān 铅 galenite, Galenitum, 467, 526

qiān chuí gāo 千捶膏, Thoroughly Pounded Paste, 75, 744

qiān dān 铅丹 minium, Minium, 728

qiān fěn 铅粉 processed galenite, Galenitum Praeparatum, 98, 445

qiān jīn sǎn 千金散, Thousand Gold Pieces Powder, 213

qiān jīn wěi jīng tāng 千金苇茎汤, Thousand Gold Pieces Phragmites Decoction, 15, 59, 373, 693

qiān jīn yào fāng 千金要方 (*Thousand Gold Pieces Prescriptions*), full title *bèi jí qiān jīn yào fāng* 备急千金要方, 41, 91, 200, 254, 268, 324, 394, 612, 675, 686, 696

qiān lǐ guāng 千里光 climbing groundsel, Senecionis Scandentis Herba, 68, 721

qiān mín tāng 千缗汤, Thousand Strings of Cash Decoction, 439

qiān nián jiàn 千年健 homalomena, Homalomenae Rhizoma, 139, 722

qiān niú zǐ 牵牛子 morning glory, Pharbitidis Semen, 98, 171, 182, 215, 411, 438, 445, 460, 666, 722

qiān rì chuāng 千日疮, thousand-day sore, 609

qiān zhèng 牵正, Pull Aright, 125, 689

qiān zhèng sǎn 牵正散, Pull Aright Powder, 125, 140, 689, 740

qián 钱, mace, 382

qián 钱, qian, 475

qián dǐng 前顶, GV-21, Before the Vertex, 586, 654, 694, 703, 749

qián gǔ 前谷, SI-2, Front Valley, 263, 281, 542, 747

qián hú 前胡 peucedanum, Peucedani Radix, 5, 47, 64, 624, 625, 686, 688, 725

qián sōu 前溲, urine, 642

qián yáng 潜阳, subduing yang, 585

qián yáng xī fēng 潜阳熄风, subduing yang and extinguishing wind, 585

qián yīn 前阴, anterior yin, 9

qián zhèn 潜镇, subduing and settling, 585

qiàn 欠, yawning, 704

qiàn cǎo gēn 茜草根 madder, Rubiae Radix, 20, 34, 70, 97, 390, 493, 512, 572, 724

qiàn shēn 欠伸, yawning, 704

qiàn shí 芡实 euryale, Euryales Semen, 11, 12, 57, 308, 334, 496, 518, 727

qiāng bàng pú bò tāng 羌蒡蒲薄汤, Notopterygium, Arctium, Dandelion, and Mint Decoction, 501

qiāng huó 羌活 notopterygium, Notopterygii Rhizoma, 11, 14, 22, 55, 102, 103, 116, 139, 154, 184, 191, 240, 247, 500–502, 546, 562, 654, 680, 681, 720

qiāng huó bài dú tāng 羌活败毒汤, Notopterygium Toxin-Vanquishing Decoction, 682, 684

qiāng huó chú shī tāng 羌活除湿汤, Notopterygium Dampness-Eliminating Decoction, 734

qiāng huó fáng fēng tāng 羌活防风汤, Notopterygium and Ledebouriella Decoction, 682

qiāng huó fù zǐ tāng 羌活附子汤, Notopterygium and Aconite Decoction, 506

qiāng huó shèng shī tāng 羌活胜湿汤, Notopterygium Dampness-Overcoming Decoction, 14, 79, 103, 114, 287, 530, 588, 680, 684, 734

qiāng lán tāng 羌蓝汤, Notopterygium and Isatis Root Decoction, 729

qiāng láng 蜣螂 dung beetle, Catharsius, 138, 139, 725

qiáng jiān 强间, GV-18, Unyielding Space, 749

qiáng wēi gēn 蔷薇根 multiflora rose root, Rosae Multiflorae Radix, 401

qiáng yīn 强阴, strengthening yin, 584

qiáng zhí 强直, rigid, 508

qiáng zhōng 强中, rigid center, 508

qiào 窍, orifice, 421

qiào hé tāng 翘荷汤, Forsythia and Mint Decoction, 734

qiē 切, cutting, 106

qié zi jí 茄子疾, eggplant disease, 169

qiè mài 切脉, feel the pulse, 197

qiè zhěn 切诊, palpation, 427

qīn xí 侵袭, assail, 11

qín 秦, Qin, 481

qín bàn wán 芩半丸, Scutellaria and Pinellia Pill, 277

qín bù dān 芩部丹, Scutellaria, Stemona, and Salvia Elixir, 738

qín jiāo 秦艽 large gentian, Gentianae Macrophyllae Radix, 72, 139, 167, 263, 451, 722

qín jiāo biē jiǎ sǎn 秦艽鳖甲散, Large Gentian and Turtle Shell Powder, 176, 572, 693, 731

qín jiāo dì huáng tāng 秦艽地黄汤, Large Gentian and Rehmannia Decoction, 535

qín jiāo fú léi tāng 秦艽扶赢汤, Large Gentian Emaciation Decoction, 731

qín lián èr chén tāng 芩连二陈汤, Scutellaria and Coptis Two Matured Ingredients Decoction, 243, 442, 737

qín lián èr mǔ wán 芩连二母丸, Scutellaria, Coptis, Anemarrhena, and Fritillaria Pill, 30, 37, 737

qín lián píng wèi tāng 芩连平胃散, Scutellaria and Coptis Stomach-Clearing Decoction, 705

qín lián sì wù tāng 芩连四物汤, Scutellaria and Coptis Four Agents Decoction, 30, 730

qín pí 秦皮 ash, Fraxini Cortex, 68, 338, 721

qìn dīng xíng pí nèi zhēn 揿钉型皮内针, thumb-tack intradermal needle, 612

qīng 青, green-blue, 248

qīng 清法, clearing, 64

qīng 清, Qing, 481

qīng 清, clear, 64

qīng cǎo 青草, green herbs, 248

qīng cháng rùn zào 清肠润燥, clearing the intestines and moistening dryness, 71

qīng cháng yǐn 清肠饮, Intestine-Clearing Beverage, 743

qīng chǎo 清炒, plain stir-frying, 445

qīng dài 青带, green-blue vaginal discharge, 248

qīng dài 青黛 indigo, Indigo Pulverata Levis, 67, 201, 319, 419, 721

qīng dài gāo 青黛膏, Indigo Paste, 445

qīng dài sǎn 青黛散, Indigo Powder, 59, 117, 225, 238, 338, 516, 546, 586, 668, 671, 686, 705, 744

qīng dài tāng 清带汤, Discharge-Clearing Decoction, 743

qīng dǎn lì shī tāng 清胆利湿汤, Gallbladder-Clearing Dampness-Disinhibiting Decoction, 733

qīng dǎn tāng 清胆汤, Gallbladder-Clearing Decoction, 476

qīng dǎn xíng qì tāng 清胆行气汤, Gallbladder-Clearing Qi-Moving Decoction, 735

qīng é wán 青娥丸, Young Maid Pill, 4, 329, 332, 370

qīng fèi huà tán wán 清肺化痰丸, Lung-Clearing Phlegm-Transforming Pill, 738

qīng fèi rùn zào 清肺润燥, clearing the lung and moistening dryness, 72

qīng fèi tāng 清肺汤, Lung-Clearing Decoction, 535, 738

qīng fèi yǐn 清肺饮, Lung-Clearing Beverage, 22, 443

qīng fèi yǐn zǐ 清肺饮子, Lung-Clearing Drink, 148, 607, 626, 731

qīng fèi zhǐ ké 清肺止咳, clearing the lung and suppressing cough, 72

qīng fěn 轻粉 calomel, Calomelas, 98, 319, 412, 727

qīng fēng 青风, green-blue wind, 248

qīng fēng nèi zhàng 青风内障, green-blue wind internal obstruction, 248

qīng fēng téng 青风藤 Orient vine, Sinomenii seu Sabiae Caulis et Rhizoma, 139, 722

qīng gān huǒ 清肝火, clearing liver fire, 71

qīng gān lú huì wán 清肝芦荟丸, Liver-Clearing Aloe Pill, 243, 533, 534

qīng gān shèn shī tāng 清肝渗湿汤, Liver-Clearing Dampness-Percolating Decoction, 733

qīng gān xiè huǒ 清肝泻火, clearing the liver and draining fire, 72

qīng gān yǐn jīng tāng 清乾引经汤, Liver-Clearing Channel-Conducting Decoction, 390

qīng gé wán 青蛤丸, Indigo and Clamshell Pill, 356

qīng gōng 清宫, clearing the palace, 72

qīng gōng tāng 清宫汤, Palace-Clearing Decoction, 71, 294, 693, 730

qīng gǔ sǎn 清骨散, Bone-Clearing Powder, 72, 572, 613, 655, 731

qīng hǎi wán 清海丸, Clear Sea Pill, 360

qīng hāo 青蒿 sweet wormwood, Artemisiae Apiaceae seu Annuae Herba, 68, 69, 72, 255, 277, 281, 282, 587, 649, 664, 721

qīng hāo biē jiǎ tāng 青蒿鳖甲汤, Sweet Wormwood and Turtle Shell Decoction, 72, 281, 282, 649, 731

qīng huà yǐn 清化饮, Clearing Transforming Beverage, 349, 702

qīng jì 轻剂, light formula, 346

qīng jiě piàn 清解片, Clearing Resolution Tablet, 730

qīng jīn 青筋, vein, 654

qīng jīn 清金, clearing metal, 71

qīng jīn huà tán tāng 清金化痰汤, Metal-Clearing Phlegm-Transforming Decoction, 356, 738

qīng jīn jiàng huǒ 清金降火, clearing metal and downbearing fire, 71

qīng jīn sǎn 青金散, Indigo and Gold Powder, 636

qīng jīng 青睛, dark of the eye, 118

qīng jīng tāng 清经汤, Channel-Clearing Decoction, 31

qīng jīng tāng (sǎn) 清经汤（散）, Channel-Clearing (Menses-Clearing) Decoction (Powder), 731

qīng kōng gāo 清空膏, Clear Sky Paste, 111, 287, 288, 687

qīng lěng yuān 清冷渊, TB-11, Clear Cold Abyss, 748

qīng lì 清利, clearing and disinhibiting, 65

qīng liáng gān lù yǐn 清凉甘露饮, Cool Clearing Sweet Dew Beverage, 76

qīng liáng gāo 清凉膏, Cool Clearing Paste, 744

qīng liáng yǐn 清凉饮, Cool Clearing Beverage, 104

qīng lín wán 青麟丸, Green-Blue Unicorn Pill, 733

qīng líng 青灵, HT-2, Green-Blue Spirit, 540, 746

qīng luò yǐn 清络饮, Network-Clearing Beverage, 69, 730

qīng máng 青盲, clear-eye blindness, 64

qīng mù xiāng 青木香 vladimiria, Vladimiriae Radix, 493, 724

qīng níng wán 清宁丸, Clear and Quiet Pill, 731, 733

qīng pí 青皮 unripe tangerine peel, Citri Exocarpium Immaturum, 19, 50, 55, 217, 223, 234, 262, 363, 397, 475, 478, 483, 490, 493, 546, 574, 685, 695, 712, 723

qīng pí chú shī yǐn 清脾除湿饮, Spleen-Clearing Dampness-Eliminating Beverage, 285

qīng pí yǐn 清脾饮, Spleen-Clearing Beverage, 317, 732

qīng qì 清气, clear qi, 72

qīng qì 清气, clearing qi, 71

qīng qì bù shēng 清气不升, clear qi failing to bear upward, 72

qīng qì fèn rè 清气分热, clearing qi-aspect heat, 71

qīng qì huà tán wán 清气化痰丸, Qi-Clearing Phlegm-Transforming Pill, 70, 282, 670, 738

qīng qì rè 清气热, clearing qi heat, 71

qīng qiào 清窍, clear orifice, 72

qīng rè 清热, clearing heat, 66

qīng rè gù jīng tāng 清热固经汤, Heat-Clearing Channel-Securing (Menses-Securing) Decoction, 31, 743

qīng rè huà shī 清热化湿, clearing heat and transforming dampness, 70

qīng rè huà tán 清热化痰, clearing heat and transforming phlegm, 70

qīng rè huà tán kāi qiào 清热化痰开窍, clearing heat, transforming phlegm, and opening the orifices, 70

qīng rè jiě biǎo 清热解表, clearing heat and resolving the exterior, 69

qīng rè jiě dú 清热解毒, clearing heat and resolving toxin, 70

qīng rè jiě shǔ 清热解暑, clearing heat and resolving summerheat, 69

qīng rè kāi qiào 清热开窍, clearing heat and opening the orifices, 69

qīng rè lì shī 清热利湿, clearing heat and disinhibiting dampness, 68

qīng rè qù shī 清热祛湿, clearing heat and dispelling dampness, 69

qīng rè tōng lín 清热通淋, clearing heat and freeing strangury, 69

qīng rè xī fēng 清热熄风, clearing heat and extinguishing wind, 69

qīng rè xiè huǒ 清热泻火, clearing heat and draining fire, 69

qīng rè zhǐ bēng tāng 清热止崩汤, Heat-Clearing Uterine Bleeding Decoction, 743

qīng rè zhǐ xuè 清热止血, clearing heat and stanching bleeding, 70

qīng shàng juān tòng tāng 清上蠲痛汤, Upper-Body-Clearing Pain-Alleviating Decoction, 740

qīng shàng wán 清上丸, Upper-Body-Clearing Pill, 436

qīng shī rè 清湿热, clearing damp-heat, 66

qīng shǔ lì shī 清暑利湿, clearing summerheat and disinhibiting dampness, 71

qīng shǔ yì qì 清暑益气, clearing summerheat and boosting qi, 71

qīng shǔ yì qì tāng 清暑益气汤, Summerheat-Clearing Qi-Boosting Decoction, 71, 455, 588, 591, 730

qīng sù fèi qì 清肃肺气, clearing and depurating lung qi, 64

qīng tuǐ yá gān 青腿牙疳, green-leg gan of the teeth and gums, 248

qīng wèi jiàng nì 清胃降逆, clearing the stomach and downbearing counterflow, 72

qīng wèi sǎn 清胃散, Stomach-Clearing Powder, 158, 190, 198, 239, 367, 566, 577, 621, 656, 687, 731

qīng wèi tāng 清胃汤, Stomach-Clearing Decoction, 15, 439, 620

qīng wēn bài dú yǐn 清瘟败毒饮, Scourge-Clearing Toxin-Vanquishing Beverage, 6, 65, 73, 388, 474, 514, 611, 664, 730

qīng xiāng zǐ 青葙子 celosia, Celosiae Argenteae Semen, 67, 720

qīng xīn 清心, clearing the heart, 71

qīng xīn dí rè 清心涤热, clearing the heart and flushing heat, 71

qīng xīn huǒ 清心火, clearing heart fire, 66

qīng xīn kāi qiào 清心开窍, clearing the heart and opening the orifices, 71

qīng xīn lián zǐ yǐn 清心莲子饮, Heart-Clearing Lotus Seed Beverage, 147, 731

qīng xīn xiè huǒ 清心泻火, clearing the heart and draining fire, 71

qīng xīn yì shèn 清心益肾, clearing the heart and boosting the kidney, 71

qīng xū rè 清虚热, clearing vacuity heat, 72

qīng xuān fèi qì 轻宣肺气, diffusing lung qi with lightness, 128

qīng xuān rùn zào 轻宣润燥, moistening dryness by light diffusion, 398

qīng xuàn yǐn 清眩饮, Dizziness-Clearing Beverage, 731

qīng xuè 圊血, latrine bleeding, 341

qīng xuè rè 清血热, clearing blood heat, 65

qīng yān lì gé tāng 清咽利膈汤, Throat-Clearing Diaphragm-Disinhibiting Decoction, 14, 581, 586, 612, 671

qīng yān rùn zào tāng 清咽润噪汤, Throat-Clearing Dryness-Moistening Decoction, 619

qīng yān yǎng yíng tāng 清咽养营汤, Throat-Clearing Construction-Nourishing Decoction, 734

qīng yáng 清阳, clear yang, 72

qīng yáng bù shēng 清阳不升, clear yang failing to bear upward, 72

qīng yáng (qì) bù shēng 清阳（或气）不升, nonupbearing of clear yang (or qi), 413

qīng yāo tāng 轻腰汤, Lumbus-Lightening Decoction, 326

qīng yè dǎn 青叶胆 pretty swertia, Swertiae Pulchellae Herba, 68, 721

qīng yí èr hào 清胰二号, Pancreas-Clearing Formula No.2, 731

qīng yí yī hào 清胰一号, Pancreas-Clearing Formula No.1, 731

qīng yíng 清营, clearing construction, 65

qīng yíng liáng xuè 清营凉血, clearing construction and cooling the blood, 66

qīng yíng tāng 清营汤, Construction-Clearing Decoction, 65, 69, 202, 388, 431, 455, 589, 591, 693, 730

qīng yíng xiè rè 清营泄热, clearing construction and discharging heat, 66

qīng yù nǎi gān 青芋艿干 dried taro, Colocasiae Tuber Exsiccatum, 544

qīng zàng fǔ rè 清脏腑热, clearing bowel and visceral heat, 65

qīng zàng fǔ rè 清脏腑热, clearing organ heat, 71

qīng zào 清燥, clearing dryness, 66

qīng zào jiù fèi 清燥救肺, clearing dryness and rescuing the lung, 66 *qīng zào jiù fèi tāng* 清燥救肺汤, Dryness-Clearing Lung-Rescuing Decoction, 49, 66, 72, 155, 156, 161, 291, 348, 366, 379, 398, 625, 659, 678, 695, 715, 734

qīng zhèn tāng 清震汤, Clearing Invigoration Decoction, 612

qīng zhōng tāng 清中汤, Center-Clearing Decoction, 186, 314, 442

qīng zhōu bái wán zǐ 青州白丸子, Qingzhou White Pill, 739

qīng zǐ 青紫, bruise, 51

qíng 情, affect, 7

qíng lián jú rú tāng 芩连橘茹汤, Scutellaria, Coptis, Tangerine Peel, and Bamboo Shavings Decoction, 736

qíng zhì 情志, emotion, 172

qíng zhì nèi shāng 情志内伤, affect-mind internal damage, 7

qíng zhì yù jié 情志郁结, affect-mind binding depression, 7

qíng zhì yù jié 情志郁结, affects causing binding depression, 7

Qingzhou White Pill, *qīng zhōu bái wán zǐ* 青州白丸子, 739

qióng yù gāo 琼玉膏, Fine Jade Paste, 603, 734

qiū xū 丘墟, GB-40, Hill Ruins, 3, 4, 19, 20, 90, 118, 137, 189, 215, 216, 236, 255, 296, 342, 344, 355, 394, 446, 474, 521, 538, 548, 567, 748

qiū zào 秋燥, autumn dryness, 12

qiú 鼽, sniveling, 543

qiú bí 鼽鼻, sniveling nose, 543

qiú hòu 球后, Back of the Ball, 521, 568, 586

qiú shuǐ 鼽水, watery sniveling, 669

qū 驱, expel, 181

qū 祛, dispel, 136

qū 麹, leaven, 342

qū 麹, medicated leaven, 388

qū bìn 曲鬓, GB-7, Temporal Hairline Curve, 219, 748

qū chā 曲差, BL-4, Deviating Turn, 747

qū chí 曲池, LI-11, Pool at the Bend, 2, 5, 6, 8, 13–16, 22, 25, 29–31, 39, 40, 44, 60–63, 65, 66, 69–76, 89, 91, 99, 103, 105, 109–113, 117, 118, 120, 127, 129, 137–140, 146, 147, 149, 151, 155, 156, 158, 167, 168, 171, 174, 178, 184, 186, 190, 197, 201, 203, 216, 225, 235, 239, 241, 244, 260, 276–278, 280–285, 287–292, 294, 295, 298, 301, 302, 318–320, 337–339, 341, 342, 347, 349, 357, 364, 366, 370, 374, 380, 382–384, 386, 390, 394, 398, 403, 405, 422, 426, 427, 434, 437–439, 443, 450, 455, 457, 458, 462, 466, 493, 501, 516, 520–522, 530, 540, 544, 546, 547, 560, 567, 569, 578, 579, 585–591, 601, 607, 611, 613, 624, 637, 652, 665, 673, 674, 677, 679, 680, 683–689, 693, 694, 700–703, 710, 712, 713, 716, 746

qū chóng 驱虫, expelling worms, 182

qū fēng chú shī 祛风除湿, dispelling wind and eliminating dampness, 139

qū fēng huà tán 祛风化痰, dispelling wind and transforming phlegm, 140

qū fēng jiě jìng 祛风解痉, dispelling wind and resolving tetany, 140

qū fēng sàn rě sǎn 驱风散, Wind-Expelling Powder, 198

qū fēng sàn rè yǐn zǐ 驱风散热饮子, Wind-Expelling Heat-Dissipating Drink, 495, 685, 740

qū fēng shèng shī 祛风胜湿, dispelling wind and overcoming dampness, 140

qū fēng yǎng xuè 祛风养血, dispelling wind and nourishing the blood, 140

qū fēng yī zì sǎn 驱风一字散, Wind-Expelling One Zi Powder, 320, 718

qū fēng 祛风, dispelling wind, 139

qū gǔ 曲骨, CV-2, Curved Bone, 221, 297, 308, 332, 453, 497, 522, 643, 701, 749

qū hán huà tán 祛寒化痰, dispelling cold and transforming phlegm, 136

qū huí tāng èr hào 驱蛔汤二号, Roundworm-Expelling Decoction No.2, 737

qū mài 瞿麦, dianthus, Dianthi Herba, 21, 69, 98, 136, 723

qū mài zhǐ zhú wán 麹麦枳术丸, Medicated Leaven, Barley Sprout, Unripe Bitter Orange, and Ovate Atractylodes Pill, 736

qū niè zhǐ zhú wán 麹蘖枳术丸, Medicated Leaven, Barley Sprout, Unripe Bitter Orange, and Ovate Atractylodes Pill, 736

qū quán 曲泉, LR-8, Spring at the Bend, 28, 69, 111, 226, 256, 283, 289, 297, 300, 320, 337, 365, 403, 415, 447, 452, 456, 457, 468, 484, 487, 489, 506, 516, 566, 568, 637, 641, 667, 711, 748

qū shī 祛湿, dispelling dampness, 137

qū tán 祛痰, dispelling phlegm, 137

qū tán wán 祛痰丸, Phlegm-Expelling Pill, 612

qū tāo tāng 驱绦汤, Tapeworm-Expelling Decoction, 737

qū tòng sǎn 趋痛散, Pain-Chasing Powder, 451

qū xié 祛邪, dispelling evil, 137

qū xié fú zhèng 祛邪扶正, dispelling evil and supporting right, 137

qū yū huó xuè 祛瘀活血, dispelling stasis and quickening the blood, 137

qū yū xiāo zhǒng 祛瘀消肿, dispelling stasis and dispersing swelling, 137

qū yū zhǐ xuè 祛瘀止血, dispelling stasis and stanching bleeding, 139

qū yuán 曲垣, SI-13, Crooked Wall, 747

qū zé 曲泽, PC-3, Marsh at the Bend, 25, 30, 34, 65, 70, 99, 289, 455, 540, 589, 590, 637, 748

qū zhú wán 麹术丸, Medicated Leaven and Atractylodes Pill, 4, 63

qú 麹, leaven, 342

qú 麹, medicated leaven, 388

qǔ yuān tāng 取渊汤, Deep-Source Decoction, 120

qù huǒ dú 去火毒, eliminating fire toxin, 171

qù lái tāng 去来汤, Coming and Going Decoction, 91

Index 870

qù lái xīn tòng 去来心痛, coming and going heart pain, 91

qù yū shēng xīn 去瘀生新, eliminating stasis and engendering the new, 171

qù yù chén cuò 去宛陈莝, eliminating depression and stale water, 171

quán biān chuāng 裙边疮, skirt-hem sore, 536

quán chì 颧赤, reddening of the cheeks, 494

quán gǔ 颧骨, cheek bone, 57

quán hóng 颧红, reddening of the cheeks, 494

quán liáo 颧膠, SI-18, Cheek Bone-Hole, 194, 253, 747

quán lù wán 全鹿丸, Whole Deer Pill, 742

quán máo dào chā 拳毛倒插, ingrown eyelash, 300

quán máo dào jié 拳毛倒睫, ingrown eyelash, 300

quán shēn 拳参 bistort, Polygoni Bistortae Rhizoma, 68, 721

quán shēng bái zhú sǎn 全生白术散, Life-for-All Ovate Atractylodes Powder, 50, 461, 600

quán xiē 全蝎 scorpion, Buthus, 54, 56, 74, 140, 146, 150, 417, 526, 541, 662, 726

Quartz Album, *bái shí yīng* 白石英, white quartz, 53

quē pén 缺盆, ST-12, Empty Basin, 220, 222, 252–254, 712, 746

quē rǔ 缺乳, scant breast milk, 513

què 阙, gate tower, 240

què 阙, glabella, 242

què bān 雀斑, freckle, 226

què máng 雀盲, sparrow blindness, 549

què mù 雀目, sparrow vision, 549

què shàng 阙上, upper gate tower, 640

què zhōng 阙中, glabella, 242

què zhōng 阙中, middle gate tower, 394

què zhuó mài 雀啄脉, pecking sparrow pulse, 429

Quiet Sleep, *ān mián* 安眠, 83, 281, 409

quilled cinnamon, *guān guì* 官桂, Cinnamomi Cortex Tubiformis, 45, 328

Quincke's edema*, 494

quinsy*, 612, 671

quisqualis, *shǐ jūn zǐ* 使君子, Quisqualis Fructus, 182, 183, 445, 509, 724

Quisqualis and Rhubarb Powder, *shǐ jūn zǐ dà huáng fěn* 使君子大黄粉, 737

Quisqualis Fructus, *shǐ jūn zǐ* 使君子, quisqualis, 182, 183, 445, 509, 724

Quisqualis Powder, *shǐ jūn zǐ sǎn* 使君子散, 696, 737

qì bù shè xuè 气不摄血, qi failing to contain the blood, 479

qīng rè xiè huǒ jiě dú 清热泻火解毒, clearing heat, draining fire, and resolving toxin, 70

radish, *lái fú* 莱菔, Raphani Radix, 527

radish seed, *lái fú zǐ* 莱菔子, Raphani Semen, 5, 141, 216, 418, 512, 589, 724

Radish Seed and Magnolia Bark Bind-Freeing Decoction, *lái pò tōng jié tāng* 莱朴通结汤, 732

radius*, 11

ramie, *zhù má gēn* 苎麻根, Boehmeriae Radix, 724

Ramie (Boehmeria) Decoction, *zhù gēn tāng* 苎根汤, 741

rán gǔ 然骨, blazing bone, 23

rán gǔ 然谷, KI-2, Blazing Valley, 16, 28–31, 36, 72, 76, 97, 99, 122, 152, 156, 158, 160, 161, 164, 168, 174–176, 180, 199, 203, 220, 229, 237, 277, 282, 283, 292, 294, 296, 332, 336, 348, 349, 360, 390, 391, 393, 410, 455, 456, 461, 462, 535, 552, 566, 567, 572, 582, 591, 597, 607, 613, 614, 641, 642, 647–649, 702, 709, 714–716, 747

rǎn tāi 染苔, stained fur, 569

ranula*, 440

Ranunculi Japonici Herba et Radix, *máo gèn* 毛茛, Japanese ranunculus, 388, 728

rǎo 扰, harass, 254

Raphani Radix, *lái fú* 莱菔, radish, 527

Raphani Semen, *lái fú zǐ* 莱菔子, radish seed, 5, 141, 216, 418, 512, 589, 724

Raw Aconite Powder, *shēng fù sǎn* 生附散, 86

raw arisaema, *shēng nán xīng* 生南星, Arisaematis Rhizoma Crudum, 243, 439, 460, 690

raw astragalus, *shēng huáng qí* 生黄芪, Astragali (seu Hedysari) Radix Cruda, 259

raw licorice, *shēng gān cǎo* 生甘草, Glycyrrhizae Radix Cruda, 17, 116, 175, 263, 310, 422, 439, 499, 516, 621

raw myrrh, *shēng mò yào* 生没药, Myrrha Cruda, 138, 724

raw pinellia, *shēng bàn xià* 生半夏, Pinelliae Tuber Crudum, 243, 464

Raw Rhinoceros Horn Powder, *shēng xī jiǎo sǎn* 生犀角散, 693

raw rhubarb, *shēng dà huáng* 生大黄, Rhei Rhizoma Crudum, 430, 460, 676, 722

raw sanguisorba, *shēng dì yú* 生地榆, Sanguisorbae Radix Cruda, 338

raw tortoise plastron, *shēng guī bǎn* 生龟版, Testudinis Plastrum Crudum, 415

raw typha pollen, *shēng pú huáng* 生蒲黄, Typhae Pollen Crudum, 586

raw white peony, *shēng bái sháo yào* 生白芍药, Paeoniae Radix Alba Cruda, 256

raw wild aconite, *shēng cǎo wū* 生草乌, Aconiti Tsao-Wu-Tou Tuber Crudum, 460

rè 热, heat, 275

rè 热, heat effusion, 199, 278

rè 热, hot, 292

rè bì 热闭, heat block, 276

rè bì 热痹, heat impediment, 280

rè bì 热秘, heat constipation, 277

rè bì jìng jué 热闭痉厥, heat-block tetanic reversal, 276

rè bìng 热病, febrile disease, 196

rè bìng 热病, heat disease, 278

rè chuǎn 热喘, heat panting, 281

rè chuāng 热疮, heat sore, 283

rè dú 热毒, heat toxin, 284

rè dú xià xuè 热毒下血, heat toxin precipitation of blood, 284

rè è 热呃, heat hiccough, 280

rè fú chōng rèn 热伏冲任, deep-lying heat in the thoroughfare and controlling vessels, 120

rè gān 热疳, heat gan, 280

rè hàn 热汗, heat sweating, 283

rè huò luàn 热霍乱, heat cholera, 276

rè jí shēng fēng 热极生风, extreme heat engendering wind, 188

rè jí shēng hán 热极生寒, extreme heat engendering cold, 188

rè jì 热剂, hot formula, 292

rè jié 热结, heat bind, 276

rè jié cháng wèi 热结肠胃, gastrointestinal heat bind, 240

rè jié cháng wèi 热结肠胃, heat binding in the stomach and intestines, 276

rè jié páng guāng 热结膀胱, bladder heat bind, 22

rè jié páng guāng 热结膀胱, heat binding in the bladder, 276

rè jié páng liú 热结旁流, heat bind with circumfluence, 276

rè jié xià jiāo 热结下焦, lower burner heat bind, 368

rè jié xiōng 热结胸, heat chest bind, 276

rè jué 热厥, heat reversal, 283

rè jué xīn tòng 热厥心痛, heat reversal heart pain, 283

rè kě qù han 热可去寒, hot [medicinals] can eliminate cold, 293

rè lèi 热泪, heat tearing, 283

rè lì 热痢, heat dysentery, 278

rè lín 热淋, heat strangury, 283

rè nüè 热疟, heat malaria, 281

rè ǒu 热呕, heat vomiting, 284

rè pò dà cháng 热迫大肠, heat distressing the large intestine, 278

rè qì huò luàn 热气霍乱, heat qi cholera, 282

rè rù xīn bāo 热入心包, heat entering the pericardium, 279

rè rù xuè fèn 热入血分, heat entering the blood aspect, 279

rè rù xuè shì 热入血室, heat entering the blood chamber, 279

rè rù yíng xuè 热入营血, heat entering construction-blood, 279

rè shāng fèi luò 热伤肺络, heat damaging the network vessels of the lung, 277

rè shāng jīn mài 热伤筋脉, heat damaging the sinews, 277

rè shāng qì 热伤气, heat damages qi, 277

rè shāng shén míng 热伤神明, heat damaging the spirit light, 277

rè shēn jué shēn 热深厥深, severe heat and severe reversal, 528

rè shèng dòng fēng 热盛动风, exuberant heat stirring wind, 189

rè shèng qì fèn 热盛气分, exuberant qi-aspect heat, 190

rè shèng zé zhǒng 热胜则肿, when heat prevails, there is swelling, 672

rè shí jié xiōng 热实结胸, heat repletion chest bind, 282

rè sòu 热嗽, heat cough, 277

rè tán 热痰, heat phlegm, 282

rè wú fàn rè 热无犯热, do not use heat against heat, 144

rè xián 热痫, heat epilepsy, 279

rè xiāo 热哮, heat wheezing, 284

rè xié 热邪, heat evil, 279

rè xié chuán lǐ 热邪传里, heat evil passing into the interior, 280

rè xié yōng fèi 热邪壅肺, heat evil congesting the lung, 280

rè xié zǔ fèi 热邪阻肺, heat evil obstructing the lung, 280

rè xiè 热泄, heat diarrhea, 278

rè xiè 热泻, heat diarrhea, 278

rè xīn tòng 热心痛, heat heart pain, 280

rè yè tí 热夜啼, heat night crying, 281

rè yīn rè yòng 热因热用, treating heat with heat, 626

rè yīn rè yòng 寒因寒用, treating cold with cold, 626

rè yù 热郁, heat depression, 278

rè yù tāng 热郁汤, Heat Depression Decoction, 278

rè yùn 热熨, hot pack METHOD@refs 1, 293

rè zhàng 热胀, heat distention, 278

rè zhě hán zhī 热者寒之, heat is treated with cold, 281

rè zhèng 热证, heat pattern, 281

rè zhòng 热中, heat stroke, 283

rè zhuó shèn yīn 热灼肾阴, heat scorching kidney yin, 283

Realgar, *xióng huáng* 雄黄, realgar, 98, 241, 383, 395, 458, 667, 690, 710, 727

realgar, *xióng huáng* 雄黄, Realgar, 98, 241, 383, 395, 458, 667, 690, 710, 727

Realgar Toxin-Resolving Pill, *xióng huáng jiě dú wán* 雄黄解毒丸, 170

Rectifying Poria (Hoelen) Decoction, *lǐ líng tāng* 理苓汤, 733

Rectum-Lifting Powder, *tí gāng sǎn* 提肛散, 493

Red Brocade Tablet, *jǐn hóng piàn* 锦红片, 743

red ginseng, *hóng shēn* 红参, Ginseng Radix Rubra, 593, 726

Red Oil Paste, *hóng yóu gāo* 红油膏, 17

red peony, *chì sháo yào* 赤芍药, Paeoniae Radix Rubra, 17, 30, 34, 58, 67, 70, 116, 137, 139, 140, 150, 181, 227, 386, 390, 395, 430, 462, 463, 467, 497, 548, 679, 721

Red Spirit Elixir, *hóng líng dān* 红灵丹, 740

Red Spirit Wine, *hóng líng jiǔ* 红灵酒, 231

red tangerine peel, *jú hóng* 橘红, Citri Exocarpium Rubrum, 95, 136, 448, 493, 723 red upborne elixir, *hóng shēng* 红升, Hydrogyrum Oxydatum Crudum Rubrum, 171

Red Upborne Elixir, *hóng shēng dān* 红升丹, 385, 744

Red-Abducting Powder, *dǎo chì sǎn* 导赤散, 36, 41, 189, 230, 238, 263, 264, 281, 283, 284, 400, 541, 542, 583, 619, 687, 731

Red-Abducting Qi-Coordinating Decoction, *dǎo chì chéng qì tāng* 导赤承气汤, 731

Redness-Severing Pill, *duàn hóng wán* 断红丸, 143

refined mirabilite, *xuán míng fěn* 玄明粉, Mirabilitum Depuratum, 44, 460, 722

rehmannia, *dì huáng* 地黄, Rehmanniae Radix, 172, 175, 176, 336, 352, 398, 455, 464

Rehmannia and Lycium Root Bark Decoction, *liǎng dì tāng* 两地汤, 31, 360, 649, 731

Rehmannia Drink, *dì huáng yǐn zǐ* 地黄饮子, 289, 368, 740, 742

Rehmannia Pill, *dì huáng wán* 地黄丸, 742

Rehmannia Powder, *dì huáng sǎn* 地黄散, 403

Rehmanniae Radix, *dì huáng* 地黄, rehmannia, 172, 175, 176, 336, 352, 398, 455, 464

Rehmanniae Radix Conquita, *shú dì huáng* 熟地黄, cooked rehmannia, 28, 37, 39, 47, 88, 140, 161, 175, 225, 298, 310, 333, 458, 459, 467, 504, 526, 537, 570, 584, 593, 595, 596, 620, 651, 727

Rehmanniae Radix Exsiccata, *gān dì huáng* 干地黄, dried rehmannia, 20, 67, 256, 526, 557, 720

Rehmanniae Radix Exsiccata seu Recens, *shēng dì huáng* 生地黄, dried/fresh rehmannia, 19, 28, 30, 65, 70, 88, 108, 116, 122, 154, 174–176, 256, 259, 277, 298, 310, 390, 391, 399, 415, 416, 422, 450, 462, 467, 495, 508, 516, 519, 526, 577, 581, 584, 586, 595, 597, 601, 604, 655, 679

Rehmanniae Radix Recens, *xiān dì huáng* 鲜地黄, fresh rehmannia, 67, 116, 720

Rejuvenation Elixir, *huán shào dān* 还少丹, 297, 742

rén bù 人部, human level, 293

rén shēn 人参 ginseng, Ginseng Radix, 47, 84, 183, 223, 236, 251, 255, 259, 270, 325, 334, 345, 384, 392, 395, 411, 448, 450, 455–457, 480, 495, 499, 503, 504, 525, 527, 572, 593–595, 600, 612, 649, 651, 661, 698, 713, 716, 726

rén shēn bài dú sǎn 人参败毒散, Ginseng Toxin-Vanquishing Powder, 258, 730

rén shēn gé jiè sǎn 人参蛤蚧散, Ginseng and Gecko Powder, 629, 741

rén shēn gù běn wán 人参固本丸, Ginseng Root-Securing Pill, 175, 378, 742

rén shēn guī pí wán 人参归脾丸, Ginseng Spleen-Returning Pill, 271

rén shēn hú táo tāng 人参胡桃汤, Ginseng and Walnut Decoction, 741

rén shēn huáng qí sǎn 人参黄芪散, Ginseng and Astragalus Powder, 175, 742

rén shēn jiàn pí wán 人参健脾丸, Ginseng Spleen-Fortifying Pill, 741

rén shēn jiàn zhōng tāng 人参建中汤, Ginseng Center-Fortifying Decoction, 713

rén shēn lú 人参芦 ginseng top, Ginseng Rhizoma, 170, 511, 727

rén shēn qǐ pí wán 人参启脾丸, Ginseng Spleen-Arousing Pill, 736

rén shēn qīng fèi tāng 人参清肺汤, Ginseng Lung-Clearing Decoction, 143

rén shēn tāng 人参汤, Ginseng Decoction, 654, 735

rén shēn wèi fēng tāng 人参胃风汤, Ginseng Stomach Wind Decoction, 318

rén shēn yǎng róng tāng 人参养荣汤, Ginseng Construction-Nourishing Decoction, 26, 27, 32, 38, 40, 116, 143, 150, 174, 213, 271, 449, 456, 461, 650, 675

rén shēn yǎng róng tāng (wán) 人参养荣汤（丸）, Ginseng Construction-Nourishing Decoction (Pill), 540

rén shēn zī bǔ piàn 人参滋补片, Enriching Ginseng Tablet, 739

rén shì bù xǐng 人事不省, loss of consciousness, 367

rén shuǐ 壬水, S9-water, 511

rén yíng 人迎, ST-9, Man's Prognosis, 222, 226, 586, 746

rén yíng 人迎, man's prognosis, 387

rén yíng mài 人迎脉, man's prognosis pulse, 387

rén zhōng 人中, GV-26, Human Center, 6, 14, 15, 19, 32, 63, 88, 178, 231, 232, 301, 394, 408, 420, 434, 437, 448, 454, 458, 696

rén zhōng 人中, human center, 293

rén zhōng 人中, philtrum, 432

rén zhōng dīng 人中疔, human-center clove sore, 293

rén-shēn yǎng róng tāng (wán) 人参养荣汤（丸）, Ginseng Construction-Nourishing Decoction (Pill), 741

rěn dōng téng 忍冬藤 lonicera stem and leaf, Lonicerae Caulis et Folium, 67, 116, 540, 721

rèn mài 任脉, CV, 107

rèn mài 任脉, conception vessel, 92

rèn mài 任脉, controlling vessel, 98

rèn shēn 妊娠, pregnancy, 460

rèn shēn chuǎn 妊娠喘, panting in pregnancy, 428

rèn shēn chuāng yáng 妊娠疮疡, sores in pregnancy, 546

rèn shēn dú yào shāng tāi 妊娠毒药伤胎, damage to the fetus by toxic medicinals in pregnancy, 108

rèn shēn fēng jìng 妊娠风痉, wind tetany in pregnancy, 693

rèn shēn fù tòng 妊娠腹痛, abdominal pain in pregnancy, 2

rèn shēn mài 妊娠脉, pregnancy pulse, 461

rèn shēn ǒu tù 妊娠呕吐, vomiting pregnancy, 657

rèn shēn shù duò tāi 妊娠数堕胎, multiple abortion, 403

rèn shēn xián zhèng 妊娠痫症, eclampsia, 167

rèn shēn xiǎo biàn bù lì 妊娠小便不利, inhibited urination in pregnancy, 302 *rèn shēn xiǎo biàn bù tōng* 妊娠小便不通, urinary stoppage in pregnancy, 641

rèn shēn xīn fù zhàng mǎn 妊娠心腹胀满, distention and fullness in the heart [region] and abdomen in pregnancy, 143

rèn shēn xīn fù zhàng mǎn 妊娠心腹胀满, fullness and distention in the heart [region] and abdomen during pregnancy, 231

rèn shēn xuàn yūn 妊娠眩晕, dizziness in pregnancy, 144

rèn shēn yāo tòng 妊娠腰痛, lumbar pain in pregnancy, 370

rèn shēn yào jì 妊娠药忌, contraindications of medicinals in pregnancy, 97

rèn shēn yí niào 妊娠遗尿, enuresis in pregnancy, 177

rèn shēn zhǒng zhàng 妊娠肿胀, swelling and distention in pregnancy, 600

rèn shēn zhòng fēng 妊娠中风, wind stroke in pregnancy, 692

rèn zǐ 妊子, pregnancy, 460

Renewal Powder, *zài zào sǎn* 再造散, 11, 730

retained placenta*, 503

retina*, 657

    pigmentary degeneration of, 291, 549

Return Again Elixir, *lái fù dān* 来复丹, 330, 443, 590, 665

Return-of-Spring Elixir, *huí chūn dān* 回春丹, 740

Reversal Powder, *diān dǎo sǎn* 颠倒散, 5, 149, 676, 744

rhagadia mammae*, 412

Rhapontici seu Echinopis Radix, *lòu lú* 漏芦, rhaponticum/echinops, 68, 227, 384, 386, 721

rhaponticum/echinops, *lòu lú* 漏芦, Rhapontici seu Echinopis Radix, 68, 227, 384, 386, 721

Rhei Rhizoma, *dà huáng* 大黄, rhubarb, 7, 17, 19, 24, 34, 50, 51, 72, 84, 93, 130, 182, 215, 255, 261, 281, 298, 311, 357, 390, 397, 434, 445, 459, 460, 502, 544, 548, 573, 577, 613, 619, 627, 664, 722

Rhei Rhizoma Crudum, *shēng dà huáng* 生大黄, raw rhubarb, 430, 460, 676, 722

rheumatism*, 684

rhinitis*, 260

    allergic, 543

    atrophic, 49, 695

    chronic, 120, 378

Rhinoceros Bezoar Pill, *xī huáng wán* 犀黄丸, 737

rhinoceros horn, *xī jiǎo* 犀角, Rhinocerotis Cornu, 67, 209, 245, 411, 422, 525, 548, 619, 720

Rhinoceros Horn and Rehmannia Decoction, *xī jiǎo dì huáng tāng* 犀角地黄汤, 24, 25, 30, 33, 51, 63, 76, 99, 102, 177, 202, 315, 390, 393, 431, 447, 567, 637, 693, 730

Rhinoceros Horn and Rehmannia Network-Clearing Beverage, *xī dì qīng luò yǐn* 犀地清络饮, 730

Rhinoceros Horn Powder, *xī jiǎo sǎn* 犀角散, 731

Rhinocerotis Cornu, *xī jiǎo* 犀角, rhinoceros horn, 67, 209, 245, 411, 422, 525, 548, 619, 720

Rhododendri Daurici Folium, *mǎn shān hóng* 满山红, Daurian rhododendron, 624, 726

Rhois Galla, *wǔ bèi zǐ* 五倍子, sumac gallnut, 466, 518, 567, 572, 675, 709, 727

rhubarb, *dà huáng* 大黄, Rhei Rhizoma, 7, 17, 19, 24, 34, 50, 51, 72, 84, 93, 130, 182, 215, 255, 261, 281, 298, 311, 357, 390, 397, 434, 445, 459, 460, 502, 544, 548, 573, 577, 613, 619, 627, 664, 722

Rhubarb and Aconite Decoction, *dà huáng fù zǐ tāng* 大黄附子汤, 24, 311, 664, 731

Rhubarb and Coptis Heart-Draining Decoction, *dà huáng huáng lián xiè xīn tāng* 大黄黄连泻心汤, 600

Rhubarb and Licorice Decoction, *dà huáng gān cǎo tāng* 大黄甘草汤, 284

Rhubarb and Moutan Decoction, *dà huáng mǔ dān pí tāng* 大黄牡丹皮汤, 318, 671, 743

Rhubarb and Moutan Decoction, *dà huáng mǔ dān tāng* 大黄牡丹汤, 459

Rhubarb and Niter Decoction, *dà huáng xiāo shí tāng* 大黄硝石汤, 111

Rhubarb and Tangkuei Powder, *dà huáng dāng guī sǎn* 大黄当归散, 33

Rhubarb and Wingless Cockroach Pill, *dà huáng zhè chóng wán* 大黄䗪虫丸, 24, 34, 152, 173, 646, 737

rì bū (suǒ) cháo rè 日晡（所）潮热, late afternoon tidal heat [effusion], 340

rì yuè 日月, GB-24, Sun and Moon, 8, 20, 88, 91, 112, 219, 235, 302, 357, 480, 590, 658, 748

riboflavin deficiency*, 516

rice bean, *chì xiǎo dòu* 赤小豆, Phaseoli Calcarati Semen, 40, 136, 164, 666, 671, 723

Rice Bean and Tangkuei Powder, *chì xiǎo dòu dāng guī sǎn* 赤小豆当归散, 743

rice sprout, *gǔ yá* 谷芽, Oryzae Fructus Germinatus, 23, 141, 420, 499, 563, 724

rice-paper plant pith, *tōng cǎo* 通草, Tetrapanacis Medulla, 66, 98, 136, 227, 434, 480, 723

Right-Restoring [Life Gate] Beverage, *yòu guī yǐn* 右归饮, 369, 594, 646, 742

Right-Restoring [Life Gate] Pill, *yòu guī wán* 右归丸, 160, 164, 180, 291, 296, 310, 331, 332, 335, 393, 523, 524, 549, 596, 646, 660, 742

Rock of Taishan Fetus-Quieting Powder, *tài shān pán shí sǎn* 泰山磐石散, 741

rohdea root, *wàn nián qīng gēn* 万年青根, Rohdeae Rhizoma et Radix, 68, 721

Rohdeae Rhizoma et Radix, *wàn nián qīng gēn* 万年青根, rohdea root, 68, 721

róng kū 荣枯, luxuriance and witheredness, 381

root poria, *fú shén* 茯神, Poria cum Pini Radice, 60, 122, 256, 262, 392, 490, 654, 726

Root Poria Powder, *fú shén sǎn* 茯神散, 235

Root-Securing Flood-Stanching Decoction, *gù běn zhǐ bēng tāng* 固本止崩汤, 212, 743

Root-Securing Pill, *gù běn wán* 固本丸, 325

roripa, *hān cài* 葐菜, Rorippae Herba seu Flos, 624, 625, 725

Rorippae Herba seu Flos, *hān cài* 蔊菜, rorippa, 624, 625, 725

rosacea*, 149

Rosae Chinensis Flos et Fructus, *yuè jì huā* 月季花, China tea rose, 138, 725

Rosae Flos, *méi guī huā* 玫瑰花, rose, 493, 724

Rosae Laevigatae Fructus, *jīn yīng zǐ* 金樱子, Cherokee rose fruit, 12, 308, 496, 518, 727

Rosae Multiflorae Radix, *qiáng wēi gēn* 蔷薇根, multiflora rose root, 401

rose, *méi guī huā* 玫瑰花, Rosae Flos, 493, 724

rose-of-Sharon, *mù jǐn huā* 木槿花, Hibisci Syriaci Flos, 728

rose-of-Sharon root bark, *mù jǐn pí* 木槿皮, Hibisci Syriaci Radicis Cortex, 728

rosin, *sōng xiāng* 松香, Pini Resina, 728

róu cì (jìng) 柔痉, soft tetany, 544

róu gān 柔肝, emolliating the liver, 172

ròu 肉, flesh, 210

ròu bì 肉痹, flesh impediment, 210

ròu cì 肉刺, corn, 99

ròu cōng róng 肉苁蓉 cistanche, Cistanches Caulis, 78, 222, 298, 310, 332, 338, 367, 511, 593, 596, 675, 727

ròu cōng róng wán 肉苁蓉丸, Cistanche Pill, 86

ròu cōng róng wán 苁蓉丸, Cistanche Pill, 508

ròu còu 肉腠, interstices of the flesh, 317

ròu dòu kòu 肉豆蔻 nutmeg, Myristicae Semen, 12, 80, 141, 316, 318, 454, 508, 518, 727

ròu fēn 肉分, flesh divide, 210

ròu gē da 肉疙瘩, elevated scar, 171

ròu guì 肉桂 cinnamon bark, Cinnamomi Cortex, 48, 81, 84, 98, 182, 196, 243, 316, 326, 331, 332, 335, 338, 393, 411, 425, 428, 450, 467, 488, 489, 502–504, 526, 562, 564, 596, 660, 662, 679, 696, 716, 723

ròu liú 肉瘤, flesh tumor, 211

ròu lún 肉轮, flesh wheel, 211

ròu tuō 肉脱, desertion of the flesh, 124

ròu wěi 肉痿, flesh wilting, 211

ròu yǐng 肉瘿, flesh goiter, 210

Rough and Ready Three Decoction, *sān ào tāng* 三拗汤, 291, 368, 684, 729

Roundworm-Expelling Decoction No.2, *qū huí tāng èr hào* 驱蛔汤二号, 737

Roundworm-Quieting Powder, *ān huí sǎn* 安蛔散, 510

Rousing Spirit Elixir, *zhèn líng dān* 震灵丹, 325, 519

rú mài 濡脉, soggy pulse, 544

rú shèng jīn dāo sǎn 如圣金刀散, Sagacious Incised Wound Powder, 298, 744

rú shèng sǎn 如圣散, Sagacious Powder, 170

rú xiè 濡泻, soggy diarrhea, 544

rú yì jīn huáng sǎn 如意金黄散, Agreeable Golden Yellow Powder, 497, 585, 670, 744

rú yín nèi zhàng 如银内障, silvery internal obstruction, 532

rǔ dú 乳毒, mammary toxin sore, 386

rǔ é 乳蛾, baby moth, 14

rǔ é 乳蛾, nipple moth, 412

rǔ fā 乳发, effusion of the breast, 169

rǔ fáng 乳房, breast, 50

rǔ gān 乳疳, mammary gan, 385

rǔ gēn 乳根, ST-18, Breast Root, 227, 228, 248, 386, 483, 513, 746

rǔ hé 乳核, breast node, 50

rǔ hé 乳核, mammary node, 385

rǔ jī 乳积, milk accumulation, 395

rǔ jū 乳疽, mammary flat-abscess, 385

rǔ láo 乳痨, mammary consumption, 385

rǔ lì 乳栗, mammary chestnut, 385

rǔ lòu 乳漏, mammary fistula, 385

rǔ nǜ 乳衄, spontaneous bleeding of the nipple, 566

rǔ pǐ 乳癖, mammary aggregation, 385

rǔ shǎo 乳少, scant breast milk, 513

rǔ shí jī zhì 乳食积滞, feeding accumulation, 197

rǔ shí jī zhì 乳食积滞, milk accumulation, 395

rǔ tán 乳痰, mammary phlegm [node], 385

rǔ tóu 乳头, nipple, 412

rǔ tóu fēng 乳头风, nipple wind, 412

rǔ tóu pò suì 乳头破碎, cracked nipple, 104

rǔ xiǎn 乳癣, suckling lichen, 585

rǔ xiāng 乳香 frankincense, Olibanum, 104, 137, 138, 503, 540, 574, 696, 724

rǔ yán 乳岩, mammary rock, 385

rǔ yōng 乳痈, mammary welling-abscess, 386

rǔ yūn 乳晕, areola, 10

rǔ zhī bù tōng 乳汁不通, breast milk stoppage, 50

rǔ zhī bù xià 乳汁不下, breast milk stoppage, 50

rǔ zhī bù xíng 乳汁不行, breast milk stoppage, 50

rǔ zhī shǎo 乳汁少, scant breast milk, 513

rǔ zhōng 乳中, ST-17, Breast Center, 746

rǔ zhōng jié hé 乳中结核, node in the breast, 412

rù chuāng 蓐（褥）疮, bedsore, 17

rù fēng 蓐风, childbed wind, 60

rù jīng 入经, channel entry, 56

rù lǐ 入里, enter the interior, 176

rù lǐ 入里, pass into the interior, 429

rù zào fǔ nì 润燥腐腻, moistness, dryness, putridity, and sliminess, 398

ruǎn gāo 软膏, ointment, 419

ruǎn jiān 软坚, softening hardness, 544

ruǎn jiān sàn jié 软坚散结, softening hardness and dissipating binds, 544

ruǎn lè 软肋, soft ribs, 544

Rub-On Medicinal Formula, *cā yào fāng* 擦药方, 691

Rubi Fructus, *fù pén zǐ* 覆盆子, rubus, 12, 229, 496, 518, 548, 727

Rubiae Radix, *qiàn cǎo gēn* 茜草根, madder, 20, 34, 70, 97, 390, 493, 512, 572, 724

rubus, *fù pén zǐ* 覆盆子, Rubi Fructus, 12, 229, 496, 518, 548, 727

ruì fà 锐发, ear lock, 166

ruì gǔ 锐骨, protuberant bone, 468

ruì zì 锐眦, outer canthus, 422

Rumicis Madaio Radix, *tŭ dà huáng* 土大黄, Madaio dock root, 116, 569

Rumicis Radix Recens, *yáng tí gēn* 羊蹄根, dock root, 724

rùn 润, moisten, 398

rùn cháng 润肠, moistening the intestines, 398

rùn cháng tāng 润肠汤, Intestine-Moistening Decoction, 315, 565, 732

rùn cháng wán 润肠丸, Intestine-Moistening Pill, 399, 683, 732

rùn fèi 润肺, moistening the lung, 398

rùn fèi huà tán 润肺化痰, moistening the lung and transforming phlegm, 398

rùn fèi sǎn 润肺散, Lung-Moistening Powder, 739

rùn jī gāo 润肌膏, Flesh-Moistening Paste, 586, 676

rùn shén sǎn 润神散, Spirit-Moistening Powder, 97

rùn xià 润下, moist precipitation, 399

rùn zào 润燥, moistening dryness, 398

rùn zào ān tāi tāng 润燥安胎汤, Dryness-Moistening Fetus-Quieting Decoction, 734

rùn zào huà tán 润燥化痰, moistening dryness and transforming phlegm, 398

Running Piglet Decoction, *bēn tún tāng* 奔豚汤, 510

ruò mài 弱脉, weak pulse, 669

Rushing Respiration Decoction, *xī bēn tāng* 息贲汤, 510

rú mén shì qīn 儒门事亲 (*Confucian Filiality*), Jīn (1115–1234), Zhāng Cóng-Zhèng 张从正 [Zǐ-Hé 子和], 181

Saccharon Granulatum, *shā táng* 沙糖, granulated sugar, 511

Saccharon Granulatum Album, *bái shā táng* 白沙糖, white sugar, 45

Safeguard Unlimited Efficacy Elixir, *bǎo ān wàn líng dān* 保安万灵丹, 417, 431

saffron, *zàng hóng huā* 藏红花, Croci Stigma, 98, 138, 387, 724

Sagacious Confucius' Pillow Elixir, *kǒng shèng zhěn zhōng dān* 孔圣枕中丹, 739

Sagacious Cure Decoction, *shèng yù tāng* 圣愈汤, 39, 159, 741

Sagacious Incised Wound Powder, *rú shèng jīn dāo sǎn* 如圣金刀散, 298, 744

Sagacious Powder, *rú shèng sǎn* 如圣散, 170

Sagacious Three Powder, *sān shèng sǎn* 三圣散, 743

Sagacious Two Powder, *èr shèng sǎn* 二圣散, 743

Sages' Aid Records (*shèng jì zǒng lù*) 圣济总录, 1111–1117 (Sòng), Government publication, 86

Sal, *shí yán* 石盐, salt, 401

Sal, *yán* 盐, salt, 383

sal ammoniac, *náo shā* 硇砂, Sal Ammoniacum, 98, 728

Sal Ammoniac Decocted Pill, *náo shā jiān wán* 硇砂煎丸, 77

Sal Ammoniac Powder, *náo shā sǎn* 硇砂散, 166

Sal Ammoniacum, *náo shā* 硇砂, sal ammoniac, 98, 728

salt, *shí yán* 石盐, Sal, 401

salt, *yán* 盐, Sal, 383

salted aconite, *xián fù zi* 咸附子, Aconiti Tuber Laterale Salsum, 367, 660, 723

salvia, *dān shēn* 丹参, Salviae Miltiorrhizae Radix, 17, 20, 28, 34, 37, 137, 138, 227, 262, 493, 516, 526, 540, 586, 724

Salvia Beverage, *dān shēn yǐn* 丹参饮, 300, 484, 737

Salviae Chinensis Herba, *shí jiàn chuān* 石见穿, Chinese sage, 139, 725

Salviae Miltiorrhizae Radix, *dān shēn* 丹参, salvia, 17, 20, 28, 34, 37, 137, 138, 227, 262, 493, 516, 526, 540, 586, 724

sān ào tāng 三拗汤, Rough and Ready Three Decoction, 291, 368, 684, 729

sān bǎo 三宝, three gems, 609

sān bì tāng 三痹汤, Three Impediment Decoction, 734

sān bǔ wán 三补丸, Triple Supplementation Pill, 63

sān bù jiǔ hòu 三部九候, three positions and nine indicators, 610

sān cái bǔ xiè 三才补泻, heaven, human, and earth supplementation and drainage, 285

sān cái fēng suǐ dān 三才封髓丹, Heaven, Human, and Earth Marrow-Retaining Elixir, 524, 739

sān cái tāng 三才汤, Heaven, Human, and Earth Decoction, 742

sān céng huí xiāng wán 三层茴香丸, Three-Option Anise Pill, 735

sān chóng bìng 三虫病, three worm diseases, 610

sān guó 三国, Three Kingdoms, 610

sān huā shén yòu wán 三花神佑丸, Three Flowers Spirit Protection Pill, 213, 442, 732

sān huà tāng 三化汤, Three Transformations Decoction, 631

sān huáng bǎo là wán 三黄宝腊丸, Three Yellow Jewels Wax Pill, 737

sān huáng là wán 三黄腊丸, Three Yellows Wax Pill, 737

sān huáng shí gāo tāng 三黄石膏汤, Three Yellows and Gypsum Decoction, 70, 500, 664, 730

sān huáng sì wù tāng 三黄四物汤, Three Yellows Four Agents Decoction, 102, 730

sān huáng tāng 三黄汤, Three Yellows Decoction, 320, 640, 670

sān huáng xǐ jì 三黄洗剂, Three Yellows Wash Preparation, 445, 744

sān huáng xiè xīn tāng 三黄泻心汤, Three Yellows Heart-Draining Decoction, 147, 282, 497, 636

sān huáng zhǐ zhú wán 三黄枳术丸, Three Yellows Bitter Orange and Ovate Atractylodes Pill, 277, 736

sān jiā jiǎn zhèng qì sǎn 三加减正气散, Third Variant Qi-Righting Powder, 733

sān jiǎ fù mài tāng 三甲复脉汤, Triple-Armored Pulse-Restorative Decoction, 526, 740

sān jiān 三间, LI-3, Third Space, 746

sān jiāo 三焦, TB, 604

sān jiāo 三焦, triple burner, 627

sān jiāo biàn zhèng 三焦辨证, triple burner pattern identification, 628

sān jiāo jīng 三焦经, triple burner channel, 628

sān jiāo ké 三焦咳, triple burner cough, 628

sān jiāo shí rè 三焦实热, triple burner repletion heat, 628

sān jiāo shū 三焦俞, BL-22, Triple Burner Transport, 15, 22, 37, 87, 91, 117, 149, 152, 182, 224, 228, 269, 301, 302, 334, 379, 449, 453, 457, 485, 537, 559, 601, 608, 663, 666, 668, 694, 703, 716, 747

sān jiāo xū hán 三焦虚寒, triple burner vacuity cold, 628

sān jiāo zhǔ jué dú 三焦主决渎, triple burner governs the sluices, 628

sān jiǎo jiǔ 三角灸, Moxibustion Triangle, 226

sān jīn tāng 三金汤, Golden Three Decoction, 733

sān léng 三棱 sparganium, Sparganii Rhizoma, 34, 98, 138, 182, 411, 512, 544, 574, 724

sān léng tāng 三棱汤, Sparganium Decoction, 737

sān léng zhēn 三棱针, three-edged needle, 609

sān máo 三毛, three hairs, 610

sān miào sǎn 三妙散, Mysterious Three Powder, 45, 117, 733

sān miào wán 三妙丸, Mysterious Three Pill, 225, 528, 686, 733

sān pǐn 三品, three grades, 609

sān pǐn yī tiáo qiāng 三品一条枪, Three-Shot Gun, 290, 744

sān qī 三七 notoginseng, Notoginseng Radix, 34, 137, 139, 540, 569, 602, 629, 724

sān qí 三奇, three mysteries, 610

sān rén tāng 三仁汤, Three Kernels Decoction, 23, 66, 69, 111, 118, 228, 297, 539, 675, 733

sān rì nüè 三日疟, quartan malaria, 490

sān shēng yǐn 三生饮, Three Raw Agents Beverage, 739

sān shèng sǎn 三圣散, Sagacious Three Powder, 743

sān shí sǎn 三石散, Three Stones Powder, 516, 671

sān wù bái sǎn 三物白散, Three Agents White Powder, 85, 731

sān wù bèi jí wán 三物备急丸, Three Agents Emergency Pill, 664, 731

sān wù xiāng rú yǐn 三物香薷饮, Three-Agent Elsholtzia Powder, 729

sān wù xiǎo bái sǎn 三物小白散, Three Agents Little White Powder, 732

sān xiāo 三消, three dispersions, 609

sān xiāo yǐn 三消饮, Three Dispersers Beverage, 514, 736

sān yáng 三阳, third yang channel, 607

sān yáng 三阳, triple yang, 628

sān yáng bìng 三阳病, triple-yang disease, 628

sān yáng hé bìng 三阳合病, triple-yang combination disease, 628

sān yáng jīng nüè 三阳经疟, triple-yang channel malaria, 628

sān yáng luò 三阳络, TB-8, Three Yang Connection, 748

sān yáng tóu tòng 三阳头痛, triple-yang headache, 628

sān yī chéng qì tāng 三一承气汤, Three-in-One Qi-Coordinating Decoction, 712, 731

sān yīn 三阴, third yin channel, 607

sān yīn 三阴, triple yin, 628

sān yīn 三因, three causes [of disease], 609

sān yīn bìng 三阴病, triple-yin disease, 628

sān yīn fāng 三因方 (*Three Causes Formulary*), full title *sān yīn jí yī bìng zhèng fāng lùn* 三因极一病症方论, 242

sān yīn jí yī bìng zhèng fāng lùn 三因极一病症方论 (*Unified Treatise on Diseases, Patterns, and Remedies According to the Three Causes*), 1174 (Sòng), Chén Yán 陈言 [Wú Zé 无择], 46, 217, 243, 508, 542, 576, 609

sān yīn jiāo 三阴交, SP-6, Three Yin Intersection, 8, 11, 14, 15, 19, 21–31, 33–41, 44, 45, 47, 51, 53, 54, 57–60, 62–64, 66, 69–71, 74, 76, 79–81, 83, 84, 86, 88, 89, 91, 93, 94, 97, 99, 103, 109–112, 115, 117–119, 123, 127–129, 138, 140, 145, 147–149, 151, 154–162, 164, 167, 168, 174–178, 180, 194, 196, 199, 201, 202, 211, 212, 217, 218, 220, 221, 223–227, 229, 230, 233–237, 239–241, 251, 256, 260, 261, 263, 265–269, 271, 273–275, 278, 279, 282–284, 288–292, 294, 296, 297, 300–302, 307, 308, 310, 314, 317–320, 330–336, 338, 339, 342, 348, 349, 352, 353, 355–362, 364–366, 368–370, 380, 381, 383, 385, 390–393, 400, 401, 403, 410, 413, 415, 416, 418, 422, 424, 426, 427, 431, 434, 435, 437, 447–458, 461, 462, 465–468, 477–485, 488–490, 493, 495, 497, 499, 503, 511, 514–516, 518, 520–522, 524–526, 533, 535, 537, 540, 542, 546, 552, 554, 557, 560, 561, 563–568, 570–572, 577, 579, 581, 584–586, 588, 591, 594–597, 600, 601, 603, 604, 607, 608, 613, 631, 637, 638, 640–642, 646–650, 652, 656, 661–663, 665, 667, 673–677, 679, 683–686, 688–690, 694, 700–703, 709–716, 746

sān yīn nüè 三阴疟, triple-yin malaria, 628

sān yīn tóu tòng 三阴头痛, triple-yin headache, 628

sān zǐ tāng 三子汤, Three-Seed Decoction, 87

sān zǐ yǎng qīn tāng 三子养亲汤, Three-Seed Filial Devotion Decoction, 141, 142, 216, 414, 435, 739

sǎn 散, powder, 458

sǎn cì 散刺, diffuse pricking, 128

sǎn jì 散剂, powder preparation, 458

sàn 散, dissipate, 142

sàn hán huà tán 散寒化痰, dissipating cold and transforming phlegm, 142

sàn huǒ tāng 散火汤, Fire-Dissipating Decoction, 110

sàn jié dìng téng tāng 散结定疼汤, Bind-Dissipating Pain-Relieving Decoction, 300, 737

sàn mài 散脉, dissipated pulse, 142

sàn mài 散脉, scattered pulse, 514

sàn piān tāng 散偏汤, Hemilateral Headache Decoction, 288

sàn yū gé gēn tāng 散瘀葛根汤, Stasis-Dissipating Pueraria Decoction, 571

sàn yū hé shāng tāng 散瘀和伤汤, Stasis-Dissipating Injury Decoction, 745

sàn zhǒng kuì jiān tāng 散肿溃坚汤, Swelling-Dispersing Hardness-Breaking Decoction, 737

sandalwood, *tán xiāng* 檀香, Santali Lignum, 493, 724

sāng bái pí 桑白皮 mulberry root bark, Mori Radicis Cortex, 64, 70, 153, 199, 228, 282, 388, 394, 624, 676, 725

sāng bái pí tāng 桑白皮汤, Mulberry Root Bark Decoction, 285, 438, 675, 738

sang jì shēng 桑寄生 mistletoe, Loranthi scu Visci Ramus, 139, 297, 352, 370, 456, 488, 722

sāng jú yǐn 桑菊饮, Mulberry Leaf and Chrysanthemum Beverage, 91, 103, 158, 184, 203, 291, 405, 414, 501, 687, 693, 729

sāng piāo xiāo 桑螵蛸 mantis egg-case, Mantidis Oötheca, 11, 12, 177, 229, 308, 496, 511, 518, 727

sāng piāo xiāo sǎn 桑螵蛸散, Mantis Egg-Case Powder, 12, 148, 174, 176, 177, 308, 449, 465, 496, 518, 743

sāng shèn 桑椹 mulberry, Mori Fructus, 37, 172, 352, 593, 597, 727

sāng shèn zǐ gāo 桑椹子膏, Mulberry Paste, 245, 742

sāng xìng tāng 桑杏汤, Mulberry Leaf and Apricot Kernel Decoction, 12, 101, 128, 155, 156, 158, 181, 398, 659, 734

sāng yè 桑叶 mulberry leaf, Mori Folium, 103, 107, 184, 420, 501, 526, 591, 686, 720

sāng zhī 桑枝 mulberry twig, Mori Ramulus, 116, 139, 263, 722

sāng zhī hǔ zhàng tāng 桑枝虎杖汤, Mulberry Twig and Bushy Knotweed Decoction, 734

sanguisorba, *dì yú* 地榆, Sanguisorbae Radix, 28, 30, 51, 338, 548, 569, 724

Sanguisorba Pill, *dì yú wán* 地榆丸, 742

Sanguisorba Powder, *dì yú sǎn* 地榆散, 462, 743

Sanguisorbae Radix, *dì yú* 地榆, sanguisorba, 28, 30, 51, 338, 548, 569, 724

Sanguisorbae Radix Cruda, *shēng dì yú* 生地榆, raw sanguisorba, 338

Santali Lignum, *tán xiāng* 檀香, sandalwood, 493, 724

sāo wèi 臊味, animal odor, 9

sào yǎng 瘙痒, itching, 320

sappan, *sū mù* 苏木, Sappan Lignum, 98, 138, 725

Sappan Lignum, *sū mù* 苏木, sappan, 98, 138, 725

sarcandra, *jiǔ jié chá* 九节茶, Sarcandrae Ramulus et Folium, 68, 721

Sarcandrae Ramulus et Folium, *jiǔ jié chá* 九节茶, sarcandra, 68, 721

Sargassi Herba, *hǎi zǎo* 海藻, sargassum, 30, 141, 243, 367, 511, 544, 624, 725

sargassum, *hǎi zǎo* 海藻, Sargassi Herba, 30, 141, 243, 367, 511, 544, 624, 725

Sargassum Jade Flask Decoction, *hǎi zǎo yù hú tāng* 海藻玉壶汤, 19, 141, 210, 243, 244, 480, 544, 737

sargentodoxa, *dà xuè téng* 大血藤, Sargentodoxae Caulis, 68, 721

Sargentodoxae Caulis, *dà xuè téng* 大血藤, sargentodoxa, 68, 721

saussurea, *mù xiāng* 木香, Saussureae (seu Vladimiriae) Radix, 38, 47, 80, 141, 223, 257, 317, 318, 338, 361, 384, 392, 398, 454, 480, 483, 493, 581, 588, 596, 694, 723

Saussurea and Amomum Six Gentlemen Decoction, *xiāng shā liù jūn zǐ tāng* 香砂六君子汤, 4, 10, 23, 47, 143, 223, 231, 393, 418, 457, 463, 487, 554, 561, 565, 575, 741

Saussurea and Amomum Six Gentlemen Pill, *xiāng shā liù jūn zǐ wán* 香砂六君子丸, 741

Saussurea and Amomum Stomach-Calming Pill, *xiāng shā píng wèi wán* 香砂平胃丸, 736

Saussurea and Amomum Two Matured Ingredients Decoction, *xiāng shā èr chén tāng* 香砂二陈汤, 738

Saussurea and Areca Pill, *mù xiāng bīng láng wán* 木香槟榔丸, 217, 240, 277, 426, 481, 549, 736

Saussurea and Coptis Pig's Stomach Pill, *xiāng lián zhū dǔ wán* 香连猪肚丸, 647

Saussurea and Coptis Pill, *xiāng lián wán* 香连丸, 110, 278, 312, 588, 645, 731

Saussurea and Magnolia Bark Pill, *xiāng pò wán* 香朴丸, 736

Saussurea Qi Flow Beverage, *mù xiāng liú qì yǐn* 木香流气饮, 116, 481

Saussurea Qi-Breaking Powder, *mù xiāng pò qì sǎn* 木香破气散, 481

Saussurea Qi-Normalizing Decoction, *mù xiāng shùn qì tāng* 木香顺气汤, 19, 483

Saussurea Qi-Normalizing Pill, *mù xiāng shùn qì wán* 木香顺气丸, 735

Saussurea Qi-Normalizing Powder, *mù xiāng shùn qì sǎn* 木香顺气散, 735

Saussurea Qi-Regulating Powder, *mù xiāng tiáo qì sǎn* 木香调气散, 74, 480

Saussurea Stagnation-Abducting Pill, *mù xiāng dǎo zhì wán* 木香导滞丸, 736

Saussurea, Amomum, Unripe Bitter Orange, and Ovate Atractylodes Pill, *xiāng shā zhǐ zhú wán* 香砂枳术丸, 216, 218, 736

Saussureae (seu Vladimiriae) Radix, *mù xiāng* 木香, saussurea, 38, 47, 80, 141, 223, 257, 317, 318, 338, 361, 384, 392, 398, 454, 480, 483, 493, 581, 588, 596, 694, 723

Saussureae Radix, *guǎng mù xiāng* 广木香, costusroot, 490, 493, 723

Saxifragae Herba, *hǔ ěr cǎo* 虎耳草, saxifrage, 68, 721

saxifrage, *hǔ ěr cǎo* 虎耳草, Saxifragae Herba, 68, 721

scabies*, 513

Scallion and Fermented Soybean Decoction, *cōng chǐ tāng* 葱豉汤, 12, 681, 729

scallion juice, *cōng zhī* 葱汁, Allii Fistulosi Herbae Succus, 307

scallion white, *cōng bái* 葱白, Allii Fistulosi Bulbus, 176, 422, 500, 502, 681, 720

Scallion White Seven-Ingredient Beverage, *cōng bái qī wèi yǐn* 葱白七味饮, 416, 729

scallion white with root, *lián xū cōng bái* 连须葱白, Allii Fistulosi Bulbus cum Radice, 228, 502

Scallion with Root Decoction, *lián xū cōng bái tāng* 连须葱白汤, 729

Scallion Yang-Freeing Decoction Plus Pig's Bile, *bái tōng jiā zhū dǎn zhī tāng* 白通加猪胆汁汤, 735

Scallion Yang-Freeing Decoction, *bái tōng tāng* 白通汤, 626, 735

Scallion, Fermented Soybean, and Platycodon Decoction, *cōng chǐ jié gěng tāng* 葱豉桔梗汤, 729

scapula*, 530

scarlet fever*, 25, 178, 664

schizonepeta, *jīng jiè* 荆芥, Schizonepetae Herba et Flos, 102, 184, 244, 338, 412, 422, 430, 449, 497, 500–502, 548, 599, 681, 712, 713, 720

Schizonepeta and Ledebouriella Decoction, *jīng fáng tāng* 荆防汤, 729

Schizonepeta and Ledebouriella Four Agents Decoction, *jīng fáng sì wù tāng* 荆防四物汤, 452

Schizonepeta and Ledebouriella Toxin-Vanquishing Powder, *jīng fáng bài dú sǎn* 荆防败毒散, 62, 91, 145, 184, 187, 303, 449, 502, 612, 681, 684, 729

Schizonepeta and Scutellaria Four Agents Decoction, *jīng qín sì wù tāng* 荆芩四物汤, 730

schizonepeta spike, *jīng jiè suì* 荆芥穗, Schizonepetae Flos, 320, 439, 549

Schizonepetae Flos, *jīng jiè suì* 荆芥穗, schizonepeta spike, 320, 439, 549

Schizonepetae Herba et Flos, *jīng jiè* 荆芥, schizonepeta, 102, 184, 244, 338, 412, 422, 430, 449, 497, 500–502, 548, 599, 681, 712, 713, 720

Schizonepetae Herba et Flos Carbonisatae, *jīng jiè tàn* 荆芥炭, charred schizonepeta, 586

schisandra, *wǔ wèi zǐ* 五味子, Schisandrae Fructus, 12, 47, 95, 96, 104, 175, 222, 230, 272, 333, 378, 409, 490, 502, 504, 512, 518, 537, 566, 571, 596, 599, 614, 651, 700, 709, 715, 726, 727

Schisandra Decoction, *wǔ wèi zǐ tāng* 五味子汤, 95, 376, 743

Schisandra Powder, *wǔ wèi zǐ sǎn* 五味子散, 477

Schisandrae Fructus, *wǔ wèi zǐ* 五味子, schisandra, 12, 47, 95, 96, 104, 175, 222, 230, 272, 333, 378, 409, 490, 502, 504, 512, 518, 537, 566, 571, 596, 599, 614, 651, 700, 709, 715, 726, 727

schistosomiasis*, 28, 616
  chronic, 28

schizophrenia*, 433, 437

sciatica*, 295

Scolopendra, *wú gōng* 蜈蚣, centipede, 54, 74, 98, 140, 146, 434, 726

scorpion, *quán xiē* 全蝎, Buthus, 54, 56, 74, 140, 146, 150, 417, 526, 541, 662, 726

scorpion tail, *xiē shāo* 蝎梢, Buthi Caudex, 562, 652

Scourge-Averting Powder, *bì wēn sǎn* 避瘟散, 590

Scourge-Clearing Toxin-Vanquishing Beverage, *qīng wēn bài dú yǐn* 清瘟败毒饮, 6, 65, 73, 388, 474, 514, 611, 664, 730

Scourge-Repelling Elixir, *bì wēn dān* 辟瘟丹, 171

Scrofula Internal Dispersion Pill, *nèi xiāo luǒ lì wán* 内消瘰疬丸, 141, 544, 737

Scrofula-Dispersing Pill, *xiāo luǒ wán* 消瘰丸, 142, 737

scrophularia, *xuán shēn* 玄参, Scrophulariae Radix, 65, 67, 108, 120, 174, 175, 298, 336, 368, 394, 399, 415, 422, 430, 459, 508, 511, 526, 541, 577, 597, 611, 612, 676, 686, 688, 714, 720

Scrophularia and Cimicifuga Decoction, *xuán shēn shēng má tāng* 玄参升麻汤, 548, 731

Scrophularia Toxin-Resolving Decoction, *xuán shēn jiě dú tāng* 玄参解毒汤, 731

Scrophulariae Radix, *xuán shēn* 玄参, scrophularia, 65, 67, 108, 120, 174, 175, 298, 336, 368, 394, 399, 415, 422, 430, 459, 508, 511, 526, 541, 577, 597, 611, 612, 676, 686, 688, 714, 720

scrub typhus*, 250

scurvy*, 249

scutellaria, *huáng qín* 黄芩, Scutellariae Radix, 20, 30, 65–67, 70, 81, 82, 115, 116, 153, 189, 191, 199, 230, 243, 255, 257, 259, 282, 303, 310, 317, 319, 338, 339, 357, 358, 372, 386, 388, 390, 394, 397, 414, 419, 421, 428, 439, 440, 457, 459, 466, 500, 501, 527, 538, 548, 569, 577, 587, 588, 637, 686, 690, 695, 709, 720

Scutellaria and Coptis Four Agents Decoction, *qín lián sì wù tāng* 芩连四物汤, 30, 730

Scutellaria and Coptis Stomach-Clearing Decoction, *qín lián píng wèi tāng* 芩连平胃散, 705

Scutellaria and Coptis Two Matured Ingredients Decoction, *qín lián èr chén tāng* 芩连二陈汤, 243, 442, 737

Scutellaria and Pinellia Pill, *qín bàn wán* 芩半丸, 277

Scutellaria and Talcum Decoction, *huáng qín huá shí tāng* 黄芩滑石汤, 733

Scutellaria Decoction Wash Formula, *huáng qín tāng xǐ fāng* 黄芩汤洗方, 744

Scutellaria Decoction, *huáng qín tāng* 黄芩汤, 71, 278, 731

Scutellaria, Coptis, Anemarrhena, and Fritillaria Pill, *qín lián èr mǔ wán* 芩连二母丸, 30, 37, 737

Scutellaria, Coptis, Tangerine Peel, and Bamboo Shavings Decoction, *qíng lián jú rú tāng* 芩连橘茹汤, 736

Scutellaria, Stemona, and Salvia Elixir, *qín bù dān* 芩部丹, 738

Scutellariae Barbatae Herba, *bàn zhī lián* 半枝莲, bearded scutellaria, 68, 76, 700, 721

Scutellariae Radix, *huáng qín* 黄芩, scutellaria, 20, 30, 65–67, 70, 81, 82, 115, 116, 153, 189, 191, 199, 230, 243, 255, 257, 259, 282, 303, 310, 317, 319, 338, 339, 357, 358, 372, 386, 388, 390, 394, 397, 414, 419, 421, 428, 439, 440, 457, 459, 466, 500, 501, 527, 538, 548, 569, 577, 587, 588, 637, 686, 690, 695, 709, 720

Scutellariae Radix Veta, *kū qín* 枯芩, old scutellaria, 690

sè cháng 涩肠, astringing the intestines, 12

sè cháng gù tuō 涩肠固脱, astringing the intestines and stemming desertion, 12

sè cháng zhǐ xiè 涩肠止泻, astringing the intestines and checking diarrhea, 12

sè jì 涩剂, astringent formula, 11

sè jīng 涩精, astringing essence, 11

sè jīng zhǐ yí 涩精止遗, astringing essence and checking seminal emission and enuresis, 11

sè kě qù tuō 涩可去脱, astringent [medicinals] can eliminate desertion, 11

sè mài 涩脉, rough pulse, 509

sè yìn sāi yòng 塞因塞用, treating the stopped by stopping, 627

sè zé 色泽, complexion, 92

Sea Source, *hǎi quán* 海泉, 37, 158, 174, 348, 607

seal's genitals, *hǎi gǒu shèn* 海狗肾, Callorhini seu Phocae Testis et Penis, 511

Second Variant Qi-Righting Powder, *èr jiā jiǎn zhèng qì sǎn* 二加减正气散, 732

Secret Treasure of the Orchid Chamber (*lán shì mì cáng*) 兰室秘藏, 1276, Lǐ Gǎo 李杲 [Dōng-Yuán 东垣], 393

Sedi Sarmentosi Herba, *shí zhǐ jiǎ* 石指甲, hanging stonecrop, 68, 357, 700, 721

selaginella, *juǎn bǎi* 卷柏, Selaginellae Herba, 724

Selaginellae Herba, *juǎn bǎi* 卷柏, selaginella, 724

semiaquilegia tuber, *tiān kuí zǐ* 天葵子, Semiaquilegiae Tuber, 68, 721

Semiaquilegiae Tuber, *tiān kuí zǐ* 天葵子, semiaquilegia tuber, 68, 721

Senecionis Scandentis Herba, *qiān lǐ guāng* 千里光, climbing groundsel, 68, 721

senna, *fān xiè yè* 番泻叶, Sennae Folium, 84, 460, 722

Sennae Folium, *fān xiè yè* 番泻叶, senna, 84, 460, 722

Sepiae seu Sepiellae Os, *hǎi piāo xiāo* 海螵蛸, cuttlefish bone, 478, 502, 511, 518, 572, 581, 727

Sepiae seu Sepiellae Os Calcinatum, *duàn wū zéi gǔ* 煅乌贼骨, calcined cuttlefish bone, 57, 334

septicemia*, 76

serissa, *bái mǎ gǔ* 白马骨, Serissae Herba, 68, 721

Serissae Herba, *bái mǎ gǔ* 白马骨, serissa, 68, 721

Serpentis Exuviae, *shé tuì* 蛇蜕, snake slough, 98, 139, 722

sesame oil, *má yóu* 麻油, Sesami Seminis Oleum, 51

Sesami Semen Atrum, *hēi zhī má* 黑脂麻, black sesame, 28, 108, 127, 398, 593, 727

Sesami Seminis Oleum, *má yóu* 麻油, sesame oil, 51

Seven Pinches Powder, *qī lí sǎn* 七厘散, 137, 138, 337, 737

Seven Qi Decoction, *qī qì tāng* 七气汤, 485

Seven-Gem Powder, *qī zhēn sǎn* 七珍散, 453

Seven-Ingredient Ovate Atractylodes Powder, *qī wèi bái zhú sǎn* 七味白术散, 600, 608, 741

Seven-Jewel Beard-Blackening Elixir, *qī bǎo měi rán dān* 七宝美髯丹, 4, 742

Seven-Jewel Powder, *qī bǎo sǎn* 七宝散, 500, 732

Sevenfold Processed Cyperus Pill, *qī zhì xiāng fù wán* 七制香附丸, 36, 484

shā 痧, sand, 512

shā chóng 杀虫, killing worms, 336

shā dú 痧毒, sand toxin, 512

shā jīn 痧筋, sand veins, 512

shā kuài 痧块, sand lump, 512

shā lín 砂淋, sand strangury, 512

shā qì 痧气, sand qi, 512

shā rén 砂仁 amomum, Amomi Semen seu Fructus, 10, 45, 80, 103, 105, 141, 224, 257, 437, 443, 450, 454, 512, 561, 564, 625, 669, 722

shā shēn 沙参 adenophora/glehnia, Adenophorae seu Glehniae Radix, 88, 108, 175, 310, 395, 398, 416, 515, 565, 581, 589, 593, 625, 679, 686, 727

shā shēn mài dōng tāng 沙参麦冬汤, Adenophora/Glehnia and Ophiopogon Decoction, 72, 108, 181, 237, 387, 398, 416, 607, 646, 714, 734

shā shí lín 砂石淋, sand strangury, 512

shā táng 沙糖 granulated sugar, Saccharon Granulatum, 511

shā yuàn zǐ 沙苑子 complanate astragalus seed, Astragali Complanati Semen, 11, 297, 584, 593, 727

shā zhàng 痧胀, sand distention, 512

shān cí gū 山慈姑 shancigu, Shancigu Bulbus, 68, 291, 544, 685, 721

shān dào nián hāo 山道年蒿 Levant wormseed flower and leaf, Artemisiae Cinae Flos et Folium, 183, 509

shān dòu gēn 山豆根 bushy sophora, Sophorae Subprostratae Radix, 68, 420, 721

shān gēn 山根, mountain root, 399

shān kuò 山廓, mountain rampart, 399

shān lán zhàng qì 山岚瘴气, mountain forest miasmic qi, 399

shān yáng jiǎo 山羊角 goral horn, Naemorhedi Goral Cornu, 54, 726

shān yào 山药 dioscorea, Dioscoreae Rhizoma, 12, 47, 141, 175, 223, 251, 267, 308, 496, 504, 563, 564, 572, 574, 593, 596, 600, 615, 726

shān zhā 山楂 crataegus, Crataegi Fructus, 107, 141, 216, 217, 418, 420, 450, 499, 514, 548, 573, 606, 724

shān zhā tàn 山楂炭 charred crataegus, Crataegi Fructus Carbonisatus, 139 *shān zhī pí* 山栀皮 gardenia husk, Gardeniae Epicarpium, 234

shān zhī zǐ 山栀子 gardenia, Gardeniae Fructus, 20, 21, 67, 69–71, 81, 105, 116, 189, 230, 238, 263, 303, 310, 357, 386, 390, 414, 439, 462, 493, 500, 501, 526, 538, 539, 547, 548, 574, 577, 588, 589, 638, 656, 673, 714, 720

shān zhōng 膻中, CV-17, Chest Center, 8, 13, 19, 25, 26, 33, 34, 58, 64, 72, 81, 82, 87, 115, 118, 123, 127, 139, 141, 142, 146, 153, 156, 158, 164, 186, 202, 210, 223, 227, 228, 230, 235, 253, 261, 263, 265, 266, 269, 273, 274, 277, 280, 285, 302, 343, 349, 366, 379, 383, 385, 386, 418, 426, 427, 433–435, 437, 438, 443, 445, 448, 452, 462, 475, 477, 478, 480, 482–484, 499, 506, 513, 522, 537, 539, 570, 571, 578, 581, 587, 588, 614, 625, 629, 646, 648, 649, 656, 661, 665, 666, 668, 683, 715, 749

shān zhōng 膻中, chest center, 57

shān zhū yú 山茱萸 cornus, Corni Fructus, 11, 39, 47, 96, 175, 176, 310, 336, 352, 458, 467, 504, 518, 526, 548, 596, 709, 727

shǎn 熌, scalding, 513

shǎn cuò yāo tòng 闪挫腰痛, wrenched lumbus pain, 696

shǎn guàn 闪罐, flash-cupping, 209

shàn 疝, mounting, 399

shàn 疝, shan, 528

shàn cuàn néng zǒu 善窜能走, mobile and penetrating, 398

shàn jī 善饥, rapid hungering, 492

shàn jiǎ 疝瘕, mounting-conglomeration, 400

shàn jiǎ 瘕疝, conglomeration-mounting, 94

shàn qì 疝气, mounting qi, 400

shàn qì tòng 疝气痛, mounting qi pain, 400

shàn tài xī 善太息, frequent sighing, 229

shàn zǒu 善走, mobile, 398

shancigu, *shān cí gū* 山慈姑, Shancigu Bulbus, 68, 291, 544, 685, 721

Shancigu Bulbus, *shān cí gū* 山慈姑, shancigu, 68, 291, 544, 685, 721

shāng 伤, damage, 108

shāng 商, Shang, 528

shāng fēng 伤风, wind damage, 683

shāng fēng ké sòu 伤风咳嗽, wind damage cough, 684

shāng fēng ké sòu tūn jì 伤风咳嗽吞剂, Wind-Damage Cough Swill-Down Pill, 738

shāng hán 伤寒, cold damage, 78

shāng hán biǎo zhèng 伤寒表证, cold damage exterior pattern, 78

shāng hán lǐ zhèng 伤寒里证, cold damage interior pattern, 78

shāng hán lùn 伤寒论 (*On Cold Damage*), Eastern Hàn, Zhāng Jī 张机 [Zhòng-Jǐng 仲景], 9, 20, 25, 57, 78, 152, 157, 186, 242, 246, 247, 249, 254, 276, 279, 306, 322, 341, 344, 345, 383, 396, 412, 415, 427, 505, 506, 509, 510, 532, 534, 545, 567, 576, 583, 584, 628, 639, 652, 666, 680, 683, 692–694, 698

shāng hán míng lǐ lùn 伤寒明理论 (*Clear Rationale of Cold Damage*), 1156 (Jīn), Chéng Wú-Jǐ 成无己, 308

shāng hán quán shēng jí 伤寒全生集 (*Cold Damage Life-for-All Collection*), Míng, Táo Jié-Ān 陶节庵, 24

shāng hán xù shuǐ zhèng 伤寒蓄水证, cold damage water amassment pattern, 79

shāng hán xù xuè zhèng 伤寒蓄血证, cold damage blood amassment pattern, 78

shāng hán zá bìng lùn 伤寒杂病论 (*On Cold Damage and Miscellaneous Diseases*), Eastern Hàn, Zhāng Jī 张机 [Zhòng-Jǐng 仲景], 318, 658

shāng jīn 伤津, damage to liquid, 108

shāng jiǔ 伤酒, liquor damage, 348

shāng jiǔ tóu tòng 伤酒头痛, liquor damage headache, 349

shāng lù 商陆 phytolacca, Phytolaccae Radix, 460, 574, 722

shāng miàn shí 伤面食, noodle-type food damage, 413

shāng qiū 商丘, SP-5, Shang Hill, 63, 80, 84, 112, 115, 197, 210, 211, 237, 239, 290, 337, 342, 359, 452, 489, 520, 557, 656, 684, 693, 746

shāng qū 商曲, KI-17, Shang Bend, 748

shāng ròu shí 伤肉食, meat-type food damage, 388

shāng shī yāo tòng 伤湿腰痛, dampness damage lumbar pain, 113

shāng shī zhǐ tòng gāo 伤湿止痛膏, Dampness Damage Pain-Relieving Plaster, 745

shāng shī zì hàn 伤湿自汗, dampness damage spontaneous sweating, 114

shāng shí 伤食, food damage, 216

shāng shí tóu tòng 伤食头痛, food damage headache, 216

shāng shí xiè 伤食泻, food damage diarrhea, 216

shāng shǔ 伤暑, summerheat damage, 587

shāng yáng 伤阳, damage to yang, 108

shāng yáng 商阳, LI-1, Shang Yang, 14, 63, 75, 103, 112, 129, 147, 158, 184, 190, 277, 281, 283, 374, 398, 420, 438, 520, 546, 547, 561, 590, 611, 620, 746

shāng yīn 伤阴, damage to yin, 108

shāng zào ké sòu 伤燥咳嗽, dryness damage cough, 154

shàng 上, upper body, 639

shàng bāo xià chuí 上胞下垂, drooping of the upper eyelid, 150

shàng bìng qǔ xià 上病取下, treating upper body disease through the lower body, 627

shàng guān 上关, GB-3, Upper Gate, 194, 222, 253, 748

shàng hán xià rè 上寒下热, upper body cold and lower body heat, 639

shàng héng gǔ 上横骨, upper transverse bone, 640

shàng jiāo 上焦, upper burner, 640

shàng jiāo rú wù 上焦如雾, upper burner is like a mist, 640

shàng jiāo zhǔ nà 上焦主纳, upper burner governs intake, 640

shàng jù xū 上巨虚, ST-37, Upper Great Hollow, 2, 3, 15, 28, 29, 40, 70, 72, 73, 77, 78, 80, 89, 111, 117, 127, 164, 168, 174, 190, 197, 215–217, 226, 254, 276–278, 284, 294, 298, 302, 312, 318, 319, 338–340, 369, 396, 415, 426, 434, 477, 544, 581, 585, 589, 645–647, 656, 658, 664, 673, 683, 746

shàng lián 上廉, LI-9, Upper Ridge, 746

shàng liáo 上髎, BL-31, Upper Bone-Hole, 220, 747

shàng qì 上气, qi ascent, 476

shàng qiào 上窍, upper orifices, 640

shàng rè xià hán 上热下寒, upper body heat and lower body cold, 639

shàng wǎn 上脘, CV-13, Upper Stomach Duct, 4, 29, 87, 157, 222, 252, 390, 436, 578, 749

shàng xià pèi xué fǎ 上下配穴法, combining upper and lower body points, 91

shàng xiāo 上消, upper dispersion, 640

shàng xīng 上星, GV-23, Upper Star, 50, 62, 92, 120, 258, 260, 320, 348, 379, 405, 414, 415, 478, 495, 521, 544, 586, 654, 678, 685, 688, 749

shàng yán 上炎, flame upward, 209

shàng yán 上炎, upflame, 639

shàng zhōng xià tōng yòng tòng fēng fāng 上中下通用痛风方, Upper, Middle, and Lower Body General-Use Wind Pain Formula, 734

shāo 烧, burn, 51

shāo cún xìng 烧存性, burning preserving nature, 52

shāo cún xìng 烧存性, nature-preservative burning, 405

shāo shān huǒ 烧山火, burning mountain fire method, 51

shāo shāng 烧伤, burn, 51

sháo yào 芍药 peony, Paeoniae Radix, 11, 72, 255, 319, 493, 500, 704

sháo yào gān cǎo tāng 芍药甘草汤, Peony and Licorice Decoction, 415

sháo yào tāng 芍药汤, Peony Decoction, 110, 426, 731

shǎo qì 少气, shortage of qi, 529

shǎo shí 少食, reduced food intake, 496

shào chōng 少冲, HT-9, Lesser Surge, 25, 65, 73, 99, 147, 263, 264, 281, 294, 400, 420, 437, 455, 538, 547, 585, 747

shào fǔ 少府, HT-8, Lesser Mansion, 29, 65, 74, 117, 123, 147, 155, 156, 168, 180, 203, 241, 244, 261, 263, 264, 269, 281, 282, 292, 294, 296, 332, 333, 336, 364, 386, 391, 392, 400, 401, 415, 416, 436, 437, 456, 495, 516, 524, 542, 567, 572, 597, 613, 641, 642, 648, 649, 652, 654, 686–688, 700, 714, 716, 747

shào fù 少腹, lesser abdomen, 343

shào fù tòng 少腹痛, lesser-abdominal pain, 343

shào fù zhú yū tāng 少腹逐瘀汤, Lesser Abdomen Stasis-Expelling Decoction, 26, 32, 35, 36, 94, 737

shào hǎi 少海, HT-3, Lesser Sea, 138, 142, 515, 540, 637, 747

shào huǒ 少火, lesser fire, 343

shào shāng 少商, LU-11, Lesser Shang, 5, 14, 62, 63, 66, 73, 90, 92, 103, 129, 147, 149, 156, 158, 184, 190, 201–203, 207, 216, 237, 261, 277, 280–283, 285, 291, 301, 348, 374, 378, 386, 394, 405, 414–416, 420, 438, 495, 501, 515, 519, 520, 522, 547, 569, 611, 620, 649, 685–688, 703, 715, 746

shào yáng 少阳, lesser yang, 343

shào yáng bìng 少阳病, lesser yang disease, 343

shào yáng jīng 少阳经, lesser yang channel, 343

shào yáng tóu tòng 少阳头痛, lesser yang headache, 344

shào yīn 少阴, lesser yin, 344

shào yīn bìng 少阴病, lesser yin disease, 344

shào yīn jīng 少阴经, lesser yin channel, 344

shào yīn tóu tòng 少阴头痛, lesser yin headache, 345

shào zé 少泽, SI-1, Lesser Marsh, 227, 228, 252, 386, 420, 513, 522, 542, 654, 747

shaved cinnamon bark, *guì xīn* 桂心, Cinnamomi Cortex Rasus, 242, 343

shé 舌, tongue, 615

shé biān 舌边, tongue margins, 619

shé biān chǐ hén 舌边齿痕, dental impressions on the margins of the tongue, 122

shé chàn 舌颤, trembling tongue, 627

shé chuáng zǐ 蛇床子 cnidium seed, Cnidii Monnieri Fructus, 116, 225, 424, 468, 516, 709, 712, 728

shé chuáng zǐ chōng xǐ jì 蛇床子冲洗剂, Cnidium Seed Rinse, 745

shé chuáng zǐ sǎn 蛇床子散, Cnidium Seed Powder, 112, 240, 468, 513, 516, 744

shé dàn 舌淡, pale tongue, 426

shé duǎn 舌短, contracted tongue, 97

shé hóng 舌红, red tongue, 496

shé jiǎn (jiǎn) 舌謇（蹇）, sluggish tongue, 541

shé jiàng 舌绛, crimson tongue, 105

shé jùn 舌菌, tongue mushroom, 619

shé liè 舌裂, fissured tongue, 204

shé lín 蛇鳞, snake scales, 543

shé má 舌麻, numbness of the tongue, 417

shé méi 蛇莓 snake strawberry, Duchesneae Herba, 68, 721

shé miàn rú jìng 舌面如镜, mirror-like tongue, 396

shé nèn 舌嫩, tender-soft tongue, 605

shé nǜ 舌衄, spontaneous bleeding of the tongue, 566

shé pàng 舌胖, enlarged tongue, 174

shé qǐ máng cì 舌起芒刺, prickly tongue, 463

shé qiáng 舌强, stiff tongue, 572

shé shàng qǐ máng cì 舌上起芒刺, prickly tongue, 463

shé shé 蛇舌, snake tongue, 543

shé shēn 蛇身, snake body, 543

shé shén 舌神, tongue spirit, 619

shé shēng pào 舌生泡, tongue blister, 615

shé shī 蛇虱, snake lice, 543

shé shòu biě 舌瘦瘪, shrunken tongue, 530

shé tāi 舌苔, tongue coating, 617

shé tāi gān zào 舌苔干燥, dry tongue fur, 158

shé tāi jiāo huáng 舌苔焦黄, burnt-yellow tongue fur, 52

shé tǐ 舌体, tongue body, 615

shé tǐ 蛇体, snake body, 543

shé tuì 蛇蜕 snake slough, Serpentis Exuviae, 98, 139, 722

shé wāi (kuāi) 舌歪, deviated tongue, 125

shé wéi xīn miáo 舌为心苗, tongue is the sprout of the heart, 619

shé wěi 舌痿, limp tongue, 347

shé yán 舌岩, tongue rock, 619

shé zhěn 舌诊, tongue examination, 617

shé zhí 舌质, tongue body, 615

shé zhí nèn hung 舌质嫩红, tender-red tongue, 605

shé zǐ 舌紫, purple tongue, 474

shé zòng 舌纵, protracted tongue, 468

shě mài cóng zhèng 舍脉从证, precedence of signs over the pulse, 458

shě tāi 舌苔, tongue fur, 617

shě zhèng cóng mài 舍证从脉, precedence of pulse over signs, 458

shè 摄, contain, 97

shè 射, shoot, 529

shè gān 射干 belamcanda, Belamcandae Rhizoma, 68, 368, 480, 611, 686, 688, 721

shè gān má huáng tāng 射干麻黄汤, Belamcanda and Ephedra Decoction, 87, 663, 677, 739

shè nà shèn qì 摄纳肾气, promoting absorption of qi by the kidney, 467

shè xiāng 麝香 musk, Moschus, 98, 243, 392, 398, 420, 449, 726

shè xuè 摄血, containing the blood, 97

shēn fù lóng mǔ tāng 参附龙牡汤, Ginseng, Aconite, Dragon Bone, and Oyster Shell Decoction, 59, 232, 735

shēn fù tāng 参附汤, Ginseng and Aconite Decoction, 27, 59, 62, 83, 84, 232, 335, 448, 629, 631, 690, 699, 702, 713, 735

shēn jiè sǎn 参蚧散, Ginseng with Gecko Powder, 335, 741

shēn jīn cǎo 伸筋草 ground pine, Lycopodii Clavati Herba cum Radice, 140, 569, 722

shēn jīn téng 伸筋藤 Chinese tinospora, Tinosporae Sinensis Caulis, 140, 722

shēn líng bái zhú sǎn 参苓白术散, Ginseng, Poria (Hoelen), and Ovate Atractylodes Powder, 163, 197, 237, 238, 393, 395, 486, 557, 558, 562–565, 601, 679, 741

shēn lú yǐn 参芦饮, Ginseng Tops Beverage, 170, 743

shēn mài 申脉, BL-62, Extending Vessel, 90, 93, 178, 255, 288, 296, 330, 341, 366, 425, 440, 519, 567, 690, 701, 747

shēn rè 身热, generalized heat [effusion], 240

shēn rè 身热, hot body, 292

shēn rè bù (wài) yáng 身热不（外）扬, unsurfaced heat, 638

shēn rè qǐ fú 身热起伏, fluctuating generalized heat [effusion], 213

shēn shé 伸舌, extended tongue, 183

shēn sū yǐn 参苏饮, Ginseng and Perilla Beverage, 47, 51, 428, 517, 730

shēn tǐ chén zhòng 身体沉重, heavy body, 286

shēn tòng 身痛, generalized pain, 240

shēn tòng zhú yū tāng 身痛逐瘀汤, Generalized Pain Stasis-Expelling Decoction, 138, 737

shēn zhě zhèn qì tnag1 参赭镇气汤, Codonopsis and Hematite Qi-Settling Decoction, 736

shēn zhòng 身重, generalized heaviness, 240

shēn zhòng 身重, heavy body, 286

shēn zhù 身柱, GV-12, Body Pillar, 14, 15, 61, 74, 75, 201, 296, 366, 383, 427, 677, 683, 693, 749

shén 神, spirit, 550

shén bù shǒu shè 神不守舍, spirit failing to keep to its abode, 551

shén cáng 神藏, KI-25, Spirit Storehouse, 748

shén dào 神道, GV-11, Spirit Path, 749

shén fēng 神封, KI-23, Spirit Seal, 748

shén gāo 神膏, spirit jelly, 551

shén hūn 神昏, clouded spirit, 75

shén mén 神门, HT-7, Spirit Gate, 5, 6, 11, 19, 25, 29–31, 35, 39, 41, 43, 58, 75, 87–91, 99, 113, 117, 123, 129, 147, 153, 155, 159, 160, 162, 168, 177, 178, 180, 203, 210, 223, 230, 232, 235, 236, 261, 263–272, 274, 275, 281, 282, 294, 296, 297, 301, 302, 308, 330, 331, 333, 335, 336, 345, 365, 386, 392, 410, 413, 416, 418, 420, 434, 436, 437, 448, 449, 451, 452, 457, 461, 467, 478, 484, 488, 514, 521, 524–526, 537, 548, 551, 572, 589–591, 594, 597, 604, 610, 613, 614, 638, 642, 648, 649, 651, 652, 655, 661, 665, 668, 673, 675, 686, 687, 694, 700, 701, 714, 716, 747

shén míng 神明, spirit light, 551

shén nóng běn cǎo jīng 神农本草经 (*Divine Husbandman's Herbal Foundation Canon*), 241, 290, 609

shén pí 神疲, lassitude of spirit, 340

shén pí fá lì 神疲乏力, fatigued spirit and lack of strength, 195

shén pí fá lì 神疲乏力, lassitude of spirit and lack of strength, 340

shén qì 神气, spirit qi, 551

shén qì bù zú 神气不足, insufficiency of spirit qi, 310

shén qíng 神情, spirit-affect, 551

shén qū 神麴 medicated leaven, Massa Medicata Fermentata, 141, 216, 223, 287, 388, 418, 450, 499, 514, 573, 724

shén qū wán 神麴丸, Medicated Leaven Pill, 739

shén què 神阙, CV-8, Spirit Gate Tower, 74, 77, 78, 82–86, 105, 127, 152, 168, 212, 231, 232, 289, 314, 338, 342, 425, 448, 453, 489, 504, 521, 625, 631, 646, 651, 664, 690, 699, 709, 749

shén shuǐ 神水, spirit water, 551

shén sī bù shuǎng 神思不爽, ungratifying thought, 637

shén táng 神堂, BL-44, Spirit Hall, 747

shén tíng 神庭, GV-24, Spirit Court, 192, 219, 222, 702, 749

shén xī dān 神犀丹, Spirit-Like Rhinoceros Horn Elixir, 6, 65, 69, 388, 740

shén xiān huó mìng tāng 神仙活命汤, Spirit Immortal Life-Giving Decoction, 129

shén xiào huáng qí tāng 神效黄芪汤, Wondrous Effect Astragalus Decoction, 210, 489, 564

shén yìng jīng 神应经 (*Wondrous Response Canon*), Míng, Chén Huì 陈会, 180

shén yìng xiāo fēng sǎn 神应消风散, Wondrous Response Wind-Dispersing Powder, 417, 431

shén yìng yǎng zhēn dān 神应养真丹, Wondrous Response True-Nourishing Elixir, 243

shéň zhì 神志, spirit-mind, 551

shén zhì hūn hú 神志昏糊, clouded spirit-mind, 75

shén zhì hūn luàn 神志昏乱, confused spirit-mind, 93

shén zhū 神珠, spirit ball, 551

shén zhú sǎn 神术散, Wondrous Atractylodes Powder, 218, 729, 732

shèn 肾, KI, 324

shèn 肾, kidney, 324

shèn 渗, percolate, 430

shèn bì 肾痹, kidney impediment, 328

shèn bìng 肾病, kidney disease, 325

shèn bù nà qì 肾不纳气, qi absorption failure, 475

shèn bù nà qì 肾气, kidney failing to absorb qi, 326

shèn cáng jīng 肾藏精, kidney stores essence, 330

shèn cáng zhì 肾藏志, kidney stores mind, 331

shèn chōng zé suǐ shí 肾充则髓实, when the kidney is full, marrow is replete, 672

shèn chóng 肾虫, kidney worm, 334

shèn chóng bìng 肾虫病, kidney worm disease, 334

shèn chuǎn 肾喘, kidney panting, 329

shèn gān 肾疳, gan of the kidney, 237

shèn gān 肾疳, kidney gan, 327

shèn hé páng guāng 肾合膀胱, kidney is connected with the bladder, 328

shèn huǒ piān kàng 肾火偏亢, hyperactive kidney fire, 294

shèn jī 肾积, kidney accumulation, 325

shèn jiān dòng qì 肾间动气, stirring qi in the kidney region, 574

shèn jīng 肾经, kidney channel, 325

shèn jīng 肾精, kidney essence, 326

shèn jīng bù zú 肾精不足, insufficiency of kidney essence, 309

shèn jīng ké sòu 肾经咳嗽, kidney channel cough, 325

shèn jīng nüè 肾经疟, kidney channel malaria, 325

shèn jué tóu tòng 肾厥头痛, kidney reversal headache, 330

shèn kāi qiào yú ěr 肾开窍於耳, kidney opens at the ears, 329

shèn kāi qiào yú èr yīn 肾开窍於二阴, kidney opens at the two yin, 329

shèn ké 肾咳, kidney cough, 325

shèn kuī 肾亏, kidney depletion, 325

shèn mài chén 肾脉沉, kidney pulse is sunken, 329

shèn náng 肾囊, scrotum, 516

shèn náng fēng 肾囊风, kidney sac wind, 330

shèn náng fēng 肾囊风, scrotal wind, 516

shèn náng yōng 肾囊痈, scrotal welling-abscess, 516

shèn qì 肾气, kidney qi, 329

shèn qì bù gù 肾气不固, insecurity of kidney qi, 308

shèn qì tōng yú ěr 肾气通于耳, kidney qi flows to the ears, 329

shèn qì wán 肾气丸, Kidney Qi Pill, 46, 379, 441, 452, 512, 641, 647, 667, 742

shèn qì xū 肾气虚, kidney qi vacuity, 329

shèn qì yóu fēng 肾气游风, kidney qi wandering wind, 330

shèn qiào 肾窍, orifices of the kidney, 421

shèn shēng gǔ suǐ 肾生骨髓, kidney engenders bone and marrow, 326

shèn shū 肾俞, BL-23, Kidney Transport, 4, 11, 15, 16, 22, 23, 26, 27, 29, 36, 39, 41, 45, 47, 59–61, 64, 78, 80–86, 88, 89, 91, 94, 96, 105, 114, 115, 117, 119, 127, 137, 140, 147, 149, 151, 152, 156–158, 160, 163, 164, 167–169, 174, 175, 177, 180, 196, 199, 210, 222, 224, 225, 227–230, 239, 240, 256, 263, 265, 266, 268, 283, 288, 291, 292, 294, 296, 297, 301, 302, 308, 310, 312, 314, 318, 325, 326, 329, 331–337, 340, 342, 345, 347–349, 352, 355, 359, 360, 366, 368–370, 374, 379, 381, 385, 393, 401, 406, 410, 413, 415, 425, 426, 434, 449, 452–454, 456, 457, 461, 462, 465–467, 474, 477, 482, 484, 489, 495, 497, 500, 513, 515, 516, 518, 521, 523–525, 529, 534, 537, 538, 542, 547, 549, 559, 563, 567–569, 571, 579, 584, 586, 594–597, 600, 604, 607, 608, 612, 614, 630, 631, 636, 638, 640–643, 647–649, 651, 652, 654, 660–662, 664, 666, 668, 675, 684, 688, 690, 693, 703, 713–716, 747

shèn shuǐ 肾水, kidney water, 334

shèn shuǐ 肾水, kidney-water, 334

shèn shuǐ bù zú 肾水不足, insufficiency of kidney water, 310

shèn shī 渗湿, percolating dampness, 430

shèn wéi qì zhī běn 肾为气之本, kidney is the root of qi, 328

shèn wéi tuò 肾为唾, kidney forms spittle, 327

shèn wéi xiān tiān zhī běn 肾为先天之本, kidney is the root of earlier heaven, 328

shèn wěi 肾痿, kidney wilting, 334

shèn wù zào 肾恶燥, kidney is averse to dryness, 328

shèn xiāo 肾消, kidney dispersion, 326

shèn xiāo 肾哮, kidney wheezing, 334

shèn xiè 肾泄, kidney diarrhea, 325

shèn xū 肾虚, kidney vacuity, 331

shèn xū bù nà qì 肾虚不纳气, vacuous kidney failing to absorb qi, 653

shèn xū bù yùn 肾虚不孕, kidney vacuity infertility, 332

shèn xū dài xià 肾虚带下, kidney vacuity vaginal discharge, 333

shèn xū ěr lóng 肾虚耳聋, kidney vacuity deafness, 331

shèn xū ěr míng 肾虚耳鸣, kidney vacuity tinnitus, 333

shèn xū huá tāi 肾虚滑胎, kidney vacuity habitual miscarriage, 331

shèn xū jīng bì 肾虚经闭, kidney vacuity menstrual block, 332

shèn xū jīng xíng hòu qī 肾虚经行后期, kidney vacuity delayed menstruation, 331

shèn xū shuǐ fàn 肾虚水泛, kidney vacuity water flood, 334

shèn xū tóu tòng 肾虚头痛, kidney vacuity headache, 331

shèn xū xuàn yūn 肾虚眩晕, kidney vacuity dizziness, 331

shèn xū yá tòng 肾虚牙痛, kidney vacuity toothache, 333

shèn xū yāo tòng 肾虚腰痛, kidney vacuity lumbar pain, 332

shèn xū yí jīng 肾虚遗精, kidney vacuity seminal emission, 333

shèn xū yuè jīng guò shǎo 肾虚月经过少, kidney vacuity scant menstruation, 332

shèn yán 肾岩, kidney rock, 330

shèn yáng 肾阳, kidney yang, 334

shèn yáng shuāi wēi 肾阳衰微, debilitation of kidney yang, 119

shèn yáng xū 肾阳虚, kidney yang vacuity, 334

shèn yáng xū shuǐ fàn 肾阳虚水泛, kidney yang vacuity water flood, 335

shèn yīn kū hé 肾阴枯涸, desiccation of kidney yin, 124

shèn yīn 肾阴, kidney yin, 335

shèn yīn bù zú 肾阴不足, insufficiency of kidney yin, 310

shèn yīn kuī xū 肾阴亏虚, kidney yin depletion, 335

shèn yīn xū 肾阴虚, kidney yin vacuity, 336

shèn yīn yáng liáng xū 肾阴阳两虚, dual vacuity of kidney yin and yang, 160

shèn yīn, shèn yáng 肾阴、肾阳, kidney yin and kidney yang, 335

shèn yǔ páng guāng xiāng biǎo lǐ 肾与膀胱相表里, kidney stands in interior-exterior relationship with the bladder, 330

shèn zhàng 肾胀, kidney distention, 326

shèn zhě cóng zhī 甚者从之, severe conditions are treated by coaction, 527

shèn zhě shuǐ zàng, zhǔ jīn yè 肾者水脏，主津液, kidney is the water viscus; it governs fluids, 328

shèn zhě wèi zhī guān 肾者胃之关, kidney is the gate of the stomach, 328

shèn zhě, zuò qiáng zhī guān, jì qiǎo chū yān 肾者，作强之官，伎巧出焉, kidney holds the office of labor, whence agility emanates, 328

shèn zhī fǔ 肾之府, house of the kidney, 293

shèn zhǔ bì cáng 肾主闭藏, kidney governs storage, 327

shèn zhǔ ěr 肾主耳, kidney governs the ears, 327

shèn zhǔ gǔ, shēng suǐ 肾主骨，生髓, kidney governs the bones and engenders marrow, 327

shèn zhǔ jì qiǎo 肾主伎巧, kidney governs agility, 327

shèn zhǔ kāi hé 肾主开阖, kidney governs opening and closing, 327

shèn zhǔ kǒng 肾主恐, kidney governs fear, 327

shèn zhǔ nà qì 肾主纳气, kidney governs qi absorption, 327

shèn zhǔ shēng zhí 肾主生殖, kidney governs reproduction, 327

shèn zhǔ shuǐ 肾主水, kidney governs water, 327

shèn zhǔ xiān tiān 肾主先天, kidney governs earlier heaven, 327

shèn zhǔ zhé 肾主蛰, kidney governs hibernation, 327

shèn zhuó 肾着, kidney fixity, 326

shèn zhuó tāng 肾着汤, Kidney Fixity Decoction, 22, 326, 425, 733

shèn, qí chōng zài gǔ 肾，其充在骨, kidney, its fullness is in the bone, 329

shèn, qí huá zài fà 肾，其华在发, kidney, its bloom is in the hair [of the head], 328

shēng 生, crude, 105

shēng 生, engender, 174

shēng 生, raw, 492

shēng 生, unprocessed, 638

shēng 升, sheng, 529

shēng 升, upbear, 638

shēng bái sháo yào 生白芍药 raw white peony, Paeoniae Radix Alba Cruda, 256

shēng bàn xià 生半夏 raw pinellia, Pinelliae Tuber Crudum, 243, 464

shēng cǎo wū 生草乌 raw wild aconite, Aconiti Tsao-Wu-Tou Tuber Crudum, 460

shēng dà huáng 生大黄 raw rhubarb, Rhei Rhizoma Crudum, 430, 460, 676, 722

shēng dān 升丹 upborne elixir, Sublimatum Triplex, 383, 727

shēng dì huáng 生地黄 dried/fresh rehmannia, Rehmanniae Radix Exsiccata seu Recens, 19, 28, 30, 65, 70, 88, 108, 116, 122, 154, 174–176, 256, 259, 277, 298, 310, 390, 391, 399, 415, 416, 422, 450, 462, 467, 495, 508, 516, 519, 526, 577, 581, 584, 586, 595, 597, 601, 604, 655, 679

shēng dì yú 生地榆 raw sanguisorba, Sanguisorbae Radix Cruda, 338

shēng dòng 升动, upbearing and stirring, 638

shēng fú yào 升浮药, upfloater, 639

shēng fù sǎn 生附散, Raw Aconite Powder, 86

shēng gān cǎo 生甘草 raw licorice, Glycyrrhizae Radix Cruda, 17, 116, 175, 263, 310, 422, 439, 499, 516, 621

shēng guī bǎn 生龟版 raw tortoise plastron, Testudinis Plastrum Crudum, 415 *shēng huà tāng* 生化汤, Engendering Transformation Decoction, 182, 300, 447–450, 454, 455, 457, 503, 737

shēng huà zhī yuán 脾为生化之源, source of engendering transformation, 548

shēng huáng qí 生黄芪 raw astragalus, Astragali (seu Hedysari) Radix Cruda, 259

shēng jī 生肌, engendering flesh, 174

shēng jī sǎn 生肌散, Flesh-Engendering Powder, 187, 259, 385, 528, 540, 565, 744

shēng jī yù hóng gāo 生肌玉红膏, Flesh-Engendering Jade and Red Paste, 17, 187, 231, 259, 412, 540, 565, 744

shēng jì 升剂, upbearing formula, 638

shēng jiāng 生姜 fresh ginger, Zingiberis Rhizoma Recens, 11, 70, 84, 95, 128, 201, 230, 243, 255, 256, 319, 343, 358, 397, 417, 426, 443, 448, 454, 464, 500–502, 527, 547, 574, 578, 581, 661, 663, 681, 683, 720

shēng jiāng xiè xīn tāng 生姜泻心汤, Fresh Ginger Heart-Draining Decoction, 732

shēng jiàng 升降, bearing, 16

shēng jiàng fú chén 升降浮沉, bearing, 16

shēng jīn 生津, engendering liquid, 174

shēng jǔ 升举, upraise, 640

shēng kě qù jiàng 升可去降, upbearing [medicinals] can eliminate downbearing, 638

shēng lóng gǔ 生龙骨 crude dragon bone, Mastodi Ossis Fossilia Cruda, 225, 585

shēng má 升麻 cimicifuga, Cimicifugae Rhizoma, 17, 55, 334, 338, 339, 415, 454, 466, 546, 600, 638, 647, 653, 686, 699, 709, 712, 720

shēng má gāo 升麻膏, Cimicifuga Paste, 384

shēng má gé gēn tāng 升麻葛根汤, Cimicifuga and Pueraria Decoction, 198, 422, 729

shēng má huáng qí tāng 升麻黄芪汤, Gastrodia and Astragalus Decoction, 15

shēng má xiāo dú yǐn 升麻消毒饮, Cimicifuga Toxin-Dispersing Beverage, 705

shēng mài sǎn 生脉散, Pulse-Engendering Powder, 47, 59, 161, 175, 239, 265, 272, 376, 428, 455, 469, 502, 586, 651, 683, 702, 709, 742

shēng mò yào 生没药 raw myrrh, Myrrha Cruda, 138, 724

shēng mǔ lì 生牡蛎 crude oyster shell, Ostreae Concha Cruda, 54, 146, 225, 256, 726

shēng nán xīng 生南星 raw arisaema, Arisaematis Rhizoma Crudum, 243, 439, 460, 690

shēng pú huáng 生蒲黄 raw typha pollen, Typhae Pollen Crudum, 586

shēng rú zhuài jù 声如拽锯, sound like the rasping of a saw, 548

shēng shān zhī 生山栀 fresh gardenia, Gardeniae Fructus Recens, 116

shēng shí gāo 生石膏 crude gypsum, Gypsum Crudum, 67, 422, 720

shēng shí jué míng 生石决明 crude abalone shell, Haliotidis Concha Cruda, 146, 225, 585

shēng suǐ yù lín dān 生髓育麟丹, Marrow-Engendering Unicorn-Fostering Elixir, 513

shēng tí 升提, uplift, 639

shēng tí zhōng qì 升提中气, uplifting center qi, 639

shēng tiě luò yǐn 生铁落饮, Iron Flakes Beverage, 386, 437, 700, 739

shēng xī jiǎo sǎn 生犀角散, Raw Rhinoceros Horn Powder, 693

shēng xiàn tāng 升陷汤, Fall-Upbearing Decoction, 639, 741

shēng yáng chú shī fáng fēng tāng 升阳除湿防风汤, Yang-Upbearing Dampness-Eliminating Ledebouriella Decoction, 319

shēng yáng sàn huǒ tāng 升阳散火汤, Yang-Upbearing Fire-Dissipating Decoction, 46

shēng yáng yì wèi tāng 升阳益胃汤, Yang-Upbearing Stomach-Boosting Decoction, 73, 648, 741

shēng yīn 声音, voice, 657

shēng yīn sī yǎ 声音嘶哑, hoarse voice, 291

shěng fēng tāng 省风汤, Awake-From-Wind Decoction, 417

shèng 胜, prevalence, 463

shèng 盛, exuberance, 188

shèng jì zǒng lù 圣济总录 (*Sages' Aid Records*), 1111–1117 (Sòng), Government publication, 86

shèng qì 生气, vital qi, 657

shèng shī 胜湿, overcoming dampness, 422

shèng shī tāng 胜湿汤, Dampness-Overcoming Decoction, 599

shèng shuāi 盛衰, exuberance and debilitation, 188

shèng yù tāng 圣愈汤, Sagacious Cure Decoction, 39, 159, 741

shī 湿, damp, 109

shī 湿, dampness, 113

shī bì 湿痹, damp impediment, 112

shī chòu 尸臭, cadaverous odor, 53

shī chuāng 湿疮, damp sores, 116

shī cóng hán huà 湿从寒化, dampness forming with cold, 114

shī cóng rè huà 湿从热化, dampness forming with heat, 114

shī dú 湿毒, damp toxin, 117

shī dú chuāng 湿毒疮, damp toxin sore, 117

shī dú dài xià 湿毒带下, damp toxin vaginal discharge, 117

shī dú liú zhù 湿毒流注, damp toxin streaming sore, 117

shī dú xià xuè 湿毒下血, damp toxin precipitation of blood, 117

shī è rè fú 湿遏热伏, dampness trapping hidden heat, 114

shī huò luàn 湿霍乱, damp cholera, 109

shī jì 湿剂, moist formula, 398

shī jiǎo qì 湿脚气, damp leg qi, 112

shī jiè 湿疥, damp scab, 116

shī jīng 失精, seminal loss, 525

shī jìng 湿痉, damp tetany, 117

shī jué 尸厥, deathlike reversal, 119

shī ké 湿咳, damp cough, 109

shī kě qù kū 湿可去枯, moist [medicinals] can eliminate desiccation, 398

shī kùn pí tǔ 湿困脾土, dampness encumbering spleen-earth, 114

shī kùn pí yáng 湿困脾阳, dampness encumbering spleen yang, 114

shī làn 湿烂, damp ulceration, 118

shī mián 失眠, Insomnia, 333

shī mián 失眠, insomnia, 308

shī nüè 湿疟, damp malaria, 113

shī qì 失气, passing of flatus, 429

shī qiàn 失欠, yawning, 704

shī rè 湿热, damp-heat, 109

shī rè fù tòng 湿热腹痛, damp-heat abdominal pain, 110

shī rè huáng dǎn 湿热黄疸, damp-heat jaundice, 111

shī rè lì 湿热痢, damp-heat dysentery, 110

shī rè liú liàn qì fèn 湿热留恋气分, damp-heat lodged in the qi aspect, 111

shī rè liú liàn sān jiāo 湿热留恋三焦, damp-heat lodged in the triple burner, 111

shī rè nèi yùn 湿热内蕴, damp-heat brewing internally, 110

shī rè shàn 湿热疝, damp-heat mounting, 111

shī rè tiáo biàn 湿热条辨 (*Systematized Identification of Damp-Heat*), 1831 (Qīng), Xuē Xuě 薛雪, 659

shī rè tóu tòng 湿热头痛, damp-heat headache, 111

shī rè wěi 湿热痿, damp-heat wilting, 112

shī rè xià zhù 湿热下注, damp-heat pouring downward, 111

shī rè xià zhù 湿热下注, downpour of damp-heat, 146

shī rè xià zhù dà cháng 湿热下注大肠, damp-heat pouring down into the large intestine, 111

shī rè xià zhù dà cháng 湿热下注大肠, downpour of damp-heat into the large intestine, 146

shī rè xià zhù páng guāng 湿热下注膀胱, damp-heat pouring down into the bladder, 111

shī rè xià zhù páng guāng 湿热下注膀胱, downpour of damp-heat into the bladder, 146

shī rè xié tòng 湿热胁痛, damp-heat rib-side pain, 111

shī rè xuàn yūn 湿热眩晕, damp-heat dizziness, 110

shī rè xuiè 湿热泻, damp-heat diarrhea, 110

shī rè yāo tòng 湿热腰痛, damp-heat lumbar pain, 111

shī rè yí jīng 湿热遗精, damp-heat seminal emission, 112

shī rè yùn jié gān dǎn 湿热蕴结肝胆, damp-heat brewing in the liver and gallbladder, 110

shī rè yùn jié páng guāng 湿热蕴结膀胱, damp-heat brewing in the bladder, 110

shī rè yùn pí 湿热蕴脾, damp-heat brewing in the spleen, 110

shī rè zǔ zhì pí wèi 湿热阻滞脾胃, damp-heat obstructing the spleen and stomach, 111

shī róng 失荣, loss-of-luxuriance, 367

shī shén 失神, spiritlessness, 551

shī shēng bù yǔ 失声不语, loss of voice, 368

shī shèng zé rú xiè 湿胜则濡泻, when dampness prevails, there is soft stool diarrhea, 672

shī shèng zé yáng wēi 湿胜则阳微, when dampness prevails, yang is debilitated, 672

shī sōu 失溲, urinary incontinence, 640

shī sòu 湿嗽, damp cough, 109

shī tán 湿痰, damp phlegm, 115

shī tán jiǎo qì 湿痰脚气, damp phlegm leg qi, 115

shī tán liú zhù 湿痰流注, damp phlegm streaming sore, 115

shī tán wěi 湿痰痿, damp phlegm wilting, 116

shī tán xuàn yūn 湿痰眩晕, damp phlegm dizziness, 115

shī tán yāo tòng 湿痰腰痛, damp phlegm lumbar pain, 115

shī wēn 湿温, damp warmth, 118

shī xiǎn 湿癣, damp lichen, 112

shī xiào sǎn 失笑散, Sudden Smile Powder, 35, 59, 138, 212, 228, 447, 452, 571, 737

shī xiào wán 失笑丸, Sudden Smile Pill, 224, 732

shī xié 湿邪, dampness evil, 114

shī xiè 湿泻, damp diarrhea, 109

shī xīn fēng 失心风, lost heart wind, 368

shī xuè 失血, blood loss, 32

shī xuè xuàn yūn 失血眩晕, blood loss dizziness, 32

shī yāo tòng 湿腰痛, damp lumbar pain, 113

shī yīn 失音, loss of voice, 368

shī yīn bù yǔ 失音不语, loss of voice, 368

shī yíng 失营, loss-of-construction, 367

shī yù 湿郁, damp depression, 109

shī yù rè fú 湿郁热伏, depressed dampness and hidden (deep-lying) heat, 122

shī yù tāng 湿郁汤, Damp Depression Decoction, 109

shī zhǒng 湿肿, damp swelling, 116

shī zhòng 湿中, dampness stroke, 114

shī zhù 尸注, corpse influx, 100

shī zhuó 湿浊, damp turbidity, 118

shī zǔ 湿阻, damp obstruction, 115

shī zǔ qì fèn 湿阻气分, dampness obstructing the qi aspect, 114

shī zǔ qì fèn 湿阻气分, qi-aspect damp obstruction, 476

shī zǔ zhōng jiāo 湿阻中焦, center burner damp obstruction, 54

shī zǔ zhōng jiāo 湿阻中焦, dampness obstructing the center burner, 114

shí 食, food, 214

shí 实, repletion, 498

shí bì 实秘, repletion constipation, 498

shí bǔ wán 十补丸, Ten Supplements Pill, 742

shí bù xià 食不下, inability to get food down, 298

shí chāng pú 石菖蒲 acorus, Acori Rhizoma, 10, 122, 222, 223, 331, 420, 433, 476, 526, 540, 541, 625, 638, 673, 709, 722, 726 *shí chuǎn* 实喘, repletion panting, 499

shí dà gōng láo yè 十大功劳叶 mahonia, Mahoniae Folium, 67, 720

shí dào ái èr hào fāng 食道癌二号方, Esophageal Cancer No.2 Formula, 745

shí dào ái yī hào fāng 食道癌一号方, Esophageal Cancer No.1 Formula, 745

shí dòu 食窦, SP-17, Food Hole, 746

shí dú 时毒, seasonal toxin, 517

shí é 石蛾, stone moth, 581

shí è 实呃, repletion hiccough, 499

shí èr guān 十二官, twelve officials, 633

shí èr jì 十二剂, twelve formula types, 633

shí èr jīng bié 十二经别, twelve channel divergences, 633

shí èr jīng jīn 十二经筋, twelve channel sinews, 633

shí èr jīng mài 十二经脉, twelve channels, 633

shí èr jīng zhī hǎi 十二经之海, sea of the twelve channels, 517

shí èr jǐng xué 十二井穴, Twelve Well Points, 33, 63, 65, 69, 74, 76, 118, 147, 152, 279, 364, 403, 624, 665, 690, 694, 699

shí èr pí bù 十二皮部, twelve cutaneous regions, 633

shí èr yuán 十二原, twelve sources, 633

shí èr yuán xué 十二原穴, twelve source points, 633

shí gān 食疳, food gan, 217

shí gāo 石膏 gypsum, Gypsum, 49, 53, 65, 67, 70, 71, 110, 239, 259, 281, 319, 339, 412, 439, 460, 500, 546, 577, 588, 589, 688, 695, 699, 720

shí gāo tāng 石膏汤, Gypsum Decoction, 730

shí gāo zhī mǔ tāng 石膏知母汤, Gypsum and Anemarrhena Decoction, 587

shí guài mài 十怪脉, ten strange pulses, 606

shí guān 石关, KI-18, Stone Pass, 78, 664, 748

shí hòu kùn dùn 食后困顿, drowsiness after eating, 150

shí hú 石斛 dendrobium, Dendrobii Caulis, 65, 174, 175, 395, 511, 565, 581, 589, 593, 597, 600, 727

shí hú míng mù wán 石斛明目丸, Dendrobium Eye Brightener Pill, 742

shí hú yè guāng wán 石斛夜光丸, Dendrobium Night Vision Pill, 742

shí huī 石灰 limestone, Calx, 569, 620, 728

shí huī sǎn 十灰散, Ten Cinders Powder, 233

shí huī sǎn (wán) 十灰散（丸）, Ten Cinders Powder (Pill), 738

shí huī wán 十灰丸, Ten Cinders Pill, 569

shí huǒ 实火, repletion fire, 498

shí jī 食积, food accumulation, 215

shí jī fù tòng 食积腹痛, food accumulation abdominal pain, 215

shí jī ké sòu 食积咳嗽, food accumulation cough, 215

shí jī ǒu tù 食积呕吐, food accumulation vomiting, 215

shí jī tán sòu 食积痰嗽, food accumulation phlegm cough, 215

shí jī xié tòng 食积胁痛, food accumulation rib-side pain, 215

shí jì 十剂, ten formula types, 605

shí jiàn chuān 石见穿 Chinese sage, Salviae Chinensis Herba, 139, 725

shí jiǔ wèi 十九畏, nineteen fears, 411

shí jué 食厥, food reversal, 218

shí jué míng 石决明 abalone shell, Haliotidis Concha, 53, 54, 230, 495, 511, 538, 676, 726

shí jué míng sǎn 石决明散, Abalone Shell Powder, 195, 500, 740

shí ké 食咳, food cough, 215

shí láo gān huáng 食劳疳黄, food taxation gan yellowing, 218

shí lián zǐ 石莲子 lotus fruit, Nelumbinis Fructus, 82

shí lín 石淋, stone strangury, 582

shí liú huáng 石硫黄 sulfur, Sulphur, 98, 154, 171, 411, 458, 676, 727

shí liú pí 石榴皮 pomegranate rind, Granati Pericarpium, 183, 298, 318, 445, 518, 727

shí mài 实脉, replete pulse, 498

shí mén 石门, CV-5, Stone Gate, 8, 91, 431, 749

shí nüè 食疟, food malaria, 217

shí ǒu 食呕, food vomiting, 218

shí pí yǐn 实脾饮, Spleen-Firming Beverage, 28, 114, 151, 287, 301, 467, 559, 661, 666, 669, 703, 709, 716, 733

shí pǐ 实痞, repletion glomus, 498

shí qì 时气, seasonal qi, 517

shí quán dà bǔ tāng 十全大补汤, Perfect Major Supplementation Decoction, 26, 27, 40, 198, 412, 449, 451, 453, 503, 528, 540, 599, 615, 649, 653, 661, 709, 741

shí rè 实热, repletion heat, 499

shí rù jí tù 食入即吐, immediate vomiting of ingested food, 295

shí sān guǐ xué 十三鬼穴, Thirteen Ghost Points, 608

shí sān guǐ xué 十三鬼穴, thirteen ghost points, 695

shí shuǐ 石水, stone water, 582

shí sì jīng 十四经, fourteen channels, 226

shí sì jīng jīng xué 十四经经穴, fourteen-channel point, 226

shí sì jīng xué 十四经穴, fourteen-channel point, 226

shí tán 食痰, food-phlegm, 218

shí wéi 石韦 pyrrosia, Pyrrosiae Folium, 69, 107, 136, 723

shí wéi sǎn 石韦散, Pyrrosia Powder, 21, 68, 544, 733

shí wèi wēn dǎn tāng 十味温胆汤, Ten-Ingredient Gallbladder-Warming Decoction, 236, 739

shí wèi xiāng rú yǐn 十味香薷饮, Ten-Ingredient Elsholtzia Beverage, 730

shí wèn 十问, ten questions, 606

shí wǔ luò 十五络, fifteen network vessels, 199

shí xiāng wán 十香丸, Ten Fragrances Pill, 736

shí xié 实邪, repletion evil, 498

shí xié 时邪, seasonal evil, 517

shí xiè 食泄, food diarrhea, 217

shí xíng 时行, seasonal current, 517

shí xíng bào ké 时行暴咳, fulminant seasonal cough, 233

shí xíng hán yì 时行寒疫, seasonal cold epidemic, 517

shí xíng sòu 时行嗽, seasonal cough, 517

shí xuān 十宣, Ten Diffusing Points, 6, 25, 70, 74, 75, 88, 92, 111, 156, 197, 283, 384, 448, 450, 455, 521, 547, 586, 589–591, 687, 693, 694, 702

shí yán 石盐 salt, Sal, 401

shí yàn dān 石燕丹, Spirifer Fossil Elixir, 195

shí yī wèi wēn dǎn tāng 十一味温胆汤, Eleven-Ingredient Gallbladder-Warming Decoction, 739

shí yì 时疫, seasonal epidemic, 517

shí yì lì 时疫痢, seasonal epidemic dysentery, 517

shí yù 食郁, food depression, 217

shí yù 食欲, appetite, 10

shí yù bù zhèn 食欲不振, poor appetite, 446

shí yù jiǎn tuì 食欲减退, poor appetite, 446

shí yù tāng 食郁汤, Food Depression Decoction, 217

shí zǎo tāng 十枣汤, Ten Jujubes Decoction, 182, 214, 441, 732

shí zé xiè qí zǐ 实则泻其子, repletion is treated by draining the child, 499

shí zé xiè zhī 实则泻之, repletion is treated by draining, 499

shí zhàng 食胀, food distention, 217

shí zhàng 实胀, repletion distention, 498

shí zhēn tāng 十珍汤, Ten-Gem Decoction, 495

shí zhèng 实证, repletion pattern, 499

shí zhǐ jiǎ 石指甲 hanging stonecrop, Sedi Sarmentosi Herba, 68, 357, 700, 721

shí zhì 食滞, food stagnation, 218

shí zhì wǎn (guǎn) tòng 食滞脘痛, food stagnation stomach duct pain, 218

shí zhì wèi wǎn (guǎn) 食滞胃脘, food stagnating in the stomach duct, 218

shí zhōng jiā xū 实中夹虚, repletion with vacuity complication, 500

shí zhǒng 实肿, repletion swelling, 500

shí zhòng 食中, food stroke, 218

shí zǐ jì ní tāng 石子荠苨汤, Gypsum and Apricot-Leaved Adenophora Decoction, 508

shí zì jiǔ 十字灸, cross moxa, 80, 105, 109, 647

shǐ 使, courier, 102

shǐ 矢, stool, 582

shǐ 屎, stool, 582

shǐ guó gōng jìn jiǔ fāng 史国公浸酒方, Statesman Shi's Wine-Steeped Formula, 288, 734

shǐ jūn zǐ 使君子 quisqualis, Quisqualis Fructus, 182, 183, 445, 509, 724

shǐ jūn zǐ dà huáng fěn 使君子大黄粉, Quisqualis and Rhubarb Powder, 737

shǐ jūn zǐ sǎn 使君子散, Quisqualis Powder, 696, 737

shǐ qì 矢气, fecal qi, 197

shǐ qì 矢气, flatus, 210

shì bǐng 柿饼 dried persimmon, Kaki Fructus Exsiccatus, 231

shì chì rú bái 视赤如白, seeing red as white, 519

shì dì 柿蒂 persimmon calyx, Kaki Calyx, 493, 499, 649, 724

shì dì tāng 柿蒂汤, Persimmon Decoction, 736

shì qián sǎn 柿钱散, Gingerless Clove and Persimmon Powder, 736

shì shí yì wù 嗜食异物, perverted appetite, 431

shì shuāng 柿霜 persimmon frost, Kaki Saccharum, 231

shì shuì 嗜睡, somnolence, 545

shì wù yì sè 视物易色, seeing things in changed colors, 519

shì yī 视衣, visual lining, 657

shì yī wéi èr 视一为二, double vision, 145

shì yī wéi èr 视一为二, seeing one as two, 519

shì zhān hūn miǎo 视瞻昏渺, indistinct vision, 299

shì zhān yǒu sè 视瞻有色, tinted vision, 614

Shielding Brightness, *yì míng* 翳明, 586

shingles*, 241

shock*, 124, 195, 232

    hemorrhagic, 478

    postpartum, 448

shōu 收, contraction, 97

shōu yǐn 收引, contracture and tautness, 97

shóu 熟, prepared, 463

shǒu ér bù zǒu 守而不走, static, 570

shǒu fǎ 手法, manipulation, 387

shǒu jué yīn xīn bāo jīng 手厥阴心包经, PC, 429

shǒu jué yīn xīn bāo jīng 手厥阴心包经, hand reverting yin pericardium channel, 253

shǒu niān sǎn 手拈散, Instant Relief Powder, 571, 737

shǒu sā yí niào 手撒遗尿, limp hands and enuresis, 347

shǒu sān lǐ 手三里, LI-10, Arm Three Li, 103, 139, 142, 171, 211, 515, 520, 540, 679, 746

shǒu sān yáng jīng 手三阳经, three yang channels of the hand, 610

shǒu sān yīn jīng 手三阴经, three yin channels of the hand, 611

shǒu shào yáng sān jiāo jīng 手少阳三焦经, TB, 604

shǒu shào yáng sān jiāo jīng 手少阳三焦经, hand lesser yang triple burner channel, 252

shǒu shào yīn xīn jīng 手少阴心经, HT, 293

shǒu shào yīn xīn jīng 手少阴心经, hand lesser yin heart channel, 253

shǒu tài yáng xiǎo cháng jīng 手太阳小肠经, SI, 531

shǒu tài yáng xiǎo cháng jīng 手太阳小肠经, hand greater yang small intestine channel, 252

shǒu tài yīn fèi jīng 手太阴肺经, LU, 369

shǒu tài yīn fèi jīng 手太阴肺经, hand greater yin lung channel, 252

shǒu wū yán shòu dān 首乌延寿丹, Flowery Knotweed Life-Extending Elixir, 245, 251

shǒu wǔ lǐ 手五里, LI-13, (Arm) Five Li, 746

shǒu yáng míng dà cháng jīng 手阳明大肠经, LI, 345

shǒu yáng míng dà cháng jīng 手阳明大肠经, hand yang brightness large intestine channel, 254

shǒu zú hán 手足寒, cold extremities, 81

shǒu zú hàn 手足汗, sweating hands and feet, 599

shǒu zú jué lěng 手足厥冷, reversal cold of the extremities, 505

shǒu zú jué nì 手足厥逆, reverse-flow of the extremities, 506

shǒu zú nì lěng 手足逆冷, counterflow cold of the extremities, 102

shǒu zú qīng lěng 手足清冷, cold extremities, 81

shǒu zú xīn rè 手足心热, heat in the (heart of the) palms and soles, 280

shòu chéng zhī guān 受盛之官, office of reception, 419

shòu pí jiān 寿脾煎, Spleen Longevity Brew, 537

shòu shì bǎo yuán 寿世保元 (*Prolonging Life and Preserving the Origin*), 17th century (Míng), Gōng Tíng-Xián 龚廷贤, 199

shòu tāi wán 寿胎丸, Fetal Longevity Pill, 199, 331, 574, 742

shòu tái gǔ 寿台骨, longevity platform bone, 366

Shoulder Front, *jiān qián*, 530

shū 腧（俞、输）, acupuncture point, 6

shū 疏, course, 102

shū 舒, soothe, 545

shū biǎo 疏表, coursing the exterior, 103

shū biǎo huà shī 疏表化湿, coursing the exterior and transforming dampness, 103

shū cì 输刺, transport needling, 625

shū fēng 疏风, coursing wind, 103

shū fēng xiè rè 疏风泄热, coursing wind and discharging heat, 103

shū fēng yǎng xuè tāng 疏风养血汤, Wind-Coursing Blood-Nourishing Decoction, 740

shū fǔ 俞府, KI-27, Transport Mansion, 748

shū gān 疏肝, coursing the liver, 103

shū gān 舒肝, soothe the liver, 545

shū gān jiě yù 疏肝解郁, coursing the liver and resolving depression, 103

shū gān jiě yù tāng 疏肝解郁汤, Liver-Coursing Depression-Resolving Decoction, 353, 736

shū gān lǐ qì 疏肝理气, coursing the liver and rectifying qi, 103

shū gān sǎn 疏肝散, Liver-Coursing Powder, 356

shū gān wán 舒肝丸, Liver-Soothing Pill, 102, 736

shū gēn bái pí 樗根白皮 ailanthus root bark, Ailanthi Altissimae Radicis Cortex, 572

shū jīn huó xuè piàn 舒筋活血片, Sinew-Soothing Blood-Quickening Tablet, 737

shū jīn huó xuè xǐ fāng 舒筋活血洗方, Sinew-Soothing Blood-Quickening Wash Formula, 745

shū jīn tāng 舒筋汤, Sinew-Soothing Decoction, 105, 734

shū mù pèi xué fǎ 俞募配穴法, combining front and back points, 88

shū mù pèi xué fǎ 俞募配穴法, combining transport and alarm points, 91

shū qì sǎn 舒气散, Qi-Smoothing Powder, 736

shū sàn fēng rè 疏散风热, coursing and dissipating wind-heat, 102

shū sàn wài fēng 疏散外风, coursing and dissipating external wind, 102

shū shù pí pí 樗树根皮丸, Ailanthus Root Bark Pill, 572

shū xué 俞穴, transport point, 625

shū xué 腧穴, transport point, 625

shū xué 输穴, stream point, 584

shū xué 输穴, transport point, 625

shū yù lǐ qì 疏郁理气, coursing depression and rectifying qi, 102

shū záo yǐn zi 疏凿饮子, Coursing and Piercing Drink, 302

shū zhāng jìn zhēn fǎ 舒张进针法, skin-spreading needle insertion, 535

shú dì huáng 熟地黄 cooked rehmannia, Rehmanniae Radix Conquita, 28, 37, 39, 47, 88, 140, 161, 175, 225, 298, 310, 333, 458, 459, 467, 504, 526, 537, 570, 584, 593, 595, 596, 620, 651, 727

shú fù zǐ 熟附子 cooked aconite, Aconiti Tuber Laterale Conquitum, 11, 48, 660, 663, 723

shǔ 暑, summerheat, 587

shǔ 属, home, 292

shǔ bìng 暑病, summerheat disease, 588

shǔ fēng 暑风, summerheat-wind, 591

shǔ fēng chéng jīng 暑风成惊, summerheat-wind turning into fright, 591

shǔ hàn 蜀汉, Shu Han, 531

shǔ huò luàn 暑霍乱, summerheat cholera, 587

shǔ jìng 暑痉, summerheat tetany, 591

shǔ jué 暑厥, summerheat reversal, 590

shǔ ké 暑咳, summerheat cough, 587

shǔ lì 暑痢, summerheat dysentery, 588

shǔ nüè 暑疟, summerheat malaria, 590

shǔ qī 蜀漆 dichroa leaf, Dichroae Folium, 170, 197, 510, 727

shǔ rè 暑热, summerheat-heat, 589

shǔ rè xié tòng 暑热胁痛, summerheat-heat rib-side pain, 589

shǔ shā 暑痧, summerheat sand, 590

shǔ shī 暑湿, summerheat-damp, 587

shǔ shī liú zhù 暑湿流注, summerheat-damp streaming sore, 588

shǔ shī xuàn yūn 暑湿眩晕, summerheat-damp dizziness, 588

shǔ shī zhèng qì wán 暑湿正气丸, Summerheat-Damp Qi-Righting Pill, 732

shǔ wēn 暑温, summerheat warmth, 591

shǔ xī 鼠蹊, groin, 249

shǔ xián 暑痫, summerheat epilepsy, 589

shǔ xiè 暑泄, summerheat diarrhea, 588

shǔ yù wán 薯蓣丸, Dioscorea Pill, 741

shù 束, fetter, 199

shù dí 漱涤, mouth wash, 401

shù gǔ 束骨, BL-65, Bundle Bone, 89, 259, 747

shù gǔ 束骨, bundle bone, 51

shù kòu 漱口, mouth wash, 401

shù zhuì tāi 数坠胎, habitual miscarriage, 251

shuāi 衰, debilitation, 119

shuāi jié 衰竭, exhaust, 181

shuāi zhě bǔ zhī 衰者补之, debility is treated by supplementing, 119

shuài gǔ 率谷, GB-8, Valley Lead, 89, 219, 258, 260, 288, 344, 506, 519, 748

shuāng 霜, frost, 231

shuāng jiě tōng shèng sǎn 双解通圣散, Double Resolution Sage-Inspired Powder, 330

shuāng shǒu jìn zhēn fǎ 双手进针法, two-handed needle insertion, 635

shuǐ 水, water, 665

shuǐ bù hán mù 水不涵木, water failing to moisten wood, 667

shuǐ bù huà qì 水不化气, water failing to transform into qi, 667

shuǐ bù jì huǒ 水不济火, water failing to help fire, 667

shuǐ chuǎn 水喘, water panting, 667

shuǐ dào 水道, ST-28, Waterway, 94, 418, 667, 746

shuǐ dòu 水痘, chicken pox, 59

shuǐ dú 水毒, water toxin, 669

shuǐ fàn wán 水泛丸, water pill, 668

shuǐ fēi 水飞, water-grinding, 667

shuǐ fēn 水分, CV-9, Water Divide, 37, 105, 109, 117, 168, 182, 224, 228, 301, 334, 335, 379, 418, 457, 485, 537, 559, 600, 608, 612, 661–663, 666–668, 694, 703, 716, 749

shuǐ gōu 水沟, GV-26, Water Trough, 4, 6, 33, 69, 71, 74, 75, 86, 117, 118, 147, 156, 178, 203, 212, 218, 260, 263, 281, 282, 296, 343, 366, 384, 386, 392, 400, 437, 442, 478, 482, 485, 504, 521, 522, 567, 589, 590, 624, 631, 646, 655, 690, 694, 699, 703, 709, 749

shuǐ gǔ 水鼓, water drum, 666

shuǐ gǔ 水臌, water drum distention, 667

shuǐ gǔ 水谷, food, 214

shuǐ gǔ 水谷, grain and water, 245

shuǐ gǔ 水蛊, water gu, 667

shuǐ gǔ bù bié 水谷不别, nonseparation of grain and water, 413

shuǐ gǔ bù huà 水谷不化, nontransformation of grain and water, 413

shuǐ gǔ zhī hǎi 水谷之海, sea of grain and water, 517

shuǐ gǔ zhī jīng wēi 水谷之精微, essence of grain and water, 179

shuǐ hán shè fèi 水寒射肺, water-cold shooting into the lung, 666

shuǐ huǒ bù jì 水火不济, fire and water failing to aid each other, 201

shuǐ huǒ tàng shāng 水火烫伤, burns and scalds, 52

shuǐ huǒ xiāng jì 水火相济, fire and water aid each other, 201

shuǐ huǒ zhī zàng 水火之脏, viscus of fire and water, 656

shuǐ huǒ zhì 水火制, fire and water processing, 201

shuǐ jié xiōng 水结胸, water chest bind, 665

shuǐ jīng gāo 水晶膏, Water Crystal Paste, 21, 53

shuǐ kuī huǒ wàng 水亏火旺, depleted water and effulgent fire, 122

shuǐ kuī huǒ yán 水亏火炎, depleted water and flaming fire, 122

shuǐ kuò 水廓, water rampart, 668

shuǐ lù èr xiān dān 水陆二仙丹, Land and Water Two Immortals Elixir, 743

shuǐ lún 水轮, water wheel, 669

shuǐ nì 水逆, water counterflow, 666

shuǐ niú jiǎo 水牛角 water buffalo horn, Bubali Cornu, 67, 720

shuǐ piǎo 水漂, long rinsing, 367

shuǐ qì 水气, water qi, 668

shuǐ qì jié xiōng 水气结胸, water qi chest bind, 668

shuǐ qì líng xīn 水气凌心, water qi intimidating the heart, 668

shuǐ quán 水泉, KI-5, Water Spring, 31, 160, 332, 333, 393, 701, 747

shuǐ quán 水泉, urine, 642

shuǐ rè jié xiōng 水热结胸, water-heat chest bind, 667

shuǐ shàn 水疝, water mounting, 667

shuǐ shī 水湿, water-damp, 666

shuǐ tú 水突, ST-10, Water Prominence, 746

shuǐ tǔ bù fú 水土不服, failure to acclimatize to a new environment, 195

shuǐ wán 水丸, water pill, 668

shuǐ xiè 水泄, water diarrhea, 666

shuǐ xiè 水泻, water diarrhea, 666

shuǐ xìng liú xià 水性流下, water by nature flows downward, 665

shuǐ yè hùn zhuó 水液混浊, turbid water humor, 632

shuǐ yín 水银 mercury, Hydrargyrum, 98, 171, 383, 411

shuǐ yǐn 水饮, water-rheum, 668

shuǐ zàng 水脏, water viscus, 669

shuǐ zhàng 水胀, water distention, 666

shuǐ zhì 水制, water processing, 668

shuǐ zhì 水蛭 leech, Hirudo seu Whitmania, 98, 138, 724

shuǐ zhǒng 水肿, water swelling, 668

shuǐ zì chuāng 水渍疮, water-soaking sore, 668

shuì mián 睡眠, sleep, 536

shuì mián bù ān 睡眠不安, unquiet sleep, 638

shuì mián bù níng 睡眠不宁, unquiet sleep, 638

shuì shí kǒu jiǎo liú xián 睡时口角流涎, drooling from the corner of the mouth during sleep, 150

shuì wò bù níng 睡卧不宁, unquiet sleep, 638

shǔn rǔ 吮乳, suckle, 585

shùn jīng tāng 顺经汤, Menstruation-Normalizing Decoction, 390

shùn qì 顺气, normalizing qi, 414

shùn qì dǎo tán tāng 顺气导痰汤, Qi-Normalizing Phlegm-Abducting Decoction, 414, 694, 739

shùn qì hé zhōng tāng 顺气和中汤, Qi-Normalizing Center-Harmonizing Decoction, 741

shùn qì huà tán 顺气化痰, normalizing qi and transforming phlegm, 414

shùn qì xiāo shí huà tán wán 顺气消食化痰丸, Qi-Normalizing Food-Dispersing Phlegm-Transforming Pill, 141, 739

shùn qì yǎng xuè tāng 顺气养血汤, Qi-Normalizing Blood-Nourishing Decoction, 696

shùn zhèng 顺证, favorable pattern (sign), 196

shuò mài 数脉, rapid pulse, 492

shuǐ pào 水（疱）泡, vesicle, 654

shuǐ pào 水疱（泡）, blister, 23

shuǐ rù zé tù 水入则吐, immediate vomiting of ingested fluids, 295

shèn náng 肾囊, kidney sac, 330

shòu lěng gān 瘦冷疳, lean cold gan, 342

shí sì jīng fā huī 十四经发挥 (*Elaboration of the Fourteen Channels*), 1341 (Yuán), Huá Shòu 滑寿 [Bó-Rén 伯仁], 226

shǒu wǔ zú dào 手舞足蹈, flailing of the arms and legs, 209

SI-1, *shào zé* 少泽, Lesser Marsh, 227, 228, 252, 386, 420, 513, 522, 542, 654, 747

SI-2, *qián gǔ* 前谷, Front Valley, 263, 281, 542, 747

SI-3, *hòu xī* 后溪, Back Ravine, 8, 40, 50, 61, 74, 82, 83, 89, 90, 92, 93, 95, 105, 113, 114, 138, 174, 178, 185, 194, 197, 240, 244, 247, 255, 260, 269, 272, 275, 281, 287, 289, 295, 317, 336, 341, 342, 358, 366, 383, 391, 394, 399, 409, 410, 415, 439, 440, 454, 489, 506, 508, 519–521, 530, 540, 542, 544, 572, 588–591, 595, 597, 604, 648, 650, 651, 656, 664, 679, 681, 683, 684, 686, 687, 690, 693, 701–703, 713–716, 747

SI-4, *wàn gǔ* 腕骨, Wrist Bone, 90, 296, 521, 548, 747

SI-5, *yáng gǔ* 阳谷, Yang Valley, 61, 137, 567, 747

SI-6, *yǎng lǎo* 养老, Nursing the Aged, 291, 530, 549, 747

SI-7, *zhī zhèng* 支正, Branch to the Correct, 90, 408, 747

SI-8, *xiǎo hǎi* 小海, Small Sea, 75, 137, 567, 637, 747

SI-9, *jiān zhēn* 肩贞, True Shoulder, 137, 341, 530, 567, 747

SI-10, *nào shū* 臑俞, Upper Arm Transport, 295, 342, 521, 530, 747

SI-11, *tiān zōng* 天宗, Celestial Gathering, 61, 462, 521, 530, 747

SI-12, *bǐng fēng* 秉风, Grasping the Wind, 220, 253, 254, 747

SI-13, *qū yuán* 曲垣, Crooked Wall, 747

SI-14, *jiān wài shū* 肩外俞, Outer Shoulder Transport, 105, 747

SI-15, *jiān zhōng shū* 肩中俞, Central Shoulder Transport, 747

SI-16, *tiān chuāng* 天窗, Celestial Window, 747

SI-17, *tiān róng* 天容, Celestial Countenance, 30, 89, 210, 220, 480, 521, 689, 747

SI-18, *quán liáo* 颧髎, Cheek Bone-Hole, 194, 253, 747

SI-19, *tīng gōng* 听宫, Auditory Palace, 89, 119, 167, 220, 253, 260, 330, 521, 566, 614, 747

sī 思, thought, 609

sī guā 丝瓜藤 luffa stem, Luffae Caulis, 121

sī guā luò 丝瓜络 loofah, Luffae Fasciculus Vascularis, 417, 569, 589, 728

sī shà 嘶嘎, hoarse voice, 291

sī zé qì jié 思则气结, thought causes qi to bind, 609

sī zhú kōng 丝竹空, TB-23, Silk Bamboo Hole, 150, 253, 500, 586, 682, 748

sǐ tāi bù xià 死胎不下, retention of dead fetus, 502

sǐ xuè xié tòng 死血胁痛, dead blood rib-side pain, 118

sì bái 四白, ST-2, Four Whites, 125, 140, 194, 289, 568, 689, 746

sì dà 四大, four greatnesses, 226

sì dú 四渎, TB-9, Four Rivers, 520, 748

sì fèng 四缝, Four Seams, 60, 61, 237, 239, 522, 557

sì guān 四关, four gates, 225

sì hǎi 四海, four seas, 226

sì hǎi shū yù wán 四海舒郁丸, Four Seas Depression-Soothing Pill, 244, 480, 737

sì huā 四花, Four Flowers, 26, 227, 648, 649

sì jí 四极, four extremities, 225

sì jiā jiǎn zhèng qì sǎn 四加减正气散, Fourth Variant Qi-Righting Powder, 732

sì jūn zǐ tāng 四君子汤, Four Gentlemen Decoction, 172, 178, 223, 228, 267, 401, 486, 488, 562, 563, 594–596, 666, 741

sì líng sǎn 四苓散, Poria (Hoelen) Four Powder, 640, 663, 733

sì mǎn 四满, KI-14, Fourfold Fullness, 34, 35, 748

sì miào tāng 四妙汤, Mysterious Four Decoction, 743

sì miào wán 四妙丸, Mysterious Four Pill, 733

sì miào yǒng ān tāng 四妙勇安汤, Mysterious Four Resting Hero Decoction, 540, 743

sì mò tāng 四磨汤, Four Milled Ingredients Decoction, 477

sì mò yǐn 四磨饮, Four Milled Ingredients Beverage, 481, 482, 736

sì nì jiā rén shēn tāng 四逆加人参汤, Counterflow Cold Decoction Plus Ginseng, 84, 735

sì nì sǎn 四逆散, Counterflow Cold Powder, 19, 103, 123, 283, 297, 361, 362, 475, 483, 505, 732

sì nì tāng 四逆汤, Counterflow Cold Decoction, 74, 77, 85, 87, 130, 292, 345, 488, 504, 505, 735

sì qī tāng 四七汤, Four-Seven Decoction, 19, 157, 256, 736

sì qì 四气, four qi, 226

sì sè sǎn 四色散, Four Colors Powder, 63, 198

sì shén cōng 四神聪, Alert Spirit Quartet, 11, 25, 178, 236, 259, 261, 271, 333, 365, 413, 457, 506, 520, 537, 638, 652, 654, 673, 716 *sì shén wán* 四神丸, Four Spirits Pill, 312, 325, 335, 647, 660, 742

sì shēng wán 四生丸, Four Fresh Agents Pill, 738

sì shòu yǐn 四兽饮, Four Animals Decoction, 399

sì téng tāng 四藤汤, Four Stems Decoction, 737

sì wān fēng 四弯风, four bends wind, 225

sì wèi xiāng rú yǐn 四味香薷饮, Four-Ingredient Elsholtzia Beverage, 729

sì wù huà yù tāng 四物化郁汤, Four Agents Depression-Transforming Decoction, 27

sì wù jiā huáng qín huáng lián tāng 四物加黄芩黄连汤, Four Agents Decoction Plus Scutellaria and Coptis, 730

sì wù tāng 四物汤, Four Agents Decoction, 30, 37–40, 152, 153, 167, 243, 251, 261, 266, 288, 320, 322, 352, 370, 390, 391, 451, 452, 455, 456, 466, 474, 484, 595, 599, 606, 612, 646, 647, 654, 670, 696, 714, 715, 741

sì wù tāng jiā wèi fāng 四物汤加味方, Supplemented Four Agents Decoction Formula, 741

sì xìng 四性, four natures, 226

sì yīn jiān 四阴煎, Four Yin Brew, 416

sì yīn tāng 四阴汤, Four-Yin Decoction, 734

sì yǐn 四饮, four rheums, 226

sì zhěn 四诊, four examinations, 225

sì zhī bù wēn 四肢不温, lack of warmth in the extremities, 338

sì zhī jū jí 四肢拘急, hypertonicity of the limbs, 294

sì zhī jué lěng 四肢厥冷, reversal cold of the limbs, 505

sì zhī jué nì 四肢厥逆, reverse-flow of the limbs, 506

sì zhī kùn juàn 四肢困倦, fatigued cumbersome limbs, 195

sì zhī nì lěng 四肢逆冷, counterflow cold of the limbs, 102

sì zhī qiàn wēn 四肢欠温, lack of warmth in the extremities, 338

sì zhī tòng 四肢痛, pain in the limbs, 425

sì zǒng xué 四总穴, four command points, 225

Sichuan coptis, *chuān huáng lián* 川黄连, Coptidis Rhizoma Sichuanensis, 439

Sichuan Coptis and Bitter Orange Decoction, *chuān lián zhǐ ké tāng* 川连枳壳汤, 199

Sichuan fritillaria, *chuān bèi mǔ* 川贝母, Fritillariae Cirrhosae Bulbus, 175, 282, 480, 624, 714, 725

Sichuan saussurea, *chuān mù xiāng* 川木香, Vladimiriae Souliei Radix, 493, 723

siegesbeckia, *xī xiān* 豨莶, Siegesbeckiae Herba, 116, 139, 722

Siegesbeckia and Clerodendron Pill, *xī tóng wán* 豨桐丸, 734

Siegesbeckia and Clerodendron Wind-Damp Tablet, *fēng shī xī tóng piàn* 风湿豨桐片, 734

Siegesbeckiae Herba, *xī xiān* 豨莶, siegesbeckia, 116, 139, 722

silk tree bark, *hé huān pí* 合欢皮, Albizziae Cortex, 491, 537, 726

silk tree flower, *hé huān huā* 合欢花, Albizziae Flos, 234, 310

silkworm, *bái jiāng cán* 白僵蚕, Bombyx Batryticatus, 5, 54, 74, 76, 140, 150, 167, 456, 526, 690, 726

silkworm droppings, *yuán cán shā* 原蚕沙, Bombycis Excrementum, 139, 722

Silkworm Droppings Decoction, *cán shǐ tāng* 蚕矢汤, 733

Sinew-Soothing Blood-Quickening Tablet, *shū jīn huó xuè piàn* 舒筋活血片, 737

Sinew-Soothing Blood-Quickening Wash Formula, *shū jīn huó xuè xǐ fāng* 舒筋活血洗方, 745

Sinew-Soothing Decoction, *shū jīn tāng* 舒筋汤, 105, 734

Sinew-Strengthening Blood-Nourishing Decoction, *zhuàng jīn yǎng xuè tāng* 壮筋养血汤, 337, 567

Single Sage Powder, *dú shèng sǎn* 独圣散, 582

Single-Armored Pulse-Restorative Decoction, *yī jiǎ fù mài tāng* 一甲复脉汤, 742

Sinomenii seu Sabiae Caulis et Rhizoma, *qīng fēng téng* 青风藤, Orient vine, 139, 722

sinusitis*

    chronic paranasal sinusitis, 310

    paranasal, 120, 260, 543

Six Gentlemen Decoction, *liù jūn zǐ tāng* 六君子汤, 63, 115, 146, 153, 163, 199, 215, 378, 440, 441, 486, 489, 537, 549, 562–564, 627, 647, 650, 651, 666, 669, 709, 740

Six Gentlemen Metal and Water Brew, *jīn shuǐ liù jūn jiān* 金水六君煎, 63, 440, 596, 603, 738

Six Harmonizations Decoction, *liù hé tāng* 六和汤, 591, 732

Six Milled Ingredients Decoction, *liù mò tāng* 六磨汤, 127, 130, 479, 735

Six Pillars Beverage, *liù zhù yǐn* 六柱饮, 196

Six Quietings Brew, *liù ān jiān* 六安煎, 738

Six Spirits Pill, *liù shén wán* 六神丸, 612, 743

Six-Ingredient Decoction, *liù wèi tāng* 六味汤, 547

Six-Ingredient Elsholtzia Beverage, *liù wèi xiāng rú yǐn* 六味香薷饮, 587, 591, 729

Six-Ingredient Pill, *liù wèi wán* 六味丸, 217, 331, 647

Six-Ingredient Rehmannia Decoction, *liù wèi dì huáng tāng* 六味地黄汤, 27, 36, 95, 309, 332, 713

Six-Ingredient Rehmannia Pill, *liù wèi dì huáng wán* 六味地黄丸, 9, 104, 105, 151, 153, 156–158, 177, 181, 198, 203, 222, 229, 238, 239, 251, 288, 291, 314, 319, 327, 331–333, 336, 360, 367, 369, 401, 409, 426, 453, 462, 497, 502, 515, 528, 538, 540, 541, 566, 567, 569, 594, 599, 604, 611, 614, 636, 651, 714, 715, 742

Six-Ingredient Yang-Returning Beverage, *liù wèi huí yáng yǐn* 六味回阳饮, 648, 713

Six-to-One Powder, *liù yī sǎn* 六一散, 71, 221, 418, 587–590, 730

Sleeping Dragon Elixir, *wò lóng dān* 卧龙丹, 740

small aconite, *cè zǐ* 侧子, Aconiti Tuber Laterale Parvum, 97

small gleditsia, *zhū yá zào* 猪牙皂, Gleditsiae Fructus Parvus, 243, 690

Smilacis Glabrae Rhizoma, *tǔ fú líng* 土茯苓, smooth greenbrier root, 68, 540, 584, 685, 691, 721

smithsonite, *lú gān shí* 炉甘石, Smithsonitum, 53, 636, 667, 713, 728

Smithsonitum, *lú gān shí* 炉甘石, smithsonite, 53, 636, 667, 713, 728

Smooth Greenbrier Mixture, *tǔ fú líng hé jì* 土茯苓合剂, 494

smooth greenbrier root, *tǔ fú líng* 土茯苓, Smilacis Glabrae Rhizoma, 68, 540, 584, 685, 691, 721

snake slough, *shé tuì* 蛇蜕, Serpentis Exuviae, 98, 139, 722

snake strawberry, *shé méi* 蛇莓, Duchesneae Herba, 68, 721

Snow Soup Decoction, *xuě gēng tāng* 雪羹汤, 738

sophora flower, *huái huā* 槐花, Sophorae Flos, 466, 566, 567, 569, 724

Sophora Flower Powder, *huái huā sǎn* 槐花散, 40, 117, 738

Sophora Fruit Pill, *huái jiǎo wán* 槐角丸, 318, 738

sophora twigs, *huái zhī* 槐枝, Sophorae Ramulus, 196

Sophorae Flavescentis Radix, *kǔ shēn* 苦参, flavescent sophora, 66, 67, 116, 225, 338, 353, 395, 424, 468, 720

Sophorae Flos, *huái huā* 槐花, sophora flower, 466, 566, 567, 569, 724

Sophorae Fructus Carbonisatus, *huái jiǎo tàn* 槐角炭, charred sophora fruit, 317

Sophorae Ramulus, *huái zhī* 槐枝, sophora twigs, 196

Sophorae Subprostratae Radix, *shān dòu gēn* 山豆根, bushy sophora, 68, 420, 721

Solani Lyrati Herba, *bái máo téng* 白毛藤, climbing nightshade, 68, 721

Solani Nigri Herba, *lóng kuí* 龙葵, black nightshade, 68, 721

Solitary Yin, *dú yīn* 独阴, 128, 503, 542

Solomon's seal, *yù zhú* 玉竹, Polygonati Yuzhu Rhizoma, 88, 108, 175, 176, 581, 593, 597, 727

Solomon's Seal Variant Decoction, *jiā jiǎn wēi ruí tāng* 加减葳蕤汤, 176, 729

Song to Elucidate Mysteries (*biāo yōu fù*) 标幽赋, Jīn-Yuán (1115–1368), Dòu Jié 窦杰 [Hàn-Qīng 汉卿], 225, 419

Song-Shi Pig's Stomach Pill, *sōng shí zhū dǔ wán* 松石猪肚丸, 743

sōng jié 松节 knotty pine wood, Pini Lignum Nodi, 139, 722

sōng pí xiǎn 松皮癣, pine bark lichen, 444

sōng shí zhū dǔ wán 松石猪肚丸, Song-Shi Pig's Stomach Pill, 743

sōng xiāng 松香 rosin, Pini Resina, 728

sòng 宋, Song, 545

sòng zǐ dān 送子丹, Child-Delivering Elixir, 741

Sore-Healing Beverage, *xiāo chuāng yǐn* 消疮饮, 744

Sore-Toxin Pill, *chuāng dú wán* 疮毒丸, 743

sōu 溲, urine, 642

sōu fēng zhú hán 搜风逐寒, tracking wind and expelling cold, 621

sōu xuè 溲血, bloody urine, 41

sòu xuè 嗽血, coughing of blood, 101

Soul-Quieting Decoction, *ān hún tāng* 安魂汤, 60

southern fangji, *guǎng fáng jǐ* 广防己, Aristolochiae Fangchi Radix, 139, 722

SP-1, *yǐn bái* 隐白, Hidden White, 29–32, 35, 41, 90, 161, 169, 199, 212, 222, 233, 289, 386, 414, 420, 448, 478, 520, 522, 551, 557, 566, 570, 595, 603, 746

SP-2, *dà dū* 大都, Great Metropolis, 54, 61, 212, 233, 281, 395, 487, 489, 604, 746

SP-3, *tài bái* 太白, Supreme White, 41, 43, 61, 64, 70, 90, 109, 161, 163, 216, 223, 224, 228, 251, 256, 271, 282, 287, 319, 361, 378–380, 400, 435, 441, 453, 477, 483, 486, 488, 489, 519, 520, 548, 557, 562, 595, 596, 603, 604, 625, 639, 746

SP-4, *gōng sūn* 公孙, Yellow Emperor, 3, 4, 28, 63, 77, 81, 83, 85–87, 90, 92, 141, 156, 164, 186, 197, 215, 216, 218, 314, 349, 353, 358, 362, 408, 425, 426, 437, 442, 443, 478, 487, 490, 499, 510, 519, 522, 551, 557–559, 562, 564, 565, 571, 575, 577–579, 608, 633, 647, 663, 669, 673, 703, 710, 746

SP-5, *shāng qiū* 商丘, Shang Hill, 63, 80, 84, 112, 115, 197, 210, 211, 237, 239, 290, 337, 342, 359, 452, 489, 520, 557, 656, 684, 693, 746

SP-6, *sān yīn jiāo* 三阴交, Three Yin Intersection, 8, 11, 14, 15, 19, 21–31, 33–41, 44, 45, 47, 51, 53, 54, 57–60, 62–64, 66, 69–71, 74, 76, 79–81, 83, 84, 86, 88, 89, 91, 93, 94, 97, 99, 103, 109–112, 115, 117–119, 123, 127–129, 138, 140, 145, 147–149, 151, 154–162, 164, 167, 168, 174–178, 180, 194, 196, 199, 201, 202, 211, 212, 217, 218, 220, 221, 223–227, 229, 230, 233–237, 239–241, 251, 256, 260, 261, 263, 265–269, 271, 273–275, 278, 279, 282–284, 288–292, 294, 296, 297, 300–302, 307, 308, 310, 314, 317–320, 330–336, 338, 339, 342, 348, 349, 352, 353, 355–362, 364–366, 368–370, 380, 381, 383, 385, 390–393, 400, 401, 403, 410, 413, 415, 416, 418, 422, 424, 426, 427, 431, 434, 435, 437, 447–458, 461, 462, 465–468, 477–485, 488–490, 493, 495, 497, 499, 503, 511, 514–516, 518, 520–522, 524–526, 533, 535, 537, 540, 542, 546, 552, 554, 557, 560, 561, 563–568, 570–572, 577, 579, 581, 584–586, 588, 591, 594–597, 600, 601, 603, 604, 607, 608, 613, 631, 637, 638, 640–642, 646–650, 652, 656, 661–663, 665, 667, 673–677, 679, 683–686, 688–690, 694, 700–703, 709–716, 746

SP-7, *lòu gǔ* 漏谷, Leaking Valley, 746

SP-8, *dì jī* 地机, Earth's Crux, 26, 31, 34–36, 94, 212, 227, 233, 279, 300, 353, 393, 431, 447, 450, 451, 483, 484, 503, 520, 540, 661, 746

SP-9, *yīn líng quán* 阴陵泉, Yin Mound Spring, 1, 2, 8, 21, 22, 36, 37, 40, 63, 66, 69–71, 76, 78–80, 84, 86, 88, 94, 103, 104, 109–118, 127, 138–140, 145,

149, 151, 167, 180, 182, 186, 210, 211, 221, 224, 228, 229, 240, 241, 257, 260, 276, 278, 282, 283, 287, 288, 296, 297, 301, 302, 308, 319, 320, 327, 335, 337, 342, 343, 347, 349, 353, 357, 359, 370, 383, 395, 401, 410, 418, 422, 424, 425, 434–436, 440–442, 452, 457, 462, 466, 468, 485, 489, 493, 498, 499, 506, 511, 516, 520, 522, 525, 529, 530, 533, 540, 542, 546, 547, 550, 554, 559, 560, 563–565, 579, 582, 585, 586, 588, 589, 600, 604, 608, 636, 637, 640, 641, 656, 658, 663, 665–668, 675, 677, 680, 684, 686, 691, 693, 694, 700, 701, 703, 710–713, 716, 746

SP-10, *xuè hǎi* 血海, Sea of Blood, 15, 21, 22, 24–37, 39–41, 59, 62, 63, 75, 93, 97, 99, 113, 117, 138, 139, 145, 149, 151, 152, 154, 162, 164, 167, 174, 199, 212, 227, 230, 233, 239, 241, 251, 269, 271, 273, 274, 279, 291, 300, 314, 319, 348, 349, 353, 356, 359, 390, 391, 418, 431, 447, 449–452, 454, 456, 457, 468, 482–484, 487, 489, 497, 503, 511, 516, 517, 522, 540, 561, 563, 567, 568, 570, 571, 586, 589, 591, 601, 607, 608, 613, 642, 649, 655, 656, 661, 665, 674, 683, 684, 686, 688, 689, 696, 702, 746

SP-11, *jī mén* 箕门, Winnower Gate, 520, 610, 746

SP-12, *chōng mén* 冲门, Surging Gate, 35, 57, 221, 233, 241, 746

SP-13, *fǔ shè* 府舍, Bowel Abode, 221, 746

SP-14, *fù jié* 腹结, Abdominal Bind, 2, 72, 127, 164, 277, 298, 318, 339, 544, 585, 673, 746

SP-15, *dà hèng* 大横, Great Horizontal, 28, 64, 77, 83, 85, 183, 479, 509, 667, 746

SP-16, *fù āi* 腹哀, Abdominal Lament, 746

SP-17, *shí dòu* 食窦, Food Hole, 746

SP-18, *tiān xī* 天溪, Celestial Ravine, 746

SP-19, *xiōng xiāng* 胸乡, Chest Village, 746

SP-20, *zhōu róng* 周荣, All-Round Flourishing, 746

SP-21, *dà bāo* 大包, Great Embracement, 26, 118, 248, 408, 746

Spanish needles, *guǐ zhēn cǎo* 鬼针草, Bidentis Bipinnatae Herba, 68, 721

Spare-the-Knife Powder, *dài dāo sǎn* 代刀散, 743

Sparganii Rhizoma, *sān léng* 三棱, sparganium, 34, 98, 138, 182, 411, 512, 544, 574, 724

sparganium, *sān léng* 三棱, Sparganii Rhizoma, 34, 98, 138, 182, 411, 512, 544, 574, 724

Sparganium Decoction, *sān léng tāng* 三棱汤, 737

spasm of the vesical sphincter*, 148

spasm*
clonic, 631

Special Achievement Powder, *yì gōng sǎn* 异功散, 450, 451, 648, 741

spider, *zhī zhū* 蜘蛛, Aranea, 98

spider nevi*, 496

spindle tree wings, *guǐ jiàn yǔ* 鬼箭羽, Euonymi Lignum Suberalatum, 139, 338, 725

spiny jujube, *suān zǎo rén* 酸枣仁, Ziziphi Spinosi Semen, 37, 122, 222, 230, 236, 309, 359, 433, 458, 490, 526, 557, 655, 726

Spiny Jujube Decoction, *suān zǎo rén tāng* 酸枣仁汤, 230, 739

spiny jujube kernel, *suān zǎo rén* 酸枣仁, Ziziphi Spinosi Semen, 60

Spirifer Fossil Elixir, *shí yàn dān* 石燕丹, 195

Spirit Immortal Life-Giving Decoction, *shén xiān huó mìng tāng* 神仙活命汤, 129

Spirit-Like Rhinoceros Horn Elixir, *shén xī dān* 神犀丹, 6, 65, 69, 388, 740

Spirit-Moistening Powder, *rùn shén sǎn* 润神散, 97

Spirit-Quieting Engendering Transformation Decoction, *ān shén shēng huà tāng* 安神生化汤, 455

Spirit-Quieting Mind-Stabilizing Pill, *ān shén dìng zhì wán* 安神定志丸, 230, 268, 538, 739

Spirit-Quieting Pill, *ān shén wán* 安神丸, 491, 739

Spleen Longevity Brew, *shòu pí jiān* 寿脾煎, 537

Spleen-Arousing Pill, *qǐ pí sǎn* 启脾散, 736

Spleen-Arousing Pill, *qǐ pí wán* 启脾丸, 197

Spleen-Arousing Pill, *xǐng pí wán* 醒脾丸, 61

Spleen-Clearing Beverage, *qīng pí yǐn* 清脾饮, 317, 732

Spleen-Clearing Dampness-Eliminating Beverage, *qīng pí chú shī yǐn* 清脾除湿饮, 285

Spleen-Draining Powder, *xiè pí sǎn* 泻脾散, 731

Spleen-Effusing Decoction Plus Ovate Atractylodes, *yuè bì jiā zhú tāng* 越婢加术汤, 287

Spleen-Effusing Decoction Plus Pinellia, *yuè bì jiā bàn xià tāng* 越婢加半夏汤, 285, 469, 739

Spleen-Effusing Decoction, *yuè bì tāng* 越婢汤, 301, 669, 694, 703, 729

Spleen-Firming Beverage, *shí pí yǐn* 实脾饮, 28, 114, 151, 287, 301, 467, 559, 661, 666, 669, 703, 709, 716, 733

Spleen-Fortifying Pill, *jiàn pí wán* 健脾丸, 141, 224, 736

Spleen-Kidney Supplementation Pill, *pí shèn shuāng bǔ wán* 脾肾双补丸, 742

Spleen Returning Decoction, *guī pí tāng* 归脾汤, 32, 37–39, 41, 161, 162, 211, 223, 251, 265, 268, 271, 272, 289, 296, 311, 367, 409, 417, 427, 453, 461, 489, 502, 537, 551, 556, 561, 562, 595, 604, 646, 648, 651, 685, 694, 711, 741

Spleen-Returning Pill, *guī pí wán* 归脾丸, 348

Spleen-Warming Decoction, *wēn pí tāng* 温脾汤, 182, 338, 425, 732

splenomegaly in malaria*, 399

splenomegaly*, 399, 544

spondylosis*, 295

Spring Pond Decoction, *chūn zé tāng* 春泽汤, 733

ST-1, *chéng qì* 承泣, Tear Container, 64, 89, 406, 495, 585, 586, 746

ST-2, *sì bái* 四白, Four Whites, 125, 140, 194, 289, 568, 689, 746

ST-3, *jù liáo* 巨髎, Great Bone-Hole, 45, 521, 746

ST-4, *dì cāng* 地仓, Earth Granary, 73, 89, 125, 140, 183, 254, 289, 426, 446, 509, 610, 689, 696, 746

ST-5, *dà yíng* 大迎, Great Reception, 142, 220, 222, 515, 521, 610, 746

ST-6, *jiá chē* 颊车, Cheek Carriage, 73, 89, 125, 140, 178, 189, 194, 222, 289, 366, 403, 446, 485, 521, 522, 611, 620, 621, 689, 690, 693, 746

ST-7, *xià guān* 下关, Below the Joint, 73, 89, 178, 194, 220, 366, 403, 485, 521, 620, 621, 690, 693, 746

ST-8, *tóu wéi* 头维, Head Corner, 32, 73, 79, 99, 153, 192, 194, 202, 216, 219, 223, 247, 259, 287, 301, 433–437, 440, 441, 487, 519, 539, 588, 684, 687, 691, 699, 746

ST-9, *rén yíng* 人迎, Man's Prognosis, 222, 226, 586, 746

ST-10, *shuǐ tú* 水突, Water Prominence, 746

ST-11, *qì shè* 气舍, Qi Abode, 746

ST-12, *quē pén* 缺盆, Empty Basin, 220, 222, 252–254, 712, 746

ST-13, *qì hù* 气户, Qi Door, 39, 254, 332, 746

ST-14, *kù fáng* 库房, Storeroom, 746

ST-15, *wū yì* 屋翳, Roof, 385, 746

ST-16, *yīng chuāng* 膺窗, Breast Window, 386, 418, 746

ST-17, *rǔ zhōng* 乳中, Breast Center, 746

ST-18, *rǔ gēn* 乳根, Breast Root, 227, 228, 248, 386, 483, 513, 746

ST-19, *bù róng* 不容, Not Contained, 746

ST-20, *chéng mǎn* 承满, Assuming Fullness, 746

ST-21, *liáng mén* 梁门, Beam Gate, 80, 87, 111, 164, 168, 207, 215, 217, 218, 224, 521, 580, 581, 746

ST-22, *guān mén* 关门, Pass Gate, 746

ST-23, *tài yǐ* 太乙, Supreme Unity, 746

ST-24, *huá ròu mén* 滑肉门, Slippery Flesh Gate, 746

ST-25, *tiān shū* 天枢, Celestial Pivot, 1, 3, 4, 8, 15, 26, 28, 29, 35, 36, 40, 47, 54, 61–64, 70, 72, 73, 77, 78, 80, 83, 86, 89, 91, 94, 105, 109–111, 114–117, 127, 136, 141, 151, 153, 157, 168, 174, 186, 196, 197, 212, 215–218, 224, 234, 235, 247, 256, 257, 267, 276–278, 280, 281, 284, 289, 290, 298, 300–302, 312, 314, 316, 318, 325, 335, 338–340, 349, 361, 383, 395, 401, 415, 418, 425, 434, 436, 438–442, 447, 450, 451, 454, 457, 462, 477, 479, 480, 482–485, 487, 498, 499, 509, 510, 522, 540, 554, 555, 558, 559, 561, 562, 564, 565, 570, 579, 581, 585, 588, 589, 601, 612, 631, 633, 645–647, 656, 664, 666, 678, 683, 684, 703, 710, 713, 716, 746

ST-26, *wài líng* 外陵, Outer Mound, 746

ST-27, *dà jù* 大巨, Great Gigantic, 746

ST-28, *shuǐ dào* 水道, Waterway, 94, 418, 667, 746

ST-29, *guī lái* 归来, Return, 26, 35, 36, 94, 226, 300, 332, 447, 483, 484, 524, 643, 661, 746

ST-30, *qì chōng* 气冲, Qi Thoroughfare, 35, 57, 111, 212, 222, 226, 233, 241, 424, 435, 450, 484, 503, 609, 746

ST-31, *bì guān* 髀关, Thigh Joint, 61, 222, 679, 746

ST-32, *fú tù* 伏兔, Crouching Rabbit, 222, 342, 520, 746

ST-33, *yīn shì* 阴市, Yin Market, 289, 337, 418, 746

ST-34, *liáng qiū* 梁丘, Beam Hill, 29, 73, 104, 137, 186, 215, 218, 296, 337, 386, 390, 520, 521, 567, 673, 679, 746

ST-35, *dú bí* 犊鼻, Calf's Nose, 337, 520, 746

ST-36, *zú sān lǐ* 足三里, Leg Three Li, 1, 3–5, 8, 11, 14–17, 19, 20, 26–30, 32, 33, 36–41, 44, 47, 55, 57–64, 66, 69–74, 76, 77, 79–89, 91, 94–97, 99, 103, 105, 109–115, 117–120, 123, 127–129, 136, 139–141, 145, 146, 149–151, 153, 154, 156, 157, 159–164, 167, 168, 174, 175, 177, 183, 185, 186, 189, 190, 192, 194, 196, 197, 199, 202, 210–212, 215–218, 221–231, 234–237, 239–241, 247, 251, 255–257, 260, 265–272, 276, 278, 280–284, 287–289, 291, 292, 296, 297, 300–302, 308–310, 312, 314, 316, 318–320, 325, 329, 332–337, 339–343, 349, 352, 357–362, 365, 369, 370, 378–380, 382, 385, 386, 391–393, 395, 396, 400, 401, 403, 408, 410, 415, 416, 418, 425–427, 430, 433–443, 445, 447–458, 461, 462, 465, 466, 477–480, 482–490, 493, 498, 499, 503, 504, 506, 509–511, 513, 515, 516, 519–525, 529, 530, 533, 537, 539, 540, 544, 547, 549–551, 554, 555, 557–566, 568, 570, 571, 575, 577–581, 585–591, 594–597, 600, 601, 603, 604, 606–608, 612–614, 620, 624, 625, 627, 629, 630, 633, 636–641, 645–650, 652, 661–666, 668, 673–680, 684–686, 689, 690, 693–696, 699–703, 709–716, 746

ST-37, *shàng jù xū* 上巨虚, Upper Great Hollow, 2, 3, 15, 28, 29, 40, 70, 72, 73, 77, 78, 80, 89, 111, 117, 127, 164, 168, 174, 190, 197, 215–217, 226, 254, 276–278, 284, 294, 298, 302, 312, 318, 319, 338–340, 369, 396, 415, 426, 434, 477, 544, 581, 585, 589, 645–647, 656, 658, 664, 673, 683, 746

ST-38, *tiáo kǒu* 条口, Ribbon Opening, 341, 342, 446, 530, 746

ST-39, *xià jù xū* 下巨虚, Lower Great Hollow, 89, 226, 263, 281, 369, 390, 746

ST-40, *fēng lóng* 丰隆, Bountiful Bulge, 4, 6, 14, 15, 58, 59, 63, 65, 70, 74, 78, 84, 87, 88, 90, 99, 109, 115, 116, 119, 123, 129, 136, 140–142, 153, 178, 186, 192, 203, 210, 216, 223, 224, 230, 235, 240, 247, 251, 257, 260, 269, 277, 280–282, 285, 287, 288, 291, 297, 301, 386, 394, 400, 408, 418, 425, 433–443, 445, 448, 457, 477, 478, 499, 507, 511, 515, 537, 539, 540, 544, 550, 562, 565, 568, 578, 588, 591, 596, 603, 608, 611, 614, 624, 625, 631, 650, 656, 663, 664, 666, 673, 677, 681, 683–685, 690, 691, 694, 746

ST-41, *jiě xī* 解溪, Ravine Divide, 80, 90, 99, 112, 115, 137, 153, 192, 223, 258, 296, 309, 342, 395, 433, 434, 436, 441, 519, 520, 567, 652, 679, 683, 691, 746

ST-42, *chōng yáng* 冲阳, Surging Yang, 90, 222, 289, 548, 610, 689, 699, 746

ST-43, *xiàn gǔ* 陷谷, Sunken Valley, 14, 54, 73, 283, 396, 520, 547, 561, 652, 665, 688, 746

ST-44, *nèi tíng* 内庭, Inner Court, 2, 4, 5, 8, 14, 15, 28–31, 63, 66, 70–73, 87, 89, 91, 109–112, 127,

129, 149, 158, 164, 168, 175, 186, 189, 190, 194, 197, 202, 203, 217, 239, 241, 276–284, 288, 290, 292, 294, 299, 302, 312, 314, 338, 342, 349, 358, 382, 386, 390, 395, 400, 414, 415, 426, 436, 437, 439, 442, 443, 448, 455, 499, 504, 515, 519, 520, 546, 547, 560, 564, 566, 567, 570, 577, 578, 580, 581, 585, 586, 588, 589, 601, 607, 611, 613, 614, 620, 621, 641, 652, 667, 686, 687, 693, 699, 700, 710, 715, 746

ST-45, *lì duì* 厉兑, Severe Mouth, 148, 186, 189, 268, 269, 279, 281, 283, 314, 333, 413–415, 420, 520, 538, 577, 699, 746

stalactite, *zhōng rǔ shí* 钟乳石, Stalactitum, 467, 526, 624, 726

Stalactitum, *zhōng rǔ shí* 钟乳石, stalactite, 467, 526, 624, 726

Stalactitum Pulveratum, *zhōng rǔ fěn* 钟乳粉, powdered stalactite, 624, 726

star anise, *bā jiǎo huí xiāng* 八角茴香, Anisi Stellati Fructus, 222, 600, 660, 723

star jasmine stem, *luò shí téng* 络石藤, Trachelospermi Caulis, 139, 256, 722

Stasis-Dispersing Beverage, *xiāo yū yǐn* 消瘀饮, 570

Stasis-Dissipating Injury Decoction, *sàn yū hé shāng tāng* 散瘀和伤汤, 745

Stasis-Dissipating Pueraria Decoction, *sàn yū gé gēn tāng* 散瘀葛根汤, 571

Stasis-Freeing Brew, *tōng yū jiān* 通瘀煎, 33, 34, 738

Stasis-Precipitating Decoction, *xià yū xuè tāng* 下瘀血汤, 118, 738

Statesman Shi's Wine-Steeped Formula, *shǐ guó gōng jìn jiǔ fāng* 史国公浸酒方, 288, 734

Statesman Wine, *guó gōng jiǔ* 国公酒, 734

Steady Gait Hidden Tiger Pill, *jiàn bù hǔ qián wán* 健步虎潜丸, 742

Stellariae Lanceolatae Radix, *yín chái hú* 银柴胡, lanceolate stellaria, 68, 72, 281, 282, 649, 722

Stellerae seu Euphorbiae Radix, *láng dú* 狼毒, Chinese wolfsbane, 411, 728

stemona, *bǎi bù* 百部, Stemonae Radix, 95, 183, 445, 468, 624, 714, 725

Stemona Enema, *bǎi bù guàn cháng jì* 百部灌肠剂, 737

Stemona Metal-Clearing Decoction, *bǎi bù qīng jīn tāng* 百部清金汤, 97

Stemona Paste, *bǎi bù gāo* 百部膏, 603

Stemonae Radix, *bǎi bù* 百部, stemona, 95, 183, 445, 468, 624, 714, 725

Stephaniae Tetrandrae Radix, *fěn fáng jǐ* 粉防己, mealy fangji, 139, 722

sterculia, *pàng dà hǎi* 胖大海, Sterculiae Semen, 291, 368

sterculia, *pàng dà hài* 胖大海, Sterculiae Semen, 624, 725

Sterculiae Semen, *pàng dà hǎi* 胖大海, sterculia, 291, 368

Sterculiae Semen, *pàng dà hài* 胖大海, sterculia, 624, 725

sternum*, 50

stinkbug, *jiǔ xiāng chóng* 九香虫, Aspongopus, 493, 724

Stomach Gate Brew, *wèi guān jiān* 胃关煎, 348, 735

stomach ulcer*, 63, 580

Stomach Wind Decoction, *wèi fēng tāng* 胃风汤, 318, 581

Stomach-Boosting Decoction, *yì wèi tāng* 益胃汤, 285, 678, 734

Stomach-Calming Poria (Hoelen) Five Decoction, *wèi líng tāng* 胃苓汤, 1, 79, 109, 113, 114, 151, 217, 302, 339, 348, 467, 556, 563, 608, 666, 711, 732

Stomach-Calming Powder, *píng wèi sǎn* 平胃散, 19, 109, 114, 153, 154, 197, 216, 218, 257, 384, 395, 418, 435, 498, 539, 563, 633, 665, 732

Stomach-Clearing Decoction, *qīng wèi tāng* 清胃汤, 15, 439, 620

Stomach-Clearing Powder, *qīng wèi sǎn* 清胃散, 158, 190, 198, 239, 367, 566, 577, 621, 656, 687, 731

Stomach-Nourishing Decoction, *yǎng wèi tāng* 养胃汤, 581, 597, 734

Stomach-Quieting Beverage, *ān wèi yǐn* 安胃饮, 280

Stomach-Regulating Qi-Coordinating Decoction, *tiáo wèi chéng qì tāng* 调胃承气汤, 54, 84, 127, 157, 314, 426, 459, 613, 731

Stomach-Warming Beverage, *wēn wèi yǐn* 温胃饮, 63, 648

stomatitis*
aphthous, 400

Stone-Expelling Decoction, *pái shí tāng* 排石汤, 733

Stone-Transforming Powder, *huà shí sǎn* 化石散, 733

strabismus*, 568

Straitened Spleen Hemp Seed Pill, *pí yuē má rén wán* 脾约麻仁丸, 289

Stream-Reducing Pill, *suō quán wán* 缩泉丸, 12, 23, 176, 308, 496, 640, 743

Striped Dragon Pill, *bān lóng wán* 斑龙丸, 523, 741

styloid process of the ulna*, 468

Styrax Liquidus, *sū hé xiāng* 苏合香, liquid storax, 10, 420, 485, 726

sū hé xiāng 苏合香 liquid storax, Styrax Liquidus, 10, 420, 485, 726

sū hé xiāng wán 苏合香丸, Liquid Storax Pill, 74, 86, 88, 152, 182, 228, 300, 384, 394, 590, 624, 629, 690, 740

sū mù 苏木 sappan, Sappan Lignum, 98, 138, 725

sū tíng gǔn tán wán 苏葶滚痰丸, Perilla Seed and Tingli Phlegm-Rolling Pill, 441

sū yè tāng 苏叶汤, Perilla Leaf Decoction, 620

sū zǐ 苏子 perilla seed, Perillae Semen, 625

sū zǐ jiàng qì tāng 苏子降气汤, Perilla Fruit Qi-Downbearing Decoction, 439, 477

sū zǐ jiàng qì tāng 苏子降气汤, Perilla Seed Qi-Downbearing Decoction, 145, 362, 477, 736

sū zǐ xìng zǐ tāng 苏子杏子汤, Perilla Seed and Apricot Seed Decoction, 372 *sù chuāng* 粟疮, millet sores, 395

sù jí 宿疾, abiding ailment, 3

sù jí 宿疾, long-standing ailment, 367

sù jiàng 肃降, depurative downbearing, 123

sù liáo 素髎, GV-25, White Bone-Hole, 32, 33, 212, 232, 478, 504, 521, 646, 674, 699, 709, 749

sù shí 宿食, abiding food, 3

sù wèn 素问 (*Elementary Questions*), first part of *huáng dì nèi jīng* 黄帝内经, 4, 13, 19–22, 25, 31, 47, 49, 53, 55–58, 67, 76–78, 80, 82, 85, 93, 100, 108, 114, 120, 123, 142, 144, 163, 171, 173, 179, 180, 185, 190, 200, 204, 205, 207–209, 213, 214, 216, 221, 229, 232, 233, 235, 251, 260, 263–265, 270, 272, 281, 283, 284, 286, 288, 295, 307, 308, 311, 313, 316–319, 327–331, 336, 340, 347, 341, 343, 349–351, 356, 358–361, 364, 367, 371, 373–379, 383, 384, 395, 400, 404, 408, 411, 419–421, 425, 428, 431, 444, 461, 469, 472, 473, 486, 488, 495, 498–499, 505, 506, 508, 514, 515, 525, 527, 529, 534–536, 543, 551–554, 557, 558, 560, 561, 578, 581–583, 586, 587, 592, 599, 600, 602, 610, 621, 622, 626–627, 630, 632, 639, 643, 647, 653–655, 658, 672–674, 678, 680, 681, 685, 691, 694, 700, 703, 706, 708, 716, 717

sù yì 宿翳, residual screen, 500

suān 酸, soreness, 546

suān 酸, twinge, 634

suān 酸（痠）, sore, 545

suān 酸, sour, 548

suān 酸, sourness, 548

suān jiāng 酸浆 lantern plant, Physalis Alkekengi Herba, 68, 721

suān rù gān 酸入肝, sourness enters the liver, 548

suān tòng 酸痛, aching pain, 4

suān tòng 酸痛, soreness, 546

suān tòng 酸痛, sore, 545

suān zǎo rén 酸枣仁 spiny jujube kernel, Ziziphi Spinosi Semen, 60

suān zǎo rén 酸枣仁 spiny jujube, Ziziphi Spinosi Semen, 37, 122, 222, 230, 236, 309, 359, 433, 458, 490, 526, 557, 655, 726

suān zǎo rén tāng 酸枣仁汤, Spiny Jujube Decoction, 230, 739

suàn ní 蒜泥 mashed garlic, Allii Sativi Bulbus Pulpatus, 388, 389

suàn zhī 蒜汁 garlic juice, Allii Sativi Bulbi Succus, 307

subarachnoid hemorrhage*, 44, 586

Sublimatum Triplex, *shēng dān* 升丹, upborne elixir, 383, 727

sublimed arsenic, *pī shuāng* 砒霜, Arsenicum Sublimatum, 411

submaxillaritis*
suppurative, 611

Substitute Dead-On Pill, *dài dǐ dàng wán* 代抵当丸, 37, 149, 542, 737

Succinum, *hǔ pò* 琥珀, amber, 153, 230, 262, 433, 490, 602, 726

Sudden Smile Pill, *shī xiào wán* 失笑丸, 224, 732

Sudden Smile Powder, *shī xiào sǎn* 失笑散, 35, 59, 138, 212, 228, 447, 452, 571, 737

suí 隋, Sui, 587

suǐ hǎi 髓海, sea of marrow, 517

suǐ hǎi kōng xū 髓海空虚, emptiness of the sea of marrow, 172

suǐ zhī fǔ 髓之府, house of the marrow, 293

Suis Adeps, *zhū zhī gāo* 猪脂膏, pork lard, 653

Suis Bilis, *zhū dǎn zhī* 猪胆汁, pig's bile, 624, 725

Suis Glandula Thyroidea, *zhū yè* 猪靥, pig's thyroid gland, 30, 243

Suis Iecur, *zhū gān* 猪肝, pig's liver, 291

Suis Spinae Medulla, *zhū jǐ suǐ* 猪脊髓, pig's spine marrow, 64, 333

sulcus nasolabialis, 432

sulfur, *shí liú huáng* 石硫黄, Sulphur, 98, 154, 171, 411, 458, 676, 727

Sulfur and Scallion Topical Application, *liú cōng fū jì* 硫葱敷剂, 744

Sulphur, *shí liú huáng* 石硫黄, sulfur, 98, 154, 171, 411, 458, 676, 727

sumac gallnut, *wǔ bèi zǐ* 五倍子, Rhois Galla, 466, 518, 567, 572, 675, 709, 727

Sumac Gallnut Powder, *wǔ bèi zǐ sǎn* 五倍子散, 744

Summerheat-Clearing Qi-Boosting Decoction, *qīng shǔ yì qì tāng* 清暑益气汤, 71, 455, 588, 591, 730

Summerheat-Damp Qi-Righting Pill, *shǔ shī zhèng qì wán* 暑湿正气丸, 732

sun spurge, *zé qī* 泽漆, Euphorbiae Helioscopiae Herba, 136, 723

sūn luò 孙络, grandchild network vessel, 245

sūn mài 孙脉, grandchild vessel, 245

sūn xiè 飧泄, swill diarrhea, 601

sūn xiè 飧泻, swill diarrhea, 601

sǔn 损, detriment, 124

suō jiǎo cháng yōng 缩脚肠痈, leg-flexing intestinal welling-abscess, 342

suō jiǎo liú zhù 缩脚流注, leg-flexing streaming sore, 342

suō luó zǐ 娑罗子 horse chestnut, Aesculi Fructus, 493, 724

suō niào 缩尿, reducing urine, 496

suō pí yǐn 缩脾饮, Amomum Splenic Beverage, 348, 732

suō quán wán 缩泉丸, Stream-Reducing Pill, 12, 23, 176, 308, 496, 640, 743

suō yáng 缩阳, retracted genitals, 503

suō yīn 缩阴, retracted genitals, 503

suǒ hóu fēng 锁喉风, throat-locking wind, 612

suǒ yáng 锁阳 cynomorium, Cynomorii Caulis, 310, 593, 679, 727

suǒ yǐ zài wán 所以载丸, Wherewithal-to-Bear Pill, 742

suǒ zài 所载, bearing, 17

superciliary arch*, 191

Supplemented Atractylodes Paste, *jiā wèi cāng zhú gāo* 加味苍术膏, 173

Supplemented Center-Rectifying Decoction, *jiā wèi lǐ zhōng tāng* 加味理中汤, 603

Supplemented Cyperus and Perilla Powder, *jiā wèi xiāng sū sǎn* 加味香苏散, 729

Supplemented Ephedra, Apricot Kernel, Gypsum, and Licorice Decoction, *jiā wèi má xìng shí gān tāng* 加味麻杏石甘汤, 189, 303, 677, 729

Supplemented Four Agents Decoction Formula, *sì wù tāng jiā wèi fāng* 四物汤加味方, 741

Supplemented Free Wanderer Powder, *jiā wèi xiāo yáo sǎn* 加味逍遥散, 123, 640

Supplemented Gallbladder-Warming Decoction, *jiā wèi wēn dǎn tāng* 加味温胆汤, 739

Supplemented Kidney Qi Pill, *jiā wèi shèn qì wán* 加味肾气丸, 742

Supplemented Lindera Decoction, *jiā wèi wū yào tāng* 加味乌药汤, 484, 735

Supplemented Metal Strength Pill, *jiā wèi jīn gāng wán* 加味金刚丸, 742

Supplemented Mind-Stabilizing Pill, *jiā wèi dìng zhì wán* 加味定志丸, 739

Supplemented Mysterious Two Powder, *jiā wèi èr miào sǎn* 加味二妙散, 111, 112, 337

Supplemented Pulsatilla Decoction, *jiā wèi bái tóu wēng tāng* 加味白头翁汤, 731

Supplemented Rough and Ready Three Decoction, *jiā wèi sān ào tāng* 加味三拗汤, 83

Supplemented Six-Ingredient Rehmannia Pill, *jiā wèi liù wèi dì huáng wán* 加味六味地黄丸, 226, 620

Supplemented Tangkuei and Peony Powder, *jiā wèi dāng guī sháo yào sǎn* 加味当归芍药散, 741

Supplemented White-Draining Powder, *jiā wèi xiè bái sǎn* 加味泻白散, 469

Supplemented Yellow Earth Decoction, *jiā wèi huáng tǔ tāng* 加味黄土汤, 743

suppurative orchitis*, 671

Supreme Jewel Elixir, *zhì bǎo dān* 至宝丹, 69, 88, 171, 197, 624, 631, 690, 740

Sweeping Down Decoction, *jiàn líng tāng* 建瓴汤, 53, 740

sweet apricot kernel, *tián xìng rén* 甜杏仁, Armeniacae Semen Dulce, 624, 725

Sweet Dew Beverage, *gān lù yǐn* 甘露饮, 239, 367, 547, 620, 731

Sweet Dew Toxin-Dispersing Elixir, *gān lù xiāo dú dān* 甘露消毒丹, 66, 69, 70, 117, 118, 167, 177, 297, 539, 733

Sweet Relief Decoction, *gān huǎn tāng* 甘缓汤, 480

sweet wormwood, *qīng hāo* 青蒿, Artemisiae Apiaceae seu Annuae Herba, 68, 69, 72, 255, 277, 281, 282, 587, 649, 664, 721

Sweet Wormwood and Scutellaria Gallbladder-Clearing Decoction, *hāo qín qīng dǎn tāng* 蒿芩清胆汤, 235, 538, 587, 733

Sweet Wormwood and Turtle Shell Decoction, *qīng hāo biē jiǎ tāng* 青蒿鳖甲汤, 72, 281, 282, 649, 731

Swelling-Dispersing Hardness-Breaking Decoction, *sàn zhǒng kuì jiān tāng* 散肿溃坚汤, 737

Swertiae Pulchellae Herba, *qīng yè dǎn* 青叶胆, pretty swertia, 68, 721

swim bladder, *yú biào* 鱼鳔, Piscis Vesica Aeris, 333

sword bean, *dāo dòu* 刀豆, Canavaliae Semen, 493

sword bean pod, *dāo dòu ké* 刀豆壳, Canavaliae Legumen, 724

syncope*
postpartum, 448

syphilis*, 494

Systematized Identification of Damp-Heat (*shī rè tiáo biàn*) 湿热条辨, 1831 (Qīng), Xuē Xuě 薛雪, 659

Systematized Identification of Warm Diseases (*wēn bìng tiáo biàn*) 温病条辨, 1798 (Qīng), Wú Táng 吴瑭 [Jú-Tōng 鞠通], 186, 276, 659

Systematized Patterns with Clear-Cut Treatments (*lèi zhèng zhì cái*) 类证治裁, 1839 (Qīng), Lín Pèi-Qín 林佩琴, 172, 362, 646

T₁, 550

tā yǎng tāng 塌痒汤, Itch-Soothing Decoction, 241

Tabanus, *méng chóng* 虻虫, tabanus, 98, 138, 724

tabanus, *méng chóng* 虻虫, Tabanus, 98, 138, 724

tachycardia*, 261, 336

taeniasis*, 298

Tai Yi Plaster, *tài yǐ gāo* 太乙膏, 187

tāi 胎, fetal, 197

tāi 胎, fetus, 199

tāi bù zhèng 胎不正, malposition of fetus, 384

tāi chì 胎赤, fetal redness, 198

tāi dǎn 胎疸, fetal jaundice, 198

tāi dòng 胎动, stirring fetus, 574

tāi dòng bù ān 胎动不安, stirring fetus, 574

tāi dú 胎毒, fetal toxin, 199

tāi féi 胎肥, fetal obesity, 198

tāi fēng 胎风, fetal wind, 199

tāi gòu 苔垢, grimy tongue fur, 249

tāi gòu 胎垢, fetal grime, 198

tāi huáng 胎黄, fetal jaundice, 198

tāi jīng 胎惊, fetal fright, 198

tāi lòu 胎漏, fetal spotting, 198

tāi qì 胎气, fetal qi, 198

tāi qì shàng bī 胎气上逼, fetal qi forcing upward, 198

tāi qì shàng bī 胎气上逼, upward forcing of fetal qi, 640

tāi qiè 胎怯, fetal timidity, 199

tāi rè dān dú 胎热丹毒, fetal heat cinnabar toxin, 198

tāi rè 胎热, fetal heat, 198

tāi rùn 苔润, moist tongue fur, 399

tāi ruò 胎弱, fetal feebleness, 197

tāi shàn 胎疝, fetal mounting, 198

tāi shòu 胎瘦, fetal emaciation, 197

tāi shuǐ 胎水, fetal water, 199

tāi sǐ bù xià 胎死不下, retention of dead fetus, 502

tāi sǐ fù zhōng 胎死腹中, death in utero, 119

tāi wèi bù zhèng 胎位不正, malposition of fetus, 384

tāi xián 胎痫, fetal epilepsy, 197

tāi xiǎn 胎癣, fetal lichen, 198

tāi yī bù xià 胎衣不下, retention of the afterbirth, 503

tāi yuán 胎元, fetal origin, 198

tāi yuán yǐn 胎元饮, Fetal Origin Beverage, 38, 199, 574

tāi yùn 胎孕, pregnancy, 460

tāi zào 苔燥, dry tongue fur, 158

tài 态, bearing, 16

tài bái 太白, SP-3, Supreme White, 41, 43, 61, 64, 70, 90, 109, 161, 163, 216, 223, 224, 228, 251, 256, 271, 282, 287, 319, 361, 378–380, 400, 435, 441, 453, 477, 483, 486, 488, 489, 519, 520, 548, 557, 562, 595, 596, 603, 604, 625, 639, 746

tài chōng 太冲, LR-3, Supreme Surge, 4, 6, 11, 14, 19, 20, 24–26, 28–37, 39, 40, 43, 53, 57–59, 61, 62, 64, 66, 69–72, 74, 82, 89, 90, 94, 99, 103, 109, 111, 118, 119, 123, 127, 128, 138, 140, 146, 147, 151, 152, 156–158, 161, 162, 164, 167, 175, 176, 178, 194, 201, 202, 210, 212, 215, 217, 218, 223, 225–230, 233–235, 241, 251, 256, 257, 259, 261, 266, 269, 273, 274, 279, 280, 284, 288, 290–292, 294, 296, 297, 300, 302, 314, 316, 319, 320, 333, 336, 337, 347–349, 352, 353, 355–362, 364–366, 382, 385, 390–393, 403, 415, 416, 424, 426, 434, 437, 438, 442, 447–449, 451–454, 456–458, 462, 468, 475, 477–485, 490, 493, 495, 499, 503, 504, 506, 511, 513, 515, 516, 524, 533, 534, 537, 538, 540, 548, 552, 554, 561, 564, 566–570, 579, 581, 585, 586, 591, 596, 597, 601, 607, 608, 610, 613, 614, 627, 640, 652, 654, 656, 658, 661, 665, 677, 683, 689–691, 693, 694, 696, 699–702, 711, 713, 714, 716, 748

tài shān pán shí sǎn 泰山磐石散, Rock of Taishan Fetus-Quieting Powder, 741

tài xī 太息, great respiration, 248

tài xī 太溪, KI-3, Great Ravine, 4, 11, 14, 23, 26, 28–31, 36, 41, 43, 45, 47, 54, 59, 61, 69, 70, 72, 84, 86, 88–90, 95–97, 105, 111, 117, 119, 123, 128, 151, 152, 154–156, 158, 160, 161, 163, 164, 167, 168, 174–177, 180, 197, 199, 201, 203, 222, 225, 229, 230, 237, 239, 256, 260, 263, 266–268, 275, 277, 282, 283, 285, 288–292, 294, 296, 302, 308, 310, 312, 314, 320, 327, 329, 331–337, 345, 347, 349, 352, 355, 360, 364–366, 368–370, 378–381, 391, 393, 398, 401, 410, 413, 415, 416, 425, 426, 449, 450, 453, 456, 461, 462, 465–467, 474, 485, 495, 500, 513, 515, 518, 521–525, 529, 547–549, 552, 559, 566, 567, 569, 570, 579, 580, 582, 584–586, 591, 594, 596, 597, 600, 603, 604, 607, 608, 610, 611, 614, 620, 630, 636, 640–643, 647–652, 660, 689, 701, 703, 711, 713–716, 747

tài yáng 太阳, Greater Yang, 11, 50, 62, 63, 79, 88, 89, 92, 111, 129, 181, 194, 217, 247, 258, 260, 287, 288, 301, 320, 344, 365, 395, 435, 437, 440, 462, 478, 495, 506, 520, 568, 586, 610, 681–687, 689, 691, 694

tài yáng 太阳, greater yang, 245

tài yáng biǎo zhèng 太阳表证, greater yang exterior pattern, 247

tài yáng bìng 太阳病, greater yang disease, 246

tài yáng fǔ bìng 太阳腑病, greater yang bowel disease, 245

tài yáng jīng 太阳经, greater yang channel, 245

tài yáng jīng bìng 太阳经病, greater yang channel disease, 245

tài yáng tóu tòng 太阳头痛, greater yang headache, 247

tài yī 太医, supreme physician, 597

tài yǐ 太乙, ST-23, Supreme Unity, 746

tài yǐ gāo 太乙膏, Tai Yi Plaster, 187

tài yīn 太阴, greater yin, 247

tài yīn bìng 太阴病, greater yin disease, 247

tài yīn jīng 太阴经, greater yin channel, 247

tài yīn tóu tòng 太阴头痛, greater yin headache, 247

tài yuān 太渊, LU-9, Great Abyss, 30, 43, 47, 70, 72, 83, 90, 92, 96, 97, 109, 146, 161, 163, 177, 207, 216, 224, 228, 237, 251, 257, 267, 301, 368, 378–380, 435, 441, 453, 467, 477, 486, 489, 515, 520, 530, 548, 550, 562, 570, 571, 589, 590, 595, 596, 603, 625, 630, 633, 639, 640, 651, 654, 663, 666, 675, 678, 683, 702, 703, 714, 715, 746

tài zǐ shēn 太子参 pseudostellaria, Pseudostellariae Radix, 108, 175, 593, 726

Talcum, *huá shí* 滑石, talcum, 17, 21, 22, 66, 69, 93, 115, 136, 463, 573, 667, 723

talcum, *huá shí* 滑石, Talcum, 17, 21, 22, 66, 69, 93, 115, 136, 463, 573, 667, 723

Tamaricis Ramulus et Folium, *chēng liǔ* 柽柳, tamarisk, 422, 501, 681, 720

tamarisk, *chēng liǔ* 柽柳, Tamaricis Ramulus et Folium, 422, 501, 681, 720

tān huàn 瘫痪, paralysis, 428

tán 痰, phlegm, 432

tán bāo 痰包, phlegm pouch, 440

tán bì 痰闭, phlegm block, 433

tán bì 痰秘, phlegm constipation, 434

tán chuǎn 痰喘, phlegm panting, 439

tán è 痰呃, phlegm hiccough, 438

tán hé 痰核, phlegm node, 439

tán huǒ 痰火, phlegm-fire, 436

tán huǒ cì (jìng) 痰火痓(痉), phlegm-fire tetany, 437

tán huǒ ěr míng 痰火耳鸣, phlegm-fire tinnitus, 437

tán huǒ rǎo xīn 痰火扰心, phlegm-fire harassing the heart, 436

tán huǒ tóu tòng 痰火头痛, phlegm-fire headache, 437

tán huǒ xuàn yūn 痰火眩晕, phlegm-fire dizziness, 436

tán huǒ zhēng chōng 痰火怔忡, phlegm-fire fearful throbbing, 436

tán jī 痰积, phlegm accumulation, 433

tán jī ǒu tù 痰积呕吐, phlegm accumulation vomiting, 433

tán jī xiè xiè 痰积泄泻, phlegm accumulation diarrhea, 433

tán jué 痰厥, phlegm reversal, 440

tán jué tóu tòng 痰厥头痛, phlegm reversal headache, 440

tán ké 痰咳, phlegm cough, 434

tán lì 痰疬, phlegm scrofula, 442

tán liú jīng luò 痰留经络, phlegm lodged in the channels, 438

tán liú xiōng xié 痰留胸胁, phlegm lodged in the chest and rib-side, 438

tán liú zhī tǐ 痰留肢体, phlegm lodged in the limbs, 438

tán méng xīn bāo 痰蒙心包, phlegm clouding the pericardium, 433

tán mí 痰迷, confounding phlegm, 93

tán mí xīn qiào 痰迷心窍, phlegm confounding the orifices of the heart, 433

tán míng 痰鸣, phlegm rale, 440

tán nüè 痰疟, phlegm malaria, 439

tán ǒu 痰呕, phlegm vomiting, 443

tán pǐ 痰痞, phlegm glomus, 437

tán pì 痰癖, phlegm aggregation, 433

tán qì hù jié 痰气互结, phlegm and qi binding together, 433

tán qì jiāo zǔ 痰气交阻, phlegm and qi obstructing each other, 433

tán qì yù jié 痰气郁结, binding depression of phlegm and qi, 19

tán rè 痰热, phlegm-heat, 437

tán rè jié xiōng 痰热结胸, phlegm-heat chest bind, 437

tán rè yōng fèi 痰热壅肺, phlegm-heat congesting the lung, 437

tán rè zǔ fèi 痰热阻肺, phlegm-heat obstructing the lung, 437

tán shī 痰湿, phlegm-damp, 435

tán shī bù yùn 痰湿不孕, phlegm-damp infertility, 435

tán shī ké sòu 痰湿咳嗽, phlegm-damp cough, 435

tán shī tóu tòng 痰湿头痛, phlegm-damp headache, 435

tán shī zǔ fèi 痰湿阻肺, phlegm-damp obstructing the lung, 435

tán shí mài 弹石脉, flicking stone pulse, 211

tán sòu 痰嗽, phlegm cough, 434

tán xián 痰痫, phlegm epilepsy, 436

tán xián 痰涎, phlegm-drool, 436

tán xián yōng shèng 痰涎壅盛, phlegm-drool congestion, 436

tán xiāng 檀香 sandalwood, Santali Lignum, 493, 724

tán xiāo 痰哮, phlegm wheezing, 443

tán xiè 痰泻, phlegm diarrhea, 435

tán yǐn 痰饮, phlegm-rheum, 440

tán yǐn chuǎn jí 痰饮喘急, phlegm-rheum rapid panting, 441

tán yǐn fù tòng 痰饮腹痛, phlegm-rheum abdominal pain, 440

tán yǐn ké sòu 痰饮咳嗽, phlegm-rheum cough, 441

tán yǐn ǒu tù 痰饮呕吐, phlegm-rheum vomiting, 442

tán yǐn wán 痰饮丸, Phlegm-Rheum Pill, 224, 663, 739

tán yǐn wèi wǎn (guǎn) tòng 痰饮胃脘痛, phlegm-rheum stomach duct pain, 441

tán yǐn wù hán 痰饮恶寒, phlegm-rheum aversion to cold, 441

tán yǐn xié tòng 痰饮胁痛, phlegm-rheum rib-side pain, 441

tán yǐn xuàn yūn 痰饮眩晕, phlegm-rheum dizziness, 441

tán yōng yí jīng 痰壅遗精, phlegm congestion seminal emission, 434

tán yù 痰郁, phlegm depression, 435

tán yù tāng 痰郁汤, Phlegm Depression Decoction, 435

tán zhēn 弹针, needle flicking, 406

tán zhèng 痰证, phlegm pattern, 439

tán zhèng zì hàn 痰证自汗, phlegm-pattern spontaneous sweating, 439

tán zhì è zǔ 痰滞恶阻, phlegm stagnation malign obstruction, 442

tán zhòng 痰中, phlegm stroke, 442

tán zhuó 痰浊, phlegm turbidity, 442

tán zhuó méng bì xīn bāo 痰浊蒙蔽心包, phlegm turbidity clouding the pericardium, 442

tán zhuó nèi bì 痰浊内闭, internal phlegm turbidity block, 316

tán zhuó shàng rǎo 痰浊上扰, phlegm turbidity harassing the upper body, 442

tán zhuó zǔ fèi 痰浊阻肺, phlegm turbidity obstructing the lung, 443

tán zǔ fèi luò 痰阻肺络, phlegm obstructing the network vessels of the lung, 439

tán zǔ xīn qiào 痰阻心窍, phlegm obstructing the orifices of the heart, 439

tàn tù 探吐, mechanical ejection, 388

tàn xī 叹息, sighing, 531

tāng jì 汤剂, decoction, 119

táng 唐, Tang, 602

táng jiāng jì 糖浆剂, syrup, 601

táng xiè 溏泄, sloppy diarrhea, 540

tàng shāng 烫伤, scald, 513

tangerine leaf, *jú yè* 橘叶, Citri Folium, 493, 723

tangerine peel, *chén pí* 陈皮, Citri Exocarpium, 5, 20, 38, 47, 80, 128, 129, 141, 153, 224, 230, 234, 256, 257, 272, 315, 317, 318, 401, 410, 418, 421, 430, 439, 454, 457, 475, 483, 493, 499, 542, 563, 577, 578, 581, 596, 625, 684, 695, 723

Tangerine Peel and Apricot Kernel Pill, *jú xìng wán* 橘杏丸, 477

Tangerine Peel and Bamboo Shavings Decoction, *jú pí zhú rú tāng* 橘皮竹茹汤, 156, 280, 736

Tangerine Peel Decocted Pill, *jú pí jiān wán* 橘皮煎丸, 485

Tangerine Peel, Pinellia, Unripe Bitter Orange, and Ovate Atractylodes Pill, *jú bàn zhǐ zhú wán* 橘半枳术丸, 736

tangerine pip, *jú hé* 橘核, Citri Semen, 19, 291, 385, 493, 606, 671, 723

Tangerine Pip Pill, *jú hé wán* 橘核丸, 51, 111, 399, 511, 735

tangerine pith, *jú luò* 橘络, Citri Fructus Fasciculus Vascularis, 417, 493, 723

tangkuei, *dāng guī* 当归, Angelicae Sinensis Radix, 17, 19, 28, 34, 37, 39, 58, 60, 93, 95, 103, 104, 116, 120, 139, 140, 154, 161, 172, 175, 227, 234, 259, 272, 309, 310, 315, 338, 352, 386, 390, 391, 398, 415, 428, 431, 448, 449, 467, 493, 495, 503, 516, 526, 588, 593, 595, 600, 613, 651, 661, 662, 666, 670, 674, 679, 727

Tangkuei and Astragalus Center-Fortifying Decoction, *guī qí jiàn zhōng tāng* 归芪建中汤, 650, 741

Tangkuei and Goat Meat Decoction, *dāng guī yáng ròu tāng* 当归羊肉汤, 741

Tangkuei and Peony Powder, *dāng guī sháo yào sǎn* 当归芍药散, 741

Tangkuei and Peony Six Gentlemen Pill, *guī sháo liù jūn wán* 归芍六君丸, 741

Tangkuei and Pueraria Decoction, *guī gé tāng* 归葛汤, 729

Tangkuei and Rehmannia Beverage, *dāng guī dì huáng yǐn* 当归地黄饮, 332, 333

Tangkuei Beverage, *dāng guī yǐn* 当归饮, 468

Tangkuei Blood-Quickening Decoction, *dāng guī huó xuè tāng* 当归活血汤, 737

Tangkuei Blood-Supplementing Decoction, *dāng guī bǔ xuè tāng* 当归补血汤, 25, 37–39, 152, 161, 171, 457, 566, 607, 646, 652, 741

tangkuei body, *dāng guī shēn* 当归身, Angelicae Sinensis Radicis Corpus, 256

Tangkuei Center-Fortifying Decoction, *dāng guī jiàn zhōng tāng* 当归建中汤, 38, 39, 94, 477, 734

Tangkuei Counterflow Cold Decoction Plus Evodia and Fresh Ginger, *dāng guī sì nì jiā wú zhū yú shēng jiāng tāng* 当归四逆加吴茱萸生姜汤, 735

Tangkuei Counterflow Cold Decoction, *dāng guī sì nì tāng* 当归四逆汤, 50, 85, 228, 231, 343, 504, 662, 711, 735

Tangkuei Decoction, *dāng guī tāng* 当归汤, 32

Tangkuei Drink, *dāng guī yǐn zǐ* 当归饮子, 117, 145, 422

tangkuei fine root, *dāng guī xū* 当归须, Angelicae Sinensis Radicis Tenuis, 356, 390

Tangkuei Pain-Assuaging Decoction, *dāng guī niān tòng tāng* 当归拈痛汤, 342, 347, 733

Tangkuei Powder, *dāng guī sǎn* 当归散, 571

Tangkuei Six Yellows Decoction, *dāng guī liù huáng tāng* 当归六黄汤, 40, 95, 176, 410, 599, 701, 715, 731

tangkuei tails, *dāng guī wěi* 当归尾, Angelicae Sinensis Radicis Extremitas, 27, 439

Tangkuei, Fresh Ginger, and Goat Meat Decoction, *dāng guī shēng jiāng yáng ròu tāng* 当归生姜羊肉汤, 741

Tangkuei, Gentian, and Aloe Pill, *dāng guī lóng huì wán* 当归龙荟丸, 158, 278, 297, 356, 365, 459, 549, 552, 566, 700, 713, 731

Tangkuei, Peony, and Rehmannia Decoction, *guī sháo dì huáng tāng* 归芍地黄汤, 741

táo dào 陶道, GV-13, Kiln Path, 8, 82, 197, 219, 383, 384, 394, 399, 439, 550, 590, 604, 650, 664, 690, 749

táo hé chéng qì tāng 桃核承气汤, Peach Kernel Qi-Coordinating Decoction, 24, 25, 36, 78, 182, 245, 316, 570, 571, 738

táo hóng sì wù tāng 桃红四物汤, Peach Kernel and Carthamus Four Agents Decoction, 24, 34, 36, 37, 138, 316, 540, 608, 738

táo huā sǎn 桃花散, Peach Blossom Powder, 25, 330, 745

táo huā tāng 桃花汤, Peach Blossom Decoction, 174, 742

táo huā xiǎn 桃花癣, peach-blossom lichen, 429

táo rén 桃仁 peach kernel, Persicae Semen, 20, 27, 34, 50, 59, 137–140, 182, 227, 356, 415, 428, 451, 512, 513, 571, 588, 679, 696, 724

táo rén chéng qì tāng 桃仁承气汤, Peach Kernel Qi-Coordinating Decoction, 34, 738

táo rén hóng huā jiān 桃仁红花煎, Peach Kernel and Carthamus Brew, 269, 273, 484

tapeworm infestation*, 298

Tapeworm-Expelling Decoction, *qū tāo tāng* 驱绦汤, 737

Taraxaci Herba cum Radice, *pú gōng yīng* 蒲公英, dandelion, 17, 67, 69, 70, 93, 120, 214, 282, 386, 440, 459, 501, 606, 685, 691, 721

TB-1, *guān chōng* 关冲, Passage Hub, 14, 152, 167, 384, 394, 403, 420, 547, 590, 611, 715, 748

TB-2, *yè mén* 液门, Humor Gate, 37, 155, 156, 158, 160, 174, 239, 294, 302, 336, 344, 348, 378, 455, 456, 462, 547, 589, 607, 611, 701, 715, 748

TB-3, *zhōng zhǔ* 中渚, Central Islet, 119, 160, 166, 167, 260, 288, 296, 330, 336, 348, 474, 566, 614, 658, 666, 748

TB-4, *yáng chí* 阳池, Yang Pool, 20, 90, 137, 231, 255, 289, 296, 344, 394, 521, 530, 548, 567, 748

TB-5, *wài guān* 外关, Outer Pass, 8, 14, 19, 61–63, 66, 69, 70, 72, 73, 82, 87, 89, 90, 92, 103, 105, 111, 112, 117, 119, 138–140, 145, 158, 166, 167, 184, 192, 194, 203, 218, 241, 247, 255, 258, 260, 283, 289, 295, 296, 301, 319, 320, 337, 342, 370, 374, 391, 403, 405, 408, 416, 437, 446, 448, 450, 452, 454, 456, 458, 474, 480, 482, 499, 501, 515, 516, 520, 530, 540, 544, 547, 568, 580, 586, 591, 620,

621, 631, 643, 665, 674, 677, 679, 680, 682, 683, 685–689, 693, 694, 703, 713, 748

TB-6, *zhī gōu* 支沟, Branch Ditch, 8, 19, 31, 34, 64, 88, 91, 112, 118, 127, 189, 190, 210, 215, 229, 233–235, 241, 280, 289, 290, 294, 302, 314, 338, 356, 357, 359, 362, 374, 426, 434, 475, 477, 478, 480, 482, 483, 485, 515, 519, 522, 585, 590, 631, 656, 658, 674, 683, 700, 703, 748

TB-7, *huì zōng* 会宗, Convergence and Gathering, 748

TB-8, *sān yáng luò* 三阳络, Three Yang Connection, 748

TB-9, *sì dú* 四渎, Four Rivers, 520, 748

TB-10, *tiān jǐng* 天井, Celestial Well, 137, 142, 295, 442, 515, 521, 567, 637, 748

TB-11, *qīng lěng yuān* 清冷渊, Clear Cold Abyss, 748

TB-12, *xiāo luò* 消泺, Dispersing Riverbed, 748

TB-13, *nào huì* 臑会, Upper Arm Convergence, 30, 210, 480, 748

TB-14, *jiān liáo* 肩髎, Shoulder Bone-Hole, 61, 89, 137, 289, 295, 342, 521, 530, 567, 748

TB-15, *tiān liáo* 天髎, Celestial Bone-Hole, 748

TB-16, *tiān yǒu* 天牖, Celestial Window, 748

TB-17, *yì fēng* 醫风, Wind Screen, 11, 73, 89, 105, 119, 125, 129, 140, 142, 160, 166, 167, 194, 220, 260, 289, 320, 329, 336, 348, 403, 474, 515, 521, 566, 614, 658, 689, 748

TB-18, *qì mài* 瘈脉, Tugging Vessel, 748

TB-19, *lú xī* 颅息, Skull Rest, 748

TB-20, *jiǎo sūn* 角孙, Angle Vertex, 500, 748

TB-21, *ěr mén* 耳门, Ear Gate, 119, 166, 167, 260, 474, 488, 521, 610, 614, 748

TB-22, *hé liáo* 和髎, Harmony Bone-Hole, 748

TB-23, *sī zhú kōng* 丝竹空, Silk Bamboo Hole, 150, 253, 500, 586, 682, 748

tè dìng xué zǔ xuǎn xué 特定穴组选穴, selection of special group points, 523

Tea-Blended Chrysanthemum Powder, *jú huā chá tiáo sǎn* 菊花茶调散, 740

Tea-Blended Ligusticum (Cnidium Root) Powder, *chuān xiōng chá tiáo sǎn* 川芎茶调散, 682, 683, 740

temporal bone*, 92

Ten Cinders Pill, *shí huī wán* 十灰丸, 569

Ten Cinders Powder (Pill), *shí huī sǎn (wán)* 十灰散（丸）, 738

Ten Cinders Powder, *shí huī sǎn* 十灰散, 233

Ten Diffusing Points, *shí xuān* 十宣, 6, 25, 70, 74, 75, 88, 92, 111, 156, 197, 283, 384, 448, 450, 455, 521, 547, 586, 589–591, 687, 693, 694, 702

Ten Fragrances Pill, *shí xiāng wán* 十香丸, 736

Ten Jujubes Decoction, *shí zǎo tāng* 十枣汤, 182, 214, 441, 732

Ten Supplements Pill, *shí bǔ wán* 十补丸, 742

Ten-Gem Decoction, *shí zhēn tāng* 十珍汤, 495

Ten-Ingredient Elsholtzia Beverage, *shí wèi xiāng rú yǐn* 十味香薷饮, 730

Ten-Ingredient Gallbladder-Warming Decoction, *shí wèi wēn dǎn tāng* 十味温胆汤, 236, 739

tender bamboo leaf (lophatherum), *zhú yè xīn* 竹叶心, Lophatheri Folium Immaturum, 65

téng 疼, pain, 423

téng tòng 疼痛, pain, 423

Terra Flava Usta, *fú lóng gān* 伏龙肝, oven earth, 311, 556, 569, 573, 666, 724

Testudinis Plastri Gelatinum, *guī bǎn jiāo* 龟版胶, tortoise plastron glue, 243, 593, 727

Testudinis Plastrum, *guī bǎn* 龟版, tortoise plastron, 53, 98, 175, 176, 310, 336, 352, 511, 524, 526, 593, 597, 614, 727

Testudinis Plastrum Crudum, *shēng guī bǎn* 生龟版, raw tortoise plastron, 415

tetanus*, 10, 366

Tetany-Relieving Powder, *zhǐ jìng sǎn* 止痉散, 456, 740

Tetrapanacis Medulla, *tōng cǎo* 通草, rice-paper plant pith, 66, 98, 136, 227, 434, 480, 723

Thalictri Rhizoma et Radix, *mǎ wěi lián* 马尾连, meadow rue, 67, 720

Third Variant Qi-Righting Powder, *sān jiā jiǎn zhèng qì sǎn* 三加减正气散, 733

thirteen ghost points, *shí sān guǐ xué* 十三鬼穴, 695

thoracic vertebra*

first, 550

Thorough Clearing Beverage, *kuò qīng yǐn* 廓清饮, 733

Thorough Knowledge of Medicine (*yī guàn*) 医贯, 1687 (Qīng), Zhào Xiàn-Kě 赵献可, 113

Thoroughfare-Quieting Decoction, *ān chōng tāng* 安冲汤, 603

Thoroughfare-Securing Decoction, *gù chōng tāng* 固冲汤, 478, 743

Thoroughly Pounded Paste, *qiān chuí gāo* 千捶膏, 75, 744

Thousand Gold Pieces Phragmites Decoction, *qiān jīn wěi jīng tāng* 千金苇茎汤, 15, 59, 373, 693

Thousand Gold Pieces Powder, *qiān jīn sǎn* 千金散, 213

Thousand Gold Pieces Prescriptions (*qiān jīn yào fāng*) 千金要方, full title *bèi jí qiān jīn yào fāng* 备急千金要方, 41, 91, 200, 254, 268, 324, 394, 612, 675, 686, 696

Thousand Gold Pieces Prescriptions for Emergencies (*bèi jí qiān jīn yào fāng*) 备急千金要方, 7th century (Táng), Sūn Sī-Miǎo 孙思邈, 243

Thousand Strings of Cash Decoction, *qiān mín tāng* 千缗汤, 439

Three Agents Emergency Pill, *sān wù bèi jí wán* 三物备急丸, 664, 731

Three Agents Little White Powder, *sān wù xiǎo bái sǎn* 三物小白散, 732

Three Agents White Powder, *sān wù bái sǎn* 三物白散, 85, 731

Three Causes Formulary (*sān yīn fāng*) 三因方, full title *sān yīn jí yī bìng zhèng fāng lùn* 三因极一病症方论, 242

Three Dispersers Beverage, *sān xiāo yǐn* 三消饮, 514, 736

Three Flowers Spirit Protection Pill, *sān huā shén yòu wán* 三花神佑丸, 213, 442, 732

Three Impediment Decoction, *sān bì tāng* 三痹汤, 734

Three Kernels Decoction, *sān rén tāng* 三仁汤, 23, 66, 69, 111, 118, 228, 297, 539, 675, 733

Three Raw Agents Beverage, *sān shēng yǐn* 三生饮, 739

Three Stones Powder, *sān shí sǎn* 三石散, 516, 671

Three Transformations Decoction, *sān huà tāng* 三化汤, 631

Three Yellow Jewels Wax Pill, *sān huáng bǎo là wán* 三黄宝腊丸, 737

Three Yellows and Gypsum Decoction, *sān huáng shí gāo tāng* 三黄石膏汤, 70, 500, 664, 730

Three Yellows Bitter Orange and Ovate Atractylodes Pill, *sān huáng zhǐ zhú wán* 三黄枳术丸, 277, 736

Three Yellows Decoction, *sān huáng tāng* 三黄汤, 320, 640, 670

Three Yellows Four Agents Decoction, *sān huáng sì wù tāng* 三黄四物汤, 102, 730

Three Yellows Heart-Draining Decoction, *sān huáng xiè xīn tāng* 三黄泻心汤, 147, 282, 497, 636

Three Yellows Wash Preparation, *sān huáng xǐ jì* 三黄洗剂, 445, 744

Three Yellows Wax Pill, *sān huáng là wán* 三黄腊丸, 737

Three-Agent Elsholtzia Powder, *sān wù xiāng rú yǐn* 三物香薷饮, 729

Three-in-One Qi-Coordinating Decoction, *sān yī chéng qì tāng* 三一承气汤, 712, 731

Three-Option Anise Pill, *sān céng huí xiāng wán* 三层茴香丸, 735

Three-Seed Decoction, *sān zǐ tāng* 三子汤, 87

Three-Seed Filial Devotion Decoction, *sān zǐ yǎng qīn tāng* 三子养亲汤, 141, 142, 216, 414, 435, 739

Three-Shot Gun, *sān pǐn yī tiáo qiāng* 三品一条枪, 290, 744

Throat Insufflation Powder, *chuī hóu sǎn* 吹喉散, 310

Throat-Clearing Construction-Nourishing Decoction, *qīng yān yǎng yíng tāng* 清咽养营汤, 734

Throat-Clearing Diaphragm-Disinhibiting Decoction, *qīng yān lì gé tāng* 清咽利膈汤, 14, 581, 586, 612, 671

Throat-Clearing Dryness-Moistening Decoction, *qīng yān rùn zào tāng* 清咽润噪汤, 619

thromboangiitis*, 540

thrombosis of the central artery of the retina*, 586

thrombosis*
   cerebral, 692

thrombotic angiitis*, 540

Thumb Bone Hollow, *dà gǔ kōng* 大骨空, 93, 195, 500, 586, 636

thunder god vine, *léi gōng téng* 雷公藤, Tripterygii Wilfordi Radix, Folium et Flos, 140, 722

thyrocele*, 544

thyroid adenoma*, 243

thyroid tumor*, 210

tí chā bǔ xiè 提插补泻, lifting and thrusting supplementation and drainage, 346

tí chā fǎ 提插法, lifting and thrusting, 346

tí gāng sǎn 提肛散, Rectum-Lifting Powder, 493

tí niē jìn zhēn fǎ 提捏进针法, pinch-and-lift needle insertion, 444

tí nóng qū fǔ 提脓祛腐, raising pus and dispelling putridity, 492

tǐ 体, constitutional body, 95

tǐ chòu 体臭, body odor, 41

tì 涕, nasal mucus, 405

tì 涕, snivel, 543

tì wéi fèi yè 涕为肺液, snivel is the humor of the lung, 544

tiān 天, heaven, 285

tiān bù 天部, heaven level, 286

tiān chí 天池, PC-1, Celestial Pool, 216, 220, 748

tiān chōng 天冲, GB-9, Celestial Hub, 748

tiān chuāng 天窗, SI-16, Celestial Window, 747

tiān dǐng 天鼎, LI-17, Celestial Tripod, 30, 129, 210, 480, 746

tiān fǔ 天府, LU-3, Celestial Storehouse, 414, 678, 746

tiān gān dì zhī 天干地支, heavenly stems and earthly branches, 286

tiān guǐ 天癸, heavenly tenth, 286

tiān guǐ 天癸, tian-gui, 613

tiān huā 天花, smallpox, 543

tiān huā fěn 天花粉 trichosanthes root, Trichosanthis Radix, 67, 82, 108, 450, 463, 581, 679, 685, 686, 720

tiān jǐng 天井, TB-10, Celestial Well, 137, 142, 295, 442, 515, 521, 567, 637, 748

tiān jiǔ 天灸, natural moxibustion, 405

tiān kuí zǐ 天葵子 semiaquilegia tuber, Semiaquilegiae Tuber, 68, 721

tiān kuò 天廓, heaven rampart, 286

tiān liáo 天髎, TB-15, Celestial Bone-Hole, 748

tiān luó sǎn 天罗散, Luffa Stem Powder, 121

tiān má 天麻 gastrodia, Gastrodiae Rhizoma, 53, 54, 56, 225, 257, 417, 690, 726

tiān má gōu téng yǐn 天麻钩藤饮, Gastrodia and Uncaria Beverage, 11, 178, 292, 365, 417, 526, 568, 574, 689, 716, 740

tiān má wán 天麻丸, Gastrodia Pill, 691

tiān mén dōng 天门冬 asparagus, Asparagi Tuber, 88, 336, 385, 409, 495, 593, 597, 727

tiān nán xīng 天南星 arisaema, Arisaematis Rhizoma, 97, 572, 623, 625, 638, 725

tiān nán xīng wán 天南星丸, Arisaema Pill, 739

tiān pào chuāng 天泡疮, heaven-borne blisters, 285

tiān qiáo mài gēn 天荞麦根 wild buckwheat root, Fagopyri Cymosi Radix et Rhizoma, 68, 469, 721

tiān quán 天泉, PC-2, Celestial Spring, 748

tiān rén dì 天人地, heaven, human, and earth, 285

tiān rén dì sān cái bǔ xiè 天人地三才补泻, heaven, human, and earth supplementation and drainage, 285

tiān rén xiāng yìng 天人相应, heaven and man are mutually responsive, 285

tiān róng 天容, SI-17, Celestial Countenance, 30, 89, 210, 220, 480, 521, 689, 747

tiān shū 天枢, ST-25, Celestial Pivot, 1, 3, 4, 8, 15, 26, 28, 29, 35, 36, 40, 47, 54, 61–64, 70, 72, 73, 77, 78, 80, 83, 86, 89, 91, 94, 105, 109–111, 114–117, 127, 136, 141, 151, 153, 157, 168, 174, 186, 196, 197, 212, 215–218, 224, 234, 235, 247, 256, 257, 267, 276–278, 280, 281, 284, 289, 290, 298, 300–302, 312, 314, 316, 318, 325, 335, 338–340, 349, 361, 383, 395, 401, 415, 418, 425, 434, 436, 438–442, 447, 450, 451, 454, 457, 462, 477, 479, 480, 482–485, 487, 498, 499, 509, 510, 522, 540, 554, 555, 558, 559, 561, 562, 564, 565, 570, 579, 581, 585, 588, 589, 601, 612, 631, 633, 645–647, 656, 664, 666, 678, 683, 684, 703, 710, 713, 716, 746

tiān tái wū yào sǎn 天台乌药散, Tiantai Lindera Powder, 83, 425, 736

tiān tíng 天庭, celestial court, 54

tiān tú 天突, CV-22, Celestial Chimney, 13, 14, 19, 30, 87, 92, 93, 109, 115, 123, 129, 153, 156, 158, 164, 210, 277, 282, 291, 292, 368, 398, 433, 435, 439, 440, 443, 445, 477, 480, 506, 521, 522, 544, 547, 611, 624, 681, 684, 689, 749

tiān wáng bǔ xīn dān 天王补心丹, Celestial Emperor Heart-Supplementing Elixir, 37, 244, 261, 266, 336, 525, 537, 701, 739

tiān xī 天溪, SP-18, Celestial Ravine, 746

tiān xiān téng sǎn 天仙藤散, Aristolochia Stem Powder, 454, 601

tiān xíng 天行, heaven current, 285

tiān xíng chì yán 天行赤眼, heaven-current red eye, 285

tiān xíng sòu 天行嗽, heaven-current cough, 285

tiān xíng wēn yì 天行温疫, heaven-current warm epidemic, 285

tiān xióng 天雄 tianxiong aconite, Aconiti Tuber Laterale Tianxiong, 23, 97

tiān yǒu 天牖, TB-16, Celestial Window, 748

tiān zhú huáng 天竹黄 bamboo sugar, Bambusae Concretio Silicea, 140, 214, 541, 624, 725

tiān zhù 天柱, BL-10, Celestial Pillar, 89, 105, 120, 168, 247, 259, 629, 747

tiān zhù dǎo 天柱倒, tumbled celestial pillar, 632

tiān zōng 天宗, SI-11, Celestial Gathering, 61, 462, 521, 530, 747

tián xìng rén 甜杏仁 sweet apricot kernel, Armeniacae Semen Dulce, 624, 725

Tiantai Lindera Powder, *tiān tái wū yào sǎn* 天台乌药散, 83, 425, 736

tianxiong aconite, *tiān xióng* 天雄, Aconiti Tuber Laterale Tianxiong, 23, 97

tiāo cì chū xuè 挑刺出血, pick to bleed, 444

tiāo cì fàng xuè 挑刺放血, pick to bleed, 444

tiāo zhēn liáo fǎ 挑针疗法, needle-picking therapy, 407

tiāo zhì 挑痔, hemorrhoid point picking, 290

tiāo zhì liáo fǎ 挑治疗法, picking therapy, 444

tiāo zhì liáo fǎ 挑痔疗法, hemorrhoid point picking, 290

tiāo zhì zhì fǎ 挑治痔法, hemorrhoid point picking, 290

tiáo 调, regulate, 498

tiáo fū 调敷, apply mixed, 10

tiáo gān sǎn 调肝散, Liver-Regulating Powder, 658, 736

tiáo gān tāng 调肝汤, Liver-Regulating Decoction, 360

tiáo hé 调和, harmonize, 255

tiáo hé cháng wèi 调和肠胃, gastrointestinal harmonization, 240

tiáo hé cháng wèi 调和肠胃, harmonizing the stomach and intestines, 257

tiáo hé gān pí 调和肝脾, harmonizing the liver and spleen, 256

tiáo hé gān pí 调和肝脾, liver spleen harmonization, 362

tiáo hé gān wèi 调和肝胃, harmonizing the liver and stomach, 256

tiáo hé pí wèi 调和脾胃, harmonizing the spleen and stomach, 257

tiáo hé pí wèi 调和脾胃, spleen-stomach harmonization, 561

tiáo hé yíng wèi 调和营卫, harmonizing construction and defense, 255

tiáo jīng 调经, regulating menstruation, 498

tiáo jīng sǎn 调经散, Channel-Regulating Powder, 456

tiáo kǒu 条口, ST-38, Ribbon Opening, 341, 342, 446, 530, 746

tiáo qì 调气, regulating qi, 498

tiáo wèi chéng qì tāng 调胃承气汤, Stomach-Regulating Qi-Coordinating Decoction, 54, 84, 127, 157, 314, 426, 459, 613, 731

tiáo yíng yǐn 调营饮, Construction-Regulating Beverage, 151, 467

tiáo yuán shèn qì tāng 调元肾气丸, Origin-Regulating Kidney Qi Pill, 745

tibia*, 658

tiě dí wán 铁笛丸, Iron Flute Pill, 729

tiě luò 铁落 iron flakes, Ferri Frusta, 54, 526, 585, 726

tiě xiàn 铁苋 copperleaf, Acalyphae Herba, 724

tiger bone, *hǔ gǔ* 虎骨, Tigris Os, 45, 139, 397, 722

Tiger Bone Four Jin Pill, *hǔ gǔ sì jīn wán* 虎骨四斤丸, 337

tiger bone glue, *hǔ gǔ jiāo* 虎骨胶, Tigris Gelatinum Ossis, 243

Tiger Bone Powder, *hǔ gǔ sǎn* 虎骨散, 45

Tigris Gelatinum Ossis, *hǔ gǔ jiāo* 虎骨胶, tiger bone glue, 243

Tigris Os, *hǔ gǔ* 虎骨, tiger bone, 45, 139, 397, 722

Tin-Like Powder, *xí lèi sǎn* 锡类散, 615, 744

Tincture of Golden Larch (root) Bark, *tǔ jǐn pí dīng* 土槿皮酊, 689

tinea corporis*, 76, 689

tinea cruris*, 710

tinea favosa*, 196

tinea manus*, 244

tinea pedis*, 221

tinea versicolor*, 473

tīng gōng 听宫, SI-19, Auditory Palace, 89, 119, 167, 220, 253, 260, 330, 521, 566, 614, 747

tīng huì 听会, GB-2, Auditory Convergence, 75, 89, 119, 160, 166, 167, 296, 320, 330, 336, 348, 474, 521, 566, 614, 658, 748

tíng 庭, court, 104

tíng 停, collect, 87

tíng ěr 聤耳, purulent ear, 474

tíng lì dà zǎo xiè fèi tāng 葶苈大枣泻肺汤, Tingli and Jujube Lung-Draining Decoction, 130, 438, 468, 469, 506, 738

tíng lì zǐ 葶苈子 tingli, Descurainiae seu Lepidii Semen, 12, 70, 130, 232, 282, 438, 624, 625, 667, 725

tíng yǐn xī jì 停饮心悸, collecting rheum heart palpitations, 87

tíng yǐn xié tòng 停饮胁痛, collecting rheum rib-side pain, 87

tíng yǐn xuàn yūn 停饮眩晕, collecting rheum dizziness, 87

tǐng cháng 挺长, persistent erection, 430

tingli, *tíng lì zǐ* 葶苈子, Descurainiae seu Lepidii Semen, 12, 70, 130, 232, 282, 438, 624, 625, 667, 725

Tingli and Jujube Lung-Draining Decoction, *tíng lì dà zǎo xiè fèi tāng* 葶苈大枣泻肺汤, 130, 438, 468, 469, 506, 738

tinospora tuber, *jīn guǒ lǎn* 金果榄, Tinosporae Tuber, 68, 721

Tinosporae Sinensis Caulis, *shēn jīn téng* 伸筋藤, Chinese tinospora, 140, 722

Tinosporae Tuber, *jīn guǒ lǎn* 金果榄, tinospora tuber, 68, 721

Tip of the Ear, *ěr jiān* 耳尖, 585

Tip of the Elbow, *zhǒu jiān* 肘尖, 142, 171, 442, 515, 544

toad venom, *chán sū* 蟾酥, Bufonis Venenum, 728

Toad Venom Pill, *chán sū wán* 蟾酥丸, 315

Toilette Pill, *gēng yī wán* 更衣丸, 459, 732

tōng 通, free, 226

tōng 通, restore flow, 502

tōng 通, unstop, 638

tōng bì 通闭, freeing blocks, 227

tōng cǎo 通草 rice-paper plant pith, Tetrapanacis Medulla, 66, 98, 136, 227, 434, 480, 723

tōng gǔ (fù) 通谷 (腹), KI-20, Open Valley, 748

tōng gǔ (zú) 通谷 (足), BL-66, (Foot) Valley Passage, 747

tōng guān sǎn 通关散, Gate-Freeing Powder, 740

tōng jì 通剂, freeing formula, 227

tōng jīng 通经, freeing menstruation, 227

tōng jīng 通经, freeing the channels, 228

tōng jīng 通经, promoting menstruation, 467

tōng jīng dǎo zhì tāng 通经导滞汤, Channel-Freeing Stagnation-Abducting Decoction, 571

tōng jīng huó luò 通经活络, freeing the channels and quickening the network vessels, 228

tōng jīng huó luò tāng 通经活络汤, Channel-Freeing Network-Quickening Decoction, 736

tōng kě qù zhì 通可去滞, freeing [medicinals] can eliminate stagnation, 227

tōng lǐ 通里, HT-5, Connecting Li, 39, 58, 69, 71, 90, 140, 223, 230, 268, 289, 294, 302, 365, 383, 408, 427, 449, 451, 455, 521, 538, 540, 572, 573, 589, 597, 629, 683, 701, 747

tōng luò 通络, freeing the network vessels, 228

tōng mài 通脉, freeing the vessels, 228

tōng mài sì nì tāng 通脉四逆汤, Vessel-Freeing Counterflow Cold Decoction, 64, 79, 85, 228, 505, 711, 735

tōng qì 通气, freeing qi, 228

tōng qì sàn jiān wán 通气散坚丸, Qi-Freeing Hardness-Dissipating Pill, 486

tōng qiào 通窍, freeing the orifices, 228

tōng qiào huó xuè tāng 通窍活血汤, Orifice-Freeing Blood-Quickening Decoction, 571, 738

tōng rǔ 通乳, freeing milk, 227

tōng rǔ dān 通乳丹, Lactation Elixir, 513, 741

tōng tiān 通天, BL-7, Celestial Connection, 120, 520, 747

tōng xuān lǐ fèi wán 通宣理肺丸, Diffusing-Freeing Lung-Rectifying Pill, 738

tōng yáng 通阳, freeing yang, 228

tōng yīn tōng yòng 通因通用, treating the free by freeing, 626

tōng yōu tāng 通幽汤, Dark-Gate–Freeing Decoction, 164

tōng yū jiān 通瘀煎, Stasis-Freeing Brew, 33, 34, 738

tóng biàn 童便 child's urine, Infantis Urina, 201, 567

tóng bìng yì zhì 同病异治, unlike treatment of like disease, 638

tóng jīng xiāng yìng qǔ xué fǎ 同经相应取穴法, selection of same-name channel points of corresponding location, 523

tóng míng jīng 同名经, same-name channel, 512

tóng míng jīng pèi xué fǎ 同名经配穴法, combining same-name channel points, 89

tóng míng jīng xuǎn xué 同名经选穴, selection of same-name channel points, 523

tóng rén 瞳仁, pupil, 473

tóng shēn cùn 同身寸, body-inch, 41

tóng shén 瞳神, pupil spirit, 473

tóng yóu 桐油 tung-oil, Aleuritis Seminis Oleum, 445

tóng zǐ 瞳子, pupil, 473

tóng zǐ liáo 瞳子髎, GB-1, Pupil Bone-Hole, 64, 93, 150, 195, 252, 320, 395, 495, 520, 568, 748

tòng 痛, pain, 423

tòng 痛, sore, 545

tòng 痛, soreness, 546

tòng bì 痛痹, painful impediment, 424

tòng fēng 痛风, pain wind, 426

tòng jīng 痛经, menstrual pain, 392

tòng rú dāo cì 痛如刀刺, pain like the stabbing of a knife, 426

tòng rú dāo gē 痛如刀割, pain like the cutting of a knife, 426

tòng rú zhuī cì 痛如锥刺, pain like the piercing of an awl, 426

tòng xiè yào fāng 痛泻要方, Pain and Diarrhea Formula, 19, 256, 361, 479, 732

tonsillitis*, 14
  acute, 659
  chronic, 581

tonsils*
  pharyngeal, 612

toosendan, *chuān liàn zǐ* 川楝子, Toosendan Fructus, 19, 103, 183, 256, 310, 334, 343, 390, 400, 483, 493, 509, 542, 581, 589, 666, 671, 723

Toosendan Fructus, *chuān liàn zǐ* 川楝子, toosendan, 19, 103, 183, 256, 310, 334, 343, 390, 400, 483, 493, 509, 542, 581, 589, 666, 671, 723

Toosendan Powder, *jīn líng zǐ sǎn* 金铃子散, 19, 27, 280, 354, 478, 483, 735

tooth niter, *yá xiāo* 牙硝, Nitrum Dentatum, 411

Topical Bone-Joining Powder, *wài fū jiē gǔ sǎn* 外敷接骨散, 745

torreya, *fěi zǐ* 榧子, Torreyae Semen, 183, 509, 724

Torreya and Aspidium Decoction, *fěi zǐ guàn zhòng tāng* 榧子贯众汤, 737

Torreyae Semen, *fěi zǐ* 榧子, torreya, 183, 509, 724

tortoise plastron, *guī bǎn* 龟版, Testudinis Plastrum, 53, 98, 175, 176, 310, 336, 352, 511, 524, 526, 593, 597, 614, 727

Tortoise Plastron and Ailanthus Bark Pill, *guī shū wán* 龟樗丸, 115

Tortoise Plastron and Deerhorn Two Immortals Glue, *guī lù èr xiān jiāo* 龟鹿二仙胶, 741

tortoise plastron glue, *guī bǎn jiāo* 龟版胶, Testudinis Plastri Gelatinum, 243, 593, 727

tóu 头, head, 258

tóu fà 头发, hair, 251

tóu fēng 头风, head wind, 259

tóu fēng bái xiè 头风白屑, head-wind white scaling, 260

tóu hàn 头汗, sweating head, 599

tóu lín qì (头)临泣, GB-15, (Head) Overlooking Tears, 150, 219, 495, 520, 682, 748

tóu miàn chuāng 头面疮, sore of the head or face, 546

tóu nǎo kōng tòng 头脑空痛, empty pain in the head, 173

tóu pí zhēn 头皮针, scalp acupuncture, 513

tóu piān tòng 头偏痛, hemilateral headache, 288

tóu qiào yīn 头窍阴, GB-11, Head Orifice Yin, 219, 748

tóu rè 头热, hot head, 292

tóu shēn kūn zhòng 头身困重, heavy cumbersome head and body, 287

tóu suǐ 头髓, head marrow, 259

tóu téng 头疼, headache, 258

tóu tòng 头痛, headache, 258

tóu tòng rú chè 头痛如掣, headache with pulling sensation, 259

tóu tòng rú chè 头痛如掣, iron-band headache, 320

tóu wéi 头维, ST-8, Head Corner, 32, 73, 79, 99, 153, 192, 194, 202, 216, 219, 223, 247, 259, 287, 301, 433–437, 440, 441, 487, 519, 539, 588, 684, 687, 691, 699, 746

tóu xiàng qiáng tòng 头项强痛, headache and stiff painful nape, 259

tóu yáo 头摇, shaking of the head, 528

tóu yūn 头晕, dizzy head, 144

tóu zhàng 头胀, distention in the head, 143

tóu zhàng 头胀, sensation of pressure in the head, 525

tóu zhēn liáo fǎ 头针疗法, scalp acupuncture, 513

tóu zhòng 头重, heavy-headedness, 287

tóu zhòng rú guǒ 头重如裹, bag-over-the-head sensation, 15

tóu zhòng rú guǒ 头重如裹, head heavy as if swathed, 259

tòu 透, outthrust, 422

tòu bān 透斑, outthrusting macules, 422

tòu biǎo 透表, outthrusting the exterior, 422

tòu nóng sǎn 透脓散, Pus-Outthrusting Powder, 187, 323, 744

tòu tiān liáng 透天凉, heaven-penetrating cooling method, 286

tòu xué 透穴, joining points, 322

tòu xué 透穴, point joining, 446

tòu zhěn 透疹, outthrusting papules, 422

toxemia*, 148, 153, 195, 202, 648

toxic encephalopathy*, 692

Toxin-Diffusing Exterior-Effusing Decoction, *xuān dú fā biǎo tāng* 宣毒发表汤, 387, 422, 729

Toxin-Dispersing Rhinoceros Beverage, *xiāo dú xī jiāo yǐn* 消毒犀角饮, 497

Toxin-Vanquishing Powder, *bài dú sǎn* 败毒散, 517, 688

Trachelospermi Caulis, *luò shí téng* 络石藤, star jasmine stem, 139, 256, 722

trachoma*, 430

Trachycarpi Stipulae Fibra, *zōng lǘ pí* 棕榈皮, trachycarpus, 569, 724

Trachycarpi Stipulae Fibra Veta, *chén zōng pí* 陈棕皮, old trachycarpus, 53

trachycarpus, *zōng lǘ pí* 棕榈皮, Trachycarpi Stipulae Fibra, 569, 724

tragus*, 166, 211, 429

Transforming Yellow Decoction, *yì huáng tāng* 易黄汤, 743

Tremor-Stabilizing Pill, *dìng zhèn wán* 定振丸, 365

Tribuli Fructus, *cì jí lí* 刺蒺藜, tribulus, 5, 53, 54, 234, 308, 320, 461, 518, 726

tribulus, *cì jí lí* 刺蒺藜, Tribuli Fructus, 5, 53, 54, 234, 308, 320, 461, 518, 726

Trichomonas Cleansing Pill, *méi dī jīng wán* 霉滴净丸, 745

trichomonas vaginitis*, 468

trichosanthes, *guā lóu* 栝楼, Trichosanthis Fructus, 201, 230, 282, 376, 388, 398, 399, 614, 624, 625, 725

Trichosanthes and Arctium Decoction, *guā lóu niú bàng tāng* 瓜蒌牛蒡汤, 386, 743

Trichosanthes and Cinnamon Twig Decoction, *guā lóu guì zhī tāng* 栝楼桂枝汤, 544

Trichosanthes and Unripe Bitter Orange Decoction, *guā lóu zhǐ shí tāng* 栝楼枳实汤, 735

trichosanthes rind, *guā lóu pí* 栝楼皮, Trichosanthis Pericarpium, 70, 107, 624, 725

trichosanthes root, *tiān huā fěn* 天花粉, Trichosanthis Radix, 67, 82, 108, 450, 463, 581, 679, 685, 686, 720

trichosanthes seed, *guā lóu zǐ* 栝楼子, Trichosanthis Semen, 372, 399, 624, 637, 725

trichosanthes seed frost, *guā lóu rén shuāng* 栝楼仁霜, Trichosanthis Seminis Pulvis, 127, 231

Trichosanthes, Chinese Chive, and Pinellia Decoction, *guā lóu xiè bái bàn xià tāng* 栝楼薤白半夏汤, 58, 59, 735

Trichosanthes, Chinese Chive, and White Liquor Decoction, *guā lóu xiè bái bái jiǔ tāng* 栝楼薤白白酒汤, 58, 228, 273, 735

Trichosanthis Fructus, *guā lóu* 栝楼, trichosanthes, 201, 230, 282, 376, 388, 398, 399, 614, 624, 625, 725

Trichosanthis Pericarpium, *guā lóu pí* 栝楼皮, trichosanthes rind, 70, 107, 624, 725

Trichosanthis Radix, *tiān huā fěn* 天花粉, trichosanthes root, 67, 82, 108, 450, 463, 581, 679, 685, 686, 720

Trichosanthis Semen, *guā lóu zǐ* 栝楼子, trichosanthes seed, 372, 399, 624, 637, 725

Trichosanthis Seminis Pulvis, *guā lóu rén shuāng* 栝楼仁霜, trichosanthes seed frost, 127, 231

Triple Supplementation Pill, *sān bǔ wán* 三补丸, 63

Triple-Armored Pulse-Restorative Decoction, *sān jiǎ fù mài tāng* 三甲复脉汤, 526, 740

Tripterygii Wilfordi Radix, Folium et Flos, *léi gōng téng* 雷公藤, thunder god vine, 140, 722

trismus*, 73

Tritici Semen Leve, *fú xiǎo mài* 浮小麦, light wheat, 95, 410, 518, 651, 727

trochanter*
   great, 607

Trogopteri seu Pteromydis Excrementum, *wǔ líng zhī* 五灵脂, flying squirrel's droppings, 137, 138, 397, 411, 448, 467, 574, 724

Trollii Flos, *jīn lián huā* 金莲花, globeflower, 68, 721

Troop-Marching Powder, *xíng jūn sǎn* 行军散, 740

True Jade Pill, *yù zhēn wán* 玉真丸, 330

True Jade Powder, *yù zhēn sǎn* 玉真散, 74, 140, 366, 740

True Man Viscus-Nourishing Decoction, *zhēn rén yǎng zàng tāng* 真人养脏汤, 12, 318, 742

True Warrior Decoction, *zhēn wǔ tāng* 真武汤, 266, 287, 301, 322, 329, 335, 341, 345, 441, 488, 541, 608, 661, 666–668, 711, 716, 733

True-Securing Decoction, *gù zhēn tāng* 固真汤, 122

True-Securing Pill, *gù zhēn wán* 固真丸, 743

Truly Wondrous Powder, *dì qí sǎn* 的奇散, 449

tsaoko, *cǎo guǒ* 草果, Amomi Tsao-Ko Fructus, 45, 113, 217, 317, 574, 625, 722

Tsaoko Pill, *dòu kòu wán* 豆蔻丸, 77, 314, 581

tū chuāng 秃疮, bald scalp sore, 16

tū chuāng yóu 秃疮油, Bald Sores Oil, 16

tǔ 土, earth, 167

tǔ bèi mǔ 土贝母 bolbosteema, Bolbosteematis Tuber, 291

tǔ bù zhì shuǐ 土不制水, earth failing to dam water, 167

tǔ chǎo 土炒, stir-frying with earth, 573

tǔ dà huáng 土大黄 Madaio dock root, Rumicis Madaio Radix, 116, 569

tǔ fú líng 土茯苓 smooth greenbrier root, Smilacis Glabrae Rhizoma, 68, 540, 584, 685, 691, 721

tǔ fú líng hé jì 土茯苓合剂, Smooth Greenbrier Mixture, 494

tǔ jǐn pí dīng 土槿皮酊, Tincture of Golden Larch (root) Bark, 689

tǔ jīng pí 土荆皮 golden larch (root) bark, Pseudolaricis Kaempferi Cortex (Radicis), 41, 728

tǔ niú xī 土牛膝 native achyranthes, Achyranthis Radix, 138, 459, 724

tǔ nòng shé 吐弄舌, protrusion and worrying of the tongue, 468

tǔ shēng wàn wù 土生万物, earth engenders the myriad things, 167

tǔ xǐ wēn zào 土喜温燥, earth likes warmth and dryness, 167

tǔ xián mò 吐涎沫, ejection of foamy drool, 170

tù 吐, eject, 170

tù chún 兔唇, harelip, 255

tù fǎ 吐法, ejection, 170

tù fǎ 吐法, emesis, 172

tù huí 吐蛔, roundworm vomiting, 510

tù qīng shuǐ 吐清水, vomiting of clear water, 657

tù sī zǐ 菟丝子 cuscuta, Cuscutae Semen, 310, 518, 529, 572, 593, 614, 727

tù sī zǐ wán 菟丝子丸, Cuscuta Seed Pill, 180, 523, 636, 743

tù suān 吐酸, acid vomiting, 4

tù tán xián 吐痰涎, eject phlegm-drool, 170

tù xuè 吐血, blood ejection, 29

tuberculosis, 616

tuberculosis of lymph node*, 515

tuberculosis of testis*, 671

tuberculosis of the bone*, 213

tuberculosis of the breast*, 385

tuberculosis of the joints*, 213

tuberculosis of the urinary tract*, 583

tuberculosis*, 377, 641, 646
  active, 290
  intestinal, 110
  pulmonary, 97, 336, 380, 530, 615, 714

tuberculous goiter*, 210

tuī guàn fǎ 推罐法, push-cupping, 474

tuī ná 推拿, tui-na, 631

tuī qì fǎ 推气法, qi-pushing method, 482

tuí 瘣, prominence, 466

tuí shàn 癞疝, bulging mounting, 51

tuí shàn 瘣疝, prominent mounting, 467

tuí (tuì) 癞, bulging, 51

tuǐ tòng 腿痛, leg pain, 342

tuì rè 退热, abating heat, 1

tuì rè sǎn 退热散, Heat-Abating Powder, 731

tuì zhēn 退针, needle retraction, 407

tumor of the tongue*, 619

tumor of the urethra*, 148

tumor of thyroid*, 243

tumor*
  brain, 260
  cystic, 632
  malign, 367

tūn suān 吞酸, acid regurgitation, 4

tūn suān 吞酸, swallowing of upflowing acid, 598

tung-oil, *tóng yóu* 桐油, Aleuritis Seminis Oleum, 445

tuō 脱, desertion, 124

tuō dú tòu nóng 托毒透脓, expressing toxin and out-thrusting pus, 183

tuō fǎ 托法, expression, 183

tuō gāng 脱肛, anal desertion, 8

tuō gāng 脱肛, prolapse of the rectum, 465

tuō gāng zhì 脱肛痔, rectal prolapse hemorrhoids, 492

tuō huā jiān 脱花煎, Falling Flower Brew, 503

tuō hàn 脱汗, desertion sweating, 124

tuō jiè 脱胯, dislocation, 136

tuō jiù 脱臼, dislocation, 136

tuō jū 脱疽, sloughing flat-abscess, 540

tuō ké náng yōng 脱壳囊痈, shell-bursting scrotal welling-abscess, 529

tuō ké rǔ yōng 脱壳乳痈, shell-bursting mammary welling-abscess, 529

tuō lǐ dìng tòng tāng 托里定痛汤, Internal Expression and Pain-Relieving Decoction, 744

tuō lǐ tòu nóng tāng 托里透脓汤, Internal Expression Pus-Expelling Decoction, 116, 744

tuō lǐ xiāo dú sǎn 托里消毒散, Internal Expression Toxin-Dispersing Powder, 9, 153, 259, 744

tuō lì huáng 脱力黄, strength desertion yellowing, 584

tuō náng 脱囊, sloughing scrotum, 540

tuō qì 脱气, deserting qi, 124

tuō ròu pò jiǒng (jùn) 脱肉破䐃, shedding of flesh and loss of bulk, 528

tuō xuè 脱血, blood desertion, 27

tuō yè 脱液, humor desertion, 293

tuō zhèng 脱证, desertion pattern, 124

tuó sēng gāo 陀僧膏, Litharge Paste, 298, 745

tuò 唾, spittle, 552

tuò wéi shèn yè 唾为肾液, spittle is the humor of the kidney, 552

tuò xuè 唾血, spitting of blood, 551

tuò yè 唾液, spittle humor, 552

tureric, *jiāng huáng* 姜黄, Curcumae Longae Rhizoma, 138, 427, 724

turtle shell, *biē jiǎ* 鳖甲, Amydae Carapax, 72, 98, 175, 176, 218, 277, 336, 352, 399, 460, 544, 593, 597, 727

Turtle Shell and Rehmannia Decoction, *biē jiǎ dì huáng tāng* 鳖甲地黄汤, 97

Turtle Shell Decocted Pill, *biē jiǎ jiān wán* 鳖甲煎丸, 26, 138, 140, 737

Turtle Shell Drink, *biē jiǎ yǐn zǐ* 鳖甲饮子, 737

turtle shell glue, *biē jiǎ jiāo* 鳖甲胶, Amydae Carapacis Gelatinum, 243, 593, 727

Turtle Shell Powder, *biē jiǎ sǎn* 鳖甲散, 237, 363

turtle's blood, *biē xuè* 鳖血, Amydae Sanguis, 397

Tussilaginis Flos, *kuǎn dōng huā* 款冬花, tussilago, 56, 95, 267, 434, 464, 527, 624, 625, 725

tussilago, *kuǎn dōng huā* 款冬花, Tussilaginis Flos, 56, 95, 267, 434, 464, 527, 624, 625, 725

Twelve Well Points, *shí èr jǐng xué* 十二井穴, 33, 63, 65, 69, 74, 76, 118, 147, 152, 279, 364, 403, 624, 665, 690, 694, 699

Two Immortals Decoction, *èr xiān tāng* 二仙汤, 741

Two Matured Ingredients Decoction, *èr chén tāng* 二陈汤, 101, 115, 116, 128, 153, 199, 216, 217, 240, 257, 400, 417, 419, 434, 435, 437, 439–443, 453, 457, 515, 625, 738

Two Matured Ingredients Stomach-Calming Powder, *èr chén píng wèi sǎn* 二陈平胃散, 638, 673

Two Spirits Pill, *èr shén wán* 二神丸, 742

Two Whites, *èr bái* 二白, 289, 656

Two-Ingredient Ginseng and Sappan Beverage, *èr wèi shēn sū yǐn* 二味参苏饮, 665

Two-Ingredient Toxin-Drawing Powder, *èr wèi bá dú sǎn* 二味拔毒散, 395

typha pollen, *pú huáng* 蒲黄, Typhae Pollen, 21, 30, 34, 56, 59, 137, 139, 464, 567, 569, 724

Typhae Pollen, *pú huáng* 蒲黄, typha pollen, 21, 30, 34, 56, 59, 137, 139, 464, 567, 569, 724

Typhae Pollen Crudum, *shēng pú huáng* 生蒲黄, raw typha pollen, 586

typhoid fever*, 118

Typhonii Gigantei Tuber, *yǔ bái fù* 禹白附, giant typhonium tuber, 623, 725

typhus*
exanthematous, 664
scrub, 250

tài píng shèng huì fāng 太平圣惠方 (*Great Peace Sagacious Benevolence Formulary*), 992 (Sòng), Wáng Huái-Yĭn 王怀隐 et. al. ed., 363, 508, 693

tí hú jiē gài fă 提壶揭盖法, raising the pot and removing the lid, 492

tú dīng xíng pí nèi zhēn 图钉型皮内针, drawing-pin intradermal needle, 147

ulcer*
gastric, 63, 483
stomach, 580
ulceration of the lower leg*, 528
ulcerative colitis*, 28
ulcers of digestive tract*, 123
Ulmi Fructus Praeparatio, *wú yí* 芜荑, elm cake, 183, 724
Ulmi Pumilae Cortex, *yú bái pí* 榆白皮, dwarf elm bark, 370
ulna*
styloid process of, 468
uncaria, *gōu téng* 钩藤, Uncariae Ramulus cum Unco, 7, 53, 54, 65, 146, 176, 225, 230, 452, 453, 526, 562, 591, 652, 726
Uncaria Beverage, *gōu téng yĭn* 钩藤饮, 140, 279, 740
Uncaria Decoction, *gōu téng tāng* 钩藤汤, 740
Uncaria Powder, *gōu téng săn* 钩藤散, 292, 739
Uncariae Ramulus cum Unco, *gōu téng* 钩藤, uncaria, 7, 53, 54, 65, 146, 176, 225, 230, 452, 453, 526, 562, 591, 652, 726
Unctuous Strangury Decoction, *gāo lín tāng* 膏淋汤, 743
Unicorn-Rearing Pill, *yù lín zhū* 毓麟珠, 332
Unified Treatise on Diseases, Patterns, and Remedies According to the Three Causes (*sān yīn jí yī bìng zhèng fāng lùn*) 三因极一病症方论, 1174 (Sòng), Chén Yán 陈言 [Wú Zé 无择], 46, 217, 243, 508, 542, 576, 609
Universal Aid Formulary (*pŭ jì fāng*) 普济方, 1406 (Míng), Téng Hóng 滕弘 et al. ed., 281
Universal Aid Toxin-Dispersing Beverage Minus Cimicifuga, Bupleurum, Scutellaria, & Coptis, *pŭ jì xiāo dú yĭn qù shēng má chái hú huáng qín huáng lián fāng* 普济消毒饮去升麻柴胡黄芩黄连方, 730
Universal Aid Toxin-Dispersing Beverage, *pŭ jì xiāo dú yĭn* 普济消毒饮, 63, 323, 387, 403, 612, 664, 691, 730
Unlimited Efficacy Elixir, *wàn líng dān* 万灵丹, 315, 744
unripe bitter orange, *zhĭ shí* 枳实, Aurantii Fructus Immaturus, 17, 50, 72, 98, 141, 216, 217, 255, 257, 276, 357, 417, 419, 434, 459, 493, 544, 564, 630, 723

Unripe Bitter Orange and Glomus-Dispersing Pill, *zhĭ shí xiāo pĭ wán* 枳实消痞丸, 224, 498, 558, 736
Unripe Bitter Orange and Ovate Atractylodes Pill, *zhĭ zhú wán* 枳术丸, 633, 736
Unripe Bitter Orange and Ovate Atractylodes Variant Decoction, *jiā jiăn zhĭ zhú tāng* 加减枳术汤, 562
Unripe Bitter Orange Center-Rectifying Pill, *zhĭ shí lĭ zhōng wán* 枳实理中丸, 85, 242, 735
Unripe Bitter Orange Stagnation-Abducting Pill, *zhĭ shí dăo zhì wán* 枳实导滞丸, 3, 15, 110, 141, 215, 239, 426, 626, 736
Unripe Bitter Orange, Chinese Chive, and Cinnamon Twig Decoction, *zhĭ shí xiè bái guì zhī tāng* 枳实薤白桂枝汤, 59, 736
unripe chebule, *zàng qīng guŏ* 藏青果, Chebulae Fructus Immaturus, 68, 721
unripe tangerine peel, *qīng pí* 青皮, Citri Exocarpium Immaturum, 19, 50, 55, 217, 223, 234, 262, 363, 397, 475, 478, 483, 490, 493, 546, 574, 685, 695, 712, 723
upborne elixir, *shēng dān* 升丹, Sublimatum Triplex, 383, 727
upper respiratory tract infection*, 659
Upper, Middle, and Lower Body General-Use Wind Pain Formula, *shàng zhōng xià tōng yòng tòng fēng fāng* 上中下通用痛风方, 734
Upper-Body-Clearing Pain-Alleviating Decoction, *qīng shàng juān tòng tāng* 清上蠲痛汤, 740
Upper-Body-Clearing Pill, *qīng shàng wán* 清上丸, 436
urethral injury*, 148
urethrostenosis*, 148
urinary calculus*, 21, 148
urinary tract infection*, 583
acute, 21
urinary tract*
inflammation of, 641
Ursi Fel, *xióng dăn* 熊胆, bear's gall, 68, 721
urticaria*, 145
giant, 494
uterine bleeding
dysfunctional, 30
uterine bleeding*, 212

vaccaria, *wáng bù liú xíng* 王不留行, Vaccariae Semen, 138, 227, 513, 725
Vaccariae Semen, *wáng bù liú xíng* 王不留行, vaccaria, 138, 227, 513, 725
vaginitis*, 468
senile, 468
valve*
ileocecal, 515
varicosity*, 534, 632
vascular nevus*, 32
vasomotor collapse*
postpartum, 448

velvet deerhorn, *lù róng* 鹿茸, Cervi Cornu Parvum, 45, 229, 511, 593, 651, 726

Velvet Deerhorn Four Jin Pill, *lù róng sì jīn wán* 鹿茸四斤丸, 337

Velvet Deerhorn Pill, *lù róng wán* 鹿茸丸, 508

Velvet Deerhorn Supplementing and Astringing Pill, *lù róng bǔ sè wán* 鹿茸补涩丸, 641

vena cava*
  inferior, 272
  superior, 272

Veratri Radix et Rhizoma, *lí lú* 藜芦, veratrum, 98, 170, 727

veratrum, *lí lú* 藜芦, Veratri Radix et Rhizoma, 98, 170, 727

verbena, *mǎ biān cǎo* 马鞭草, Verbenae Herba (cum Radice), 138, 725

Verbenae Herba (cum Radice), *mǎ biān cǎo* 马鞭草, verbena, 138, 725

verruca vulgaris*, 665

verruca*, 384

vertex cranii*, 654

vertigo*
  otogenic, 443

Vespae Nidus, *lù fēng fáng* 露蜂房, hornet's nest, 298, 449, 728

Vespertilionis Excrementum, *yè míng shā* 夜明砂, bat's droppings, 139, 291, 725

Vessel's Root, *mài gēn* 脉根, 540

Vessel-Freeing Counterflow Cold Decoction, *tōng mài sì nì tāng* 通脉四逆汤, 64, 79, 85, 228, 505, 711, 735

vicarious menstruation*, 102

Vincent's angina*, 474

Vinegar Soaking Formula, *cù pào fāng* 醋泡方, 11, 221, 244

Violae Herba cum Radice, *dì dīng* 地丁, violet, 67, 588, 721

Violae Yedoensis Herba cum Radice, *zǐ huā dì dīng* 紫花地丁, Yedo violet, 67, 691, 721

violet, *dì dīng* 地丁, Violae Herba cum Radice, 67, 588, 721

vitamin A deficiency*, 549

vitamin B deficiency*, 616

vitamin B$_1$ deficiency*, 112, 154, 342

vitex, *màn jīng zǐ* 蔓荆子, Viticis Fructus, 17, 55, 420, 488, 680, 686, 720

Viticis Fructus, *màn jīng zǐ* 蔓荆子, vitex, 17, 55, 420, 488, 680, 686, 720

vitiligo*, 676

vitreous humor*, 551

vladimiria, *qīng mù xiāng* 青木香, Vladimiriae Radix, 493, 724

Vladimiriae Radix, *qīng mù xiāng* 青木香, vladimiria, 493, 724

Vladimiriae Souliei Radix, *chuān mù xiāng* 川木香, Sichuan saussurea, 493, 723

wǎ léng zǐ 瓦楞子 ark shell, Arcae Concha, 59, 478, 581, 728

wài 外, external, 185

wài 外, outer body, 422

wài chuī 外吹, external blowing, 185

wài chuī rǔ yōng 外吹乳痈, external blowing mammary welling-abscess, 185

wài fū gāo jì 外敷膏剂, topically applied paste, 621

wài fū jiē gǔ sǎn 外敷接骨散, Topical Bone-Joining Powder, 745

wài fǔ gǔ 外辅骨, outer assisting bone, 422

wài gǎn 外感, external contraction, 185

wài gǎn bù dé wò 外感不得卧, external contraction sleeplessness, 186

wài gǎn rè bìng 外感热病, externally contracted heat (febrile) disease, 186

wài gǎn rè bìng biàn zhèng 外感热病辨证, externally contracted heat (febrile) disease pattern identification, 186

wài gǎn wèi wǎn (guǎn) tòng 外感胃脘痛, external contraction stomach duct pain, 186

wài gǎn yāo tòng 外感腰痛, external contraction lumbar pain, 185

wài guān 外关, TB-5, Outer Pass, 8, 14, 19, 61–63, 66, 69, 70, 72, 73, 82, 87, 89, 90, 92, 103, 105, 111, 112, 117, 119, 138–140, 145, 158, 166, 167, 184, 192, 194, 203, 218, 241, 247, 255, 258, 260, 283, 289, 295, 296, 301, 319, 320, 337, 342, 370, 374, 391, 403, 405, 408, 416, 437, 446, 448, 450, 452, 454, 456, 458, 474, 480, 482, 499, 501, 515, 516, 520, 530, 540, 544, 547, 568, 580, 586, 591, 620, 621, 631, 643, 665, 674, 677, 679, 680, 682, 683, 685–689, 693, 694, 703, 713, 748

wài hán 外寒, external cold, 185

wài hán fàn wèi 外寒犯胃, external cold invading the stomach, 185

wài kē chán sū wán 外科蟾酥丸, External Medicine Toad Venom Pill, 744

wài kē dà chéng 外科大成 (*Great Compendium of External Medicine*), 1665 (Qīng), Qí Kūn 祁坤, 303, 528

wài kē shū yào 外科枢要 (*Pivot of External Medicine*), 1571 (Míng), Xuē Jǐ 薛己 [Lì-Zhāi 立斋], 46

wài kē zhèng zhì quán shēng jí 外科证治全生集 (*Life-for-All Compendium of External Medicine, Patterns and Treatment*), 1740 (Qīng), Wáng Wéi-Dé 王维德 [Hóng-Xù 洪绪], 46

wài kē zhèng zōng 外科正宗 (*Orthodox External Medicine*), 1617 (Qīng), Chén Shí-Gōng 陈实功, 210, 670

wài kē 外科, external medicine, 187

wài líng 外陵, ST-26, Outer Mound, 746

wài qiū 外丘, GB-36, Outer Hill, 748

wài shāng 外伤, external injury, 186

wài shāng 外伤, trauma, 626

wài shāng yāo tòng 外伤腰痛, external injury lumbar pain, 186

wài shèn 外肾, external kidney, 186

wài shèn diào tòng 外肾吊痛, painful pendulous external kidney, 424

wài shèn suō rù 外肾缩入, retracted external kidney, 503

wài tái mì yào 外台秘要 (*Essential Secrets from Outside the Metropolis*), 752 (Táng), Wáng Táo 王焘, 142

wài xié 外邪, external evil, 186

wài yīn 外因, external cause, 185

wài yōng 外痈, external welling-abscess, 187

wài zhàng 外障, external obstruction, 187

wài zì 外眦, outer canthus, 422

walnut, *hú táo rén* 胡桃仁, Juglandis Semen, 97, 467, 526, 593, 596, 726

wān zhēn 弯针, bent needle, 18

wán 丸, pill, 444

wán bì 顽痹, insensitive impediment, 308

wán dài tāng 完带汤, Discharge-Ceasing Decoction, 563, 677, 743

wán gǔ 完骨, GB-12, Completion Bone, 219, 247, 748

wán gǔ 完骨, completion bone, 92

wán gǔ bù huà 完谷不化, nontransformation of food, 413

wán jì 丸剂, pill, 444

wǎn fā 晚发, late emergence, 340

wǎn fù zhuì zhàng 脘腹坠胀, sagging distention in the stomach duct and abdomen, 511

wǎn wǎn 宛宛, depression, 123

wǎn (guǎn) 脘, stomach duct, 576

wàn gǔ 腕骨, SI-4, Wrist Bone, 90, 296, 521, 548, 747

wàn líng dān 万灵丹, Unlimited Efficacy Elixir, 315, 744

wàn nián qīng gēn 万年青根 rohdea root, Rohdeae Rhizoma et Radix, 68, 721

wàn yìng gāo 万应膏, Myriad Applications Paste, 745

wàn yìng wán 万应丸, Myriad Applications Pill, 509, 695, 737

wandering pain*, 517

Wang's Coptis and Magnolia Bark Beverage, *wáng shì lián pò yǐn* 王氏连朴饮, 2

Wang's Summerheat-Clearing Qi-Boosting Decoction, *wáng shì qīng shǔ yì qì tāng* 王氏清暑益气汤, 69, 488, 589, 591, 613, 730

wáng 亡, collapse, 87

wáng bù liú xíng 王不留行 vaccaria, Vaccariae Semen, 138, 227, 513, 725

wáng gōng 王宫, king's palace, 336

wáng jīn yè 亡津液, fluid collapse, 213

wáng shì lián pò yǐn 王氏连朴饮, Wang's Coptis and Magnolia Bark Beverage, 2

wáng shì qīng shǔ yì qì tāng 王氏清暑益气汤, Wang's Summerheat-Clearing Qi-Boosting Decoction, 69, 488, 589, 591, 613, 730

wáng xuè 亡血, blood collapse, 26

wáng yáng 亡阳, yang collapse, 699

wáng yáng xū tuō 亡阳虚脱, yang-collapse vacuity desertion, 699

wáng yīn 亡阴, yin collapse, 709

wáng yīn xū tuō 亡阴虚脱, yin-collapse vacuity desertion, 709

wǎng lái hán rè 往来寒热, alternating fever and chills, 8

wǎng lái hán rè 往来寒热, alternating heat [effusion] and [aversion to] cold, 8

wǎng qiú zhǒu 网球肘, tennis elbow, 605

wàng 旺, effulgent, 168

wàng sè shí fǎ 望色十法, ten-principle inspection of the complexion, 605

wàng xíng 妄行, frenetic movement, 229

wàng zhěn 望诊, inspection, 308

wàng zhěn 望诊, looking examination, 367

wàng zhěn 望诊, visual examination, 657

Warlord's Troop-Marching Powder, *wǔ hóu xíng jūn sǎn* 武侯行军散, 740

Warp and Weft of Warm Heat (*wēn rè jīng wěi*) 温热经纬, 1852 (Qīng), Wáng Mèng-Yīng 王孟英, 659

wart*, 384
    common, 665

water buffalo horn, *shuǐ niú jiǎo* 水牛角, Bubali Cornu, 67, 720

water chestnut, *bí qí* 荸荠, Heleocharitis Cormus, 624, 725

Water Controller Yu Powder, *yǔ gōng sǎn* 禹功散, 667, 732

Water Crystal Paste, *shuǐ jīng gāo* 水晶膏, 21, 53

Water-Abducting Poria (Hoelen) Decoction, *dǎo shuǐ fú líng tāng* 导水茯苓汤, 733

Water-Enriching Liver-Clearing Beverage, *zī shuǐ qīng gān yǐn* 滋水清肝饮, 656

Water-Enriching Liver-Clearing Beverage, *zī shuǐ qīng gān yǐn* 滋水清肝饮, 742

Water-Transforming Seed-Planting Decoction, *huà shuǐ zhòng zǐ tāng* 化水种子汤, 741

watermelon, *xī guā* 西瓜, Citrulli Fructus, 67, 231, 720

watermelon frost, *xī guā shuāng* 西瓜霜, Mirabiliti et Citrulli Praeparatio, 67, 720

watermelon rind, *xī guā pí* 西瓜皮, Citrulli Exocarpium, 67, 589, 720

wax gourd rind, *dōng guā pí* 冬瓜皮, Benincasae Exocarpium, 136, 723

wax gourd seed, *dōng guā zǐ* 冬瓜子, Benincasae Semen, 136, 282, 625, 723

weed soot, *bǎi cǎo shuāng* 百草霜, Herbarum Ustarum Fuligo, 724

wèi hán è zǔ 胃寒恶阻, stomach cold malign obstruction, 575

wèi rè è zǔ 胃热恶阻, stomach heat malign obstruction, 577

wēi 煨, roasting, 508

wēi chǎo 微炒, light stir-frying, 346

wēi líng xiān 威灵仙 clematis, Clematidis Radix, 45, 139, 227, 722

wēi líng xiān wán 威灵仙丸, Clematis Pill, 477

wēi mài 微脉, faint pulse, 195

wēi xǐ wán 威喜丸, Powerful Happiness Pill, 743

wēi zhě nì zhī 微者逆之, mild conditions are treated by counteraction, 395

wéi bāo 维胞, Holding the Uterus, 711

wéi dào 维道 GB-28, Linking Path, 242, 711, 748

wéi zhēn fǎ 围针法, encirclement needling, 173

wěi 痿, atony, 12

wěi 痿, wei, 670

wěi 痿, wilting, 678

wěi bì 痿痹, wilting-impediment, 679

wěi bì 痿躄, crippling wilt, 105

wěi gǔ 尾骨, tail bone, 602

wěi jīng tāng 苇茎汤, Phragmites Stem Decoction, 743

wěi líng cài 委陵菜 Chinese silverweed, Potentillae Chinensis Radix seu Herba cum Radice, 68, 721

wěi yáng 委阳, BL-39, Bend Yang, 22, 117, 369, 449, 582, 661, 703, 716, 747

wěi zhèng 痿证, wilting pattern, 679

wěi zhōng 委中, BL-40, Bend Center, 4, 5, 11, 14, 15, 17, 25, 34, 36, 39, 44, 62, 63, 70, 73, 75, 80, 89, 99, 111, 113–115, 137, 145, 152, 154, 160, 225, 292, 296, 302, 327, 330, 332, 336, 337, 342, 347, 369, 370, 382, 415, 422, 427, 450, 453, 455, 462, 484, 540, 546, 559, 566, 567, 571, 589, 590, 597, 637, 651, 658, 665, 676, 684, 688, 696, 710, 747

wěi zhōng dú 委中毒, bend-center toxin [sore], 17

wěi zhōng yōng 委中痈, bend-center welling-abscess, 18

wèi 胃, ST, 569

wèi 胃, gastric, 239

wèi 胃, gastro-, 239

wèi 胃, stomach, 575

wèi 味, flavor, 210

wèi 卫, defense, 121

wèi 魏, Wei, 670

wèi biǎo 卫表, defensive exterior, 121

wèi biǎo bù gù 卫表不固, insecurity of the defensive exterior, 308

wèi bìng 胃病, stomach disease, 575

wèi bù hé 胃不和, disharmony of the stomach, 135

wèi bù hé 胃不和, gastric disharmony, 239

wèi bù hé 胃不和, stomach disharmony, 576

wèi bù hé bù dé wò 胃不和不得卧, stomach disharmony sleeplessness, 576

wèi bù hé wò bù ān 胃不和卧不安, unquiet sleep due to stomach disharmony, 638

wèi bù hé zé wò bù ān 胃不和则卧不安, when the stomach is in disharmony, there is unquiet sleep, 673

wèi cāng 胃仓, BL-50, Stomach Granary, 747

wèi cháng zhàng qì 胃肠胀气, gastrointestinal qi distention, 240

wèi dāi 胃呆, torpid stomach, 621

wèi fǎn 胃反, stomach reflux, 579

wèi fèn 卫分, defense aspect, 121

wèi fèn zhèng 卫分证, defense-aspect pattern, 121

wèi fēng 胃风, stomach wind, 581

wèi fēng tāng 胃风汤, Stomach Wind Decoction, 318, 581

wèi guān jiān 胃关煎, Stomach Gate Brew, 348, 735

wèi hán 胃寒, stomach cold, 575

wèi hán cháng rè 胃寒肠热, stomach cold and intestinal heat, 575

wèi hán è nì 胃寒呃逆, stomach cold hiccough, 575

wèi huǒ 胃火, stomach fire, 576

wèi huǒ chì shèng 胃火炽盛, intense stomach fire, 310

wèi huǒ yá tòng 胃火牙痛, stomach fire toothache, 577

wèi jiā 胃家, stomach domain, 576

wèi jiā shí 胃家实, stomach domain repletion, 576

wèi jīn 胃津, stomach liquid, 578

wèi jīng 胃经, stomach channel, 575

wèi ké 胃咳, stomach cough, 575

wèi kǒu 胃口, appetite, 10

wèi kǒu bù hǎo 胃口不好, poor appetite, 446

wèi líng tāng 胃苓汤, Stomach-Calming Poria (Hoelen) Five Decoction, 1, 79, 109, 113, 114, 151, 217, 302, 339, 348, 467, 556, 563, 608, 666, 711, 732

wèi nà bù jiā 胃纳不佳, poor stomach intake, 447

wèi nà dāi zhì 胃纳呆滞, torpid stomach intake, 621

wèi nà jiǎn shǎo 胃纳减少, reduced food intake, 496

wèi qì 胃气, stomach qi, 578

wèi qì 卫气, defense qi, 121

wèi qì bù gù 卫气不固, insecurity of defense qi, 307

wèi qì bù hé 胃气不和, disharmony of stomach qi, 135

wèi qì bù jiàng 胃气不降, nondownbearing of stomach qi, 413

wèi qì nì 胃气逆, counterflow stomach qi, 102

wèi qì ruò 胃气弱, weak stomach qi, 669

wèi qì shàng nì 胃气上逆, stomach qi ascending counterflow, 578

wèi qì tòng 胃气痛, stomach qi pain, 579

wèi qì xū 胃气虚, stomach qi vacuity, 579

wèi qì xū hán 胃气虚寒, stomach qi vacuity cold, 579

wèi qì yīn liǎng xū 胃气阴两虚, dual vacuity of stomach qi and yin, 161

wèi qì yíng xuè 卫气营血, defense, qi, construction, and blood, 121

wèi qì yíng xuè 卫气营血, four aspects, 225

wèi qì yíng xuè biàn zhèng 卫气营血辨证, four-aspect pattern identification, 225

wèi qì zhì 胃气滞, stomach qi stagnation, 579

wèi qì zhǔ jiàng 胃气主降, stomach qi governs downbearing, 579

wèi qiáng pí ruò 胃强脾弱, strong stomach and weak spleen, 584

wèi rè 胃热, stomach heat, 577

wèi rè è nì 胃热呃逆, stomach heat hiccough, 577

wèi rè shā gǔ 胃热杀谷, stomach heat with rapid digestion, 577

wèi rè yōng shèng 胃热壅盛, exuberant stomach heat, 190

wèi ruò è zǔ 胃弱恶阻, weak stomach malign obstruction, 669

wèi shī hé jiàng 胃失和降, impaired harmonious downbearing of the stomach, 295

wèi shī hé jiàng 胃失和降, impairment of gastric harmony and downbearing, 295

wèi shí 胃实, stomach repletion, 580

wèi shí è nì 胃实呃逆, stomach repletion hiccough, 580

wèi shí hán 胃实寒, stomach repletion cold, 580

wèi shū 胃俞, BL-21, Stomach Transport, 1, 3, 4, 15, 17, 27, 29, 33, 37–41, 47, 55, 73, 80, 84, 87–89, 91, 97, 127, 128, 156, 161, 164, 174, 175, 197, 199, 215, 216, 218, 223, 224, 237, 251, 256, 257, 309, 312, 314, 316, 333, 339, 349, 359, 361, 370, 379, 415, 416, 418, 447, 449, 457, 477, 486, 487, 489, 499, 503, 537, 557, 561–565, 575, 577–579, 581, 595–597, 600, 607, 613, 620, 638, 639, 645–647, 661–663, 666, 669, 673, 679, 711, 714, 715, 747

wèi tòng 胃痛, gastric pain, 239

wèi tòng 胃痛, stomach pain, 578

wèi wǎn (guǎn) 胃脘, stomach duct, 576

wèi wǎn (guǎn) 胃脘, venter, 654

wèi wǎn (guǎn) nèi yōng 胃脘内痈, internal welling-abscess of the stomach duct, 317

wèi wǎn (guǎn) téng tòng 胃脘疼痛, stomach duct pain, 576

wèi wǎn (guǎn) tòng 胃脘痛, stomach duct pain, 576

wèi wǎn (guǎn) yōng 胃脘痈, stomach duct welling-abscess, 576

wèi wǎn (guǎn) yōng 胃脘痈, welling-abscess of the stomach duct, 670

wèi wéi shuǐ gǔ zhī hǎi 胃为水谷之海, stomach is the sea of grain and water, 577

wèi xiāo 胃消, gastric dispersion, 239

wèi xiāo 胃消, stomach dispersion, 576

wèi xīn tòng 胃心痛, stomach heart pain, 577

wèi xū 胃虚, stomach vacuity, 580

wèi xū è nì 胃虚呃逆, stomach vacuity hiccough, 581

wèi xū hán 胃虚寒, stomach vacuity cold, 580

wèi yáng 胃阳, stomach yang, 581

wèi yáng bù gù 卫阳不固, insecurity of defensive yang, 307

wèi yáng xū 胃阳虚, stomach yang vacuity, 581

wèi yīn 胃阴, stomach yin, 581

wèi yīn bù zú 胃阴不足, insufficiency of stomach yin, 310

wèi yīn kuī xū 胃阴亏虚, stomach yin depletion, 581

wèi yīn xū 胃阴虚, stomach yin vacuity, 581

wèi yōng 胃痈, stomach welling-abscess, 581

wèi yōng 胃痈, welling-abscess of the stomach, 670

wèi zhī 胃汁, gastric juices, 239

wèi zhī 胃汁, stomach juices, 578

wèi zhī dà luò 胃之大络, great network vessel of the stomach, 248

wèi zhì 胃滞, gastric stagnation, 239

wèi zhì 胃滞, stomach stagnation, 580

wèi zhōng rè 胃中热, heat in the stomach, 280

wèi zhōng zào shǐ 胃中燥矢, dry stool in the stomach, 157

wèi zhǔ fǔ shóu 胃主腐熟, stomach governs decomposition, 577

wèi zhǔ jiàng zhuó 胃主降浊, stomach governs downbearing of the turbid, 577

wèi zhǔ shòu nà 胃主受纳, stomach governs intake, 577

wèi, shén, gēn 胃、神、根, stomach, spirit, and root, 580

Well-Tried Flooding Formula, *bēng zhèng jí yàn fāng* 崩证极验方, 743

wēn 温, warm, 658

wēn 温, warmth, 664

wēn bìng 温病, warm disease, 658

wēn bìng tiáo biàn 温病条辨 (*Systematized Identification of Warm Diseases*), 1798 (Qīng), Wú Táng 吴瑭 [Jú-Tōng 鞠通], 186, 276, 659

wēn bǔ mìng mén 温补命门, warming and supplementing the life gate, 660

wēn bǔ shèn yáng 温补肾阳, warming and supplementing kidney yang, 660

wēn dǎn ān shén 温胆安神, warming the gallbladder and quieting the spirit, 662

wēn dǎn tāng 温胆汤, Gallbladder-Warming Decoction, 70, 123, 223, 230, 236, 358, 417, 418, 437, 537, 539, 541, 578, 614, 662, 738

wēn dú 温毒, warm toxin, 664

wēn fǎ 温法, warming, 660

wēn fèi huà tán 温肺化痰, warming the lung and transforming phlegm, 662

wēn fèi huà yǐn 温肺化饮, warming the lung and transforming rheum, 662

wēn fèi zhǐ liú dān 温肺止流丹, Lung-Warming Nose-Drying Elixir, 739

wēn fèi zhú yǐn 温肺逐饮, warming the lung and expelling rheum, 662

wēn huà 温化, warming and transforming, 661

wēn huà hán tán 温化寒痰, warming and transforming cold phlegm, 661

wēn huà hán yǐn 温化寒饮, warming and transforming cold rheum, 661

wēn huà qū yū 温化祛瘀, warming and transforming static blood, 661

wēn huà shuǐ shī 温化水湿, warming and transforming water-damp, 661

wēn huáng 瘟黄, scourge jaundice, 514

wēn jīng qū hán 温经祛寒, warming the channels and dispelling cold, 662

wēn jīng sàn hán 温经散寒, warming the channels and dissipating cold, 662

wēn jīng tāng 温经汤, Channel-Warming (Menses-Warming) Decoction, 26, 93, 326, 735 *wēn jiǔ qì* 温灸器, moxa burner, 401

wēn kāi 温开, warm opening, 664

wēn liū 温溜, LI-7, Warm Dwelling, 386, 746

wēn nüè 温疟, warm malaria, 664

wēn pí 温脾, warming the spleen, 663

wēn pí tāng 温脾汤, Spleen-Warming Decoction, 182, 338, 425, 732

wēn rè 温热, warm heat, 660

wēn rè bìng 温热病, warm heat disease, 660

wēn rè jīng wěi 温热经纬 (*Warp and Weft of Warm Heat*), 1852 (Qīng), Wáng Mèng-Yīng 王孟英, 659

wēn rè lùn 温热论 (*On Warm Heat*), 1746, Qīng, Gù Jǐng-Wén 顾景文, 186, 279, 382, 581, 622, 659

wēn shā 瘟痧, scourge sand, 515

wēn shèn 温肾, warming the kidney, 662

wēn shèn lì shuǐ 温肾利水, warming the kidney and disinhibiting water, 662

wēn shèn nà qì 温肾纳气, warming the kidney to promote qi absorption, 662

wēn shuǐ zàng 温水脏, warming the water viscus, 663

wēn wèi 温胃, warming the stomach, 663

wēn wèi jiàn zhōng 温胃健中, warming the stomach and fortifying the center, 663

wēn wèi sàn hán 温胃散寒, warming the stomach and dissipating cold, 663

wēn wèi yǐn 温胃饮, Stomach-Warming Beverage, 63, 648

wēn wèi zhǐ ǒu 温胃止呕, warming the stomach and checking vomiting, 663

wēn xià 温下, warm precipitation, 664

wēn xié 温邪, warm evil, 659

wēn xié fàn fèi 温邪犯肺, invasion of the lung by a warm evil, 319

wēn xié fàn fèi 温邪犯肺, warm evil invading the lung, 659

wēn xīn yáng 温心阳, warming heart yang, 661

wēn xuè 温血, warming the blood, 661

wēn yáng huà yǐn 温阳化饮, warming yang and transforming rheum, 663

wēn yáng lì shuǐ 温阳利湿, warming yang and disinhibiting dampness, 663

wēn yì 温疫, warm epidemic, 659

wēn yì lùn 温疫论 (*On Warm Epidemics*), 1642 (Míng), Wú Yǒu-Xìng 吴有性 [Yòu-Kě 又可], 276, 658

wēn zào 温燥, warm dryness, 659

wēn zhēn 温针, warm needling, 664

wēn zhōng qū hán 温中祛寒, warming the center and dispelling cold, 661

wēn zhōng sàn hán 温中散寒, warming the center and dissipating cold, 661

wén huǒ 文火, civil flame, 63

wén wǔ tāng 文武膏, Mulberry Paste, 742

wén zhěn 闻诊, audio-olfactory examination, 12

wén zhěn 闻诊, listening and smelling, 349

wèn zhěn 问诊, inquiry, 303

Wheezing and Panting External Application Formula, *xiāo chuǎn fù zhì fāng* 哮喘敷治方, 744

Wherewithal-to-Bear Pill, *suǒ yǐ zài wán* 所以载丸, 742

White Discharge Tablet, *bái dài piàn* 白带片, 743

white downborne elixir, *bái jiàng dān* 白降丹, Praeparatio Sublimata Alba, 171, 383

White Downborne Elixir, *bái jiàng dān* 白降丹, 744

White Jade Plaster, *bái yù gāo* 白玉膏, 528

white mustard, *bái jiè zǐ* 白芥子, Brassicae Albae Semen, 104, 388, 389, 433, 434, 438, 624, 625, 725

White Patch Tablet, *bái bó piàn* 白驳片, 676

white peony, *bái sháo yào* 白芍药, Paeoniae Radix Alba, 17, 19, 28, 36, 37, 39, 95, 103, 116, 140, 154, 172, 175–177, 227, 246, 256, 259, 309, 310, 315, 352, 363, 390, 391, 397, 416, 425, 428, 495, 498, 502, 516, 537, 546, 548, 566, 567, 580, 588, 593, 613, 620, 661, 662, 674, 709, 713, 715, 727

white pepper, *bái hú jiāo* 白胡椒, Piperis Fructus Albicatus, 402

white perilla bark, *bái sū pí* 白苏皮, Perillae Albae Cortex, 66

white perilla leaf, *bái sū yè* 白苏叶, Perillae Albae Folium, 47

white perilla seed, *bái sū zǐ* 白苏子, Perillae Albae Semen, 17, 64, 145

white poria, *bái fú líng* 白茯苓, Poria Alba, 141, 394

white quartz, *bái shí yīng* 白石英, Quartz Album, 53

white sliced aconite, *bái fù piàn* 白附片, Aconiti Tuber Laterale Album, 660, 723

white sugar, *bái shā táng* 白沙糖, Saccharon Granulatum Album, 45

white tangerine peel, *jú bái* 橘白, Citri Exocarpium Album, 493, 723

White Tiger Decoction Plus Cinnamon Twig, *bái hǔ jiā guì zhī tāng* 白虎加桂枝汤, 664, 730

White Tiger Decoction Plus Ginseng, *bái hǔ jiā rén shēn tāng* 白虎加人参汤, 455, 588, 591, 601, 640, 701, 730

White Tiger Decoction Plus Rehmannia, *bái hǔ jiā dì huáng tāng* 白虎加地黄汤, 730

White Tiger Decoction, *bái hǔ tāng* 白虎汤, 54, 71, 73, 202, 203, 281, 283, 431, 505, 589, 591, 607, 626, 698, 699, 701, 730

White Tiger Qi-Coordinating Decoction, *bái hǔ chéng qì tāng* 白虎承气汤, 731

White-Diffusing Qi-Coordinating Decoction, *xuān bái chéng qì tāng* 宣白承气汤, 731

White-Draining Origin-Boosting Powder, *xiè bái yì yuán sǎn* 泻白益元散, 587

White-Draining Powder, *xiè bái sǎn* 泻白散, 15, 72, 101, 147, 201, 238, 277, 280, 329, 372, 374, 674, 677, 695, 731

Whiteness-Dispersing Beverage, *xiāo bái yǐn* 消白饮, 733

Whole Deer Pill, *quán lù wán* 全鹿丸, 742

wild aconite, *cǎo wū tóu* 草乌头, Aconiti Tsao-Wu-Tou Tuber, 411, 660, 723

wild buckwheat root, *tiān qiáo mài gēn* 天荞麦根, Fagopyri Cymosi Radix et Rhizoma, 68, 469, 721

wild chrysanthemum flower, *yě jú huā* 野菊花, Chrysanthemi Indicae seu Borealis Flos, 686, 720

Willow Flower Powder, *liǔ huā sǎn* 柳花散, 615

Wind-Coursing Blood-Nourishing Decoction, *shū fēng yǎng xuè tāng* 疏风养血汤, 740

Wind-Damage Cough Swill-Down Pill, *shāng fēng ké sòu tūn jì* 伤风咳嗽吞剂, 738

Wind-Dispersing Blood-Nourishing Decoction, *xiāo fēng yǎng xuè tāng* 消风养血汤, 740

Wind-Dispersing Powder, *xiāo fēng sǎn* 消风散, 145, 260, 395, 494, 591, 671, 676, 686, 688, 740

Wind-Dispersing Red-Abducting Decoction, *xiāo fēng dǎo chì tāng* 消风导赤汤, 586

Wind-Eliminating Boosting Decoction, *chú fēng yì sǔn tāng* 除风益损汤, 740

Wind-Eliminating Spleen-Clearing Beverage, *chú fēng qīng pí yǐn* 除风清脾饮, 395, 691

Wind-Expelling Heat-Dissipating Drink, *qū fēng sàn rè yǐn zǐ* 驱风散热饮子, 495, 685, 740

Wind-Expelling One Zi Powder, *qū fēng yī zì sǎn* 驱风一字散, 320, 718

Wind-Expelling Powder, *pái fēng sǎn* 排风散, 689

Wind-Expelling Powder, *qū fēng sàn rě* 驱风散, 198

Wind-Smoothing Powder, *yùn fēng sǎn* 熨风散, 744

wingless cockroach, *zhè chóng* 蟅虫, Eupolyphaga seu Opisthoplatia, 34, 50, 138, 182, 540, 724

Wings of the Golden Coffer (*jīn guì yì*) 金匮翼, 1768 (Qīng), Lóng Zài-Jīng 龙在泾, 693

Wings to the Classified Canon (*lèi jīng fù yì*) 类经附翼, 1624 (Míng), Zhāng Jiè-Bīn 张介宾 (Jīng-Yuè 景岳), 20

wò bù ān 卧不安, unquiet sleep, 638

wò lóng dān 卧龙丹, Sleeping Dragon Elixir, 740

Wondrous Atractylodes Powder, *shén zhú sǎn* 神术散, 218, 729, 732

Wondrous Effect Astragalus Decoction, *shén xiào huáng qí tāng* 神效黄芪汤, 210, 489, 564

Wondrous Response Canon (*shén yìng jīng*) 神应经, Míng, Chén Huì 陈会, 180

Wondrous Response True-Nourishing Elixir, *shén yìng yǎng zhēn dān* 神应养真丹, 243

Wondrous Response Wind-Dispersing Powder, *shén yìng xiāo fēng sǎn* 神应消风散, 417, 431

Wondrous Six Powder, *liù shén sǎn* 六神散, 740

Wood-Quelling Pill, *fā mù wán* 伐木丸, 737

woody fangji, *mù fáng jǐ* 木防己, Cocculi Radix, 139, 722

Woody Fangji Decoction, *mù fáng jǐ tāng* 木防己汤, 120, 468, 733

Woody Fangji Variant Decoction, *jiā jiǎn mù fáng jǐ tāng* 加减木防己汤, 733

Worm-Expelling Pill, *zhuī chóng wán* 追虫丸, 696, 737

Worm-Transforming Pill, *huà chóng wán* 化虫丸, 64, 172, 426, 445, 509, 695, 696, 737

wū jī bái fèng wán 乌鸡白凤丸, Black Chicken and White Phoenix Pill, 741

wū lòu mài 屋漏脉, leaking roof pulse, 341

wū lún chì yūn 乌轮赤晕, red areola surrounding the dark of the eye, 494

wū méi 乌梅 mume, Mume Fructus, 80, 82, 417, 462, 510, 518, 548, 599, 604, 612, 712, 727

wū méi wán 乌梅丸, Mume Pill, 64, 228, 509, 510, 695, 696, 737

wū shé 乌蛇 black-striped snake, Zaocys, 139, 722

wū tóu chì shí zhī wán 乌头赤石脂丸, Aconite Main Tuber and Halloysite Pill, 58

wū tóu guì zhī tāng 乌头桂枝汤, Aconite Main Tuber and Cinnamon Twig Decoction, 735

wū tóu jiān 乌头煎, Aconite Main Tuber Brew, 505

wū tóu tāng 乌头汤, Aconite Main Tuber Decoction, 662, 735

wū yào 乌药 lindera, Linderae Radix, 19, 83, 103, 493, 572, 694, 724

wū yào sǎn 乌药散, Lindera Powder, 736

wū yào tāng 乌药汤, Lindera Decoction, 736

wū yī 巫医, shaman healer, 528

wū yì 屋翳, ST-15, Roof, 385, 746

wū zhū 乌珠, dark of the eye, 118

wú 吴, Wu, 697

wú bān hén jiǔ 无瘢痕灸, nonscarring moxibustion, 413

wú bǐ shān yào wán 无比山药丸, Matchless Dioscorea Pill, 41

wú fàn wèi qì 无犯胃气, do not harm stomach qi, 144

wú gōng 蜈蚣 centipede, Scolopendra, 54, 74, 98, 140, 146, 434, 726

wú hàn 无汗, absence of sweating, 3

wú lì 无力, forceless, 222

wú lì 无力, lack of strength, 338

wú mèng ér yí 无梦而遗, seminal emission without dreaming, 525

wú míng zhǒng dú 无名肿毒, innominate toxin swelling, 303

wú tóu jū 无头疽, headless flat-abscess, 259

wú yí 芜荑 elm cake, Ulmi Fructus Praeparatio, 183, 724

wú zhū yú 吴茱萸 evodia, Evodiae Fructus, 84, 256, 343, 363, 400, 447, 450, 506, 542, 561, 578, 581, 649, 660, 663, 723

wú zhū yú jiā fù zǐ tāng 吴茱萸加附子汤, Evodia Decoction with Aconite Decoction, 735

wú zhū yú tāng 吴茱萸汤, Evodia Decoction, 81, 83, 87, 156, 170, 343, 506, 578, 662, 663, 735

wǔ bǎo sǎn 五宝散, Five-Jewel Powder, 586, 744

wǔ bèi zǐ 五倍子 sumac gallnut, Rhois Galla, 466, 518, 567, 572, 675, 709, 727

wǔ bèi zǐ sǎn 五倍子散, Sumac Gallnut Powder, 744

wǔ bì 五痹, five impediments, 205

wŭ bì tāng 五痹汤, Five Impediments Decoction, 45, 210, 328, 358, 654, 734

wŭ bù nán 五不男, five unmanlinesses, 208

wŭ bù nŭ 五不女, five unwomanlinesses, 208

wŭ chí 五迟, five slownesses, 207

wŭ chù 五处, BL-5, Fifth Place, 520, 747

wŭ dài 五代, Five Dynasties, 204

wŭ fú huà dú dān 五福化毒丹, Five Happinesses Toxin-Transforming Elixir, 238

wŭ gān 五疳, five gan, 204

wŭ gēng (jīng) sòu 五更嗽, fifth-watch cough, 199

wŭ gēng (jīng) xiè 五更泄, fifth-watch diarrhea, 199

wŭ guān 五官, five offices, 205

wŭ hóu xíng jūn săn 武侯行军散, Warlord's Troop-Marching Powder, 740

wŭ hòu cháo rè 午后潮热, postmeridian tidal heat [effusion], 447

wŭ hŭ tāng 五虎汤, Five Tigers Decoction, 443

wŭ hŭ zhuī fēng săn 五虎追风散, Five-Tigers-Chasing-the-Wind Powder, 74, 140, 366, 740

wŭ huáng săn 五黄散, Five Yellows Powder, 745

wŭ huŏ 武火, martial flame, 387

wŭ jī 五积, five accumulations, 204

wŭ jī săn 五积散, Five Accumulations Powder, 80, 82, 104, 186, 216, 516, 606, 730

wŭ jiā jiăn zhèng qì săn 五加减正气散, Fifth Variant Qi-Righting Powder, 732

wŭ jiā pí 五加皮 acanthopanax, Acanthopanacis Radicis Cortex, 139, 722

wŭ láo 五劳, five taxations, 207

wŭ láo qī shāng 五劳七伤, five taxations and seven damages, 207

wŭ láo suŏ shāng 五劳所伤, damage by the five taxations, 108

wŭ lì huí chūn dān 五粒回春丹, Five Grains Return-of-Spring Elixir, 171

wŭ lín 五淋, five stranguries, 207

wŭ lín săn 五淋散, Five Stranguries Powder, 283, 583, 733

wŭ líng săn 五苓散, Poria (Hoelen) Five Powder, 79, 110, 117, 136, 151, 170, 179, 224, 232, 245, 348, 400, 541, 588, 600, 647, 663, 666–669, 694, 716, 733

wŭ líng zhī 五灵脂 flying squirrel's droppings, Trogopteri seu Pteromydis Excrementum, 137, 138, 397, 411, 448, 467, 574, 724

wŭ lún 五轮, five wheels, 209

wŭ mò yĭn zĭ 五磨饮子, Five Milled Ingredients Drink, 426, 736

wŭ pí săn 五皮散, Five-Peel Powder, 136

wŭ pí săn (yĭn) 五皮散（饮）, Five-Peel Powder (Beverage), 733

wŭ pí yĭn 五皮饮, Five-Peel Beverage, 153, 239, 608, 669

wŭ rén tāng 五仁汤, Five Kernels Decoction, 732

wŭ rén wán 五仁丸, Five Kernels Pill, 399, 646, 732

wŭ rù 五入, five entries, 204

wŭ ruăn 五软, five limpnesses, 205

wŭ sè 五色, five colors, 204

wŭ sè zhŭ bìng 五色主病, disease correspondences of the five colors, 134

wŭ shén tāng 五神汤, Five Spirits Decoction, 744

wŭ shēng 五声, five voices, 209

wŭ shí jiān 五十肩, fifty-year-old's shoulder, 200

wŭ shū 五枢, GB-27, Fifth Pivot, 242, 748

wŭ shū pèi xué fă 五输配穴法, combining transport points, 91

wŭ shū xué 五俞穴, five transport points, 207

wŭ shū xué 五腧穴, five transport points, 207

wŭ shū xué 五输穴, five transport points, 207

wŭ shuĭ 五水, five waters, 209

wŭ wĕi tāng 五痿汤, Five Wiltings Decoction, 733

wŭ wèi 五味, five flavors, 204

wŭ wèi suŏ rù 五味所入, five-flavor entries, 204

wŭ wèi xiāo dú yĭn 五味消毒饮, Five-Ingredient Toxin-Dispersing Beverage, 75, 76, 636, 691, 744

wŭ wèi zĭ 五味子 schisandra, Schisandrae Fructus, 12, 47, 95, 96, 104, 175, 222, 230, 272, 333, 378, 409, 490, 502, 504, 512, 518, 537, 566, 571, 596, 599, 614, 651, 700, 709, 715, 726, 727

wŭ wèi zĭ săn 五味子散, Schisandra Powder, 477

wŭ wèi zĭ tāng 五味子汤, Schisandra Decoction, 95, 376, 743

wŭ wŭ dān 五五丹, Five-to-Five Elixir, 187, 259, 492, 744

wŭ wù 五恶, five aversions, 204

wŭ wù xiāng rú yĭn 五物香薷饮, Five Agents Elsholtzia Beverage, 729

wŭ xié 五邪, five evils, 204

wŭ xīn 五心, five hearts, 205

wŭ xīn fán rè 五心烦热, vexing heat in the five hearts, 655

wŭ xíng 五行, five phases, 205

wŭ xiù 五臭, five odors, 205

wŭ yí 五宜, five proprieties, 207

wŭ yì 五液, five humors, 205

wŭ yùn liù qì 五运六气, five movements and six qi, 205

wŭ yùn liù qì 五运六气, five periods and six qi, 205

wŭ zàng 五脏, five viscera, 208

wŭ zàng bì 五脏痹, impediments of the five viscera, 296

wŭ zàng bì 五脏痹, visceral impediment, 656

wŭ zàng huà yè 五脏化液, five viscera form humors, 209

wŭ zàng liù fŭ ké 五脏六腑咳, five viscera and six bowels cough, 208

wŭ zàng liù fŭ ké 五脏六腑咳, organ cough, 421

wŭ zàng suŏ wù 五脏所恶, aversions of the five viscera, 13

wŭ zàng suŏ zhŭ 五脏所主, governings of the five viscera, 244

wŭ zàng xì jiē shŭ yú xīn 五脏系皆属于心, ties of the five viscera home to the heart, 614

wŭ zhī ān zhōng yĭn 五汁安中饮, Five Juices Center-Quieting Beverage, 164 *wŭ zhī yĭn* 五汁饮, Five Juices Beverage, 607, 734

wŭ zhì 五志, five minds, 205

wŭ zhì guò jí 五志过极, excess among the five minds, 181

wŭ zhì huà huŏ 五志化火, five minds forming fire, 205

wŭ zhŭ 五主, five governings, 205

wŭ zhù xué 五柱穴, Five Pillar Points, 2, 5, 61, 73, 207, 562, 647

wŭ zĭ bŭ shèn wán 五子补肾丸, Five-Seed Kidney-Supplementing Pill, 742

wŭ zĭ yăn zōng wán 五子衍宗丸, Five-Seed Progeny Pill, 461, 523, 742

wù fēng 恶风, aversion to wind, 13

wù guāng xiū míng 恶光羞明, aversion to light, 13

wù guāng xiū míng 恶光羞明, photophobia, 443

wù hán 恶寒, aversion to cold, 13

wù hán fā rè 恶寒发热, heat [effusion] and [aversion to] cold, 279

wù jĭ wán 戊己丸, Fifth and Sixth Heavenly Stem Pill, 109, 732

wù jiàn dēng huŏ 恶见灯火, aversion to lights and fire, 13

wù rè 恶热, aversion to heat, 13

wù shí 恶食, aversion to food, 13

wù táng 鹜溏, duck's slop, 163

wù tŭ 戊土, S5-earth, 511

wèi nüè 胃疟, stomach malaria, 578

wēn 瘟, scourge, 514

wēn yì 瘟疫, scourge epidemic, 514

Xanthii Fructus, *cāng ĕr zĭ* 苍耳子, xanthium, 120, 121, 681, 686, 720

xanthium, *cāng ĕr zĭ* 苍耳子, Xanthii Fructus, 120, 121, 681, 686, 720

Xanthium Powder, *cāng ĕr săn* 苍耳散, 740

Xanthium Powder, *cāng ĕr zĭ săn* 苍耳子散, 120, 740

xī 膝, knee, 336

xī bēn 息贲, rushing respiration, 510

xī bēn tāng 息贲汤, Rushing Respiration Decoction, 510

xī dì qīng luò yĭn 犀地清络饮, Rhinoceros Horn and Rehmannia Network-Clearing Beverage, 730

xī fēng 熄风, extinguishing wind, 187

xī fēng huà tán 熄风化痰, extinguishing wind and transforming phlegm, 188

xī guā 西瓜 watermelon, Citrulli Fructus, 67, 231, 720

xī guā pí 西瓜皮 watermelon rind, Citrulli Exocarpium, 67, 589, 720

xī guā shuāng 西瓜霜 watermelon frost, Mirabiliti et Citrulli Praeparatio, 67, 720

xī guān 膝关, LR-7, Knee Joint, 337, 748

xī hàn 西汉, Western (Former) Han, 671

xī huáng wán 犀黄丸, Rhinoceros Bezoar Pill, 737

xī jiăo 犀角 rhinoceros horn, Rhinocerotis Cornu, 67, 209, 245, 411, 422, 525, 548, 619, 720

xī jiăo dì huáng tāng 犀角地黄汤, Rhinoceros Horn and Rehmannia Decoction, 24, 25, 30, 33, 51, 63, 76, 99, 102, 177, 202, 315, 390, 393, 431, 447, 567, 637, 693, 730

xī jiăo săn 犀角散, Rhinoceros Horn Powder, 731

xī jiĕ 膝解, knee joint, 337

xī jìn 西晋, Western Jin, 671

xī mén 吸门, breath gate, 50

xī mén 郄门, PC-4, Cleft Gate, 29, 30, 58, 70, 89, 129, 265, 268, 294, 314, 343, 390, 416, 427, 440, 452, 522, 538, 566, 567, 570, 608, 629, 668, 675, 748

xī tóng wán 豨桐丸, Siegesbeckia and Clerodendron Pill, 734

xī tòng 膝痛, knee pain, 337

xī wèi 西魏, Western Wei, 671

xī xiān 豨莶 siegesbeckia, Siegesbeckiae Herba, 116, 139, 722

xī xián săn 稀涎散, Drool-Thinning Powder, 170, 743

xī yăn 膝眼, Eye of the Knee, 104, 137, 296, 337, 521, 567

xī yăn fēng 膝眼风, knee's eye wind, 337

xī yáng guān 膝阳关, GB-33, Knee Yang Joint, 61, 104, 137, 154, 296, 337, 521, 567, 748

xī yáng shēn 西洋参 American ginseng, Panacis Quinquefolii Radix, 175, 593, 726

xī yóu fēng 膝游风, wandering knee wind, 658

xī zhōu 西周, Western Zhou, 671

xí 袭, assail, 11

xí lèi săn 锡类散, Tin-Like Powder, 615, 744

xĭ 喜, joy, 323

xĭ 洗, washing, 665

xĭ àn 喜按, like pressure, 346

xĭ lĕng 喜冷, like cold, 346

xĭ lĕng yĭn 喜冷饮, liking for cool drinks, 347

xĭ rè 喜热, like heat, 346

xĭ xīn săn 洗心散, Heart-Washing Powder, 202, 740

xĭ xīn yĭn 徙薪饮, Firewood-Removing Beverage, 29

xĭ zé qì huăn 喜则气缓, joy causes qi to slacken, 323

xì 系, tie, 614

xì mài 细脉, fine pulse, 200

xì xīn 细辛 asarum, Asiasari Herba cum Radice, 11, 17, 55, 243, 262, 311, 326, 343, 405, 438, 660, 664, 681, 723

xì xīn săn 细辛散, Asarum Powder, 620

xì xué 郄穴, cleft point, 73

xiā yóu mài 虾游脉, darting shrimp pulse, 118

xiá bái 侠白, LU-4, Guarding White, 520, 746

xiá xī 侠溪, GB-43, Pinched Ravine, 11, 20, 66, 93, 119, 147, 158, 167, 175, 176, 235, 240, 241, 263, 281, 292, 337, 344, 355, 356, 359, 364–366, 462, 495, 511, 519, 538, 568, 585, 601, 614, 656, 658, 689, 713, 748

xià 夏, Xia, 698

xià 下, lower body, 368

xià 下, precipitate, 459

xià bìng qǔ shàng 下病取上, treating lower body disease through the upper body, 626

xià fǎ 下法, precipitation, 459

xià fú yù yú shàng zhī huǒ 下怫郁于上之火, precipitating depressed upper body fire, 459

xià gān 下疳, lower body gan, 368

xià guān 下关, ST-7, Below the Joint, 73, 89, 178, 194, 220, 366, 403, 485, 521, 620, 621, 690, 693, 746

xià hé xué 下合穴, lower uniting point, 369

xià héng gǔ 下横骨, lower transverse bone, 369

xià jí 下极, lower extreme, 369

xià jí shèn yīn 下汲肾阴, sapping of kidney yin, 512

xià jí zhī xià 下极之下, [region] below the lower extreme, 497

xià jiāo 下焦, lower burner, 368

xià jiāo rú dú 下焦如渎, lower burner is like a sluice, 369

xià jiāo shī rè 下焦湿热, lower burner damp-heat, 368

xià jiāo shī rè niào xuè 下焦湿热尿血, lower burner damp-heat bloody urine, 368

xià jiāo zhǔ chū 下焦主出, lower burner governs exit, 368

xià jù xū 下巨虚, ST-39, Lower Great Hollow, 89, 226, 263, 281, 369, 390, 746

xià kū cǎo 夏枯草 prunella, Prunellae Spica, 67, 141, 385, 459, 526, 538, 544, 685, 720

xià kū cǎo gāo 夏枯草膏, Prunella Paste, 737

xià kū cǎo tāng 夏枯草汤, Prunella Decoction, 737

xià lì 下利, diarrhea and dysentery, 126

xià lì qīng gǔ 下利清谷, clear-food diarrhea, 64

xià lián 下廉, LI-8, Lower Ridge, 542, 746

xià liáo 下髎, BL-34, Lower Bone-Hole, 118, 220, 241, 424, 468, 747

xià pò 下迫, lower body distress, 368

xià qì 下气, precipitating qi, 459

xià qiào 下窍, lower orifices, 369

xià quán 下泉, urine, 642

xià rè dú 下热毒, precipitating heat toxin, 459

xià rǔ 下乳, promote lactation, 467

xià rǔ tiān jiāng yǐn 下乳天浆饮, Celestial Fluid Lactation-Promoting Beverage, 741

xià tiān wú 夏天无 Jilong corydalis, Corydalis Decumbentis Tuber et Herba, 140, 722

xià wǎn 下脘, CV-10, Lower Stomach Duct, 2–4, 15, 141, 157, 186, 197, 207, 215–217, 237, 239, 302, 316, 426, 450, 499, 557, 564, 578, 633, 749

xià wèi cháng rè jié 下胃肠热结, precipitating gastrointestinal heat bind, 459

xià xiàn 下陷, downward fall, 146

xià xiàn 罅陷, crevice, 105

xià xiāo 下消, lower burner dispersion-thirst, 368

xià xiāo 下消, lower dispersion, 369

xià xuè 下血, precipitation of blood, 460

xià yīn 下阴, lower yin, 369

xià yū xuè tāng 下瘀血汤, Stasis-Precipitating Decoction, 118, 738

xià yuán 下元, lower origin, 369

xià yuán bù gù 下元不固, insecurity of the lower origin, 308

xià yuán kuī sǔn 下元亏损, depletion of the lower origin, 122

xià yuán xū bèi 下元虚惫, exhaustion of the lower origin, 181

xià yuán xū lěng 下元虚冷, vacuity cold of the lower origin, 646

xià zhī liú huǒ 下肢流火, lower limb fire flow, 369

xià zhù 下注, downpour, 146

xià zhù chuāng 下注疮, downpour sore, 146

xiān bǔ hòu gōng 先补后攻, supplementation followed by attack, 594

xiān dì huáng 鲜地黄 fresh rehmannia, Rehmanniae Radix Recens, 67, 116, 720

xiān fāng huó mìng yǐn 仙方活命饮, Immortal Formula Life-Giving Beverage, 62, 187, 259, 386, 427, 585, 744

xiān gōng hòu bǔ 先攻后补, attack followed by supplementation, 12

xiān hé yè 鲜荷叶 fresh lotus leaf, Nelumbinis Folium Recens, 625

xiān hè cǎo 仙鹤草 agrimony, Agrimoniae Herba, 298, 502, 519, 569, 724

xiān hè cǎo gēn yá 仙鹤草根芽 agrimony root sprout, Agrimoniae Rhizoma Pullulatum, 183

xiān jiān 先煎, predecoction, 460

xiān lú gēn 鲜芦根 fresh phragmites, Phragmititis Rhizoma Recens, 67, 282, 720

xiān máo 仙茅 curculigo, Curculiginis Rhizoma, 335, 593, 596, 727

xiān máo gēn 鲜茅根 fresh imperata, Imperatae Rhizoma Recens, 30, 703

xiān qí tāng 先期汤, Premature Periods Decoction, 730

xiān shǒu wū 鲜首乌 fresh flowery knotweed, Polygoni Multiflori Radix Recens, 399

xiān tiān 先天, congenital constitution, 94

xiān tiān 先天, earlier heaven, 166

xiān tiān zhī běn 先天之本, root of earlier heaven, 508

xiān zhào liú chǎn 先兆流产, threatened miscarriage, 609

xiān zhú yè 鲜竹叶 fresh bamboo leaf (lophatherum), Lophatheri Folium Recens, 589

xián 痫, epilepsy, 178

xián 涎, drool, 149

xián 弦, eyelid rim, 192

xián 咸, saltiness, 511

xián 咸, salty, 511

xián fù zǐ 咸附子 aconite, Aconiti Tuber Laterale Salsum, 311

xián fù zǐ 咸附子 salted aconite, Aconiti Tuber Laterale Salsum, 367, 660, 723

xián mài 弦脉, stringlike pulse, 584

xián mài 弦脉, wiry pulse, 694

xián pǐ 痃癖, strings and aggregations, 584

xián rù shèn 咸入肾, saltiness enters the kidney, 511

xián tuò 涎唾, drool-spittle, 150

xián wéi pí yè 涎为脾液, drool is the humor of the spleen, 150

xián zhèng 痫证, epilepsy pattern, 178

xiǎn 癣, lichen, 345

xiǎn yào shuǐ 癣药水, Lichen Medicinal Water, 689

xiàn gǔ 陷谷, ST-43, Sunken Valley, 14, 54, 73, 283, 396, 520, 547, 561, 652, 665, 688, 746

xiàn zhèng 陷证, fall pattern, 195

xiāng bèi yǎng yíng tāng 香贝养营汤, Cyperus and Fritillaria Construction-Nourishing Decoction, 737

xiāng bó 相搏, contend, 97

xiāng chéng 相乘, overwhelming, 422

xiāng fù zhī guān 相傅之官, office of assistant, 419

xiāng fù zǐ 香附子 cyperus, Cyperi Rhizoma, 19, 93, 103, 115, 201, 227, 384, 397, 418, 426, 428, 433, 457, 474, 475, 478, 480, 483, 493, 538, 574, 581, 647, 663, 670, 694, 723

xiāng gǎng jiǎo 香港脚, Hongkong foot, 292

xiāng jiān 相兼, combination, 88

xiāng kè 相克, restraining, 502

xiāng lián wán 香连丸, Saussurea and Coptis Pill, 110, 278, 312, 588, 645, 731

xiāng lián zhū dǔ wán 香连猪肚丸, Saussurea and Coptis Pig's Stomach Pill, 647

xiāng pò wán 香朴丸, Saussurea and Magnolia Bark Pill, 736

xiāng rú 香薷 elsholtzia, Elsholtziae Herba, 69, 587, 681, 720

xiāng rú sǎn 香薷散, Elsholtzia Powder, 729

xiāng rú tāng 香薷汤, Elsholtzia Decoction, 729

xiāng rú yǐn 香薷饮, Elsholtzia Beverage, 18, 588, 590

xiāng shā 相杀, killing, 336

xiāng shā èr chén tāng 香砂二陈汤, Saussurea and Amomum Two Matured Ingredients Decoction, 738

xiāng shā liù jūn zǐ tāng 香砂六君子汤, Saussurea and Amomum Six Gentlemen Decoction, 4, 10, 23, 47, 143, 223, 231, 393, 418, 457, 463, 487, 554, 561, 565, 575, 741

xiāng shā liù jūn zǐ wán 香砂六君子丸, Saussurea and Amomum Six Gentlemen Pill, 741

xiāng shā píng wèi wán 香砂平胃丸, Saussurea and Amomum Stomach-Calming Pill, 736

xiāng shā zhǐ zhú wán 香砂枳术丸, Saussurea, Amomum, Unripe Bitter Orange, and Ovate Atractylodes Pill, 216, 218, 736

xiāng shēng 相生, engendering, 174

xiāng shǐ 相使, empowering, 172

xiāng sū sǎn 香苏散, Cyperus and Perilla Powder, 480, 686, 729

xiāng wèi 相畏, fear, 196

xiāng wǔ 相侮, rebellion, 492

xiāng wù 相恶, aversion, 13

xiāng xū 相须, mutual need, 404

xiǎng shēng pò dí wán 响声破笛丸, Broken Flute Pill, 729

xiàng 象, sign, 531

xiàng huǒ 相火, ministerial fire, 396

xiàng huǒ wàng dòng 相火妄动, stirring of the ministerial fire, 574

xiàng pí 象皮 elephant's hide, Elephantis Corium, 728

xiàng pí gāo 象皮膏, Elephant Skin Paste, 100

xiàng qiáng 项强, rigidity of the neck, 508

xiàng zhōng jū 项中疽, mid-nape flat-abscess, 394

xiāo 消, disperse, 140

xiāo 消, dispersion, 142

xiāo 哮, wheezing, 671

xiāo bái yǐn 消白饮, Whiteness-Dispersing Beverage, 733

xiāo chuǎn 哮喘, wheezing and panting, 672

xiāo chuǎn fù zhì fāng 哮喘敷治方, Wheezing and Panting External Application Formula, 744

xiāo chuāng yǐn 消疮饮, Sore-Healing Beverage, 744

xiāo dǎo 消导, abductive dispersion, 2

xiāo dú xī jiǎo yǐn 消毒犀角饮, Toxin-Dispersing Rhinoceros Beverage, 497

xiāo fǎ 消法, dispersion, 142

xiāo fēng dǎo chì tāng 消风导赤汤, Wind-Dispersing Red-Abducting Decoction, 586

xiāo fēng sǎn 消风散, Wind-Dispersing Powder, 145, 260, 395, 494, 591, 671, 676, 686, 688, 740

xiāo fēng yǎng xuè tāng 消风养血汤, Wind-Dispersing Blood-Nourishing Decoction, 740

xiāo gān 消疳, dispersing gan, 141

xiāo gǔ shàn jī 消谷善饥, swift digestion with rapid hungering, 601

xiāo gǔ xǐ jī 消谷喜饥, swift digestion with rapid hungering, 601

xiāo kě 消渴, dispersion-thirst, 142

xiāo kě fāng 消渴方, Dispersion-Thirst Formula, 640, 734

xiāo luǒ wán 消瘰丸, Scrofula-Dispersing Pill, 142, 737

xiāo luò 消泺, TB-12, Dispersing Riverbed, 748

xiāo pǐ ē wèi wán 消痞阿魏丸, Glomus-Dispersing Asafetida Pill, 736

xiāo pǐ huà jī 消痞化积, dispersing glomus and transforming accumulations, 141

xiāo shí 消食, dispersing food, 140

xiāo shí 硝石 niter, Nitrum, 214, 383, 458, 544, 728

xiāo shí dǎo zhì 消食导滞, dispersing food and abducting stagnation, 140

xiāo shí fán shí sǎn 硝石矾石散, Niter and Alum Powder, 21, 737

xiāo shí huà tán 消食化痰, dispersing food and transforming phlegm, 141

xiāo shí huà zhì 消食化滞, dispersing food and transforming stagnation, 141

xiāo shòu 消瘦, emaciation, 171

xiāo tán 消痰, dispersing phlegm, 141

xiāo tán píng chuǎn 消痰平喘, dispersing phlegm and calming panting, 141

xiāo tán ruǎn jiān 消痰软坚, dispersing phlegm and softening hardness, 142

xiāo xīn 消心, heart dispersion, 262

xiāo yáo sǎn 逍遥散, Free Wanderer Powder, 19, 103, 202, 223, 229, 256, 315, 358, 362, 367, 385, 386, 393, 412, 478, 480, 482, 484, 493, 497, 513, 515, 524, 599, 643, 655, 656, 685, 732

xiāo yǐng luǒ tán hé 消瘿瘰痰核, dispersing goiter, scrofula, and phlegm nodes, 141

xiāo yǐng tāng 消瘿汤, Goiter-Dispersing Decoction, 737

xiāo yū yǐn 消瘀饮, Stasis-Dispersing Beverage, 570

xiāo zhēng jiǎ jī jù 消癥瘕积聚, dispersing concretions, conglomerations, accumulations, and gatherings, 140

xiāo zhèng 哮证, wheezing patterns, 672

xiāo zhì yǐn 消痔饮, Hemorrhoid-Dispersing Beverage, 744

xiǎo bàn xià jiā fú líng tāng 小半夏加茯苓汤, Minor Pinellia Decoction Plus Poria (Hoelen), 87, 442, 578, 665

xiǎo bàn xià tāng 小半夏汤, Minor Pinellia Decoction, 736

xiǎo biàn 小便, urine, 642

xiǎo biàn bù jìn 小便不禁, urinary incontinence, 640

xiǎo biàn bù lì 小便不利, inhibited urination, 301

xiǎo biàn bù shuǎng 小便不爽, ungratifying urination, 637

xiǎo biàn bù tōng 小便不通, urinary stoppage, 641

xiǎo biàn chì sè 小便赤涩, rough voidings of reddish urine, 509

xiǎo biàn chū fèn 小便出粪, stool in the urine, 582

xiǎo biàn duǎn chì 小便短赤, short voidings of reddish urine, 530

xiǎo biàn duǎn shǎo 小便短少, short voidings of scant urine, 530

xiǎo biàn hún zhuó 小便浑浊, turbid urine, 632

xiǎo biàn lín lì 小便淋沥, dribbling urination, 149

xiǎo biàn lín lì bù jìn 小便淋沥不禁, dribbling urinary incontinence, 149

xiǎo biàn pín shuò 小便频数, frequent urination, 229

xiǎo biàn qīng cháng 小便清长, long voidings of clear urine, 367

xiǎo biàn shī jìn 小便失禁, urinary incontinence, 640

xiǎo biàn shuò 小便数, frequent urination, 229

xiǎo biàn zì lì 小便自利, uninhibited urination, 637

xiǎo chái hú tāng 小柴胡汤, Minor Bupleurum Decoction, 20, 57, 255, 279, 284, 344, 362, 394, 449, 599, 683, 688, 712, 732

xiǎo chǎn 小产, miscarriage, 396

xiǎo cháng 小肠, SI, 531

xiǎo cháng 小肠, small intestine, 543

xiǎo cháng bìng 小肠病, small intestinal disease, 542

xiǎo cháng jīng 小肠经, small intestine channel, 543

xiǎo cháng ké 小肠咳, small intestinal cough, 542

xiǎo cháng qì 小肠气, small intestinal qi, 542

xiǎo cháng qì tòng 小肠气痛, small intestinal qi pain, 542

xiǎo cháng shàn 小肠疝, small intestinal mounting, 542

xiǎo cháng shí rè 小肠实热, small intestinal repletion heat, 542

xiǎo cháng shū 小肠俞, BL-27, Small Intestine Transport, 15, 36, 41, 89, 91, 509, 542, 747

xiǎo cháng xū hán 小肠虚寒, small intestinal vacuity cold, 542

xiǎo cháng yōng 小肠痈, small intestinal welling-abscess, 543

xiǎo cháng zhě, shòu chéng zhī guān yě, huà wù chū yān 小肠者，受盛之官也，化物出焉, small intestine holds the office of reception, whence the transformation of things emanates, 543

xiǎo cháng zhǔ fēn bié qīng zhuó 小肠主分别清浊, small intestine governs separation of the clear and the turbid, 543

xiǎo cháng zhǔ shòu chéng 小肠主受盛, small intestine governs reception, 543

xiǎo cháng zhǔ yè 小肠主液, small intestine governs humor, 543

xiǎo chéng qì tāng 小承气汤, Minor Qi-Coordinating Decoction, 84, 127, 239, 426, 459, 499, 613, 731

xiǎo ér 小儿, infant, 299

xiǎo ér dān dú 小儿丹毒, infantile cinnabar toxin, 299

xiǎo ér gān yǎn 小儿疳眼, child eye gan, 60

xiǎo ér huí chūn dān 小儿回春丹, Children's Return-of-Spring Elixir, 740

xiǎo ér jí bìng 小儿疾病, infants' and children's diseases, 299

xiǎo ér jīng fēng 小儿惊风, child fright wind, 60

xiǎo ér jīng jué 小儿惊厥, child fright reversal, 60

xiǎo ér kè wǔ 小儿客忤, child visiting hostility, 60

xiǎo ér lì jí 小儿痢疾, child dysentery, 60

xiǎo ér wěi zhèng 小儿痿证, child wilting pattern, 60

xiǎo ér yè tí 小儿夜啼, night crying in infants, 409

xiǎo ér zá bìng 小儿杂病, children's diseases, 60

xiǎo ér zhǐ zhěn 小儿指诊, infant's finger examination, 299

xiǎo fēn 小分, minor divide, 396

xiǎo fù 小腹, smaller abdomen, 541

xiǎo fù mǎn 小腹满, smaller-abdominal fullness, 541

xiǎo fù tòng 小腹痛, smaller-abdominal pain, 541

xiǎo gǔ kōng 小骨空, Little Finger Bone Hollow, 93, 195, 500, 586, 636

xiǎo hǎi 小海, SI-8, Small Sea, 75, 137, 567, 637, 747

xiǎo huó luò dān 小活络丹, Minor Network-Quickening Elixir, 14, 621, 734

xiǎo jì 小蓟 cephalanoplos, Cephalanoploris Herba seu Radix, 21, 30, 34, 70, 569, 724

xiǎo jì yǐn zǐ 小蓟饮子, Cephalanoplos Drink, 22, 30, 36, 41, 738

xiǎo jiàn zhōng tāng 小建中汤, Minor Center-Fortifying Decoction, 217, 487, 488, 581, 713, 735 *xiǎo jié xiōng* 小结胸, minor chest bind, 396

xiǎo jīn dān 小金丹, Minor Golden Elixir, 259, 737

xiǎo jīn qián cǎo 小金钱草 dichondra, Dichondrae Herba, 136, 723

xiǎo mài 小脉, small pulse, 543

xiǎo qīng lóng jiā shí gāo tāng 小青龙加石膏汤, Minor Green-Blue Dragon Decoction Plus Gypsum, 441, 469, 739

xiǎo qīng lóng tāng 小青龙汤, Minor Green-Blue Dragon Decoction, 78, 85, 120, 170, 246, 373, 438, 468, 550, 625, 663, 666, 667, 739

xiǎo shuǐ 小水, urine, 642

xiǎo sōu 小溲, urine, 642

xiǎo wèi dān 小胃丹, Minor Stomach Elixir, 442, 638

xiǎo wēn zhōng wán 小温中丸, Minor Center-Warming Pill, 736

xiǎo xiàn xiōng tāng 小陷胸汤, Minor Chest Bind Decoction, 189, 277, 303, 396, 738

xiǎo xù mìng tāng 小续命汤, Minor Life-Prolonging Decoction, 45, 456, 568, 631, 693, 740

xiǎo yíng jiān 小营煎, Minor Construction Brew, 94, 741

xiǎo zì 小眦, outer canthus, 422

xiē shāo 蝎梢 scorpion tail, Buthi Caudex, 562, 652

xié 邪, evil, 180

xié 邪, pathogen, 429

xié 胁, rib-side, 507

xié cì 斜刺, oblique insertion, 418

xié cì 斜刺, slanted insertion, 536

xié fēi mài 斜飞脉, oblique-running pulse, 418

xié hài kōng qiào 邪害空窍, evils harm the empty orifices, 181

xié lè téng tòng 胁肋疼痛, rib-side pain, 507

xié lè zhàng tòng 胁肋胀痛, rib-side pain and distention, 507

xié liàn xīn bāo 邪恋心包, evil lodged in the pericardium, 181

xié liú sān jiāo 邪留三焦, evil lodged in the triple burner, 181

xié qì 邪气, evil qi, 181

xié qì shèng zé shí 邪气盛则实, when evil qi is exuberant, there is repletion, 672

xié rè 邪热, evil heat, 181

xié shí 邪实, evil repletion, 181

xié shì 斜视, squint, 568

xié tòng 胁痛, rib-side pain, 507

xiè 泄, discharge, 130

xiè 泻, drain, 146

xiè 洩, discharge, 130

xiè bái 泻白, draining the white, 147

xiè bái 薤白 Chinese chive, Allii Bulbus, 398, 493, 724

xiè bái sǎn 泻白散, White-Draining Powder, 15, 72, 101, 147, 201, 238, 277, 280, 329, 372, 374, 674, 677, 695, 731

xiè bái yì yuán sǎn 泻白益元散, White-Draining Origin-Boosting Powder, 587

xiè chǐ 齘齿, grinding of the teeth, 249

xiè fǎ 泻法, drainage, 146

xiè fèi 泻肺, draining the lung, 147

xiè gān 泄肝, discharge the liver, 130

xiè gān 泻肝, draining the liver, 147

xiè gān ān shén wán 泻肝安神丸, Liver-Draining Spirit-Quieting Pill, 731

xiè huáng sǎn 泻黄散, Yellow-Draining Powder, 558, 600, 731

xiè huǒ 泻火, draining fire, 146

xiè huǒ jiě dú 泻火解毒, draining fire and resolving toxin, 147

xiè huǒ qīng fèi tāng 泻火清肺汤, Fire-Draining Lung-Clearing Decoction, 281

xiè huǒ xī fēng 泻火熄风, draining fire and extinguishing wind, 146

xiè jì 泄剂, discharging formula, 130

xiè jīng 蟹睛, crab's-eye, 104

xiè kě qù bì 泄可去闭, discharging [medicinals] can eliminate blocks, 130

xiè mù 蟹目, crab's-eye, 104

xiè pí sǎn 泻脾散, Spleen-Draining Powder, 731

xiè qīng gè bàn tāng 泻清各半汤, Green-Blue–Draining Half-and-Half Decoction, 353, 401

xiè qīng wán 泻青丸, Green-Blue–Draining Pill, 6, 51, 359, 731

xiè shī tāng 泻湿汤, Dampness-Draining Decoction, 733

xiè wèi tòu rè 泄卫透热, discharge defense and out-thrust heat, 130

xiè xià 泻下, draining precipitation, 147

xiè xiè 泄泻, diarrhea, 125

xiè xīn 泻心, draining the heart, 147

xiè xīn dǎo chì tāng 泻心导赤汤, Heart-Draining Red-Abducting Decoction, 237

xiè xīn tāng 泻心汤, Heart-Draining Decoction, 29, 189, 263, 281, 294, 459, 552, 731

xiè zhuǎ (zhǎo) 蟹爪, crab claw markings, 104

xīn 心, HT, 293

xīn 心, heart, 260

xīn 辛, acrid, 5

xīn 辛, acridity, 5

xīn 辛, pungency, 473

xīn bāo 心包, PC, 429

xīn bāo 心包, pericardium, 430

xīn bāo jīng 心包经, pericardium channel, 430

xīn bāo luò 心包络, pericardiac network [vessel], 430

xīn bāo luò hé sān jiāo 心包络合三焦, pericardium connects with the triple burner, 430

xīn bào zhèng 心包证, pericardiac pattern, 430

xīn bì 心痹, heart impediment, 265

xīn bìng 心病, heart disease, 261

xīn cáng shén 心藏神, heart stores the spirit, 272

xīn chè 心掣, pulling heart, 469

xīn chóng bìng 心虫病, heart worm disease, 273

xīn dǎn xū qiè 心胆虚怯, heart-gallbladder vacuity timidity, 264

xīn dòng jì 心动悸, stirring heart palpitations, 574

xīn fèi liǎng xū 心肺两虚, dual vacuity of the heart and lung, 161

xīn fèi qì xū 心肺气虚, heart-lung qi vacuity, 267

xīn fèi yáng xū 心肺阳虚, heart-lung yang vacuity, 267

xīn fèi yīn xū 心肺阴虚, heart-lung yin vacuity, 267

xīn fù 心腹, heart [region] and abdomen, 271

xīn fù lěng tòng 心腹冷痛, cold pain in the heart [region] and abdomen, 83

xīn fù tòng 心腹痛, pain in the heart [region] and abdomen, 425

xīn gān 心疳, gan of the heart, 237

xīn gān huǒ wàng 心肝火旺, effulgent heart-liver fire, 168

xīn gān xuè xū 心肝血虚, heart-liver blood vacuity, 266

xīn gǎn 新感, new contraction, 409

xīn gǎn wēn bìng 新感温病, new contraction warm disease, 409

xīn gǎn yǐn dòng fú xié 新感引动伏邪, new contraction stirring latent evil, 409

xīn hàn 心汗, heart sweating, 272

xīn hé mài 心合脉, heart is connected with the vessels, 265

xīn hé xiǎo cháng 心合小肠, heart is connected with the small intestine, 265

xīn huāng 心慌, flusteredness, 214

xīn huǒ 心火, heart fire, 263

xīn huǒ 心火, heart-fire, 263

xīn huǒ chì shèng 心火炽盛, intense heart fire, 310

xīn huǒ kàng shèng 心火亢盛, hyperactive heart fire, 293

xīn huǒ nèi chì 心火内炽, intense internal heart fire, 310

xīn huǒ nèi fén 心火内焚, heart fire deflagrating internally, 263

xīn huǒ shàng yán 心火上炎, heart fire flaming upward, 263

xīn huǒ shàng yán 心火上炎, upflaming heart fire, 639

xīn huǒ shèng 心火盛, exuberant heart fire, 189

xīn huǒ wàng 心火旺, effulgent heart fire, 168

xīn jī 心积, heart accumulation, 260

xīn jì 心悸, heart palpitations, 268

xīn jì 心悸, palpitations, 427

xīn jiā huáng lóng tāng 新加黄龙汤, Newly Supplemented Yellow Dragon Decoction, 732

xīn jiā xiāng rú yǐn 新加香薷饮, Newly Supplemented Elsholtzia Beverage, 591, 729

xīn jīn 辛金, S8-metal, 511

xīn jīng 心经, heart channel, 261

xīn jīng ké sòu 心经咳嗽, heart channel cough, 261

xīn kāi kǔ jiàng 辛开苦降, acrid opening and bitter downbearing, 5

xīn kāi kǔ jiàng 辛开苦降, opening with acridity and downbearing with bitterness, 421

xīn kāi kǔ xiè 辛开苦泄, acrid opening and bitter discharging, 5

xīn kāi kǔ xiè 辛开苦泄, opening with acridity and discharging with bitterness, 420

xīn kāi qiào yú shé 心开窍于舌, heart opens at the tongue, 267

xīn ké 心咳, heart cough, 261

xīn liáng jiě biǎo 辛凉解表, cool acrid exterior resolution, 99

xīn liáng jiě biǎo 辛凉解表, resolving the exterior with coolness and acridity, 501

xīn mài bì zǔ 心脉痹阻, heart vessel obstruction, 272

xīn mài hóng 心脉洪, heart pulse is surging, 270

xīn pí liǎng xu 心脾两虚, dual vacuity of the heart and spleen, 161

xīn pí liǎng xū 心脾两虚, heart-spleen vacuity, 271

xīn pí qì xū 心脾气虚, heart-spleen qi vacuity, 271

xīn pí xuè xū 心脾血虚, heart-spleen blood vacuity, 271

xīn pí yáng xū 心脾阳虚, heart-spleen yang vacuity, 271

xīn qì 心气, heart qi, 270

xīn qì bào tuō 心气暴脱, fulminant desertion of heart qi, 232

xīn qì bù gù 心气不固, insecurity of heart qi, 308

xīn qì bù níng 心气不宁, disquieting of heart qi, 142

xīn qì bù shōu 心气不收, noncontraction of heart qi, 413

xīn qì bù zú 心气不足, insufficiency of heart qi, 309

xīn qì rè 心气热, heart qi heat, 270

xīn qì shèng 心气盛, exuberant heart qi, 189

xīn qì shí 心气实, heart qi repletion, 270

xīn qì xīn xuè 心气、心血, heart qi and heart blood, 270

xīn qì xū 心气虚, heart qi vacuity, 270

xīn qì xū bù dé wò 心气虚不得卧, heart qi vacuity sleeplessness, 270

xīn qì xuè jù xū 心气血俱虚, dual vacuity of heart qi and blood, 159

xīn qì xuè liǎng xū 心气血两虚, dual vacuity of heart qi and blood, 159

xīn qì yīn liǎng xū 心气阴两虚, dual vacuity of heart qi and yin, 159

xīn qiào 心窍, orifice of the heart, 421

xīn rè 心热, heart heat, 264

xīn rè duō jīng 心热多惊, heart heat susceptibility to fright, 264

xīn rù fèi 辛入肺, acridity enters the lung, 5

xīn shàn 心疝, heart mounting, 267

xīn shén bù ān 心神不安, disquieted heart spirit, 142

xīn shén shī shǒu 心神失守, heart spirit failing to contain itself, 271

xīn shèn bù jiāo 心肾不交, breakdown of heart-kidney interaction, 50

xīn shèn bù jiāo 心肾不交, noninteraction of the heart and kidney, 413

xīn shèn qì xū 心肾气虚, heart-kidney qi vacuity, 265

xīn shèn wán 心肾丸, Heart-Kidney Pill, 651

xīn shèn xiāng jiāo 心肾相交, heart and kidney interact, 260

xīn shèn yáng xū 心肾阳虚, heart-kidney yang vacuity, 266

xīn shèn yīn xū 心肾阴虚, heart-kidney yin vacuity, 266

xīn shū 心俞, BL-15, Heart Transport, 11, 15, 33, 38, 39, 58, 59, 81, 87, 89, 91, 129, 147, 153, 159, 160, 162, 180, 222, 223, 228, 230, 232, 235, 236, 261, 263–274, 281, 282, 294, 296, 297, 301, 308, 333, 335, 336, 345, 386, 392, 410, 413, 416, 418, 427, 434, 436, 437, 448–452, 457, 461, 467, 484, 488, 514, 518, 521, 524–526, 537, 538, 551, 572, 594, 595, 597, 629, 641, 642, 651, 652, 654–656, 661, 665, 668, 675, 687, 694, 747

xīn shuǐ 心水, heart water, 273

xīn shén 心神, heart spirit, 271

xīn téng 心疼, heart pain, 268

xīn tòng 心痛, heart pain, 268

xīn tòng chè bèi 心痛彻背, heart pain stretching to the back, 268

xīn wéi hàn 心为汗, heart forms sweat, 263

xīn wěi 心痿, heart wilting, 273

xīn wèi huǒ shèng 心胃火盛, exuberant heart-stomach fire, 189

xīn wèi shí huǒ 心胃实火, heart-stomach repletion fire, 272

xīn wēn jiě biǎo 辛温解表, resolving the exterior with warmth and acridity, 501

xīn wēn jiě biǎo 辛温解表, warm acrid exterior resolution, 658

xīn wù rè 心恶热, heart is averse to heat, 265

xīn wù tòu nóng sǎn 心悟透脓散, Medical Insights Pus-Outthrusting Powder, 744

xīn xì 心系, heart tie, 272

xīn xià 心下, [region] below the heart, 497

xīn xià jí 心下急, distress below the heart, 143

xīn xià jì 心下悸, palpitations below the heart, 427

xīn xià kōng xū 心下空虚, emptiness below the heart, 172

xīn xià mǎn 心下满, fullness below the heart, 232

xīn xià nì mǎn 心下逆满, counterflow fullness below the heart, 102

xīn xià pǐ 心下痞, glomus below the heart, 242

xīn xià pǐ yìng 心下痞硬, hard glomus below the heart, 254

xīn xià tòng 心下痛, pain below the heart, 424

xīn xià zhī jié 心下支结, propping bind below the heart, 468

xīn xiōng biē mèn 心胸憋闷, stifling oppression in the heart and chest, 573

xīn xiōng yù mèn 心胸郁闷, oppression in the heart and chest, 421

xīn xū 心虚, heart vacuity, 272

xīn xū dǎn qiè 心虚胆怯, heart vacuity and gallbladder timidity, 272

xīn xuè 心血, heart blood, 261

xīn xuè bù zú 心血不足, insufficiency of heart blood, 309

xīn xuè xū 心血虚, heart blood vacuity, 261

xīn xuè xū bù dé wò 心血虚不得卧, heart blood vacuity sleeplessness, 261

xīn yáng 心阳, heart yang, 273

xīn yáng bù zhèn 心阳不振, devitalized heart yang, 125

xīn yáng shèng 心阳盛, exuberant heart yang, 189

xīn yáng xū 心阳虚, heart yang vacuity, 273

xīn yí 辛夷 magnolia flower[1], Magnoliae Flos[1], 120, 129, 405, 681, 720

xīn yí qīng fèi sǎn 辛夷清肺散, Magnolia Flower Lung-Clearing Powder, 283

xīn yí sǎn 辛夷散, Magnolia Flower Powder, 120, 405, 543, 740

xīn yīn 心阴, heart yin, 274

xīn yīn bù zú 心阴不足, insufficiency of heart yin, 309

xīn yīn xū 心阴虚, heart yin vacuity, 274

xīn yīn yáng liǎng xū 心阴阳两虚, dual vacuity of heart yin and yang, 159

xīn yīn, xīn yáng 心阴、心阳, heart yin and heart yang, 274

xīn yíng 心营, heart construction, 261

xīn yíng bù zú 心营不足, insufficiency of heart construction, 309

xīn yíng guò hào 心营过耗, excessive wearing of heart construction, 181

xīn yǔ xiǎo cháng xiāng biǎo lǐ 心与小肠相表里, heart and small intestine stand in interior-exterior relationship, 261

xīn zhàng 心胀, heart distention, 262

xīn zhě jūn zhǔ zhī guān yě, shén míng chū yān 心者，君主之官也，神明出焉, heart holds the office of monarch, whence the spirit light emanates, 265

xīn zhì jú pí zhú rú tāng 新制橘皮竹茹汤, New Tangerine Peel and Bamboo Shavings Decoction, 72

xīn zhǔ hàn 心主汗, heart governs sweat, 264

xīn zhǔ mài 心主脉, heart governs the vessels, 264

xīn zhǔ shé 心主舌, heart governs the tongue, 264

xīn zhǔ shén míng 心主神明, heart governs the spirit light, 264

xīn zhǔ xuè mài 心主血脉, heart governs the blood and vessels, 264

xīn zhǔ yán 心主言, heart governs speech, 264

xīn (huǒ) yí rè yú xiǎo cháng 心（火）移热于小肠, heart (fire) spreading heat to the small intestine, 263

xīn, qí huá zài miàn 心，其华在面, heart, its bloom is in the face, 264

xìn 囟, fontanel, 214

xìn huì 囟会, GV-22, Fontanel Meeting, 50, 260, 415, 749

xìn jiě 囟解, ununited fontanels, 638

xìn kāi bù hé 囟开不合, nonclosure of the fontanels, 412

xìn mén 囟门, fontanel gate, 214

xìn mén chí bì 囟门迟闭, retarded closure of the fontanel gate, 502

xìn mén gāo tú 囟门高凸, bulging fontanel, 51

xìn mén xià xiàn 囟门下陷, depressed fontanel gate, 122

xìn tián 囟填, bulging fontanel, 51

xìn xiàn 囟陷, depressed fontanel, 122

xìn zǎo sǎn 信枣散, Arsenic-Jujube Powder, 745

xīng wèi 腥味, fishy smell, 204

xīng xiāng tāng 星香汤, Arisaema and Saussurea Decoction, 739

xīng xīng sǎn 惺惺散, Clever Powder, 61

xíng 形, physical body, 443

xíng bì 行痹, moving impediment, 401

xíng chí 行迟, slowness to walk, 541

xíng hán 形寒, physical cold, 444

xíng hán zhī lěng 形寒肢冷, physical cold and cold limbs, 444

xíng jiān 行间, LR-2, Moving Between, 3, 4, 11, 14, 19–21, 29–32, 34–36, 40, 61, 66, 69, 72, 74, 84, 86, 93, 97, 99, 117, 119, 120, 123, 127, 147, 155, 158, 164, 167, 176, 194, 203, 218, 225, 229, 231, 233, 235, 240, 241, 263, 281, 283, 291, 292, 297, 310, 319, 349, 353, 355, 356, 358, 359, 365, 384, 386, 390–393, 403, 415, 424, 436, 437, 442, 445, 450, 462, 477, 480–485, 495, 497, 504, 511, 533, 534, 538, 542, 547, 549, 552, 566, 567, 570, 582, 586, 601, 613, 614, 620, 631, 636, 640, 656, 658, 665, 677, 689, 695, 701, 710, 711, 713, 748

xíng jūn sǎn 行军散, Troop-Marching Powder, 740

xíng qì 行气, moving qi, 401

xíng qì fǎ 行气法, qi-moving technique, 481

xíng shèng qì xū 形盛气虚, full physique with vacuous qi, 232

xíng tǐ 形体, body, 41

xíng tǐ shòu xuè 形体瘦削, emaciation, 171

xíng tǐ xiāo shòu 形体消瘦, emaciation, 171

xǐng nǎo jìng 醒脑静, Xingnaojing, 740

xǐng pí 醒脾, arousing the spleen, 10

xǐng pí wán 醒脾丸, Spleen-Arousing Pill, 61

xǐng xiāo wán 醒消丸, Awake to Dispersion Pill, 259, 744

xìng néng 性能, characteristic, 56

xìng rén 杏仁 apricot kernel, Armeniacae Semen, 56, 72, 82, 95, 127–129, 201, 228, 246, 368, 376, 398, 399, 410, 434, 513, 527, 571, 624, 625, 683, 686, 688, 703, 714, 725

xìng sū sǎn 杏苏散, Apricot Kernel and Perilla Powder, 12, 86, 102, 129, 405, 681, 690, 734

xìng wèi 性味, nature and flavor, 405

Xingnaojing, *xǐng nǎo jìng* 醒脑静, 740

xiōng 胸, chest, 57

xiōng bì 胸痹, chest impediment, 58

xiōng bì 胸痹, thoracic impediment, 608

xiōng bù 胸部, chest, 57

xiōng gāo 胸高, raised chest, 492

xiōng gé mǎn mèn 胸膈满闷, fullness and oppression in the chest and diaphragm, 231

xiōng gǔ 胸骨, chest bones, 57

xiōng guī sǎn 芎归散, Ligusticum and Tangkuei Powder, 453

xiōng mǎn 胸满, fullness in the chest, 232

xiōng mǎn 胸满, thoracic fullness, 608

xiōng mèn 胸闷, oppression in the chest, 421

xiōng pǐ 胸痞, glomus in the chest, 242

xiōng pǐ 胸痞, thoracic glomus, 608

xiōng tòng 胸痛, chest pain, 58

xiōng tòng 胸痛, thoracic pain, 609

xiōng xiāng 胸乡, SP-19, Chest Village, 746

xiōng xié 胸胁, chest and rib-side, 57

xiōng xié kǔ mǎn 胸胁苦满, chest and rib-side fullness, 57

xiōng xié kǔ mǎn 胸胁苦满, chest and rib-side suffering fullness, 57

xiōng xié kǔ mǎn 胸胁苦满, suffering of fullness in the chest and rib-side, 587

xiōng xié mǎ 胸胁支满, propping fullness in the chest and rib-side, 468

xiōng xié mǎn 胸胁满, chest and rib-side fullness, 57

xiōng xié tòng 胸胁痛, chest and rib-side pain, 57

xiōng xīn dǎo tán tāng 芎辛导痰汤, Ligusticum and Asarum Phlegm-Abducting Decoction, 260, 440

xiōng xīn tāng 芎辛汤, Ligusticum and Asarum Decoction, 79, 435

xiōng yáng 胸阳, chest yang, 59

xiōng yáng 胸阳, thoracic yang, 609

xiōng zhōng 胸中, interior of the chest, 311

xiōng zhōng fán rè 胸中烦热, heat vexation in the chest, 284

xiōng zhōng pǐ yìng 胸中痞硬, hard glomus in the chest, 254

xiōng zhú tāng 芎术汤, Ligusticum (Cnidium Root) and Atractylodes Decoction, 702

xióng dǎn 熊胆 bear's gall, Ursi Fel, 68, 721

xióng huáng 雄黄 realgar, Realgar, 98, 241, 383, 395, 458, 667, 690, 710, 727

xióng huáng jiě dú wán 雄黄解毒丸, Realgar Toxin-Resolving Pill, 170

xiòng mèn 胸闷, thoracic oppression, 609

xiphoid process*, 633

xiū gān tāng 修肝汤, Liver-Repairing Decoction, 740

xiū xī lì 休息痢, intermittent dysentery, 311

xiù 嗅, insufflate, 310

xiù bí bì yún sǎn 嗅鼻碧云散, Nasal Insufflation Jasper Clouds Powder, 744

xiù qiú fēng 绣球风, bobble wind, 41

xiǎo ér bìng yuán fāng lùn 小儿病源方论 (*Children's Diseases: Remedies and Sources*), 1254 (Sòng), Chén Wén-Zhōng 陈文中, 48

Xu's Wondrous Atractylodes Powder, *xǔ xué shì shén zhú sǎn* 许学士神术散, 732

xū 虚, vacuity, 645

xū 虚, vacuous, 653

xū bān 虚斑, vacuity macules, 650

xū bì 虚秘, vacuity constipation, 646

xū chuǎn 虚喘, vacuity panting, 650

xū è 虚呃, vacuity hiccough, 649

xū fán 虚烦, vacuity vexation, 652

xū fán bù dé mián 虚烦不得眠, vacuity vexation and sleeplessness, 652

xū fēng nèi dòng 虚风内动, vacuity wind stirring internally, 652

xū fú 虚浮, vacuity puffiness, 650

xū hán 虚寒, vacuity cold, 645

xū huáng 虚黄, vacuity jaundice, 649

xū huǒ 虚火, vacuity fire, 648

xū huǒ chuǎn jí 虚火喘急, vacuity fire rapid panting, 648

xū huǒ shàng yán 虚火上炎, upflaming vacuity fire, 639

xū huǒ shàng yán 虚火上炎, vacuity fire flaming upward, 648

xū jī lì 虚积痢, vacuity accumulation dysentery, 645

xū jìng 虚痉, vacuity tetany, 652

xū láo 虚劳, vacuity taxation, 651

xū láo dào hàn 虚劳盗汗, vacuity-taxation night sweating, 651

xū láo jīng shǎo 虚劳精少, vacuity-taxation scant semen, 652

xū láo ké sòu 虚劳咳嗽, vacuity-taxation cough, 651

xū láo yāo tòng 虚劳腰痛, vacuity-taxation lumbar pain, 651

xū lǐ 虚里, apical pulse, 9

xū lǐ 虚里, vacuous li, 653

xū lì 虚痢, vacuity dysentery, 647

xū mài 虚脉, vacuous pulse, 653

xū nüè 虚疟, vacuity malaria, 650

xū pǐ 虚痞, vacuity glomus, 648

xū rè 虚热, vacuity heat, 648

xū rè jīng xíng xiān qī 虚热经行先期, vacuity heat advanced menstruation, 649

xū shí 虚实, vacuity and repletion, 645

xū shí cuò zá 虚实错杂, vacuity-repletion complex, 650

xū sǔn 虚损, vacuity detriment, 646

xū sǔn láo shāng 虚损劳伤, vacuity-detriment taxation damage, 647

xū tán 虚痰, vacuity phlegm, 650

xū tuō 虚脱, vacuity desertion, 646

xū tuō è 虚脱呃, vacuity desertion hiccough, 646

xū xián 虚痫, vacuity epilepsy, 647

xū xiàn 虚陷, vacuity fall, 648

xū xié 虚邪, vacuity evil, 648

xū xiè 虚泻, vacuity diarrhea, 647

xū xīn tòng 虚心痛, vacuity heart pain, 648

xū xū shí shí 虚虚实实, evacuate vacuity and replenish repletion, 180

xū yáng bù liǎn 虚阳不敛, unconstrained vacuous yang, 636

xū yáng shàng fú 虚阳上浮, vacuous yang floating upward, 653

xū zhàng 虚胀, vacuity distention, 647

xū zhě bǔ qí mǔ 虚者补其母, vacuity is treated by supplementing the mother, 649

xū zhě bǔ zhī 虚者补之, vacuity is treated by supplementing, 649

xū zhèng 虚证, vacuity pattern, 650

xū zhōng jiā shí 虚中夹实, vacuity with repletion complication, 652

xū zhǒng 虚肿, vacuity swelling, 651

xū zhòng 虚中, vacuity stroke, 650

xū zuò nǔ zé 虚坐努责, vain straining, 654

xú cháng qīng 徐长卿 paniculate cynanchum, Cynanchi Paniculati Herba cum Radice, 139, 722

xú jí bǔ xiè 徐疾补泻, quick and slow supplementation and drainage, 490

xǔ xué shì shén zhú sǎn 许学士神术散, Xu's Wondrous Atractylodes Powder, 732

xù bí 嚏鼻, nasal insufflation, 405

xù duàn 续断 dipsacus, Dipsaci Radix, 251, 352, 453, 593, 727

xù duàn wán 续断丸, Dipsacus Pill, 347

xù suí zǐ 续随子 caper spurge seed, Euphorbiae Lathyridis Semen, 460, 722

xù suí zǐ wán 续随子丸, Caper Spurge Seed Pill, 732

xù xuè 蓄血, blood amassment, 24

xù xuè fā huáng 蓄血发黄, blood amassment yellowing, 24

xuān 宣, diffuse, 128

xuān bái 宣白, diffusing the white, 129

xuān bái chéng qì tāng 宣白承气汤, White-Diffusing Qi-Coordinating Decoction, 731

xuān bì tāng 宣痹汤, Impediment-Diffusing Decoction, 547

xuān dú fā biǎo tāng 宣毒发表汤, Toxin-Diffusing Exterior-Effusing Decoction, 387, 422, 729

xuān fèi 宣肺, diffusing the lung, 128

xuān fèi huà tán 宣肺化痰, diffusing the lung and transforming phlegm, 129

xuān fèi píng chuǎn 宣肺平喘, diffusing the lung and calming panting, 128

xuān fèi qū tán 宣肺祛痰, diffusing the lung and dispelling phlegm, 128

xuān jì 宣剂, diffusing formula, 128

xuān kě qù shí 轻可去实, light [medicinals] can eliminate repletion, 346

xuān kě qù yōng 宣可去壅, diffusing [medicinals] can eliminate congestion, 128

xuān míng wán 宣明丸, Brightness Pill, 730

xuān tōng 宣通, perfuse, 430

xuān tōng fèi qì 宣通肺气, diffusing lung qi, 128

xuān tōng shuǐ dào 宣通水道, freeing the waterways, 228

xuán fǔ 玄府, mysterious house (mansion), 404

xuán fù huā 旋覆花 inula flower, Inulae Flos, 17, 145, 146, 394, 578, 624, 669, 696, 725

xuán fù huā dài zhě shí tāng 旋覆花代赭石汤, Inula and Hematite Decoction, 445, 499, 578, 736

xuán fù huā tāng 旋覆花汤, Inula Decoction, 356

xuán jī 璇玑, CV-21, Jade Swivel, 15, 141, 145, 186, 197, 215, 218, 224, 426, 499, 564, 578, 645, 749

xuán lí 悬厘, GB-6, Suspended Tuft, 222, 253, 748

xuán lú 悬颅, GB-5, Suspended Skull, 748

xuán míng fěn 玄明粉 refined mirabilite, Mirabilitum Depuratum, 44, 460, 722

xuán qí fēng 悬旗风, flying flag wind, 214

xuán qí fēng 悬旗风, flying flag wind, 214

xuán qiú 悬球, suspended ball, 598

xuán shēn 玄参 scrophularia, Scrophulariae Radix, 65, 67, 108, 120, 174, 175, 298, 336, 368, 394, 399, 415, 422, 430, 459, 508, 511, 526, 541, 577, 597, 611, 612, 676, 686, 688, 714, 720

xuán shēn jiě dú tāng 玄参解毒汤, Scrophularia Toxin-Resolving Decoction, 731

xuán shēn shēng má tāng 玄参升麻汤, Scrophularia and Cimicifuga Decoction, 548, 731

xuán shū 悬枢, GV-5, Suspended Pivot, 749

xuán yǐn 悬饮, suspended rheum, 598

xuán yōng 悬壅, uvula, 644

xuán yōng chuí 悬壅垂, uvula, 644

xuán zhōng 悬钟, GB-39, Suspended Bell, 47, 61, 80, 89, 105, 112, 115, 120, 138, 154, 160, 289, 296, 329–331, 336, 342, 540, 652, 679, 748

xuǎn xué 选穴, point selection, 446

xuàn 眩, dizzy vision, 144

xuàn yūn 眩晕, dizziness, 144

xué dào 穴道, acupuncture point, 6

xué dào 穴道, point, 445

xué wèi 穴位, point, 445

xuě gēng tāng 雪羹汤, Snow Soup Decoction, 738

xuě kǒu 雪口, snow mouth, 544

xuè 血, bleed, 23

xuè bēng fù tòng 血崩腹痛, flooding with abdominal pain, 212

xuè bēng hūn àn 血崩昏暗, flooding with clouding vision, 212

xuè bì 血痹, blood impediment, 31

xuè bìng zhèng hòu 血病证候, blood disease pattern, 28

xuè bù guī jīng 血不归经, blood failing to stay in the channels, 29

xuè bù xún jīng 血不循经, blood failing to stay in the channels, 29

xuè bù yǎng jīn 血不养筋, blood failing to nourish the sinews, 29

xuè fèn 血分, blood aspect, 25

xuè fèn rè dú 血分热毒, blood-aspect heat toxin, 25

xuè fèn zhèng 血分证, blood-aspect pattern, 25

xuè fǔ zhú yū tāng 血府逐瘀汤, House of Blood Stasis-Expelling Decoction, 34, 35, 59, 230, 260, 273, 297, 417, 484, 570, 571, 586, 608, 613, 738

xuè gǔ 血鼓, blood drum, 28

xuè gǔ 血臌, blood drum distention, 28

xuè gǔ 血蛊, blood gu, 30

xuè guàn tóng shén 血灌瞳神, blood pouring into the pupil spirit, 33

xuè hǎi 血海, SP-10, Sea of Blood, 15, 21, 22, 24–37, 39–41, 59, 62, 63, 75, 93, 97, 99, 113, 117, 138, 139, 145, 149, 151, 152, 154, 162, 164, 167, 174, 199, 212, 227, 230, 233, 239, 241, 251, 269, 271, 273, 274, 279, 291, 300, 314, 319, 348, 349, 353, 356, 359, 390, 391, 418, 431, 447, 449–452, 454, 456, 457, 468, 482–484, 487, 489, 497, 503, 511, 516, 517, 522, 540, 561, 563, 567, 568, 570, 571, 586, 589, 591, 601, 607, 608, 613, 642, 649, 655, 656, 661, 665, 674, 683, 684, 686, 688, 689, 696, 702, 746

xuè hǎi 血海, sea of blood, 517

xuè hǎi kōng xū 血海空虚, emptiness of the sea of blood, 172

xuè hán 血寒, blood cold, 25

xuè hán jīng xíng hòu qī 血寒经行后期, blood cold delayed menstruation, 25

xuè hán yuè jīng guò shǎo 血寒月经过少, blood cold scant menstruation, 26

xuè jī 血积, blood accumulation, 24

xuè jiàn 血箭, blood arrow, 25

xuè jié 血竭 dragon's blood, Daemonoropis Draconis Resina, 728

xuè jié xiōng 血结胸, blood chest bind, 25

xuè jué 血厥, blood reversal, 33

xuè kě 血渴, blood thirst, 37

xuè kū 血枯, blood desiccation, 27

xuè kū jīng bì 血枯经闭, blood desiccation menstrual block, 27

xuè kuài 血块, clot, 74

xuè kuī jīng bì 血亏经闭, blood depletion menstrual block, 26

xuè lì 血痢, blood dysentery, 28

xuè lín 血淋, blood strangury, 36

xuè liú 血瘤, blood tumor, 37

xuè lún 血轮, blood wheel, 40

xuè luò 血络, blood network vessel, 33

xuè mǔ kuài 血母块, mother's blood lump, 399

xuè rè 血热, blood heat, 30

xuè rè bēng lòu 血热崩漏, blood heat flooding and spotting, 31

xuè rè huá tāi 血热滑胎, blood heat habitual miscarriage, 31

xuè rè jīng xíng xiān qī 血热经行先期, blood heat advanced menstruation, 30

xuè rè wàng xíng 血热妄行, frenetic blood heat, 229

xuè rè wàng xíng 血热妄行, frenetic movement of hot blood, 229

xuè rè yuè jīng guò duō 血热月经过多, blood heat profuse menstruation, 31

xuè ròu yǒu qíng zhī pǐn 血肉有情之品, medicinal with an affinity to flesh and blood, 389

xuè shàn 血疝, blood mounting, 32

xuè shì 血室, blood chamber, 25

xuè suí qì xiàn 血随气陷, blood falling with qi, 29

xuè tuō 血脱, blood desertion, 27

xuè tuō qì tuō 血脱气脱, blood desertion with qi desertion, 27 *xuè wéi qì zhī mǔ* 血为气之母, blood is the mother of qi, 32

xuè wèi 穴位, acupuncture point, 6

xuè xū 血虚, blood vacuity, 37

xuè xū bì 血虚痹, blood vacuity impediment, 39

xuè xū bù yùn 血虚不孕, blood vacuity infertility, 39

xuè xū dào hàn 血虚盗汗, blood vacuity night sweating, 39

xuè xū ěr lóng 血虚耳聋, blood vacuity deafness, 38

xuè xū fā rè 血虚发热, blood vacuity heat effusion, 39

xuè xū fù tòng 血虚腹痛, blood vacuity abdominal pain, 38

xuè xū huá tāi 血虚滑胎, blood vacuity habitual miscarriage, 38

xuè xū jīng xíng hòu qī 血虚经行后期, blood vacuity delayed menstruation, 38

xuè xū rè 血虚热, blood vacuity heat effusion, 39

xuè xū shēng fēng 血虚生风, blood vacuity engendering wind, 38

xuè xū tóu tòng 血虚头痛, blood vacuity headache, 38

xuè xū wěi 血虚痿, blood vacuity wilting, 40

xuè xū xīn jì 血虚心悸, blood vacuity heart palpitations, 39

xuè xū xuàn yūn 血虚眩晕, blood vacuity dizziness, 38

xuè xū yāo tòng 血虚腰痛, blood vacuity lumbar pain, 39

xuè xū yuè jīng guò shǎo 血虚月经过少, blood vacuity scant menstruation, 39

xuè xū zì hàn 血虚自汗, blood vacuity spontaneous sweating, 40

xuè yì 血溢, blood spillage, 33

xuè yǐng 血瘿, blood goiter, 30

xuè yū 血瘀, blood stasis, 34

xuè yū bēng lòu 血瘀崩漏, blood stasis flooding and spotting, 35

xuè yū bù yùn 血瘀不孕, blood stasis infertility, 35

xuè yū jīng xíng hòu qī 血瘀经行后期, blood stasis delayed menstruation, 34

xuè yū tòng jīng 血瘀痛经, blood stasis menstrual pain, 35

xuè yū wěi 血瘀痿, blood stasis wilting, 36

xuè yū yāo tòng 血瘀腰痛, blood stasis lumbar pain, 35

xuè yū yuè jīng guò shǎo 血瘀月经过少, blood stasis scant menstruation, 35

xuè yú 血余 hair, Hominis Crinis, 653

xuè yú tàn 血余炭 charred hair, Hominis Crinis Carbonisatus, 567, 724

xuè yù 血郁, blood depression, 27

xuè yù tāng 血郁汤, Blood Depression Decoction, 27

xuè zào 血燥, blood dryness, 28

xuè zào shēng fēng 血燥生风, blood dryness engendering wind, 28

xuè zhēng 血癥, blood concretion, 26

xuè zhèng 血证, blood pattern, 33

xuè zhèng lùn 血证论 (*On Blood Patterns*), 1884 (Qīng), Táng Róng-Chuān 唐容川, 152, 181

xuè zhī fǔ 血之府, house of the blood, 293

xuè zhì 血痣, blood mole, 32

xuè zhì 血痔, bleeding hemorrhoids, 23

xuè zhì fù tòng 血滞腹痛, blood stagnation abdominal pain, 33

xuè zhì jīng bì 血滞经闭, blood stagnation menstrual block, 33

xuè zhǒng 血肿, blood swelling, 36

xuè (xiě) 血, blood, 24

xūn 薰, fume, 233

xūn xǐ 熏洗, steam-wash, 572

xūn zhēng 薰蒸, swelter, 601

xún 循, channel rubbing, 56

xún gǔ fēng 寻骨风 mollissima, Aristolochiae Mollissimae Rhizoma seu Herba, 139, 722

xún jīng qǔ xué 循经取穴, selection of points on the affected channel, 522

xún shè fǎ 循摄法, channel-freeing manipulation, 56

xún yī mō chuáng 循衣摸床, carphology, 54

xún yī mō chuáng 循衣摸床, picking at bedclothes, 444

xìn mén bù hé, nonclosure of the fontanel gate, 412

yā dǎn zǐ 鸦胆子 brucea, Bruceae Fructus, 68, 183, 445, 665, 721

yā táng 鸭溏, duck's slop, 163

yā zhí cǎo 鸭跖草 dayflower, Commelinae Herba, 67, 69, 720

yá 牙, tooth, 619

yá chē 牙车, tooth carriage, 620

yá chǐ 牙齿, tooth, 619

yá chǐ fú dòng 牙齿浮动, loosening of the teeth, 367

yá chǐ gān kū 牙齿干枯, desiccated teeth, 124

yá chǐ gān zào 牙齿干燥, dry teeth, 157

yá chǐ gān zào rú kū gǔ 牙齿干燥如枯骨, teeth dry as desiccated bones, 605

yá chǐ kū gǎo 牙齿枯槁, desiccated teeth, 124

yá chǐ sōng dòng 牙齿松动, loosening of the teeth, 367

yá chuáng 牙床, tooth bed, 620

yá gān 牙疳, gan of the teeth and gums, 238

yá guān jǐn bì 牙关紧闭, clenched jaw, 73

yá tòng 牙痛, toothache, 619

yá xiāo 牙硝 tooth niter, Nitrum Dentatum, 411

yá xuān 牙宣, gaping gums, 239

yá yín 牙龈, gum, 250

yá yín 牙龂, gum, 250

yá yín chū xuè 牙龈出血, bleeding gums, 23

yá yín xuān lù 牙龈宣露, gaping gums, 239

yǎ mén 哑门, GV-15, Mute's Gate, 291, 368, 410, 573, 749

yān 咽, pharynx, 432

yān 咽, throat, 611

yān gān 咽干, dry pharynx, 156

yān hóu 咽喉, throat, 611

yān hóu téng tòng 咽喉疼痛, sore throat, 547

yān hóu tòng 咽喉痛, sore throat, 547

yān hóu zào tòng 咽喉燥痛, sore dry throat, 546

yān hóu zhǒng tòng 咽喉肿痛, sore swollen throat, 547

yān yì tòng 咽嗌痛, sore throat, 547

yán 岩, rock, 508

yán 颜, face, 193

yán 颜, forehead, 222

yán 研, grinding, 249

yán 盐 salt, Sal, 383

yán hú suǒ 延胡索 corydalis, Corydalis Tuber, 19, 103, 137, 138, 227, 361, 363, 397, 431, 464, 493, 561, 574, 581, 696, 724

yán hú suǒ tāng 延胡索汤, Corydalis Decoction, 738

yán mò 研末, grinding, 249

yán tāng tàn tù fāng 盐汤探吐方, Mechanical Ejection Brine, 743

yán xiāo 盐哮, salt wheezing, 511

yán yǔ bù néng 言语不能, loss of speech, 368

yán yǔ cuò luàn 言语错乱, deranged speech, 123

yán yǔ jiǎn (jiǎn) sè 言语謇（蹇）涩, sluggish speech, 541

yán zhì 盐炙, mix-frying with brine, 396

yǎn 眼, eye, 190

yǎn bāo tán hé 眼胞痰核, phlegm node of the eyelid, 439

yǎn chī 眼眵, eye discharge, 192

yǎn dān 眼丹, cinnabar eye, 62

yǎn dāo mài 偃刀脉, upturned knife pulse, 640

yǎn jiǎn 眼睑, eyelid, 192

yǎn jīng 眼睛, eye, 190

yǎn jīng hóng zhǒng tòng 眼睛红肿痛, red sore swollen eyes, 496

yǎn xì 眼系, eye tie, 192

yǎn xián 眼弦, eyelid rim, 192

yǎn xián chì làn 眼弦赤烂, ulceration of the eyelid rim, 636

yàn fāng 验方, empirical formula, 172

yàn shí 厌食, aversion to food, 13

Yang Dawn Decoction, *yáng dàn* 阳旦汤, 729

Yang-Returning Emergency Decoction, *huí yáng jiù jí tāng* 回阳救急汤, 735

Yang-Returning Jade Dragon Paste, *huí yáng yù lóng gāo* 回阳玉龙膏, 104, 744

Yang-Returning Root-Reviving Decoction, *huí yáng fǎn běn tāng* 回阳返本汤, 735

Yang-Righting Powder, *zhèng yáng sǎn* 正阳散, 735

Yang-Supplementing Five-Returning Decoction, *bǔ yáng huán wǔ tāng* 补阳还五汤, 289, 454, 568, 737

Yang-Upbearing Dampness-Eliminating Ledebouriella Decoction, *shēng yáng chú shī fáng fēng tāng* 升阳除湿防风汤, 319

Yang-Upbearing Fire-Dissipating Decoction, *shēng yáng sàn huǒ tāng* 升阳散火汤, 46

Yang-Upbearing Stomach-Boosting Decoction, *shēng yáng yì wèi tāng* 升阳益胃汤, 73, 648, 741

yáng 阳, yang, 698

yáng bái 阳白, GB-14, Yang White, 89, 125, 140, 150, 194, 253, 258, 520, 586, 689, 748

yáng bān 阳斑, yang macules, 700

yáng bìng 阳病, yang disease, 699

yáng bìng zhì yīn 阳病治阴, yang disease is treated through yin, 699

yáng chí 阳池, TB-4, Yang Pool, 20, 90, 137, 231, 255, 289, 296, 344, 394, 521, 530, 548, 567, 748

yáng dàn 阳旦汤, Yang Dawn Decoction, 729

yáng fǔ 阳辅, GB-38, Yang Assistance, 20, 61, 142, 515, 748

yáng gāng 阳纲, BL-48, Yang Headrope, 747

yáng gǔ 阳谷, SI-5, Yang Valley, 61, 137, 567, 747

yáng hé jiě níng gāo 阳和解凝膏, Harmonious Yang Decongealing Plaster, 45, 46, 210, 243, 259, 315, 744

yáng hé tāng 阳和汤, Harmonious Yang Decoction, 44, 46, 213, 259, 315, 540, 744

yáng huáng 阳黄, yang jaundice, 699

yáng jiāo 阳交, GB-35, Yang Intersection, 748

yáng jié 阳结, yang bind, 698

yáng jīn huā 洋金花 datura flower, Daturae Flos, 624, 725

yáng jīng 阳经, yang channel, 699

yáng jìng 阳痉, yang tetany, 702

yáng jué 阳厥, yang reversal, 700

yáng líng quán 阳陵泉, GB-34, Yang Mound Spring, 3, 4, 6, 11, 14, 19, 20, 26, 30, 31, 47, 51, 57, 61, 66, 75, 80, 88, 89, 93, 104, 110, 112, 115, 118, 120, 123, 127, 138, 139, 147, 151, 154, 157, 158, 164, 166, 167, 169, 178, 194, 202, 203, 215–217, 229, 230, 234–236, 240, 241, 256, 257, 263, 268, 269, 281, 288, 289, 293, 296, 297, 302, 310, 314, 330, 337, 342, 349, 355–359, 361, 362, 366, 369, 374, 382, 393, 395, 445, 450, 452, 453, 456–458, 462, 474, 475, 478, 480, 482–485, 504, 511, 516, 519–522, 530, 534, 538, 540, 546, 554, 561, 564, 586, 587, 589–591, 597, 606, 614, 637, 641, 650, 654, 656, 658, 679, 683, 689, 695, 700, 710, 713, 748

yáng luò 阳络, yang network vessel, 700

yáng luò shāng zé xuè wài yì 阳络伤则血外溢, when yang network vessels are damaged, blood spills out, 673

yáng mài 阳脉, yang vessel, 704

yáng mài zhī hǎi 阳脉之海, sea of the yang vessels, 517

yáng méi chuāng 杨梅疮, red bayberry sore, 494

yáng méi yī jì sǎn 杨梅一剂散, One-Packet Red Bayberry Powder, 494

yáng míng 阳明, yang brightness, 698

yáng míng bìng 阳明病, yang brightness disease, 698

yáng míng fǔ zhèng 阳明腑证, yang brightness bowel pattern, 698

yáng míng jīng 阳明经, yang brightness channel, 698

yáng míng jīng zhèng 阳明经证, yang brightness channel pattern, 698

yáng míng tóu tòng 阳明头痛, yang brightness headache, 699

yáng míng xù xuè 阳明蓄血, yang brightness blood amassment, 698

yáng qǐ shí 阳起石 actinolite, Actinolitum, 53, 511, 593, 727

yáng qì 阳气, yang qi, 700

yáng qì shèng 阳气盛, exuberant yang qi, 190

yáng qiáng 阳强, persistent erection, 430

yáng qiáng 阳强, yang rigidity, 700

yáng qiáng bù dǎo 阳强不倒, persistent erection, 430

yáng qiāo (qiāo) mài 阳跷（跷）脉, YAS, 704

yáng qiāo (qiāo) mài 阳跷（跷）脉, yang springing vessel, 701

yáng rè 阳热, yang heat, 699

yáng shā yīn cáng 阳杀阴藏, when yang abates, yin hides, 673

yáng shèn 羊肾 goat's kidney, Caprae seu Ovis Renes, 333

yáng shēng yīn zhǎng 阳生阴长, when yang arises, yin grows, 673

yáng shēng yú yīn 阳生于阴, yang is engendered by yin, 699

yáng shèng 阳盛, exuberant yang, 190

yáng shèng gé yīn 阳盛格阴, exuberant yang repelling yin, 190

yáng shèng yīn shāng 阳盛阴伤, exuberant yang damages yin, 190

yáng shèng zé nèi hán 阴盛则内寒, when yin is exuberant, there is internal cold, 674

yáng shèng zé rè 阳胜则热, when yang prevails, there is heat, 673

yáng shèng zé wài rè 阳盛则外热, when yang is exuberant, there is external heat, 673

yáng shèng zé yīn bìng 阳胜则阴病, when yang prevails, yin ails, 673

yáng shì bù jǔ 阳事不举, yang rising failure, 701

yáng shǒu zhí zú 扬手踯足, flailing of the arms and legs, 209

yáng shǔ 阳暑, yang summerheat, 701

yáng shuǐ 阳水, yang water, 703

yáng sǔn jí yīn 阳损及阴, detriment to yang affects yin, 124

yáng suō 阳缩, retracted genitals, 503

yáng tí gēn 羊蹄根 dock root, Rumicis Radix Recens, 724

yáng tí gēn sǎn 羊蹄根散, Curled Dock Root Powder, 744

yáng tuó 阳脱, yang desertion, 699

yáng wéi mài 阳维脉, YAL, 698

yáng wéi mài 阳维脉, yang linking vessel, 700

yáng wěi 阳痿, impotence, 296

yáng wěi 阳痿, yang wilt, 703

yáng wěi 阳萎, yang wilt, 703

yáng xī 阳溪, LI-5, Yang Ravine, 137, 296, 520, 521, 567, 621, 679, 746

yáng xián 阳痫, yang epilepsy, 699

yáng xián fēng 羊痫风, epilepsy, 178

yáng xié 阳邪, yang evil, 699

yáng xū 阳虚, yang vacuity, 702

yáng xū shuǐ fàn 阳虚水泛, yang vacuity water flood, 703

yáng xū tóu tòng 阳虚头痛, yang vacuity headache, 702

yáng xū xuàn yūn 阳虚眩晕, yang vacuity dizziness, 702

yáng xū yīn shèng 阳虚阴盛, yang vacuity with yin exuberance, 703

yáng xū zé wài hán 阳虚则外寒, when yang is vacuous, there is external cold, 673

yáng xū zì hàn 阳虚自汗, yang vacuity spontaneous sweating, 702

yáng zhèng 阳证, yang pattern, 700

yáng zhèng fā bān 阳证发斑, yang-pattern macules, 700

yáng zhèng sì yīn 阳证似阴, yang pattern resembling yin, 700

yáng zhōng zhī yáng 阳中之阳, yang within yang, 703

yáng zhōng zhī yīn 阳中之阴, yin within yang, 716

yǎng 养, nourish, 415

yǎng gān 养肝, nourishing the liver, 416

yǎng jīn yè 养津液, nourishing the fluids, 416

yǎng jīng zhòng yù tāng 养精种玉汤, Essence-Nourishing Jade-Planting Decoction, 39

yǎng lǎo 养老, SI-6, Nursing the Aged, 291, 530, 549, 747

yǎng róng zhuàng shèn tāng 养荣壮肾汤, Construction-Nourishing Kidney-Invigorating Decoction, 453

yǎng wèi 养胃, nourishing the stomach, 416

yǎng wèi tāng 养胃汤, Stomach-Nourishing Decoction, 581, 597, 734

yǎng xīn ān shén 养心安神, nourishing the heart and quieting the spirit, 416

yǎng xīn tāng 养心汤, Heart-Nourishing Decoction, 270, 451, 594, 694, 739

yǎng xuè 养血, nourishing the blood, 415

yǎng xuè dāng guī dì huáng tāng 养血当归地黄汤, Blood-Nourishing Tangkuei and Rehmannia Decoction, 568

yǎng xuè jiě biǎo 养血解表, nourishing the blood and resolving the exterior, 415

yǎng xuè róu gān 养血柔肝, nourishing the blood and emolliating the liver, 415

yǎng xuè rùn fū yǐn 养血润肤饮, Blood-Nourishing Skin-Moistening Beverage, 173

yǎng xuè rùn zào 养血润燥, nourishing the blood and moistening dryness, 415

yǎng yīn 养阴, nourishing yin, 416

yǎng yīn jiě biǎo 养阴解表, nourishing yin and resolving the exterior, 416

yǎng yīn qīng fèi 养阴清肺, nourishing yin and clearing the lung, 416

yǎng yīn qīng fèi tāng 养阴清肺汤, Yin-Nourishing Lung-Clearing Decoction, 129, 156, 158, 178, 394, 416, 674, 676, 715, 734 *yǎng yīn rùn zào* 养阴润燥, nourishing yin and moistening dryness, 416

yāo 腰, lumbus, 370

yāo bèi tòng 腰背痛, lumbar and back pain, 370

yāo jǐ tòng 腰脊痛, pain in the lumbar spine, 425

yāo rú shéng shù 腰如绳束, waist as if girthed with rope, 658

yāo sè 夭色, perished complexion, 430

yāo shū 腰俞, GV-2, Lumbar Transport, 749

yāo suān 腰酸, aching lumbus, 4

yāo suān tuǐ ruǎn 腰酸腿软, aching lumbus and limp legs, 4

yāo suān xī ruǎn 腰酸膝软, aching lumbus and limp knees, 4

yāo suān zú ruǎn 腰酸足软, aching lumbus and limp legs, 4

yāo tòng 腰痛, lumbar pain, 370

yāo tuǐ suān ruǎn 腰腿酸软, limp aching lumbus and legs, 347

yāo wéi shèn zhī fǔ 腰为肾之府, lumbus is the house of kidney, 370

yāo xī ruǎn ruò 腰膝软弱, limp lumbus and knees, 347

yāo xī suān lěng 腰膝酸冷, cold aching lumbus and knees, 77

yāo xī suān ruǎn 腰膝酸软, limp aching lumbus and knees, 347

yāo xī wěi ruǎn 腰膝痿软, limp wilting lumbus and knees, 348

yāo xī wěi ruò 腰膝痿弱, weak wilting lumbus and knees, 669

yāo xī wú lì 腰膝无力, lack of strength in the lumbus and knees, 338

yāo yǎn 腰眼, Lumbar Eye, 360

yāo yáng guān 腰阳关, GV-3, Lumbar Yang Pass, 11, 14, 15, 39, 80, 114, 115, 137, 160, 296, 302, 326, 330, 332, 336, 347, 366, 370, 453, 462, 521, 559, 567, 571, 597, 651, 684, 696, 749

yáo zhēn 摇针, needle waggling, 408

yǎo gǔ jū 咬骨疽, bone-eating flat-abscess, 44

yǎo yá 咬牙, grinding of the teeth, 249

yào 药, agent, 7

yào 药, drug, 150

yào 药, medicine, 389

yào 药, medicinal, 388

yào cái 药材, medicinal materials, 389

yào gāo 药膏, medicinal paste, 389

yào jiǔ 药酒, medicinal wine, 389

yào lù 药露, medicinal dew, 388

yào wù fā pào jiǔ 药物发泡灸, medicinal-induced blister moxibustion, 388

yào xiàn yǐn liú 药线引流, medicated thread drainage, 388

yē gé 噎膈, dysphagia-occlusion, 163

yě jú huā 野菊花 wild chrysanthemum flower, Chrysanthemi Indicae seu Borealis Flos, 686, 720

yè 液, humor, 293

yè hàn 腋汗, sweating armpits, 599

yè hé huā 夜合花 dwarf magnolia, Magnoliae Coco Flos, 491, 726

yè jiān duō niào 夜间多尿, nocturia, 412

yè jiān duō niào 夜间多尿, profuse urination at night, 465

yè jiāo téng 夜交藤 flowery knotweed stem, Polygoni Multiflori Caulis, 490, 537, 593, 726, 727

yè máng 夜盲, night blindness, 409

yè mén 液门, TB-2, Humor Gate, 37, 155, 156, 158, 160, 174, 239, 294, 302, 336, 344, 348, 378, 455, 456, 462, 547, 589, 607, 611, 701, 715, 748

yè mèng guǐ jiāo 夜梦鬼交, dreaming of intercourse with ghosts, 148

yè míng shā 夜明砂 bat's droppings, Vespertilionis Excrementum, 139, 291, 725

yè shuì bù ān 夜睡不安, unquiet sleep, 638

yè sòu 夜嗽, night cough, 409

yè wǎn gāng yǎng 夜晚肛痒, nighttime anal itch, 410

yè wò bù ān 夜卧不安, unquiet sleep, 638

Yedo violet, *zǐ huā dì dīng* 紫花地丁, Violae Yedoensis Herba cum Radice, 67, 691, 721

Yellow Dragon Decoction, *huáng lóng tāng* 黄龙汤, 24, 532, 732

Yellow Earth Decoction, *huáng tǔ tāng* 黄土汤, 28, 143, 314, 556, 738

yellow jessamine, *gōu wěn* 钩吻, Gelsemii Herba, 97

yellow upborne elixir, *huáng shēng* 黄升, Hydrogyrum Oxydatum Crudum Aureum, 445

yellow wax, *huáng là* 黄腊, Cera Aurea, 57

Yellow-Boosting Powder, *yì huáng sǎn* 益黄散, 742

Yellow-Draining Powder, *xiè huáng sǎn* 泻黄散, 558, 600, 731

yī chún shèng yì 医醇賸义 (*Enriching the Meaning of the Wine of Medicine*), 1863 (Qīng), Fèi Bó-Xióng 费伯雄, 363

yī fāng jí jiě 医方集解 (*Medical Formulas Gathered and Explained*), 1682 (Qīng), Wāng Áng 汪昂, 691

yī fāng kǎo 医方考 (*Medical Remedies Researched*), 1584 (Míng), Wú Kūn 吴昆, 553

yī fú sǎn 一服散, One Dose Powder, 743

yī guàn 医贯 (*Thorough Knowledge of Medicine*), 1687 (Qīng), Zhào Xiàn-Kě 赵献可, 113

yī guàn jiān 一贯煎, All-the-Way-Through Brew, 144, 151, 228, 244, 256, 310, 314, 467, 647, 701, 742

yī hào xiǎn yào shuǐ 一号癣药水, No.1 Lichen Medicinal Water, 710

yī jiā jiǎn zhèng qì sǎn 一加减正气散, First Variant Qi-Righting Powder, 732

yī jiǎ fù mài tāng 一甲复脉汤, Single-Armored Pulse-Restorative Decoction, 742

yī qì 噫气, belching, 17

yī sǎo guāng 一扫光, Gone-in-One-Sweep, 744

yī shù 医述 (*Account of Medicine*), 1826 (Qīng), Chéng Wén-Yòu 程文囿, 366

yī xī 譩譆, BL-45, Yi Xi, 747

yī xué 医学, medicine, 389

yī xué zhèng zhuàn 医学正传 (*Orthodox Tradition of Medicine*), 1515 (Míng), Yú Tuán 虞抟, 231, 428, 672

yī yīn jiān 一阴煎, All Yin Brew, 450, 701

yī zōng bì dú 医宗必读 (*Indispensable Medical Reading*), 1637 (Míng), Lǐ Zhōng-Zǐ 李中梓 [Shì-Cái 土材], 380, 671, 703

yī zōng jīn jiàn 医宗金鉴 (*Golden Mirror of Medicine*), 1742 (Qīng), Wú Qiān 吴谦 ed., 17, 60, 232, 259, 386, 395, 461, 482, 678

yí 颐, jowl, 323

yí 颐, lower cheek, 369

yí jīng 遗精, seminal emission, 524

yí niào 遗尿, enuresis, 176

yí niào 遗溺, enuresis, 176

yí táng 饴糖 malt sugar, Granorum Saccharon, 148, 511, 580, 593, 600, 602, 726

yǐ mù 乙木, S2-wood, 511

yǐ zì tāng 乙字汤, One Zi Decoction, 718

yì 益, boost, 47

yì 翳, eye screen, 192

yì 疫, epidemic disease, 177

yì bìng tóng zhì 异病同治, like treatment of unlike disease, 346

yì chòu 腋臭, armpit odor, 10

yì dú lì 疫毒痢, epidemic toxin dysentery, 178

yì fēng 翳风, TB-17, Wind Screen, 11, 73, 89, 105, 119, 125, 129, 140, 142, 160, 166, 167, 194, 220, 260, 289, 320, 329, 336, 348, 403, 474, 515, 521, 566, 614, 658, 689, 748

yì fū fǎ 一夫法, hand standard, 254

yì gān 抑肝, repress the liver, 500

yì gān 嗌干, dry throat, 157

yì gōng sǎn 异功散, Special Achievement Powder, 450, 451, 648, 741

yì hóu shā 疫喉痧, epidemic throat sand, 177

yì huáng sǎn 益黄散, Yellow-Boosting Powder, 742

yì huáng tāng 易黄汤, Transforming Yellow Decoction, 743

yì huǒ shēng tǔ 益火生土, boosting fire and engendering earth, 47

yì huǒ xiāo yīn 益火消阴, boosting fire and dispersing yin, 47

yì huǒ zhī yuán yǐ xiāo yīn yì 益火之原以消阴翳, boosting the source of fire to disperse the shroud of yin, 47

yì jī 易饥, rapid hungering, 492

yì jīng 易惊, susceptibility to fright, 598

yì jīng xuǎn xué 异经选穴, selection of opposite-channel points, 521

yì ké 疫咳, epidemic cough, 177

yì lì 疫痢, epidemic dysentery, 177

yì lì 疫疠, epidemic pestilence, 177

yì lì zhī qì 疫疠之气, epidemic pestilential qi, 177

yì míng 翳明, Shielding Brightness, 586

yì mǔ cǎo 益母草 leonurus, Leonuri Herba, 34, 94, 137, 138, 431, 448, 724

yì mǔ cǎo gāo 益母草膏, Leonurus (Motherwort) Paste, 35

yì mǔ shèng jīn dān 益母胜金丹, Leonurus (Motherwort) Metal-Overcoming Elixir, 738

yì nù 易怒, irascibility, 320

yì nüè 疫疟, epidemic malaria, 177

yì pí 益脾, boosting the spleen, 48

yì qì 异气, abnormal qi, 3

yì qì 噫气, eructation, 178

yì qì cōng míng tāng 益气聪明汤, Qi-Boosting Sharp and Bright Decoction, 741

yì qì dǎo niào tāng 益气导尿汤, Qi-Boosting Urine-Abducting Decoction, 529

yì qì hé wèi 益气和胃, boosting qi and harmonizing the stomach, 47

yì qì jiě biǎo 益气解表, boosting qi and resolving the exterior, 47

yì qì shēng jīn 益气生津, boosting qi and engendering liquid, 47

yì qì zhǐ lín tāng 益气止淋汤, Qi-Boosting Strangury-Checking Decoction, 583

yì shè 意舍, BL-49, Reflection Abode, 747

yì wèi 益胃, boosting the stomach, 48

yì wèi tāng 益胃汤, Stomach-Boosting Decoction, 285, 678, 734

yì xuè rùn cháng wán 益血润肠丸, Blood-Boosting Intestine-Moistening Pill, 127

yì yáng 一阳, first yang [channel], 203

yì yǐ fù zǐ bài jiàng sǎn 薏苡附子败酱散, Coix, Aconite, and Baijiang Powder, 318, 743

yì yǐ gēn 薏苡根 coix root, Coicis Radix, 136, 723

yì yǐ rén 薏苡仁 coix, Coicis Semen, 69, 84, 98, 136, 223, 251, 434, 600, 671, 723

yì yǐ rén tāng 薏苡仁汤, Coix Decoction, 734

yì yǐ zhú yè sǎn 薏苡竹叶散, Coix and Bamboo Leaf Powder, 733

yì yīn 益阴, boosting yin, 48

yì yīn 一阴, first yin [channel], 203

yì yīn 溢饮, spillage rheum, 550

yì yuán sǎn 益元散, Origin-Boosting Powder, 36, 179, 590, 713, 730

yì yuán tāng 益元汤, Origin-Boosting Decoction, 735

yì zào 嗌燥, dry throat, 157

yì zhì rén 益智仁 alpinia, Alpiniae Oxyphyllae Fructus, 12, 177, 223, 335, 454, 496, 593, 727

yin tǐng cháng 阴挺长, persistent erection, 430

Yin-Enriching Clearing Transforming Pill, *zī yīn qīng huà wán* 滋阴清化丸, 201, 409

Yin-Enriching Dampness-Eliminating Decoction, *zī yīn chú shī tāng* 滋阴除湿汤, 671

Yin-Enriching Fire-Downbearing Decoction, *zī yīn jiàng huǒ tāng* 滋阴降火汤, 551, 731

Yin-Enriching Major Supplementation Pill, *zī yīn dà bǔ wán* 滋阴大补丸, 742

Yin-Forming Brew, *huà yīn jiān* 化阴煎, 733

Yin-Nourishing Lung-Clearing Decoction, *yǎng yīn qīng fèi tāng* 养阴清肺汤, 129, 156, 158, 178, 394, 416, 674, 676, 715, 734

Yin-Rectifying Brew, *lǐ yīn jiān* 理阴煎, 63, 82, 425, 646, 735

Yin-Safeguarding Brew, *bǎo yīn jiān* 保阴煎, 31, 199, 431, 574, 701

Yin-Securing Brew, *gù yīn jiān* 固阴煎, 331, 332, 369, 393

Yin-Supplementing Pill, *bǔ yīn wán* 补阴丸, 40

yīn 阴, yin, 705

yīn 瘖, loss of voice, 368

yīn 喑, loss of voice, 368

yīn bān 阴斑, yin macules, 710

yīn bāo 阴包, LR-9, Yin Bladder, 748

yīn bìng 阴病, yin disease, 709

yīn bìng 瘖病, loss of voice, 368

yīn bìng zhì yáng 阴病治阳, yin disease is treated through yang, 709

yīn bó yáng bié 阴搏阳别, yin beating differently from yang, 708

yīn bù néng yán 瘖不能言, loss of voice, 368

yīn chén hāo 茵陈蒿 capillaris, Artemisiae Capillaris Herba, 69, 116, 136, 198, 357, 589, 723

yīn chén hāo tāng 茵陈蒿汤, Capillaris Decoction, 66, 69, 70, 79, 111, 112, 151, 198, 357, 570, 700, 733

yīn chén sì nì tāng 茵陈四逆汤, Capillaris Counter-flow Cold Decoction, 735

yīn chén wǔ líng sǎn 茵陈五苓散, Capillaris and Poria (Hoelen) Five Powder, 495, 564, 733

yīn chén zhú fù tāng 茵陈术附汤, Capillaris, Atractylodes, and Aconite Decoction, 710, 735

yīn chuāng 阴疮, yin sore, 712

yīn chuī 阴吹, vaginal flatus, 653

yīn dì zhì yí 因地制宜, act(ion) according to place, 5

yīn dū 阴都, KI-19, Yin Metropolis, 748

yīn gǔ 阴谷, KI-10, Yin Valley, 22, 41, 149, 289, 301, 302, 360, 431, 453, 461, 589, 637, 647, 711, 748

yīn gǔ 阴股, yin of the thigh, 711

yīn hán 阴寒, genital cold, 240

yīn hán 阴寒, yin cold, 709

yīn hán níng jié 阴寒凝结, congealing yin cold, 94

yīn hàn 阴汗, genital sweating, 241

yīn hàn 阴汗, yin sweating, 713

yīn hù 阴户, yin door, 709

yīn hù zhǒng tòng 阴户肿痛, painful swelling of the yin door, 424

yīn huáng 阴黄, yin jaundice, 710

yīn huǒ 阴火, yin fire, 710

yīn jiāo 阴交, CV-7, Yin Intersection, 27, 332, 643, 749

yīn jié 阴结, yin bind, 709

yīn jié yáng tuō 阴竭阳脱, exhaustion of yin and desertion of yang, 181

yīn jīng 阴经, yin channel, 709

yīn jīng 阴茎, penis, 430

yīn jìng 阴痉, yin tetany, 713

yīn jū 阴疽, yin flat-abscess, 710

yīn kuī huǒ wàng 阴亏火旺, effulgent yin depletion fire, 168

yīn lěng 阴冷, yin cold, 709

yīn lián 阴廉, LR-11, Yin Corner, 749

yīn líng quán 阴陵泉, SP-9, Yin Mound Spring, 1, 2, 8, 21, 22, 36, 37, 40, 63, 66, 69–71, 76, 78–80, 84, 86, 88, 94, 103, 104, 109–118, 127, 138–140, 145, 149, 151, 167, 180, 182, 186, 210, 211, 221, 224, 228, 229, 240, 241, 257, 260, 276, 278, 282, 283, 287, 288, 296, 297, 301, 302, 308, 319, 320, 327, 335, 337, 342, 343, 347, 349, 353, 357, 359, 370, 383, 395, 401, 410, 418, 422, 424, 425, 434–436, 440–442, 452, 457, 462, 466, 468, 485, 489, 493, 498, 499, 506, 511, 516, 520, 522, 525, 529, 530, 533, 540, 542, 546, 547, 550, 554, 559, 560, 563–565, 579, 582, 585, 586, 588, 589, 600, 604, 608, 636, 637, 640, 641, 656, 658, 663, 665–668, 675, 677, 680, 684, 686, 691, 693, 694, 700, 701, 703, 710–713, 716, 746

yīn luǎn 阴卵, testicle, 606

yīn mài 阴脉, yin vessel, 716

yīn mài zhī hǎi 阴脉之海, sea of the yin vessels, 517

yīn mén 殷门, BL-37, Gate of Abundance, 61, 111, 370, 658, 747

yīn náng 阴囊, scrotum, 516

yīn náng 阴囊, yin sac, 712

yīn náng sāo yǎng 阴囊瘙痒, scrotal itch, 515, 712

yīn nì 阴䘌, invisible worm sore of the genitals, 320

yīn píng yáng mì 阴平阳秘, when yin is calm and yang is sound, 673

yīn qì 阴器, yin organs, 711

yīn qì 阴气, yin qi, 712

yīn qì bù yòng 阴器不用, ineffectiveness of the yin organ, 299

yīn qiáng 阴强, persistent erection, 430

yīn qiáng 阴强, yin rigidity, 712

yīn qiáng bù dǎo 阴强不倒, persistent erection, 430

yīn qiāo (qiáo) mài 阴跷（蹺）脉, YIS, 717

yīn qiāo (qiáo) mài 阴跷（蹺）脉, yin springing vessel, 712

yīn qié 阴茄, eggplant yin, 169

yīn rén zhì yí 因人制宜, act(ion) according to person, 5

yīn shàn 阴疝, yin mounting, 711

yīn shēng yú yáng 阴生于阳, yin is engendered by yang, 710

yīn shèng 阴盛, exuberant yin, 190

yīn shèng gé yáng 阴盛格阳, exuberant yin repelling yang, 190

yīn shèng nèi hán 阴盛内寒, exuberant internal yin cold, 189

yīn shèng yáng shuāi 阴盛阳衰, yin exuberance with yang debilitation, 710

yīn shèng yáng xū 阴盛阳虚, yin exuberance with yang vacuity, 710 *yīn shèng zé hán* 阴胜则寒, when yin prevails, there is cold, 674

yīn shèng zé hán 阴盛则寒, when yin is exuberant, there is cold, 673

yīn shèng zé yáng bìng 阴胜则阳病, when yin prevails, yang ails, 674

yīn shī chuāng 阴虱疮, pubic louse sore, 468

yīn shí 阴蚀, genital erosion, 241

yīn shí zhì yí 因时制宜, act(ion) according to time, 5

yīn shì 阴市, ST-33, Yin Market, 289, 337, 418, 746

yīn shǔ 阴暑, yin summerheat, 713

yīn shuǐ 阴水, yin water, 716

yīn sǔn jí yáng 阴损及阳, detriment to yin affects yang, 124

yīn suō 阴缩, retracted genitals, 503

yīn tiān 阴天, yin-type weather, 714

yīn tǐng 阴挺, persistent erection, 430

yīn tǐng 阴挺, vaginal protrusion, 654

yīn tǐng 阴挺, yin protrusion, 712

yīn tóu 阴头, glans penis, 242

yīn tóu 阴头, yin head, 710

yīn tóu yōng 阴头痈, yin head welling-abscess, 710

yīn tuí 阴癫, yin bulging, 709

yīn tuō 阴脱, yin desertion, 709

yīn wéi mài 阴维脉, YIL, 705

yīn wéi mài 阴维脉, yin linking vessel, 710

yīn wěi 阴痿, impotence, 296

yīn xī 阴郄, HT-6, Yin Cleft, 40, 72, 95, 97, 176, 210, 237, 269, 272, 275, 336, 341, 410, 448, 454, 463, 489, 521, 572, 589, 590, 595, 597, 648, 651, 690, 702, 713–716, 747

yīn xián 阴痫, yin epilepsy, 709

yīn xiǎn 阴癣, yin lichen, 710

yīn xié 阴邪, yin evil, 710

yīn xū 阴虚, yin vacuity, 714

yīn xū cháo rè 阴虚潮热, yin vacuity tidal heat [effusion], 715

yīn xū chuǎn 阴虚喘, yin vacuity panting, 715

yīn xū dào hàn 阴虚盗汗, yin vacuity night sweating, 715

yīn xū fā rè 阴虚发热, yin vacuity heat effusion, 714

yīn xū fèi zào 阴虚肺燥, yin vacuity lung dryness, 714

yīn xū hóu bì 阴虚喉痹, yin vacuity throat impediment, 715

yīn xū hóu xiǎn 阴虚喉癣, yin vacuity throat lichen, 715

yīn xū huǒ shèng 阴虚火盛, exuberant yin vacuity fire, 190

yīn xū huǒ wàng 阴虚火旺, effulgent yin vacuity fire, 168

yīn xū huǒ wàng 阴虚火旺, yin vacuity fire effulgence, 714

yīn xū tóu tòng 阴虚头痛, yin vacuity headache, 714

yīn xū wěi 阴虚痿, yin vacuity wilting, 715

yīn xū wèi wǎn (guǎn) tòng 阴虚胃脘痛, yin vacuity stomach duct pain, 715

yīn xū xuè rè 阴虚血热, yin vacuity blood heat, 714

yīn xū yáng fú 阴虚阳浮, yin vacuity with floating yang, 716

yīn xū yáng kàng 阴虚阳亢, yin vacuity with yang hyperactivity, 716

yīn xū zé nèi rè 阴虚则内热, when yin is vacuous, there is internal heat, 674

yīn xuè 阴血, yin-blood, 709

yīn xuè kuī xū 阴血亏虚, yin-blood depletion, 709

yīn yǎ 音哑, loss of voice, 368

yīn yáng 阴阳, yin and yang, 705

yīn yáng 阴阳, yin-yang, 717

yīn yáng hù gēn 阴阳互根, yin and yang are rooted in each other, 707

yīn yáng kě fēn ér bù kě lí 阴阳可分而不可离, yin and yang are divisible but inseparable, 707

yīn yáng lí jué 阴阳离决, separation of yin and yang, 525

yīn yáng liǎng xū 阴阳两虚, dual vacuity of yin and yang, 163

yīn yáng shī tiáo 阴阳失调, yin-yang disharmony, 717

yīn yáng xiāng hù yī cún 阴阳相互依存, interdependence of yin and yang, 311

yīn yáng xiāng hù yī cún 阴阳相互依存, yin and yang are interdependent, 707

yīn yáng xiāo zhǎng 阴阳消长, waxing and waning of yin and yang, 669

yīn yáng zhì yuē 阴阳制约, yin and yang counterbalance each other, 708

yīn yáng zhuǎn huà 阴阳转化, mutual convertibility of yin and yang, 403

yīn yǎng 阴痒, pudendal itch, 468

yīn yè 阴液, yin humor, 710

yīn yūn tāng 氤氲汤, Misty Decoction, 395

yīn zhèng 阴证, yin pattern, 711

yīn zhèng fā bān 阴证发斑, yin-pattern macules, 711

yīn zhèng shāng hán 阴证伤寒, yin-pattern cold damage, 711

yīn zhèng sì yáng 阴证似阳, yin pattern resembling yang, 711

yīn zhì 阴痔, yin pile, 711

yīn zhōng zhī yáng 阴中之阳, yang within yin, 703

yīn zhōng zhī yīn 阴中之阴, yin within yin, 717

yīn zòng 阴纵, yin protraction, 711

yín 龈, gum, 250

yín 淫, excess, 181

yín chái hú 银柴胡 lanceolate stellaria, Stellariae Lanceolatae Radix, 68, 72, 281, 282, 649, 722

yín fèn 营分, construction aspect, 96

yín huáng piàn 银黄片, Lonicera and Scutellaria Tablet, 731

yín jiāo 龈交, GV-28, Gum Intersection, 749

yín qì 淫气, excess, 181

yín qiào mǎ bó sǎn 银翘马勃散, Lonicera, Forsythia, and Puffball Powder, 729 *yín qiào sǎn* 银翘散, Lonicera and Forsythia Powder, 59, 69, 91, 103, 118, 178, 184, 320, 387, 469, 501, 547, 586, 591, 611, 620, 686–688, 691, 693, 729

yín qiào tāng 银翘汤, Lonicera and Forsythia Decoction, 729

yín wěi hé jì 银苇合剂, Lonicera and Phragmites Mixture, 282, 625

yín xìng wú yōu sǎn 银杏无忧散, Mercury and Apricot Kernel Carefree Powder, 468

yín yáng huò 淫羊藿 epimedium, Epimedii Herba, 298, 335, 397, 593, 596, 679, 727

yǐn 饮, beverage, 18

yǐn 饮, rheum, 506

yǐn 引, conductor, 92

yǐn bái 隐白, SP-1, Hidden White, 29–32, 35, 41, 90, 161, 169, 199, 212, 222, 233, 289, 386, 414, 420, 448, 478, 520, 522, 551, 557, 566, 570, 595, 603, 746

yǐn huǒ guī yuán 引火归原, returning fire to its source, 504

yǐn jīng yào 引经药, channel conductor, 55

yǐn pì 饮癖, rheum aggregation, 506

yǐn piàn 饮片, decocting pieces, 119

yǐn shí 饮食, food, 214

yǐn shí shǎo sī 饮食少思, little thought of food and drink, 351

yǐn shí shī tiáo 饮食失调, dietary irregularities, 126

yǐn shǒu 引手, rebounding, 492

yǐn tòng 隐痛, dull pain, 163

yǐn xié yōng fèi 饮邪壅肺, rheum evil congesting the lung, 506

yǐn yào 引药, conductor, 92

yǐn zhēn 引针, needle extraction, 406

yǐn zhēn 引针, needle removal, 407

yǐn zhěn 瘾疹, dormant papules, 145

yǐn zǐ 饮子, drink, 149

yǐn zi= 引子, conductor, 92

yìn táng 印堂, Hall of Impression, 6, 83, 89, 92, 120, 149, 281, 349, 409, 448, 543, 681, 686, 687, 691, 699

yìn táng 印堂, glabella, 242

yìn táng 印堂, hall of impression, 252

yīng chuāng 膺窗, ST-16, Breast Window, 386, 418, 746

yīng sù ké 罂粟壳 poppy husk, Papaveris Pericarpium, 12, 95, 318, 518, 727

yíng 营, construction, 96

yíng fèn zhèng 营分证, construction-aspect pattern, 96

yíng fēng liú lèi 迎风流泪, tearing on exposure to wind, 605

yíng qì 营气, construction qi, 96

yíng suí bǔ xiè 迎随补泻, directional supplementation and drainage, 129

yíng wèi bù hé 营卫不和, construction-defense disharmony, 96

yíng wèi qì xuè 营卫气血, construction, defense, qi, and blood, 96

yíng xiāng 迎香, LI-20, Welcome Fragrance, 5, 75, 89, 92, 120, 149, 194, 260, 348, 378, 405, 521, 522, 543, 674, 681, 686, 688, 746

yíng xué 荥穴, spring point, 567

yǐng 瘿, goiter, 243

yìng zhǐ 应指, rebounding, 492

yōng 痈, welling-abscess, 670

yōng zhǒng 痈肿, swollen welling-abscess, 601

yōng zhǒng 痈肿, welling-abscess swelling, 671

yōng 壅, congest, 94

yǒng quán 涌泉, KI-1, Gushing Spring, 6, 32, 33, 47, 53, 63, 74, 81, 88, 123, 156, 160, 176, 178, 203, 212, 225, 231, 232, 256, 282, 283, 289, 292, 294, 319, 320, 331, 333, 336, 337, 343, 345, 364, 366, 384, 391, 401, 410, 413, 415, 420, 425, 437, 448, 452, 456, 458, 467, 478, 495, 504, 506, 511, 534, 537, 547, 566–568, 572, 597, 620, 641, 646, 648, 649, 654, 656, 683, 690, 699, 709, 714–716, 747

yǒng tù fǎ 涌吐法, ejection, 170

yǒng zhǒng 臃肿, grossness, 249

yòng yào 用药, medication, 388

yōu 忧, anxiety, 9

yōu mén 幽门, KI-21, Dark Gate, 748

yōu mén 幽门, dark gate, 118

yóu 疣, wart, 665

yóu chuāng 疣疮, wart, 665

yóu dāng guī 油当归 oily tangkuei, Angelicae Sinensis Radix Pinguis, 399

yóu fēng 油风, glossy scalp wind, 243

yóu fēng 游风, wandering wind, 658

yóu gāo 油膏, oil paste, 419

yóu hàn 油汗, oily sweat, 419

yóu huī zhǐ jiǎ 油灰指甲, oily ashen nail, 419

yóu zhì 油炙, mix-frying with fat, 397

yǒu gēn 有根, presence of root, 463

yǒu lì 有力, forceful, 222

yǒu shén 有神, presence of spirit, 463

yǒu tóu jū 有头疽, headed flat-abscess, 259

yǒu wèi 有胃, presence of stomach, 463

yǒu yú 有余, superabundance, 592

yòu guī wán 右归丸, Right-Restoring [Life Gate] Pill, 160, 164, 180, 291, 296, 310, 331, 332, 335, 393, 523, 524, 549, 596, 646, 660, 742

yòu guī yǐn 右归饮, Right-Restoring [Life Gate] Beverage, 369, 594, 646, 742

yòu kē zhǔn shéng 幼科准绳 (*Level-Line of Pediatrics*), full title *yòu kē zhèng zhì zhǔn shéng* 幼科证治准绳, 81, 82

yòu yòu jí chéng 幼幼集成 (*Young Child Compendium*), 1750 (Qīng), Chén Fù-Zhèng 陈复正, 299

Young Child Compendium (*yòu yòu jí chéng*) 幼幼集成, 1750 (Qīng), Chén Fù-Zhèng 陈复正, 299

Young Dragon Pill, *zǐ lóng wán* 子龙丸, 732

Young Maid Pill, *qīng é wán* 青娥丸, 4, 329, 332, 370

yū 瘀, stasis, 570

yū bān 瘀斑, stasis macule, 570

yū diǎn 瘀点, stasis speckle, 570

yū è 瘀呃, stasis hiccough, 570

yū kuài 瘀块, stasis clot, 570

yū rè 瘀热, stasis heat, 570

yū rè zài lǐ 瘀热在里, stasis heat in the interior, 570

yū tòng 瘀痛, stasis pain, 570

yū xuè 瘀血, static blood, 570

yū xuè fā huáng 瘀血发黄, static blood yellowing, 571

yū xuè fù tòng 瘀血腹痛, static blood abdominal pain, 570

yū xuè guàn yǎn jīng fāng 瘀血灌眼睛方, Eye Stasis Formula, 730

yū xuè ké 瘀血咳, static blood cough, 570

yū xuè liú zhù 瘀血流注, static blood streaming sore, 571

yū xuè tóu tòng 瘀血头痛, static blood headache, 571

yū xuè wèi wǎn (guǎn) tòng 瘀血胃脘痛, static blood stomach duct pain, 571

yū xuè yāo tòng 瘀血腰痛, static blood lumbar pain, 571

yū zhǒng 瘀肿, stasis swelling, 570

yú 鱼, fish, 203

yú bái pí 榆白皮 dwarf elm bark, Ulmi Pumilae Cortex, 370

yú biào 鱼鳔 swim bladder, Piscis Vesica Aeris, 333

yú jì 鱼际, LU-10, Fish Border, 14, 65, 70, 72, 91, 97, 147, 156, 158, 176, 184, 190, 201, 207, 237, 277, 280, 281, 285, 291, 292, 336, 356, 374, 393, 416, 501, 520, 547, 572, 603, 611, 613, 640, 665, 686, 688, 695, 714–716, 746

yú jì 鱼际, fish's margin, 204

yú kǒu 鱼口, fish mouth, 204

yú luò 鱼络, fish network vessels, 204

yú nǎo shí 鱼脑石 otolith, Pseudosciaenae Otolithum, 310, 405

yú rè 余热, residual heat, 500

yú xiáng mài 鱼翔脉, waving fish pulse, 669

yú xīng cǎo 鱼腥草 houttuynia, Houttuyniae Herba cum Radice, 64, 68, 69, 118, 282, 388, 469, 686, 721

yú yāo 鱼腰, Fish's Lumbus, 150, 259, 714

yǔ bái fù 禹白附 giant typhonium tuber, Typhonii Gigantei Tuber, 623, 725

yǔ chí 语迟, slowness to speak, 540

yǔ gōng sǎn 禹功散, Water Controller Yu Powder, 667, 732

yǔ shēng zhòng zhuó 语声重浊, deep turbid voice, 121

yǔ yán cuò luàn 语言错乱, deranged speech, 123

yǔ yán diān dǎo 语言颠倒, topsy-turvy speech, 621

yǔ yú liáng 禹余粮 limonite, Limonitum, 12, 318, 518, 519, 727

yù 郁, depressed, 122

yù 郁, depression, 123

yù 育, foster, 224

yù dài wán 愈带丸, Discharge-Curing Pill, 743

yù hóng gāo 玉红膏, Jade and Red Paste, 744

yù hú wán 玉壶丸, Jade Flask Pill, 478

yù hù 玉户, jade doors, 322

yù huǒ 郁火, depressed fire, 122

yù jīn 郁金 curcuma, Curcumae Tuber, 19, 27, 138, 223, 234, 262, 356, 357, 385, 393, 411, 434, 475, 480, 483, 493, 538, 586, 670, 724

yù jīng 玉茎, jade stem, 322

yù lǐ rén 郁李仁 bush cherry kernel, Pruni Japonicae Semen, 460, 462, 722

yù lín zhū 毓麟珠, Unicorn-Rearing Pill, 332

yù lù sǎn 玉露散, Jade Dew Powder, 187, 494, 540, 744

yù mén 玉门, jade gates, 322

yù mén bù bì 玉门不闭, nonclosure of the jade gate, 412

yù mǐ xū 玉米须 corn silk, Mays Stylus, 136, 723

yù nǚ jiān 玉女煎, Jade Lady Brew, 172, 190, 202, 239, 414, 431, 566, 577, 621, 687, 714, 731

yù píng fēng sǎn 玉屏风散, Jade Wind-Barrier Powder, 95, 378, 489, 527, 702, 742

yù quán sǎn 玉泉散, Jade Spring Powder, 455

yù rè yí jīng 郁热遗精, depressed heat seminal emission, 122

yù róng wán 玉容丸, Jade Countenance Pill, 226

yù shū dān 玉枢丹, Jade Pivot Elixir, 152, 171, 578, 590, 740

yù táng 玉堂, CV-18, Jade Hall, 749

yù yè tāng 玉液汤, Jade Humor Decoction, 734

yù yī 御医, imperial physician, 296

yù yīn 育阴, fostering yin, 224

yù yīn qián yáng 育阴潜阳, fostering yin and subduing yang, 225

yù yuàn yún qì sǎn 御苑匀气散, Imperial Garden Qi-Evening Powder, 238

yù zhēn sǎn 玉真散, True Jade Powder, 74, 140, 366, 740

yù zhēn wán 玉真丸, True Jade Pill, 330

yù zhěn 玉枕, BL-9, Jade Pillow, 259, 747

yù zhěn gǔ 玉枕骨, jade pillow bone, 322

yù zhěn gǔ 玉枕骨, occipital bone, 419

yù zhèng 郁证, depression pattern, 123

yù zhōng 彧中, KI-26, Lively Center, 748

yù zhú 玉竹 Solomon's seal, Polygonati Yuzhu Rhizoma, 88, 108, 175, 176, 581, 593, 597, 727

yù zhú sǎn 玉烛散, Jade Candle Powder, 28, 732

yuān yè 渊腋, GB-22, Armpit Abyss, 748

yuán 元, Yuan, 717

yuán 元, origin, 421

yuán cán shā 原蚕沙 silkworm droppings, Bombycis Excrementum, 139, 722

yuán fǔ 元府, original house (mansion), 421

yuán huā 芫花 genkwa, Daphnes Genkwa Flos, 44, 97, 182, 460, 574, 722

yuán luò pèi xué fǎ 原络配穴法, combining source and network points, 90

yuán qì 元气, original qi, 421

yuán qì 原气, source qi, 548

yuán qì dà xū 元气大虚, major vacuity of original qi, 383

yuán qì xū ruò 元气虚弱, original qi vacuity, 421

yuán shén zhī fǔ 元神之府, house of the original spirit, 293

yuán tǔ gù tāi tāng 援土固胎汤, Earth-Rescuing Fetus-Securing Decoction, 742

yuán xiǎn 圆癣, coin lichen, 76

yuán xué 原穴, source point, 548

yuán yáng 元阳, original yang, 421

yuán yì 圆翳, coin screen, 76

yuán yīn 元阴, original yin, 421

yuǎn bù xuǎn xué 远部选穴, selection of distant points, 519

yuǎn dào cì 远道刺, distant needling, 143

yuǎn dào qǔ xué 远道取穴, selection of distant points, 519

yuǎn dào xuǎn xué 远道选穴, selection of distant points, 519

yuǎn jìn pèi xué fǎ 远近配穴法, combining local and distant points, 88

yuǎn xuè 远血, distal bleeding, 142

yuǎn zhì 远志 polygala, Polygalae Radix, 20, 60, 222, 331, 392, 433, 476, 490, 540, 557, 654, 709, 726

yuǎn zhì wán 远志丸, Polygala Pill, 739

yuē shù 约束, retainer, 502

yuè bì jiā bàn xià tāng 越婢加半夏汤, Spleen-Effusing Decoction Plus Pinellia, 285, 469, 739

yuè bì jiā zhú tāng 越婢加术汤, Spleen-Effusing Decoction Plus Ovate Atractylodes, 287

yuè bì tāng 越婢汤, Spleen-Effusing Decoction, 301, 669, 694, 703, 729

yuè huá wán 月华丸, Moonlight Pill, 379, 742

yuè jì huā 月季花 China tea rose, Rosae Chinensis Flos et Fructus, 138, 725

yuè jīng 月经, menstrual flow, 390

yuè jīng 月经, menstruation, 393

yuè jīng bù lì 月经不利, inhibited menstruation, 301

yuè jīng bù tiáo 月经不调, menstrual irregularities, 391

yuè jīng chuán 越经传, skipping channels, 536

yuè jīng guò duō 月经过多, profuse menstruation, 465

yuè jīng guò shǎo 月经过少, scant menstruation, 513

yuè jīng hòu qī 月经后期, delayed menstruation, 121

yuè jīng sè shǎo 月经涩少, scant inhibited menstruation, 513

yuè jīng xiān hòu wú dìng qī 月经先后无定期, menstruation at irregular intervals, 393

yuè jīng xiān qī 月经先期, advanced menstruation, 7

yuè jú wán 越鞠丸, Depression-Overcoming Pill, 19, 244, 736

yuè lòu 月漏, menstrual spotting, 393

yuè shuǐ bù duàn 月水不断, persistent menstrual flow, 431

yuè shuǐ bù jué 月水不绝, persistent menstrual flow, 431

yuè shuǐ bù lì 月水不利, inhibited menstruation, 301

yūn 晕, dizzy head, 144

yūn dǎo 晕倒, faint, 195

yūn jué 晕厥, faint, 195

yūn zhēn 晕针, needle sickness, 407

yún mén 云门, LU-2, Cloud Gate, 746

yùn 蕴, brew, 50

yùn fǎ 熨法, hot pack [method], 293

yùn fēng sǎn 熨风散, Wind-Smoothing Powder, 744

yùn pí 运脾, moving the spleen, 401

yùn qì xié tòng 运气胁痛, moving qi rib-side pain, 401

yùn qì xué shuō 运气学说, doctrine of periods and qi, 144

yáng hàn 阳汗, yang sweating, 701

yáng xū fā rè 阳虚发热, yang vacuity heat effusion, 702

yī mén fǎ lǜ 医门法律 (*Axioms of Medicine*), 1658, Qīng, Yù Chāng 喻昌, 582

yī xué rù mén 医学入门 (*Gateway to Medicine*), 1515 (Míng), Lǐ Yán 李延, 317, 435, 550, 600, 614, 671

yī xué xīn wù 医学心悟 (*Medical Insights*), 1732 (Qīng), Chéng Guó-Péng 程国彭, 245, 587

zá bìng 杂病, miscellaneous disease, 396

zá bìng yuán liú xī zhú 杂病源流犀烛 (*Incisive Light on the Source of Miscellaneous Disease*), 1773 (Qīng), Shěn Jīn-Áo 沈金鳌, 45, 191, 683

zá qì 杂气, miscellaneous qi, 396

zá zhèng 杂症, miscellaneous disease, 396

zài zào sǎn 再造散, Renewal Powder, 11, 730

zǎn zhú 攒竹, BL-2, Bamboo Gathering, 27, 62, 93, 125, 140, 150, 192, 194, 195, 259, 260, 289, 290, 331, 349, 395, 406, 500, 521, 568, 586, 689, 714, 747

zàn yù dān 赞育丹, Procreation Elixir, 296, 742

zàng 脏, viscus, 656

zàng dú 脏毒, visceral toxin, 656

zàng fǔ 脏腑, bowels and viscera, 49

zàng fǔ 脏腑, organ, 421

zàng fǔ 脏腑, viscera, 655

zàng fǔ biàn zhèng 脏腑辨证, bowel and visceral pattern identification, 48

zàng fǔ biàn zhèng 脏腑辨证, organ pattern identification, 421

zàng fǔ jīng zhèng 脏腑惊证, bowel and visceral fright pattern, 48

zàng fǔ jīng zhèng 脏腑惊证, organ fright pattern, 421

zàng fǔ zhī qì 脏腑之气, bowel and visceral qi, 49

zàng fǔ zhī qì 脏腑之气, organ qi, 421

zàng hóng huā 藏红花 saffron, Croci Stigma, 98, 138, 387, 724

zàng lián wán 脏连丸, Pig's Intestines and Coptis Pill, 143, 290, 656, 738

zàng qīng guǒ 藏青果 unripe chebule, Chebulae Fructus Immaturus, 68, 721 *zàng xiàng* 脏象, visceral manifestation, 656

zàng zào 脏躁, visceral agitation, 655

Zanthoxyli Pericarpium, *huā jiāo* 花椒, zanthoxylum, 225, 242, 320, 405, 468, 513, 620, 660, 662, 723

Zanthoxyli Radix, *huā jiāo gēn* 花椒根, zanthoxylum root, 36

Zanthoxyli Semen, *jiāo mù* 椒目, zanthoxylum seed, 660, 723

zanthoxylum, *huā jiāo* 花椒, Zanthoxyli Pericarpium, 225, 242, 320, 405, 468, 513, 620, 660, 662, 723

zanthoxylum root, *huā jiāo gēn* 花椒根, Zanthoxyli Radix, 36

zanthoxylum seed, *jiāo mù* 椒目, Zanthoxyli Semen, 660, 723

zǎo fán wán 枣矾丸, Jujube and Melanterite Pill, 737

zǎo ní 枣泥 jujube paste, Ziziphi Fructus Pasta, 251

zǎo xiè 早泄, premature ejaculation, 461

zǎo xiū 蚤休 paris, Paridis Rhizoma, 67, 721

zào 躁, agitation, 7

zào 燥, dry, 152

zào 燥, dryness, 154

zào fán 躁烦, agitated vexation, 7

zào huǒ 燥火, dryness-fire, 155

zào huǒ xuàn yūn 燥火眩晕, dryness-fire dizziness, 155

zào jì 燥剂, dry formula, 153

zào jiá 皂荚 gleditsia, Gleditsiae Fructus, 5, 170, 214, 244, 405, 419, 434, 624, 625, 725, 727

zào jiǎo cì 皂角刺 gleditsia thorn, Gleditsiae Spina, 315, 398, 516, 624, 725

zào jiǎo kǔ shēn wán 皂角苦参丸, Gleditsia and Flavescent Sophora Pill, 395

zào jìng 燥痉, dryness tetany, 156

zào kě qù shī 燥可去湿, dry [medicinals] can eliminate dampness, 154

zào qì 燥气, dryness qi, 156

zào qì shāng fèi 燥气伤肺, damage to the lung by the dryness qi, 108

zào qì shāng fèi 燥气伤肺, dryness qi damaging the lung, 156

zào rè 燥热, dryness-heat, 155

zào rè fàn fèi 燥热犯肺, dryness-heat invading the lung, 155

zào rè huà tán 燥湿化痰, drying dampness and transforming phlegm, 153

zào rè ké sòu 燥热咳嗽, dryness-heat cough, 155

zào rè shāng fèi 燥热伤肺, dryness-heat damaging the lung, 155

zào rè wěi 燥热痿, dryness-heat wilting, 155

zào shèng zé gān 燥胜则干, when dryness prevails, there is aridity, 672

zào shī 燥湿, drying dampness, 153

zào shī hé wèi 燥湿和胃, drying dampness and harmonizing the stomach, 153

zào shī hé zhōng 燥湿和中, drying dampness and harmonizing the center, 153

zào tán 燥痰, dryness phlegm, 156

zào xié 燥邪, dryness evil, 154

zào xié fàn fèi 燥邪犯肺, dryness evil invading the lung, 154

Zaocys, *wū shé* 乌蛇, black-striped snake, 139, 722

zé kuò 泽廓, marsh rampart, 387

zé lán 泽兰 lycopus, Lycopi Herba, 34, 116, 137, 138, 356, 725

zé qī 泽漆 sun spurge, Euphorbiae Helioscopiae Herba, 136, 723

zé xiè 泽泻 alisma, Alismatis Rhizoma, 21, 30, 47, 56, 136, 224, 230, 238, 243, 390, 394, 397, 410, 434, 463, 666, 679, 703, 716, 723

zé xiè tāng 泽泻汤, Alisma Decoction, 87

Zedoariae Rhizoma, *é zhú* 莪术, zedoary, 34, 98, 116, 138, 182, 385, 544, 574, 724

zedoary, *é zhú* 莪术, Zedoariae Rhizoma, 34, 98, 116, 138, 182, 385, 544, 574, 724

zēng 增, increase, 298

zēng hán 憎寒, abhorrence of cold, 2

zēng shuǐ xíng zhōu 增水行舟, increasing water to move the ship, 298

zēng shuǐ xíng zhōu 增水行舟, refloating the grounded ship, 497

zēng sǔn bā wù tāng 增损八物汤, Modified Eight Agents Decoction, 692

zēng yè 增液, increasing humor, 298

zēng yè chéng qì tāng 增液承气汤, Humor-Increasing Qi-Coordinating Decoction, 298, 532, 732

zēng yè rùn xià 增液润下, humor-increasing moist precipitation, 293

zēng yè tāng 增液汤, Humor-Increasing Decoction, 108, 127, 298, 416, 597, 607, 734

zhā qū píng wèi sǎn 楂麯平胃散, Crataegus and Medicated Leaven Stomach-Calming Powder, 736

zhà sāi 痄腮, mumps, 403

zhān yán 谵言, delirious speech, 122

zhān yǔ 谵语, delirious speech, 122

zhàn guó 战国, Warring States, 665

zhàn hán 战寒, shivering, 529

zhàn hàn 战汗, shiver sweating, 529

zhàn lì 战栗, shivering, 529

Zhang's Clear View of Medicine (*zhāng shì yī tōng*) 张氏医通, 1695 (Qīng), Zhāng Lù 张璐 [Lù-Yù 路玉], 217, 240, 337, 495, 510, 535

zhāng kǒu tái jiān 张口抬肩, gaping mouth and raised shoulders, 239

zhāng mén 章门, LR-13, Camphorwood Gate, 1, 4, 8, 19, 37, 61, 62, 64, 78–80, 91, 109, 114, 151, 156, 161–163, 174, 196, 197, 217, 220, 233, 237, 242, 256, 271, 272, 301, 312, 314, 318, 325, 340, 349, 361, 384, 399, 401, 410, 418, 436, 479, 482, 487, 498, 499, 509, 521, 522, 537, 544, 554, 555, 557, 558, 561–565, 579, 581, 588, 596, 600, 612, 647, 669, 673, 710, 711, 716, 749

zhāng nǎo 樟脑 camphor, Camphora, 389, 398, 728

zhāng shì yī tōng 张氏医通 (*Zhang's Clear View of Medicine*), 1695 (Qīng), Zhāng Lù 张璐 [Lù-Yù 路玉], 217, 240, 337, 495, 510, 535

zhǎng xīn dú 掌心毒, palm heart toxin sore, 427

zhǎng xīn fēng 掌心风, palm heart wind, 427

zhàng 胀, distention, 143

zhàng bìng 胀病, distention disease, 143

zhàng nüè 瘴疟, miasmic malaria, 394

zhàng qì 气胀, distention qi, 143

zhàng tòng 胀痛, distending pain, 143

zhǎo jiǎ sè bù róng 爪甲不荣, lusterless nails, 381

zhǎo wéi jīn zhī yú 爪为筋之馀, nails are the surplus of the sinews, 405

zhǎo (zhuǎ) 爪, nail, 405

zhǎo (zhuǎ) qiè jìn zhēn fǎ 爪切进针法, nail press needle insertion, 405

zhào hǎi 照海, KI-6, Shining Sea, 12–14, 28–31, 47, 59, 60, 69, 71, 72, 78, 88, 90, 91, 93, 95–97, 111, 119, 122, 127–129, 148, 152, 154–156, 158, 160, 161, 163, 164, 168, 174–176, 178, 180, 186, 201–203, 226, 229, 235, 237, 239, 256, 267, 268, 275, 277, 282, 283, 285, 288–292, 294, 296, 299, 302, 314, 319, 320, 331–333, 336, 337, 339, 348, 349, 355, 360, 365, 368, 369, 372, 374, 378–380, 390, 391, 398, 401, 409, 410, 415, 416, 425, 438, 446, 450, 452, 455–457, 461, 462, 466, 468, 495, 516, 521, 524, 525, 535, 537, 538, 547, 552, 565–569, 572, 577, 580–582, 585, 587–589, 591, 596, 597, 601, 603, 607, 611, 613, 614, 640, 641, 643, 646–649, 652, 664, 701, 703, 712, 714–716, 747

zhé jīn 辄筋, GB-23, Sinew Seat, 748

zhé zhēn 折针, needle breakage, 406

zhè bèi mǔ 浙贝母 Zhejiang fritillaria, Fritillariae Verticillatae Bulbus, 70, 385, 387, 544, 624, 688, 725

zhè chóng 蟅虫 wingless cockroach, Eupolyphaga seu Opisthoplatia, 34, 50, 138, 182, 540, 724

Zhejiang fritillaria, *zhè bèi mǔ* 浙贝母, Fritillariae Verticillatae Bulbus, 70, 385, 387, 544, 624, 688, 725

zhēn 针, needle, 406

zhēn 真, true, 629

zhēn 鍼, needle, 406

zhēn cì bǔ xiè fǎ 针刺补泻法, supplementation and drainage needling, 593

zhēn cì má zuì 针刺麻醉, acuanesthesia, 5

zhēn cì shǒu fǎ 针刺手法, needle manipulation (technique), 407

zhēn gǎn 针感, needle sensation, 407

zhēn hán jiǎ rè 真寒假热, true cold and false heat, 629

zhēn jīng pò sǔn 真睛破损, true eye damage, 629

zhēn jiǔ 针灸, acupuncture, 5

zhēn jiǔ 针灸, acumoxatherapy, 5

zhēn jiǔ dà chéng 针灸大成 (*Great Compendium of Acupuncture and Moxibustion*), 1601 (Míng), Yáng Jì-Zhōu 杨继洲, 225

zhēn qì 真气, true qi, 630

zhēn rè jiǎ hán 真热假寒, true heat and false cold, 629

zhēn rén yǎng zàng tāng 真人养脏汤, True Man Viscus-Nourishing Decoction, 12, 318, 742

zhēn shí jiǎ xū 真实假虚, true repletion and false vacuity, 630

zhēn tóu tòng 真头痛, true headache, 629

zhēn wǔ tāng 真武汤, True Warrior Decoction, 266, 287, 301, 322, 329, 335, 341, 345, 441, 488, 541, 608, 661, 666–668, 711, 716, 733

zhēn xīn tòng 真心痛, true heart pain, 629

zhēn xū jiǎ shí 真虚假实, true vacuity and false repletion, 630

zhēn yǎn 针眼, sty, 585

zhēn yáng 真阳, true yang, 631

zhēn yáng bù zú 真阳不足, insufficiency of true yang, 310

zhēn yīn 真阴, true yin, 631

zhēn yīn bù zú 真阴不足, insufficiency of true yin, 310

zhēn yuán 真元, true origin, 629

zhēn yuán bù zú 真元不足, insufficiency of the true origin, 310

zhēn yuán hào sǔn chuǎn 真元耗损喘, true origin vacuity panting, 629

zhēn yuán xià xū 真元下虚, vacuity of the true origin in the lower body, 650

zhēn zàng mài 真脏脉, true visceral pulse, 630

zhēn zàng sè 真脏色, true visceral complexion, 630

zhēn zhòng fēng 真中风, true wind stroke, 631

zhēn zhū 珍珠 pearl, Margarita, 54, 249, 490, 726

zhēn zhū mǔ 珍珠母 mother-of-pearl, Concha Margaritifera, 53, 54, 230, 434, 490, 526, 538, 539, 585, 726

zhēn zhū mǔ wán 珍珠母丸, Mother-of-Pearl Pill, 365, 739

zhēn zhū sǎn 真珠散, Pearl Powder, 32

zhěn 疹, papule, 428

zhěn duàn 诊断, diagnosis, 125

zhěn gǔ 枕骨, occipital bone, 419

zhěn gǔ 枕骨, pillow bone, 444

zhěn xìn 枕囟, pillow fontanel, 444

zhěn zhǐ wén 诊指纹, finger vein examination, 200

zhěn zhōng dān 枕中丹, Pillow Elixir, 739

zhèn 镇, settle, 525

zhèn gān xī fēng 镇肝熄风, settling the liver and extinguishing wind, 526

zhèn gān xī fēng tāng 镇肝熄风汤, Liver-Settling Wind-Extinguishing Decoction, 53, 364, 689, 716, 740

zhèn jīng ān shén 镇惊安神, settling fright and quieting the spirit, 526

zhèn jìng 镇痉, settling tetany, 526

zhèn lì 振栗, shivering, 529

zhèn líng dān 震灵丹, Rousing Spirit Elixir, 325, 519

zhèn nà 镇纳, settling and absorption, 525

zhèn nì bái hǔ tāng 镇逆白虎汤, Counterflow-Settling White Tiger Decoction, 730 *zhèn qián* 镇潜, settling and subduing, 526

zhèn shèn jué míng wán 镇肾决明丸, Kidney-Settling Abalone Shell Pill, 104

zhēng 蒸, steam, 571

zhēng 蒸, steaming, 572

zhēng 癥, concretion, 92

zhēng bìng 蒸病, steaming disease, 572

zhēng chōng 怔忡, fearful throbbing, 196

zhēng jiǎ jī jù 癥瘕积聚, concretions and gatherings, 92

zhēng jiǎ jī jù 癥瘕积聚, concretions, conglomerations, accumulations, and gatherings, 92

zhēng lù 蒸露, distillation, 143

zhěng tǐ guān 整体观, holism, 292

zhěng tǐ guān niàn 整体观念, holism, 292

zhèng 证, pattern, 429

zhèng 证, sign, 531

zhèng 正, right, 507

zhèng cháng mài 正常脉, normal pulse, 414

zhèng cháng shé tāi 正常舌苔, normal tongue fur, 414

zhèng gǔ 正骨, bone righting, 45

zhèng gǔ tàng yào 正骨烫药, Bone-Righting Hot Pack, 745

zhèng gǔ zǐ jīn dān 正骨紫金丹, Bone-Righting Purple Gold Elixir, 45, 337

zhèng hòu 证候, pattern, 429

zhèng hòu 证候, sign, 531

zhèng jīng 正经, regular channel, 497

zhèng qì 正气, right qi, 507

zhèng qì 正气, righting qi, 507

zhèng qì tāng 正气汤, Qi-Righting Decoction, 702

zhèng qì tiān xiāng sǎn 正气天香散, Qi-Righting Lindera and Cyperus Powder, 736

zhèng róng tāng 正容汤, Face-Righting Decoction, 568, 569, 689

zhèng sè 正色, right complexion, 507

zhèng shēng 郑声, mussitation, 403

zhèng shuǐ 正水, regular water, 498

zhèng tóu tòng 正头痛, ambilateral headache, 8

zhèng tóu tòng 正头痛, medial headache, 388

zhèng xū xié shí 正虚邪实, right vacuity and evil repletion, 507

zhèng yáng sǎn 正阳散, Yang-Righting Powder, 735

zhèng yīn mài zhì 症因脉治 (*Pathoconditions, Causes, Pulses, and Treatments*), 1641 (Míng), Qín Jǐng-Míng 秦景明, 58, 313, 356, 372, 628, 704

zhèng yíng 正营, GB-17, Upright Construction, 748

zhèng zhì 正治, straight treatment, 583

zhèng zhì yào jué 证治要诀 (*Essential Rhymes for Patterns and Treatment*), Míng (1368–1644), Dài Sī-Gōng 戴思恭 [Yuán-Lǐ 原礼], 529

zhèng zhì zhǔn shéng 证治准绳 (*Level-Line of Pattern Identification and Treatment*), 1602 (Míng), Wáng Kěn-Táng 王肯堂, 299, 368, 384, 557, 568, 704

zhī 支, branch, 50

zhī 支, propping, 467

zhī 汁, juice, 323

zhī 肢, limb, 347

zhī bǎi bā wèi wán 知柏八味丸, Anemarrhena and Phellodendron Eight-Ingredient Pill, 147, 176, 288, 296, 330, 331, 355, 476, 583, 641, 714

zhī bǎi dì huáng tāng 知柏地黄汤, Anemarrhena, Phellodendron, and Rehmannia Decoction, 36

zhī bǎi dì huáng wán 知柏地黄丸, Anemarrhena, Phellodendron, and Rehmannia Pill, 14, 33, 41, 76, 104, 167, 181, 230, 292, 294, 336, 415, 474, 495, 512, 547, 566, 574, 597, 611, 615, 648, 715, 731

zhī bǎi sì wù tāng 知柏四物汤, Anemarrhena and Phellodendron Four Agents Decoction, 38

zhī fēng wán 蜘蜂丸, Agelena and Hornet's Nest Pill, 298

zhī gōu 支沟, TB-6, Branch Ditch, 8, 19, 31, 34, 64, 88, 91, 112, 118, 127, 189, 190, 210, 215, 229, 233–235, 241, 280, 289, 290, 294, 302, 314, 338, 356, 357, 359, 362, 374, 426, 434, 475, 477, 478, 480, 482, 483, 485, 515, 519, 522, 585, 590, 631, 656, 658, 674, 683, 700, 703, 748

zhī jī bù shí 知饥不食, no desire to eat despite hunger, 412

zhī jié tòng 肢节痛, limb joint pain, 347

zhī juàn fá lì 肢倦乏力, fatigued limbs and lack of strength, 195

zhī jué 肢厥, limb reversal, 347

zhī lěng 肢冷, cold limbs, 82

zhī lián èr chén tāng 栀连二陈汤, Gardenia and Coptis Two Matured Ingredients Decoction, 4, 211, 443

zhī liú 脂瘤, fatty tumor, 196

zhī mǎn 支满, propping fullness, 468

zhī mǔ 知母 anemarrhena, Anemarrhenae Rhizoma, 65, 67, 71, 104, 127, 154, 176, 239, 281, 282, 326, 331, 388, 397, 422, 456, 495, 527, 546, 589, 649, 679, 695, 720

zhī mǔ yǐn 知母饮, Anemarrhena Beverage, 731

zhī tǐ kūn zhòng 肢体困重, heavy cumbersome limbs, 287

zhī yǐn 支饮, propping rheum, 468

zhī zhèng 支正, SI-7, Branch to the Correct, 90, 408, 747

zhī zhū 蜘蛛 spider, Aranea, 98

zhī zhū gǔ 蜘蛛鼓, spider drum, 550

zhī zǐ 栀子 gardenia, Gardeniae Fructus, 524

zhī zǐ bǎi pí tāng 栀子柏皮汤, Gardenia and Phellodendron Decoction, 198, 700, 731

zhī zǐ chǐ tāng 栀子豉汤, Gardenia and Fermented Soybean Decoction, 71, 284, 303, 652, 730

zhī zǐ dà huáng tāng 栀子大黄汤, Gardenia and Rhubarb Decoction, 349

zhī zǐ gān cǎo chǐ tāng 栀子甘草豉汤, Gardenia, Licorice, and Fermented Soybean Decoction, 730

zhī zǐ hòu pò tāng 栀子厚朴汤, Gardenia and Magnolia Bark Decoction, 730 *zhī zǐ qīng gān tāng* 栀子清肝汤, Gardenia Liver-Clearing Decoction, 166, 244

zhī zǐ shēng jiāng chǐ tāng 栀子生姜豉汤, Gardenia, Fresh Ginger, and Fermented Soybean Decoction, 730

zhí cì 直刺, perpendicular insertion, 430

zhí jiē jiǔ 直接灸, direct moxibustion, 129

zhí shì 直视, forward-staring eyes, 224

zhí zhòng 直中, direct strike, 129

zhí zhòng sān yīn 直中三阴, direct strike on the triple yin, 130

zhí zhòng yīn jīng 直中阴经, direct strike on the yin channels, 130

zhǐ cùn fǎ 指寸法, finger standard, 200

zhǐ dài 止带, checking vaginal discharge, 57

zhǐ dài fāng 止带方, Discharge-Checking Formula, 118

zhǐ dài piàn 止带片, Discharge-Checking Tablet, 57, 743

zhǐ hàn sǎn 止汗散, Perspiration-Checking Powder, 454, 742

zhǐ jiǎ 指甲, nail, 405

zhǐ jìng 止痉, checking tetany, 57

zhǐ jìng sǎn 止痉散, Tetany-Relieving Powder, 456, 740

zhǐ jú tāng 枳橘汤, Bitter Orange and Tangerine Peel Decoction, 481

zhǐ jù zǐ 枳椇子 honey tree fruit, Hoveniae Fructus seu Semen, 415

zhǐ ké 枳壳 bitter orange, Aurantii Fructus, 19, 47, 50, 153, 217, 234, 317, 318, 415, 421, 437, 439, 466, 477, 483, 493, 538, 573, 588, 669, 709, 723

zhǐ ké sǎn 枳壳散, Bitter Orange Powder, 736

zhǐ mí fú líng wán 指迷茯苓丸, Pathfinder Poria (Hoelen) Pill, 14, 439, 441, 738

zhǐ ǒu 止呕, checking vomiting, 57

zhǐ qiè jìn zhēn fǎ 指切进针法, finger-press needle insertion, 200

zhǐ sān guān 指三关, three bars of the finger, 609

zhǐ shí 枳实 unripe bitter orange, Aurantii Fructus Immaturus, 17, 50, 72, 98, 141, 216, 217, 255, 257, 276, 357, 417, 419, 434, 459, 493, 544, 564, 630, 723

zhǐ shí dǎo zhì wán 枳实导滞丸, Unripe Bitter Orange Stagnation-Abducting Pill, 3, 15, 110, 141, 215, 239, 426, 626, 736

zhǐ shí lǐ zhōng wán 枳实理中丸, Unripe Bitter Orange Center-Rectifying Pill, 85, 242, 735

zhǐ shí xiāo pǐ wán 枳实消痞丸, Unripe Bitter Orange and Glomus-Dispersing Pill, 224, 498, 558, 736

zhǐ shí xiè bái guì zhī tāng 枳实薤白桂枝汤, Unripe Bitter Orange, Chinese Chive, and Cinnamon Twig Decoction, 59, 736

zhǐ sòu huà tán dìng chuǎn wán 止嗽化痰定喘丸, Cough-Suppressing Phlegm-Transforming Panting-Stabilizing Pill, 738

zhǐ sòu sǎn 止嗽散, Cough-Stopping Powder, 84, 99, 129, 625, 682, 684, 738

zhǐ xiè 止泻, checking diarrhea, 56

zhǐ xuè 止血, stanching bleeding, 569

zhǐ xuè fěn 止血粉, Blood-Stanching Powder, 738

zhǐ xuè sǎn 止血散, Blood-Stanching Powder, 745

zhǐ xuè tāng 止血汤, Blood-Stanching Decoction, 738

zhǐ ya 指压, shiatsu, 529

zhǐ yǎng 止痒, Itch Reliever, 113, 117, 422, 516, 522, 561, 591, 674, 686, 688

zhǐ yǎng xué 止痒穴, Itch Reliever, 145

zhǐ zhēn 指针, acupressure, 5

zhǐ zhú wán 枳术丸, Unripe Bitter Orange and Ovate Atractylodes Pill, 633, 736

zhì 滞, stagnant, 569

zhì 滞, stagnation, 569

zhì 志, mind, 395

zhì 痣, mole, 399

zhì 痔, hemorrhoid, 289

zhì 痔, pile, 444

zhì 炙, mix-frying, 396

zhì bǎo dān 至宝丹, Supreme Jewel Elixir, 69, 88, 171, 197, 624, 631, 690, 740

zhì běn 治本, treating the root, 626

zhì biān 秩边, BL-54, Sequential Limit, 89, 137, 290, 480, 567, 688, 747

zhì biāo 治标, treating the tip, 627

zhì bìng bì qiú yú běn 治病必求于本, to treat disease, it is necessary to seek its root, 621

zhì chǎn 滞产, delivery stagnation, 122

zhì chuāng 痔疮, hemorrhoid, 289

zhì chuāng 痔疮, pile, 444

zhì fǎ 治法, method of treatment, 394

zhì fǎ 疗法, method of treatment, 394

zhì fēng huà tán 治风化痰, controlling wind and transforming phlegm, 98

zhì fēng xiān zhì xuè, xuè xíng fēng zì miè 治风先治血，血行风自灭, to treat wind, first treat the blood; when the blood moves, wind naturally disappears, 621

zhì fù nèi chóng fāng 治腹内虫方, Abdominal Worm Formula, 737

zhì gān cǎo tāng 炙甘草汤, Honey-Fried Licorice Decoction, 59, 159, 160, 269, 270, 594, 741

zhì hé shǒu wū 制何首乌 processed flowery knotweed, Polygoni Multiflori Radix Praeparatum, 604

zhì jì 制剂, preparation, 463

zhì jì 制剂, preparation of medicinals, 463

zhì liáo 治疗, treatment, 627

zhì nóng xiōng fāng 治脓胸方, Pyothorax Formula, 743

zhì nüè 治疟, controlling malaria, 98

zhì shì 志室, BL-52, Will Chamber, 4, 89, 97, 148, 160, 222, 266, 288, 294, 308, 332, 333, 336, 347, 352, 360, 453, 461, 513, 518, 521, 524, 525, 569, 584, 594, 597, 647, 651, 716, 747

zhì shuāng 制霜, frosting, 231

zhì wèi bìng 治未病, treating disease before it arises, 626

zhì xià 滞下, stagnant diarrhea, 569

zhì yáng 至阳, GV-9, Extremity of Yang, 151, 174, 349, 384, 564, 700, 749

zhì yǐ nǎo fāng 治乙脑方, Encephalitis Formula, 731

zhì yīn 至阴, BL-67, Reaching Yin, 82, 128, 219, 385, 420, 747

zhì zé 治则, principle of treatment, 463

zhì zhēn 滞针, stuck needle, 585

zhì zhōng tāng 治中汤, Center-Ordering Decoction, 3, 77, 216, 648, 735

zhì zhuó gù běn wán 治浊固本丸, Anti-Turbidity Root-Securing Pill, 179

zhōng 中, center, 54

zhōng 中, middle, 394

zhōng cǎo yào 中草药, Chinese medicinals and herbs, 61

zhōng chōng 中冲, PC-9, Central Hub, 25, 65, 73, 99, 147, 203, 218, 263, 281, 294, 384, 400, 408, 420, 427, 437, 442, 455, 485, 567, 589, 590, 631, 748

zhōng dū 中都, LR-6, Central Metropolis, 19, 296, 431, 481, 748

zhōng dú 中渎, GB-32, Central River, 19, 89, 519, 748

zhōng fēng 中封, LR-4, Mound Center, 61, 511, 542, 667, 748

zhōng fǔ 中府, LU-1, Central Treasury, 8, 91, 142, 203, 219, 261, 439, 587, 746

zhōng hán 中寒, center cold, 54

zhōng jí 中极, CV-3, Central Pole, 7, 8, 21–23, 26, 33–36, 68, 69, 71, 80, 84, 86, 89, 91, 93, 94, 111, 112, 118, 149, 151, 177, 180, 199, 219–221, 227, 229, 240, 241, 282, 283, 297, 300–302, 308, 317, 331, 332, 353, 393, 424, 431, 447, 449–451, 456, 457, 465, 468, 483–485, 497, 503, 516, 518, 522, 533, 541, 542, 582, 589, 597, 604, 631, 636, 640, 641, 643, 661, 667, 675, 701, 711, 713, 749

zhōng jiāo 中焦, center burner, 54

zhōng jiāo 中焦, middle burner, 394

zhōng jiāo rú ōu 中焦如沤, center burner is like foam, 54

zhōng jiāo shī rè 中焦湿热, center burner damp-heat, 54

zhōng jiāo zhǔ huà 中焦主化, center burner governs transformation, 54

zhōng jīng zhī fǔ 中精之腑, bowel of center essence, 49

zhōng kuí 中魁, Central Eminence, 164, 579

zhōng liáo 中膠, BL-33, Central Bone-Hole, 747

zhōng lǚ shū 中膂俞, BL-29, Central Backbone Transport, 747

zhōng mǎn fēn xiāo tāng 中满分消汤, Center Fullness Separating and Dispersing Decoction, 80

zhōng mǎn fēn xiāo wán 中满分消丸, Center Fullness Separating and Dispersing Pill, 151, 278, 733

zhōng mǎn zhě xiè zhī yú nèi 中满者泻之于内, center fullness is treated by draining the inner body, 55

zhōng qì 中气, center qi, 55

zhōng qì bù zú 中气不足, insufficiency of center qi, 309

zhōng qì xià xiàn 中气下陷, center qi fall, 55

zhōng qīng zhī fǔ 中清之腑, bowel of center clearness, 49

zhōng quán 中泉, Central Spring, 61

zhōng rǔ fěn 钟乳粉 powdered stalactite, Stalactitum Pulveratum, 624, 726

zhōng rǔ shí 钟乳石 stalactite, Stalactitum, 467, 526, 624, 726

zhōng shū 中枢, GV-7, Central Pivot, 749

zhōng tíng 中庭, CV-16, Center Palace, 749

zhōng wǎn 中脘, CV-12, Center Stomach Duct, 2–4, 6, 8, 17, 20, 28, 29, 32, 38, 41, 54, 55, 59, 61–64, 66, 70, 73, 77, 79–89, 94, 99, 109–111, 113–115, 117–119, 127, 136, 141, 142, 145, 151–153, 156, 157, 161, 163, 164, 168, 174, 186, 189, 196, 203, 207, 210–212, 215–218, 222–224, 230, 235, 237, 240, 242, 247, 251, 252, 256, 257, 260, 268, 272, 278, 284, 287, 291, 301, 302, 309, 312, 314, 318, 325, 339, 340, 343, 349, 358, 361, 362, 383, 390, 394–396, 401, 403, 410, 414, 418, 425, 433–443, 445, 447, 448, 450, 457, 462, 477–480, 482, 487, 488, 490, 498, 503, 506, 509, 510, 521, 522, 537, 539, 540, 549–551, 554, 555, 557–559, 561–566, 571, 575, 577–581, 585, 587–589, 591, 595, 596, 603, 604, 608, 612–614, 633, 638, 645, 647, 649, 650, 658, 662–669, 671, 673, 678, 679, 684, 685, 691, 694, 703, 709, 713, 716, 749

zhōng xiāo 中消, center dispersion, 54

zhōng yáng bù zhèn 中阳不振, devitalized center yang, 125

zhōng yáng bù zú 中阳不足, insufficiency of center yang, 309

zhōng yào 中药, Chinese medicinal, 61

zhōng zàng jīng 中藏经 (*Central Treasury Canon*), 2nd century (Eastern Hàn), attributed to Huà Tuó 华佗 (?), 86, 205

zhōng zhèng zhī guān 中正之官, office of justice, 419

zhōng zhǐ tóng shēn cùn 中指同身寸, middle finger body-inch, 394

zhōng zhǔ 中渚, TB-3, Central Islet, 119, 160, 166, 167, 260, 288, 296, 330, 336, 348, 474, 566, 614, 658, 666, 748

zhōng zhù 中注, KI-15, Central Flow, 748

zhǒng 肿, swelling, 600

zhǒng dú 肿毒, toxin swelling, 621

zhòng 中, strike, 584

zhòng 中, stroke, 584

zhòng 重, heaviness, 286

zhòng 重, heavy, 286

zhòng è 中恶, malignity stroke, 384

zhòng fēng 中风, wind strike, 691

zhòng fēng 中风, wind stroke, 691

zhòng fēng bì zhèng 中风闭证, wind stroke block pattern, 692

zhòng fēng tuō zhèng 中风脱证, wind stroke desertion pattern, 692

zhòng fǔ 中腑, bowel stroke, 49

zhòng jì 重剂, heavy formula, 287

zhòng jīng 中经, channel stroke, 56

zhòng jīng luò 中经络, channel and network stroke, 55

zhòng kě qù qiè 重可去怯, heavy [medicinals] can eliminate timidity, 288

zhòng luò 中络, network stroke, 409

zhòng rén 中人, strike-on-person, 584

zhòng shēn 重身, pregnancy, 460

zhòng shǔ 中暑, summerheat stroke, 590

zhòng shǔ xuàn yūn 中暑眩晕, summerheat stroke dizziness, 590

zhòng tīng 重听, hearing impairment, 260

zhòng tòng 重痛, heavy pain, 288

zhòng zàng 中脏, visceral stroke, 656

zhòng zàng fǔ 中脏腑, bowel and visceral stroke, 49

zhòng zàng fǔ 中脏腑, organ stroke, 421

zhòng zhèn ān shén 重镇安神, quieting the spirit with heavy settlers, 491

zhòng zhèn yào 重镇药, heavy settler, 288

zhōu 周, Zhou, 718

zhōu bì 周痹, generalized impediment, 240

zhōu chē (jū) wán 舟车丸, Boats and Carts Pill, 151, 182, 732

zhōu róng 周荣, SP-20, All-Round Flourishing, 746

zhōu shēn tòng 周身痛, generalized pain, 240

zhǒu hòu bèi jí fāng 肘后备急方 (*Emergency Standby Remedies*), Gě Hóng 葛洪 (281–341, Jìn)281–341, 58, 83, 106, 384

zhǒu jiān 肘尖, Tip of the Elbow, 142, 171, 442, 515, 544

zhǒu láo 肘劳, elbow taxation, 170

zhǒu liáo 肘髎, LI-12, Elbow Bone-Hole, 520, 746

zhòu jiǎo 皱脚, wrinkly foot, 696

Zhu Dan-Xi's Damp Phlegm Formula, *zhū dān xī zhì shī tán fāng* 朱丹溪治湿痰方, 93

zhu hán kāi qiào 逐寒开窍, expelling cold and opening the orifices, 182

zhū dān xī zhì shī tán fāng 朱丹溪治湿痰方, Zhu Dan-Xi's Damp Phlegm Formula, 93

zhū dǎn zhī 猪胆汁 pig's bile, Suis Bilis, 624, 725

zhū dǔ wán 猪肚丸, Pig's Stomach Pill, 122, 743

zhū fú shén 朱茯神 cinnabar root poria, Poria cum Pini Radice et Cinnabare, 433

zhū gān 猪肝 pig's liver, Suis Iecur, 291

zhū gě xíng jūn sǎn 诸葛行军散, Zhuge's Troop-Marching Powder, 740

zhū huáng sǎn 珠黄散, Pearl and Bezoar Powder, 744

zhū jǐ suǐ 猪脊髓 pig's spine marrow, Suis Spinae Medulla, 64, 333

zhū líng 猪苓 polyporus, Polyporus, 21, 136, 153, 224, 230, 390, 410, 434, 666, 723

zhu líng sǎn 猪苓散, Polyporus Powder, 239

zhū líng tāng 猪苓汤, Polyporus Decoction, 176, 467, 541, 733

zhū líng wán 猪苓丸, Polyporus Pill, 434

zhū shā 朱砂 cinnabar, Cinnabaris, 148, 230, 249, 262, 287, 288, 383, 392, 490, 524, 526, 585, 602, 667, 675, 726

zhū shā ān shén wán 朱砂安神丸, Cinnabar Spirit-Quieting Pill, 39, 61, 274, 310, 525, 537, 538, 604, 701, 739

zhū yá zào 猪牙皂 small gleditsia, Gleditsiae Fructus Parvus, 243, 690

zhū yáng zhī huì 诸阳之会, confluence of the yang [channels], 92

zhū yè 猪靥 pig's thyroid gland, Suis Glandula Thyroidea, 30, 243

zhū zàng wán 猪脏丸, Pig's Intestine Pill, 738

zhū zhī gāo 猪脂膏 pork lard, Suis Adeps, 653

zhú 逐, expel, 181

zhú bīn 筑宾, KI-9, Guest House, 28, 75, 748

zhú fù tāng 术附汤, Ovate Atractylodes and Aconite Decoction, 80, 588, 733

zhú hán 攻逐寒积, expelling cold accumulations, 182

zhú hán dàng jīng tāng 逐寒荡惊汤, Cold-Dispelling Fright-Assuaging Decoction, 735

zhú lì 竹沥 dried bamboo sap, Bambusae Succus Exsiccatus, 84, 116, 178, 282, 434, 448, 624, 637, 725

zhú lì dá tán wán 竹沥达痰丸, Bamboo Sap Phlegm-Outthrusting Pill, 738

zhú lì yùn tán wán 竹沥运痰丸, Dried Bamboo Sap Phlegm-Moving Pill, 433

zhú nì tāi 浊腻苔, turbid slimy tongue fur, 632

zhú rú 竹茹 bamboo shavings, Bambusae Caulis in Taeniam, 20, 256, 257, 434, 440, 526, 574, 577, 578, 624, 709, 725

zhú rú tāng 竹茹汤, Bamboo Shavings Decoction, 284, 736

zhú shuǐ 逐水, expelling water, 182

zhú tán 逐痰, expelling phlegm, 182

zhú yè 竹叶 bamboo leaf, Bambusae Folium, 67, 720

zhú yè huáng qí tāng 竹叶黄芪汤, Bamboo Leaf and Astragalus Decoction, 259

zhú yè liǔ bàng tāng 竹叶柳蒡汤, Bamboo Leaf, Tamarisk, and Arctium Decoction, 422, 729

zhú yè shí gāo tāng 竹叶石膏汤, Bamboo Leaf and Gypsum Decoction, 108, 155, 157, 221, 284, 415, 499, 558, 590, 599, 730

zhú yè tāng 竹叶汤, Bamboo Leaf Decoction, 458, 652, 731

zhú yè xīn 竹叶心 tender bamboo leaf (lophatherum), Lophatheri Folium Immaturum, 65

zhú yū 逐瘀, expelling stasis, 182

zhǔ 主, chief, 60

zhǔ 主, govern, 244

zhǔ 主, governor, 245

zhǔ 煮, boiling, 44

zhǔ fǔ zuǒ yǐn 主辅佐引, chief, support, assistant, and conductor, 60

zhǔ fǔ zuǒ yǐn 主辅佐引, medicinal roles, 389

zhǔ kè pèi xué fǎ 主客配穴法, combining guest and host points, 88

zhǔ sè 主色, governing complexion, 244

zhǔ zhì 主治, indication, 299

zhù 注, influx, 300

zhù 疰, infixation, 300

zhù chē wán 驻车丸, Carriage-Halting Pill, 174, 312, 742

zhù gēn tāng 苎根汤, Ramie (Boehmeria) Decoction, 741

zhù gǔ 杼骨, shuttle bone, 531

zhù jiě shāng hán lùn 注解伤寒论 (*Annotated Cold Damage*), 1144 (Jīn), Chéng Wú-Jǐ 成无己, 583

zhù jǐng wán 驻景丸, Long Vistas Pill, 406

zhù jǐng wán jiā jiǎn fāng 驻景丸加减方, Long Vistas Pill Variant Formula, 64, 742

zhù má gēn 苎麻根 ramie, Boehmeriae Radix, 724

zhù shè jì 注射剂, injection fluid, 303

zhù shè yì 注射液, injection fluid, 303

zhù xià 注夏, summer influx, 592

zhù xià 注下, downpour diarrhea, 146

zhù xià 疰夏, summer infixation, 592

zhù xiè 注泻, outpour diarrhea, 422

zhù xīn tòng 注心痛, influx heart pain, 300

zhù yáng 助阳, assisting yang, 11

zhù yáng 助阳, reinforcing yang, 498

zhù yáng jiě biǎo 助阳解表, assisting yang and resolving the exterior, 11

zhuǎn bāo 转胞, shifted bladder, 529

zhuǎn dāi dān 转呆丹, Dementia-Shifting Elixir, 122

zhuǎn dòu mài 转豆脉, spinning bean pulse, 550

zhuǎn huà 转化, conversion, 99

zhuǎn jīn 转筋, cramp, 104

zhuǎn tāi fāng 转胎方, Fetus-Turning Formula, 384, 741

zhuǎn wán mài 转丸脉, spinning pill pulse, 550

zhuǎn zhēn 转针, needle rotation, 407

zhuàng 壮, invigorate, 319

zhuàng huǒ 壮火, invigorating fire, 319

zhuàng huǒ 壮火, vigorous fire, 655

zhuàng jīn yǎng xuè tāng 壮筋养血汤, Sinew-Strengthening Blood-Nourishing Decoction, 337, 567

zhuàng rè 壮热, vigorous heat [effusion], 655

zhuàng shuǐ zhī zhǔ yǐ zhì yáng guāng 壮水之主以制阳光, invigorating the governor of water to restrain the brilliance of yang, 319

zhuàng shuǐ zhì yáng 壮水制阳, invigorating water to restrain yang, 319

zhuàng yáng 壮阳, invigorating yang, 319

Zhuge's Troop-Marching Powder, *zhū gě xíng jūn sǎn* 诸葛行军散, 740

zhuī 追, expel, 181

zhuī chóng wán 追虫丸, Worm-Expelling Pill, 696, 737

zhuō 顀, facial prominence, 194

zhuó 浊, turbid, 632

zhuó 浊, turbidity, 632

zhuó 灼, scorch, 514

zhuó bì 着痹, fixed impediment, 209

zhuó bì yàn fāng 着痹验方, Fixed Impediment Empirical Formula, 138

zhuó qì 浊气, turbid qi, 632

zhuó qì bù jiàng 浊气不降, turbid qi failing to bear downward, 632

zhuó qì guī xīn 浊气归心, turbid qi goes to the heart, 632

zhuó qiào 浊窍, turbid orifices, 632

zhuó rè 灼热, scorching heat, 514

zhuó tòng 灼痛, scorching pain, 514

zhuó xié hài qīng 浊邪害清, turbid evils harm the clear, 632

zhuó yīn 浊阴, turbid yin, 632

zhuó yīn bù jiàng 浊阴不降, turbid yin failing to bear downward, 632

zhū bìng yuán hòu lùn 诸病源候论 (*Origin and Indicators of Disease*), 610 (Suí), Cháo Yuán-Fāng 巢元方, 6, 51, 122, 149, 150, 154, 178, 189, 298, 302, 311, 363, 367, 370, 412, 444, 451, 485, 497, 513, 526, 572, 583, 610, 632, 636, 641, 651, 658, 667, 677, 684, 692

zī 滋, enrich, 175

zī bǔ gān shèn 滋补肝肾, enriching (and supplementing) the liver and kidney, 175

zī bǔ piàn 滋补片, Enriching Supplementation Tablet, 739

zī cuì yǐn 滋膵饮, Pancreas-Enriching Beverage, 369

zī róng huó luò tāng 滋荣活络汤, Construction-Enriching Network-Quickening Decoction, 457

zī róng yì qì fù shén tāng 滋荣益气复神汤, Construction-Enriching Qi-Boosting Spirit-Returning Decoction, 455

zī shèn gù chōng tāng 滋肾固冲汤, Kidney-Enriching Thoroughfare-Securing Decoction, 743

zī shèn tōng guān wán 滋肾通关丸, Kidney-Enriching Gate-Opening Pill, 203

zī shèn wán 滋肾丸, Kidney-Enriching Pill, 122, 649, 733

zī shēng wán 资生丸, Life-Promoting Pill, 741

zī shuǐ hán mù 滋水涵木, enriching water to moisten wood, 175

zī shuǐ qīng gān yǐn 滋水清肝饮, Water-Enriching Liver-Clearing Beverage, 656

zī tài 姿态, bearing, 16

zī yǎng gān shèn 滋养肝肾, enriching (and nourishing) the liver and kidney, 175

zī yǎng wèi yīn 滋养胃阴, enriching (and nourishing) stomach yin, 175

zī yīn 滋阴, enriching yin, 175

zī yīn bǔ shèn 滋阴补肾, enriching yin and supplementing the kidney, 176

zī yīn chú shī tāng 滋阴除湿汤, Yin-Enriching Dampness-Eliminating Decoction, 671 *zī yīn dà bǔ wán* 滋阴大补丸, Yin-Enriching Major Supplementation Pill, 742

zī yīn jiàng huǒ 滋阴降火, enriching yin and down-bearing fire, 176

zī yīn jiàng huǒ tāng 滋阴降火汤, Yin-Enriching Fire-Downbearing Decoction, 551, 731

zī yīn jiě biǎo 滋阴解表, enriching yin and resolving the exterior, 176

zī yīn lì shī 滋阴利湿, enriching yin and disinhibiting dampness, 176

zī yīn píng gān qián yáng 滋阴平肝潜阳, enriching yin, calming the liver, and subduing yang, 176

zī yīn qīng huà wán 滋阴清化丸, Yin-Enriching Clearing Transforming Pill, 201, 409

zī yīn qīng rè 滋阴清热, enriching yin and clearing heat, 175

zī yīn rùn zào 滋阴润燥, enriching yin and moistening dryness, 176

zī yīn shū gān 滋阴疏肝, enriching yin and coursing the liver, 176

zī yīn xī fēng 滋阴熄风, enriching yin and extinguishing wind, 176

zī yīn yì qì 滋阴益气, enriching yin and boosting qi, 175

zī yīn zhì huǒ 滋阴制火, enriching yin to restrain fire, 176

zī zào yǎng yíng tāng 滋燥养营汤, Dryness-Enriching Construction-Nourishing Decoction, 28, 741

zǐ bái diàn fēng 紫白癜风, purple and white patch wind, 473

zǐ bèi 紫贝 purple cowrie, Mauritiae, Erosariae seu Cypraeae Testa, 54, 726

zǐ cǎo 紫草 puccoon, Lithospermi, Macrotomiae, seu Onosmatis Radix, 30, 67, 387, 459, 637, 683, 721

zǐ cháng bù shōu 子肠不收, prolapse of the uterus, 466

zǐ fán 子烦, vexation of pregnancy, 655

zǐ gōng 子宫, Infant's Palace, 39, 332, 466, 711, 712

zǐ gōng 子宫, uterus, 643

zǐ gōng 子宫, womb, 695

zǐ gōng 紫宫, CV-19, Purple Palace, 749

zǐ gōng tuō chuí 子宫脱垂, prolapse of the uterus, 466

zǐ gōng xià chuí 子宫下垂, prolapse of the uterus, 466

zǐ hé chē 紫河车 placenta, Hominis Placenta, 222, 298, 310, 511, 593, 726

zǐ huā dì dīng 紫花地丁 Yedo violet, Violae Yedoensis Herba cum Radice, 67, 691, 721

zǐ jīn fěn 紫金粉, Purple Gold Powder, 740

zǐ jīn niú 紫金牛 Japanese ardisia, Ardisiae Japonicae Caulis et Folium, 624, 725

zǐ jīng pí sǎn 紫荆皮散, Cercis Powder, 745

zǐ lín 子淋, strangury of pregnancy, 583

zǐ lóng wán 子龙丸, Young Dragon Pill, 732

zǐ mǎn 子满, fullness of pregnancy, 232

zǐ mén 子门, infant's gate, 300

zǐ qì 子气, pregnancy qi, 461

zǐ shí yīng 紫石英 amethyst/fluorite, Amethystum seu Fluoritum, 467, 490, 519, 526, 726

zǐ shuǐ qīng gān yǐn 滋水清肝饮, Water-Enriching Liver-Clearing Beverage, 742

zǐ sòu 子嗽, cough of pregnancy, 101

zǐ sū 紫苏 perilla leaf, Perillae Folium, Caulis et Calyx, 449

zǐ sū 紫苏 perilla, Perillae Folium, Caulis et Calyx, 128, 256, 681, 720

zǐ sū ān tāi yǐn 紫苏安胎饮, Perilla Leaf Fetus-Quieting Beverage, 736

zǐ sū gěng 紫苏梗 perilla stem, Perillae Caulis, 19, 386, 540, 681, 720

zǐ sū yè 紫苏叶 perilla leaf, Perillae Folium, 82, 103, 107, 176, 184, 454, 500, 501, 547, 577, 681, 720

zǐ sū yè 紫苏叶 perilla, Perillae Folium, 502

zǐ sū zǐ 紫苏子 perilla seed, Perillae Fructus, 145, 146, 439, 624, 625, 703, 725

zǐ wǎn 紫菀 aster, Asteris Radix et Rhizoma, 95, 267, 397, 434, 624, 625, 725

zǐ wǎn tāng 紫菀汤, Aster Decoction, 267, 739

zǐ wǔ liú zhù 子午流注, midday-midnight point selection, 394

zǐ wǔ liú zhù 子午流注, stem and branch point selection, 572

zǐ xián 子痫, eclampsia, 167

zǐ xián 子痫, epilepsy of pregnancy, 178

zǐ xuě 紫雪, Purple Snow, 450, 637

zǐ xuě dān 紫雪丹, Purple Snow Elixir, 65, 69, 88, 156, 171, 177, 202, 394, 589, 693, 740

zǐ xuě sǎn 紫雪散, Purple Snow Powder, 198

zǐ yōng 子痈, welling-abscess of the testicle, 671

zǐ yún gāo 紫云膏, Purple Clouds Plaster, 745

zǐ zhǒng 子肿, swelling of pregnancy, 600

zǐ zhū 紫珠 beauty-berry leaf, Callicarpae Folium, 724

zì 眦, canthus, 54

zì 字, zi, 718

zì hàn 自汗, spontaneous sweating, 567

zì jiǔ 自灸, natural moxibustion, 405

zì lòu 眦漏, weeping canthus, 669

zì rán tóng 自然铜 pyrite, Pyritum, 53, 138, 725

zì xià lì 自下利, spontaneous diarrhea, 567

Zingiberis Rhizoma, *jiāng* 姜, ginger, 154, 217

Zingiberis Rhizoma Exsiccatum, *gān jiāng* 干姜, dried ginger, 5, 12, 23, 84, 94, 98, 128, 136, 182, 196, 228, 242, 257, 272, 292, 293, 343, 345, 393, 425, 426, 438, 455, 456, 463, 469, 504, 612, 625, 649, 660, 662, 663, 679, 723

Zingiberis Rhizoma Recens, *shēng jiāng* 生姜, fresh ginger, 11, 70, 84, 95, 128, 201, 230, 243, 255, 256, 319, 343, 358, 397, 417, 426, 443, 448, 454, 464, 500–502, 527, 547, 574, 578, 581, 661, 663, 681, 683, 720

Zingiberis Rhizoma Tostum, *páo jiāng* 炮姜, blast-fried ginger, 26, 139, 199, 417, 431, 503, 556, 562, 564, 569, 660, 662, 723

Zingiberis Rhizomatis Cortex, *jiāng pí* 姜皮, ginger skin, 153, 262, 681, 720

Zingiberis Rhizomatis Succus, *jiāng zhī* 姜汁, ginger juice, 116, 448

Ziziphi Fructus, *dà zǎo* 大枣, jujube, 11, 96, 217, 255, 358, 499, 580, 593, 600, 726

Ziziphi Fructus Ater, *hēi zǎo* 黑枣, black jujube, 667

Ziziphi Fructus Pasta, *zǎo ní* 枣泥, jujube paste, 251

Ziziphi Spinosi Semen, *suān zǎo rén* 酸枣仁, spiny jujube, 37, 122, 222, 230, 236, 309, 359, 433, 458, 490, 526, 557, 655, 726

Ziziphi Spinosi Semen, *suān zǎo rén* 酸枣仁, spiny jujube kernel, 60

zōng jīn 宗筋, ancestral sinew, 9

zōng jīn chí zòng 宗筋弛纵, slackness of the ancestral sinew, 536

zōng jīn suǒ jù 宗筋所聚, gathering place of the ancestral sinews, 240

zōng lǘ pí 棕榈皮 trachycarpus, Trachycarpi Stipulae Fibra, 569, 724

zōng mài 宗脉, ancestral vessels, 9

zōng mài suǒ jù 宗脉所聚, gathering place of the ancestral vessels, 240

zōng qì 宗气, ancestral qi, 9

zōng qì 宗气, gathering qi, 240

zòng tíng bù shōu 纵挺不收, persistent erection, 430

Zosterae Marinae Herba, *hǎi dài* 海带, eelgrass, 624, 725

zǒu cuàn 走窜, mobile and penetrating, 398

zǒu ér bù shǒu 走而不守, mobile, 398

zǒu fāng yī 走方医, itinerant healer, 321

zǒu guàn 走罐, slide-cupping, 539

zǒu huáng 走黄, running yellow, 510

zǒu mǎ gān 走马疳, galloping gan, 236

zǒu mǎ yá gān 走马牙疳, galloping gan of the teeth and gums, 236

zú gēn tòng 足跟痛, heel pain, 288

zú héng zhǒng 足胻肿, swelling of the feet and lower legs, 601

zú jué yīn gān jīng 足厥阴肝经, LR, 369

zú jué yīn gān jīng 足厥阴肝经, foot reverting yin liver channel, 221

zú lín qì 足临泣, GB-41, Foot Overlooking Tears, 8, 33, 75, 89, 90, 93, 112, 142, 162, 195, 220, 221, 231, 320, 386, 474, 500, 515, 606, 716, 748

zú qiào yīn 足窍阴, GB-44, Foot Orifice Yin, 75, 147, 148, 220, 333, 413, 420, 521, 538, 546, 748

zú sān lǐ 足三里, ST-36, Leg Three Li, 1, 3–5, 8, 11, 14–17, 19, 20, 26–30, 32, 33, 36–41, 44, 47, 55, 57–64, 66, 69–74, 76, 77, 79–89, 91, 94–97, 99, 103, 105, 109–115, 117–120, 123, 127–129, 136, 139–141, 145, 146, 149–151, 153, 154, 156, 157, 159–164, 167, 168, 174, 175, 177, 183, 185, 186, 189, 190, 192, 194, 196, 197, 199, 202, 210–212, 215–218, 221–231, 234–237, 239–241, 247, 251, 255–257, 260, 265–272, 276, 278, 280–284, 287–289, 291, 292, 296, 297, 300–302, 308–310, 312, 314, 316, 318–320, 325, 329, 332–337, 339–343, 349, 352, 357–362, 365, 369, 370, 378–380, 382, 385, 386, 391–393, 395, 396, 400, 401, 403, 408, 410, 415, 416, 418, 425–427, 430, 433–443, 445, 447–458, 461, 462, 465, 466, 477–480, 482–490, 493, 498, 499, 503, 504, 506, 509–511, 513, 515, 516, 519–525, 529, 530, 533, 537, 539, 540, 544, 547, 549–551, 554, 555, 557–566, 568, 570, 571, 575, 577–581, 585–591, 594–597, 600, 601, 603, 604, 606–608, 612–614, 620, 624, 625, 627, 629, 630, 633, 636–641, 645–650, 652, 661–666, 668, 673–680, 684–686, 689, 690, 693–696, 699–703, 709–716, 746

zú sān yáng jīng 足三阳经, three yang channels of the foot, 610

zú sān yīn jīng 足三阴经, three yin channels of the foot, 610

zú shào yáng dǎn jīng 足少阳胆经, GB, 240

zú shào yáng dǎn jīng 足少阳胆经, foot lesser yang gallbladder channel, 219

zú shào yīn shèn jīng 足少阴肾经, KI, 324

zú shào yīn shèn jīng 足少阴肾经, foot lesser yin kidney channel, 220

zú tài yáng páng guāng jīng 足太阳膀胱经, BL, 20

zú tài yáng páng guāng jīng 足太阳膀胱经, foot greater yang bladder channel, 218

zú tài yīn pí jīng 足太阴脾经, SP, 549

zú tài yīn pí jīng 足太阴脾经, foot greater yin spleen channel, 219

zú wǔ lǐ 足五里, LR-10, Foot Five Li, 610, 748

zú xīn tòng 足心痛, pain in the heart of the sole, 425

zú xīn tòng 足心痛, pain in the soles of the foot, 425

zú yáng míng nüè 足阳明疟, foot yang brightness malaria, 221

zú yáng míng wèi jīng 足阳明胃经, ST, 569

zú yáng míng wèi jīng 足阳明胃经, foot yang brightness stomach channel, 221

zú zhǒng 足肿, swelling of the feet, 601

zǔ 阻, obstruct, 418

zuǐ chún 嘴唇, lip, 348

zuì xiāng yù xiè 醉乡玉屑, Enchanted Land Jade Shavings, 732

zuǒ 佐, assistant, 11

zuǒ guī wán 左归丸, Left-Restoring [Kidney Yin] Pill, 160, 256, 310, 329, 331, 332, 352, 360, 524, 528, 714, 742

zuǒ guī yǐn 左归饮, Left-Restoring [Kidney Yin] Beverage, 369, 594, 742

zuǒ jīn wán 左金丸, Left-Running Metal Pill, 4, 19, 20, 24, 63, 202, 362, 461, 478, 549, 578, 731

zuǒ shèn yòu mìng 左肾右命, kidney is on the left and the life [gate] is on right, 328

zuǒ yòu pèi xué fǎ 左右配穴法, combining left and right points, 88

zuò bǎn chuāng 坐板疮, seat sores, 517

zuò bǎn gǔ 坐板骨, seat board bone, 517

zuò guàn fǎ 坐罐法, stationary cupping, 571

zuò qiáng zhī guān 作强之官, office of labor, 419

zygomatic bone*, 57